Visit our website

to find out about other books from W.B. Saunders
and our sister companies in Harcourt Health Sciences

Register free at
www.harcourt-international.com

and you will get

- the latest information on new books, journals and electronic products in your chosen subject areas

- the choice of e-mail or post alerts or both, when there are any new books in your chosen areas

- news of special offers and promotions

- information about products from all Harcourt Health Sciences' companies including W. B. Saunders, Churchill Livingstone, and Mosby

You will also find an easily searchable catalogue, online ordering, information on our extensive list of journals...and much more!

Visit the Harcourt Health Sciences website today!

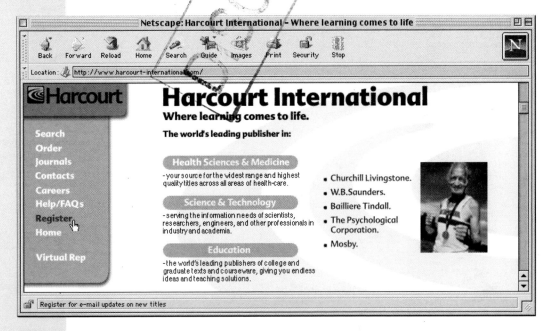

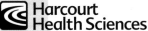
Harcourt
Health Sciences

Surgery of the Liver and Biliary Tract

Volume I

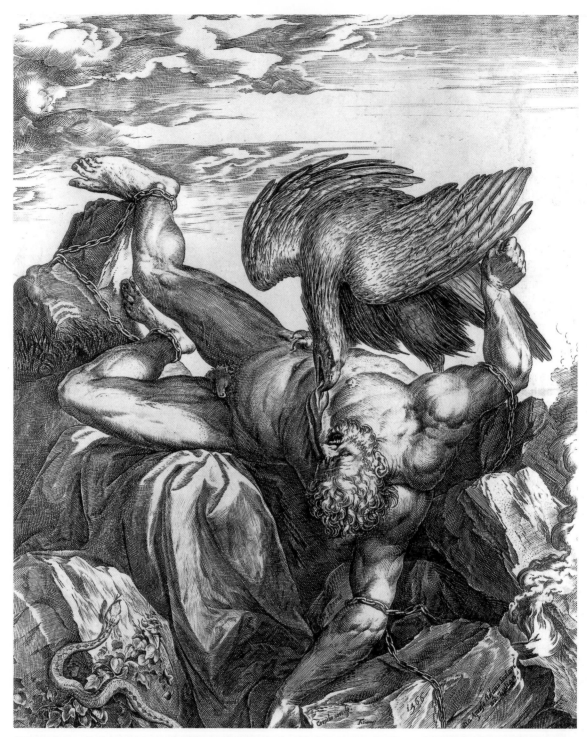

Prometheus, chained to the rocky Mount Caucasus, has his liver eaten by the eagle of Zeus. (Engraving, 1566, possibly after a work by Titian. Reproduced by permission of the Hulton Getty Picture Collection, London)

Commissioning Editor: Miranda Bromage
Project Manager: Ian Stoneham
Project Controller: Helen Sofio
Proof-reader: J. Ian Ross

Surgery of the Liver and Biliary Tract

Third Edition

EDITED BY

L. H. Blumgart BDS MD DSc(Hon) FACS FRCS(Eng, Edin) FRCPS(Glas)

Enid A. Haupt Chair in Surgery,
Chief, Hepatobiliary Service,
Director, Hepatobiliary Disease Management Program,
Memorial Sloan-Kettering Cancer Center;
Professor of Surgery,
Weill Medical College of Cornell University,
New York, NY, USA

and

Y. Fong MD FACS

Attending Surgeon,
Memorial Sloan-Kettering Cancer Center;
Professor of Surgery,
Weill Medical College of Cornell University,
New York, NY, USA

Volume I

 W. B. SAUNDERS COMPANY LTD

London • Edinburgh • New York • Philadelphia • St Louis • Sydney • Toronto 2000

W.B. SAUNDERS
An imprint of Harcourt Publishers Limited

© Harcourt Publishers Limited 2000

Ⓢ is a registered trademark of Harcourt Publishers Limited

The rights of L. H. Blumgart and Y. Fong to be identified as the editors of
this work has been asserted by them in accordance with the Copyright,
Designs and Patents Act 1988

First edition 1988
Second edition 1994
Third edition 2000
Reprinted 2001

ISBN 0-7020-25011

British Library Cataloguing in Publication Data
A catalogue record for this book is available from the British Library

Library of Congress Cataloging-in-Publication Data
A catalog record for this book is available from the Library of Congress

Note
Medical knowledge is constantly changing. As new information becomes
available, changes in treatment, procedures, equipment and the use of
drugs become necessary. The editors and the publishers have taken care
to ensure that the information given in this text is accurate and up to
date. However, readers are strongly advised to confirm that the
information, especially with regard to drug usage, complies with the
latest legislation and standards of practice.

Printed in the United Kingdom

The
Publisher's
policy is to use
**paper manufactured
from sustainable forests**

I

Contents

SECTION 12: CIRRHOSIS AND PORTAL HYPERTENSION

SECTION 14: LIVER TRANSPLANTATION

Contributors

Andreas Adam MB BS FRCP FRCR FRCS
Professor of Interventional Radiology,
Department of Radiology,
St Thomas' Hospital,
London, UK

Tim Akhurst MBBS FRACP
Research Associate,
Department of Radiology, Nuclear Medicine Service,
Memorial Sloan-Kettering Cancer Center,
New York, NY, USA

H. Richard Alexander MD
Head, Surgical Metabolism Section,
Surgery Branch,
National Cancer Institute,
National Institute of Health,
Bethesda, MA, USA

David J. Allison BSc MD MRCP FRCR
Director of Diagnostic Radiology,
Department of Imaging,
Imperial College School of Medicine,
Hammersmith Hospital,
London, UK

Marjorie E. M. Allison BSc MD FRCP
Senior Research Fellow,
Medical Education Unit,
University of Glasgow,
Glasgow, UK

Annelore K. Altendorf-Hofmann MD PhD
Professor of Theoretical Surgery,
Abteilung fur Aligemeine und Viszerale Chirurgie,
Friedrich-Schiller Universität Jena,
Jena, Germany

Farin Amersi MD
General Surgery Resident,
Post Doctoral Fellow,
Dumont-University of California at Los Angeles Liver
    Transplant Center,
Los Angeles, CA, USA

Daniel Azoulay MD
Hepatobiliary Surgeon,
Centre Hepatobiliaire,
Hôpital Paul Brousse,
Villejuif, France

Francesco Azzaroli MD
Dipartimento di Medicina Interna e Gastroenterologia,
Università di Bologna,
Bologna, Italy

David L Bartlett MD
Senior Investigator,
National Cancer Institute,
National Institute of Health;
Assistant Professor,
USUHS,
Bethesda, MD, USA

Franco Bazzoli MD
Associate Professor of Gastroenterology,
Dipartimento di Medicina Interna e Gastroenterologia,
Università di Bologna,
Bologna, Italy

Robert M. Beazley MD
Professor of Surgery and Chief,
Section of Surgical Oncology and Endocrinology,
Boston University Medical Center,
Boston, MA, USA

Christoph D. Becker MD
Chargé de cours,
Department of Radiology,
Geneva University Hospital,
Geneva, Switzerland

Ian J. Beckingham MD
Consultant Hepatobiliary and Laparoscopic Surgeon,
Department of Surgery,
University Hospital,
Nottingham, UK

Jacques Belghiti MD
Professor and Chairman,
Department of Digestive Surgery,
Hôpital Beaujon,
Clichy, France

Jean-Pierre Benhamou MD
Professor Emeritus of Hepatology and Gastroenterology,
University of Paris,
Service of Hepatology,
Hôpital Beaujon,
Clichy, France

Irving S. Benjamin BSc MB ChB MD FRCS(GLAS & ENG)
Professor of Surgery,
Guy's, King's & St Thomas' School of Medicine,
King's College Hospital,
London, UK

George Berci MD FACS FRCSEd(Hon)
Clinical Professor of Surgery,
Director of Surgical Endoscopy Research,
Department of Surgery,
Cedars-Sinai Medical Center,
Los Angeles, CA, USA

Thomas V. Berne MD FACS
Professor of Surgery,
Department of Surgery,
Los Angeles County–University of Southern California
   Medical Center,
Los Angeles, CA, USA

Kenneth F. Binmoeller MD
Associate Professor of Medicine and Surgery,
University of California at San Diego,
San Diego, CA, USA

Henri Bismuth MD FACS(HON)
Professor and Head,
Department of Surgery,
Hôpital Paul Brousse,
Villejuif, France

Martin J. K. Blomley MA MB MRCP FRCR
Senior Lecturer and Honorary Consultant,
Department of Imaging,
Imperial College School of Medicine,
Hammersmith Hospital,
London, UK

Stephen R. Bloom MA MD DSC FRCPath FRCP
Head of Division of Investigative Science,
Endocrine Unit,
Imperial College School of Medicine,
London, UK

Leslie H. Blumgart BDS MD DSC(Hon) FACS FRCS(Eng,
Edin) FRCPS(Glas)
Enid A. Haupt Chair in Surgery,
Chief, Hepatobiliary Service,
Director, Hepatobiliary Disease Management Program,
Memorial Sloan-Kettering Cancer Center;
Professor of Surgery,
Weill Medical College of Cornell University,
New York, NY, USA

Giacomo Borgonovo MD
Professor of Surgery,
Dipartimento di Discipline Chirurgiche e Metodologie
   Integrate,
Università di Genova,
Genova, Italy

Philippus C. Bornman FRCS(Edin) MMED(surg)
Professor of Surgery,
Department of Surgery,
Groote Schuur Hospital,
Cape Town, South Africa

Murray F. Brennan MD
Benno C. Schmidt Chair in Clinical Oncology,
Chairman, Department of Surgery,
Memorial Sloan-Kettering Cancer Center;
Professor of Surgery,
Weill Medical College of Cornell University,
New York, NY, USA

Lynn A. Brody MD
Clinical Assistant Radiologist,
Memorial Sloan-Kettering Cancer Center;
Clinical Assistant Professor of Radiology,
Weill Medical College of Cornell University,
New York , NY, USA

Christophe E. Broelsch MD
Professor of Surgery and Chairman,
Department of General Surgery and Transplantation,
University Hospital Essen,
Essen, Germany

Thomas A. Broughan MD
Professor and Chairman,
Department of Surgery,
Health Sciences Center,
University of Oklahoma,
Tulsa, OK, USA

Karen T. Brown MD
Associate Attending Radiologist,
Memorial Sloan-Kettering Cancer Center;
Associate Professor of Radiology,
Weill Medical College of Cornell University,
New York, NY, USA

Melissa L. Brown MS RD/LD CNSD
Clinical Dietitian,
Department of Nutrition and Dietetics,
University of Illinois at Chicago Medical Center,
Chicago, IL, USA

Andrew K. Burroughs MB ChB(Hon) FRCP
Consultant Physician and Hepatologist,
Liver Transplantation and Hepatobiliary Medicine,
Royal Free Hospital,
London, UK

Ronald W. Busuttil MD PhD
Professor and Chief, Surgery, Liver and Pancreas
  Transplantation,
University of California at Los Angeles Medical Center,
Los Angeles, CA, USA

Sir Roy Y. Calne FRS
Emeritus Professor of Surgery,
University of Cambridge,
Cambridge, UK

David L. Carr-Locke MB BChir FRCP FACG DRCOE
Director of Endoscopy and Associate Professor of
  Medicine,
Endoscopy Center,
Brigham and Women's Hospital,
Harvard Medical School,
Boston, MA, USA

Adrian Casavilla MD DPhil
Associate Professor of Surgery,
University of Pittsburgh,
Pittsburgh, PA, USA;
Assistant Professor of Surgery,
University of Buenos Aires;
Chief of Liver Unit,
Hospital Churruca Visca,
Buenos Aires, Argentina

Denis Castaing MD
Professor of Hepatobiliary Surgery,
Centre Hepatobiliaire,
Hôpital Paul Brousse,
Villejuif, France

Ronald S. Chamberlain MD
Assistant Attending Surgeon,
Montefiore Medical Center;
Assistant Professor of Surgery,
Albert Einstein Medical College,
New York, NY, USA

David O. Cosgrove MA FRCP FRCR
Professor of Clinical Ultrasound,
Department of Imaging,
Imperial College School of Medicine,
Hammersmith Hospital,
London, UK

Sir Alfred Cuschieri MD ChM FRSEd FRCS(Eng)
FRCPS(Glas) FRCSI FRSE
Professor of Surgery,
Department of Surgery and Molecular Oncology,
Ninewells Hospital and Medical School,
Dundee, UK

Abraham Czerniak MD FACS
Professor of Surgery,
Department of Surgery,
The E. Wolfson Medical Center,
Sackler School of Medicine,
Holon, Israel

Douglas R. DeCorato MD
Assistant Attending Radiologist,
Memorial Sloan-Kettering Cancer Center;
Assistant Professor of Radiology,
Weill Medical College of Cornell University,
New York, NY, USA

Ronald P. DeMatteo MD
Assistant Attending Surgeon,
Memorial Sloan-Kettering Cancer Center;
Assistant Professor of Surgery,
Weill Medical College at Cornell University,
New York, NY, USA

Achilles A. Demetriou MD PhD FACS
Chairman,
Department of Surgery,
Cedars-Sinai Medical Center,
Los Angeles, CA, USA

Arthur J. Donovan MD
Emeritus Professor of Surgery,
University of Southern California,
Los Angeles, CA, USA

R. Hermon Dowling MD FRCP
Professor of Gastroenterology,
Guy's King's and St Thomas' School of Medicine,
St Thomas' Hospital,
London, UK

Robert J. Eckersley PhD
Clinical Scientist,
Department of Imaging,
Imperial College School of Medicine,
Hammersmith Hospital,
London, UK

Serge Erlinger MD
Professor of Hepatology and Gastroenterology,
Hôpital Beaujon,
University of Paris,
Paris, France

Sheung-Tat Fan MBBS MS MD FRCS(Glas) FACS FCSHK
FHKAM
Professor of Surgery,
Department of Surgery,
University of Hong Kong Medical Centre,
Queen Mary Hospital,
Hong Kong, China

Olivier Farges MD
Professor of Diagnostic Radiology,
Hepatobiliary and Liver Transplant Centre,
Hôpital Paul Brousse,
Villejuif, France

Douglas G. Farmer MD
Assistant Professor of Surgery,
Division of Liver and Pancreas Transplantation,
University of California at Los Angeles,
Los Angeles, CA, USA

Nelson Fausto MD
Professor and Chairman,
Department of Pathology,
University of Washington School of Medicine,
Seattle, WA, USA

Annie H. Fecteau MD FRCS(C)
Assistant Professor of Surgery,
Department of Surgery,
Hospital for Sick Children,
Toronto, Ontario, Canada

David V. Feliciano MD
Professor of Surgery,
Emory University School of Medicine;
Chief of Surgery,
Grady Memorial Hospital,
Atlanta, GA, USA

Mary Fischer MD
Associate Attending Anesthesiologist,
Memorial Sloan-Kettering Cancer Center;
Associate Professor of Anesthesiology,
Weill Medical College of Cornell University,
New York, NY, USA

Yuman Fong MD FACS
Attending Surgeon,
Memorial Sloan-Kettering Cancer Center;
Professor of Surgery,
Weill Medical College of Cornell University,
New York, NY, USA

Dominique Franco MD
Professor of Digestive Surgery,
University of Paris,
Hôpital Antoine Béclère,
Paris, France

Jonathan W. Freeman MB ChB FRCA
Consultant Liver Transplant Anesthetist and Intensivist,
Divisional Director,
University Hospital and Selly Oak Hospital,
Birmingham, UK

O. James Garden BSc MB ChB MD FRCS(Glas) FRCS(Edin)
Regius Professor of Clinical Surgery,
Department of Clinical and Surgical Sciences,
Royal Infirmary,
Edinburgh, UK

Philippe Gertsch MD FMH(Surg) FCS HK
Professor of Surgery,
Department of Surgery,
Ospedale de San Giovanni,
Bellinzona, Switzerland

George I. Getrajdman MD
Associate Attending Radiologist,
Memorial Sloan-Kettering Cancer Center;
Associate Professor of Radiology,
Weill Medical College of Cornell University,
New York, NY, USA

Robert N. Gibson MBBS FRACR DDU
Associate Professor of Radiology,
University of Melbourne,
Royal Melbourne Hospital,
Melbourne, VA, Australia

Robert M. Girard MD FRCSC
Professor of Surgery,
Department of Surgery,
Université de Montreal,
Hôpital Maisonneuve-Rosemont,
Montreal, Canada

Dermot C. Gleeson MD BSc FRCP
Consultant Hepatologist,
Gastroenterology and Liver Unit,
Royal Hallamshire Hospital,
Central Sheffield University Hospitals,
Sheffield,
UK

Marvin L. Gliedman MD
Professor and Past Chairman,
Albert Einstein College of Medicine,
Montefiore Medical Centre,
New York, NY, USA

Robert D. Gordon MD
Medical Director: Transplantation,
Roche Laboratories Inc,
Kingsland,
Nutley, NJ, USA

John Goulis MD
Clinical Research Fellow,
Liver Transplantation and Hepatobiliary Medicine,
Royal Free Hospital,
London, UK

Gian Luca Grazi MD
Assistant Professor,
Surgical Unit,
University of Bologna,
Bologna, Italy

Sanjay Gupta MB BS MS FRCS
Lecturer in Surgery,
Academic Department of Surgery,
Guy's King's & St Thomas' School of Medicine,
King's College Hospital,
London, UK

Nicholas S. Hadjis MD
Formerly Assistant Professor,
Department of Surgery,
University of Saskatchewan,
Royal University Hospital,
Saskatoon, Saskatchewan, Canada

Ulrich Hanack MD
Senior Resident in Surgery,
Klinik für Transplantationschirurgie,
Georg-August-Universität Göttingen,
Göttingen, Germany

Lucy E. Hann MD
Associate Attending Radiologist,
Memorial Sloan-Kettering Cancer Center;
Associate Professor of Radiology,
Weill Medical College of Cornell University,
New York, NY, USA

W. Scott Helton MD
Chief,
General Surgery,
University of Illinois at Chicago Medical Center,
Chicago, IL, USA

Anne P. Hemingway BSC MB BS DMRD FRCP FRCR
Consultant Radiologist,
Directorate of Imaging,
Hammersmith Hospital,
London, UK

J. Michael Henderson MB Chb FRCS(Edin) FACS
Chairman of General Surgery,
Cleveland Clinic Foundation,
Cleveland, OH, USA

Robert E. Hermann MD
Emeritus Chairman,
Department of General Surgery,
Cleveland Clinic Foundation,
Cleveland, OH, USA

Edward R. Howard MS FRCS(Eng & Edin)
Professor of Paediatric Hepatobiliary Surgery,
Department of Surgery,
King's College Hospital,
London, UK

Thomas J. Hugh MD FRACS
Consultant Surgeon,
Royal North Shore Hospital,
Sydney, NSW, Australia

Nicholas C. A. Hunt BSC MBBS MRCPath
Clinical Lecturer in Pathology,
Nuffield Department of Clinical Laboratory Sciences,
University of Oxford and John Radcliffe Hospital,
Oxford, UK

Duane G. Hutson MD
Professor of Surgery,
Miami University School of Medicine,
Miami, FL, USA

Clement W. Imrie BSC MB ChB FRCS
Consultant Surgeon,
Glasgow Royal Infirmary,
Glasgow, UK

James E. Jackson MB BS MCRP FRCR
Consultant in Charge of Vascular and Non-vascular
  Interventional Radiology,
Imperial College School of Medicine,
Hammersmith Hospital,
London, UK

William R. Jarnagin MD
Assistant Attending Surgeon,
Memorial Sloan-Kettering Cancer Center;
Assistant Professor of Surgery,
Weill Medical College of Cornell University,
New York, NY, USA

Roger L. Jenkins MD FACS
Chief of Hepatobiliary Surgery,
Lahey Clinic Medical Center,
Burlington, MA, USA

Alan G. Johnson MChir FRCS
Professor of Surgery,
Department of Surgical and Anesthetic Sciences,
University of Sheffield,
Royal Hallamshire Hospital,
Sheffield, UK

Philip J. Johnson MD FRCP
Professor and Chairman,
Department of Clinical Oncology,
Prince of Wales Hospital,
The Chinese University of Hong Kong,
Hong Kong, China

Ronald N. Kaleya MD FACS
Attending Surgeon,
Montefiore Medical Center;
Associate Professor,
Albert Einstein College of Medicine,
New York, NY, USA

Junichi Kamiya MD
Associate Professor of Surgery,
The First Department of Surgery,
Nagoya University School of Medicine,
Nagoya, Japan

Nancy E. Kemeny MD
Attending Physician,
Memorial Sloan-Kettering Cancer Center;
Professor of Medicine,
Weill Medical College of Cornell University,
New York, NY, USA

Juichi Kitagawa MD
Lecturer of Surgery,
The First Department of Surgery,
Nagoya University School of Medicine,
Nagoya, Japan

Stuart J. Knechtle MD
Associate Professor of Surgery,
University of Wisconsin Medical School,
Madison, WI, USA

Jake E. J. Krige MB ChB FRCS FCS(SA)
Associate Professor of Surgery,
Department of Surgery,
University of Cape Town Medical School,
Cape Town, South Africa

Robert C. Kurtz MD
Chief, Gastroenterology and Nutrition Service,
Department of Medicine,
Memorial Sloan-Kettering Cancer Center;
Professor of Clinical Medicine,
Weill Medical College of Cornell University,
New York, NY, USA

Hanke Lang MD
Klinik und Poliklinik für Allgemein und
   Transplantationschirurgie,
Universitätsklinikum Essen,
Essen, Germany

Michael P. LaQuaglia MD
Chief, Pediatric Surgery,
Memorial Sloan-Kettering Cancer Center;
Professor of Surgery,
Weill Medical College of Cornell University,
New York, NY, USA

Steven M. Larson MD
Chief, Nuclear Medicine Service,
Department of Radiology,
Director, Laurent and Alberta Gerschel PET Center,
Memorial Sloan-Kettering Cancer Center;
Professor of Medicine,
Weill Medical College of Cornell University,
New York, NY, USA

Nicholas F. LaRusso MD
Chairman,
Department of Internal Medicine,
Mayo Clinic,
Rochester, MN, USA

Joseph W. Y. Lau MD FRCS (Edin, Glas & Eng) FRACS FACS
Professor and Chairman,
Department of Surgery,
Chinese University of Hong Kong,
Prince of Wales Hospital,
Hong Kong, China

Bernard Launois MD
Professor of Surgery,
Faculte de Médecine,
Université de Rennes,
Centre Medico-Clinisurgical St Vincent,
St Gregoire, France

Steven K. Libutti MD
Senior Investigator,
Surgery Branch, National Cancer Institiute,
National Health Institute,
Bethesda, MA, USA

Charles Lightdale MD
Director, Clinical Gastroenterology,
Columbia Presbetarian Hospital,
Professor of Clinical Medicine,
Columbia University College of Physicians and Surgeons,
New York, NY, USA

Pamela A. Lipsett MD
Fellowship Director,
Surgical Critical Care,
John Hopkins Medical Centre,
Baltimore, MD, USA

Alan S. Livingstone MD FACS
Professor and Chairman,
Chief, Division of Surgical Oncology,
Daughtry Family Department of Surgery,
Sylvester Cancer Center;
University of Miami School of Medicine,
Miami, FL, USA

Jeremy P. A. Lodge MD FRCS
Consultant in Hepatobiliary and Transplant Surgery,
Hepatobiliary Unit,
St James's University Hospital,
Leeds, UK

Stephen V. Lynch FRACS MBBS
Associate Professor of Surgery,
Princess Alexandra Hospital,
Brisbane, NSW, Australia

James O'D. McGee MD, PhD, FRCPath
Professor and Head,
Nuffield Department of Radiology,
John Radcliffe Hospital,
Oxford, UK

Paul McMaster MA MB ChM FRCS FICS
Professor of Hepatobiliary Surgery,
Liver Unit,
Queen Elizabeth Hospital,
Birmingham, UK

Lindsay Machan MD FRCP(C)
Joachim Burhenne Scholar in Abdominal Radiology,
Department of Radiology,
University of British Columbia Hospital,
Vancouver, BC, Canada

Ali W. Majeed MD FRCS
Senior Lecturer in Surgery,
Royal Hallamshire Hospital,
Sheffield, UK

Pietro E. Majno MD FRCS(Eng)
Chef de Clinique Scientifique,
Transplantation Unit,
Department of Surgery,
University Hospitals of Geneva,
Geneva, Switzerland

Masatoshi Makuuchi MD PhD
Professor and Chairman,
Department of Hepato-biliary-pancreatic and Transplant
  Surgery,
Faculty of Medicine,
University of Tokyo,
Tokyo, Japan

Massimo Malago MD
Oberaret Director of Transplantation and Hepato
  Pancreatico Biliary Surgery,
Klinik und Poliklinik für Allgemein und
  Transplantationschirurgie,
Universitätsklinikum Essen,
Essen, Germany

Dominique Mariette MD
Department of General and Digestive Surgery,
Hôpital Antoine Béclère,
Clamart, France

Robert T. Mathie BSc(Hons) PhD
Senior Lecturer in Surgical Physiology,
Division of Surgery, Anaesthetics and Intensive Care,
Imperial College School of Medicine,
Hammersmith Hospital,
London, UK

Alighieri Mazziotti MD
Professor and Chief of Surgery,
Surgical Unit,
University of Bologna,
S. Orsola Hospital,
Bologna, Italy

Jose A. Melendez MD
Associate Attending Anaesthesiologist,
Memorial Sloan-Kettering Cancer Center;
Associate Professor of Anesthesiology,
Weill Medical College of Cornell University,
New York, NY, USA

Yves Menu MD
Professor of Radiology,
Hôpital Beaujon
Clichy, France

Miroslav N. Milicevic MD PhD FACS
Professor of Surgery,
Institute for Digestive Diseases,
The First Surgical Clinic,
University Clinical Center Belgrade (KCS),
Belgrade, Federal Republic of Yugoslavia

Lyle L. Moldawer PhD
Professor of Surgery,
Department of Surgery,
University of Florida College of Medicine,
Gainesville, FL, USA

Nicholas G. Moss BSC PLO
Research Associate Professor,
Department of Cell and Molecular Physiology,
University of North Carolina at Chapel Hill,
Chapel Hill, NC, USA

Joanne Moysey MB ChB FRCA
Specialist Registrar in Anaesthesia,
Featherstone Department of Anaesthetics and Intensive
  Care,
Queen Elizabeth Hospital,
Birmingham, UK

Masato Nagino MD PhD
Associate Professor Surgery,
The First Department of Surgery,
Nagoya University School of Medicine,
Nagoya, Japan

David M. Nargorney MD
Consultant, Division of Gastroenterologic and General
  Surgery,
Mayo Clinic and Mayo Foundation;
Professor of Surgery,
Mayo Medical School,
Rochester, MN, USA

James Neuberger DM FRCP
Professor of Medicine,
Liver Unit,
Queen Elizabeth Hospital,
Birmingham, UK

Yuji Nimura MD PHD
Professor and Chairman of Surgery,
The First Department of Surgery,
Nagoya University School of Medicine,
Nagoya, Japan

Risteárd Ó Laoide MB MRCPI FRCR FFR(RCSI)
Consultant Radiologist,
Department of Radiology,
St Vincent's University Hospital,
Dublin, Ireland

Mark S. Orloff MD
Associate Professor of Surgery,
Department of Surgery,
Strong Memorial Hospital,
Rochester, NY, USA

Marshall J. Orloff MD
Professor of Surgery,
University of Califonia Medical Center,
Los Angeles, CA, USA

H. Leon Pachter MD
Professor of Surgery and Interim Chairman,
Department of Surgery,
New York University School of Medicine,
New York, NY, USA

George V. Papatheodoridis MD
Clinical Research Fellow,
Liver Transplantation and Hepatobiliary Medicine,
Royal Free Hospital,
London, UK

Philip B. Paty MD
Associate Attending Surgeon,
Memorial Sloan-Kettering Cancer Center;
Associate Professor of Surgery,
Weill Medical College of Cornell University,
New York, NY, USA

Henry A. Pitt MD
Chairman,
Department of Surgery,
Medical College of Wisconsin,
Milwaukee, WI, USA

James J. Pomposelli MD PhD
Transplantation and Hepatobiliary Fellow,
Beth Israel Deaconess Medical Center,
Boston, MA, USA

Ian M. Pope MD FRCS
Specialist Surgical Registrar,
The Royal Infirmary,
Edinburgh, UK

Graeme J. Poston MB MS FRCS(Eng) FRCS(Edin)
Consultant Surgeon and Chief,
Hepatobiliary Service,
Royal Liverpool University Hospital,
Liverpool, UK

Richard T. Prall MD
Instructor of Internal Medicine,
Fellow, Division of Gastroenterology and Hepatology,
Mayo Clinic,
Rochester, MN, USA

Fabio Procacciante MD
Professor of Surgery,
Seconda Clinica Chirurgica,
Università Degli Studi di Roma 'La Sapienza',
Rome, Italy

Thanjavur S. Ravikumar MD FACS
Professor and Chairman of Surgery,
Department of Surgery,
Albert Einstein College of Medicine,
Montefiore Medical Centre,
New York, NY, USA

Ravindra Kadiyala Venkata MS McH
Assistant Professor,
Department of Surgery,
St John's Medical College Hospital,
Bangalore, India

Jürg Reichen MD
Professor of Medicine,
Department of Clinical Pharmacology,
University of Berne,
Berne, Switzerland

Giorgio Ribotta MD
Professor of Surgery,
VI Clinica Chirurgica,
Università Degli Studi Di Roma 'La Sapienza',
Roma, Italy

Layton F. Rikkers MD
A. R. Curreri Professor and Chairman,
Department of Surgery,
University of Wisconsin,
Madison, WI, USA

Burckhardt Ringe MD
Professor of Surgery,
Klinik für Transplantationschirurgie,
Georg-August-Universität Göttingen,
Göttingen, Germany

Stephen M. Riordan MD FRACP
Staff Specialist in Hepatology,
The Prince of Wales Hospital,
Sydney, NSW, Australia

Enrico Roda MD
Professor of Medicine,
Departimento di Medicina Interna e Gastroenterolgia,
Università di Bologna,
Bologna, Italy

Mary E. Roddie BMedSci MRCP FRCR
Consultant Radiologist,
Department of Imaging,
Charing Cross Hospital,
London, UK

Brian J. Rowlands MD FRCS FACS
Professor of Surgery,
Section of Surgery,
Queen's Medical Centre,
University Hospital,
Nottingham, UK

Jacek Rozga MD PhD
Associate Professor of Surgery,
Liver Support Research Laboratory,
Cedars-Sinai Medical Center,
Los Angeles, CA, USA

Edward Russell MD FACR
Professor and Director of Diagnostic Radiology,
Department of Radiology,
University of Miami School of Medicine,
Miami, FL, USA

Pierre F. Saldinger MD
Surgical Director,
Liver and Gastrointestinal Cancer Program,
Beth Israel Deaconess Medical Center;
Assistant Professor of Surgery,
Harvard Medical School,
Boston MA, USA

Didier Samuel MD
Professor of Hepatology,
Centre Hepatobiliaire,
Hôpital Paul Brousse,
Paris, France

J. Philip Sandblom MD PhD
Professor Emeritus of Surgery and Former President,
University of Lund,
Lund, Switzerland

Tsuyoshi Sano MD PhD
Assistant Professor of Surgery,
The First Department of Surgery,
Nagoya University School of Medicine,
Nagoya, Japan

Johannes Scheele MD
Absteilungsdirektor,
Abteilung für Aligemeine und Viszerale Chirurgie,
Friendrich-Schiller Universitat Jena,
Jena, Germany

Frank Peter Schulze MD
Resident in Surgery,
Georg-August-Universität Göttingen,
Klinik für Transplantationschirurige,
Göttingen, Germany

Lawrence H. Schwartz MD
Associate Professor of Radiology,
Department of Radiology,
Memorial Sloan-Kettering Cancer Center,
New York, NY, USA

Arjun Shankar-Chowdhury MD FRCS
Lecturer in Surgery,
Department of Surgery,
Royal Free and University Medical School,
London, UK

Sir Robert Shields MD, DSC, FRCS
Emeritus Professor of Surgery,
Department of Surgery,
The Royal Liverpool University Hospital,
Liverpool, UK

Elin R Sigurdson MD PhD
Member,
Fox Chase Cancer Center,
Philadelphia, PA, USA

Claude Smadja MD PhD
Professor of Digestive Surgery,
Department of General and Digestive Surgery,
University of Paris,
Hôpital Antoine Béclère,
Clamart, France

Nib Soehendra MD
Professor of Surgery,
Department of Endoscopic Surgery,
University Hospital of Hamburg,
Hamburg, Germany

Kaumudi Somnay MD
Assistant Professor of Medicine,
Johns Hopkins University School of Medicine,
Baltimore, MD, USA

Karl Søndenaa MD
Consultant HPB-Surgery,
Department of Surgery,
Rogaland Central Hospital,
Stavanger, Norway

Nathaniel J. Soper MD FACS
Professor of Surgery,
Washington University School of Medicine,
St Louis, MO, USA

Eric van Sonnenberg MD
Radiologist,
Brigham & Women's Hospital;
Professor of Radiology,
Harvard Medical School;
Chief of Radiology,
Dana Farber Cancer Institute;
Boston, MA, USA

Odd Søreide MD
Professor of Surgery,
Department of Surgery B,
National Hospital (Rikshospitalet),
University of Oslo,
Oslo, Norway

Richard Stangl MD PhD
Lecturer in Surgery,
Friendlich-Alexander University,
Erlangen, Germany

Sarah A. Stanley MA MB BChir MRCP
Clinical Research Fellow,
Endocrine Unit,
Imperial College School of Medicine,
London, UK

Thomas E. Starzl MD PhD
Professor of Surgery,
Department of Surgery,
University of Pittsburgh Medical Centre,
Pittsburgh, PA, USA

Peter D. Stevens MD
Assistant Professor of Clinical Medicine,
Columbia University College of Physicians and Surgeons,
New York, NY, USA

Russell W. Strong MB BS FRCS FRACS FACS FRACDS
Professor of Surgery,
Princess Alexandra Hospital,
Brisbane, NSW, Australia

John A. Summerfield MD FRCP
Professor of Medicine,
Department of Medicine,
Imperial College School of Medicine,
St Mary's Hospital,
London, UK

Tadatoshi Takayama MD PhD
Associate Professor,
Department of Hepato-biliary-pancreatic and
  Transplantation Surgery,
Faculty of Medicine,
University of Tokyo,
Tokyo, Japan

Irving Taylor MD CHM FRCS
Professor of Surgery and Chairman,
Academic Division of Surgical Specialists,
Royal Free and University College Medical School,
London, UK

John Terblanche CHM FCS(SA) FRCS(Eng)
Professor of Surgery and Head,
Department of Surgery,
University of Cape Town,
Groote Schuur Hospital,
Cape Town, South Africa

Onno T. Terpstra MD PhD FRCS
Professor and Head of Surgery,
Department of Surgery,
Leiden University Medical Centre,
Leiden, The Netherlands

Philip G. Thomas MS FACS
Professor of Surgery,
Unit of Hepatobiliary Surgery and Organ
   Transplantation,
St John's Medical College Hospital,
Bangalore, India

James Toouli MBBS BMedSci FRACS PhD
Professor of Surgery,
Department of General and Digestive Surgery,
Flinders Medical Centre,
Adelaide, SA, Australia

Robert A. Underwood MD
Research Fellow,
Washington University School of Medicine,
St Louis, MO, USA

Jean-Nicolas Vauthey MD FACS
Associate Professor and Chief,
Liver Service,
University of Texas M. D. Anderson Cancer Center,
Houston, TX, USA

Christian H. Wakefield BSc MBBS MD FRCS(Eng)
Lecturer in Surgery,
Department of Clincial and Surgical Sciences,
Royal Infirmary,
Edinburgh, Scotland

Antony M. Wheatley BSc(Hons) PhD
Professor of Physiology,
Department of Physiology,
School of Medical Sciences,
University of Otago,
Dunedin, New Zealand

Russell H. Wiesner MD
Professor of Medicine,
Director of Liver Transplantation,
Mayo Clinic,
Rochester, MN, USA

Roger Williams CBE MD FRCP FRCS FRCPE FRACP FMedSci
   FACP(Hon)
Professor and Director,
Institute of Hepatology,
University College London Medical School,
London, UK

John Wong MD PhD FRACS FACS
Professor of Surgery,
Department of Surgery,
University of Hong Kong Medical Centre,
Queen Mary Hospital,
Hong Kong, China

Arthur Zimmermann MD
Professor of Pathology,
Institute of Pathology,
University of Berne,
Berne, Germany

Heinz Zimmermann MD
Chief, Trauma and Emergency Unit,
Inselspital,
University of Bern,
Bern, Switzerland

Preface

In the preparation of the third edition of this book, I have invited Dr Yuman Fong to join me as co-editor. Together we have maintained the general format of comprehensively covering the surgical aspects of the management of liver and biliary tract disorders. In addition, we include a CD-ROM illustrating some of the key surgical procedures.

All of the contributors, who represent a cross-section of those involved in the specialty management of liver and biliary tract disease, have been asked to discuss their subject from the point of view of surgical management and to relate their views to the opinions of others. In many instances, authors with conflicting opinions have been chosen so as to allow the reader an opportunity to assess the views of enthusiasts with different approaches to the same problem. In some instances, deliberate overlap between chapters has been encouraged, firstly to allow each contribution to be an encapsulated account which stands on its own for the reader who wishes to consult the book as a reference, and secondly to allow the display of different nuances of approach to particularly difficult problems. Balancing chapters are inserted in an attempt to draw together a rational approach for the utilization of diagnostic imaging modalities and to correlate the extraordinary advances that have taken place.

There have been very extensive modifications and additions throughout this edition. Indeed, Dr Fong and I have had the feeling that we have been editing an entirely new book. Some chapters which previously stood alone have now been combined. For example, the chapters on the surgical and radiologic anatomy of the liver and of the biliary tract were separate contributions in the last edition but are now amalgamated into one comprehensive chapter.

We have included considerable detail recognizing the importance of laparoscopic diagnostic and surgical procedures and of the newer techniques of tumor ablation. Importantly, the operative descriptions have been extended so that the book has major sections that can be read more as an atlas of technique. Almost all of the previous contributions have been updated to take into account recent advances in the biological understanding of disease processes and of the newer diagnostic and therapeutic modalities.

The initial section of the book is devoted to the applied anatomy of the liver and biliary tract including its radiological demonstrations. Throughout the anatomical contributions of Claude Couinaud are recognized, the liver anatomy and nomenclature of the various operative approaches being generally according to his description. Normal function and pathophysiological aspects are covered with particular reference to measurement techniques and to the response not only of the liver and biliary tract but also of the patient to disease. The molecular and genetic basis of liver regeneration and of hepatobiliary disease is included. Perioperative and operative diagnostic approaches are again fully covered and the text has been expanded to include important new developments in nuclear medicine, computed tomography, and magnetic resonance imaging.

All aspects of diagnostic and therapeutic approaches to gallstones, biliary strictures, and liver and biliary cancer are discussed and interventional endoscopic and radiological approaches are argued in relation to surgical techniques.

There is a full discussion and illustrated description of the operative approaches to biliary disease with special emphasis on the management of gallstones, biliary strictures and fistula, and of biliary and periampullary and pancreatic cancer. Liver and biliary infections due to pyogenic organisms and parasitic infestations are detailed. Liver and biliary cysts and their surgical management are fully described, as is the management of injuries to the liver and associated biliary ducts, arteries, and veins. An entire section covering biliary tumors and primary and secondary liver tumors has been specially updated and the differences in approach in the Western world and Asia extensively described. There is a particular recognition of the major contribution of Japanese surgeons to the field.

Recent years have seen extraordinary refinement in the operative techniques pertaining to liver resection and these are covered in special detail. Newly introduced approaches and the importance of conserving blood loss in major liver resective surgery and of intraoperative ultrasonographically guided operation are detailed.

Cirrhosis of the liver and the management of portal hypertension including operative descriptive techniques for the control of variceal hemorrhage, are extensively discussed and such recent advances as, for example, the place of radiologic intervention are included. The management of liver failure and the treatment of ascites and fulminant hepatic failure are covered. The entire section on liver transplantation, its complications and results has been expanded to cover new developments in the field.

In short, we have attempted to include all aspects of anatomy, pathology, diagnosis, and surgically related therapeutic approaches to liver and biliary tract disorders, and to provide a text which will be of value not only to the trainee surgeon and the established specialist, but also to the interested specialist in the important related disciplines concerned with the management of diseases of the liver and biliary system. We have attempted throughout to enlist new contributors and to give latitude to conflicting opinions and yet provide guidance so as to allow the reader to form an individual approach based on contemporary attitudes.

I sincerely hope this book proves of value not only as an account of the current "state-of-the-art" in the surgical aspects of liver and biliary disease but also act as stimulus to those interested in further study of the very many unresolved problems which await investigation. When I wrote the preface to the last edition, I mentioned that hepatobiliary surgery had come of age and that it deserved specialty recognition. There is no doubt that this has come to pass and that it is now widely recognized that refined hepatobiliary surgery requires special training.

L. H. Blumgart
New York, 2000

Acknowledgments

We are deeply grateful to all who have contributed to this publication. Our colleagues in surgery, internal medicine, radiology, endoscopy, pathology and anesthesiology all responded enthusiastically and added the weight of their experience. We are especially grateful to them for adding the spice of differing opinion and the aroma of international practice to the basic flavor of the work.

Particular thanks are due to the members of our own staff and colleagues at Memorial Sloan-Kettering Cancer Center, New York, who have contributed and assisted us in the preparation of this work.

In the first edition, the illustrative work in the book was of uniform character and nearly all the drawings were done by Mr Doig Simmonds, medical illustrator at the Royal Postgraduate Medical School at Hammersmith Hospital, London. However, many of these have now been modified.

There are extensive new illustrations that have been contributed by Mr Philip Wilson of London who, in discussion with us, has produced a remarkable series of drawings.

Editorial assistance has been carried out entirely by Ms Maria Reyes who has very efficiently undertaken the major task of gathering contributions and of coordinating with the publishers, the artist and ourselves. She has also provided considerable help in proofreading. We are extremely grateful to her for a major task, which she has discharged with expertise.

Finally, our thanks and appreciation are due to our new publisher, Harcourt Health Sciences and in particular to Mr Sean Duggan of London who has kept contact with us in New York.

L. H. Blumgart
Y. Fong

Anatomy and pathophysiology

Surgical and radiologic anatomy of the liver and biliary tract

L.H. BLUMGART AND L.E. HANN

Precise knowledge of the anatomy of the liver, biliary tract and pancreas, and the related blood vessels and the lymphatic drainage are essential for the performance of liver, biliary and pancreatic surgery.

THE LIVER

The liver lies under cover of the lower ribs closely applied to the undersurface of the diaphragm and astride the vena cava posteriorly. Most of the liver bulk lies to the right of the midline where the lower border coincides with the right costal margin but extends as a wedge to the left of the midline between the anterior surface of the stomach and the left dome of the diaphragm. The upper surface is boldly convex, molded to the diaphragm, and the surface projection on the anterior body wall extends up to the fourth intercostal space on the right and the fifth space on the left. The convexity of the upper surface slopes down to a posterior surface, which is triangular in outline. The liver is invested with peritoneum except on the posterior surface where the peritoneum reflects onto the diaphragm forming the right and left triangular ligaments. The undersurface of the liver is concave and extends down to a sharp anterior border. The posterior surface of the liver is triangular in outline with its base to the right and here the liver lying between the upper and lower leaves of the triangular ligaments is bare and devoid of peritoneum. The anterior border lies undercover of the right costal margin lateral to the right rectus abdominis muscle, but slopes upward to the left across the epigastrium. Anteriorly the convex surface of the liver lies comfortably against the concavity of the diaphragm and is attached to it by the falciform ligament, left triangular ligament and the upper layer of the right triangular ligament.

RETROHEPATIC INFERIOR VENA CAVA

The inferior vena cava runs on the right of the aorta, on the bodies of the lumbar vertebrae, diverging somewhat from it as it passes upwards. Inferior to the liver it lies behind the duodenum and head of the pancreas as a retroperitoneal structure passing upwards behind the Foramen of Winslow posterior to the right hilar structures of the liver. The renal veins lie in front of the arteries and join the inferior vena cava at almost a right angle on the left and obliquely on the right. Behind the liver the inferior vena cava is embraced in a groove on its posterior surface (Figs 1.1, 1.2). The inferior vena cava comes to lie on the right crus of the diaphragm behind the bare area of the liver and then extends to the central tendon of the diaphragm which it pierces on a level with the body of T8, somewhat behind and higher than the commencement of the abdominal aorta. As it courses upward it is separated from the right crus of the diaphragm by the right celiac ganglion and higher up by the right phrenic artery. The right adrenal vein is a short vessel that enters the inferior vena cava behind the bare area (Fig. 1.1). It is important to recognize that there may be a small accessory adrenal vein on the right that enters into the confluence of the right renal vein and the inferior vena cava. The lumbar veins drain posterolaterally into the inferior vena cava below the level of the renal veins, but above this level there are usually no vena caval tributaries posteriorly.

HEPATIC VEINS

The *hepatic veins* (Figs 1.3, 1.4, 1.5) drain directly from the upper part of the posterior surface of the liver at a somewhat oblique angle directly into the vena cava. The right hepatic vein, somewhat larger than the left and middle hepatic veins, has a short extrahepatic course of usually some 1 cm. The left and middle hepatic veins may drain separately into the

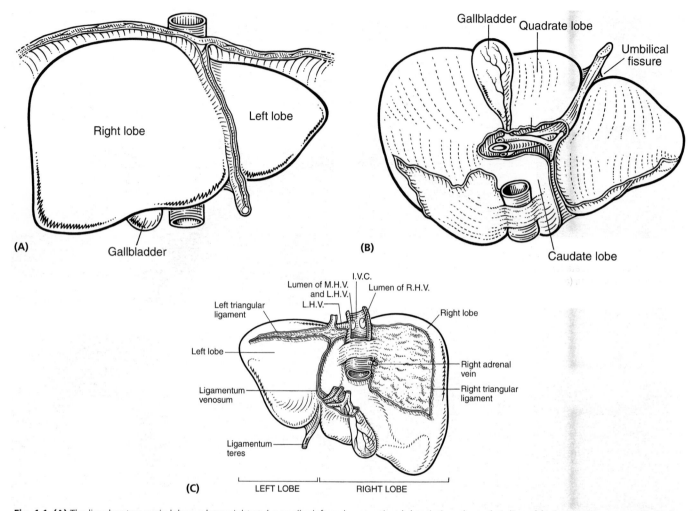

Fig. 1.1 (A) The liver has two main lobes, a large right and a smaller left and conventional description places their line of fusion on the upper surface of the liver along the attachment of the falciform ligament at the inferior extent of which the ligamentum teres enters the umbilical fissure. **(B)** On the inferior surface of the right lobe is the transverse hilar fissure which constitutes the posterior limit of this lobe. The portion of the right lobe located anterior to the fissure is called the quadrate lobe limited on the left by the umbilical fissure and on the right by the gallbladder fossa. Posterior to the hilar transverse fissure is a fourth lobe, the caudate lobe. This lobe hugs the inferior vena cava and extends upwards on its left side. Thus, the liver is comprised of two main lobes and two smaller lobes which are separated by visible well defined fissures on the liver surface. **(C)** The inferior vena cava lies snugly in a deep grove within the bare area; the hepatic veins opening directly into it. Within this bare area the right suprarenal gland lies adjacent to the inferior vena cava and the adrenal vein drains into the right of the inferior vena cava. The remainder of the bare area of liver is directly in contact with the diaphragm. To the left of the inferior vena cava the caudate lobe slopes upward from the inferior to the posterior surface of the liver and is demarcated on the left by a fissure within which lies the ligamentum venosum. The gastrohepatic omentum is attached to the ligamentum venosum placing the caudate lobe within the lesser sac of the peritoneum but the left lobe of the liver anteriorly in the supracolic compartment of the peritoneal cavity. The posterior surface of the left lobe is narrow, there being a very fine bare area on this side. As the vena cava traverses upwards in the groove on the posterior surface of the liver it is shielded on the right side by a layer of fibrous tissue passing from the posterior edge of the liver backwards toward the lumbar vertebrae and fanning out posteriorly especially in the upper part. Behind the inferior vena cava a prolongation of this fibrous layer joins a less marked fibrous extension from the lateral edge of the caudate lobe. This layer of fibrous tissue, sometimes called the ligament of the vena cava, must be divided on the right to allow surgical exposure of the inferior vena cava and the hepatic veins and on the left to allow mobilization of the caudate lobe. Occasionally, the liver tissue embraces the vena cava completely so that it runs within a tunnel of parenchyma. RHV, right hepatic vein. MHV, middle hepatic vein. LHV, left hepatic vein.

inferior vena cava but are frequently joined after a short extrahepatic course to form a common venous channel some 2 cm in length which traverses to the left part of the anterior surface of the inferior vena cava below the diaphragm (Figs 1.3, 1.5). It should be appreciated that there are additional hepatic veins to the three major hepatic veins. The umbilical vein is single, in most cases, running beneath the falciform ligament between the middle and left hepatic veins and emptying into the terminal portion of the left hepatic vein although rarely into the middle hepatic vein or directly into the confluence of the middle and left hepatic veins.

Additional posterior inferior draining hepatic veins with a short course into the anterior surface of the inferior vena cava are encountered, and may be large (Fig. 1.4).

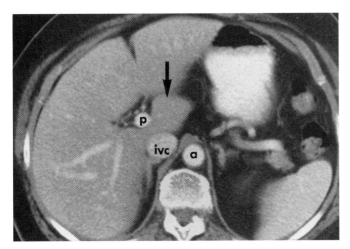

Fig. 1.2 Contrast-enhanced CT image of the liver shows the intimate relationship of the caudate lobe (arrow), inferior vena cava (ivc) and portal vein (p), and aorta (a).

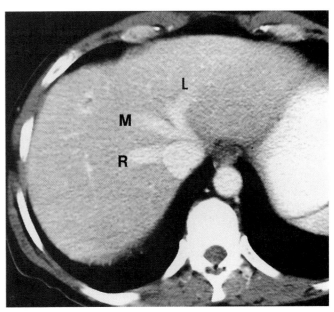

(A)

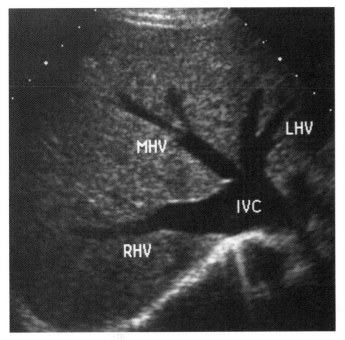

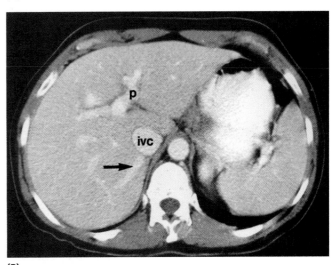

(B)

Fig. 1.4 An inferior accessory right hepatic vein shown by CT scan. **(A)** The hepatic venous confluence with left (L), middle (M) and right (R) hepatic veins. **(B)** An additional inferior accessory right hepatic vein (arrow) enters the inferior vena cava (ivc) separately at a lower level (p, portal vein).

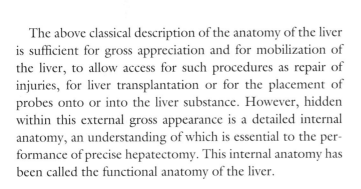

Fig. 1.3 Transverse sonogram of the hepatic vein confluence. Right hepatic vein (RHV), middle hepatic vein (MHV), left hepatic vein (LHV) and inferior vena cava (IVC).

The above classical description of the anatomy of the liver is sufficient for gross appreciation and for mobilization of the liver, to allow access for such procedures as repair of injuries, for liver transplantation or for the placement of probes onto or into the liver substance. However, hidden within this external gross appearance is a detailed internal anatomy, an understanding of which is essential to the performance of precise hepatectomy. This internal anatomy has been called the functional anatomy of the liver.

FUNCTIONAL SURGICAL ANATOMY

The internal architecture of the liver is composed of *a series of segments combining to form sectors separated by scissurae containing the hepatic veins* (Fig. 1.6). Together or separately they constitute the visible lobes described above.

The internal architecture of the liver has been clarified by the publications of McIndoe and Counseller (1927), Ton That Tung (1939), Hjörstjö (1931), Healey and Schroy (1953),

Goldsmith and Woodburne (1957), Couinaud (1957) and by Bismuth et al (1982). The description of Couinaud is the most complete and exact and also the most useful for the operating surgeon and this is the description which will be used throughout this book. Essentially, *the three main hepatic veins within the scissurae divide the liver into four sectors each of which receives a portal pedicle* with alternation between the hepatic veins and portal pedicles. The main portal scissura contains the middle hepatic vein and progresses from the middle of the gallbladder bed anteriorly to the left of the vena cava posteriorly. The right and left liver, demarcated by the main portal scissura, are independent in terms of portal and arterial vascularization and of biliary drainage (Fig. 1.7).

These right and left livers are themselves divided into two by the remaining portal scissurae. These four subdivisions are referred to as segments in the description of Goldsmith and Woodburne (1957) but in Couinaud's nomenclature (1957) are termed *sectors* (Figs 1.6, 1.7).

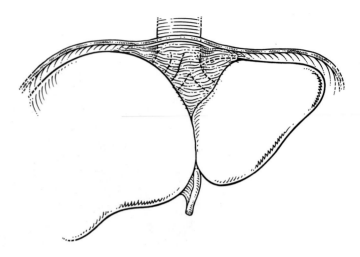

Fig. 1.5 The anterior surface of the major extrahepatic veins and the inferior vena cava are retroperitoneal and masked behind the layers of the falciform ligament as it splits and passes to the right and left triangular ligaments.

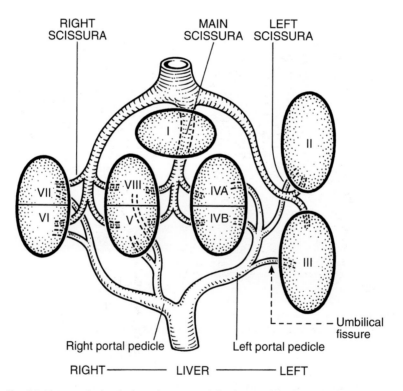

Fig. 1.6 The portal vein, the hepatic artery and the draining bile ducts are distributed within the liver in a beautifully symmetrical pedicular pattern which belies the asymmetric external appearance. Each Segment I–VIII is supplied by a portal triad composed of a branch of the portal vein and hepatic artery and drained by a tributary of the right or left main hepatic ducts. The four sectors demarcated by the three main hepatic veins are called the portal sectors, these portions of parenchyma being supplied by independent portal pedicles. The hepatic veins run between the sectors in the portal scissurae while the scissurae containing portal pedicles are called the hepatic scissurae. The umbilical fissure corresponds to an hepatic scissurae. So it is, that the internal architecture of the liver consists of two livers, or hemilivers, the right and the left liver separated by the main portal scissura also known as Cantlie's line. It is preferable to call them the right and left liver rather than the right and left lobes for this last nomenclature is erroneous there being no visible mark that permits identification of a true hemiliver.

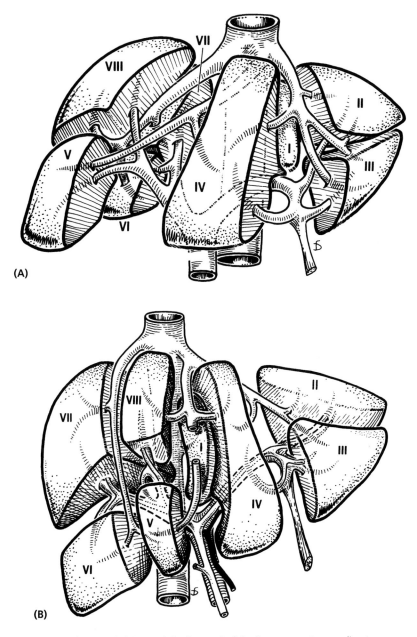

Fig. 1.7 The functional division of the liver and of the liver segments according to Couinaud's nomenclature. **(A)** As seen in the patient; **(B)** in the ex-vivo position (see text).

The right portal scissura separating the right liver into two sectors – anteromedial or anterior and posterolateral or posterior – is almost in the frontal plane with the body supine. The right hepatic vein runs within the right scissura.

The left portal scissura divides the left liver into two sectors superior and posterior. The left portal scissura is not within the umbilical fissure since this fissure is not a portal scissura and, indeed, contains a portal pedicle. The left portal scissura is, in fact, located posterior to the ligamentum teres and within the left lobe of the liver along the course of the left hepatic vein. Thus, the anterior sector of the left

liver is composed of a part of the right lobe which is to the left of the main portal scissura and of the anterior part of the left lobe (Figs 1.6, 1.7).

At the hilus of the liver the right portal triad pursues a short course of approximately 1 to 1.5 cm before entering the substance of the right hemiliver (Fig. 1.8). On the left side, however, the portal triad crosses over some 3 to 4 cm beneath the quadrate lobe embraced in a peritoneal sheath at the upper end of the gastrohepatic ligament and separated from the under surface of the quadrate lobe by connective tissue (the hilar plate). This prolongation of the left

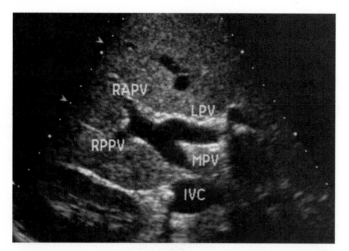

Fig. 1.8 Transverse sonogram at the level of the portal vein bifurcation. The main portal vein (MPV) bifurcates into the left (LPV) and right portal veins. The right portal vein bifurcates shortly into the right anterior (RAPV) and right posterior (RPPV) branches but the left portal vein has a longer horizontal course within the hilar plate. The inferior vena cava (IVC) is seen posteriorly.

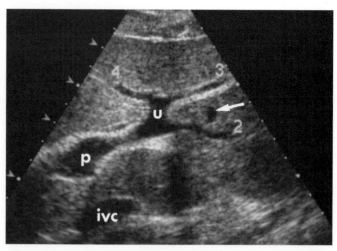

Fig. 1.9 Transverse sonogram shows the branching pattern of the left portal vein (p) which courses horizontally and then into the umbilical fissure. The umbilical portion of the left portal vein (u) gives branches to the left hepatic Segments (II, III and IV). Left hepatic vein (arrow) and inferior vena cava (ivc) are also shown.

portal pedicle turns anteriorly and caudally within the umbilical fissure giving branches of supply to Segments II, III and recurrent branches to Segment IV (Figs 1.6, 1.9). Beneath the quadrate lobe the pedicle is composed of the left branch of the portal vein and the left hepatic duct but it is joined at the base of the umbilical fissure by the left branch of the hepatic artery.

The branching of the portal pedicle at the hilus (Figs. 1.6, 1.8, 1.9, 1.10), the distribution of the branches to the caudate lobe (segment I) on the right and left side, and the distribution to the segments of the right (Segments V–VIII) and left (Segments II–IV) hemiliver follow a remarkably symmetrical pattern and, as described by Scheele (1994), allows separation of Segment IV into Segment IVa superiorly and Segment IVb inferiorly (Fig. 1.6). This arrangement of subsegments mimics the distribution to Segments V and VIII on the right side. The umbilical vein provides drainage of, at least, parts of Segment IVb after ligation of the middle hepatic vein and is important in the performance of segmental resection.

The caudate lobe (segment I) is the dorsal portion of the liver lying posteriorly and embracing the retrohepatic inferior vena cava. It should be clearly appreciated that the lobe lies between major vascular structures – the inferior vena cava posteriorly and the left portal triad inferiorly and the inferior vena cava and the middle and left hepatic veins superiorly (Figs 1.11, 1.12).

The portion of the caudate on the right is variable but is usually quite small. The anterior surface *within the parenchyma* is covered by the posterior surface of Segment

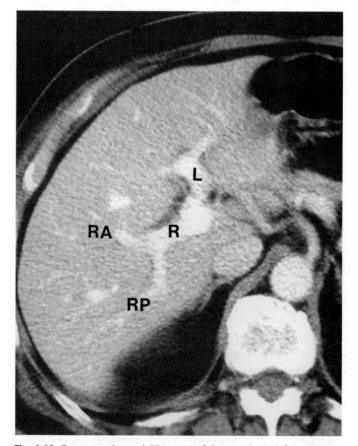

Fig. 1.10 Contrast-enhanced CT images of the portal vein bifurcation. L, left portal vein; R, right portal vein; RA, right anterior portal vein; RP, right posterior portal vein.

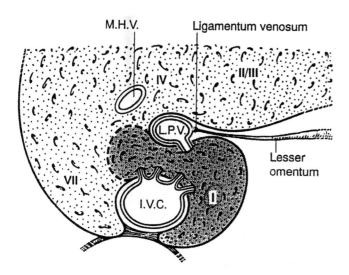

Fig. 1.11 The main bulk of the caudate lobe (Segment I) (shaded) lies to the left of the inferior vena cava (IVC) – the left and inferior margins being free in the lesser omental bursa. The gastrohepatic (lesser) omentum separates the left portion of the caudate from Segments II and III of the liver as it passes between them to be attached to the ligamentum venosum. The left portion of the caudate lobe inferiorly traverses to the right between the portal vein (LPV) and inferior vena cava as the caudate process where it fuses with the right lobe of the liver. Note the position of the middle hepatic vein (MHV).

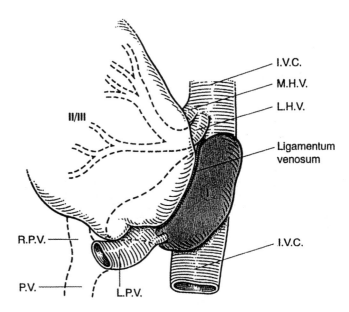

Fig. 1.12 The caudate lobe (shaded): segments II and III rotated to the patient's right. Superiorly the left portion of the caudate lobe is linked by a deep anterior portion which is embedded in the parenchyma immediately under the middle hepatic vein (MHV) reaching inferiorly to the posterior margin of the hilus of the liver and fusing antero-laterally to the inferior vena cava (IVC) on the right side to Segments VI and VII of the right liver. The major blood supply arises from the left branch of the left portal vein (LPV) and the left hepatic artery close to the base of the umbilical fissure of the liver. The hepatic veins (MHV, LHV) are short in course and drain from the caudate directly into the anterior and left aspect of the vena cava. LHV, left hepatic vein. RPV, right portal vein. PV, main trunk of portal vein.

IV, the limit being an oblique plane slanting from the left portal vein to the left hepatic vein. Thus, there is a caudate lobe (Segment I) with a constantly present left portion and a right portion of variable size (Figs 1.11, 1.12).

The caudate lobe is supplied by blood vessels and drained by biliary tributaries both from the right and left portal triad. Small vessels from the portal vein and tributaries joining the biliary ducts are also found, usually two on the left side and one on the right. The right portion of the caudate lobe including the caudate process predominantly receives portal venous blood from the right portal vein or the bifurcation of the main portal vein whereas on the left side the portal supply arises from the left branch of the portal vein almost exclusively. Similarly, the arterial supply and biliary drainage of the right portion is most commonly associated with the right posterior sectoral vessels or pedicle and the left portion with the left main vessels.

The hepatic venous drainage of the caudate is unique in that it is the only hepatic segment draining directly into the inferior vena cava. These veins can sometimes drain into the posterior aspect of the vena cava if there is a significant retrocaval caudate component.

In the usual and common circumstance the posterior edge of the caudate lobe on the left has a fibrous component which fans out attaching lightly to the crural area of the diaphragm but importantly extending posteriorly

behind the vena cava to link with a similar component of fibrous tissue protruding from the posterior surface of Segment VII and embracing the vena cava (Figs 1.1C, 1.11). It is important to note that in up to 50% of patients this ligament is replaced, in whole or in part, by hepatic tissue and the caudate may thus completely encircle the IVC and contact Segment VII on the right side. A significant retrocaval component may prevent a left-sided approach to the caudate veins. The caudal margin of the caudate lobe has a papillary process which on occasion may attach to the rest of the lobe via a narrow connection. It is bulky in 27% of cases and can be mistaken for an enlarged lymph node on computed tomography (CT) scan (Fig. 1.13).

To summarize: (1) The liver is divided into two hemi-livers by the main hepatic scissura within which runs the middle hepatic vein. (2) The left liver is divided into two sectors by the left portal scissura within which the left hepatic vein runs (Fig. 1.6). The posterior sector is comprised of only one segment, Segment II, which is the posterior part of the left lobe. This is the only sector which is comprised of one segment. The anterior sector is divided by

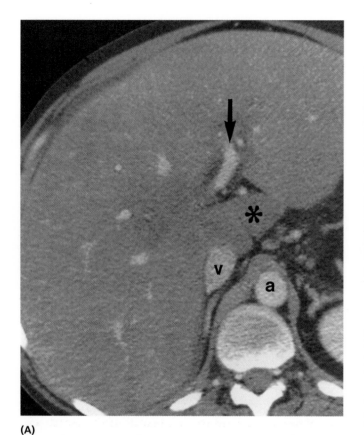

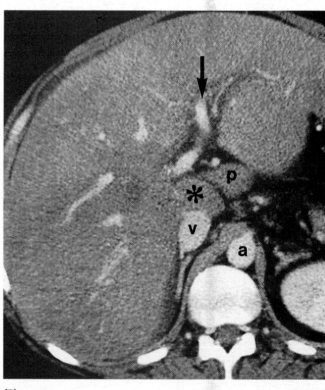

(A)

(B)

Fig. 1.13 CT images of the caudate lobe with papillary process. **(A)** Caudate (asterisk) positioned between the left portal vein (arrow) and inferior vena cava (v). Aorta (a). **(B)** Papillary process of the caudate (p) represents the lower medial extension of the caudate (asterisk) and may mimic a periportal lymph node.

the umbilical fissure into two segments, a medial segment (the quadrate lobe) (Segment IV) and a lateral segment (Segment III) which is the anterior part of the left lobe. (3) The right liver is divided into two sectors by the right portal scissura containing the right hepatic vein. Each of these two sectors is divided into two segments; an anterior sector (Segment V inferiorly and Segment VIII superiorly) and a posterior sector – (Segment VI inferiorly and Segment VII superiorly) (Figs. 1.6, 1.7). (4) Segment I (the caudate lobe) lies posteriorly embracing the vena cava, its intra-parenchymal anterior surface abutting the posterior surface of segment IV and merging with Segments VI and VII on the right (Figs 1.11, 1.14). Further details of segmental anatomy important in sectoral or segmental resection are described in Chapter 83.

SURGICAL IMPLICATIONS AND EXPOSURE

All methods for precise partial hepatectomy depend upon control of the inflow vasculature and draining bile ducts and of the outflow hepatic veins to the portion of liver to be excised whether this be a segment, subsegment or an entire lobe. The remnant remaining after partial hepatectomy

must be provided with an excellent portal venous and hepatic arterial supply and biliary drainage and an unimpeded hepatic venous outflow. Under such circumstances hepatic regeneration is usually prompt. The classification of the various partial hepatic resection procedures, incisions and exposure, necessary mobilization of the liver and the methods of control of the structures within the portal triads and of the hepatic veins is described in detail in Chapter 83.

THE BILIARY TRACT

Biliary exposure and precise dissection are the most important steps in any biliary operative procedure. A thorough anatomical knowledge is essential if optimal results are to be obtained.

INTRAHEPATIC BILE DUCT ANATOMY

The right liver and the left liver are respectively drained by the right and the left hepatic ducts whereas the dorsal lobe (caudate lobe) is drained by several ducts joining both the

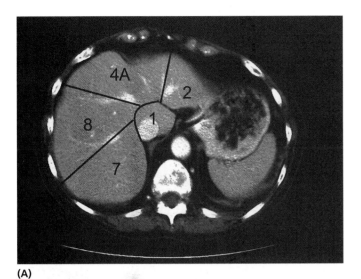

(A)

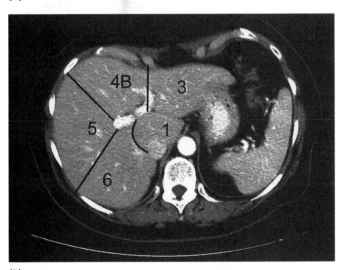

(B)

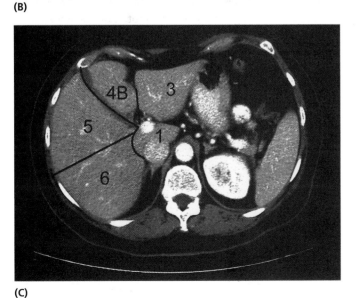

(C)

Fig. 1.14 Hepatic segmental anatomy as shown by CT. **(A)** At the level of the hepatic veins. **(B)** At the portal vein bifurcation. **(C)** Below the hepatic hilus (see text).

right and left hepatic ducts. The intrahepatic ducts are tributaries of the corresponding hepatic ducts which form part of the major portal triads which penetrate the liver invaginating Glisson's capsule at the hilus. Bile ducts are usually located above the corresponding portal branches whereas hepatic arterial branches are situated inferiorly to the veins. Each branch of the intra-hepatic portal veins corresponds to one or two bile ducts tributaries joining to form the right and left hepatic ductal systems converging at the liver hilus to constitute the common hepatic duct. The umbilical fissure divides the left liver passing between segment III and segment IV where it may be bridged by a tongue of liver tissue. The ligamentum teres passes through the umbilical fissure to join the left branch of the portal vein (Fig. 1.1).

The left hepatic duct drains the three segments (II, III and IV) which constitute the left liver (Fig. 1.15).

The duct draining Segment III is located slightly behind the left horn of the umbilical recessus. It is joined by the tributary from Segment IVB to form the left duct which is similarly joined by the duct of Segment II and the duct of Segment IVA at the point where the left branch of the portal vein turns forward and caudally. The left hepatic duct traverses beneath the left liver at the base of Segment IV, just above and behind the left branch of the portal vein, crosses the anterior edge of that vein and joins the right hepatic duct to constitute the hepatic ductal confluence. In its transverse portion it receives one to three small branches from Segment IV.

The right hepatic duct drains Segments V, VI, VII and VIII and arises from the junction of two main sectoral ductal tributaries (Fig. 1.16). The posterior or lateral duct and the anterior or medial duct are each accompanied by its corresponding vein. The right posterior sectoral duct has an almost *horizontal* course and is constituted by the confluence of the ducts of segments VI and VII (Figs 1.15, 1.16). The duct then runs to join the right anterior sectoral duct as it descends in a *vertical* manner. The right anterior sectoral duct is formed by the confluence of the ducts draining Segments V and VIII. Its main trunk is located to the left of the right anterior sectoral branch of the portal vein, which pursues an ascending course. The junction of these two main right biliary channels usually takes place above the right branch of the portal vein.

The right hepatic duct is short and joins the left hepatic duct to constitute the confluence lying in front of the right portal vein and forming the common hepatic duct.

The caudate lobe (Segment I) has its own biliary drainage (Healey & Schroy 1953). The caudate lobe is divided into right and left portions and a caudate process. In 44% of individuals, three separate ducts drain these three parts of the lobe, while in 26% there is a common duct between the

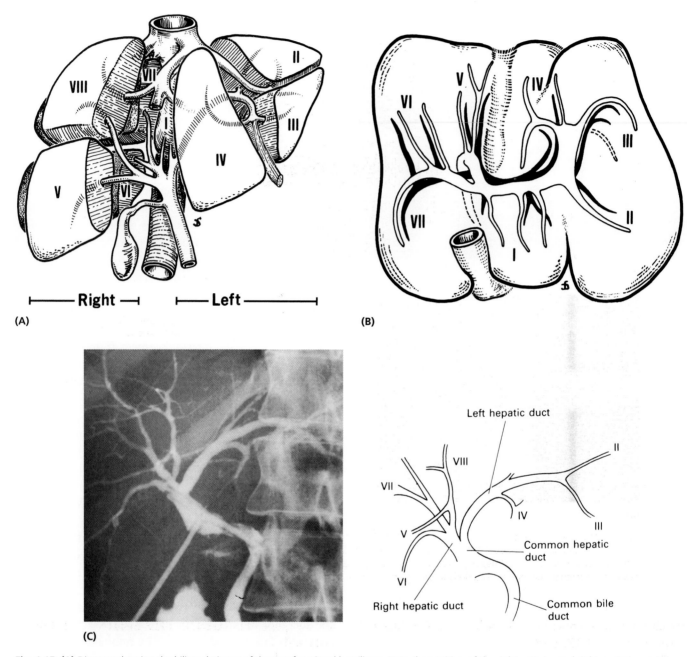

Fig. 1.15 (A) Diagram showing the biliary drainage of the two functional hemilivers. Note the position of the right anterior and right posterior sectors. The caudate lobe drains into the right and left ductal system. **(B)** Diagram showing the inferior aspect of the liver. The biliary tract is represented in black and the portal branches in white. Note the biliary drainage of segment IV. Segment VIII is not represented because of its cephalad location. **(C)** T-tube cholangiogram showing the most common arrangement of hepatic ducts.

right portion of the caudate lobe proper and the caudate process and an independent duct draining the left part of the caudate lobe. The site of drainage of these ducts is variable. In 78% of cases, drainage of the caudate lobe is into both right and left hepatic ducts but in 15% drainage is by the left hepatic ductal system only. In about 7% the drainage is into the right hepatic system.

EXTRAHEPATIC BILIARY AND VASCULAR ANATOMY

The extrahepatic bile ducts are represented by the extrahepatic segments of the right and left hepatic ducts joining to form the biliary confluence and the main biliary channel draining to the duodenum. The accessory biliary apparatus,

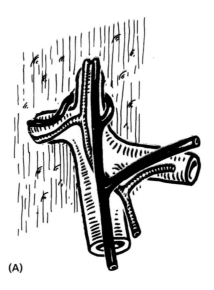

(A)

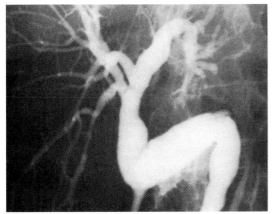

(B)

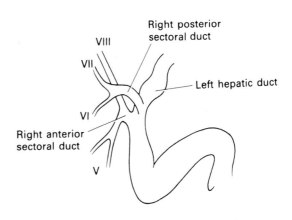

Fig 1.16 (A) Biliary and vascular anatomy of the right liver. Note the horizontal course of the posterior sectoral duct and the vertical course of the anterior sectoral duct. **(B)** Transtubal cholangiogram showing a common normal variant where the right posterior sectoral duct drains into the left hepatic duct. In this case the posterior duct is anterior to the posterior sectoral duct. Frequently in this variant the posterior duct passes posteriorly to the anterior sectoral pedicle.

which constitutes a reservoir, comprises the gallbladder and cystic duct (Figs 1.17, 1.18).

The confluence of the right and left hepatic ducts takes place at the right of the hilar fissure of the liver anterior to the portal venous bifurcation and overlying the origin of the right branch of the portal vein (Fig. 1.17). The extrahepatic segment of the right duct is short but the left duct has *a much longer extrahepatic course*. The biliary confluence is separated from the posterior aspect of the quadrate lobe of the liver by the hilar plate, which is the fusion of connective tissue enclosing the biliary and vascular elements with Glisson's capsule (Fig. 1.19). Because of the absence of any vascular interposition, it is possible to open the connective tissue constituting the hilar plate at the inferior border of the quadrate lobe and by elevating it to display the biliary convergence and left hepatic duct (Fig. 1.20).

THE MAIN BILE DUCT, THE SPHINCTER OF ODDI

The main bile duct (Fig. 1.17), the mean diameter of which is about 6 mm, is divided into two segments: the upper segment is called the common hepatic duct and is situated above the cystic duct, which joins it to form the common bile duct (Fig. 1.18). The common duct courses downwards anterior to the portal vein in the free edge of the lesser omentum and is closely applied to the hepatic artery which runs upwards on its left, giving rise to the right branch of the hepatic artery which crosses the main bile duct usually posteriorly, though in about 20% of cases anteriorly. The cystic artery, arising from the right branch of the hepatic artery, may cross the common hepatic duct posteriorly or anteriorly. The common hepatic duct constitutes the

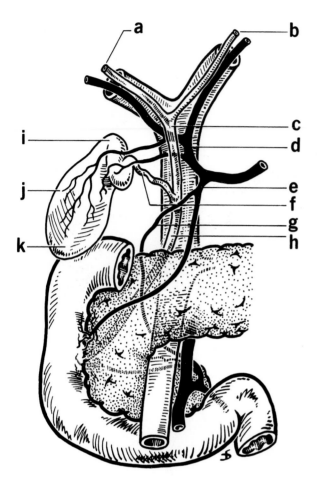

Fig. 1.17 Anterior aspect of the biliary anatomy: a, right hepatic duct; b, left hepatic duct; c common hepatic duct; d, hepatic artery; e, gastroduodenal artery; f, cystic duct; g, retroduodenal artery; h, common bile duct; i, neck of the gallbladder; j, body of the gallbladder; k, fundus of the gallbladder. Note particularly the situation of the hepatic bile duct confluence anterior to the right branch of the portal vein, the posterior course of the cystic artery behind the common hepatic duct and the relationship of the neck of the gallbladder to the right branch of the hepatic artery.

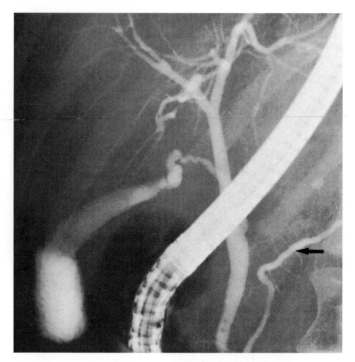

Fig. 1.18 Endoscopic retrograde choledochopancreatogram showing the pancreatic duct (arrow), gallbladder and biliary tree.

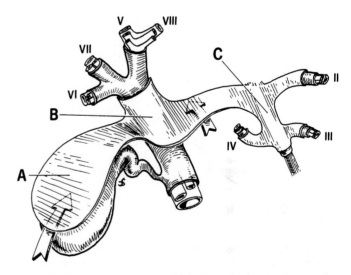

Fig. 1.19 Sketch of the anatomy of the plate system. Note the cystic plate (A) above the gallbladder, the hilar plate (B) above the biliary confluence and at the base of the quadrate lobe and the umbilical plate (C) above the umbilical portion of the portal vein. Large, curving arrows indicate the plane of dissection of the cystic plate during cholecystectomy and of the hilar plate during approaches to the left hepatic duct.

left border of the triangle of Calot, the other corners of which were originally described as the cystic duct below and the cystic artery above (Rocko et al 1981). However, the commonly accepted working definition of Calot's triangle recognizes the inferior surface of the right lobe of the liver as the upper border and the cystic duct as the lower (Wood 1979). Dissection of Calot's triangle is of key significance during cholecystectomy since in this triangle runs the cystic artery, often the right branch of the hepatic artery and occasionally a bile duct which should be displayed prior to cholecystectomy. If there is a replaced or accessory common or right hepatic artery, it usually runs behind the cystic duct to enter Calot's triangle (Fig. 1.21).

The common variations in relationship of the hepatic artery and origin and course of the cystic artery to the biliary apparatus are shown in Fig. 1.22.

Ignorance of these may provoke unexpected hemorrhage or biliary injury (Champetier et al 1982) during cholecystectomy and may result in bile duct injury during efforts to secure hemostasis.

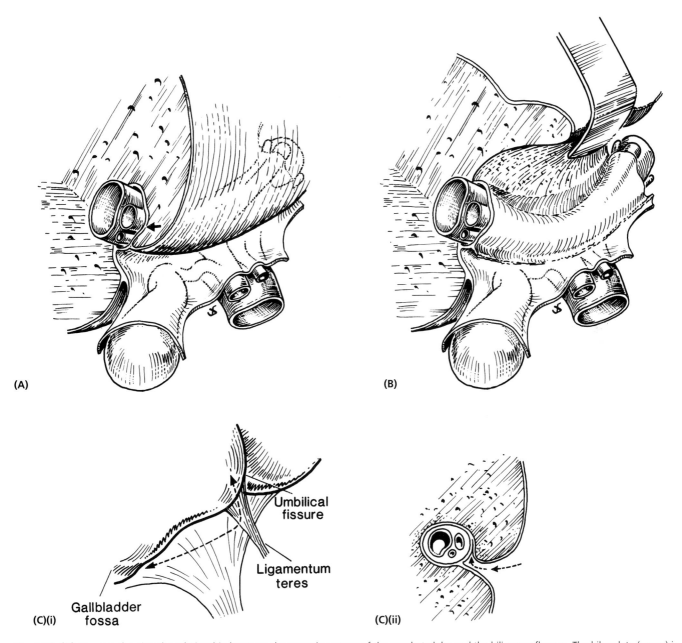

(A)

(B)

(C)(i)

Umbilical
fissure

Ligamentum
teres

Gallbladder
fossa

(C)(ii)

Fig. 1.20 (A) Diagram showing the relationship between the posterior aspect of the quadrate lobe and the biliary confluence. The hilar plate (arrow) is formed by the fusion of the connective tissue enclosing the biliary and vascular elements with Glisson's capsule. **(B)** Diagram showing the biliary confluence and left hepatic duct exposed by lifting the quadrate lobe upwards after incision of Glisson's capsule at its base. This technique (lowering of the hilar plate) (Hepp & Couinaud 1956) is generally used to display a dilated bile duct above an iatrogenic stricture or hilar cholangiocarcinoma. **(C)(i)** Sketch showing the line of incision to allow extensive mobilization of the quadrate lobe. This maneuver is of particular value for high bile duct stricture and in the presence of liver atrophy/hypertrophy. The procedure consists of lifting the quadrate lobe upwards (see parts **A** and **B** above) and then opening not only the umbilical fissure but incising the deepest portion of the gallbladder fossa. **(C)(ii)** Diagram showing incision of Glisson's capsule in order to gain access to the biliary system (arrow).

The union between the cystic duct and the common hepatic duct may be located at various levels. At its lower extrahepatic portion the common bile duct traverses the posterior aspect of the pancreas running in a groove or tunnel. The retropancreatic portion of the common bile duct approaches the second portion of the duodenum obliquely, accompanied by the terminal part of the pancreatic duct of Wirsung.

GALLBLADDER AND CYSTIC DUCT

The gallbladder is a reservoir located on the undersurface of the right lobe of the liver within the cystic fossa and separated from the hepatic parenchyma by the cystic plate, which is constituted of connective tissue closely applied to Glisson's capsule and prolonging the hilar plate (Fig. 1.19).

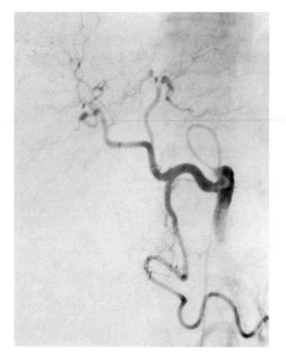

(A)

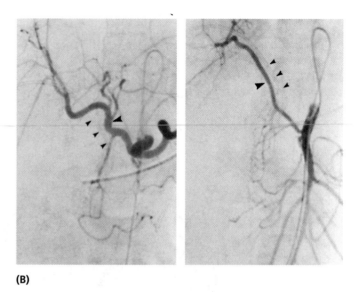

(B)

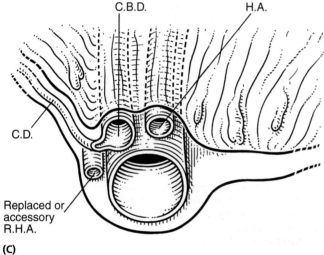

(C)

Fig. 1.21 **(A)** A replaced common hepatic artery arises from the superior mesenteric trunk. **(B)** Angiogram (Left) The hepatic artery (large arrow) arises from the celiac axis. The small arrows indicate a drainage catheter in the bile duct. (Right) An accessory right hepatic artery (large arrow) is arising from the superior mesenteric artery and lies lateral to the catheter (small arrows) in the common bile duct. **(C)** This vessel usually courses upwards in the groove posterolateral to the common bile duct (CBD), appearing on the medial side of Calot's triangle and usually running just behind the cystic duct (CD). This is common and occurs in some 25% of individuals. HA, hepatic artery.

Sometimes the gallbladder is deeply embedded in the liver but occasionally presents on a mesenteric attachment and may then be liable to volvulus. The gallbladder varies in size and consists of a fundus, a body and a neck (Fig. 1.23). The tip of the fundus usually, but not always, reaches the free edge of the liver and is closely applied to the cystic plate. The cystic fossa is a precise anterior guide mark to the main liver scissura. The neck of the gallbladder makes an angle with the fundus and creates Hartmann's pouch which may obscure the common hepatic duct and constitute a real danger point during cholecystectomy.

The cystic duct arises from the neck or infundibulum of the gallbladder and extends to join the common hepatic duct. Its lumen usually measures some 1–3 mm. Its length is variable, depending upon the type of union with the com-

mon hepatic duct. The mucosa of the cystic duct is arranged in spiral folds known as the valves of Heister (Wood 1979). While the cystic duct joins the common hepatic duct in its supraduodenal segment in 80% of cases it may extend downwards to the retroduodenal or even retropancreatic area. Occasionally the cystic duct may join the right hepatic duct or a right hepatic sectoral duct (Fig. 1.24).

BILIARY DUCTAL ANOMALIES

Full knowledge of the frequent variations from the described normal biliary anatomy is required while performing any hepatobiliary procedure.

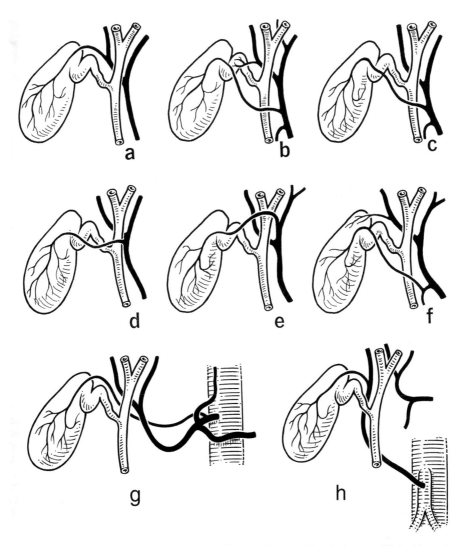

Fig. 1.22 Sketch showing the main variations of the cystic artery:(**a**) typical course, (**b**) double cystic artery, (**c**) cystic artery crossing anterior to main bile duct, (**d**) cystic artery originating from the right branch of the hepatic artery and crossing the common hepatic duct anteriorly, (**e**) cystic artery originating from the left branch of the hepatic artery, (**f**) cystic artery originating from the gastroduodenal artery, (**g**) the cystic artery may arise from the celiac axis, (**h**) the cystic artery originates from a replaced right hepatic artery.

The constitution of a normal biliary confluence by union of the right and left hepatic ducts as described above is reported in up to 72% (Healey and Schroy 1953) of cases. There is a triple confluence of the right anterior and posterior sectoral ducts and the left hepatic duct in 12% (Couinaud 1957) of cases. In addition, a right sectoral duct joins the main bile duct directly in 20% of individuals. In 16% the right anterior sectoral duct and in 4% the right posterior sectoral duct may approach the main bile duct in this fashion (Fig. 1.25A). Furthermore, in 6% a right sectoral duct may join the left hepatic duct (the posterior duct in 5% and the anterior duct in 1%) (Fig. 1.16B). In 3% there is an absence of the hepatic duct confluence and in 2% the right posterior sectoral duct may join the neck of the gallbladder

or may be entered by the cystic duct (Couinaud 1957). In any event, these multiple biliary ductal variations at the hilus are important to recognize, both in resective and reconstructive surgery of the biliary tree at the hilus and also during partial hepatectomy.

Intrahepatic bile duct variations are also common (Fig. 1.26) (Healey and Schroy 1953). The main right intrahepatic duct variations are represented by an ectopic drainage of Segment V in 9%, of Segment VI in 14%, and of Segment VIII in 20%. In addition, a subvesical duct has been described in 20 to 50% of cases. This duct, sometimes deeply embedded in the cystic plate, joins either the common hepatic duct or the right hepatic duct. This duct does not drain any specific liver territory, never communicates

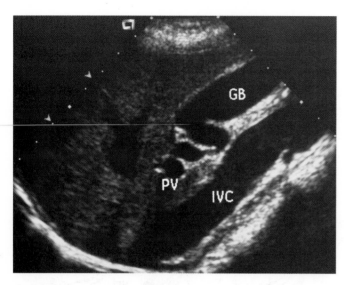

Fig. 1.23 Longitudinal sonogram shows the relationship of the liver, gallbladder (GB), portal vein (PV) and inferior vena cava (IVC).

with the gallbladder, and is not a satellite of an intrahepatic branch of the portal vein or hepatic artery. Although not of major anatomical significance, injury may occur during cholecystectomy if the cystic plate is not preserved, and this may lead to a postoperative biliary leak.

There is in 67% (Healey and Schroy 1953) of instances a classical distribution of the main left intrahepatic biliary ductal system. The main variation in this region is represented by a common union between the ducts of segments III and IV in 25%. In only 2% does the duct of segment IV join the common hepatic duct independently.

Several anomalies of drainage of the intrahepatic ducts into the neck of the gallbladder or cystic duct have been reported (Couinaud 1957, Albaret et al 1981) (Fig. 1.27) and these must be kept in mind during cholecystectomy.

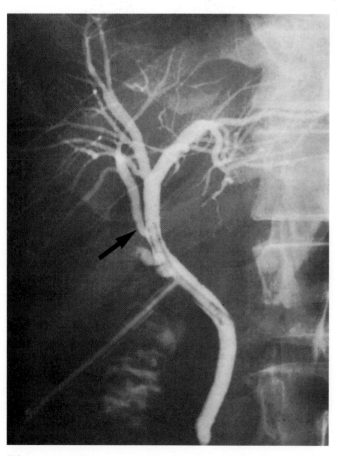

(A)

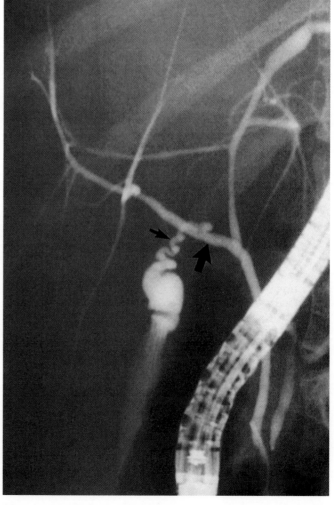

(B)

Fig. 1.24 (A) T-tube cholangiogram showing a very low insertion of a right sectoral duct into the common hepatic duct (arrow). **(B)** Endoscopic retrograde choledochopancreatograph showing low right sectoral duct (large arrow) into which is draining the cystic duct (small arrow), an uncommon but important normal variant.

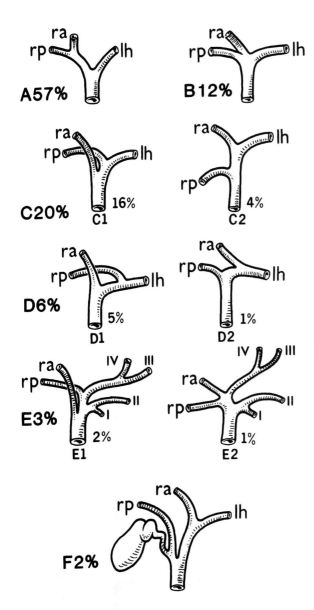

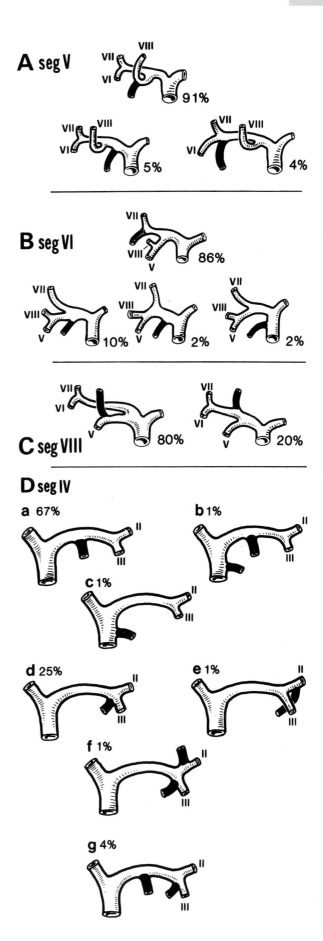

Fig. 1.25 Main variations of the hepatic duct confluence (Couinaud 1957). **(A)** typical anatomy of the confluence, **(B)** triple confluence, **(C)** ectopic drainage of a right sectoral duct into the common hepatic duct (C1, right anterior duct draining into the common hepatic duct; C2, right posterior ducts draining into the common hepatic duct), **(D)** ectopic drainage of a right sectoral duct into the left hepatic ductal system (D1, right posterior sectoral duct draining into the left hepatic ductal system; D2, right anterior sectoral duct draining into the left hepatic ductal system), **(E)** absence of the hepatic duct confluence, **(F)** absence of right hepatic duct and ectopic drainage of the right posterior duct into the cystic duct.

Fig. 1.26 A sketch to show the main variations of the intrahepatic ductal system: **(A)** variations of Segment V, **(B)** variations of Segment VI, **(C)** variations of Segment VIII, **(D)** variations of Segment IV. Note that there is no variation of drainage of Segments II, III and VII.

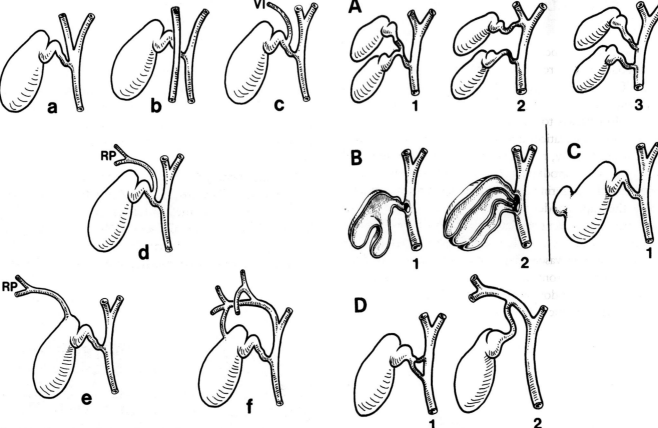

Fig. 1.27 The main variations of ectopic drainage of the intrahepatic ducts into the gallbladder and cystic duct: **(a)** drainage of the cystic duct into the biliary confluence, **(b)** drainage of cystic duct into the left hepatic duct associated with no biliary confluence, **(c)** drainage of segment VI duct into the cystic duct, **(d)** drainage of the right posterior sectoral duct into the cystic duct, **(e)** drainage of the distal part of the right posterior sectoral duct into the neck of the gallbladder, **(f)** drainage of the proximal part of the right posterior sectoral duct into the body of the gallbladder.

Fig. 1.28a Main variations in gallbladder and cystic duct anatomy: **(A)** bilobed gallbladder, **(B)** septum of the gallbladder, **(C)** diverticulum of the gallbladder, **(D)** variations in cystic ductal anatomy.

Fig. 1.28b Different types of union of the cystic duct and common hepatic duct: **(a)** angular union, **(b)** parallel union, **(c)** spiral union.

ANOMALIES OF THE ACCESSORY BILIARY APPARATUS

A number of anomalies have been described (Gross 1936) (Fig. 1.28a). While rare, agenesis of the gallbladder (Boyden 1926, Rogers et al 1975, Rachad-Mohassel et al 1973), bilobar gallbladders with a single cystic duct but two fundi (Hobby 1970) and duplication of the gallbladder with two cystic ducts have all been described. Finally, a double cystic duct may drain a unilocular gallbladder (Perelman 1961). Congenital diverticulum of the gallbladder with a muscular wall is also to be found (Eelkema et al 1958).

More frequently reported are anomalies of position of the gallbladder, which may lie either in an intrahepatic position completely surrounded by normal liver tissue or may be found on the left of the liver (Newcombe and Henley 1964).

The mode of union of the cystic duct with the common hepatic duct may be angular, parallel or spiral (Fig. 1.28b). An angular union is the most frequent and is found in 75% of patients (Kune 1970). The cystic duct may run a parallel course to the common hepatic duct in 20%, with connective tissue ensheathing both ducts. Finally, the cystic duct may approach the common bile duct in a spiral fashion. The absence of a cystic duct is probably an acquired anomaly representing a choledochocholecystic fistula.

BILE DUCT BLOOD SUPPLY

The bile duct may be divided into three segments: hilar, supraduodenal and retropancreatic (lower common bile duct). The blood supply of the supraduodenal duct is essentially axial (Fig. 1.29) (Northover and Terblanche 1979). Most vessels to the supraduodenal duct arise from the superior pancreaticoduodenal artery, the right branch of the hepatic artery, the cystic artery, the gastroduodenal artery and the retroduodenal artery. On average, eight small arteries measuring each about 0.3 mm in diameter supply the supraduodenal duct. The most important of these vessels run along the lateral borders of the duct and have been called the 3 o'clock and 9 o'clock arteries. Of the blood vessels vascularizing the supraduodenal duct, 60% runs upwards from the major inferior vessels, and only 38% of arteries run downwards, originating from the right branch of the hepatic artery and other vessels. Only 2% of the arterial supply is non-axial, arising directly from the main trunk of the hepatic artery as it courses up parallel to the main biliary channel. The hilar ducts receive a copious supply of arterial blood from surrounding vessels, forming a rich network on the surface of the ducts in continuity with the plexus around the supraduodenal duct. The source of blood supply of the retropancreatic common bile duct is from the retroduodenal artery, which provides multiple small vessels running around the duct to form a mural plexus.

The veins draining the bile ducts are satellites to the corresponding described arteries, draining into 3 o'clock and 9 o'clock veins along the borders of the common biliary channel. Veins draining the gallbladder empty into this venous system and not directly into the portal vein. The biliary tree seems to have its own portal venous pathway to the liver.

THE ANATOMY OF BILIARY EXPOSURE

BILIARY-VASCULAR SHEATHS AND EXPOSURE OF THE HEPATIC BILE DUCT CONFLUENCE

The fusion of Glisson's capsule with the connective tissue sheaths surrounding the biliary and vascular elements at the inferior aspect of the liver constitute the plate system (Figs 1.19, 1.20), which includes the hilar plate above the biliary confluence, the cystic plate related to the gallbladder, and the umbilical plate situated above the umbilical portion of the left portal vein (Couinaud 1957).

Hepp and Couinaud (1956) described a technique where, by lifting the quadrate lobe upwards and incising the Glisson's capsule at its base, a good exposure of the hepatic hilar structures could be obtained (Figs 1.20A & B). This technique was referred to as lowering of the hilar plate. It can be carried out with safety since there is only exceptionally (in 1% of cases) any vascular interposition between the hilar plate and the inferior aspect of the liver. This maneuver is of particular value in exposing the extrahepatic segment of the left hepatic duct since it has a long course beneath the quadrate lobe. It is not as effective in exposing the extrahepatic right duct or its secondary branches, which are short. The technique is of major importance for the identification of proximal biliary mucosa during bile duct repair following injury. Basically, an incision is required at the posterior edge of the quadrate lobe where Glisson's capsule is attached to the hilar plate (Fig. 1.20B and Chapter 30). The upper surface of the hilar plate can then be separated from the hepatic

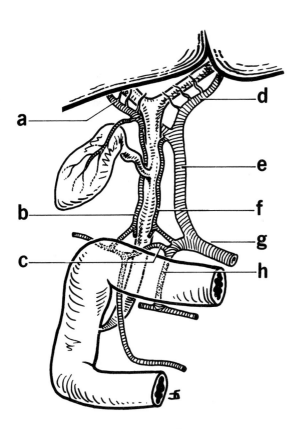

Fig. 1.29 The bile duct blood supply. Note the axial arrangement of the vasculature of the supraduodenal portion of the main bile duct and the rich network enclosing the right and left hepatic ducts: (a) right branch of the hepatic artery; (b) 9 o'clock artery; (c) retroduodenal artery; (d) left branch of the hepatic artery; (e) hepatic artery; (f) 3 o'clock artery; (g) common hepatic artery; (h) gastroduodenal artery.

parenchyma and, by lifting the quadrate lobe upwards, display of the hepatic duct convergence, which is *always* extra-hepatic, is effected. Bile duct incision then allows performance of a mucosa-to-mucosa anastomosis. In some rare instances it may be hazardous to approach the biliary confluence in this manner, especially when anatomical deformity has been created by atrophy/hypertrophy of liver lobes and in patients where there appears to be a very deep hilus which is displaced upwards and rotated laterally. Frequently, by a simultaneous opening of the deepest portion of the gallbladder fossa and the umbilical fissure (Fig. 1.20C), a good exposure of the biliary duct confluence and especially the right hepatic duct can be obtained without the necessity for full hepatotomy.

THE UMBILICAL FISSURE AND THE SEGMENT III (LIGAMENTUM TERES) APPROACH

The round ligament, which is the remnant of the obliterated umbilical veins, runs through the umbilical fissure to connect with the left branch of the portal vein within the umbilical fissure. The round ligament is sometimes deeply embedded in the umbilical fissure. The ligament joins the termination of the left portal vein at which point prolongations containing channels which are elements of the left portal system course into the liver. The bile ducts of the left lobe of the liver (Figs 1.30 and 1.31A) are located above the left branch of the portal vein and lying behind these prolongations, whereas the corresponding artery is situated below the vein. Dissection of the round ligament on its *left* side and division of one or two vascular prolongations to Segment III allows display of the pedicle or anterior branch of the duct of Segment III (Fig. 1.31B). In the event of biliary obstruction with intrahepatic biliary ductal dilatation, the Segment III duct is generally easily located above the left branch of the portal vein.

It is often preferable to split the normal liver tissue just to the left of the umbilical fissure in order to widen the fissure further. This allows access to the ductal system without the necessity to divide any elements of the portal blood supply to Segment III (Fig. 1.32).

SURGICAL APPROACHES TO THE RIGHT HEPATIC BILIARY DUCTAL SYSTEM

Because of the lack of precise anatomical guide-marks, exposure of the right intrahepatic ductal system is much more hazardous and imprecise than the left. In some cases of hilar cholangiocarcinoma the planned surgical procedure (partial hepatectomy or Segment III duct bypass) appears impossible at operation. In such a critical operative situa-

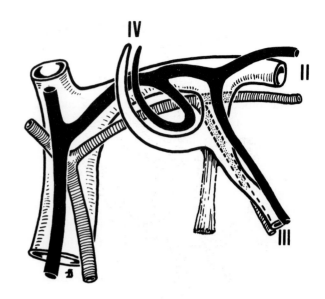

Fig. 1.30 Biliary and vascular anatomy of the left liver. Note the location of the segment III duct above the corresponding vein. The anterior branch of the segment IV duct is not represented.

tion, intrahepatic right ductal system drainage is an option. Anatomically, the anterior sectoral duct and its branches run on the left side of the corresponding portal vein. In essence, the end of the liver scissura within which lies the right branch of the portal vein is opened over a short distance. The anterior sectoral duct is displayed on the left aspect of the vein. The dilated duct is opened longitudinally and anastomosed to a Roux-en-Y loop of jejunum (Fig. 1.33). Although this technique is rarely used, it may be of value in selected cases (see Chapter 54).

An alternative method is to open into the segment V duct through the gallbladder fossa. The authors seldom use this approach and prefer the anterior sectoral duct approach.

EXPOSURE OF THE BILE DUCTS BY LIVER RESECTION

This chapter does not detail exposure of the bile ducts by resection of liver substance. In essence a segment of the left lobe may be amputated to expose the Segments II or III ducts, or a similar procedure carried out after removal of the inferior tip of the right lobe. Finally, in some instances removal of the quadrate lobe may be carried out to effect exposure of the biliary confluence. This procedure really represents a simple extension of the mobilization of the quadrate lobe after opening of the principal scissura and the umbilical fissure as described above.

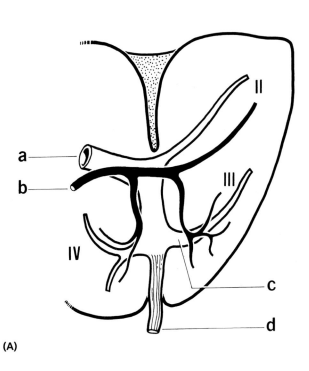

(A)

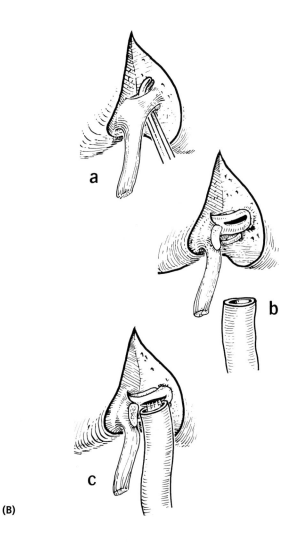

(B)

Fig. 1.31 (A) The biliary and vascular anatomy of the left liver. Note the relationship of the left horn of the umbilical recess with the segment III ductal system: (a) left portal vein; (b) left hepatic duct; (c) Segment III system, note the duct (black) lies adjacent to the portal venous branch indicated; (d) ligamentum teres. **(B)** Segment III ductal approach: (a) exposure of the left horn of the umbilical recess; (b) division of the left horn of the umbilical recess including Segment III portal vein branches. Exposure and opening of Segment III duct: (c) hepaticojejunostomy to the Segment III ductal system (see also Ch. 30).

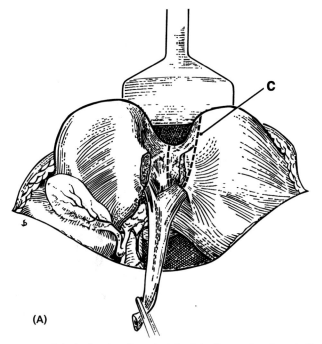

(A)

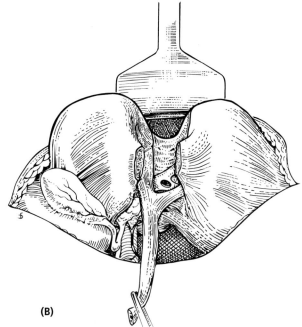

(B)

Fig. 1.32 (A) The liver is split to the left of the ligamentum teres in the umbilical fissure. It may be necessary to remove a small wedge of liver tissue (a). **(B)** The Segment III duct is exposed at the base of the liver split above and behind its accompanying vein and is ready for anastomosis (see also Ch. 30).

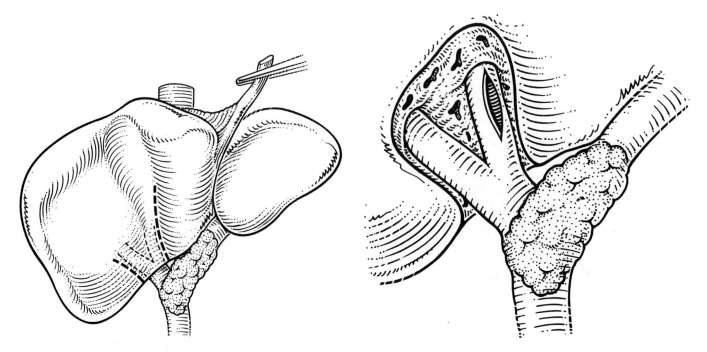

Fig. 1.33 Anterior sectoral approach. If necessary, the liver substance is opened over a short distance in the line of the right anterior sectoral pedicle. The duct is displayed anterior and to the left side of the corresponding vein. This can be facilitated using a posterior pedicular approach as described by Launois (see Ch. 83).

EXTRAHEPATIC VASCULATURE

THE CELIAC ACCESS AND THE BLOOD SUPPLY OF LIVER, BILIARY TRACT AND PANCREAS

The usual description of the arterial blood supply of the liver, biliary system and pancreas are found in only some 60% of specimens (Figs 1.34, 1.35, 1.36).

The right and the left hepatic artery, the former in the right of the hilus of the liver and the latter in the left at the base of the umbilical fissure become enclosed in the sheath of peritoneum forming the right and left portal triads and in this sheath further branching to the right anterior and posterior sectors of the liver and on the left to Segments II, III and IV take place within the respective pedicles which also come to enclose the portal vein branches and the tributary bile ducts from these sectors and segments (see above). The arterial supply of the common bile duct is described above and arises from branches of the hepatic artery and the gastroduodenal artery and the pancreaticoduodenal arcades.

For practical surgical issues, the most important relationships in the anatomy of the pancreas concern the arterial blood supply and the venous drainage.

The dorsal pancreatic artery is a major branch, usually arising from the splenic artery, but it can arise directly from the hepatic. It is important to establish the site of origin of the distal pancreatic artery when splenectomy is performed, by proximal arterial ligation, to avoid distal pancreatic necrosis. The superior mesenteric artery arises from the aorta posteriorly behind the pancreas and runs forward and upward to run first behind and then to the left of the superior mesenteric vein (Fig. 1.35).

VARIATIONS IN THE HEPATIC ARTERY

As a result of the complex embryological development of the celiac axis and superior mesenteric artery there are wide variations in the arterial supply of the liver (Fig. 1.37). These variations are important to both the angiographer and surgeon. Failure to demonstrate all arteries feeding the liver at angiography may not only result in errors of diagnosis but may also seriously mislead the surgeon or the interventional radiologist. In the majority of cases the hepatic artery arises from the celiac axis as described above but it may be entirely replaced by a common hepatic artery taking origin from the superior mesenteric artery. In this instance the hepatic artery passes lateral to the portal vein and lies posterior and lateral to the common bile duct in the hepatoduodenal ligament where it is susceptible to operative injury if not recognized. This applies to a replaced or to an accessory hepatic artery (see below). Other variations in the origin of the common hepatic artery include its origin from the aorta and the persistence of a primitive embryological link between the celiac and superior mesenteric systems.

These variations are of considerable importance in controlling the arterial blood supply to the liver during hepatic resection or enucleative procedures, in the performance of devascularization of the liver, in the placement of intra-arterial hepatic infusional devices, and in the resection of the head of the pancreas.

THE PORTAL VEIN

The portal vein (Fig. 1.38) is formed behind the neck of the pancreas by confluence of the superior mesenteric and splenic veins (see also Fig. 1.39).

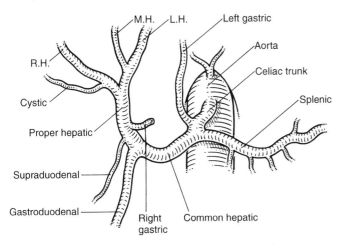

Fig. 1.34 The celiac trunk is a short thick artery originating from the aorta just below the aortic hiatus of the diaphragm and extending horizontally and forwards above the pancreas where it divides into the left gastric, the common hepatic and the splenic arteries. An inferior phrenic artery, usually arising from the aorta or the splenic artery, occasionally arises from the celiac trunk. The left gastric artery curves toward the stomach and extends along its lesser curve forming anastomoses with the right gastric artery. The splenic artery, the largest of the three celiac branches, takes a tortuous course to the left behind and along the upper border of the pancreas and at the hilus of the spleen breaks into a number of terminal branches. The splenic artery usually approaches and runs, superiorly, to the splenic vein. An uncommon but dangerous abnormality can occur when the splenic artery runs inferiorly and behind the splenic vein close to the splenic vein–mesenteric vein confluence. The left gastroepiploic artery and the short gastric arteries take origin from one of these terminal branches. The common hepatic artery passes forward into the retroperitoneum and then curves to the right to enter the right margin of the lesser omentum just above the pancreas and then ascends approaching the common bile duct on its left side and running usually anterior to the portal vein. As it turns upward just above the pancreas it gives rise to the gastroduodenal artery (which may also originate from the right hepatic artery). This descends to supply the anterior, superior and posterior surfaces of the first inch of the duodenum. The gastroduodenal artery can be duplicate and often has a small branch running with it toward the pylorus. The right gastric artery passes to the left along the lesser curve of the stomach and anastomosis is as described to the left gastric artery. The continuation of the common hepatic artery beyond the origin of the gastroduodenal artery and right gastric artery is known as the proper hepatic artery and usually soon divides into a right and left branch. The left branch extends vertically directly toward the base of the umbilical fissure and usually gives off a branch known as the middle hepatic artery (MH) which is directed toward the right of the umbilical fissure and is destined to supply the quadrate lobe (Segment IV) of the liver. A further branch of the left hepatic artery (LH) courses to the left to supply the caudate lobe and further smaller caudate branches arise from the left and right hepatic artery. The right hepatic artery usually passes behind the common hepatic duct and enters the cystic triangle of Calot but in some cases it passes in front of the bile duct and this is of importance in surgical exposure of the common bile duct. The cystic artery usually arises from the right hepatic artery but has many variations which are described above.

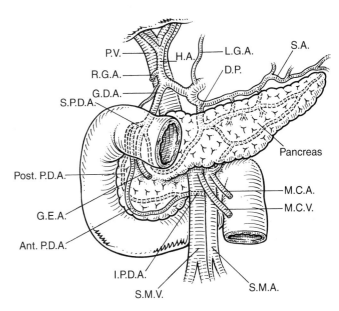

Fig. 1.35 The primary arteries supplying the pancreas are the gastroduodenal artery (GDA) which arises usually from the common hepatic artery (HA) as it crosses the portal vein above the pancreas proper and the dorsal pancreatic artery (DP) arising from the splenic artery (SA). The superior pancreaticoduodenal arteries (SPDA) arise from the gastroduodenal artery and join the inferior pancreaticoduodenal arteries (IPDA) from the superior mesenteric artery (SMA) forming two arcades along the anterior and posterior aspects of the head of the pancreas. The gastroduodenal artery after giving rise to the pancreaticoduodenal artery (PDA) passes forward and to the left as the right gastroepiploic artery (GEA). The gastroduodenal artery is a good landmark for the identification of the portal vein above the pancreas, and surgical division of the gastroduodenal just at its origin from the common hepatic artery gives much greater access to the anterior surface of the portal vein at this site. The right gastric artery (RGA) also usually arises from the common hepatic artery, just distal to the gastroduodenal, but it can arise from various sites. The gastroduodenal artery commonly divides into a larger right gastroepiploic artery (GEA) and smaller superior pancreaticoduodenal artery (SPDA). The right gastroepiploic runs forward between the first part of the duodenum and pancreas. The superior pancreaticoduodenal artery divides into anterior and posterior branches. The anterior superior pancreaticoduodenal artery continues downward on the anterior surface of the head of the pancreas to anastomose with the inferior pancreaticoduodenal artery which arises from the superior mesenteric artery. The posterior superior pancreaticoduodenal artery behaves similarly. SMV, superior mesenteric vein. SMA, superior mesenteric artery. MCA, middle colic artery. MCV, middle colic vein.

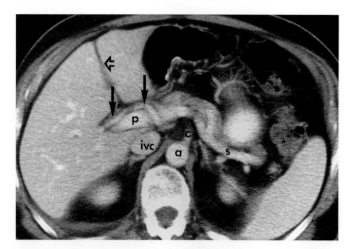

Fig. 1.36 Computed tomography (CT) image of the main portal vein shows the hepatic artery (arrows) coursing anterior to the portal vein (p). The interlobar fissure (open arrow), splenic vein (s), celiac axis (c), aorta (a), and inferior vena cava (ivc) are also shown.

The venous drainage of the pancreas runs in the main parallel to the arterial supply. There are anterior and posterior superior and inferior pancreaticoduodenal veins which drain to the portal vein and the superior mesenteric vein, respectively. The left gastric vein and the inferior mesenteric vein usually drain into the splenic vein, but can drain directly into the portal while the various small splenic tributaries drain directly to the splenic vein.

The anatomical relationship of the pancreas to the superior mesenteric vein, the splenic vein and the portal vein (Fig. 1.38) are important in pancreaticoduodenectomy (Ch. 56). The uncinate process can extend behind the superior mesenteric vein to well behind the superior mesenteric artery (Fig. 1.35). Access to the portal vein behind the pancreas is usually obtained from below by elevating the pancreas from the surface of the superior mesenteric vein just before it joins the splenic vein. With the exception of the inferior pancreaticoduodenal veins, which enter the superior mesenteric vein at the inferior border of the pancreas, it is uncommon to see branches from the pancreas run directly posteriorly into the superior mesenteric vein. Fixation here is usually by some inflammatory or neoplastic process. Superiorly the portal vein runs behind the pancreas and is identified first in the gap between the curvature of the splenic vein, the splenic artery, the common hepatic artery and the gastroduodenal artery. Division of the gastroduodenal artery will provide much greater access to the superior surface of the portal vein. If difficulty is encountered in this area, division of the common bile duct, usually above the cystic duct can provide excellent access to the right lateral aspect and anterior surface of the portal vein. The superior mesenteric artery can be approached posteriorly behind the

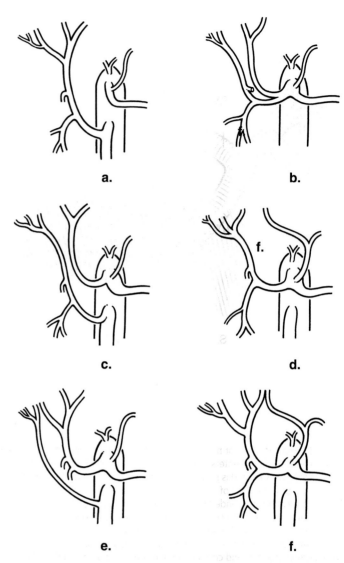

Fig. 1.37 In some 25% of individuals the right hepatic artery arises partially or completely from the superior mesenteric artery (**a**, **c**, **e**) and in a similar proportion of patients the left hepatic artery may be partially or completely replaced by a branch arising from the left gastric artery and coursing through the gastrohepatic omentum to enter the liver at the base of the umbilical fissure (**d**, **f**). Rarely the right or left hepatic arteries originate independently from the celiac trunk or branch after a very short common hepatic artery origin from the celiac (**b**, **c**). The gastroduodenal artery may originate from the right hepatic artery (**b**, **c**).

pancreas above the point at which it is embraced by the uncinate process at the origin from the aorta. This plan can allow dissection of the most proximal part of the superior mesenteric artery from behind.

Occasionally the middle colic artery and other vessels of supply to the colon can arise from the more proximal superior mesenteric artery, such that they actually pass through the pancreas. This abnormality should be carefully searched for. Division of the middle colic artery is usually, however,

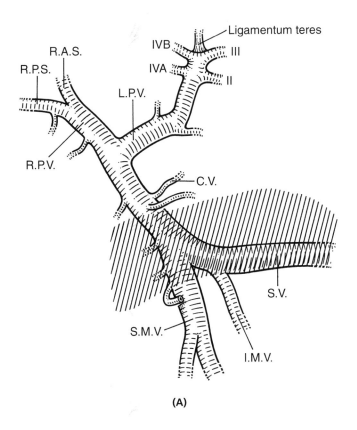

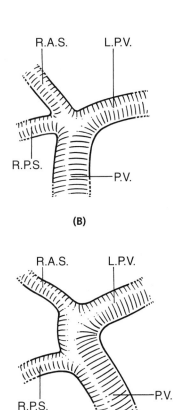

Fig. 1.38 (A) The superior mesenteric vein (SMV) at the root of the lesser omentum is usually a single trunk but two, or sometimes even three, branches may unite as the vessel enters the tunnel beneath the neck of the pancreas (shaded) to form a superior mesenteric trunk. This trunk ascends behind the neck of the pancreas and is joined by the splenic vein (SV) which enters it from the left to form the portal vein which emerges from the retroperitoneal upper border of the neck of the pancreas and ascends toward the liver within the free edge of the lesser omentum lying behind the bile duct and the hepatic artery and surrounded by the lymphatics and nodes of the lesser omentum. During this course it receives blood through the coronary vein (CV) which communicates with esophageal venous collaterals which in turn connect with the gastric vein and the esophageal plexus. Sometimes a separate right gastric vein enters the portal vein in this area. A superior pancreaticoduodenal vein often enters the portal just above the level of the pancreas and several smaller veins enter the superior mesenteric and portal vein from its right side beneath the neck of the pancreas. As the portal vein ascends behind the common bile duct and common hepatic duct it approaches the hilus of the liver and bifurcates into two branches, a larger right (RPV) and a smaller left (LPV). The branch on the left courses below the left hepatic duct to enter the umbilical fissure in company with the left hepatic artery and subsequently branches to supply to the left liver Segments II, III and IV. Just before its entry into the umbilical fissure it gives off a major caudate vein (Segment I) which runs posteriorly and laterally to the left and sometimes this vein consist of two or more branches. The right portal branch which is much shorter in length before its entry into the liver divides at the extremity of the hilus into the right anterior (RAS) and posterior (RPS) sectoral branches and is accompanied by the respective arterial branches and biliary tributaries. **(B)** This division of the portal vein may, however, arise more proximally and, indeed, the right anterior and posterior sectoral portal vein may arise independently from the portal venous trunk **(C)**.

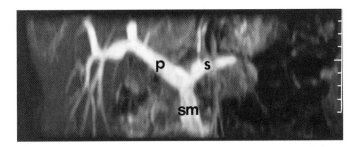

Fig. 1.39 Magnetic resonance image of the splenoportal confluence, post contrast T1 3-D gradient echo coronal maximum intensity projection (MIP). Splenic vein (s), portal vein (p), superior mesenteric vein (sm).

not a problem, as the colon has other multiple blood supplies.

Important to the surgeon is the direct relationship of the head of the pancreas to the duodenum and posteriorly to the right renal vein, the anterior surface of the inferior vena cava, and of the neck and body of the pancreas posteriorly to the superior mesenteric artery, and the splenic vessels and their branches, the left renal vein and more laterally, the left kidney.

The right gastroepiploic vein commonly drains into the anterior surface of the superior mesenteric vein just at the inferior border of the pancreas. This can often be involved as can the anterior branch of the inferior pancreaticoduodenal vein by tumor. The middle colic vein may join at this point. In mobilizing the superior mesenteric vein, these vessels are ligated so as to avoid bothersome hemorrhage. Abnormalities of the inferior vena cava are uncommon with duplication of the vena cava and a left-sided vena cava seen rarely.

There are several rare congenital anomalies of the portal vein which are of surgical significance (Figs 1.40, 1.41, 1.42, 1.43).

These anomalies are of very considerable significance. Performance of right hepatic resection, with division of what appears to be the right portal vein can in fact deprive the entire liver of blood. This surgical error is usually followed by the death of the patient. The portal venous blood supply is, of course, derived from the venous drainage of the stomach, small bowel, spleen, and pancreas, and this drainage is of importance in considering the surgery of the pancreas (and in patients with portal hypertension) and is described in detail along with the description of the anatomy of the pancreas.

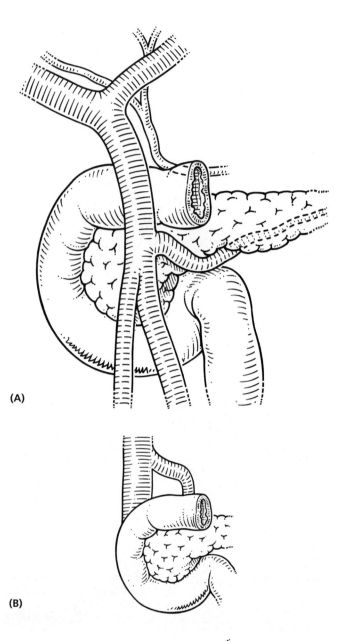

(A)

(B)

(C)

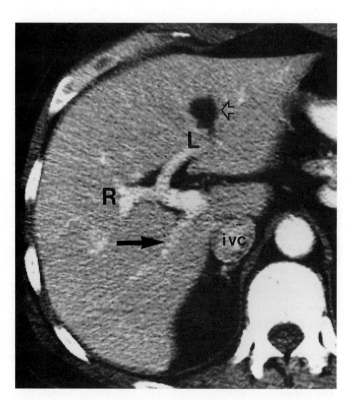

Fig. 1.40 CT image of variant portal vein branching. The right posterior portal vein (arrow) has a separate early origin from the main portal vein. The right anterior portal vein (R) and the left main portal vein (L) share a common trunk. Fissure of the ligamentum teres is seen anteriorly (open arrow).

Fig. 1.41 (A) There may be an abnormal position of the portal vein anterior to the head of the pancreas and the duodenum. **(B)** Another rare but interesting anomaly is the entrance of the portal vein into the inferior vena cava and **(C)** very rarely the entrance of a pulmonary vein into the portal vein, although the authors have never encountered this.

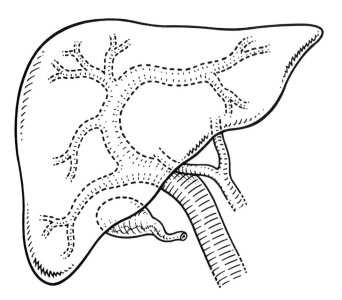

Fig. 1.42 There may be congenital absence of the left branch of the portal vein as described by Couinaud, the right branch then coursing through the right lobe of the liver supplying it and curving within the liver substance to supply the left lobe – which is in such instances – usually somewhat smaller than normal.

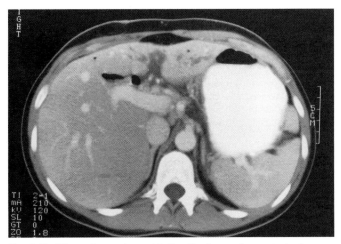

Fig. 1.43 CT scan in a patient with Caroli's disease demonstrates large right portal trunk. The left branch of the portal vein is absent – findings confirmed at operation for left hepatic lobectomy.

THE PANCREAS

The pancreas is a posteriorly situated retroperitoneal organ draped across the major vessels and the vertebral column (Fig. 1.44). The organ is composed of a head, neck and body, the head being encompassed by the duodenum and the tail resting in the splenic hilum (Fig. 1.45). Usually four to six inches in length, the relative dimensions have recently been evaluated. The mean weight is 91.8 g (range

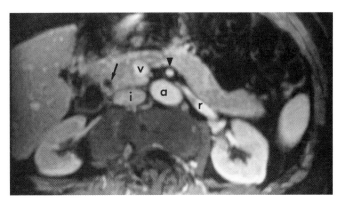

Fig. 1.44 Magnetic resonance image of the pancreas, oblique axial reconstruction T1 3D gradient echo technique. Aorta (a), inferior vena cava (i), common bile duct (arrow), inferior mesenteric vein at the splenoportal confluence (v), superior mesenteric artery (arrowhead) and left renal vein (r).

40.9–182 g). To the right of the common bile duct the average weight of the pancreas is 11.4% of the total weight; the portion lateral to the portal vein averaging 56.4% of the total weight. The pancreatic capsule is loosely attached to the surface of the pancreas and is contiguous with the anterior layer of the mesocolon, such that it can, if necessary, be dissected in continuity. The mesenteric attachments to the pancreas tend to be contiguous (Fig. 1.46).

THE PANCREATIC DUCT

A duct (the Duct of Wirsung) beginning in the distal tail as a confluence of small ductules runs through the body to the head, where it usually passes downward and backward in close juxtaposition to the common bile duct (Fig. 1.45).

The sphincter of Oddi (Fig. 1.47) has been thoroughly studied and consists of a unique cluster of smooth muscle fibers distinguishable from the adjacent smooth muscle of the duodenal wall.

The papilla of Vater at the termination of the common bile duct is a small nipple-like structure protruding into the duodenal lumen and marked by a longitudinal fold of duodenal mucosa. The duct of Wirsung as it runs down parallel with the common bile duct for some 2 cm joins it within the sphincter segment in some 70 to 85% of cases, enters the duodenum independently in 10 to 13% of patients and in only 2% is replaced by the duct of Santorini (Fig. 1.45). Throughout the pancreas are scattered the islands or islets of Langerhans, which provide the endocrine component of the gland.

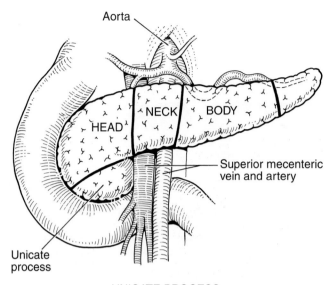

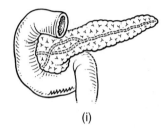
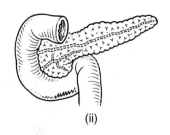

(C)

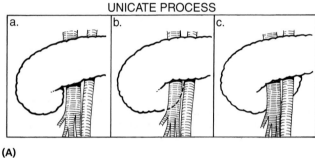

(A)

POSITION OF THE COMMON BILE DUCT

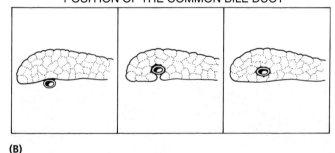

(B)

Fig. 1.45 **(A)** The head of the pancreas is somewhat globular with an extension, the uncinate process, which curves behind the superior mesenteric vessels. The uncinate process may finish even before it embraces the superior mesenteric vein (a) or it may pass completely behind between the aorta and the left of the patient's superior mesenteric artery (b, c). All variations are commonly seen. Posteriorly the head of the pancreas lies in juxtaposition to the inferior vena cava at the level of the entry of the left and right renal veins. The head of the pancreas forms a narrow neck in front of the superior mesenteric and splenic vein confluence. The neck joins to the body of the gland which forms a narrow tail. **(B)** The common bile duct (CBD) passes through the pancreas either directly in the substance of the gland or initially with a posterior groove. **(C)** The duct of Wirsung courses from left to right within the pancreas, curves downwards approaching the common bile duct, and runs parallel with but separated from it by the transampullary septum to enter the duodenum some 7–10 cm distal to the pylorus at the papilla of Vater after traversing the sphincter of Oddi. An accessory duct (the duct of Santorini) runs more proximally in the head of the pancreas and usually terminates in the duodenum at an accessory papilla. Multiple variations of the ductal system occur depending on the extent of development of the accessory duct of Santorini, such that on rare occasions the accessory duct can enter the duodenum inferior to the main duct. (i) It can be in communication with the main duct directly, or (ii) it can occur in duplicate version known as pancreas divisum. The duct of Santorini draining the body and tail of the organ and the duct of Wirsung, the head and the uncinate process.

ANNULAR PANCREAS

Annular pancreas is the development of a ring of pancreatic tissue, which surrounds and often embraces the duodenum. This may contain a large duct and can be firmly affixed to the duodenal musculature. The duodenum beneath this annulus is often stenosed, such that dividing this ring does not always relieve chronic duodenal obstruction. This accounts for the common process of applying duodeno-jejunostomy to relieve strictures caused by such an annulus (see below).

THE LYMPHATIC DRAINAGE

Liver

The lymphatic drainage of the gallbladder is mainly to nodes in the hepatoduodenal ligament and along the hepatic artery and is shown in Fig. 1.49A.

Pancreas

The lymphatic drainage of the pancreas is predominantly to the nodes that lie in juxtaposition to the arteries and veins (Fig. 1.49B).

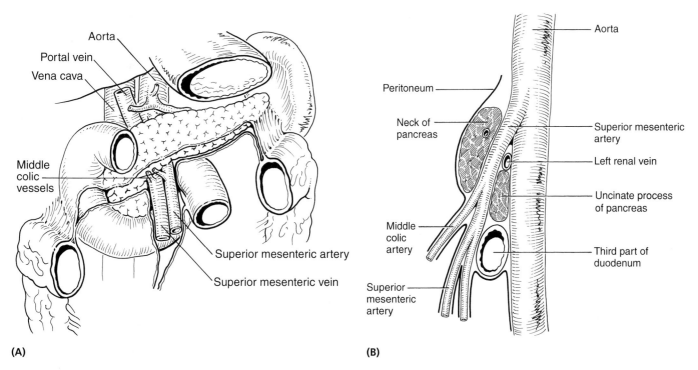

(A)   **(B)**

Fig. 1.46 (A) The anterior surface of the pancreas which is covered by the posterior layer of the omental bursa or lesser peritoneal sac, can itself often be obliterated by adhesions. The transverse mesocolon arises from the lower border of the pancreas and envelops the middle colic vessels as they arise from the superior mesenteric vessels just beneath the pancreatic neck. **(B)** The relationship of the pancreatic neck and uncinate process to the aorta and superior mesenteric artery. Note the position of the left renal vein and duodenum.

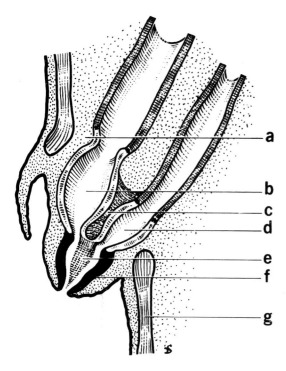

Fig. 1.47 Schematic representation of the sphincter of Oddi: (a) notch; (b) biliary sphincter; (c) transampullary septum; (d) pancreatic sphincter; (e) membranous septum of Boyden; (f) common sphincter; (g) smooth muscle of duodenal wall.

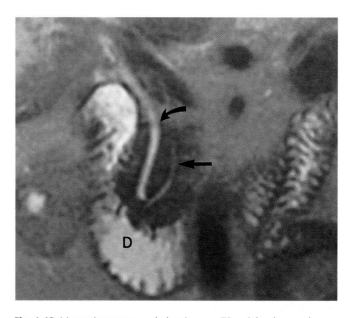

Fig. 1.48 Magnetic resonance cholangiogram, T2 weighted coronal (SSFSE) image at the level of the ampulla, shows the duodenum (D) and the pancreatic head with common bile duct (curved arrow), and pancreatic duct (straight arrow).

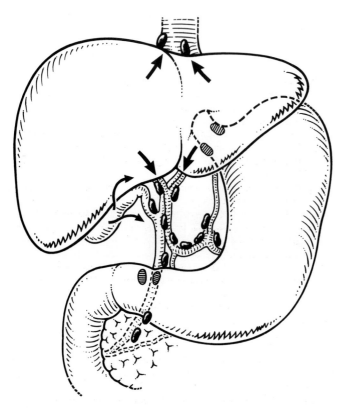

Fig. 1.49A The liver drains principally to hepatoduodenal nodes at the hilus and along the hepatic artery and portal vein. The gallbladder drains partly to the liver but also via the cystic node to nodes of the hepatoduodenal ligament and to suprapancreatic nodes.

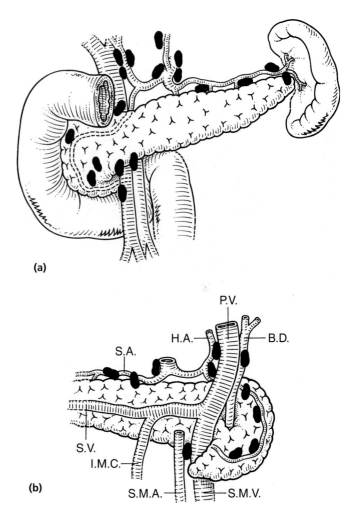

(a)

P.V.

H.A. — — B.D.

S.A.

S.V.

I.M.C. —

(b)

S.M.A. — — S.M.V.

Fig. 1.49B (a) Numerous nodes lie along the superior mesenteric vein, along the borders of the pancreas, draining back into the splenic hilar nodes, along the superior border of the pancreas, to the superior pancreatic nodes, and then to the celiac trunk and nodes at the base of the common hepatic artery. A large node commonly lodges in intimate association with the surface of the superior border of the pancreas and the right side of the common hepatic artery. This node often needs to be dissected and elevated to gain access to the anterior surface of the portal vein. Removal of this node often improves access, as does division of the gastroduodenal artery. **(b)** Posterior pancreaticoduodenal nodes lie along the posterior pancreatic duodenal arterial arcade.

LYMPH NODE METASTASIS AND CARCINOMA OF THE HEAD OF THE PANCREAS

The majority of patients who have carcinoma of the head of the pancreas have nodal positivity in the infra-pyloric nodes, the common hepatic lymph nodes, the lymph nodes along the splenic artery or the lymph nodes in the hepatoduodenal ligament. However, the most common are posterior pancreaticoduodenal lymph nodes, comprising 50–60% of all lymph nodes positive for carcinoma of the head of the pancreas. Other common sites are along the superior mesenteric artery and the para-aortic and anterior pancreaticoduodenal areas. Again, in order of frequency, it is the anterior and posterior duodenal lymph nodes that are most commonly involved.

In carcinoma of the distal bile duct or of the ampulla of Vater, the two most common sites for nodal involvement are the suprapyloric and the posterior pancreatic lymph nodes. It is, therefore, important to maximize staging so that at the time of resection an adequate dissection of the lymph nodes posterior to the pancreas will be performed. This is best done by dissection that begins on the anterior surface of the right renal veins, elevates the tissue in front of

the vena cava and the left renal vein across to the aorta. The delivery of this soft tissue is not difficult and will maximize the likelihood of identifying nodes that can be expected to be positive.

NERVE SUPPLY TO THE LIVER AND PANCREAS (Fig. 1.50)

The nerve supply is from branches of the celiac ganglion and is composed of sympathetic and parasympathetic elements.

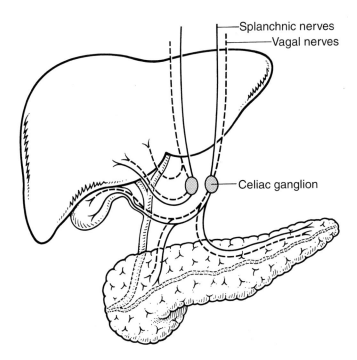

— Splanchnic nerves
— Vagal nerves

— Celiac ganglion

Fig. 1.50 Note the distribution of sympathetic and parasympathetic nerves to the liver and pancreas from the celiac ganglion mainly in association with major arteries.

REFERENCES

Albaret P, Chevalier J M, Cronier P, Enon B, Moreau O, Pillet J 1981 A propos des caneaux hépatiques directement abouchés dans la voie biliaire accessorie. Annales de Chirurgie 35: 88–92

Bismuth H, Houssin D, Castaing D 1982 Major and minor segmentectomies – 'règlèes' – in liver surgery. World Journal of Surgery 6: 10–24

Boyden E A 1926 The accessory gallbladder. An embryological and comparative study of aberrant biliary vesicles occurring in man and the domestic mammals. American Journal of Anatomy 38: 177–231

Boyden E A 1957 The anatomy of the choledochoduodenal junction in man. Surgery, Gynecology and Obstetrics 104: 641–652

Champetier J, Davin J L, Yver R, Vigneau B, Letoublon C 1982 Aberrant biliary ducts (vasa aberrantia): Surgical implications. Anatomica Clinica 4: 137–145

Couinaud C 1957 Le Foi. Etudes anatomogiques et chirurgicales. Masson, Paris

Delmont J 1979 Le sphincter d'Oddi: anatomie traditionelle et fonctionnelle. Gastroentrologie Clinique et Biologique 3: 157–165

Eelkema H H, Staar G F, Good C A 1958 Partial duplication of the gallbladder, diverticulum type. Report of a case. Radiology 70: 410–412

Gelfand D W 1983 Plain fil radiographic anatomy of the liver. In: Herlinger H, Lunderquist A, Wallace S (eds) Clinical radiology of the liver. Marcel Dekker, New York

Goldsmith N A, Woodburne R T 1957 Surgical anatomy pertaining to liver resection. Surgery, Gynecology and Obstetrics 195: 310–318

Gross R E 1936 Congenital abnormalities of the gallbladder. A review of 148 cases with report of a double gallbladder. Archives of Surgery 32: 131–162

Hand B H 1973 Anatomy and function of the extrahepatic biliary system. Clinics in Gastroenterology 2: 3–29

Healey J E, Schroy P C 1953 Anatomy of the biliary ducts within the human liver. Analysis of the prevailing pattern of branchings and the major variations of the biliary ducts. American Medical Association Archives of Surgery 66: 599–616

Hepp J, Couinaud C 1956 L'abord et l'utilisation du canal hepatique gauche dans les reparations de la voie biliare principale. Presse Medicale 64: 947–948

Hjörtsjö C H 1931 The topography of the intrahepatic duct systems. Acta Anatomica 11: 599–615

Hobby J A E 1970 Bilobed gallbladder. British Journal of Surgery 57: 870–872

Kune G A 1970 The influence of structure and function in the surgery of the biliary tract. Annals of the Royal College of Surgeons of England 47: 78–91

McIndoe A H, Counseller V X 1927 A report on the bilaterality of the liver. Archives of Surgery 15: 589

Newcombe J F, Henley F A 1964 Left-sided gallbladder. A review of the literature and a report of a case associated with hepatic duct carcinoma. Archives of Surgery 88: 494–497

Northover J M A, Terblanche J 1979 A new look at the arterial blood supply of the bile duct in man and its surgical implications. British Journal of Surgery 66: 379–384

Perelman H 1961 Cystic duct reduplication. Journal of the American Medical Association 175: 710–711

Rachad-Mohassel M A, Baghieri F, Maghsandi H, Nik Akhtar B 1973 Duplication de la vésicule biliaire. Archives Francais des Maldies de l'Appareil Digestif 62: 679–683

Rocko J M, Swan K G, Di Gioia J M 1981 Calot's triangle revisited. Surgery, Gynecology and Obstetrics 153: 410–414

Rogers H I, Crews R D, Kalser M H 1975 Congenital absence of the gallbladder with choledocholithiasis. Literature review and discussion of mechanisms. Gastroenterology 48: 524–529

Ton That Tung 1939 La vascularisation veineuse du foie et ses applications aux resections hepatiques. Thèse Hanoi

Ton That Tung 1979 Les resections majeures et mineures du foie. Masson, Paris.

Wood D 1979 Eponyms in biliary tract surgery. American Journal of Surgery 138: 746–754

2

Assessment of liver function in the surgical patient

H. ZIMMERMANN, J. REICHEN

INTRODUCTION

Preoperative assessment of liver function and prediction of postoperative remaining functional liver parenchymal mass and its reserve is of paramount importance to minimize the surgical risk. Liver failure is the major cause of death after hepatectomy especially in patients with liver cirrhosis and jaundice (Elias et al 1995, Nagino et al 1993, Didolkar et al 1989, Koperna et al 1998). Such an assessment should be able to evaluate hepatic function with just a few specific and simple tests. Unfortunately, none of the tests which we will discuss below meet these criteria and very few of them have been unambiguously validated in prospective studies. The liver exerts a wide variety of functions, including carbohydrate, lipid and protein metabolism, metabolism and storage of vitamins, production of bile, detoxification and excretion of endo- and xenobiotics. Although many of these different aspects of hepatic function can and have been used to assess functional reserve, few are used in everyday clinical practice. As a matter of fact, many commonly used 'liver tests' measure neither liver function nor are they specific for the liver. This holds particularly true for serum enzyme activities such as those of transaminases and of alkaline phosphatase.

One can arbitrarily divide liver tests into search tests, diagnostic tests and quantitative tests (Table 2.1). Search tests answer the question 'is liver disease present' while diagnostic tests give clues as to its etiology, e.g. serologic testing for hepatitis B markers or testing for mitochondrial antibodies in primary biliary cirrhosis. Finally, quantitative tests attempt to measure functional reserve and are particularly suited for prognostication and assessment of therapeutic effects. As will be seen, the border between these categories is not unambiguous and many search tests will give indications about functional reserve either alone or in combination with other tests.

Table 2.1 Liver tests

SEARCH TESTS

Test	Function/event measured
Serum bilirubin	Uptake, conjugation, excretion
Serum bile acids	Excretion, shunting
Alkaline phosphatase	Cholestasis
Gamma-glutamyl transpeptidase	Cholestasis, enzyme induction, alcohol abuse
5'-Nucleotidase	Cholestasis
Transaminases	Necrosis
Coagulation factors, prothrombin time	Synthesis
Albumin	Synthesis

DIAGNOSTIC TESTS

Test	Disease tested
Hepatitis A IgM	Acute hepatitis A
HBs, anti-HBs, anti-HBc etc.	Hepatitis B
Anti-HCV	Hepatitis C
Antimitochondrial antibodies	Primary biliary cirrhosis
Antineutrophil antibodies	Primary sclerosing cholangitis
ANA, ASM, anti-LKM	Autoimmune hepatitis
Iron, binding capacity, ferritin	Hemochromatosis
Alpha-1-antitrypsin	Alpha-1-antitrypsin deficiency
Ceruloplasmin, urine copper	Wilson's disease

QUANTITATIVE TESTS

Test	Function tested
Aminopyrine breath test	Microsomal function
Antipyrine clearance	Microsomal function
Caffeine clearance	Microsomal function
Lidocaine clearance (MEGX)	Microsomal function
Methacetin breath test	Microsomal function
Galactose elimination capacity (GEC)	Cytosolic function
Low dose galactose clearance	Hepatic perfusion
Sorbitol clearance	Hepatic perfusion
ICG disappearance	Hepatic perfusion, anion excretion
BSP clearance	Hepatic perfusion, anion excretion
Albumin synthesis	Synthetic function
Urea synthesis	Synthetic function
'Redox potential'	Mitochondrial function
^{99m}Tc-GSA	Functioning hepatocyte mass

This chapter gives an overview of some of the most commonly used liver tests; it will focus only on the search and quantitative tests and their combination into prognostic scores.

SEARCH TESTS

Search tests (Table 2.1) include the standard 'liver function' tests such as total bilirubin, serum transaminases, serum alkaline phosphatase, gamma-glutamyl transpeptidase, serum albumin and prothrombin time. Neither is a true measure of liver function since an activity or concentration of some substance in blood is measured. Serum concentration is the amount (A) of the substance present in its volume of distribution (V_d) where A obviously is the difference between production (P) and elimination (E):

$$[c] = A/V_d = (P - E)/V_d \qquad [1]$$

Equation 1 demonstrates the difficulties in interpreting a level as a measure of function, since most often neither the volume of distribution nor the processes leading to formation and elimination are known. Moreover, to be a true liver function test, the substance under investigation should be produced and/or eliminated only in the liver. This is clearly not the case. Thus for example bilirubin concentration can also be affected by nonhepatic processes such as hemolysis and prothrombin time depends on the formation of vitamin K by intestinal bacteria.

BILIRUBIN

Unconjugated bilirubin is the main degradation product of heme formed in the reticulo-endothelial system of the spleen, bone marrow and liver; 75 to 80% of bilirubin is derived from hemoglobin of senescent erythrocytes, the remainder being due to the catabolism of heme of myoglobin and shorter-lived hepatic hemoproteins, in particular cytochrome P450. Unconjugated bilirubin is highly water-insoluble and tightly bound to albumin. Hepatic metabolism of bilirubin is shown in Figure 2.1: unconjugated bilirubin is taken up from plasma by a carrier-mediated transport process into the hepatocyte and some of it returns unaltered back into the circulation. In the cytosol it is bound by cytosolic binding proteins, in particular ligandin, before being conjugated in the smooth endoplasmic reticulum by UDP-glucuronyl transferase to bilirubin mono- and diglucuronide; a minor proportion is conjugated with other sugars. The bilirubin conjugates are then excreted via a second carrier protein into the canalicular lumen and a small portion refluxes back into plasma (Fig. 2.1). In the intes-

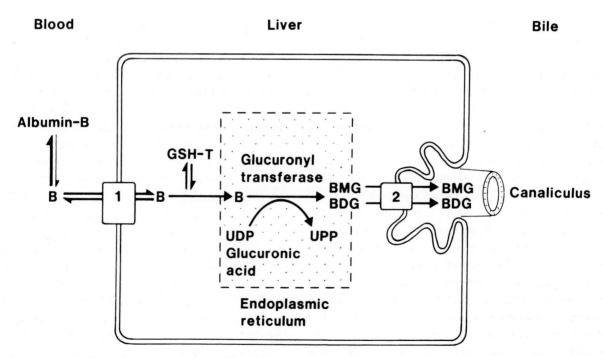

Fig. 2.1 Bilirubin metabolism in the hepatocyte. Unconjugated bilirubin (B) is tightly bound to albumin in plasma; it is transported across the sinusoidal membrane by a distinct carrier protein (1); in the cytosol, (B) is bound to glutathione transferases (GSH-T), in particular ligandin. It enters the endoplasmic reticulum, where it is conjugated by (UDP)-glucuronyltransferase to bilirubin mono- (BMG) and diglucuronide (BDG) which are then excreted via a second carrier protein (2) into the canalicular lumen.

tine, bilirubin is degraded to urobilinogen and further degradation products which give the stool its particular color. Most of it is excreted in the feces and 10 to 15% is absorbed into the portal circulation. In the serum of normal individuals < 5% of bilirubin is conjugated. The water-soluble conjugated bilirubin can be excreted in the urine but normal urine is free of bile pigment. Determinations of urine urobilinogen and urine bilirubin as screening tests for liver disease are not worthwhile because of the high proportion of false-negative results.

The scheme in Figure 2.1 indicates that a variety of hepatic and extrahepatic factors can affect serum bilirubin concentration (Table 2.2). In the routine clinical laboratory, total and direct reacting bilirubin are determined; the latter does not correspond to conjugated bilirubin since the reaction is relatively unspecific (De Cock et al 1988). Conjugated bilirubin can be accurately assessed by high performance liquid chromatography; this has been found highly specific for cholestatic liver disease (VanHootegem et al 1985, Sieg et al 1990), but this method is usually not available in clinical practice. After long-standing cholestasis, bilirubin becomes covalently bound to serum albumin C, the so-called delta-bilirubin (Weiss et al 1983). This fraction disappears from serum with the half-life of albumin (20 d); this phenomenon accounts for the slow resolution of jaundice after relief of long-standing obstruction in spite of otherwise normal liver function. In patients with severe extrahepatic bacterial infection and jaundice conjugated bilirubin is often increased with normal or only modest increase in levels of alkaline phosphatase and transaminases (Zimmermann et al 1979). This cholestasis may be due to a selective defect in the excretion of conjugated bilirubin, but the exact mechanism of hepatic injury is not known (Miller et al 1976, Zimmermann et al 1979).

Bilirubin levels are neither very sensitive nor very specific in detecting liver disease. Thus, an elevation of direct reacting bilirubin does not differentiate between intra- and extrahepatic cholestasis. Moreover, in localized biliary obstruction (e.g. intrahepatic gallstones or tumors, sclerosing cholangitis, primary biliary cirrhosis) bilirubin can be normal for a long time due to the large functional reserve capacity of the nonobstructed parenchyma. A range of situations not directly related to biliary integrity can lead to bilirubin elevation in the postoperative period (Table 2.2). These include sepsis (Miller et al 1976, Wood et al 1979), the syndrome of benign postoperative cholestasis (Caroli et al 1950, Schmid et al 1965) and prolonged (2–3 weeks) total parenteral nutrition (Stanko et al 1987). Bilirubin may be abnormal after an uncomplicated cholecystectomy in a significant percentage of patients for up to 1 year (Harada et al 1977). Increased serum bilirubin postoperatively does

Table 24.2 Disorders of bilirubin metabolism

Type	Mechanism	Examples
Unconjugated	Overproduction	Hemolysis
		Ineffective erythropoiesis
		Extravasation of blood
		Prolonged fasting
	Decreased uptake	Sepsis
		Drugs
		M. Gilbert
	Decreased conjugation	Crigler Najjar syndrome I/II
		M. Gilbert
		Newborn
		Drugs
		Cirrhosis, hepatitis
Conjugated	Decreased secretion	Dubin-Johnson syndrome
		Rotor syndrome
		Cholestasis of pregnancy
		Benign recurrent intrahepatic cholestasis
		Drugs
		Cirrhosis, hepatitis
	Obstruction	Gallstones
		Strictures
		Tumors
		Biliary atresia

not always indicate a complication (Didolkar et al 1989, Ekberg et al 1986). Of particular concern is the elevation of serum bilirubin in patients after portacaval shunt surgery: an increase above 85 gmols/L (5 mg/dl) was always associated with either portal vein thrombosis or a marked change in sinusoidal pressure (Vo & Rikkers 1985).

The presence of cholestasis with increased serum bilirubin and alkaline phosphatase is associated with increased complication rate and mortality after hepatectomy (Didolkar et al 1989, Gavelli et al 1993, Lau et al 1997a,b). Total serum bilirubin but not transaminase, alkaline phosphatase, serum albumin or presence of cirrhosis may predict postoperative complications after major hepatic resections (Sitzmann & Greene 1994). However, after extended right hepatectomies others found no differences in morbidity or mortality whether serum total bilirubin was increased or not (Miyagawa et al 1994). In contrast to partial drainage complete surgical biliary decompression of obstructive jaundice normalize bilirubin, serum alkaline phosphatase, AST and ALT by six weeks (Watanapa 1996).

While bilirubin is not a good screening test, it carries some prognostic significance; this was recognized by Sherlock as early as 1946 (Sherlock 1946) and has been confirmed in many studies since (Schlichting et al 1983a, Adson et al 1984, Christensen et al 1984, Gines et al 1987). This seems to be particularly true for patients with primary biliary cirrhosis where with two consecutive bilirubin levels above 34 mols/L (2 mg/dl), 102 mols/L (6 mg/dl) and 170 mols/L (10 mg/dl) a mean survival of 49, 25 and 17 months, respectively, was observed (Shapiro et al 1979). Also, in patients with liver cirrhosis 1 year before death bilirubin was markedly increased together with a decrease in prothrombin time, albumin and cholesterol 1 year before death (Christensen et al 1985a,b). Serum bilirubin is part of many general and disease-specific scores, including the Child classification (vide infra).

SERUM BILE ACIDS (see also Ch. 8)

In the liver cholesterol is degraded to bile acids; the two primary bile acids formed, cholate and chenodeoxycholate, are conjugated within the hepatocyte to glycine or taurine forming four conjugated bile acids and are excreted into bile (Fig. 2.2). In the gut, they undergo different modifications by intestinal bacteria including deconjugation and dehydroxylation, the latter leading to formation of the secondary bile acids deoxycholate and lithocholate. Bile acids are reabsorbed passively in the jejunum and actively in the ileum. Since hepatic extraction of bile acids from portal blood and liver artery is incomplete—averaging 50 to 90% in man depending on the bile acid species studied (Angelin et al 1982, Miescher et al 1983)—a minor part escapes into the systemic circulation. In the fasting state serum concentration is much lower than after eating. The metabolism of bile acids was reviewed by (Hofmann 1983). Bile acids are important in fat digestion but also potent toxins (reviewed by Schoelmerich & Straub 1992). The organisms have elaborated an ingenious system to keep them where they are used and can do no harm, i.e. within the biliary system and the intestinal lumen (Fig. 2.2).

It is evident from Figure 2.2 that three processes are the main determinants of serum bile acid levels, i.e. intestinal absorption, hepatic extraction and canalicular secretion. In chronic liver disease, three processes could theoretically lead to increased serum bile acid levels; portosystemic shunting

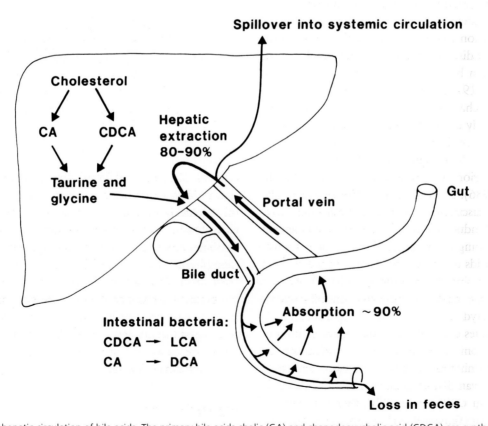

Fig. 2.2 The enterohepatic circulation of bile acids. The primary bile acids cholic (CA) and chenodeoxycholic acid (CDCA) are synthesized from cholesterol and conjugated with taurine or glycine. They are secreted into the canaliculus; after storage in the gallbladder, bile acids reach the intestine where intestinal bacteria can lead to deconjugation and dehydroxylation. The latter leads to formation of the secondary bile acids deoxycholic acid (DCA) and lithocholic acid (LGA). Bile acids are efficiently reabsorbed, passively in the jejunum and actively in the ileum. Fecal bile acid loss is restored by de novo synthesis. Reabsorbed bile acids reach the hepatocyte via the portal circulation. They are efficiently extracted from portal blood via a sodium-coupled, active transport system and undergo the cycle again. Since hepatic extraction is incomplete, some spillover into the systemic circulation occurs even under normal circumstances.

and/or a decrease in hepatic extraction capacity and cholestasis (i.e. failure of secretion). All mechanisms have been found operative in different forms of liver disease. Thus, serum bile acid concentrations correlate with porto-systemic shunting in experimental animals (Reichen et al 1988) and in man (Ohkubo et al 1984) with liver cirrhosis. Bile acids are one of the earliest indicators of cholestasis pregnancy (Lunzer et al 1986) and benign recurrent intra-hepatic cholestasis (Summerfield et al 1981, Bijleveld et al 1989). Serum bile acids are quite useful in differentiating between hepatobiliary disease and congenital hyperbilirubin-emia, in particular Gilbert's syndrome, serum bile acid levels being uniformly normal in the latter (Vierling et al 1982).

Initial reports were enthusiastic that either fasting (Korman et al 1974, Barnes et al 1975, Osuga et al 1977) or 2-h post-prandial (Kaplowitz et al 1973, Jones et al 1981) bile acid levels are very sensitive indicators of liver damage. Theoretically, postprandial serum bile acid measurements should be more sensitive than fasting levels since there is a larger load after gallbladder contraction and mixing of intestinal contents; however, in clinical practice it was found that postprandial levels were equal (Mannes et al 1982) or inferior (Festi et al 1983, van Blankenstein et al 1983) to fasting levels.

There is no question that serum bile acid determination can detect mild liver disease even when other standard liver tests including serum bilirubin are normal (Bloomer et al 1976, Milstein et al 1976, Skrede et al 1978, Douglas et al 1981, Simko & Michael 1986). Of particular interest for the surgeon is a study demonstrating that serum bile acids can detect inactive liver cirrhosis with normal transaminases with a sensitivity of > 90% (Mannes et al 1982).

The test is superior to serum enzymes and albumin (Greenfield et al 1986). In alcoholic liver disease, serum bile acids were found to discriminate between acute alcohol intoxication and alcohol-induced structural liver disease (Joelsson et al 1984). This finding is not universal, AST being as sensitive as serum bile acids in one study (Ferraris et al 1983); in another study, transaminases were more sensitive but less specific than serum bile acids in the detection of cirrhosis (Tobiasson & Boeryd 1980), in partial agreement with another study (Mannes et al 1982). However, not all biopsy-proven cases of chronic liver disease can be identified by serum bile acid determinations although they were more sensitive than bilirubin (van Blankenstein et al 1983). When bile acids are analyzed in conjunction with other conventional liver tests, they do not (Winkel et al 1975, Sher 1977) or only marginally increase discriminatory power (Linnet and Andersen 1983). Sensitivity and specificity of serum bile acid levels in different disease states are compiled in Table 2.3.

Serum bile acid levels also carry prognostic information for short-term survival in patients with cirrhosis (Mannes et

Table 2.3 Sensitivity and—where available—specificity of total serum bile acid levels in different settings.

Patient group F/PP	Sensitivity (%)	Specificity (%)	Authors
Mild liver disease			
F	100		Simko & Michael 1986
F	90		Greenfield et al 1986
F	48		Ferraris et al 1983
PP	80		Greenfield et al 1986
PP	3–23		Van Blankenstein et al 1983
Chronic active hepatitis/compensated cirrhosis			
F	93		Ferraris et al 1983
F	82		Poupon et al 1978
PP	90		Collins et al 1979
PP	85		Poupon et al 1987
Compensated cirrhosis			
F	93		Mannes et al 1982
F	75		Ohkubo et al 1984
PP	93		Mannes et al 1982
Decompensated cirrhosis			
F	100		Joelsson et al 1983
F	100		Joelsson et al 1984
Unselected populations Medical Unit*			
F	78	93	Ferraris et al 1983

Only publications reporting total serum bile acid levels, determined either enzymatically or by radioimmunological methods, are reported. F/PP refers to bile acid levels obtained either fasting or 2 h postprandially.
* In this study, predictive values based on the prevalence of hepatobiliary diseases could be calculated. In a GI unit (with a high prevalence of hepatobiliary diseases) the positive and negative predictive values of an abnormal fasting bile acid level were 94 and 74%, respectively. In contrast, in a medical unit with a low prevalence of hepatobiliary disease the positive predictive value dropped to 10%.

al 1986, Siciliano et al 1989). The prognostic information contained in serum bile acid levels is independent of that of the Child classification and adds prognostic value to the latter (Mannes et al 1986). Elevation of serum bile acids has been reported to herald decompensation much earlier than bilirubin or albumin (Kishimoto et al 1985).

In conclusion, serum bile acid levels are a useful, albeit not perfect screening tool for the presence of structural liver disease. They are helpful in determining the hepatic origin of elevated bilirubin and/or alkaline phosphatase levels and finally, they appear to be a useful adjunct in prognostication of cirrhotic liver disease.

SERUM ENZYMES

The determination of serum enzyme activities has been useful in the diagnosis of chronic liver disease over the past 50 years (Zieve & Hill 1955, Wroblewski 1959, Zimmermann & West 1963). Diagnostic accuracy has been found to be only 14% in one study (Baron 1970) but in others it was

60–70% (Solberg et al 1975, Winkel et al 1975), the most important variables being AST and alkaline phosphatase. In asymptomatic patients with elevated serum liver enzymes, the number of false positives may be reduced by ultrasound examination (Ekberg et al 1986). Albeit imperfect, serum activity determination of transaminases, alkaline phosphatase and gamma-glutamyltranspeptidase remains the mainstay in screening for hepatobiliary disease.

Alkaline phosphatase

Alkaline phosphatase is expressed in liver, bone, intestine, placenta, kidney and leukocytes. Three different isoenzymes coded by separate genes can be identified in serum, an unspecific form derived from liver, bone and kidney and isoenzymes derived from placenta and intestine. Some publications have demonstrated that isoenzyme determinations could differentiate between alkaline phosphatase from bone and liver (Epstein et al 1984) and even between parenchymatous and cholestatic liver disease (Domar et al 1988). In particular, a high molecular weight enzyme has been found to be a good marker of cholestatic liver disease (Price et al 1972, Crofton et al 1979). However, separation of different isoenzymes is not performed in most routine clinical laboratories since this does not add to the discriminatory power (Winkelman et al 1972). Clinically the most important differentiation is between skeletal and hepatic origin; this is best achieved by simultaneous determination of gamma-glutamyltranspeptidase and/or serum bile acids.

Elevated alkaline phosphatase in serum is found in patients with bone, liver and neoplastic disorders. The elevation of alkaline phosphatase in hepatobiliary disease is due to increased synthesis (Kaplan & Righetti 1970, Seetharam et al 1986) perhaps stimulated by bile acids (Hatoff et al 1979). This explains why, in patients with acute biliary obstruction, the elevation of alkaline phosphatase often lags behind the onset of symptoms and even jaundice. Although an elevated hepatic alkaline phosphatase indicates cholestasis unspecific elevations are often seen; therefore, it has been suggested that it may behave as an acute phase reactant (Brensilver & Kaplan 1975). In patients with unrelieved bile duct obstruction limited to one lobe of the liver it was found that the initial rise of serum alkaline phosphatase gradually decreased and returned to normal, parallel with the atrophy of the liver segment subjected to bile stasis (Hadjis et al 1990).

A much debated indication for alkaline phosphatase determination is the detection of primary hepatic tumors and metastases. Alkaline phosphatase is not useful as a screening test for metastatic disease in colorectal cancer (Jonsson et al 1984, Nishio et al 1986, Christensen et al 1987, Lin & Lin 1991, Rocklin et al 1991, Osanaga et al 1992) other cancers

from the digestive tract (Osanaga et al 1992) and breast cancer (Karmen et al 1984) (Clark et al 1988). In bronchogenic carcinoma, in contrast, alkaline phosphatase levels were elevated in most patients with liver metastases but the finding was not specific (Margolis et al 1974). Transaminases and alkaline phosphatase were normal in > 30% of patients with CT-proven hepatic metastases from different origins (Ottmar et al 1989). Whether determination of specific isoenzymes increases sensitivity in detecting metastases and hepatocellular carcinoma remains to be determined. Encouraging reports have been reported when only the high molecular weight form, also termed alpha-1-fraction, was determined (Viot et al 1981, Burlina et al 1983, Bukofzer et al 1988); however, the specificity appears to be lacking (Viot et al 1983). After resection of colorectal carcinoma alkaline phosphatase is elevated in only about 20% of patients with secondary liver metastasis whereas CEA is elevated in most cases (Rocklin et al 1991). In this study, omission of the conventional liver function tests would have led to missing of delaying diagnosis of liver metastasis in only 2% (Rocklin et al 1991).

The level of alkaline phosphatase is not an indicator of function and in most circumstances bears no prognostic significance. Exceptions are some scores where alkaline phosphatase seems to convey prognostic information together with other parameters in primary sclerosing cholangitis (Farrant et al 1991) and alcoholic hepatitis (Orrego et al 1983); the latter may be an expression of the fact that the cholestatic form of alcoholic hepatitis has a poor prognosis per se (Nissenbaum et al 1990). In colorectal metastases, patients with elevated alkaline phosphatase fare worse than those with normal levels (Klompje et al 1987). After bilioenteric anastomosis for benign bile duct stricture alkaline phosphatase is always elevated (Nealon & Urrutia 1996).

Alkaline phosphatase levels are nonspecific indicators of cholestatic liver disease; together with the determination of hepatic enzymes of more specific hepatic origin such as 5′-Nucleotidase or gamma-glutamyltranspeptidase or with serum bile acids it is assured a place as a potent screening test. However, it does not assess function and therefore has no prognostic significance.

Other indicators of cholestasis

Since alkaline phosphatase lacks specificity for the liver, other enzymes have been proposed as markers of cholestasis. The best introduced and the only ones which will be considered here are gamma-glutamyltranspeptidase and 5′-Nucleotidase.

Gamma-glutamyltranspeptidase (GGT) occurs in many organs besides the liver; these include the kidneys, seminal vesicles, spleen, pancreas, heart and brain (Naftalin et al

1969). Aside from liver disease, it is also elevated in renal failure, pancreatic disease, myocardial infarction, diabetes (Rosalki et al 1970) and some other diseases (Goldberg & Martin 1975). Even more cumbersome is the fact that its activity is induced by a variety of drugs and by ethanol in the absence of any evidence of hepatotoxicity leading to false positive results (Knight & Haymond 1981). It remains a valuable tool, nevertheless, since it permits determination as to whether an alkaline phosphatase level is of hepatic or osseous origin (Lum & Gambino 1972) and is a better indicator of obstruction in children since, in contrast to alkaline phosphatase, its activity is not age-dependent (Knight & Haymond 1981).

GGT increases markedly (up to 40-fold) in mechanical bile duct obstruction; it has been proposed that the ALT/GGT ratio was better able to differentiate between obstructive jaundice and hepatitis than alkaline phosphatase or any of the enzymes taken alone (Aronson et al 1965). The bilirubin/GGT ratio has some prognostic value in cirrhotic patients (Poynard et al 1984). GGT may be of value in the diagnosis of acute obstruction and cholecystitis where it is almost universally elevated (Lum & Gambino 1972, Whitfield et al 1972) in contrast to alkaline phosphatase, since alkaline phosphatase elevations require de novo synthesis of the enzyme and therefore often lag behind the onset of acute obstruction (vide supra). However, the lack of specificity has to be taken into account when interpreting an elevated GGT level (Whitfield et al 1972).

Together with aspartate aminotransferase and median corpuscular volume (MCV) GGT is a sensitive, albeit nonspecific indicator of chronic alcohol abuse (Lai et al 1982, Eriksen et al 1984, Nilssen et al 1992). However, it can be elevated even after sporadic acute alcohol intake (Zein & Discombre 1970) and, conversely, is not a reliable indicator of alcohol intake in heavy drinkers (Evans et al 1984, Orrego et al 1985). Finally, GGT determination may be superior to alkaline phosphatase in detecting liver metastases (Osanaga et al 1992).

Besides the liver, 5′-Nucleotidase is found in the intestine, brain, heart, blood vessels and pancreas. Nevertheless, elevations of 5′-Nucleotidase appear to occur uniquely in liver disease (Young 1958, Kowlessar et al 1961, Hill & Sammons 1967). It is therefore useful in determining whether the origin of an elevated alkaline phosphatase is due to liver or bone disease and it has been found to be more useful in detecting hepatic metastases than either alkaline phosphatase or GGT (Kim et al 1977).

Both GGT and 5′-Nucleotidase are of value to affirm the hepatic origin of an elevated alkaline phosphatase. Neither is an ideal screening test, carries any prognostic information or gives clues as to functional reserve.

Transaminases

Determination of transaminase activity was introduced into clinical medicine in 1955 (Karmen et al 1955); they are time-proven indicators of ongoing hepatocellular necrosis (Table 2.1). Alanine aminotransferase (ALT, previously called glutamate pyruvate transaminase, GPT) is a cytosolic enzyme while aspartate aminotransferase (AST, formerly glutamate oxalate transaminase, GOT) is 80% mitochondrial and 20% cytosolic in origin. AST is not liver specific since it also occurs in heart, muscle, kidney, erythrocytes and brain; in contrast, ALT is localized mainly in the liver and therefore quite liver specific. There is some activity in muscle and ALT can be elevated after severe crush injury.

The level of transaminase elevation bears no prognostic significance since there is no correlation with the extent of necrosis (Schneider et al 1980, Sahdew et al 1991) or severity of the liver disease (Fig. 2.3). Accordingly, transaminase levels bear no prognostic significance and do not correlate with functional impairment.

Transaminases have been found to be useful screening tools for the presence of traumatic liver injury in pediatric (Hennes et al 1990) and adult patients (Sahdew et al 1991). In children, levels above 200 and 100 IU/L for AST and

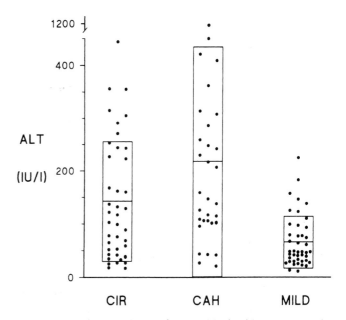

Fig. 2.3 Serum alanine aminotransferase activity (ALT) in 110 consecutive patients with unclear transaminase elevations undergoing liver biopsy. Based on liver biopsy the patients were classified as having cirrhosis (CIR), chronic active hepatitis (CAH) or mild liver disease, the latter including nonalcoholic steatosis, nonspecific portal inflammation and normal histology. There was no significant difference between the three groups by analysis of variance. From A. Gyger, MD thesis, Berne, Switzerland (unpublished observations).

ALT, respectively, predicted hepatic trauma and correlated with injury (Qidman et al 1984); in adults, the cut-off was 130 IU/L for AST but did not correlate with the severity of hepatic trauma.

Aspartate aminotransferase and ALT should be performed simultaneously since ALT can confirm the hepatic origin of the less specific but more sensitive AST. Moreover, the ratio of AST:ALT may give some clues as to the etiology of the liver disease, since in alcoholic liver disease this ratio is > 2 in 90% of patients (Cohen & Kaplan 1979, Salaspuro 1987, Williams & Hoofnagle 1988). This is due to a decrease of ALT in the liver of alcoholics (Matloff et al 1980) and may be related to pyridoxal deficiency (Lumeng & Li 1974). This is not specific for alcoholic liver disease, however, and may also be found in steatosis in morbidly obese patients (Nanji et al 1989, Fletcher et al 1991).

Transaminase levels are usually less elevated in alcoholic liver disease than in viral or toxic hepatitis; very high transaminase levels in alcoholic patients are indicative of other processes, in particular acetaminophen intoxication (Seeff et al 1986). Besides viral hepatitis, transaminases can reach very high levels in congestive heart failure (Richman et al 1961, Nouel et al 1980), biliary obstruction, with or without cholangitis (Patwardhan et al 1987, Roberts-Thomson et al 1990) and in toxic hepatitis. In these entities, they typically decline very rapidly, in the case of biliary obstruction even when obstruction persists (Patwardhan et al 1987). After cholecystectomy and morphine analgesia transaminases and other enzymes may rise due to prolonged increase in intrabiliary pressure (Roberts-Thomson et al 1990).

Partial hepatectomy induces a mild increase in transaminase activity which is not increased by the Pringle maneuver (Miyagawa et al 1994, Nagasue et al 1984). After hepatic artery ligation for unresectable carcinoma, transaminases increase 5-60-fold to return to normal within 1 week (Lee 1978). High preoperative levels of ALT and alkaline phosphatase in patients with hepatocellular carcinoma indicate a significantly increased risk after hepatectomy to develop in-hospital mortality and morbidity (Noun et al 1997) and tumor recurrence (Suehiro et al 1994). In patients with cirrhosis the postoperative increase of GPT levels at day 1 and 3 is significantly higher after partial right hepatectomy than after right hepatectomy (Suehiro et al 1994). Elevated ALT levels in hepatectomized patients with hepatitis C virus (HCV)-associated cirrhosis and hepatocellular carcinoma may indicate HCC recurrence (Tarao et al 1997). In the postsurgical patient, an increase in transaminases may herald the onset of halothane hepatitis, particularly after repeated exposure (Wright et al 1975, Böttiger et al 1976); this is a rare occurrence, however, estimated at an incidence of 1:7000–36 000.

Transaminases are the time proven screening test for hepatocyte necrosis; the degree of elevation bears little diagnostic and no prognostic information. The finding of elevated transaminases should lead to more intensive investigations using other diagnostic tests (Table 2.1) to find the reason for hepatocellular necrosis and diagnostic scores or quantitative tests to assess the severity of the functional impairment.

SERUM PROTEINS

Most serum proteins are synthesized within the liver, the major exception being the immunoglobulins. Therefore, they have been used as a measure of hepatic synthetic capacity; however, many other extrahepatic factors, in particular elimination, influence the serum levels of all serum proteins (see equation 1). The most frequently used parameters of synthetic capacity are clotting factors and serum albumin.

Clotting factors

The liver is the major site of synthesis of blood clotting factors. Coagulation defects are frequent in chronic liver disease; they do not universally reflect impaired synthetic capacity but may also be related to intravascular coagulation and vitamin K malabsorption. Production of factors II, VII, IX and X are vitamin K dependent. The best studied parameter is prothrombin time; it is part of several prognostic indices (vide infra) and determined serially carries prognostic information on its own in e.g. paracetamol poisoning (Harrison et al 1990).

Individual clotting factors have also been evaluated as diagnostic tools; thus factor VII was found to be an excellent measure of hepatic synthetic function (Green et al 1976). Factor V is used to predict timing of liver transplantation in fulminant hepatic failure (Bismuth et al 1986). Factor V levels are also good predictors of survival in liver transplantation in adults and children (Stock et al 1987). Fibrinogen levels are usually normal or slightly elevated in mild liver disease but markedly decreased in massive hepatocellular damage (Ratnoff 1975). There is disagreement as to whether or not preoperative coagulation abnormalities predict intraoperative blood loss, blood product use and survival in liver transplantation (Mariette et al 1997, Bontempo et al 1985, Ritter et al 1989). Bleeding after liver biopsy cannot be predicted from measurements of peripheral coagulation (Ewe 1981).

Determination of the prothrombin time is routine; its value should be incorporated into diagnostic scores where appropriate (vide infra).

Albumin

Like clotting factors, albumin is synthesized exclusively in the liver. Its serum concentration is dependent upon the volume of distribution and there can be extrahepatic loss leading to low albumin levels in the absence of structural liver disease. Albumin is not a very sensitive indicator of synthetic function since a 50% reduction in synthesis rate induces only a 20% fall in serum levels (Skrede et al 1973). Because of its relatively long half-life of 20 days it does not indicate synthetic function in acute liver disease. Hypoalbuminemia is found not only in chronic liver disease and hepatic malignancy but also in many non-hepatic diseases such as renal disease, protein malnutrition, protein-losing enteropathy, burns and others (Andersson 1976). In chronic liver disease, once extra-hepatic losses are excluded, albumin carries prognostic information, particularly when incorporated into a score (Zimmerer et al 1996).

Prealbumin may be a more sensitive indicator than albumin and other conventional liver function tests (Hutchinson et al 1981) (Joelsson et al 1983, Teppo & Maury 1983, Rondana et al 1987). It correlates with the Child classification and galactose elimination capacity (Rondana et al 1987) but it has yet to prove its superiority to albumin determinations.

Albumin level is a poor screening test but should be measured where there is a suspicion of malnutrition and/or chronic liver disease. When incorporated into scores, it carries prognostic information in cirrhotic liver disease.

QUANTITATIVE LIVER FUNCTION TESTS

Patients with abnormal standard liver function tests do not necessarily have any significant loss of hepatic function; therefore, the prognostic value of conventional liver tests is virtually nil. It has been proposed that dynamic or quantitative liver function tests could detect functional impairment and hepatic failure more accurately and be helpful in prognosis (Lotterer et al 1997). This rationale is sound since patients with, for example, liver cirrhosis die predominantly of hepatic failure (Baker et al 1959, Schlichting et al 1983b). This is particularly well illustrated by an old study on the natural history of varices (Fig. 2.4) which shows that the mortality was the same in patients who bled from their varices as in those who did not (Baker et al 1959). However, quantitative liver function tests have only partially fulfilled this promise. Some of these quantitative or dynamic liver function tests permit grouping of patients according to their prognosis (Bircher et al 1973, Lindskov 1982a, Henry et al

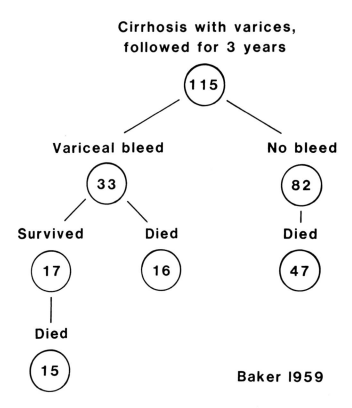

Fig. 2.4 The natural history of esophageal varices during a 3-year follow-up. Redrawn with permission from Baker et al (1959).

1985, Villeneuve et al 1986, Pomier Layrargues et al 1988, Poulson & Loft 1988, Merkel et al 1989, Merkel et al 1992); however, it remains unclear whether these tests are superior to simple scoring systems (Villeneuve et al 1986) as long as none of the quantitative liver function tests has been evaluated in a prospective fashion on a sufficient number of patients in the settings of surgery.

We have proposed that their main strength may be when they are used in a serial fashion. Thus, hepatic function declines in a predictable fashion in a rat model of biliary cirrhosis; this decline has a very high negative predictive value, an attractive feature when considering the timing of transplantation (Gross et al 1987). This concept has been confirmed in patients with primary biliary cirrhosis (Reichen et al 1991) and chronic active hepatitis (Aebli & Reichen 1991). Such a feature could also be helpful when assessing the value of novel forms of treatment (Williams & Farrell 1989) and serve as a surrogate endpoint in randomized clinical trials.

Most dynamic liver function tests rely on the clearance principle (Rowland et al 1973, Wilkinson & Shand 1975): hepatic clearance (Cl) is the product of flow (Q) and extraction (E):

$$Cl = Q \bullet E \qquad [2]$$

Equation 2 indicates that a substance will behave differently depending on whether its extraction is high or low: with a high extraction, clearance will approach blood flow (flow-limited clearance) while with a low extraction it will be flow-independent and measure the process being responsible for its clearance. Since most of these processes are enzymatic (e.g. cytochrome P450-mediated metabolism), this regime is called enzyme-limited (Wilkinson & Shand 1975). A measure of these processes is the intrinsic clearance (Cl_{int}) which is defined as the ratio of the maximal reaction velocity (V_{max}) and the affinity (K_m):

$$Cl_{int} = V_{max}/K_m \qquad [3]$$

Equation 2 can then be rewritten as

$$Cl = (Q \bullet Cl_{int})/(Q + Cl_{int}) \qquad [4]$$

Intrinsic clearance cannot be measured unambiguously in man; investigators have estimated it by combining equations 2 and 4 and solving it for Cl_{int} (Poupon et al 1981, Barbare et al 1985). This is mathematically correct but does not estimate true intrinsic clearance since extraction is flow-dependent; thus, these values are correct for the given flow but do not permit appreciation of the true value of intrinsic clearance.

In cirrhosis, at least in the end-stage of the disease, portal flow is reduced; considering equation 2 one would then predict that the clearance of flow-limited compounds should be affected more than that of enzyme-limited compounds. However, it was found that there was no difference in impairment between the clearance of enzyme- and flow-limited drugs (Branch et al 1976, Colli et al 1988); this apparent paradox has been explained by the intact cell theory (Wood et al 1979) which states that a reduced number of intrinsically normal hepatocytes are only partially perfused owing to hemodynamic alterations. This theory has been proven for some (Reichen et al 1987a,b, Kawasaki et al 1992) but not all (Reichen et al 1987a,b, Ohara et al 1992) hepatic functions. Particularly in the rat model of biliary cirrhosis, the sick cell hypothesis C which states that a given function expressed per hepatocyte is reduced C applies (Ohara et al 1992). The application of classic pharmacokinetic theory as given by equation 4 to patients with liver disease is fraught with hazards (Huet & Villeneuve 1983) since many enzymatic and hemodynamic phenomena contribute to the reduced hepatic function in chronic liver disease. Thus, besides portosystemic shunting (Wood et al 1979, Poupon et al 1981, Pomier-Layrargues et al 1986) sinusoidal capillarization (Huet et al 1982, Reichen et al 1988) contributes to decreased clearance. In a comprehensive study, investigating all hemodynamic and enzymatic aspects, sinusoidal capillarization was found to be the main determinant of galactose and aminopyrine elimination (vide infra) while anatomic shunts were the main predictors of bile acid clearance (Reichen et al 1988).

Given these uncertainties as well as the many different aspects of hepatic function (Table 2.1) it is quite clear that there will never be *the* test of hepatic function. Some of the quantitative tests discussed in the following section have proven their value in certain clinical situations; whether they are superior to the scores reviewed in paragraph IV remains to be shown. In the opinion of these reviewers, the following can be stated about quantitative liver function tests:

1. No one test can express hepatic function.
2. Qualitative tests are not useful in differential diagnosis; they may be of use in separating patients into prognostic groups, however.
3. The main strength of quantitative tests will be their serial application where they can be used to assess the success of therapeutic interventions and where they could serve as surrogate end-points in clinical trials.
4. Quantitative tests are a useful tool in clinical investigation to further our understanding of derangement of hepatic function in chronic liver disease.

TESTS OF MICROSOMAL FUNCTION

Many model compounds have been proposed as measures of microsomal function; the best are tests based on the clearance of antipyrine, aminopyrine, caffeine and lidocaine. They are the only ones which will be considered here. The main drawback of all these tests is that the cytochrome P450 system which they probe (Table 2.1) is subject to a wide variety of environmental and hormonal influences. Thus, enzyme inducers affect the clearance of antipyrine or aminopyrine while smoking profoundly affects caffeine clearance. Since many drugs are used in patients with chronic liver disease, serial observations may be hampered by such influences. Their main popularity relies on their relative ease of performance.

Antipyrine clearance and aminopyrine breath test

Antipyrine (phenazone) and aminopyrine (amidopyrine, dimethylaminoantipyrine) are closely related pyrazolone derivatives formerly used as antipyretics. Antipyrine is the oldest model drug to probe the function of the cytochrome P450 system (Brodie & Axelrod 1950). It probes similar but not equal isoenzymes of cytochrome P450 as does aminopyrine. Nevertheless, their metabolism is sufficiently similar to review them together. In clinical practice they have about the same prognostic value.

Aminopyrine is a popular test compound since its metabolism is usually assessed by a breath test after administration of [14]C- or ^{13}C-dimethyl-aminopyrine; the labeled methyl groups are metabolically cleaved by cytochrome P450 and convened within the liver to labeled CO_2 which can be assessed in exhaled air by liquid scintillation counting or mass spectrometry. Unfortunately, investigators have used a wide variety of experimental protocols for drug administration (tracer only or tracer with mass; per-oral or intravenous) and to express their results (cumulative exhalation, single time points, decay constant in breath, V_{max} peak exhalation rate). Schoeller et al (1982) proposed the 30 min value as the best way to express data; this has been confirmed by others (Miotti et al 1988).

The aminopyrine breath test is affected by enzyme inducers and inhibitors: it is induced by ethanol, diphenylhydantoin, phenobarbital and rifampicin, inhibited by allopurinol, cimetidine, contraceptive steroids, omeprazole, pesticides and ethanol. There is probably a small decrease with age (Pirotte & El Allaf 1983, Schnegg & Lauterburg 1986).

The aminopyrine breath test was introduced into clinical medicine with the idea of a noninvasive screening test for severe liver disease (Hepner & Vessell 1975, Bircher et al 1976). In a variety of situations it has been proven superior to standard liver tests in predicting outcome, among others in alcoholic hepatitis (Schneider et al 1980), paracetamol poisoning (Saunders et al 1980), surgical interventions in patients with cirrhosis (Gill et al 1983) and chronic active hepatitis (Lashner et al 1988). It has been useful to predict severity of histological lesions in chronic active hepatitis (Monroe et al 1982), alcoholic liver disease (Saunders et al 1980, Pauwels et al 1982) and to differentiate between chronic hepatitis and cirrhosis (Hepner & Vessell 1975, Bircher et al 1976). These encouraging results have not been uniformly confirmed; thus, some investigators did not find the aminopyrine breath test to be superior to standard liver function tests (Galizzi et al 1978, Carlisle et al 1979, Morelli et al 1981) or to the Child–Pugh classification (Beuers et al 1991). In particular, it failed to predict histologic severity in primary biliary cirrhosis (Galizzi et al 1978, Baker et al 1987) or outcome in bypass surgery for morbid obesity (Baker et al 1983). Combination with other tests has been shown to improve sensitivity in some studies, e.g. with serum albumin (Henry et al 1985) or antithrombin III (Rodzynek et al 1986). These conflicting results are not surprising since, at least in animal models, it has now been quite clearly demonstrated that aminopyrine depends on hepatocellular mass which can be long maintained in the evolution of cirrhosis (Reichen et al 1987a,b).

The main use for quantitative liver function tests should be in prognostication. Villeneuve et al (1986) found the aminopyrine breath test to reliably predict prognosis in patients with cirrhosis but found that the Child score gave identical prognostic information; yet another study found the Child score to be superior to the aminopyrine breath test (Albers et al 1989). However, multivariate analysis of the parameters of the Child score and aminopyrine breath test found the presence of ascites and aminopyrine breath test to be the best predictors of survival (Adler et al 1990). In the most recent study, Merkel and colleagues followed a large, well characterized population for up to 4 years and found that etiology of cirrhosis, aminopyrine breath test and Child score predicted death from liver failure with 94% sensitivity and 88% specificity (Merkel et al 1992) (Fig. 2.5). In recent study, the ABT was inferior to ICG clearance in predicting outcome in surgical patients (Fan et al 1995, Lau et al 1997a,b). Portacaval shunting induces a marked decrease in microsomal function and the preoperative ABT value predicts 1-year survival (Horsmans et al 1993).

In patients with cholestatic disease the aminopyrine breath test was not different from normal individuals and was not useful in identifying the presence of cirrhosis in cholestatic patients (Baker et al 1987), probably because decreased microsomal enzyme function assessed by this test is a late feature of cholestatic liver disease. After general surgical procedures aminopyrine or antipyrine test results either are unchanged (Baker et al 1983), slightly increased (Loft et al 1985) or decreased (Pessayre et al 1978). The aminopyrine breath test is not affected by portacaval shunts (Pomier-Layrargues et al 1986).

The pharmacokinetic properties of *antipyrine* have recently been reviewed (St Peter & Awni 1991). It is a safe, time-proven model compound with excellent absorption after oral administration; antipyrine plasma clearance

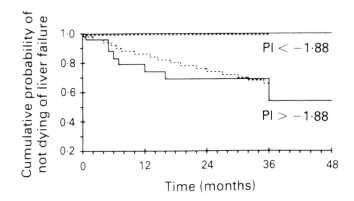

Fig. 2.5 Cumulative probability of not dying from liver failure according to a prognostic index taking into account Child–Pugh score, aminopyrine breath test and etiology of the disease. The solid lines are derived from the test set, the dotted lines from the training set. Reproduced with permission from Merkel et al (1992).

reflects microsomal P450 activity. It can easily be measured in saliva, even with a one time sample (Poulson & Loft 1988). Inhibition and induction are similar to those with aminopyrine and are reviewed by Poulson & Loft (1988) and Reichen (Reichen 1995).

Antipyrine parallels functional impairment as assessed by conventional parameters (Andreasen et al 1974, Branch et al 1976) and correlates partly with severity of histological disease (Farrell et al 1978, Sotaniemi et al 1986). In stable patients after liver transplantation oxidative drug metabolism is not different from normal individuals as assessed by the saliva antipyrine test (Mehta et al 1986). The same holds true for patients with extensive liver metastatic disease (Robertz-Vaupel et al 1992).

There are few data on the prognostic properties of antipyrine clearance determinations. It was found to be a predictor of outcome in obstructive jaundice (McPherson et al 1985) but others could not confirm this (Elfstrom & Lindgren 1974, St Peter & Awni 1991). Presumably it has the same prognostic power as the aminopyrine breath test; the latter has displaced antipyrine clearance determinations since it is perceived to be easier to perform. In patients with liver metastasis from primary colorectal cancer, even when the liver was largely replaced by neoplastic tissue, antipyrine clearance was normal (Grieco et al 1992).

We conclude that single determinations of aminopyrine N-demethylation are of prognostic value in some, but not all chronic liver diseases; combination with other aspects of liver function may improve its prognostic power. The value of serial determinations and/or the incorporation of aminopyrine in time-dependent Cox models may considerably improve its prognostic yield.

Caffeine clearance

Caffeine is a substrate for cytochrome P450 isoenzymes different from those responsible for aminopyrine/antipyrine metabolism (Axelrod & Reichenthal 1953, Wietholtz et al 1981). Determination of caffeine clearance (Desmond et al 1980) and of fasting caffeine plasma levels (Wahländer et al 1985) have been proposed as quantitative tests of liver function. Caffeine clearance is induced in smokers even in the presence of liver disease (Renner et al 1984, Joeres et al 1988) and declines with advanced age. Decreased elimination of caffeine is seen by some drugs like cimetidine (Broughton & Rogers 1981). The recent introduction of a simple assay which can be performed in any clinical chemistry laboratory (McDonagh et al 1991) should facilitate its use in clinical practice. Because caffeine is only 30% protein-bound and has a low hepatic extraction ratio, hepatic clearance is mostly independent of liver blood flow but dependent on

decrease of the caffeine metabolizing enzymes and the 'functioning hepatocyte mass' (Scott et al 1988).

However, there is marked overlap in caffeine clearance between patients with structural liver disease and normal volunteers; only decompensated liver cirrhosis was associated with decreased caffeine clearance (Scott et al 1988). Caffeine clearance seems not to be superior to antipyrine clearance in discriminatory power (Marchesini et al 1988, Shrestha et al 1997) and correlates well with the aminopyrine breath test (Jost et al 1987). Caffeine clearance was not useful in a small series of patients to detect complications after liver transplantation (Nagel et al 1990). There are as yet no other data on the prognostic significance, if any, of caffeine clearance.

At the present time, caffeine clearance determination cannot be recommended as a routine tool for follow-up. The innocuousness of the substance and its ease of assay make it an attractive candidate as a model drug; however, clearly more data are needed to evaluate its prognostic value.

Lidocaine

Lidocaine clearance gives similar diagnostic information to antipyrine or indocyanine green clearance, with respect to severity of liver disease (Forrest et al 1977, Colli et al 1988). It does not predict outcome of portacaval shunt surgery with respect to survival or the development of hepatic encephalopathy, the Pugh score being clearly superior in this (Dubois et al 1993, Pomier-Layrargues et al 1988). The clearance of lidocaine is flow-dependent and influenced by complex distribution phenomena; this difficulty has been overcome by a simple test proposed recently, namely measurement of the main metabolite, mono-ethylglycinexylide (MEGX) (Oellerich et al 1989). In this study, the MEGX test, performed on liver donors, was able to predict the outcome of liver transplantation; however, others disagree (Dette et al 1997, Balderson et al 1992, Zotz et al 1997, Fairchild et al 1996). Oellerich et al reported it to be a good short-term prognosticator in patients with cirrhosis awaiting liver transplantation (Oellerich et al 1991a, Oellerich et al 1991b). In children MEGX formation was able to predict severity of hepatic disease (Gremse et al 1990).

Time will tell whether this test will outperform the more established quantitative liver function tests (Maynard et al 1997, Kim et al 1997). Its attractiveness lies in its ease of assay; however it is not without side effects and its prognostic significance has not been universally accepted (Reichen 1995). Recently a low dose MEGX test was proposed which gives identical results but has fewer side effects (Reichel et al 1997). The pharmacokinetics basis of the test is much more complicated than that of, e.g. aminopyrine or antipyrine

(Reichen 1993) and, therefore, the proposed single point measurements are liable to introduce systematic errors. The data on selection of organ donors and prediction of survival in patients awaiting transplantation from Hannover, Germany, were encouraging but could not be confirmed by other groups yet.

TESTS OF METABOLIC CAPACITY

The liver has many other metabolic tasks in addition to drug metabolism. Different aspects have been used to assess hepatic function. Their advantage may lie in the fact that in contrast to cytochrome P450-dependent tests they are less susceptible to environmental influences.

Galactose elimination capacity

In the liver galactose is phosphorylated and then converted to glucose. The rate limiting step in galactose elimination capacity is the phosphorylation of galactose to galactose-1-phosphate by the enzyme galactokinase. The elimination capacity is determined after a saturating dose of galactose given i.v. or p.o. This test is different from low-dose galactose clearance, which has been proposed as a measure of hepatic blood flow (Henderson et al 1982, Schirmer et al 1986). Galactokinase is genetically heterogeneous and low activity can be due to such genetic differences rather than to the presence of liver disease. Moreover, there is considerable extrahepatic metabolism (Lindskov et al 1983). Determination of galactose elimination capacity is rather cumbersome requiring repeated blood sampling (Tygstrup 1963); however, a galactose breath test has been described and validated (Shreeve et al 1976, Grimm et al 1980).

Galactose elimination capacity is not useful as a screening test to detect minor functional impairment (Tygstrup 1963, Lindskov 1982a). It is of some prognostic value in patients with cirrhosis (Lindskov 1982b) and adds to the prognostic information contained in the Child classification (Hultcrantz et al 1986). In contrast to standard liver function tests, galactose elimination capacity C together with age C was able to predict development of portosystemic encephalopathy after shunt surgery (Kardel et al 1975). Galactose elimination capacity was maintained after distal splenorenal but not after central portacaval shunts (Henderson et al 1982). It was also used to monitor liver function in patients with portal hypertension either after sclerotherapy or distal splenorenal shunt; liver function improved in the sclerotherapy group but not in the shunt group (Warren et al 1986). In post-transplant patients galactose elimination capacity was found to be of no value in detecting complications (Nagel et al 1990).

We submit that the main value of galactose elimination capacity—perhaps as that of all quantitative tests—remains in serial determinations. Single point determinations test introduces in patients with more advanced liver disease considerable error (Fabbri et al 1997). In rats with biliary obstruction, galactose elimination capacity declines predictably with time; this decline predicts death with a high negative predictive value (Gross et al 1987). In fulminant hepatic failure, galactose elimination capacity, determined at diagnosis, was of some prognostic value but there was overlap between survivors and nonsurvivors (Ranek et al 1976); however, all patients with a decrease in galactose elimination capacity died, an outcome which could not be predicted by standard liver function tests (Ranek et al 1976). In primary biliary cirrhosis, an individual, but predictable decline could be observed (Fig. 2.6) which allowed prediction of death with high accuracy (Reichen et al 1991). In contrast, in alcoholic cirrhosis a predictable decline was only observed in patients who continued to drink (Marchesini et al 1990); in abstinent alcoholic and nonalcoholic cirrhosis the pattern of evolution was not predictable. In chronic active hepatitis, only a decrease in galactose elimination capacity predicted an unfavorable outcome while conventional liver tests had no prognostic value (Aebli & Reichen 1991).

Galactose elimination capacity is of no value in the detection of clinically inapparent liver disease; it contains some prognostic information, however, in particular in hepatic fulminant failure and assessing patients for portacaval shunt surgery. Its main strength is its independence of environmental factors and—at least in some diseases—its predictable decline with time. It remains to be determined by

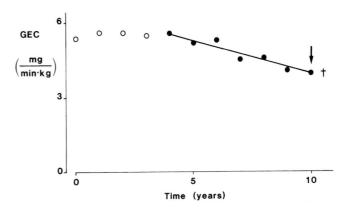

Fig. 2.6 Evolution of the galactose elimination capacity in a patient with primary biliary cirrhosis. After a period of stable liver function (o) galactose elimination capacity starts to decline (•). Death was predicted as the time at which the regression line reached a value of 4. Reproduced with permission from Reichen et al (1991).

prospective studies whether it is superior to scores or other quantitative liver function tests.

Other metabolic tests

Ozawa has proposed that *mitochondrial function* is a limiting factor affecting survival in cirrhotics undergoing hepatic resection. Indeed, this group was able to demonstrate that a simple glucose load correlated with hepatic energy charge and was of predictive value in partial hepatectomy (Ozawa et al 1976). Similarly the ketone body ratio (acetoacetate/ beta-hydroxybutyrate) was found to predict the postoperative course (Ukikusa et al 1981, Asano et al 1983). The same group has recently proposed a redox tolerance index calculated from glucose levels and ketone body ratio (Mori et al 1990). This test was also found to be an indicator of primary graft nonfunction after liver transplantation (Gubernatis et al 1989).

Hepatic enzymes incorporate NH_3 and the amino groups of amino acids into urea. The rate of urea production is proportional to protein intake in normal individuals. The maximal rate of *urea synthesis* (MRUS) is used by some investigators (Rudman et al 1973); in the natural course of cirrhosis it declines before hyperammonemia occurs and encephalopathy becomes manifest when it is reduced to < 70%. It was also suggested that in shunt surgery MRUS could identify patients at greater risk of developing encephalopathy (Rudman et al 1973). It was very sensitive in the detection of functional impairment in animal models (Fischer-Nielsen et al 1990). Urea synthesis remains inducible even in cirrhosis (Hamberg et al 1992); moreover, data on the prognostic capacity of this test in man have yet to be generated.

Protein synthesis has been measured by various means (Rotschild et al 1972, Pirwitz 1979, Ballmer et al 1990). In particular, a recently described method of measuring albumin synthesis with stable isotopes (Ballmer et al 1990) may be well suited to allow assessment of this important aspect of hepatic function. Whether this will provide any advantage over the more established function tests remains to be determined.

Nuclear magnetic resonance spectroscopy is a promising new technique permitting direct insight into biochemical processes; it permits easy estimation of energy-rich phosphates and permits observations of differences in phosphorus spectra (Oberhaensli et al 1986, Angus et al 1990). The diagnostic accuracy has not yet been scrutinized. Dynamic NMR spectroscopy appears more promising, after for example, a fructose load which induces ATP depletion and allows metabolism of energy-rich phosphates and phosphate monoesters to be followed noninvasively (Oberhaensli et al 1990); indeed, several aspects of fructose metabolism assayed by dynamic magnetic resonance spectroscopy after a fructose load correlated well with galactose elimination capacity and Child classification (Dufour et al 1992). This procedure requires expensive equipment, however, and whether it will offer any advantage over more simple tests appears dubious.

CLEARANCE OF ORGANIC ANIONIC DYES

The assessment of the clearance of these compounds, in particular of sulfobromophthalein (BSP) and indocyanine green (ICG) has initially been introduced as a measure of hepatic perfusion. This aspect will not be covered in this chapter. Suffice to say that in end-stage cirrhosis the extraction of these compounds gets too low to reliably calculate perfusion by the Fick principle. For this reason, they should be replaced by carbohydrates such as low-dose galactose (Henderson et al 1982) or sorbitol (Zeeh et al 1988) the extraction of which is better maintained even in end-stage cirrhosis.

Sulfobromophthalein (BSP)

BSP was the first compound used to estimate hepatic clearance (Rosenthal & White 1924) and Bradley et al (1945) introduced it as a measure of hepatic blood flow. Because of severe anaphylactic reactions it is rarely used now. Sulfobromophthalein is a dye which is taken up by the liver cells, conjugated with glutathione and excreted into bile (Reichen 1995). It discriminates between cirrhotic and noncirrhotic liver disease (Wardle et al 1980, Cozzolino et al 1983). It has been found to be a good predictor of resectability of hepatocellular carcinoma (Lee et al 1985) and has been found to be helpful in predicting the outcome of portosystemic shunt surgery by some (Douglass & Snell 1950, Blakemore 1952, Barker & Reemtsma 1960, Satterfield et al 1965, Hsu 1972) but not all (Ellis et al 1956, Hallenbeck et al 1959, Sedgwick & Hume 1959) investigators. It has been proposed that adequate kinetic analysis could estimate partial hepatic functions, in particular uptake, excretion and conjugation (Molino et al 1978). BSP was the best test to differentiate congenital biliary atresia from neonatal hepatitis in children (Matsusue et al 1984). It appears doubtful that this test has a great future with the exception perhaps of assessing the efficacy of novel anticholestatic drugs (Poupon et al 1987, Cotting et al 1990).

Indocyanine green (ICG)

The dye indocyanine green is removed by the liver by a carrier-mediated mechanism and excreted unchanged into bile. Its main advantage over sulfobromophthalein lies in the fact that it is not metabolized and disappears much more rapidly from blood. Because of this high degree of hepatic clearance ICG clearance is used to estimate hepatic function; the use of ICG as a means to estimate hepatic blood flow will not be considered here. Anaphylactoid reactions have rarely been observed (Speich et al 1988) but are related to dose and speed of injection rather than to a true immunological mechanism. Therefore, the substance can still be considered to be reasonably safe.

Some measure of ICG clearance, be it elimination rate constant, half-life, 15 min retention or 'intrinsic clearance' has been found to add prognostic information to the Child score in some (Barbare et al 1985, Merkel et al 1991, Oellerich et al 1991a, Oellerich et al 1991b) but not all (Albers et al 1989, Merkel et al 1989) studies. It was able to discern between cirrhotic and noncirrhotic stages in patients with primary biliary cirrhosis (Vaubourdolle et al 1991). Indocyanine green clearance was the only test which was useful to predict hospital mortality (Fan et al 1995, Lau et al 1997a,b) and survival in cirrhotic patients with hepatic resection (Hemming et al 1992, Yasui et al 1995). In cirrhotic patients an ICG retention of 14% at 15 min was the cut-off level separating survivors from nonsurvivors (Fan et al 1995). ICG-R_{max} was related to the volume of the liver remnant after hepatectomy and thereby reliably predicting outcome (Noguchi et al 1990). ICG-R_{max} of the remnant liver of > 0.8 µg/kg/min/cm³ predicted fair morphological regeneration but no functional recovery while an ICG-R_{max} < 0.5 µg/kg/min/cm³ predicted functional deterioration of the remnant liver. Accuracy for prediction of long-term prognosis was 100% in both retrospectively and prospectively evaluated cases (Noguchi et al 1990). It was suggested that small hepatocellular carcinoma in cirrhotic patients with normal bilirubin and with an ICG_{15} of 10 to 15% could safely be resected. In patients with ICG_{15} of 10 to 15% resection should be limited to left lobectomy or right monosegmentectomy, with ICG_{15} of 20 to 29% to subsegmentectomy (segment of Couinaud), with ICG_{15} of 30 to 39% to a limited resection, and with ICG_{15} of > 40% to enucleation. Using this decision scheme the authors achieved excellent mortality and survival rates even in cirrhotic patients (Makuuchi et al 1993, Kawasaki et al 1995). However, in contrast standard right hepatectomy in cirrhotic patients with ICG_{15} < 20% could be performed without increased mortality to resection in noncirrhotic patients (Suehiro et al 1994) or hepatic resection with ICG_{15} of 22.3% was performed with no mortality (Miyagawa et al 1994). ICG was not able to predict outcome with respect to survival or encephalopathy in portosystemic shunt surgery (Pomier Layrargues et al 1988).

Complications after hepatic resection could be predicted by the evolution of ICG clearance on the third operative day (Matsumata et al 1987, Kanematsu et al 1989). Rejection after liver transplantation also correlated with ICG clearance (Clements et al 1988). Prolonged halothane anesthesia compared to isoflurane depressed liver function as assessed by ICG clearance (Murray et al 1992). After portal vein embolization ICG was used to estimate hepatic lobar function (Uesaka et al 1996).

ICG is still a useful compound for the estimation of hepatic blood flow in patients with compensated liver disease (i.e. a maintained extraction). Most studies do not indicate that it significantly adds prognostic information.

Technetium-99m-galactosyl human serum albumin (^{99m}Tc-GSA)

Technetium-99m-diethylenetriaminpentaacetic acid-galactosyl human serum albumin (Tc-GSA) is a new liver scintigraphy agent (Pimstone et al 1994, Kwon et al 1997, Kwon et al 1995). Tc-GSA binds to the receptors for asialoglycoproteins (ASPG) in the sinusoidal membrane of hepatocytes. The ASGP receptors decrease in patients with chronic liver disease (Sawamura et al 1984). The maximal removal rate of Tc-GSA (GSA-R_{max}) is calculated and is low in such patients (Kwon et al 1997). Preliminary data indicate that extended hepatectomies in patients with low GSA-R_{max} are at high-risk. Further data will show whether Tc-GSA may be a reliable method for estimating the functioning hepatocyte mass or useful for predicting postoperative complications.

PROGNOSTIC SCORES

A bewildering number of general and disease-specific scores has been proposed to classify patients with chronic liver disease according to their surgical risk (Table 2.4). One of the first scores was introduced by Wantz and Payne as early as 1947 to assess the risk of portosystemic shunt surgery (Wantz & Payne 1961); the most popular of these scores is the one proposed by Child and Turcotte (Child & Turcotte 1964) which was later modified in different ways.

The advantage of these scores is that they are usually based on easily obtained clinical signs and routine laboratory values. The combination of different aspects of the disease (e.g. in the Child score excretory function, synthetic function, portal hypertension) should really assess global function better than any single dynamic test probing only a partial aspect of hepatic function and its derangement in disease.

Scores are usually derived by multiple logistic regression analysis on a large patient population; the best method is the risk analysis according to Cox (1972); recently, time-dependent Cox models have been introduced which will further refine the prognostic information by taking into account the individual evolution of patients (Christensen et al 1986). Such models are valid for the population from which they were derived. To be generally applicable, they should be validated on an independent population. Initially, investigators often use the split sample technique to validate their statistical analysis; this does not completely fulfill the criterion for general applicability. Table 2.4 indicates which scores have been validated on independent samples.

GENERAL SCORES

The Child score and its variants

The Child–Turcotte score (Child & Turcotte 1964) or its modification by Pugh et al (1973) were devised to assess hepatocellular function in patients considered for portocaval shunts. We give preference to the Pugh modification since it replaces the original 'nutritional state' criterion in the Child classification by the more objective prothrombin time; the Pugh modification is shown in Table 2.5. This score has proven its prognostic significance in many prospective (Foster et al 1971, Campbell et al 1973, Turcotte & Lambert 1973, Cameron et al 1979, Dowling 1979, Smith et al 1980, Cello et al 1981, Beuers et al 1991) and randomized trials (Resnick et al 1969, Conn 1981, Langer et al 1985, Harley et al 1986, Teres et al 1987, Grace et al 1988, Henderson et al 1990) on the value of portosystemic shunt surgery but also in conservatively treated cirrhotic patients (Christensen et al 1984, Villeneuve et al 1986, Infante-Rivard et al 1987). However, it was shown that it was not useful for deciding who should have a portosystemic shunt or conservative treatment (Resnick et al 1974).

The classification into Child's A, B and C patients is not uniformly applied; Conn has discussed in depth the different ways to allocate patients to the different grades (Conn 1981). When the parameters of the Child classification are subjected to logistic regression analysis, not all parameters are necessarily selected and other combinations may give

Table 2.4 Different general and disease-specific scores used to quantitate hepatic function and to assess prognosis in patients with chronic liver disease

GENERAL SCORES	
Score	Parameters used
Child–Turcotte*	Bilirubin, albumin, ascites, encephalopathy, nutrition
Child–Pugh*	Bilirubin, albumin, ascites, encephalopathy, prothrombin time
Paul Brousse	Bilirubin, albumin, ascites, encephalopathy, prothrombin time and factor II
Schlichting	Sex, age, prothrombin time, acetylcholinesterase, several bioptic features
Maddrey*	Bilirubin, prothrombin time
Tanaka	Heavy alcohol consumption, age

DISEASE-SPECIFIC SCORES		
Authors	Disease	Parameters used
Orrego et al 1983	Alcoholic	Encephalopathy, collateral circulation, edema, ascites, spider nevi, weakness, anorexia, prothrombin time, hematocrit, albumin, bilirubin, alkaline phosphatase
Maddrey et al 1978*	Alcoholic	Weighted bilirubin and prothrombin time
Gluud et al 1988	Alcoholic	Child plus wedged hepatic vein pressure and size of esophageal varices
Dickson et al 1989*	PBC	Age, edema, bilirubin, albumin, prothrombin time
Christensen et al 1984	PBC	Age, albumin, bilirubin, presence of cirrhosis and central cholestasis on biopsy
Helzberg et al 1987	PSC	Hepatomegaly, serum bilirubin
Wiesner et al 1989	PSC	Age, bilirubin, hemoglobin, associated inflammatory bowel disease, histologic stage
Farrant et al 1991	PSC	Hepatomegaly, splenomegaly, serum alkaline phosphatase, histologic stage, age
Okuda et al 1985	HCC	Tumour size, ascites, bilirubin, albumin
Calvet et al 1990	HCC	Age, ascites, BUN, serum sodium, GGT, bilirubin, tumor size, toxic syndrome, metastases

* Indicates scores which have been validated in independent samples.

Table 2.5 Pugh's modification of the Child score to assess severity of cirrhosis

	Points		
Parameter	1	2	3
Albumin (g/dl)	> 3.5	2.8–3.5	< 3.5
Bilirubin (µmol/1)	< 25	25–40	> 40
Bilirubin (mg/dl)	< 2	2–3	> 3*
Prothrombin time (s above normal)	< 4	4–6	> 6
Prothrombin levels, %	> 64	40–65	< 40*
Ascites	None	Mild Controlled	Moderate Refractory*
Encephalopathy (grade)	0 None	I–II Minimal	III–IV Advanced*

In the original Child–Turcotte classification, nutrition (good=1; moderate=2, poor=3) had been used instead of the prothrombin time.
Most authors place patients with 5–7 points in grade A, 8–10 points in grade B and 11–15 points in grade C. Numeric expression of the results is preferable to avoid the controversies in reporting the Child score.
* Alternatively used. For further details see text.

better prognostic information (Schlichting et al 1983a, Christensen et al 1986, Gines et al 1987). Probably the best way to express the Child classification is not to allocate patients to classes but to use the numerical score as computed from the five parameters given in Table 2.5 (Ohmann et al 1990). A further refinement has been achieved by using the parameters derived from a logistic regression model (Infante-Rivard et al 1987); in this way, a sensitivity and specificity of 80% respectively could be obtained (Fig. 2.7). It remains to be demonstrated on an unrelated sample whether these computations add significantly to the numeric score.

Mortality and survival rates after hepatectomy was shown to be higher in patients in Child class B/C compared to A (Franco et al 1990, Nonami et al 1997), however, even in Child class B mortality is not necessarily due to an increased incidence of hepatic failure (Chou et al 1994). Since survival is not affected in Child class A, cirrhosis per se does not affect mortality (Vauthey et al 1995). Age is not taken into account in Child classification; this may be of relevance since elderly patients were shown to be at higher risk than younger patients in the same Child classification (Yanaga et al 1988).

The Child score, albeit well accepted, is less than perfect (Zimmerer et al 1996). Not all investigators found it useful in predicting outcome for portosystemic shunt surgery (Resnick et al 1974). Conn has analyzed nine randomized trials on shunt surgery encompassing 976 patients (Conn 1981); the mortality in the different trials for classes A, B and C ranged from 0 to 8%, 4 to 30% and 10 to 70%, respectively (Fig. 2.8).

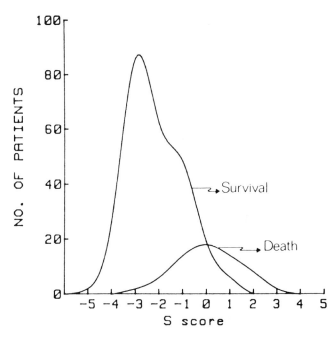

Fig. 2.7 Distribution of patients with liver cirrhosis surviving or succumbing to their disease as a function of a weighted Child–Pugh score. Reproduced with permission from Infante-Rivard et al (1987).

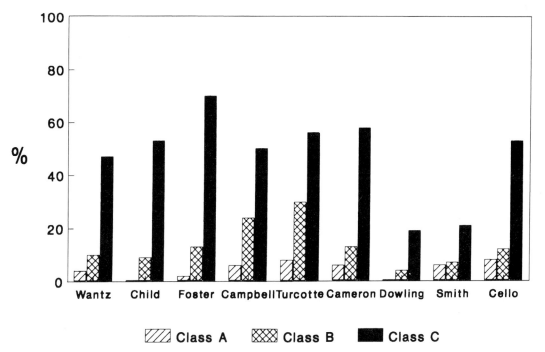

Fig. 2.8 Mortality (%) in 976 patients from nine trials on portosystemic shunt surgery according to Child classification. Redrawn with permission from the review by Conn (1981).

There are also some features which are quite subjective; thus, nutrition as in the original Child score is not clearly defined. The presence of ascites or encephalopathy is also difficult to grade and may depend on the clinical situation. Thus, in a patient with one episode of severe encephalopathy after a variceal bleed the presence of encephalopathy carries less ominous significance than the presence of mild encephalopathy in a stable patient on a protein-restricted diet (Conn 1981).

Other general scores

The Paul Brousse classification system for cirrhotic patients, a modification of the Child score, has been introduced in France and applied to patients undergoing portacaval shunts (Adam et al 1992). It gives one point each if the following conditions are met: presence of clinical ascites, encephalopathy (disorientation to time and space and/or asterixis), bilirubin > 30 μmol/L, albumin < 3 g/100 ml, prothrombin time (factor II) and factor V < 60%, and two points if prothrombin time (factor II) and factor V are < 40%. Patients with 0 points are considered grade A, those with 1 or 2 points B and those with over 2 points grade C. Whether this is superior to the Child–Pugh score has not been determined.

In a multivariate analysis of 51 variables in 488 patients, eight variables were found to be significantly associated with 5-year survival: sex, age, prothrombin time, acetylcholinesterase, eosinophils in the liver biopsy, liver cell necrosis, inflammation in connective tissue and efferent veins in parenchymal nodules (Schlichting et al 1983a); an even more elaborate score was later developed from a subset of the original patients and tested on an independent sample (Christensen et al 1986). This score appears less attractive since it relies heavily on data obtained at liver biopsy which cannot be obtained in all patients and certainly not for updating the score after, for example, a therapeutic intervention.

Tanaka found age at onset and a history of heavy alcohol consumption to be the best predictors of outcome (Tanaka et al 1987). A more complicated analysis by D'Amico et al (1986) of 1155 consecutive patients found different indicators to predict 6-year survival for compensated and decompensated disease; also, some disease specific markers entered into the final prognostic score. Christensen et al (1989) found that coma (when bleeding), ascites, prothrombin time and serum creatinine predicted survival in patients with the first variceal bleed; Gines et al (1987) used serum bilirubin, prothrombin time, sex, age, serum alkaline phosphatase and hepatic stigmata to predict survival. All these scores share some similarities with the Child classification and none has undergone validation on an independent sample.

DISEASE SPECIFIC SCORES

Alcoholic liver disease

The Maddrey score (Maddrey et al 1978) was initially designed to assess survival in patients with alcoholic hepatitis but has also been used in other groups (Theodossi et al 1982, Sauerbruch et al 1988). A more elaborate score, the CCLI (combined clinical and laboratory index; see Table 2.4) has been proposed by Orrego et al (1983).

Neither has undergone testing in independent populations; the Maddrey score has been used in randomized controlled trials where the control group confirmed the prognosis initially predicted (Ramond et al 1992). Gluud et al (1988) found that the addition of the size of esophageal varices and of wedged hepatic vein pressure improved upon the Child score in patients with alcoholic liver disease.

Primary biliary cirrhosis

Although rare, primary biliary cirrhosis is a prime indication for liver transplantation; therefore, it is not surprising that different prognostic indicators for this disease have been developed. The value of serum bilirubin (Shapiro et al 1979) and galactose elimination capacity (Reichen et al 1991) have been considered in earlier paragraphs. The value of serial quantitative liver function tests especially in early disease stage has been questioned (Schonfeld et al 1997). Christensen et al (1985) developed a prognostic indicator based on bilirubin, age, albumin and presence of cirrhosis and central cholestasis on biopsy. The best model is that proposed by Dickson et al (1989). It considers age, albumin, bilirubin, prothrombin time and presence of edema (Table 2.4). Its main advantage over the Christensen model is that it does not require a liver biopsy. It has been validated in different independent samples from different continents (Grambsch et al 1989, Bonsel et al 1990, Reichen et al 1991, Klion et al 1992) and can also be used serially to assess the evolution of disease (Klion et al 1992).

Primary sclerosing cholangitis

Three different models (Helzberg et al 1987, Wiesner et al 1989, Farrant et al 1991) have been proposed (Table 2.4); the Mayo score has been validated and refined (Dickson et al 1992). The models by Farrant et al and Wiesner et al require liver biopsy information, while that from Yale (Helzberg et al 1987) relies only on the presence of hepatomegaly and serum bilirubin.

Hepatocellular carcinoma

Most authors use the Child classification to assess surgical risk prior to hepatic resection or other treatment modalities. Indeed, in a variety of scores one or the other of the Child criteria were selected by multiple regression analysis.

The best characterized score is that introduced by Okuda et al (1985) which takes into account three parameters of the Cox model (serum bilirubin, albumin and presence of ascites) and tumor size (Table 2.4). Although widely used, the Okuda score has never been subjected to independent validation. A quite complicated score has recently been proposed by Calvet et al (1990) which may be more representative for this tumor in Western populations. The Calvet score includes age, ascites, BUN, serum sodium, GGT, bilirubin, tumor size, toxic syndrome and metastases. However, validation is also required in independent samples for this score. Yamanaka et al (1994) proposed a refined score. Abnormal ICG retention and oral glucose tolerance test were selected as variables to separate survivors from nonsurvivors. To predict liver failure after hepatectomy in patients with carcinoma of the biliary tract another system was suggested: postoperative hepatocellular failure was predicted with 83% specificity and 96% sensitivity by resection rate, oral glucose tolerance test, cholangitis, pancreatoduodenectomy and ICG (Nagino et al 1993).

SPECIAL CONSIDERATIONS OF LIVER FUNCTION AFTER PARTIAL HEPATECTOMY

Estimation of remaining functional parenchyma

The following formula (Bismuth et al 1986) was suggested to estimate the amount of functional parenchyma remaining after resection (M_r):

$$M_r = M_e / M_t \times PBC$$

where M_e is the quantity of functional liver removed, M_t the total quantity of functional liver and PBC the Paul Brousse Hospital classification as mentioned above. However, postoperative mortality or complications are not dependent on the amount or resected parenchyma alone. In the study by Bismuth et al (1986) mortality was 5% even after minimal resection. To avoid postoperative liver failure others have suggested that more than 30% of functional liver volume should be left (Soyer et al 1992) and no mortality was observed when the estimated liver volume was greater than 35%.

Cohnert et al proposed the liver resection index (LRI) based on ABT, parenchymal hepatic resection rate (PHRR) and tumor volume/liver volume to predicte fatal postoperative complications (Cohnert et al 1997). This index has to be evaluated by other groups.

Evolution of liver tests after hepatectomy

Postoperative biochemical changes are difficult to interpret due to factors like patients with no or underlying liver disease, blood transfusion and postoperative complications (Didolkar et al 1989, Sitzmann & Greene 1994, Zoli et al 1986). In uncomplicated resection (no underlying liver disease, no blood or plasma transfusion and temporary pedicle inflow occlusion) postoperative changes of the most commonly used conventional liver tests have been studied (Vauthey et al 1995, Bolder et al 1993). Alkaline phophatase and GGT may be elevated for up to 3 months after surgery (Vauthey et al 1995). Postoperative changes of bile acids, transaminases, bilirubin and prothrombin time appear to depend on the amount of resected parenchyma and not only on complicating factors as mentioned above.

CONCLUSIONS

For the surgeon, it is of paramount importance to reliably detect the presence of liver disease not only in liver-related (Lee et al 1985, Bismuth et al 1986, Neuberger et al 1986) but also in general surgery (Gayer & Sohmer 1955, Lindenmuth & Eisenberg 1963, Garrison et al 1984, Tinkoff et al 1990) so as to avoid unnecessary complications when operating on patients with liver cirrhosis. In the last decade perioperative and postoperative morbidity and mortality decreased steadily to low levels in most series (Adam et al 1997, Chan et al 1998, Ohlsson et al 1998, Brancatisano et al 1998). Because surgeons still rely more or less on the same liver function tests as used for the last 20–30 years one has to conclude that probably surgical skills, better perioperative care and better selection of patients are more important factors which led to the impressive results than determination of liver function (Shimada et al 1998, Taylor et al 1997, Yamaoka et al 1992, Kin et al 1998). To this effect, the use of standard liver function tests such as transaminases, alkaline phosphatase, bilirubin, clotting factors and albumin are usually adequate, although far from perfect. Their sometimes unsatisfactory sensitivity can be improved by incorporating serum bile acid levels into the screening protocol.

When the presence of liver disease e.g. liver cirrhosis and biliary obstruction has been detected, a diagnosis should be obtained by judicious use of diagnostic tests, imaging techniques and liver biopsy. However, none of these procedures will reliably assess the severity of disease. This can be adequately assessed in daily clinical practice by the use of general or disease-specific scores. Quantitative tests convey similar, and sometimes more accurate, prognostic information than scores. They certainly have improved our understanding of factors leading to hepatocellular dysfunction and will therefore be used by academic surgeons, in particular in evaluating the effect of therapeutic interventions. Prospective studies on large numbers of patients using dynamic tests and/or scores are needed to achieve the goal of predicting postoperative liver function objectively. For the time being, their use in daily practice is not required.

ACKNOWLEDGMENTS

The authors were supported by grants from the Swiss National Foundation for Scientific Research (No. 32-50886.97 to HZ and 32-30168.90 to JR). The authors wish to thank Ms M. Kappeler for the artwork.

REFERENCES

Abraham S C, Furth E E 1995 Receiver operating characteristic analysis of serum chemical parameters as tests of liver transplant rejection and correlation with histology. Transplantation 59: 740–6

Adam R, Diamond T, Bismuth H 1992 Partial portocaval shunt: Renaissance of an old concept. Surgery 111: 610–6

Adam R, Bismuth H, Castaing D, Waechter F, Navarro F, Abascal A, Majno P, Engerran L 1997 Repeat hepatectomy for colorectal liver metastases. Annals of Surgery 225: 51–62

Adler M, VanLaethem J, Gilbert A, Gelin M, Bourgeois N, Vereerstraeten P C 1990 Factors influencing survival at one year in patients with nonbiliary hepatic parenchymal cirrhosis. Digestive Diseases and Sciences 35: 1–5

Adson M, van Heerden J, Ilstrup D 1984 The distal splenorenal shunt. Archives of Surgery 119: 609–14

Aebli N, Reichen J 1991 (The prognostic value of the serial determination of galactose elimination capacity in chronic active hepatitis). Schweizerische Medizinische Wochenschrift 121: 970–6

Albers I, Hartmann H, Bircher J, Creutzfeldt W 1989 Superiority of the Child–Pugh classification to quantitative liver function tests for assessing prognosis of liver cirrhosis. Scandinavian Journal of Gastroenterology 24: 269–76

Andersson L O 1976 Transport proteins. I. Serum albumin. In: Blomback B, Hanson L A, (eds) Plasma proteins. John Wiley, Chichester, p 43–72

Andreasen P, Ranek L, Statland B, Tygstrup N 1974 Clearance of antipyrine. Dependence of quantitative liver function. European Journal of Clinical Investigation 4: 129–34

Angelin B, Bjoerkhem I, Einarsson K, Ewerth S 1982 Hepatic uptake of bile acids in man. Fasting and postprandial concentrations of individual bile acids in portal venous and systemic blood serum. Journal of Clinical Investigation 70: 724–31

Angus P W, Dixon R M, Rajagopalan B, Ryley N G, Simpson K J, Peters T J, Jewell D P, Radda G K 1990 A study of patients with alcoholic liver disease by 31P nuclear magnetic resonance spectroscopy. Clinical Science 78: 33–8

Aronson K F, Hanson A, Nosslin B 1965 The value of Gamma-glutamyl transpeptidase in differentiating viral hepatitis from obstructive jaundice. A statistical comparison with alkaline phosphatase. Acta Chirurgica Scandinavica 130: 92–9

Asano M, Ozawa K, Tobe T 1983 Postoperative prognosis as related to blood ketone body ratios in hepatectomized patients. European Surgical Research 15: 302–11

Axelrod J, Reichenthal J 1953 The fate of caffeine in man and a method for its determination in biological material. Journal of Pharmacology 107: 519–23

Baker A L, Krager P S, Glagov S, Schoeller D 1983 Aminopyrine breath test. Prospective comparison with liver histology and liver chemistry tests following jejunoileal bypass performed for refractory obesity. Digestive Diseases and Sciences 28: 405–10

Baker A L, Krager P S, Kotake A N, Schoeller D A 1987 The aminopyrine breath test does not correlate with histologic disease severity in patients with cholestasis. Hepatology 7: 464–7

Baker L A, Smith C, Lieberman G 1959 The natural history of esophageal varices. American Journal of Medicine 26: 228–37

Balderson G A, Potter J M, Hickman P E, Chen Y, Lynch S V, Strong R W 1992 MEGX as a test of donor liver function. Transplantation Proceedings 24: 1960–1961

Ballmer P, McNurlan M, Milne E, Heys S, Buchan V, Calder A, Garlick P 1990 Measurement of albumin synthesis in humans: a new approach employing stable isotopes. American Journal of Physiology 259: E797–E803

Barbare J C, Poupon R E, Jaillon P, Prod'homme S, Darnis F 1985 Intrinsic hepatic clearance and Child–Turcotte classification for assessment of liver function in cirrhosis. Journal of Hepatology 1: 253–9

Barker H G, Reemtsma K 1960 The portacaval shunt operation in patients with cirrhosis and ascites. Surgery 48: 142–54

Barnes S, Gallo G A, Trash D B, Morris J S 1975 Diagnostic value of serum bile acid estimations in liver disease. Journal of Clinical Pathology 28: 506–9

Baron D N 1970 A critical look at the value of biochemical liver function tests with special reference to discriminant function analysis. Annals of Clinical Biochemistry 7: 100–12

Beuers U, Jager F, Wahllander A, Ansari H, Kirsch C M 1991 Prognostic value of the intravenous 14C-aminopyrine breath test compared to the Child–Pugh score and serum bile acids in 84 cirrhotic patients. Digestion 50: 212–8

Bijleveld C M, Vonk R J, Kuipers F, Havinga R, Boverhof R, Koopman B J, Wolthers B G, Fernandes J 1989 Benign recurrent intrahepatic cholestasis: altered bile acid metabolism. Gastroenterology 97: 427–32

Bircher J, Blankart R, Halpern A, Haecki W, Laissue J A, Preisig R 1973 Criteria for assessment of functional impairment in patients with cirrhosis of the liver. European Journal of Clinical Investigation 3: 72–85

Bircher J, Kuefer A, Gikalov I, Preisig R 1976 Aminopyrine demethylation measured by breath analysis in cirrhosis. Clinical and Pharmacological Therapy 20: 484–92

Bismuth H, Houssin D, Ornowski J, Meriggi F 1986 Liver resections in cirrhotic patients: a western experience. World Journal of Surgery 10: 311–7

Blakemore A H 1952 Portacaval shunting for portal hypertension. Surgery, Gynecology and Obstetrics 94: 443–8

Bloomer J R, Allen R M, Klatskin G 1976 Serum bile acids in primary biliary cirrhosis. Archives of Internal Medicine 136: 57–61

Bolder U, Tacke J, Imhoff M, Lohlein D 1993 Postoperative course of functional and cellular variables in liver resection. Scandinavian Journal of Gastroenterology 28: 949–57

Bonsel G, Klompmaker I, Vantveer F, Habbema J D, Sloof M J 1990 Use of prognostic models for assessment of value of liver transplantation in primary biliary cirrhosis. Lancet 335: 493–7

Bontempo F A, Lewis J H, Van Thiel D H, et al 1985 The relation of preoperative coagulation findings to diagnosis, blood usage, and survival in adult liver transplantation. Transplantation 39: 532–6

Böttiger L E, Dalen E, Hallen B 1976 Halothane-induced liver damage: An analysis of the material reported to the Swedish Adverse Drug Reaction Committee, 1966–1973 Acta Anaesthesiologica Scandinavica 20: 40–6

Bradley S, Ingelfinger F, Bradley G, Currey J 1945 The estimation of hepatic blood flow in man. Journal of Clinical Investigation 24: 890–7

Brancatisano R, Isla A, Habib N 1998 Is radical hepatic surgery safe? American Journal of Surgery 175: 161–163

Branch R, James J, Read A 1976 The clearance of antipyrine and indocyanine green in normal subjects and in patients with chronic liver disease. Clinical Pharmacology and Therapy 20: 81–9

Brensilver H L, Kaplan M M 1975 Significance of elevated liver alkaline phosphatase in serum. Gastroenterology 68: 1556–62

Brodie B, Axelrod J 1950 The fate of antipyrine in man. Journal of Pharmacology and Experimental Therapeutics 98: 97–104

Broughton L J, Rogers H J 1981 Decreased systemic clearance of caffeine due to cimetidine. British Journal of Clinical Pharmacology 12: 155–9

Bukofzer S, Kew M C, Rowe P 1988 The prevalence of variant alkaline phosphatase in hepatocellular carcinoma in southern African blacks. Cancer 62: 978–81

Burlina A, Plebani M, Dechecchi C, Zaninotto M, Farinati F, Naccarato R 1983 Occurrence of an atypical alkaline phosphatase fraction ('biliary') in primary liver cancer. Clinical Biochemistry 16: 346–9

Calvet X, Bruix J, Gines P, Bru C, Sole M, Vilana R, Rodes J 1990 Prognostic factors of hepatocellular carcinoma in the West: a multivariate analysis in 206 patients. Hepatology 12: 753–60

Cameron J L, Zuideman G D, Smith G W, et al 1979 Mesocaval shunts for the control of bleeding esophageal varices. Surgery 85: 257–62

Campbell D P, Parker D E, Anagnostopoulos C E 1973 Survival prediction in portacaval shunts: a computerized statistical analysis. American Journal of Surgery 126: 748–51

Carlisle R, Galambos J, Warren D 1979 The relationship between conventional liver tests, quantitative function tests, and histopathology in cirrhosis. Digestive Diseases and Sciences 24: 358–62

Caroli J, Paraf A, Champeau J, et al 1950 Les icterese de la gastrectomie. Arch.Mal.App.Dig. 39: 1057–85

Cayer D, Sohmer MF 1955 Surgery in patients with cirrhosis. Archives of Surgery 71: 828–838

Cello J P, Deveney K E, Trunkey D D, et al 1981 Factors influencing survival after therapeutic shunts. American Journal of Surgery 141: 257–65

Chan A C, Blumgart L H, Wuest D L, Melendez J A, Fong Y 1998 Use of preoperative autologous blood donation in liver resections for colorectal metastases. American Journal of Surgery 175: 461–465

Child C G, Turcotte J G 1964 Surgery and portal hypertension. In: Child CG (ed) The liver and portal hypertension. W.B. Saunders, Philadelphia, p 50–1

Chou F F, Sheen Chen S M, Chen C L, Chen Y S, Chen M J 1994 Prognostic factors after hepatectomy for hepatocellular carcinoma. Hepatogastroenterology. 41: 419–23

Christensen E, Schlichting P, Fauerholdt L, Gluud C, Andersen P, Juhl E, Poulsen H, Tygstrup N 1984 Copenhagen study group for liver diseases: Prognostic value of Child-Turcotte criteria in medically treated cirrhosis. Hepatology 4: 430–5

Christensen E, Neuberger J, Crowe J, Altman D, Popper H, Portman B, Doniach D, Ranek L, Tiegstrup N, Williams R 1985a Beneficial effect of azathioprine and prediction of prognosis in primary biliary cirrhosis. Gastroenterology 89: 1084–91

Christensen E, Schlichting P, Fauerholdt L, Juhl E, Poulsen H, Tygstrup N, The Copenhagen Study Group for Liver Diseases 1985b Changes of laboratory variables with time in cirrhosis: prognostic and therapeutic significance. Hepatology 5: 843–53

Christensen E, Schlichting P, Amdersen P, Fauerholdt L, Schou G, Pedersen B, Juhl E, Poulsen H, Tygstrup N 1986 Updating prognosis and therapeutic effect evaluation in cirrhosis with cox's multiple regression model for time-dependent variables. Scandinavian Journal of Gastroenterology 21: 163–74

Christensen M, Jacobsen P M 1987 Efficiency of composite tests in gastrointestinal cancer Preoperative prediction of liver metastases by scintigraphy, alkaline phosphatase, and carcinoembryonic antigen. Scandinavian Journal of Gastroenterology 22: 273–8

Christensen E, Krintel J, Hansen S, Johansen J, Juhl E 1989 Prognosis after the first episode of gastrointestinal bleeding or coma in cirrhosis. Scandinavian Journal of Gastroenterology 24: 999–1006

Clark C P, Foreman M L, Peters G N, Cheek J H, Sparkman R S 1988 Efficacy of peroperative liver function tests and ultrasound in detecting hepatic metastasis in carcinoma of the breast. Surgery, Gynecology and Obstetrics 167: 510–4

Clements D, McMaster P, Elias E 1988 Indocyanine green clearance in acute rejection after liver transplantation. Transplantation 46: 383–5

Cohen J A, Kaplan M M 1979 The SGOT/SGPT ratio—an indicator of alcoholic liver disease. Digestive Diseases and Sciences 24: 835–8

Cohnert T U, Rau H G, Buttler E, Hernandez-Richter T, Sauter G, Reuter C, Schildberg F W 1997 Preoperative risk assessment of hepatic resection for malignant disease. World Journal of Surgery 21: 396–401

Colli A, Buccino G, Cocciolo M, Parravicini R, Scaltrini G 1988 Disposition of a flow-limited drug (lidocaine) and a metabolic capacity-limited drug (theophylline) in liver cirrhosis. Clinical Pharmacology and Therapy 44: 642–9

Collins D M, Van Tongeren A, Cook H B, Campbell C B 1979 Serum bile acids and routine liver function tests in patients with chronic liver disease and cholestasis. New Zealand Medical Journal 89: 432–434

Conn H O 1981 A peek at the Child–Turcotte classification. Hepatology 1: 673–6

Cotting J, Lentze M, Reichen J 1990 Effects of ursodeoxycholic acid therapy on nutrition and liver function in patients with cystic fibrosis and long-standing cholestasis. Gut 31: 918–21

Cox D 1972 Regression models and life-tables. Journal of the Royal Statistical Society (B) 34: 187–202

Cozzolino G, Lonardo A, Francica G, Amendola F, Cacciatore L 1983 Differential diagnosis between hepatic cirrhosis and chronic active hepatitis: specificity and sensitivity of physical and laboratory findings in a series from the Mediterranean area. American Journal of Gastroenterology 78: 442–5

Crofton P M, Elton R A, Smith A F 1979 High molecular weight alkaline phosphatase, a clinical study. Clinica Chimica Acta 98: 263–75

D'Amico G, Morabito A, Pagliaro L, Marubini E 1986 Survival and prognostic indicators in compensated and decompensated cirrhosis. Digestive Diseases and Sciences 31: 468–75

De Cock K M, Niland J C, Lu H P, Rahimian A, Edwards V, Shriver K, Govindarajan S, Redeker A G 1988 Experience with human immunodeficiency virus infection in patients with hepatitis B virus and hepatitis delta virus infections in Los Angeles, 1977–1985 American Journal of Epidemiology 127: 1250–60

Desmond P V, Patwardhan R V, Johnson R F, Schenker S 1980 Impaired elimination of caffeine in cirrhosis. Digestive Diseases and Sciences 25: 193–7

Dette K, Knoop M, Langrehr J M, Haller G, Steinmueller T, Guckelberger O, Horch D, Haeusler M, Neuhaus P 1997 Donor MEGX test fails to predict graft function after orthotopic liver transplant. Transplantation Proceedings 29: 376–377

Dickson E R, Grambsch P M, Fleming T R, Fisher L D, Langworthy A 1989 Prognosis in primary biliary cirrhosis: Model for decision making. Hepatology 10: 1–7

Dickson E R, Murtaugh P A, Wiesner R H, Grambsch P M, Fleming T R, Ludwig J, LaRusso N F, Malinchoc M, Chapman R W, Kaplan M M, et al 1992 Primary sclerosing cholangitis: Refinement and validation of survival models. Gastroenterology 103: 1893–901

Didolkar M S, Fitzpatrick J L, Elias E G, Whitley N, Keramati B, Suter C M, Brown S 1989 Risk factors before hepatectomy, hepatic function after hepatectomy and computed tomographic changes as indicators of mortality from hepatic failure. Surgery, Gynecology and Obstetrics 169: 17–26

Domar U, Danielsson A, Hirano K, Stigbrand T 1988 Alkaline phosphatase isozymes in non-malignant intestinal and hepatic diseases. Scandinavian Journal of Gastroenterology 23: 793–800

Douglas J G, Beckett G J, Nimmo I A, Finlayson N D C, Percy-Robb I W 1981 Clinical value of bile salt tests in anicteric liver disease. Gut 22: 141–8

Douglass B E, Snell A M 1950 Portal cirrhosis: An analysis of 444 cases with notes on modern methods of treatment. Gastroenterology 15: 407–25

Dowling J B 1979 Ten years experience with mesocaval grafts. Surgery, Gynecology and Obstetrics 149: 518–22

Dubois A, Dauzat M, Pignodel C, Pomier-Layrargues G, Marty-Double C, Lopez F M, Janbon C 1993 Portal hypertension in lymphoproliferative and myeloproliferative disorders: Hemodynamic and histological correlations. Hepatology 17: 246–50

Dufour J, Stoupis C, Lazeyras F, Vock P, Terrier F, Reichen J 1992 Alterations in hepatic fructose metabolism in cirrhotic patients demonstrated by dynamic ^{31}phosphorus spectroscopy. Hepatology 15: 835–42

Ekberg H, Tranberg K G, Andersson R, Jeppsson B, Bengmark S 1986 Major liver resection: perioperative course and management. Surgery 100: 1–8

Ekberg O, Aspelin P 1986 Ultrasonography in asymptomatic patients with abnormal biochemical liver tests. Scandinavian Journal of Gastroenterology 21: 573–6

Elfstrom J, Lindgren S 1974 Disappearance of phenazone from plasma in patients with obstructive jaundice. European Journal of Clinical Pharmacology 7: 467–71

Elias D, Lasser P, Rougier P, Ducreux M, Bognel C, Roche A 1995 Frequency, technical aspects, results, and indications of major hepatectomy after prolonged intra-arterial hepatic chemotherapy for initially unresectable hepatic tumors. Journal of the American College of Surgeons 180: 213–9

Ellis D S, Linton R R, Jones C M 1956 Effect of venous shunt surgery on liver function in patients with portal hypertension; follow-up study of 125 patients operated on in last 10 years. New England Journal of Medicine 254: 931–6

Epstein E, Kiechle F L, Zak B 1984 Use of alkaline phosphatase isoenzyme analysis in the evaluation of cholestatic liver disease. Annals of Clinical and Laboratory Science 14: 292–7

Eriksen J, Staun Olsen P, Thomsen C 1984 Gamma-glutamyltrans-peptidase aspartate aminotransferase and erythrocyte mean corpuscular volume as indicators of alcohol consumption in liver disease. Scandinavian Journal of Gastroenterology 19: 813–9

Evans J, Ogston S, Guthrie A, Johnston B, McKechnie L 1984 The relationship between liver function tests and alcohol intake in patients admitted to an alcoholism unit. Annals of Clinical Biochemistry 21: 261–7

Ewe K 1981 Bleeding after liver biopsy does not correlate with indices of peripheral coagulation. Digestive Diseases and Sciences 26: 388–93

Fabbri A, Bianchi G, Brizi M, Zoli M, Marchesini G 1997 Uncertainty in liver function assessment on the basis of single-point galactose concentration. Digestion 58: 379–383

Fairchild R, Solomon H, Contis J, Kaminski D 1996 Prognostic value of the monoethylglycinexylidide liver function test in assessing donor liver suitability. Archives of Surgery 131: 1099–1002

Fan S T, Lai E C, Lo C M, Ng I O, Wong J 1995 Hospital mortality of major hepatectomy for hepatocellular carcinoma associated with cirrhosis. Archives of Surgery 130: 198–203

Farrant J, Hayllar K, Wilkinson M, Karani J, Portmann B, Westaby D, Williams R 1991 Natural history and prognostic variables in primary sclerosing cholangitis. Gastroenterology 100: 1710–7

Farrell G C, Cooksley W G E, Hart P, Powell W L 1978 Drug metabolism in liver disease. Identification of patients with impaired hepatic drug metabolism. Gastroenterology 75: 580–8

Ferraris R, Colombatti G, Fiorentini M T, Carosso R, Arossa W, De La P M 1983 Diagnostic value of serum bile acids and routine liver function tests in hepatobiliary diseases. Sensitivity, specificity, and predictive value. Digestive Diseases and Sciences 28: 129–36

Festi D, Morselli Labate A M, Roda A, Bazzoli F, Frabboni R, Rucci P, Taroni F, Aldini R, Roda E, Barbara L 1983 Diagnostic effectiveness of serum bile acids in liver diseases as evaluated by multivariate statistical methods. Hepatology 3: 707–13

Fischer-Nielsen A, Poulsen H, Hansen B, Hage E, Keiding S 1990 CCl4 cirrhosis in rats: Irreversible histologic changes and differentiated functional impairment. Journal of Hepatology 12: 110–7

Fletcher L M, Kwoh Gain I, Powell E E, Powell L W, Halliday J W 1991 Markers of chronic alcohol ingestion in patients with nonalcoholic steatohepatitis: an aid to diagnosis. Hepatology 13: 455–9

Forrest J A, Finlayson N D, Adjepon-Yamoah K, Prescott L 1977 Antipyrine, paracetamol, and lignocaine elimination in chronic liver disease. British Medical Journal 1(6073): 1384–1387

Foster J H, Ellison L H, Donovan T J, et al 1971 Quantity and quality of survival after portosystemic shunts. American Journal of Surgery 121: 490–501

Franco D, Capussotti L, Smadja C, Bouzari H, Meakins J, Kemeny F, Grange D, Dellepiane M 1990 Resection of hepatocellular carcinomas. Results in 72 European patients with cirrhosis. Gastroenterology. 98: 733–738

Galizzi J, Long R G, Billing B H, Sherlock S 1978 Assessment of the [^{14}C]-aminopyrine breath test in liver disease. Gut 19: 40–45

Garrison R, Cryer H, Howard D, Polk H 1984 Clarification of risk factors for abdominal operations in patients with hepatic cirrhosis. Annals of Surgery 199: 648–655

Gavelli A, Ghiglione B, Huguet C 1993 (Risk factors of hepatectomies: results of a multivariate study. Apropos of 113 cases). Annales de Chirurgie 47: 586–591

Gill R A, Goodman M W, Golfus G R, Onstad G R, Bubrick M P 1983 Aminopyrine breath test predicts surgical risk for patients with liver disease. Annals of Surgery 198: 701–704

Gines P, Quintero E, Arroyo V, Teres J, Bruguera M, Rimola A, Caballeria J, Rodes J, Rozman C 1987 Compensated cirrhosis: Natural history and prognostic factors. Hepatology 7: 122–128

Gluud C, Henriksen J H, Nielsen G 1988 Copenhagen study group for liver diseases: Prognostic indicators in alcoholic cirrhotic men. Hepatology 8: 222–227

Goldberg D M, Martin J V 1975 Role of Gamma-glutamyl transpeptidase activity in the diagnosis of hepatobiliary disease. Digestion 12: 232–246

Grace N D, Conn H O, Resnick R H, et al 1988 Distal splenorenal vs. portal-systemic shunts after hemorrhage from varices: A randomized controlled trial. Hepatology 8: 1275–1481

Grambsch P M, Dickson E R, Kaplan M, Lesage G, Fleming T R, Langworthy A L 1989 Extramural cross-validation of the Mayo primary biliary cirrhosis survival model establishes its generalizability. Hepatology 10: 846–850

Green G, Poller L, Thomson J M, Dymock I W 1976 Factor VII as a marker of hepatocellular synthetic function in liver disease. Journal of Clinical Pathology 29: 971–975

Greenfield S, Soloway R, Carithers R, Soper K, Silva de Barros S, Balistreri W 1986 Evaluation of postprandial serum bile acid response as a test of hepatic function. Digestive Diseases and Sciences 31: 785–791

Gremse A, A-Kader H, Schroeder T J, Balisteri W F 1990 Assessment of lidocaine metabolite formation as a quantitative liver function test in children. Hepatology 12: 565–569

Grieco A, Barone C, Coletta P, Castellano R, Ragazzoni E, Cassano A, Astone A, Gambassi G 1992 Antipyrine metabolism in patients with liver metastases from colorectal cancer. Cancer 70: 1477–1482

Grimm L, Bircher J, Preisig R 1980 The galactose breath test. Modification of the method and comparison with galactose elimination capacity and plasma disappearance of bromsulphthalein. Zeitschrift fur Gastroenterologie 18: 45–56

Gross J, Reichen J, Zeltner T, Zimmermann A 1987 The evolution of changes in quantitative liver function tests in a rat model of cirrhosis: correlation with morphometric measurement of hepatocyte mass. Hepatology 7: 457–463

Gubernatis G, Bornscheuer A, Taki Y, et al 1989 Total oxygen consumption, ketone body ratio and a special score as early indicators of irreversible liver allograft dysfunction. Transplantation Proceedings 21: 2279–2281

Hadjis N S, Blenkharn J I, Hatzis G, Adam A, Beacham J, Blumgart L H 1990 Patterns of serum alkaline phosphatase activity in unilateral hepatic duct obstruction: a clinical and experimental study. Surgery 107: 193–200

Hallenbeck G A, Comess M S, Wollaeger E E, Gage R P 1959 Bleeding varices due to cirrhosis. Survival after (1) nonsurgical treatment, (2) splenectomy with or without omentopexy, and (3) portacaval or splenorenal shunt. Archives of Surgery 78: 774–784

Hamberg O, Nielsen K, Vilstrup H 1992 Effects of an increase in protein intake on hepatic efficacy for urea synthesis in healthy subjects and in patients with cirrhosis. Journal of Hepatology 14: 237–243

Harada T, Sugaya H, Maehara M, Kimura K, Hisauchi T, Tajima Y, Ohya G, Kubo T, Unuma T 1977 A follow-up study of liver function tests after surgical treatment for gallstone diseases. Gastroenterol Jpn. 12: 446–454

Harley H A, Morgan T, Redeker A, Reynolds T, Villamil F, Weiner J, Yellin A 1986 Results of a randomized trial of end-to-side portacaval shunt and distal splenorenal shunt in alcoholic liver disease and variceal bleeding. Gastroenterology 91: 802–8

Harrison P, O'Grady J, Keays R, Alexander G J, Williams R 1990 Serial prothrombin time as prognostic indicator in paracetamol induced fulminant hepatic failure. British Medical Journal 301: 964–966

Hatoff D E, Hardison W G M 1979 Induced synthesis of alkaline phosphatase by bile acids in rat liver cell culture. Gastroenterology 77: 1062–7

Helzberg J H, Petersen J M, Boyer J L 1987 Improved survival with primary sclerosing cholangitis. A review of clinicopathological festures and comparison of symptomatic and asymptomatic patients. Gastroenterology 92: 1869–75

Hemming A W, Scudamore C H, Shackleton C R, Pudek M, Erb S R 1992 Indocyanine green clearance as a predictor of successful hepatic resection in cirrhotic patients. American Journal of Surgery 163: 515–8

Henderson J M, Kutner M H, Bain R P 1982a First-order clearance of plasma galactose: the effect of liver disease. Gastroenterology. 83: 1090–6

Henderson J M, Millikan W J, Wright L, et al 1982b Quantitative estimation of metabolic and hemodynamic hepatic function: The effect of shunt surgery. Surgical Gastroenterology 1: 77–85

Henderson J M, Kuttner M, Millikan W, et al 1990 Endoscopic variceal sclerosis compared with distal splenorenal shunt to prevent recurrent variceal bleeding in cirrhosis: a prospective, randomized trial. Annals of Internal Medicine 112: 262–9

Hennes H M, Smith D S, Schneider K, Hegenbarth M A, Duma M A, Jona J Z 1990 Elevated liver transaminase levels in children with blunt abdominal trauma: a predictor of liver injury. Pediatrics 86: 87–90

Henry D A, Kitchingman G, Langman M J 1985 (^{14}C)Aminopyrine breath analysis and conventional biochemical tests as predictors of survival in cirrhosis. Digestive Diseases and Sciences 30: 813–8

Hepner G, Vessell E 1975 Quantitative assessment of hepatic function by breath analysis after oral administration of [^{14}C]aminopyrine. Annals of Internal Medicine 83: 632–8

Hill P G, Sammons H G 1967 An assessment of 5′-nucleotidase as a liver function test. Quarterly Journal of Medicine 36: 457–68

Hofmann A F 1983 The enterohepatic circulation of bile acids in health and disease. In: Sleisenger M H, Fordtran J S (eds) Gastrointestinal disease. Pathophysiology, diagnosis, management. 3rd edn. W.B. Saunders, Philadelphia, vol I, p 115–131

Horsmans Y, Lejeune D, Geubel A P, Otte J B, Pauwels S 1993 Hepatic [C-14]aminopyrine demethylation capacity after portocaval shunting—comparative study in patients with and without arterialization of portal vein. Digestive Diseases and Sciences 38: 2177–82

Hsu K Y 1972 Portal systemic shunt for portal hypertension: Importance of bromosulphalein retention for prediction of survival. Annals of Surgery 175: 569–76

Huet P, Villeneuve J 1983 Determinants of drug disposition in patients with cirrhosis. Hepatology 3: 913–8

Huet P M, Goresky C A, Villeneuve J P, Marleau D, Lough JO 1982 Assessment of liver microcirculation in human cirrhosis. Journal of Clinical Investigation 70: 1234–44

Hultcrantz R, Glaumann H, Lindberg G, Nilsson L H 1986 Liver investigation in 149 asymptomatic patients with moderately elevated activities of serum aminotransferases. Scandinavian Journal of Gastroenterology 21: 109–13

Hutchinson D R, Halliwell R P, Smith M G, Parke D V 1981 Serum prealbumin as an index of liver function in human hepatobiliary disease. Clinica Chimica Acta 114: 69–74

Infante-Rivard C, Esnaola S, Villeneuve J P 1987 Clinical and statistical validity of conventional prognostic factors in predicting short-term survival among cirrhotics. Hepatology 7: 660–4

Joelsson B, Hultberg B, Alwmark A, Gullstrand P, Bengmark S 1983 Total serum bile acids, gamma-glutamyl transferase, prealbumin, and tyrosine: sensitive serum markers of hepatic dysfunction in alcoholic liver cirrhosis. Scandinavian Journal of Gastroenterology 18: 497–501

Joelsson B, Hultberg B, Isaksson A, Alwmark A, Gullstrand P, Bengmark S 1984 Total fasting serum bile acids and beta-hexosaminidase in alcoholic liver disease. Clinica Chimica Acta 136: 203–9

Joeres R, Klinker H, Heusler H, Epping J, Zilly W, Richter E 1988 Influence of smoking on caffeine elimination in healthy volunteers and in patients with alcoholic liver cirrhosis. Hepatology 8: 575–9

Jones M B, Weinstock S, Koretz R L, Lewin K J, Higgins J, Gitnick G L 1981 Clinical value of serum bile acid levels in chronic hepatitis. Digestive Diseases and Sciences 26: 978–83

Jonsson P E, Bengtsson G, Carlsson G, Jonson G, Tryding N 1984 Value of serum-5-nucleotidase, alkaline phosphatase and gamma-glutamyl transferase for prediction of liver metastases preoperatively in colorectal cancer. Acta Chirurgica Scandinavica 150: 419–23

Jost G, Wahllander A, von Mandach U, Preisig R 1987 Overnight salivary caffeine clearance: a liver function test suitable for routine use. Hepatology 7: 338–44

Kanematsu T, Sonoda T, Yasunaga C, Takenaka K, Shirabe K, Sugimachi K 1989 Morphologic and functional changes in the remnant liver following resection for cirrhosis or chronic hepatitis. American Journal of Surgical Pathology 13: 776–81

Kaplan M M, Righetti A 1970 Induction of rat liver alkaline phosphatase: the mechanism of the serum elevation in bile duct obstruction. Journal of Clinical Investigation 49: 508–16

Kaplowitz N, Kok E, Javitt N B 1973 Postprandial serum bile acid for the detection of hepatobiliary disease. Journal of the American Medical Association 225: 292–3

Kardel T, Ramsoe K, Norby Rasmussen S 1975 Preoperative liver function tests correlated with encephalopathy after porta-caval anastomosis. Scandinavian Journal of Gastroenterology 10: 29–32

Karmen A, Wroblewski F, LaDue J 1955 Transaminase activity in human blood. Journal of Clinical Investigation 34: 126–33

Karmen C, Mayne P D, Foo A Y, Parbhoo S, Rosalki SB 1984 Measurement of biliary alkaline phosphatase by mini-column chromatography and by electrophoresis and its application to the detection of liver metastases in patients with breast cancer. Journal of Clinical Pathology 37: 212–7

Kawasaki S, Imamura H, Bandai Y, Sanjo K, Idezuki Y 1992 Direct evidence for the intact hepatocyte theory in patients with liver cirrhosis. Gastroenterology 102: 1351–5

Kawasaki S, Makuuchi M, Miyagawa S, Kakazu T, Hayashi K, Kasai H, Miwa S, Hui A M, Nishimaki K 1995 Results of hepatic resection for hepatocellular carcinoma. World Journal of Surgery 19: 31–34

Kim N K, Yasmineh W G, Freier E F, et al 1977 Value of alkaline phosphatase, 5′-nucleotidase, Gamma-glutamyl-transferase and glutamate dehydrogenase activity measurements (single or combined) in serum in diagnosis of metastasis to the liver. Clinical Chemistry 23: 2034–8

Kim Y K, Nakano H, Yamaguchi M, Kumada K, Takeuchi S, Kitamura N, Takahashi H, Hasebe S, Midorikawa T, Sanada Y 1997 Jun. Prediction of postoperative decompensated liver function by technetium-99m galactosyl-human serum albumin liver scintigraphy in patients with hepatocellular carcinoma complicating chronic liver disease. British Journal of Surgery 84: 793–796

Kin T, Nakajima Y, Kanehiro H, Hisanaga M, Ohyama T, Nishio K, Sho M, Nagao M, Nakano H 1998 Repeat hepatectomy for recurrent colorectal metastases. World Journal of Surgery 22: 1087–1091

Kishimoto Y, Hijiya S, Takeda I 1985 Clinical significance of fasting serum bile acid in the long-term observation of chronic liver disease. American Journal of Gastroenterology 80: 136–8

Klion F M, Fabry T L, Palmer M, Schaffner F 1992 Prediction of survival of patients with primary biliary cirrhosis. Gastroenterology 102: 310–3

Klompje J, Petrelli N J, Herrera L, Mittelman A 1987 The prognostic value of preoperative alkaline phosphatase for resection of solitary liver metastasis from colorectal carcinoma. European Journal of Surgical Oncology 13: 345–7

Knight J A, Haymond R E 1981 Gamma-glutamyltransferase and alkaline phosphatase activities compared in serum of normal children and children with liver disease. Clinical Chemistry 27: 48–51

Koperna T, Kisser M, Schulz F 1998 Hepatic resection in the elderly. World Journal of Surgery 22: 406–412

Korman M G, Hofmann A F, Summerskill W H J 1974 Assessment of activity in chronic active liver disease—serum bile acids compared with conventional tests and histology. New England Journal of Medicine 290: 1399–402

Kowlessar O D, Haeffner L J, Riley E M, Sleisenger M H 1961 Comparative study of serum leucine aminopeptidase, 5-nucleotidase and non-specific alkaline phosphatase in diseases affecting the pancreas, hepatobiliary tree and bone. American Journal of Medicine 31: 231–7

Kwon A H, Ha-Kawa S K, Uetsuji S, Kamiyama Y, Tanaka Y 1995 Use of technetium 99m diethylenetriamine-pentaacetic acid-galactosyl-human serum albumin liver scintigraphy in the evaluation of preoperative and postoperative hepatic functional reserve for hepatectomy. Surgery 117: 429–434

Kwon A H, Ha-Kawa S K, Uetsuji S, Inoue T, Matsui Y, Kamiyama Y 1997 Preoperative determination of the surgical procedure for hepatectomy using technetium-99m-galactosyl human serum albumin (99mTc-GSA) liver scintigraphy. Hepatology 25: 426–429

Lai C, Ng R, Lok A S 1982 The diagnostic value of the ratio of serum gamma-glutamyl transpeptidase to alkaline phosphatase in alcoholic liver disease. Scandinavian Journal of Gastroenterology 17: 41–7

Langer B, Taylor B, Mackenzie D, Gilas T, Stone R, Blendis L 1985 Further report of a prospective randomized trial comparing distal splenorenal shunt with end-to-side portacaval shunt. Gastroenterology 88: 424–9

Lashner B A, Jonas R B, Tang H S, Evans A A, Ozeran S E, Baker A L 1988 Chronic hepatitis: Disease factors at diagnosis predictive of mortality. American Journal of Medicine 85: 609–14

Lau H, Man K, Fan ST, Yu W C, Lo C M, Wong J 1997a Evaluation of preoperative hepatic function in patients with hepatocellular carcinoma undergoing hepatectomy. British Journal of Surgery 84: 1255–1259

Lau W, Leung K, Leung T W, Liew C T, Chan M S, Yu S C, Li A K 1997b A logical approach to hepatocellular carcinoma presenting with jaundice. Annals of Surgery 225: 281–5

Lee C S, Chao C C, Lin T Y 1985 Partial hepatectomy on cirrhotic liver with a right lateral tumor. Surgery 98: 942–8

Lee Y T 1978 Liver function tests after ligation of hepatic artery. Journal of Surgical Oncology 10: 305–20

Lin H H, Lin D Y 1991 Is preoperative ultrasound cancer survey necessary in patients with normal liver function tests. Journal of Clinical Gastroenterology 13: 108–10

Lindenmuth W W, Eisenberg M M 1963 The surgical risk in cirrhosis of the liver. Archives of Surgery 86: 235–42

Lindskov J 1982a The quantitative liver function as measured by the galactose elimination capacity. II. Prognostic value and changes during disease in patients with cirrhosis. Acta Medica Scandinavica 212: 303–8

Lindskov J 1982b The quantitative liver function as measured by the galactose elimination capacity. I. Diagnostic value and relations to clinical, biochemical, and histological findings in patients with steatosis and patients with cirrhosis. Acta Medica Scandinavica 212: 295–302

Lindskov J, Ranek L, Tygstrup N, Winkler K 1983 Splanchnic galactose uptake in patients with cirrhosis during continuous infusion. Clinical Physiology 3: 179–85

Linnet K, Andersen J R 1983 Differential diagnostic value in hepatobiliary disease of serum conjugated bile acid concentrations and some routine liver tests assessed by discriminant analysis. Clinica Chimica Acta 127: 217–28

Loft S, Boel J, Kyst A, Rasmussen B, Hansen S H, Dossing M 1985 Increased hepatic microsomal enzyme activity after surgery under halothane or spinal anesthesia. Anesthesiology 62: 11–16

Lotterer E, Hogel J, Gaus W, Fleig W E, Bircher J 1997 Quantitative liver function tests as surrogate markers for end-points in controlled clinical trials: a retrospective feasibility study [see comments]. Hepatology 26: 1426–1433

Lum G, Gambino R 1972 Serum gamma-glutamyl transpeptidase activity as an indicator of disease of liver, pancreas, or bone. Clinical Chemistry 18: 358–62

Lumeng L, Li T K 1974 Vitamin B6 metabolism in chronic alcohol abuse. Pyridoxal phosphate synthesis and degradation in human erythrocytes. Journal of Clinical Investigation 53: 693–704

Lunzer M, Barnes P, Byth K, O'Halloran M 1986 Serum bile acid concentrations during pregnancy and their relationship to obstetric cholestasis. Gastroenterology 91: 825–9

Maddrey W C, Boitnott J K, Bedine M S 1978 Corticosteroid therapy of alcoholic hepatitis. Gastroenterology 75: 169–73

Makuuchi M, Kosuge T, Takayama T, Yamazaki S, Kakazu T, Miyagawa S, Kawasaki S 1993 Surgery for small liver cancers. Seminars in Surgical Oncology 9: 298–304

Mannes G A, Stellaard F, Paumgartner G 1982 Increased serum bile acids in cirrhosis with normal transaminases. Digestion 25: 217–21

Mannes G, Thieme C, Stellaard F, Wang T, Sauerbruch T, Paumgartner G 1986 Prognostic significance of serum bile acids in cirrhosis. Hepatology 6: 50–3

Marchesini G, Checchia G A, Grossi G, Lolli R, Bianchi G P, Zoli M, Pisi E 1988 Caffeine intake, fasting plasma caffeine and caffeine clearance in patients with liver diseases. Liver 8: 241–6

Marchesini G, Fabbri A, Bugianesi E, Bianchi G, Marchi E, Zoli M, Pisi E 1990 Analysis of the deterioration rates of liver function in cirrhosis, based on galactose elimination capacity. Liver 10: 65–71

Margolis R, Hansen H H, Muggia F M, Kanhouwa S 1974 Diagnosis of liver metastases in bronchogenic carcinoma. A comparative study of liver scans, function tests, and peritoneoscopy with liver biopsy in 111 patients. Cancer 34: 1825–9

Mariette D, Smadja C, Naveau S, Borgonovo G, Vons C, Franco D 1997 Preoperative predictors of blood transfusion in liver resection for tumor. American Journal of Surgery 173: 275–279

Matloff D S, Selinger M J, Kaplan M M 1980 Hepatic transaminase activity in alcoholic liver disease. Gastroenterology 78: 1389–92

Matsumata T, Kanematsu T, Yoshida Y, Furuta T, Yanaga K, Sugimachi K 1987 The indocyanine green test enables prediction of postoperative complications after hepatic resection. World Journal of Surgery 11: 678–81

Matsusue S, Kashihara S, Maetani S 1984 Differentiation of congenital biliary atresia and neonatal hepatitis by statistical methods. Progress in Pediatric Surgery 17: 189–99

Maynard N D, Bihari D J, Dalton R N, Beale R, Smithies M N, Mason R C 1997 Liver function and splanchnic ischemia in critically ill patients. Chest 111: 180–187

McDonagh J E, Nathan V V, Bonavia I C, Moyle G R, Tanner A R 1991 Caffeine clearance by enzyme multiplied immunoassay technique: a simple, inexpensive, and useful indicator of liver function. Gut 32: 681–4

McPherson G A D, Benjamin I S, Boobis A R, Blumgart L H 1985 Antipyrine elimination in patients with obstructive jaundice: a predictor of outcome. American Journal of Surgery 149: 140–3

Mehta M U, Venkataramanan R, Burckart G J, Ptachcinski R J, Yang S L, Gray J A, Van Thiel D H, Starzl T E 1986 Antipyrine kinetics in liver disease and liver transplantation. Clinical Pharmacology and Therapeutics 39: 372–377

Merkel C, Bolognesi M, Finucci G F, Angeli P, Caregaro L, Rondana M, Gatta A 1989 Indocyanine green intrinsic hepatic clearance as a prognostic index of survival in patients with cirrhosis. Journal of Hepatology 9: 16–22

Merkel C, Gatta A, Zoli M, Bolognesi M, Angeli P, Iervese T, Marchesini G, Ruol A 1991 Prognostic value of galactose elimination capacity—aminopyrine breath test—and ICG clearance in patients with cirrhosis. Comparison with the Pugh score. Digestive Diseases and Sciences 36: 1197–203

Merkel C, Bolognesi M, Bellon S, Honisch B, Lampe H, Angeli P, Gatta A 1992 Aminopyrine breath test in the prognostic evaluation of patients with cirrhosis. Gut 33: 836–42

Miescher G, Paumgartner G, Preisig R 1983 Portal-systemic spill-over of bile acids: A study of mechanisms using ursodeoxycholic acid. European Journal of Clinical Investigation 13: 439–45

Miller D J, Keeton G R, Webber B L, Saunders S J 1976 Jaundice in severe bacterial infection. Gastroenterology 71: 94–7

Milstein H J, Bloomer J R, Klatskin G 1976 Serum bile acids in alcoholic liver disease: comparison with histological features of the disease. American Journal of Digestive Diseases 21: 281–5

Miotti T, Bircher J, Preisig R 1988 The 30-minute aminopyrine breath test: optimization of sampling times after intravenous administration of ^{14}C-aminopyrine. Digestion 39: 241–250

Miyagawa S, Makuuchi M, Kawasaki S, Kakazu T 1994 Changes in serum amylase level following hepatic resection in chronic liver disease. Archives of Surgery 129: 634–8

Molino G, Milanese M, Villa A, Cavanna A, Gaidano G 1978 Discrimination of hepatobiliary diseases by the evaluation of bromsulfophthalein blood kinetics. Journal of Laboratory and Clinical Medicine 91: 396–408

Monroe P S, Baker A L, Schneider J F, Krager P S, Klein P D, Schoeller D 1982 The aminopyrine breath test and serum bile acids reflect histologic severity in chronic hepatitis. Hepatology. 2: 317–22

Morelli A, Narducci F, Pelli M A, Farroni F, Vedovelli A 1981 The relationship between aminopyrine breath test and severity of liver disease in cirrhosis. American Journal of Gastroenterology 76: 110–3

Mori K, Ozawa K, Yamamoto Y, Maki A, Shimahara Y, Kobayashi N, Yamaoka Y, Kumada K 1990 Response of hepatic mitochondrial redox state to oral glucose load. Redox tolerance test as a new predictor of surgical risk in hepatectomy. Annals of Surgery 211: 438–46

Murray J M, Rowlands B J, Trinick T R 1992 Indocyanine green clearance and hepatic function during and after prolonged anaesthesia: comparison of halothane with isoflurane. British Journal of Anaesthesia 68: 168–171

Naftalin L, Child V J, Morley D A 1969 Observations on the site of origin of serum Gamma-glutamyl transpeptidase. Clinica Chimica Acta 26: 297–300

Nagasue N, Yukaya H, Suehiro S, Ogawa Y 1984 Tolerance of the cirrhotic liver to normothermic ischemia. A clinical study of 15 patients. American Journal of Surgery 147: 772–5

Nagel R, Dirix L, Hayllar K, Preisig R, Tredger J, Williams R 1990 Use of quantitative liver function tests—caffeine clearance and galactose elimination capacity—after orthotopic liver transplantation. Journal of Hepatology 10: 144–8

Nagino M, Nimura Y, Hayakawa N, Kamiya J, Kondo S, Sasaki R, Hamajima N 1993 Logistic regression and discriminant analyses of hepatic failure after liver resection for carcinoma of the biliary tract. World Journal of Surgery 17: 250–5

Nanji A A, French S W, Mendenhall C L 1989 Serum aspartate aminotransferase to alanine aminotransferase ratio in human and experimental alcoholic liver disease: relationship to histologic changes. Enzyme 41: 112–5

Nealon W H, Urrutia F 1996 Long-term follow-up after bilioenteric anastomosis for benign bile duct stricture. Annals of Surgery 223: 639–8

Neuberger J, Altman D G, Christensen E, Tygstrup N, Williams R 1986 Use of a prognostic index in evaluation of liver transplantation for primary biliary cirrhosis. Transplantation 41: 713–6

Nilssen O, Huseby N, Hoyer G, et al 1992 New alcohol markers—how useful are they in population studies: the Svalbard Study 1988–89 Alcoholism Clin Exp Res 16: 82–6

Nishio H, Sakuma T, Nakamura S, Horai T, Ikegami H, Matsuda M 1986 Diagnostic value of high molecular weight alkaline phosphatase in detection of hepatic metastasis in patients with lung cancer. Cancer 57: 1815–9

Nissenbaum M, Chedid A, Mendenhall C, Gartside P 1990 Prognostic significance of cholestatic alcoholic hepatitis. Digestive Diseases and Sciences 35: 891–6

Noguchi T, Imai T, Mizumoto R 1990 Preoperative estimation of surgical risk of hepatectomy in cirrhotic patients. Hepatogastroenterology 37: 165–71

Nonami T, Harada A, Kurokawa T, Nakao A, Takagi H 1997 Hepatic resection for hepatocellular carcinoma. American Journal of Surgery 44: 798–802

Nouel O, Henrion J, Bernuau J, Degott C, Rueff B, Benhamou J P 1980 Fulminant hepatic failure due to transient circulatory failure in patients with chronic heart disease. Digestive Diseases and Sciences 25: 49–52

Noun R, Jagot P, Farges O, Sauvanet A, Belghiti J 1997 High preoperative serum alanine transferase levels: effect on the risk of liver resection in Child grade A cirrhotic patients. World Journal of Surgery 21: 390–394

Oberhaensli R, Galloway G, Taylor D, Bore P, Radda G 1986 Assessment of human liver metabolism by phosphorus-31 magnetic resonance spectroscopy. British Journal of Radiology 59: 695–9

Oberhaensli R, Rajagopalan B, Galloway G J, Taylor D J, Radda G K 1990 Study of human liver disease with P-31 magnetic resonance spectroscopy. Gut 31: 463–7

Oellerich M, Ringe B, Gubernatis G et al 1989 Lignocaine metabolite formation as a measure of pre-transplant liver function. Lancet i: 640–642

Oellerich M, Burdelski M, Lautz H U, Binder L, Pichlmayr R 1991a Predictors of one-year pretransplant survival in patients with cirrhosis. Hepatology 14: 1029–34

Oellerich M, Burdelski M, Lautz H U, Rodeck B, Duewel J, Schulz M, Schmidt F W, Brodehl J, Pichlmayr R 1991b Assessment of pretransplant prognosis in patients with cirrhosis. Transplantation 51: 801–6

Ohara N, Schaffner T, Reichen J 1993 Structure–function relationship in secondary biliary cirrhosis in the rat: Stereologic and hemodynamic characterization of a model. Journal of Hepatology 17: 155–162

Ohkubo H, Okuda K, Iida S, Ohnishi K, Ikawa S, Makino I 1984 Role of portal and splenic vein shunts and impaired hepatic extraction in the elevated serum bile acids in liver cirrhosis. Gastroenterology 86: 514–20

Ohlsson B, Stenram U, Tranberg K G 1998 Resection of colorectal liver metastases: 25-year experience. World Journal of Surgery 22: 268–277

Ohmann C, Stoeltzing H, Wins L, Busch E, Thon K 1990 Prognostic scores in eosophageal or gastric variceal bleeding. Scandinavian Journal of Gastroenterology 25: 501–12

Okuda K, Ohtsuki T, Obata H, et al 1985 Natural history of hepatocellular carcinoma and prognosis in relation to treatment. Study of 850 patients. Cancer 56: 918–28

Orrego H, Israel Y, Blake J, Medline A 1983 Assessment of prognostic factors in alcoholic liver disease: Toward a global quantitative expression of severity. Hepatology 3: 896–905

Orrego H, Blake J, Israel Y 1985 Relationship between gamma-glutamyl-transpeptidase and mean urinary alcohol levels in alcoholic while drinking and after alcohol withdrawal. Alcoholism 9: 10–3

Osanaga E, Larre Borges A, Sanguinetti J, Mancusso G, Lopez A, Larreborges U 1992 (Comparative study between alkaline phosphatase and gamma- glutamyltranspeptidase in the diagnosis of hepatic metastases). Journal de Chirurgie 1985: 17–20

Osuga T, Mitamura K, Mashige F, Imai K 1977 Evaluation of fluorimetrically estimated serum bile acid in liver disease. Clinica Chimica Acta 75: 81–90

Ottmar M D, Gonda R L, Jr., Leithauser K J, Gutierrez O H 1989 Liver function tests in patients with computed tomography demonstrated hepatic metastasis. Gastrointestinal Radiology 14: 55–8

Ozawa K, Ida T, Yamada T, Honjo I 1976 Significance of glucose tolerance as prognostic sign in hepatectomized patients. American Journal of Surgery 131: 541–6

Patwardhan R, Smith O, Farmelant M 1987 Serum transaminase levels and cholescintigraphic abnormalities in acute biliary tract obstruction. Archives of Internal Medicine 147: 1249–53

Pauwels S, Geubel A P, Dive C, Beckers C 1982 Breath $^{14}CO_2$ after intravenous administration of (^{14}C)aminopyrine in liver diseases. Digestive Diseases and Sciences 27: 49–56

Pessayre D, Allemand H, Benoist C, Afifi F, Francois M, Henhamon J P 1978 Effect of surgery under general anaesthesia on antipyrine metabolism. British Journal of Clinical Pharmacology 6: 505–13

Pimstone N R, Stadalnik R C, Vera D R, Hutak D P, Trudeau W L 1994 Evaluation of hepatocellular function by way of receptor- mediated uptake of a technetium-99m-labeled asialoglycoprotein analog. Hepatology 20: 917–23

Pirotte J, El Allaf D 1983 Effect of age and sex on the N-demethylation rate of 14C-aminopyrine studied by the breath test. Digestion 28: 210–5

Pirwitz B 1979 The testing of liver function by means of radioactive 75Se- selenium-methionine. Materia Medica Polonz 11: 360–6

Pomier-Layrargues G, Huet P, Villeneuve J, Marleau D 1986 Effect of portacaval shunt on drug disposition in patients with cirrhosis. Gastroenterology 91: 163–7

Pomier-Layrargues G, Huet P M, Infante Rivard C, Villeneuve J P, Marleau D, Duguay L, Tanguay S, Lavoie P 1988 Prognostic value of indocyanine green and lidocaine kinetics for survival and chronic hepatic encephalopathy in cirrhotic patients following elective end-to-side portacaval shunt. Hepatology 8: 1506–10

Poulson H E, Loft S 1988 Antipyrine as a model drug to study hepatic drug-metabolizing capacity. Journal of Hepatology 6: 374–82

Poupon R, Lebrec D, LeQuernec L, Darnis F 1981 Mechanisms for reduced hepatic clearance and elevated plasma levels of bile acids in cirrhosis. A study in patients with an end-to-side portacaval shunt. Gastroenterology 80: 1438–44

Poupon R, Chretien Y, Poupon R E, Ballet F, Calmus Y, Darnis F 1987 Is ursodeoxycholic acid an effective treatment for primary biliary cirrhosis? Lancet i: 834–6

Poynard T, Zourabichvili O, Hilpert G, Naveau S, Poitrine A, Benatar C, Chaput J C 1984 Prognostic value of total serum bilirubin/gamma-glutamyl transpeptidase ratio in cirrhotic patients. Hepatology 4: 324–7

Price C P, Hill P G, Sammons H G 1972 The nature of the alkaline phosphatases of bile. Journal of Clinical Pathology 25: 149–54

Pugh R N H, Murray-Lyon I M, Dawson J L, Pietroni M C, Williams R 1973 Transsection of the oesophagus for bleeding oesophageal varices. British Journal of Surgery 60: 646–9

Ramond M J, Poynard T, Rueff B, Mathurin P, Theodore C, Chaput J C, Benhamou J P 1992 A randomized trial of prednisolone in patients with severe alcoholic hepatitis. New England Journal of Medicine 326: 507–12

Ranek L, Andreasen P B, Tygstrup N 1976 Galactose elimination capacity as a prognostic index in patients with fulminant liver failure. Gut 17: 959–64

Ratnoff O D 1975 Disordered hemostasis in hepatic disease. In: Schiff L (ed) Diseases of the liver. Lippincottt, Philadelphia, p 183–203

Reichel C, Nacke A, Sudhop T, Wienkoop G, Luers C, Hahn C, Pohl C, Spengler U, Sauerbruch T 1997 The low-dose monoethyl-glycinexylidide test: assessment of liver function with fewer side effects. Hepatology 25: 1323–1327

Reichen J 1993 MEGX test in hepatology: The long-sought, ultimate quantitative liver function test? Journal of Hepatology 19: 4–7

Reichen J 1995 Assessment of hepatic function with xenobiotics. Seminars in Liver Diseases 15: 189–201

Reichen J, Arts B, Schafroth U, Zimmermann A, Zeltner T, Zysset T 1987a Aminopyrine N-demethylation by rats with liver cirrhosis: Evidence for the intact cell hypothesis. A morphometric-functional study. Gastroenterology 93: 719–26

Reichen J, Hoilien C, Le M, Jones R H 1987b Decreased uptake of taurocholate and of ouabain by hepatocytes isolated from cirrhotic rat liver. Hepatology 7: 67–70

Reichen J, Egger B, Ohara N, Zeltner T, Zysset T, Zimmermann A 1988 Determinants of hepatic functions in liver cirrhosis in the rat: a multivariate analysis. Journal of Clinical Investigation 82: 2069–76

Reichen J, Widmer T, Cotting J 1991 Accurate prediction of death by serial determination of galactose elimination capacity in primary biliary cirrhosis: a comparison with the Mayo model. Hepatology 14: 504–10

Renner E, Wietholtz H, Huguenin P, Arnaud M J, Preisig R 1984 Caffeine: a model compound for measuring liver function. Hepatology 4: 38–46

Resnick R H, Chalmers T C, Ishihara A M, Garceau A J, Callow A D, Schimmel E M, O'Hara E T 1969 A controlled study of the prophylactic portacaval shunt. A final report. Annals of Internal Medicine 70: 675–88

Resnick R H, Iber F L, Ishihara A M, Chalmers T C, Zimmermann H 1974 A controlled study of therapeutic portocaval shunt. Gastroenterology 67: 843–57

Richman S, Delman A, Grob D 1961 Alterations in indices of liver function in congestive heart failure with particular reference to serum enzymes. American Journal of Medicine 30: 211–25

Ritter D M, Rettke S R, Lunn R J, Bowie E J, Ilstrup D 1989 Preoperative coagulation screen does not predict intraoperative blood product requirements in orthotopic liver transplantation. Transplantation Proceedings 21: 3533–4

Roberts-Thomson I C, Jonsson J R, Frewin D B, Coates G C 1990 Sympathetic activation: a mechanism for morphine induced pain and rises in liver enzymes after cholecystectomy. Gut 31: 217–21

Robertz-Vaupel G M, Lindecken K D, Edeki T, Funke C, Belwon S, Dengler H J 1992 Disposition of antipyrine in patients with extensive metastatic liver disease. European Journal of Clinical Pharmacology 42: 465–9

Rocklin M S, Senagore A J, Talbott T M 1991 Role of carcinoembryonic antigen and liver function tests in the detection of recurrent colorectal carcinoma. Diseases of the Colon and Rectum 34: 794–7

Rodzynek J J, Preux C, Leautaud P, Abramovici J, Di Paolo A, Delcourt A 1986 Diagnostic value of antithrombin III and aminopyrine breath test in liver disease. Archives of Internal Medicine 146: 677–80

Rondana M, Milani L, Merkel C, Caregaro L, Gatta A 1987 Value of prealbumin plasma levels as liver test. Digestion 37: 72–8

Rosalki S B, Rau D, Lehmann D, Prentice M 1970 Determination of gamma-glutamyl transpeptidase activity and its clinical applications. Annals of Clinical Biochemistry 7: 143–7

Rosenthal S M, White E C 1924 Studies in hepatic function. VI. A. The pharmocological behavior of certain phthalein dyes. B. The value of selected phthalein compounds in the estimation of hepatic function. J Pharma Exper Ther 24: 265

Rotschild M A, Oratz M, Schreiber S S 1972 Albumin synthesis. New England Journal of Medicine 286: 748–57

Rowland M, Benet L, Graham G 1973 Clearance concepts in pharmacokinetics. Journal of Pharmacokinetics and Biopharmaceutics 1: 123–36

Rudman D, DiFulco T J, Galambos J T, Smith R B, Salam A A, Warren W D 1973 Maximal rates of excretion and synthesis of urea in normal and cirrhotic subjects. Journal of Clinical Investigation 52: 2241–9

Sahdew P, Meadow E, Garramone R R, Schwartz R J, Steelman S R, Jacobs L M 1991 Evaluation of liver function tests in screening for intra-abdominal injuries. Annals of Emergency Medicine 20: 838–41

Salaspuro M 1987 Use of enzymes for the diagnosis of alcohol-related organ damage. Enzyme 37: 87–107

Satterfield J V, Mullican L V, Butcher H R, Jr 1965 Esophageal varices, comparison of operative and nonoperative treatment. Archives of Surgery 90: 666–72

Sauerbruch T, Ansari H, Wotzka R, Soehandra H, Köpcke W 1988 Prognose-Parameter bei Leberzirrhose, Varizenblutung und Sklerosierungstherapie. Deutsche Medizinische Wochenschrift 113: 11–4

Saunders J, Wright N, Lewis K 1980 Predicting outcome of paracetamol poisoning by using [^{14}C]-aminopyrine breath test. British Medical Journal i: 279–80

Saunders J B, Lewis K O, Paton A 1980 Early diagnosis of alcoholic cirrhosis by the aminopyrine breath test. Gastroenterology 79: 112–4

Sawamura T, Nakada H, Hazama H, Shiozaki Y, Sameshima Y, Tashiro Y 1984 Hyperasialoglycoproteinemia in patients with chronic liver diseases and/or liver cell carcinoma. Gastroenterology 87: 1217–21

Schirmer W J, Townsend M C, Schirmer J M, Hampton W W, Fry D E 1986 Galactose clearance as an estimate of effective hepatic blood flow: validation and limitations. Journal of Surgical Research 41: 543–56

Schlichting P, Christensen E, Andersen P K, Fauerholdt L, Juhl E, Poulsen H, Tygstrup N 1983a. Prognostic factors in cirrhosis identified by Cox's regression model. Hepatology 3: 889–95

Schlichting P, Christensen E, Fauerholdt L, Poulsen H, Juhl E, Tygstrup N 1983b. Main causes of death in cirrhosis. Scandinavian Journal of Gastroenterology 18: 881–8

Schmid M, Hefti M, Gattiker R, Kistler H, Senning A 1965 Benign postoperative intrahepatic cholestasis. New England Journal of Medicine 272: 545–50

Schnegg M, Lauterburg B H 1986 Quantitative liver function in the elderly assessed by galactose elimination capacity, aminopyrine demethylation and caffeine clearance. Journal of Hepatology 3: 164–71

Schneider J F, Baker A L, Haines N W, Hatfield G, Boyer J L 1980 Aminopyrine N-demethylation: a prognostic test of liver function in patients with alcoholic liver disease. Gastroenterology 79: 1145–50

Schoeller D, Baker A, Monroe P, Krager P, Schneider J 1982 Comparison of different methods expressing results of the aminopyrine breath test. Hepatology 2: 455–462

Schoelmerich J, Straub R 1992 Mechanisms of bile salt toxicity. In: Lentze M J, Reichen J (eds) Paediatric cholestasis. Novel approaches to treatment. Kluwer Academic Publishers, Dordrecht, p 83–103

Schonfeld J, Breuer N, Zotz R B, Beste M, Goebell H 1997 Serial quantitative liver function tests in patients with primary biliary cirrhosis: a prospective long-term study. Digestion 58: 396–401

Scott N R, Stambuk D, Chakraborty J, Marks V, Morgan MY 1988 Caffeine clearance and biotransformation in patients with chronic liver disease. Clinical Science 74: 377–84

Sedgwick C E, Hume H A 1959 Analysis of forty-two shunt procedures for portal hypertension. Archives of Surgery 78: 359–63

Seeff L B, Cuccherini B A, Zimmermann H J, Adler E, Benjamin S B 1986 Acetaminophen hepatotoxicity in alcoholics. A therapeutic misadventure. Annals of Internal Medicine 104: 399–404

Seetharam S, Sussman N L, Komoda T, et al 1986 The mechanism of elevated alkaline activity after bile duct ligation in the rat. Hepatology 6: 374

Shapiro J M, Smith H, Schaffner F 1979 Serum bilirubin: A prognostic factor in primary biliary cirrhosis. Gut 20: 137–40

Sher P P 1977 Diagnostic effectiveness of biochemical liver-function tests, as evaluated by discriminant function analysis. Clinical Chemistry 23: 627–30

Sherlock S 1946 Biochemical investigations in liver disease; some correlations with hepatic histology. Journal of Pathological Bacteriology 58: 523–44

Shimada M, Takenaka K, Taguchi K, Fujiwara Y, Gion T, Kajiyama K, Maeda T, Shirabe K, Yanaga K, Sugimachi K 1998 Prognostic factors after repeat hepatectomy for recurrent hepatocellular carcinoma. Annals of Surgery 227: 80–85

Shreeve W W, Shoop J D, Ott D G, McInteer B B 1976 Test for alcoholic cirrhosis by conversion of (^{14}C) or (^{13}C) galactose to expired CO^2 Gastroenterology 71: 98–101

Shrestha R, McKinley C, Showalter R, Wilner K, Marsano L, Vivian B, Everson G T 1997 Quantitative liver function tests define the functional severity of liver disease in early-stage cirrhosis. Liver Transplantation Surgery 3: 166–173

Siciliano M, Barbesino G, Marra L, Milani A, Rossi L 1989 Long-term prognostic value of serum bile acids in liver cirrhosis: a prospective study. Zeitschrift fur Gastroenterologie 27: 653–6

Sieg A, Koenig R, Ulrich D, Fevery J 1990 Subfractionation of serum bilirubins by alkaline methanolysis and thin-layer chromatography: an aid in the differential diagnosis of icteric diseases. Journal of Hepatology 11: 159–64

Simko V, Michael S 1986 Bile acid levels in diagnosing mild liver disease. Fasting and postcholecystokinetic values. Archives of Internal Medicine 146: 695–7

Sitzmann J V, Greene P S 1994 Perioperative predictors of morbidity following hepatic resection for neoplasm. A multivariate analysis of a single surgeon experience with 105 patients. Annals of Surgery 219: 13–7

Skrede S, Blomhoff J P, Elgjo K, Gjone E 1973 Biochemical tests in evaluation of liver function. Scandinavian Journal of Gastroenterology 8 (supplement 19): 37–46

Skrede S, Solberg H E, Blomhoff J P, Gjone E 1978 Bile acids measured in serum during fasting as a test for liver disease. Clinical Chemistry 24: 1095–9

Smith R B 3d, Warren W D, Salam A A, Millikan W J, Ansley J D, Galambos J T, Kutner M, Bain R P 1980 Dacron interposition shunts for portal hypertension. An analysis of morbidity correlates. Annals of Surgery 192: 9–17

Solberg H E, Skrede S, Blomhoff J P 1975 Diagnosis of liver disease by laboratory results and discriminant analysis: Identification of best combination of laboratory tests. Scandinavian Journal of Clinical and Laboratory Investigation 35: 713–21

Sotaniemi E A, Niemela O, Risteli L, Stenback F, Pelkonen R O, Lahtela J T, Risteli J 1986 Fibrotic process and drug metabolism in alcoholic liver disease. Clinical Pharmacology and Therapeutics 40: 46–55

Soyer P, Roche A, Elias D, Levesque M 1992 Hepatic metastases from colorectal cancer: influence of hepatic volumetric analysis on surgical decision making. Radiology 184: 695–7

Speich R, Saesseli B, Hoffmann U, Neftel K, Reichen J 1988 Anaphylactoid reactions after indocyanine-green administration. Annals of Internal Medicine 109: 345–6

St Peter J V, Awni W M 1991 Quantifying hepatic function in the presence of liver disease with phenazone (antipyrine) and its metabolites. Clinical Pharmacokinetics 20: 50–65

Stanko R T, Nathan G, Mendelow H, Adibi S 1987 Development of hepatic cholestasis and fibrosis in patients with massive loss of intestine supported by prolonged parenteral nutrition. Gastroenterology 92: 197–202

Stock P G, Estrin J A, Fryd D S, Payne W D, Belani K G, Elick B A, Najarian J S, Ascher N L 1987 Prognostic perioperative factors predicting the outcome of liver transplantation. Transplantation Proceedings 19: 2427–8

Suehiro T, Sugimachi K, Matsumata T, Itasaka H, Taketomi A, Maeda T 1994 Protein induced by vitamin K absence or antagonist II as a prognostic marker in hepatocellular carcinoma. Comparison with alpha-fetoprotein. Cancer 73: 2464–71

Summerfield J A, Kirk A P, Chitranukroh A, Billing B H 1981 A distinctive pattern of serum bile acid and bilirubin concentrations in benign recurrent intrahepatic cholestasis. Hepatogastroenterology 28: 139–42

Tanaka R, Itoshima T, Nagashima H 1987 Follow-up study of 582 liver cirrhosis patients for 26 years in Japan. Liver 7: 316–24

Tarao K, Takemiya S, Tamai S, Sugimasa Y, Ohkawa S, Akaike M, Tanabe H, Shimizu A, Yoshida M, Kakita A 1997 Relationship between the recurrence of hepatocellular carcinoma (HCC) and serum alanine aminotransferase levels in hepatectomized patients with hepatitis C virus-associated cirrhosis and HCC. Cancer 79: 688–694

Taylor M, Forster J, Langer B, Taylor B R, Greig P D, Mahut C 1997 A study of prognostic factors for hepatic resection for colorectal metastases. American Journal of Surgery 173: 467–471

Teppo A M, Maury C P J 1983 Serum prealbumin, transferrin and immunoglobulins in fatty liver, alcoholic cirrhosis and primary biliary cirrhosis. Clinica Chimica Acta 129: 279–86

Teres J, Baroni R, Bordas J, Visa J, Pera C, Rodes J 1987 Randomized trial of portacaval shunt, stapling transection and endoscopic sclerotherapy in uncontrolled variceal bleeding. Journal of Hepatology 4: 159–67

Theodossi A, Eddleston A, Williams R 1982 Controlled trial of methylprednisolone therapy in severe acute alcoholic hepatitis. Gut 23: 75–9

Tinkoff G, Rhodes M, Diamond D, Lucke J 1990 Cirrhosis in the trauma victim. Effect on mortality rates. Annals of Surgery 211: 172–7

Tobiasson B, Boeryd B 1980 Serum cholic acid conjugates and standard liver function tests in various morphological stages of alcoholic liver disease. Scandinavian Journal of Gastroenterology 15: 657–63

Turcotte J G, Lambert M J 1973 Variceal hemorrhage, hepatic cirrhosis, and portocaval shunts. Surgery 73: 810–7

Tygstrup N 1963 Determination of the hepatic galactose elimination capacity after a single intravenous injection in man. Acta Physiologica Scandinavica 58: 162–72

Uesaka K, Nimura Y, Nagino M 1996 Jan. Changes in hepatic lobar function after right portal vein embolization. An appraisal by biliary indocyanine green excretion. Annals of Surgery 223: 77–83

Ukikusa M, Ozawa K, Shimahara Y, Asano M, Nakatani T, Tobe T 1981 Changes in blood ketone body ratio: their significance after major hepatic resection. Archives of Surgery 116: 781–5

van Blankenstein M, Frenkel M, van den B J W, ten Kate F J, Bosman Jacobs E P, Touw Blommesteyn A C 1983 Endogenous bile acid tolerance test for liver function. Digestive Diseases and Sciences 28: 137–44

VanHootegem P, Fevery J, Blanckaert N 1985 Serum bilirubins in hepatobiliary disease: Comparison with other liver function tests and changes in the postobstructive period. Hepatology 5: 112–7

Vaubourdolle M, Gufflet V, Chazouilleres O, Giboudeau J, Poupon R 1991 Indocyanine green-sulfobromophthalein pharmacokinetics for diagnosing primary biliary cirrhosis and assessing histological severity. Clinical Chemistry 37: 1688–900

Vauthey J N, Klimstra D, Franceschi D, Tao Y, Fortner J, Blumgart L, Brennan M 1995 Factors affecting long-term outcome after hepatic resection for hepatocellular carcinoma. American Journal of Surgery 169: 28–34

Vierling J M, Berk P D, Hofmann A F, Martin J, Wolkoff A W, Scharschmidt B F 1982 Normal fasting-state levels of serum cholyl-conjugated bile acids in Gilbert's syndrome: an aid to the diagnosis. Hepatology 2: 340–3

Villeneuve J P, Infante Rivard C, Ampelas M, Pomier Layrargues G, Huet P M, Marleau D 1986 Prognostic value of the aminopyrine breath test in cirrhotic patients. Hepatology 6: 928–31

Viot M, Thyss A, Viot G, Ramaioli A, Cambon P, Schneider M, Lalanne C M 1981 Comparative study of gamma glutamyl transferase, alkaline phosphatase and its alpha 1 isoenzyme as biological indicators of liver metastases. Clinica Chimica Acta 115: 349–58

Viot M, Thyss A, Schneider M, Viot G, Ramaioli A, Cambon P, Lalanne C M 1983 Alpha-1 isoenzyme of alkaline phosphatases. Clinical importance and value for the detection of liver metastases. Cancer 52: 140–5

Vo N, Rikkers L 1985 Hyperbilirubinemia following distal spleno-renal shunt. Archives of Surgery 120: 301–5

Wahlländer A, Renner E, Preisig R 1985 Fasting plasma caffeine concentration. A guide to the severity of chronic liver disease. Scandinavian Journal of Gastroenterology 20: 1133–41

Wantz G E, Payne M A 1961 Experience with portacaval shunt for portal hypertension. New England Journal of Medicine 265: 721–8

Wardle N, Anderson A, James O 1980 Kupffer cell phagocytosis in relation to BSP clearance in liver and inflammatory bowel diseases. Digestive Diseases and Sciences 25: 414–9

Warren W, Galambos J, Riepe S, Henderson W, Brooks W, Salam A, Millikan W, J, , Kutner M 1986 Distal splenorenal shunt versus endoscopic sclerotherapy for long-term management of variceal bleeding. Annals of Surgery 203: 454–62

Watanapa P 1996 Recovery patterns of liver function after complete and partial surgical biliary decompression. American Journal of Surgery 171: 230–4

Weiss J S, Gautam A, Lauff J J, Sundberg M W, Jatlow P, Boyer J L, Seligson D 1983 The clinical importance of a protein-bound fraction of serum bilirubin in patients with hyperbilirubinemia. New England Journal of Medicine 309: 147–50

Whitfield J B, Pounder R E, Neale G, Moss D W 1972 Serum Gamma-glutamyl transpeptidase activity in liver disease. Gut 13: 702–8

Wiesner R H, Grambsch P M, Dickson E R, Ludwig J, MacCarty R L, Hunter E B, Fleming T R, Fisher L D, Beaver S J, LaRusso N F 1989 Primary sclerosing cholangitis: natural history, prognostic factors and survival analysis. Hepatology 10: 430–6

Wietholtz H, Voegelin M, Arnaud M J, Bircher J, Preisig R 1981 Assessment of the cytochrome P-448 dependent liver enzyme system by a caffeine breath test. European Journal of Clinical Pharmacology 21: 53–9

Wilkinson G, Shand D 1975 A physiologic approach to hepatic drug clearance. Clinical Pharmacological Therapy 18: 377–90

Williams A L B, Hoofnagle J H 1988 Ratio of serum aspartate to alanine aminotransferase in chronic hepatitis. Gastroenterology 95: 734–9

Williams S, Farrell G 1989 Serial antipyrine clearance studies detect altered hepatic metabolic function during spontaneous and interferon-induced changes in chronic hepatitis b disease activity. Hepatology 10: 192–7

Winkel P, Ramsoe K, Lyngbye J, Tygstrup N 1975 Diagnostic value of routine liver tests. Clinical Chemistry 21: 71–5

Winkelman J, Nadler S, Demteriou J, Pileggi VJ 1972 The clinical usefulness of alkaline phophatase isoenzyme determinations. American Journal of Clinical Pathology 57: 625–34

Wood A J J, Villeneuve J P, Branch R A, Rogers L W, Shand D G 1979 Intact hepatocyte theory of impaired drug metabolism in experimental cirrhosis in the rat. Gastroenterology 76: 1358–62

Wright R, Eade O E, Chisholm M, Hawksley M, Lloyd B, Moles T M, Edwards J T, Gardner M J 1975 Controlled prospective study of the effect on liver function of multiple exposure to halothane. Lancet i: 817–21

Wroblewski F 1959 The clinical significance of transaminase activities of serum. American Journal of Medicine 27: 911–23

Yamanaka N, Okamoto E, Oriyama T, Fujimoto J, Furukawa K, Kawamura E, Tanaka T, Tomoda F 1994 A prediction scoring system to select the surgical treatment of liver cancer. Further refinement based on 10 years of use. Annals of Surgery 219: 342–6

Yamaoka Y, Kumada K, Ino K, Takayasu T, Shimahara Y, Mori K, Tanaka A, Morimoto T, Taki Y, Washida M 1992 Liver resection for hepatocellular carcinoma (HCC) with direct removal of tumor thrombi in the main portal vein. World Journal of Surgery 16: 1172–1176

Yanaga K, Kanematsu T, Takenaka K, Matsumata T, Yoshida Y, Sugimachi K 1988 Hepatic resection for hepatocellular carcinoma in elderly patients. American Journal of Surgery 155: 238–41

Yasui M, Harada A, Torii A, Nakao A, Nonami T, Takagi H 1995 Impaired liver function and long-term prognosis after hepatectomy for hepatocellular carcinoma. World Journal of Surgery 19: 439–43

Young I I 1958 Serum 5-Nucleotidase: Characterization and evaluation in disease states. Annals of the New York Academy of Sciences 75: 357–62

Zeeh J, Lange H, Bosch J, Pohl S, Loesgen H, Eggers R, Navasa M, Chesta J, Bircher J 1988 Steady-state extrarenal sorbitol clearance as a measure of hepatic plasma flow. Gastroenterology 95: 749–59

Zein M, Discombre G 1970 Serum gamma-glutamyl transpeptidase as a diagnostic. Lancet ii: 748–9

Zieve L, Hill E 1955 An evaluation of factors influencing the discriminative effectiveness of a group of liver function tests. II. Normal limits of eleven representative hepatic tests. Journal of Laboratory and Clinical Medicine 28: 766–84

Zimmerer J, Haubitz I, Mainos D, Hadass H, Tittor W 1996 Survival in alcoholic liver cirrhosis: prognostic value of portal pressure, size of esophageal varices and biochemical data. Comparison with Child classification. Zeitschrift fur Gastroenterologie 34: 421–7

Zimmermann H J, West M 1963 Serum enzyme levels in the diagnosis of hepatic disease. American Journal of Gastroenterology 387–404

Zimmermann H J, Fang M, Utili R, Seeff L B, Hoofnagle J H 1979 Jaundice due to bacterial infections. Gastroenterology 77: 362–72

Zoli M, Marchesini G, Melli A, Viti G, Marra A, Marrano D, Pisi E 1986 Evaluation of liver volume and liver function following hepatic resection in man. Liver 6: 286–91

Zotz R B, von Schonfeld J, Erhard J, Breuer N, Lange R, Beste M, Goebell H, Eigler F W 1997 Value of an extended monoethylglycinexylidide formation test and other dynamic liver function tests in liver transplant donors. Transplantation 63: 538–541

Liver hyperplasia, hypertrophy and atrophy, and the molecular basis of liver regeneration

3

N. FAUSTO, N.S. HADJIS, Y. FONG

INTRODUCTION

Compensatory enlargement of liver tissue as a response to partial resection for damage of liver tissue has clear surgical implications. Such 'regeneration' of liver tissue is essential for recovery from partial hepatectomy. This phenomenon of growth of the remnant after partial resection has been described in many species (Fishback 1929, Higgins & Anderson 1931, Higgins et al 1932, Grindlay & Bollman 1952, Yokoyama et al 1953, Pack et al 1962). As far as can be assessed from published works (Bucher 1963), there is no known species or strain in which uncomplicated surgical resection of a substantial part of the liver is not attended by enlargement of the remnant. The nature of the phenomenon, first described about a century ago (Ponfick 1889, Von Meister 1894) is comparable in different species and in different circumstances and there is now little conflict about the morphologic (Brues & Marble 1937, Harkness 1952, Grisham 1962) and biochemical changes which have been found (MacManus et al 1973, Baserga 1974, Lewan et al 1977, McGowan & Fausto 1978).

Virchow's concept of hypertrophy distinguished between the increase in mass of an organ by increase in cell size and by increase in cell number. Since then, the term 'hypertrophy' has come to imply increase in mass due to increase in cell size without an increase in genetic substance. By contrast, the term 'hyperplasia' indicates an increase in mass due to cell division and increase in cell numbers.

Following acute loss of liver substance through injury or surgical resection, the restoration of liver mass to its former size involves a combination of hyperplasia and hypertrophy. However, adaptive hepatic growth is basically a hyperplastic process, although in this chapter the term 'hypertrophy' will be retained for descriptive purposes.

Hepatic atrophy also has important surgical implications.

Such loss in hepatic mass may result from disease processes that cause vascular compromise or biliary obstruction. Unilobar atrophy will usually lead to contralateral hypertrophy/hyperplasia. Such combined atrophy and contralateral hypertrophy has characteristic anatomic and radiologic appearances. The classic appearance of atrophic changes will be described below. Recognizing these not only provides important diagnostic information concerning the responsible clinical entity but also is important in planning the technical aspects of liver resection.

This chapter will first describe the cellular and molecular changes in hepatic hyperplasia and regeneration. Then it will concentrate on the *clinical aspects* of lobar or segmental liver atrophy and concomitant hypertrophy (hyperplasia) of the unaffected parenchyma. It is this 'atrophy–hypertrophy complex' that gives rise to particular diagnostic problems and accounts for the management difficulties associated with many liver disease processes.

The liver has the unique capacity to regulate its growth and mass. In humans as well as in rodents used for laboratory research, the liver of the newborn is a proliferative organ in which hepatocytes actively replicate (Fausto & Webber 1994, Fausto et al 1995). Hepatocyte replication terminates in a few months (humans) or weeks (2–3 weeks for rats and mice) after birth and remains very low throughout adult life. It has been estimated that adult livers have one mitotic figure in 10 000–20 000 cells (Bucher & Malt 1971). Because mitosis proper constitutes a short portion of the cell replication process, the actual number of replicating hepatocytes in adult livers is probably around 0.1%. In the neonatal period hepatocyte proliferation is associated with the expression of at least one important growth factor, namely transforming growth factor alpha (TGF-α). As hepatocyte replication decreases to the very low rates of the adult liver, the levels of hepatic TGF-α also decrease and are barely detectable (Fausto & Webber 1994, Fausto et al

1995). TGF-α, as well as other growth factors, is transiently expressed in short-liver proliferative responses in the adult liver, such as liver regeneration after partial hepatectomy (Fausto 1991, Webber et al 1994, Michalopoulos & DeFrances 1997). However, if TGF-α is constitutively expressed, it causes the development of hepatocellular adenomas and carcinomas. This was clearly demonstrated in transgenic mouse lines that contained an inserted human TGF-α gene in the germ line and constitutively overexpressed TGF-α in the liver. At approximately 12–15 months of age approximately 90% of these mice developed liver tumors (Lee et al 1992). This example underscores the notion that factors that can induce liver growth are tightly regulated: they are highly expressed in postnatal liver, repressed in adult normal liver, transiently increased in regulated hyperplastic responses, and constitutively expressed in neoplastic growth.

HYPERTROPHY AND LIVER REGENERATION

THE SET POINT FOR LIVER GROWTH PROCESSES

Hepatocytes, the main cellular elements of the liver (constituting approximately 65% of the cells and 95% of hepatic mass), are highly differentiated but not terminally differentiated cells. That is, although normally quiescent, these cells have not lost the capacity to proliferate (Fausto & Webber 1994, Michalopoulos & DeFrance 1997). Of major importance both for research and clinical practice is that the growth responses of the adult liver, excluding neoplasia, are highly regulated and self-limited. The healthy adult liver rapidly responds to changes in functional mass. If, on the contrary, hepatic mass is in excess of functional needs, growth does not take place and liver mass may decrease by programmed cell death (apoptosis) of hepatocytes (Columbano & Shinozuka 1996). The set point for growth is the optimal liver mass/body mass, a ratio that is established at the end of the postnatal period and remains relatively constant throughout adult life in an intact non-diseased liver (Fausto & Webber 1994). Clinical conditions in which regulated liver growth are observed include: regeneration after partial hepatectomy or acute necrogenic liver injury, growth of small-for-size transplants (Van Thiel et al 1987, Francavilla et al 1994a,b), growth of split liver transplants and the growth of both donor and transplanted liver in living donor transplantation. In all of these cases, livers that are less than optimal in size grow to reach the appropriate set point. Decreases in liver mass or absence of

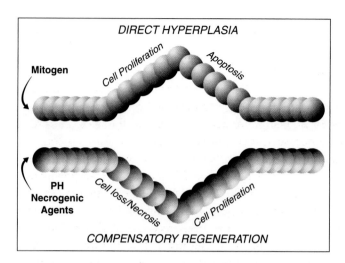

Fig. 3.1 Regulation of hepatocyte proliferation. The figure shows two opposite processes of regulation of hepatic mass. In response to decreased mass caused by partial hepatectomy or massive acute cell death, hepatocytes readily proliferate to compensate for the loss of tissue or cells (lower diagram). A similar situation exists in small-for-size transplants (small organ in a large recipient, split transplants, living donor transplantation). The upper diagram illustrates a situation in which cell proliferation is induced in the liver by mitogenic drugs in humans. In this case, the increased liver mass does not persist if the mitogenic agents are discontinued. The liver decreases in mass and regains its normal mass by a process of programmed cell death (apoptosis). (Reprinted with permission from Columbano & Shinozuka 1996).

growth are observed in large-for-size transplants (Kam et al 1987) and in non-surgical conditions involving drug-induced hyperplasia. In drug-induced hyperplasia the termination of drug administration is followed by liver mass decrease and return to normal values (Fig. 3.1).

CELLULAR AND HISTOLOGIC ASPECTS OF LIVER REGENERATION

Hepatocyte proliferation and turnover occur in a complex spatial pattern, which has not yet been fully elucidated, and which may not only depend on growth stimulating signals, but also on the cells' position and polarity in a plate and in the lobule, on their age and history, on the positions and functions of neighboring littoral cells, and on the interactions with the extracellular matrix. Thus it has been shown that, in the normal young adult rat liver, 80% of BrdU-labeled cells are located in lobular zone 1 (the periportal zone), and only about 2% in the pericentral zone 3, whereas labeled Kupffer cells appear to be distributed randomly or at least less typical (Jezequel et al 1991). The spatial relationship between proliferating hepatocytes and Kupffer cells is not yet clear, as arguments relating to such an association have been favored (Jezequel et al 1991) and refuted

(Zajicek et al 1988). It is however agreed that a local prolif-eration of Kupffer cells, and not only of hepatocytes, does occur after partial hepatectomy (Bouwens et al 1984), but it appears to lag behind the parenchymal cells (Karran & McLaren 1985). Except for cells in the M phase it is difficult or impossible to identify morphologically individual hepato-cytes as being proliferative without the aid of distinct methods, such as labeling using ^{3}H-Tdr or BrdU incorpora-tion, or immunohistochemical visualization of proliferation-associated antigens (such as PCNA or Ki-67) or polymerase alpha (Seki et al 1990). When testing ultrastructural features of proliferating hepatocytes using anti-DNA-polymerase alpha antibodies it has been recognized that polymerase alpha appears in the nuclei just before the onset of DNA synthesis, and reaches a maximum level at the late S or G_2 phases (Nakamura et al 1984).

With regard to positional fate of resting and proliferating hepatocytes within a lobule, it has been proposed that these cells, like littoral cells, may continuously 'stream' from the portal tracts towards the terminal hepatic veins along puta-tive trajectories averaged as a 'tissue radius.' According to this view, cells become older as a function of their position away from their postulated periportal origin, and it has been estimated that the portofugal shift occurs at a speed of about 2 mm per day (Schwartz-Arad et al 1989). Concomitantly, the ploidy of hepatocyte nuclei appears to increase, as older cells tend to accumulate DNA rather than to divide (Zajicek et al 1989), resulting in some sort of DNA 'amplification' in lobular zones 1 and 2, but a subse-quent 'deamplification' and reduction in ploidy in lobular zone 3 (Zajicek & Schwartz-Arad 1990). Hence DNA syn-thesis is not equal to cell production, and considerable frac-tions of newly formed DNA may be stored in polyploid hepatocytes, of which four categories are identified, one being characterized by a binuclear and octoploid phenotype (Papa et al 1987).

In a regenerative response reaction, rat hepatocytes appear to proliferate continuously, offspring cells may then enter the next DNA synthesis cycle, with another temporal gap (G_1, 6–8 h) between a previous mitosis and the next S phase. Restoration of liver mass to preoperative levels will take about 2 weeks in the rat after two-thirds hepatectomy.

Even though, under resting conditions, the majority of hepatocytes in cycle are located in lobular zone 1, partial hepatectomy is followed by an influx of cells into S phase which reveals a spatial maximum in the lobular areas imme-diately adjacent to the portal tracts (Rabes et al 1976). Maximum influx into S phase is found here at 34 h but in the perivenous parts of the lobule at 40 h. Thus, some sort of a spatial gradient (or wave) is observed, the causes of which are still not clearly known. However, construction of

overall lobular gradients and of gradients on a still smaller scale may be related to uncoupling of intercellular junctions, which occurs in an asynchronous way as well (Meyer et al 1981). It has been shown that gap junction-mediated coupling of hepatocytes, which is extensive in the quiescent hepatocyte population under normal resting conditions is markedly reduced during regeneration (Traub et al 1983). Decoupling asynchrony or heterogeneity may play a role in the formation of microgradients of intercellular signaling substances, and in the production of still hypothetical signal waves, whereas a closing of junctions (i.e. coupling) may prevent signal dissipation, leading to a highly efficient regulatory system. One candidate of a signal making part of coupling-mediated microcircuits may be $5',5''-p^1,p^4$-tetraphosphate (Ap_4A), a nucleotide which seems to act as a ligand for DNA polymerase alpha and as a primer for DNA synthesis (Yamaguchi et al 1985). The intracellular concen-tration of Ap_4A is inversely related to cellular doubling time and correlated positively with hepatic regenerative capacity.

MOLECULAR MECHANISMS OF LIVER REGENERATION

Understanding the molecular mechanisms that regulate liver regeneration is of enormous scientific and clinical importance. The analysis of these mechanisms is intimately linked to efforts to understand cell cycle regulation in com-plex mammalian organs and regulation defects that may cause neoplasia. There is an urgent need for clinical thera-pies that would enhance regulated hepatocyte replication in acute liver failure, in liver transplantation (i.e. 'small-for-size transplants,' split transplants, living donor partial hepatec-tomy and transplants) as well as in cell and gene therapy strategies that require cell proliferation. Most of our knowl-edge about the molecular mechanisms that regulate hepatic growth derive from experimental studies of liver regenera-tion induced by either partial hepatectomy (removal of 68% of the liver in rats and slightly less in mice) or acute chemi-cal injury (carbon tetrachloride being the most common agent) (Grisham 1962, Wright & Alison 1984, Bucher 1995). There is every reason to believe that the conclusions reached in studies involving these experimental models are applicable to humans with only small variations.

Liver regeneration after partial hepatectomy is a growth response that culminates in hepatocyte replication. This process has several important biological characteristics: (a) it is a process of compensatory hyperplasia rather than true regeneration in that removed parts do not grow back but instead the liver remnant increases in mass; (b) the process depends on the replication of differentiated hepato-cytes (diploid, tetraploid, even octoploid cells) and does not involve precursor ('stem cells') cells or oval cells; (c) replication of hepatocytes proceeds in a synchronous wave and is followed (approximately 1 day later) by replication of non-parenchymal cells; (d) growth terminates when liver mass reaches normal values, within about ±10% of the original liver mass.

Because DNA replication in hepatocytes is a synchronized process and is preceded by a prereplicative stage (12–14 h in rats, 24–30 h in mice) it has been possible to map out the major events of cell-cycle activation and replication in hepatocytes during liver regeneration. During the last few years the major focus of these studies has been: (a) the analysis of the expression of proto-oncogenes and growth factors, (b) the activation of cell-replication-related transcription factors, and more recently; (c) the role of cytokines, mainly tumor necrosis factor (TNF) and Interleukin-6 (IL-6). It is likely that in the near future new emphasis will be given to studies involving oxygen free radicals, adhesion molecules and protease activation at the initiation of liver regeneration. The molecular analysis of liver regeneration has been greatly aided by the development of genetically modified mice which overexpress a specific gene (transgenic mice) or have a specific gene deleted or inactivated (knockout mice). Important transgenic models have included the generation of mice that overexpress growth factors (TGF-α and hepatocyle growth factor (HGF)), proto-oncogenes and cell-cycle genes (c-myc,

p21) and knockout mice with functional deletions of TNF receptors, IL-6 and inducible nitric oxide synthase, among others (Fausto et al 1995, Diehl & Rai 1996, Pistoi & Morello 1996, Taub 1996). Some knockout mice that lack genes of importance for liver regeneration die during the embryonic period. The most interesting examples are mice that lack HGF, c-jun knockout mice, epidermal growth factor receptor (EGFR) knockout mice, which die either prenatally or a week or so postnatally (Miettinen et al 1995, Sibilia & Wagner 1995, Threadgill et al 1995), and mice lacking the p65 component of the transcription factor NFκ (see below) which die with massive hepatic apoptosis at 14–16 day of embryonic development (Beg et al 1995, Beg & Baltimore 1996).

Gene expression during liver regeneration: proto-oncogenes and growth factors

Gene expression during liver regeneration can be divided into several phases (Fig. 3.2). The immediate early gene phase consists of the expression of transcriptionally regulated genes that do not require protein synthesis for activation. They can respond rapidly to mitogenic stimuli but their expression is generally short-lived. The first described members of immediate early genes were the proto-oncogenes c-fos, c-jun and c-myc (Thompson et al 1986). Detailed studies involving subtraction hybridization tech-

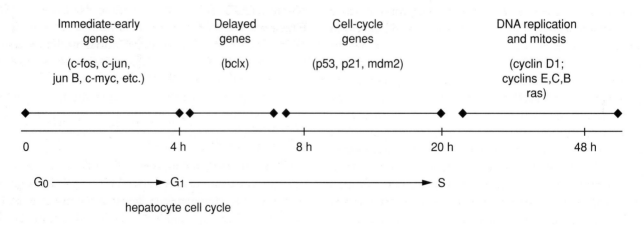

Fig. 3.2 Sequence of gene activation in the regenerating liver. The figure illustrates the various phases of gene activation during liver regeneration after partial hepatectomy. The times of expression for the various genes is approximate and represents the response to partial hepatectomy in rats. The first phase in which immediate-early genes are expressed involves 70 or more genes and includes proto-oncogenes, transcription factors, adhesion molecules, proteases among other. Among delayed-immediate genes in the antiapoptotic gene bclx. In the regenerating liver, activators of the cell cycle such as mdm2 and cyclin D1 as well as cell-cycle inhibitor genes such as p53 and p21 are expressed transiently. Cyclin D1 may be an important gene connecting cell cycle progression with DNA replication in hepatocytes.

niques have now demonstrated that almost 70 genes may be involved in this process (Mohn et al 1991, Haber et al 1993, Diamond et al 1994). An issue of major interest is to determine which among these genes is essential for hepatocyte replication. Among immediate delayed genes (Fig. 3.2), an interesting component is bcl-X (Kren et al 1995, Tzung et al 1997), an antiapoptotic gene present in hepatocytes (in the liver bcl-2, the major antiapoptotic gene in most other tissues) is expressed mostly in biliary cells rather than hepatocytes (Fig. 3.2). The expression of cell cycle genes at the G_1 phase of the cell-cycle (Thompson et al 1986, Albrecht et al 1993, Loyer et al 1994, Trembley et al 1994, Fan et al 1995, Kren & Steer 1996, Loyer et al 1996, Timchenko et al 1996) during liver regeneration is characterized by the expression of both cell cycle stimulators (mdm2, cyclin D1) as well as inhibitors of the cell cycle (p53, p21). Expression of these genes is sequential and transient. This pattern of expression is probably a key element that regulates and self-limits the growth process.

Several growth factors including HGF, EGF, TGF-α, acidic fibroblast growth factor, heparin binding EGF and keratinocyte growth factor are capable of stimulating DNA replication of hepatocytes in primary cultures (Fausto & Webber 1994, Bucher 1995, Michalopoulos & DeFrances 1997). Among these, HGF and TGF-α are the most important ones and are associated with regenerative processes in vivo. HGF (also known as Scatter Factor) has a characteristic kringle-containing structure similar to that of plasminogen. It increases in the blood very rapidly after partial hepatectomy and is produced by non-parenchymal liver cells several hours later (Matsumoto & Nakamura 1992, Zarneagar & Michalopoulos 1995). This peptide is found in precursor (single chain, unable-to-bind receptors) or active form (2-chain peptide) in the blood, but it is still uncertain what are the proportions of circulating active and inactive HGF (Arakaki et al 1995). In addition to its mitogenic properties of hepatocytes and many other cell types (epithelial, endothelial etc.) HGF has mitogenic and morphogenic activity (Matsumoto & Nakaaura 1992, Zarnegar & Michalopoulos 1995). In addition to its production in the liver, it is synthesized by mesenchymal cells of most tissues. Although it seem that HGF would be an attractive candidate to stimulate liver regeneration in clinical settings, caution should be raised because the amounts of HGF in the blood are greatly increased in acute liver failure and can be elevated in liver injury not involving regeneration (Gohda et al 1990, Tsubouchi et al 1991). An interesting possibility for modulating hepatocyte replication may be the modulation of signal transduction through the proto-oncogene c-met, the receptor for HGF.

TGF-α is produced by hepatocytes during development, regeneration and carcinogenesis (Webber et al 1994, Fausto et al 1995). Its receptor is EGFR, that is, the same receptor as EGF (Derynck 1992). TGF-α is found as a diffusable growth factor that acts in an autocrine way in hepatocytes or as a larger peptide precursor anchored in the plasma membrane. The anchored form is active and can bind to cells that contain EGFR (hepatocytes have an abundant amount of EGFR in their plasma membrane. The anchored form is active and can bind to cells that contain EGFR (hepatocytes have an abundant amount of EGFR in their plasma membrane). This type of bound ligand/receptor interaction induces both growth through the activation of EGFR signal transduction as well as cell adhesion by docking the 2 cells together ('juxtacrine' effect).

A major puzzle regarding the effects of HGF and TGF-α on hepatocyte replication is that while very efficient stimulators of DNA replication for hepatocytes in culture, their in vivo effects (directly infused into portal or mesenteric veins) is much less impressive (Liu et al 1994, Webber et al 1994, Webber et al 1998). Thus, while it is possible to obtain enhanced hepatocyte cell proliferation in hepatocytes of normal mice by in vivo HGF injection or infusion, the dosages needed are extremely high and administration of the factor has to be prolonged or repeated (Fujiwara et al 1993, Patijn et al 1998). The answer to this puzzle appears to be that hepatocytes need to be 'primed' to become competent to respond to these factors (Webber et al 1994, Webber et al 1998). Priming may represent the passage of quiescent hepatocytes from the G_0 (resting) phase to the cell cycle proper (G_1 phase). This phase corresponds to the activation of immediate early genes and is modulated by the activation of 4 transcription factors : NFκB, STAT3, AP1, and C/EBP (Cressman et al 1995, FitzGerald et al 1995, Soriano et al 1995, Diehl & Rai 1996, Taub 1996). All of these factors are important for liver regeneration and at least NFκB and STAT3 are required for normal regeneration.

The initiation of liver regeneration: transcription factors and cytokines

NFκB is a heterodimeric transcription factor which in the liver is formed by the p65 (also known as RelA) and p50 subunits (Baeuerle & Baltimore 1996, Ghosh et al 1998). The active factor (p65/p50) is activated within the first hour after partial hepatectomy and remains high for only 3–4 hours (Cressman et al 1994, FitzGerald et al 1995). Activation consists of the release of an inhibitor (IκB release requires its phosphorylation and degradation. Active NFκB migrates to the nucleus and binds to a large number of genes, which contain NFκB recognition sequences, initiating the transactivation of these genes. Target genes for NFκB include adhesion molecules, antiapoptotic genes, and cytokines among others (Baeuerle & Baltimore 1996, Ghosh et al 1998). The cytokine IL-6 is transactivated by NFκB and is in itself a potent stimulator of the transcription factor STAT3 (Libermann & Baltimore 1990). This factor is a member of the Stimulators of Transduction and Activator of Transcription family of genes, which transmit signals from the cell membrane directly into the nucleus (Heinrich et al 1998). Genes activated by STAT3 include cyclin D1 and probably other cell-cycle genes (Cressman et al 1996).

Studies by two groups of investigators using mice deficient for tumor necrosis factor receptor type 1 (TNFR1) or for IL-6 demonstrated that animals that lack either of these genes have a very high mortality after partial hepatectomy and that the survivors have deficient regeneration (Cressman et al 1996, Yamada et al 1997, Yamada & Fausto 1998, Yamada et al 1998). These studies were preceded by data showing that antibodies to TNF can inhibit liver regeneration (Akerman et al 1992, Diehl et al 1994) and that TNF is a potent activator of liver NFκB (FitzGerald et al 1995). Taken together these studies have established a sequence of events triggered by TNF by which liver regeneration can be initiated:

$$TNF \rightarrow TNFR1 \rightarrow NF\kappa B \rightarrow IL\text{-}6 \rightarrow STAT3 \rightarrow cyclin\ D1...$$
$$DNA\ replication$$

It has also been established that: (a) both TNF and IL-6 rise very rapidly but transiently in the liver and blood after partial hepatectomy (Akerman et al 1992, Trautwein et al 1996, Yamada et al 1997, Yamada et al 1998); (b) the mitogenic activity of TNF is signaled through type 1 but not type 2 TNF receptors (Yamada et al 1997, Yamada & Fausto 1998, Yamada et al 1998); (c) the mortality of mice that lack either TNFR1 or IL-6 is associated with extensive lipid accumulation in hepatocytes (Cressman et al 1996, Yamada et al 1997, Yamada et al 1998); (d) a single IL-6 injection before partial hepatectomy is capable of restoring normal liver regeneration to TNFR1 or IL-6 knockout mice; (e) IL-6 injection in either TNFR1 or IL-6 knockout mice causes STAT3 binding which is not detectable in these animals after partial hepatectomy (Cressman et al 1996, Yamada et al 1997). Recent data have shown that inducible nitric oxide synthase (iNOS) is an important hepatoprotective factor during liver regeneration (Rai et al 1998). Mice that lack a functional iNOS gene have deficient regeneration associated with activation of caspase 3, hepatocyte apoptosis and liver failure. In these animals induction of TNF and IL-

6 as well as activation of NFκB and STAT3 after partial hepatectomy are not altered. It is then plausible that nitric oxide may function to protect hepatocytes against the potential toxic effect TNF (Rai et al 1998).

Conclusions and prospects

Although chapters on liver regeneration usually state that the mechanisms that initiate liver regeneration are unknown, much knowledge has been gained about these mechanisms and new information is rapidly accumulating. It is probably more accurate to say that the mechanisms that initiate liver regeneration are being identified. The separation of events into a priming phase, which is necessary but not sufficient for hepatocyte replication, and a cell-cycle progression phase provides a useful context in which to place these studies. The priming response involving the cytokines TNF and IL-6 make hepatocytes capable of responding to growth factors (HGF, TGF-α). Growth factors make cells progress through the cell cycle and replicate (Fig. 3.3). This sequence of events is strengthened by the recent demonstration that TNF greatly potentiates the effects of growth factors on hepatocyte replication in vivo (Webber et al 1998). Genetically altered mouse models have provided key insights into the process of liver regeneration and progress is bound to increase steadily with the development of new mice strains deficient in proto-oncogenes, growth factors, transcription factors, cytokines and

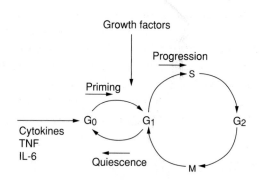

Fig. 3.3 Multistep model of liver regeneration. The figure indicates that hepatocyte replication requires 2 steps: priming and progression. In the priming phase, the transcription factors NFκB and STAT3 are activated by posttranslation mechanisms. These and other transcription factors (AP1 and C/EBP) participate in the activation of immediate-early genes, and make hepatocytes sensitive to the effect of growth factors such as HGF and TGF-α. The growth factors are necessary to make hepatocytes progress through the cell cycle and replicate. The priming phase is mediated by the cytokines TNF and IL-6 also with the involvement of nitric oxide. The priming phase is necessary but not sufficient for DNA replication and may be reversible.

proteases, which are important for liver regeneration. Clinical application of these findings will become even more feasible as this work progresses.

ATROPHY

ETIOLOGY

Many cases of lobar or segmental liver atrophy have been reported in association with primary hepatocellular disease, predominantly cirrhosis (Ham 1979), affecting the entire liver and, therefore, of little surgical significance since the disease process is by definition irreversible. Furthermore, the atrophy–hypertrophy complex is usually absent in these cases.

The most common causes of the atrophy–hypertrophy complex encountered in surgical practice are bile duct obstruction or portal venous occlusion, or both, to the atrophied area (Braasch et al 1972, Longmire & Tompkins 1975, Bismuth & Malt 1979, Takayasu et al 1986, Hadjis et al 1986b, 1989). Other causes include occlusion of the hepatic veins (Meyer 1950, Galloway et al 1973) and space-occupying hepatic lesions, notably hydatid disease and hepatocellular carcinoma, compressing or invading vascular channels from without (Hueston 1953, Lorigan et al 1988, Ham 1990). In one series, 78 cases of liver atrophy seen by Hadjis et al (1994) over a period of 8 years, 64 had biliary obstruction in association with benign or malignant bile duct strictures. Specifically, the incidence of atrophy in this review of 235 patients with hilar cholangiocarcinoma was 23%, with about half of the patients with atrophy having concomitant ipsilateral portal venous occlusion. Similar figures have been reported from other centers with a special interest in the subject (Nesbit et al 1988, Ham 1990). In Hadjis' series (1994) and that of Bismuth (1982), post-cholecystectomy bile duct strictures head the list of benign causes, with an incidence of atrophy of 10 to 15% (Fig. 3.4).

PATHOGENESIS

Although the concept that obliteration of individual branches of the portal vein induces atrophy of the corresponding parts of the hepatic parenchyma ('portal atrophy') was discussed as early as 1858 (Frerichs 1861), the matter remained in dispute until the classical experimental work of Rous and Larimore (1920a). Others, subsequently, have confirmed the invariable liver atrophy associated with deprivation of portal blood flow in many species (Schalm et al 1956, Steiner & Martines Batiz 1961, Starzl et al 1976,

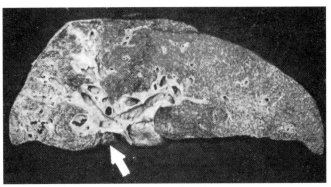

(A)

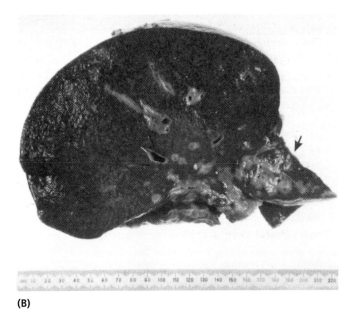

(B)

Fig. 3.4 (A) Coronal section of a liver specimen from a patient with benign duct stricture who died of liver failure. There is gross atrophy of the right liver (arrow), with evident fibrosis, and marked left liver hypertrophy. **(B)** Coronal section of a liver specimen from a patient with hilar cholangiocarcinoma, showing marked left lobe atrophy (arrow) and compensatory enlargement of the right lobe.

Putnam et al 1976). Regarding its pathogenesis, the consensus is that portal blood controls hepatocyte size, and the lack of it results in loss of hepatocyte cytoplasmic mass (Rous & Larimore 1920a, Weinbren 1964, Weinbren & Tarsh 1964, Starzl et al 1976, Dubuisson et al 1982a) by mechanisms as not yet fully defined (Cole et al 1971, Pfeifer 1978, 1982). Some investigators have shown ligation of the portal vein to be associated with hepatocyte necrosis (Steiner & Martines Batiz 1962, Kerr 1971, Rozga et al 1985), but the contribution of that process to the striking reduction in lobe size observed after portal venous ligation is likely to be, if anything, very limited.

In contrast to the predictable response of portal venous occlusion, the magnitude of the response to bile duct obstruction differs substantially among species (Harley & Barratt 1901, McMaster & Rous 1921, Stewart et al 1937, Steiner & Martines Batiz 1961, Braasch et al 1972), and this has been attributed to the variation in bile production (Rous & Larimore 1920b). The pathogenesis of liver atrophy after biliary obstruction ('biliary atrophy'), was first studied experimentally by Nasse (1894) and later by Harley and Barratt (1901), Rous and Larimore (1920b) and McMaster and Rous (1921). Benz et al (1952) reported seven cases of left lobe atrophy secondary to bile duct obstruction and considered, on the limited anatomical evidence, that this was effected by compression of the long, slender left branch of the portal vein by the dilated left hepatic duct. They reasoned that this accounted for the more common involvement of the left lobe, at least with biliary atrophy. However, Hadjis et al (1994) found that right and left lobe atrophy occurs with equal frequency. Moreover, in 15 cases of left lobe atrophy, with angiographic information, no vascular compression was observed that was unaccountable by direct tumor involvement.

Rous and Larimore (1920b) postulated that biliary atrophy was mediated by deflection of the portal venous stream consequent upon the increased intrabiliary pressure. Experimental data on atrophy after biliary obstruction suggest a reduction in the number of hepatocytes and atrophy of the hepatic lobules (Harley & Barratt 1901, Swanson et al 1967, Johnstone & Lee 1976), but a decrease in the size of individual hepatocytes, that would have to be present if reduced portal blood flow were an important factor in the pathogenesis of biliary atrophy, is less well-documented. Hadjis and Keith (1992) have tested the hypothesis of Roux and Larimore in an experimental model in the rabbit by constructing a totally diverting portacaval shunt and synchronously ligating a segmental duct draining 80% of the liver. Biliary atrophy developed to a degree comparable with that observed in the presence of intact portal flow. It seems that segmental duct obstruction exerts its deleterious effect directly.

ATROPHY AS A STIMULUS FOR COMPENSATORY HYPERTROPHY

Portal vein occlusion results in atrophy of the affected hepatocytes and striking hyperplasia of cells enjoying an intact portal flow. The compensatory cellular proliferation initiated by atrophied hepatocytes is reproducible and comparable in time and intensity with the adaptive DNA synthetic response observed after liver resection (Weinbren & Tarsh 1964). Although striking structural changes have been

described in hepatocytes deprived of portal blood, among them depletion of the rough endoplasmic reticulum and reduction in the membrane-bound polyribosomes (Putnam et al 1976, Starzl et al 1976), the mechanism by which atrophy initiates compensatory hepatic DNA synthesis is unclear. Since there is no significant reduction in total DNA in the lobes deprived of portal flow, it has been postulated that the regeneration of the mitotic stimulus does not depend on reduced nuclear material but that it is likely that a cytoplasmic component, within the atrophying hepatocyte, is involved in the production of the initiating signal that results in DNA synthesis (Weinbren & Tarsh 1964). Unlike the hepatocytes, the Kupffer cells appear not to be affected by portoprivation either in number or function (Dubuisson et al 1982a,b, Edgcomb et al 1982).

Bile duct obstruction may also result in similar morphological changes in the liver. The effects of prohibition of bile flow depend on the level of obstruction. Obstruction below the confluence of the hepatic ducts results in enlargement of the entire liver. By contrast, lobar or segmental duct obstruction leads, like portal venous occlusion, to atrophy of the affected liver and compensatory hyperplasia of the remaining parenchyma with unimpaired bile drainage (Rous & Larimore 1920b, Ogawa et al 1960, Braasch et al 1972, Longmire & Tompkins 1975). However, hepatocyte loss rather than hepatocyte atrophy occurs. The microscopic picture of biliary atrophy, unlike portal atrophy, includes ductular proliferation and periportal fibrosis with expansion of the portal tracts and destruction of adjacent liver cells (Rous & Larimore 1920b, Weinbren et al 1985). The remaining hepatocytes may show variable degrees of atrophy, but in general the size of the hepatocytes does not correlate with the degree of lobar atrophy (Benz et al 1952). Indeed, in a morphometric study of biliary atrophy, there was no statistically significant difference in the hepatocyte size between the atrophied and hypertrophied lobes (Hadjis et al 1991). Hadjis & Keith (1991) have compared, in an experimental model in the rabbit, the pathophysiological sequelae after segmental portal venous occlusion or bile duct obstruction, to 80% of the liver. Both procedures induce significant liver atrophy and compensatory hyperplasia that are of comparable magnitude; liver function, which is initially deranged, is fully restored, without the development of portal hypertension in either group.

The *clinical situation*, however, is often more complex. Lobar biliary atrophy can be asymptomatic until such time as the contralateral hepatic duct also becomes obstructed. With the two lobes sequentially obstructed and 'disadvantaged' (Schalm et al 1956), the loss of hepatocytes consequent to the expanding portal tracts generates the stimulus for compensatory hyperplasia that affects the hepatocytes of both lobes. Given time, the hepatocytes of the atrophied lobe as well as those of the contralateral lobe become hyperplastic, even if the former cells were previously atrophied (Weinbren et al 1985). The microscopic picture confirms experimental data that bile duct obstruction does not inhibit hepatocyte proliferation (Weinbren 1953, Swanson et al 1967), and supports existing experimental evidence that hepatocyte protein synthesis controlling atrophy or hypertrophy and DNA synthesis leading to hyperplasia are independent processes, i.e. atrophic hepatocytes can also be hyperplastic (Fisher et al 1962, Sigel et al 1967, Weinbren et al 1972, Starzl et al 1976, Weinbren 1982).

Clinical aspects of atrophy/hypertrophy complex

The clinical presentation depends on the underlying cause of atrophy. Most patients with lobar atrophy associated with bile duct obstruction present with jaundice. The shortest interval that we have encountered between the time a bile duct injury was recorded and the subsequent diagnosis of atrophy is 1 year. However, this is likely to be an overestimate of the time required for atrophy to develop since its prompt diagnosis is an unusual event. In our experience, unless one is aware of its existence, lobar atrophy may be missed even at operation. Of the laboratory tests, the serum alkaline phosphatase is of interest. Although the enzyme is invariably raised in the presence of obstructive jaundice, anicteric patients with unilateral hepatic duct obstruction show an early rise (an important diagnostic feature), but as atrophy is gradually established serum enzyme levels return to normal values (Hadjis et al 1990).

With malignant obstruction, lobar atrophy is commonly associated with a neoplasm arising in one hepatic duct (Ch. 54). This results in atrophy of the affected liver, although the patient may remain asymptomatic or with non-specific constitutional complaints. In time, the tumor grows into the contralateral duct leading to the development of jaundice (Marshall 1932). Although the incidence of lobar atrophy (indicating initial unilateral hepatic duct obstruction) in hilar cholangiocarcinoma is about 25% (Carr et al 1985, Nesbit et al 1988, Ham 1990), only two of 116 patients with this disease studied by the authors were diagnosed during the anicteric phase when the tumor was limited to one hepatic duct, and in both cases the lesions were resected (Hadjis et al 1987). It is conceivable that an awareness of lobar atrophy as a feature of hilar biliary obstruction might result in earlier diagnosis and a higher resectability rate of neoplastic lesions.

Inadvertent damage to a bile duct, be it sectoral or lobar, during biliary operations is the most common cause of atrophy in patients with benign biliary disease (Ch. 49).

However, where recurrent pyogenic cholangitis is prevalent, intrahepatic stones are just as important a cause (Chen et al 1984, Fan et al 1990). Reconstructive surgery at the hilum may be followed by atrophy if anastomotic repair is complicated by recurrent, fibrous stenosis of one or other hepatic duct. Atrophy may also complicate a particular surgical procedure. Hadjis et al (1994) reported that six of 22 patients with postcholecystectomy bile duct stricture reoperated on after a previous mucosal-graft procedure (Ch. 49) were found to have gross lobar atrophy. On the other hand, of 48 patients with a stricture of the same cause who had not been treated by this procedure, only five were found to have atrophy. The number of previous explorations was similar in the two groups. It is possible that the pulling up of the jejunal loop into the liver obstructs side ducts leading to atrophy. Lobar atrophy consequent on portal venous occlusion may be asymptomatic, for example, after injury to the portal vein during cholecystectomy (Blumgart et al 1984), or the patient may complain of symptoms associated with a space-occupying hepatic lesion that is obstructing a branch of the portal vein causing atrophy.

Liver atrophy as part of the atrophy–hypertrophy complex is associated with particular diagnostic problems which may be clinical or radiological. Of 48 cases with the atrophy/hypertrophy complex, ten presented with a palpable abdominal mass: seven in the epigastrium, the result of right lobe atrophy with compensatory enlargement of the left lobe producing a 'mass' effect, and three below the right hypochondrium indicating the obverse (Hadjis et al 1986b). Three of the 'masses' were thought on referral to be neoplastic. It is important that patients with a history of jaundice and previous biliary surgery presenting with an epigastric or right subcostal mass are investigated with the possibility in mind that this may be the result of lobar hypertrophy. This mass effect in not unique to biliary atrophy; portal venous obstruction, hepatic venous occlusion, and ischemic liver necrosis may all lead to and present as an undiagnosed abdominal mass (Tsuzuki et al 1973, Hadjis et al 1986b). In most cases of Budd–Chiari syndrome both lobes are affected, so that the compensatory enlargement of the caudate lobe (Rensing et al 1984), which drains directly into the inferior vena cava (Tavill et al 1975), can be mistaken for a liver tumor (Wilkinson & Sherlock 1984) (Fig. 3.5). If one of the main hepatic veins remains patent, disparity develops between the right and left liver (Meyer 1950, Galloway et al 1973). It is noteworthy that the palpable mass in liver atrophy represents the functionally competent or least impaired hepatic parenchyma.

Further diagnostic confusion can result from gross hypertrophy of the left liver misinterpreted as splenomegaly and from the appearance of a radioisotope liver scan obtained to inves-

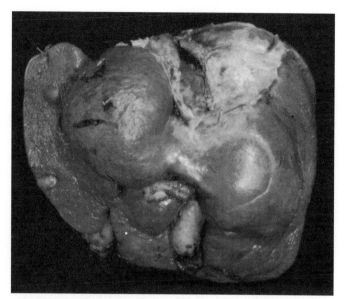

Fig. 3.5 Gross liver specimen of a patient with Budd–Chiari syndrome. The right and left lobes are small; the caudate lobe is grossly hypertrophied.

tigate suspected hepatobiliary disease or an abdominal mass. Depending on the degree that hepatocytes and Kupffer cells have been replaced by periportal fibrosis, the atrophied lobe or segment may imitate a 'cold' area on the scan and be erroneously interpreted as a space-occupying lesion with metastases (mass) (Ham 1979, Makler et al 1980, Hadjis et al 1986b).

RADIOLOGICAL DIAGNOSIS OF ATROPHY

The diagnosis of liver atrophy can be made preoperatively by several radiological modalities, a reduction in lobe size being the common finding. Computed tomography (CT) scanning (Ch. 15) is probably the best single non-invasive investigation in revealing atrophy, particularly left liver atrophy (Carr et al 1985) (Fig. 3.6A–C). It is less accurate in the diagnosis of right liver atrophy, but this should always be suspected whenever there is marked left-sided hypertrophy. Since the line between the gallbladder fossa and the inferior vena cava demarcates the left from the right liver, atrophy of the right liver is likely to be missed in rare cases where the

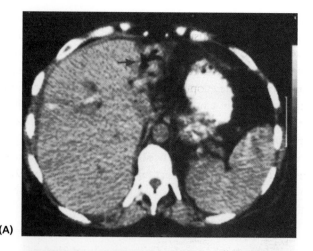

(A)

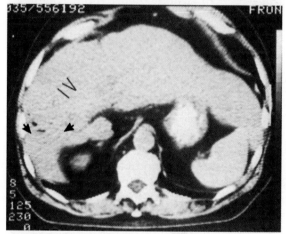

(B)

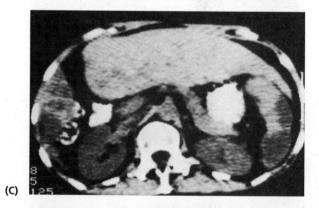

(C)

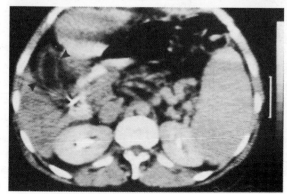

(D)

Fig. 3.6 (A) Computerized tomography (CT) scan illustrating gross atrophy of the left lobe with dilated ducts (arrow), in a patient with postcholecystectomy bile duct stricture. **(B)** CT scan showing marked right liver atrophy and considerable hypertrophy of segment IV and the left lobe, in a patient with benign stricture of the right hepatic duct. **(C)** CT appearance of gross hypertrophy of the left lobe in a patient with right liver atrophy due to occlusion of the right branch of the portal vein by hepatocellular carcinoma. **(D)** CT scan of a patient with left-sided gallbladder and a very small right liver. The quadrate lobe (segment IV) and the left lobe, on either side of the gallbladder (arrow), were misinterpreted to be the right and left liver.

gallbladder is attached to the left liver (Fig. 3.6D). Segmental atrophy is usually indicated by a concave change in the outline of the liver over the affected segment. Finally, the altered anatomical relations of the hilar structures consequent on the development of the atrophy/hypertrophy complex can be shown on CT.

Percutaneous cholangiography (PTC) (Ch. 17) is complementary to CT scanning. The intrahepatic ducts of the affected lobe appear crowded together and may or may not be dilated even in the presence of obstruction (Ham 1979,

Myracle et al 1981; Hadjis et al 1986) (Fig. 3.7A). Percutaneous cholangiography is more sensitive than CT in showing segmental and right liver atrophy provided that all ducts have been outlined (Fig. 3.7B,C). The hypertrophied lobe extends across the midline, and the relevant hepatic duct may or may not be obstructed. Angiography demonstrated tortuous vessels clustered together and provides information on the underlying cause of atrophy (Ham 1979) (Fig. 3.8). Ultrasonography does have the potential of accurately diagnosing every case of lobar atrophy and it can point to its cause.

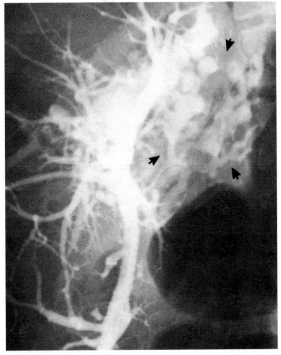

(A)

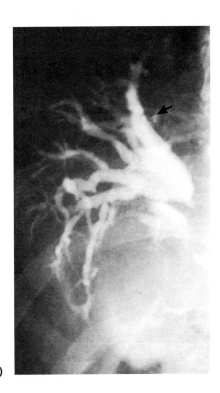

(B)

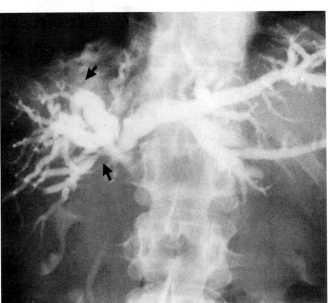

(C)

Fig. 3.7 (A) Percutaneous cholangiogram of a patient with hilar cholangiocarcinoma showing crowding of the intrahepatic ducts in the left lobe (arrow) indicative of atrophy. The right lobe is enlarged. **(B)** Percutaneous cholangiogram of the right hepatic ductal system. The superior ducts are crowded (arrow), a sign consistent with segmental atrophy. **(C)** Percutaneous cholangiogram of a patient with hilar cholangiocarcinoma. Gross atrophy of the right liver is indicated by the crowding of the intrahepatic ducts (arrows). There is hypertrophy of the left liver.

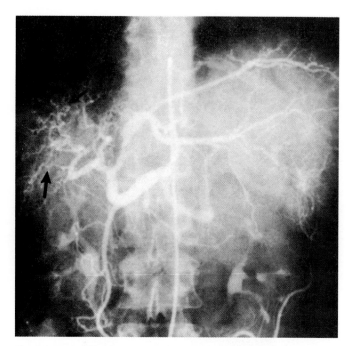

Fig. 3.8 Typical angiographic appearance of atrophy (same case as in Fig. 3.7C). Note the crowded, tortuous arteries in the right liver (arrows); there is evident hypertrophy of the left liver with enlarged arteries.

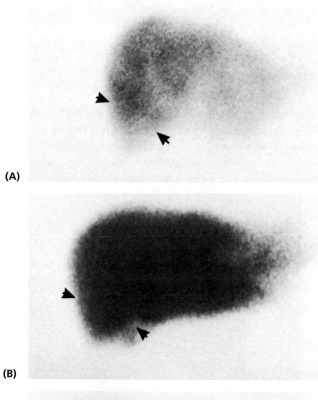

(A)

(B)

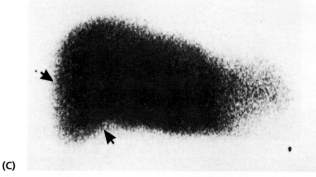

(C)

Fig. 3.9 Patient with postcholecystectomy stricture of the common hepatic duct and occlusion of the right branch of the portal vein, shown angiographically. **(A)** HIDA scan before repair of the stricture. There is reduced uptake of the radionuclide by the whole liver. The right liver appears to be small (arrows). **(B)** HIDA scan 6 months after repair of the stricture. The right liver remains small (arrows), but the uptake is normal. The left liver is hypertrophied. **(C)** Sulphur colloid scan showing normal function of the atrophied right liver (arrows).

Liver scintigraphy (Ch. 14) contributes significantly to the diagnosis of liver atrophy. The uptake curve of a HIDA scan gives an indication of parenchymal dysfunction. Based on experimental evidence that portoprivation is compatible with normal uptake of HIDA and colloid preparation by hepatocytes and Kupffer cells respectively, and given the pronounced destruction of hepatocytes and Kupffer cells common to atrophy, consequent on biliary obstruction but absent in atrophy associated with portoprivation, Hadjis et al (1994) used a combination of HIDA and colloid scans to differentiate the two conditions. As would have been predicted, a small lobe with normal uptake of both radionuclides is indicative of portal atrophy (Fig. 3.9). By contrast, the scintigraphy picture of biliary atrophy reflects the variable degree of hepatocyte and Kupffer cell replacement by proliferating ductular cells and fibrosis. Reduced, patchy uptake of both HIDA and colloid characterizes cases of moderate severity (Fig. 3.10), but with marked fibrosis there may be no uptake at all (Ham 1979, Makler et al 1980) (Figs 3.11 and 3.12). With ipsilateral occlusion of the portal vein as well as the bile duct, the scintigraphic findings are those of bilary atrophy.

SURGICAL IMPLICATIONS

The management of patients with liver lobe disparity consequent on atrophy, as exemplified by the atrophy/ hypertrophy complex, calls for an understanding of the anatomical and functional changes associated with this condition. An appreciation of these changes is particularly important whenever operation is required to relieve symptoms usually related to bile duct disease.

The surgical problems relate to the functional reserve of the atrophied liver are enhanced by poor access to the ducts. Although 30% of normal parenchyma is compatible with

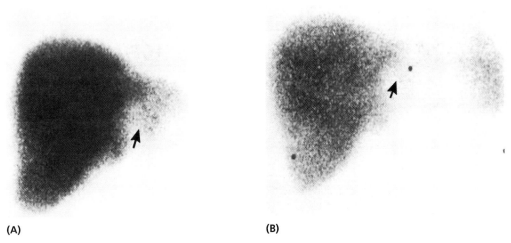

(A) **(B)**

Fig. 3.10 Patient with hilar cholangiocarcinoma and left lobe atrophy. Note the reduced uptake of the tracer in **(A)** the HIDA scan (arrow) and **(B)** the colloid scan (arrow).

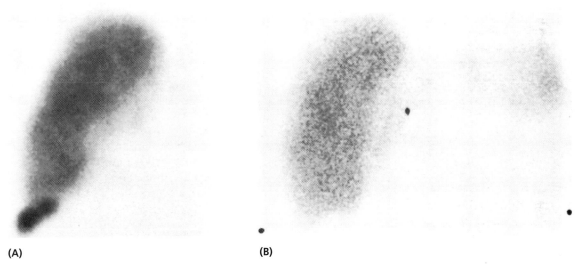

(A) **(B)**

Fig. 3.11 Patient with hilar cholangiocarcinoma and left lobe atrophy. There is no radionuclide uptake by the atrophied lobe in either **(A)** the HIDA scan or **(B)** the colloid scan.

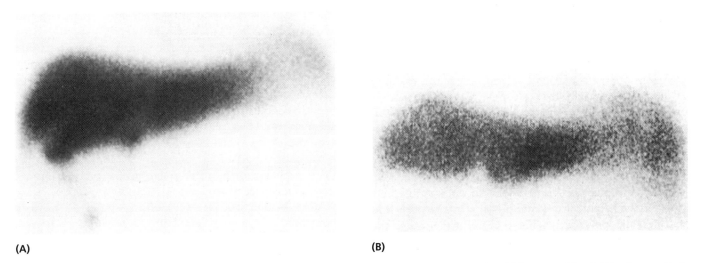

(A) **(B)**

Fig. 3.12 Patient with right liver atrophy due to benign stricture of the right hepatic duct. There is no uptake of **(A)** HIDA or **(B)** colloid by the atrophied liver. Segment IV and the left lobe are markedly hypertrophic.

normal serum bilirubin (Bismuth & Malt 1979), the functional capacity of an atrophied lobe to relieve jaundice after drainage is doubtful. Likewise, the presence of lobar atrophy precludes resection of an otherwise resectable lesion sited in the contralateral lobe and requiring lobectomy. The functional results of biliary decompression of atrophied lobes experimentally and by doing HIDA and colloid scans before and after surgery has been studied. Unequivocally, relief of segmental ductal obstruction does not reverse the process of atrophy; the affected liver continues to atrophy in the absence of obstruction (Fig. 3.13). Drainage of an atrophied lobe associated with ipsilateral portal venous occlusion and obstruction below the confluence of the hepatic ducts may increase its functional capacity (Fig. 3.9).

Operative difficulties emanate from the distorted configuration of the liver and the tendency of the hypertrophying lobe to rotate and extend across the midline, particularly with right liver atrophy (Ch. 49). Vessels and ducts conform to this spatial lobar rearrangement with the following consequences: (1) the portal vein lies more superficially and is at risk of being injured; (2) the portal venous branches develop an anterior relation to the bile duct, making access to these ducts exceedingly difficult. In effect, the hilar structures come to course obliquely upwards; the hepatic artery and portal vein anteriorly and the bile duct posteriorly (Fig. 3.14). Furthermore, the atrophied right liver tends to be hidden high and posteriorly under the costal margin, hampering mobilization while the convex edge of the hypertrophied left liver extends forwards and downwards in an overhanging fashion with the hilar structures obscured beneath it. Similar anatomical changes in the vascular and ductal channels occur after partial hepatectomy, and any future approach, for example, to correct a post-traumatic bile duct stricture, will be confounded by the same problems of access.

In general, the primary pathology, whether benign or malignant, the site of atrophy, and the nature and severity of symptoms are the main factors determining the options of treatment. The demonstration of atrophy does not imply irresectability of a neoplastic lesion provided there is no

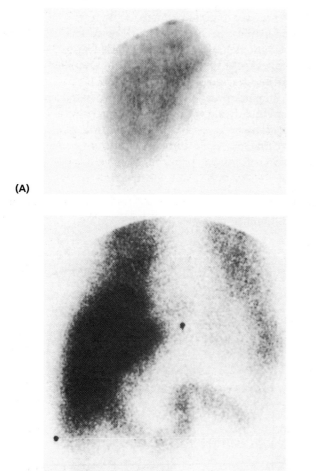

(A)

(C)

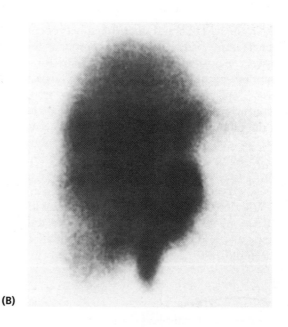

(B)

Fig. 3.13 Patient with postcholecystectomy high bile duct stricture and left lobe atrophy. **(A)** HIDA scan before repair of the stricture. The uptake by the right lobe is reduced. There is no function in the left lobe. **(B)** HIDA scan 18 months after repair of the stricture. The function of the right lobe has returned to normal, but the left lobe remains 'silent.' (The patency of the anastomosis was confirmed by cholangiography.) **(C)** Colloid scan confirming the findings on HIDA (HIDA tracer is present in the bowel).

Fig. 3.14 (A) Schematic drawing depicting normal anatomical relations of liver segments of vascular and ductal structures, with the common bile duct anterior to the portal vein. **(B)** Schematic representation of the altered relation of vessels and duct as seen with right liver atrophy/left liver hypertrophy. The rotation of the hilar structures has caused the portal vein to lie ventral to the duct.

vascular or second-order duct involvement in the contralateral lobe. With left liver hypertrophy associated with malignant obstruction, the options of palliation available include percutaneous, endoscopic or surgical intubation and formal anastomosis to the left ducts either by the round ligament or by a left intrahepatic hepaticojejunostomy. Access to the right ductal system is normally poor because of the short extrahepatic course of the right hepatic duct and anatomical inaccessibility of the segmental ducts; hypertrophy of the right lobe accentuates these problems. Intubation or intrahepatic hepaticojejunostomy to the right liver may be considered, although the latter procedure may not completely relieve symptoms where second-order ducts are involved or when a substantial part of the parenchyma drains into the left duct; such variations of drainage occur in about 30% of cases (Healey & Schroy 1953).

With benign disease, every effort should be made to construct a hilar mucosa-to-mucosa anastomosis because intrahepatic biliary–enteric anastomoses away from the hilum tend to have a higher rate of stricture recurrence. Interventional radiology has a place in the treatment of these patients, especially when combined with initial surgical repair (Czerniak et al 1986). Where atrophy is secondary to unilateral hepatic duct obstruction, and provided that the contralateral lobe functions normally, expectant therapy may be warranted (Hadjis et al 1986a). Episodes of cholangitis and pain should be treated with antibiotics and analgesics.

Finally, liver lobe disparity associated with biliary disease nearly always indicates hilar pathology. Preoperative diag-

nosis is important and should be precise in every case so that operative difficulties are anticipated and a clear plan of action is formulated. However, liver atrophy secondary to bile duct obstruction is usually indicative of advanced disease, diagnostic delay or therapeutic mismanagement. Therapy, whether curative or palliative, is usually complicated and good results are correspondingly difficult to obtain.

REFERENCES

Akerman P, Cote P, Yang S Q et al 1992 Antibodies to tumor necrosis factor-α inhibit liver regeneration after partial hepatectomy. American Journal of Physiology 263: G579–G585

Albrecht J H, Hoffman J, Kren B et al 1993 Cyclin and cyclin-dependent kinase 1 mRNA expression in models of regenerating liver and human liver diseases. American Journal of Physiology 265: G579–G585

Arakaki N, Kawakami K, Nakamura O et al 1995 Evidence of the presence of an inactive precursor of human hepatocyte growth factor in plasma and sera of patients with liver diseases. Hepatology 22: 1728: 1734

Baeuerle P and Baltimore D 1996 NF-κB: ten years after. Cell 87: 13–20

Baserga R 1974 Non-histone chromosomal proteins in normal and abnormal growth. Life Sciences 15: 1057–1071

Beg A A, Sha W C, Bronson R T et al 1995 Embryonic lethality and liver degeneration in mice lacking the RelA component of NF-κB. Nature 376: 167–170

Beg A A, Baltimore D 1996 An essential role for MF-κB in preventing TNF-alpha-induced cell death. Science 274: 782–784

Benz E J, Baggenstoss A H, Wollaeger E E 1952 Atrophy of the left lobe of the liver. Archives of Pathology 53: 315–330

Bismuth H, Malt RA 1979 Carcinoma of the biliary tract. New Engl Journal Med. 301: 704–706

Bismuth H 1982 Postoperative strictures of the bile duct. In: Blumgart L H (Ed.) The biliary tract, pp. 209–218. Edinburgh: Churchill Livingstone

Blumgart L H, Kelley C J, Benjamin I S 1984 Benign bile duct stricture following cholecystectomy: critical factors in management. British Journal of Surgery 71: 836–843

Bouwens L, Baekeland M, Wisse E 1984 Importance of local proliferation in the expanding Kupffer cell population of rat liver after zymogen stimulation and partial hepatectomy. Hepatology 4: 213–219

Braasch J W, Whitcomb F F, Watkins E, Maguire R R, Khazei A M 1972 Segmental obstruction of the bile duct. Surgery, Gynecology and Obstetrics 134: 915–920

Brues A M, Marble B B 1937 An analysis of mitosis in liver restoration. Journal of Experimental Medicine 65: 15–27

Bucher N L 1963 Regeneration of the mammalian liver. International Review of Cytology 15: 245

Bucher N L, Malt R A 1971 Regeneration of liver and kidney. Boston, Little, Brown and Co. pp 55–57

Bucher N L 1995 Liver regeneration: then and now. In: Jirtle R (Ed.) Liver Regeneration and Carcinogenesis: Molecular and Cellular Mechanisms, pp. 1–25. San Diego: Academic Press

Carr D, Hadjis N, Banks H L, Hemingway A, Blumgart L H 1985 Computed tomography of hilar cholangiocarcinoma. American Journal of Roentgenology 145: 53–56

Chen H H, Zhang W, Wang S S 1984 Twenty-two year experience with the diagnosis and treatment of intrahepatic calculi. Surgery, Gynecology and Obstetrics 159: 519–524

Cole S, Matter A, Karnovsky M 1971 Autophagic vacuoles in experimental atrophy. Experimental and Molecular Pathology 14: 158–175

Columbano A, Shinozuka H 1996 Liver regeneration versus direct hyperplasia. FASEB Journal 10: 1118–1128

Cressman D E, Greenbaum L E, Haber B A et al 1994 Rapid activation of post-hepatectomy factor/nuclear factor κB in hepatocytes, a primary response in regenerating liver. Journal of Biological Chemistry 269: 30429–30435

Cressman D E, Diamond R H, Taub R. 1995 Rapid activation of the Stat3 transcription complex in liver regeneration. Hepatology 21: 1443–1449

Cressman D E, Greenbaum L E, DeAngelis R A et al 1996 Liver failure and defective hepatocyte regeneration in interleukin-6-deficient mice. Science 274: 1379–1383

Czerniak A, Soreide O, Gibson R 1986 Liver atrophy complicating benign bile duct strictures. Surgical and interventional radiological approaches. American Journal of Surgery 152: 294–300

Derynck R 1992 The physiology of transforming growth factor-alpha. Advances in Cancer Research 58: 27–52

Diamond R H, Cressman D E, Laz T M et al 1994 PRL-1, a unique nuclear protein tyrosine phosphatase, affects cell growth. Molecular and Cellular Biology 14: 3752–3762

Diehl A M, Yin M, Fleckenstein J et al 1994 Tumor necrosis factor-alpha induces c-jun during the regenerative response to liver injury. American Journal of Physiology 267: G552–G561

Diehl A M, Rai R M 1996 Regulation of signal transduction during liver regeneration. FASEB Journal 10: 215–227

Dubuisson L, Bioulac P, Aric J, Balabaud C 1982a Hepatocyte ultrastructure in rats with portacaval shunt. Digestive Diseases & Sciences 27: 1003–1010

Dubuisson L, Bioulac-Sage P, Hemet J, Dubois J P, Balabaud C 1982b Ultrastructure of sinusoidal cells in rats with long term portacaval shunt. In: Knook DL and Wisse E (Eds.) Sinusoidal liver cells, pp. 109–116. Amsterdam: Elsevier

Edgcomb L, Knol J A, Strodel W E, Exkhauser F E 1982 Differential effects of portal diversion on hepatocyte function (HF) and hepatic reticuloendothelial cells (HRSE) activity in the dog. Journal of Surgical Research 33: 233–244

Fan G, Xu R, Wessendorf M W et al 1995 Modulation of retinoblastoma and retinoblastoma-related proteins in regenerating rat liver and primary hepatocytes. Cell Growth & Differentiation 6: 1463–1476

Fan S T, Choi T K, Chan F, Lai E, Wong J 1990 Role of computed tomography in the management of recurrent pyogenic cholangitis. Australian and New Zealand Journal of Surgery 60: 599–605

Fausto N 1991 Growth factors in liver development, regeneration and carcinogenesis. Prog.Growth.Factor.Res. 3: 219–234

Fausto N, Webber E M 1994 Liver regeneration. In: Arias I M, Boyer J L, Fausto N, Jakoby W, Schachter D, Hafritz D (eds.) The Liver Biology and Pathobiology, pp. 1059–1084. New York: Raven Press, Ltd

Fausto N, Laird A D, Webber E M 1995 Role of grown factors and cytokines in hepatic regeneration. FASEB Journal 9: 1527–1536

Fishback F C 1929 A morphologic study of regeneration of the liver after partial removal. Archives of Pathology 7: 955–977

Fisher B, Lee S, Fisher E, Saffer E 1962 Liver regeneration following portacaval shunt. Surgery 52: 88–102

FitzGerald M, Webber E, Donovan J R et al 1995 Rapid DNA binding by nuclear factor κB in hepatocytes at the start of liver regeneration. Cell Growth & Differentiation 6: 417–427

Francavilla A, Porter K A, Benichou J, Jones A F, Starzl T 1978 Liver regeneration in dogs: morphologic and chemical changes. Journal of Surgical Research 25: 409–419

Francavilla A, Ove P, Polimeno L 1994a Regulation of liver size and regeneration: importance in liver transplantation. Transplantation Proceedings 20: 494–497

Francavilla A, Zeng Q H, Polimeno L 1994b Small-for-size liver transplanted into larger recipient: a model of hepatic regeneration. Hepatology 19: 210–216

Frerichs F T 1861 Diseases of the liver. The Syndham Society, London, Vol II, p 369

Fujiwara K, Nagoshi S, Ohno A et al 1993 Stimulation of liver growth by exogenous human hepatocyte growth factor in normal and partially hepatectomized rats. Hepatology 18: 1443–1449

Galloway S, Casarella W, Price J 1973 Unilobar veno-occlusive disease of the liver. American Journal of Roentgenology 119: 89–94

Ghosh S, May M J, Kopp E B 1998 NF-κB and Re1 proteins: evolutionarily conserved mediators of immune responses. Annual Review of Immunology 16: 225–260

Gohda E, Yamasaki T, Tsubouchi H et al 1990 Biological and immunological properties of human hepatocyte growth factor from plasma of patients with fulminant hepatic failure. Biochimica et Biophysica Acta 1053: 21–26

Grindlay J H, Bollman J L 1952 Regeneration of the liver in the dog after partial hepatectomy. Surgery, Gynecology and Obstetrics 94: 491–496

Grisham J W 1962 A morphologic study of deoxyribonucleic acid synthesis and cell proliferation in regenerating rat liver; autoradiography with thymidine-H3. Cancer Research 22: 842–849

Haber A H, Mohn K L, Diamond R H et al 1993 Induction patterns of 70 genes during nine days after hepatectomy define the temporal course of liver regeneration. Journal of Clinical Investigations 91: 1319–1326

Hadjis N S, Carr D, Banks L, Gibson R, Blumgart L H 1986a Expectant management of patients with unilateral hepatic duct obstruction and liver atrophy. Gut 27, 1223–1227

Hadjis N S, Hemingway A, Carr D, Blumgart L H 1986b Liver lobe disparity consequent upon atrophy. Diagnostic, operative and therapeutic considerations. Journal of Hepatology 3: 285–293

Hadjis N S, Carr D, Hatzis G, Benjamin I S, Hemingway A, Blumgart L H 1987 Anicteric presentation of hilar cholangiocarcinoma. Anatomical and pathological considerations. Digestive Surgery 4: 119–122

Hadjis N S, Adam A, Gibson R, Blenkharn J I, Benjamin I, Blumgart L H 1989 Nonoperative approach to hilar cancer determined by the atrophy-hypertrophy complex. American Journal of Surgery 157: 395–399

Hadjis N S, Blenkharn J I, Hatzis G, Adam A, Beacham J, Blumgart L H

1990 Patterns of serum alkaline phosphatase activity in unilateral hepatic duct obstruction. A clinical and experimental study. Surgery 107: 193–200

Hadjis N S, Keith R 1991 Significant liver atrophy and hepatocyte hyperplasia are induced by segmental biliary obstruction. Clinical and Investigative Medicine 14: A51

Hadjis N S, Blenkharn J I, Hatzis G, Guzail M, Benjamin I S 1991 Pathological and hemodynamic sequelae of unilobar bilairy. Surgery 109: 671–676

Hadjis N S, Keith R 1992 Liver atrophy induced by selective bile duct obstruction is independent of portal blood flow. Surgical Forum 43: 177–178

Hadjis N S, Schweizer W, Blumgart L H 1994 Liver hyperplasia, hypertrophy and atrophy: clinical relevance. In: Blumgart L H (Ed.) Surgery of the Liver and Biliary Tract, 2nd edn. pp. 83–94. Edinburgh: Churchill Livingstone

Ham J M 1990 Lobar and segmental atrophy of the liver. World Journal of Surgery 14: 457–462

Ham J M 1979 Partial and complete atrophy affecting hepatic segments and lobes. British Journal of Surgery 66: 333–337

Harkness R D 1952 The spatial distribution of dividing cells in the liver of the rat after partial hepatectomy. Journal of Physiology 116: 373–379

Harley V, Barrat W 1901 The experimental production of hepatic cirrhosis. Journal of Pathology and Bacteriology 7: 203–213

Healey J, Schroy P 1953 The anatomy of the bile ducts within the human liver; an analysis of the prevailing patterns of branching and their major variants. Archives of Surgery 66, 599–616

Heinrich P C, Behrman I, Muller-Newen G et al 1998 Interleukin-6-type cytokine signalling through the gp130/Jak/STAT pathway. Biochemical Journal 334: 297–314

Heinrich PC, Behrman I, Muller-Newen G et al 1998 Interleukin-6-type cytokine signalling through the gp130/Jak/STAT pathway. Biochemical Journal 334: 297–314

Higgins G M, Anderson R M 1931 Experimental pathology of the liver. I. Restoration of the liver of the white rat following partial surgical removal. Archives of Pathology 12: 186–202

Higgins G M, Mann F C, Priestley J T 1932 Restoration of the liver of the domestic fowl. Archives of Pathology 14: 491–497

Hueston J 1953 The production of liver lobe atrophy by hydatid cysts. British Journal of Surgery 41: 427–430

Jezequel A M, Paolucci F, Benedetti et al 1991 Enumeration of S-phase cells in normal rat liver by immunohistochemistry using bromodeoxyuridine-antibromodeoxyuridine system. Digestive Diseases & Sciences 36: 482–484

Johnstone J M S, Lee E G 1976 A quantitative assessment of the structural changes in the rat's liver following obstruction of the common bile duct. British Journal of Surgery 66: 333–337

Kam I, Lynch S, Svanas et al 1987 Evidence that host size determines liver size: studies in dogs receiving orthotopic liver transplants. Hepatology 7, 362–366

Kam I, Lynch S, Svanas G et al 1987 Evidence that host size determines liver size: studies in dogs receiving orthotopic liver transplants. Hepatology 7: 362–366

Karran S, McLaren M 1985 Physical aspects of hepatic regeneration. In: Wright R (ed.) Liver and biliary disease, 2nd edn. pp. 233–250. London: Baillière and Tindall

Kerr J F R 1971 'Shrinkage necrosis' a distinct model of cellular death. Journal of Pathology 105: 13–20

Kren, B.T. and Steer, C.J. (1996) Posttranscriptional regulation of gene expression in liver regeneration: role of mRNA stability. FASEB Journal 10, 559–573.

Kren, B T and Steer C J (1996) Posttranscriptional regulation of gene expression in liver regeneration: role of mRNA stability. FASEB Journal 10: 559–573.

Kren B T, Trembley J H, Behrens T et al 1995 Modulation of apoptosis-associated genes bcl-2, bcl-x and bax during liver regeneration. Hepatology 22: 487a

Lee G H, Merlino G, Fausto N 1992 Development of liver tumors in transforming growth factor alpha transgenic mice. Cancer Research 52: 5162–5180

Leffert H L, Koch K S, Lad P J et al 1988 Hepatocyte regeneration, replication, and differentiation. In: Arias I M, Jakoby W, Popper H et al (eds.) The liver: biology and pathobiology, 2nd edn. pp. 833–850. New York: Raven Press

Lewan L, Ynger T, Engelbrecht 1977 The biochemistry of the regenerating liver. International Journal of Biochemistry 8: 477–487

Libermann T A, Baltimore D 1990 Activation of interleukin-6 gene expression through the NF-κB transcription factor. Molecular and Cellular Biology 10: 2327–2334

Liu M-L, Mars WM, Zarnegar et al 1994 Collagenase pretreatment and the mitogenic effects of hepatocyte growth factor and transforming growth factor-alpha in adult rat liver. Hepatology 19: 1521–1527

Longmire W P and Tompkins R G 1975 Lesions of the segmental and lobar hepatic ducts. Annals of Surgery 182: 478–495

Lorigan J G, Charnsangaver C, Carrasco C H, Richli W R 1988 Atrophy with compensatory hypertrophy of the liver in hepatic neoplasms: radiologic findings. American Journal of Roentgenology 150: 1291–1295

Loyer P, Cariou S, Glaise D et al 1996 Growth factor dependence of progression through G1 and S phases of adult rat hepatocytes in vitro. Journal of Biological Chemistry 271: 11484–11492

Loyer P, Glaise D, Cariou S et al 1994 Expression and activation of cdks (1 and 2) and cyclins in the cell cycle progression during liver regeneration. Journal of Biologial Chemistry 269: 2491–2500

MacManus J P, Braceland B M, Youdale T, Whitfield J F 1973 Adrenergic antagonists, and a possible link between the increase in cyclic adenosine 3′,5′-monophosphate and DNA synthesis during liver regeneration. Journal of Cellular Physiology 82, 157–164

Makler P T, Lewis E, Cantor, Charkes N D, Malmud L S 1980 Nonvisualization of the left lobe of the liver due to atrophy or aplasia. Clinical Nuclear Medicine 5: 63–65

Marshall J M 1932 Tumors of the bile ducts. Surg Gyn Obstet 54: 6–12

Matsumoto K, Nakamura T 1992 Hepatocyte growth factor: molecular structure, roles in liver regeneration, and other biological functions. Critical Reviews in Oncogenesis 3, 27–54

McGowan J, Fausto N 1978 Ornithine decarboxylase activity and the onset of deoxyribonucleic acid synthesis in regenerating liver. Biochemical Journal 170: 123–127

McMaster P, Rous P 1921 The biliary obstruction required to produce jaundice. Journal of Experimental Medicine 33, 731–750

Meyer D, Yansey S B, Revel J-P 1981 Intercellular communication in normal and regenerating rat liver: a quantitative analysis. Journal of Cell Biology 91: 505–523

Meyer W W 1950 Unilaterale leberschwunde oder lappenhypolasien de leber? Virchows Archiv 319: 127–230

Michalopoulos G K, DeFrances M C 1997 Liver regeneration. Science 276: 60–66

Miettinen P J, Berger J E, Meneses et al 1995 Epithelial immaturity and multiorgan failure in mice lacking epidermal growth factor receptor. Nature 376: 337–341

Mohn K L, Laz T M, Hsu J-C et al 1991 The immediate-early growth response in regenerating liver and insulin-stimulated H-35 cells; comparison with serum-stimulated 3T3 cells and identification of 41 novel immediate-early genes. Molecular and Cellular Biology 11, 381–390

Myracle W W, Stadalnik R C, Blaisdell F W, Farkas J P, Matin P 1981 Segmental biliary obstruction: diagnostic significance of bile duct crowing. American Journal of Roentgenology 137: 169–171

Nakamura H, Morita T, Masaki S et al 1984 Intercellular localization and metabolism of DNA polymerase alpha in human cells visualized with monoclonal antibody. Experimental Cell Research 151: 123–133

Nasse 1894 Ueber experimente an der leber und den gallenwegen. Archiv fur Klinische Chirurgie 48: 885–893

Nesbit G M, Johnson C, James E et al 1988 Cholangiocarcinoma: diagnosis and evaluation of resectability by CT and sonography as procedures complementary to cholangiography. American Journal of Roentgenology 151: 933–938

Ogawa T, Jefferson N C, Necheles 1960 Comparative study of bile drainage in dogs and man. American Journal of Surgery 99: 57–62

Ogilvy C S, Pakzaban P, Lee J M 1993 Oculomotor nerve cavernous angioma in a patient with Roberts syndrome. Surgical Neurology 40: 39–42

Pack G T, Islami A H, Hubbard J C, Brashfield R D 1962 Regeneration of human liver after major hepatectomy. Surgery 52: 617–623

Papa S, Capitani S, Mattetucci A et al 1987 Flow cytometric analysis of isolated rate liver nuclei during growth. Cytometry 8: 595–598

Patijn G A, Lieber A, Schowalter D B et al 1998 Hepatocyte growth factor induces hepatocyte proliferation in vivo and allows for efficient retroviral-mediated gene transfer in mice. Hepatology 28: 707–716

Pfeifer U 1978 Inhibition by insulin of the formation of autophagic vacuoles in rat liver. A morphometric approach to the kinetics of intracellular degradation by autophagy. Journal of Cell Biology 75: 152–167

Pfeifer U 1982 Kinetic and subcellular aspects of hypertrophy and atrophy. Review of Experimental Pathology 23: 1–45

Pistoi S, Morello D 1996 Prometheus' myth revisited: transgenic mice as a powerful tool to study liver regeneration. FASEB Journal 10, 819–828

Ponfick E 1889 Experimentelle Beitrage zur Pathologie der Leber. Archiv fur Pathologische Anatomie 188: 209–249

Putnam C W, Porter K A, Starzl T E 1976 Hepatic encephalopathy and light and electron micrographic changes of the baboon liver after portal diversion. Annals of Surgery 184: 155–161

Rabes H M, Wirsching R, Tuczek H V, Iseler G 1976 Analysis of cell cycle compartments of hepatocytes after partial hepatectomy. Cell and Tissue Kinetics 9: 517–532

Rai R M, Lee F Y J, Rosen A et al 1998 Impaired liver regeneration in inducible nitric oxide synthase-deficient mice. Proceedings of the National Academy of Sciences 95: 13829–13834

Rensing U, Wimmer B, Lesch R, Wenz W 1984 Budd-Chiari-Stuart-Bras syndrome: clinical, sonographic, radiological re-examination in occlusive diseases of hepatic veins. Hepato-Gastroenterology 31: 218–226

Rous P, Larimore L D 1920a Relation of the portal blood to liver maintenance. Journal of Experimental Medicine 31: 609–632

Rous P, Larimore L D 1920b The biliary factor in liver lesions. Journal of Experimental Medicine 32, 249–272

Rozga J, Jeppson B, Bengmark S 1985 Hepatotrophic factors in liver growth and atrophy. British Journal of Experimental Pathology 66: 669–678

Schalm L, Bax H, Mansesn B 1956 Atrophy of the liver after occlusion of the bile ducts or portal vein and compensatory hypertrophy of the unoccluded portion and its clinical importance. Gastroenterology 31: 131–155

Schwartz-Arad D, Zajicek G, Bartfeld E 1989 The streaming liver. IV: DNA content of hepatocyte increases with its age. Liver 9: 93–99

Seki S, Sakaguchi H, Kawakita N et al 1990 Identification of fine structure of proliferating hepatocytes in malignant and nonmalignant liver diseases by use of a monoclonal antibody against DNA polymerase alpha. Human Pathology 21, 1020–1030

Sibilia M, Wagner E 1995 Strain-dependent epithelial defects in mice lacking the EGF receptor. Science 269: 234–238

Sigel B, Baldia L B, Menduke H, Feigl P 1967 Independence of hyperplastic and hypertrophic responses in liver regeneration. Surgery, Gynecology and Obstetrics 125: 95–100

Soriano H, Bilyeu T A, Juan T S et al 1995 DNA binding by C/EBP

proteins correlates with hepatocyte proliferation. In Vitro Cellular and Development Biology Animal 31: 703–709

Starzl T E, Watanabe K, Porter K A, Putnam C W 1976 Effects of insulin, glucagon, and insulin/glucagon infusions in liver morphology and cell division after complete portacaval shunt in dogs. Lancet i: 821–825

Steiner P E, Martinez Batiz J 1962 Effects on the rat liver of bile duct, portal vein and hepatic artery ligations. American Journal of Pathology 39: 257–289

Stewart H L, Cantarow A, Morgan D R 1937 Changes in the liver of the cat following ligation of simple hepatic ducts. Archives of Pathology 23: 641–652

Swanson E A, Millians W S, Sotus P C, Skandalakis J E 1967 Liver cell regeneration and degeneration after lobar biliary obstruction in dogs. American Journal of Gastroenterology 47: 280–286

Takayasu K, Muramatsu Y, Shima Y et al 1986 Hepatic lobar atrophy following obstruction of the ipsilateral portal vein from hilar cholangiocarcinoma. Radiology 160: 389–393

Taub R 1996 Transcriptional control of liver regeneration. FASEB Journal 10: 413–427

Tavill A, Wood E J, Kreel L, Jones E A, Gregory M, Sherlock S 1975 The Budd-Chiari syndrome: correlation between hepatic scintigraphy and the clinical radiological and pathological findings in nineteen cases of hepatic venous outflow obstruction. Gastroenterology 68: 509–518

Thompson N L, Mead J E, Braun L et al 1986 Sequential protooncogene expression during rat liver regeneration. Cancer Research 46: 3111–3117

Threadgill D, Dulgosz A, Hansen L A et al 1995 Targeted disruption of mouse EGF receptor: effect of genetic background on mutant phenotype. Science 269: 230–234

Timchenko N A, Wilde M, Nakanishi et al 1996 CCAAT/enhancer-binding protein alpha (C/EBP alpha) inhibits cell proliferation through the p21 (WAF-i CIP-1/SDI-1) protein. Genes & Development 10: 804–815

Traub O, Druge P M, Willecke K 1983 Degradation and resynthesis of gap junction protein in plasma membranes of regenerating liver after partial hepatectomy or cholestasis. Proceedings of the National Academy of Sciences of the United States of America 80: 755–759

Trautwein C, Rakemann T, Niehof M, Rose-John S, Manns M P 1996 Acute-phase response factor, increased binding, and target gene transcription during liver regeneration. Gastroenterology 110: 1854–1862

Trembley J H, Kren B T, Steer C J 1994 Postranscriptional regulation of cyclin B messenger RNA expression in the regenerating rat liver. Cell Growth & Differentiation 5: 99–108

Tsubouchi H, Niitani Y, Hirono S et al 1991 Levels of human hepatocyte growth factor in serum of patients with various liver diseases determined by an enzyme-linked immunosorbent assay. Hepatology 13: 1–5

Tsuzuki T G, Hoshino Y, Uchiyama T, Kitazima M, Mikata A, Matsuki S 1973 Compensatory hypertrophy of the lateral quadrant of the left hepatic lobe due to atrophy of the rest of the liver, appearing as a mass in the left upper quadrant of the abdomen: a case report. Annals of Surgery 177: 406–410

Tzung S P, Fausto N, Hockenbery D M 1997 Expression of Bcl-2 family during liver regeneration and identification of Bcl-x as a delayed early response gene. American Journal of Pathology 145: 398–408

van Thiel D H, Gavaler J S, Kam I et al 1987 Rapid growth of an intact human liver transplanted into a recipient larger than the donor. Gastroenterology 93: 1414–1419

Von Meister V 1894 Recreation des Lebergewebes nach Abtragung ganzer Leberlappen. Bietrage zur Pathologischen Anatomie und zur Allgemeinen Pathologie 15: 1

Webber E, Wu J, Wang L et al 1994 Overexpression of transforming growth factor-alpha causes liver enlargement and increased hepatocyte proliferation in transgenic mice. American Journal of Pathology 145: 398–408

Webber E M, Bruix J, Pierce R H et al 1998 Tumor necrosis factor primes hepatocytes for DNA replication in the rat. Hepatology 28: 1226–1234

Weinbren K 1953 Effect of bile duct obstruction on regeneration of the rat's liver. British Journal of Experimental Pathology 36: 583–591

Weinbren K 1964 Experimental diffuse nodular hepatic hyperplasia. Toxicologic Pathology 10: 81–92

Weinbren K, Stirling G A, Washington S L A 1972 The development of proliferative response in liver parenchyma deprived of portal blood flow. British Journal of Experimental Pathology 53: 54–58

Weinbren K 1982 The portal blood supply and regeneration of the rat's liver. British Journal of Experimental Pathology 36, 583–591

Weinbren K, Hadjis N S, Blumgart L H 1985 Structural aspects of the liver in patients with biliary disease and portal hypertension. Journal of Clinical Pathology 38: 1013–1020

Weinbren K, Tarsh E 1964 The mitotic response in the rat liver after different regenerative stimuli. British Journal of Experimental Pathology 53: 54–58

Wilkinson M, Sherlock S 1984 A case of ascites. Hospital Update 10: 712–726

Wright N, Alison M 1984 The liver. In: Wright N and Alison M (Eds.) The Biology of Epithelial Cell Populations, pp. 880–980. Oxford: Clarendon Press

Yamada H, Webber E, Kirillova I et al 1998 Analysis of liver regeneration in mice lacking type 1 or type 2 tumor necrosis factor receptor: requirement for type 1 but not type 2 receptor. Hepatology 28: 959–970

Yamada Y, Kirillova I, Peschon J J, Fausto N 1997 Initiation of liver growth by tumor necrosis factor: deficient liver regeneration in mice lacking type I tumor necrosis factor receptor. Proceedings of the National Academy of Sciences of the United States of America 94: 1441–1446

Yamada Y, Fausto N 1998 Deficient liver regeneration after carbon tetrachloride injury in mice lacking type 1 but not type 2 tumor necrosis factor receptor. American Journal of Pathology 152: 1577–1589

Yamaguchi N, Kodama M, Ueda K 1985 Diadenosine tetraphosphate as a signal molecule linked with the functional state of the rat liver. Gastroenterology 89: 723–731

Yokoyama H O, Wilson M E, Tsuboi K K, Stowell R E 1953 Regeneration of mouse liver after partial hepatectomy. Cancer Research 13: 80–85

Zajicek G, Ariel I, Arber N 1988 The streaming liver. III: Littoral cells accompany the streaming hepatocyte. Liver 8, 213–218

Zajicek G, Schwartz-Arad D, Bartfeld E 1989 The streaming liver. V: Time and age-dependent changes of hepatocyte DNA content following partial hepatectomy. Liver 9: 164–171

Zajicek G, Schwartz-Arad D 1990 Streaming liver. VII: DNA turnover in acinus zone-3. Liver 10: 137–140

Zarnegar R, Michalopoulos G K 1995 The many faces of hepatocyte growth factor: from hepatopoiesis to hematopoiesis. Journal of Cellular Biology 129: 1177–1180

Liver blood flow: physiology, measurement and clinical relevance

4

R.T. MATHIE, A.M. WHEATLEY

The hepatic circulation is both large and complex. This chapter describes the nature and physiological control of the liver's blood supply, outlines the techniques used for its measurement in experimental animals and in man, and explores its importance in a variety of clinical situations.

PHYSIOLOGY

LIVER BLOOD SUPPLY

The liver normally receives about one quarter of the total cardiac output, and obtains its supply from two main sources, the hepatic artery and the portal vein. Mixing of arterial and portal blood takes place in the sinusoids which are drained by the hepatic venous system into the inferior vena cava.

Hepatic artery

The hepatic arterioles empty directly or via a peribiliary plexus into the sinusoids and terminal portal venules. Direct artery to hepatic vein connections do not usually exist, but may arise in some liver diseases such as cirrhosis. Reduction of pressure in the arterial system towards that existing in the portal circulation is achieved mainly by: (1) the presinusoidal arteriolar resistance (especially that provided by the peribiliary plexus), and (2) the intermittent closure of the arterioles, which effectively shields the portal bloodstream from the arterial pressure (Rappaport 1973).

The hepatic artery normally supplies about 30 ml/min per 100 g liver tissue, approximately 25% of the total blood flow to the liver. However, it may provide up to 30–50% of the liver's normal oxygen requirement, largely because the arterial blood has a greater oxygen content than portal blood (see below). The intrahepatic bile ducts are probably exclusively perfused by hepatic arterial blood via the peribiliary plexus.

A large number of smaller arteries provides a small blood supply to the liver and, in the event of hepatic arterial occlusion, they are a potent source for the formation of a collateral circulation. Following hepatic arterial ligation, the major potential arterial collaterals arise from the inferior phrenic arteries, which can develop connections with hepatic arteries within the liver, and from the gastroduodenal arteries, which derive blood flow from the superior mesenteric artery and supply the liver via the peribiliary arterial plexus around the intrahepatic bile ducts (Rappaport & Schneiderman 1976). The precise nature of the functional collateral supply after hepatic arterial ligation is dependent on the site of occlusion: if the common hepatic artery is interrupted, revascularization occurs through both major routes indicated above; if only the right or left hepatic artery is interrupted, however, intrahepatic translobar anastomoses re-establish arterial flow in the ligated system (Mays & Wheeler 1974). Ligation of the proper hepatic arteries leads to revascularization solely via a hypertrophied inferior phrenic circulation (Jefferson et al 1956). Clearly therefore, complete long-term dearterialization of the liver by any form of arterial vascular occlusion is extremely unlikely.

Portal vein

The tributaries of the portal vein collect the venous outflow from the entire prehepatic splanchnic vascular bed, i.e. the intestinal tract from the lower esophagus to the rectum plus the pancreas and spleen. The portal vein normally carries about 75% of the total blood flow to the liver, or 90 ml/min per 100 g liver weight. Normal portal pressure is in the region of 5–8 mmHg. Portal blood is postcapillary and therefore partly deoxygenated but, because of its large volume flow rate, may supply 50–70% of the liver's normal oxygen requirement. Hepatic oxygen supply may be at risk if portal blood flow is significantly reduced, but the effect is minimized by an increase in oxygen extraction from the hepatic arterial blood and/or by an increase in the arterial blood flow rate to the liver (see below).

Hepatic veins

The hepatic venous system is the final common pathway of hepatic arterial and portal venous blood after sinusoidal mixing in the normal liver. It is thus the drainage tract of the entire splanchnic circulation. A total liver blood flow of 1.5 L/min would be considered the normal value in healthy men of average weight, but the range is quite wide (1–2 L/min). The free pressure in a hepatic vein is 1–2 mmHg. Wedged hepatic venous pressure is a useful method of estimating sinusoidal pressure, and may also be an indicator of portal venous pressure (Boyer et al 1977).

Hepatic venous blood is normally about two-thirds saturated with oxygen; this may be markedly reduced during periods of low delivery of oxygen to the liver, when an increased proportion of the available supply is extracted by the liver cells. Under normal conditions, the liver accounts for some 20% of the total oxygen consumption of the body.

CONTROL OF LIVER BLOOD FLOW

The majority of investigations responsible for the information outlined in this section have been carried out in experimental animals rather than in man, while human studies have largely concentrated on the changes in the hepatic circulation in disease.

The control of liver blood flow takes place in four distinct areas: the hepatic arterioles, the portal venules, the hepatic venules, and the arterioles of the prehepatic splanchnic bed. The arterial blood supply of the liver is subject to active control by the normal array of factors influencing the peripheral vasculature, including endothelium-derived nitric oxide (NO) (Pannen & Bauer 1998). The portal venous blood supply normally encounters minimal resistance in the portal venules or in the hepatic sinusoids, and is therefore effectively controlled outside the liver by the action of the arterial resistance vessels within the organs of the digestive tract and spleen.

Intrahepatic vascular resistance in health

In the majority of species, intrahepatic vascular resistance (IHVR) would appear to be located at the level of the portal venules (pre-sinusoidal) and/or sinusoids (Sherman et al 1996, Shibayama & Nakata 1985, Zhang et al 1994, Zhang et al 1995). In dogs and cats, however, IHVR is located at the level of hepatic venules (post-sinusoidal), at least under resting conditions (Lautt et al 1986, Lautt et al 1987), whereas it may be shifted to pre-sinusoidal sites during neural stimulation (Greenway & Lautt 1970, Legare & Lautt 1987). Sinusoidal contraction in response to the vasoconstrictor endothelin-1 (ET-1) has been observed despite their lack of smooth muscle (Zhang et al 1994, Zhang et al 1995, Bauer et al 1994, Bauer et al 1995, Okumura et al 1994). This contractility is mainly attributed to hepatic stellate cells (HSC, also called Ito cells, lipocytes and fat-storing cells) which are distinguished by autofluorescence derived from their intracellular vitamin A (Zhang et al 1994, Suematsu et al 1995). In many aspects HSC are analogous to pericytes in that they have perisinusoidal and intrahepatocellular branching processes containing smooth muscle-specific intermediate desmin-like and actin-like filaments which encircle neighboring sinusoids (Greenwel et al 1991, Martinez-Hernandez 1985, Martinez-Hernandez & Amenta 1993). Available evidence suggests that HSC have contractile properties which can be modulated by vasoactive substances (e.g. nitric oxide, carbon monoxide, and prostaglandin $F_{2\alpha}$, angiotensin, thrombin, ET) in either the normal state or in liver injury (Zhang et al 1994, Suematsu et al 1995, Rockey et al 1992, Rockey & Weisiger 1996, Pinzani et al 1992). Studies using intra vital fluorescent microscopy (IVFM) have demonstrated that the sites of sinusoidal dilation and constriction is co-localized with that of an autofluorescent-vitamin A substance (Zhang et al 1994, Zhang et al 1995, Suematsu et al 1995, Suematsu et al 1996). Thus, HSC cells acting as liver-specific pericytes (Martinez-Hernandez 1985, Martinez-Hernandez & Amenta 1993, Friedman 1997) may play a crucial role in modulating IHVR and blood flow especially at the sinusoidal level (Pannen et al 1996, Zhang et al 1994, Zhang et al 1995, Bauer et al 1994, Okumura et al 1994, Pannen et al 1996). Fresh evidence also shows that endothelium-derived NO in the hepatic sinusoids may modulate portal resistance under physiological circumstances (Bauer et al 1997, Shah et al 1997). Derangements in such control mechanisms are now believed to contribute importantly to the hemodynamic abnormalities of portal hypertension (see below).

RELATIONSHIP BETWEEN HEPATIC ARTERY AND PORTAL VEIN BLOOD FLOW

Studies of the individual control mechanisms of the hepatic arterial and portal venous circulations are complicated by the existence of a hemodynamic interaction between the two bloodstreams within the liver, formerly termed the 'reciprocal relationship' between arterial and portal flow. Many workers have demonstrated an increase in hepatic arterial blood flow after portal flow reduction (e.g. Schenk et al 1962, Kock et al 1972, Mathie et al 1980a), but the converse (i.e. an increase in portal flow after arterial flow reduction) has rarely been observed (Mathie 1997). The ability of the hepatic artery to respond acutely to changes in portal flow is now referred to as the 'hepatic arterial buffer response' (Lautt 1981). Hepatic arterial hyperemia following loss of portal inflow is unable to provide complete hemodynamic compensation (Mathie & Blumgart 1983a), but may be of importance in conditions such as portal hypertension (see below). A number of experimental studies support the view that adenosine, accumulating in the liver as a result of reduced hepatic outflow or released from the walls of blood vessels in response to partial tissue hypoxia, has a significant role in the regulation of the buffer response (Lautt & Legare 1985, Mathie & Alexander 1990). The demonstration of receptors mediating dilatation to adenosine in the hepatic arterial vascular bed reinforces this view (Mathie et al 1991a). Such receptors may be envisaged as existing within the vasoregulatory area of the arteriole, illustrated in Fig. 4.1.

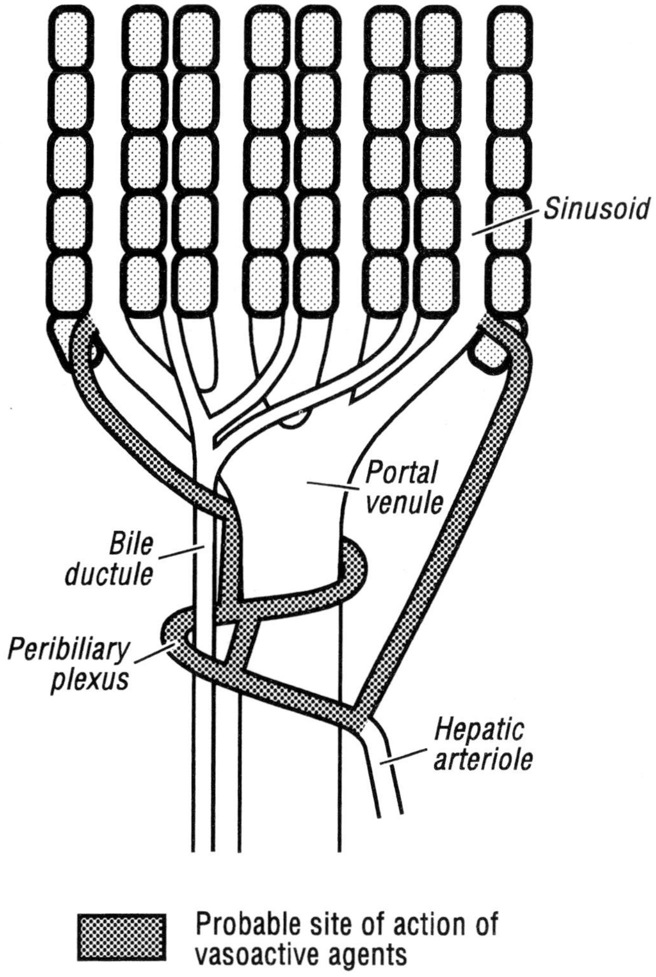

METABOLISM

The presumption that hepatic arterial blood flow is linked to liver metabolism has been challenged now for some time (Lautt 1983, Mathie & Blumgart 1983a). It has been shown, for example, that neither altered oxygen supply nor bile secretion cause a dependent change in arterial flow (Lautt 1983), and it has been concluded that the hepatic artery acts as a buffer to prevent significant changes in total liver blood flow, thereby tending to maintain a constant level of hepatic clearance of blood-borne drugs and hormones. Thus the hepatic artery may uniquely be regarded as subservient to the metabolic requirements of the entire organism rather than to those of the perfused tissue. As stated previously, however, the hepatic artery is still highly important for the supply of oxygen to the liver and biliary system, and uptake may increase according to local requirements, particularly in situations of low portal blood flow; by contrast, its blood flow *control* appears to be independent of the oxygen demands of the liver.

BLOOD GAS TENSIONS

Several experimental studies have clarified the influence of arterial blood gas tensions and pH on the hepatic circulation. Hypercarbia ($PaCO_2 > 70$ mmHg) increases portal venous flow and decreases hepatic arterial flow in dogs (Hughes et al 1979a), while hypocarbia ($PaCO_2 < 30$ mmHg) decreases both (Hughes et al 1979b). Systemic hypoxia ($PaCO_2 < 70$ mmHg) causes a fall in arterial flow but no change in the portal venous contribution (Hughes et al 1979c). The hepatic hemodynamic reaction to metabolic acidosis is similar to that induced by hypercarbia, while metabolic alkalosis has little biologically significant effect (Hughes et al 1980b). The mechanisms for these responses are not totally understood, although it is evident that the sympathetic nervous system is responsible for the hepatic arterial vasoconstriction observed in both hypercarbia and hypoxia (Mathie & Blumgart 1983b).

Sinusoid

Portal venule

Bile ductule

Peribiliary plexus

Hepatic arteriole

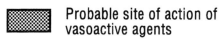 **Probable site of action of vasoactive agents**

Fig. 4.1 Diagrammatic representation of the microvascular bed of the liver, showing the anatomical association between hepatic arterioles, portal venules and bile ductules. The probable site of action of vasoactive agents on the hepatic arterial circulation is indicated.

SYMPATHETIC NERVOUS SYSTEM

Denervation experiments have shown that the sympathetic nervous system is not involved in basal arterial tone in the liver (Mathie & Blumgart 1983b). Hepatic sympathetic nervous stimulation, however, causes hepatic arterial vasoconstriction and reduced blood flow, but this is not maintained and autoregulatory escape occurs (Greenway & Stark 1971); portal pressure rises due to an increase in portal venous resistance, but portal flow does not decrease unless there is a decrease in intestinal or splenic blood flow caused by simultaneous sympathetic stimulation of these vascular beds. The liver is a significant blood reservoir and 50% of its blood volume may be mobilized by nerve stimulation (Greenway & Lautt 1989).

Both α- and β-adrenergic receptors exist in the hepatic artery; the portal venous system is thought to contain only α-receptors (Richardson & Withrington 1981). In vivo, the hemodynamic response to noradrenaline is very similar to that produced by nerve stimulation. The effect of adrenaline is complicated by the dose-dependency of its action on α- and β-receptors: at low doses, hepatic and mesenteric arterial vasodilatation predominate, whereas at high doses vasoconstriction occurs in both the hepatic arterial and portal venous vascular beds as well as in the mesenteric circulation (Greenway & Stark 1971, Richardson & Withrington 1981).

OTHER ENDOGENOUS VASOACTIVE AGENTS

As reviewed by Greenway and Lautt (1989), a variety of endogenous agents have an effect on hepatic hemodynamics. Hepatic blood flow is profoundly increased by glucagon; the flow increase is a consequence of its strong vasodilatory action on the mesenteric vasculature and a lesser vasodilatory influence on the hepatic arterial system. Insulin has little hemodynamic effect on the hepatic circulation. Histamine causes hepatic arterial dilatation and, in the dog only, hepatic venous constriction or outflow block. Bradykinin is a potent hepatic arterial vasodilator but has little effect on the portal venous system. The hepatic arterial vascular bed is dilated by the majority of prostaglandins. Prostacyclin does not affect hepatic arterial flow, but increases portal blood flow through a vasodilator effect on the prehepatic vascular bed. NO causes vasodilatation in both the hepatic arterial and mesenteric vascular beds (see above). Each of the gut hormones gastrin, secretin, cholecystokinin and vasoactive intestinal peptide causes vasodilatation of the hepatic artery.

Angiotensin decreases both hepatic arterial and portal blood flows, and indeed is one of the few substances to produce a significant vasoconstrictor effect on the hepatic artery. The vasoconstrictor peptides, endothelins, in addition to exerting a powerful and prolonged generalized systemic constriction (Miller et al 1989, Zhang et al 1994) have a direct effect on the hepatic blood flow. ETs reduce hepatic perfusion (Kurihara et al 1992), increase portal pressure (Tran-Thi et al 1993, Tanaka et al 1994, Isales et al 1993, Bauer et al 1994) and reduce sinusoidal diameter (Bauer et al 1994, Okumura et al 1994, Zhang et al 1994). Vasopressin decreases portal flow and pressure by mesenteric arterial vasoconstriction, but has variable effects on the hepatic artery. 5-Hydroxytryptamine (5-HT, serotonin) is believed to mediate vasoconstriction of portal radicals, and has thus been targeted as a substance involved in the maintenance of portal hypertension (see below).

An interesting phenomenon is that intraportal administration of exogenous vasoactive agents affects hepatic arterial resistance (Lautt et al 1984). The mechanisms underlying this intrahepatic transvascular effect are not understood, but it is evident that the vasoactive constituents in portal blood have access to the arterial resistance sites within the liver. The close anatomical association between arterioles and venules (Fig. 4.1) could permit this, and may thus be a means by which hepatic arterial blood flow is finely controlled by endogenous agents such as gut hormones.

ANESTHETIC AGENTS

Most investigations into the effects of general anesthetic agents on liver blood flow have concentrated attention on halothane, though the newer products have been the subject of rather more recent studies. Both hepatic arterial and portal venous blood flow decrease passively in parallel with cardiac output during halothane inhalation, with little change in vascular resistance (Thulin et al 1975, Hughes et al 1980a). Hepatic oxygen consumption is not diminished by halothane because of a marked increase in the oxygen extraction rate from the reduced blood supply (Andreen et al 1975). Enflurane has been found to have somewhat similar effects to those of halothane, although there is a decrease in hepatic arterial vascular resistance as part of a generalized decrease in peripheral vascular resistance (Hughes et al 1980a). Both cyclopropane and methoxyflurane reduce liver blood flow, mainly by increasing the mesenteric vascular resistance (Batchelder & Cooperman 1975). Nitrous oxide in concentrations of 30–70% reduces both hepatic artery and portal vein flow, possibly as a result of a generalized stimulatory action on α-adrenergic receptors (Thomson et al 1982). Isoflurane appears to have minimal effects on hepatic arterial and portal venous flows (Nagano et al 1988). The intravenous agent fentanyl may have little effect on prehepatic splanchnic blood flow (Nagano et al 1988), while thiopentone in low doses vasoconstricts both the hepatic arterial and mesenteric vascular beds (Thomson et al 1986).

MEASUREMENT OF LIVER BLOOD FLOW

Many different techniques have been employed in attempts to measure hepatic blood flow in experimental animals and in humans. The earliest workers (Burton-Opitz 1910, 1911, MacLeod & Pearce 1914), approached the problem using direct invasive techniques such as intravascular devices or venous outflow collection, which had no application in clinical investigations. Later developments allowed an indirect determination of blood flow by the use of a variety of indicator clearance techniques which could also be applied to the clinical situation, though with diminished accuracy in the presence of liver disease. More sophisticated technology now enables liver blood flow or tissue perfusion to be determined either directly or indirectly in animals or in humans with greater accuracy and fewer difficulties than before. Methods will be discussed under three broad headings: (1) flow in single blood vessels, (2) total liver blood flow, and (3) hepatic tissue perfusion; those techniques *currently* employed for experimental and clinical investigations are further listed in Table 4.1.

Table 4.1 Summary of methods currently used for measuring liver blood flow

Flow in single vessels
Electromagnetic flowmeter
Doppler ultrasound

Total liver blood flow
Clearance techniques
Hepatocyte excretion
    Indocyanine green
    Galactose
Reticulo-endothelial uptake
    Sulfur colloid (^{99m}Tc)
Indicator dilution
    Red blood cells (^{51}Cr)
    Serum albumin (^{131}I, ^{99m}Tc)
Indicator fractionation
    Microspheres (various labels)

Hepatic tissue perfusion
Inert gas clearance
    Krypton (^{85}Kr)
    Xenon (^{133}Xe)
    Hydrogen
Laser Doppler Flowmetry

1. FLOW IN SINGLE VESSELS

Electromagnetic flowmeter

The direct and continuous measurement of both hepatic arterial and portal venous blood flows with electromagnetic flow probes remains the best available means of assessing individual vessel flow. Although the technique has found widespread application in experiments using large animals, its use in clinical situations has been limited both by the relatively extensive vascular dissection required for placement of the probes and by the overestimation of true hepatic tissue blood flow which occurs in the presence of portal-systemic shunts. Using this method, Schenk and colleagues (1962) found total liver blood flow in anesthetized subjects to be approximately 1 L/min, of which about 25% was supplied by the hepatic artery. Subsequent clinical studies have concentrated on hemodynamic investigations of liver diseases such as cirrhosis. Electromagnetic probes have been used intraoperatively to assess the hemodynamic status of the liver immediately following transplantation (Takaoka et al 1990). A typical experimental preparation utilizing electromagnetic flow probes is illustrated in Fig. 4.2.

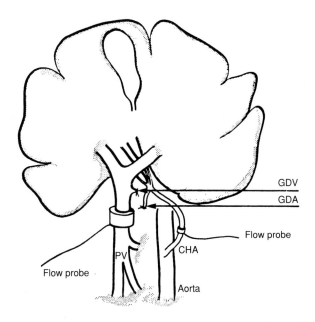

Fig. 4.2 Experimental arrangement for measuring liver blood flow in the dog with electromagnetic flow probes. Probes are placed around the portal vein (PV) and common hepatic artery (CHA). The gastroduodenal vein (GDV) and gastroduodenal artery (GDA) are ligated as illustrated, to ensure that the flows measured by the probes are those which actually perfuse the liver.

Doppler ultrasound

Real-time measurement of blood flow by Doppler ultrasonic devices has been one of the major advances in diagnostic radiology. The principle of flow estimation by Doppler flowmetry is simple, flow being a product of the average velocity of the blood measured in the vessel of interest and the cross-sectional area of the vessel. Two forms of Doppler ultrasound devices exist. The first consists of a flowmeter with an ultrasonic probe which is placed directly on the vessel; measurement with such a device is invasive. The second consists of a combined image scanner and flowmeter (duplex) with which flow in a vessel can be measured transcutaneously and thus non-invasively.

(i) Invasive. As the ultrasonic probes are fitted directly to the vessel, flow measurements are relatively easy to perform, as has been demonstrated in an animal model (Ohnishi et al 1987). Such systems have been used successfully in the intra-operative (Henderson et al 1991) and postoperative measurement (up to 7 days) of portal venous and hepatic arterial blood flow in liver transplant patients (Payen et al 1990). In the latter study, total liver blood flow values in the region of 1350–2050 ml/min were found in those patients without signs of complications.

(ii) Noninvasive. In experiments performed on anesthetized dogs, good correlation between portal venous flow measured by a transcutaneous Doppler duplex system and electromagnetic flow probes fitted to the portal vein was found (Dauzat & Layrargues 1989). Clinically, however, fully quantitative hepatic blood flow measurements, especially in the portal vein, using transcutaneous Doppler ultrasound devices remain difficult to achieve with confidence (Burns et al 1987). Applications of the technique include postoperative hemodynamic assessment of portal-systemic shunt procedures such is TIPS (Fung et al 1998) (Ch. 101) and in the diagnosis of cirrhosis and portal hypertension (Iwao et al 1997). There is controversy, however, whether such measurement is a useful parameter for discriminating patients with cirrhosis (Dinc et al 1998) — and see later discussions. In normal subjects, portal blood flow of 600–900 ml/min has been reported (Moriyasu et al 1986, Brown et al 1989), while blood flow in the common hepatic artery was reported to be approximately 250 ml/min (Nakamura et al 1989). The use of color Doppler has improved the suitability of the Doppler method for routine clinical use (Rosemurgy et al 1997). The recent availability of ultrasound echo-enhancing materials such as the galactose-based microbubble agent Levovist (Ernst et al 1996) may further improve the precision of hepatic blood flow measurement, as well as imaging, using the Doppler technique.

2. TOTAL LIVER BLOOD FLOW

Clearance techniques

First applied to man by Bradley and colleagues in 1945, indirect clearance methods of liver blood flow measurement are based on the Fick Principle, which allows an assessment of organ blood flow by determining both the rate of removal of a substance and the arteriovenous concentration difference across the organ. The flow measurement obtained by Bradley's group depended on the fact that intravenously injected Bromsulphthalein (BSP) is removed from the bloodstream entirely by the hepatocytes into the bile. They derived a value for the rate of hepatic BSP removal indirectly by determining the rate of intravenous infusion of dye that maintained the arterial concentration at a constant level; by also measuring the arteriovenous concentration difference of BSP, they were thus able to calculate total hepatic blood flow. The mean value obtained in a group of normal subjects was 1.5 L/min.

Since 1945, this technique has been used extensively for hepatic blood flow measurement, sometimes substituting BSP with other substances dependent on hepatocyte extraction into bile such as indocyanine green (ICG) (Caesar et al 1961). None of these substances actually achieves complete hepatic removal, and so hepatic vein cannulation is necessary to allow the calculation of the true extraction efficiency. Many investigators are now utilizing a simplified version of the original method, in which ICG is administered as a bolus instead of an infusion and hepatic extraction efficiency is determined from an analysis of the clearance curve derived from blood samples taken from a peripheral vein instead of the hepatic vein (Grainger et al 1983). Two other hepatic clearance techniques have been employed: colloidal clearance by the hepatic Kupffer cells (Dobson & Jones 1952), and hepatocyte removal of galactose (Keiding 1988) or highly extracted drugs such as propranolol (George 1979); the more complete hepatic extraction of these substances overcomes the need to cannulate a hepatic vein in patients with normal liver function.

Though the clearance methods may be accurate in normal subjects, problems arise in patients with liver disease, when there may be reduced cellular uptake and a variable degree of extrahepatic removal of the marker. There may also be vascular shunts within or around the liver, allowing bypass of the liver cells. In these circumstances, the clearance techniques become increasingly useful as tests of hepatic *function* rather than blood flow. There remains considerable doubt whether these techniques are capable of identifying patients with cirrhosis and/or fibrosis (Gadano et al 1997). Indeed, in view of similar concerns over Doppler ultrasound (see above), the question arises that there may be little or no significant difference in total hepatic blood flow actually to detect between cirrhotic and normal subjects. The measurable hemodynamic abnormalities that may occur in cirrhotic individuals are discussed in more detail later in this chapter.

Developed about 15 years ago, a modification of the colloid extraction method allows the derivation of the ratio of hepatic arterial to total liver blood flow, termed the hepatic perfusion index. The basis of the technique is the ability to determine by dynamic scintigraphy the temporal separation of accumulating hepatic activity from the arterial and portal supplies following the intravenous administration of a bolus of ^{99m}Tc sulfur colloid (Fleming et al 1981, Parkin et al 1983). The method, though prone to some inaccuracy, has been applied, for example, to the hemodynamic study of patients with cirrhosis and of those with liver tumor (see below).

Indicator dilution

Reichman et al (1958) were the first to apply an indicator dilution technique to the measurement of total liver blood flow in humans. The method involves the hepatic arterial or portal venous injection of a labeled substance that is not removed by the liver (red blood cells or serum albumin), and either measuring the changes in hepatic vein concentration by blood sampling, or monitoring the hepatic isotope activity with an external detector. Portal vein flow may be determined separately using a modification of this technique, by sampling portal blood after splenic vein or superior mesenteric artery injection (Chiandussi et al 1968, Huet et al 1973). Hepatic artery flow may then be calculated as the difference between total hepatic and portal flows. In addition, a modified thermal dilution technique has been used to measure portal blood flow in man (Biber et al 1983). Indicator dilution methods suffer from the problem of overestimating true blood flow to hepatic tissue when intra- or extra-hepatic shunts are present, though it has proved possible to measure azygous blood flow by thermal dilution in patients with cirrhosis (Bosch & Groszmann 1984).

Indicator fractionation

Sapirstein (1956) was responsible for developing a method for the measurement of the distribution of cardiac output using this principle. Substances used originally included ^{42}K

and ^{86}Rb, but now radioactive (or colored) microspheres enjoy widespread application for experimental investigations of the peripheral circulation in experimental animals. The hepatic arterial blood flow is conveniently determined by this method, but the portal flow contribution is found indirectly by addition of the flow values in the prehepatic splanchnic organs. Examination of the intrahepatic distribution of microspheres provides a means of assessing the pattern of arterial flow in different regions of the liver (Greenway & Oshiro 1972). Since the microsphere method requires the post-mortem removal of the organs of interest for radioactivity or colorimetric measurement, the additional determination of tissue weight enables flow per gram (i.e. tissue perfusion) to be calculated. Microspheres may be employed to determine the extent of portal-systemic shunts, by measuring the fractional distribution in liver with respect to systemic (lung) activity following portal vein injection.

3. HEPATIC TISSUE PERFUSION

Inert gas clearance

This technique allows the direct measurement of hepatic tissue perfusion (expressed in ml/min per unit weight of liver) derived from the combined arterial and portal supply (Leiberman et al 1978a). The method, using either krypton (^{85}Kr) or xenon (^{133}Xe), requires only the measurement of the rate of clearance of gas after its injection into the hepatic blood supply. Following its injection and rapid diffusion throughout the liver, the gas clears from the tissue into the blood, and is almost completely eliminated from the body after a single passage through the lungs. The clearance rate, monitored by a suitable radioactivity detector positioned over the liver, is proportional to hepatic tissue perfusion, which may be calculated using a standard formula (Leiberman et al 1978a). The β-emissions of ^{85}Kr may be recorded by a Geiger-Müller tube or semiconductor (silicon) detector placed on or immediately above the exposed liver surface, or the γ-emissions of ^{133}Xe may be monitored transcutaneously by a single scintillation crystal or a γ-camera; the latter device allows simultaneous measurement of hepatic tissue perfusion in many regions of interest. Inert gas techniques involve minimal trauma to the subject being investigated and their accuracy is not markedly affected by the presence of hepatic cellular disease or non-perfusion shunts. The first workers to use the method in the hepatic circulation were Aronsen et al (1966), who recorded the γ-emissions of ^{133}Xe after the injection of a saline solution of the isotope into the portal vein. Some investigators have employed H_2 gas inhalation and measured its hepatic clearance with one or more platinum needle detectors placed within the liver parenchyma. However, errors from this approach arise both from the gas inhalation procedure and from the local tissue trauma caused by needle insertion into the liver.

Laser Doppler flowmetry

One of the most recent methods to be employed in the measurement of hepatic perfusion is laser Doppler flowmetry (LDF). In this technique, the surface of the liver is illuminated with a low-powered laser of fixed frequency. A portion of the light interacts with moving red blood cells and its frequency is Doppler-shifted and back-scattered to the detector. A flow-dependent output is extracted from the power and frequency distribution of Doppler-shifted signals from the tissue. Linearity of the LDF signal from the liver with total organ perfusion has been demonstrated (Shepherd et al 1983, 1987, Almond & Wheatley 1992) and the technique has been shown to be sensitive to rapid changes in organ flow (Almond & Wheatley 1992). In the rat, the technique provides a good measure of hepatic perfusion in vivo (Wheatley et al 1993). Laser Doppler flowmetry has also been successfully used to assess liver blood flow (LBF) during shock and resuscitation (Wang et al 1995) and during drug-induced changes in LBF in the rat (Kurihara et al 1992). For reasons not fully understood, LDF may not be appropriate to measure LBF in the pig liver due to the fact that the LDF signal from the liver surface is more sensitive to changes in hepatic arterial (HA) than portal venous (PV) blood flow (Wheatley & Hickman 1995). Nonetheless, the technique has been successfully applied to measure LBF during liver transplantation in humans (Seifalian et al 1997). One of the major drawbacks of the technique is that, due to the small volume of tissue interrogated by the laser, the LDF signal cannot be quantified. The development of laser Doppler perfusion imaging devices, which estimate tissue perfusion by scanning an area of tissue using a laser, may well overcome this problem of signal calibration (Wardell et al 1993).

In vivo fluorescent microscopy

Investigations of microhemodynamics in the liver can be achieved using in vivo or IVFM. Using this technique, individual sinusoids and terminal venules can be visualized as well as changes in their diameters and the velocities with which erythrocytes pass through them (Menger & Messmer 1991). From a hemodynamic point of view, IVFM is not without its problems of interpretation (Sherman et al 1990). In perfused liver, a 2.5-fold increase in portal venous blood flow has been found to be associated with only a 22% increase in sinusoidal red blood cell velocity, suggesting that changes in portal venous blood flow have only a minor effect on the capillary transit time (Sherman et al 1996). However, in the regenerating liver, a 50% increase in portal venous blood flow resulted in a similar (66%) increase in sinusoidal red blood cell velocity (Wheatley et al 1996, Zhang et al 1997).

New and future developments

PV blood flow measured by non-invasive magnetic resonance imaging (MRI) has been found to correlate well with flow measured by Doppler ultrasound flowprobes (Pelc et al 1992). Subsequently, the technique has been used to measure PV blood flow in human liver transplantation candidates (Kuo et al 1995). Further methodology improvements in MRI (such as dynamic contrast-enhanced enhancement) and in other techniques such as positron emission tomography (PET) may lead to their increasing use in the study of hepatic hemodynamics in humans.

CLINICAL RELEVANCE

HEMORRHAGIC SHOCK, HYPOPERFUSION AND ISCHEMIA-REPERFUSION INJURY

Much has been written about the effect of hemorrhage and shock on the hepatic circulation, particularly in experimental animals. Total liver blood flow decreases approximately in relation to the severity of the hemorrhagic hypotension. Portal venous blood flow decreases in parallel to cardiac output but, in common with the coronary, pulmonary and cerebral circulations, hepatic arterial flow does not fall until quite severely low blood pressures are reached. As a result, the hepatic oxygen supply tends to be maintained, though oxygen extraction greatly increases in order to preserve normal total oxygen consumption (Smith et al 1979). Hepatic outflow block has been reported to occur with retransfusion of the shed blood after hemorrhagic hypotension, but this phenomenon appears to be a feature rather specific to the hepatic venous anatomy of the dog, and is a complication that would arise rarely in the clinical situation.

Clinically, ischemic hepatitis or shock liver has long been recognized following cardiogenic or hemorrhagic shock (Birgens et al 1978, Bynum et al 1979). Hepatic dysfunction caused by hepatic hypoperfusion is characterized morphologically by centrilobular necrosis and clinically with abdominal pain, cholestatic jaundice, and marked elevation of serum transaminases. Gottlieb et al (1983) showed that hepatic dysfunction in man following trauma was related to reduced hepatic blood flow rate. They found that hepatic blood flow was markedly reduced after injury and that, although total splanchnic oxygen delivery was decreased, oxygen consumption remained normal due to increased extraction.

More recently, hemorrhagic shock has been recognized to result in generalized vascular endothelial dysfunction and impaired endothelial biosynthesis of NO, a situation that almost certainly includes the liver. Endothelial NO that continues to be expressed by the liver is believed to protect against the initial hepatic injury arising from severe hemorrhage. By contrast, more prolonged hemorrhagic shock (of greater than about 6 hours' duration) induces greatly increased production of NO due to activation of an inducible NO synthase enzyme in hepatocytes and Kupffer cells; such conditions probably yield the cytotoxic product peroxynitrite, with resulting loss of hepatic vascular tone and tissue integrity (Peitzman et al 1995).

Survival has been documented following portal vein ligation carried out to control hemorrhage after traumatic injury (Pachter et al 1979) or following temporary portal occlusion during difficult biliary tract surgery. Similarly, survival after hepatic artery ligation for either trauma, aneurysm, hemobilia, or neoplasms has been long described (Rappaport & Schneiderman 1976). However, the outcome after ligation of either the portal vein or the hepatic artery in the face of shock, infection or concomitant organ failure is much less certain.

In the transplantation era, the consequences of ischemia and reperfusion for the liver have become increasingly investigated and understood. The damage to the hepatic endothelium and parenchyma that results from post-ischemic reperfusion is caused by a number of inter-related phenomena, including the action of locally liberated oxygen-derived free radicals and excess formation of vasoconstrictor agents (Wendon 1999). As in hemorrhagic shock, outlined above, endogenous NO tends to protect the liver in the early reperfusion period following hepatic ischemia (Wang et al 1995, Shimamura et al 1996).

LIVER ATROPHY (see also Ch. 3)

Alterations in liver blood flow which significantly reduce either the volume flow or the composition or concentration of hepatotrophic substances result in liver atrophy. The degree of atrophy is dependent upon the degree of blood flow deprivation. Atrophy of the liver resulting from reduced blood flow may either be segmental, lobar or diffuse and results from a sustained reduction in either portal venous or hepatic artery blood flow, or both.

Atrophy and fatty degeneration of the canine liver after

total portal diversion through an Eck fistula was initially reported over a century ago (Hahn et al 1893). Numerous experimental studies in a variety of species have confirmed that both partial and complete diversion of portal vein blood flow from the liver results in atrophy. Complete portal venous flow diversion with interruption of all portal venous collaterals results in more profound liver atrophy than the partial deviation of portal venous flow resulting from side-to-side portacaval anastomoses (Bollman 1961). An accurate quantitative relationship for the degree of liver atrophy relative to the reduction of portal venous blood flow remains to be determined, primarily because changes in both volume flow and composition of portal blood are involved, but also because of attendant changes in hepatic arterial flow.

There is accumulating evidence that liver atrophy following portal diversion is not the result of a decrease in absolute volume flow but the consequence of the effective loss of hepatotrophic constituents in the portal blood. Rats subjected to portal flow diversion with portacaval transposition underwent a decrease in relative liver weight (Guest et al 1977), despite the effective preservation of portal perfusion from the inferior vena cava (Ryan et al 1978). Dogs with 'partial portacaval transposition' (Marchioro et al 1967) or 'splanchnic flow division' (Starzl et al 1973, 1975) revealed atrophy in those liver lobes deprived of pancreatic venous drainage, although normal tissue perfusion was demonstrated in all regions of the liver (Mathie et al 1979). Thus liver size depends critically on its portal circulation, but this is due predominantly to the quality of the blood it supplies to the liver rather than the quantity of flow it provides.

The fate of the liver after ligation of the hepatic artery depends largely upon the extent of a functional collateral arterial circulation (Rappaport & Schneiderman 1976). If collaterals are few, liver infarction and necrosis may occur after hepatic artery ligation and may result in death. However, with an adequate collateral supply, hepatic artery ligation results only in transient ischemic changes in the periphery of the hepatic acinus (zone 3). Atrophy after hepatic artery ligation occurs grossly in liver segments which have sufficient collateral supply to prevent complete necrosis but insufficient collaterals to compensate completely for arterial ligation. The effects of hepatic artery interruption are compounded by low portal venous blood flow and oxygen saturation, superimposed infection, and complicated by species-specific differences (Rappaport & Schneiderman 1976). Histologically, arterial obstruction rapidly causes ischemic changes with mitochondrial swelling, cell membrane disruption, platelet aggregation , and widening of the spaces of Disse (Mallet-Guy et al 1972).

LIVER RESECTION AND REGENERATION
(see also Chs 3 and 83)

The adult liver exhibits a remarkable potential to restore its cellular mass in response to injury by hepatocyte hyperplasia; thus following the removal of two-thirds of liver mass in the rat by partial hepatectomy (PH), both liver mass and function are fully recovered by 2–3 weeks. In the early stages of regeneration as a consequence of hepatocyte division, clusters of hepatocytes develop with a reduced distribution of sinusoids (Martinez-Hernandez & Amenta 1995). The hemodynamic sequelae of hepatocyte hyperplasia has only relatively recently received attention. A number of studies in man have confirmed that hepatic regeneration of the normal in situ liver remnant proceeds rapidly following partial hepatic resection (Aronsen et al 1970, Blumgart et al 1971).

The effect of partial liver resection in experimental animals on portal pressure is still not fully clarified. The majority of studies indicate that major resection is associated with a significant and persistent rise in portal pressure (Lee et al 1987, Wu et al 1993, Morsiani et al 1995).

Partial liver resection without devascularization would normally be expected to produce little change in total blood flow to the liver. This occurs because the major contributor to total flow, the portal vein, is affected less by events taking place within the liver than by control mechanisms in the arterial resistance vessels of the prehepatic splanchnic bed. Because essentially the same total blood flow is therefore redistributed to a smaller mass of liver tissue, a corresponding increase in tissue perfusion (ml/min per unit tissue weight) would be anticipated in the non-resected remnant. Experimental studies support these expectations; an increase in hepatic tissue perfusion was observed in rats immediately following two-thirds hepatectomy (Rice et al 1977, Wheatley et al 1993, Wu et al 1993). This rise in hepatic perfusion is due primarily to portal venous inflow (Wu et al, 1993) as hepatic arterial bood flow is low and hepatic arterial resistance is high even 24 hours after partial hepatectomy in the rat (Lee et al 1993, Wheatley et al 1996). Similar studies in patients demonstrated an immediate increase in tissue perfusion of approximately 120% in the remnant (Mathie & Blumgart 1982) The processes of revascularization of the regenerating liver require further elucidation.

The significance of blood flow in relation to liver regeneration has frequently been debated during the 55 years since Mann (1944) suggested that regenerative hyperplasia of the liver after partial resection was a function of portal blood flow and that the process could be prevented by portal flow diversion. As discussed elsewhere (Ch. 3), however, it is now believed that regenerative hyperplasia is not dependent on either the increase in tissue perfusion normally seen after partial hepatectomy or, in contrast to the requirements for the prevention of liver atrophy, the direct supply of portal venous blood to the liver cells (Blumgart 1978). The most important evidence to uphold this hypothesis arises from studies of hepatic hemodynamics and metabolic activity in rats (Guest et al 1977, Ryan et al 1978): regenerative hyperplasia takes place normally following partial liver resection in portacavally transposed animals, in which there is no direct supply of portal blood or the usual posthepatectomy rise in hepatic tissue perfusion.

BLOOD FLOW IN HEPATIC TUMORS

For many years it has been recognized that primary and secondary tumors of the liver are perfused almost exclusively with arterial blood (Breedis & Young 1954). On the basis that the tumor-bearing liver is therefore likely to possess a raised arterial component of hepatic blood flow, several investigators have attempted to achieve differential diagnosis of patients by measuring the proportion of the hepatic arterial contribution to total flow, adopting either the hepatic perfusion index obtained by scintigraphy (Leveson et al 1985) or the Doppler perfusion index obtained by ultrasound (Leen et al 1991a). Such measurements have indeed demonstrated an increased hepatic arterial contribution in patients with confirmed liver metastases compared to normal subjects. However, a decrease in portal venous flow has also been noted, an effect possibly due to the presence of a humoral splanchnic vasoconstrictor agent; the raised hepatic arterial flow may therefore be a buffer response to reduced portal inflow. The results in a third group of patients with colorectal cancer, but in whom no hepatic metastases were detected at laparotomy, overlapped those of the other groups; it was proposed that this third group may have had a high incidence of occult liver metastases responsible for the detected hemodynamic alterations (Leen et al 1991b). Duplex/color Doppler sonography of the Doppler perfusion index has recently been shown to be more sensitive in the detection of colorectal liver metastases than computed tomography, conventional ultrasound or laparotomy alone (Leen et al 1995).

Enhanced targeted drug therapy for liver tumors by blood flow manipulation has been achieved by the application of the vasoconstrictors adrenaline, phenylephrine or angiotensin: improved cytotoxic drug delivery to tumor-bearing regions in man and experimental animals has been indicated (Bloom et al 1987, Goldberg et al 1991, Hemingway et al 1991). This approach is based on the fact that the neovasculature of tumor tissue appears to be devoid of smooth muscle and thus unreactive to vasoconstrictor agents, enabling increased delivery of chemotherapeutic drugs. Biodegradable microspheres have also been used for enhancing targeted therapy: they cause temporary blood flow interruption, resulting in improved uptake of chemotherapeutic agents in tumor tissue and consequent reduced systemic toxicity (Ball 1991).

BILE DUCT OBSTRUCTION (see also Ch. 7)

Bile duct obstruction can significantly affect hepatic hemodynamics. In general, liver blood flow is reduced in the presence of chronic biliary obstruction. Indeed, reduction of liver blood flow in this setting may contribute to hepatic dysfunction. Conversely, *acute* increases in bile duct pressure following obstruction result in a reactive increase in liver blood flow which may represent an attempt by the liver to maintain adequate function against an increase in the pressure gradient opposing secretion and excretion of bile. Most evidence suggests that the hemodynamic response of the liver to biliary obstruction is related, directly or indirectly, to changes in bile duct pressure. Hepatic haemodynamics after complete bile duct obstruction are unaffected acutely (<4 h) unless bile duct pressure is increased abruptly. Nagorney et al (1982) showed that acute serial increases in bile duct pressure in dogs with complete bile duct obstruction increased hepatic arterial blood flow by 250% but did not affect portal venous blood flow.

Chronic bile duct obstruction is associated with a decrease in total liver blood flow. In addition, dilatation of the sinusoids and elevation of portal pressure in dogs was noted after 4 weeks of complete bile duct obstruction (Ohlsson et al 1970). Relief of long-term obstruction is not associated with a return of normal hemodynamics, suggesting irreversible intrahepatic vascular damage (Aronsen et al 1969). Indeed, Aronsen (1968) further showed that a 23% reduction in effective liver blood flow persisted for 1–5 years after operative decompression in patients with choledocholithiasis and jaundice if cholestasis was evident more than 2 weeks preoperatively. Hunt (1979) serially measured liver blood flow daily for 1 week following bile duct ligation in rats, using the ^{133}Xe clearance technique to document the early hemodynamic response. Total liver blood flow decreased steadily after the first postoperative day to a plateau level of approximately 50% of the preoperative value 5 days after operation. More recently, Mathie et al (1988) confirmed the decrease in total liver blood flow following bile duct ligation and extended Hunt's findings by measuring the individual portal venous and hepatic arterial components of liver blood flow. Using electromagnetic flow meters in dogs with complete bile duct ligation, hepatic arterial and portal venous blood flow were observed to decrease by 36 and

44%, respectively. Moreover, they showed a 200% increase in intrahepatic portal resistance but a lesser increase in hepatic arterial resistance. Similarly, Bosch et al (1983) have demonstrated that dogs with chronic bile duct ligation had decreased portal venous flow, and had developed sinusoidal portal hypertension and extensive portal-systemic shunting.

The precise mechanism for reduction in liver blood flow following chronic bile duct obstruction is unknown. Although increased portal vascular resistance is the agreed underlying cause, the primary site of this resistance change has been considered to be presinusoidal (Reuter & Chuang 1976), sinusoidal (Bosch et al 1983), or postsinusoidal (Tamakuma et al 1975). Bosch and colleagues (1983) also showed the development of significant portal-systemic shunting with an inverse correlation between shunting and portal venous blood flow, suggesting that the reduced portal flow was related to a large fraction of the portal inflow being diverted through portal-systemic collaterals. Both Bosch et al (1983) and Ohlsson (1972) have demonstrated that the site of shunting is predominantly extrahepatic.

Clinically, hemodynamic abnormalities associated with chronic biliary obstruction are encountered in two situations: portal hypertension associated with secondary biliary fibrosis; and shock following biliary tract decompression. Approximately 20% of patients with prolonged biliary obstruction develop clinically significant portal hypertension (Sedgwick et al 1966, Adson & Wychulis 1968, Blumgart et al 1984). The operative risk of biliary decompression in these patients is significant. Technical difficulties of stricture repair (dense fibrous adhesions, hilar ductal involvement, infection) are compounded with the risk of hemorrhage from subhepatic and periductal varices and the potential of postoperative liver failure. These complex problems warrant a careful and thorough preoperative evaluation. Decisions on surgical decompression of either the biliary or the portal system must be based on the exclusion of hepatic failure from other causes. Portal-systemic shunts may be performed prior to biliary decompression in patients with bleeding esophageal varices or previous intraoperative hemorrhage which precluded successful stricture repair (Sedgwick et al 1966, Adson & Wychulis 1968).

In addition to the hemodynamic consequences of chronic bile duct obstruction, sudden decompression of the obstructed biliary tree may also have profound hemodynamic effects. Tamakuma et al (1975) have studied the significance of clinical shock following biliary decompression. They noted that hypotension and shock could develop in the immediate postoperative period following biliary decompression, even though no apparent cause of shock, such as hemorrhage, infection or cardiac failure, was evident. They hypothesized that factors associated with sudden release of biliary obstruction and establishment of biliary drainage might affect both hepatic and systemic hemodynamics. They showed that biliary decompression resulted in an abrupt decrease in wedged hepatic vein pressure, portal vein pressure, and arterial pressure within 30 min of decompression. Similarly, Steer et al (1968) reported that rapid needle decompression of an obstructed biliary tree in jaundiced dogs induced a decreased arterial pressure, central venous pressure, and portal venous pressure within 1 h, and concluded that sudden decompression of chronic biliary obstruction permitted sequestration of fluid within the liver, leading to a decrease in the effective circulating plasma volume, resulting in hypotension.

PORTAL HYPERTENSION

Hemodynamics

Portal hypertension is a state of sustained increase in the intraluminal pressure of the portal vein and its collaterals. A mean pressure > 12 mmHg would generally be accepted as qualifying for the definition; variceal bleeding does not occur at a pressure of less than this value (Garcia-Tsao et al 1985). Hemodynamic factors which influence portal hypertension are best understood by application of the pressure-flow-resistance relationship to the portal venous system. Thus, portal pressure depends upon two basic components: portal blood flow and hepatic portal vascular resistance. Portal hypertension may therefore result from a significant increase either in hepatic portal inflow from the prehepatic splanchnic vasculature or in intrahepatic portal resistance, or both. Although simple in concept, multiple factors may influence both components of the system and thus the pathophysiology of portal hypertension.

The hemodynamics of portal hypertension, for example in cirrhosis, are characterized by raised portal pressure, diminished hepatic portal blood flow and an extensive extrahepatic collateral venous network supplied by a hyperdynamic splanchnic and systemic circulation. The traditional view of the source of raised portal pressure is fibrotic encroachment around portal radicles leading to increased intrahepatic portal resistance. In cirrhotic patients, extrahepatic shunts may account for at least 50% of the portal flow, while up to 80% of portal flow actually reaching the liver has been observed to bypass the sinusoidal vascular bed via intrahepatic shunts (Okuda et al 1977). The magnitude of extrahepatic shunt flow in cirrhotics has been measured directly by thermal dilution assessment of azygous blood flow: a value some 300 ml/min greater than in patients without portal hypertension was noted (Bosch & Groszmann 1984). The hepatic artery probably provides a greater relative contribution to the total liver blood flow in cirrhotics than in normal subjects, though it has also been demonstrated that up to 33% of the arterial blood may flow through intrahepatic shunts to the systemic venous circulation (Groszmann et al 1977).

The direction of portal blood flow has been postulated as both a consequence of and a contributor to the pathophysiology of portal hypertension. The progression of intrahepatic disease and increasing sinusoidal pressure has been considered as offering the potential for reversed blood flow in the portal vein, which would therefore be diverted away from the liver and accelerate the disease by depriving the liver of nutrient flow (Warren & Muller 1959). However, reversed (or hepatofugal) portal vein flow has actually been demonstrated in only a very small percentage of patients: hemodynamic information from 273 cirrhotic patients collected from the literature 25 years ago revealed no case of spontaneous flow reversal (Moreno et al 1975), while more recently Gaiani and colleagues (1991) reported an incidence of only 3.1% in a sample of 228 patients.

In the past decade, considerable attention has been paid to the hyperdynamic hemodynamic condition associated with portal hypertension, founded on the hypothesis that the low peripheral vascular resistance may be caused by the stimulated production of an endogenous vasodilator. It was suggested that NO (induced by endotoxemia) may be the substance concerned (Vallance & Moncada 1991). There was swift initial experimental evidence for this: for example, Pizcueta et al (1992) demonstrated an increase in systemic and splanchnic vascular resistance in cirrhotic rats following the administration of an NO inhibitor. The weight of evidence currently favors the view that NO is indeed implicated in the hemodynamic alterations associated with cirrhosis and portal hypertension, though it is increasingly apparent that it is the decompensated end-stage of the cirrhotic condition that is most strongly associated with both endotoxemia (Lee et al 1995) and a hyperdynamic circulation involving NO (Niederberger et al 1995). A consensus view of the prehepatic splanchnic circulation has emerged in which the activity of constitutive NO synthase appears to be upregulated in discrete anatomical locations, such as in the endothelium of the mesenteric artery and in the esophageal, gastric and jejunal mucosa (Mathie 1999).

Intrahepatic vascular resistance in liver cirrhosis

Liver cirrhosis occurs in response to chronic liver injury and is primarily characterized by a disruption of hepatic architecture, with the development of fibrous septa, and abnormal nodules and circulation leading to a sustained increase in portal vascular resistance and portal pressure. In addition, both afferent (portal venules and hepatic arterioles) and efferent (hepatic venules) vessels can be found within the fibrous septa (Kelty et al 1950). In cirrhosis, striking changes in space of Disse occur including excessive accumulation of collagen, leading to the collagenization of the space of Disse and Ito cell activation (Greenwel et al 1991, Martinez-Hernandez 1985, Martinez-Hernandez & Amenta 1993). Likewise, the sinusoidal endothelial cells are deranged during cirrhosis with defenestration (loss of endothelial cell pores) and with the appearance of basement membrane a phenomenon termed 'capillarization' (Varin & Huet 1985). In the cirrhotic liver, the sites of vascular resistance are still unclear; however, since portal and hepatic venules can both be found within the fibrous septa, constriction or distortion of portal venules, hepatic venules or both may be involved (Kelty et al 1950).

Until quite recently, conventional wisdom had it that the elevated IHVR in cirrhosis was immutable. The balance of evidence now suggests that it can be reduced pharmacologically with vasodilators (Bhathal & Grossman 1985,

Reichen & Le 1986). It has been shown that IHVR can be marginally reduced by prostaglandin E₂ (Ballet 1991) and isoprenaline and more substantially by nitroprusside, papaverine and verapamil (Ballet 1991, Bhathal & Grossman 1985, Reichen & Le 1986). In addition, Groszmann and co-workers have reported that intravenous nitroglycerin caused a 24% fall in IHVR in cirrhotic patients (Orrego et al 1981) (see below).

In alcoholic patients, a significant correlation between the extent of HSC activation and the level of portal vascular resistance has been found (Rockey & Chung 1995). The mechanisms of initiation and perpetuation of HSC activation are not fully understood but several factors have been implicated such as inflammatory mediators, cytokines and growth factors (Greenwel et al 1991, Friedman 1997, Friedman 1993, Gandhi et al 1994) and ET (Rockey & Weisiger 1996, Rockey et al 1998, Pinzani et al 1996). ET-induced contractility of isolated HSC increases in proportion to the degree of HSC activation and with progressive liver injury and is most prominent in the cirrhotic liver,

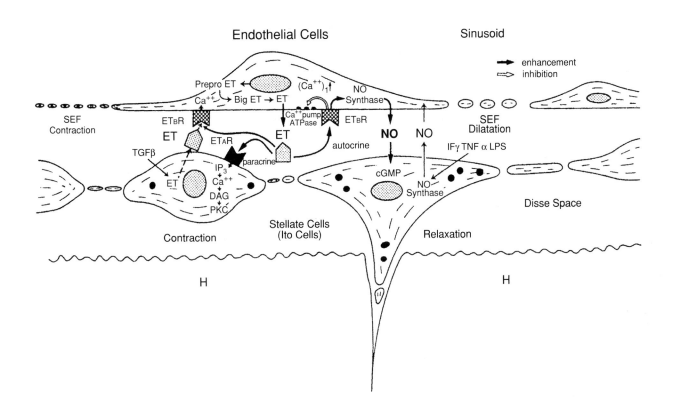

Fig. 4.3 Local regulatory mechanisms of hepatic sinusoidal microcirculation. IP₃, inositol triphosphate; DAG, diacylglycerol; PKC, protein kinase C; TGFβ, transforming growth factor β; ET, endothelin; ETAR, endothelin A receptor; ETBR, endothelin B receptor; [Ca⁺⁺], concentration of intracytoplasmic free calcium ion; NO, nitric oxide; cGMP, cyclic guanylic monophosphate; IF γ, interferon γ; TNFα, tumor necrosis factor α; SEF, sinusoidal endothelial fenestrae; H, hepatocyte; LPS, lipopolysaccharide.

induced by carbon tetrachloride (Rockey & Weisiger 1996). In human liver cirrhosis, an overexpression of ET-1 has been found (Rockey & Weisiger 1996, Housset et al 1993) which is believed to contribute to the elevated IHVR probably by increased HSC contraction (Rockey & Weisiger 1996, Housset et al 1993). Both ET-1 and its receptors (ET_A and ET_B) are detected on all cell types in rat liver but they are far more numerous on Ito cells than on other hepatic cells especially in the cirrhosis subject (Rockey et al 1998, Pinzani et al 1996, Leivas et al 1995). In the rat, ET-1 induced hepatic sinusoidal contractility is enhanced in the ethanol-induced fatty but not in the cirrhotic liver indicating that ET-1 may be involved in the regulation of sinusoidal flow in the early stage of liver cirrhosis (Bauer et al 1995). In addition, the effects of ET-1 on hepatic hemodynamics are blunted in advanced cirrhosis (Rockey & Weisiger 1996, Leivas et al 1995). The reasons for these phenomena are not understood.

Recent evidence points to a *decrease* in endothelial NO synthesis/release by the liver (Gupta et al 1998, Rockey & Chung 1998), with an associated increase in portal vascular resistance that may be potentiated by the interplay of increased ET-1 expression both by hepatic endothelial and by HSC cells (Pinzani et al 1996). The interplay between NO, ET and other local regulatory mechanisms controlling sinusoidal hemodynamics is depicted in Figure 4.3. Groszmann (1990) suggested that the increased mesenteric blood flow in the hyperdynamic stage of portal hypertension may be relatively less important than the elevated intrahepatic portal resistance in maintaining raised portal pressure—the above recent findings are testimony to the validity of this hypothesis. The splanchnic vasodilatory state nevertheless clearly serves to increase flow in the extrahepatic collateral circulation, promoting its tendency to hemorrhage.

Treatment

The ultimate goal of medical and surgical management of portal hypertension is to improve patient survival by the reduction of pressure and flow in extrahepatic variceal vessels (esophageal and gastric), whilst ensuring adequate portal flow to the liver. Portal-systemic shunting and pharmacological reduction of portal flow can provide effective decompression but both necessarily entail further hepatic porto-privation. Surgical relief of portal hypertension may be achieved by one of the many portal-systemic shunt procedures (Ch. 100). First performed experimentally over a century ago by Nikolai Eck, the initial clinical application of the portacaval shunt was reported 50 years later (Whipple 1945). The hemodynamic consequences of shunt surgery are complex, and depend upon the particular shunt performed, the nature and severity of the disease, and the pre-existing hemodynamic conditions in the individual patient. End-to-side portacaval shunt diverts all portal blood flow away from the liver, while less severe procedures reduce portal flow in proportion to the degree to which the shunt reduces portal pressure. The hepatic artery flow may increase by up to 100%, but even a maximal flow increase can usually only partly compensate for loss of portal flow (Mathie & Blumgart 1983a); hepatic oxygen consumption tends to be maintained, however, but at the expense of increased oxygen extraction from the available arterial supply.

Total portacaval shunt is extremely effective in reducing portal pressure, and indeed is the most successful treatment for the prevention of bleeding from esophageal varices. However, as this form of shunt deprives the liver entirely of inflow from the portal venous system and allows splanchnic venous blood to reach the systemic circulation directly, liver failure and encephalopathy are common complications of the operation (Ch. 102). Such problems led to the search for alternative operations which would not compromise the liver in this way, and the side-to-side, the mesocaval (Ch. 104), and the proximal or distal splenorenal shunts (Ch. 103) and other variants have all enjoyed a degree of clinical popularity. Direct portal-hepatic venous recanalization by the angiographic application of a transjugular intrahepatic portasystemic stent shunt (TIPS), first reported by Rössle et al (1989), is currently an important treatment modality for recurrent variceal bleeding in patients who are refractory to conservative medical management (Iannitti & Henderson 1997) (Ch. 101).

Many studies have attempted to utilize pre- or intraoperative hemodynamic parameters to predict morbidity and mortality in patients undergoing portal-systemic shunts for portal hypertension, as discussed above. In general, measurement of portal and hepatic arterial blood flows has not been additive in patient evaluation (Gadano et al 1997) nor predictive of survival from portal-systemic shunt surgery (Ch. 102). However, a raised hepatic perfusion index (i.e. increased ratio of hepatic arterial blood flow compared with total liver blood flow) has been observed to correlate with worsening liver status (Shikare et al 1996). Nearly a quarter of a century ago, one investigation suggested that additional hemodynamic data may have prognostic value for survival and encephalopathy (Burchell et al 1976). These authors retrospectively correlated immediate intraoperative changes in hepatic artery blood flow with early postoperative deaths and encephalopathy in patients with portacaval shunts, and found that over 90% of those who had an increase in flow of < 100 ml/min subsequently died or developed encephalopathy. Intraoperative data have been utilized by others to predict hepatic hemodynamics after a total portacaval shunt, and shown to provide some practical benefit: by measuring hepatic tissue perfusion before and after temporary portal vein occlusion, Leiberman et al (1978b) and Mathie et al (1980b) were able to distinguish patients who showed a marked decrease in liver perfusion and who were therefore not given a total shunt, but a side-to-side or a distal splenorenal shunt instead. Routine surgical intervention for the treatment of portal hypertension has today dropped out of favor in most centers, in response to the increased application of alternative procedures such as TIPS or esophageal variceal sclerotherapy or transection, or the more conservative pharmacological therapy. Thus, hemodynamic abnormalities do exist and can be detected in cirrhotic subjects, though the ability to detect this is dependent on the severity of disease and the specific technique of measurement employed. A related, more contentious, issue is whether routine measurement of hepatic blood flow or perfusion makes an important impact on patient management.

Pharmacological reduction of portal hypertension was initially based largely on an attempt to diminish hepatic portal inflow from the mesenteric vascular bed by the use of vasoconstrictor agents. This approach was introduced by the seminal study of Lebrec and his colleagues in 1981, some years before the recognition even of the existence of the hyperdynamic circulatory condition associated with cirrhosis. They showed that the β-adrenoceptor antagonist propranolol, at doses that decrease the heart rate by 25%, significantly reduced the risk of re-bleeding in cirrhotic patients who were otherwise in good condition. Propranolol is believed to exert its action by two mechanisms: decreasing cardiac output as a result of β_1-adrenergic cardiac receptor blockade, as well as an antagonism of β_2-adrenoceptors in the splanchnic vasculature, leaving unopposed the vasoconstrictive influence of α-adrenergic receptors. Both mechanisms decrease portal flow and thus portal pressure. Results from subsequent studies did not universally support Lebrec's original data (Burroughs et al 1983), but the efficacy of propranolol in the prevention of variceal rebleeding is now widely accepted (McCormick et al 1998).

Many studies have followed, using different vasoconstrictor agents, for example vasopressin (Bosch et al 1988) and somatostatin (Kravetz et al 1984) or its analogue octreotide (Møller et al 1997). Vasopressin causes generalized peripheral vasoconstriction, whereas the effect of somatostatin is specific to the splanchnic vascular bed and is the result both of an inhibition of glucagon release and direct vasoconstriction. Somatostatin is at least as effective as vasopressin in controlling bleeding, with fewer side-effects, and may be the agent of choice in the acute management of variceal hemorrhage. There is also evidence to suggest that 5-HT plays a significant role in maintaining raised portal pressure, and smooth muscle 5-HT-receptor antagonists have been shown to lower the pressure in cirrhosis (Hadengue et al 1987, Mastaï et al 1989).

Recent interest has been shown in an alternative pharmacological approach (Ch. 95), which reflects earlier discussion on the control of intrahepatic portal resistance. Arising from investigations which established that certain vasodilators are able to reduce portal resistance in the cirrhotic liver (Bhathal & Grossman 1985, Reichen & Le 1986, Navasa et al 1989, Reichen 1990), it became evident that there exists in the portal bed of cirrhotic liver a component that can be pharmacologically modulated (see discussion above). The nitro-vasodilators isosorbide dinitrate and mononitrate were observed to lower the portal pressure in portal hypertensive animals (Blei & Gottstein 1986) and increase hepatic (but not azygous) blood flow in cirrhotic patients (Navasa et al 1989), suggesting that they may act by reducing intrahepatic portal vascular resistance. Application of nitroglycerin by transdermal tape to cirrhotic patients resulted in a reduction in portal pressure without affecting hepatic blood flow (Iwao et al 1991). Given the modern concept of hepatic sinusoidal tone and its controlling mechanisms involving NO and ET-1 (see earlier discussion), it is now clear that the rationale for the success of this therapeutic approach is as a provider of supplementary NO. Moreover, an ET receptor antagonist has very recently been reported to reduce portal pressure in cirrhotic rats by nearly 30% (Reichen et al 1998). Conceptually, the application of an agent which selectively reduces intrahepatic portal resistance but does not directly affect splanchnic or collateral resistance is highly attractive, since reduction of hepatic portal flow can thus be avoided. Combination therapy using the long-acting nitro-vasodilator molsidomine plus propranolol has been found by some researchers (Hori et al 1996) but not others (García-Pagán et al 1996) to be a more effective portal hypotensive regimen than β-blockade alone. It is nevertheless currently considered that propranolol might optimally be combined with a nitro-vasodilator in the prevention of primary variceal bleeding (Lebrec 1997).

HUMAN LIVER TRANSPLANTATION : HEMODYNAMIC STUDIES

Initial investigations have revealed that orthotopic liver transplantation (OLT) (Ch. 109) leads to a rapid normalization of portal pressure but that the reversal of splanchnic and systemic hemodynamic abnormalities remains incomplete (see Henderson, 1993 for review). Thus, it has been shown that total hepatic blood flow (THBF) remains elevated up to 6 months after OLT (Hadengue et al 1993, Henderson et al 1989, Navasa et al 1993) with PV blood flow accounting for the majority of the elevated flow (Henderson 1992, Henderson et al 1993, Paulsen & Klintmalm 1992). Portal-systemic collateral blood vessels (Chezmar et al 1992) and portal-systemic collateral blood flow (Navasa et al 1993) have also been reported after OLT. Ligation of these portal-systemic collateral pathways has been shown to increase PV blood flow (Fujimoto et al 1995). Initial data on changes in systemic hemodynamics have been more equivocal, with cardiac output reported to remain elevated (Hadengue et al 1993) or to return to the normal range after OLT (Navasa et al 1993). Recently, Gadano and co-workers (1995) have emphasized that factors such as anemia and sepsis may account for the deranged hemodynamics after OLT.

EFFECT OF LIVER TRANSPLANTATION ON LBF

The publication by Henderson and co-workers (1989) that LBF remains elevated for a prolonged period after liver transplantation represents one of the most important findings in the field of hepatic hemodynamics in the past 10 years. It indicated that basal LBF may be under direct sympathetic control, which, following OLT, is lost allowing LBF to rise to a higher level. From a physiological standpoint, the hemodynamic consequences of OLT per se in human patients is difficult to interpret because (i) it is obviously not possible to include a control group of patients in any study, (ii) the patients receive immunosuppressive drugs which are known to have vasoactivity (for example, cyclosporin is a hypertensive agent), and (iii) the patients may in addition be given vasodilators to control systemic hypertension after OLT. Nonetheless, the theory that OLT may have a direct effect on LBF is contrary to the currently accepted understanding of hepatic hemodynamics, namely that basal LBF is not under neural control (see Lautt (1980) and Richardson and Withrington (1981) for reviews of nervous control of LBF). However, as the latter hypothesis is mainly based on the fact that acute surgical denervation of the liver (i) leaves unstimulated LBF unchanged (Ginsburg et al 1952, Cohn & Kountz 1963, Mundschau et al 1966, Lautt 1977, Mathie et al 1980a, Mathie & Blumgart 1983b) and (ii) blocks the transient increase in hepatic arterial vascular resistance which occurs with bilateral occlusion of the carotid arteries in adrenalectomized animals (Greenway et al 1967), the results may be open to question. Possible shortcomings of such acute liver denervation experiments are that the animal has a limited time to recover from a major surgical intervention involving considerable manipulation of the liver and that there is no guarantee that complete hepatic denervation has been achieved.

Animal studies

Until recently, very few studies on the effect of OLT on systemic or hepatic hemodynamics have been performed. Some time ago it was, however, shown in a small number of dogs that LBF after OLT remained constant for up to 3 weeks (Groth et al 1968). More recently, Chaland and co-workers (1990) found that cardiac output was elevated

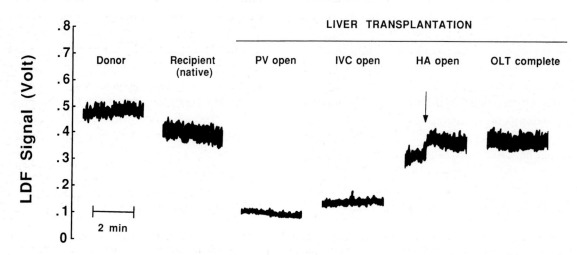

Fig. 4.4 Laser doppler flowmetry (LDF) measurements during a single liver transplantation operation in the rat. The point at which the hepatic artery was opened is shown by the arrow. Reproduced from Wheatley and Zhao 1993 with permission.

1 week after OLT. It should be noted that the results of neither of these studies can be considered physiological; in the former immunosuppression was given and in the latter pathophysiological changes to the liver including hepatic enlargement with lobular necrosis and elevated portal pressure were in evidence.

Measurement of graft reperfusion during the rat OLT operation has been performed using LDF (Wheatley &

Zhao 1993) (Fig. 4.4). LDF provided an excellent measure of hepatic perfusion throughout the OLT operation and was especially effective in demonstrating that rearterialization of the graft had been achieved. The final LDF signal from the graft was not significantly different from that of either the donor liver or the native liver of the recipient, indicating that in the early phases after OLT, total LBF is in the normal range (Wheatley & Zhao 1993).

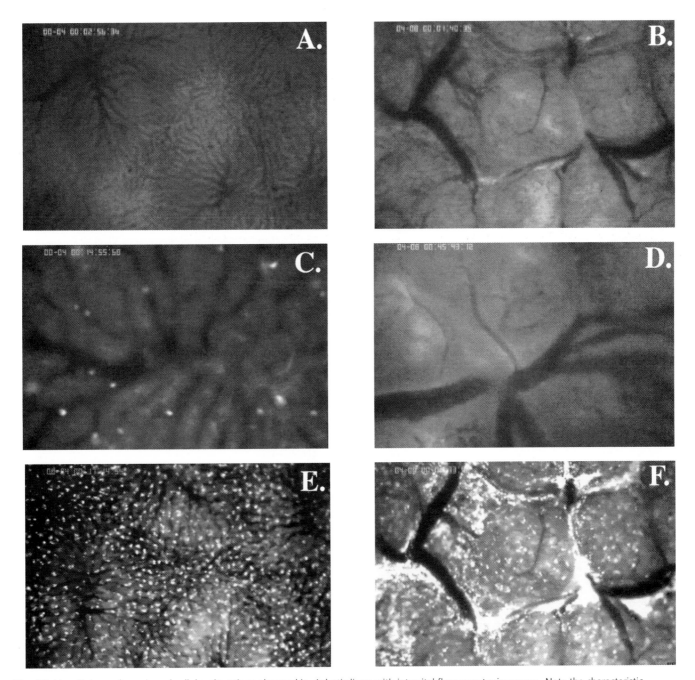

Fig. 4.5 Hepatic hemodynamic and cellular alterations observed in cirrhotic livers with intravital fluorescent microscopy. Note the characteristic alterations in cirrhotic livers with regard to distention of the central veins (**A** control vs. **B** cirrhotic), reduction in number of sinusoids directly feeding into to the central veins (**C** control vs. **D** cirrhotic), and movement of hepatic stellate cells (as measured by their vitamin A auto-fluorescence) from a homogenous distribution in control livers (**E**) to a heterogeneous distribution focused around and along fibrous bands connecting the central veins (**F**).

Long-term hemodynamic effects

Initial experiments on anesthetized animals 4 weeks after OLT indicated that LBF measured by the ^{133}Xe clearance technique was not significantly different from control (Wheatley et al 1993). Subsequently, it has been shown that if an all-suture OLT technique is used, LBF and cardiac output are normal in conscious animals 3 months after OLT (Kuznetsova et al 1995). These results indicate (i) that liver transplantation is unlikely to have any effect on hepatic hemodynamics, and (ii) that the sympathetic nervous system does not play a dominant role in the maintenance of basal hepatic hemodynamics. If, however, cuff anastomoses are used in the OLT operation, the animals develop hyperkinetic circulation with increased cardiac index and HA blood flow and decreased PV blood flow, most probably due to the development of PSS in excess of 50% (Kuznetsova et al 1995). The importance of PSS in hemodynamic changes after OLT has been emphasized recently by the report that in human transplant patients without pre-existing PSS (e.g. acute hepatic failure) both systemic and hepatic hemodynamics are normal after OLT (Gadano et al 1995). However, when the patients have pre-existing portal systemic shunts before OLT (e.g. cirrhosis) (Fig. 4.5), altered hemodynamics are likely to persist for some time after OLT (Gadano et al 1995). In a recent study, OLT in rats with established portal systemic shunting led to the reversal of the abnormal hemodynamics in the majority of animals (Zhang et al 1999). The mechanisms underlying the gradual return to normal LBF and cardiac output are not understood.

REFERENCES

Adson M A, Wychulis A R 1968 Portal hypertension in secondary biliary cirrhosis. Archives of Surgery 96: 604–612

Almond N E, Wheatley A M 1992 Measurement of hepatic perfusion in the rat by laser Doppler flowmetry. American Journal of Physiology 262: G203–G209

Andreen M, Irestedt L, Thulin L 1975 The effect of controlled halothane anaesthesia on splanchnic oxygen consumption in the dog. Acta Anaesthesiologica Scandinavica 19: 238–244

Aronsen K F 1968 Late effects of biliary stasis on the effective liver blood flow. Acta Chirurgica Scandinavica 134: 278–281

Aronsen K F, Ericsson B, Fajgelj A, Lindell S E 1966 The clearance of ^{133}Xenon from the liver after intraportal injection in man. Nuclear Medicine 5: 241–245

Aronsen K F, Nylander G, Ohlsson E G 1969 Liver blood flow studies during and after various periods of total biliary obstruction in the dog. Acta Chirurgica Scandinavica 135: 55–59

Aronsen K F, Ericsson B, Nosslin B, Nylander G, Phil B, Waldeskog B 1970 Evaluation of hepatic regeneration by scintillation scanning, cholangiography and angiography in man. Annals of Surgery 171: 567–574

Ball A B S 1991 Regional chemotherapy for colorectal hepatic metastases using degradable starch microspheres. A review. Acta Oncologica 30: 309–313

Ballet F 1991 Hepatic resistance in isolated perfused normal and cirrhotic liver. In: Ballet F, Thurman R G (eds) Research in perfused liver. INSERM/John Libbey, p 339–360

Batchelder B M, Cooperman L H 1975 Effects of anesthetics on splanchnic circulation and metabolism. Surgical Clinics of North America 55: 787–794

Bauer C, Walcher F, Kalweit U, Larsen R, Marzi I 1997 Role of nitric oxide in the regulation of the hepatic microcirculation in vivo. Journal of Hepatology 27: 1089–1095

Bauer M, Zhang J X, Bauer I et al 1994 ET-1 induced alterations of hepatic microcirculation: sinusoidal and extrasinusoidal sites of action. American Journal of Physiology 267: G143–G149

Bauer M, Paquette N, Zhang J et al 1995 Chronic ethanol consumption increases hepatic sinusoidal contractile response to endothelin-1 in the rat. Hepatology 22: 1565–1576.

Bhathal P S, Grossman H J 1985 Reduction of the increased portal vascular resistance of the isolated perfused cirrhotic rat liver by vasodilators. Journal of Hepatology 1: 325–337

Biber, Holm C, Winsö O et al 1983 Portal blood flow in man during surgery, measured by a modification of the continuous thermodilution method. Scandinavian Journal of Gastroenterology 18: 233–239

Birgens H S, Henriksen J, Matzen P, Poulsen H 1978 The shock liver. Acta Medica Scandinavia 204: 417–421

Blei A R, Gottstein J 1986 Isosorbide dinitrate in experimental portal hypertension: a study of factors that modulate the hemodynamic response. Hepatology 6: 107–111

Blei A T, Gareia-Tsao G, Groszmann R J et al 1987 Hemodynamic evaluation of isosorbide dinitrate in alcoholic cirrhosis: Pharmacokinetic–hemodynamic interactions. Gastroenterology 93: 576–583

Bloom N D, Kroop E, Sadjadi M, Jacobs R, Ramaswamy G, Ackerman N B 1987 Enhancement of tumor blood flow and tumoricidal effect of doxorubicin by intraportal epinephrine in experimental liver metastasis. Archives of Surgery 122: 1269–1272

Blumgart L H 1978 Liver atrophy, hypertrophy and regenerative hyperplasia in the rat: the relevance of blood flow. In: Ciba Foundation Symposium 55 (new series): Hepatotrophic factors. Elsevier Excerpta Medica, Amsterdam, p 181–215

Blumgart L H, Leach K G, Karran S J 1971 Observations on liver regeneration after right hepatic lobectomy. Gut 12: 922–928

Blumgart L H, Kelley C J, Benjamin I S 1984 Benign bile duct stricture following cholecystectomy: Critical factors in management. British Journal of Surgery 71: 836–843

Bollman J L 1961 The animal with an Eck fistula. Physiological Reviews 41: 607–621

Bosch J, Groszmann R J 1984 Measurement of azygous venous blood flow by a continuous thermal dilution technique: an index of blood flow through gastroesophageal collaterals in cirrhosis. Hepatology 4: 424–429

Bosch J, Enriquez R, Groszmann R J, Storer E H 1983 Chronic bile duct ligation in the dog: Hemodynamic characterization of a portal hypertensive model. Hepatology 3: 1002–1007

Bosch J, Bordas J M, Mastai R et al 1988 Effects of vasopressin on the intravariceal pressure in patients with cirrhosis: Comparison with the effects on portal pressure. Hepatology 8: 861–865

Boyer T D, Triger D R, Horisawa M, Redeker A G, Reynolds T B 1977 Direct transhepatic measurement of portal vein pressure using a thin needle. Comparison with wedged hepatic vein pressure. Gastroenterology 72: 584–589

Bradley S E, Ingelfinger F J, Bradley G P, Curry J J 1945 The estimation of hepatic blood flow in man. Journal of Clinical Investigation 24: 890–897

Breedis C, Young G 1954 The blood supply of neoplasms in the liver. American Journal of Pathology 30: 969–985

Brown H S, Halliwell M, Qamar M, Read A E, Evans J M, Wells P N T

1989 Measurement of normal portal venous blood flow by Doppler ultrasound. Gut 30: 503–509

Burchell A R, Moreno A H, Panke W F, Nealon T F 1976 Hepatic artery flow improvement after portacaval shunt: A single hemodynamic clinical correlate. Annals of Surgery 184: 289–302

Burns P, Taylor K, Blei A T 1987 Doppler flowmetry and portal hypertension. Gastroenterology 92: 824–826

Burroughs A K, Jenkins W J, Sherlock S et al 1983 Controlled trial of propranolol for the prevention of recurrent variceal hemorrhage in patients with cirrhosis. New England Journal of Medicine 309: 1539–1542

Burton-Opitz R 1910 The vascularity of the liver. I. The flow of blood in the hepatic artery. Quarterly Journal of Experimental Physiology 3: 297–313

Burton-Opitz R 1911 The vascularity of the liver. IV. The magnitude of the portal inflow. Quarterly Journal of Experimental Physiology 4: 113–125

Bynum T E, Boitnott J K, Maddrey W C 1979 Ischaemic hepatitis. Digestive Diseases and Sciences 24: 129–135

Caesar J, Shaldon S, Chiandussi L, Guevara L, Sherlock S 1961 The use of indocyanine green in the measurement of hepatic blood flow and as a test of hepatic function. Clinical Science 21: 43–57

Chaland P, Braillon A, Gaudin C et al 1990 Orthotopic liver transplantation with hepatic artery anastomoses. Transplantation 49: 675–678

Chezmar J L, Redvanly R D, Nelson R C, Henderson J M 1992 Persistence of portal systemic collaterals and splenomegaly on CT scan after orthotopic liver transplantation. American Journal of Roentgenology Radium Therapy Nuclear Medicine 159: 317–320

Chiandussi L, Greco F, Sardi G, Vaccarino A, Ferraris C M, Curti B 1968 Estimation of hepatic arterial and portal venous blood flow by direct catheterisation of the vena porta through the umbilical cord in man. Acta Hepatosplenologica 15: 166–171

Cohn R, Kountz S 1963 Factors influencing control of arterial circulation in the liver of the dog. American Journal of Physiology 205: 1260–1264.

Dauzat M, Layrargues G P 1989 Portal vein blood flow measurements using pulsed Doppler and electromagnetic flowmetry in dogs: A comparative study. Gastroenterology 96: 913–919

Dinc H, Sari A, Resit-Gumele H, Cihanyurdu N, Baki A 1998 Portal and splanchnic haemodynamics in patients with advanced post-hepatitic cirrhosis and in healthy adults. Assessment with duplex Doppler ultrasound. Acta Radiology 39: 152–156

Dobson E L, Jones H B 1952 The behaviour of intravenously injected particulate material. Its rate of disappearance from the blood stream as a measure of liver blood flow. Acta Medica Scandinavica (Supplementum) 273: 1–71

Ernst H, Hahn E G, Balzer T, Schlief R, Heyder N 1996 Color doppler ultrasound of liver lesions: signal enhancement after intravenous injection of the ultrasound contrast agent Levovist. Journal of Clinical Ultrasound 24: 31–35

Fleming J S, Humphries N L M, Karran S J, Goddard B A, Ackery D M 1981 In vivo assessment of hepatic-arterial and portal-venous components of liver perfusion: Concise communication. Journal of Nuclear Medicine 22: 18–21

Friedman S L 1993 The cellular basis of hepatic fibrosis. Mechanisms and treatment strategies. New England Journal of Medicine 119: 1828–1835

Friedman S L 1997 Molecular mechanisms of hepatic fibrosis and principles of therapy. Journal of Gastroenterology 32: 424–430

Fujimoto M, Moriyasu F, Nada T et al 1995 Influence of spontaneous portosystemic collateral pathways on portal hemodynamics in living-related liver transplantation in children: Doppler ultrasonographic study. Transplantation 60: 41–45

Fung Y, Glajchen N, Shapiro R S, Wolf D C, Cooper J M 1998 Portal vein velocities measured by ultrasound: usefulness for evaluating shunt functioning following TIPS. Abdominal Imaging 23: 511–514

Gadano A, Hadengue A, Widmann J J et al 1995 Hemodynamics after orthotopic liver transplantation: Study of associated factors and long-term effects. Hepatology 22: 458–465

Gadano G, Hadengue A, Vachiery F et al 1997 Relationship between hepatic blood flow, liver tests, haemodynamic values and clinical characteristics in patients with chronic liver disease. Journal of Gastroenterology and Hepatology 12: 167–171

Gaiani S, Bolondi L, Li Bassi S, Zironi G, Siringo S, Barbara L 1991 Prevalence of spontaneous, hepatofugal portal flow in liver cirrhosis. Gastroenterology 100: 160–167

Gandhi C R, Berkowitz D E, Watkins, W D 1994 Endothelins. Biochemistry and pathophysiologic actions. Anesthesiology 80: 892–905

García-Pagán J C, Escorsell A, Feu F et al 1996 Propranolol plus molsidomine vs propranolol alone in the treatment of portal hypertension in patients with cirrhosis. Journal of Hepatology 24: 430–435

Garcia-Tsao G, Groszmann R J, Fisher R L, Conn H O, Atterbury C E, Glickman M 1985 Portal pressure, presence of gastroesophageal varices and variceal bleeding. Hepatology 5: 419–424

George C F 1979 Drug kinetics and hepatic blood flow. Clinical Pharmacokinetics 4: 433–448

Ginsburg M, Grayson J, Johnson D H 1952 The nervous regulation of liver blood flow. Proceedings of the Physiological Society 17: 74P–75P

Goldberg J A, Murray T, Kerr D J et al 1991 The use of angiotensin II as a potential method of targeting cytotoxic microspheres in patients with intrahepatic tumour. British Journal of Cancer 63: 308–310

Gottlieb M E, Sarfeh I J, Stratton H, Goldman M L Newell J C, Shah D M 1983 Hepatic perfusion and splanchnic oxygen consumption in patients post injury. Journal of Trauma 23: 836–843

Grainger S L, Keeling P W N, Brown I M H, Marigold J H, Thompson R P H 1983 Clearance and non-invasive determination of the hepatic extraction of indocyanine green in baboons and man. Clinical Science 64: 207–212

Greenway C V, Lawson A E, Mellander S 1967 The effects of stimulation of the hepatic nerves, infusions of noradrenaline and occlusion of the carotid arteries on liver blood flow in the anaesthetised cat. Journal of Physiology 192: 21–41

Greenway C V, Stark R D 1971 Hepatic vascular bed. Physiological Reviews 51: 23–65

Greenway C V, Lautt W W 1970 Effects of hepatic venous pressure on transsinusoidal fluid transfer in the liver of the anesthetized cat. Circulation Research 26: 697–703

Greenway C V, Oshiro G 1972 Intrahepatic distribution of portal and hepatic arterial blood flows in anaesthetized cats and dogs and the effects of portal occlusion, raised venous pressure and histamine. Journal of Physiology (London) 227: 473–485

Greenway C V, Lautt W W 1989 Hepatic circulation. In: Schultz S G, Wood J D, Rauner B B (eds) Handbook of physiology—The gastrointestinal system 1. American Physiological Society, Oxford University Press, New York, p 1519–1564

Greenwel P, Schwartz M, Rosas M, Peyrol S, Grimaud J A, Rojkind M 1991 Characterization of fat-storing cell lines derived from normal and CCl_4–cirrhotic livers. Differences in the production of interleukin-6. Laboratory Investigation 65: 644–653

Groszmann R J 1990 Pathophysiology of portal hypertension. In: Gentilini P, Arias I M, Arroyo V, Schrier R W (eds) Liver diseases and renal complications. Raven Press, New York, p 165–173

Groszmann RJ, Kravetz D, Parysow O 1977 Intrahepatic arteriovenous shunting in cirrhosis of the liver. Gastroenterology 73: 201–204

Groth C G, Porter K A, Otte J B et al 1968 Studies of blood flow and ultrastructural changes in rejecting and nonrejecting canine orthotopic liver homografts. Surgery 63: 658–668

Guest J, Ryan C J, Benjamin I S, Blumgart L H 1977 Portacaval transposition and subsequent partial hepatectomy in the rat: effects on liver atrophy, hypertrophy and regenerative hyperplasia. British Journal of Experimental Pathology 58: 140–146

Gupta T K, Toruner M, Chung M K, Groszmann R J 1998 Endothelial dysfunction and decreased production of nitric oxide in the intrahepatic microcirculation of cirrhotic rats. Hepatology 28: 926–931

Hadengue A, Lee S S, Moreau R, Braillon A, Lebrec D 1987 Beneficial hemodynamic effects of ketanserin in patients with cirrhosis: possible role of serotinergic mechanisms in portal hypertension. Hepatology 7: 644–647

Hadengue A, Moreau R, Sogni P et al 1991 High cardiac output after liver transplantation (OLT) is due to persistent portasystemic collateral and elevated hepatic blood flow. Hepatology 14: 57A

Hadengue A, Lebrec D, Moreau R et al 1993 Persistence of systemic and splanchnic hyperkinetic circulation in liver transplant patients. Hepatology 17: 175–178

Hahn M, Massen O, Nencki M, Pawlow J 1893 Die Eck'sche Fistel zwischen der unteren Hohlvene und der Pfortader und ihre Folgen für den Organismus. Archiv für Experimentelle Pathologie und Pharmakologie 32: 161–210

Hemingway D M, Cooke T G, Chang D, Grime S J, Jenkins S A 1991 The effects of intra-arterial vasoconstrictors on the distribution of a radiolabelled low molecular weight marker in an experimental model of liver tumour. British Journal of Cancer 63: 495–498

Henderson J M 1993 Abnormal splanchnic and systemic hemodynamics of end-stage liver disease: what happens after liver transplantation? Hepatology 17: 514–516

Henderson J M, Millikan W J, Hooks M, Noe B, Kutner M H, Warren W D 1989 Increased galactose clearance after liver transplantation: A measure of increased blood flow through the denervated liver? Hepatology 10: 288–291

Henderson J M, Gilmore G T, Galloway J R, Dodson T F 1991 Hepatic artery flow increases intraoperatively during liver transplantation in response to portal vein flow reduction. Hepatology 14: 48A

Henderson J M, Gilmore G T, Mackay G J, Galloway J R, Dodson T F, Kutner M H 1992a Hemodynamics during liver transplantation: the interactions between cardiac output and portal venous and hepatic arterial blood flows. Hepatology 16: 715–718

Henderson J M, Mackay G J, Hooks M et al 1992b High cardiac output of advanced liver disease persists after orthotopic liver transplantation. Hepatology 15: 258–262

Hori N, Okanoue T, Sawa Y, Mori T, Kashima K 1996 Haemodynamic effects of combined treatment with molsidomine and propranolol on portal hypertension in conscious and unrestrained cirrhotic rats. Journal of Gastroenterology and Hepatology 11: 985–992

Housset C, Rockey D C, Bissell D M 1993 Endothelin receptors in rat liver: lipocytes as a contractile target for endothelin 1. Proceedings of the National Academy of Science USA 90: 9266–9270

Huet P M, Lavoie P, Viallet A 1973 Simultaneous estimation of hepatic and portal blood flows by an indicator dilution technique. Journal of Laboratory and Clinical Medicine 82: 836–846

Hughes R L, Mathie R T, Campbell D, Fitch W 1979a The effect of hypercarbia on hepatic blood flow and oxygen consumption in the greyhound. British Journal of Anaesthesia 51: 289–296

Hughes R L, Mathie R T, Fitch W, Campbell D 1979b Liver blood flow and oxygen consumption during hypocapnia and IPPV in the greyhound. Journal of Applied Physiology 47: 290–295

Hughes R L Mathie R T, Campbell D, Fitch W 1979c Systemic hypoxia and hyperoxia, and liver blood flow and oxygen consumption in talc greyhound. Pflügers Archiv 381: 151–157

Hughes R L, Campbell D, Fitch W 1980a Effects of enflurane and halothane on liver blood flow and oxygen consumption in the greyhound. British Journal of Anaesthesia 52: 1079–1086

Hughes R L, Mathie R T, Fitch W, Campbell D 1980b Liver blood flow and oxygen consumption during metabolic acidosis and alkalosis in the greyhound. Clinical Science 60: 355–361

Hunt D R 1979 Changes in liver blood flow with development of biliary obstruction in the rat. Australian and New Zealand Journal of Surgery 49: 733–737

Iannitti D A, Henderson J M 1997 Surgery in portal hypertension. Baillières Clinical Gastroenterology 11: 351–364

Isales C M, Nathanson M H, Bruck R 1993 Endothelin-1 induces cholestasis which is mediated by an increase in portal pressure. Biochemical Biophysical Research Communications 191: 1244–1251

Iwao T, Toyonaga A, Sumino M et al 1991 Hemodynamic study during transdermal application of nitroglycerin tape in patients with cirrhosis. Hepatology 13: 124–128

Iwao T, Toyonaga A, Oho K et al 1997 Value of Doppler ultrasound parameters of portal vein and hepatic artery in the diagnosis of cirrhosis and portal hypertension. American Journal of Gastroenterology 92: 1012–1017

Jefferson N C, Hassan M I, Popper H L, Necheles H 1956 Formation of effective collateral circulation following excision of hepatic artery. American Journal of Physiology 184: 589–592

Keiding S 1988 Galactose clearance measurements and liver blood flow. Gastroenterology 94: 477–481

Kelty R H, Baggenstoss A H, Butt H R 1950 The relation of the regenerated liver nodule to the vascular bed in cirrhosis. Gastroenterology 15: 285–295

Kock N G, Hahnloser P, Roding B, Schenk W G 1972 Interaction between portal venous and hepatic arterial blood flow: An experimental study in the dog. Surgery 72: 414–419

Kravetz D, Bosch J, Teres J, Bruix J, Rimola A, Rodes J 1984 Comparison of intravenous somatostatin and vasopressin infusions in treatment of acute variceal hemorrhage. Hepatology 4: 442–446

Kuo P C, King L, Alfrey E J, Jeffery R B, Garcia G, Dafoe D C 1995 Magnetic resonance imaging and hepatic hemodynamics: Correlation with metabolic function in liver transplantation candidates. Surgery 117: 373–379

Kurihara T, Akimoto M, Kurokawa K et al 1992 Relationship between endothelin and thromboxane A2 in rat liver microcirculation. Life Science 51: PL281–5

Kuznetsova L V, Zhao D, Wheatley A M 1995 Effect of orthotopic liver transplantation on systemic and splanchnic hemodynamics in conscious rat. American Journal of Physiology 269: G153–G159

Lautt, W W 1977 Effect of stimulation of hepatic nerves on hepatic O_2 uptake and blood flow. American Journal of Physiology 232: H652–H656

Lautt W W 1980 Hepatic nerves: A review of their functions and effects. Canada Journal of Physiology and Pharmacology 58: 105–123.

Lautt W W 1981 Role and control of the hepatic artery. In: Lautt W W (ed) Hepatic circulation in health and disease. Raven Press, New York, p 203–226

Lautt W W 1983 Relationship between hepatic blood flow and overall metabolism: the hepatic arterial buffer response. Federation Proceedings 42: 1662–1666

Lautt W W, Legare D J 1985 The use of 8-phenyltheophylline as a competitive antagonist of adenosine and an inhibitor of the intrinsic regulatory mechanism of the hepatic artery. Canadian Journal of Physiology and Pharmacology 63: 711–722

Lautt W W, Legare D J, Daniels T R 1984 The comparative effects of substances via the hepatic artery or portal vein on hepatic arterial resistance, liver blood volume and hepatic extraction in cats. Hepatology 4: 927–932

Lautt W W, Greenway C V, Legare D J, Weisman H 1986 Localization of intrahepatic portal vascular resistance. American Journal of Physiology 251: G375–G381

Lautt W W, Greenway C V, Legare D J 1987 Effect of hepatic nerves, norepinephrine, angiotensin, and elevated central venous pressure on postsinusoidal resistance sites and intrahepatic pressures in cats. Microvascular Research 33: 50–61

Lebrec D 1997 Pharmacotherapeutic agents in the treatment of portal hypertension. Journal of Gastroenterology and Hepatology 12: 159–166

Lebrec D, Poynard T, Hillon P, Benhamou J-P 1981 Propranolol for prevention of recurrent gastrointestinal bleeding in patients with cirrhosis. A controlled study. New England Journal of Medicine 305: 1371–1374

Lee F Y, Wang S S, Yang M C M et al 1995 Peripheral endotoxemia and hyperdynamic circulation of rats with intrahepatic or extrahepatic portal hypertension. Hepatology 22: 257A

Lee S, Hadengue A, Girod C, Braillon A, Lebrec D 1987 Reduction of intrahepatic vascular space in the pathogenesis of portal hypertension. Gastroenterology 157–161

Leen E, Goldberg J A, Robertson J, Sutherland G R, McArdle C S 1991a The use of Duplex sonography in the detection of colorectal hepatic metastases. British Journal of Cancer 63: 323–325

Leen E, Goldberg J A, Robertson J et al 1991b Detection of hepatic metastases using Duplex/color Doppler sonography. Annals of Surgery 214: 599–604

Leen E, Angerson W J, Wotherspoon H, Moule B, Cooke T G, McArdle C S 1995 Detection of colorectal liver metastases: comparison of laparotomy, CT, US, and Doppler perfusion index and evaluation of postoperative follow-up results. Radiology 195: 113–116

Legare D J, Lautt W W 1987 Hepatic venous resistance site in the dog: localization and validation of intrahepatic pressure measurements. Canadian Journal of Physiology and Pharmacology 65: 352–359

Leiberman D P, Mathie R T, Harper A M, Blumgart L H 1978a The hepatic arterial and portal venous circulations of the liver studied with a krypton-85 clearance technique. Journal of Surgical Research 25: 154–162

Leiberman D P, Mathie R T, Harper A M, Blumgart L H 1978b An isotope clearance method for measurement of liver blood flow during portasystemic shunt in man. British Journal of Surgery 65: 578–580

Leivas A, Jimenez W, Lamas S et al 1995 Endothelin-1 does not play a major role in the homeostasis of arterial pressure in cirrhotic rats with ascites. Gastroenterology 108: 1842–1848

Leveson S H, Wiggins P A, Giles G R, Parkin A, Robinson P J 1985 Deranged liver blood flow patterns in the detection of liver metastases. British Journal of Surgery 72: 128–130

MacLeod J J R, Pearce R G 1914 The outflow of blood from the liver as affected by variations in the condition of the portal vein and hepatic artery. American Journal of Physiology 35: 87–105

Mallet-Guy Y, Paillot J M, Switalska C, Mallet-Guy P 1972 Note sur les lésions ultrastructurales immédiates du foie après clampage expérimental de l'artère hépatique. Lyon Chirurgical 68: 170–175

Mann F C 1944 The William Henry Welch Lectures: II. Restoration and pathologic reactions of the liver. Journal of Mount Sinai Hospital 11: 65–74

Marchioro T L Porter K A, Brown B 1, Otte J-B, Starzl T E 1967 The effect of partial portacaval transposition on the canine liver. Surgery 61: 723–732

Martinez-Hernandez A 1985 The hepatic extracellular matrix. II. Electron immunohistochemical studies in rats with CCl_4–induced cirrhosis. Laboratory Investigation 53: 166–186

Martinez-Hernandez A, Amenta P S 1993 The hepatic extracellular matrix. I. Components and distribution in normal liver [editorial]. Virchow Archives — A, Pathology Anatomy and Histopathology 423, 1–11.

Martinez-Hernandez A, Amenta P S 1995 The extracellular matrix in hepatic regeneration. FASEB Journal 9: 1401–1410

Mastaï R, Rocheleau B, Huet P-M 1989 Serotonin blockade in conscious, unrestrained cirrhotic dogs with portal hypertension. Hepatology 9: 265–268

Mathie R T 1997 Hepatic haemodynamics during and after brief occlusion of the hepatic artery. Hepatology Research 8: 198–206

Mathie R T 1999 The hepatic haemodynamic effects of nitric oxide. In:

Mathie R T, Griffith T M (eds) The Haemodynamic Effects of Nitric Oxide. Imperial College Press, London, p 292–317

Mathie R T, Blumgart L H 1982 Hepatic tissue perfusion studies during partial hepatectomy in man. Surgical Gastroenterology 1: 297–302

Mathie R T, Blumgart L H 1983a The hepatic haemodynamic response to acute portal venous blood flow reductions in the dog. Pflügers Archiv 399: 223–227

Mathie R T, Blumgart L H 1983b Effect of denervation on the hepatic haemodynamic response to hypercapnia and hypoxia in the dog. Pflügers Archiv 397: 152–157

Mathie R T, Alexander B 1990 The role of adenosine in the hyperaemic response of the hepatic artery to portal venous occlusion (the 'buffer response'). British Journal of Pharmacology 100: 626–630

Mathie R T, Leiberman D P, Harper A M, Blumgart L H 1977 The solubility of ^{85}Krypton in the regenerating liver of the rat. British Journal of Experimental Pathology 58: 231–235

Mathie R T, Leiberman D P, Harper A M, Blumgart L H 1979 The role of blood flow in the control of liver size. Journal of Surgical Research 27: 139–144

Mathie R T, Lam P H M, Harper A M, Blumgart L H 1980a The hepatic arterial blood flow response to portal vein occlusion in the dog: The effect of hepatic denervation. Pflügers Archiv 386: 77–83

Mathie R T, Toouli J, Smith A, Harper A M, Blumgart L H 1980b Hepatic tissue perfusion studies during distal splenorenal shunt. American Journal of Surgery 140: 384–386

Mathie R T, Nagorney D M, Lewis M H, Blumgart L H 1988 Hepatic hemodynamics after chronic obstruction of the biliary tract in the dog. Surgery, Gynecology and Obstetrics 166: 125–130

Mathie R T, Alexander B, Ralevic V, Burnstock G 1991a Adenosine-induced dilatation of the rabbit hepatic arterial vasculature is mediated by A_2–purinoceptors. British Journal of Pharmacology 103: 1103–1107

Mays E T, Wheeler C S 1974 Demonstration of collateral arterial flow after interruption of hepatic arteries in man. New England Journal of Medicine 290: 993–996

McCormick P A, Patch D, Greenslade L, Chin J, McIntyre N, Burroughs A K 1998 Clinical vs haemodynamic response to drugs in portal hypertension. Journal of Hepatology 28: 1015–1019

Menger M D, Messmer K 1991 In vivo fluorescent microscopy for quantitative analysis of the hepatic microcirculation in hamsters and rats. European Surgical Research 23: 158–169

Miller W L, Redfield M M, Burnett J C 1989 Integrated cardiac, renal, and endocrine actions of endothelin. Journal of Clinical Investment 83: 317–320.

Møller S, Brinch K, Henriksen J H, Becker U 1997 Effect of octreotide on systemic, central, and splanchnic haemodynamics in cirrhosis. Journal of Hepatology 26: 1026–1033

Moreno A H, Burchell A R, Reddy R V, Steen J A, Panke W F, Nealon T F 1975 Spontaneous reversal of portal blood flow: The call for and against its occurrence in patients with cirrhosis of the liver. Annals of Surgery 181: 346–358

Moriyasu F, Ban N, Nishida O et al 1986 Clinical application of an ultrasonic Duplex system in the quantitative measurement of portal blood flow. Journal of Clinical Ultrasound 14: 579–588

Morsiani E, Mazzoni M, Aleotti A, Gorini P, Ricci D 1995 Increased sinusoidal wall permeability and liver fatty change after two-thirds hepatectomy: an ultrastructural study in the rat. Hepatology 21: 539–544

Mundschau G A, Zimmerman S W, Gildersleeve J W, Murphy Q R 1966 Hepatic and mesenteric artery resistances after sinoaortic denervation and hemorrhage. American Journal of Physiology 211: 77–82

Nagano K, Gelman S, Parks D, Henderson T, Lowery T 1988 Hepatic oxygen supply–demand relationship during anaesthesia in the pig. Anesthesiology 69: A440

Nagorney D M, Mathie R T, Lygidakis N J, Blumgart L H 1982 Bile duct pressure as a modulator of liver blood flow after common bile duct obstruction. Surgical Forum 33: 206–208

Nakamura T, Moriyasu F, Ban N et al 1989 Quantitative measurement of abdominal arterial blood flow using image-directed Doppler ultrasonography: superior mesenteric, splenic and common hepatic arterial blood flow in normal adults. Journal of Clinical Ultrasound 17: 261–268

Navasa M, Chesta J, Bosch J, Rodes J 1989 Reduction of portal pressure by isosorbide-5-mononitrate in patients with cirrhosis. Gastroenterology 96: 1110–1118

Navasa M, Feu F, Bosch J et al 1991 Systemic, splanchnic and humoral changes after orthotopic liver transplantation (OLT) in cirrhosis. Journal of Hepatology 13 (Supplement 2): S55

Navasa M, Feu F, Garcia-Pagan J C et al 1993 Hemodynamic and humoral changes after liver transplantation in patients with cirrhosis. Hepatology 17: 355–360

Niederberger M, Martin P-Y, Ginès P et al 1995 Normalization of nitric oxide production corrects arterial vasodilation and hyperdynamic circulation in cirrhotic rats. Gastroenterology 109: 1624–1630

Ohlsson E G 1972 The arterial circulation in the liver after total biliary obstruction in dogs. Acta Chirurgica Scandinavica 138: 1–58

Ohlsson E G, Rutherford R B, Boitnott J I C, Haalebos M M P, Zuidema G D 1970 Changes in portal circulation after biliary obstruction in dogs. American Journal of Surgery 120: 16–22

Ohnishi K, Saito M, Sato S et al 1987 Portal hemodynamics in idiopathic portal hypertension (Banti's syndrome). Gastroenterology 92: 751–758

Okuda IC, Suzuki K, Musha H, Arimizu N 1977 Percutaneous transhepatic catheterization of the portal vein for the study of portal hemodynamics and shunts. A preliminary report. Gastroenterology 73: 279–284

Okumura S, Takei Y, Kawano S, Nagano K, Masuda E, Goto M, Tsuji S, Michida T, Chen S S, Kashiwagi T, Fusamoto H, Kamada T, Sato N 1994 Vasoactive effect of endothelin-1 on rat liver in vivo. Hepatology 19: 155–161

Orrego H, Blendis L M, Crossley I R, Medline A, Macdonald A, Ritchie S, Israel Y 1981. Correlation of intrahepatic pressure with collagen in the Disse space and hepatomegaly in humans and in the rat. Gastroenterology 80: 546–556

Pachter H L, Drager S, Godfrey N, LeFleur R 1979 Traumatic injuries of the portal vein: The role of acute ligation. Annals of Surgery 189: 383–385

Pannen B H J, Bauer M 1998 Differential regulation of hepatic arterial and portal venous vascular resistance by nitric oxide and carbon monoxide in rats. Life Science 62: 2025–2033

Pannen B H J, Bauer M, Zhang J X, Robotham J L, Clemens M G 1996 Endotoxin pretreatment enhances portal venous contractile response to endothelin-1. American Journal of Physiology 270: H7–15

Parkin A, Robinson P J, Baxter P, Leveson S H, Wiggins P A, Giles G R 1983 Liver perfusion scintigraphy—method, normal range and laparotomy correlation in 100 patients. Nuclear Medicine Communications 4: 395–402

Paulsen A W, Klintmalm G B G 1992 Direct measurement of hepatic blood flow in native and transplanted organs, with accompanying systemic hemodynamics. Hepatology 16: 100–111.

Payen D M, Fratacci M D, Dupuy P et al 1990 Portal and hepatic arterial blood flow measurements of human transplanted liver by implanted Doppler probes: Interest for early complications and nutrition. Surgery 107: 417–427

Peitzman A B, Billiar T R, Harbrecht B G, Kelly E, Odekwu A O, Simmons R L 1995 Hemorrhagic shock. Current Problems in Surgery 32: 925–1002

Pelc L C, Pelc N J, Rayhill S C et al 1992 Arterial and venous blood flow: non-invasive quantitation with MR imaging. Radiology 185: 809–812

Pinzani M, Failli P, Ruocco C et al 1992 Fat-storing cells as liver-specific pericytes. Spatial dynamics of agonist-stimulated intracellular calcium transients. Journal of Clinical Investigations 90: 642–646

Pinzani M, Milani S, De Franco R et al 1996 Endothelin-1 is overexpressed in human cirrhotic liver and exerts multiple effects on activated hepatic stellate cells. Gastroenterology 110: 534–548

Pizcueta P, Pique J M, Fernandez M et al 1992 Modulation of the hyperdynamic circulation of cirrhotic rats by nitric oxide inhibition. Gastroenterology 103: 1909–1915

Rappaport A M 1973 The microcirculatory hepatic unit. Microvascular Research 6: 212–228

Rappaport A M, Schneiderman J H 1976 The function of the hepatic artery. Reviews of Physiology, Biochemistry and Pharmacology 76: 129–175

Reichen J 1990 Liver function and pharmacological considerations in pathogenesis and treatment of portal hypertension. Hepatology 11: 1066–1078

Reichen J, Le M 1986 Verapamil favorably influences hepatic microvascular exchange and function in rats with cirrhosis of the liver. Journal of Clinical Investigation 78: 448–455

Reichen J, Gerbes A L, Steiner M J, Sägesser H, Clozel M 1998 The effect of endothelin and its antagonist Bosentan on hemodynamics and microvascular exchange in cirrhotic rat liver. Journal of Hepatology 28: 1020–1030

Reichman S, Davis W D, Storaasli J P, Gorlin R 1958 Measurement of hepatic blood flow by indicator dilution techniques. Journal of Clinical Investigation 37: 1848–1856

Reuter S R, Chuang V P 1976 The location of increased resistance to portal blood flow in obstructive jaundice. Investigative Radiology 11: 54–59

Rice G C, Leiberman D P, Mathie R T, Ryan C J, Harper A M, Blumgart L H 1977 Liver tissue blood flow measured by ^{85}Kr clearance in the anaesthetized rat before and after partial hepatectomy. British Journal of Experimental Pathology 58: 243–250

Richardson P D I, Withrington P G 1981 Liver blood flow. II. Effects of drugs and hormones on liver blood flow. Gastroenterology 81: 356–375

Rockey D C, Chung J J 1995 Inducible nitric oxide synthase in rat hepatic lipocytes and the effect of nitric oxide on lipocyte contractility. Journal of Clinical Investigation 95: 1199–1206

Rockey D C, Weisiger R A 1996 Endothelin induced contractility of stellate cells from normal and cirrhotic rat liver: implications for regulation of portal pressure and resistance. Hepatology 24: 233–240

Rockey D C, Chung J J 1998 Reduced nitric oxide production by endothelial cells in cirrhotic rat liver: endothelial dysfunction in portal hypertension. Gastroenterology 114: 344–351

Rockey D C, Boyles J K, Gabbiani G, Friedman S L 1992 Rat hepatic lipocytes express smooth muscle actin upon activation in vivo and in culture. Journal Submicrosc Cyto & Path, 24: 193–203

Rockey D C, Fouassier L, Chung J J, Carayon A, Vallee P, Rey C, Housset C 1998 Cellular localization of endothelin-1 and increased production in liver injury in the rat — potential for autocrine and paracrine effects on stellate cells. Hepatology 27: 472–480

Rosemurgy A S, Zervos E F, Goode S E, Black T J, Zwiebel B R 1997 Differential effects on portal and effective hepatic blood flow. A comparison between transjugular intrahepatic portasystemic shunt and small diameter H-graft portacaval shunt. Annals of Surgery 225: 607–608

Rössle M, Richter G M, Nöldge G, Palmaz J C, Wenz W, Gerok W 1989 New non-operative treatment for variceal haemorrhage. Lancet ii: 153

Ryan C J, Guest J, Harper A M, Blumgart L H 1978 Liver blood flow measurement in the portacavally transposed rat before and after partial hepatectomy. British Journal of Experimental Pathology 59: 111–115

Sapirstein L A 1956 Fractionation of the cardiac output of rats with isotopic potassium. Circulation Research 4: 689–692

Schenk W G, McDonald J C, McDonald K, Drapanas T 1962 Direct measurement of hepatic blood flow in surgical patients: with related observations on hepatic flow dynamics in experimental animals. Annals of Surgery 156: 463–469

Sedgwick C E, Poulantzas J K, Kune G A 1966 Management of portal hypertension secondary to bile duct strictures: Review of 18 cases with splenorenal shunt. Annals of Surgery 163: 949–953

Seifalian A M, Mallet S V, Rolles K, Davidson B R 1997 Hepatic microcirculation during human orthotopic liver transplantation. British Journal of Surgery 84: 1391–1395

Shah V, Haddad F G, García-Cardeña G et al 1997 Liver sinusoidal endothelial cells are responsible for nitric oxide modulation of resistance in the hepatic sinusoids. Journal of Clinical Investigation 100: 2923–2930

Shepherd A P, Riedel G L, Ward W F 1983 Laser Doppler measurements of blood flow within the intestinal wall and on the surface of the liver. In: Koo A, Lam S K, Smaje L H (eds) Microcirculation of the alimentary tract. World Scientific Publishing Company, Singapore, p 115–129

Shepherd A P, Riedel G L, Kiel J W, Haumschild D J, Maxwell L C 1987 Evaluation of an infrared laser-Doppler blood flowmeter. American Journal of Physiology 252: G832–G839

Sherman I A, Pappas S C, Fisher M M 1990 Hepatic microvascular changes associated with development of liver fibrosis and cirrhosis. American Journal of Physiology 258: H460–H465

Sherman I A, Dlugosz J A, Barker F, Sadeghi F M, Pang K S 1996 Dynamics of arterial and portal venous flow interactions in perfused rat liver: An intravital microscopic study. American Journal of Physiology 271: G201–G210

Shibayama Y, Nakata K 1985 Localization of increased hepatic vascular resistance in liver cirrhosis. Hepatology 5: 643–648

Shikare S V, Bashir K, Abraham P, Tilve G H 1996 Hepatic perfusion index in portal hypertension of cirrhotic and non-cirrhotic aetiologies. Nuclear Medicine Communications 17: 520–522

Shimamura T, Zhu Y, Zhang S et al 1996 Nitric oxide down-regulates endothelin production during ischemia and reperfusion of canine livers. Hepatology 24: 579A

Smith A, Mathie R T, Hughes R L, Harper A M, Blumgart L H 1979 Effect of haemorrhagic hypotension on liver blood flow and oxygen consumption in the dog. Gut 20: A454

Starzl T E, Francavilla A, Halgrimson C G 1973 The origin, hormonal nature and action of hepatotrophic substances in portal venous blood. Surgery, Gynecology and Obstetrics 137: 179–199

Starzl T E, Porter K A, Kashiwagi N, Lee I Y, Russell W J I, Putnam C W 1975 The effect of diabetes mellitus on portal blood hepatotrophic factors in dogs. Surgery, Gynecology and Obstetrics 140: 549–562

Steer M L, Thomas A N, Rosson C T, Ketchum S A, Hali A D 1968 Chronic biliary obstruction: Hemodynamic effects of decompression. Surgical Forum 19: 342–344

Suematsu M, Goda N, Sano T, Kashiwagi S, Egawa T, Shinoda Y, Ishimura Y 1995 Carbon monoxide: an endogenous modulator of sinusoidal tone in the perfused rat liver [see comments]. Journal of Clinical Investigation 96: 2431–2437

Suematsu M, Wakabayashi Y, Ishimura Y 1996 Gaseous monoxides: a new class of microvascular regulator in the liver. Cardiovascular Research 32: 679–686

Takaoka F, Brown M R, Ramsay M A E, Paulsen A W, Brajtbord D, Klintmalm G B 1990 Intraoperative evaluation of Eurocollins and University of Wisconsin preservation solutions in patients undergoing hepatic transplantation. Transplantation 49: 544–547

Tamakuma S, Wada N, Ishiyama M et al 1975 Relationship between hepatic hemodynamics and biliary pressure in dogs: Its significance in clinical shock following biliary decompression. Japanese Journal of Surgery 5: 255–268

Tanaka A, Katagiri K, Hoshino M, Hayakawa T, Tsukada K, Takeuchi T

1994 Endothelin-1 stimulates bile acid secretion and vesicular transport in the isolated perfused rat liver. American Journal of Physiology 266: G324–G329

Thomson I A, Hughes R L, Fitch W, Campbell D 1982 Effects of nitrous oxide on liver haemodynamics and oxygen consumption in the greyhound. Anaesthesia 37: 548–553

Thomson I A, Fitch W, Hughes R L, Campbell D, Watson R 1986 Effects of certain i.v. anaesthetics on liver blood flow and hepatic oxygen consumption in the greyhound. British Journal of Anaesthesia 58: 69–80

Thulin L, Andreen M, Irestedt L 1975 Effect of controlled halothane anaesthesia on splanchnic blood flow and cardiac output in the dog. Acta Anaesthesiologica Scandinavica 19: 146–153

Tran-Thi T A, Kawada N, Decker K 1993 Regulation of endothelin-1 action on the perfused rat liver. FEBS Letter 318: 353–357

Vallance P, Moncada S 1991 Hyperdynamic circulation in cirrhosis: A role for nitric oxide? Lancet 337: 776–778

Varin F, Huet P M 1985 Hepatic microcirculation in the perfused cirrhotic rat liver. Journal of Clinical Investigations 76: 1904–1912

Wang Y, Mathews W R, Guido D M, Farhood A, Jaeschke H 1995 Inhibition of nitric oxide synthesis aggravates reperfusion injury after hepatic ischemia and endotoxemia. Shock 4: 282–288

Wardell K, Jakobsson A, Nilsson G E 1993 Laser Doppler perfusion imaging by dynamic light scattering. IEEE Transactions on Biomedical Engineering 40: 309–316

Warren W D, Muller W H 1959 A classification of some hemodynamic changes in cirrhosis and their surgical significance. Annals of Surgery 150: 413–427

Wendon J A 1999 Local consequences of reperfusion in the liver. In: Grace P A, Mathie R T (eds) Ischaemia–Reperfusion Injury. Blackwell Science, Oxford, p 56–64

Wheatley A M, Zhao D 1993 Intraoperative assessment by laser Doppler flowmetry of hepatic perfusion during orthotopic liver transplantation in the rat. Transplantation, 56: 1315–1318

Wheatley A M, Hickman R 1995 The influence of flow and hematocrit on the laser Doppler flux signal from the surface of the perfused pig liver. Microcirculation 2: 19–25

Wheatley A M, Almond N E, Stuart E T, Zhao D 1993a Interpretation of the laser Doppler signal from the liver of the rat. Microvascular. Research 45: 290–301

Wheatley A M, Stuart E T, Zhao D, Zimmermann A, Gassel H-J, Blumgart L H 1993b Effect of orthotopic liver transplantation and chemical denervation of the liver on hepatic hemodynamics in the rat. Journal of Hepatology 19: 442–450

Wheatley A M, Kuznetsova L V, Lagger H, Sadeghi F, Pang K S, Sherman I A 1996 Altered hemodynamics during hepatic regeneration in the adult rat. Hepatology 24: 144A

Whipple A O 1945 The problem of portal hypertension in relation to the hepatosplenopathies. Annals of Surgery 122: 449–475

Wu Y, Campbell K A, Sitzmann J V 1993 Hormonal and splanchnic hemodynamic alterations following hepatic resection. Surgical Research 44–48

Zhang J X, Pegoli W, Jr, Clemens M G 1994 Endothelin-1 induces direct constriction of hepatic sinusoids. American Journal of Physiology 266: G624–632

Zhang J X, Bauer M, Clemens M G 1995 Vessel- and target cell-specific actions of endothelin-1 and endothelin-3 in rat liver. American Journal of Physiology 269: G269–277

Zhang X Y, Kuznetsova L V, Richter S, Wheatley A M 1997 Involvement of endothelin in changes to the hepatic microcirculation in the regenerating rat liver. Hepatology 26: 276A

Zhang XY, Kuznetsova L V, Francis R B, Wheatley A M 1999 Hepatic haemodynamics following orthotopic liver transplantation in the rat. In Press

Bile secretion

S. ERLINGER

Bile secretion is one of the major functions of the liver. Bile is an aqueous solution of organic and inorganic compounds. Bile acids, bile pigments, cholesterol and phospholipids are the chief organic compounds. Bile also contains small amounts of protein. Because of the peculiar aggregation properties of the bile acids, which readily form micelles at physiological concentrations, bile is more complex than most other secretions, especially with regard to the osmotic properties of its constituents. Bile formed by the hepatocytes is secreted into the bile canaliculi. It is then modfied during its passage in the bile ductules and ducts, and in the gallbladder, where water and inorganic electrolytes are reabsorbed by the cholangiocytes, with as a result, concentration of the organic constituents. In this chapter, the cellular mechanisms of bile secretion and the alterations leading to cholestasis will be reviewed. Detailed references may be found in recent reviews (Trauner et al 1998, Erlinger 1999).

BILE COMPOSITION

In general, inorganic electrolytes are present in common duct bile at concentrations closely reflecting those in plasma (Table 5.1). However, bile concentrations of sodium, potassium, calcium, and bicarbonate may be appreciably higher than in plasma, while the chloride level may be lower.

In spite of these variations, bile osmolality, as measured by freezing point depression, is usually approximately 300 mosmol/kg and it varies in parallel with plasma osmolality. The total osmotic activity is accounted for only by the inorganic electrolytes because it is generally assumed that bile acids, which are in micellar form, have little or no osmotic activity in final bile.

The concentration of bicarbonate in bile is often higher than that in plasma. This may be due to bicarbonate transport mechanisms, which are present in the hepatocytes, and in the bile ductules and ducts, in response to secretin (see below).

The major organic constituents of bile are the conjugated bile acids, the bile pigments, cholesterol and phospholipids. The concentration and physiochemical properties of these compounds, which are important for the understanding of cholesterol and pigment gallstone formation, will be discussed in Chapter 31.

Table 5.1 Flow and electrolyte concentrations of hepatic bile

Species	Flow ($\mu l\ min^{-1}\ kg^{-1}$)	Concentration (mmol/L)						
		Na^+	K^+	Ca^{2+}	Mg^{2+}	Cl^-	HCO_3^-	Bile acids
Man	1.5–15.4	132–165	4.2–5.6	0.6–2.4	0.7–1.5	96–126	17–55	3–45
Dog	10	141–230	4.5–11.9	1.5–6.9	1.1–2.7	31–107	14–61	16–187
Sheep	9.4	159.6	5.3	—	—	95	21.2	42.5
Rabbit	90	148–156	3.6–6.7	1.3–3.3	0.15–0.35	77–99	40–63	6–24
Rat	30–150	157–166	5.8–6.4	—	—	94–98	22–26	8–25
Guinea pig	115.9	175	6.3	—	—	69	49–65	—

Numbers indicate range or means of published values.

STRUCTURE–FUNCTION RELATIONSHIPS IN THE BILIARY SYSTEM

Bile is secreted primarily by the hepatocytes into bile canaliculi which are formed by a groove of the lateral plasma membrane between two hepatocytes and are about 1 μm in diameter (Fig. 5.1). The membrane forms numerous microvilli which increase the surface area.

The bile canalicular membrane represents about 13% of the hepatocyte plasma membrane. The bile canaliculi connect to bile ducts, lined by biliary epithelial cells or cholangiocytes. The smallest bile duct, the ductule, connects the canaliculus with the portal (interlobular) bile ducts. The interlobular bile ducts drain into larger bile ducts which form the intra- and extrahepatic biliary tree (Fig. 5.2). With respect to bile secretion, the liver may be regarded as an epithelium transporting a variety of substrates from blood to bile. This vectorial transport is made possible by the high degree of polarization of the hepatocyte plasma membrane. As in other transporting epithelia, the canalicular lumen is sealed by intercellular junctions.

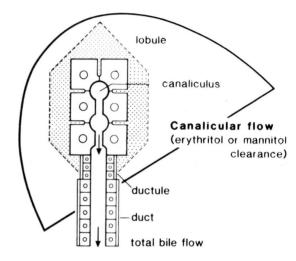

Fig. 5.2 Schematic diagram of the biliary system.

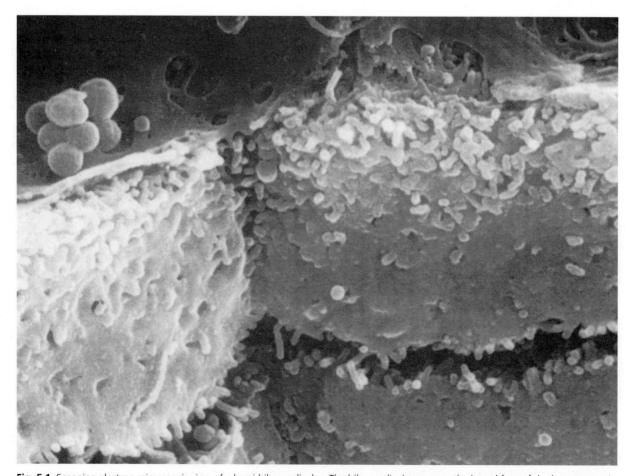

Fig. 5.1 Scanning electron microscopic view of a hemi-bile canaliculus. The bile canaliculus runs on the lateral face of the hepatocyte. At the top, the sinusoid with red cells.

THE POLARIZATION OF THE HEPATOCYTE PLASMA MEMBRANE

Three domains of the hepatocyte plasma membrane may be recognized: sinusoidal (facing the blood sinusoids), lateral (or intercellular) and canalicular. They demonstrate important morphological, biochemical and enzymatic differences. The sinusoidal and lateral membrane includes the sodium pump (Na$^+$, K$^+$-ATPase) and proteins that serve as carriers for the uptake of substrates (bile acids, bilirubin, drugs) from blood into the hepatocytes. The canalicular membrane includes carriers for the secretion of substrates from the hepatocyte into the canalicular lumen. Alkaline phosphatase, whose role in transport and bile secretion is not known, is also located on the canalicular membrane.

THE TIGHT JUNCTION AND THE PARACELLULAR PATHWAY

A substrate in plasma can enter canalicular bile in one of two ways: by the transcellular pathway (entering the hepatocyte through the sinusoidal membrane, crossing the hepatocyte and entering the canaliculus through the canalicular membrane) or by the paracellular pathway. In the latter case, the solute crosses the intercellular junction. The junction includes the tight junction, which is a sealing structure between the lumen of the bile canaliculus and the intercellular space and, hence, the sinusoidal blood. Tight junctions differ among epithelia. In impermeable epithelia (such as the toad bladder), the tight junction provides a high transepithelial resistance to the movement of water and ions (and, hence, to electrical current) whereas in relatively permeable epithelia (such as the gallbladder, intestine or proximal kidney tubule), the tight junction is 'leaky' permitting some passage of water and ions with, as a result, a low electrical resistance. The liver is of an intermediate type and there is evidence for a paracellular ion and fluid flux into bile which could play an important role in choleresis and possibly cholestasis.

THE HEPATOCYTE CYTOSKELETON

The canaliculus is surrounded by a narrow zone of organelle-poor cytoplasm, known as a pericanalicular ectoplasm, where actin microfilaments, 7 nm in diameter, are particularly present. They form a pericanalicular network, insert in the intercellular junction and extend into the microvilli where they appear to insert on the inner part of the membrane. They may have a key role in maintaining the shape of the cell, particularly its microvilli. Agents that interfere with the structure and function of microfilaments affect bile flow, which suggests a role for these organelles in secretion.

Microtubules, which are 24 nm in diameter, are more randomly distributed within the liver cell cytoplasm than are microfilaments. They play a role in the intracellular (vesicular) transport and secretion by the liver cell of proteins and lipoproteins. Antimicrotubular agents may also affect bile formation (see below).

CANALICULAR BILE FLOW

The maximal bile secretory pressure (about 25–30 cmH$_2$O) exceeds the sinusoidal perfusion pressure (about 5–10 cmH$_2$O): this excludes hydrostatic filtration as an important mechanism of canalicular bile secretion. Canalicular bile flow is regarded mainly as an osmotic water flow in response to active, solute transport. The major solutes serving as driving forces for canalicular bile flow are bile acids (bile acid-dependent flow) and glutathione (bile acid-independent flow) (Fig. 5.3).

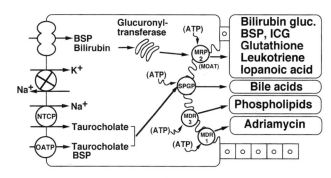

Fig. 5.3 Schematic representation of the mechanisms of bile secretion.

ESTIMATION OF CANALICULAR BILE FLOW

Canalicular bile flow may be estimated by measuring the biliary clearance of nonmetabolized solutes that enter canalicular bile by passive processes and are neither secreted nor reabsorbed by the biliary epithelium (Fig. 5.2). The most widely used of such solutes are erythritol and mannitol (labelled with ^{14}C). In brief, when injected into the systemic circulation, the biliary secretion rate of such a solute during a steady state should depend on the permeability of the canaliculus and on canalicular bile flow. The biliary clearance (C) is calculated as C = F × [B]/[P] where F is bile flow, [B] and [P] the biliary and plasma concentrations respectively. The technique implies that the selected solute: (1) is unable to cross the biliary epithelium; (2) has a permeability in the canaliculi high enough to achieve diffusion equilibrium at the highest rates of canalicular flow. Depending on the species, erythritol (MW 122) and mannitol (MW 182) meet these requirements.

BILE ACID TRANSPORT AND BILE ACID-DEPENDENT SECRETION

About 30 g (50 mmol) of bile acids circulate between the intestine and the liver each day. This efficient entero-hepatic circulation is possible because of active transport systems located on hepatocytes and enterocytes.

In hepatocytes, two baso-lateral (sinusoidal) transport systems responsible for the *uptake* of bile acids from sinusoidal blood have been identified by expression-cloning techniques in *Xenopus laevis* oocytes (Hagenbuch & Meier 1996, Muller & Jansen 1998). The first uptake system, the Na-taurocholate co-transporting polypeptide (NTCP* in humans) is a symport (co-transport) of sodium and taurocholate. Its mRNA has been cloned both in rat and in man. In man, the 1.599 bp mRNA encodes for a 38 kDa polypeptide. The gene is located on chromosome 14. This system probably accounts for the major part of conjugated bile acid uptake. The system is energized by the sodium gradient provided by the Na⁺,K⁺-ATPase located on the baso-lateral membrane.

The second uptake mechanism is a sodium-independent system named OATP (organic anion transporting polypeptide). It transports taurocholate and organic anions, like bromosulfophthalein (BSP) or bilirubin. Its mRNA has been cloned in the rat and in man. In man, the mRNA has 2010 bp and encodes for a 59 kDa polypeptide. The gene is located on chromosome 12 (Hagenbuch & Meier 1996, Muller & Jansen 1998).

The *intracellular transport* of bile acids from the sinusoidal to the canalicular pole of the hepatocyte occurs mostly by protein binding and diffusion throughout the cytosol. The major bile acid binding proteins are the glutathione-transferases and binders I and II (Stolz et al 1989, Erlinger 1993).

Several lines of evidence support the view that a vesicular system derived from the Golgi apparatus is involved in the intracellular transport or in the canalicular secretion of bile acids. An interaction of bile acids with intracellular vesicles has been observed by immunoperoxidase and by immunofluorescence. It has also been observed repeatedly that

colchicine, a well known inhibitor of microtubule function, inhibited the biliary secretion of bile acids. Rather than being involved in intracellular transport of bile acids per se, one can propose the hypothesis that these vesicles, derived from the Golgi apparatus, could play a role in regulation of canalicular excretion by a mechanism of vesicle recycling (Erlinger 1996, Boyer & Soroka 1995). In brief, this process includes: (a) endocytic retrieval of canalicular carriers toward an endosomal intracellular compartment; (b) exocytic insertion of carriers into the canalicular membrane, when needed by an increased load of bile acids (for example after a meal). Such a cycle, postulated for other transport systems, could provide a rapid regulation system for canalicular secretion of bile acids.

Canalicular secretion of bile acids is mediated apparently by two transport systems. The major one is an ATP-dependent system identified on canalicular membrane vesicles. The protein responsible, named sister P-glycoprotein (or SPGP) (Gerloff et al 1998) belongs to the ABC (ATP-binding cassette)-protein family. The second is an electrogenic system energized by the membrane potential. The protein involved has not yet been identified.

An apparently linear relationship between bile acid secretion rate and bile flow has been demonstrated in many animal species, including man (Fig. 5.4). The slope of the regression line between bile flow and bile acid secretion (usually 7–12 µl/µmol) is generally termed apparent choleretic activity.

The hypothesis that bile acids increase bile flow by providing an osmotic driving force for water and electrolytes was proposed by Sperber. However, because bile acids are in micellar form in bile, most osmotic activity must be accounted for by their counter-ions (or cations accompanying the bile acid anions to maintain electroneutrality).

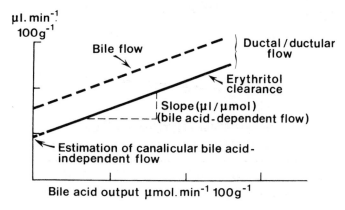

Fig. 5.4 Relationship between bile flow (- - -), [¹⁴C]erythritol clearance (——) and bile acid secretion in cholecystectomized patients with T-tubes in the common bile duct.

---

* Abbreviations of protein names are usually designated with capitals in humans (NTCP) and lower case letters (ntcp) in animals.

HYPERCHOLERETIC BILE ACIDS AND THE CHOLE-HEPATIC SHUNT HYPOTHESIS

Ursodeoxycholic acid (3α,7β-dihydroxycholanoic acid, the 7β epimer of cheno-deoxycholic acid), a bile acid which is widely used in the treatment of cholestatic liver disease, has a much more pronounced choleretic effect than taurocholate (Dumont et al 1980) or even than its own conjugate, tauroursodeoxycholate (Fig. 5.5). Several other bile acids have been shown to have a similar hypercholeretic effect for example, 23-norursodeoxycholate or 23-norchenodeoxycholate. In all cases, hypercholeresis is associated with a marked stimulation of bicarbonate concentration and secretion into bile.

The mechanism of this curious phenomenon is not yet established. At present, the best explanation is probably the so-called chole-hepatic shunt hypothesis, proposed by Hofmann and colleagues (Yoon et al 1986). According to this hypothesis, ursodeoxycholate is transported into bile in part in the unconjugated form. It becomes protonated in the biliary lumen into ursodeoxycholic acid. The proton comes from H_2CO_3 and the process generates one bicarbonate ion which is secreted into bile. The protonated ursodeoxycholic acid is lipid soluble and readily absorbed by the biliary epithelial cells into the peribiliary vascular plexus and returns to the hepatocyte which re-secretes it into bile. The bile acid does not appear in final bile, but, at each cycle, one bicarbonate is secreted and stimulates bile flow (Fig. 5.6). Other explanations have been proposed, involving

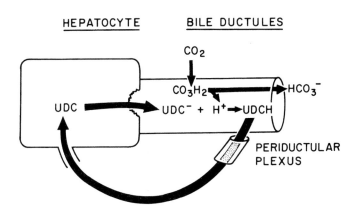

Fig. 5.6 The chole-hepatic shunt hypothesis. See text for explanation.

hepatocytic mechanisms, including stimulation of the Na^+/H^+ exchange in the plasma membrane. This hypothesis rests on the observation that amiloride, an inhibitor of the Na^+/H^+ exhanger, inhibits ursodeoxycholate-induced choleresis. Direct proof, however, is not available.

BILE ACID-INDEPENDENT FLOW

The mechanisms of formation of the canalicular bile acid-independent flow have been controversial for a long time. This component of bile flow is usually estimated by extrapolating the regression line between canalicular bile flow and bile acid secretion for a zero bile acid secretion (Fig. 5.4). It is now clear that a major driving force for this component of bile flow is the secretion of glutathione (or glutathione conjugates). The two major pieces of evidence for this view are: (1) there is a significant correlation between the magnitude of bile acid-independent flow and the biliary excretion of glutathione in the rat in various experimental situations (Ballatori & Truong 1989); (2) in TR⁻ rats, which have an inherited defect in organic anion secretion into bile, bile acid-independent flow is markedly reduced (Jansen & Elferink 1993); in parallel, glutathione is virtually absent from their bile (Jansen & Elferink 1993). It is interesting that in man, after liver transplantation, bile acid-independent flow is also decreased and biliary glutathione concentration is very low (Durand & Erlinger, unpublished observations).

BILIRUBIN AND ORGANIC ANION TRANSPORT

The uptake of bilirubin and other organic anions is mediated by one or several proteins. Three putative carrier proteins have been identified: bilitranslocase, the organic anion

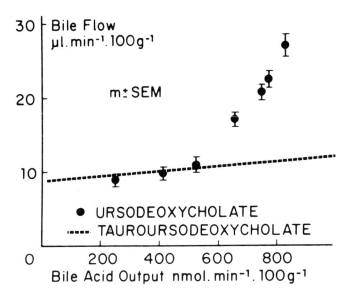

Fig. 5.5 Hypercholeretic effect of ursodeoxycholate. Bile flow induced by ursodeoxycholate, at high bile acid outputs in bile, far exceeds that induced by tauroursodeoxycholate.

binding protein and the BSP-bilirubin binding protein (Stremmel et al 1993). These proteins appear different but further precise characterization will have to await molecular cloning.

In the cytosol, bilirubin is bound to several proteins, mostly glutathione transferase, and is transferred toward the endoplasmic reticulum where it is transformed into several conjugates. The predominant conjugate is bilirubin diglucuronide, which is water soluble and secreted into bile. The enzyme bilirubin uridine diphosphate glucuronosyl transferase is now well characterized and several mutations resulting in unconjugated hyperbilirubinemia (Crigler-Najjar & Gilbert syndromes) have been identified (Jansen 1996).

Secretion of bilirubin diglucuronide into bile through the canalicular membrane is mediated by a carrier named canalicular multiple organic anion transporter (cMOAT), or MRP2, or leukotriene export carrier (LEC) (because it also transports cysteinyl leukotrienes). It is reponsible for biliary secretion of bilirubin diglucuronide, BSP and other anionic dyes, biliary opacifying agents, glutathione and glutathione-conjugates, leukotrienes and probably other organic compounds. It is an active system requiring ATP. A recent study has convincingly demonstrated that the protein belongs to the MRP (for multidrug resistance protein) family, and has a molecular weight of 190 kDa. This family also includes MDR1 and MDR3, also located on the canalicular membrane and responsible for biliary excretion of cationic anticancer drugs (MDR1) and phospholipids (MDR3) (see below). They all possess an ATP-binding cassette.

The cMOAT (or MRP2) is defective in three strains of rats having conjugated hyperbilirubinemia: the TR⁻ rat, the Groningen yellow rat (GY) and the Eisai hyperbilirubinemic rat (EHBR) (Paulusma et al 1997). These mutant rats are animal models of the Dubin–Johnson syndrome in man, a benign disease also characterized by conjugated hyperbilirubinemia. The Dubin–Johnson syndrome is due to a mutation of the human MRP2 (Kartenbeck et al 1996, Paulusma et al 1997).

PHOSPHOLIPID TRANSPORT

Phospholipid excretion into bile is not a purely passive process. It requires an ATP-dependent mechanism. The mdr2 protein (which is the murine equivalent of the human MDR3) is clearly involved in this process. Mice in which both alleles of the mdr2 gene had been inactivated (mdr2−/− 'knock out' mice) had virtually no detectable phospholipid in bile, in spite of a *normal* bile acid excretion (Smit et al 1993). Cholesterol secretion was decreased, but not abolished.

Most interestingly, these mice had hepatic biochemical and histological abnormalities, with increased serum activities of aminotransferases, alkaline phosphatase and γ-glutamyl transferase and, histologically, portal fibrosis and inflammation, bile ductular proliferation, and eventually biliary cirrhosis (Smit et al 1993, Mauad et al 1994). Hypothetically, liver damage in these animals could be due to toxicity of phospholipid-free bile acid micelles on the membranes of hepatocyte and/or biliary epithelial cells. One form of progressive familial intrahepatic cholestasis leading to biliary cirrhosis in children is due to mutations of the human MDR3 (Deleuze et al 1996, De Vree et al 1998).

CATIONIC DRUG TRANSPORT

A third member of the MDR proteins family, MDR1, present on the canalicular membrane, mediates the excretion into bile of cationic anticancer drugs, such as adriamycin or daunomycin (Gatmaitan & Arias 1995). Overexpression of this protein explains, at least in part, the resistance of most hepatocellular carcinomas to chemotherapy.

The major transport systems of the hepatocyte are represented schematically in Figure 5.7.

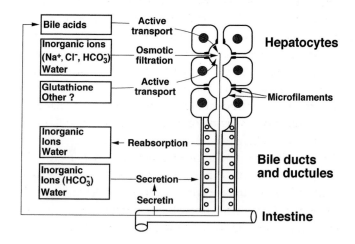

Fig. 5.7 Schematic representation of the hepatocyte transport systems.

ROLE OF DUCTULES AND DUCTS

REABSORPTION

The biliary channels (bile ductules and ducts) may reabsorb water and electrolytes. It has been known for a long time that, after cholecystectomy in the dog (and probably also in man), 'hepatic bile' was concentrated to approximately the same extent as normal gallbladder bile. This implies that there is reabsorption of water (and electrolytes) by the bile ducts or ductules.

SECRETION

Under normal conditions, there is a net secretion of water and ions in the biliary tree (Fig. 5.4). This secretion has been well studied after bile duct ligation in the rat, which induces a proliferation of bile ductules. After bile duct ligation, bile flow increases progressively. The increase is proportional to the number of γ-GT-positive cells (biliary epithelial cells). This increase in flow is largely due to secretion of bicarbonate and water, and is strongly stimulated by *secretin* (Alpini et al 1988, 1989). The molecular mechanism of this secretion has been clarified recently by the demonstration of the CFTR (Cystic Fibrosis Transmembrane conductance Regulator) on the apical membrane of biliary epithelial cells, both in rats and in humans (McGill et al 1992, Fitz et al 1993, Cohn et al 1993). This protein acts as a chloride channel and is activated by cAMP. Upon the action of secretin, which binds to a receptor on the basolateral membrane of the cell there is stimulation of cAMP formation and activation of CFTR. This leads to chloride extrusion out of the cell. This, in turn, could stimulate a HCO_3^-/Cl^- exchanger also present on the luminal membrane of biliary cells (Roberts et al 1997) and account for bicarbonate secretion. Secretin has also been shown to stimulate the extrusion of acidic vesicles at the basolateral pole of the biliary cell but the contribution of this process to bicarbonate secretion remains to be clarified.

The secretory activity of the bile ductules and ducts explains the choleresis that occurs in certain diseases. Elevated bile flow has been recorded in patients with cirrhosis, other chronic liver diseases associated with ductular proliferation, and in congenital dilatation of the intrahepatic biliary tree (Caroli's syndrome). An augmented surface of the biliary epithelium is common to these conditions.

MECHANISMS OF CHOLESTASIS

Cholestasis is defined as a diminution (or cessation) of bile flow and is subdivided as extrahepatic and intrahepatic (Fig. 5.8). *Extrahepatic cholestasis* is the result of mechanical obstruction of the extrahepatic bile ducts usually by a gallstone or a tumor. *Intrahepatic cholestasis* may be the result of two different mechanisms: (i) mechanical obstruction of intrahepatic bile ducts, for example by lesions of interlobu-

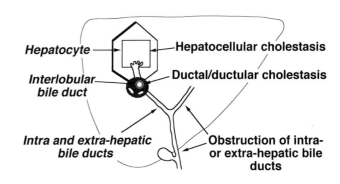

Fig. 5.8 The different types of cholestasis.

lar bile ducts (in primary biliary cirrhosis), a primary or secondary liver tumour, granulomas, infiltration by lymphoma or any other space-occupying lesion; (ii) disturbance of canalicular bile flow, for example during viral or drug-induced hepatitis, drug-induced cholestasis, or genetic cholestasis.

Cholestasis must be distinguished from necrosis during liver parenchymal disease: both can occur separately or together. For instance, during viral hepatitis, necrosis can occur alone (anicteric hepatitis), or in association with cholestasis (common acute hepatitis with jaundice), while cholestasis can occur alone or predominantly (cholestatic hepatitis).

EXTRAHEPATIC CHOLESTASIS

Common bile duct ligation in the rat is the most widely used experimental model of extrahepatic cholestasis. Bile duct ligation induces a dilatation of bile canaliculi, with a loss of microvilli, and alterations of intercellular junctions. These alterations lead to an increase in canalicular permeability (Erlinger 1999) and allow a 'regurgitation' of bile constituents into hepatic lymph and blood.

In addition to canalicular modifications, bile duct ligation induces profound modifications in hepatocytes. The polarity of the plasma membrane is modified with a redistribution of various enzymes and carriers from the canalicular (apical) to the sinusoidal and lateral (baso-lateral) pole of the cell (Erlinger 1999). Because of this inverse polarity of the cell, substrates normally secreted into bile may be, in part, re-secreted into blood after their entry into the hepatocyte. This could contribute to cholestasis. In bile duct obstructed rats, there is a reduced expression of the carriers responsible for bile acid uptake, ntcp (Gartung et al 1996) and oatp1 (Dumont et al 1997). The reduced expression is due to a decreased transcription, because mRNA levels are decreased in parallel to proteins. This down-regulation could, in part, prevent the accumulation of potentially toxic bile acids and organic anions within the hepatocytes. There is also a down-regulation of the cmoat (mrp2) which could contribute to impaired biliary excretion (Trauner et al 1997). Hepatocyte metabolism is modified, with an increased production of alkaline phosphatase and cholesterol; this explains, in part, the increased serum alkaline phosphatase activity and hypercholesterolemia.

When biliary obstruction is prolonged, it leads, in animals and in man, to bile ductular proliferation, fibrosis and, ultimately, to secondary biliary cirrhosis (Kountouras et al 1984). The precise mechanisms of ductular proliferation and fibrosis are not known. Proliferated bile ductules secrete, like normal ones, a bicarbonate rich solution (see above). This secretion accounts for the markedly increased bile flow observed in patients with cirrhosis or congenital hepatic fibrosis. Secondary biliary cirrhosis is also responsible for portal hypertension and a hyperdynamic circulation (Lee et al 1986).

In animals, the changes observed after biliary obstruction, including biliary cirrhosis and portal hypertension, are reversible when obstruction is relieved and an adequate biliary drainage is restored (Zimmermann et al 1992). It has been suggested that this may also occur in man (Blumgart 1978).

INTRAHEPATIC CHOLESTASIS

Intrahepatic cholestasis may be due to obstruction of intrahepatic bile ducts or to alteration of bile secretion by the hepatocytes (hepatocellular cholestasis).

Obstruction of intrahepatic bile ducts

The mechanisms of cholestasis due to obstruction of intrahepatic bile ducts are basically the same as those of extrahepatic obstruction, with the remarkable exception of *cystic fibrosis*. In cystic fibrosis, it is most likely that the function of CFTR is impaired, with a decrease of chloride and bicarbonate secretion (Colombo et al 1998). This leads to a decrease of ductular/ductal bile flow. The decreased bile flow probably plays a role in the hepatic disease of cystic fibrosis. The decreased bile flow leads to mucous precipitation and obstruction of small bile ducts. Obstruction is followed by ductular proliferation, inflammation and focal fibrosis, leading to focal biliary cirrhosis. This may progress to (diffuse) secondary biliary cirrhosis (Colombo et al 1998). Extrahepatic bile duct lesions, with a cholangiographic appearance resembling sclerosing cholangitis, have also been reported (Waters et al 1995). The clinical and biochemical abnormalities are improved by ursodeoxycholic acid (Colombo et al 1998, 1996).

Hepatocellular cholestasis

Impairment of bile secretion by the hepatocytes may be due to hemodynamic disturbances or alteration of any of the steps of hepatic transport: the sinusoidal, intracellular or canalicular steps.

Hemodynamic alterations

The maximal biliary pressure (or bile secretory pressure) is about 20 mmHg. It is markedly higher than the sinusoidal perfusion pressure (3–5 mmHg). This explains why, clinically, there is usually no cholestasis in spite of wide variations of sinusoidal perfusion pressure or hepatic blood flow, except when there is marked hepatic ischemia and liver cell necrosis. However, experimentally, when hepatic vein pressure is abruptly increased, bile flow decreases markedly (Preisig et al 1972). This is probably due to an increase in hepatic vein pressure above bile secretory pressure. This may explain the increased serum alkaline phosphatase and activity, and occasional cholestatic jaundice observed in patients with cardiac failure or the Budd–Chiari syndrome.

Baso-lateral membrane alterations

In several models of cholestasis, Na^+,K^+-ATPase activity is decreased: this has been reported in cholestasis induced by ethinyl estradiol, chlorpromazine, monohydroxy bile acids and other bile acids (Erlinger 1999). The number of enzyme sites and protein mass appear unaltered (Erlinger 1999). The decreased enzyme activity has been explained by a decreased membrane fluidity, probably related to an increased cholesterol content of the plasma membrane (Erlinger 1999).

In addition to the decreased Na^+,K^+-ATPase activity, estrogen cholestasis in rats is associated with a decreased Na^+-dependent and Na^+-independent taurocholate uptake and a decreased expression of the Na^+-dependent and Na^+-independent taurocholate transporters ntcp and oatp (Simon et al 1996). This is due to a decreased transcription, because ntcp and oatp mRNA levels are also decreased (Simon et al 1996). There may be generalized abnormalities in sinusoidal membrane properties and function in this model.

Intracellular alterations

Interference with bile acid binding *cytosolic proteins*, for example by indomethacin, decreases bile acid secretion and may thus induce cholestasis.

Functional and morphological evidence suggest that alterations of the *cytoskeleton* are involved in cholestasis. *Microtubule* inhibitors, like colchicine and vinblastine, decrease bile acid-induced bile flow and bile acid secretion after a bile acid load (Crawford et al 1988). Microtubules are known to be involved in vesicle movement within the cells. It is thought that a microtubule-dependent vesicular mechanism is involved in the regulation of canalicular transporters (Erlinger 1996, Boyer & Soroka 1995).

Microfilament poisons, such as phallodin and cytochalasin B, also induce cholestasis in experimental animals (Phillips et al 1986). Microfilaments are thought to play a role in canalicular contractions. Interference with microfilament function could lead to canalicular 'paralysis' and to a decrease of bile flow (Phillips et al 1986). It has been proposed that cholestasis induced by some drugs like norethandrolone (Phillips et al 1978) and cholestasis associated with North American Indian cirrhosis (Weber et al 1981) may be related to microfilament dysfunction. Direct evidence for this proposal is lacking.

An increase in *intracellular ionized calcium* concentration has been found in isolated rat hepatocytes exposed to lithocholate and taurolithocholate, two potent cholestatic agents (Anwer et al 1988, Combettes et al 1988). This increased calcium concentration is due to the release of calcium stored in the endosplasmic reticulum calcium stores (Combettes et al 1989). Thus alterations in intracellular calcium may play a role in cholestasis; however, the exact mechanism is unclear.

Canalicular alterations

There is considerable evidence that cholestasis, in particular estrogen-induced cholestasis, is associated with a *decreased biliary secretory capacity* for a variety of organic anions including bile salts, bilirubin and bromosulfophthalein (Bossard et al 1993). Estrogen-induced cholestasis is associated with a decrease of ATP-dependent canalicular taurocholate transport (Bossard et al 1993) and with a decrease of ATP-dependent transport of organic anions (like S-(2,4-dinitrophenyl) glutathione) (Bossard et al 1993), known to be mediated by the cMOAT. The availability of molecular probes has allowed demonstration of a decrease of mrp2 protein expression in cholestasis induced by ethinyl-estradiol, endotoxin and common bile duct ligation (Trauner et al 1997). Down-regulation of mrp2 expression probably accounts for the decreased canalicular secretion of organic anions in these models of cholestasis. One form of progressive familial intrahepatic cholestasis is due to a mutation of the gene of the canalicular bile acid transporter, SPGP, leading to the absence of the transporter on the canalicular membrane (Jansen et al 1998).

Taurolithocholate-induced cholestasis was initially thought to be related *to bile canalicular precipitation* of this poorly water soluble bile acid. The canalicular precipitate was later shown to be made predominantly of cholesterol. Whether this plays a role in cholestasis remains to be demonstrated. Canalicular precipitation has also been proposed as a mechanism for cholestasis induced by protoporphyrin (Berenson et al 1990) and bile acid glucuronides and sulfates (Bellentani et al 1990), but the causal relationship beween precipitation ('bile thrombi') and cholestasis remains unproven.

An impairment of *phospholipid secretion* is responsible for a form of progressive familial intrahepatic cholestasis (see above).

Paracellular permeability

An increased permeability of the paracellular (tight junction) pathway, with possible regurgitation of bile constituents into plasma, has been observed in several models of cholestasis. This increased permeability is usually assessed by an increased biliary clearance of large inert solutes such as sucrose, by permeation of horseradish peroxidase or lanthanum, and by demonstration of morphologic alterations of the tight junctions (Erlinger 1999). However, extrahepatic cholestasis is also associated with increased permeability of the paracellular pathway, which is clearly a consequence of the obstruction in this model, not a cause. Thus, one may propose that increased tight junction permeability is probably, in most situations, a secondary phenomenon, a consequence of cholestasis, rather than an initiating process. Nevertheless, by allowing some regurgitation of biliary constituents into blood, it may contribute to the clinical or biochemical signs of cholestasis.

Mixed hepatocellular and ductular lesions may be observed in some cases of drug-induced cholestasis. Experimentally, α-naphthyl isothiocyanate (ANIT) induces both hepatocytic and cholangiocytic lesions. It has been proposed that the lesions of cholangiocytes could be mediated by exposure to high concentrations of ANIT: ANIT forms a conjugate with glutathione which is excreted into bile through the cmoat. Once in bile, the conjugate dissociates into glutathione and ANIT, which is possibly responsible for cholangiocyte toxicity (Mehendale et al 1994).

CHOLERETICS: MECHANISMS OF ACTION

A choleretic drug might act by one of several possible mechanisms: (i) concentrative (usually active) secretion into bile canaliculi followed by osmotic filtration of water and electrolytes. This process may be conveniently called 'bile acid-like choleresis' and operate for most commercial choleretics. However, this type of choleresis is not accompanied by an increase in biliary lipid secretion, in contrast to the choleresis induced by physiological bile acids. (ii) Stimulation of 'bile acid-independent mechanisms' as with phenobarbital and other drugs (spironolactone or clofibrate in the rat) that are microsomal enzyme inducers. (iii) Stimulation of secretion by the ductules or ducts, for example with secretin.

There is no evidence that any of these choleretics are of therepeutic value in patients with cholestasis, with the possible exception of phenobarbitone (phenobarbital) in children with intrahepatic cholestasis. Ursodeoxycholic acid is of proven benefit in primary biliary cirrhosis (Poupon et al 1997) (and possibly other cholestatic diseases). Its main mechanism of action is probably related to its lack of detergent effect (in contrast to physiological bile acids) rather than to its choleretic potential.

BILIARY SECRETION IN MAN

Although the existence of most of the processes described previously has been inferred from animal studies, similar processes may well operate in man (Fig. 5.9). Patients with T-tubes in the common bile duct show a linear relationship between bile flow (and erythritol or mannitol clearance) and bile acid secretion rate, with a mean of 11 μl of canalicular bile secreted per μmol of bile acids. When the enterohepatic

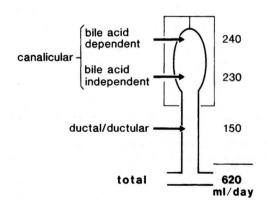

Fig. 5.9 Bile secretion in man. From data collected in cholecystectomized patients with T-tubes in the common bile duct.

circulation is intact, a mean of approximately 15 μmol of bile acids is secreted per min, which gives a mean flow associated with bile acids of 0.15–0.16 ml/min. The estimated canalicular bile acid-independent flow is 0.16–0.17 ml/min, and the estimated ductular/ductal secretions is about 0.11 ml/min. The daily hepatic bile production under these circumstances (i.e. after cholecystectomy) is therefore approximately 600 ml.

SUMMARY

Bile is an isotonic aqueous solution of bile acids, cholesterol, phospholipids, bile pigments and inorganic electrolytes. It is secreted by the hepatocytes into the bile canaliculi and modifed in the bile ductules or ducts. The three main processes identified in the generation of bile flow are schematized in Figure 5.3. They are defined as follows:

1. Active transport (concentrative) of bile acids from blood into bile canaliculi. This is responsible for the bile acid-dependent canalicular bile flow. Coupling between water flow and bile acid secretion is probably effected mainly through an osmotic mechanism. There is evidence that water flows (at least in part) through the interhepatocytic junctions. The vectorial transport of bile acids by the hepatocyte is effected by sinusoidal (NTCP and OATP) and canalicular (SPGP) transporters. The bile acid-dependent flow accounts for 30 to 60% of spontaneous basal bile flow.
2. A canalicular, bile acid-independent secretion, mostly due to secretion of glutathione into bile. This fraction of the bile flow represents 30 to 60% of basal bile flow. Normal canalicular bile flow also depends on the integrity of intracellular cytoskeletal organelles, mostly microfilaments.
3. Reabsorption and secretion of fluid and inorganic electrolytes by the ductules and ducts. Secretion chiefly occurs in response to secretin (by a mechanism mediated by CFTR) and represents 30% of basal bile flow.

Cholestasis may be extrahepatic or intrahepatic. Extrahepatic cholestasis results from mechanical obstruction of extrahepatic bile ducts, usually by a stone or a tumour. Intrahepatic cholestasis may be the result of:

1. Mechanical obstruction of intrahepatic bile ducts (such as in primary biliary cirrhosis)
2. Alteration of the flow-generating systems by the hepatocytes (due, for instance, to a virus or a drug). The basis of this alteration might be an interference with the sodium

pump (Na+,K+-ATPase) or other membrane transporters in hepatocytes, an alteration of the permeability of the biliary system (possibly of the paracellular pathway), a lesion of the cytoskeleton, alterations in intracellular calcium, and, in some cases, mutations of the genes coding for hepatocytic transporters.

REFERENCES

Alpini G, Lenzi R, Zhai W R, Sarkozi L, Tavoloni N 1988 Biliary physiology in rats with bile ductular cell hyperplasia. Journal of Clinical Investigation 81: 569–578

Alpini G, Lenzi R, Zhai W R, Slott P A, Liu M H, Sarkozi L, Tavoloni N 1989 Bile secretory function of intrahepatic biliary epithelium in the rat. American Journal of Physiology 257: G124–G133

Anwer M S, Engelking L R, Nolan K, Sullivan D, Zimniak P, Lester R 1988 Hepatotoxic bile acids increase cytosolic Ca++ activity of isolated rat hepatocytes. Hepatology 8: 887–891

Ballatori N, Truong A T 1989 Relation between biliary glutathione excretion and bile acid-independent bile flow. American Journal of Physiology 256: G22–G30

Bellentani S, Armocida C, Pecorari M, Saccocio G, Marcheginano P, Angeloni A, Manenti F, Ricci G L 1990 The role of calcium precipitation in the sulfoglycolithocholate-induced cholestasis of the bile fistula hamster. Journal of Hepatology 10: 356–360

Berenson M M, Gunther C, Samowitz W S, Bjorkman D J 1990 Formation of biliary thrombi in protoporphyrin-induced cholestasis in perfused rat liver. Hepatology 11: 757–763

Blumgart L H 1978 Biliary tract obstruction – new approaches to old problems. American Journal of Surgery 135: 19–31

Bossard R, Stieger B, O'Neill B, Fricker G, Meier P J 1993 Ethinylestradiol treatment induces multiple canalicular membrane transport alterations in rat liver. Journal of Clinical Investigation 91: 2714–2720

Boyer J L, Soroka C J 1995 Vesicle targeting to the apical domain regulates bile excretory function in isolated rat hepatocyte couplets. Gastroenterology 109: 1600–11

Cohn J A, Strong T V, Picciotto M R, Nairn A C, Collins F S, Fitz J G 1993 Localization of the cystic fibrosis transmembrane conductance regulator in human bile duct epithelial cells. Gastroenterology 105: 1857–1864

Colombo C, Battezzati P M, Podda M, Bettinardi N, Giunta A, and the Italian group of the study of ursodeoxycholic acid in cystic fibrosis 1996 Ursodeoxycholic acid for liver disease associated with cystic fibrosis: a double-blind multicenter trial. Hepatology 23: 1484–1490

Colombo C, Battezzati PM, Strazzabosco M, Podda M 1998 Liver and biliary problems in cystic fibrosis. Seminars Liver in Disease 18: 227–235

Combettes L, Dumont M, Berthon B, Erlinger S, Claret M 1988 Release of calcium from the endoplasmic reticulum by bile acids in rat liver cells. Journal of Biological Chemistry 263: 2299–2303

Combettes L, Berthon B, Doucet E, Erlinger S, Claret M 1989 Characteristics of bile acid-mediated Ca2+ release from permeabilized liver cells and liver microsomes. Journal of Biological Chemistry 264: 157–167

Crawford J M, Berken C A, Gollan J L 1988 Role of the hepatocyte microtubular system in the excretion of bile salts and biliary lipid: implications for intracellular vesicular transport. Journal of Lipid Research 29: 144–156

De Vree J M L, Jacquemin E, Sturm E et al 1998 Mutations in the MDR3 gene cause progressive familial intrahepatic cholestasis. Proceedings National Academy of Sciences of the USA 95: 282–287

Deleuze J F, Jacquemin E, Dubuisson C, Cresteil D, Dumont M, Erlinger S, Bernard O, Hadchouel M 1996 Defect of multidrug-resistance 3 gene expression in a subtype of progressive familial intrahepatic cholestasis. Hepatology 23: 904–908

Dumont M, Jacquemin E, D'Hont C, Descout C, Cresteil D, Haouzi D, Desrochers M, Stieger B, Hadchouel M, Erlinger S 1997 Expression of the liver Na+–independent organic anion transporting polypeptide (oatp-1) in rats with bile duct ligation. Journal of Hepatology 27: 1051–1056

Dumont M, Uchman S, Erlinger S 1980 Hypercholeresis induced by ursodeoxycholic acid and 7-ketolithocholic acid in the rat: possible role of bicarbonate transport. Gastroenterology 79: 82–9

Erlinger S 1993 Intracellular events in bile acid transport by the liver. In Tavoloni N and Berk P D (eds) Hepatic Transport and Bile Secretion. Physiology and Pathophysiology, New York: Raven Press, 467–475

Erlinger S 1996 Do intracellular organelles have any role in transport of bile acids by the hepatocytes? Journal of Hepatology 24: 88–93

Erlinger S 1999 Cholestasis. In: Schiff E R, Sorrell M F, Maddrey W C (eds) Diseases of the Liver, 8th edn. Lippincott-Raven, Philadelphia, 611–629

Fitz J G, Basavappa S, McGill J M, Melhus O, Cohn J A 1993 Regulation of membrane chloride currents in rat bile duct epithelial cells. Journal of Clinical Investigation 91: 319–328

Gartung C, Ananthanarayanan M, Rahman M A, Schuele S, Nundy S, Soroka C J, Stolz A, Suchy F J, Boyer J L 1996 Down-regulation of expression and function of the rat liver Na+/bile acid cotransporter in extrahepatic cholestasis. Gastroenterology 110: 199–209

Gatmaitan Z C, Arias I M 1995 ATP-dependent transport systems in the canalicular membrane of the hepatocyte. Physiological Reviews 75: 261–275

Gerloff T, Stieger B, Hagenbuch B, Madon J, Landmann L, Roth J, Hofmann A F, Meier P J 1998 The sister of P-glycoprotein represents the canalicular bile salt export pump of mammalian liver. Journal of Bioliology Chemistry 273: 10046–10050

Hagenbuch B, Meier P J 1996 Sinusoidal (basolateral) bile salt uptake systems of hepatocytes. Seminars in Liver Disease 16: 129–136

Jansen P, Hooiveld G, Koning H et al 1998 The SPGP gene, encoding the canalicular bile acid transporting protein SPGP/cBST, is not expressed in a subgroup of patients with progressive familial intrahepatic cholestasis (PFIC-2). Journal of Hepatology 28: (suppl 1): 42 (abst)

Jansen P L M, Oude Elferink R P J 1993 Defective hepatic anion secretion in mutant TR- rats. In: Tavoloni N, Berk P D (eds) Hepatic Transport and Bile Secretion. Physiology and Pathophysiology. Raven Press, New York, 721–732

Jansen P L M 1996 Genetic diseases of bilirubin metabolism: the inherited unconjugated hyperbilirubinemias. Journal of Hepatology 25: 398–404

Kartenbeck J, Leuschner U, Mayer R, Keppler D 1996 Absence of the canalicular isoform of the MRP gene-encoded conjugate export pump from the hepatocytes in Dubin–Johnson syndrome. Hepatology 23: 1061–6

Kountouras J, Billing B H, Scheuer P J 1984 Prolonged bile duct obstruction: a new experimental model for cirrhosis in the rat. British Journal of Experimental Pathology 65: 305–311

Lee S S, Girod C, Braillon A, Hadengue A, Lebrec D 1986 Hemodynamic characterization of chronic bile duct-ligated rats: effect of pentobarbital sodium. American Journal of Physiology 251: G176–G180

Mauad T H, van Nieuwkerk C M J, Dingemans K P, Smit J M J, Schinkel A H Notenboom R G E, van den Bergh Weerman M A, Verkruisen R P, Groen A K, Oude Elferink R P J, van der Valk M A, Borst P, Offerhaus G J A 1994 Mice with homozygous disruption of the mdr2 p-glycoprotein gene: a novel animal model for studies of nonsuppurative inflammatory cholangitis and hepatocarcinogenesis. American Journal of Pathology 145: 1237–1245

McGill J M, Basavappa S, Fitz J G 1992 Characterization of high-conductance anion channels in rat bile duct epithelial cells. American Journal of Physiology 262: G703–G710

Mehendale H M, Roth R A, Gandolfi A J, Klaunig J E, Lemasters J J, Curtis LR 1994 Novel mechanisms in chemically induced hepatotoxicity. FASEB Journal 8: 1285–1295

Muller M, Jansen P L M 1998 The secretory function of the liver: new aspects of hepatobiliary transport. Journal of Hepatology 28: 344–354

Paulusma C C, Bosma P J, Guido J, Zaman R, Conny T, Bakker M, Otter M, Scheffet G L, Scheper RJ, Borst P,Oude Elferink R P J 1996 Congenital jaundice in rats with a mutation in a multidrug resistance-associated protein gene. Science 271: 1126–1128

Paulusma C C, Kool M, Bosma P J, Scheffer J L, Borg F, Scheper R J, Tytgat G N J, Borst P, Baas F, Oude Elferink R P J 1997 A mutation in the human canalicular multispecific organic anion transporter gene causes the Dubin–Johnson syndrome. Hepatology 25: 1539–42

Phillips M J, Oda M, Fumatsu K 1978 Evidence for microfilament involvement in norethandrolone-induced intrahepatic cholestasis. American Journal of Pathology 93: 729–739

Phillips M J, Poucell S, Oda M 1986 Biology of disease. Mechanisms of cholestasis. Laboratory Investigation 54: 593–608

Poupon R E, Lindor K D, Cauch-Dudek K, Dicson E R, Poupon R, Heathcote J 1997 Combined analysis of randomized controlled trials of ursodeoxycholic acid in primary biliary cirrhosis. Gastroenterology 113: 884–890

Preisig R, Bircher J, Paumgartner G 1972 Physiologic and patho-physiologic aspects of the hepatic hemodynamics.In: Popper H and Schaffner F (eds). Progress in Liver Diseases. Grune & Stratton, New York and London, 4: 201–216

Roberts S K, Ludwig J, Larusso N F 1997 The pathobiology of biliary epithelia. Gastroenterology 112: 269–279

Simon F R, Fortune J, Iwahashi M, Gartung C, Wolkoff A, Sutherland E 1996 Ethinyl estradiol cholestasis involves alterations in expression of liver sinusoidal transporters. American Journal of Physiology 271: G1043–G1052

Smit J J M, Schinkel A H, Oude Elferink R P J, Groen A K, Wagenäar E, van Deemter L, Mol C A A M, Ottenhof R, van der Lugt N M T, van Roon M A, van der Valk A, Offerhaus G J A, Berns A J M, Borst P 1993 Homozygous disruption of the murine mdr2 p-glycoprotein gene leads to a complete absence of phospholipid from bile and to liver disease. Cell 75: 451–462

Stolz A, Takikawa H, Ookhtens M, Kaplowitz N 1989 The role of cytoplasmic proteins in hepatic bile acid transport. Annual Review of Physiology 51: 161–176

Stremmel W, Tiribelli C, Vyska K 1993 Multiplicity of sinusoidal membrane carrier systems of organic anions. In: Tavoloni N, Berk PD (eds) Hepatic Transport and Bile Secretion. Physiology and Pathophysiology. Raven Press, New York, 225–234

Trauner M, Arrese M, Soroka C J, Ananthanarayanan M, Koeppel T A, Schlosser S F, Suchy F J, Keppler D, Boyer J L 1997 The rat canalicular conjugate export pump (Mrp2) is down-regulated in intrahepatic and obstructive cholestasis. Gastroenterology 113: 255–264

Trauner M, Meyer P J, Boyer J L 1998 Molecular pathogenesis of cholestasis. New England Journal of Medicine 339: 1217–1227

Waters D L, Dorney S F A, Gruca M A, Martin H C O, Howman-Giles R, Kan A E, De Silva M, Gaskin K J 1995 Hepatobiliary disease in cystic fibrosis patients with pancreatic sufficiency. Hepatology 21: 963–969

Weber A M, Tuchweber B, Yousef I, Brochu P, Turgeon C, Gabbiani G, Morin C L, Roy C C 1981 Severe familial cholestasis in North American Indian children; a clinical model of microfilament dysfunction? Gastroenterology 81: 653–662

Yoon Y B, Hagey L R, Hofmann A F, Gurantz D, Michelotti E L, Steinbach JH 1986 Effect of side-chain shortening on the physiologic properties of bile acids: hepatic transport and effect on biliary secretion of 23-nor-ursodeoxycholate in rodents. Gastroenterology 90: 837–52

Zimmermann H, Reichen J, Zimmermann A, Sagesser H, Thenisch B, Höflin F 1992 Reversibility of secondary biliary fibrosis by biliodigestive anastomosis in the rat. Gastroenterology 103: 579–589

The function of the biliary tract and factors in the production of biliary pain

6

J. TOOULI

INTRODUCTION

The liver and the biliary tract are mentioned in the earliest recorded observations of man (Glenn & Grafe 1966). The Babylonians (2000 BC) described the gallbladder, cystic, hepatic and common bile ducts but their role in digestion was not appreciated. In 1543 Vesalius reported the presence of a membrane near the distal end of the common bile duct thought to impede reflux of duodenal contents into the bile duct, and in 1879 this structure was described as a sphincter and named after Rugero Oddi who in 1887 published a detailed description of its anatomy (Oddi 1887). In 1928 Ivy and Oldberg reported the successful extraction from hog duodenal mucosa of the hormone cholecystokinin which was shown to contract the gallbladder and reduce sphincter of Oddi resistance. These and subsequent studies firmly established that an intimate relationship existed between gallbladder contraction, sphincter of Oddi function and the flow of bile into the duodenum.

ANATOMY

EMBRYOLOGY

Embryological studies have demonstrated that the gallbladder and bile ducts arise from the caudal portion of a diverticular anlage that originates from the ventral floor of the foregut. The pancreas develops from two foregut buds in the region of the future duodenum. In 1957 Boyden confirmed that the distal muscularis propria of the bile duct and pancreatic duct are independent from duodenal musculature. In studies of the human fetus he showed that the sphincter of Oddi musculature arises de novo from mesenchyme, appearing approximately 5 weeks after the intestinal musculature.

MORPHOLOGY

Bile from the hepatocytes is secreted into canaliculi which communicate with numerous interlobular ducts, which in turn drain into two main hepatic ducts. The main right and left hepatic ducts fuse at the porta hepatis into the common hepatic duct and the cystic duct joins the common hepatic duct at a variable distance caudal to the porta hepatis to form the common bile duct.

The human gallbladder is a pear-shaped sac nestled along a fossa on the right inferior surface of the liver. The gallbladder is divided anatomically into the blunt ended fundus, the body and the neck, which leads to the cystic duct. A sacculation at the neck of the gallbladder is known as Hartman's pouch. The cystic duct is of variable length, usually joining the common hepatic duct at an acute angle to form the common bile duct.

The common bile duct (Ch. 1) passes dorsal to the first part of the duodenum lying in a groove either within or posterior to the head of the pancreas and enters the second part of the duodenum through the major duodenal papilla in association with the pancreatic duct of Wirsung. The junction of the terminal common bile duct, pancreatic duct and duodenum at the papilla assumes one of three configurations that may be likened to a Y, V or U. In approximately 70% of subjects the ducts open into a common channel and thus have a Y configuration. This common channel drains into the duodenum through a single orifice on the duodenal papilla of Vater. In approximately 20% of subjects the common channel is almost nonexistent and the two ducts have a common V shape opening on the papilla. In 10% of subjects the common bile duct and pancreatic duct have separate openings on the tip of the papilla; these openings lie adjacent to each other and give a U-shaped configuration. The terminal parts of the common bile duct and pancreatic duct, the common channel and major duodenal papilla of Vater are invested by varying thickness of smooth muscle and together form the sphincter or Oddi segment.

The major part of the human sphincter of Oddi lies within the duodenal wall, and anatomically has been shown to be distinctly separate from it. Boyden (1937), in a series of publications on the anatomy of the sphincter of Oddi, described distinct sphincters at the terminal end of the common bile duct (sphincter choledochus), the terminal end of the pancreatic duct (sphincter pancreaticus) and the common channel (sphincter ampullae). However more recently Hand (1963) using a combination of radiological, duct cast techniques and histological sectioning methods, did not distinguish separate sphincters. Hand concluded from his human autopsy studies that the common bile duct and pancreatic duct become fused in a common connective tissue sheath outside the duodenal wall and pass together through a slit in the duodenal muscle known as the 'choledochal window'. The lumina, however, do not join at this level but are separated by a thick muscular septum. In most subjects fusion of the two lumina occurs in the submucosal layer of the duodenum to form a common channel varying in length between 2 and 17 mm. Before entering the duodenum each duct becomes completely surrounded by circular muscle, some of which forms a figure of eight pattern around the two ducts. The point at which the smooth muscle starts on each duct is readily identified radiologically as a notch (Fig. 6.1). Distal to the notch each lumen becomes narrow as it traverses the duodenal wall, this narrowing being associated with a thickening of the duct wall due to smooth muscle, connective tissue and mucous glands. As the ducts pass through the duodenal wall longitudinal muscle fibers interdigitate between the circular ductular muscle fibers and the duodenal muscle. The ducts emerge from the duodenal muscle layers to have a course of variable length through the duodenal submucosa before opening on to the papilla of Vater; throughout this submucosal course, the ducts are ensheathed by circularly orientated smooth muscle (Fig. 6.2). Manometric studies in man support Hand's description of the sphincter of Oddi in that separate sphincteric zones have not been identified (Toouli et al 1982a).

The mucosa of the human sphincter of Oddi segment is lined by columnar epithelium and contains numerous mucus-secreting glands. The mucosa is thrown into longitudinal folds likened to mucosal valvules (Tansy et al 1975). These folds are least marked proximally and increase distally becoming maximal in the common channel. The mucosal folds may occasionally be seen projecting through the orifice of the duodenal papilla.

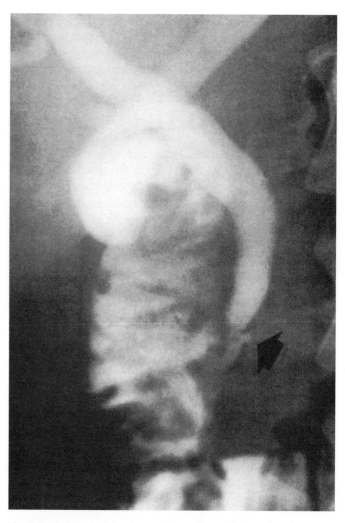

Fig. 6.1 Choledochogram demonstrating the notch (arrow) at the terminal end of the bile duct. This notch identifies the uppermost margin of the sphincter of Oddi. Reproduced with permission from the publishers, Butterworth, London, and the British Journal of Surgery 71: 251–256.

INNERVATION

The gallbladder and extrahepatic bile ducts are supplied by both extrinsic sympathetic and parasympathetic nerves. The celiac ganglia contribute both motor and sensory nerves made up of sympathetic fibers which originate in the T7 to T10 spinal segments. Nerve fibers from both vagal nerves merge to form the hepatic plexus which supplies parasympathetic motor nerves to the extrahepatic biliary system (Burnett et al 1964).

Intrinsic nerve plexuses are found throughout the extrahepatic biliary system. The plexuses contain cells with histological features consistent with ganglia and are believed to be analogous to the submucosal and muscular plexuses of the gut. Histochemical labeling has shown

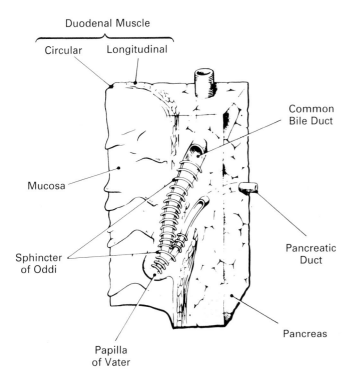

Fig. 6.2 Diagram of the human sphincter of Oddi demonstrating the circular smooth muscle which surrounds the terminal common bile duct and pancreatic duct. The length of the sphincter along the pancreatic duct is shorter than the length investing the terminal common bile duct. The major part of the sphincter lies within the duodenal wall and enters the duodenum through a slit in the duodenal muscle.

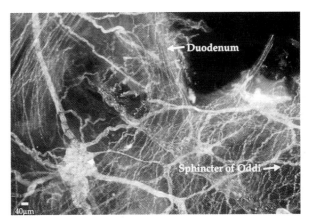

Fig. 6.3 Peptidergic neurones in the sphincter region.

that the gallbladder is richly supplied with both andrenergic and cholinergic ganglia. In addition, studies (Sundler et al 1977, Wen-Qin & Gabella 1983) have shown the presence of immunoreactive peptidergic nerves which label with vasoactive intestinal polypeptide (VIP). The sphincter of Oddi has a rich ganglionic plexus which appears to have a predominance of cholinergic ganglia and a smaller number of andrenergic ganglia. Immunohistochemical studies from our laboratory have demonstrated the presence of a wide range of peptidergic neurones in the sphincter region (Fig. 6.3). These include galanin, substance P and somatostatin-containing nerves. In addition, the inhibitory transmitter nitric oxide has been demonstrated in nerves to the sphincter and is thought to have an important function in modulating sphincter relaxation. The nerves in the sphincter region have been demonstrated to communicate with the proximal biliary tract, the gallbladder and the duodenum (Padbury et al 1993, Saccone et al 1994).

METHODS OF STUDY

A number of different techniques have been used in the study of biliary physiology and pathophysiology, and the following is an overview of some of the most useful methods.

RADIOGRAPHY

Historically, cholecystography had been used extensively for the study of gallbladder motility. Estimations of gallbladder volumes were made and the effects of ingested food substances, intravenous injection of gastrointestinal hormones, and parasympathetic and sympathetic nerve stimulation recorded. The kinetics of common bile duct sphincter of Oddi motility were studied by infusing the contrast medium into the biliary system via a tube inserted in the common bile duct and making a continuous record by cineradiography (Caroli et al 1960). These techniques have been replaced by new methods which provide more accurate and reproducible data.

MANOMETRY

Measurement of pressure changes from within the extrahepatic biliary system has been the basic investigation for understanding biliary dynamics. Intraluminal gall bladder pressures have been recorded with the cystic duct either patent or occluded in both anesthetized and awake animals. Intraluminal gallbladder pressures have also been recorded in anesthetized humans undergoing surgery for gallbladder disease, and the effect of intravenously administered drugs on the gallbladder pressures determined (Csendes & Sepulvela 1980).

Pressure measurements from the bile ducts have been obtained in animals and man anesthetized or awake by inserting a tube into the bile duct area. Pressures have been read visually from fluid-filled manometers or recorded by a transducer linked to a polygraph (Hess 1979). Investigators have determined the opening, passage and closing pressures of the sphincter of Oddi by either increasing or decreasing the height of the fluid reservoir connected in series with the tube inside the bile duct. From measurements of common bile duct pressure inferences were drawn about sphincter of Oddi function (Cushieri et al 1972).

Accurate direct pressure measurements from the sphincter of Oddi became possible by miniaturization of manometry catheters and the development of manometric systems of low compliance. A triple lumen constantly perfused catheter is inserted into the sphincter of Oddi segment and intraluminal pressure changes reflecting the activity of the sphincter recorded (Geenen et al 1980). These pressure measurements are made in awake humans under mild sedation by introducing the catheter into the papilla of Vater via an endoscope (Fig. 6.4). In addition, prolonged sphincter of Oddi manometric studies may be conducted in patients with a T-tube in the bile duct following duct exploration for stones. A manometry catheter may be passed down the T-tube and its recording ports positioned to record from the sphincter or Oddi. Studies up to 8 h in length may be conducted 1–2 weeks after the surgery and prior to removal of the T-tube (Worthley et al 1989). Similarly in animals manometry catheters are positioned within the sphincter of Oddi segment either through the bile duct or from the duodenum.

Perfusion manometry may produce artefact due to the fluid infusion. Therefore solid state manometric catheters have been developed. In studies where this technology has been compared to perfusion manometry, pressure measurements have been similar, hence dispelling fears that perfusion manometry may produce artefact. Whilst solid state manometry is appealing, the catheters are expensive and currently do not have the capacity to record from multiple sites.

ELECTROMYOGRAPHY

Extacellular bioplar or monopolar electrodes sutured to the outside surface of the biliary tract have been used to record contractile activity from both animals and man (Sarles et al 1975). Studies have shown that the biliary tree, like the rest of the gastrointestinal tract, is characterized by two basic types of myelectrical activity, i.e. slow regular changes in membrane potential known as 'slow waves' and rapid

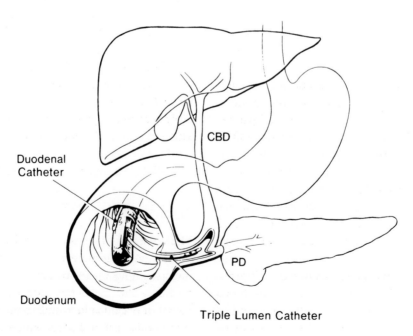

Fig. 6.4 Diagram illustrating endoscopic sphincter of Oddi manometry. A triple lumen catheter is inserted into either the common bile duct or the pancreatic duct and withdrawn so that all the three lumens are stationed within the sphincter. A separate single lumen catheter records duodenal pressure. Reproduced with permission from the publishers, Butterworth, London and the British Journal of Surgery (1984) 71: 251–256.

depolarization spikes called 'spike bursts' (Honda et al 1982). In general, spike bursts are virtually always associated with a phasic smooth muscle contraction and as such reflect intraluminal pressure changes.

RADIOISOTOPE IMAGING

A variety of ^{99m}Tc IDA (iminodiacetic acid) compounds are cleared through the liver into bile after intravenous administration (Ch. 16). ^{99m}Tc gives off 140 Kev gamma photons that are ideally suited for imaging and counting by a gamma camera. These properties of the ^{99m}Tc IDA compounds have been used to image the gallbladder by producing temporal profiles monitoring of gallbladder filling and emptying can be studied (Shaffer et al 1980). Adaptation of those techniques to the study of bile flow through the bile duct in postcholecystectomy subjects also has been possible (Roberts-Thomson et al 1986). A major advantage of the isotope method is its noninvasive nature, which makes it suitable for use in humans. Close correlation with manometric studies of the sphincter of Oddi has been reported (Corazziari et al 1994, Sostre et al 1992).

ULTRASONOGRAPHY (Ch. 15)

An important use of ultrasonography has been in the determination of gallbladder volume. In order to calculate gallbladder volume at a point in time, the maximal length and corresponding transverse diameter of the gallbladder are determined. Volume then is calculated from the ultrasound images as the sum of a series of cylinders (Everson et al 1980). Repeated measurements of gallbladder volume determine changes with various stimuli. In addition, ultrasonography has been used to evaluate bile duct and pancreatic duct diameter in patients suspected of sphincter of Oddi dysfunction. In patients with biliary type symptoms, real time sonography has been used to measure bile duct diameter before and after a fatty meal stimulus of 3.3 ml/kg corn oil (Lipomul). Normally, duct diameter should decrease as the sphincter relaxes. An abnormal response is diagnosed if duct diameter does not change or increases (Darweesh et al 1988).

In patients being investigated for causes of idiopathic recurrent pancreatitis, the diameter of the pancreatic duct is measured before and after secretin (1 μg/kg) infusion. A normal response comprises an increase in duct diameter with a rapid return to normal within 30 minutes. If the duct remains dilated (i.e. 1.5 mm), sphincter of Oddi dysfunction is suspected as the possible cause of pancreatitis (Bolondi et al 1984).

PHYSIOLOGY

GALLBLADDER

Fluid transport and its regulation

Studies in animals and man have demonstrated that the gallbladder concentrates hepatic bile by selective reabsorption of bile constituents. However, in addition, studies have shown that both under physiological and pathological conditions reversal of fluid transport across the gallbladder mucosa occurs and net secretion into the gallbladder lumen results. Sodium and chloride ions are absorbed from the gallbladder lumen by both active and passive transport mechanisms. Water absorption is thought to be passive and secondary to active solute movement resulting from osmotic equilibration of transported solute within the epithelium. The secretion of water and electrolytes by the gallbladder mucosa is an active process which can take place against hydrostatic and osmotic gradients (Wood & Svanvik 1983).

Animal in vitro and in vivo studies have demonstrated that a number of gastrointestinal peptides affect gallbladder fluid transport. Cyclic AMP acts as a second messenger for the effects of several mediators and has been implicated in sodium and chloride transport in rabbit and necturus gallbladder. Vasoactive inhibitory polypeptide (VIP) and secretin have been shown to modify gallbladder fluid transport at concentrations which suggest a physiological role. However, other peptides such as glucagon, cholecystokinin, neurotensin, bombesin, motilin and somatostatin, which have been shown to enhance absorption in vitro, may act to potentiate or inhibit the effects of the major peptides (Wood et al 1982).

Application of prostaglandins of the E and F series to in vitro animal gallbladder preparations have demonstrated inhibition of fluid absorption by arachidonic acid (Thornell et al 1979). In animal studies bile salts, female sex hormones and autonomic nerve stimulation also have been shown to influence fluid transport.

During fasting the normal gallbladder absorbs fluid at a rate corresponding to one third of the fasting gallbladder volume. After feeding there is reversal of the direction of gallbladder transport from a net absorption to a net secretion into the gallbladder lumen. The net water transport across the gallbladder wall may be influenced by both humoral factors and autonomic nerves. During inflammation of the gallbladder, often associated with cystic duct obstruction, the absorptive capacity of the gallbladder mucosa is lost and net secretion into the lumen results, producing a hydrops. This pathological effect appears to be mediated by prostaglandin release due to formation of lysolecithin by hydrolysis of phospholipid in the gallbladder. This process can be reversed by indomethacin, supporting the belief that at least part of the change in fluid transport may result from endogenous prostaglandin formation.

Gallbladder motility

Estimations of human fasting gallbladder volume by ultrasound techniques have shown a mean volume of approximately 17 ml in normal subjects. In the past it was thought that the gallbladder volume gradually increased during fasting until the mean maximal volume was reached and only emptied after a food stimulus. However, studies in dogs (Takahashi et al 1982b) and opossums have shown that the gallbladder contracts up to 40% of maximal contractile capacity during the interdigestive period, and that these gallbladder contractions occur during phase II of the migrating motor complex (MMC). The periodic gallbladder contractions during fasting empty concentrated viscous bile and enable gallbladder refilling with dilute hepatic bile. Studies in man using ultrasound estimation of gallbladder volume confirm that a similar cyclical pattern of gallbladder volume changes occur in man, in association with phase III of the MMC (Toouli et al 1986). The controlling mechanism which produces gallbladder volume changes during fasting is unknown. A potential candidate is motilin, a hormone produced by the mucosa of proximal small intestine. Serum motilin levels show cyclic changes during MMC cycles with the peak values preceding phase III MMC activity. In animal studies motilin has been shown to produce gallbladder contraction (Takahashi et al 1982b).

The flow of bile into the gallbladder is modulated by hepatic secretory pressure, sphincter of Oddi tone and cystic duct resistance. Only 50% of secreted hepatic bile enters the gallbladder during fasting, the remaining bile passing into the duodenum without concentration by the gallbladder. Gallbladder emptying produced by a meal of exogenous cholecystokinin occurs as a slow steady contraction which delivers bile into the duodenum for 20 min or longer while generating an intraluminal gallbladder pressure that is generally only a few cmH$_2$O above that in the common bile duct. The slow emptying of the gallbladder is typical of a graded tonic smooth-muscle contraction such as that which occurs in the fundus of the stomach during gastric emptying of liquids.

The ability of a fatty meal to elicit gallbladder contraction has been well documented in man and a number of animal species. Proteins entering the duodenum also produce gallbladder contraction but carbohydrates have only a minimal effect. Endogenous cholecystokinin is released from the mucosa of proximal small intestine and studies which measure serum CCK levels by radio-immunoassay have shown that gallbladder contraction induced by intraduodenal infusion of fat correlates directly with the level of circulating CCK (Weiner et al 1981).

The role of autonomic nerves in regulating gallbladder volume is not clear. In one study increased fasting volume of the human gallbladder was demonstrated after vagotomy (Johnson & Boyden 1952). A number of studies have investigated the effect of vagal stimulation and vagotomy on gallbladder contractility (Benevantano & Rosen 1969), but the results generally have been inconclusive. Similarly, studies of sympathetic innervation have produced inconstant and variable findings, and the role of the sympathetic autonomic nervous system in gallbladder motility requires further study (Persson 1972).

CYSTIC DUCT

Accumulating evidence suggests that the cystic duct is not merely a passive conduit between the gallbladder and the common bile duct, but may play an active role in the flow of bile into and out of the gallbladder. Histologically an anatomically prominent sphincter, as described by Lutken, does not appear to be present; however, a thin layer of smooth muscle is evident in the wall of the duct and, along with the prominent mucosal folds which make up the valves of Heister, the cystic duct may act as a variable resistor to flow.

Flow studies in dogs have demonstrated resistance to flow across the cystic duct, the resistance being equal whether perfusion was carried either into or out of the gallbladder (Scott & Otto 1979). Significant reductions in flow were induced following systemic intravenous or local intra-arterial injection of morphine, adrenalin or cholecystokinin, suggesting that the cystic duct performs like a sphincter in modulating flow through its lumen. Studies in the prairie dog gallstone model have shown that cystic duct resistance to flow increases prior to gallstone formation in these animals (Pitt et al 1981a). These studies suggest that abnormalities in cystic duct formation may be implicated in the pathophysiology of gallstone formation.

COMMON BILE DUCT

The role of the common bile duct in the control of bile flow has been confused due to anatomical differences in species studied. As in the cystic duct, histological studies in man have demonstrated only thin longitudinally orientated layers of smooth muscle within the walls of the common bile duct (Toouli & Watts 1971). The major tissue component appears to be elastic fibers. However, in other species such as in sheep, the common bile duct is invested with circularly orientated smooth muscle which exhibits peristaltic activity.

The weight of evidence suggests that the human common bile duct does not have a primary propulsile function. However, the elastic fibers and the longitudinally orientated smooth muscle provide a tonic pressure that may help overcome the tonic resistance of the sphincter of Oddi.

The diameter of the human common bile duct before and after cholecystectomy has been the subject of controversy. Part of the controversy has been due to methodology used in determining duct size. It has become quite obvious that duct size as determined by ultrasonography cannot be equated to duct size determined by endoscopic retrograde cholangiography or intraoperative extraluminal measurements. Ultrasound measurement records the non distended lumen, whereas at ERCP contrast produces dispersion. Intraoperative measurements include wall thickness. In general the normal diameter of the common bile duct as determined by ultrasound is less than 6 mm, by retrograde cholangiography less than 10 mm, and by intraoperative extraluminal measurements less than 12 mm. What has become clear from recent studies, however, is that the common bile duct does not increase in diameter significantly following cholecystectomy (Le Quesne et al 1959, Hunt & Scott 1989). The major cause of dilated common bile duct is increased intraluminal pressure which generally is produced by either primary or secondary obstruction at the sphincter of Oddi.

SPHINCTER OF ODDI

The mechanism by which the sphincter of Oddi controls the flow of the bile and pancreatic secretion has been clarified by studies in animals and man which have evaluated sphincter of Oddi function by sophisticated direct and indirect techniques. These studies have shown that sphincter of Oddi motility differs from one species to another, largely reflecting the anatomical variability between species. Thus, whilst many commonalities exist, one has to be circumspect in translating animal data directly into the motility and function of the human sphincter of Oddi.

Sphincter of Oddi motility studies in animals

In vivo studies in dogs, cats, rabbits, monkeys and opossums have demonstrated that the sphincter of Oddi exhibits muscle contractions which are independent of duodenal activity. The results from the dog studies suggested that the sphincter of Oddi has a milking effect on bile, thus propelling small volumes of fluid from the common bile duct into the duodenum (Watts & Dunphy 1966). Manometric and electromyographic studies of the opossum sphincter of Oddi demonstrated phasic contractions which propagate along the entire length from the cephalic to the caudal end (Toouli et al 1983a). The common bile duct and pancreatic duct proximal to the sphincter do not demonstrate spontaneous motor activity.

Analysis of simultaneous cineradiography, transsphincteric flow and electromyographic recordings from the

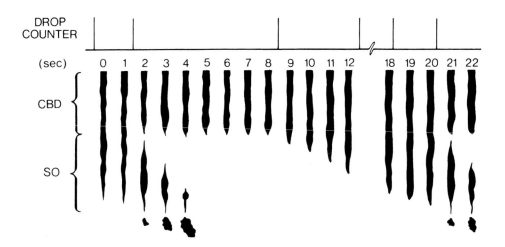

Fig. 6.5 Schematic representation of images from a cineradiographic recording illustrating flow through the sphincter of Oddi (SO). Contrast flowed into the common bile duct (CBD) at a rate of approx 6 drops/min (0.1 ml/min) from a reservoir and each drop is indicated by a vertical line. In this example contrast flows into the CBD and fills the SO segment. A phasic contraction begins at the junction of the CBD and SO, expelling contrast into the duodenum. Simultaneously flow from the CBD is interrupted and there is no flow from the reservoir into the CBD. On completion of the SO phasic contraction the SO segment relaxes and fluid passes from the CBD into the SO. The cycle then repeats itself. J.C.I. 1987 71: 208–220.

opossum sphincter of Oddi has demonstrated the effect of the phasic contractions on flow of bile into the duodenum (Fig. 6.5). The predominant mechanism of common bile duct emptying in the opossum is the antegrade sphincter of Oddi phasic contraction. A wave of contraction begins at the junction of the common bile duct and sphincter of Oddi stripping the contents of the sphincter of Oddi segment into the duodenum. During the period of sphincter of Oddi contraction, flow into the common bile duct ceases and there is no flow from the common bile duct into the sphincter of Oddi segment. Next, the sphincter of Oddi relaxes and passive flow of bile occurs from the common bile duct into the sphincter of Oddi segment. After filling of the sphincter of Oddi segment, a wave of contraction again begins at the junction of the common bile duct and sphincter segment and the cycle repeats itself. The overall effect of the phasic contractions is to promote flow from the common bile duct into the duodenum. During sphincter contraction, or systole, flow from the common bile duct into the sphincter of Oddi segment stops and flow into the sphincter segment occurs only during sphincter relaxation or diastole. Increasing the frequency of sphincter contractions by administering the sphincter agonists phenylephrine (50 µg/kg i.v.) and bethanechol (30 µg/kg i.v.) decreased the diastolic interval between contractions and decreased the time available for passive flow of fluid from the common bile duct into the sphincter segment. Initially, an increase in the frequency of sphincter phasic contractions produced an increase of flow across the sphincter. However, as the frequency of contractions increases further, flow decreases due to the decrease in the diastolic interval. When the frequency of contractions exceeds eight per minute, the diastolic interval is abolished and there is no flow across the sphincter of Oddi segment of the opossum.

Following the ingestion of a meal, neuronal and hormonal stimuli influence the motor activity of the sphincter of Oddi and the hormone cholecystokinin plays a major role in the control of this activity. Its mechanisms of action on the sphincter or Oddi has been studied in the cat (Behar & Biancani 1980). In this animal, an intravenous bolus of cholecystokinin inhibited the phasic contractions and produced a fall in sphincter tone. Following administration of the neurotoxin tetrodotoxin, cholecystokinin administration no longer produced inhibition, but instead caused contraction in the sphincter of Oddi. The investigators concluded that cholecystokinin produces its effect by stimulation of nonadrenergic noncholingeric inhibitory neurones, this effect overriding a lesser, direct smooth muscle stimulatory action of the hormone.

Neurohistochemical studies have demonstrated both adrenergic and cholinergic neurones within the sphincter of Oddi and experiments in animals have determined the pharmacological effects of histamine, cholinergic and adrenergic stimulation on the sphincter muscle (Toouli et al 1983a). However, the physiological significance of these drug actions on the sphincter of Oddi requires further investigation.

The function of the vagus nerve in sphincter of Oddi physiology remains obscure. Studies in dogs suggested that following vagal transection the resistance to flow across the sphincter of Oddi is decreased (Pitt et al 1981b). However, in the prairie dog increased resistance to flow through the sphincter of Oddi occurs after truncal vagotomy. Results from vagal stimulation studies have failed to define clearly the role of the vagus in biliary dynamics.

Studies carried out in opossums with chronically implanted electrodes positioned in the sphincter of Oddi and the small intestine have demonstrated that the phasic activity of the sphincter of Oddi is omnipresent (Honda et al 1982). However, the frequency of the phasic contractions varies periodically during fasting. Four phases which are analogous to the phases of the intestinal interdigestive migrating motor complexes have been described for the sphincter of Oddi. Food ingestion and the intravenous infusion of cholecystokinin and pentagastrin abolish the periodic nature of the interdigestive sphincter of Oddi contractions, and in this species ingested food produced an increase in contractile frequency which increased flow of bile into the duodenum. The physiological function of the periodic sphincter of Oddi contractions during fasting might be similar to that proposed for intestinal migrating motor complexes and that is to act as a housekeeper to eliminate any debris which may accumulate at the lower end of the bile duct. In addition, this activity of the sphincter may modulate the volume of bile passing into either the duodenum or gallbladder during fasting.

The Australian possum sphincter of Oddi demonstrates an activity which is different to that of the American opossum, but similar to the human sphincter. In this species, inhibition of sphincter phasic contractions promotes flow of the bile. This inhibition is mediated by neural release of nitric oxide (Baker et al 1993).

Sphincter of Oddi motility in man

Cineradiographic studies of the human sphincter of Oddi exhibit rhythmic contractions which propel contrast into the duodenum (Hess 1979). Sphincter of Oddi pressure studies conducted at the time of biliary tract surgery demonstrated variations in pressure thought to be the manometric equivalent of the cineradiographic contractions (Cushieri et al 1972). Resistance to outflow of fluid from the common bile duct into the duodenum also was demonstrated by the intraoperative studies. This resistance was reduced after administration of cholecystokinin octapeptide or smooth muscle relaxants such as amylnitrite (Butsch et al 1936).

Manometric recordings from within the sphincter of Oddi segment (Geenen et al 1980) have demonstrated that the human sphincter of Oddi is characterized by prominent phasic contractions superimposed on a basal sphincter of Oddi pressure 3 mmHg above the pressure in the common bile duct and pancreatic duct (Fig. 6.6). The amplitude of the phasic contractions is approximately 130 mmHg and the mean frequency is four per minute. Analysis of the direction of propagation of the phasic contractions during a continuous 3-min period demonstrated that the majority of contractions (60%) are orientated in an antegrade direction from the common bile duct towards the duodenum. A smaller number of contractions occurred either simultaneously (24%) or had a retrograde orientation (15%). Intravenous bolus injection of cholecystokinin octapeptide (20 ng/kg) normally produces inhibition of the phasic contractions and a fall in the basal sphincter of Oddi pressure (Fig 6.7). Table 6.1 shows the pressures recorded from the sphincter of Oddi of normal subjects. Studies from patients with T-tubes inserted in the common bile duct following bile duct exploration (Worthley et al 1989) have shown that the frequency of sphincter of Oddi phasic contractions during fasting exhibits a periodicity in relation to duodenal migrating motor complexes, similar to that demonstrated in the opossum (Fig. 6.8).

Following the ingestion of a meal, bile flow across the sphincter of Oddi is promoted by inhibition or reduction in the amplitude of the phasic contractions and a fall in the sphincter of Oddi basal pressure. This effect on the human sphincter of Oddi is similar to that following intravenous injection of the cholecystokinin octapeptide. Consequently in man, unlike the American opossum, bile flow occurs mainly between sphincter of Oddi phasic contractions during the period of diastole. The phasic contractions do propel small volumes of bile into the duodenum, but this is not the major means by which bile flow occurs. The phasic contractions in man may function to prevent reflux of duodenal contents into either the bile or pancreatic ducts, and to maintain the ducts free of small debris. In order to promote flow across the human sphincter of Oddi, inhibition or reduction of the phasic contractions and a fall in basal pressure is necessary.

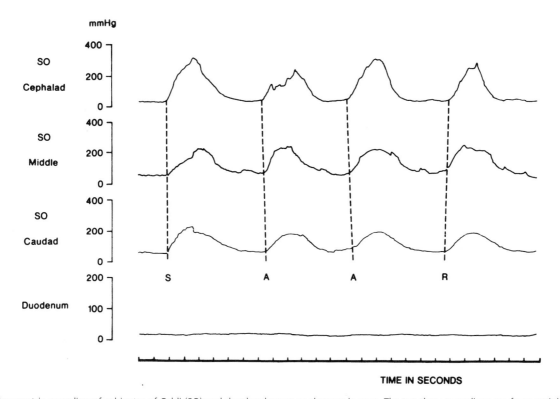

Fig. 6.6 Manometric recording of sphincter of Oddi (SO) and duodenal pressure changes in man. The top three recordings are from a triple lumen catheter stationed in the SO. The SO recording sizes are spaced 2 mm apart. A line is drawn at the commencement of each phasic wave starting from the cephalic recording site to the caudal recording site. The phasic contractions show simultaneous (S), antegrade (A) and retrograde (R) orientations and are independent of duodenal pressure changes.

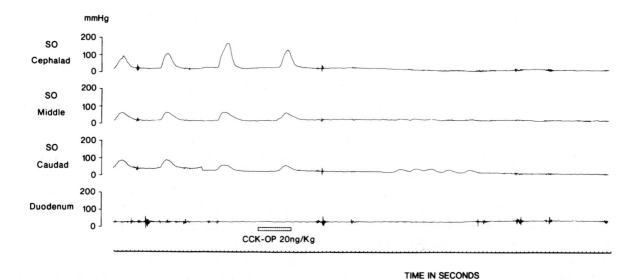

Fig. 6.7 Manometric recording showing the effect of a bolus i.v. injection of cholecystokinin-octapeptide (CCK-OP) on sphincter of Oddi (SO) phasic contractions. CCK-OP caused inhibition of the SO phasic contractions and no change in duodenal pressure. Reproduced with permission from the publishers, Butterworth, London, and The British Journal of Surgery (1984) 71: 251–256.

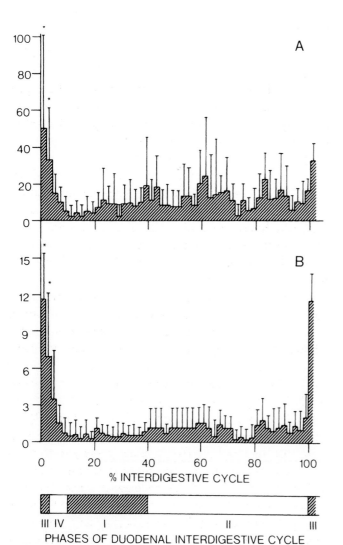

Table 6.1 SO pressures

| | Normal | | Abnormal |
	Median	Range	
Basal Pressure (mmHg)	15	3–35	> 40
Amplitude (mmHg)	135	95–195	> 300
Frequency (n/min)	4	2–6	> 7
Sequences			
Antegrade %	80	12–100	
Simultaneous %	13	0–50	
Retrograde %	9	0–50	> 50
CCK 20 ng/kg		Inhibits	Contracts

OVERVIEW OF BILIARY TRACT PHYSIOLOGY

In humans during fasting periods approximately 50% of secreted hepatic bile is stored in the gallbladder whilst the remaining bile passes into the duodenum. The contractile activity of the sphincter of Oddi appears to modulate bile flow and either diverts small volumes into the gallbladder or promotes its flow into the duodenum. This function of the sphincter of Oddi is controlled by the sphincter of Oddi basal pressure and the prominent phasic contractions which

Fig. 6.8 Histograms of duodenal wave **(A)** amplitude and **(B)** frequency over 100% of the interdigestive cycle. The interdigestive cycle is divided into 2% intervals and values expressed as the mean (SD) for six patients. Duodenal activity is separated into four phases and is recorded at the bottom of the figure. *A significant difference compared with Phases I and II. Reproduced with permission from The British Journal of Surgery 1989; 76: 709–714.

may be antegrade in direction and thus propel small volumes of fluid into the duodenum, or retrograde and simultaneous which inhibit flow. Most of the flow across the sphincter occurs in between the sphincter contractions. The cystic duct generates a small resistance which can readily be overcome either by strong sphincter of Oddi contractions or in reverse by the tonic contractions of the gallbladder. Bile stored in the gallbladder is concentrated by absorption of water and electrolytes. Both the gallbladder and sphincter of Oddi demonstrate a periodicity respectively with regard to volume changes and frequency of phasic contractions. This periodicity is related to the duodenal migrating motor complexes and its role might be as a housekeeper in eliminating small microcrystals which may develop in supersaturated fasting bile.

Following a meal, neuronal and hormonal stimuli produce slow gallbladder contraction, a reduction in sphincter of Oddi basal pressure and inhibition of the sphincter of Oddi contractions. These responses of the sphincter allow flow of bile into the duodenum actively propeled by pressure generated from the gallbladder and hepatic secretion of bile.

PATHOPHYSIOLOGY—PRODUCTION OF BILIARY PAIN

Biliary pain characteristically is felt in the epigastrium and radiates to the right hypochondrium and to the right subscapular region (Doran 1967). The pain is erroneously labeled as a colic, although it is most commonly constant in nature with only minor fluctuations in intensity. Occasionally the site of the pain may differ from its classical position and be felt in the chest, left hypochondrium or lower abdomen. Pain originates from inflammation of the gallbladder and cystic duct, from distention of the gallbladder or bile duct and from direct irritation of the sphincter of Oddi.

The commonest and most readily understood cause of biliary pain is that which occurs in association with gallstones. Gallbladder stones impact in Hartman's pouch to produce obstruction of the cystic duct, thereby causing stasis of gallbladder bile. This initiating factor sets into motion a train of events in which prostaglandins appear to have an important role. Transport of fluid across the gallbladder mucosa is reversed, distention of the gallbladder and inflammation occurs and biliary pain of a visceral nature is felt. In most people the pain resolves spontaneously within hours, and this is due to relief of the cystic duct obstruction. Administration of a prostaglandin synthetase inhibitor, such as indomethacin, appears to promote early resolution of the symptoms (Thornell et al 1979). If the cystic duct obstruction is not relieved, the inflammatory process continues leading to acute cholecystitis with involvement of the parietal peritoneum in the right hypochondrium and pain of somatic origin is experienced.

When a stone migrates into or originates in the bile duct, obstruction of bile outflow may result if the stone impacts at the lower end of the common bile duct. Acute obstruction of the bile duct causes bile duct distention which gives rise to biliary pain. Similar pain may be produced inadvertently in patients with a T-tube in the common bile duct following bile duct exploration, if fluid is rapidly infused through the T-tube into the bile duct to produce acute distention.

The pathophysiology of noncalculous biliary pain is not as readily understood and the mechanisms by which such pain may originate remain the subject of investigation and controversy. A major problem in understanding noncalculous biliary pain has been the lack of objective evidence to incriminate biliary pathology as the cause.

GALLBLADDER DYSKINESIA

Abnormalities of gallbladder contraction are postulated to comprise either decreased contraction (hypokinesia) or excessive contraction (hyperkinesia) with or without production of biliary pain. Diagnosis of gallbladder dyskinesia has centered upon the visualization of the gallbladder either by contrast or isotope, followed by the administration of a standard stimulus such as cholecystokinin.

A large number of studies (Valberg et al 1971, Goldstein et al 1974, Dunn et al 1974) assessed gallbladder pain following a bolus injection of cholecystokinin octapeptide. A positive diagnosis was made if the injection reproduced the patient's pain. Analysis of the studies, however, has shown a strong placebo effect and lack of reproducibility, hence they have gone out of favour.

One of the first studies to provide objective and reproducible measurement of gallbladder emptying in patients with clinically diagnosed gallbladder dyskinesia used a scintigraphic technique and infusion of cholecystokinin octapeptide at a dose shown not to produce pain (Yap et al 1991). In this study, the gallbladder ejection fraction (GBEF) in response to a 45-min infusion of CCK-OP, was determined for a group of normal individuals (Fig. 6.9) and a normal value of > 40% defined. Patients with a GBEF less than 40% were randomized to either cholecystectomy or follow up. Patients undergoing cholecystectomy had histological abnormalities of the gallbladder consistent with chronic cholecystitis and were symptom free at 3 years following cholecystectomy. The control patients continued to experience pain and most have subsequently undergone

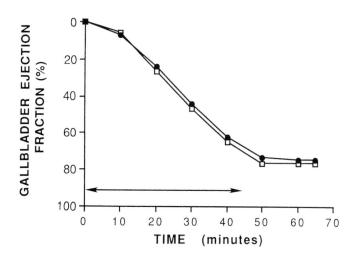

Fig. 6.9 Comparison of the effect of a 45-min infusion of CCK on 20 normal volunteers on repeated testing. Mean gallbladder ejection fractions are indicated as solid circles from the first test and as squares for the repeat test. Arrow indicates the duration of CCK infusion. The GBEF is highly reproducible. Reproduced with permission from Gastroenterology (1991) 101: 786–793.

cholecystectomy. This objective investigation selects a group of patients with gallbladder dyskinesia who respond to cholecystectomy.

CYSTIC DUCT STUMP SYNDROME

Episodes of recurrent biliary pain occurring after cholecystectomy have been attributed in a small number of patients to continuing or recurrent disease in the cystic duct stump. A long cystic duct stump per se does not appear to be the cause of pain. However, stump neuromas, persistent chronic inflammation around a nonabsorbable suture have all been associated with recurrent postcholecystectomy biliary pain. To date there are no investigations which allow diagnosis of this entity prior to surgery; thus laparotomy and excision of the stump is performed usually on clinical suspicion.

SPHINCTER OF ODDI DYSFUNCTION

Dysfunction of sphincter of Oddi motility may be responsible for the production of biliary pain in patients who have previously had cholecystectomy performed for calculous or noncalculous biliary disease. In addition, sphincter of Oddi dysfunction may contribute to noncalculous gallbladder disease, the formation of primary common bile duct stones and be associated with recurrent pancreatitis. Diagnosis of sphincter of Oddi dysfunction has lacked objectivity and pain provocative tests such as the morphine-neostigmine test have not lived up to early expectations. Endoscopic

sphincter of Oddi manometry has provided the most objective method for evaluating sphincter of Oddi activity (Toouli 1984). Based on the endoscopic manometric data, sphincter of Oddi disorders are categorized into two major groups (Table 6.2):

Table 6.2 SO dysfunction	
Stenosis	• Basal pressure 40 mmHg
Dyskinesia	• Frequency 7/min
	• Intermittent rise in basal pressure
	• Retrograde contractions 50%
	• Paradoxical CCK-OP response

1. Sphincter of Oddi stenosis

Manometrically this group of patients is characterized by an abnormally elevated sphincter of Oddi basal pressure suggestive of stenosis (Fig. 6.10). The sphincter stenosis may produce increased resistance to flow through the sphincter giving rise to biliary type pain or pancreatitis. Although correlative pathological evidence is lacking, it is postulated that the sphincter of Oddi of these patients may be narrowed by a fibrotic stenosis, smooth muscle hypertrophy or mucosal hyperplasia.

2. Sphincter of Oddi dyskinesia

An abnormally functioning sphincter of Oddi is characterized manometrically by one or more of the following findings:

a. *Excessive retrograde contractions*
In control subjects the majority of the sphincter of Oddi phasic waves have an antegrade orientation towards the duodenum. When the percentage of retrograde contractions exceeds 50%, flow through the sphincter of Oddi may be impeded, giving rise to a relative obstruction to outflow that may produce bile duct distention and pain (Toouli et al 1982a).

b. *Rapid phasic contraction frequency*
Spontaneously occurring bursts of rapid phasic contractions or spasm may also produce acute obstruction to outflow resulting in bile duct distention and pain (Toouli et al 1983b). The obstruction results from a decrease in the diastolic interval between rapidly contacting phasic waves.

c. *Paradoxical response to cholecystokinin*
Cholecystokinin normally produces inhibition of the sphincter of Oddi phasic contractions with decrease in resistance to flow from the bile duct into the duodenum.

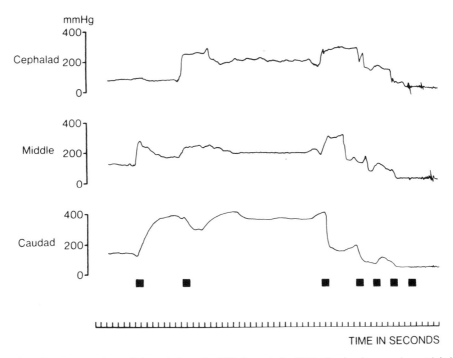

Fig. 6.10 Manometric recording showing a station pull through from the CBD through the SO to the duodenum using a triple lumen catheter. The square marks indicate withdrawal of the triple lumen catheter by 2 mm steps. A high basal pressure is demonstrated in all three lumens as the catheter is being withdrawn through a high pressure zone.

In a group of patients with suspected sphincter of Oddi dysfunction a paradoxical response to cholecystokinin-octapeptide administration was noted, giving rise to increase in contraction frequency instead of the expected inhibition. If this response were to occur following meal-stimulated release of cholecystokinin, flow of bile would be impeded giving rise to bile duct distention and pain.

The reproducibility of manometry in diagnosing sphincter of Oddi dysfunction was evaluated in 12 patients who had manometry repeated at 3-month intervals (Thune et al 1991). The diagnosis of sphincter stenosis, as demonstrated by a high basal pressure or normal motility were highly reproducible. However, the diagnosis of dyskinesia showed variation and is consistent with the belief that this entity may be intermittent and occur following provocative stimuli such as opiate-containing medications, stress or different food substances.

TREATMENT OF PATIENTS WITH SUSPECTED SPHINCTER OF ODDI DYSFUNCTION

Smooth muscle relaxants have been used without success in the treatment of patients with suspected sphincter of Oddi dysfunction. If medical therapy were to have a place in the management of the patients then it is expected that it might be most effective in the patients with the dyskinetic dis-

orders and not those patients with a structural stenosis. However, the symptoms experienced by the patients with sphincter of Oddi dyskinesia tend to be episodic with variable intervals of time between attacks of pain. Therefore, an effective medication would need to be rapidly absorbed and effective in aborting an episode of pain.

Intrasphincteric injection of botulinum toxin administered via an endoscope approach has been used to treat patients with biliary type pain due to sphincter of Oddi dysfunction (Pasricha et al 1994). The toxin inhibits cholinergic nerves and has been shown to produce sphincter relaxation (Sand et al 1993). However, its effect is short lasting and is unlikely to be useful for long term therapy of patients with sphincter of Oddi dysfunction.

A structural stenosis of the sphincter of Oddi might best be treated by division of the sphincter either endoscopically or by transduodenal operation. In a prospective randomized study, the effect of endoscopic sphincterotomy in the treatment of patients with suspected sphincter of Oddi dysfunction was evaluated (Geenen et al 1984). Post-cholecystectomy patients were selected for the study on the basis of clinical symptoms suggestive of biliary disease plus one or both objective signs of common bile duct dilatation and/or liver function test abnormality with episodes of pain. All patients underwent endoscopic manometry; as part of their diagnostic work-up; however, the manometric findings were not used to determine treatment. Twenty-two patients were randomized to endoscopic sphincterotomy and 23 patients served as controls. Neither group of patients were told whether a sphincterotomy was performed as the endoscope and papillotome were introduced into all patients whilst under sedation. Follow-up of symptoms was carried out prospectively for a period of 4 years. The results revealed that ten out of 11 patients with an abnormally elevated sphincter of Oddi basal pressure became totally asymptomatic, whilst only three of the 12 controls with this manometric abnormality responded. Eleven patients with manometric findings suggestive of sphincter of Oddi dyskinesia did not improve significantly when compared to 11 controls with this disorder.

Long-term results from two surgical studies (Moody et al 1983, Nardi et al 1983) in which patients underwent transduodenal sphincteroplasty and transampullary septectomy for treatment of chronic incapacitating upper abdominal pain also suggest that division of the sphincter of Oddi may alleviate pain in patients having a stenosis of the sphincter of Oddi. These results support the hypothesis that dysfunction of the sphincter of Oddi produces recurrent episodes of biliary pain, and it appears that endoscopic manometric assessment of sphincter of Oddi activity offers an objective method for selecting patients for treatment by either endoscopic or transduodenal division of the sphincter of Oddi.

In patients with sphincter of Oddi dysfunction producing recurrent pancreatitis, the finding of manometric pancreatic sphincter stenosis also has been shown to predict those patients who will improve following division of the sphincter of Oddi (Toouli et al 1996). In this group of patients, the sphincter division is best performed via an open operative approach in which both the biliary and pancreatic components of the sphincter of Oddi are divided.

SUMMARY

The biliary tract is made up of well orchestrated components which act in concert to control flow of bile from the ducts and gallbladder into the duodenum. These components exhibit characteristic motility which is modulated by extrinsic and intrinsic nerves and circulating hormones. The most common pathological conditions giving rise to pain from the biliary tract are associated with inflammation secondary to stone formation. However, motility disorders of the gallbladder and sphincter of Oddi explain the etiology of noncalculous biliary symptoms and in a subgroup of patients episodes of recurrent pancreatitis. Specific investi-

gations for the diagnosis of these conditions has been developed and long term clinical studies have shown that effective therapy now exists.

REFERENCES

Baker R A, Saccone G T P, Toouli J 1993 Nitric oxide mediates nonadrenergic, noncholinergic neural relaxation of the sphincter of Oddi of the Australian brush tailed possum. Gastroenterology 105: 1746–1753

Behar J, Biancani P 1980 Effect of cholecystokinin and the octapeptide of cholecystokinin on the feline sphincter of Oddi and gallbladder. Mechanisms of action. Journal of Clinical Investigation 66: 1231–1239

Benevantano T C, Rosen R G 1969 The physiological effect of acute vagal section of canine biliary dynamics. Journal of Surgical Research 9: 331–334

Bolandi L, Gaiani S, Gullo, Lobo G 1984 Secretin administration induces dilatation of the main pancreatic duct. Digestive Diseases Sciences 29: 802–808

Boyden E A 1937 The sphincter of Oddi in man and certain representative mammals. Surgery 1: 24–37

Boyden E A 1957 The anatomy of the choledochoduodenal junction in man. Surgery, Gynecology and Obstetrics 104: 641–652

Burnett W, Gairns F W, Bacsich 1964 Some observations on the innervation of the extrahepatic biliary system in man. Annals of Surgery 159: 8–26

Butsch W L, McGowan J M, Waslters W 1936 Clinical studies on the influence of certain drugs in relation to bliary pain and to the variations in intrabiliary pressure. Surgery, Gynecology and Obstetrics 63: 451–456

Caroli J, Porcher P, Pequignot G, Delattre M 1960 Contribution of cineradiography to study of the function of the human biliary tract. American Journal of Digestive Diseases 5: 677–696

Corazziari E, Cicala M, Habib F I, Scopinaro F, Fiocca F, Palotta N, Viscardi A, Vognoni A, Torsoli A 1994. Hepatoduodenal bile transit in cholecystectomised subjects. Relationship with sphincter of Oddi function and diagnostic value. Digestive Diseases Science 39 (9): 1985–1993

Csendes A, Sepulveda A 1980 Intraluminal gallbladder pressure measurements in patient with chronic or acute cholecystitis. American Journal of Surgery 139: 383–384

Cushieri A, Hughes J H, Cohen M 1972 Biliary pressure studies during cholecystectomy. British Journal of Surgery 59: 267–273

Darweesh R M A, Dodds W J, Hogan W J 1988 Efficacy of quantitative hepatobiliary scintigraphy and fatty meal sonography for evaluating patients with suspected partial common bile duct obstruction. Gastroenterology 94: 779–786

Doran F S 1967 The sites to which pain is referred from the common bile duct in man and its implication for the theory of referred pain. British Journal of Surgery 54: 599–606

Dunn F H, Christensen E C, Reynolds J et al 1974 Cholecystokinin cholecystography. Journal of the American Medical Association 228: 997–999

Everson G T, Baverman D Z, Johnson M L, Kern F Jr 1980 A critical evaluation of real-time utrasonography for the study of gallbladder volumes and contraction. Gastroenterology 79: 40–46

Geenen J E, Hogan W J, Dodds W J, Stewart E T, Arndorfer R C 1980 Intraluminal pressure recording from the human sphincter of Oddi. Gastroenterology 78: 317–324

Geenen J E, Hogan W J H, Dodds W J, Toouli J, Venu R P 1989 The efficacy of endoscopic sphincterotomy in post-cholecystectomy patients with sphincter of Oddi dysfunction. New England Journal of Medicine 320: 82–87

Glenn F, Grafe W R Jr 1966 Historical events in biliary tract surgery. Archives of Surgery 93: 848–852

Goldstein F, Grunt R, Magulies M 1974 Cholecystokinin cholestography in the differential diagnosis of acalculous gallbladder disease. American Journal of Digestive Diseases 19: 835–839

Hand B H 1963 An anatomical study of the choledochoduodenal area. British Journal of Surgery 50: 486–494

Hess W 1979 Physiology of the sphincter of Oddi. In: Classen M, Geenen J, Kawai K (eds) The papilla Vateri and its diseases. Proceedings of the International Workshop of the World Congress of Gastroenterology held in Madrid 1978. Verlag Gerhard Witzshock Kohn: 14–21

Honda R, Toouli J, Dodds W J, Sarna S, Hogan W J, Itoh Z 1982 Relationship of sphincter of Oddi spike bursts to gastro-intestinal myoelectric activity in conscious opossums. Journal of Clinical Investigation 69: 770–778

Hunt D R, Scott A J 1989 Changes in bile duct diameter after cholecystectomy: 1–5 year perioperative study. Gastroenterology 97: 1485–1488

Ivy A C, Oldberg E 1928 A hormone mechanism for gallbladder contraction and evacuation. American Journal of Physiology 86: 599–613

Johnson F E, Boyden E A 1952 The effect of double vagotomy on the motor activity of the human gallbladder. Surgery 32: 591–601

Le Quesne L P, Wihtsid C G, Hand B T 1959 The common bile duct after cholecystectomy. British Medical Journal 1: 329–332

Moody F G, Becker J M, Potts J R 1983 Transduodenal sphincterotoplasty and transampullary septectomy for postcholecystectomy pain. Annals of Surgery 197: 627–636

Nardi G L, Michelassi F, Zannini P 1983 Transduodenal sphincteroplasty 5–25 year follow-up of 89 patients. Annals of Surgery 198: 453–461

Oddi R 1887 D'une disposition a sphincter speciale de l'ouverture du canal cholidoque. Archives of Italian Biology 8: 317–322

Padbury T T A, Furness J B, Baker R A, Toouli J, Messenger J P 1993 Projection of nerve cells from the duodenum to the sphincter of Oddi and gallbladder of the Australian possum. Gastroenterology: 104: 130–136

Pasricha P J, Miskovsky E P, Kalloo A N 1994 Intrasphincteric injection of botulinum toxin for suspected sphincter of Oddi dysfunction. Gut 35: 1319–1321

Persson C G A 1972 Adreno receptors in the gall bladder. Acta Pharmacologia 32: 177–185

Pitt H A, Roslyn J J, Kuchenbocker S L, Doty J F, DenBensten L 1981a The role of cystic duct resistance in the pathogenesis of cholesterol gallstones. Journal of Surgical Research 30: 508–514

Pitt H A, Doty J E, Roslyn J J, DenBesten L 1981b The role of altered extrahepatic biliary function in the pathogenesis of gallstones after vagotomy. Surgery 90: 418–425

Roberts-Thomson I C, Toouli J, Blanchett W, Lichtenstein M, Andrews J T 1986. Assessment of bile flow by radioscintigraphy in patients with biliary-type pain after cholecystectomy. Australian and New Zealand Journal of Medicine 16: 788–793

Saccone G T P, Harvey J R, Baker R A, Toouli J 1994 Intramural neural pathways between the duodenum and sphincter of Oddi in the Australian Brush-tailed possum in vivo. Journal of Physiology 481(2): 447–456

Sand J, Nordback I, Koskinen M, Matikainen M, Lindholm T S 1993 Nifedipine for suspected type II sphincter of Oddi dyskinesia. American Journal of Gastroenterology 88: 530–535

Sarles J C, Midejean A, Devaux M A 1975 Electromyography of the sphincter of Oddi. American Journal of Gastroenterology 63: 221–231

Scott G W, Otto W J 1979 Resistance and sphincter-like properties of the cystic duct. Surgery, Gynecology and Obstetrics 149: 177–182

Shaffer E A, McOrmond P, Duggan H 1980 Quantitative cholescintigraphy: assessment of gallbladder filling and emptying and duodenogastric reflux. Gastroenterology 79: 899–906

Sostre S, Kalloo A N, Spiegler E J, Camargo E E, Wagner Jr H N 1992. A non-invasive test of sphincter of Oddi dysfunction in postcholecystectomy patients. The scintigraphic score. Journal of Nuclear Medicine 33(6): 1216–1224

Sundler F, Alumets J, Hakanson R, Ingemansson S, Fahrenkrug J, Schaffalitzky O B 1977 VIP innervation of the gallbladder. Gastroenterology 72: 1375–1377

Takahashi I, Nakaya M, Suzuki T, Itoh Z 1982a Postprandial changes in contractile activity and bile concentration in gallbladder of the dog. American Journal of Physiology 6: G366–NG371

Takahashi I, Suzuki T, Aizawa, Itoh Z 1982b Comparison of gallbladder contractions induced by motilin and cholecystokinin in dogs. Gastroenterology 82: 419–N424

Tansy M F, Salkin L, Innes D L, Martin J S, Kendall F M, Litwack D 1975 The mucosal lining of the intramural common bile duct as a determinant of ductal opening pressure. American Journal of Digestive Disease 20: 613–625

Thornell E, Jansson R, Kral J G, Svanvik J 1979 Inhibition of prostaglandin synthesis as a treatment of biliary pain. Lancet i: 584

Thune A, Scicchitano J, Roberts-Thomson I, Toouli J 1991 Reproducibility of endoscopic sphincter of Oddi manometry. Digestive Diseases Sciences 36: 1401–1405

Toouli J 1984 Sphincter of Oddi motility. British Journal of Surgery 71: 251–256

Toouli J, Watts J McK 1971 In vitro motility studies on the canine and human extrahepatic biliary tracts. Australian and New Zealand Journal of Surgery 40: 380–387

Toouli J, Dodds W J, Honda R, Hogan W J 1981 Effect of histamine on motor function of opossum sphincter of Oddi. American Journal of Physiology 241: G122–G128

Toouli J, Geenen J E, Hogan W J, Dodds W J, Arndorfer R C 1982a Sphincter of Oddi motor activity: A comparison between patients with common bile duct stones and controls. Gastroenterology 82: 111–117

Toouli J, Hogan W J, Geenen J E, Dodds W J, Arndorfer R C 1982b Action of cholecystokinin octapeptide on sphincter of Oddi basal pressure and phasic wave activity in humans. Surgery 92: 497–503

Toouli J, Dods W J, Honda R, et al 1983a Motor function of the Opossum sphincter of Oddi. Journal of Clinical Investigation 71: 208–220

Toouli J, Roberts-Thomson I, Dent J, Watts J 1983b Endoscopic biliary manometry in patients with suspected sphincter of Oddi dysfunction. Gastroenterology 84: 1335

Toouli J, Bushell M, Stevenson G, Dent J, Wycherley A, Iannos J 1986 Gallbladder emptying in man related to fasting duodenal migrating motor contractions. Australian and New Zealand Journal of Surgery 56: 147–151

Toouli J, Di Francesco V, Saccone G T P, Kollias J, Schloithe A, Shanks N 1996 Division of the sphincter of Oddi for treatment of dysfunction associated with recurrent pancreatitis. British Journal of Surgery 83: 1205–1210

Valberg L S, Jabbari M, Kerr J W, Curtis A C, Ramchard S, Prentice R S A 1971. Biliary pain in the absence of gallstones. Gastroenterology 60: 1020–1026

Watts J McK, Dunphy J E 1966 The role of the common bile duct in biliary dynamics. Surgery, Gynecology and Obstetrics 122: 1207–1281

Weiner I, Kazutomo I, Fagan C J, Lilja P, Watson L C, Thompson J C 1981 Release of cholecystokinin in man, correlation of blood levels with gallbladder contraction. Annals of Surgery 194: 321–327

Wen-Qin Cai, Gabella G 1983 Innervation of the gallbladder and biliary pathways in the guinea pig. Journal of Anatomy 136: 97–109

Wood J R, Svanvik J 1983 Gallbladder water and electrolyte transport and its regulation. Gut 24: 579–593

Wood J R, Brennan L J, Hombrey J M, McLoughlin T A 1982 Effects of regulatory peptides on gallbladder function. Scandinavian Journal of Gastroenterology 17: (suppl) 78

Worthley C S, Baker R A, Iannos J, Saccone G T P, Toouli J 1989 Human fasting and post-prandial sphincter of Oddi motility. British Journal of Surgery 76: 709–714

Yap L, McKenzie J, Wycherley A, Toouli J 1991 Gallbladder ejection fraction for acalculous gallbladder pain. Gastroenterology 101: 786–793

Biliary tract obstruction – pathophysiology

7

I.S. BENJAMIN AND S. GUPTA

DEFINITION

Obstruction of the biliary tract in one of its many forms is a problem frequently encountered by the general surgeon. While clearly the most obvious presentation of biliary tract obstruction is obstructive jaundice such as that due to tumor or to choledocholithiasis, there has been increasing recognition of the more subtle forms of this entity. Clear understanding of the problem demands a broader view of biliary tract obstruction than that presented by the jaundiced patient. We have previously proposed (Benjamin 1983) a classification which has proved useful in practice, and which recognizes four categories of biliary obstruction:

- Type I *Complete obstruction*, producing jaundice
- Type II *Intermittent obstruction*, which produces symptoms and typical biochemical changes, but may or may not be associated with attacks of clinical jaundice.
- Type III *Chronic incomplete obstruction*, with or without classic symptoms or the observation of biochemical changes, which will eventually produce pathological changes in the bile ducts or the liver.
- Type IV *Segmental obstruction*, in which one or more anatomical segments of the intrahepatic biliary tree are obstructed. In its turn, this segmental obstruction may take the form of complete, intermittent, or chronic incomplete obstruction, as defined above.

Advances in biliary tract imaging have allowed increasing recognition of these categories, and these are further discussed in Ch. 21. It is inappropriate to attempt comprehensive listing of the specific causes of these types of obstruction, but it may be helpful in forming a concept of the categories to refer to the examples of lesions typically associated with them shown in Table 7.1.

Table 7.1 Lesions commonly associated with biliary tract obstruction

Type I   Complete obstruction

    Tumors, especially of the pancreatic head
    Ligation of the common bile duct
    Cholangiocarcinoma
    Parenchymal liver tumors, primary or secondary

Type II   Intermittent obstruction

    Choledocholithiasis
    Periampullary tumors
    Duodenal diverticula
    Papillomas of the bile duct
    Choledochal cyst
    Polycystic liver disease
    Intrabiliary parasites
    Hemobilia

Type III   Chronic incomplete obstruction

    Strictures of the common bile duct
        Congenital
        Traumatic (iatrogenic)
        Sclerosing cholangitis
        Post-radiotherapy
    Stenosed biliary-enteric anastomoses
    Chronic pancreatitis
    Cystic fibrosis
    Stenosis of the sphincter of Oddi
    ?Dyskinesia (sphincter of Oddi dysfunction)

Type IV   Segmental obstruction

    Traumatic (including iatrogenic)
    Hepatodocholithiasis
    Sclerosing cholangitis
    Cholangiocarcinoma

The aim of this chapter is to review some of the pathophysiological effects of biliary tract obstruction, and to discuss their relevance to the clinical situation and to the therapeutic options available to the surgeon.

PHYSICAL EFFECTS

INCREASED PRESSURE

The normal secretory pressure of bile is 120–250 mm of water (Papageorgiou & Lynn 1985) and secretion ceases when biliary pressure exceeds 300 mm of water (Csendes et al 1988). Following total bile duct obstruction the common bile duct pressure stabilizes at about 300 mm of water (Hallenbeck 1967), at which time inhibition of the various elements of bile production commences. Cholesterol and phospholipid secretion are more readily reduced by high pressure than bile salt secretion, so that the composition of hepatic bile is altered and becomes less lithogenic (Strasburg et al 1971). The reduction in bile salt dependent canalicular bile flow under high pressure conditions results in inhibition of bile salt synthesis. Following relief of obstruction and return to normal pressure, the recovery of secretion of cholesterol and phospholipid is more rapid than that of bile salts so that bile becomes more lithogenic during this period. Some of these observations may be relevant to the clinical situations in which intermittent or incomplete obstruction occur. Manometric studies in man show that common bile duct pressures may intermittently rise above the maximal secretory pressure for bile, resulting in fluctuations in lithogenicity of the bile.

High biliary pressures causing bacterial reflux into lymphatic and venous systems (cholangiovenous reflux) are important. Huang et al (1969) demonstrated lymphatic and venous bacterial reflux in a canine model when biliary pressures exceeded 250 mm of water. Indeed Lygidakis and Brummelkamp (1985) showed good correlation between severity and mortality of cholangitis with increased biliary pressures. Forceful injection of contrast during direct cholangiography may also cause bacteremia (Yoshimoto et al 1989). Biliary decompression can therefore be an important therapeutic issue in the management of this condition.

Complete obstruction of the main extrahepatic bile ducts or of a major segmental duct will normally lead to proximal dilatation of the bile duct or of intrahepatic biliary radicles. However, this is not invariably the case, and the degree of dilatation will depend on the extent and the duration of obstruction, and also on the capacity of the bile ducts and surrounding hepatic parenchyma to expand. The lack of intrahepatic ductal dilatation constitutes a pitfall in the radiological diagnosis of biliary obstruction, and in particular in the use of ultrasound to distinguish between intrahepatic and extrahepatic cholestasis (Ch. 13). In a series of 200 cases of proven biliary obstruction studied at Mount Sinai Hospital in New York, 16 showed no evidence of ductal dilatation (Beinart et al 1981). Such findings should alert the clinician to the possibility of either secondary hepatic fibrosis or cirrhosis, or to co-existing unrelated hepatic parenchymal disease (such as alcoholic or post-hepatitic cirrhosis). Chronic obstruction which has undergone a slow evolution may fail to produce significant proximal dilatation, particularly when associated with marked chronic cholangitis and ductal fibrosis.

HEPATIC BLOOD FLOW (see also Ch. 4)

Argument from first principles would suggest that total hepatic tissue perfusion might be reduced in the face of increasing hydrostatic pressure within the liver due to increased intra-ductal pressure and ductal dilatation. However, actual clinical evidence of this is negligible, and experimental studies are conflicting. Following bile duct ligation in the rat, one group has shown decreased liver blood flow (Hunt 1979), while other workers have shown no such change in the dog (Hall et al 1977). Work from our own laboratories has shown that in the dog increases in bile duct pressure up to 25 mmHg have no perceptible effect, while increases between 25 and 45 mmHg result in a linear increase of hepatic arterial flow, reaching a maximum of 3.5 times the resting value (Nagorney et al 1982). These changes were not accompanied by a significant change in portal venous flow. The mechanism of these changes has not been determined, but may be related to the 'buffer response' induced by reduction of portal venous perfusion in man and other species (Lautt 1981, Alexander et al 1989).

Alterations in hepatic tissue perfusion may be of some importance in relation to liver resection. Liver resection in the presence of obstructive jaundice carries a higher risk, and it may be that some of this risk relates to secondary hepatocellular dysfunction which may be compounded by reduced hepatic tissue perfusion. Animal and human models have demonstrated that biliary obstruction causes an exaggerated hypotensive response to minimal losses in blood volume (Williams et al 1960, Cattel and Birnstingl 1967). This is perhaps mediated by a blunted response to vasoactive substances (Bomzon et al 1978). Unfortunately, clinical studies are difficult to undertake in this area (Mathie and Blumgart 1972).

PAIN

'Painless' progressive jaundice is the clinical hallmark of malignant biliary tract obstruction, but a history of abdominal pain is by no means uncommon in such patients. Pain was a feature in 27 of 94 patients with hilar cholangiocarcinoma studied at Hammersmith Hospital (Blumgart et al

1984b). Similarly, 11 of 19 patients with carcinoma of the gallbladder had pain as a presenting feature, and in six this was typical of biliary 'colic'. The origin of pain in biliary obstruction may be distension of the gallbladder or bile duct or may be associated with stretching of the liver capsule in cases of rapidly progressive obstruction. Nevertheless, severe pain of a spasmodic nature is more characteristic of calculous obstruction than of malignancy. This subject, and the more difficult subject of pain due to biliary dyskinesia, is covered in more detail in Ch. 6.

PATHOLOGICAL EFFECTS

BILE DUCTS AND CANALICULI

The ravages brought about by unrelieved biliary tract obstruction on the liver and biliary system begin at the level of the bile duct canaliculi. The canaliculus is formed by a groove in the lateral plasma membranes of two adjacent hepatocytes and is a tubular structure about one micron in diameter penetrating the hepatocyte plate. It is flanked on both sides by tight junctions which are continuous intercellular contacts defining the borders of the canaliculus. It now appears that there is a correlation between the degree of cholestasis and disruption of these tight junctions, and this is true for both extrahepatic and intrahepatic cholestasis (Rahner et al 1996). It is, however, unclear whether an injury results from increased hydrostatic pressure in a closed canalicular space that forces the tight junctions to open, intrahepatic inflammation, accumulation of toxic bile compounds such as lithocholate, or other metabolic changes (Anderson 1996). The hepatocyte plasma membrane projects into the canalicular lumen as numerous microvilli. This membrane is a highly active structure involved in complex mechanisms for production of both bile salt dependent and bile salt independent bile flow (Ch. 5).

In both extrahepatic and intrahepatic cholestasis the bile canaliculi become dilated and the microvilli distorted and swollen (Schaffner & Popper 1985). Bile pigment 'thrombi' may be seen in the canaliculi and in the adjacent hepatocytes. If cholestasis is prolonged, there is an apparent proliferation of the canaliculi, with an increase in length and tortuosity. It is interesting that all of these changes can be induced not only by ligation of the bile duct in experimental animals but also by injection or feeding of lithocholic acid (Schaffner & Javitt 1966), and in both cases the pathological effects may be initiated by high local concentrations of bile salts at the canalicular membrane (Schaffner et al 1971). Thus it may be difficult in some cases for the histopathologist to distinguish between intra- and extrahepatic cholestasis in a biopsy specimen.

Reabsorption of bile constituents from the ductules leads to a marked inflammatory reaction in the portal tracts, with a polymorphonuclear leukocyte infiltrate. This 'acute cholangiolitis' does not necessarily imply ascending bacterial infection, but is a tissue reaction to an irritant chemical stimulus. These cholangiolitic changes are followed by increased fibrogenesis with deposition of reticulin fibers and eventually of collagen bundles.

In the hepatocytes of the periportal zones both bilirubin and bile acid retention occur, and both exert toxic effects within the hepatocyte. The maximum damage to hepatocytes occurs at the biliary pole, and may be related to the tissue bile salt content (Greim 1972). Bile salts in particular cause both inhibition of cytochrome P450 and transformation into the inactive cytochrome P420 (Schaffner & Popper 1985). Both smooth and rough endoplasmic reticulum are disrupted and canalicular membrane components become solubilized, which explains in part the increased release of canalicular alkaline phosphatase into the bloodstream. Cytoplasmic hyaline deposits are seen, and feathery degeneration may eventually proceed to destruction of the hepatocytes around the portal tracts associated with leukocyte infiltration, the so-called 'biliary piecemeal necrosis'. Experimental observations have shown that if obstruction is relieved within two weeks these morphological changes are readily reversible, and that the appearance of the mitochondrial cristae may be useful in assessing this reversibility (Yokoi 1983). However, the exact mechanisms for bile salt damage to hepatocytes remains undetermined (Hoffman 1992).

FIBROTIC CHANGES

If obstruction continues the reticulin laid down in the periportal areas matures to type I collagen, causing scarring fibrosis around the bile ducts, which may further aggravate the cholestasis. The extrahepatic ducts are also subject to these changes, and mucosal atrophy and squamous metaplasia followed by inflammatory infiltration and fibrosis in the sub-epithelial layers of the ducts may supervene, particularly in the presence of superadded infection and the presence of foreign material, including biliary stents (Karsten et al 1991).

When the intrahepatic fibrotic changes have progressed beyond this point, mechanical obstruction to sinusoidal flow may result in secondary portal hypertension. Fibrous septa may ultimately produce a severe perilobular fibrosis, but the lobular architecture of the liver is usually well preserved and only proceeds to a true pattern of secondary biliary cirrhosis as a late event. Because of this, we believe that many of the fibrotic changes are at least potentially reversible, and have observed a return to near normality of liver architecture on biopsy following relief of biliary obstruction (Blumgart 1978). Interestingly some of these fibrotic changes are preventable by the somatostatin analogue octreotide (Tracy et al 1993) and alpha interferons (Muriel 1996) in animal models although the clinical significance of these findings is yet to be evaluated. Since it takes weeks to months of biliary obstruction to produce this degree of fibrosis, this situation is more likely to arise with chronic incomplete obstruction which does not produce a clamant clinical picture of obstructive jaundice. It is thus important that the clinician should not lightly accept continuing incomplete obstruction, since cholangitic and fibrotic changes may be progressing relentlessly with little biochemical or clinical evidence, but may yet be arrested or reversed by complete and adequate biliary drainage (Ch. 49).

Benign iatrogenic biliary strictures, which are often chronic and incomplete, have a high association with portal hypertension (Ch. 49). In a report from the Lahey Clinic, 19% of patients with biliary strictures had some degree of portal hypertension (Sedgwick et al 1966). At Hammersmith Hospital 14% of patients with iatrogenic biliary strictures had portal hypertension on referral, as evidenced by endoscopic, radiological or operative findings (Blumgart et al 1984a). Some authors have reported such changes as early as two years from the onset of obstruction (Kune 1972), but in our experience portal hypertension has been related to the length of history. The median duration of obstruction in 11 patients in our series with portal hypertension was 48 months, significantly higher than that in 67 patients without portal hypertension (15.5 months). Moreover, all the patients with portal hypertension gave a history of frequent and severe episodes of cholangitis, while only 16 of 67 patients without portal hypertension gave this history. These findings appeared also to be significantly related to the number of previous operations, which in turn influenced the occurrence of major infective episodes by the time of presentation (Blumgart et al 1984a). A related observation has been that in our experience portal hypertension was significantly more common in patients with high (Bismuth III–IV) strictures (nine of 44) than in those with low (Bismuth I–II) lesions (two of 41) (Kelley et al 1986). The relationship to atrophy/hyperplasia will be discussed later.

It should be noted in passing that iatrogenic bile duct strictures may also be associated with direct operative damage to the hepatic arteries or portal veins (Ch. 49), and such damage to the portal vein may result in portal hypertension.

Since the management of this type of portal hypertension may be different from that caused by hepatic fibrosis, it is important to consider this variant during the investigation of such patients.

CHOLANGITIS

Although the neutrophil infiltrate associated with cholangiolitis is primarily part of a chemical reaction associated with biliary obstruction, and does not imply bacterial infection in the presence of biliary stasis secondary bacterial colonization may produce the additional element of infective cholangitis. Although classically referred to as 'ascending' cholangitis, the actual mechanism for entry of bacteria into the unoperated biliary tract may not always be clear. The normal biliary tree does not harbor bacteria. The sphincter of Oddi guards the bile duct from entry of bacteria and constant bile flow and biliary IgA secretion ensure biliary sterility. Organisms are found in the bile in approximately one-third of patients with malignant biliary tract obstruction, but in the presence of previous biliary surgery, instrumentation, intubation or biliary-enteric anastomosis, this rate may be much higher (McPherson et al 1982b, Brody et al 1998). The highest rate of bile colonization is found in patients with choledocholithiasis or with benign bile duct strictures, where as many as 80% of patients may have positive cultures (Jackaman et al 1980). Following biliary intubation our own early data showed colonization of transhepatic biliary tubes in every case, with polymicrobial growth in 79% (McPherson et al 1982b). This type of contamination may go on to produce serious invasive sepsis. A recent large retrospective study however failed to show an increased rate of infective complications in patients with obstructive jaundice undergoing major surgical procedures despite a high rate of biliary bacterial contamination following preoperative biliary drainage in these patients (Karsten et al 1996). The group in Nagoya (Nagino et al 1995a) have routinely employed multiple percutaneous drainage catheters in preparing jaundiced patients for resection, and usually avoid serious septic complications. When segmental cholangitis occurs, they perform additional hepatic duct puncture and drainage (see also Ch. 54).

In the presence of acute cholangitis, there is marked portal edema and neutrophil leukocyte infiltration not only around the ductules but also between the epithelial cells. In severe infection microabscesses may form leading to progressive duct destruction. The perilobular fibrotic changes already described become more marked in the presence of superadded infection.

The combination of bacterial colonization and bile stasis may also be important in the pathogenesis of choledocholithiasis. The commonest organisms isolated from bile are *Escherichia coli*, *Enterococcus* and other gram-negative coliforms. *Escherichia coli* is a producer of β-glucuronidase which may lead to deconjugation of bilirubin in bile. This may lead to the formation of primary common bile duct stones with a high bile pigment content, and indeed the formation of such stones has been shown to correlate with the presence of *Escherichia coli* in the bile duct (Saharia et al 1977). The mechanism for this is not entirely clear. One hypothesis relates the presence of enteric organisms which produce β-glucuronidase to the deconjugation of bilirubin and the formation of calcium bilirubinate deposits (Maki 1966). This hypothesis has not been clearly proven in man, and there is evidence from clinical studies in a large series of patients that this may not be the case (Aloj et al 1989). Moreover, in an experimental model of chronic biliary stricture in the dog, no relationship was found between the level of β-glucuronidase and unconjugated bilirubin in the bile, despite the formation of sludge and stones above the stricture (Aloj 1993). The presence of bacteria may, however, act as a nidus for the nucleation of ductal stones: foreign material such as non-absorbable sutures within the biliary tree can certainly do so. Nonetheless, the most potent clinical situation for the production of such stones is that of chronic obstruction due to an incomplete stricture and more particularly to partial stenosis of a biliary-enteric stoma such as a hepaticojejunostomy or choledochoduodenostomy. In contrast, an adequately draining stoma rarely if ever produces cholangitis and primary duct stones, even in the presence of free reflux of intestinal content across the anastomosis.

ATROPHY

Although the early stages of unilateral hepatic duct obstruction may produce enlargement of the obstructed lobe, the characteristic effect is fibrosis and cellular atrophy of the obstructed liver parenchyma with compensatory hyperplasia of the unaffected segments of the liver (Ch. 3). Indeed, a grossly hyperplastic left lobe palpable in the epigastrium in association with unilateral obstruction and right lobe atrophy may be misinterpreted as a hepatic tumor. Such unilateral or segmental ductal obstruction may fail to produce jaundice in the presence of the normal contralateral lobe. Thus four cases in a series of 116 patients with hilar cholangiocarcinoma were anicteric at presentation because of asymmetrical ductal obstruction: three of these patients were not jaundiced on admission despite obstruction of more than 70% of the liver. Such lobar or segmental atrophy can be demonstrated radiologically in some 20% of patients with hilar cholangiocarcinoma (Carr et al 1985). Similar

phenomena are seen in some cases of iatrogenic biliary injury (Hadjis et al 1991) and sclerosing cholangitis (Hadjis et al 1989a).

The mechanism of the atrophy–hyperplasia complex remains somewhat obscure. The secondary effects of obstruction of the bile duct on hepatocytes have already been considered, and certainly the hepatocyte necrosis produced by local bile salt effects may be sufficient to trigger the well-recognized though incompletely explained compensatory hyperplastic response in the unobstructed liver segments. Secondary effects on portal blood flow may also be important, since portal factors are at least permissive and possibly regulatory in the control of hepatocyte growth (Bucher & McGowan 1985).

The practical importance of lobar atrophy in a surgical context lies in the fact that an atrophic liver lobe may be inadequate to support life following resection of normal or hyperplastic liver tissue (Hadjis et al 1989b), and moreover biliary drainage of such an obstructed lobe may also fail to produce resolution of jaundice. Nimura's group (Uesaka et al 1996) showed that indocyanine green (ICG) excretion via an external biliary catheter in the bile of obstructed lobes was impaired in patients with malignant biliary obstruction reflecting the lobar cellular level of ATP. This was improved by contralateral portal venous embolization. The surgical importance of these phenomena is considered in more detail elsewhere (Ch. 54).

BIOCHEMICAL EFFECTS

BILIRUBIN

With complete biliary outflow obstruction serum total bilirubin levels typically increase by 25–43 μmol/L/day (Schiff 1993). As serum conjugated bilirubin concentrations increase, glomerular filtration and excretion of conjugated bilirubin also increase resulting in plateauing of serum bilirubin levels. Conjugated hyperbilirubinemia is the classic biochemical feature of obstructive jaundice. However, in complex cases with prolonged partial obstruction, functional effects on the hepatocytes may produce a mixed biochemical picture, with elevation of circulating unconjugated bilirubin. This diagnostic conundrum stems from the fact already noted that the basic lesion of cholestasis at the subcellular level is similar irrespective of the mechanical or metabolic nature of the agent producing cholestasis (Schaffner & Popper 1985). Cholestasis is defined as 'bile secretory failure of the liver cell with concomitant accumulation of bile constituents in the blood' (Desmet 1979).

There must therefore exist a pathway for regurgitation of accumulated bile constituents from the biliary compartment to the bloodstream. The mechanism for this is complex: it is probable that the early stages of obstruction produce biliary-lymphatic regurgitation, and that, as the pressure rises, biliary-venous regurgitation supervenes, but much of this pathway remains speculative. In addition to the intercellular escape, transhepatocytic regurgitation by means of reversal of the secretory polarity of the hepatocyte has been proposed (Desmet 1979). Finally, as a late event dilated canaliculi and inspissated bile thrombi may rupture into the sinusoids by necrosis of surrounding liver cells.

Even the actual mechanisms of transport of conjugated bilirubin within the hepatocyte and its secretion into the canaliculus are incompletely understood. Although the secretory mechanisms for bile acids and for bilirubin and a variety of exogenous organic anions (such as bromsulphthalein and some dyes used in cholecystography) are functionally distinct, they are not entirely independent. This is considered further below.

It must be stated again that segmental or lobar obstruction even to a very major degree may fail to produce jaundice in the presence of one or more functioning and possibly hyperplastic liver segments. Nonetheless, a completely normal plasma bilirubin is the exception in any case of extrahepatic biliary obstruction.

ALKALINE PHOSPHATASE

When the obvious pitfalls of sources of alkaline phosphatase apart from the liver and biliary tract are excluded, elevation of this enzyme is the most widely used and probably the most sensitive indicator of biliary tract obstruction. Certainly high levels of alkaline phosphatase are found in patients with complete obstruction and elevation of this enzyme may be the only biochemical indicator of incomplete or segmental obstruction. However, the true situation is more complex than this. Elevation of serum alkaline phosphatase is not entirely due to true regurgitation from the biliary compartment. Acute obstruction of the bile duct causes a prompt increase in hepatic synthesis of alkaline phosphatase (Kaplan et al 1983), and the sinusoidal cell membranes become histochemically strongly positive for the enzyme. There is a large and complex literature on the isoenzymes of alkaline phosphatase in patients with liver disease. However, it appears certain that there are two principal fractions of alkaline phosphatase found in bile: one fraction is derived from the liver cell, and the other only appears when there is obstruction to the flow of bile (Price & Sammons 1974). It has been suggested that this second component may allow better differentiation of patients with

extrahepatic obstruction from those with intrahepatic cholestasis than total levels of the enzyme. Moreover, there is now considerable evidence that the large molecular size isoenzyme which appears in cholestasis is actually of hepatocyte origin and is attached to circulating membrane fragments which also contain a number of other enzymes, including 5′-nucleotidase, gammaglutamyl transpeptidase and lipoprotein X (Desmet 1979, Price & Alberti 1985). These large enzyme-containing membrane fragments are probably released from the liver cell as one of the local effects of the detergent action of bile salts.

While elevation of alkaline phosphatase is a sensitive marker of biliary obstruction, its return to normal following relief of obstruction is extremely variable. Long after the hyperbilirubinemia has subsided levels of alkaline phosphatase may remain two or more times higher than normal despite an apparently satisfactory clinical outcome (Smith 1978, Way et al 1981). The reason for this persistence is not always clear, but in using HIDA scanning (Ch. 14) to assess the long-term patency of biliary-enteric anastomosis in the follow-up of patients who have had repair of bile duct strictures, we have observed a number of patients in whom elevated alkaline phosphatase is associated with minor segmental obstruction or established lobar atrophy, in the presence of adequately functioning biliary-enteric drainage. Thus while alkaline phosphatase is a useful and sensitive test in the follow-up of such patients, it is not always necessary to proceed to invasive investigation on the basis of continued stable elevation (Ch. 49).

PROTEIN SYNTHESIS

The liver occupies a central role in protein synthesis, and albumin is quantitatively the most important plasma protein synthesized by the liver. However, because of the long half-life of albumin in the circulation (20 days) only minimal changes may occur secondary to the hepatocyte damage produced by biliary tract obstruction. Younes et al (1991) reported no significant hypoalbuminemia in bile duct ligated rats until two weeks after ligation and hypoalbuminemia was not reversed within 2 weeks after decompression despite all other biochemical and metabolic parameters returning to normal levels. Nonetheless, since biliary obstruction is frequently associated with other factors, such as malignancy and inadequate nutrition, hypoalbuminemia remains an important feature of the patient with biliary obstruction. Moreover, several studies have now shown that low serum albumin levels represent a significant risk factor in the patient undergoing major biliary surgery (Blamey et al 1983, Dixon et al 1983).

As an acute marker of hepatic protein synthesis, serum

prealbumin is more valuable since the half-life of this protein in the circulation is 1.9 days. This factor and others have been shown to be important prognostic markers in obstructive jaundice (Halliday et al 1988): this is considered in more detail in the chapter on nutrition (Ch. 26). Retinol-binding protein and transferrin have similar characteristics.

A most important aspect of protein synthesis relates to the role of the liver in the maintenance of the normal blood coagulation process (Ch. 11). Thus fibrinogen, prothrombin and Factor VII may all be affected in severe and prolonged obstructive jaundice. Of course, the major deficit in most cases of biliary obstruction relates to failure of vitamin K absorption due to absence of bile salts from the intestine. In cases of long-standing biliary obstruction with severe secondary hepatocyte malfunction, coagulopathy may fail to be corrected by parenteral administration of vitamin K. This should alert the clinician to the possibility of severe secondary changes or pre-existing alcoholic or other parenchymal liver disease.

LIPIDS

Cholesterol levels may be elevated in long-standing biliary obstruction. A number of alterations in low density lipoproteins have been observed, but these appear to be neither of great specific diagnostic value nor of major functional importance. The abnormal low density lipoprotein X has already been referred to above in relation to the membrane fragments associated with high molecular weight alkaline phosphatase. While this has been suggested as a valuable test in differentiating between intrahepatic and extrahepatic cholestasis, not all workers have found this to be so (Harry et al 1985). Scriven et al (1994) have shown a fall in plasma and tissue polyunsaturated fatty acids along with the substrates for eicosanoid production and suggested this may explain some of the reticuloendothelial system dysfunction in extrahepatic cholestasis. There have also been recent reports of depressed production of interleukin-2 and intereukin-1 in patients with obstructive jaundice (Haga et al 1989).

CARBOHYDRATE METABOLISM

Younes et al (1991) found significantly decreased glucose levels in a rodent model of biliary obstruction compared to pair fed controls. Abnormal glucose tolerance may be seen in patients with impaired liver function, and impaired gluconeogenesis has been found after bile duct ligation in the rat (Lee et al 1972). This has been confirmed in patients with biliary tract obstruction due to malignancy, but it is suggested that the malignant disease might be the primary mechanism and that biliary tract obstruction causes no further deterioration in glucose tolerance in these patients (Flannigan 1986).

BILE SALT CIRCULATION

The enterohepatic circulation of bile salts is completely interrupted by total biliary tract obstruction, and this may lead to gross elevation of serum bile acid levels, up to 60 times normal (Neale et al 1971). This is associated with a decrease in hepatic synthesis of bile acids, increased urinary excretion and the formation of abnormal bile acids by the liver (including ursodeoxycholate), which are more easily excreted in the urine than the normal bile acids. The role of the bile acids in producing hepatocellular damage at the canalicular level has already been noted. Bile salts have also been strongly implicated in the genesis of pruritus, a concept strongly supported by the therapeutic success of cholestyramine. However, the exact nature of the effector mechanism remains unclear. Clements et al (1994) found increased blood histamine levels and decreased mast cell histamine content in animals with obstructive jaundice. These results demonstrate that mast cells degranulate in biliary obstruction with consequent release of histamine into the systemic circulation, which may play an important role in the pruritus of cholestasis.

There are two important consequences of these liver/bile salt relationships. Firstly, by virtue of its emulsifying properties the absence of bile salts from the intestine is associated with altered small bowel microflora, altered gut mucosal barrier and increased absorption of endotoxin (Ch. 5). Secondly, following external biliary drainage the secretion of bile is under an altered physiological drive, which may be modified by administration of oral bile salts. These aspects are considered below.

OTHER FUNCTIONAL EFFECTS

HEPATOCYTE FUNCTION

It has already been noted that severe and prolonged biliary tract obstruction has effects on hepatocytes which may be reflected in gross biochemical abnormalities such as hypoalbuminemia and unconjugated hyperbilirubinemia. However, these are relatively non-specific and insensitive tests of 'liver function' and apart from their relationships with malnourishment and malignancy do not appear to have specific prognostic value. Bromsulphthalein, galactose, and indocyanine green elimination tests have not been widely used in biliary tract obstruction.

More recently the value of drugs as quantitative indicators of hepatic function has been recognized (Branch 1982) and the long-term objective must be to produce for hepatology the equivalent of the nephrologist's ability to measure renal blood flow, glomerular filtration rate and tubular function. Various approaches have been adopted (Ch. 2). Japanese surgeons have extensively reported on the use of ICG excretion and clearance as a marker of hepatocyte function preoperatively, including selective excretion into segmental biliary drainage catheters (Uesaka et al 1996). They have demonstrated improvement in ICG clearance after selective portal venous embolization of the contralateral lobe, as well as evidence of changes in segmental mass on CT scanning (Nagino et al 1995b). Logistical regression analysis of factors affecting post-resection liver failure showed impaired ICG clearance, impaired glucose tolerance and pre-operative cholangitis to be significant (Nagino et al 1993).

Elimination of aminopyrine by N-demethylation is a sensitive and quantitative indicator of hepatic microsomal function: its elimination may be estimated by breath analysis after oral administration of ^{14}C-aminopyrine, the aminopyrine breath test. Gill and his colleagues (1983) demonstrated that the aminopyrine breath test could predict the surgical risk in patients with known liver disease undergoing major surgery. Monroe and his colleagues (1982) also showed that the aminopyrine breath test reflects histological severity in patients with chronic hepatitis. Antipyrine (phenazone) is a minor analgesic which is eliminated by oxidation within the hepatocytes, and its clearance has been shown to correlate well with cytochrome P450 levels in the liver (McPherson et al 1982a). Because of the known effects of obstructive jaundice on cytochrome P450, antipyrine elimination is a particularly appropriate means of assessing hepatic function in the jaundiced patient. Our studies show that antipyrine clearance was significantly impaired in patients with obstructive jaundice, and moreover that antipyrine clearance was better correlated with the subsequent rate of fall of plasma bilirubin following relief of obstruction than were standard liver function tests. Moreover, the degree of impairment of antipyrine clearance was significantly related to the risk of surgical mortality in a series of patients with obstructive jaundice (McPherson et al 1985).

The effect of biliary obstruction on hepatocyte function are aggravated by the presence of infection. Nagano et al (1994) showed increased loss of hepatic mitochondrial phosphorylating capacity in rats with bile duct ligation after introduction of *Escherichia coli* into the biliary tree.

ENDOTOXEMIA AND RETICULO-ENDOTHELIAL FUNCTION

Endotoxin is the lipopolysaccharide derived from the cell walls of Gram-negative bacteria present in the gut. Normally only minute amounts of endotoxin enter the portal circulation and these traces are cleared by the hepatic reticulo-endothelial system. In obstructive jaundice endotoxin has been found in the peripheral circulation in up to 50% of patients (Bailey 1976) and plays a central role in its pathophysiology (Clements et al 1998). Circulating endotoxin has widespread systemic pathological effects, which are reviewed elsewhere (Ch. 9): these include renal vasoconstriction, redistribution of intrarenal blood flow away from the cortex, release of vasoactive cytokines and activation of complement, leukocytes, macrophages and platelets resulting in a tendency to disseminated intra-vascular coagulation. There is increasing evidence implicating the systemic cytokine response in the pathophysiology of obstructive jaundice (Kimmings et al 1995). The multi-organ dysfunction seen in obstructive jaundice is most likely an indirect effect of endotoxin, stimulating cytokine release from cells of the mononuclear phagocytic system resulting in a systemic inflammatory response typified by microcirculatory disruption, decreased oxygen delivery and ultimately multiple organ dysfunction syndrome (MODS). Experimental evidence has shown three main sources of this endotoxemia. Firstly, the absence of bile salts from the small intestine encourages endotoxin production both by loss of a specific binding function of bile salts, and by alteration of the small bowel microflora. Secondly, this effect is compounded by an actual increase in the rate of absorption from the intestine (Ingoldby 1980). Morphological changes have been reported in the small bowel mucosa, which may contribute to a general breakdown of gastrointestinal barrier function and consequently promote bacterial translocation and ensuing endotoxemia (Deitch et al 1990, Ding et al 1994, Clements et al 1996). Recently Welsh et al (1998) demonstrated an impaired gut barrier function in patients with obstructive jaundice and reported an increased intestinal permeability. This was found to be associated with local immune cell and enterocyte activation. Finally, depressed hepatic reticulo-endothelial cell function results in decreased clearance of absorbed endotoxin from the portal circulation.

External biliary drainage has not been shown to reduce the mortality from acute renal failure following surgery for obstructive jaundice, and this may be partly because it fails to correct the lack of bile salts in the small intestine. Administration of bile salts in rats (Bailey 1976) and in man (Cahill 1983) significantly reduced the incidence of endotoxemia. However, the use of preoperative bowel preparation or of the anti-endotoxin polymixin B had no significant effect on endotoxemia, although some changes in renal function were observed in each case (Hunt & Blumgart 1982, Ingoldby et al 1984). Gouma and his colleagues (1986) showed that endotoxemia in rats with biliary obstruction was significantly reduced after internal biliary drainage, while both portal and systemic endotoxemia persisted after external drainage. There is thus an increasing body of evidence to suggest the prime importance of bile salts in the gut in the management of patients with biliary obstruction. However, another controled study of preoperative ursodeoxycholic acid administration in jaundiced patients showed a reduction in portal (but not systemic) endotoxemia, but no significant effect on renal function or serum FDP levels, nor on the outcome of surgery. However, preoperative elevated FDP levels were associated with postoperative mortality (Thompson et al 1986). These differences are probably related to the differing detergent and bile-binding capacities of the different bile salts (Pain & Bailey 1988).

It remains uncertain whether *internal* biliary drainage has a significant effect on the clinical outcome. Some recent reports have revealed decreased perioperative morbidity for patients undergoing endoscopic biliary drainage before surgery (Lygidakis et al 1987, Trede and Schwall 1988, Marcus et al 1998) although other studies do not support these findings (Karsten et al 1996, Lai et al 1994).

There have always been technical problems in endotoxin research, because detection of endotoxin was formerly difficult and largely qualitative. Roughneen and his colleagues (1988a), using the quantitative chromogenic endotoxin assay, failed to show any clear correlation between portal or systemic endotoxemia and intestinal bile salts in bile duct ligated rats, implicating other factors in the development of endotoxemia in obstructive jaundice. Moreover, by performing choledocho-vesical fistulae as well as bile duct ligation followed by choledocho-vesical and choledocho-duodenal anastomoses in rats, they found that only the animals with ligated bile ducts showed systemic endotoxemia and increased mortality from intravenous lead acetate (Diamond et al 1990). These results suggest that biliary obstruction and its relief per se may be more important than changes in intestinal bile salts in the development and reversal of endotoxemia. The difference between these findings and those of Gouma et al (1986, 1987), who used an external biliary fistula as one of their models, may be due to infection in the presence of external fistulae, one of the major clinical problems with external biliary catheter drainage (McPherson et al 1982b; Blenkharn et al 1984). Clements et al (1998) recently reported usage of 'EndoCab'

enzyme linked immunosorbent assay (ELISA) as a novel, sensitive and specific method of endotoxin detection which measures endogenous IgG antibody to the inner core region of circulating endotoxin. They clearly demonstrated a central role for endotoxin in the pathophysiology of obstructive jaundice in rats. The subject of endotoxemia is covered in greater depth in Ch. 9.

IMMUNOLOGICAL EFFECTS

It is well recognized that extrahepatic biliary obstruction induces specific and non-specific depression of host immune status although the mechanisms for this are not very clear. Many reports of cellular immune dysfunction have been published and Greve et al (1990) suggested that depression of T-cell function was direct effect of systemic endotoxemia. It has also been shown that T-cell mitogen suppression occurs as a secondary effect of bacterial translocation (Deitch et al 1991). A defect in cell-mediated immunity was reflected by diminished skin test reactivity in Halliday's study of nutritional assessment in jaundiced patients (Halliday et al 1988). Thompson et al (1990) showed that in rats following bile duct ligation T-cell reactivity to PHA stimulation in vitro was diminished in proportion to the duration of obstructive jaundice. Fourteen days of internal drainage was required to return lymphocyte function to normal, and moreover internal drainage was more effective than external in restoring normality. The same group had also shown impaired lymphoproliferative response to tumor antigen and reduced natural killer (NK) cell toxicity to a tumor cell line in vitro (Roughneen et al 1988b).

We undertook studies in man to examine T-cell responsiveness and to determine whether any changes found were due to an intrinsic cellular defect, or caused by some transferable factor in the 'jaundiced' serum environment (Pace et al 1991). Cells and serum were respectively cryopreserved and frozen from patients with obstructive jaundice, and from the same patients six weeks after relief of obstruction by surgical or other means. The cells and serum from these two occasions were then incubated in various combinations with each other, with control serum, with cells and serum from normal volunteers, and in fetal calf serum. We in fact failed to show any significant depression of T-cell responsiveness to PHA stimulation, and in particular no effect of jaundiced serum on normal or convalescent cells. It is not clear why these results are different from those of Thompson et al (1990).

There is also increasing evidence showing impaired mononuclear phagocytic system function in obstructive jaundice (Megison et al 1991, Scott-Conner & Grogan 1994). Sung et al (1995) demonstrated decreased biliary IgA secretion in patients with biliary obstruction and suggested this might facilitate bacterial colonization and the development of acute cholangitis. Bemelmans et al (1996) recently reported elevated tumor necrosis factor (TNF) and soluble TNF receptors (sTNFr) in mice with biliary obstruction. Furthermore sTNFr concentrations rather than TNF showed a good correlation with mortality after surgery in obstructive jaundice, and reduction of sTNFr by lactulose reduced mortality, while anti-TNF antibodies were ineffective.

The area of immunostimulation in jaundiced patients has not been widely studied. However, recent studies from India have shown significantly increased survival and lower septic complication rates in both jaundiced patients and laboratory rats after treatment with the Ayurvedic medicine *Tinospora cordifolia* (Bapat et al 1990, Dahanukar et al 1990). This is a plant which has been used in the traditional Ayurvedic system of medicine for many centuries, including for patients with jaundice. The observation that an aqueous extract of this plant has significant effects in restoring immune function is an important one and requires further studies and confirmation in vitro.

CHANGES AFTER RELIEF OF OBSTRUCTION

Following relief of biliary tract obstruction, whether surgical or by means of interventional radiological or endoscopic techniques, a return to normal biliary secretion, liver structure and function might be anticipated. However, these events do not occur at a predictable or constant rate, and the important features of each will be considered below.

BILE SECRETION

Bile secretion following relief of obstruction is readily observed after insertion of an external percutaneous transhepatic biliary drain. There is frequently a prompt and major choleresis, and bile volumes may exceed four liters per day. Failure to replace the large fluid and electrolyte losses at this time may result in dehydration and electrolyte depletion with a metabolic acidosis. While sometimes this may necessitate intravenous fluid replacement, it may be sufficient to administer an oral electrolyte solution. The replacement of bile salts, if desired, may also be undertaken in the form of commercially available capsule preparations. An alternative is to return the patient's own bile by means of a nasogastric tube or by adding it to drinks to disguise the taste, but these methods are often not acceptable to the patient, and may result in biliary gastritis or esophagitis.

During the first few days of biliary drainage the bile produced is of low bilirubin and bile salt concentration, although the total bilirubin and bile salt output may be high because of the large volume. This is partly due to a slow return of the impaired liver to normal function, and partly to loss of the enterohepatic circulation of bile salts. In experimental animals external diversion of bile produces a decrease in the bile salt dependent canalicular flow within 30 minutes. This is promptly restored to normal by intravenous infusion of low concentrations of bile acids, which are taken up very rapidly from the plasma, 60 to 90% being cleared at the first passage through the liver (Heaton 1985). While it is known that bile salts thus stimulate the bile salt dependent component of canalicular flow, it is less widely appreciated that bile salts also stimulate more rapid excretion of bilirubin (Goresky et al 1974). We have examined this phenomenon in jaundiced patients following external tubal biliary drainage: oral administration of ursodeoxycholic acid in a dose of 300 mg four times daily increased not only total bile flow but also excretion of bilirubin and bilirubin clearance. This may provide a further rationale for administration of bile salts in patients in whom external biliary decompression is necessary, and who have no endogenous intestinal bile salts.

RECOVERY OF FUNCTION

In the majority of cases, plasma bilirubin begins to fall promptly after insertion of a drainage catheter or an internal biliary bypass procedure and this is accompanied by clinical improvement. However, return of hepatocyte function to normal is not instantaneous. We examined plasma antipyrine clearance serially after surgical relief of obstructive jaundice in a group of patients in whom the postoperative clinical course was uncomplicated. The return of antipyrine clearance to normal was not seen until 6 weeks after relief of obstruction and the time taken to recover did not correlate well with other standard preoperative liver function tests nor with postoperative changes in these tests (Thompson et al 1985). Koyama et al (1981) have also suggested that preoperative biliary decompression may have to be continued for at least 6 weeks to allow recovery of hepatocellular function. Furthermore, excretion of antibiotics in the bile, severely impaired or even absent in the presence of total biliary obstruction, was still greatly reduced up to 3 weeks after external tubal drainage (Blenkharn et al 1985). Thus if the beneficial effects of preoperative biliary drainage in reducing the morbidity of subsequent surgery rely upon a return to normal hepatocyte function, a period of drainage of up to 6 weeks may be required to achieve this effect. There is no information on the equivalent time taken for return of reticulo-endothelial function.

These results apply to uncomplicated biliary obstruction, but other factors may have a further adverse influence on recovery. In dogs, infection of the obstructed biliary tract results in impaired biliary mannitol clearance and bilirubin UDP-glucuronyl transferase activity of the liver after relief of biliary obstruction (Higashino & Nagakawa 1985), so that pre-existing cholangitis may be a significant complicating factor. Moreover, in patients with severely impaired hepatic function following long-standing biliary obstruction, one should anticipate slow bilirubin clearance as well as impairment of the more subtle forms of hepatocyte function for many weeks after biliary decompression. This may be particularly important when relief of obstruction is accompanied by resection of liver tissue as in patients with obstructive jaundice due to hilar cholangiocarcinoma.

STRUCTURAL CHANGES

There has been little study of the physiology of the intra- and extrahepatic bile ducts after decompression. One study has demonstrated return to near normal bile duct diameter 24 h after decompression by a variety of methods (Scudamore et al 1985). Certainly ultrasonographic evidence shows that the extrahepatic bile ducts display rapid fluctuations in size with intermittent obstruction. However, it has not been our experience in patients with long-standing biliary obstruction to see a rapid return to normal diameter of the intrahepatic bile ducts. These bile ducts, which have been subject to edema, inflammatory infiltration, cholangitis and fibrotic change, are likely to retain some rigidity for a considerable time after decompression. Indeed, there is evidence of continued poor emptying and intrahepatic ductal abnormalities on barium studies even several months after choledochoduodenostomy for long-standing biliary obstruction (Lygidakis 1981). In this study some patients had barium retained in the biliary tree up to one month after ingestion. Karsten et al (1991) reported structural changes in the extrahepatic ducts secondary to biliary stenting. Marked thickening of the duct walls with the lumen approximating the stent calibre, and extensive mucosal ulceration with epithelial denudation was observed in such patients. Histologically there was severe acute inflammatory infiltrate with marked fibrosis of the duct walls.

As regards reversal of intrahepatic fibrotic changes following drainage, it is difficult to obtain clear clinical evidence since this would rely upon serial liver biopsies in asymptomatic patients. Nevertheless, we have seen at least one patient with biliary obstruction and associated fibrosis in whom the fibrotic changes had resolved to normality on a subsequent biopsy. If such fibrotic changes, so long as they

remain short of true secondary biliary cirrhosis, remain reversible by adequate drainage, then it is also possible that portal hypertension secondary to such fibrosis may be improved with adequate drainage and obviate the need for definitive treatment of the portal hypertension. Thus it is probably sensible in difficult cases with long-standing obstruction and portal hypertension to ensure complete biliary decompression by the safest means and if necessary to treat associated varices by sclerotherapy, and to pursue an expectant policy in anticipation of a progressive fall in portal pressure as the liver changes resolve. Nonetheless, these patients with chronic biliary obstruction and consequent portal hypertension remain the highest risk group of patients with biliary obstruction, and pose both the most complex operative technical problems and the most difficult clinical decisions (Blumgart et al 1984a, Ch. 49).

REFERENCES

Alexander B, Blumgart L H, Mathie R T 1989 The effect of propranolol on the hepatic arterial buffer response to portal occlusion in the dog. British Journal of Pharmacology 96: 356–362

Aloj G 1993 Relationships amongst bile stasis, sepsis and choledocholithiasis: clinical and experimental studies. PhD Thesis, University of London

Aloj G, Li S K, Bianco C, Benjamin I S 1989 Infected common duct bile is not associated with bilirubin deconjugation in man. Gut 30: A744

Anderson J M 1996 Leaky junctions and cholestasis: a tight correlation (editorial). Gastroenterology 110: 1662–1664

Bailey M E 1976 Endotoxin, bile salts, and renal function in obstructive jaundice. British Journal of Surgery 63: 774–778

Bapat R, Rege N, Koti R, Desai N, Dahanukar S 1990 Improved survival in surgical jaundice with *Tinospora cordifolia*, an immunomodulator. HPB Surgery 2 (Suppl): 210

Beinart C, Efremedis S, Cohen B, Mitty H A 1981 Obstruction without dilation. Importance in evaluating jaundice. Journal of the American Medical Association 245: 353–356

Bemelmans M H, Greve J W, Gouma D J, Buurman W A 1996 Increased concentration of tumour necrosis factor (TNF) and soluble TNF receptors in biliary obstruction in mice; soluble TNF receptors as prognostic factors for mortality. Gut 38: 447–453

Benjamin I S 1983 Biliary tract obstruction. Surgical Gastroenterology 2: 105–120

Blamey S L, Feavon K C N, Gilmour W H, Osborne D H, Carter D C 1983 Prediction of risk in biliary surgery. British Journal of Surgery 70: 535–538

Blenkharn J I, McPherson G A D, Blumgart L H 1984 Septic complications of percutaneous transhepatic biliary drainage. Evaluation of a new closed drainage system. American Journal of Surgery 147: 318–321

Blenkharn J I, Habib N, Mok D, John L, McPherson G A D, Gibson R, Blumgart L H, Benjamin IS 1985 Decreased biliary excretion of piperacillin following percutaneous relief of extrahepatic obstructive jaundice. Antimicrobial Agents and Chemotherapy 28: 778–780

Blumgart L H 1978 Biliary tract obstruction—new approaches to old problems. American Journal of Surgery 135: 19–31

Blumgart L H, Kelley C J, Benjamin I S 1984a Benign bile duct stricture following cholecystectomy: critical factors in management. British Journal of Surgery 71: 836–843

Blumgart L H, Benjamin I S, Hadjis N S, Beazley R M 1984b Surgical approaches to cholangiocarcinoma at the confluence of hepatic ducts. Lancet i: 66–70

Bomzon L, Wilton P B, McCalden T 1978 Impaired skeletal muscle vasomotor response to infused noradrenaline in baboons with obstructive jaundice. Clinical Sciences & Molecular Medicine 55: 109–112

Branch R A 1982 Drugs as indicators of hepatic function. Hepatology 2: 97–105

Brody L A, Brown K T, Getrajdman G I, Kannegieter L S, Brown A E, Fong Y, Blumgart L H 1998 Clinical factors associated with positive bile cultures during primary percutaneous biliary drainage. Journal of Vascular and Interventional Radiology 9(4): 572–578

Bucher N L R, McGowan J A 1985 Regulatory mechanisms in hepatic regeneration. In: Wright R, Alberti K G M M, Karran S, Millward-Sadler G D T (eds) Liver and biliary disease: Pathophysiology, diagnosis, management, 2nd edn. Saunders, London, ch.11, 251–265

Cahill C J 1983 Prevention of postoperative renal failure in patients with obstructive jaundice—the role of bile salts. British Journal of Surgery 70: 590–595

Carr D, Hadjis N S, Banks L, Hemingway A, Blumgart L H 1985 Computed tomography of hilar cholangiocarcinoma. American Journal of Radiology 145: 53–56

Cattel W, Birnstingl M 1967 Blood-volume and hypotension in obstructive jaundice. British Journal of Surgery 54: 272–278

Clements W D, O'Rourke D M, Rowlands B J, Ennis M 1994 The role of mast cell activation in cholestatic pruritus. Agents & Action 41 spec No: C30–C31

Clements W D, Parks R, Erwin P, Halliday M I, Barr J, Rowlands B J 1996 Role of gut in the pathophysiology of extrahepatic biliary obstruction. Gut 39: 587–593

Clements W D, Erwin P, McCaigue M D, Halliday I, Barclay G R, Rowlands B J 1998 Conclusive evidence of endotoxaemia in biliary obstruction. Gut 42(2): 293–299

Csendes A, Sepulveda A, Burdiles P, Braghetto I, Bastias J, Schutte H, Diaz J C, Yarmuch J, Maluenda F 1988 Common bile duct pressures in patients with common bile duct stones with or without acute suppurative cholangitis. Archives of Surgery 123: 697–699

Dahanukar S, Rege N, Bapat R 1990 Immunosuppression in surgical jaundice. HPB Surgery 2(Suppl): 38

Deitch E A, Sittig K, Li M, Berg R, Specian R D 1990 Obstructive jaundice promotes bacterial translocation from the gut. American Journal of Surgery 159: 79–84

Deitch E A, Xu D Z, Qi L, Berg R D 1991 Bacterial translocation from the gut impairs systemic immunity. Surgery 109: 269–276

Desmet V J 1979 Cholestasis: extrahepatic obstruction and secondary biliary cirrhosis. In: McSween RNM, Anthony PP, Scheuer PJ (eds) Pathology of the liver. Churchill Livingstone, London, ch 13, 272–305

Diamond T, Dolan S, Thompson R L E, Rowlands B J 1990 Development and reversal of endotoxaemia and endotoxin-related death in obstructive jaundice. Surgery 108: 370–375

Ding J W, Andersson R, Soltesz V, Willen R, Bengmark S 1994 Obstructive jaundice impairs reticuloendothelial function and promotes bacterial translocation in the rat. Journal of Surgical Research 57: 238–245

Dixon J M, Armstrong C P, Duffy S W, Davies G C 1983 Factors affecting morbidity and mortality after surgery for obstructive jaundice: a review of 373 patients. Gut 24: 845–852

Flannigan M 1986 Glucose metabolism in obstructive jaundice. MS Thesis, University of London

Gill R A, Goodman M W, Golfus G R, Onstad G R, Bubrick M P 1983 Aminopyrine breath test predicts surgical risk for patients with liver disease. Annals of Surgery 198: 701–704

Goresky C A, Haddad H H, Kluger W S, Nadleau B E, Bach G G 1974 The enhancement of maximal bilirubin excretion with taurocholate-induced increment in bile flow. Canadian Journal of Physiological Pharmacology 52: 389–403

Gouma D J, Coelho J C U, Fisher J D, Schlegal J F, Li Y F, Moody F G 1986 Endotoxemia after relief of biliary obstruction by internal and external drainage in rats. American Journal of Surgery 151: 476–479

Gouma D J, Coelho J C U, Schlegal J F, Yong F L, Moody F G 1987 The effect of preoperative internal and external biliary drainage on mortality of jaundiced rats. Archives of Surgery 122: 731–734

Greim H 1972 Mechanism of cholestasis: 6. Bile acids in human livers with or without biliary obstruction. Gastroenterology 63: 846

Greve J W, Gouma D J, Soeters P B, Buurman W A 1990 Suppression of cellular immunity in obstructive jaundice is caused by endotoxins: a study with germ free rats. Gastroenterology 77: 478–485

Haga Y, Sakamoto K, Hiroshi E 1989 Changes in the production of interleukin-1 and interleukin-2 associated with obstructive jaundice and biliary drainage in patients with gastrointestinal cancer. Surgery 106: 842–848

Hadjis N S, Adam A, Blenkharn J I, Hatzis G, Benjamin I S, Blumgart L H 1989a Primary sclerosing cholangitis associated with liver atrophy. American Journal of Surgery 158: 43–47

Hadjis N S, Adam A, Gibson R N, Blenkharn J I, Benjamin I S, Blumgart L H 1989b Nonoperative approach to hilar cancer determined by the atrophy-hypertrophy complex. American Journal of Surgery 157: 395–399

Hadjis N S, Blenkharn J I, Hatzis G, Demianiuk C, Guzail M, Benjamin I S 1991 Pathologic and hemodynamic sequelae of unilobar biliary obstruction and associated liver atrophy. Surgery 109: 671–676

Hall L, Bergen A, Henriken J E 1977 Blood flow in normal and cholestatic dogs as measured by intraparenchymal injection of Xenon-133. European Surgical Research 9: 357–363

Hallenbeck, G A 1967 Biliary and pancreatic intraductal pressure. In: Code C F (ed) The Handbook of Physiology, Section 6, The alimentary canal, secretion, Vol II. American Physiological Society, Washington, DC pp 1007–1025

Halliday A W, Benjamin I S, Blumgart L H 1988 Nutritional risk factors in major hepatobiliary surgery. Journal of Parenteral & Enteral Nutrition 12: 43–48

Harry D S, Owen J S, McIntyre N 1985 Plasma lipoproteins and the liver. In: Wright R, Albert K G M M, Karran S, Millward-Sadler G D T (eds) Liver and biliary disease: Pathophysiology, diagnosis, management, 2nd edn. Saunders, London, ch. 4, 65–85

Heaton K W 1985 Bile salts. In: Wright R, Albert K G M M, Karran S, Millward-Sadler G D T (eds) Liver and biliary disease: Pathophysiology, diagnosis, management, 2nd edn. Saunders, London, ch. 13, 277–299

Higashino Y, Nagakawa N 1985 Influence of biliary tract infection on bile secretion in dogs after relief from obstructive jaundice. Italian Journal of Surgical Science 15: 111

Hoffman A F 1992 Bile acids in liver and biliary disease. In: Milward-Sadler G H, Wright R, Arthur M J P (eds) Wright's liver and biliary disease, WB Saunders, London

Huang T, Bass J A, Williams R D 1969 The significance of biliary pressure in cholangitis. Archives of Surgery 98: 629–632

Hunt D R 1979 Changes in liver blood flow with development of biliary obstruction in the rat. Australian and New Zealand Journal of Surgery 49: 733–737

Hunt D R, Blumgart L H 1982 Sodium homeostasis with obstructive jaundice: a randomized trial of preoperative bowel preparation. Chirurgia Epatobiliare 1: 99–102

Ingoldby C J H 1980 The value of polymyxin B in endotoxaemia due to experimental obstructive jaundice and mesenteric ischaemia. British Journal of Surgery 67: 565–567

Ingoldby C J H, McPherson G A D, Blumgart L H 1984 Endotoxemia in human obstructive jaundice: effect of Polymyxin B. American Journal of Surgery 144: 766–771

Jackaman F R, Hilson G R F, Lord Smith of Marlow 1980 Bile bacteria in patients with benign bile duct stricture. British Journal of Surgery 67: 329–332

Kaplan M M, Ohkubo A, Quarone E G, Szetu D 1983 Increased synthesis of rat liver alkaline phosphatase by bile duct ligation. Hepatology 3: 368–376

Karsten T M, Coene P, Gulik T, Bosma A, Marle J, James J, Lygidakis N J, Klopper P J, Heyde M 1991 Morphological changes of extrahepatic bile ducts during obstruction and subsequent decompression by endoprosthesis. Surgery 111: 562–568

Karsten T M, Allema J, Reinders M, Gulik T M, Wit L T, Verbeek P C M, Huibregtse K, Tytgat GNJ, Gouma DJ 1996 Preoperative biliary drainage, colonisation of bile and postoperative complications in patients with tumors of the pancreatic head: a retrospective analysis of 241 consecutive patients. European Journal of Surgery 162: 881–888

Kelley C J, Benjamin, I S, Blumgart, L H 1986 Portal hypertension and post-cholecystectomy biliary strictures. Digestive Surgery 3: 292–296

Kimmings AN, Deventer SJH, Obertop H, Rauws EAJ, Gouma DJ 1995 Inflammatory and immunologic effects of obstructive jaundice: pathogenesis and treatment. Journal of American College of Surgeons 181: 567–581

Koyama K, Takagi Y, Ito K, Sato T 1981 Experimental and clinical studies on the effect of biliary drainage in obstructive jaundice. American Journal of Surgery 142: 293–299

Kune G A (ed) 1972 Current practice of biliary surgery. Little Brown, Boston

Lai E C S, Mok F P T, Fan S T, Lo C M, Chu K M, Liu C L, Wong J 1994 Preoperative endoscopic drainage for malignant obstructive jaundice. British Journal of Surgery 81: 1195–1198

Lautt W W 1981 In: Hepatic circulation in health and disease. Lautt WW (ed) Raven Press, New York, 203–220

Lee E, Ross B D, Haines J R 1972 The effect of experimental bile duct obstruction on critical biosynthetic function of the liver. British Journal of Surgery 59: 564–568

Lygidakis N J 1981 Histological changes and intrahepatic biliary abnormalities in extrahepatic biliary tract obstruction. Surgery, Gynecology and Obstetrics 153: 532–536

Lygidakis N J, Brummelkamp W H 1985 The significance of intrabiliary pressure in acute cholangitis. Surgery, Gynaecology & Obstetrics 161: 465–469

Lygidakis N J, van der Heyde M N, Lubbers M J 1987 Evaluation of preoperative biliary drainage in the surgical management of pancreatic head carcinoma. Acta Chirurgia Scandinavia 153: 665–668

McPherson G A D, Benjamin I S, Boobis A R, Brodie M J, Hampden C, Blumgart L H 1982a Antipyrine elimination as a dynamic test of hepatic functional integrity in obstructive jaundice. Gut 23: 737–738

McPherson G A D, Blenkharn J I, Nathanson B, Bowley N B, Benjamin I S, Blumgart L H 1982b Significance of bacteria in external biliary drainage systems: a possible role for antisepsis. Journal of Clinical Surgery 1: 22–26

McPherson G A D, Benjamin I S, Boobis A R, Blumgart L H 1985 Antipyrine elimination in patients with obstructive jaundice: a predictor of outcome. American Journal of Surgery 149: 140–143

Marcus S G, Dobryansky M, Shamamian P, Cohen H, Gouge T H, Pachter H L, Eng K 1998 Endoscopic biliary drainage before pancreaticoduodenectomy for periampullary malignancies. Journal of Clinical Gastroenterology 26: 125–129

Maki T 1966 Pathogenesis of calcium bilirubinate gallstones: role of E. coli betaglucuronidase and coagulation by inorganic ions, polyelectrolytes and agitation. Annals of Surgery 164: 90

Mathie R T, Blumgart L H 1972 Hepatic tissue perfusion studies during partial hepatectomy in man. Surgical Gastroenterology 1: 297–302

Megison S M, Dunn C W, Horton J W, Chao H 1991 Effects of relief of biliary obstruction on mononuclear phagocytic system function and cell mediated immunity. British Journal of Surgery 78: 568–571

Monroe P S, Baker A L, Schneider J F, Krager P S, Klein P D, Schoeller D 1982 The aminopyrine breath test and serum bile acids reflect histologic severity in chronic hepatitis. Hepatology 2: 317–322

Muriel P 1996 Alpha-interferon prevents liver collagen deposition and damage induced by prolonged bile duct obstruction in the rat. Journal of Hepatology 24(5): 614–621

Nagano I, Kato S, Nimura Y, Wakabayashi T 1994 Hepatic mitochondrial changes in experimental obstructive jaundice complicated by biliary infection. Hepato-Gastroenterology 41: 432–437

Nagino M, Nimura Y, Hayakawa N, Kamiya J, Kondo S, Sasaki R, Hamajima N 1993 Logistical regression and discriminant analyses of hepatic failure after liver resection for carcinoma of the biliary tract. World Journal of Surgery 17: 250–255

Nagino M, Nimura Y, Kamiya J, Kondo S, Kanai M, Miyachi M, Yamamoto H, Hayakawa N 1995a Preoperative management of hilar cholangiocarcinoma. Journal of HPB Surgery 2: 215–223

Nagino M, Nimura Y, Kamiya J, Kondo S, Uesaka K, Kin Y, Hayakawa N, Yamamoto H 1995b Changes in hepatic lobe volume in biliary tract cancer patients after right portal vein embolization. Hepatology 21: 434–439

Nagorney D M, Mathie R T, Lygidakis N J, Blumgart L H 1982 Bile duct pressure as a modulator of liver blood flow after common bile duct obstruction. Surgical Forum 33: 206–208

Neale G, Lewis B, Weaver V, Panvelliwalla D 1971 Serum bile acids in liver disease. Gut 12: 145–152

Pace R F, Gonzaga R, Kaminski E, Hodgson H J F, Benjamin I S 1991 Human lymphocyte responsiveness is not enhanced by relief of biliary obstruction: an in-vitro study. Canadian Journal of Surgery 34: 123–127

Pain J A, Bailey M E 1988 Prevention of endotoxaemia in destructive jaundice – a comparative study of bile salts. HPB Surgery 1: 21–27

Papageorgiou G, Lynn J A 1985 Physiology of the extrahepatic biliary tree. In: Wright R, Albert K G M M, Karran S, Millward-Sadler G D T (eds) Liver and biliary disease: Pathophysiology, diagnosis, management, 2nd edn. WB Saunders, London, ch. 11, 267–276

Price C P, Sammons H G 1974 The nature of the serum alkaline phosphatases in liver disease. Journal of Clinical Pathology 27: 392–398

Price C P, Alberti K G M M 1985 Biochemical assessment of liver function. In: Wright R, Alberti K G M M, Karran S, Millward-Sadler G D T (eds) Liver and biliary disease: Pathophysiology, diagnosis, management, 2nd edn. WB Saunders, London, ch. 18, 455–493

Rahner C, Steiger B, Landmann L 1996 Structure–function correlation of tight junctional impairment after intrahepatic and extrahepatic cholestasis in rat liver. Gastroenterology 110: 1564–1578

Roughneen P T, Kumar S C, Pellis N R, Rowlands B J 1988a Endotoxemia and cholestasis. Surgery, Gynecology & Obstetrics 167: 205–210

Roughneen P T, Kulkarni S, Kumar S C, Kulkarni A D, Fanslow W, Pellis N R, Rowlands B J 1988b The influence of hepatocellular function on NK and T cell tumoricidal activity. Surgery 104: 888–893

Saharia P C, Zuidema G D, Cameron J L 1977 Primary common duct stones. Annals of Surgery 185: 598–604

Schaffner F, Javitt N H 1966 Morphologic changes in hamster livers during intrahepatic cholestasis induced by taurolithocholate. Laboratory Investigations 15: 1783–1966

Schaffner F, Popper H 1985 Classification and mechanism of cholestasis. In Wright R, Albert K G M M, Karran S, Millward-Sadler D G T (eds) Liver and biliary disease: Pathophysiology, diagnosis, management, 2nd edn. WB Saunders, London, ch. 15, pp 359–386

Schaffner F, Bacchin P G, Hutterer F, Scharnbeck H H, Sarkozi L L, Denk H, Popper H 1971 Mechanism of cholestasis: 4. Structural and biochemical changes in the liver and serum of rats after bile duct ligation. Gastroenterology 60: 888–897

Schiff L 1993 Jaundice: a clinical approach. In Schiff L, Schiff E R (eds) Diseases of the liver. JB Lippincott, Philadelphia, pp 334–342

Scott-Conner C E, Grogan J B 1994 The pathophysiology of biliary obstruction and its effect on phagocytic and immune function. Journal of Surgical Research 57: 316–336

Scriven M W, Horrobin D F, Puntis M C 1994 Study of plasma and red cell phospholipid fatty acids in extrahepatic cholestatic jaundice. Gut 35(7): 987–990

Scudamore C H, Azad A, Cooperberg P 1985 The changes of the intra and extrahepatic bile duct diameter after decompression. Italian Journal of Surgical Science 15: 110

Sedgwick C E, Poulantzas J K, Kune G A 1966 Management of portal hypertension secondary to bile duct stenosis: review of 18 cases with splenorenal shunt. Annals of Surgery 163: 949–953

Smith, Lord 1978 Injuries of the liver, biliary tree and pancreas. British Journal of Surgery 65: 673–677

Strasburg S M, Dorne B C, Redinger R N, Small D N, Egdall R H 1971 Effect of alteration of biliary pressure on bile composition – a method for study: primate biliary physiology. V. Gastroenterology 61: 357–362

Sung J J Y, Leung J C K, Tsui C P, Chung S C S, Lai K N 1995 Biliary IgA secretion in obstructive jaundice: the effects of endoscopic drainage. Gastrointestinal Endoscopy 42: 439–444

Thompson J N, Pickford M, Tsang V, Aslam M, McPherson G A D, Benjamin I S, Blumgart L H 1985 Recovery of plasma antipyrine clearance following surgical relief of obstructive jaundice. Italian Journal of Science 15: 111

Thompson J N, Cohen J, Blenkharn J I, McConnell J S, Matkin J, Blumgart L H 1986 A randomized clinical trial of preoperative oral ursodeoxycholic acid in obstructive jaundice. British Journal of Surgery 73: 634–636

Thompson R L E, Hoper M, Diamond T, Rowlands B J 1990 Development and reversibility of T lymphocyte dysfunction in experimental obstructive jaundice. British Journal of Surgery 77: 1229–1232

Tracy T F Jr, Tector A J, Goerke M E, Kitchen S, Lagunoff D 1993 Somatostatin analogue (octreotide) inhibits bile duct epithelial cell proliferation and fibrosis after extrahepatic biliary obstruction. American Journal of Pathology 143: 1574–1578

Trede M, Schwall G 1988 The complications of pancreatectomy. Annals of Surgery 207: 39–47

Uesaka K, Nimura Y, Nagino M 1996 Changes in hepatic lobar function after right portal vein embolization. Annals of Surgery 223: 77–83

Way L W, Bernhoft R A, Thomas J M 1981 Biliary stricture. Surgical Clinics of North America 61: 963–972

Welsh F K, Ramsden C W, MacLennan K, Sheridan M B, Barclay G R, Guillou P J, Reynolds J V 1998 Increased intestinal permeability and altered mucosal immunity in cholestatic jaundice. Annals of Surgery 227: 205–212

Williams R D, Elliot D W, Zollinger R M 1960 The effect of hypotension in obstructive jaundice. Archives of Surgery 81: 334–340

Yokoi H 1983 Morphological changes of the liver in obstructive jaundice and its reversibility—with special reference to morphometric analysis of ultrastructure of the liver in dogs. Acta Hepatologica 24: 1381–1391

Yoshimoto H, Ikeda S, Tanaka M, Matsumoto S 1989 Relationship of biliary pressure to cholangiovenous reflux during endoscopic retrograde balloon catheter cholangiography. Digestive Diseases and Sciences 34: 16–20

Younes R N, Vydelingum N A, Derooij P, Scognamiglio F, Andrade L, Posner M C, Brennan M F 1991 Metabolic alterations in obstructive jaundice: effect of duration of jaundice and bile-duct decompression. HPB Surgery 5: 35–48

Infections in hepatic, biliary and pancreatic surgery

8

J.E.J. KRIGE AND P.C. BORNMAN

INTRODUCTION

Intra-abdominal sepsis and its systemic consequences constitute a major cause of morbidity and mortality in patients undergoing complex operation for disease of the liver, biliary tract and pancreas. Part of the immune system of the body and much of the reticulo-endothelial system is found in the liver and spleen, organs which are reduced or removed during operation. In addition, disease processes such as jaundice, cirrhosis or tumor may further compromise the immune system. Furthermore the use of radiological and endoscopic biliary intervention has increased the susceptibility to sepsis and thus complicate or compromise the safety of operative procedures.

This chapter reviews the current concepts on host defense mechanisms, interacting pathophysiological processes, the bacteriological spectrum, risk factors which predispose to infective complications after liver and biliary surgery and the use of appropriate antibiotic therapy. The pathogenesis of sepsis and current role of antibiotic therapy in severe pancreatitis and the management of septic complications after pancreatic surgery are also examined.

HOST DEFENSE MECHANISMS IN THE LIVER AND BILIARY TRACT

The biliary tract has several defense mechanisms against bacterial invasion (Sung et al 1992a) (Table 8.1). These include (1) anatomical barriers (the sphincter of Oddi and tight junctions between hepatocytes), (2) physical mechanisms (bile flow and biliary mucus), (3) chemical factors (bile salts), and (4) immunological protection (Küpffer cells and immunoglobulins).

Table 8.1 Hepato-biliary defense mechanisms

Anatomical barriers
- sphincter of Oddi
- hepatic tight junctions

Physical mechanisms
- bile flow
- mucus

Chemical factors
- bile salts

Immunological defense
- Küpffer cells
- IgA
- complement
- fibronectin

ANATOMICAL BARRIERS

Bacteria can reach the biliary tract either directly from the duodenum by passing through the ampulla of Vater or indirectly from the gut via the portal venous blood. Under normal circumstances, the sphincter of Oddi provides an effective mechanical barrier which prevents bacteria and toxins from entering the biliary system. Ascending infections from the intestine can, however, occur as a result of cannulation of the bile duct, of a disrupted sphincter of Oddi following endoscopic sphincterotomy, a biliary enteric anastomosis or endoscopic placement of biliary stents (Yu et al 1996, Lee & Chung 1997). Direct contamination can also occur in patients with a T-tube in situ, or after placement of a percutaneous transhepatic biliary drain.

Hepatic tight junctions seal bile canaliculi from liver sinusoids. Their integrity is essential in preventing flux of bacteria between blood and bile. Tight junction permeability is influenced by bile acids and intrabiliary pressure (Sung et al 1992a). Cholangitis and increased biliary pressure may result in cholangiovenous reflux which is an important mechanism in the development of septicemia.

PHYSICAL MECHANISMS

Unimpeded flow of bile clears bacteria from the biliary tract, preventing bacteria from colonizing the biliary mucosa (Sung et al 1992b). The columnar epithelium of the extra-hepatic bile ducts secretes a water-insoluble mucus which covers the mucosa and provides a mechanical barrier against bacterial adherence, colonization and invasion, and in addition retains secretory immunoglobulin A within the mucus.

CHEMICAL FACTORS

Bile salts exhibit bacteriostatic and bactericidal properties *in vitro* (Stewart et al 1986). Hydrophobic bile salts in particular have a strong antibacterial effect (Sung et al 1993). In the presence of lecithin (the predominant phospholipid in human bile), however, the antibacterial properties of bile salts are markedly reduced. Bile salts and phospholipids form mixed micelles which result in inward projection of the hydrophobic portion of the molecule. This diminishes the detergent effect of bile salts and their antibacterial effect. Several types of enteric bacteria are inhibited by bile salts. The inhibition contributes to the maintenance of the enteric bacterial ecology, and decreases the risk of bacterial translocation. In addition the trophic action of bile on intestinal mucosa improves the integrity of the gut barrier. The anti-endotoxin effect produced by bile acids in the intestine blocks the absorption of endotoxin and contributes to the maintenance of host integrity. This inhibitory effect of bile acids on bacterial growth may also prevent infection (Stewart et al 1986).

IMMUNOLOGICAL DEFENSE

Küpffer cells, together with other phagocytic cells of the liver such as sinusoidal lining cells, constitute more than 85% of all fixed macrophages of the reticulo-endothelial system and have a major responsibility in host defense (Wang et al 1993a,b, Kimmings et al 1995). The preferential location of Küpffer cells in the periportal region of the sinusoid allows blood entering the sinusoid to be 'filtered'. The functions of Küpffer cells include phagocytosis of particulate matter, detoxification of endotoxin, secretion of mediators, regulation of the hepatic microcirculation, processing of antigens, as well as uptake and catabolism of lipids and glycoproteins. Besides their phagocytic function, Küpffer cells also function as antigen-presenting cells for the induction of T-lymphocyte response and the release of cytokines such as interleukins, interferons and tumor necrosis factor (Laskin 1990) (Ch. 9) which are important components of the host defense mechanism. Küpffer cell function is depressed in obstructive jaundice (Clements et al 1996). The diminished phagocytic capacity correlates inversely with plasma bilirubin levels, duration of jaundice, endotoxin and anticore glycolipid concentration (Kimmings et al 1995).

A variety of substances, including biliary proteins and glycoproteins are secreted by the liver. The predominant immunoglobulin in bile is secretory immunoglobulin A (IgA), which is excreted into bile by receptor-mediated transport across the biliary epithelium, particularly in the gallbladder (Sung et al 1992a). IgA-producing lymphoid cells also occur in the mucosa of bile ducts. Secretory IgA forms part of the local humoral luminal defense mechanism both in the intestine and the biliary tract. The beneficial effects of IgA include enhancement of the barrier function of the intestinal epithelium by antigen binding, and binding and prevention of bacteria from attachment to and penetration of epithelial cells (Scott-Conner & Grogan 1994). In patients with biliary obstruction, the excretion of IgA in bile is suppressed. IgA excretion recovers after removal of the obstruction. IgA-deficient individuals however do not have a markedly raised incidence of biliary tract infections. Fibronectin, an opsonic glycoprotein and other opsonins such as biliary complement are additional specific defense mechanisms effective against bacterial infection in the biliary tract (Wilton et al 1987).

BACTERIAL TRANSLOCATION

In jaundiced patients with an obstructed biliary system and a competent sphincter of Oddi, translocation of bacteria from the ileum and colon can occur (van den Hazel et al 1994a,b). Bacteria migrate from the gut via the portal vein to the liver, appearing in the bile by a paracellular route (Sung et al 1991). The increased biliary pressure caused by obstruction disrupts the tight junctions that form the barrier between the sinusoids (Disse's space) and the biliary canaliculi (Robenek et al 1980). Several other factors facilitate bacterial translocation. Colonization of the gut by non-pathogenic obligate anaerobic organisms (10^2–10^3 more than other bacteria) prevents other bacteria from binding to the mucosa and reduces bacterial overgrowth (Steffen & Berg 1983). Alterations in the composition of gut flora as a result of antibiotic use, intestinal stasis or altered nutrition may promote translocation (Kueppers et al 1993). The bowel mucosa and mucus layer, normally an efficient barrier, becomes permeable as a result of direct injury to the enterocytes or reduced blood flow to the intestine, as may occur in hemorrhagic shock or thermal injury (Herndon &

Ziegler 1993, Tokay et al 1993) or during total parenteral nutrition, when gut mucosal atrophy occurs (Shou et al 1994). Translocating bacteria may escape phagocytosis when the immune system is depressed. Various chemotherapeutic drugs and steroids promote translocation. Experimentally athymic mice have translocation to 50% of mesenteric lymph nodes (Owens & Berg 1980), suggesting that T-lymphocytes play a role. IgA secreted into the intestinal lumen also serves as a first line of defense against bacterial invasion (Alverdy et al 1985). In animals with obstructive jaundice, increased permeability of the intestinal wall (Parks et al 1996) and bacterial overgrowth in the gut result in a raised incidence of bactibilia (Deitch et al 1990). While Küpffer cells normally remove bacteria from the portal blood, the clearance capacity of Küpffer cells is lower in jaundiced animals than in non-jaundiced controls (Sung et al 1991).

BILIARY BACTERIOLOGY

Under normal circumstances the bile, biliary tree and liver are sterile. A variety of factors predispose the biliary tract to bacterial proliferation. Biliary stasis, obstruction to normal bile flow and foreign bodies within the bile duct are important factors determining the type and degree of bacterial colonization. In general, the most severe septic complications occur when biliary obstruction is complete and bacterial counts are high (Pitt & Couse 1990).

The endogenous biliary pathogens present in infected bile are predominantly gram-negative enteric aerobes including *Escherichia coli*, *Klebsiella* and *Proteus* (Lee & Chung 1997). *Pseudomonas aeruginosa* is uncommon except after interventional endoscopic biliary procedures. Anaerobes are found infrequently in patients at low risk for biliary sepsis. Fastidious culture techniques, however, reveal *Bacteroides fragilis* with increasing frequency in elderly patients, with cholangitis or those undergoing complex revisionary biliary surgery. Although the pathogenicity of *Enterococcus faecalis* in biliary infection has been questioned, this organism is usually isolated in association with anaerobic organisms suggesting that enterococci may play a synergistic role. An increasing incidence of staphylococcal wound infection has been identified in patients with jaundice and diabetes undergoing biliary surgery. Infected bile is usually polymicrobial and a single species is recovered in only a third of patients with biliary infection (Leung et al 1994).

Anaerobes are seldom isolated from patients with chronic cholecystitis and cholelithiasis (Krige et al 1992b). Even in patients with acute cholecystitis anaerobes are infrequently cultured except in the most severe forms such as empyema and emphysematous cholecystitis (Doty & Pitt 1986). In comparison, anaerobes have been isolated from 25 to 30% of patients with cholangitis secondary to choledocholithiasis. Anaerobes are also more common in elderly patients and in those with complex biliary problems and indwelling tubes (Van den Hazel et al 1994a,b).

Thompson et al (1994) and Lipsett and Pitt (1990) have reported an increase in isolates of *Pseudomonas*, *Serratia*, *Streptococcus* and *Enterobacter* in patients treated for biliary tract infections. The continued prevalence of *E. coli*, *Klebsiella*, and enterococci in reports from other hospitals suggests that such changes in bacteriology are probably related to differences in antibiotic practice, an increasing cohort of patients with previously treated recurrent cholangitis, endoscopic or transhepatic manipulations, indwelling stents and more patients with malignant obstruction being treated at tertiary referral institutions (Lee & Chung 1997). Patients with malignant obstruction have significantly more isolates with *Klebsiella*, *Enterobacter*, *Streptococcus* and *Candida* than do patients with benign obstruction (Thompson et al 1994).

RISK FACTORS FOR INFECTIOUS COMPLICATIONS IN BILIARY TRACT SURGERY

The risk of postoperative septic complications is mostly determined by the presence of bacteria in bile and it is therefore important that patients at risk for bactibilia should be identified early in order to institute prophylactic antibiotics. The incidence of bactibilia in low-risk patients undergoing elective cholecystectomy ranges from 10 to 15% (Reiss et al 1982, Lewis et al 1987, Wells et al 1989), increases substantially in patients with either nonfunctioning gallbladders or acute cholecystitis (Reiss et al 1982, Grant et al 1992).

Several risk factors for bactibilia have been identified (Reiss et al 1982, Wells et al 1989, Thompson et al 1990). These include patients over the age of 70 years, associated cholangitis, common bile duct stones, acute cholecystitis and nonfunctioning gallbladders (Reiss et al 1982, Wells et al 1989, Thompson et al 1990, Landau et al 1992). The presence of biliary drains or stents or biliary-enteric anastomoses also considerably increase the risk of ascending infection from the intestine to the biliary tract (Sung et al 1992b). Similarly, other factors, such as diabetes mellitus and immunosuppression increase the risk. Foreign materials have been shown to promote bactibilia and subsequent septic complications, significantly reducing the minimum bacterial inoculum required to initiate and maintain biliary sepsis in experimental studies (Yu et al 1996).

Bacterial cultures from gallbladder bile or the gallbladder wall are positive in two-thirds of patients (Claesson et al 1986) with acute cholecystitis. Bactibilia has been reported in 81% of patients with acute cholecystitis who underwent operation within 2 days of the onset of symptoms, while positive cultures decreased to 50–65% after longer preoperative intervals (Claesson et al 1986). In patients with common bile duct stones and acute suppurative cholangitis, bacterial cultures from bile are positive in 95% of specimens (Lee & Chung 1997).

Bactibilia is the most important factor in the development of postoperative septic complications in high risk patients (Table 8.2). In a prospective study in 800 consecutive cholecystectomies, a close correlation was found between positive bile cultures and the incidence of septic complications (Reiss et al 1982). Both postoperative wound infection and septicemia are frequently caused by the same bacteria, cultured from bile specimens taken during biliary operation in high risk patients (Lewis et al 1987, Wells et al 1989). Contamination of the wound with infected bile is a major cause of both postoperative wound infection and intraabdominal sepsis. In high risk patients enteric bacterial translocation due to an impaired RES and gut barrier function, as occurs in obstructive jaundice, is the commonest cause of bactibilia. In contrast in low risk patients, with sterile bile at the time of operation, exogenous bacterial contamination from the patient's own skin flora constitutes the major cause of post-operative wound infection.

Table 8.2 Risk factors for septic complications in biliary tract surgery

- Bactibilia
- Biliary obstruction
- Age (> 70 years)
- Acute cholecystitis
- Common bile duct stones
- Non-functioning gallbladder
- Diabetes mellitus
- Foreign material (stents/tubes)

SEPTIC COMPLICATIONS RELATED TO BILIARY OBSTRUCTION

Infections associated with biliary obstruction are unique in the sense that there are additional risk factors specifically related to the jaundice and its underlying causes and effects (Ch. 7). Patients with obstructive jaundice are frequently in their seventh or eighth decade and often have associated cardiovascular and renal disease. Those with malignant biliary obstruction have the added burden of malnutrition and poor wound healing, which is prevalent in carcinoma of the pancreas where cachexia factors are responsible for severe weight loss (Wigmore et al 1997). Jaundice per se increases the susceptibility to sepsis, a subject which has been intensively studied and reviewed in recent years (Clements et al 1993, Bornman & Krige 1997). The serum bilirubin level, which reflects the severity of the jaundice, is an important predictor of septic complications. The mechanisms by which obstructive jaundice increases the risk of sepsis are now well defined. The anti-endotoxin effects of bile salts in the gastrointestinal tract is lost and allows increased absorption of endotoxins into the portal circulation (Bailey 1976). The associated impaired Küpffer cell phagocytic function in the liver (Clements et al 1993a,b) results in spillover of endotoxins in the systemic circulation. This systemic endotoxemia activates the inflammatory response resulting in a cascade of events which includes reduced production of anti-endotoxin secretory immunoglobulin A from the liver, depression of monocellular phagocytic function, deficient cell-mediated and humoral immunity, changes in mucosal permeability (Bjarnason et al 1995, Parks et al 1996) and reduced blood flow to the gut.

PRE-OPERATIVE BILIARY DRAINAGE

While the concept of biliary drainage to reduce operative mortality in patients with biliary tract obstruction dates back to 1935 (Whipple et al 1935) it was the advent of radiological biliary intervention in the 1970s which ushered in the modern era of pre-operative biliary drainage (Nakayama et al 1978). However, controlled trials have shown that pre-operative biliary drainage is associated with increased morbidity related to excessive bile loss and risk of sepsis associated with external catheter drainage (Hatfield et al 1982, McPherson et al 1984, Smith et al 1984, Pitt et al 1985). In addition the problem of increased costs, mainly due to prolonged hospital stay, was emphasized by Pitt et al (1985).

Clinical trials have not specifically addressed the potential advantage of endoscopic internal biliary stenting which has been available for the last 20 years. Internal drainage has the advantage of avoiding external bile losses and overcomes the problem of endotoxemia by re-introducing bile into the gut and allows flexibility in the timing of surgery. Küpffer cell function and the gut mucosal barrier dysfunction (Parks et al 1996) takes 4–6 weeks to recover. Both these defense mechanisms are important to avoid renal dysfunction and sepsis.

Experimentally internal drainage is better than external

drainage (Gouma et al 1987) and a non-randomized trial (Trede & Schwall 1988) showed a reduction in postoperative complications after internal drainage. However this has not been confirmed in a prospective randomized trial in a group of patients with both high and low malignant bile duct obstruction (Lai et al 1994) in whom a high incidence of endoscopic related sepsis particularly occurred in patients with malignant hilar obstruction. The problem of stent sepsis and associated morbidity has been further emphasized in a recent prospective audit from the Memorial Sloan Kettering Clinic New York in a homogeneous group of patients with proximal cholangiocarcinoma (Hochwald et al 1999) (Table 8.3). Patients with stents had a significantly increased risk of bactibilia and infectious complications. Most of the infections were due to organisms cultured in the bile. Stenting did not reduce the incidence of other complications nor was there a reduction in the mortality rate. The concern that liver resection may be accompanied by an increased mortality if done in the presence of obstructive jaundice was not evident in this study (Ch. 54). Virtually all patients with biliary stents will eventually have organisms in their bile as a result of ascending colonization particularly if the stent protrudes into the duodenum (Karsten et al 1996). Bacterial beta glucoronidase predisposes to sludge which in turn forms a nidus for infection (Yu et al 1996).

An important aspect of pre-operative biliary drainage is the associated septic morbidity which occurs when there is failure to establish adequate drainage after insertion of a stent or catheter. This is a particular problem in high bile duct obstructions with second order hepatic duct involvement. The risk of sepsis in undrained segments of the liver is high and often impossible to eradicate, jeopardizing the chances of a curative operation. In this regard it is probably safer to use the percutaneous rather than the endoscopic stents (Nimura et al 1990, Bismuth et al 1992) which avoid the indiscriminate introduction of contrast into segments that are not drained by the procedure.

Routine use of preoperative stenting is not required and should be restricted to patients with pre-existing cholangitis or those in whom renal impairment does not respond to conservative measures. Careful attention to rehydration, the use of prophylactic antibiotics, correction of coagulopathy with vitamin K or fresh frozen plasma and perhaps oral bile salts and lactulose administration are sufficient preparation to minimize complications after major surgery (Bornman & Krige 1997). The practice of pre-operative biliary drainage will however probably continue in many parts of the world as most patients are referred to surgical units by endoscopists with stents already in place as part of the initial diagnostic work-up. Constraints on the availability of operating room time is another reason why stents are used to delay definitive surgery.

ANTIBIOTIC THERAPY IN BILIARY SURGERY

The routine use of therapeutic systemic antibiotics in patients with established biliary sepsis is standard practise. Similarly, the use of prophylactic antibiotics is advisable in patients with bactibilia at the time of operation, and in patients undergoing endoscopic retrograde cholangiography or non-operative biliary manipulation. To achieve maximal beneficial effect, antibiotic prophylaxis, which provides effective tissue concentrations, is necessary before wound contamination occurs or therapeutic intervention is initiated. A definitive microbiological diagnosis in patients with biliary infection is however limited by delay in operative bile culture results and the low incidence of positive blood cultures. While the choice of antibiotic prophylaxis is usually empiric, antibiotic administration is governed by the following principles which include the identification of:

(i)   the subgroup of patients at risk for bactibilia
(ii) the resident biliary microflora
(iii) the therapeutic efficacy of antimicrobial agents in the biliary tract.

The choice of an appropriate antibiotic for either prophylaxis or treatment of biliary infection is generally based on the antibacterial spectrum, serum and tissue concentrations, biliary penetration, toxicity and cost. Biliary secretion of various antibiotics and their metabolites depends on molecular weight, polarity and hepatic metabolism. Compounds with a molecular weight below 500 to 600 are excreted predominantly in the urine while those of a higher molecular weight

Table 8.3 Infectious complications after biliary stenting

Type (n)*	No Stent (n = 29)	Stent (n = 42)	p-Value
Wound infection	4	12	0.10
Intra-abdominal abscess	4	5	ns
Pneumonia	1	3	ns
Cholangitis	–	4	ns
Clostridium difficile	1	4	ns
Candida esophagitis	1	–	ns
Total (n)*	11	28	< 0.05
Total (%)**	28	52	< 0.05

*Patients can be listed in more than one category if more than one complication has occurred
**Percent of patients with an infectious complication

Hochwald et al 1999

are excreted in bile. In acute cholangitis, hepatic excretion of bile may be markedly impaired or absent depending on the severity of the biliary obstruction. While high biliary excretion levels may have theoretical advantages, other pharmacokinetic properties are more important and superior prophylactic agents include those which provide increased serum and wound concentrations during surgery.

Other considerations when selecting antibiotic therapy include the type, susceptibility and minimum inhibitory concentration relative to the bacteria responsible. Intercurrent illness such as renal or hepatic dysfunction that impact on the safety of the antibiotic when administered at appropriate dosage are also important. The timing of antibiotic administration is crucial, and to be effective, prophylactic antibiotics should be given pre-operatively before wound contamination. There is no benefit in continuing therapy for extended periods after the initial dose in elective biliary surgery; single dose pre-operative administration reduces the risk of drug toxicity and the development of resistant organisms.

Initial antibiotic therapy should include cover for enteric gram-negative organisms, anaerobes and enterococci. Penicillin derivatives including mezlocillin, piperacillin, imipenem and the combination drugs, ampicillin-sulbactam and ticarcillin-clavulanic acid each provide adequate single-drug cover. Aminoglycosides provide excellent cover against the gram-negative aerobes including *Escherichia coli* and *Klebsiella*. In addition, the combination of a penicillin, such as ampicillin, with an aminoglycoside is synergistic against enterococci. However, major concerns about compromising renal function in elderly, jaundiced patients receiving aminoglycosides has led to the evaluation of alternative non-nephrotoxic antibiotics. Options include ureidopenicillins, third-generation cephalosporins, monobactam agents such as imipenem, or combinations of penicillins or cephalosporins with agents that prolong or increase their activity such as clavulanic acid or sulbactam. Antibiotics with enhanced biliary excretion (i.e. cefamandole, moxalactam, cefoperazone) have been associated with antibiotic-related diarrhea and coagulation defects due to interruption of normal colonic flora. Most authorities agree that broad-spectrum antibiotic cover of gram-negative aerobes, anaerobes, and enterococci should be utilized in patients with cholangitis. The current cephalosporins do not provide adequate cover for enterococci, nor do many of the newer agents adequately cover anaerobes. The newer penicillin derivatives provide adequate cover against both anaerobes and enterococci. The choice of antibiotic regimen must be based on characteristics of both the patient and the infection as well as the toxicity of the therapy, pending definitive drainage of the obstructed biliary tract.

ABDOMINAL SEPSIS FOLLOWING MAJOR LIVER RESECTION

CLINICAL BACKGROUND

Although liver resection is now performed with increasing safety, morbidity is still substantial, with postoperative complications occurring in 10 to 40% of patients (Rees et al 1996, Strong et al 1994, Tsao et al 1994, Brancatisano et al 1998) and up to 47% in the elderly (Fong et al 1997). The most serious complications that occur after hepatectomy are abdominal sepsis, hepatorenal failure, liver decompensation, bile leaks and bleeding (Rees et al 1997, Finch et al 1998, Lise et al 1998, Melendez et al 1998).

Septic complications represent the most frequent cause of morbidity following liver resection (Melendez et al 1998). The reported incidence of bacterial infection varies from 4 to 20%. This constitutes 30 to 50% of all postoperative complications and is responsible for up to 40% of postoperative deaths (Ekberg et al 1986, Fortner & Rinser 1990, Melendez et al 1998). Fortner et al (1978) described a 20% (22/108) incidence of subphrenic abscesses and Andersson et al (1990a,b) reported an 8% (11/138) incidence of intraabdominal abscess after major liver resection. Culture-proven intraabdominal fluid collections occur in 13–30% of patients after hepatic resection (Yanaga et al 1986, Pace et al 1989). Mortality due to abdominal sepsis after major hepatectomy is ultimately caused by multiple system organ failure (Yanaga et al 1986, Andersson et al 1990a,b).

RISK FACTORS AND CAUSATIVE BACTERIA

Ischemic tissue at the resection line following extensive liver resection is an important local factor predisposing to intraabdominal septic complications (Yanaga et al 1986). In addition, the presence of free intraperitoneal blood and bile, if contaminated by bacteria, aggravates the outcome (Andersson et al 1989) by impairing peritoneal phagocyte function (Andersson et al 1990b). Trauma, cholangiocarcinoma, biliary obstruction, preoperative biliary stenting and the presence of a biliary-enteric anastomosis are associated with higher postoperative intraabdominal sepsis rates, as are extensive resections (Yanaga et al 1986, Pace et al 1989, Andersson et al 1990a, Hochwald et al 1999). Other variables significantly correlating with the development of abdominal sepsis following hepatectomy were age > 60 years, long operation time, amount of blood transfused, major intraoperative bleeding, reoperation for hemorrhage, long postoperative stay and prolonged abdominal drainage.

Most of these parameters merely reflect the extent and magnitude of the liver resection and the decreased resistance of the body. Bacteria of gut origin dominate culture findings obtained from the abdominal cavity in patients with intraperitoneal sepsis following hepatectomy. Most frequently *Escherichia coli* and *Enterococcus* are cultured, but a broad spectrum of enteric bacteria are represented and in 50 to 75% multiple bacteria are cultured (Pace et al 1989, Wang et al 1992).

CHANGES IN HOST DEFENSE FOLLOWING HEPATECTOMY

The decrease in RES function following liver resection is primarily attributable to the decrease in reticuloendothelial cell volume, paralleling the extent of liver resection. No signs of depression of RES activity in the remaining healthy liver tissue have been observed, despite the impaired resistance to a septic challenge (Vo & Chi 1988, Andersson & Foss 1991). However, hepatectomy decreases RES clearance of endotoxin, which is already impaired in the diseased liver. Hepatectomy also induces changes in circulatory factors regulating RES function such as a decrease in the glycoprotein fibronectin (Kwon et al 1990). Furthermore, major hepatectomy leads to a decrease in the production of hepatic bile. This decrease results in several potentially negative effects, as bile in the intestine exerts a trophic stimulus on the gut mucosa (Borghi et al 1991), binds intraluminal endotoxin, thus preventing endotoxemia (Cahill et al 1987) and regulates intestinal bacterial composition and bacterial adhesion (Dahlgren et al 1986).

PATHOPHYSIOLOGICAL MECHANISMS

The frequent finding of bacteria of gut origin in the abdominal cavity and blood following major liver resection suggests that enteric bacterial translocation plays an important role. The definition of translocation includes not only bacteria but also endotoxin and other particles (Alexander et al 1990). The process of enteric bacterial translocation is complex and depends upon both local and systemic factors. Experimentally, enteric bacterial translocation to mesenteric lymph nodes and blood is demonstrated in the early phase following major liver resection in the rat, with an incidence proportional to the amount of liver removed (Wang et al 1992). Major liver resection results in morphological changes in the intestine within hours of the operation. Thus, small intestinal mucosal mass and microvillous height decrease and protein content in enterocytes and bile secretion from the liver remnant are reduced. Simultaneously, a decrease in microcirculatory flow to the intestine and an overgrowth and colonization of *Escherichia coli* in the distal small intestine are observed (Wang et al 1993a,b).

Furthermore, experimental hepatectomy in the rat results in impaired intestinal motility, correlating with enteric bacterial overgrowth, reduction in intramucosal and intraluminal pH in the gastrointestinal tract. These changes promote and further disturb enteric bacterial ecology. An altered membrane permeability and increased bacterial adherence to the intestinal mucosa is also noted (Wang et al 1993a,b). The enteric bacterial overgrowth can destroy intestinal mucosa by the direct effect of bacterial proteases on specific microvillous membrane proteins (Riepe et al 1980) or by other changes of the intracellular biochemistry (Batt et al 1984). Microvillous alterations may explain why both bacteria and endotoxin attach to the enterocyte surface and either penetrate through apparently morphologically intact intestinal epithelial cells (Alexander et al 1990) or are phagocytosed by submucosal macrophages (Well et al 1988).

INTRAABDOMINAL SEPSIS AFTER LIVER TRAUMA (see also Ch. 68)

After exsanguination, intraperitoneal sepsis is the commonest cause of early death after liver trauma and is the major cause of late morbidity (Scott et al 1988, Krige et al 1997). Factors associated with an increased incidence of intraabdominal sepsis following liver injury are listed in Table 8.4.

There is experimental evidence identifying the adjuvant effect of hemoglobin in the development of intraabdominal sepsis. Hemoglobin reduces normal tolerance to bacterial contamination by the inhibition of bacterial absorption from the peritoneal cavity, inhibition of polymorphonuclear leukocyte chemotaxis, and intracellular killing or by a direct enhancement of bacterial growth. In addition to the adjuvant effect of hemoglobin, blood transfusion may result in impaired immune function. Blood transfusions have been linked with stimulation of suppressor T-cells, impaired cell-mediated immunity and macrophage function and suppres-

Table 8.4 Factors associated with increased risk of intraabdominal sepsis following liver injury

Major liver injury
Blood transfusion
Liver packs
Splenectomy
Colonic injury
> 3 abdominal organs injured
Shock on admission
Gunshot wounds
Open drainage of the abdomen

sion of lymphocyte proliferation. Major blood loss and prolonged hypotension may lead to hypothermia, poor tissue perfusion, and ineffective distribution of antibiotics. Resulting undrained hematomas shield bacteria from host defenses and antibiotics.

The judicious use of therapeutic perihepatic packing to provide tamponade for control of bleeding in complex liver trauma has evolved as an acceptable and recognized emergency measure (Krige et al 1992a). However, sepsis is a major source of morbidity following packing (Krige 1991). In one study septic complications ensued in 6 of 25 patients who had been packed at some time during their treatment (Hollands & Little 1989). In a group of patients from New York with predominantly penetrating trauma, the infection rate was significantly increased in patients submitted to packing (83%), compared to a similar group (20%) who had debridement-resection without packing (Ivatury et al 1986). Patients who had bowel or bile leaks or were packed for more than 72 hours or required repacking, invariably became septic (Krige et al 1997). Current recommendations are to remove the packs within 48 hours after correction of coagulation and metabolic abnormalities and, if possible, to avoid repacking. In liver injuries with gross bowel contamination or bile leaks identified during operation in whom packing is unavoidable, packs should be retrieved at relaparotomy within 24 hours (Krige et al 1992a).

PANCREATIC SEPSIS

Pancreatic sepsis is most commonly encountered as a complication of severe pancreatitis. In centers where operations on the pancreas are frequently performed sepsis remains the most important cause of post-operative morbidity and mortality.

PANCREATITIS

Sepsis is the most devastating complication of severe necrotizing pancreatitis and is responsible for 80% of late deaths. Considerable progress has been made in the understanding of the pathogenesis, pathology, diagnosis and management of pancreatic sepsis. Pancreatic sepsis occurs almost exclusively when pancreatitis is complicated by pancreatic and peripancreatic necrosis. Reports from the Ulm group showed that the risk of sepsis increases proportionately to the extent of pancreatic necrosis (Beger et al 1986, Block et al 1986, Rau et al 1998) although this association has not been confirmed in a study from Boston (Tenner et al 1997).

The incidence of sepsis in severe pancreatitis is approximately 30% (Widdison & Karanjia 1993). Sepsis usually occurs more than a week after a severe attack and the incidence progressively increases with time and may be as high as 70% at 3 weeks (Beger et al 1986). However, in studies where sepsis is diligently sought by fine needle aspiration, early sepsis is more frequently detected (Gerzof et al 1987).

Pathogenesis

Bacterial contamination of pancreatic necrosis is usually due to translocation of gut organisms (Medich et al 1993). Support for this hypothesis is based on experimental data (Widdison et al 1994, Foitzik et al 1995) and the fact that the majority of organisms cultured from infected necrosis are of gut origin (Büchler et al 1992) (Table 8.5). The beneficial effects of selective gut decontamination (Foitzik et al 1995, Luiten et al 1995) and early feeding which prevents the breakdown of the gut mucosal barrier (Kimmings et al 1995) provide indirect evidence for gut derived organisms being implicated as the major source of pancreatic sepsis. However, when anaerobic bacteria are cultured from pancreatic sepsis, the spectrum resembles that found in bile (Widdison & Karanjia 1993). In gallstone pancreatitis cultures from infected necrosis show a significantly greater incidence of gram negative organisms while in alcohol induced pancreatitis, gram positive bacteria are more prevalent (Räty et al 1998). Fungal infections (eg. *Candida*) and *Pseudomonas* related sepsis occur during the late stages, a problem commonly encountered in intensive care units. Polymicrobial infections are more commonly found in pancreatic abscesses than in infected pancreatic necrosis (Bittner et al 1987).

Table 8.5 Frequency of bacteria in pancreatic infection

Escherichia coli	26%
Pseudomonas sp.	16%
Staphylococcus aureus	15%
Klebsiella sp.	10%
Proteus sp.	10%
Streptococcus faecalis	4%
Enterobacter sp.	3%
Anaerobes	16%

Büchler et al 1992a

Confirmation of sepsis

While sterile necrosis is regarded as a relatively benign condition, there is general agreement that early surgery is mandatory in patients with infected necrosis (Beger et al 1986, Bradley & Allen 1991). Pancreatic sepsis is suspected and sought when there is persistence of organ failure, associated with features of systemic infection (temperature of 38–39°C and white blood count of > 20 000/mm³) (Lankisch & Banks 1998). These parameters and other septic markers are not, however, sufficiently reliable on their own to dictate management strategies. Although the severity of pancreatitis as measured by Ranson's criteria or the APACHE II scoring system (Ranson et al 1985, Bradley & Allen 1991, Rattner et al 1992) is associated with a higher risk of infection, the sensitivity and specificity of these parameters are generally poor. This also applies to markers of necrosis including C-reactive protein, (Büchler et al 1986, Rattner et al 1992, Widdison & Karanjia 1993) and extent of pancreatic necrosis as determined by CT scanning (Ranson et al 1985, Bradley & Allen 1991).

Blood cultures may be helpful if gram negative organisms are grown although bacteremia from a pancreatic abscess may be intermittent and transient (Widdison & Karanjia 1993). The most definitive diagnosis of infected necrosis is made by direct culture of necrotic material either by percutaneous aspiration (Gerzof et al 1987, Rau et al 1998) or during surgery. A positive gram stain or culture on fine needle aspiration is now widely used as a mandate for surgical intervention. Concern, however, has been expressed in a recent French study (Paye et al 1998) that fine needle aspiration and catheter drainage may introduce sepsis, and that the outcome of the aspirate (whether positive or negative) does not predict the outcome nor the need for surgical intervention.

Antibiotic prophylaxis

The value of prophylactic antibiotics to reduce the incidence of sepsis in pancreatitis has been debated for more than two decades. Early reports including randomized studies (Howes et al 1975, Finch et al 1976) did not support the routine use of prophylactic antibiotics although the potential benefit of antibiotics may have been masked by the inclusion of patients with mild pancreatitis and the use of inappropriate antibiotics such as ampicillin which have poor penetration properties (Roberts & Williams 1979, Trudel et al 1994). In recent years the use of antibiotics has been revisited. Büchler et al (1992a,b) studying human pancreatic tissue levels of ten bactericidal antibiotics demonstrated the limitations of many commonly used antibiotics. Experimental and clinical studies have assessed the penetration capabilities of newer generation antibiotics in the pancreas and peripancreatic necrotic tissue and determined the spectrum of organisms and their sensitivity to antibiotic treatment (Bradley 1989, Powell et al 1998). Current information indicates that third generation cephalosporins, piperacillin, mezlocillin, 4-quinolones (ciprofloxacin and oflaxacin) imipenem and metronidazole achieve the best therapeutic pancreatic tissue concentrations (Powell et al 1998). However, these observations may not necessarily apply in the clinical setting. Antibiotics which are usually excreted via the pancreatic duct may not reach the avascular extrapancreatic necrosis when infected by translocation of organisms from the gut. Moreover, local and systemic antibacterial clearance is impaired in acute pancreatitis (Gianotti et al 1995) and factors such as prolonged parenteral feeding compromise local gut immunity, promote gut overgrowth with translocation of bacteria (Alverdy et al 1988) and impair remote immunity (Kudsk et al 1996).

Recent controlled trials (Table 8.6) evaluating prophylactic antibiotic therapy in patients with severe pancreatitis have shown a trend in reducing morbidity and mortality. In

Table 8.6 Prospective controlled trials on prophylactic antibiotic therapy in severe pancreatitis

Author	Antibiotic regime	Number	Sepsis Pancreas	Other	Mortality
Pederzoli et al 1993	Imipenem 0.5 g 8 hourly	41	5*	6	3
	Controls	33	10*	16	4
Sainio et al 1995	Cefuroxime 4.5 g/day	30	9	21	1*
	Controls: antibiotic when clinically indicated	30	12	32	7†
Delcenserie et al 1996	Ceftazidine, amikacin, metronidazole	11	0	0	0
	Controls	12	4	3	3
Luiten et al 1995	Selective decontamination	50	3	NS	11‡
	Controls	53	10	NS	18

*$p < 0.01$, †$p < 0.03$, ‡$p < 0.048$ (adjusted for Imrie score & Balthazar grade)
NS not stated

a multicentre study using imipenem (0.5 g intravenously 8 hourly for 14 days) Pederzoli et al (1993) demonstrated a significant reduction in infected pancreatic necrosis and non-pancreatic infections ($p < 0.01$). The incidence of infected necrosis in the treatment group, however, was still 36% and in those with > 50% necrosis there was no reduction in the number of patients with multi-organ failure or those requiring surgery or mortality. The higher number of patients in the subgroup with > 50% necrosis in the treatment group may have obscured a survival benefit.

A study by a Finnish group (Sainio et al 1995) using intravenous cefuroxime as prophylaxis (1.5 g three times a day from admission until clinical recovery and normalization of C-reactive protein concentration) came to a different conclusion. No difference was noted in the rate of pancreatic infection between the two groups although cefuroxime reduced infection rate due to a marked fall in the incidence of urinary tract infections. Interestingly the most common organism cultured from the urine was *Staphylococcus epidermis* which was also frequently cultured in pancreatic necrotic tissue. The benefits achieved therefore are surprising since *Staphylococcus epidermis* is not particularly sensitive to cefuroxime. The number of patients requiring surgery and mortality, however, was significantly reduced. Five of the seven deaths in the non-treated group were due to verified sepsis, three of whom had proven pancreatic sepsis. The reduction of mortality also became more significant considering that an appreciable number of patients in the non-treatment group received antibiotics during the course of the study. The authors concluded that cefuroxime given early in necrotizing pancreatitis is beneficial and may reduce mortality, probably by decreasing the frequency of sepsis.

A randomized study from France (Delcenserie et al 1996) which included only 23 patients in which the treated group received ceftazidine, amikacin and metronidazole for 10 days, showed a remarkably lower sepsis rate when compared to controls. This however did not translate into a reduction in mortality.

On the assumption that selective gut decontamination prevents translocation of gut organisms a Dutch group (Luiten et al 1995) compared a comprehensive oral antimicrobial regime of coliston, amphotericin and norfloxacin combined with intravenous cefotaxime to a control group who received antibiotics only when there was concurrent infection. This is the largest randomized study reported to date and included 103 patients with severe pancreatitis determined by multiple laboratory criteria (Imrie score) and contrast enhanced computed tomography using the Balthazar grading system. While the overall mortality was not significantly reduced (22% treated group; 35% controls), deaths due to gram-negative pancreatic sepsis was substantially

reduced. Also, when allowing for differences in disease severity, multivariate analysis suggested a significant survival benefit following gut decontamination. There was no difference in the number of patients requiring surgery although more laparotomies were performed per patient in the control group. As in the Finnish study (Sainio et al 1995) the results in this trial should be interpreted with caution because an unspecified number of patients in the control group received antibiotic therapy at some stage of the disease.

There is still insufficient data to indicate which antibiotic is the best for the prevention of sepsis. Results of a recent randomized study would seem to favour imipenem over peflexacin despite the fact that the latter has a better pancreatic tissue penetration and a wider spectrum of action (Bassi et al 1998).

The difficulties in performing randomized trials in this complex disease should not be underestimated. The number of eligible patients are small and there are many confounding variables which may influence the outcome. The need for therapeutic antibiotics at various stages of the disease also clouds the outcome of these studies. The case for the routine use of prophylactic antibiotics in severe pancreatitis rests at best on retrospective observations of reduction in infections in units which have changed to a liberal antibiotic policy (Ho & Frey 1997) and the favourable trends in small randomized studies (Pederzoli et al 1993, Luiten et al 1995, Sainio et al 1995, Delcenserie et al 1996). Larger randomized trials will be required to convince the sceptics (Barie 1996, Banks 1997) especially when considering that drug resistant pathogens are a major problem in many intensive care units. Such studies will be difficult to mount as it has been calculated that to show a clear benefit each study will require over 300 patients. Accrual to clinical trials is likely to be slow as most clinical practices routinely use antibiotic prophylaxis (Powell et al 1998).

Treatment

Surgical treatment in severe pancreatitis is largely governed by the nature and extent of the necrotic process. Total necrosis of the pancreas is rare but areas of focal necrosis are not infrequently encountered. Damage to the main pancreatic duct is common in these cases, and may be responsible for continuing necrosis and sepsis (Baron et al 1996, Kozarek 1996). More commonly the necrosis is extra-pancreatic with preservation of the central core of the gland (Nordback et al 1985, Bradley 1993). In severe cases the necrosis may extend along the entire retroperitoneal space and mesentery of small and large bowel.

Differences between infected necrosis and pancreatic abscess have also been emphasized (Bittner et al 1987,

Bradley 1993). Pancreatic abscess is defined as a circumscribed intra-abdominal collection of pus, closely associated to the pancreas and containing little necrotic material. Generally pancreatic abscesses occur later than infected necrosis, usually > 4 weeks after the onset of pancreatitis. Two types of pancreatic abscesses are recognized; (a) those that occur after focal pancreatic or peripancreatic necrosis with secondary liquifaction and eventual infection and (b) secondary infection of a pancreatic pseudocyst occurring in patients with chronic pancreatitis (Lankisch & Banks 1998). Compared with infected necrosis, pancreatic abscesses are seen after less severe attacks of pancreatitis and have a lower mortality (Bittner et al 1987). The type of organisms cultured in pancreatic abscesses is also different from infected necrosis and tends to be polymicrobial (Widdison & Karanjia 1993). Other than prognosis, the importance of differentiating between infected necrosis and pancreatic abscess relates to differences in treatment strategy. The results of pancreatic abscesses treated by percutaneous radiological drainage or surgical drainage through a limited approach are appreciably better than in pancreatic necrosis. It must be stressed that it is not always easy to distinguish between infected necrosis and pancreatic abscess as the former may merge inperceptibly with the latter. Computerized tomography may underestimate the amount of debris within the fluid collection and in such cases the term organized pancreatic necrosis has been suggested (Baron et al 1996).

The management of infected pancreatic necrosis is more complicated. Catheter drainage is usually a temporary measure and only achieves effective drainage of the fluid component of the infected necrotizing process (Rattner et al 1992). Operation often requires extensive necrosectomy with the associated hazards of bleeding and bowel fistula. There are three conventional surgical approaches to the management of infected necrosis: (a) 'open abdomen' with packing and planned re-exploration (Davidson and Bradley III 1981, Sarr et al 1991, Bradley 1994, Bosscha et al 1998, Branum et al 1998). (b) 'closed approach' with free drainage (Warshaw and Jin 1985) and (c) closure with suitable drains allowing continuous lavage (Beger et al 1998). The two latter approaches are followed by either planned re-exploration (Sarr et al 1991) or relook on demand. Each of these approaches has strong proponents (Rau et al 1997); the open technique is regarded as an easy method to perform repeat necrosectomy (which is often necessary) while others argue that the closed technique is easier to manage (for nursing) with less risk of bowel fistula. There are also different approaches to making the abdominal incision. Those who prefer a midline incision believe that the exposure provides better access of extensive retroperitoneal necrosis and also allows easier placement of stomas, feeding tubes and drains (Urbach & Marshall 1996). The transverse subcostal incision however, may cause less respiratory compromise and is more suitable when the 'open abdomen' technique is used (Bradley 1994). Limited flank incisions with a retroperitoneal approach can be used when the infected process is localized (Fagniez et al 1989).

Strict adherence to prescribed diagnostic and treatment strategies in the individual patient is often difficult. Good clinical practise should allow flexibility in management and as such the sensible use of all available diagnostic and treatment modalities may ultimately achieve the best results. Thus rather than performing early urgent surgery, patients with proven sepsis may be best served by an initial period of supportive treatment with appropriate antibiotics followed by the placement of a CT guided percutaneous catheter when necrosis is associated with an appreciable fluid collection. Adopting this approach early surgery may be deferred and lessen the need for extensive necrosectomy at a later stage. Newer approaches with limited interventional procedures such as endoscopic drainage (Baron et al 1996) or intra-operative or laparoscopic necrosectomy via the catheter drainage site hold promise but need further evaluation. These lesser procedures could be used as an adjunct to radiological drainage which has proved to be successful after open necrosectomy operations (Lee et al 1992).

The notion that sterile necrosis is a benign disease which rarely requires surgical intervention while infected necrosis should always undergo surgical necrosectomy should now be challenged. There is cumulative evidence that sterile necrosis is as lethal as infected necrosis when associated with multi-organ failure (Karimgani et al 1992, Rattner et al 1992, Rau et al 1995). Although there is no evidence yet that surgery is beneficial for sterile necrosis, few would withhold exploratory laparotomy in patients who deteriorate despite intensive supportive therapy. Warshaw & Jin (1996) have also identified a subgroup of cases with sterile necrosis who will ultimately require surgery several weeks or months later for ongoing pain, inability to eat, weight loss, recurrent hospitalization and loss of work.

PANCREATIC OPERATIONS
(see also Chs 55, 56)

Although the overall mortality of pancreatic resection has decreased to less than 5% the morbidity remains in the region of 30%. Sepsis forms a major component of postoperative complications and is mainly due to anastomotic leakage. The risk of leakage is highest at the pancreatic–intestinal anastomosis with a reported incidence ranging from 5 to 30% (Trede & Carter 1997). Despite numerous modifications of the anastomotic technique no specific method is superior and the single most important factor remains the expertise of the surgeon (Trede & Schwall 1988).

The presentation of a pancreatic leak depends on whether there is a major disruption which usually presents early with a high output fistula or a smaller leak which typically presents 5 to 10 days after the operation. In the latter the onset may be insidious with the patient making a slow recovery. The leak may remain subclinical. A high nasogastric drainage output, prolonged ileus and a low grade temperature with positive septic markers should raise the suspicion of a leak. The diagnosis of a pancreatic anastomotic leak is often under-reported, and is overlooked and diagnosed as pancreatitis or a pancreatic abscess.

COMPUTED TOMOGRAPHY (CT)

Computed tomography (CT) scan is the best investigation to delineate the nature and extent of necrosis and also allows accurate placement of drainage catheters. Percutaneous drainage is the most widely used method of draining localized peripancreatic collections and abscesses. In cases with a major leak, surgery may be required at an early stage to establish adequate drainage. At the time of re-laparotomy the surgeon has to make a critical decision whether the pancreatic stump should be removed as a life saving measure (Trede & Carter 1997). The decision is usually easy when there is a major disruption of the anastomosis particularly when the pancreatic stump is soft. Most patients will develop a prolonged ileus requiring TPN or enteral feeding via a naso-jejunal or feeding jejunostomy tube. The use of somatostatin which is reported to reduce the risk of postoperative fistulae (Büchler et al 1992a,b, Montorsi et al 1995) can be used to hasten resolution of the fistula.

The organisms cultured when sepsis occurs after pancreatic resection are invariably of gut origin. The empiric use of a broad spectrum antibiotic covering both aerobic and anaerobic bacteria is usually appropriate until culture results are obtained. Microbiological cultures demonstrate multiple bacterial growth in at least half of patients and represent a spectrum of enteric bacteria with *Escherichia coli*, *Enterococcus*, *Klebsiela* and *Pseudomonas* species dominating (Warshaw & Jin 1985). In addition, anaerobic bacteria such as *Bacteroides* and *Clostridium* species have been encountered.

CONCLUSION

An improved understanding of the defense mechanisms and pathophysiology of sepsis and multiple organ failure related to hepatobiliary and pancreatic surgery has emerged in the last two decades. The protective role of hepatic Küppfer cells, the barrier function of the gastrointestinal tract in the prevention of translocation of enteric bacteria and the products of activated macrophages are the fundamental components of the current paradigm (Reynolds et al 1998). Protocols designed to prevent the complications associated with obstructive jaundice, the introduction of early enteral feeding, appropriate antibiotic therapy and the use of selective gut decontamination have reduced the incidence of hepatobiliary infection (Nathens & Marshall 1999). The role of preoperative endoscopic biliary drainage remains controversial. Subspecialization and the establishment of multidisciplinary hepatobiliary units have had a major impact on outcome.

REFERENCES

Alexander J W, Boyce S T, Babcock G F 1990 The process of microbial translocation. Annals of Surgery 212: 496–511

Alverdy J C, Aoys E, Moss G S 1985 The effect of parenteral nutrition on gastrointestinal immunity. Annals of Surgery 202: 681–684

Alverdy J C, Aoys E, Moss G S 1988 Total parenteral nutrition promotes bacterial translocation from the gut. Surgery 104: 185–190

Andersson R, Foss A 1991 Abdominal sepsis following liver resection in the rat. Hepatogastroenterology 38: 547–549

Andersson R, Tranberg K-G, Alwmark A, Bengmark S 1989 Factors influencing the outcome of *E. coli* peritonitis in rats. Acta Chirurgica Scandinavica 55: 155–157

Andersson R, Saarela A, Tranberg K-G, Bengmark S 1990a Intraabdominal abscess formation after major liver resection. Acta Chirurgica Scandinavica 56: 707–710

Andersson R, Willen R, Massa G, Tranberg K-G, Karlen B, Bengmark S 1990b Effect of bile on peritoneal morphology in *Escherichia coli* peritonitis. Scandinavian Journal of Gastroenterology 25: 405–411

Bailey M E 1976 Endotoxin, bile salts and renal function in obstructive jaundice. British Journal of Surgery 63: 774–778

Banks P A 1997 Practice guidelines in acute pancreatitis. American Journal of Gastroenterology 92: 377–386

Barie P S 1996 A critical review of antibiotic prophylaxis in severe acute pancreatitis. American Journal of Surgery 172: 38–43

Baron T H, Thaggard W G, Morgan D E, Stanley R J 1996 Endoscopic therapy or organized pancreatic necrosis. Gastroenterology 111: 755–764

Batt R M, Carter M W, Peters T J 1984 Biochemical changes in the jejunal mucosa of dogs with a naturally occurring enteropathy associated with bacterial overgrowth. Gut 25: 816–823

Bassi C, Falconi M, Talamini G, Uomo G 1998 Controlled clinical trial of pefloxacin versus imipenem in severe acute pancreatitis. Gastroenterology 115: 1513–1517

Beger H G, Bittner R, Block S, Büchler M 1986 Bacterial contamination of pancreatic necrosis. A prospective clinical study. Gastroenterology 91: 433–438

Beger H G, Büchler M, Bittner R, Block S, Nevalinen T, Roscher R 1998

Necrosectomy and postoperative local lavage in necrotizing pancreatitis. British Journal of Surgery 75: 207–212

Bismuth H, Nakache R, Diamond T 1992 Management strategies in resection for hilar cholangiocarcinoma. Annals of Surgery 215: 31–38

Bittner R, Block S, Büchler M, Beger H G 1987 Pancreatic abscess and infected pancreatic necrosis. Different local septic complications in acute pancreatitis. Digestive Diseases and Sciences 1082–1087

Bjarnason I, MacPherson A, Hollander D 1995 Intestinal permeability: an overview. Gastroenterology 108: 1566–1581

Block S, Maier W, Bittner R, Buchler M, Malfertheimer P, Beger H G 1986 Identification of pancreas necrosis in severe acute pancreatitis: Imaging procedures versus clinical staging. Gut 27: 1035–1042

Borghi A F, Petrino R, Vargoni A, Fronticelli C M, Gentilli S 1991 Modifications of the trophism of intestinal mucosa after intestinal and bilio-pancreatic diversion in the rat. Italian Journal of Gastroenterology 23: 202–207

Bornman P C and Krige J E J 1997 Surgical palliation of pancreatic and periampullary tumours. In: Trede M, Carter DC (eds) Surgery of the Pancreas 2nd edn. Churchill Livingstone, London, pp 533–550

Bosscha K, Hulstaert P F, Hennipman A, Visser M R, Gooszen H G et al 1998 Fulminant acute pancreatitis and infected necrosis: Results of open management of the abdomen and 'planned' reoperations. Journal of the American College of Surgeons 187: 255–262

Bradley E L. 1989 Antibiotics in acute pancreatitis. Current status and future directions. American Journal of Surgery 158: 472–478

Bradley E L, Allen K 1991 A prospective longitudinal study of observation versus surgical intervention in the management of necrotizing pancreatitis. American Journal of Surgery 161: 19–25

Bradley E L, III 1993 A clinically based classification system for acute pancreatitis. Summary of the International Symposium on Acute Pancreatitis, Atlanta GA, September 1992. Archives of Surgery 128: 586–590

Bradley E L, III 1994 Surgical indications and techniques in necrotising pancreatitis. In: Bradley EL (ed) Acute pancreatitis: diagnosis and therapy. Raven, New York, pp 105–117

Brancatisano R, Isla A, Habib N 1998 Is radical hepatic surgery safe? American Journal of Surgery 175: 161–163

Branum G, Galloway J, Hirchowitz W, Fendley M, Hunter J 1998 Pancreatic necrosis: results of necrosectomy, packing and ultimate closure over drains. Annals of Surgery 227: 870–877

Büchler M, Malfertheimer P, Schoetensack C, Uhl W, Beger H G 1986 Sensitivity of antiproteases, complement factors and c-reactive protein in detecting pancreatic necrosis. Results of a prospective clinical trial. International Journal of Pancreatology 1: 227–235

Büchler M, Malfertheimer P, Friess H, Isenmann R, Vaneke E, Grimm H 1992a Human pancreatic tissue concentration of bactericidal antibiotics. Gastroenterology 103: 1902–1908

Büchler M, Friess H, Klempa I 1992b. Role of octreotide in the prevention of post-operative complications following pancreatic resection. American Journal of Surgery 163: 125–134

Cahill C J, Pain I H, Bailey M E 1987 Bile salts, endotoxin and renal function in obstructive jaundice. Surgery, Gynecology and Obstetrics 165: 519–522

Claesson B E B, Holmiund D E W, Matzsch T W 1986 Microflora of the gallbladder related to duration of acute cholecystitis. Surgery, Gynecology and Obstetrics 162: 531–535

Clements W D B, Halliday M I, McCaigue M, Barclay R J, Rowlands B J 1993a Effects of extrahepatic obstructive jaundice on Küpffer cell clearance capacity. Archives of Surgery 128: 200–205

Clements W D B, Diamond T, McCrory D C, Rowlands B J 1993b Biliary drainage in obstructive jaundice: experimental and clinical aspects. British Journal of Surgery 80: 834–842

Clements W D B, McCaigue M, Erwin P, Halliday I, Rowlands B J 1996 Biliary decompression promotes Küpffer cell recovery in obstructive jaundice. Gut 38: 925–931

Dahlgren U I H, Svanvik J, Svanborg-Eden C 1986 Antibodies to Escherichia coli and anti-adhesive activity impaired serum, hepatic and gallbladder bile samples. Scandinavian Journal of Immunology 24: 251–260

Davidson E D and Bradley E L III 1981 'Marsupialization' in the treatment of pancreatic abscess. Surgery 89: 252–256

Deitch E A, Sittig K, Ma L, Berg R, Specian R D 1990 Obstructive jaundice promotes bacterial translocation from the gut. American Journal of Surgery 159: 79–84

Delcenserie R, Yzet T, Ducroix J P 1996 Prophylactic antibiotic in treatment of severe acute alcoholic pancreatitis. Pancreas 13: 198–201

Doty J E, Pitt H A 1986 Management of empyema of the gallbladder. Infections in Surgery 5: 271–297

Ekberg H, Tranberg K-G, Andersson R, Jeppsson B, Bengmark S 1986 Major liver resection: perioperative course and management. Surgery 100: 1–7

Fagniez P L, Rotman N, Kracht M 1989 Direct retroperitoneal approach to necrosis in severe acute pancreatitis. British Journal of Surgery 76: 264–267

Finch W T, Sawyers J L, Schenker S 1976 A prospective study to determine the efficacy of antibiotics in acute pancreatitis. Annals of Surgery 183: 667–671

Finch M D, Crosbie J L, Currie E, Garden O J 1998 An 8-year experience of hepatic resection: indications and outcome. British Journal of Surgery 85: 315–319

Foitzik T, Fernandez-del Castiuo C, Ferraro M J, Mithofer K, Rattner D W, Warshaw A L 1995 Pathogenesis and prevention of early pancreatic infection in experimental acute necrotizing pancreatitis. Annals of Surgery 222: 179–185

Fong Y, Brennan M F, Brown K, Heffernan N, Blumgart L H 1996 Drainage is unnecessary after elective liver resection. The American Journal of Surgery 171: 158–162

Fong Y, Brennan M F, Cohen A M, Herrernan N, Freiman A, Blumgart L H 1997 Liver resection in the elderly. British Journal of Surgery 84: 1386–1390

Fortner J G, Rinser R M 1990 Hepatic resection in the elderly. Annals of Surgery 211: 141–145

Fortner J G, Kim D K, MacLean B J 1978 Major hepatic resection for neoplasia: personal experience in 108 patients. Annals of Surgery 188: 363–371

Gerzof S G, Banks P A, Robbins A H, Johnson W C, Spechler S J, Wetzner S M et al 1987 Early diagnosis of pancreatic infection by computed tomography-guided aspiration. Gastroenterology 93: 1315–1320

Gianotti L, Solomonkin J S, Munda R, Alexander J W 1995 Failure of local and systemic bacterial clearance in rates with acute pancreatitis. Pancreas 10: 78–84

Gouma D J, Coelho J C U, Schlegel J F, Li Y F, Moody F G 1987 The effect of preoperative internal and external biliary drainage on mortality of jaundiced rats. Archives of Surgery 122: 731–733

Grant M D, Jones R C, Wilson S E 1992 Single-dose cephalosporine prophylaxis in high-risk patients undergoing surgical treatment of the biliary tract. Surgery, Gynecology and Obstetrics 174: 347–354

Hatfield A R W, Terblanche J, Fataar S, Kernoff L, Tobias R, Girdwood A H, Harries-Jones P, Marks I N 1982 Preoperative external biliary drainage in obstructive jaundice. The Lancet ii: 896–898

Herndon D N, Ziegler S T 1993 Bacterial translocation after thermal injury. Critical Care Medicine 21: S50–S54

Hochwald S N, Burke E C, Jarnagin W R, Fong Y, Blumgart L H 1999 Preoperative biliary stenting is associated with increased post-operative infectious complications in proximal cholangiocarcinoma. Archives of Surgery (in press)

Ho H S and Frey C F 1997 The role of antibiotic prophylaxis in severe acute pancreatitis. Archives of Surgery 132: 487–493

Hollands M J, Little J M 1989 Perihepatic packing: its role in the management of liver trauma. Australian and New Zealand Journal of Surgery 59: 21–24

Howes R, Zuidema G D, Cameron J L 1975 Evaluation of prophylactic antibiotics in acute pancreatitis. Journal of Surgical Research 18: 197–200

Isenmann R and Büchler M W 1994 Infection and acute pancreatitis. British Journal of Surgery 81: 1707–1708

Ivatury R R, Nallathambi M, Gundoz T 1986 Liver packing for uncontrolled haemorrhage. A reappraisal. Journal of Trauma 26: 744–753

Karimgani I, Porter K A, Langevin E, Banks P A 1992 Prognostic factors in sterile pancreatic necrosis. Gastroenterology 103: 1636–1640

Karsten T M, Allema J H, Reinders M et al 1996 Preoperative biliary drainage, colonisation of bile and postoperative complications in patients with tumors of the pancreatic head: A retrospective analysis of 241 consecutive patients. European Journal of Surgery 1623: 881–888

Kimmings A N, Sander J H van Deventer, Obertop H, Rauws E A J, Gouma D J 1995 Inflammatory and immunologic effects of obstructive jaundice: pathogenesis and treatment. Journal of the American College of Surgeons 181: 567–576

Kozarek R A 1996 Endotherapy for organized pancreatic necrosis: Perspective on skunk-poking. Gastroenterology 111: 820–822

Krige J E J 1991 Perihepatic packing in the management of liver trauma. HPB Surgery 3: 141–144

Krige J E J, Bornman P C, Terblanche J 1992a Therapeutic perihepatic packing in complex liver trauma. British Journal of Surgery 79: 43–46

Krige J E J, Isaacs S, Stapleton G N, McNally J 1992b Prospective, randomized study comparing amoxycillin-clavulanic acid and cefamandole for the prevention of wound infection in high-risk patients undergoing elective biliary surgery. Journal of Hospital Infection (Suppl A) 33–41

Krige J E J, Bornman P C, Terblanche J 1997 Liver trauma in 446 patients. South African Journal of Surgery 35: 10–15

Kudsk K A, Li J, Regegar K B 1996 Loss of upper respiratory tract immunity with parenteral feeding. Annals of Surgery 223: 629–638

Kueppers P M, Miller T A, Chen C-Y 1993 Effect of total parenteral nutrition plus morphine on bacterial translocation in rats. Annals of Surgery 217: 286–292

Kwon A H, Inada Y, Uetsuji S, Yamamura M, Hioki K, Yamamoto M 1990 Response of fibronectin to liver regeneration after hepatectomy. Hepatology 11: 593–598

Lai E C S, Mok F P T, Fan S T, Lo C M, Chu K M, Liu C L, Wong J 1994 Preoperative endoscopic drainage for malignant obstructive jaundice. British Journal of Surgery 81: 1195–1198

Landau O, Kott I, Deutsch A A, Stelman E, Reiss R 1992 Multifactorial analysis of septic bile and septic complications in biliary surgery. World Journal of Surgery 16: 962–965

Lankisch P G, Banks P A 1998 Acute pancreatitis: Springer-Verlag, New York, pp 145–182

Laskin D L 1990 Non-parenchymal cells and hepatotoxicity. Seminars in Liver Disease 10: 293–304

Lee M J, Rattner D W, Legemate D A, Saim S, Dawson S L, Hahn P F et al 1992 Acute complicated pancreatitis: redefining the role of interventional radiology. Radiology 183: 171–174

Lee D W H, Chung S C S 1997 Biliary infection. Baillière's Clinical Gastroenterology 11: 707–724

Leung J W C, Ling T K W, Chan R C Y, Cheung S W, Lai C W, Sung J J Y, Chung S C S, Cheng A F B 1994 Antibiotics, biliary sepsis and bile duct stones. Gastrointestinal Endoscopy 40: 716–721

Lewis R T, Goodall R G, Marien B, Park M, Lloyd-Smith W, Wigand F M 1987 Biliary bacteria, antibiotic use, and wound infection in surgery of the gallbladder and common bile duct. Archives of Surgery 122: 44–47

Lipsett P A, Pitt H A 1990 Acute cholangitis. Surgical Clinics of North America 70: 1297–1312

Lise M, Bacchetti S, Da Pian P, Nitti D, Pilati P L, Pigato P 1998 Prognostic factors affecting long term outcome after liver resection for hepatocellular carcinoma. Cancer 82: 1028–1036

Luiten E J, Hop W C J, Lange J F, Bruining H A 1995 Controlled clinical trial of selective decontamination for the treatment of severe acute pancreatitis. Annals of Surgery 222: 57–65

Maluenda F, Csendes A, Burdiles P, Diaz J 1989 Bacteriological study of choledochal bile in patients with common bile duct stones, with or without acute suppurative cholangitis. HepatoGastroenterology 36: 132–135

McPherson G A D, Benjamin I S, Hodgson H J F, Bowley N B, Allison D J 1984 Preoperative percutaneous transhepatic biliary drainage: the results of a controlled trial. British Journal of Surgery 71: 371–375

Medich D S, Lee T J, Melham M F 1993 Pathogenesis of pancreatic sepsis. American Journal of Surgery 165: 46–52

Melendez J A, Arslan V, Fischer M, Wuest D, Jarnagin W R, Fong Y, Blumgart L H 1998 Perioperative outcomes of major hepatic resections under low central venous pressure anesthesia: blood loss, blood transfusion, and the risk of postoperative renal dysfunction. Journal of the American College of Surgeons 187: 620–625

Montorsi M, Zago M, Mosca F 1995 Efficacy of octreotide in the prevention of pancreatic fistula after elective pancreatic resections: a prospective, controlled randomised clinical trial: Surgery 117: 1023–1027

Nakayama T, Ekeda A, Okuda K 1978 Percutaneous transhepatic drainage of the biliary tract: Technique and results of 104 cases. Gastroenterology 74: 554–559

Nathens A B, Marshall J C 1999 Selective decontamination of the digestive tract in surgical patients. Archives of Surgery 134: 170–176

Nimura Y, Hayakawa N, Kamiya J, Kondo S, Shinoya S 1990 Hepatic segmentectomy with caudate lobe resection for bile duct carcinoma of the hepatic hilus. World Journal of Surgery 14: 535–544

Nolan I P 1981 Endotoxin, reticuloendothelial function and liver injury. Hepatology 1: 458–465

Nordback I, Pessi T, Auvinen O, Autio V 1985 Determination of necrosis in necrotizing pancreatitis. British Journal of Surgery 72: 870–877

Owens W E, Berg R D 1980 Bacterial translocation from the gastrointestinal tract of athymic (nu/nu) mice. Infection and Immunity 27: 461–467

Pace R F, Blenkhan J I, Edwards W J, Orloff M, Blumgart L H, Benjamin I S 1989 Intraabdominal sepsis after hepatic resection. Annals of Surgery 209: 302–306

Parks R W, Clements W D B, Smye M G, Pope C, Rowlands B J, Diamond T 1996 Intestinal barrier dysfunction in clinical and experimental obstructive jaundice and its reversal by internal biliary drainage. British Journal of Surgery 83: 1345–1349

Paye F, Rotman N, Radier C, Nouira R, Fagniez P L 1998 Percutaneous aspiration for bacteriological studies in patients with necrotizing pancreatitis. British Journal of Surgery 85: 755–759

Pederzoli P, Bassi C, Vesentini S, Campedelli A 1993 A randomized multicenter clinical trial of antibiotic prophylaxis of septic complications in acute necrotizing pancreatitis with imipenem. Surgery, Gynecology & Obstetrics 176: 480–483

Pitt H A, Couse N R 1990 Biliary sepsis and toxic cholangitis. In: Moody F G (ed) Surgical treatment of digestive disease, 2nd edn. Year Book Medical Publishers, Chicago, pp 332–350

Pitt H A, Gomes A S, Lois J F, Mann L L 1985 Does preoperative percutaneous biliary drainage reduce operative risk or increase hospital cost. Annals of Surgery 201: 545–553

Powell J J, Miles R, Siriwardena A K 1998 Antibiotic prophylaxis in the initial management of severe acute pancreatitis. British Journal of Surgery 85: 582–587

Ranson J H C, Balthazar E, Caccavale R, Cooper M 1985 Computed tomography and the prediction of pancreatic abscess in acute pancreatitis. Annals of Surgery 201: 656–663

Rattner D W, Legermate D A, Lee M J, Mueller P R, Warshaw A L 1992

Early surgical debridement of symptomatic pancreatic necrosis is beneficial irrespective of infection. The American Journal of Surgery 163: 105–109

Räty S, Sand J, Nordback 1998 Difference in microbes contaminating pancreatic necrosis in biliary and alcoholic pancreatitis. International Journal of Pancreatology 24: 187–191

Rau B, Pralle U, Uhl W, Schoenberg M H, Beger H G 1995 Management of sterile necrosis in instances of severe acute pancreatitis. Journal American College of Surgeons 181: 279–288

Rau B, Uhl W, Buchler M W, Beger H G 1997 Surgical treatment of infected necrosis. World Journal of Surgery 21: 155–161

Rau B, Pralle U, Mayer J M, Beger H G 1998 Role of ultrasonographically guided fine-needle aspiration cytology in the diagnosis of infected pancreatic necrosis. British Journal of Surgery 85: 170–184

Rees M, Plant G, Wells J, Bygrave S 1996 One hundred and fifty hepatic resections: evolution of technique towards bloodless surgery. British Journal of Surgery 83: 1526–1529

Rees M, Plant G, Bygrave S 1997 Late results justify resection for multiple hepatic metastases from colorectal cancer. British Journal of Surgery 84: 1136–1140

Reiss R, Eliashiv A, Deutsch A A 1982 Septic complications of bile cultures in 800 consecutive cholecystectomies. World Journal of Surgery 6: 195–199

Reynolds J V, Murchan P, Keane F B V, Taller W A 1998 Impaired gut barrier function and sepsis in experimental obstructive jaundice. Journal of the Irish College of Physicians and Surgeons 27: 94–101

Riepe S P, Goldstein J, Alpers B H 1980 Effect of secreted bactericides proteases on human intestinal brush border hydrolases. Journal of Clinical Investigation 66: 314–322

Robenek H, Herwig J, Themann H 1980 The morphologic characteristics of intracellular junctions between normal human liver cells and cells from patients with extrahepatic cholestasis. American Journal of Pathology 100: 93–114

Roberts E A, Williams R J 1979 Ampicillin concentrations in pancreatic fluid bile obtained at endoscopic retrograde cholangiopancreatography (ERCP). Scandinavian Journal of Gastroenterology 14: 669–672

Sainio V, Kemppainene E, Puolakkainen P, Taavitsainen M 1995 Early antibiotic treatment in acute necrotising pancreatitis. Lancet 346: 663–666

Sarr M G, Nagorney D M, Mucha P, Farnell M B, Johnson C D 1991 Acute necrotizing pancreatitis: management by planned, staged pancreatic necrosectomy debridement and delayed primary wound closure over drains. British Journal of Surgery 78: 576–581

Scott C M, Grassberger R C, Heeran T F, Williams L E, Hirsch E F 1988 Intraabdominal sepsis after hepatic trauma. American Journal of Surgery 155: 284–288

Scott-Connor C E H, Grogan J B 1994 The pathophysiology of biliary obstruction and its effect on phagocytic and immune function. Journal of Surgical Research 57: 316–336

Shou J, Lappin J, Minnard E A, Daly J M 1994 Total parenteral nutrition, bacterial translocation and host immune function. American Journal of Surgery 167: 145–150

Smith R C, Pooley M, George C R P, Faithful R 1984 Preoperative percutaneous transhepatic internal drainage in obstructive jaundice: a randomized controlled trial examining renal function. Surgery 96: 641–647

Steffen E, Berg R D 1983 Relationship between cecal population levels of indigenous bacteria and translocation to the mesenteric lymph nodes. Infection and Immunity 39: 1252–1259

Stewart L, Pellegrini C A, Way L W 1986 Antibacterial activity of bile acids against common biliary tract organisms. Surgical Forum 37: 157–159

Strong R W, Lynch S V, Wall D R, Ong T H 1994 The safety of elective liver resection in a special unit. Australian and New Zealand Journal of Surgery 64: 530–534

Sung J Y, Shaffer E A, Olson M E, Leung J W C, Lam K, Costerton J W 1991 Bacterial invasion of the biliary system by way of the portal-venous system. Hepatology 14: 313–317

Sung J Y, Costerton J W, Shaffer E A 1992a Defense system in the biliary tract against baterial infection. Digestive Diseases and Sciences 37: 689–696

Sung J Y, Leung J W C, Shaffer E A, Lam K, Olson M E, Costerton J W 1992b Ascending infection of the biliary tract after surgical sphincterotomy and biliary stenting. Journal of Gastroenterology and Hepatology 7: 240–245

Sung J Y, Shaffer E A, Costerton J W 1993 Antibacterial activity of bile salts against common biliary pathogens. Effects of hydrophobicity of the molecule and in the presence of phospholipids. Digestive Diseases and Sciences 38: 2104–2112

Tenner S, Sica G, Hughes M, Noordhoek E, Feng S 1997 Relationship of necrosis to organ failure in severe acute pancreatitis. Gastroenterology 113: 899–903

Thompson J E, Bennion R S, Doty J E, Muller E I L, Pitt H A 1990 Predictive factors for bactibilia in acute cholecystitis. Archives of Surgery 125: 261–264

Thompson J E, Bennion R S, Pitt H A 1994 An analysis of infectious failures in acute cholangitis. HPB Surgery 8: 139–144

Tokay R, Ziegler S T, Traber D L 1993 Postburn gastrointestinal vasoconstriction increases bacterial and endotoxin translocation. Journal of Applied Physiology 74: 1521–1527

Trede M, Schwall G 1988 The complications of pancreatectomy. Annals of Surgery 207: 39–47

Trede M, Carter D C 1997 The complications of pancreatoduodenectomy and their management. In: Trede M, Carter D C (eds) Surgery of the pancreas 2nd edn. Churchill Livingstone, pp 675–691

Trudel J L, Wittnich C, Brown R A 1994 Antibiotic bio-availability in acute experimental pancreatitis. Journal of the American College of Surgeons 178: 475–479

Tsao J I, Loftuf J P, Nagorney D M, Adson M A, Ilstrup D M 1994 Trends in morbidity and mortality of hepatic resection for malignancy. A matched comparative analysis. Annals of Surgery 220: 199–205

Urbach D R and Marshall J C 1996 Pancreatic abscess and infected pancreatic necrosis. Current Opinions in Surgical Infections 4: 57–66

Van den Hazel S J, Speelman P, Tytgat G N J, Dankert J, van Leeuwen D J 1994a The pathogenesis of bacterial cholangitis. European Journal of Gastroenterology and Hepatology 6: 1053–1057

Van den Hazel S J, Speelman P, Tytgat G N J, Dankert J, van Leeuwen D J 1994b Role of antibiotics in the treatment and prevention of acute and recurrent cholangitis. Clinical Infectious Diseases 19: 279–286

Vo N M, Chi D S 1988 Effect of hepatectomy on the reticuloendothelial system of septic rats. Journal of Trauma 28: 852–854

Wang X D, Andersson R, Soltesz V, Bengmark S 1992 Bacterial translocation after major hepatectomy in patients and rats. Archives of Surgery 127: 1101–1106

Wang X D, Andersson R, Ding J, Norgren L, Bengmark S 1993a Reticuloendothelial system function following acute liver failure induced by 90% hepatectomy in the rat. HPB Surgery 6: 151–162

Wang X D, Ar'Rajab A, Andersson R 1993b The influence of surgically induced acute liver failure on the intestine in the rat. Scandinavian Journal of Gastroenterology 28: 31–40

Warshaw A L, Jin G 1985 Improved survival in 43 patients with pancreatic abscess. Annals of Surgery 202: 408–415

Well C L, Maddaus M A, Simmons R L 1988 Proposed mechanisms for the translocation of intestinal bacteria. Reviews of Infectious Diseases 10: 958–979

Wells G R, Taylor E W, Lindsay G, Morton L 1989 Relationship between bile colonisation, high-risk factors and postoperative sepsis in patients undergoing biliary tract operations while receiving a prophylactic antibiotic. British Journal of Surgery 76: 374–377

Whipple A O, Parsons W B, Mullins C R 1935 Treatment of carcinoma of the ampulla of Vater. Annals of Surgery 102: 763–779

Widdison A L and Karanjia N D 1993 Pancreatic infection complicating acute pancreatitis. British Journal of Surgery 80: 148–154

Widdison A L, Karanija N D, Reber H A 1994 Routes of spread of pathogens into the pancreas in a feline model of acute pancreatitis. Gut 36: 1306–1310

Wigmore S J, Plester C G, Ross J A, Fearon K C H 1997 Contribution of anorexia and hypermetabolism to weight loss in anicteric patients with pancreatic cancer. British Journal of Surgery 84: 196–197

Wilton P B, Daimasso A P, O'Connor Allen M 1987 Complement in local biliary tract defense: dissociation between bile complement and acute phase reactants in cholecystitis. Journal of Surgical Research 42: 434–439

Yanaga K, Kanematsu T, Sugimachi K, Takenaka K 1986 Intraperitoneal septic complications after hepatectomy. Annals of Surgery 203: 148–152

Yu J L, Andersson R, Ljungh A 1996 Infections associated with biliary drains. Scandinavian Journal of Gastroenterology 31: 625–630

Endotoxin and cytokines in liver and biliary tract disease

9

L.L. MOLDAWER

INTRODUCTION

In this chapter, the role endotoxin and proinflammatory cytokines play in the normal physiology and the pathophysiology of the liver and biliary tract are reviewed, with special reference to surgical practice. The field has moved explosively in the past three years, and there have been several key discoveries, which are directly salient to this review and to surgical practice. The putative signal transduction protein of the endotoxin receptor has been recently identified (Toll-like receptor (TLR) 2), and novel roles for cytokines such as interleukin-6 (IL-6), tumor necrosis factor α (TNFα) and Fas ligand in normal liver physiology and pathophysiology have been identified. More importantly, anti-cytokine and cytokine therapies have begun to enter clinical trials as adjunct therapies for chronic hepatitis, obstructive jaundice, and hepatic regeneration. This review will focus primarily on several new advances in our understanding of the role played by endotoxin and cytokines in normal liver physiology, and in the response to surgical injury, viral infections and chronic liver and bile duct inflammation.

ENDOTOXIN—STRUCTURE AND BIOLOGICAL ACTIVITY

It has been known for at least a century that endotoxin, or its purified lipopolysaccharide, has a wide range of harmful biological activities when introduced into vertebrates (for review see Zivot and Hoffman, 1995). However, it has only been in the past decade that research has begun to elucidate the mechanisms by which the host recognizes endotoxin, and the innate immune responses that ensue. Although endotoxin has been implicated in both the beneficial and injurious host responses to Gram negative infections, the exact role of endotoxin in the pathogenesis of human disease remains uncertain. Furthermore, similarities in host responses to endotoxin, and to bacterial exotoxins, or the glycoconjugates of Gram positive bacterial and fungal infections suggest that the host innate immune system has evolved to respond consistently to microbial invasion, regardless of its antigenic source (Fearon and Locksley, 1996).

Endotoxin is the major constituent of the outer cell wall of Gram negative bacteria, and can comprise up to 65% by weight of the total bacterium. Endotoxin is shed spontaneously from the cell walls of living bacteria, and is released in copious amounts upon cell death and cell lysis. Endotoxin is comprised of three major components comprising an inner lipid A, an intermediate R-core oligosaccharide and an outer O-polysaccharide (Figure 9.1). The inner lipid A portion is generally conserved, whereas the structure of the O-polysaccharide is unique for each strain of bacteria, and represents the primary immunogenic 'O' antigen. There is often less variability in the 'R'-core oligosaccharide which is exposed in rough forms of Gram negative bacteria and is often conserved. The internal lipid A moiety is poorly antigenic, but appears to possess the toxic properties of endotoxin. Binding of endotoxin to serum proteins and its activation of host immunity through its cellular receptor(s) is mediated predominantly via the lipid A moiety (Ulevitch and Tobias, 1999; Raetz et al. 1991).

The host response to endotoxin is immediate (within minutes), dose dependent, and affects all organ and tissue systems (Table 9.1). It is in general difficult to make general statements regarding the nature of the host responses to endotoxin, in part because of differences in endotoxin sensitivity by various species, the bacterial sources of endotoxin and their method of purification, the route of endotoxin administration, and the prior immunological status of the host which may lead to either the development of tolerance, or to priming. High dose administration of endotoxin in rodents and primates reproduces the toxic effects of Gram negative bacteria administration, characterized by hemodynamic collapse, shock, organ failure and death (Fischer et al. 1991; Beutler et al. 1985). Low dose administration of endotoxin, as has been frequently conducted in human volunteers (Fong et al. 1990; Michie et al. 1988), produces a variety of constitutional responses consistent with a mild infectious process, including fever, myalgia, tachycardia, occasional hypotension, transient leukopenia followed by

---

Table 9.1 Biological actions of endotoxin

Fever
- direct effect on hypothalamus, via prostaglandins
- indirect effect mediated by local IL-1 and IL-6 production.

Hemodynamic effects
- vasoconstriction
  - direct effect
  - secondary sympathetic neurogenic activity
  - indirectly by catecholamine and prostaglandin release
- vasodilatation
  - secondary to tissue hypoperfusion caused by vasoconstriction, endothelial injury and reduced cardiac output
  - indirectly caused by complement activation, neutrophil degranulation, prostacyclin and prostaglandin release, nitric oxide production
  - produces pooling of blood in pulmonary and splanchnic vascular beds with hypotensive shock

Endothelial cell injury
- probable direct cell membrane damage by endotoxin at high concentrations
- prostaglandins, prostacyclin, procoagulants (e.g. tissue factor, factor V) and plasminogen activator inhibitor-1 (PAI-1) release upregulation of adherence molecules with neutrophil adherence
- indirectly through TNFα release

Intravascular coagulation
- direct activation of the intrinsic and extrinsic pathways
- indirectly by release of tissue factor from monocytes and endothelial cells

Complement activation (antibody-independent)
- classical pathway activation (lipid A)
- alternative pathway activation (polysaccharide, fraction)

White blood cell effects
- transient leucocytopenia followed by leukocytosis, primarily a neutrophilia
- sustained monocytopenia and lymphopenia
- direct and indirect neutrophil activation and cytokine release including tumor necrosis factor α (TNFα), interleukins 1-α, 1-β, 6 and 8, colony stimulating factors (CSF), platelet activating factor (PAF), procoagulants, prostanoids and leukotrienes

Platelet effects
- platelet aggregation and release of active constituents, direct effect of endotoxin and indirectly by release of platelet activating factor (PAF) from monocytes/macrophages
- thrombocytopenia, probably secondary to platelet aggregation and intravascular coagulation

Activation of reticulo-endothelial system
- direct effect on tissue macrophages with release of secondary inflammatory mediators
- indirectly by proinflammatory cytokine release

Immunological effects
- specific B cell antibody response to endotoxin antigens especially potent 'O' antigen
- nonspecific polyclonal B cell stimulation, indirectly by cytokines in response to IL-6, IL-11 release
- T cell/macrophage regulation of antibody responses
- B cells release of colony stimulating factors (CSF)

Endocrine and metabolic responses
- increased resting energy expenditure
- increased plasma growth hormone, ACTH, and cortisol
- increased lipolysis with raised plasma free fatty acid levels
- alterations in carbohydrate metabolism, increased gluconeogenesis, glycogenolysis
- decreased albumin synthesis, increased acute phase response protein production mediated by IL-6, and to a lesser extent, TNFα and IL-1

Organ specific injury
- primarily lung, liver and kidney
- secondary to microvascular effects and secondary cytokine release by infiltrating inflammatory cells.

Table 9.1 Biological responses to low dose endotoxin in human volunteers

Constitutional responses[1]	*Hemodynamic responses*
Fever (38°–39°C)	Tachycardia (90–105 beats/min)[2]
headache	Transient hypertension (increasing to 90–100 mmHg)[1]
chills	
myalgia,	*Leukocyte responses*
photophobia	Transient neutropenia (<2000 cells/μL)[1]
nausea, vomiting	Sustained delayed neutrophilia (>8000 cells/μL)[3]
	Sustained lymphopenia and monocytopenia[3]
Cytokine/hormone responses	*Metabolic responses*
TNFα (50–200 pg/ml)[1]	Resting energy expenditure (20% increase)[1]
IL-6 (100–500 pg/ml)[1]	Increased FFA concentration and appearance
IL-1ra (100 ng/ml)[3]	Increased amino acid release and splanchnic uptake
sTNFR (5–10 ng/ml)[3]	Increased whole body and skeletal muscle protein
ACTH (80–120 pg/ml)[1]	breakdown
Cortisol (350–500 ng/ml)[2]	Increased gluconeogenesis and glucose oxidation
Epinephrine (50–60 pg/ml)[1]	
Norepinephrine (375–450 pg/ml)[1]	

From Fong et al. 1990 and Van Zee et al. 1992
[1] of four hours or less duration
[2] of six to 12 hours duration
[3] of six to 24 hours duration

neutrophilia, and a hepatic acute phase response (Table 9.2).

Because of the wide range of biological activities associated with endotoxin administration, it has often been difficult to separate the direct and indirect effects of endotoxin on host responses. Although the host responses to endotoxin are likely to be dose-dependent, there is growing appreciation that a large number of the phenomena associated with systemic endotoxin administration are probably secondary to the host innate immune response, and are not due to direct interactions between endotoxin and cell membranes or secretory proteins (Ulevitch and Tobias, 1999; Fearon and Locksley, 1996). Endotoxin may activate complement directly, however, both through the classical and alternative pathways, and at high doses may produce direct endothelial injury. But there is growing appreciation that the majority of host responses to endotoxin are not mediated directly, but through the release of humoral factors, including proinflammatory cytokines.

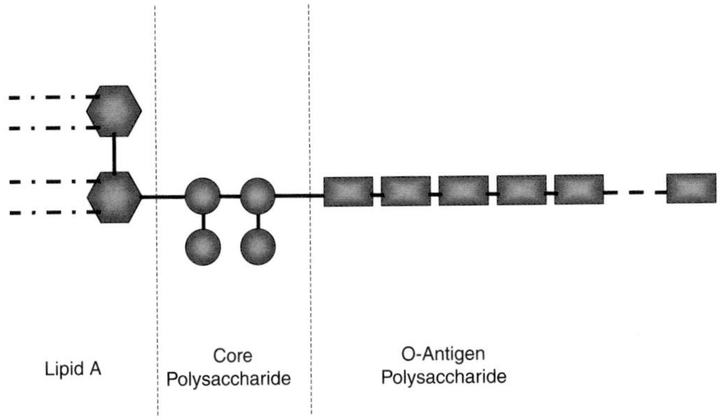

ENDOTOXIN BINDING PROTEINS AND SIGNAL TRANSDUCTION

The presence of endotoxin in biological fluids is detected readily by the innate immune system. This detection process of microbial cell products represents the first line of defense against microbial invasion (Fearon and Locksley, 1996). Picogram per ml concentrations of endotoxin in the plasma will elicit profound biological responses in mammals. The presence of endotoxin in the plasma and lymphatic system is initially recognized by serum proteins and lipoproteins which initiates their recognition and activation by the innate immune response.

Although the chemical structure of endotoxin has been known for several decades, the molecular basis for this recognition of endotoxin by the innate immune system has only begun to be resolved in the past few years (Ulevitch and Tobias, 1999; Ulevitch, 1993). The innate immune system relies on cell surface receptors and hepatic secretory proteins, primarily opsonins, to recognize carbohydrate, but also lipid, protein and DNA structures indicative of a microbial infection. The first step in the recognition of endotoxin by the innate immune system is its binding to a hepatic secretory protein, called lipopolysaccharide binding protein or LBP (Figure 9.2). LBP is a member of a group of homologous lipid binding proteins that function as lipid transfer proteins

Lipid A   Core Polysaccharide   O-Antigen Polysaccharide

Fig. 9.1 Schematic representation of the structure of endotoxin.

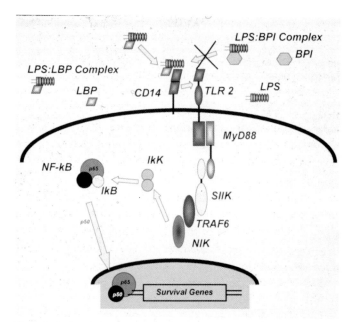

Fig. 9.2 Endotoxin binding proteins and signal transduction. Endotoxin in body fluids is rapidly recognized by endotoxin-binding proteins and lipoproteins. The balance between LBP and BPI and/or HDL determines whether endotoxin in body fluids is detected by macrophages and other effector cells of the innate immune system. LBP–endotoxin complexes bind to CD14 and interact with a TLR2 membrane protein that activates intracellular and IL-1 receptor associated kinase that transduces an NF-KB activation signal.

(Wright et al. 1989, Tobias et al. 1986, 1989). Secreted by the liver and found in human blood in 2–20 μg/ml concentrations (Calvano et al. 1994, Opal et al. 1994a), LBP binds avidly to the lipid A moiety of endotoxin and mediates its transfer to the cell surface endotoxin receptor, CD14. Although CD14 functions as a ligand binding protein for endotoxin–LBP complexes, CD14 is bound to the cell membrane through a glycosylphosphatidyl-inositol anchor and lacks an intracellular domain capable of transducing a signal. Thus, LBP–endotoxin complexes binding to CD14 are insufficient in themselves to transduce a signal.

Identification of the signal-transducing component of a CD14 bipartite complex has been recently accomplished. The putative signal transducing protein has been identified as a member of a family of *Toll*-like receptors (TLR), specifically TLR2 (Kirschning et al. 1998, Yang et al. 1998). This membrane-associated protein appears to physically interact with the CD14, LBP-endotoxin complex, and transduces a signal through a related IL-1 receptor associated kinase (IRAK), leading to NF-κB activation (Yang et al. 1999, Zhang et al. 1999). Although it is presently not known how CD14-dependent signaling is integrated from the cell surface, via TLR2, the confirmation of TLR2 as the signaling complex is important because it identifies signal transduc-

tion pathways and potential therapeutic targets. There remain several unresolved issues concerning the role played by other members of the TLR family, particularly TLR4 in endotoxin signaling. For example, endotoxin resistance in the murine C3H/HeJ strain of mice appears to be governed by a mutation in the mouse TLR4 gene, which is structurally distinct from the murine TLR2 gene (Hoshino et al. 1999).

The presence of LBP in the plasma increases the sensitivity of cells bearing CD14 to endotoxin by at least a thousand fold. From a teleological approach, this has distinct advantages. Endotoxin can be detected and innate immunity activated early in response to Gram negative infections, prior to bacterial overgrowth and colonization. However, increasing the sensitivity and the magnitude of the innate immune response to endotoxin can have devastating pathological consequences if the appearance of endotoxin is significant, as may occur during sepsis or when gastrointestinal integrity is lost. These pathological consequences include loss of vascular integrity and shock, organ failure and death. The organism has necessarily evolved several mechanisms to reduce the likelihood of an exaggerated endotoxin-induced signal, particularly after induction of the innate immune response. This latter response is aimed at modulating the magnitude and duration of the innate immune response to endotoxin.

High density lipoproteins can bind endotoxin in serum and may play a role in protecting against endotoxinemia (Cue et al. 1994, Levine et al. 1993). Administration of reconstituted HDL protects animals from experimental endotoxinemia. One additional endogenous mechanism to suppress endotoxin responsiveness is through the release of an LBP-homologous protein called 'bactericidal permeability inducing' protein, or BPI. BPI is a 55–60 kDa protein structurally similar to LBP. It binds endotoxin through its lipid A moiety, but the resulting BPI–endotoxin complexes do not bind to CD14 and transduce a signal (Elsbach, 1998). Rather, BPI acts as an endogenous endotoxin inhibitor. In addition, BPI released from activated neutrophils can bind directly to endotoxin being expressed on the surface of Gram negative bacteria and is both growth arresting and cytolytic for the bacteria.

BPI is stored in the granules of neutrophils and is released on neutrophil activation and degranulation. In the healthy adult, BPI levels in the serum are very low (15–50 ng/ml), but concentrations rise in response to an inflammatory or endotexemic challenge (Calvano et al. 1994). In contrast, LBP concentrations are several logs higher in the healthy adult (2–20 μg/ml) and increase modestly in response to inflammation. Opal and his colleagues have evaluated LBP and BPI concentrations in the plasma and the fluid from closed space infections and found that in the plasma, the ratio of LBP to BPI concentrations was nearly one thousand, and the ratio of LBP to BPI favored endotoxin signaling. However, in the closed spaces of infections infiltrated with neutrophils, BPI exceeded LBP concentrations, and BPI concentrations were directly proportional to neutrophil counts (Opal et al. 1994b). These findings suggest that in the normal healthy adult and in sepsis, the relationship between plasma LBP and BPI concentrations favors the recognition of endotoxin and activation of the innate immune response. However, in local infectious sites where neutrophil and inflammatory cell recruitment has occurred, the increased BPI response is presumably compensatory and aimed at reducing bacterial growth and the continued activation of the immune system.

Endotoxin signaling via the CD14 receptor and TLR2 involves a novel IL-1 receptor associated kinase, which activates a secondary kinase termed NIK, or NF-KB inducing kinase (Yang et al. 1999, Kirschning et al. 1998). Activation of this cascade rapidly induces the phosphorylation of additional kinases which result in NF-KB translocation and the transcription of KB dependent genes. The number of genes containing KB response elements is exceedingly large, and includes most of the proinflammatory cytokines, including tumor necrosis factor α (TNFα), interleukin (IL-)-1, IL-6, IL-8, IL-12, IL-18 and interferon γ (IFNγ) (Blackwell and Christman, 1997).

It is now recognized that the vast majority of the systemic inflammatory responses to endotoxin are mediated by the release of proinflammatory cytokines and other humoral factors, predominantly TNFα, IL-1 and IL-6, and to a lesser extent FasL (Suffredini et al. 1999, Martich et al. 1993). These proinflammatory cytokines not only globally regulate the inflammatory response to endotoxin, but also play a critical role in reprogramming the metabolic and protein synthetic responses by the liver. As will be discussed in greater detail, TNFα and IL-6 in particular play unique roles in regulating not only the hepatocyte acute phase response to endotoxin, but also in regulating hepatocyte proliferation versus apoptosis in liver regeneration (Michalopoulos and DeFrances 1997), viral hepatitis (Hayashi and Mita 1997) and toxic liver injury (McClain et al. 1999, Batey et al. 1999, Bradham et al. 1998a). FasL in contrast, is a potent inducer of hepatocyte apoptosis and has been implicated in the pathogenesis of viral hepatitis (Kondo et al. 1997, Hayashi and Mita, 1997).

Tumor necrosis factor α

TNFα is a member of a growing family of peptide mediators comprising at least fifteen cytokines (Bazzoni and Beutler 1996, Gruss and Dower 1995), including TNFβ (lympho-

toxin), Fas ligand, nerve growth factor (NGF) and CD40 ligand. With the sequencing of the human genome, additional proteins have been identified which share structural homology with TNFα and can now be classified as members of a much larger TNF superfamily, including peptides with such esoteric names as APRIL, LIGHT, TWEAK and RANKL. Although little is known about the functions of these proteins, there are several commonalities among members of this family. For example, members of the TNF superfamily are primarily homotrimeric proteins, with the exception of lymphotoxin, and exist primarily in a membrane-associated form (Bazzoni and Beutler, 1996). As a general rule, members of the TNFα family are also primarily involved in the regulation of cell proliferation and apoptosis, although several of the members, including TNFα, TNFβ, CD30L and CD40L, have proinflammatory properties .

TNFα is initially synthesized as a 26 kDa cell associated protein which is bioactive and is primarily involved in juxtacrine signaling of cytotoxicity (Kriegler et al. 1988). This 26 kDa protein is enzymatically cleaved by a matrix metalloproteinase (Moss et al. 1997, Black et al. 1997) to a 17 kDa secreted form that is released and acts in a paracrine or endocrine fashion (Figure 9.3). TNFα was characterized simultaneously as a factor that produced necrosis of tumors in vivo, and exhibited antitumor activity by inducing cell apoptosis. It has subsequently been recognized that TNFα modulates growth, differentiation, and metabolism in a variety of cell types, can produce cachexia by stimulating lipolysis and inhibiting lipoprotein lipase activity in adipocytes and stimulating hepatic lipogenesis, and can initiate apoptosis (programmed cell death) in hepatocytes and lymphoid cells (for review see Ksontini et al. 1998) (Table 9.3).

TNFα is a powerful inducer of the inflammatory response, and the inflammatory responses to TNFα are mediated both directly and through the stimulation of the expression of IL-1 and more distal proinflammatory cytokines. Secondary mediators that are known to be induced by systemically-administered TNFα are: cytokines (IL-1, IL-2, IL-4, IL-6, IL-10, IL-12, IFN-γ, TGF-β, LIF, MIF), hormones (cortisol, epinephrine, glucagon, insulin, norepinephrine), and assorted other molecules (acute-phase proteins, IL-1Ra, leukotrienes, oxygen free radicals, platelet-activating factor, prostaglandins) (Tracey and Cerami, 1996). Some of the other principle biologic effects of TNFα are listed in Table 9.3.

There is also a growing recognition that not only is TNFα involved in tissue inflammation and injury, but it also appears to be a prominent ligand for the activation of programmed cell death through apoptosis. This latter function

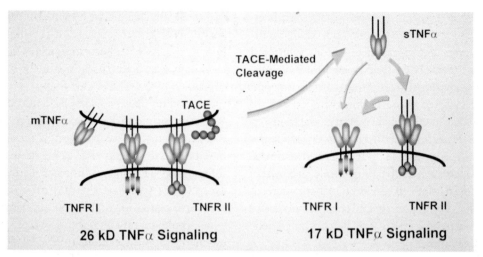

Fig. 9.3 Processing of TNFα. TNFα is initially synthesized as a 26 kDa membrane associated protein that is processed by TACE to a secreted 17 kDa homotrimer. Both cell associated and secreted molecules can bind and transduce a signal through two TNF receptors (p55, type I and p75, type II).

Table 9.3 Biological activities of TNFα

Immune cells	Non-immune cells	In vivo
Monocytes-Macrophages:	*Vascular endothelial cells:*	*CNS:*
Activate/autoinduce TNF	Modulate angiogenesis	Fever
Induce cytokines, prostaglandins	Increase permeability	Anorexia
Chemotaxis & transmigration	Antifibrinolytic/procoagulant	Altered pituitary hormone secretion
Stimulate metabolism	Suppress proliferation	
Inhibit differentiation	Rearrange cytoskeleton	*Cardiovascular:*
Suppress proliferation	Induce NO synthase	Shock
	Induce cytokines IL-1, IL-3R, G-CSF, GM-CSF	Capillary leakage
Polymorphonuclear leukocytes:	Induce prostacyclin	
Prime integrin response	Induce E-selectin, ICAM, VCAM	*Gastro-Intestinal:*
Increase phagocytic capacity		Ischemia
Enhance production of superoxide	*Fibroblasts:*	Colitis
Increase adherence to extracellular matrix	Induce proliferation	Hepatic necrosis
	Induce cytokines IL-1, IL-6, LIF	Inhibit albumin expression
	Induce metalloproteinases (MMPs)	Decrease hepatic catalase
Lymphocytes:	Suppress respiratory activity	
Induce T-cell colony formation	Inhibit collagen synthesis	*Metabolic:*
Induce superoxide in B-cells		Net lipid catabolism
Induce apoptosis in mature T-cells		Net protein catabolism
Activate cytotoxic T-cell invasiveness	*Adipocytes:*	Release stress hormone
	Enhance release of free fatty acids	Insulin resistance
	Suppress lipoprotein lipase	
		Inflammatory:
	Endocrine system:	Activate cytotoxicity
	Stimulate ACTH, prolactin	Enhance NK-cell function
	Inhibit TSH, FSH, GH	Mediate IL-2 tumor toxicity
	Enhance IL-1 inhibition of steroidogenesis	

occurs routinely during normal growth and development, but may also result from pathological conditions in which local and systemic production of TNFα is increased. Hepatocytes are particularly sensitive to TNFα induced apoptosis, especially during simultaneous transcriptional inhibition (Leist et al. 1994).

TNFα has been administered to human beings, both in low doses in human volunteers and in higher doses as part of a regional chemotherapeutic treatment plan for sarcomas and melanoma. The physiological responses to low dose TNFα administration are remarkably similar to the responses seen with low dose endotoxin administration. In human volunteers, $50\,\mu g/m^2$ of recombinant human TNFα, not unexpectedly, had profound effects. The individuals developed fevers and complained of consititutional symptoms of pain, headaches, myalgia and nausea, very similar to that seen following low dose endotoxin administration. Hematologically, the volunteers developed a rapid neutropenia followed by neutrophilia, whereas the lymphopenia and monocytopenia were sustained (van der Poll et al. 1992). Plasma IL-6 levels increased 40 fold, and the individuals developed an acute phase protein response. Prostaglandin production was markedly increased (increase in 6-ketoPGF1a) (van der Poll et al. 1991c). Metabolically, the patients exhibited increased lipolysis and glucose turnover (van der Poll et al. 1991b).

There were also significant effects on the vascular endothelium. TNFα administration induced an early activation of the fibrinolytic system within one hour, as well as activation of the coagulation system thereafter (van der Poll et al. 1991a). At much higher doses of TNFα, as are seen with the regional perfusion of limbs with cancer, the systemic release of large quantities of protein occasionally occur and the effects on the vascular endothelium are profound. Under these conditions, activation of the endothelium is evident by increased release of soluble selectins and integrins, and hemodynamic instability is often observed (Aderka et al. 1998, Zwaveling et al. 1996).

Interleukin-1

IL-1, like TNFα, is a prototypic, proinflammatory cytokine that is produced in response to endotoxin stimulation. IL-1 possesses several biological properties resulting in the increased expression of more distal proinflammatory genes. The most salient and relevant is the ability of IL-1 to initiate and sustain the expression of cyclooxygenase-type 2 (COX-2) and inducible nitric oxide (iNOS) (Dinarello, 1996). This accounts for the large amount of PGE_2 and NO produced by cells exposed to IL-1 or in animals or humans injected with IL-1. Another important proinflammatory property of IL-1 is its ability to increase IL-8 synthesis and the expression of adhesion molecules on endothelial and other cell surfaces. This property accounts for the infiltration of inflammatory and immune competent cells into the extravascular space.

There are three members of the IL-1 gene family: IL-1α, IL-1β, and IL-1 receptor antagonist (IL-1Ra). IL-1α and IL-1β are agonists and IL-1Ra is a specific receptor antagonist. The naturally occurring IL-1Ra appears to be unique in cytokine biology (Arend, 1993). The intron–exon organization of the three IL-1 genes suggests duplication of a common gene some 350 million years ago. Before this common

IL-1 gene, there may have been an ancestral gene from which acidic fibroblast growth factor (acidicFGF) evolved since IL-1 and acidFGF share significant amino acid homologies, and form an all β-pleated sheet tertiary structure. Processing of IL-1α or IL-1β to 'mature' forms of 17-kDa requires specific cellular proteases. In contrast, IL-1Ra evolved with a signal peptide and is readily transported out of the cell and termed secreted IL-1Ra (sIL-1Ra).

Even under conditions of cell stimulation, human blood monocytes do not process nor readily secrete mature IL-1α. The 31-kDa IL-1α precursor (proIL-1α) is synthesized in association with cytoskeletal structures (microtubules), which is unlike most proteins translated in the endoplasmic reticulum (Stevenson et al. 1992). ProIL-1 is fully active as a precursor (Mosley et al. 1987) and remains intracellular. The opposite is the case with the IL-1β precursor (proIL-1β) which is not fully active and a considerable amount is secreted following cleavage by a specific, intracellular cysteine protease, IL-1β converting enzyme.

Nearly all microbes and microbial products induce production of the three IL-1 family proteins but stimulants of non-microbial origin can also stimulate transcription and synthesis. Stimulants such as the complement component C5a (Schindler et al 1990), hypoxia (Ghezzi et al. 1991), adherence to surfaces (Schindler et al. 1990) or clotting of blood (Mileno et al. 1995) induce the synthesis of large amounts of IL-1 mRNA in monocytic cells without significant translation into the IL-1 protein.

Although animal experiments revealed that IL-1 was proinflammatory, a great deal of information has been learned from studies in which humans have been injected with either recombinant IL-1α or IL-1β. Humans receiving IL-1α infusions have been part of clinical trials for treating cancer or bone marrow suppression since pre-clinical studies had suggested a role for IL-1 in those conditions. The subjects were relatively stable, and although there was no reduction in tumors, faster bone marrow recovery with IL-1 treatment was reported (Smith et al. 1993). However, in patients receiving IL-1α for bone marrow stimulation, even at 30–50 ng/kg, all patients developed fever, hypotension and profound systemic, flu-like symptoms, similar to those seen after endotoxinemia (Smith et al. 1993). As can be discerned, the data provide information not available from animal studies such as myalgia and headache and loss of appetite. In addition, the exquisite sensitivity of humans to IL-1 given systemically was not appreciated from animal studies.

Interleukin-6

IL-6 is another pleiotropic cytokine produced by a wide variety of cells. It plays important roles both in regulating the innate immune response and stimulating hepatocyte proliferation. Historically, IL-6 has had several functional monikers including B cell stimulatory factor 2, interferon-β2, hepatocyte stimulating factor and 26K factor, representing its appreciable number of biological activities (Kishimoto et al. 1995). The IL-6 gene has been mapped to chromosome 7 and its product varies from 21 to 28 kDa, depending on post-translational modifications. However, IL-6 belongs to a much larger superfamily of related cytokines including leukemia inhibitory factor (LIF), oncostatin-m, ciliary neurotrophic factor (CNTF), cardiotrophin-1 and IL-11 (Taga and Kishimoto, 1997). All members of this superfamily share a modest degree of structural homology, but more importantly, all these related cytokines use a common signal transduction pathway, through gp130.

Endotoxin is a potent inducer of IL-6, although the synthesis of IL-6 appears to be more dependent upon endotoxin-induced TNFα and IL-1 synthesis, rather than by endotoxin directly (Zhang et al. 1990). The biological activities of IL-6 are numerous and can be divided into those involved in the regulation of the hematopoietic system, and those involved in activation of the innate immune response. Although IL-6 shares several biological responses with Tnfα and IL-1, IL-6 is the predominant regulator of the hepatic acute phase response, and induces hepatocyte proliferation during liver regeneration (Table 4) (Le and Vilcek 1989).

One of the more particularly interesting biological activities of IL-6 is its ability to suppress proinflammatory responses and to down-regulate TNFα, IL-1 and chemokine expression. In fact, IL-6 resists categorization as either a proinflammatory or anti-inflammatory cytokine since it possesses characteristics of both classes of cytokines. The reduction in TNFα and IL-1 synthesis in response to IL-6 is important in terms of understanding the allosteric-like regulation of TNFα and IL-1 expression, since TNFα and IL-1 are potent inducers of IL-6 expression. Pretreatment of mice with IL-6 induces survival to lethal endotoxemia, and reduces the systemic TNFα response (Yoshizawa et al. 1996, Barton and Jackson, 1993).

Many of the biological activities of IL-6 are shared by other members of the superfamily. For example, all of the cytokines have the capacity to regulate an acute phase response, but IL-11 and oncostatin M have less acute phase protein induction than IL-6 or CNTF (Taga and Kishimoto, 1997).

FasL

Fas ligand (FasL) is another member of the TNFα superfamily that is both structurally and functionally related to TNFα and other members of its superfamily. Like TNFα, FasL is synthesized and expressed first as a 40 kDa membrane associated protein, and then processed further by matrix metalloproteinases to a homotrimeric 26 kDa secreted form (Nagata and Golstein, 1995). Historically, FasL was presumed to have predominantly apoptotic inducing properties, especially for hepatocytes, and these were primarily associated with its membrane-associated form. Although it was noted that secreted FasL formed trimeric structures and retained its ability to ligate the Fas receptor, it was unclear whether soluble FasL could induce apoptosis (Schneider et al. 1998, Tanaka et al. 1995). Studies in mice in particular, suggested that the soluble forms of FasL may actually be receptor antagonists of Fas, and inhibit cell associated FasL mediated apoptosis.

The hypothesis that soluble FasL is strictly an inhibitor of Fas has recently been challenged by several groups who have reported that soluble FasL is chemotactic for neutrophils. Ottanello et al have recently demonstrated that human soluble FasL is endowed with potent chemotactic properties

Table 9.4 Overlapping biological activities of the IL-1, TNFα and IL-6

	IL-1	TNFα	IL-6
Endogenous pyrogen	Strong	Yes	Weak
Hepatic acute phase inducer	Yes	Weak	Strong
Anorexia and cachexia	Yes	Yes	Yes
Induction of the hypothalamic, pituitary, adrenal axis	Yes	Weak	Yes
Prostaglandin, nitric oxide synthesis induction	Strong	Strong	Weak
Shock producing	Yes[1]	Strong	No
NF-KB induction	Yes	Yes	No
Induction of hepatocyte apoptosis	Inhibitor	Yes[2]	No/Inhibitor
Hepatic regeneration	Weak	Strong	Strong

The terms weak and strong are relative to the other two cytokines.
[1] Shock is not irreversible with IL-1
[2] In the presence of transcriptional inhibition

for neutrophils at concentrations incapable of producing apoptosis (Ottonello et al. 1999). Furthermore, FasL did not appear to activate neutrophils, only recruit them, since neutrophil calcium flux, superoxide production, and degranulation were not affected. Other investigators have come to similar conclusions (Seino et al. 1998, Chen et al. 1998). These authors have demonstrated that these chemotactic properties are separate and distinct from the apoptosis inducing properties of FasL. The observation is significant in part because it suggests that FasL, like TNFα and other members of the superfamily, may contribute to the neutrophilic infiltration and recruitment, as part of the host inflammatory response. This is particularly relevant in viral hepatitis, where both increased FasL expression and neutrophil infiltration have been observed.

Although FasL was originally thought to be expressed only by cells of the lymphoid or myeloid lineage, including predominantly T and B cells, phagocytes and NK cells, it is now recognized that FasL can be frequently expressed by nonlymphoid cells (Liles et al. 1996) (Kiener et al. 1997). The Fas receptor, also called CD95 or Apo1, is widely expressed on a variety of cell types, including hepatocytes. The Fas receptor shares structural homology with the TNF-RI receptor (Figure 9.4). The Fas apoptotic signaling pathway, like the TNF-RI, involves activation of caspase-8 via concatemerization of FADD and TRADD. However, there has been more recent evidence that Fas signaling can also lead to proinflammatory events through the activation of NF-KB dependent pathways. NIK (NF-KB-inducing kinase), which binds to TRAF2 and stimulates NF-KB activity has been described (Malinin et al. 1997). This latter signal transduction peptide appears to be involved in both TNFα, and FasL induced pathways of NF-KB activation, and may be responsible for its chemotactic properties.

CYTOKINES AND THE LIVER

REGULATION OF CYTOKINE EXPRESSION IN THE LIVER

Cytokine production by resident cell populations in the liver contributes significantly not only to local cytokine appearance and organ homeostasis, but also to their appearance in the systemic circulation. Fong and colleagues cannulated the hepatic vein of human volunteers and examined the efflux of TNFα and IL-6 from the splanchnic bed following an intravenous endotoxin administration (Fong et al. 1990). Almost 40% of the TNFα which appeared in the systemic circulation was derived from the splanchnic bed. Not only are Kupffer

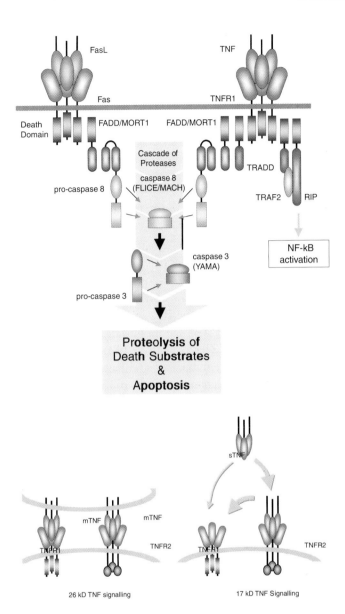

Fig. 9.4 TNF Receptor I and Fas signaling of apoptosis and NF-KB activation. TNF type I and Fas signaling share a common signal transduction pathway leading to apoptosis through caspase-8 and caspase-3. TNF type I receptor signaling leads directly to NF-KB activation through a divergent TRAF2 dependent pathway. Fas signaling can also induce NF-KB through NIK activation, but under in vivo conditions, Fas signaling is a weaker inducer of NF-KB than is TNF type I receptor.

cells a potential source of proinflammatory cytokines in the liver, but biliary epithelial cells and venous endothelial cells can make significant quantities of cytokines, especially TNFα during liver regeneration (Bradham et al. 1998b). In addition, resident and infiltrating T- and NK cells can contribute significantly to TNFα and FasL production, especially during viral-induced hepatic injury (Hayashi and Mita 1997, Fukuda et al. 1995). In fact there is some evidence that virally infected hepatocytes themselves can express TNFα directly

(Gonzalez-Amaro et al. 1994). TNFα, IL-1, IL-6 and FasL expression are all increased in the liver in response to intravenous endotoxin administration, generalized peritonitis, hepatic ischemia/reperfusion injury, infected burn injury, concanavalin A induced hepatitis, and during liver regeneration (Tannahill et al. 1999; Solorzano et al. 1997; Scotte et al. 1997; Satoh et al. 1991; Keogh et al. 1990).

Cytokines and the hepatic acute phase response

The local and systemic release of TNFα, IL-1 and IL-6 provide the increased anabolic signals to the liver to direct the increased synthesis of hepatic acute phase reactant proteins (Table 9.5). IL-1 and IL-6 in particular, act on the hypothalamic–pituitary axis to stimulate the release of corticotropin-releasing hormone, corticotropin and cortisol (Besedovsky et al. 1986, Del Rey and Besedovsky, 1992), and these serve to facilitate the mobilization of free amino acids from skeletal muscle, connective tissue and gut to the liver where amino acid uptake is enhanced. These free amino acids become the precursors for the increased protein synthesis and the altered protein synthetic pattern seen in patients with chronic inflammation, and mediated directly by IL-6, IL-1 and to a lesser extent TNFα.

These three cytokines transcriptionally suppress albumin synthesis (Hooper et al. 1981), the primary protein secretory product of the liver in the healthy adult. In fact, decreased albumin synthesis and hypoalbuminemia are well-described consequences of chronic liver disease, and the patient's plasma albumin concentration has often been predictive of adverse outcome in a variety of hospitalized patients. In addition, IL-6, IL-1 and TNFα induce the transcription of a class of heavily glycosylated secretory proteins, termed acute phase reactants. The number of acute phase reactants synthesized by the liver in response to these cytokines is quite large, and has been recently reviewed (Gabay and Kushner, 1999). As a class, the acute phase proteins have diverse biological functions, but many of these proteins are recognition molecules of the innate immune system, including C-reactive protein, MBP *(collectin)*, lipopolysaccharide binding protein, amyloid A and amyloid P (Fearon and Locksley, 1996). These proteins bind microbial polysaccharides or lipopolysaccharides and either activate complement or enhance phagocytosis. Other acute phase reactants, such as α1-antitrypsin, α1-antichymotrypsin, and tissue inhibitors of metalloproteinases (TIMPS) are protease inhibitors, while others like haptoglobin and hemopexin are antioxidants. The function of these latter two groups of acute phase reactants is to reduce local tissue damage secondary to activation of the innate immune response.

CYTOKINES AND HEPATOCYTE APOPTOSIS

Although TNFα first gained notoriety for its ability to cause necrosis of solid tumors, as well as its propensity to produce

Table 9.5 Hepatic acute phase reactant and lps recognition molecules

Molecule	Synthesis	Ligand	Function
C-reactive Protein	Hepatic acute phase reactant	Microbial polysaccharides	Complement activation, increased phagocytosis
Serum amyloid P	Hepatic acute phase reactant	Microbial cell wall polysaccharides, extra-cellular matrix proteins	Increased phagocytosis, stabilizes extracellular matrix proteins
Mannose binding protein	Hepatic secretory protein	Microbial cell wall polysaccharides	Binds collectin receptor and activates complement, increased phagocytosis
LPS binding protein	Hepatic acute phase reactant	Transfers LPS to CD14 and serum lipoproteins	Macrophage activation, enhances sensitivity to LPS
Bactericidal-permeability inducing protein (BPI)	Neutrophil granules	Binds LPS and prevents transfer to LBP/CD14	Prevents LPS induced actions
Soluble CD14	Plasma protein derived shed from monocytic cells	LPS and other microbial cell wall fragments	Enhances sensitivity to LPS, particularly in cells lacking CD14 but possessing TLR
C3	Hepatic acute phase reactant	Forms ester linkages with OH groups on proteins	Ligand attachment for CD21 and CD35

Modified from Fearon and Locksley, 1996.

endothelial injury, hypotension and shock (Beutler and Cerami, 1986), TNFα also appears to be a prominent ligand for the activation of *programmed cell death* through apoptosis.

Hepatocytes are particularly sensitive to TNFα mediated apoptosis (Leist et al. 1994) (Leist et al. 1995b). Interestingly, recent studies suggest that TNFα simultaneously invokes signaling pathways in hepatocytes that both induce and antagonize apoptosis, suggesting a delicate balance within and between TNFα signaling pathways (Beg and Baltimore, 1996) (Van et al. 1996) (Figure 9.5). Induction of TNFα's proinflammatory properties, induced in part through activation of NF-κB dependent 'survival genes', appears to directly inhibit apoptosis (Baker and Reddy, 1998). NF-κB is a ubiquitous transcription factor that plays a critical role in the cellular response to TNFα's and IL-6's signal transduction . It is comprised of two families of p50 and p65 subunits. All members of this family (NF-KB) share a conserved region of approximately 300 amino acids (Rel homology domain) important for their dimerization, nuclear translocation and DNA binding (Baeuerle, 1998). These NF-KB proteins form homo and heterodimers and their activity is modulated by interactions with inhibitory proteins of the I-κB family. Inactive NF-KB/Rel complexes bound to I-κB are located in the cytoplasm and, upon cell activation, dissociate from IkB and translocate to the nucleus where they bind the κB sites and modulate transcription of genes containing the κB sites in their promoters (Baeuerle, 1998).

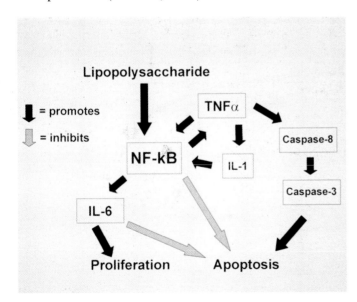

Fig. 9.5 Hepatocyte fate is determined by the balance between TNFα mediated NF-KB activation and apoptosis. TNFα signaling simultaneously activates pathways that both induce and antagonize caspase-dependent apoptosis. Drugs or agents that inhibit NF-KB activation promote apoptosis, whereas cytokines that induce NF-KB protect against TNFα mediated apoptosis.

In contrast, activation of TNFα signaling of caspase-8 and caspase-3 via TRADD/FADD leads to apoptosis through pathways shared by FasL signaling. It is the balance between these two pathways which ultimately determine whether a cell will respond to TNFα with increased proliferation, or undergo an apoptotic death (Van et al., 1996, Beg and Baltimore, 1996).

The role that specific cytokines play in the apoptotic liver injury secondary to endotoxin administration has been well characterized. Surprisingly, high dose endotoxin administration results in significant liver injury secondary to hepatocyte necrosis, although hepatocyte apoptosis is minimal (Bohlinger et al. 1996). Simultaneous inhibition of transcription, either by depleting hepatocyte nucleotides with D-galactosamine or by blocking transcription with actinomycin-D, results in 1000 fold increased sensitivity to endotoxin-induced lethality, and the hepatic injury is characterized by massive liver apoptosis (Leist et al. 1994, Leist et al. 1995b, Solorzano et al. 1997, Leist et al. 1997). The liver injury appears to be dependent primarily on TNFα expression, although FasL probably plays some contributory roles (Kondo et al. 1997). Mice lacking either TNFα or the TNF type I receptor are completely protected from endotoxin and D-galactosamine induced hepatocyte apoptosis and mortality (Leist et al. 1996, Leist et al. 1995c), whereas they are still susceptible to high dose endotoxin induced lethality (Pfeffer et al. 1993, Rothe et al. 1993). Not surprisingly, this increased apoptosis and hepatocyte injury to endotoxin can be reproduced with TNFα administration in the presence of transcriptional inhibition (Leist et al. 1995a), or by Fas agonists (Ogasawara et al. 1993). Fas agonists, like the monoclonal antibody Jo-2, apparently can induce massive hepatocyte apoptosis in the absence of transcriptional inhibition. The differential response to TNFα and FasL mediated apoptosis appears to be due to the observation that FasL is a significantly weaker inducer of NF-κB than is TNFα. IL-1 and nitric oxide protect hepatocytes from TNFα mediated apoptosis, presumably by stimulating NF-κB activation and inhibiting caspase activities (Bohlinger et al. 1995). Caspases play central roles as the 'suicide effectors' of hepatocyte apoptosis, since treatment of mice with broadacting caspase inhibitors prevent both apoptotic liver injury and mortality (Kunstle et al. 1997, Mignon et al. 1999).

ROLE OF CYTOKINES AND GROWTH FACTORS IN LIVER REGENERATION

The humoral factors, which regulate the regeneration of liver tissue after surgical injury or removal, have also been the source of significant research investigation. It has been demonstrated that humoral factors are required since hepatectomy in a rodent joined in parabiotic circulation results in proliferation and regeneration of the intact liver from the other member of the pair (Moolten and Bucher, 1967). This provides convincing evidence that some mitogenic factor or factors are released into the peritoneal or systemic circulation during liver regeneration. Studies with recombinant proteins, cytokine inhibitors and transgenic mice have now convincingly demonstrated that at least three cytokines, TNFα, IL-6 and hepatocyte growth factor, play critical roles in this regenerative process (reviewed in Michalopoulos and DeFrances, 1997). Additional cytokines, including TGFα and EGF may also play additional roles.

TNFα, in particular, appears to play a critical early role in the regenerative process. Several converging lines of evidence suggest that TNFα, and particularly its signaling through the type I receptor (p55 to p60) are essential for the regenerative process. Treatment of animals with neutralizing antibodies against TNFα delays regeneration, decreases DNA synthesis and abrogates the increases in Jun kinase, *c-jun* mRNA and nuclear AP1 activity (Yamada et al. 1997; Diehl et al. 1994). DNA synthesis is also impaired after partial hepatectomy in TNF receptor type I knockout

mice, and increases in the intracellular protein STAT3 in response to a partial hepatectomy are abrogated. Understanding whether these defects are due directly to the effects of TNFα or are mediated through TNFα-dependent IL-6 expression is not fully resolved, since treating TNF receptor type I knockout mice with exogenous IL-6 corrected this delay in regeneration.

IL-6's role in hepatic regeneration has also been clearly established. IL-6 is produced by Kupffer cells, and its secretion is stimulated by TNFα and IL-1. Plasma IL-6 concentrations increase after partial hepatectomy, peaking within 24–48 hours (Rai et al. 1996; Matsunami et al. 1992). Although it is controversial whether IL-6 is directly mitogenic for hepatocytes in culture, it is clear that IL-6 is mitogenic for biliary epithelial cells (Matsumoto et al. 1994), and the absence of IL-6 delays regeneration in vivo (Cressman et al. 1996). Hepatocyte DNA synthesis after a partial hepatectomy was suppressed in IL-6 knockout mice. Hepatocytes from these mice also failed to mount an intracellular STAT3 response, which could be corrected by injection of recombinant IL-6 (Cressman et al. 1996).

This IL-6 expression, which is required for a normal regenerative response, appears to be dependent on NF-κB translocation (Figure 9.6). It is enlightening that NF-κB dependent pathways which are required to protect hepato-

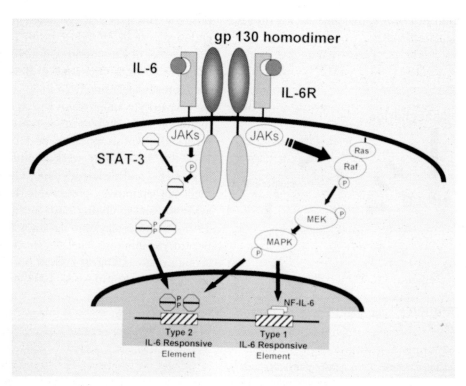

Fig. 9.6 Activation of intracellular signaling pathways during hepatic regeneration. Several pathways are activated simultaneously during hepatic regeneration. TNFα and IL-6 appear to play critical roles as signals for the induction of these pathways, and NF-KB plays a central role in the intracellular signaling.

cytes from TNFα mediated apoptosis are similar to the pathways required for the regenerative process. Evocative studies from several groups have shown that inhibition of TNFα-mediated NF-κB activation exaggerates apoptotic pathways initiated by TNFα and Fas ligand. Xu and colleagues noted that blocking NF-κB in RALA hepatocytes resulted in TNFα mediated apoptosis (Xu et al. 1998). Actinomycin D pretreatment of the same cells also promoted TNFα apoptosis, but did not prevent NF-κB translocation. Rather, actinomycin D prevented the transcription of NF-κB induced genes in response to TNFα. In addition, inhibition of NF-κB by forced overexpression of an I-κB dominant negative in the livers of mice after hepatic resection produces massive apoptosis and liver failure (Iimuro et al. 1998). Taken together, these findings suggest that blockade of NF-κB dependent transcription of 'survival genes' in hepatocytes during liver regeneration results in TNFα mediated apoptosis.

PATHOGENESIS OF ENDOTOXIN AND CYTOKINES IN LIVER AND BILIARY TRACT DISEASE

ENDOTOXEMIA AND BACTERIAL TRANSLOCATION

Bacterial translocation has been defined as the process by which viable enteric bacteria crosses the intestinal mucosal barrier to mesenteric lymph nodes and remote organs and tissues (Lemaire et al. 1997, MacFie, 1997). Since the bowel contains massive amounts of viable, pathogenic bacteria and endotoxin, several physiologic mechanisms must be disrupted for bacterial translocation to occur.

The exact mechanism(s) by which bacterial translocation occurs through the intestinal mucosa are not fully known. Electron microscopy has revealed bacteria actually penetrating epithelial cells, whereas translocation through tight junctions has not been observed (Alexander et al. 1990). Most of the bacteria are phagocytosed by macrophages, but free bacteria can be recovered from blood and lymphatics. In fact, translocation of bacteria from the gut can proceed via both the portal circulation and the lymphatics.

For bacterial translocation to occur, however, several perturbations must occur simultaneously. The presence of nonpathogenic obligate anerobic organisms, the mucosal barrier and an efficient reticuloendothelial system all act in concert to reduce the frequency of pathogenic bacterial translocation. Alterations in the composition of the gut flora due to poor nutritional status, antibiotic use, changes in bile production or intestinal stasis all predispose the patient to bacterial translocation. Similarly, drugs or diseases, which alter the integrity of the mucosal barrier, will increase the risk of bacterial translocation. For example, total parenteral nutrition which may result in gut atrophy, or direct injury secondary to hemorrhagic shock and reperfusion injury, or chemotherapeutic agents may all increase bacterial translocation. Chemotherapeutic agents may also reduce antimicrobial functions of the immune cells, and secretory IgA may be a first line of defense.

It is interesting to note that endotoxemia per se, can further promote bacterial translocation, possibly suggesting an amplification cascade. Endotoxemia frequently produces hypoperfusion of the splanchnic bed, leading to decreased perfusion of the distal ileum and cecum, and increased intestinal permeability. In mice, endotoxin administration induced bacterial translocation, which could be blocked by inhibitors of xanthine oxidase activity, suggesting an oxygen free radical component secondary to ischemia reperfusion injury (Deitch et al. 1989a, Deitch et al. 1989b, Deitch et al. 1989c). In humans, low dose endotoxin administration increases urinary excretion of orally administered D-mannitol, suggesting a reduction in gut barrier function even with modest administrations (O'Dwyer et al. 1988).

Bacterial translocation has been proposed to occur in a number of liver diseases, including obstructive jaundice, cirrhosis and portal hypertension, alcoholic hepatitis, and secondary to hepatic surgery (Campillo et al. 1999, Wang et al. 1992). Although the measurement of endotoxin in the blood of patients using the limulus lysate assay is problematic, increased appearance of endotoxin in the systemic circulation is a reproducible event. Bacterial translocation has also been implicated in pathogenesis of multisystem organ failure and sepsis in patients with liver disease. Several investigators have postulated that endotoxinemia and bacterial translocation are the 'engines' that drive the systemic inflammatory response syndrome.

Systemic endotoxemia rarely occurs in patients without liver disease or sepsis, although the portal appearance of minute amounts of endotoxin have been postulated. However, in patients with cirrhosis, alcoholic hepatitis or obstructive jaundice, systemic appearance of endotoxin has been reported in up to 70% of the patients, and increased levels frequently are associated with an adverse outcome (Hanck et al. 1998, Kimmings et al. 1995, Sheron et al. 1991, Fukui et al. 1991, Pain and Bailey 1987, Ingoldby et al. 1984). It is important to realize that the appearance of endotoxin in the systemic circulation can be the result of increased portal appearance secondary to reduced gut barrier function, as well as reduced clearance by the liver and reticuloendothelial system. One hypothesis has been that in obstructive jaundice, at least, the absence of bile secretion leads to increased portal vein endotoxemia, as internal biliary drainage and bile salts reduce the absorption of endotoxin (Kimmings et al. 1995).

The liver is the primary site of endotoxin uptake and detoxification from the blood stream. Clearance of endotoxin by the liver is greater from the portal vein than the hepatic artery. There is considerable experimental and clinical evidence to suggest that the increased systemic appearance of endotoxin seen in patients with liver and biliary tract disease is the result both of increased enteric absorption and reduced clearance from the hepatic reticuloendothelial system (Kimmings et al. 1995). Increased endotoxemia has been reported in patients with cirrhosis, acute hepatic failure, severe hepatitis B and C infections, and obstructive jaundice. In many cases, the appearance of endotoxemia in fulminant hepatic failure correlates strongly with liver disease severity, coexisting renal failure and mortality. There is a higher frequency of detecting endotoxin in the circulation of patients with cirrhosis who exhibit ascites (Ingoldby et al. 1984), renal dysfunction, and portal-caval shunting, and endotoxemia is a predictor of adverse outcome (Kimmings et al. 1995). However, endotoxin can bypass the liver directly by traversing the lymphatics. In fact, in rats subjected to a cecal ligation and puncture, endotoxin appearance in the thoracic lymph duct was several hundred fold higher than in the portal blood, suggesting that lymphatic flow may represent a significant source for the systemic circulation (Olofsson et al. 1986).

PATHOGENESIS OF PROINFLAMMATORY CYTOKINES

There is now convincing circumstantial evidence that increased TNFα and FasL-mediated apoptosis contributes to hepatocyte injury in chronic hepatitis C infections and in alcoholic hepatitis. Increased TNFα and FasL expression has been detected in liver biopsies from patients with hepatitis C infections (Larrea et al. 1996, Fukuda et al. 1995, Gonzalez-Amaro et al. 1994), presumably localized to infiltrating inflammatory cells (Kupffer, T- and NK$^+$ cells). In addition, patients with chronic hepatitis B and C often have elevated plasma TNFα concentrations, and occasionally have increased soluble Fas and FasL concentrations. Plasma concentrations of the shed TNF receptors are commonly elevated in chronic hepatitis B and C infections, and levels frequently correlate with the extent of inflammation and hepatocyte death.

Increased hepatocyte apoptosis has also been detected in livers from patients with chronic hepatitis C (Lau et al. 1998, Jiang et al. 1997). In a recent editorial, Khowdley speculated that host-driven inflammation and TNFα mediated hepatocyte injury might be the 'smoking gun' in the pathogenesis of chronic hepatitis C (Kowdley, 1999). In fact, Phase II clinical trials are currently underway with recombinant human IL-10 (a potent suppressor of TNFα synthesis) in patients with chronic hepatitis C infection who are simultaneously receiving interferon and antiviral treatments.

Similarly, plasma TNFα, IL-6 and endotoxin levels are all increased in patients with alcoholic hepatitis, and concentrations often correlate with mortality (Naveau et al. 1998, Sheron et al. 1991, Khoruts et al. 1991, Bird et al. 1990, Felver et al. 1990, McClain et al. 1986). Furthermore, peripheral blood monocytes from patients with alcoholic cirrhosis spontaneously release more TNFα and IL-6 than monocytes from healthy adults, and do so in response to ex vivo endotoxin stimulation (Schafer et al. 1995). One explanation for this increased endotoxemia and increased TNFα expression is that ethanol consumption increases the permability of the gut to bacterial products such as endotoxin, potentially inducing TNFα and FasL expression in the liver.

There have been several reports that the concentrations of TNFα, its shed receptors and IL-6 are elevated in animals and patients with obstructive jaundice (for review see Kimmings et al. 1995). In animal models of experimental biliary obstruction, increased TNF mRNA expression in the liver is increased, and plasma concentrations rise (Beierle et al. 1996). Furthermore, these animals produce more TNFα after a surgical injury than do healthy mice, and the increased production correlates with an adverse outcome (Bemelmans et al. 1993, Bemelmans et al. 1992b). In jaundiced patients with obstructive disease, elevated TNFα production by peripheral blood mononuclear cells has also been detected (Kimura et al. 1998, Puntis and Jiang, 1996a, Kakumu et al. 1990).

There is considerable controversy, however, whether the increased TNFα appearance that is seen in the circulation is biologically active, since many of the current ELISA assays detect total TNFα. The shed receptors of TNFα (p55 and p75) are natural inhibitors of TNFα bioactivity, and their concentrations also rise in patients with obstructive jaundice. Shedding of the TNF receptors may represent a protective mechanism to reduce the pathologic responses to TNFα by binding and blocking their interaction with cellular receptors (Van Zee et al. 1992). Furthermore, binding of TNFα to its shed receptor may facilitate its clearance by the kidneys (Bemelmans et al. 1994, Bemelmans et al. 1993). In mice with jaundice, the concentrations of the shed receptors are increased (Bemelmans et al. 1996), and similar findings are seen in patients with obstructive liver disease (Kimmings et al. 1995).

IL-6 concentrations are also elevated in mice with

obstructive disease (Plebani et al. 1999, Lechner et al. 1998, Bemelmans et al. 1992a). Serum IL-6 levels were also significantly higher in patients with biliary obstruction compared to control subjects (Kimura et al. 1999, Akiyama et al. 1998, Yamashiki et al. 1998, Puntis and Jiang, 1996b). In one study, serum IL-6 levels decreased significantly after drainage (Akiyama et al. 1998). Patients with elevated serum IL-6 levels were characterized by lower serum levels of total protein and albumin, higher mean age, and more frequently positive cultures of bile compared to those with lower serum IL-6 levels.

FUTURE DIRECTIONS

Although it is premature to promulgate the use of anti-endotoxin or immunoadjuvant therapies for the patient with acute and chronic liver injury, research is clearly moving in that direction. Anti-endotoxin approaches are already being used in patients with obstructive jaundice. Administration of sodium deoxycholate to patients with obstructive jaundice reduces the incidence of portal and systemic endotoxemia, presumably from its detergent effects on endotoxin and blocking endotoxin uptake (Pain et al. 1991; Pain and Bailey, 1988). Similarly, enterally administered cholestyramine, a potent endotoxin binding agent, has been shown to improve survival rates after partial hepatectomy in rodents and supporting immune responses (van et al. 1995). Even such routine procedures as bowel preparation and irrigation may reduce the number of bacteria in the gut lumen, and therefore reduce the amount of endotoxin available for absorption.

However, the greatest degree of excitement has focused on the recent availability of anti-endotoxin and anti-TNFα therapies developed by recombinant technology which are now entering the clinic for other diseases, which may be available in the near future for the patient with liver disease or injury. Two of the more attractive approaches currently under evaluation are anti-endotoxin antibodies and BPI.

Anti-endotoxin antibodies have been evaluated in patients with sepsis, generally with disappointing results (Ziegler et al. 1991). Although concerns have been raised about the neutralizing capacity and specificity of some of these antibodies (Fink, 1995), the lack of efficacy could be explained in part by the inadequate selection of patients and the timing of administration. Only a fraction of the patients receiving anti-endotoxin therapies actually were endotoxemic, and the administration of the antibody usually occurred 12–24 hours after the onset of symptomology.

An alternative approach currently in clinical trials is recombinant BPI. In human volunteers treated with low dose endotoxin, recombinant BPI administration reduced the proinflammatory cytokine responses and activation of the fibrinolytic and coagulation pathways (von der Mohlen et al. 1995). Recombinant BPI continues to be under FDA investigation for its potential use in children with meningococcal sepsis, as earlier open labeled studies suggested a significant benefit on outcome (Giroir et al. 1997). In rats subjected to a partial hepatectomy, recombinant BPI reduced liver injury and the magnitude of the inflammatory response (Kimmings et al. 1999).

A different approach has been to focus on the immunological response by blocking the actions of the proinflammatory cytokine TNFα. Either monoclonal antibodies or novel soluble TNF receptor immunoadhesins are currently in clinical trials for rheumatoid arthritis, inflammatory bowel disease, and congestive heart failure (Deswal et al. 1999; Moreland et al. 1997; Targan et al. 1997). Two, Enbrel® and Remicaid® have received FDA approval for rheumatoid arthritis and inflammatory bowel disease. Similarly, recombinant human IL-10, a potent inhibitor of TNFα synthesis, is currently in clinical trials for patients with chronic hepatitis C infection.

Several treatment modalities which offer the opportunity to interrupt the endotoxin and proinflammatory cytokine responses in liver disease remain of considerable interest. Anti-endotoxin therapies are of particular interest in obstructive jaundice and acute alcoholic hepatitis. In chronic viral hepatitis where increased TNFα and FasL mediated apoptosis are presumed to occur, enthusiasm remains for the opportunity to intervene with either immunuoadhesins or antibodies. The use of anti-inflammatory cytokines, such as IL-10, also remain a significant possibility, although the risk of added immune suppression remains a concern. However, it is clear that as our understanding of the pathogenesis of endotoxinemia in acute and chronic liver injury increases, our ability to rationally design new therapeutic interventions will increase dramatically.

REFERENCES

Aderka D, Sorkine P, Abu-Abid S et al 1998 Shedding kinetics of soluble tumor necrosis factor (TNF) receptors after systemic TNF leaking during isolated limb perfusion. Relevance to the pathophysiology of septic shock. Journal of Clinical Investigations 101: 650–659

Akiyama T, Hasegawa T, Sejima T et al 1998 Serum and bile interleukin 6 after percutaneous transhepatic cholangio-drainage. Hepatogastroenterology 45: 665–671

Alexander J W, Boyce S T, Babcock G F et al 1990 The process of microbial translocation. Annals of Surgery 212: 496–510

Arend W P 1993 Interleukin-1 receptor antagonist. Advanced Immunology 54: 167–227

Baeuerle P A 1998 IkappaB-NF-kappaB structures: at the interface of inflammation control [comment]. Cell 95: 729–731

Baker S J, Reddy E P 1998 Modulation of life and death by the TNF receptor superfamily. Oncogene 17: 3261–3270

Barton B E, Jackson J V 1993 Protective role of interleukin 6 in the lipopolysaccharide-galactosamine septic shock model. Infection and Immunity 61: 1496–1499

Batey R G, Clancy R L, Pang G T, Cao Q 1999 Alcoholic hepatitis as a T-cell mediated disorder: an hypothesis. Alcoholism, Clinical and Experimental Research 23: 1207–1209

Bazzoni F, Beutler B 1996 The tumor necrosis factor ligand and receptor families. New England Journal of Medicine 334: 1717–1723

Beg A A, Baltimore D 1996 An essential role for NF-kappaB in preventing TNF-alpha-induced cell death [see comments]. Science 274: 782–784

Beierle E A, Vauthey J N, Moldawer L L, Copeland E M 1996 Hepatic tumor necrosis factor-alpha production and distant organ dysfunction in a murine model of obstructive jaundice. American Journal of Surgery 171: 202–206

Bemelmans M H, Gouma D J, Buurman W A 1993 Influence of nephrectomy on tumor necrosis factor clearance in a murine model. Journal of Immunology 150: 2007–2017

Bemelmans M H, Gouma D J, Buurman W A 1994 Tissue distribution and clearance of soluble murine TNF receptors in mice. Cytokine. 6, 608–615

Bemelmans M H, Gouma D J, Greve J W, Buurman W A 1992a Cytokines tumor necrosis factor and interleukin-6 in experimental biliary obstruction in mice. Hepatology 15: 1132–1136

Bemelmans M H, Gouma D J, Greve J W, Buurman W A 1992b Cytokines tumor necrosis factor and interleukin-6 in experimental biliary obstructionin mice. Hepatology 15: 1132–1136

Bemelmans M H, Gouma D J, Greve J W, Buurman W A 1993 Effect of antitumour necrosis factor treatment on circulating tumour necrosis factor levels and mortality after surgery in jaundiced mice. British Journal of Surgery 80: 1055–1058

Bemelmans M H, Greve J W, Gouma D J, Buurman W A 1996 Increased concentrations of tumour necrosis factor (TNF) and soluble TNF receptors in biliary obstruction in mice; soluble TNF receptors as prognostic factors for mortality [see comments]. Gut 38: 447–453

Besedovsky H, Del Rey A, Sorkin E, Dinarello C A 1986 Immunoregulatory feedback between interleukin-1 and glucocorticoid hormones. Science 233: 652–654

Beutler B, Cerami A 1986 Cachectin and tumour necrosis factor as two sides of the same biological coin. Nature 320: 584–588

Beutler B, Milsark IW, Cerami A 1985 Passive immunization against cachectin/tumor necrosis factor protects mice from the lethal effect of endotoxin. Science 229: 869–871

Bird G L, Sheron N, Goka A K, Alexander G J, Williams R S 1990 Increased plasma tumor necrosis factor in severe alcoholic hepatitis. Annals of Internal Medicine 112: 917–920

Black R A, Ruach C T, Kozlosky C J et al 1997 A metalloproteinase disintegrin that releases tumor-necrosis factor-α from cells. Nature 385: 729–732

Blackwell T S, Christman J W 1997 The role of nuclear factor-kappa B in cytokine gene regulation. American Journal of Respiratory Cell and Molecular Biology 17: 3–9

Bohlinger I, Leist M, Barsig J, Uhlig S, Tiegs G, Wendel A 1995 Interleukin-1 and nitric oxide protect against tumor necrosis factor alpha-induced liver injury through distinct pathways. Hepatology 22: 1829–1837

Bohlinger I, Leist M, Gantner F, Angermuller S, Tiegs G, Wendel A 1996 DNA fragmentation in mouse organs during endotoxic shock. American Journal of Pathology 149: 1381–1393

Bradham C A, Plumpe J, Manns M P, Brenner D A, Trautwein C 1998a Mechanisms of hepatic toxicity. I. TNF-induced liver injury. American Journal of Physiology 275: G387–G392

Bradham C A, Plumpe J, Manns M P, Brenner D A, Trautwein C 1998b Mechanisms of hepatic toxicity. I. TNF-induced liver injury. American Journal of Physiology 275: G387–G392

Calvano S E, Thompson W A, Marra M N et al 1994 Changes in polymorphonuclear leukocyte surface and plasma bactericidal/permeability-increasing protein and plasma lipopolysaccharide binding protein during endotoxemia or sepsis. Archives of Surgery 129: 220–226

Campillo B, Pernet P, Bories P N, Richardet J P, Devanlay M, Aussel C 1999 Intestinal permeability in liver cirrhosis: relationship with severe septic complications. European Journal of Gastroenterolgy and Hepatology 11: 755–759

Chen J J, Sun Y, Nabel G J 1998 Regulation of the proinflammatory effects of Fas ligand (CD95L). Science 282: 1714–1717

Cressman D E, Greenbaum L E, DeAngelis R A et al 1996 Liver failure and defective hepatocyte regeneration in interleukin-6-deficient mice. Science 274: 1379–1383

Cue J I, DiPiro J T, Brunner L J et al 1994 Reconstituted high density lipoprotein inhibits physiologic and tumor necrosis factor alpha responses to lipopolysaccharide in rabbits. Archives of Surgery 129: 193–197

Deitch E A, Ma L, Ma W J et al 1989a Inhibition of endotoxin-induced bacterial translocation in mice. Journal of Clinical Investigations 84: 36–42

Deitch E A, Ma W J, Ma L, Berg R, Specian R D 1989b Endotoxin-induced bacterial translocation: a study of mechanisms. Surgery 106: 292–299

Deitch E A, Taylor M, Grisham M, Ma L, Bridges W, Berg R 1989c Endotoxin induces bacterial translocation and increases xanthine oxidase activity. Journal of Trauma. 29: 1679–1683

Del Rey A, Besedovsky H O 1992 Metabolic and neuroendocrine effects of pro-inflammatory cytokines. European Journal of Clinical Investigations 22 Suppl 1, 10–15

Deswal A, Bozkurt B, Seta Y 1999 Safety and efficacy of a soluble P75 tumor necrosis factor receptor (Enbrel, etanercept) in patients with advanced heart failure [see comments]. Circulation 99: 3224–3226

Diehl A M, Yin M, Fleckenstein J et al 1994 Tumor necrosis factor-alpha induces c-jun during the regenerative response to liver injury. American Journal of Physiology 267: G552–G561

Dinarello C A 1996 Biologic basis for interleukin-1 in disease. Blood 87: 2095–2147

Elsbach P 1998 The bactericidal/permeability-increasing protein (BPI) in antibacterial host defense. Journal of Leukocyte Biology 64: 14–18

Fearon D T, Locksley R M 1996 The instructive role of innate immunity in the acquired immune response. Science 272: 50–53

Felver M E, Mezey E, McGuire M et al 1990 Plasma tumor necrosis factor alpha predicts decreased long-term survival in severe alcoholic hepatitis. Alcoholism, Clinical and Experimental Research 14: 255–259

Fink M P 1995 Another negative clinical trial of a new agent for the treatment of sepsis: rethinking the process of developing adjuvant treatments for serious infections [editorial: comment]. Critical Care Medicine 23: 989

Fischer E, Marano M A, Barber A E et al 1991 Comparison between effects of interleukin-1alpha administration and sublethal endotoxemia in primates. American Journal of Physiology 261, R442–R452

Fong Y M, Marano M A, Moldawer L L et al 1990 The acute splanchnic and peripheral tissue metabolic response to endotoxin in humans. Journal of Clinical Investigations 85, 1896–1904

Fukuda R, Satoh S, Nguyen X T et al 1995 Expression rate of cytokine mRNA in the liver of chronic hepatitis C: comparison with chronic hepatitis British Journal of Gastroenterology 30: 41–47

Fukui H, Brauner B, Bode J C, Bode C 1991 Plasma endotoxin concentrations in patients with alcoholic and non-alcoholic liver disease: reevaluation with an improved chromogenic assay. Journal of Hepatology 12: 162–169

Gabay C, Kushner I 1999 Acute-phase proteins and other systemic responses to inflammation. New England Journal of Medicine 340: 448–454

Ghezzi P, Dinarello C A, Bianchi M, Rosandich M E, Repine J E, White C W 1991 Hypoxia increases production of interleukin-1 and tumor necrosis factor by human mononuclear cells. Cytokine 3: 189–194

Giroir B P, Quint P A, Barton P et al 1997 Preliminary evaluation of recombinant amino-terminal fragment of human bactericidal/permeability-increasing protein in children with severe meningococcal sepsis [see comments]. Lancet 350: 1439–1443

Gonzalez-Amaro R, Garcia-Monzon C, Garcia-Buey L et al 1994 Induction of tumor necrosis factor alpha production by human hepatocytes in chronic viral hepatitis. Journal of Experimental Medicine 179: 841–848

Gruss H J, Dower S K 1995 The TNF ligand superfamily and its relevance for human diseases. Cytokines Molecular Therapy 1: 75–105

Hanck C, Rossol S, Bocker U, Tokus M, Singer M V 1998 Presence of plasma endotoxin is correlated with tumour necrosis factor receptor levels and disease activity in alcoholic cirrhosis. Alcohol Alcohol 33: 606–608

Hayashi N, Mita E 1997 Fas system and apoptosis in viral hepatitis. Journal of Gastroenterology and Hepatology 12: S223–S226

Hooper D C, Steer C J, Dinarello C A, Peacock A C 1981 Haptoglobin and albumin synthesis in isolated rat hepatocytes. Response to potential mediators of the acute-phase reaction. Biochimica et Biophysica Acta 653: 118–129

Hoshino K, Takeuchi O, Kawai T et al 1999 Cutting edge: Toll-like receptor 4 (TLR4)-deficient mice are hyporesponsive to lipopolysaccharide: evidence for TLR4 as the Lps gene product. Journal of Immunology 162, 3749–3752

Iimuro Y, Nishiura T, Hellerbrand C et al 1998 NFkappaB prevents apoptosis and liver dysfunction during liver regeneration [published erratum appears in J Clin Invest 1998 Apr 1; 101(7): 1541]. Journal of Clinical Investigations 101: 802–811

Ingoldby C J, McPherson G A, Blumgart L H 1984 Endotoxemia in human obstructive jaundice. Effect of polymyxin B. American Journal of Surgery 147: 766–771

Jiang Z, Liu Y, Savas L, Smith L, Bonkovsky H, Baker S, Banner B 1997 Frequency and distribution of DNA fragmentation as a marker of cell death in chronic liver diseases. Virchows Archiv 431: 189–194

Kakumu S, Yoshioka K, Tsutsumi Y, Wakita T, Arao M 1990 Production of tumor necrosis factor, interleukin 1, and interferon-gamma by peripheral blood mononuclear cells from patients with primary biliary cirrhosis. Clinical Immunology and Immunopathology 56: 54–65

Keogh C, Fong Y, Marano M A et al 1990 Identification of a novel tumor necrosis factor alpha/cachectin from the livers of burned and infected rats. Archives of Surgery 125: 79–84

Khoruts A, Stahnke L, McClain C J, Logan G, Allen J I 1991 Circulating tumor necrosis factor, interleukin-1 and interleukin-6 concentrations in chronic alcoholic patients. Hepatology 13: 267–276

Kiener P A, Davis P M, Rankin B M et al 1997 Human monocytic cells contain high levels of intracellular Fas ligand: rapid release following cellular activation. Journal of Immunology 159: 1594–1598

Kimmings A N, van D S, Obertop H, Gouma D J 1999 Treatment with recombinant bactericidal/permeability-increasing protein to prevent endotoxin-induced mortality in bile duct-ligated rats. Journal of the American College of Surgery 189: 374–379

Kimmings A N, van D S, Obertop H, Rauws E A, Gouma D J 1995 Inflammatory and immunologic effects of obstructive jaundice: pathogenesis and treatment. Journal of the American College of Surgery 181: 567–581

Kimura F, Miyazaki M, Suwa T et al 1998 Hyperactive cytokine response after partial hepatectomy in patients with biliary obstruction. European Surgical Research 30: 259–267

Kimura F, Miyazaki M, Suwa T et al 1999 Serum interleukin-6 levels in patients with biliary obstruction. Hepatogastroenterology. 46: 1613–1617

Kirschning C J, Wesche H, Merrill A T, Rothe M 1998 Human toll-like receptor 2 confers responsiveness to bacterial lipopolysaccharide. Journal of Experimental Medicine 188: 2091–2097

Kishimoto T, Akira S, Narazaki M, Taga T 1995 Interleukin-6 family of cytokines and gp130. Blood 86: 1243–1254

Kondo T, Suda T, Fukuyama H, Adachi M, Nagata S 1997 Essential roles of the Fas ligand in the development of hepatitis. Nature Medic. 3: 409–413

Kowdley K V 1999 TNF-alpha in chronic hepatitis C: the smoking gun? [editorial; comment]. American Journal of Gastroenterology 94: 1132–1135

Kriegler M, Perez C, DeFay K, Albert I, Lu S D 1988 A novel form of TNF/cachectin is a cell surface cytotoxic transmembrane protein: ramifications for the complex physiology of TNF. Cell 53: 45–53

Ksontini R, MacKay S L, Moldawer L L 1998 Revisiting the role of tumor necrosis factor alpha and the response to surgical injury and inflammation. Archives of Surgery 133: 558–567

Kunstle G, Leist M, Uhlig S et al 1997 ICE-protease inhibitors block murine liver injury and apoptosis caused by CD95 or by TNF-alpha. Immunology Letters 55: 5–10

Larrea E, Garcia N, Qian C, Civeira M P, Prieto J 1996 Tumor necrosis factor alpha gene expression and the response to interferon in chronic hepatitis C. Hepatology 23: 210–217

Lau J Y, Xie X, Lai M M, Wu P C 1998 Apoptosis and viral hepatitis. Seminars in Liver Disease 18: 169–176

Le J M, Vilcek J 1989 Interleukin 6: a multifunctional cytokine regulating immune reactions and the acute phase protein response. Laboratory Investigations 61: 588–602

Lechner A J, Velasquez A, Knudsen K R, Johanns C A, Tracy T F J, Matuschak G M 1998 Cholestatic liver injury increases circulating TNF-alpha and IL-6 and mortality after Escherichia coli endotoxemia. American Journal of Respiratory and Critical Care Medicine 157: 1550–1558

Leist M, Gantner F, Bohlinger I, Germann P G, Tiegs G, Wendel A 1994 Murine hepatocyte apoptosis induced in vitro and in vivo by TNF-alpha requires transcriptional arrest. Journal of Immunology 153: 1778–1788

Leist M, Gantner F, Bohlinger I, Tiegs G, Germann P G, Wendel A 1995a Tumor necrosis factor-induced hepatocyte apoptosis precedes liver failure in experimental murine shock models. American Journal of Pathology 146: 1220–1234

Leist M, Gantner F, Bohlinger I, Tiegs G, Germann P G, Wendel A 1995b Tumor necrosis factor-induced hepatocyte apoptosis precedes liver failure in experimental murine shock models. American Journal of Pathology 146: 1220–1234

Leist M, Gantner F, Jilg S, Wendel A 1995c Activation of the 55 kDa TNF receptor is necessary and sufficient for TNF-induced liver failure, hepatocyte apoptosis, and nitrite release. Journal of Immunology 154: 1307–1316

Leist M, Gantner F, Kunstle G et al 1996 The 55-kD tumor necrosis factor receptor and CD95 independently signal murine hepatocyte apoptosis and subsequent liver failure. Molecular Medicine 2: 109–124

Leist M, Gantner F, Naumann H et al 1997 Tumor necrosis factor-induced apoptosis during the poisoning of mice with hepatotoxins. Gastroenterology 112: 923–934

Lemaire L C, van L J, Stoutenbeek C P, van D S, Wells C L, Gouma, D J 1997 Bacterial translocation in multiple organ failure: cause or epiphenomenon still unproven [see comments]. British Journal of Surgery 84: 1340–1350

Levine D M, Parker T S, Donnelly T M, Walsh A, Rubin A L 1993 In vivo protection against endotoxin by plasma high density lipoprotein. Proceedings of the National Acadmy of Science USA. 90: 12040–12044

Liles W C, Kiener P A, Ledbetter J A, Aruffo A, Klebanoff S J 1996 Differential expression of Fas (CD95) and Fas ligand on normal human phagocytes: implications for the regulation of apoptosis in neutrophils. Journal of Experimental Medicine 184: 429–440

MacFie J 1997 Bacterial translocation in surgical patients. Annals of the Royal College of Surgeons of England 79: 183–189

Malinin N L, Boldin M P, Kovalenko A W, Wallach D 1997 MAP3K-related kinase involved in NF-kB induction by TNF, CD95 and IL-1. Nature 385: 540–544

Martich G D, Boujoukos A J, Suffredini A F 1993 Response of man to endotoxin. Immunobiology 187: 403–416

Matsumoto K, Fujii H, Michalopoulos G, Fung J J, Demetris A J 1994 Human biliary epithelial cells secrete and respond to cytokines and hepatocyte growth factors in vitro: interleukin-6, hepatocyte growth factor and epidermal growth factor promote DNA synthesis in vitro. Hepatology 20: 376–382

Matsunami H, Kawasaki S, Ishizone S et al 1992 Serial changes of h-HGF and IL-6 in living-related donor liver transplantation with special reference to their relationship to intraoperative portal blood flow. Transplantation Proceedings 24: 1971–1972

McClain C J, Barve S, Deaciuc I, Kugelmas M, Hill D 1999 Cytokines in alcoholic liver disease. Seminars in Liver Disease 19: 205–219

McClain C J, Cohen D A, Dinarello C A, Cannon J G, Shedlofsky S I, Kaplan A M 1986 Serum interleukin-1 (IL-1) activity in alcoholic hepatitis. Life Sciences 39: 1479–1485

Michalopoulos G K, DeFrances M C 1997 Liver regeneration. Science 276: 60–66

Michie H R, Manogue K R, Spriggs D R et al 1988 Detection of circulating tumor necrosis factor after endotoxin administration. New England Journal of Medicine 318: 1481–1486

Mignon A, Rouquet N, Fabre M et al 1999 LPS challenge in D-galactosamine-sensitized mice accounts for caspase-dependent fulminant hepatitis, not for septic shock. American Journal of Respiratory and Critical Care Medicine 159: 1308–1315

Mileno M D, Margolis N H, Clark B D, Dinarello C A, Burke J F, Gelfand J A 1995 Coagulation of whole blood stimulates interleukin-1β gene expression. Journal of Infectious Diseases 172: 308–311

Moolten F L, Bucher N L 1967 Regeneration of rat liver: transfer of humoral agent by cross circulation. Science 158: 272–274

Moreland L W, Baumgartner S W, Schiff M H et al 1997 Treatment of rheumatoid arthritis with a recombinant human tumor necrosis factor receptor (p75)-Fc fusion protein [see comments]. New England Journal of Medicine 337: 141–147

Mosley B, Urdal D L, Prickett K S 1987 The interleukin-1 receptor binds the human interleukin-1 alpha precursor but not the interleukin-1 beta precursor. Journal of Biological Chemistry 262: 2941–2944

Moss M L, Catherine-Jin S L, Milla M E et al 1997 Cloning of a disintegrin metalloproteinase that processes precursor tumor-necrosis factor-α. Nature 385: 733–736

Nagata S, Golstein P 1995 The Fas death factor. Science 267: 1449–1455

Naveau S, Emilie D, Balian A et al 1998 Plasma levels of soluble tumor necrosis factor receptors p55 and p75 in patients with alcoholic liver disease of increasing severity. Journal of Hepatology 28: 778–784

O'Dwyer S T, Michie H R, Ziegler T R, Revhaug A, Smith R J, Wilmore D W 1988 A single dose of endotoxin increases intestinal permeability in healthy humans. Archives of Surgery 123: 1459–1464

Ogasawara J, Watanabe-Fukunaga R, Adachi M et al 1993 Lethal effect of the anti-Fas antibody in mice. Nature 364: 806–809

Olofsson P, Nylander G, Olsson P 1986 Endotoxin: routes of transport in experimental peritonitis. American Journal of Surgery 151: 443–446

Opal S M, Palardy J E, Marra M N, Fisher C J J, McKelligon B M, Scott R W 1994a Relative concentrations of endotoxin-binding proteins in body fluids during infection. Lancet 344: 429–431

Opal S M, Palardy J E, Marra M N, Fisher C J J, McKelligon B M, Scott R W 1994b Relative concentrations of endotoxin-binding proteins in body fluids during infection. Lancet 344: 429–431

Ottonello L, Tortolina G, Amelotti M, Dallegri F 1999 Soluble Fas ligand is chemotactic for human neutrophilic polymorphonuclear leukocytes. Journal of Immunology 162: 3601–3606

Pain J A, Bailey M E 1987 Measurement of operative plasma endotoxin levels in jaundiced and non-jaundiced patients. European Surgical Research 19: 207–216

Pain J A, Bailey M E 1988 Prevention of endotoxinaemia in obstructive jaundice—a comparative study of bile salts. HPB Surgery 1: 21–27

Pain J A, Cahill C J, Gilbert J M, Johnson C D, Trapnell J E, Bailey M E 1991 Prevention of postoperative renal dysfunction in patients with obstructive jaundice: a multicentre study of bile salts and lactulose. British Journal of Surgery 78: 467–469

Pfeffer K, Matsuyama T, Kundig T M et al 1993 Mice deficient for the 55 kD tumor necrosis factor receptor are resistant to endotoxic shock, yet succumb to *L. monocytogenes* infection. Cell 73: 457–467

Plebani M, Panozzo M P, Basso D, De P M, Biasin R, Infantolino D 1999 Cytokines and the progression of liver damage in experimental bile duct ligation. Clinical and Experimental Pharmacology and Physiology 26: 358–363

Puntis M C, Jiang W G 1996a Plasma cytokine levels and monocyte activation in patients with obstructive jaundice. Journal of Gastroenterology and Hepatology 11: 7–13

Puntis M C, Jiang W G 1996b Plasma cytokine levels and monocyte activation in patients with obstructive jaundice. Journal of Gastroenterology and Hepatology 11: 7–13

Raetz C R, Ulevitch R J, Wright S D, Sibley C H, Ding A, Nathan C F 1991 Gram-negative endotoxin: an extraordinary lipid with profound effects on eukaryotic signal transduction. FASEB Journal 5: 2652–2660

Rai R M, Yang S Q, McClain C, Karp C L, Klein A S, Diehl A M 1996 Kupffer cell depletion by gadolinium chloride enhances liver regeneration after partial hepatectomy in rats. American Journal of Physiology 270: G909–G918

Rothe J, Lesslauer W, Lotscher H et al 1993 Mice lacking the tumour necrosis factor receptor 1 are resistant to TNF-mediated toxicity but highly susceptible to infection by *Listeria monocytogenes*. Nature 364: 798–802

Satoh M, Adachi K, Suda T, Yamazaki M, Mizuno D 1991 TNF-driven inflammation during mouse liver regeneration after partial hepatectomy and its role in growth regulation of liver. Molecular Biotherapy 3: 136–147

Schafer C, Schips I, Landig J, Bode J C, Bode C 1995 Tumor-necrosis-factor and interleukin-6 response of peripheral blood monocytes to low concentrations of lipopolysaccharide in patients with alcoholic liver disease. Zeitschrift fur Gastroenterologie 33: 503–508

Schindler R, Clark B D, Dinarello C A 1990 Dissociation between interleukin-1 beta mRNA and protein synthesis in human peripheral blood mononuclear cells. Journal of Biological Chemistry 265: 10232–10237

Schneider P, Holler N, Bodmer J L et al 1998 Conversion of membrane-bound Fas(CD95) ligand to its soluble form is associated with downregulation of its proapoptotic activity and loss of liver toxicity. Journal of Experimental Medicine 187: 1205–1213

Scotte M, Masson S, Lyoumi S et al 1997 Cytokine gene expression in liver following minor or major hepatectomy in rat. Cytokine. 9: 859–867

Seino K, Iwabuchi K, Kayagaki N et al 1998 Chemotactic activity of soluble Fas ligand against phagocytes. Journal of Immunology 161: 4484–4488

Sheron N, Bird G, Goka J, Alexander G, Williams R 1991 Elevated plasma interleukin-6 and increased severity and mortality in alcoholic hepatitis. Clinical and Experimental Immunology 84: 449–453

Smith J W, Longo D L, Alvord W G et al 1993 The effects of treatment with interleukin-1 alpha on platelet recovery after high-dose carboplatin. New England Journal of Medicine 328, 756–761

Solorzano C C, Ksontini R, Pruitt J H et al 1997 Involvement of 26-kDa cell-associated TNF-alpha in experimental hepatitis and exacerbation of liver injury with a matrix metalloproteinase inhibitor. Journal of Immunology 158: 414–419

Stevenson F T, Torrano F, Locksley R M, Lovett D H 1992 Interleukin 1: the patterns of translation and intracellular distribution support alternative secretory mechanisms. Journal of Cellular Physiology 152: 223–231

Suffredini A F, Fantuzzi G, Badolato R, Oppenheim J J, O'Grady N P 1999 New insights into the biology of the acute phase response. Journal of Clinical Immunology 19: 203–214

Taga T, Kishimoto T 1997 Gp130 and the interleukin-6 family of cytokines. Annual Review of Immunology 15: 797–819

Tanaka M, Suda T, Takahashi T, Nagata S 1995 Expression of the functional soluble form of human fas ligand in activated lymphocytes. EMBO Journal 14, 1129–1135

Tannahill C, Fukuzuka K, Marum T et al 1999 Discordant TNFα superfamily expression in bacterial peritonitis and endotoxemic shock. Surgery 126: 349–357

Targan S R, Hanauer S B, van D S 1997 A short-term study of chimeric monoclonal antibody cA2 to tumor necrosis factor alpha for Crohn's disease. Crohn's Disease cA2 Study Group. New England Journal of Medicine 337: 1029–1035

Tobias P S, Soldau K, Ulevitch R J 1986 Isolation of a lipopolysaccharide-binding acute phase reactant from rabbit serum. Journal of Experimental Medicine 164: 777–793

Tobias P S, Soldau K, Ulevitch R J 1989 Identification of a lipid A binding site in the acute phase reactant lipopolysaccharide binding protein. Journal of Biological Chemistry 264: 10867–10871

Tracey K J, Cerami A 1996 Tumor necrosis factor: a pleiotropic cytokine and therapeutic target. Annual Review of Medicine 45: 491

Ulevitch R J 1993 Recognition of bacterial endotoxins by receptor-dependent mechanisms. Advanced Immunology 53: 267–289

Ulevitch R J, Tobias P S 1999 Recognition of gram-negative bacteria and endotoxin by the innate immune system. Current Opinions in Immunology 11: 19–22

van der Poll T, Levi M, Buller H R et al 1991a Fibrinolytic response to tumor necrosis factor in healthy subjects. Journal of Experimental Medicine 174: 729–732

van der Poll T, Romijn J A, Endert E, Borm J J, Buller H R, Sauerwein H P 1991b Tumor necrosis factor mimics the metabolic response to acute infection in healthy humans. American Journal of Physiology 261: E457–E465

van der Poll T, van Deventer S J, Buller H R, Sturk A, ten Cate J W 1991c Comparison of the early dynamics of systemic prostacyclin release after administration of tumor necrosis factor and endotoxin to healthy humans. Journal of Infectious Diseases 164: 599–601

van der Poll T, van Deventer S J, Hack C E et al 1992 Effects on leukocytes after injection of tumor necrosis factor into healthy humans. Blood 79: 693–698

Van Zee K J, Kohno T, Fischer E, Rock C S, Moldawer L L, Lowry S F 1992 Tumor necrosis factor soluble receptors circulate during experimental and clinical inflammation and can protect against excessive tumor necrosis factor alpha in vitro and in vivo. Proceedings of the National Academy of Sciences USA 89: 4845–4849

Van A D, Martin S J, Kafri T, Green D R, Verma I M 1996 Suppression of TNF-alpha-induced apoptosis by NF-kappaB [see comments]. Science 274: 787–789

van L P, Boermeester M A, Houdijk A P 1995 Pretreatment with enteral cholestyramine prevents suppression of the cellular immune system after partial hepatectomy. Annals of Surgery 221: 282–290

von der Mohlen M A, Kimmings A N, Wedel N I, Mevissen ML, Jansen J, Friedmann N, Lorenz T J, Nelson B J, White M L, Bauer R 1995 Inhibition of endotoxin-induced cytokine release and neutrophil activation in humans by use of recombinant bactericidal/permeability-increasing protein. Journal of Infectious Diseases 172: 144–151

Wang X, Andersson R, Soltesz V, Bengmark S 1992 Bacterial translocation after major hepatectomy in patients and rats. Archives of Surgery 127: 1101–1106

Wright, S D, Tobias P S, Ulevitch R J, Ramos R A 1989 Lipopolysaccharide (LPS) binding protein opsonizes LPS-bearing particles for recognition by a novel receptor on macrophages. Journal of Experimental Medicine 170: 1231–1241

Xu Y, Bialik S, Jones B E, Iimuro Y 1998 NF-kappaB inactivation converts a hepatocyte cell line TNF-alpha response from proliferation to apoptosis. American Journal of Physiology 275: C1058–C1066

Yamada Y, Kirillova I, Peschon J J, Fausto N 1997 Initiation of liver growth by tumor necrosis factor: deficient liver regeneration in mice lacking type I tumor necrosis factor receptor. Proceedings of the National Academy of Sciences USA 94: 1441–1446

Yamashiki M, Kosaka Y, Nishimura A, Watanabe S, Nomoto M, Ichida F 1998 Analysis of serum cytokine levels in primary biliary cirrhosis patients and healthy adults. Journal of Clinical Laboratory Analysis 12: 77–82

Yang R B, Mark M R, Gray A et al 1998 Toll-like receptor-2 mediates lipopolysaccharide-induced cellular signalling [see comments]. Nature 395: 284–288

Yang R B, Mark M R, Gurney A L, Godowski P J 1999 Signaling events induced by lipopolysaccharide-activated toll-like receptor 2. Journal of Immunology 163: 639–643

Yoshizawa K, Naruto M, Ida N 1996 Injection time of interleukin-6 determines fatal outcome in experimental endotoxin shock. J Interferon Cytokine Res 16: 995–1000

Zhang F X, Kirschning C J, Mancinelli R et al 1999 Bacterial lipopolysaccharide activates nuclear factor-kappaB through interleukin-1 signaling mediators in cultured human dermal endothelial cells and mononuclear phagocytes. Journal of Biological Chemistry 274: 7611–7614

Zhang Y H, Lin J X, Vilcek J 1990 Interleukin-6 induction by tumor necrosis factor and interleukin-1 in human fibroblasts involves activation of a nuclear factor binding to a kappa B-like sequence. Molecular and Cellular Biology 10: 3818–3823

Ziegler E J, Fisher C J Jr, Sprung C L et al 1991 Treatment of gram-negative bacteremia and septic shock with HA-1A human monoclonal antibody against endotoxin. A randomized, double-blind, placebo-controlled trial. The HA-1A Sepsis Study Group [see comments]. New England Journal of Medicine 324: 429–436

Zivot J B, Hoffman W D 1995 Pathogenic effects of endotoxin. New Horizons 3: 267–275

Zwaveling J H, Maring J K, Clarke F L et al 1996 High plasma tumor necrosis factor (TNF)-alpha concentrations and a sepsis-like syndrome in patients undergoing hyperthermic isolated limb perfusion with recombinant TNF-alpha, interferon-gamma, and melphalan. Critical Care in Medicine 24: 765–770

Molecular and genetic determinants of hepatobiliary and pancreatic neoplasia

10

R.P. DeMATTEO, Y. FONG

INTRODUCTION

Advances in the techniques of molecular analysis have improved the understanding of neoplastic disorders. Alterations in DNA are known to be associated with cancer. Most tumors are usually discovered late in their clinical course when they are at least 1 gram in size which is about 10^9 cells and represents approximately 30 tumor doublings. The impetus for the molecular characterization of specific tumors rests on the premise that it will: (1) facilitate the diagnosis of cancer; (2) provide prognostic information; and (3) improve treatment. The application of molecular techniques may enable earlier detection of tumors at a time when they are more responsive to available therapies. Similarly, tumor recurrence after treatment may be more readily identified. In equivocal cases, molecular markers may help distinguish neoplasia from benign disease. Molecular assays may be utilized to identify high-risk individuals or to screen relatives in cases of familial cancer. The molecular profile of a tumor may help determine its biology and predict clinical outcome. It may also predict the response of a particular tumor to surgery, chemotherapy, or radiation. In addition, molecular characterization may suggest novel treatment strategies. In this chapter, the molecular and genetic events in hepatic, biliary and pancreatic neoplasia will be summarized.

MOLECULAR EVENTS IN NEOPLASIA

Most tumors are thought to be monoclonal in origin arising from a single abnormal cell. Mutations in DNA may either be inherited from the germline or occur spontaneously in an individual as a somatic mutation. Most cancers arise from somatic mutations. Somatic mutations may be due to point mutations of the DNA sequence, gene deletion, or gene rearrangement. They may result from a chemical mutagen,

radiation, viral infection, or dietary factors. Knudson (1971) originally postulated the multihit concept of tumorigenesis. Patients with inherited retinoblastoma were proposed to carry a germline genetic mutation defect in all cells. The development of a somatic mutation would then lead to tumor formation in the cell in which it occurred. In contrast, in the sporadic form of retinoblastoma, two somatic mutations within the same cell are required making this a less common entity. Based on this concept, Vogelstein emphasized that the pathogenesis of colorectal cancer begins with the accumulation of molecular mutations within a cell that leads to cell proliferation, adenoma formation, and eventually carcinoma development (Fearon & Vogelstein 1990, Vogelstein et al 1988).

Human tumors result most commonly from mutations in both tumor suppressor genes and proto-oncogenes (Table 10.1). DNA mismatch repair genes are a third group of genes that are frequently involved and appear to cause cancer indirectly by increasing the chance of mutations in tumor suppressor genes and proto-oncogenes. A defective mismatch repair gene is responsible for hereditary non-polyposis colon cancer (HNPCC). Multiple genetic defects are

Table 10.1 Comparison of tumor suppressor genes and proto-oncogenes

Feature	Tumor suppressor gene	Proto-oncogene
Normal function	Inhibition of cell growth	Stimulation of cell growth
Normal action	Recessive	Dominant
Germline transmission of mutation	Frequent	Rare
Somatic mutation required for cancer	Yes	Yes
Number of mutant alleles in cancer	Both	One
Consequence of mutation	Loss of function	Gain of function

usually present in any given tumor. The initial mutations are the most important for our understanding of carcinogenesis. As cancers develop, they are more susceptible to additional genetic changes.

There are more than a dozen tumor suppressor genes that have been identified. Normally, they function to inhibit cellular proliferation. Tumor suppressor genes are considered 'recessive' since loss of both alleles is necessary for a mutant phenotype to occur. In familial cancer, one mutant allele is usually inherited through the germline and the other allele must be lost or undergo mutation. In sporadic cancer, there is typically either loss of one allele with mutation of the other gene copy or homozygous gene deletion. Somatic mutation may occur via point mutation (in which a single base substitution occurs resulting in a single amino acid alteration). Alternatively, chromosomal alterations (gene conversion, recombination, non-disjunction) result in a replacement of the wild type (normal) allele with a copy of the abnormal gene. The presence of two mutant alleles that are identical results in what is termed loss of heterozygosity (LOH). LOH is also seen with gene deletion. Normally, heterozygosity is present between the two copies of a gene since there are minor differences between the paternal and maternal copy of a given gene. LOH can be detected with molecular techniques.

Proto-oncogenes are normal genes that regulate cell proliferation and their activation may result in cancer. Over 100 proto-oncogenes have been identified and most human tumors have involvement of at least one. Proto-oncogene products function in cell signaling and include growth factors and their receptors, transcription factors, and other components of intracellular signaling pathways. Proto-oncogenes are considered to be 'dominant' since only one abnormal copy of the gene is required to produce a tumor. Activation confers increased cell growth and may occur in four ways. Point mutation occurs as with tumor suppressor genes. Gene amplification results in the duplication of numerous (usually greater than 100) copies of a particular gene. Amplification of n-myc occurs in neuroblastoma. Chromosomal translocation may also activate a gene and is found in leukemia and lymphoma. Insertional mutagenesis occurs when DNA is inserted near a proto-oncogene and causes its activation. The classic example of this occurs with the insertion of retroviral DNA near a proto-oncogene.

PANCREATIC ADENOCARCINOMA

Pancreatic ductal adenocarcinoma is one of the best characterized human malignancies (Lumadue et al 1995).

Table 10.2 Genetic mutations in pancreatic adenocarcinoma.

Gene	Mutation Fraction	%	Reference
K-ras	21/22	95	Almoguera et al 1988
	68/82	83	Hruban et al 1993
p53	8/14	57	Kalthoff 1993
	18/35	51	Pellegata 1994
p16	29/37	78	Caldas et al 1994b
	20/48	42	Huang 1996
DPC4	25/84	30	Hahn et al 1996

Molecular analysis has revealed that there are a variety of genetic abnormalities associated with pancreatic cancer. The majority of pancreatic tumors have activation of the K-ras oncogene and many have inactivation of the tumor suppressor genes p53, p16, or DPC4 (Table 10.2). In contrast, defects in DNA repair genes, as evidenced by microsatellite instabilities, occur less than 5% of the time (Goggins et al 1998). Cytogenetic studies have shown that DNA amplification also is not a major factor in pancreatic cancer as it occurred in only eight of 62 patients in one study (Griffin et al 1995).

K-ras

K-ras mutation is the most frequently identified genetic defect in pancreatic cancer and occurs in over 80% of cases. The K-ras gene encodes a membrane-associated guanine nucleotide-binding protein involved in signal transduction via tyrosine kinase receptors. K-ras is involved in a number of cellular functions including cell division. Mutation resulting in K-ras overexpression leads to permanent cellular proliferation. Almoguerra first reported its importance in pancreatic cancer after finding genetic alterations in 21 of 22 patients (Almoguera et al 1988). K-ras mutation in pancreatic cancer occurs primarily as a point mutation in the region of codon 12 (and occasionally codon 13) resulting in a missense mutation. This is in contrast to K-ras mutations in colorectal adenocarcinoma which occur commonly at codons 13 and 61. The most frequent mutation is a base change from guanine to adenine. However, there is considerable geographic variation in the site of mutation which suggests the importance of other genetic or environmental factors (Scarpa et al 1994). The end result is an alteration of GTPase activity which renders the oncogene constitutively active. K-ras mutation is thought to represent an early event in pancreatic neoplasia since it is found in proliferative ductal lesions, in cancer in situ, and in the majority of individual cells within a tumor (Lemoine et al 1992a).

K-ras mutation is theoretically attractive as a diagnostic marker of pancreatic cancer since it has a high prevalence, is limited to two codons making detection easier, and is an early event in carcinogenesis. Iguchi et al found K-ras mutations in the duodenal fluid in 12 of 19 patients with pancreatic cancer compared to one of 41 patients with benign pancreatic disease (Iguchi et al 1996). However, another group detected the mutation in the duodenal fluid of only 13 of 51 patients (Wilentz et al 1998). Meanwhile, Tada et al found K-ras mutations in the blood of two out of six patients with pancreatic cancer (Tada et al 1993). Examination of the stool of patients revealed K-ras mutation in two of six patients with pancreatic cancer, two of three with cholangiocarcinoma, and one of three with chronic pancreatitis (Caldas et al 1994a).

Unfortunately, the clinical use of K-ras mutation is currently limited for several reasons. It has not been shown to correlate with tumor stage or survival (Hruban RH et al 1993). K-ras mutation is not organ-specific and occurs in other tumors. There is certainly a fraction of patients with pancreatic cancer without K-ras alteration. Furthermore, it is not clear how to manage a patient with a K-ras mutation who lacks other evidence of a pancreatic cancer since it does not necessarily mean that a cancer will develop.

Another proto-oncogene that has been implicated in pancreatic cancer is c-erb-B2 (Williams et al 1991). It is a putative transmembrane growth factor. c-erb-B2 was found to be overexpressed in 17 of 87 pancreatic cancers but in only three of 14 patients with chronic pancreatitis (Hall et al 1990). Only two patients had evidence for amplification meaning that genetic mutation did not account for the increased protein production.

p53 GENE

p53 is the most commonly involved tumor suppressor gene in pancreatic adenocarcinoma and, in fact, it is the most frequently mutated gene in human cancer (Vogelstein & Kinzler 1992). The gene is situated on chromosome 17p and it encodes a DNA-binding transcriptional factor. It has numerous functions that include slowing replication and promoting apoptosis both of which are regulatory functions in tumor prevention (Kern et al 1992). Mutant p53 alleles may act in one of two ways. First, they can be recessive meaning that inactivation of both alleles is required for p53 function to be lost within a cell. In addition, they may act in a 'dominant negative' manner whereby a single mutant p53 gene inactivates the wild type p53 protein produced by the other allele in a cell which is normal. Typically, one allele is lost and the other is mutated. The most common mutation is a point mutation producing a missense. Loss of function may also occur through homozygous deletion. Unlike K-ras mutations which occur in a limited number of areas within

the gene, p53 mutations occur throughout a large expanse within the gene making detection more difficult. It is unclear when these mutations occur in the development of pancreatic cancer. p53 mutation is present in about 40% of patients with pancreatic cancer; it was detected in 29 of 71 patients in one study and in 14 of 34 cases in another (Scarpa et al 1993, Weyrer et al 1996). Its presence has been correlated with survival (Weyrer et al 1996). The existence of a p53 mutation alone is not sufficient to cause pancreatic cancer as demonstrated in transgenic mice without p53 (Donehower et al 1992).

p16 AND DPC4

The p16 tumor suppressor gene is inactivated in about 80% of patients with pancreatic cancer (Caldas et al 1994b). It is also known as p16^{INK4} and multiple tumor suppressor 1 (MTS1). It is located on chromosome 9p. Normally, p16 inhibits cyclin-dependent kinases and inhibits cell cycling. About half of the mutations are homozygous deletions.

The tumor suppressor gene DPC4 (deleted in pancreatic carcinoma, locus 4) is involved in pancreatic cancer (Hahn et al 1996). The gene is located on the 18q chromosome. Its function appears to be the regulation of the TGF-beta signaling pathway to lower cell growth. In 25 of 84 patients, there was a homozygous deletion and in 20% there is a potentially inactivating mutation. As opposed to K-ras and p53 mutations, DPC4 mutations are rarely found in other major tumors.

Other areas besides the location of known tumor suppressor genes have been found to be abnormal in pancreatic cancer. Loss of heterozygosity has been shown to occur in >40% of tumors at 1p, 6p, 6q, 8p, 10q, 12q, 13q, 21q, and 22q. These sites may represent other as yet unidentified tumor suppressor genes (Hahn et al 1995).

HEREDITARY PANCREATIC CANCER

While most pancreatic cancers occur in a sporadic fashion, there are also familial forms of the disease. In a study of 179 patients with pancreatic cancer, there was a 7.8% incidence of a family history of pancreatic cancer compared to a rate of 0.6% in controls (Ghadirian et al 1991). Several kindreds with clusters of pancreatic cancer have been identified. There has been a report of a family with a p16 mutation but none with DPC4, K-ras, or p53 mutations (Hussussian et al 1994). It is difficult to identify patients at risk for familial pancreatic cancer due to its incomplete penetrance. Patients with a positive family history may benefit from molecular screening.

Pancreatic cancer is also associated with several disease syndromes. Patients with hereditary non-polyposis colorectal cancer (HNPCC, Lynch II syndrome) are more likely to develop pancreatic cancer (Lynch et al 1996). This is an autosomal dominant condition resulting from a defect in one of several DNA mismatch repair genes. It is also associated with endometrial, ovarian, and breast cancer. Patients with hereditary pancreatitis, an autosomal dominant condition, also have an increased risk of pancreatic cancer. However, whether this results from a genetic defect or is secondary to inflammation is unclear. There is about a 7% incidence of pancreatic cancer in familial atypical mole-multiple melanoma (FAMM) (Bergman et al 1990). This syndrome is characterized by multiple nevi, atypical nevi, and melanoma and may actually be linked to a defect in p16 (Bullock et al 1999). The autosomal dominant Peutz-Jeghers syndrome is characterized by gastrointestinal hamartomas and mucocutaneous melanin deposits and confers an increased pancreatic cancer risk. Familial adenomatous polyposis has a relative risk of 4.5 for pancreatic cancer. Ataxia-telangiectasia is occasionally associated with pancreatic cancer (Giardiello et al 1993). BRCA2 is a tumor suppressor gene that is involved in breast, ovarian, prostate, and colon cancer. BRCA2 mutations accounted for three of 41 (7.3%) cases of sporadic pancreatic cancer in one population only two of 245 cases in a larger series (Goggins et al 1996).

PANCREATIC TUMOR PROGRESSION

The progression of pancreatic cancer usually involves multiple genetic events by the time it is recognized clinically. The tumor suppressor genes p16, p53, DPC4 were each inactivated in 37% of 40 patients with pancreatic cancer (Rozenblum et al 1997). Pancreatic cancer may arise and progress in a similar manner to colorectal carcinoma. The hypothesis is that ductal hyperplasia leads to ductal atypia which progresses to carcinoma in situ and then cancer (Furukawa et al 1994). K-ras mutations have been found in early duct lesions and are therefore thought to be important in tumorigenesis (Caldas et al 1994a). In patients with pancreatic cancer, there are often surrounding areas of hyperplasia with atypia and such precursor lesions usually have K-ras mutations and some have p16 defects (Moskaluk et al 1997). However, Tada found that in patients without cancer or pancreatitis, 12 of 38 patients with ductal hyperplasia had K-ras mutations. Thus, although a mutation is identified, it does not necessarily mean that the patient has or will develop pancreatic cancer (Tada et al 1996).

OTHER PANCREATIC CANCERS

There is less information regarding other types of pancreatic cancer than ductal adenocarcinoma. Intraductal papillary neoplasms (IPN) of the pancreas have been reported to have K-ras mutations in three of five cases in one study and in eight of 26 patients in another series (Sessa et al 1994, Tada et al 1991). However, no K-ras mutations were found in another report (Lemoine et al 1992b). Acinar cell carcinoma rarely has K-ras mutation. Pancreatic neuroendocrine cancer has been associated with DPC4 mutations as mutations were shown in 5 of 9 non-functioning tumors but in none of 16 insulinomas, gastrinomas, and VIPomas (Bartsch et al 1999). One group reported K-ras mutation in all four ampullary cancers that were studied (Watanabe et al 1994).

HEPATOCELLULAR CARCINOMA

Hepatocellular carcinoma (HCC) is the most common cancer of solid organs worldwide. However, unlike in pancreatic adenocarcinoma, there is a limited understanding of its molecular pathogenesis. Hepatocellular carcinoma is a heterogeneous tumor that has been found to have a variety of genetic lesions (Unsal et al 1994). It occurs most frequently in the Southeast Asia and sub-Saharan Africa but its incidence is increasing in the United States (El Serag & Mason 1999). The geographic distribution correlates with the incidence of hepatitis B virus (HBV), hepatitis C virus (HCV) infection and aflatoxin B_1 (AFB_1) exposure. It is not clear whether etiologic factors cause HCC directly or whether they act indirectly by producing chronic liver injury. Chronic liver inflammation leads to hepatocyte proliferation and cirrhosis and is a common pathway for hepatitis viral infection, alcohol intake, metabolic disorders, and other environmental agents. About 75% of all HCC is associated with cirrhosis. Genetic mutations are more likely to occur in this setting as demonstrated in animal models (Huang & Chisari 1995).

TUMOR SUPPRESSOR GENES IN HCC

Tumor suppressor gene loss or mutation has been identified in HCC. The p53 gene has been investigated extensively. Alterations in the p53 gene have been found in 30 to 60% of patients with HCC. The most common finding is a point mutation in one allele with deletion of the other copy. Over 100 mutations have been identified throughout the p53 gene (Nishida et al 1993). However, mutation in the p53 gene is most likely a late event in the pathogenesis of HCC (Teramoto et al 1994). This is supported by the finding that in one study p53 mutation was found in none of 24 well-differentiated, four of 11 moderately differentiated, and four of eight poorly differentiated HCC (Murakami et al 1991). Furthermore, patients with multifocal HCC may just have a p53 gene mutation in one of their tumors (Murakami et al 1991, Oda et al 1992).

Mutation of the p53 gene is common in patients with HCC from geographic areas with high aflatoxin B_1 (AFB_1) exposure. AFB_1 is a metabolite produced by the fungi *Aspergillus flavus* and *parasiticus*. It is found on rice, corn, and peanuts. Humans are exposed to AFB_1 by ingestion of contaminated food or products of animals that have eaten contaminated food. The risk of developing HCC is proportional to the amount of dietary intake. The estimated median toxic dose of AFB_1 for human cancer is 132 µg/kg/day (Wogan 1992). AFB is metabolized to an epoxide which may cause genetic mutations (Bailey et al 1996).

The highest exposure to AFB_1 occurs in southern Africa and southern China. In these areas, a specific mutation in the p53 gene has been identified that involves codon 249. (Table 10.3). In southern Africa, five of ten patients had a p53 gene mutation and three of them had a G to T transversion in the third nucleotide of codon 249 resulting in a substitution of arginine to serine in the p53 protein (Bressac et al 1991). In a study of 36 patients in China with HCC, 21 had a mutation in codon 249 (Scorsone et al 1992). Thirteen of the 21 patients with a codon 249 mutation had lost the other gene allele. In contrast, in the United States where AFB_1 exposure is low, the p53 mutations in HCC do not involve codon 249 (Kar et al 1993, Kazachkov et al 1996, Ozturk 1991, Ueda et al 1995). Occasional mutations are found in some, but not all, reports from Japan and Taiwan where there is low AFB_1 exposure (Nishida et al 1992, Oda et al 1992, Ozturk 1991, Sheu et al 1992).

Thus, AFB_1 is necessary for mutation in codon 249 because it rarely occurs with HBV infection alone.

Mutation in codon 249 appears to be an early event in hepatic carcinogenesis because it may be found even in normal individuals exposed to AFB_1 who do not have cirrhosis. The effects of AFB_1 are synergistic with those of HBV exposure (Aguilar et al 1994, Scorsone et al 1992). A study in Shanghai of over 18 000 men reported the interrelationship of HCC, HBV, and AFB_1 (Qian et al 1994, Ross et al 1992). Patients with AFB_1 exposure alone had a relative risk (RR) of HCC of 3.4. HBV infection resulted in a RR of 7.3. However, patients with elevated urinary aflatoxin levels and HBV infection had a RR of 59.4 for developing HCC. AFB_1 has also been shown to cause mutation of the p53 codon 249 in HepG2 human hepatocyte cell line. Diets contaminated with aflatoxins have been shown to cause HCC in a variety of animals including rodents and non-human primates. However, in four primates with AFB_1 induced HCC, there were no codon 249 mutations (Fujimoto et al 1992).

OTHER TUMOR SUPPRESSOR GENES

A number of other tumor suppressor genes have been associated with HCC. Cytogenetic analysis has revealed loss of heterozygosity of the following chromosomes (with percentage of patients affected) in patients with HCC: 1p (30%), 4 (54%), 5q (37%), 8p (40%), 10q (25%), 11p (44%), 13q (49%), 16 (48%), 17p (54%), and 22q (33%) (Geissler 1997). These sites may represent tumor suppressor genes. Loss of heterozygosity has been detected in the adenomatous polyposis coli (APC) gene in five of 29 patients with HCC (Piao et al 1997). p16 is another tumor suppressor gene that is involved in HCC. In one report, four of 26 patients with HCC had a germline mutation in p16 and three did not have cirrhosis (Chaubert et al 1997). In another study, p16 protein was not detectable in 11 of 32 HCC tumors but present in normal surrounding liver (Hui et al 1996). There were no DNA mutations detected implicating an alteration in post-transcriptional regulation of p16. BRCA2 mutation was found in three of 60 patients with HCC in another study (Katagiri et al 1996).

ONCOGENES IN HCC

Unlike in other human tumors, proto-oncogene mutation or amplification does not appear to be a major factor in the development of HCC though overexpression does play a role. The retinoblastoma (Rb) gene has loss of heterozygosity in 25 to 44% of HCC and 80% when p53 was mutated (Tabor 1994, Zhang et al 1994). In the presence of a p53

Table 10.3 Gene mutations in codon 249 of the p53 gene in HCC by exposure to aflatoxin B1

Location	p53 Mutation Total	p53 Mutation Codon 249	Reference
AFB_1 high			
Southern Africa	5/10	3/5	Bressac et al 1991
Southern Africa, Southeast Asia	—	12/72	Ozturk 1991
China	—	21/36	Scorsone et al 1992
China	9/20	9/9	Li 1993
AFB_1 low			
North America, Europe, Middle East, Japan	—	0/95	Ozturk et al 1991
Japan	49/169	7/49	Oda et al 1992
Japan	17/53	0/17	Nishida et al 1992
Taiwan	20/61	4/20	Sheu et al 1992
United States	—	0/47	Kar et al 1993
United States	5/12	0/5	Kazachkov et al 1996

Adapted with permission from Okuda and Tabor

mutation, there were six of seven patients with an Rb alteration (Murakami et al 1991). A defect in Rb may lead to unrestricted cell growth. Ras mutations are infrequent in HCC (Tsuda et al 1989). One study reported no mutations in 12 patients while a different group found two point mutations in 21 patients and a third report showed one of six to have a mutation (Ogata et al 1991, Stork et al 1991, Tada et al 1990). Overexpression of the c-myc proto-oncogene is common and was found in all 12 patients with HCC in one study (Zhang et al 1994). However, gene mutation of c-myc is rarely present (Lee et al 1988). Similar findings have been identified with c-fos as overexpression occurs commonly. The c-met proto-oncogene encodes the receptor for hepatocyte growth factor and overexpression was present in eight of 18 HCC tumors (Boix et al 1994). Patients with high c-met levels have more frequent intrahepatic metastases and shorter survival (Ueki et al 1997). Cerb-B-2 overexpression was identified in only two of 26 patients with HCC (Collier et al 1992).

HEPATITIS B VIRUS

Hepatitis B virus is a hepadnavirus that measures 3.2 kb and replicates through an RNA intermediate. There is convincing evidence that HBV infection results in HCC. First, over 80% of HCC occurs in people infected with HBV. Next, the geographic distribution of HCC correlates with the prevalence of HBV. The rate of HCC is greatest in Eastern Asia and sub-Saharan Africa which have the highest rates of chronic HBV infection. Hepatitis B virus increases the risk of HCC over 100 fold (Beasley et al 1981). Nevertheless, some data argue against a role of HBV infection in HCC. There are areas (e.g. Chile) with a high frequency of HBV infection that have a low prevalence of HCC. Also, a minority of patients with HBV infection actually develops HCC.

It is not clear whether HBV exerts a direct influence on hepatic carcinogenesis or plays an indirect role via inflammation (Fig. 10.1). Several lines of evidence favor a direct viral mechanism. Hepatitis B virus integrates into the host DNA in about 80% of patients with HCC (Brechot et al 1980, Chen et al 1982, Matsubara & Tokino 1990). However, insertional mutagenesis does not appear to contribute significantly to HCC. Integration appears to occur at variable sites and in a random manner. There have been remarkably few sites reported to be within or close to functional genes (Wang et al 1990). At the site of insertion, all patients demonstrate microdeletions of DNA and some have chromosomal translocations. Another point supporting a direct effect of HBV is that the virus may be oncogenic even in the absence of cirrhosis since HCC has been reported to occur in patients with HBV infection alone

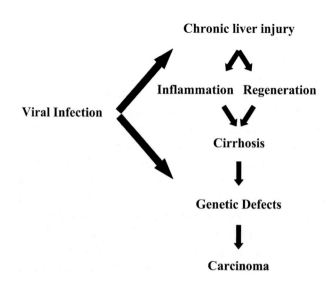

Fig. 10.1 Hypotheses of action of HBV in the pathogenesis of HCC

(Okuda et al 1982). In vitro, transfection of HBV DNA into murine hepatocytes results in malignant transformation (Hohne et al 1990).

Woodchucks and Beechey ground squirrels also get hepadnavirus associated hepatocellular carcinoma. Direct viral effects appear to be involved but they are distinct (Robinson 1994) (Table 10.4). Woodchuck hepatitis (WHV) virus infection results in insertional mutagenesis of viral DNA near the c-myc or n-myc proto-oncogene half the time and increased myc transcription (Brechot et al 1980, Edman et al 1980, Fourel et al 1990, Hsu et al 1988). Interestingly, more than 90% of infected woodchucks die of HCC but they do not get cirrhosis. In the Beechey ground squirrels, the ground squirrel hepatitis virus (GSHV) also seems to act directly in the pathogenesis of HCC. C-myc amplification occurs (Transy et al 1992). The expression of c-myc has been shown to be increased in some humans with HCC as discussed above. As in the woodchuck, the ground

Table 10.4 Comparison of hepadnavirus infections.

	Woodchuck	Squirrel	Human
Hepadnavirus	WHV	GSHV	HBV
Cirrhosis	—	—	+
HCC	> 90%	50%	15%
myc alterations			
Overexpression	+	+	+
Insertional mutagenesis	+	—	—
Amplification	—	+	—
p53 mutation	—	—	+

WHV, woodchuck hepatitis virus; GSHV, ground squirrel hepatitis virus; HBV, hepatitis B virus

squirrel does not get cirrhosis. Mutation in p53 is absent in both the woodchuck and squirrel.

In humans, the HBV X protein may also exert a direct effect in the development of HCC. Instead of inserting into cellular DNA, HBV may act through transcriptional activation of distant genes. The HBV X gene produces a protein that is a promiscuous transactivator of many gene promoters in vitro and it alters a number of nuclear transcription factors. Specifically, it has been shown to activate the oncogenes c-jun and c-fos in vitro (Natoli et al 1994). It can also bind to p53 protein in the cytoplasm and inhibits the functions of p53 both in vitro and in vivo including p53-mediated apoptosis (Wang et al 1995, Wang et al 1994). In 84% of transgenic mice engineered to express the HBV X protein, liver cancer arises after 1 year of age in the absence of inflammation or cirrhosis (Kim et al 1991, Koike et al 1994). The X protein also increases epidermal growth factor receptor expression on human hepatocellular carcinoma cells lines which allows for the action of TGF alpha which is upregulated in HBV associated HCC (Hsia et al 1992, Menzo et al 1993).

There is evidence to support an indirect mechanism for HBV to lead to HCC as well. The hypothesis is that viral infection leads to chronic liver injury which produces regeneration and inflammation. Cirrhosis is the end result and predisposes to the development of HCC (Fig. 10.1). First, the extent of inflammation in HBV infection is proportional to the risk of developing cancer as those with cirrhosis have a higher susceptibility than those with chronic active hepatitis or just HBV infection alone. Next, about 20% of patients with HCC do not have integrated HBV DNA. Even when it does occur, integration of viral DNA near a cellular gene is rarely encountered in humans infected with HBV. Also, 80% of HBV-related HCC occurs in cirrhotics. Furthermore, cirrhotic nodules within an individual liver usually have different clonality with respect to HBV sequences (Aoki & Robinson 1989). In experimental systems, HBV transgenic mice which overexpress the hepatitis B surface antigen develop regeneration and inflammation followed by cirrhosis and then progress to HCC (Chisari et al 1989). HCC has been shown to arise in regenerative nodules and there is clonality between a tumor that develops within a regenerative nodule and the surrounding adenomatous hyperplasia (Takayama et al 1990, Tsuda et al 1988).

HEPATITIS C

Hepatitis C is a 9.6 kb single-stranded RNA virus of the flavivirus family. More than half of infected patients develop chronic infection and about one-quarter progress

to cirrhosis and are at risk for HCC (Heintges & Wands 1997). Transmission occurs by the parenteral route and involves blood transfusion or contact with blood products. The molecular mechanism responsible for the development of HCC in the setting of hepatitis C infection has not been elucidated. Integration of the viral DNA does not occur into the host DNA since the RNA virus does not undergo reverse transcription into DNA. However, viral RNA and evidence for viral replication have been identified in HCC specimens (Kobayashi et al 1994). Most patients with HCC have active infection as there is detectable RNA in serum. A transcriptional activator has not been identified. Mutations in p53 have been reported in 20 of 67 patients with HCV associated HCC (Oda et al 1992). The interval between infection and the time of cirrhosis and then carcinoma is 20–30 years (Kiyosawa et al 1990). Comparisons have been made between HCC associated with HBV and HCV (Shiratori et al 1995). Overall, infection with HCV appears to produce more severe inflammation of the liver as more patients are cirrhotic (70 versus 50%) and fewer are Child's Class A (37 versus 65%). Those with HCV cirrhosis develop HCC in 75% of cases within 15 years (compared to 27% in HBV cirrhosis) (Ikeda et al 1993). Dual infection with HCV and HBV produces the highest risk of HCC in cirrhotics (Benvegnu et al 1994). As has been reported with HBV infection, there are patients with HCV infection who develop HCC without cirrhosis (De Mitri et al 1995).

METABOLIC DISEASES

The importance of cirrhosis in the development of hepatocellular carcinoma is underscored by the association of several metabolic diseases with HCC. A number of metabolic diseases are associated with cirrhosis and the development of HCC. Hemochromatosis is the most frequent metabolic disease associated with HCC. It is autosomal recessive and about 40 to 60% of patients will develop HCC (Niederau et al 1985). Before the onset of cirrhosis in these patients HCC is rare and with cirrhosis the risk of HCC is 200 times greater. Alpha 1 anti-trypsin deficiency is an autosomal recessive disorder that may result in HCC though this occurs in only 10–15% of patients and essentially only in those that are homozygous. The altered serum proteinase inhibitor accumulates in the rough endoplasmic reticulum and causes hepatitis. The relative risk of HCC is 20 and about half occur without cirrhosis (Eriksson et al 1986). The risk of HCC in the heterozygous state is not increased. Tyrosinemia is an autosomal recessive disease that carries nearly a 40% chance of HCC and patients greater than 2 years of age are at risk resulting in these patients now undergoing liver transplantation. There are only 11 reported cases of HCC in Wilson's disease (Cheng et al 1992). HCC in Type I glycogen storage disease may occur without cirrhosis.

FAMILIAL LIVER CANCER

The existence of familial liver cancer is controversial. It is difficult to distinguish genetic factors from environmental factors which are clustered such as HBV infection or AFB_1 exposure. Convincing data for a genetic predisposition to HCC is lacking and HCC is not part of any multicancer syndromes. There are two studies that suggest a genetic inheritance. In a study from China of nearly 500 families, there was an increased risk of HCC among parents and children of patients with liver cancer even when the analysis was controlled for HBV infection (Shen et al 1991). In men infected with HBV, there was a lifetime risk of 84% for developing liver cancer compared to 9% in infected males without a family history. Hepatitis B virus infected females had a 46% chance of liver cancer (versus 1%). Alberts et al (1991) studied Native Alaskans and identified five families in which one-third of the 45 cases of liver cancer occurred. In four of the families, HBV was involved. The risk of HCC in patients with the susceptible genotype was estimated at 90% compared to 9% in those without it. The median age at diagnosis of HCC in the population with the susceptible genotype was 22 years compared to 54 years in the others.

CHOLANGIOCARCINOMA

There have been few investigations into the molecular pathogenesis of cholangiocarcinoma. In a study of 63 patients with cholangiocarcinoma (of unspecified location), there were 47 (75%) patients with ras mutations, 59 (95%) with myc mutations, and 46 (73%) with erb-B-2 alterations (Voravud et al 1989). In a study of 21 intrahepatic cholangiocarcinomas, K-ras mutation was found in ten patients and p53 mutation was detected in four (Ohashi et al 1995). Another group found p53 mutations in 13 of 38 patients (Kiba et al 1993). There are also several reports of molecular analysis of extrahepatic cholangiocarcinoma. In an analysis of 15 patients, all had a codon 12 mutation in K-ras (Levi et al 1991). Watanabe et al (1994) reported K-ras mutations in all ten patients studied. There were 13 of 32 patients with extrahepatic cholangiocarcinoma who had K-ras mutation in another study (Imai et al 1994).

GALLBLADDER CANCER

Gallbladder cancer also has been found to have K-ras mutations and in one study it was present in six of 18 patients (Imai et al 1994). Other investigators demonstrated K-ras mutation in six of 11 patients (Watanabe et al 1994). In an analysis of 26 patients with early stage gallbladder cancer, there were 20 patients with normal biliary anatomy who had a 65% rate of p53 mutation and 6% prevalence of K-ras mutation (Hanada et al 1996). In addition, there were 6 patients who had an anomalous junction of the pancreaticobiliary duct and four of them had a p53 mutation and three of them had a K-ras mutation. Thus, p53 mutation occurs in early gallbladder cancer as does K-ras mutation but the latter is more common with abnormal ductal anatomy. In a report of nine patients with hyperplasia of the gallbladder, there were two patients with K-ras mutation (Tada et al 1990, Tanno et al 1998).

REFERENCES

Aguilar F, Hussain S P, Cerutti P 1993 Aflatoxin B1 induces the transversion of G→T in codon 249 of the p53 tumor suppressor gene in human hepatocytes. Proceedings of the National Academy of Sciences of the USA 90: 8586–8590

Aguilar F, Harris C C, Sun T, Hollstein M, Cerutti P 1994 Geographic variation of p53 mutational profile in nonmalignant human liver. Science 264: 1317–1319

Alberts S R, Lanier A P, McMahon B J, Harpster A, Bulkow L R et al 1991 Clustering of hepatocellular carcinoma in Alaska Native families. Genetic Epidemiology 8: 127–139

Almoguera C, Shibata D, Forrester K, Martin J, Arnheim N, Perucho M 1988 Most human carcinomas of the exocrine pancreas contain mutant c-K-ras genes. Cell 53: 549–554

Aoki N, Robinson W S 1989 State of hepatitis B viral genomes in cirrhotic and hepatocellular carcinoma nodules. Molecular Biology Medicine 6: 395–408

Bailey E A, Iyer R S, Stone M P, Harris T M, Essigmann J M 1996 Mutational properties of the primary aflatoxin B1–DNA adduct. Proceedings of the National Academy of Sciences of the USA 93: 1535–1539

Bartsch D, Hahn S A, Danichevski K D et al 1999 Mutations of the DPC4/Smad4 gene in neuroendocrine pancreatic tumors. Oncogene 18: 2367–2371

Beasley R P, Hwang L Y, Lin C C, Chien C S 1981 Hepatocellular carcinoma and hepatitis B virus. A prospective study of 22 707 men in Taiwan. Lancet 2: 1129–1133

Benvegnu L, Fattovich G, Noventa F et al 1994 Concurrent hepatitis B and C virus infection and risk of hepatocellular carcinoma in cirrhosis. A prospective study. Cancer 74: 2442–2448

Bergman W, Watson P, de Jong J, Lynch H T, Fusaro R M 1990 Systemic cancer and the FAMMM syndrome. British Journal of Cancer 61: 932–936

Boix L, Rosa J L, Ventura F 1994 c-met mRNA overexpression in human hepatocellular carcinoma. Hepatology 19: 88–91

Brechot C, Pourcel C, Louise A, Rain B, Tiollais P 1980 Presence of integrated hepatitis B virus DNA sequences in cellular DNA of human hepatocellular carcinoma. Nature 286: 533–535

Bressac B, Kew M, Wands J, Ozturk M 1991 Selective G to T mutations of p53 gene in hepatocellular carcinoma from southern Africa [see comments]. Nature 350: 429–431

Bullock G J, Green J L, Baron P L 1999 Impact of p16 expression on surgical management of malignant melanoma and pancreatic carcinoma. [Review] [39 refs]. American Journal of Surgery 177: 15–18

Caldas C, Hahn S A, da Costa L T et al 1994a Frequent somatic mutations and homozygous deletions of the p16 (MTS1) gene in pancreatic adenocarcinoma [published erratum appears in Nature Genetics 1994 8(4):410] Nature Genetics 8: 27–32

Caldas C, Hahn S A, Hruban R H, Redston M S, Yeo C J, Kern S E 1994b Detection of K-ras mutations in the stool of patients with pancreatic adenocarcinoma and pancreatic ductal hyperplasia. Cancer Research 54: 3568–3573

Chaubert P, Gayer R, Zimmermann A et al 1997 Germ-line mutations of the p16INK4(MTS1) gene occur in a subset of patients with hepatocellular carcinoma. Hepatology 25: 1376–1381

Chen D S, Hoyer B H, Nelson J, Purcell R H, Gerin J L 1982 Detection and properties of hepatitis B viral DNA in liver tissues from patients with hepatocellular carcinoma. Hepatology 2: 42s–46s

Cheng W S, Govindarajan S, Redeker A G 1992 Hepatocellular carcinoma in a case of Wilson's disease. Liver 12: 42–45

Chisari F V, Klopchin K, Moriyama T et al 1989 Molecular pathogenesis of hepatocellular carcinoma in hepatitis B virus transgenic mice. Cell 59: 1145–1156

Collier J D, Guo K, Mathew J et al 1992 c-erbB-2 oncogene expression in hepatocellular carcinoma and cholangiocarcinoma. Journal of Hepatology 14: 377–380

De Mitri M S, Poussin K, Baccarini P et al 1995 HCV-associated liver cancer without cirrhosis. Lancet 345: 413–415

Donehower L A, Harvey M, Slagle B L et al 1992 Mice deficient for p53 are developmentally normal but susceptible to spontaneous tumours. Nature 356: 215–221

Edman J C, Gray P, Valenzuela P, Rall L B, Rutter W J 1980 Integration of hepatitis B virus sequences and their expression in a human hepatoma cell. Nature 286: 535–538

El Serag H B, Mason A C 1999 Rising incidence of hepatocellular carcinoma in the United States. New England Journal of Medicine 340: 745–750

Eriksson S, Carlson J, Velez R 1986 Risk of cirrhosis and primary liver cancer in alpha 1-antitrypsin deficiency. New England Journal of Medicine 314: 736–739.

Fearon E R, Vogelstein B 1990 A genetic model for colorectal tumorigenesis. Cell 61: 759–767

Fourel G, Trepo C, Bougueleret L et al 1990 Frequent activation of N-myc genes by hepadnavirus insertion in woodchuck liver tumours. Nature 347: 294–298

Fujimoto Y, Hampton L L, Luo L D, Wirth P J, Thorgeirsson S S 1992 Low frequency of p53 gene mutation in tumors induced by aflatoxin B1 in nonhuman primates. Cancer Research 52: 1044–1046

Furukawa T, Chiba R, Kobari M, Matsuno S, Nagura H, Takahashi T 1994 Varying grades of epithelial atypia in the pancreatic ducts of humans. Classification based on morphometry and multivariate analysis and correlated with positive reactions of carcinoembryonic antigen. Archives of Pathology & Laboratory Medicine 118: 227–234

Ghadirian P, Boyle P, Simard A, Baillargeon J, Maisonneuve P, Perret C 1991 Reported family aggregation of pancreatic cancer within a population-based case-control study in the Francophone community in Montreal, Canada. International Journal of Pancreatology 10: 183–196

Giardiello F M, Offerhaus G J, Lee D H et al 1993 Increased risk of thyroid and pancreatic carcinoma in familial adenomatous polyposis. Gut 34: 1394–1396

Goggins M, Schutte M, Lu J et al 1996 Germline BRCA2 gene mutations in patients with apparently sporadic pancreatic carcinomas. Cancer Research 56: 5360–5364

Goggins M, Offerhaus G J, Hilgers W et al 1998 Pancreatic adenocarcinomas with DNA replication errors (RER+) are associated with wild-type K-ras and characteristic histopathology. Poor differentiation, a syncytial growth pattern, and pushing borders suggest RER+. American Journal of Pathology 152: 1501–1507

Griffin C A, Hruban R H, Morsberger L A et al 1995 Consistent chromosome abnormalities in adenocarcinoma of the pancreas. Cancer Research 55: 2394–2399

Hahn S A, Seymour A B, Hoque A T et al 1995 Allelotype of pancreatic adenocarcinoma using xenograft enrichment. Cancer Research 55: 4670–4675

Hahn S A, Schutte M, Hoque A T et al 1996 DPC4, a candidate tumor suppressor gene at human chromosome 18q21.1. Science 271: 350–353

Hall P A, Hughes C M, Staddon S L, Richman P I, Gullick W J, Lemoine N R 1990 The c-erb B-2 proto-oncogene in human pancreatic cancer. Journal of Pathology 161: 195–200

Hanada K, Itoh M, Fujii K, Tsuchida A, Ooishi H, Kajiyama G 1996 K-ras and p53 mutations in stage I gallbladder carcinoma with an anomalous junction of the pancreaticobiliary duct. Cancer 77: 452–458

Heintges T, Wands J R 1997 Hepatitis C virus: Epidemiology and transmission. Hepatology 26: 521–526

Hohne M, Schaefer S, Seifer M, Feitelson M A, Paul D, Gerlich W H 1990 Malignant transformation of immortalized transgenic hepatocytes after transfection with hepatitis B virus. DNA EMBO J. 9: 1137–1145

Hruban R H, Van Mansfield A D M, Offerhaus G J A et al 1993 K-ras oncogene activation in adenocarcinoma of the human pancreas. American Journal of Pathology 143: 545–554

Hsia C C, Axiotis C A, Di Bisceglie A M, Tabor E 1992 Transforming growth factor-alpha in human hepatocellular carcinoma and coexpression with hepatitis B surface antigen in adjacent liver. Cancer 70: 1049–1056

Hsu T, Moroy T, Etiemble J et al 1988 Activation of c-myc by woodchuck hepatitis virus insertion in hepatocellular carcinoma. Cell 55: 627–635

Huang S N, Chisari F V 1995 Strong, sustained hepatocellular proliferation precedes hepatocarcinogenesis in hepatitis B surface antigen transgenic mice. Hepatology 21: 620–626

Huang L, Goodrow T L, Zhang S Y, Klein-Szanto A J, Chang H, Ruggeri B A 1996 Deletion and mutation analyses of the P16/MTS-1 tumor suppressor gene in human ductal pancreatic cancer reveals a higher frequency of abnormalities in tumor-derived cell lines than in primary ductal adenocarcinomas. Cancer Research 56: 1137–1141

Hui A M, Sakamoto M, Kanai Y et al 1996 Inactivation of p16INK4 in hepatocellular carcinoma. Hepatology 24: 575–579

Hussussian C J, Struewing J P, Goldstein A M et al 1994 Germline p16 mutations in familial melanoma [see comments]. Nature Genetics 8: 15–21

Iguchi H, Sugano K, Fukayama N et al 1996 Analysis of Ki-ras codon 12 mutations in the duodenal juice of patients with pancreatic cancer. Gastroenterology 110: 221–226

Ikeda K, Saitoh S, Koida I et al 1993 A multivariate analysis of risk factors for hepatocellular carcinogenesis: a prospective observation of 795 patients with viral and alcoholic cirrhosis. Hepatology 18: 47–53

Imai M, Hoshi T, Ogawa K 1994 K-ras codon 12 mutations in biliary tract tumors detected by polymerase chain reaction denaturing gradient gel electrophoresis. Cancer 73: 2727–2733

Kalthoff H, Schmiegel W, Roeder C, Kasche D, Schmidt A, Lauer G, Thiele H G, Honold G, Pantel K, Rietmuller G 1993 p53 and K-Ras alterations in pancreatic epithelial cell lesions. Oncogene 8: 289–298

Kar S, Jaffe R, Carr B I 1993 Mutation at codon 249 of p53 gene in a human hepatoblastoma. Hepatology 18: 566–569

Katagiri T, Nakamura Y, Miki Y 1996 Mutations in the BRCA2 gene in hepatocellular carcinomas. Cancer Research 56: 4575–4577

Kazachkov Y, Khaoustov V, Yoffe B, Solomon H, Klintmalm G B, Tabor E 1996 p53 abnormalities in hepatocellular carcinoma from United States patients: analysis of all 11 exons. Carcinogenesis 17: 2207–2212

Kern S E, Pietenpol J A, Thiagalingam S, Seymour A, Kinzler K W, Vogelstein B 1992 Oncogenic forms of p53 inhibit p53-regulated gene expression. Science 256: 827–830

Kiba T, Tsuda H, Pairojkul C, Inoue S, Sugimura T, Hirohashi S 1993 Mutations of the p53 tumor suppressor gene and the ras gene family in intrahepatic cholangiocellular carcinomas in Japan and Thailand. Mol Carcinog 8: 312–318

Kim C M, Koike K, Saito I, Miyamura T, Jay G 1991 HBx gene of hepatitis B virus induces liver cancer in transgenic mice. Nature 351: 317–320

Kiyosawa K, Sodeyama T, Tanaka E, Gibo Y, Yoshizawa K et al 1990 Interrelationship of blood transfusion, non-A, non-B hepatitis and hepatocellular carcinoma: analysis by detection of antibody to hepatitis C virus. Hepatology 12: 671–675

Knudson A G 1971 Mutation and cancer: Statistical study of retinoblastoma. Proceedings of the National Academy of Sciences of the United States of America 68: 820–823

Kobayashi S, Hayashi H, Itoh Y, Asano T, Isono K 1994 Detection of minus-strand hepatitis C virus RNA in tumor tissues of hepatocellular carcinoma. Cancer 73: 48–52

Koike K, Moriya K, Iino S, Yotsuyanagi H, Endo Y et al 1994 High-level expression of hepatitis B virus HBx gene and hepatocarcinogenesis in transgenic mice. Hepatology 19: 810–819

Lee H S, Rajagopalan M S, Vyas G N 1988 A lack of direct role of hepatitis B virus in the activation of ras and c-myc oncogenes in human hepatocellular carcinogenesis. Hepatology 8: 1116–1120

Lemoine N R, Jain S, Hughes C M, Staddon S L, Maillet B et al 1992 Ki-ras oncogene activation in preinvasive pancreatic cancer. Gastroenterology 102: 230–236

Levi S, Urbano-Ispizua A, Gill R, Thomas D M, Gilbertson J et al 1991 Multiple K-ras codon 12 mutations in cholangiocarcinomas demonstrated with a sensitive polymerase chain reaction technique. Cancer Res. 51: 3497–3502

Li D, Cao Y, He L, Wang N J, Gu J R 1993 Aberrations of p53 gene in human hepatcellular carcinoma from China. Carcinogenesis 14: 169–173

Lumadue J A, Griffin C A, Osman M, Hruban R H 1995 Familial pancreatic cancer and the genetics of pancreatic cancer. Surgical Clinics of North America 75: 845–855

Lynch H T, Smyrk T, Kern S E, Hruban R H, Lightdale C J et al 1996 Familial pancreatic cancer: a review. Seminars in Oncology 23: 251–275

Matsubara K, Tokino T 1990 Integration of hepatitis B virus DNA and its implications for hepatocarcinogenesis. Molecular Biology Medicine 7: 243–260

Menzo S, Clementi M, Alfani E, Bagnarelli P, Iacovacci S et al 1993 Trans-activation of epidermal growth factor receptor gene by the hepatitis B virus X-gene product. Virology 196: 878–882

Moskaluk C A, Hruban R H, Kern S E 1997 p16 and K-ras gene mutations in the intraductal precursors of human pancreatic adenocarcinoma. Cancer Research 57: 2140–2143

Murakami Y, Hayashi K, Hirohashi S, Sekiya T 1991 Aberrations of the tumor suppressor p53 and retinoblastoma genes in human hepatocellular carcinomas. Cancer Research 51: 5520–5525

Natoli G, Avantaggiati M L, Chirillo P, Costanzo A, Artini M et al 1994 Induction of the DNA-binding activity of c-jun/c-fos heterodimers by the hepatitis B virus transactivator pX. Molecular and Cellular Biology 14: 989–998

Niederau C, Fischer R, Sonnenberg A, Stremmel W, Trampisch H J, Strohmeyer G 1985 Survival and causes of death in cirrhotic and in noncirrhotic patients with primary hemochromatosis. New England Journal of Medicine 313: 1256–1262

Nishida N, Fukuda Y, Kokuryu H et al 1992 Accumulation of allelic loss on arms of chromosomes 13q, 16q and 17p in the advanced stages of human hepatocellular carcinoma. International Journal of Cancer 51: 862–868

Nishida N, Fukuda Y, Kokuryu H et al 1993 Role and mutational heterogeneity of the p53 gene in hepatocellular carcinoma. Cancer Research 53: 368–372

Oda T, Tsuda H, Scarpa A, Sakamoto M, Hirohashi S 1992 p53 mutation spectrum in hepatocellular carcinoma. Cancer Research 52: 6358–6364

Ogata N, Kamimura T, Asakura H 1991 Point mutation, allelic loss and increased methylation of c-Ha-ras gene in human hepatocellular carcinoma. Hepatology 13: 31–37

Ohashi K, Nakajima Y, Kanehiro H et al 1995 Ki-ras mutations and p53 protein expressions in intrahepatic cholangiocarcinoma: relation to gross tumor morphology. Gastroenterology 109: 1612–1617

Okuda K, Nakashima T, Sakamoto K et al 1982 Hepatocellular carcinoma arising in noncirrhotic and highly cirrhotic livers: a comparative study of histopathology and frequency of hepatitis B markers. Cancer 49: 450–455

Okuda K, Tabor E (Eds.) Liver Cancer. Churchill Livingstone, New York

Ozturk M 1991 p53 mutation in hepatocellular carcinoma after aflatoxin exposure. Lancet 338: 1356–1359

Pellegata N S, Sessa F, Renault B, Bonato M, Leone B E, Solcia E, Ranzani G N 1994 K-ras and p53 gene mutations in pancreatic cancer: ductal and nonductal tumors progress through different genetic lesions. Cancer Research 54: 1556–1560

Piao Z, Kim H, Jeon B K, Lee W J, Park C 1997 Relationship between loss of heterozygosity of tumor suppressor genes and histologic differentiation in hepatocellular carcinoma. Cancer 80: 865–872

Qian G S, Ross R K, Yu M C et al 1994 A follow-up study of urinary markers of aflatoxin exposure and liver cancer risk in Shanghai, People's Republic of China. Cancer Epidemiology Biomarkers Prevention 3: 3–10

Robinson W S 1994 Molecular events in the pathogenesis of hepadnavirus-associated hepatocellular carcinoma. [Review] [94 refs]. Annual Review of Medicine 45: 297–323

Ross R K, Yuan J M, Yu M C et al 1992 Urinary aflatoxin biomarkers and risk of hepatocellular carcinoma. Lancet 339: 943–946

Rozenblum E, Schutte M, Goggins M et al 1997 Tumor-suppressive pathways in pancreatic carcinoma. Cancer Research 57: 1731–1734

Scarpa A, Capelli P, Mukai K et al 1993 Pancreatic adenocarcinomas frequently show p53 gene mutations. American Journal of Pathology 142: 1534–1543

Scarpa A, Capelli P, Villanueva A et al 1994 Pancreatic cancer in Europe: Ki-ras gene mutation pattern shows geographical differences. International Journal of Cancer 57: 167–171

Scorsone K A, Zhou Y Z, Butel J S, Slagle B L 1992 p53 mutations cluster at codon 249 in hepatitis B virus-positive hepatocellular carcinomas from China. Cancer Research 52: 1635–1638

Sessa F, Solcia E, Capella C et al 1994 Intraductal papillary-mucinous tumours represent a distinct group of pancreatic neoplasms: an investigation of tumour cell differentiation and K-ras, p53 and c-erbB-2 abnormalities in 26 patients. Virchows Archives 425: 357–367

Shen F M, Lee M K, Gong H M, Cai X Q, King M C 1991 Complex segregation analysis of primary hepatocellular carcinoma in Chinese families: interaction of inherited susceptibility and hepatitis B viral infection. American Journal of Human Genetics 49: 88–93

Sheu J C, Huang G T, Lee P H et al 1992 Mutation of p53 gene in hepatocellular carcinoma in Taiwan. Cancer Res 52: 6098–6100

Shiratori Y, Shiina S, Imamura M et al 1995 Characteristic difference of hepatocellular carcinoma between hepatitis B- and C-viral infection in Japan. Hepatology 22: 1027–1033

Stork P, Loda M, Bosari S, Wiley B, Poppenhusen K, Wolfe H 1991 Detection of K-ras mutations in pancreatic and hepatic neoplasms by non-isotopic mismatched polymerase chain reaction. Oncogene 6: 857–862

Tabor E 1994 Tumor suppressor genes, growth factor genes, and oncogenes in hepatitis B virus-associated hepatocellular carcinoma. [Review] [86 refs]. Journal of Medical Virology 42: 357–365

Tada M, Yokosuka O, Omata M, Ohto M, Isono K 1990 Analysis of ras gene mutations in biliary and pancreatic tumors by polymerase chain reaction and direct sequencing. Cancer 66: 930–935

Tada M, Omata M, Ohto M 1991 Ras gene mutations in intraductal papillary neoplasms of the pancreas. Analysis in five cases. Cancer 67: 634–637

Tada M, Omata M, Kawai S et al 1993 Detection of ras gene mutations in pancreatic juice and peripheral blood of patients with pancreatic adenocarcinoma. Cancer Research 53: 2472–2474

Tada M, Ohashi M, Shiratori Y et al 1996 Analysis of K-ras gene mutation in hyperplastic duct cells of the pancreas without pancreatic disease. Gastroenterology 110: 227–231

Takayama T, Makuuchi M, Hirohashi S et al 1990 Malignant transformation of adenomatous hyperplasia to hepatocellular carcinoma. Lancet 336: 1150–1153

Tanno S, Obara T, Fujii T et al 1998 Proliferative potential and K-ras mutation in epithelial hyperplasia of the gallbladder in patients with anomalous pancreaticobiliary ductal union. Cancer 83: 267–275

Teramoto T, Satonaka K, Kitazawa S, Fujimori T, Hayashi K, Maeda S 1994 p53 gene abnormalities are closely related to hepatoviral infections and occur at a late stage of hepatocarcinogenesis. Cancer Research 54: 231–235

Transy C, Fourel G, Robinson W S, Tiollais P, Marion P L, Buendia M A 1992 Frequent amplification of c-myc in ground squirrel liver tumors associated with past or ongoing infection with a hepadnavirus. Proceedings of the National Academy of Sciences of the USA 89: 3874–3878

Tsuda H, Hirohashi S, Shimosato Y, Terada M, Hasegawa H 1988 Clonal origin of atypical adenomatous hyperplasia of the liver and clonal identity with hepatocellular carcinoma. Gastroenterology 95: 1664–1666

Tsuda H, Hirohashi S, Shimosato Y, Ino Y, Yoshida T, Terada M 1989 Low incidence of point mutation of c-Ki-ras and N-ras oncogenes in human hepatocellular carcinoma. Japanese Journal of Cancer Research 80: 196–199

Ueda H, Ullrich S J, Gangemi J D et al 1995 Functional inactivation but not structural mutation of p53 causes liver cancer. Nature Genetics 9: 41–47

Ueki T, Fujimoto J, Suzuki T, Yamamoto H, Okamoto E 1997 Expression of hepatocyte growth factor and its receptor c-met proto-oncogene in hepatocellular carcinoma. Hepatology 25: 862–866

Unsal H, Yakicier C, Marcais C et al 1994 Genetic heterogeneity of hepatocellular carcinoma. Proceedings of the National Academy of Sciences of the USA 91: 822–826

Vogelstein B, Kinzler K W 1992 p53 function and dysfunction. Cell 70: 523–526

Vogelstein B, Fearon E R, Hamilton S R et al 1988 Genetic alterations during colorectal-tumor development. New England Journal of Medicine 319: 525–532

Voravud N, Foster C S, Gilbertson J A, Sikora K, Waxman J 1989 Oncogene expression in cholangiocarcinoma and in normal hepatic development. Human Pathology 20: 1163–1168

Wang J, Chenivesse X, Henglein B, Brechot C 1990 Hepatitis B virus integration in a cyclin A gene in a hepatocellular carcinoma. Nature 343: 555–557

Wang X W, Gibson M K, Vermeulen W et al 1995 Abrogation of p53-mediated apoptosis by the hepatitis B virus X gene. Cancer Research 55: 6012–6016

Wang X W, Forrester K, Yeh H, Feitelson M A, Gu J R, Harris C C 1994 Hepatitis B virus X protein inhibits p53 sequence-specific DNA binding, transcriptional activity, and association with transcription factor ERCC3. Proceedings of the National Academy of Sciences of the USA 91: 2230–2234

Watanabe M, Asaka M, Tanaka J, Kurosawa M, Kasai M, Miyazaki T 1994 Point mutation of K-ras gene codon 12 in biliary tract tumors. Gastroenterology 107: 1147–1153

Weyrer K, Feichtinger H, Haun M et al 1996 p53, Ki-ras, and DNA ploidy in human pancreatic ductal adenocarcinomas. Laboratory Investigation 74: 279–289

Wilentz R E, Chung C H, Sturm P D et al 1998 K-ras mutations in the duodenal fluid of patients with pancreatic carcinoma. Cancer 82: 96–103

Williams T M, Weiner D B, Greene M I, Maguire H C J 1991 Expression of c-erbB-2 in human pancreatic adenocarcinomas. Pathobiology 59: 46–52

Wogan G N 1992 Aflatoxins as risk factors for hepatocellular carcinoma in humans. Cancer Research 52: 2114s–2118s

Zhang X, Xu H J, Murakami Y et al 1994 Deletions of chromosome 13q, mutations in retinoblastoma 1, and retinoblastoma protein state in human hepatocellular carcinoma. Cancer Research 54: 4177–4182

Hemostasis in hepatic and biliary disorders

11

G.V. PAPATHEODORIDIS AND A.K. BURROUGHS

Hemostasis is a dynamic process that prevents the escape of blood from a damaged vessel (Fig. 11.1). Under normal physiological conditions, blood circulates through the vasculature without thrombosis or bleeding. When vessel injury occurs, platelets are activated and adhere to the damaged endothelium or subendothelium leading to the formation of the primary hemostatic plug (primary hemostasis). The exposed subendothelium also activates the coagulation cascade which ultimately leads to thrombin generation (Carr 1989). Thrombin leads to generation of fibrin, which is deposited between and attached to the platelets and strengthens the friable primary hemostatic plug. At the same time, degradation of fibrin (fibrinolysis) begins in an orderly manner to confine the hemostatic process to the site of vascular injury.

Primary hemostasis depends mainly on the number and function of platelets, while coagulation depends on the activation of several clotting factors as well as on the presence of activated platelets (Roberts et al 1998) (Fig. 11.2). The tissue factor released by the injured vessel and activated factor VII play the key role in the initiation of the coagulation cascade. This results in activation of factors X and IX; activated factor X with its co-factor V converts prothrombin (factor II) to thrombin, which subsequently activates platelets and factors V, VIII and perhaps XI. Activated factors IX and VIII recruit and activate more factor X, which again converts prothrombin to thrombin (Fig. 11.2). This secondary thrombin production is essential, since it produces large amounts of thrombin which are necessary for stable fibrin clot formation. Finally, thrombin converts fibrinogen to fibrin and activates factor XIII, which is involved in the integration of fibrin polymers into the platelet plug. Fibrinolysis is initiated by the tissue plasminogen activator (tPA), which is released from endothelial cells and converts plasminogen to active plasmin causing fibrin degradation (Fig. 11.3).

The liver has a central role in the maintenance of normal hemostatic mechanisms, so that impairment of hemostasis is

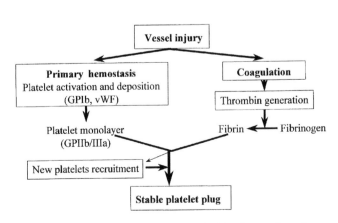

Fig. 11.1 Main hemostatic mechanisms. GPIb: (platelet membrane) glycoprotein Ib, GPIIb/IIIa: complex of the (platelet membrane) glycoproteins IIb and IIIa, vWF: von Willebrand's factor.

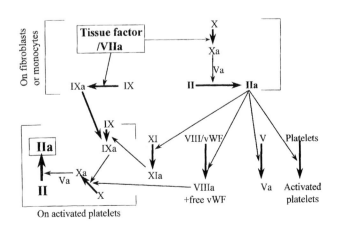

Fig. 11.2 The coagulation cascade. Roman numerals represent the corresponding coagulation factors, 'a' means activated coagulation factor, vWF: von Willebrand's factor.

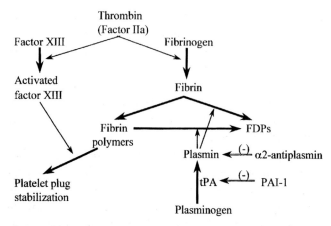

Fig. 11.3 Fibrinogenesis and fibrinolysis. FDPs: fibrin degradation products, tPA: tissue plasminogen activator, PAI-1: plasminogen activator inhibitor, (–) means inhibition

quite common in liver disease. The effect of liver disease on the hemostatic balance is complex, since the liver is responsible for the synthesis, activation, and clearance of most factors and inhibitors involved in coagulation and fibrinolysis. Moreover, thrombocytopenia and abnormal platelet function are frequently present. Thus, bleeding is a common complication and a leading cause of death in patients with advanced liver disease (Schlichting et al 1983), but thrombotic complications can also occur. Although hemostatic disorders usually accompany liver diseases with damaged hepatocytes, they may also be found in patients with extrahepatic portal hypertension (Robson et al 1993).

HEMOSTATIC FACTORS

PROCOAGULANT FACTORS

The liver is the main site of synthesis of all coagulation factors except von Willebrand's factor (vWF) (Mammen 1994). Thus, acute or chronic liver failure results in impaired synthesis of almost all coagulation factors. Factor VIII is synthesized mainly by the hepatocyte but also by many other tissues (Wion et al 1985), and so it is not reduced in liver disease. vWF is synthesized by vascular endothelial cells (Jaffe et al 1973).

Vitamin K-dependent factors

The vitamin K-dependent coagulation factors (II, VII, IX, X) belong to a unique group of calcium-binding proteins, all of which contain γ-carboxyglutamic acid. They are all synthesized in the liver in non-functional precursor forms called 'proteins induced in vitamin K absence' (PIVKA). Reduced vitamin K is necessary for the activation of the non-functional PIVKA (through carboxylation by a liver carboxylase of the N-terminal glutamic acid residues prior to glycosylation and secretion). Failure of bile salt secretion results in poor vitamin K absorption and therefore PIVKA may be produced in the presence of obstructive jaundice. PIVKA can also be detected in patients with liver disease without vitamin K deficiency suggesting an acquired defect of carboxylation (Blanchard et al 1981). The suggested mechanism is either premature release of prothrombin precursors because of hepatic necrosis or vitamin K-dependent carboxylase deficiency. Abnormal prothrombin (decarboxy-prothrombin) has been suggested as a marker of primary hepatocellular cancer (Liebman et al 1984). It is detected in the serum of most patients with hepatocellular cancer and does not disappear after vitamin K administration; its concentration is reduced by tumor resection and chemotherapy.

The vitamin K-dependent factors are the first coagulation factors that are reduced in liver disease, with factor VII (the factor with shortest half-life) being the most sensitive (Goodnight et al 1971). Declines in factors II and X levels usually follow, while factor IX concentration may be less affected (Lechner et al 1977). Recently, a genetic variation in the 3' untranslated region of the prothrombin gene was described and it was associated with increased plasma prothrombin levels and a high risk for venous thrombotic episodes (Poort et al 1996). The role of this mutation in patients with liver disease has not been studied yet.

Fibrinogen

Normal fibrinogen (factor I) concentrations are usually lower than normal in cirrhosis (Lechner et al 1977), but high levels of fibrinogen may be detected in cirrhosis, chronic hepatitis, obstructive jaundice and biliary cirrhosis and hepatoma (Soria et al 1980). High fibrinogen levels are due to abnormal non-functional fibrinogen because of defective polymerization and may be found in about 70% of patients with liver disease (Francis & Armstrong 1978, Green et al 1976a). Excess amount of low molecular weight fibrinogen (Lipinski et al 1977), abnormal α chains (Weinstein & Deykin 1978) and higher than normal sialic acid contents (Martinez et al 1978) have been described in these abnormal fibrinogen molecules. Acquired dysfibrinogenemia should be suspected in patients with prolonged thrombin time in the absence of abnormal concentrations of fibrinogen or increased fibrin degradation products (FDPs). Dysfibrinogenemia is thought to reflect the severity of liver function impairment (Green et al 1977).

Factor VIII and von Willebrand's factor

Both factor VIII and vWF concentrations are raised in chronic liver disease (Green & Rantoff 1974, Kelly et al 1985). There is a disproportionate increase in the procoagulant antigen of factor VIII and vWF (VIII:CAg & vWF:Ag) compared with the functional coagulant activities of these proteins (VIII:C & vWF: C). The interpretation of this finding is not clear. The plasma concentration of factor VIII is said to be helpful in differentiating coagulation abnormalities secondary to fulminant hepatic failure or DIC, since levels of factor VIII are low in DIC but often very high in fulminant liver failure.

PLATELETS

Platelets play a central role in hemostasis after activation by the vessel injury or the initial thrombin: (a) They form the primary hemostatic plug through aggregation and adhesion [vWF and the platelet membrane glycoprotein (GP) Ib play a central role]. (b) Their membrane offers an ideal surface for coagulation factors reactions to occur for the secondary thrombin generation. (c) Together with fibrin/fibrinogen, they form the stable hemostatic plug (the complex GPIIb/IIIa play a central role) (Ferguson et al 1998) (Fig. 11.1).

A number of platelet abnormalities have been reported in patients with chronic liver disease (Rubin et al 1979). Thrombocytopenia is one the most frequent laboratory findings in liver disease. It is often due to hypersplenism secondary to portal hypertension with enlargement and congestion of spleen which results in increased platelet sequestration and destruction (Aster 1966). However, only a few patients with thrombocytopenia due to advanced liver disease respond with an increase in production of platelets (Stein & Harker 1982). Moreover, portal decompression procedures either by surgical shunts (Mutchnick et al 1980, Soper & Rikkers 1982) or by transjugular intrahepatic portosystemic shunts (Alvarez et al 1996, Sanyal et al 1996) have not led to a consistent rise in platelet count. Therefore, other mechanisms, alone or in combination, should also be responsible. Bone marrow depression, abnormalities of primary platelet metabolism, folic acid deficiency in alcoholics, DIC, or autoimmune type thrombocytopenia have all been found in patients with liver diseases. In particular, anti-platelet antibodies and autoimmune type thrombocytopenia have been reported in patients with acute hepatitis A and B, autoimmune hepatitis or chronic hepatitis B (Landolfi et al 1980, Pfueller et al 1983), primary biliary cirrhosis (Bassendine et al 1985) and a variety of other liver diseases (Barrison et al 1981, de

Noronha et al 1991). Recently, chronic hepatitis C has been associated with autoimmune thrombocytopenia (Nagamine et al 1996) and has been found to be the cause of many cases previously labeled as 'idiopathic thrombocytopenic purpura'. The recent discovery of thrombopoietin, which is a potent stimulator of megakaryocyte growth and platelet production (de Sauvage et al 1994, Lok et al 1994) and is probably synthesized by the liver (Shimada et al 1995), has offered new explanations for the thrombocytopenia in liver disease and a possible link between liver disease and abnormal platelet growth and production. Thrombopoietin levels has been found to be low in patients with cirrhosis and to increase after liver transplantation (Peck-Radosavljevic et al 1997, Goulis et al 1999, Martin et al 1997).

Heavy alcohol intake by itself may also result in thrombocytopenia and qualitative platelet abnormalities (Cowan & Hines 1971). Profound thrombocytopenia is seen in those rare patients in whom aplastic anemia follows acute hepatitis, usually due to non-A, non-B, non-C agent. Thrombocytopenia may worsen during excessive blood transfusion for severe gastrointestinal bleeding in cirrhosis, since stored bank blood or packed red cells do not provide viable platelets nor adequate amounts of factors V or VIII. Interferon treatment may also be associated with thrombocytopenia due to bone marrow depression or rarely due to induction of autoimmune type thrombocytopenia (Shrestha et al 1995).

Various qualitative platelet defects have also been described in liver disease. Diminished clot retraction, impaired aggregation of platelets by ADP, collagen or thrombin and impaired agglutination by ristocetin have all been reported (Breddin 1962, Thomas et al 1967, Ballard & Marcus 1976, Rubin et al 1979). Platelet aggregation is frequently impaired in chronic liver disease (Ballard & Marcus 1976) and this is currently believed to be due to intrinsic platelet defects (Violi et al 1992, Laffi et al 1996, Younger et al 1997), although circulating factors such abnormal high density lipoprotein particles (apoE) have also been documented (Owen et al 1981, Desai et al 1989). Recently, an adhesion defect was reported to be more evident and consistent than the aggregation abnormalities in cirrhosis irrespective of the hematocrit (Ordinas et al 1996).

ANTICOAGULANT FACTORS

Protein C

Protein C is a vitamin K-dependent glycoprotein (Kiesel 1975, Stenflo 1975). It is so named because it was present as the third of four peaks, the others being peaks A, B and D, containing factors IX, II and X, respectively, eluted from a chromatography column used to separate vitamin K-dependent factors. It has been detected in the human hepatocyte and is presumed to be synthesized there (Wion et al 1985). It is activated by thrombin and thrombomodulin, which is contained within endothelial cells. Activated protein C inactivates factors V and VIII, thus behaving as an anticoagulant. Activated protein C also prevents the release from endothelial cells of the inhibitor of plasminogen activator, and in this way protein C promotes fibrinolysis. Deficiency of protein C may result in a thrombotic tendency. Genetic deficiency (autosomal recessive) is rare, but protein C deficiency may be detected (measured functionally or immunologically) in patients with chronic liver disease (Mannucci & Vigano 1982) and fulminant hepatic failure (Langley & Williams 1988). The low levels of protein C in liver disease usually reflect the general decrease in coagulation factors and parallel levels of factor VII (Griffin et al 1982). Warfarin treatment is very rarely required for protein C deficiency in patients with liver disease; protein C levels are usually replenished by fresh frozen plasma (Everson 1997). Genetic deficiency is treated by warfarin after replenishment of protein C levels by fresh-frozen plasma; it has been cured by liver transplantation (Casella et al 1988).

Recently, a point mutation in the factor V gene, the factor V Leiden mutation, has been described as the most frequent cause of hereditary thrombophilia (Dahlback et al 1993, Bertina et al 1994). In these patients, the abnormal factor V is resistant to cleavage by activated protein C resulting in uncontrolled hypercoagulant tendency. The factor V Leiden mutation has been associated with Budd–Chiari syndrome and hepatic vein thrombosis (Denninger et al 1995, Mahmoud et al 1995, Blanshard et al 1996) and rarely with portal vein thrombosis (Mahmoud et al 1997).

Protein S

Named after the city of Seattle where it was discovered, this vitamin K-dependent protein is synthesized chiefly by the hepatocytes (Fair & Marlar 1986), but from endothelial cells as well (Fair et al 1986). It occurs in two forms in plasma: 40% in the free form and 60% bound to C4B-binding protein. The free form is a cofactor of activated protein C that enhances its anticoagulant effect (Clousse & Comp 1986). Deficiency is rare and is associated with thrombotic episodes. Protein S levels are low in patients with liver disease and their decrease usually follows the decrease in other coagulation factors (Comp 1990).

Antithrombin III

Antithrombin III is a vitamin K-dependent glycoprotein synthesized by both hepatocytes and endothelial cells. It uses heparin as a cofactor, and forms complexes with all the serine protease coagulation factors (except factor VII) and inhibits thrombin and plasmin (Schipper & Ten Cate 1982). Thus, antithrombin III behaves as an anticoagulant. The evidence for this is supported by the observation that a small reduction of the serum antithrombin III level is associated with an increased risk of venous thrombosis and that antithrombin III replacement can be an effective treatment in cirrhotics with recurrent venous thrombosis (Carmassi et al 1995). Genetic deficiency (autosomal recessive) is rare and results in accelerated clotting. Low levels of antithrombin III are found in cirrhosis and acute hepatitis, which are thought to be due to reduced synthesis or consumption (Liebman et al 1983). However, depression of antithrombin III is usually mild to moderate in patients with liver disease and very rarely of clinical significance. Recently, antithrombin III replacement was shown to reduce hyperfibrinolysis markers (plasmin–antiplasmin complexes) in patients with liver cirrhosis (Carmassi et al 1997), but not to slow down the baseline consumptive coagulation component (Scherer et al 1997). The significance of these findings in clinical practice is still unclear.

FIBRINOLYSIS

Fibrinolysis is initiated by the tissue plasminogen activator (tPA), which converts plasminogen to active plasmin, which subsequently degrades fibrin into fibrin degradation products (FDPs) (Fig. 11.3). tPA is synthesized by and released from endothelial cells and is cleared by the liver. The activated fibrinolytic system is mainly controlled by two antifibrinolytic factors: the plasminogen activator inhibitor (PAI-1) and a plasmin inhibitor, α2-antiplasmin. Plasminogen and both antifibrinolytic factors are synthesized by the liver.

In vitro accelerated fibrinolysis in cirrhosis was first reported by Goodpasture in 1914 and subsequently by many others (Hans & Curtis 1938, Rantoff 1949, Fletcher et al 1964, De Hovi et al 1977). Accelerated fibrinolysis in acute or chronic liver disease, hepatocellular carcinoma, or obstructive jaundice is controversial and not universally accepted. However, it is a recognized phenomenon of hepatectomy and liver trauma (Ch. 68). Several mechanisms of hyperfibrinolysis have been postulated in liver disease: (a) increased levels of profibrinolytic factors (tPA) caused by reduced clearance (Fletcher et al 1964, Ogston et al 1971, Mowat et al 1974), (b) decreased levels of antifibrinolytic factors (PAI and/or antiplasmin) (Kwaan et al 1956, O'Connell et al 1964, Osman et al 1992), (c) a shift in balance between fibrinolytic and antifibrinolytic factors (Leebeek et al 1991), and (d) secondary hyperfibrinolysis due to clotting activation (Violi et al 1993) probably caused by endotoxemia (Violi et al 1995a).

Hyperfibrinolysis as defined by increases in profibrinolytic or decreases in antifibrinolytic factors appears to be a relatively common feature in patients with advanced liver cirrhosis. However, the various mechanisms which may be involved in the changes of such markers (such as decreased synthesis by the liver or impaired clearance or even loss to and/or degradation in extravascular spaces) make interpretations of the mechanisms extremely difficult. No correlation between levels of tPA and overall fibrinolytic activity as measured by dilute whole blood clot lysis time has been reported (Hersch et al 1987). We also did not find any evidence of fibrinolysis detected by thromboelastography (TEG), a test for global assessment of whole blood hemostasis, in cirrhotic patients (Ben-Ari et al 1997, Chau et al 1998, Papatheodoridis et al 1998). In one of our studies, hyperfibrinolysis was detected by TEG in only two patients after 5 days of ongoing sepsis (Papatheodoridis et al 1998).

Irrespective of their incidence, if changes in fibrinolysis occur, they have a serious impact on the hemostatic balance. Patients with congenital disorders of fibrinolysis, such as dysfibrinogenemia or homozygous deficiency of the α2-antiplasmin, experience a life-long hemophilia-like bleeding disorder. The extent to which hyperfibrinolysis contributes to the bleeding manifestations of liver disease has been assessed by several investigators with contradictory findings. A study of 861 patients with varying degrees of liver failure suggested that increased fibrinolysis increases the risk of gastrointestinal hemorrhage in patients with advanced cirrhosis (Violi et al 1992). However, in another study, accelerated fibrinolysis, as demonstrated by elevated tPA levels, was not predictive of bleeding (Boks et al 1986). In a different study, patients with abnormal clot lysis times seemed to be more susceptible to soft tissue bleeding after trauma and showed a trend towards increased intracranial bleeding but no increased susceptibility to gastrointestinal bleeding (Francis & Feinstein 1984).

DISSEMINATED INTRAVASCULAR COAGULATION

The primary abnormality in disseminated intravascular coagulation (DIC) is thrombosis (Colman et al 1972). Inappropriate thrombosis results from an inappropriate stimulus for coagulation with consumption of coagulation proteins and platelets. A compensatory fibrinolysis results. The coincidence of low clotting factor levels, hypofibrinogenemia and thrombocytopenia (common findings in chronic liver disease) has led to the belief that DIC plays a role in the hemostatic failure of liver disease. Three precipitating factors have been suggested: (a) a procoagulant factor released by necrotic hepatocytes (Verstraete et al 1974), (b) decreased levels of anticoagulants, such as antithrombin III (Bakker et al 1992), and most frequently (c) endotoxins (Wardle 1974, Wilkinson 1977, Violi et al 1995a) (Ch. 9) perhaps through endothelial procoagulant activation (Ferro et al 1997).

The presence of DIC in cirrhosis is controversial and not universally accepted. Although patients with cirrhosis have similar coagulation profiles to those found in patients with DIC, they do not have evidence of bleeding. Factor VIII:C levels have been suggested as reliable markers of increased consumption of coagulation factors, and a sudden drop was thought to support the diagnosis of DIC (Mammen 1994). Evidence for the presence of DIC in cirrhosis was supported by initial reports of a therapeutic effect of heparin in cirrhosis (Johansson 1964, Cordova et al 1982) and by the findings of elevated FDPs levels (Kelly & Tuddenham 1986). However, FDPs are only minimally elevated in patients with cirrhosis without bleeding (Mombelli et al 1988, Cioni et al 1990) and rarely present in the absence of precipitating factors such as sepsis (Violi et al 1992). In an autopsy series of 184 cases of patients with acute and/or chronic liver disease, microthrombi in more than three organs (evidence for DIC) were present in only 4 of 184 patients (Oka & Tanaka 1979). Although modern hemostatic measurements [such as thrombin/antithrombin III (TAT) complex, plasmin/α2-antiplasmin (PAP) complex, D-dimer levels] are frequently found to be elevated in liver cirrhosis (Kemkes-Matthes et al 1991, Bakker et al 1992, Kario et al 1992), they may be inferior to the conventional hemostasis parameters for the diagnosis of DIC in cirrhotic patients (Ho et al 1998).

An attractive explanation for the conflicting findings about DIC and hemostatic disorders in general in patients with advanced liver disease is that a new tenuous hemostatic balance is created with decreased control of both coagulation and fibrinolysis (Everson 1997). The balance may be disturbed by several triggering factors (infection, bleeding) towards either direction mainly resulting in consumptive coagulopathy or impaired fibrinolysis, which may manifest by hemorrhage or clotting episodes respectively.

Clinically significant DIC is rare in patients with liver disease and usually complicates severe bacterial infections or sepsis and shock. Clinically significant DIC can also develop in patients with peritoneovenous shunts (Harmon et al 1979) (Ch. 94). It is thought that thromboplastin from the ascitic fluid may activate coagulation, since filtration of the ascitic fluid prevents DIC (Parbhoo et al 1974). Therapy should, therefore, be directed toward the precipitating factors and replacing the clotting factors and inhibitors of coagulation and fibrinolysis by transfusion of fresh frozen plasma (Carr 1989). In the case of peritoneovenous shunts, shunt removal may be required. Heparin is not recommended for DIC in patients with liver disease.

CLINICAL ASPECTS OF ABNORMAL HEMOSTASIS IN LIVER AND BILIARY DISORDERS

EVALUATION OF THE RISK OF BLEEDING

Assessment of the risk of bleeding is important in the management of patients with all forms of liver disease: fulminant hepatic failure, cirrhosis and obstructive jaundice, particularly for patients undergoing diagnostic or therapeutic procedures (e.g. liver biopsy and other diagnostic and therapeutic invasive procedures, including surgery and transplantation). Evaluation of the risk of bleeding may also be important in assessing prognosis. Prothrombin time and platelet count have become the two traditional markers for bleeding risk on a historical basis mainly because they can be easily measured. However, the risk of bleeding cannot be always evaluated by routine hemostatic tests. Ewe (1981), in a study of 200 patients undergoing laparoscopic liver biopsies, found no correlation between the two traditional tests and the 'liver bleeding time'. This indicates that peripheral blood coagulation values do not reflect in vivo tissue clotting. 'Safe' values of coagulation indices have been suggested by different investigators. Sherlock and Dooley (1993) suggest needle biopsy should not be performed if the prothrombin time is more than 3 seconds longer than that of control plasma or if the platelet count is less than 80 000/ml. McVay and Toy (1990) found the frequency of bleeding complications in patients undergoing percutaneous liver biopsy with platelet counts over $50 \times 10^9/L$ was 3.4% (six of 175) with no significant difference between patients with mild hemostatic abnormalities (prothrombin times 1.1–1.5 times normal) and patients with normal parameters; malignancy was highly associated with bleeding complications. The same investigators have reported lack of increased bleeding after paracentesis and thoracentesis in patients with mild coagulation abnormalities (McVay & Toy 1991).

Burroughs et al (1988) recommend the use of the bleeding time in the assessment of bleeding risk in chronic liver diseases when the prothrombin time is not very elevated despite clinically significant hepatocellular failure. The bleeding time is the only test that represents primary hemostasis and is dependent on platelet number, size and function. It also depends on the concentration of vWF, the hematocrit, red cell deformability and the vessel wall. There is an inverse relationship between the bleeding time and a platelet count below $100 \times 10^9/L$ (Harker & Slichter 1972) but, in cirrhosis, abnormal bleeding times can be found with relatively high platelet counts, and there is not such a close correlation (Burroughs et al 1988).

Thromboelastography (TEG), first developed by Hartert in 1948, allows a global evaluation of hemostasis of whole blood. It evaluates viscoelastic properties of whole blood and is especially useful during the perioperative period (Kang et al 1985). TEG enables a global assessment of hemostatic function to be made from a single blood sample documenting the inter-reaction of platelets with the protein coagulation cascade, from the time of the initial platelet–fibrin interaction, through platelet aggregation, clot strengthening and fibrin cross-linkage right through to eventual clot lysis. The tracings generated can give information on clotting factor activity, platelet function and clinically significant fibrinolytic process within 20–30 minutes. The thromboelastograph is a small instrument, that can easily be set up in the operating, anesthetic room or ward. By virtue of having two separate channels it is possible to perform serial blood coagulation profiles. This allows coagulation to be monitored directly at regular intervals, enabling the effects of any therapeutic intervention to be assessed rapidly. We have found the TEG to be useful in the assessment and monitoring of coagulation profiles of cirrhotic patients with stable liver disease (BenAri et al 1997), variceal bleeding (Chau et al 1998), and bacterial infection (Papatheodoridis et al 1998).

When prothrombin time is above and/or platelet count below the 'traditional' thresholds prior to invasive procedures (e.g. needle liver biopsy), there is little evidence to support the use of fresh frozen plasma and/or platelets. It is advisable in such situations to obtain liver biopsy through the transjugular route (Lebrec et al 1982). Alternatively, a guided liver biopsy can be plugged with Gelfoam (Riley et al 1984, Sawyerr et al 1992). In our centre, plugged percutaneous liver biopsy is used in cases with prothrombin time between 3 and 5 s over control value and/or platelet count between 50 and $80 \times 10^9/L$ and transjugular liver biopsy in cases with worse parameters (Papatheodoridis et al 1999).

PROGNOSTIC VALUE OF COAGULATION PROTEINS

Coagulation tests are sensitive indicators of liver synthetic function and some are used as prognostic indicators. A prolonged prothrombin time not corrected by vitamin K parenteral administration indicates poor hepatic synthetic function and severe hepatocellular disease. Prothrombin time is one of the five components of the Pugh score (Pugh et al 1973). Because of its short half-life, factor VII is regarded by some as the best guide to the severity of liver disease (Green et al 1976b, Cordova et al 1986) and prognosis (Dymock et al 1975, Violi et al 1995b). Concentrations of factor V were also found to be a useful prognostic factor in chronic liver disease (Nanji & Blank 1983) and fulminant viral hepatitis (Bernau et al 1986, Bernau et al 1991), and a good marker for discrimination between acute alcoholic hepatitis and chronic alcoholic liver disease (Pereira et al 1992). Concentrations of factor V, however, were not found to be very effective in predicting the outcome of patients with paracetamol-induced fulminant hepatic failure (Izumi et al 1996). Recently in the liver transplant setting, effluent thrombomodulin levels were suggested as markers of the extent of graft preservation injury and as useful predictive markers for the early graft function (Suehiro et al 1997).

THERAPY FOR HEMOSTATIC ABNORMALITIES IN LIVER DISEASE

Vitamin K injections (10 mg daily) should be given if there is evidence of vitamin K deficiency, but should be discontinued if there is no further response after treatment for 2–3 days. Vitamin K usually corrects a prolonged prothrombin time in obstructive jaundice, but seldom in parenchymal liver disease. Whole blood or packed red blood cells should be given in severe blood loss (e.g. bleeding varices), but overtransfusion should be avoided; a common target is hemoglobin of 10 mg/dL or hematocrit of 30%. Platelet concentrates are used in patients with severe thrombocytopenia (platelet count $< 50 \times 10^9$/L) when severe complications (bleeding) occur, or before invasive procedures. Platelet transfusions are also needed in case of massive blood transfusion. Fresh frozen plasma supplies all the missing clotting factors, and it is usually used before invasive procedures and in patients with hemorrhage and coagulopathy. However, fresh frozen plasma carries the risk of transmitting unknown or undetected viruses since it is an unheated blood product; it may also be associated with fluid overload problems. All patients should be advised to avoid any drugs that can affect hemostasis (such as aspirin and non-steroidal antiinflammatory drugs, which cirrhotic patients should always avoid) for 7 days before any invasive procedure.

Recombinant activated factor VII (rFVIIa), which was developed for the treatment of hemophilia A and B patients with inhibitors against factors VIII and IX (Lusher 1996), seems to be a very promising drug for the management of hemostatic disorders in cirrhotic patients. Recently, a single dose of rFVIIa was shown to correct the prolonged prothrombin time in cirrhotics in a dose dependent manner (Bernstein et al 1997). Interestingly, another group showed that high dose of rFVIIa has platelet activity in vitro independent of tissue factor (Monroe et al 1997). We effectively used rFVIIa to correct hemostasis in a cirrhotic patient with hepatocellular cancer and to safely treat the cancer with alcohol injections (unpublished data). We observed that rFVIIa corrected not only prothrombin time but bleeding time as well. Thus, rFVIIa seems to represent a therapeutic advance, as it can correct both primary hemostasis and coagulation defects in cirrhosis, and, despite its high cost, it may find applications in routine clinical practice in the future.

Antithrombin III concentrates have been effective in DIC (Egbring et al 1981), fulminant hepatitis (Braude et al 1981) and in cirrotics with recurrent venous thrombosis (Carmassi et al 1995). Antithrombin III was found to be effective in preventing thrombosis after liver transplantation in children (Harper et al 1988), but it was ineffective in improving coagulation and fibrinolysis parameters and transfusional needs during liver transplantation in adults (Palareti et al 1991). It is essential to measure plasma thrombin–antithrombin III complex levels when antithrombin III concentrate is used.

DDAVP (desamino-D-arginylvasopressin) is a synthetic analogue of vasopressin which produces a two- to four-fold increase in plasma levels of factor VIII and vWF, presumably by release from storage sites (Mannucci et al 1981). DDAVP has been shown to shorten or normalize the bleeding time (Burroughs et al 1985, Mannucci et al 1986) and to shorten the partial thromboplastin time in cirrhosis (Agnelli et al 1995). In chronic liver disease, the use of DDAVP together with fresh frozen plasma enhances primary hemostasis which is not improved by plasma factors alone. However, a controlled clinical trial showed that DDAVP in combination with glypressin was not more effective than glypressin alone in the management of bleeding varices in cirrhotic patients (De Franchis et al 1993). Currently, there are no other prospective studies of the therapeutic benefit of DDAVP in liver disease (Mannucci 1997).

An interesting group of drugs that have been tried for the management of hemostatic disorders in liver diseases are the antifibrinolytic drugs. Two groups of antifibrinolytics are currently used: the lysine analogs (ε-aminocaproic acid and tranexamic acid) and the serine protease inhibitors (aprotinin). The lysine analogs are synthetic compounds which bind to plasminogen and plasmin (tranexamic acid is ten times more potent than ε-aminocaproic acid), while aprotinin ('Trasylol') is a natural polypeptide (from bovine lung) which inhibits plasmin, trypsin, kallikrein, and factor XIIa activation of complement. An antifibrinolytic drug may be used in case of confirmed ongoing primary fibrinolysis, but it should be avoided in case of secondary fibrinolysis due to DIC. To date, there is no randomized trial of antifibrinolytic drugs in the management of variceal bleeding in cirrhosis. Antifibrinolytics are most frequently used in the transplant setting and they are further discussed in that section.

COAGULOPATHY POST-PERITONEOVENOUS SHUNT

The development of ascites in cirrhosis is associated with poor prognosis. Treatment of ascites with diuretics can be dangerous and sometimes is not effective or is poorly tolerated. In early series, diuretics hastened death from renal failure rather than prolonged survival (Vesin 1972).

Peritoneovenous shunt (Ch. 94) restores the normal blood volume and normalizes the renal capacity to excrete salt and water and is an effective method of management of ascites. It has long been known to surgeons that blood shed into the peritoneal cavity becomes incoagulable. Such blood is immediately coagulated by soluble collagen and concurrently lysed by tPA. Large volumes of ascitic fluid infused into circulating blood is thought to simulate the fate of blood shed into the peritoneal cavity with lysis playing a major role. Post-shunt coagulopathy was thought to be due to DIC (Epstein 1982), and some recommended heparin as a prophylactic measure (Tawes et al 1981). However, DIC as a cause of post-shunt coagulopathy is not universally accepted and heparin has not proved to be effective (Harmon et al 1979).

A study by LeVeen et al (1987), found addition of ascitic fluid to normal platelet-rich plasma in vitro initiates clot lysis on TEG which was counteracted by ε-aminocaproic acid. They also found disposal of ascitic fluid at surgery prevented or ameliorated coagulopathy. Mild coagulopathy occurred only twice in 150 patients (1.3%) with only one case being clinically significant (0.6%), whereas severe post-shunt coagulopathy occurred seven times in 98 patients (7%) whose ascitic fluid was not discarded. They concluded that severe coagulopathy requires disconnection or removal of the shunt and bleeding should be treated with clotting factors and ε-aminocaproic acid. Peritoneal lavage with saline pre-

vents the recurrence of coagulopathy on reopening the shunt. Recently, Tang et al (1992) have shown that antiplatelet therapy prevents coagulopathy after ascitic reinfusion, but this is not a practical therapeutic option in patients with varices.

LIVER TRANSPLANTATION (See Chs. 107, 109, 110, 115)

The First Report of the European Liver Transplant Registry (Bismuth et al 1987) found bleeding complications to be the most frequent cause of death intraoperatively and during the first postoperative week (34%) and the second most frequent cause of death within the first 30 days. Moreover, large perioperative blood losses or large requirements of red blood cell transfusions have been associated with a high post-transplant mortality (Bontempo et al 1985, Van Thiel et al 1986, Kirby et al 1987). Recent advances in anesthetic and surgical techniques and improved graft preservation have contributed to reduced intraoperative blood loss. However, peri- and postoperative hemorrhage can still be a serious problem in orthotopic liver transplantation (OLT), which may require massive transfusion of blood and blood products.

Combinations of several mechanisms may contribute to defective hemostasis and increased bleeding:

1. Fragile and dilated collateral vessels due to pre-transplant portal hypertension which have to be dissected during the native hepatectomy. The presence of collateral circulation and previous abdominal surgery have been associated with excessive blood loss (Starzl et al 1982, Goldsmith 1983, Iwatsuki et al 1983, Barroso Garcia de Silva et al 1986, Kirby et al 1987), while a routine mini-laparotomy was not found to cause serious problems (Calne et al 1986).

2. Pre-existing hypocoagulable state. Preoperative liver synthetic function, coagulation defects and their severity and underlying diagnosis were found to correlate with intraoperative bleeding and transfusion requirements (Bontempo et al 1985, Haagsma et al 1985, Lewis et al 1988). However, such findings are not universal (Gerlach et al 1993) and no study has shown that preoperative correction of coagulopathy is associated with a decrease in intraoperative transfusion requirement. Thus, preoperative correction of coagulopathy is not routinely recommended.

3. Fibrinolysis, DIC. Several reports have suggested hyperfibrinolysis as a major cause of intraoperative bleeding (Arnoux et al 1989, Dzik et al 1988, Porte et al 1989) and antifibrinolytic drugs are used prophylactically in many centres. However, it is essential to differentiate

primary from secondary fibrinolysis. Secondary fibrinolysis follows DIC and is well documented in patients with liver disease (Carr 1989, Violi et al 1993). The above differential diagnosis is critical, since antifibrinolytics agents used for primary fibrinolysis can potentially cause disastrous thrombotic complications in patients with DIC and secondary fibrinolysis.

Traditionally, the hemostatic problems encountered during liver transplantation are divided according to the different stages of surgery: induction of anesthesia and preparation of the patient (pre-anhepatic phase), anhepatic phase, post-anhepatic and reperfusion phase and postoperative period.

Pre-anhepatic phase

In the pre-anhepatic phase, there are not usually serious changes in hemostasis (Lewis et al 1989). Hemostatic abnormalities and blood loss are strongly associated with preoperative coagulation studies (Bontempo et al 1985, Shaw et al 1985, Van Imhoff et al 1985), underlying liver disease, renal function and the presence of ascites (Haagsma et al 1985, Kirby et al 1987, Lewis et al 1987, 1988). Although a hypocoagulable state is usually present in patients with advanced liver diseases (Kang et al 1985, Lewis et al 1989), hypercoagulability may be present in the pre-anhepatic phase in patients with liver tumors (Howland et al 1974) or primary biliary cirrhosis and primary sclerosing cholangitis (BenAri et al 1997). Enhanced fibrinolysis has also been found to be a contributory factor of bleeding in cirrhotic patients (Kang et al 1987, Palareti et al 1988) in the pre-anhepatic phase.

Marked differences in transfusional needs and in pre- and intraoperative blood coagulation and fibrinolytic changes were observed between recipients with primary biliary cirrhosis and those with cirrhosis due to other etiologies (Palareti et al 1991). In the latter, increases in tissue-type plasminogen activator activity, total euglobulin fibrinolytic activity and fibrin-derived degradation products occurred earlier and were more marked, as were the signs of increased thrombin formation. These differences may be related to the findings of hypercoagulability on TEG in patients with biliary cirrhosis (Ben Ari et al 1997).

Anhepatic phase – post-anhepatic and reperfusion phase

The most significant changes in hemostasis start to occur during the anhepatic phase (usually lasts about 1 h). In patients in a pre-existing hypocoagulable state with or without hyperfibrinolysis or DIC, clotting or antifibrinolytic agents are not synthesized, while dilution, hypothermia and hypocalcemia further worsen the hemostatic profile. DIC (Flute et al 1969, Groth et al 1969, Bohmig 1977) and/or hyperfibrinolysis (Kang et al 1985, Lewis et al 1989) may also start to complicate the hemostatic problem.

Graft reperfusion during the post-anhepatic phase is associated with a major deterioration of coagulation. Reasons include DIC (Flute et al 1969, Bohmig 1977), hyperfibrinolysis (Kang et al 1987), trapping of platelets (Plevak et al 1983), dilutional effect of preservation fluid (Kang et al 1985), preservation damage (Mieny et al 1968), and humoral and metabolic factors (e.g. metabolic acidosis, cardio-vascular instability, hypocalcemia, hypothermia and hyperkalemia) (Aldrete et al 1970, Pappas et al 1971, Farman et al 1974, Gray et al 1986).

It should be noted that intraoperative and even postoperative blood loss also depend on the surgical skills, surgical and anesthetic techniques, and donor graft cold ischemia time. The quality of the donor liver is clearly a very important factor in determining coagulation abnormalities, bleeding, and, thus, mortality and overall survival (Von Kaulla et al 1966, Groth et al 1969, Bohmig 1977).

The management of coagulation in OLT is still a matter of debate among different transplant centers. Since changes in hemostasis during OLT occur rapidly, close and rapid monitoring to facilitate prompt response has been favored in many centers (Kang 1997). Platelet count monitoring during surgery is necessary and relatively easy to perform; however, routine tests of coagulation (prothrombin time, activated partial thromboplastin time) take time. TEG, which enables a global assessment of hemostasis and fibrinolysis in a relatively short time, has been used to guide replacement therapy (Kang et al 1985, Mallett & Platt 1991). However, no report has definitely proven the usefulness of coagulation monitoring, and there are certainly centers that use standard protocols for management of coagulation during OLT and do not depend on laboratory monitoring (Reyle-Hahn & Rassaint 1997).

Another area of controversy is the use of antifibrinolytic agents (Kufner 1997, Ramsay 1997). Aprotinin was initially found to decrease blood loss and blood requirements in several non-randomized, non-controlled studies (Neuhaus et al 1989, Mallett et al 1991, Patrassi et al 1994, Scudamore et al 1995). However, the use of aprotinin or of tranexamic acid was not always found to be associated with reduction in blood requirements in the subsequent randomized controlled trials (Milroy et al 1995, Boylan et al 1996, Marcel et al 1996, GarciaHuete et al 1997). Thus, the prophylactic use of antifibrinolytic agents is not generally accepted. However, such drugs may be extremely helpful in cases with excessive hemorrhage due to confirmed primary fibrinolysis (Kang et al 1987, Kaspar et al 1997). It should be noted that antifibrinolytic drugs have potential hazards which should always be considered. Potentially serious side effects include thrombotic episodes, renal dysfunction, and anaphylactic reactions. It is advised to avoid such drugs in patients with predisposition to thrombotic complications and to be cautious when treating patients with renal impairment. In our center, a pre-transplant TEG which shows hyperfibrinolysis is a contraindication to starting aprotinin infusion.

In the past, investigators who believed in the role of DIC advocated beneficial effects of intravenous heparin (Howland et al 1974), but others have questioned the role of DIC and found no beneficial effects of heparin administration (Kang et al 1985). The use of heparin is generally avoided (especially if venovenous bypass is not employed) as small amounts of heparin may lead to severe hemorrhage. Prophylactic use of antithrombin III was initially reported to correct DIC (Buller & Ten Cate 1983), but this was not confirmed later (Palareti et al 1991).

Postoperative period (see also Ch. 115)

The commonest coagulation abnormality in the post-operative period is thrombocytopenia. DIC has been suggested to explain post-transplant thrombocytopenia, as it may occur postoperatively (Bohmig 1977). It was recently reported that thrombocytopenia following OLT is associated with platelet consumption and thrombin generation; formation and lysis of thrombus following surgery was thought to be responsible (Richards et al 1997). The restored thrombopoietin production by the new liver usually results in a relatively rapid resolution of thrombocytopenia. Thrombopoietin levels increase after transplant and peak on the fifth post-transplant day with a subsequent rise of platelet count, which return to normal range within four to six days after the peak of thrombopoietin (Goulis et al 1999).

Hepatic artery thrombosis is a life-threatening complication in the post-transplant period, which necessitates retransplantation. Portal vein thrombosis is another serious complication and a substantial cause of mortality (Tzakis et al 1985). Hepatic artery thrombosis occurs more frequently in children than in adults. In children, persistent low levels of protein C have been demonstrated for 10 days postoperatively (Harper et al 1988) together with a reduction in antithrombin III and a rise in PAI levels. This is the rationale for using antithrombin III in children undergoing liver transplantation. Recently, a new syndrome of hypercoagulable state was described in patients with massive ascitic fluid

losses after OLT; thrombotic complications may develop in one to four weeks after transplant probably due to unreplaced losses of coagulation factors into the drained ascitic fluid and accumulation of thrombin in the systemic circulation (Gane et al 1995).

Auxiliary liver transplantation (Ch. 113) has the theoretical advantage of avoiding the anhepatic phase (Fortner et al 1979) and the benefit of leaving the recipient's own liver in place, which continues to synthesize clotting factors and clear degradation products throughout the operative period. However, coagulation abnormalities in the reperfusion phase are similar to those encountered in OLT (Knot et al 1988). Overall coagulation abnormalities in auxiliary liver transplantation are less than those in OLT, especially the absence of enhanced fibrinolysis, and hence reduced transfusion requirements (Terpstra et al 1988).

REFERENCES

Agnelli G, Parise P, Levi M et al 1995 Effects of desmopressin on hemostasis in patients with liver-cirrhosis. Hemostasis 25: 241–7

Aldrete J, Clapp H W, Starzl T E 1970 Body temperature changes during organ transplantation. Anaesthesia and Analgesia 49: 384–8

Alvarez O A, Lopera G A, Patel V et al 1996 Improvement of thrombocytopenia due to hypersplenism after transjugular intrahepatic portosystemic shunt placement in cirrhotic patients. American Journal of Gastroenterology 91: 134–7

Arnoux D, Boutiere B, Houvenaeghel M et al 1989 Intraoperative evolution of coagulation parameters and the tPA/PAI balance in orthotopic liver transplantation. Thrombosis Research 55: 319–28

Aster R H 1966 Pooling of platelets in the spleen: Role in the pathogenesis of 'hypersplenic' thrombocytopenia. Journal of Clinical Investigation 45: 645

Bakker C M, Knot E A R, Stibbe J et al 1992 Disseminated intravascular coagulation in liver cirrhosis. Journal of Hepatology 15: 330–5

Ballard H S & Marcus A J 1976 Platelet aggregation in portal cirrhosis. Archives of Internal Medicine 136: 316–9

Barrison I G, Knight I D, Viola L et al 1981 Platelet associated immunoglobulins in chronic liver disease. British Journal of Haematology 48: 347–50

Barroso Garcia de Silva E, Gore S M, White D J G et al 1986 An analysis of risk factors in liver transplantation. Transplant Proceedings 18: 1210–2

Bassendine M F, Collins J D, Stephenson J et al 1985 Platelet associated immunoglobulins in primary biliary cirrhosis: a cause of thrombocytopenia? Gut 26: 1074–9

BenAri Z, Panagou M, Patch D et al 1997 Hypercoagulability in patients with primary biliary cirrhosis and primary sclerosing cholangitis evaluated by thrombelastography. Journal Of Hepatology 26: 554–9

Bernuau J, Goudeau A, Poynard T et al 1986 Multivariate analysis of prognostic factors in fulminant hepatitis B. Hepatology 6: 648–51

Bernuau J, Samuel D, Durand F et al 1991 Criteria for emergency liver transplantation in patients with acute viral hepatitis and factor V (FV) below 50% of normal: a prospective study. Hepatology 14: 49A

Bernstein D E, Jeffers L, Erhardtsen E et al 1997 Recombinant factor VIIa corrects prothrombin time in cirrhotic patients: a preliminary study. Gastroenterology 113: 1930–7

Bertina R M, Koeleman P C, Koster T et al 1994 Mutation in blood coagulation factor V associated with resistance to activated protein C. Nature 369: 64–7

Bismuth H, Castaing D, Ericzon BG et al 1987 Hepatic transplantation in Europe. First report of the European Liver Transplant Registry. Lancet ii: 674–6

Blanchard RA, Furie CB, Jorgensen M et al 1981 Acquired vitamin K dependent carboxylation deficiency in liver disease. New England Journal of Medicine 305: 242–8

Blanshard C, Pasi J, Rolles K et al 1996 Acute Budd–Chiari syndrome treated by liver transplantation in a woman with homozygous factor V Leiden deficiency. European Journal of Gastroenterology & Hepatology 8: 925–7

Bohmig H J 1977 The coagulation disorder of orthotopic hepatic transplantation. Seminars in Thrombosis and Hemostasis 4: 57–82

Boks A L, Brommer E J P, Schalm S W et al 1986 Haemostasis and fibrinolysis in severe liver failure and their relation to haemorrhage. Hepatology 6: 79–86

Bontempo F A, Lewis J H, Van Thiel D H et al 1985 The relation of preoperative coagulation findings to diagnosis, blood usage, and survival in adult liver transplantation. Transplantation 39: 532–6

Boylan J F, Klinck J R, Sandler A N et al 1996 Tranexamic acid reduces blood loss, transfusion requirements, and coagulation factor use in primary orthotopic liver transplantation. Anesthesiology 85: 1043–8

Braude P, Arias J, Hughes R D et al 1981 Antithrombin III infusion during fulminant hepatic failure. Thrombosis and Hemostasis 46: 369

Breddin K 1962 Hamorrhagische Diathesen bei Lebererrkrankungen unter besonderer Berucksichtigung der Thrombocyten Function. Acta Haematologica 27: 1–16

Bullen H R & Ten Cate J W 1983 Antithrombin III infusion in patients undergoing peritovenous shunt operation: failure in the prevention of disseminated intravascular coagulation. Thrombosis and Hemostasis 49: 128–31

Burroughs A K, Mathews K, Quadira M et al 1985 Desmopressin and bleeding time in patients with cirrhosis. British Medical Journal 291: 1377–81

Burroughs A K, McCormick P A, Sprengers D 1988 Assessment of bleeding risk in chronic liver disease. Fibrinolysis 2: 56–60

Calne RY, Williams R, Rolles K 1986 Liver transplantation in the adult. World Journal of Surgery 10: 422–31

Carmassi F, Morale M, De Negri F et al 1995 Modulation of hemostatic balance with antithrombin III replacement therapy in a case of liver cirrhosis associated with recurrent venous thrombosis. Journal of Molecular Medicine 73: 89–93

Carmassi F, De Negri F, Morale M et al 1997 Antithrombotic and antifibrinolytic effects of antithrombin III replacement in liver cirrhosis. Lancet 349: 1069

Carr J M 1989 Disseminated intravascular coagulation in cirrhosis. Hepatology 10: 103–10

Casella J F, Lewis J H, Bontempo F A et al 1988 Successful treatment of homozygous protein C deficiency by hepatic transplantation. Lancet i: 435–7

Chau T N, Chan Y W, Patch D et al 1998 Thrombelastographic changes and early rebleeding in cirrhotic patients with variceal bleeding. Gut 43: 267–71

Cioni G, Cristani A, Mussini C et al 1990 Incidence and clinical significance of elevated fibrin(ogen) degradation products and/or D-dimer levels in liver cirrhosis patients. Italian Journal of Gastroenterology 22: 70–4

Clouse L H & Comp P C 1986 The regulation of hemostasis: The protein C system. New England Journal of Medicine 314: 1298–304

Comp P C 1990 Laboratory evaluation of protein S status. Seminars in Thrombosis and Hemostasis 16: 177

Colman R W, Robboy S J, Minna J D 1972 Disseminated intravascular coagulation (DIC): an approach. American Journal of Medicine 52: 679–89

Cordova C, Musca A, Violi F et al 1982 Improvement of some blood coagulation factors in cirrhotic patients treated with low doses of heparin. Scandinavian Journal of Haematology 29: 235–40

Cordova C, Violi F, Alessandri C et al 1986 Pre kallikrein factor VII as prognostic index of liver failure. American Journal of Clinical Pathology 85: 579–82

Cowan D H & Hines J D 1971 Thrombocytopenia in severe alcoholism. Annals of Internal Medicine 74: 37–43

Dahlback B, Carlsson M, Svensson P J 1993 Familial thrombophilia due to a previously unrecognized mechanism characterized by poor anticoagulant response to activated protein C: prediction of a cofactor to activated protein C. Proceedings of the National Academy of Science of the USA 90: 1004–8

De Franchis R, Arcidiacono P G, Carpinelli P G et al 1993 Randomized controlled trial of desmopressin plus terlipressin versus terlipressin alone for the treatment of acute variceal hemorrhage in cirrhotic patients. Hepatology 18: 1102–6

De Hovi A G, Ponari O, Civardi E et al 1977 Impaired fibrin formation in advanced cirrhosis. Hemostasis 6: 137–48

Denninger M-H, Beldjord K, Durand F et al 1995 Budd–Chiari syndrome and factor V Leiden mutation. Lancet 345: 525–6

de Noronha R, Taylor B A, Wild G et al 1991 Interrelationships between platelet count, platelet IgG, serum IgG, immune complexes and severity of liver disease. Clinical and Laboratory Haematology 13: 127–35

Desai K, Mistry P, Bagget C et al 1989 Inhibition of platelet aggregation by abnormal high density lipoprotein particles in plasma from patients with hepatic cirrhosis. Lancet i: 693–5

de Sauvage F J, Hass P E, Spencer S D et al 1994 Stimulation of megakaryocytopoiesis and thrombopoiesis by the c-Mpl ligand. Nature 369: 533–8

Dymock I W, Tucher J S, Woolf I L et al 1975 Coagulation studies as a prognostic index in acute liver failure. British Journal of Haematology 29: 385–95

Dzik W H, Arkin C F, Jenkins R L et al 1988 Fibrinolysis during liver transplantation in humans: role of tissue-type plasminogen activator. Blood 71: 1090–5

Egbring R, Klungemann H G, Heimberger H E et al 1981 Antithrombin III substitution in acute hepatic failure due to C14 intoxication. Hemostasis 46: 373

Epstein M 1982 Peritoneovenous shunt in the management of ascites and the hepatorenal syndrome. Gastroenterology 82: 790–9

Everson G T 1997 A hepatologist's perspective on the management of coagulation disorders before liver transplantation. Liver Transplantation and Surgery 3: 646–52

Ewe K 1981 Bleeding after liver biopsy does not correlate with indices of peripheral coagulation. Digestive Diseases and Sciences 26: 388–93

Fair D S & Marlar R A 1986 Biosynthesis and secretion of factor VII, protein C, protein S and the protein C inhibitor from a human hepatoma cell line. Blood 67: 64–77

Fair D S, Marlar R A, Wevin E G 1986 Human endothelial cells synthesize protein S. Blood 67: 1168–71

Farman J V, Lines J G, Williams R et al 1974 Liver transplantation in man. Anaesthetic and biochemical management. Anaesthesia 29: 17–32

Ferguson J J, Waly H M, Wilson J M 1998 Fundamentals of coagulation and glycoprotein IIb/IIIa receptor inhibition. American Heart Journal 135: S35–S42

Ferro D, Basili S, Lattuada A et al 1997 Systemic clotting activation by low-grade endotoxaemia in liver cirrhosis: a potential role for endothelial procoagulant activation. Italian Journal of Gastroenterology and Hepatology 29: 434–40

Fletcher A P, Biederman O, Moore D et al 1964 Abnormal plasminogen–plasmin system activity in patients with hepatic cirrhosis: its cause and consequences. Journal of Clinical Investigation 43: 681–95

Flute P T, Rake M O, Williams R 1969 Liver transplantation in man. IV. Haemorrhage and thrombosis. British Medical Journal iii: 20–3

Fortner J G, Yeh S D J, Shiu M H et al 1979 The case for and technique of heterotopic liver grafting. Transplant Proceedings 11: 269–75

Francis J L & Armstrong D J 1978 Acquired dysfibrinogenaemia in liver disease. Journal of Clinical Investigation 61: 3535–47

Francis R B & Feinstein D I 1984 Clinical significance of accelerated fibrinolysis in liver disease. Hemostasis 14: 460–5

Gane E, Langley P, Williams R 1995 Massive ascitic fluid loss and coagulation disturbances after liver-transplantation. Gastroenterology 109: 1631–8

GarciaHuete L, Domenech P, Sabate A et al 1997 The prophylactic effect of aprotinin on intraoperative bleeding in liver transplantation: A randomized clinical study. Hepatology 26: 1143–8

Gerlach H, Slama K J, Bechstein W O et al 1993 Retrospective analysis of coagulation parameters after 250 liver transplantations. Seminars in Thrombosis and Hemostasis 19: 223–32

Goldsmith M F 1983 Liver Transplantation: big business in blood. Journal of the American Medical Association 250: 2904–5

Goodnight S H, Feinstein D I, Osterub B et al 1971 Factor VII antibody neutralizing material in hereditary and acquired factor VII deficiency. Blood 38: 1

Goodpasture E W 1914 Fibrinolysis in chronic hepatic insufficiency. Bulletin of the Johns Hopkins Hospital 25: 330–6

Goulis J, Chau T N, Jordan S et al 1999 Thrombopoietin levels are low in patients with cirrhosis and thrombocytopenia and are restored after orthotopic liver transplantation. Gut (in press)

Gray T A, Buckley B M, Sealey M M et al 1986 Plasma ionised calcium monitoring during liver transplantation. Transplantation 41: 335–9

Green A F & Rantoff O D 1974 Elevated antihaemophilic factor (AHF, factor VIII) procoagulant activity and AHF-like antigen in alcoholic cirrhosis of the liver. Journal of Laboratory and Clinical Medicine 83: 189–97

Green G, Thomson J M, Dymock I W et al 1976a Abnormal fibrin polymerization in liver disease. British Journal of Haematology 34: 427–39

Green G, Poller L, Thompson J M et al 1976b Factor VII as a marker of hepatocellular biological data in liver disease. Journal of Clinical Pathology 29: 971–5

Green G, Poller L, Thompson J M et al 1977 Association of abnormal fibrin polymerization with severe liver disease. Gut 18: 909–12

Griffin J H, Mosher D F, Zimmerman T S et al 1982 Protein C, an antithrombotic protein, is reduced in hospitalized patients with intravascular coagulation. Blood 60: 261

Groth C G, Pechet L, Starzl T E 1969 Coagulation during and after orthotopic liver transplantation of the human liver. Archives of Surgery 98: 31–4

Haagsma E B, Gips C H, Wesenhagen H et al 1985 Liver disease and its effects on hemostasis during liver transportation. Liver 5: 123–8

Hans T H & Curtis F C 1938 Plasma fibrinogen response in man. Influence of the nutritional state, induced hyperpyrexia, infectious disease and liver damage. Medicine 17: 413–45

Harker L A & Slichter S J 1972 The bleeding time as a screening test for evaluation of platelet function. New England Journal of Medicine 287: 155–9

Harmon D C, Demirjlan Z, Ellman L et al 1979 Disseminated intravascular coagulation after the peritoneo-venous shunt. Annals of Internal Medicine 90: 774–6

Harper P L, Edgar P F, Luddington R J et al 1988 Protein C deficiency and portal thrombosis in liver transplantation in children. Lancet ii: 924–7

Hartert H 1948 Blutgerninnung-studien mit der Thromboelastographic, einen neven untersuchingsuer Fahren. Klinische Wochenschrift 16: 257

Hersch S L, Kunelis T, Francis RB Jr 1987 The pathogenesis of accelerated fibrinolysis in liver cirrhosis: a critical role for tissue plasminogen activator inhibitor. Blood 69: 1315–9

Ho CH, Hou MC, Lin HC et al 1998 Can the more advanced hemostatic parameters detect disseminated intravascular coagulation more accurately in liver cirrhosis? British Journal of Haematology 102: 264

Howland W S, Castro E B, Fortner J B et al 1974 Hypercoagulability. Thromboelastographic monitoring during extensive hepatic surgery. Archives of Surgery 108: 605–8

Iwatsuki S, Shaw B W Jr, Starzl T E 1983 Current status of hepatic transplantation. Seminars in Liver Disease 3: 173–80

Izumi S, Langley P G, Wendon J et al 1996 Coagulation factor V levels as a prognostic indicator in fulminant hepatic failure. Hepatology 23: 1507–11

Jaffe E A, Hoyer L W, Nachman R L 1973 Synthesis of antihaemophilic antigen by cultured human endothelial cells. Journal of Clinical Investigation 52: 2757–64

Johansson S 1964 Studies on blood coagulation factors in a case of liver cirrhosis. Remission of the haemorrhagic tendency on treatment with heparin. Acta Medica Scandinavica 175: 177–83

Kang Y 1997 Transfusion based on clinical coagulation monitoring does reduce hemorrhage during liver transplantation. Liver Transplantation and Surgery 3: 655–9

Kang Y G, Martin D J, Marquez J et al 1985 Intraoperative changes in blood coagulation and thromboelastographic monitoring in liver transplantation. Anaesthesia and Analgesia 64: 888–96

Kang Y G, Lewis J H, Navalgund A et al 1987 Epsilon-aminocaproic acid for treatment of fibrinolysis during liver transplantation. Anaesthesiology 66: 766–73

Kario K, Matsuo T, Kodama K et al 1992 Imbalance between thrombin and plasmin activity in disseminated intravascular coagulation. Hemostasis 22: 179

Kaspar M, Ramsay M A E, Nguyen A T et al 1997 Continuous small-dose tranexamic acid reduces fibrinolysis but not transfusion requirements during orthotopic liver transplantation. Anesthesia and Analgesia 85: 281–5

Kelly D A & Tuddenham E G D 1986 Hemostatic problems in liver disease. Gut 27: 339–49

Kelly D A, O'Brian F J, Hutton R A et al 1985 The effect of liver disease on factors V, VII and protein C. British Journal of Haematology 61: 541–8

Kemkes-Matthes B, Bleyl H, Matthes K J 1991 Imbalance between thrombin and plasmin activity in disseminated intravascular coagulation. Thrombosis Research 64: 253

Kiesel W 1975 Human protein C isolation, characterisation and mechanism of activation by alpha-thrombin. Journal of Clinical Investigation 64: 761–9

Kirby R M, McMaster P, Clemens D et al 1987 Orthotopic liver transplantation: postoperative complications and their management. British Journal of Surgery 74: 3–11

Knot E A R, Porte R J, Terpstra O T et al 1988 Coagulation and fibrinolysis in the first human auxiliary partial liver transplantation in Rotterdam. Fibrinolysis 2: 111–117

Kufner R P 1997 Antifibrinolytics do not reduce transfusion requirements in patients undergoing orthotopic liver transplantation. Liver Transplantation and Surgery 3: 668–74

Kwaan H C, McFadzean A J S, Cook J 1956 Plasma fibrinolytic activity in cirrhosis of the liver. Lancet i: 132–6

Landolfi R, Leone G, Fedeli G et al 1980 Platelet associated IgG in acute and chronic hepatic diseases. Scandinavian Journal of Haematology 25: 417–22

Laffi G, Cinotti S, Filimberti E et al 1996 Defective aggregation in cirrhosis is independent of in vivo platelet activation. Journal of Hepatology 24: 436–43

Langley P G & Williams R 1988 The effect of fulminant hepatic failure on protein C antigen and activity. Thrombosis and Haemostasis 59: 316–8

Lebrec D, Goldfarb G, Degott C et al 1982 Transvenous liver biopsy. An experience based on 1000 hepatic tissue samplings with this procedure. Gastroenterology 83: 338–40

Lechner K, Niessner H, Thaler E 1977 Coagulation abnormalities in patients with liver disease. Seminars in Thrombosis and Hemostasis 4: 40–56

Leebeek F W G, Kluft C, Knot E A R et al 1991 A shift in balance between profibrinolytic and antifibrinolytic factors causes enhanced fibrinolysis in cirrhosis. Gastroenterology 101: 1382–90

LeVeen H, Ahmed N, Hutto R B et al 1987 Coagulopathy post peritoneovenous shunt. Annals of Surgery 205: 305–11

Lewis J H, Bontempo F A, Cornell F W et al 1987 Blood use in liver transplantation. Transfusion 27: 222–5

Lewis J H, Bontempo F A, Cornell F W et al 1988 Blood use in transplantation: liver, heart, artificial heart and heart lung. Transplant Proceedings 20: 533–5

Lewis J H, Bontempo F A, Kang Y G et al 1989 Liver transplantation: intraoperative changes in coagulation factors in 100 first transplants. Hepatology 9: 710–14

Liebman H A, McGehee W G, Patch M J et al 1983 Severe depression of antithrombin III associated with disseminated intravascular coagulation in women with fatty liver of pregnancy. Annals of Internal Medicine 98: 330–3

Liebman H, Furie B C, Tong M et al 1984 Des-γ-carboxy (abnormal) prothrombin as a serum marker of primary hepatocellular carcinoma. New England Journal of Medicine 310: 1427–31

Lipinski B, Lipinska I, Nowak A et al 1977 Abnormal fibrinogen heterogeneity and fibrinolytic activity in advanced liver disease. Journal of Laboratory and Clinical Medicine 90: 187–94

Lok S, Kaushansky K, Holly R D et al 1994 Cloning and expression of murine thrombopoietin cDNA and stimulation of platelet in vivo. Nature 369: 565–8

Lusher J M 1996 Recombinant factor VIIa in the treatment of internal bleeding in patients with factor VIII and IX inhibitors. Hemostasis 26 (Suppl. 1): 124–30

McVay P A & Toy P T C Y 1990 Lack of increased bleeding after liver biopsy in patients with mild hemostatic abnormalities. American Journal of Clinical Pathology 94: 747–53

McVay P A & Toy P T C Y 1991 Lack of increased bleeding after paracentesis and thoracentesis in patients with mild coagulation abnormalities. Transfusion 31: 164–71

Mahmoud A E A, Wilde J T, Elias E 1995 Budd–Chiari syndrome and factor V Leiden mutation. Lancet 345: 526

Mahmoud A E A, Elias E, Beauchamp N et al 1997 Prevalence of the factor V Leiden mutation in hepatic and portal vein thrombosis. Gut 40: 798–800

Mallett S V & Platt M 1991 Role of thromboelastography in bleeding diatheses and regional anaesthesia. Lancet 338: 765–6

Mallett S V, Cox D, Burroughs A K et al 1991 Intraoperative use of trasylol (Aprotinin) in liver transplantation. Transplant International 4: 227–30

Mammen E F 1994 Coagulation defects in liver disease. Medical Clinics of North America 78: 545–54

Mannucci P M 1997 Desmopressin (DDAVP) in the treatment of bleeding disorders: the first 20 years. Blood 90: 2515–21

Mannucci P M & Vigano S 1982 Deficiency of protein C, an inhibitor of blood coagulation. Lancet ii: 463–6

Mannucci P M, Canciani M T, Rota L et al 1981 Response of factor VIII von Willebrand's factor to DDAVP in healthy subjects and patients with haemophilia A and von Willebrand's disease. British Journal of Haematology 47: 283–93

Mannucci P M, Vicentre V, Vianello L et al 1986 Controlled trial of desmopressin in liver cirrhosis and other conditions associated with a prolonged bleeding time. Blood 67: 1148–53

Marcel R J, Stegall W C, Suit C T et al 1996 Continuous small-dose aprotinin controls fibrinolysis during orthotopic liver transplantation. Anesthesia and Analgesia 82: 1122–5

Martin T G, Somberg K A, Meng G et al 1997 Thrombopoietin levels in patients with cirrhosis before and after orthotopic liver transplantation. Annals of Internal Medicine 127: 285–8

Martinez J, Palascak J E, Kwasniak D 1978 Abnormal sialic acid content of the dysfibrinogenemia associated with liver disease. Journal of Clinical Investigations 61: 535

Mieny C J, Homatas J, Moore A R et al 1968 Limiting functions of preserved liver homograft. Gastroenterology 55: 179–82

Milroy S J, Cottam S, Tan K C et al 1995 Improved haemodynamic instability with administration of aprotinin during orthotopic liver transplantation. British Journal of Anaesthesia 75: 747–51

Mombelli G, Monotti R, Haeberli A et al 1988 Low grade DIC in liver cirrhosis: fact or fiction? Thrombosis and Hemostasis 59: 345

Monroe D M, Hoffman M, Oliver J A et al 1997 Platelet activity of high-dose factor VIIa is independent of tissue factor. British Journal of Haematology 99: 542–7

Mowat N A G, Brunt P W, Ogston D 1974 The fibrinolytic enzyme system in acute and chronic liver injury. Acta Haematologica 52: 289–93

Mutchnick M G, Lerner E, Conn H O 1980 Effect of portocaval anastomosis on hypersplenism. Digestive Diseases and Science 25: 929–38

Nagamine T, Ohtuka T, Takehara K et al 1996 Thrombocytopenia associated with hepatitis C viral infection. Journal of Hepatology 24: 135–40

Nanji A A & Blank D W 1983 Clinical status as reflected in biochemical tests on patients with chronic alcoholic liver disease. Clinical Chemistry 29: 992–3

Neuhaus P, Bechstein W O, Lefebre B et al 1989 Effect of aprotinin on intraoperative bleeding and fibrinolysis in liver transplantation. Lancet 2: 924–5

O'Connell R A, Grossi C E, Rousselot L M 1964 Role of inhibitors of fibrinolysis in hepatic cirrhosis. Lancet ii: 990–1

Ogston D, Bennett N B, Ogston C M 1971 The fibrinolytic enzyme system in hepatic cirrhosis and malignant metastases. Journal of Clinical Pathology 24: 822–6

Oka F & Tanaka K 1979 Intravascular coagulation in autopsy cases with liver disease. Thrombosis and Hemostasis 42: 564–70

Ordinas A, Escolar G, Cirera I et al 1996 Existence of a platelet-adhesion defect in patients with cirrhosis independent of hematocrit: studies under flow conditions. Hepatology 24: 1137–42

Osman E, Hutton R, McIntyre N et al 1992 Fibrinolytic activity in liver disease. Gut 33 (suppl. 1): 13

Owen J S, Hutton R A, Day R C et al 1981 Platelet lipid composition and platelet aggregation in human liver disease. Journal of Lipid Research 22: 423–30

Palareti G, De Rosa V, Fortunato G et al 1988 Control of hemostasis during orthotopic liver transplantation. Fibrinolysis 2: 61–6

Palareti G, Legnani C, Maccaferri M et al 1991 Coagulation and fibrinolysis in orthotopic liver transplantation. Role of the recipient's disease and use of antithrombin III concentrates. Haemostasis 21: 68–76

Papatheodoridis G V, Patch D, Webster G J M et al 1998 Infection and hemostasis in decompensated liver cirrhosis: a prospective study. Hepatology 28 (suppl.): 454A

Papatheodoridis G V, Patch D, Watkinson A et al 1999 Transjugular liver biopsy in the nineties: a two year audit. Alimentary Pharmacology and Therapeutics (in press)

Pappas G, Palmer W M, Martineau G L et al 1971 Haemodynamic alterations caused during orthotopic liver transplantation in humans. Surgery 70: 872–5

Parbhoo S P, Ajudukiewicz A, Sherlock S 1974 Treatment of ascites by continuous ultrafiltration and reinfusion of protein concentrate. Lancet i: 949–51

Patrassi G M, Viero M, Sartori M T et al 1994 Aprotinin efficacy on intraoperative bleeding and transfusion requirements in orthotopic liver-transplantation. Transfusion 34: 507–11

Peck-Radosavljevic M, Zacherl J, Meng Y G et al 1997 Is inadequate thrombopoietin production a major cause of thrombocytopenia in cirrhosis of the liver? Journal of Hepatology 27: 127–31

Pereira L M, Langley P G, Bird G L et al 1992 Coagulation factors V and VIII in relation to severity and outcome in acute alcoholic hepatitis. Alcohol and Alcoholism 27: 55–61

Pfueller S L, Firkin B G, Kerlero de Rosbo N et al 1983 Association of increased immune complexes, platelet IgG and serum IgG in chronic active hepatitis. Clinical and Experimental Immunology 54: 655–60

Plevak D J, Halma G A, Forstrom L A et al 1983 Thrombocytopenia after liver transplantation. Transplant Proceedings 20: 630–3

Poort S R, Rosendaal F R, Reitsma P H et al 1996 A common genetic variation in the 3′-untranslated region of the prothrombin gene is associated with elevated plasma prothrombin levels and an increase in venous thrombosis. Blood 88: 3698–703

Porte R J, Bontempo F A, Knot E A R et al 1989 Systemic effects of tissue plasminogen activator-associated fibrinolysis and its relation to thrombin generation in orthotopic liver transplantation. Transplantation 47: 978–84

Pugh R N, Murray-Lyon I M, Dawson J L et al 1973 Transection of the oesophagus for bleeding oesophageal varices. British Journal of Surgery 60: 646–9

Ramsay M A E 1997 The use of antifibrinolytic agents results in a reduction in transfused blood products during liver transplantation. Liver Transplantation and Surgery 3: 665–8

Rantoff O D 1949 Studies on a proteolytic enzyme in human plasma. IV. The rate of lysis of plasma clots in normal and diseased individuals, with particular reference to the hepatic disease. Bulletin of the Johns Hopkins Hospital 84: 29–42

Reyle-Hahn M & Rassaint R 1997 Coagulation techniques are not important in directing blood product transfusion during liver transplantation. Liver Transplantation and Surgery 3: 659–63

Richards E M, Alexander G J M, Calne R Y et al 1997 Thrombocytopenia following liver transplantation is associated with platelet consumption and thrombin generation. British Journal of Haematology 98: 315–21

Riley S A, Ellis W R, Lintott D J et al 1984 Percutaneous liver biopsy with plugging of needle tract. A safe method for patients with impaired blood coagulation. Lancet ii: 436–8

Roberts H R, Monroe D M, Oliver J A et al 1998 Newer concepts of blood coagulation. Haemophilia 4: 331–4

Robson S, Kahn D, Kruskal J et al 1993 Disordered hemostasis in extrahepatic portal hypertension. Hepatology 18: 853–7

Rubin M H, Weston M J, Langley P G et al 1979 Platelets function in chronic liver disease. Digestive Diseases and Sciences 24: 197–202

Sanyal A J, Freedman A M, Purdum P P et al 1996 The hematologic consequences of transjugular intrahepatic portosystemic shunts. Hepatology 23: 32–9

Sawyerr A M, McCormick P A, Tennyson G S et al 1992 A comparison of transjugular and plugged percutaneous liver biopsy in patients with impaired coagulation. Journal of Hepatology 17: 81–5

Scherer R, Kabatnik M, Erhard J et al 1997 The influence of antithrombin III (AT III) substitution to supranormal activities on systemic procoagulant turnover in patients with end-stage chronic liver disease. Intensive Care Medicine 23: 1150–8

Schipper H G & Ten Cate J W 1982 Antithrombin III transfusion in patients with hepatic cirrhosis. British Journal of Haematology 52: 25–33

Schlichting P, Christensen E, Fauerholdt L et al 1983 Main causes of death in cirrhosis. Scandinavian Journal of Gastroenterology 18: 881–8

Scudamore C H, Randall T E, Jewesson P J et al 1995 Aprotinin reduces the need for blood products during liver-transplantation. American Journal of Surgery 169: 546–9

Shaw B W, Wood R P, Gordon R D et al 1985 Influence of selected patient variables and operative blood loss on six-month survival following liver transplantation. Seminars in Liver Disease 5: 385–93

Sherlock S & Dooley J 1993 Needle biopsy of the liver. In: Sherlock S & Dooley J (eds) Diseases of the Liver and Biliary System, 9th edn, Blackwell Scientific Publications, Oxford, pp. 33–43

Shimada Y, Kato T, Ogami K et al 1995 Production of thrombopoietin (TPO) by rat hepatocytes and hepatoma cell lines. Experimental Hematolology 23: 1388–96

Shrestha R, McKinley C, Bilir B M et al 1995 Possible idiopathic thrombocytopenic purpura associated with natural alpha interferon therapy for chronic hepatitis C infection. American Journal of Gastroenterology 90: 1146–7

Soper N J & Rikkers L F 1982 Effect of operations for variceal hemorrhage on hypersplenism. American Journal of Surgery 144: 700–3

Soria J, Soria C, Samama M et al 1980 Study of acquired dysfibrinogenaemia in liver disease. Thrombosis Research 19: 29

Sprengers E D & Kluft C 1987 Plasminogen activator inhibitors. Blood 69: 381–7

Starzl T E, Iwatsuki S, Van Thiel D H et al 1982 Evolution of liver transplantation. Hepatology 2: 614–36

Stein S & Harker L A 1982 Kinetic and functional studies of platelets, fibrinogen, and plasminogen in patients with hepatic cirrhosis. Journal of Laboratory and Clinical Medicine 99: 217–30

Stenflo J 1975 A new vitamin K dependent protein. Purification from bovine plasma and preliminary characterisation. Journal of Biological Chemistry 251: 355–63

Suehiro T, Boros P, Sheiner P et al 1997 Effluent levels of thrombomodulin predict early graft function in clinical liver transplantation. Liver 17: 224–9

Tang H H, Salem H H, Wood L J et al 1992 Coagulopathy during ascites reinfusion; prevention by antiplatelet therapy. Gastroenterology 102: 1334–9

Tawes R L, Sydorak G R, Kennedy P A et al 1981 Coagulopathy associated with peritoneovenous shunting. American Journal of Surgery 142: 51–5

Thomas D P, Ream V J, Stuart R K 1967 Platelet aggregation in patients with Laennecs cirrhosis of the liver. New England Journal of Medicine 276: 1344–8

Terpstra O T, Schalm S W, Weimar W et al 1988 Auxiliary partial liver transplantation for end-stage chronic liver disease. New England Journal of Medicine 319: 1507–11

Tzakis A G, Gordon R D, Shaw B W Jr et al 1985 Clinical presentation of hepatic artery thrombosis after liver transplantation in the cyclosporin era. Transplantation 40: 667–71

Van Thiel D H, Tarter R, Gavaler J S et al 1986 Liver transplantation in adults. An analysis of costs and benefits at the University of Pittsburgh. Gastroenterology 90: 211–6

Van Imhoff G W, Haagshma E B, Wesenhagen H et al 1985 Coagulation and bleeding during orthotopic liver transplantation. In: Gips C H & Krom R A F (eds) Progress in Liver Transplantation Martinus Nijhoff, The Hague. pp 71–84

Verstraete M, Vermylen J, Collen D 1974 Intravascular coagulation in liver disease. Annual Review of Medicine 25: 447–55

Vesin P 1972 Potassium supplements and diuretics. Lancet ii: 1262–3

Violi F, Ferro D, Basili S et al 1992 Hyperfibrinolysis increases the risk of gastrointestinal haemorrhage in patients with advanced cirrhosis. Hepatology 15: 672–6

Violi F, Leo R, Davi G et al 1992 Thombocytopenia and thrombocytopathia in liver cirrhosis. Platelets 3: 233–9

Violi F, Ferro D, Basili S et al 1993 Hyperfibrinolysis resulting from clotting activation in patients with different degrees of cirrhosis. Hepatology 17: 78–83

Violi F, Ferro D, Basili S et al 1995a Association between low-grade disseminated intravascular coagulation and endotoxemia in patients with liver-cirrhosis. Gastroenterology 109: 531–9

Violi F, Ferro D, Basili S et al 1995b Prognostic value of clotting and fibrinolytic systems in a follow-up of 165 liver cirrhotic-patients. Hepatology 22: 96–100

Von Kaulla K N, Kayne H, Von Kaulla E et al 1966 Changes in blood coagulation before and after hepatectomy or transplantation in dogs and man. Archives of Surgery 92: 71–9

Wardle E N 1974 Fibrinogen in liver disease. Archives of Surgery 109: 741–6

Weinstein M J, Deykin D 1978 Quantitative abnormality of an α chain molecular weight form in the fibrinogen of cirrhotic patients. British Journal of Haematology 40: 617–30

Wilkinson S P 1977 Endotoxins and liver disease. Scandinavian Journal of Gastroenterology 12: 385–6

Wion K L, Kelly D A, Summerfield J A et al 1985 Distribution of factor VIII mRNA and antigen in human liver and other tissues. Nature 317: 726–9

Younger H M, Hadoke P W F, Dillon J F et al 1997 Platelet function in cirrhosis and the role of humoral factors. European Journal of Gastroenterology and Hepatology 9: 989–92

Diagnostic techniques

Clinical examination and investigation

12

A. SHANKAR, I. TAYLOR

Despite the rapid increase in diagnostic modalities available to the clinician dealing with hepatobiliary disease, a detailed history and clinical examination is still important if an accurate overall assessment is to be made. This chapter will address the specific features in the history and clinical examination which are of particular importance in hepatobiliary disease in conjunction with a general overview of related investigations.

CLINICAL HISTORY

Jaundice and pain are the most common presenting complaints relating to patients with hepatobiliary disease. The cause of jaundice has been classically divided into:

Pre-hepatic—due to increased hemolysis
Hepatic—due to defective hepatic metabolism of the products of red cell breakdown
Post-hepatic—due to obstruction of the biliary tree.

This is however oversimplistic as a mixed picture is often seen especially with the latter two groups. (See also Ch. 7.)

An accurate clinical history is particularly important in differentiating the various causes of jaundice and in conjunction with examination should determine the most appropriate investigations.

The increase in foreign travel and migration throughout developed countries has led to increased exposure not only to viral hepatitis but also to an increased incidence of the rarer causes of both pre and hepatic causes of jaundice such as malaria, as well as inherited hemaglobinopathies. A family history is also important with regard to other familial disorders which may cause jaundice, such as Gilbert's syndrome, Wilson's disease and autoimmune conditions which may lead to chronic active hepatitis or primary biliary cirrhosis.

Particular attention should be paid to identifying groups at particular risk of contracting infective viral hepatitis such as intravenous drug abusers, homosexuals, needle stick injuries, contact with jaundiced individuals and rarely patients who have received blood transfusions.

Given that some drugs and enviromental hepatotoxins may cause hemolysis a careful drug and occupational history should also be sought. Excess alcohol intake is especially important and a detailed history should be taken from the patient, general practitioner and relatives.

The typical complaints associated with obstructive jaundice are of dark urine, pale stools and pruritus. Whether or not this is associated with pain or rigors is important and should be included in the history. Recurrent episodes of right upper quadrant or epigastric pain often associated with the intake of a fatty meal is highly suggestive of biliary disease and if combined with an episode of jaundice and rigors implies an attack of cholangitis. Although jaundice if painless or associated with pain radiating to the back, is highly suggestive of pancreatic pathology, such symptoms are also found in patients with gallstones. Fluctuating levels of jaundice suggests intermittent obstruction which may occur with temporary retention of a stone at the ampulla of Vater or may represent intrahepatic cholestasis or Gilbert's syndrome. This may rarely occur with either pancreatic cancer or cholangiocarcinoma.

Pruritus may be present in all types of jaundice, usually generalized and particularly affects the palms and soles of the feet. Excessive pruritus in middle aged women associated with jaundice is suggestive of primary biliary cirrhosis.

The systemic features of malignancy should be sought such as weight loss, anemia and anorexia, especially if of short duration. These symptoms in conjunction with painless jaundice are highly suspicious of neoplasia of the head of the pancreas.

PHYSICAL EXAMINATION

GENERAL INSPECTION

Although many patients with hepatobiliary disease may be asymptomatic the stigmata of liver disease should be sought. These include:

An *altered level of conciousness* may occur in advanced liver disease due to neuropsychiatric complications.

Jaundice or icterus is the staining of tissues, especially the sclera, with bilirubin and other pigments such as biliverdin. Jaundice becomes clinically detectable when the serum bilirubin exceeds 3 mg per 100 ml and as the level raises so does the level of pigmentation.

Other skin changes commonly found in association with liver disease include *spider nevi* (Fig. 12.1) which are telangectatic lesions consisting of a central arteriole with radiating small vessels. They are also commonly found in normal subjects especially during childhood and pregnancy. The classical feature of spider naevi is that they blanch on pressure and refill via the central arteriole on release of pressure. The distribution of spider nevi in association with liver disease is in the chest and upper body. Increase in the number, size and appearance in later life are suggestive of liver disease. Spontaneous bruising of the skin and bleeding around venepuncture sites may occur in liver disease due to failure of production of clotting factors.

Slate-gray discoloration of the skin is found in association with hemochromatosis, whilst flushing of the palms, *palmar erythema*, is also associated with liver disease (Fig. 12.2). *Palmar erythema* particularly affects the thenar and hypothenar eminences and the bases of the fingers. Also affecting the palms of the hands are Dupytrens contractures, thickenings in the *palmar fascia*, which can be found in association with liver disease especially when due to alcohol (Fig. 12.3). *Xanthomas*, which are cholesterol deposits, can be found in the palmar creases or above the eyes in patients with primary biliary cirrhosis. In the late stages of hepatic failure patients may develop a *flapping tremor* when the hands are outstretched. *Kaiser-Fleisher* rings are areas of

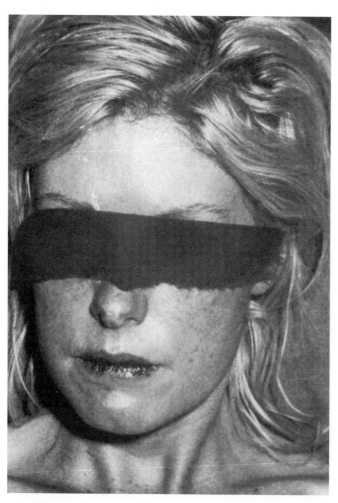

Fig. 12.1 Spider naevi affecting the face and chest wall.

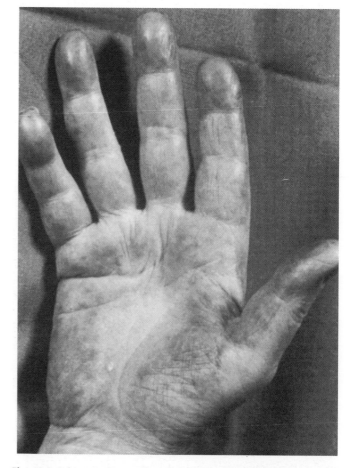

Fig. 12.2 Palmar erythema affecting the thenar and hypothenar eminences.

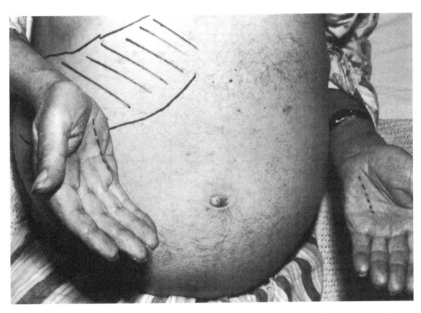

Fig. 12.3 Hepatomegaly and Dupuytren's contracture in a patient with extensive cirrhosis.

copper deposition found in the cornea of patients with Wilson's disease. Nail changes are not uncommon features of liver disease. These consist of either *clubbing* or white nails (*leuconychia*) (Fig. 12.4), the latter seen particularly in primary biliary cirrhosis.

Superficial glandular changes which occur with liver disease include *parotid enlargement*, which is usually painless and bilateral and usually found in association with alcohol related liver disease, *testicular atrophy* and *gynecomastia*.

Gynecomastia is probably due to either altered estrogen metabolism or spironolactone therapy and is usually bilateral and associated with areolar pigmentation (Fig. 12.5).

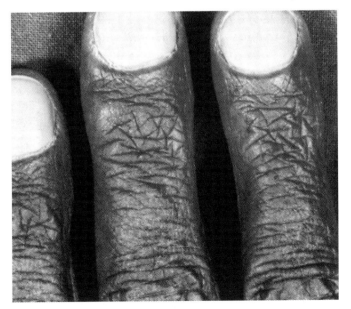

Fig. 12.4 Leuconychia (white nails) in a patient with cirrhosis.

Altered levels of fluids and electrolytes in conjunction with hypoproteinemia may lead to *peripheral edema*. Poorly nourished alcoholics often manifest *peripheral neuropathies* which include parasthesia, loss of sensation to pin prick and light touch and absent ankle jerks.

INSPECTION OF THE ABDOMEN

Rarely on inspection of the abdomen there may be evidence of portosystemic anastamosis secondary to portal hypertension. Here the portal circulation joins the systemic circulation via the left branch of the portal vein which then communicates with the superficial veins via the umbilical vein leading to the classical *caput medusae*. These veins radiate out from the umbilicus with blood flowing outwards. Another rarer site of portosystemic anastamosis is at the anus giving rise to hemorrhoidal varices. Bruising of the abdomen is frequently observed due to abnormal clotting and an increased tendency to trauma (especially in alcoholic cirrhosis).

ASCITES

Ascites is the presence of a pathological amount of fluid within the peritoneal cavity and is a common feature of liver disease. On lateral inspection, the abdomen is distended, with the maximal circumference above the level of the umbilicus, which is often everted (Fig. 12.6). Clinical confirmation of ascites is achieved by eliciting shifting dullness on percussion and a fluid 'thrill' on tapping the flanks.

The cause of the ascites in patients with cirrhosis is due to

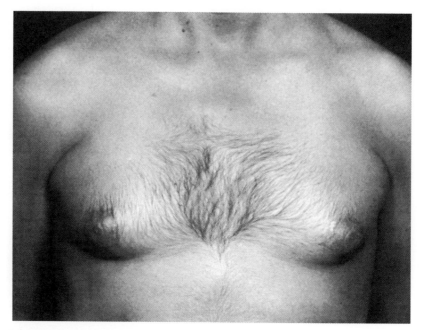

Fig. 12.5 Bilateral gynecomastia in a patient with alcoholic liver disease.

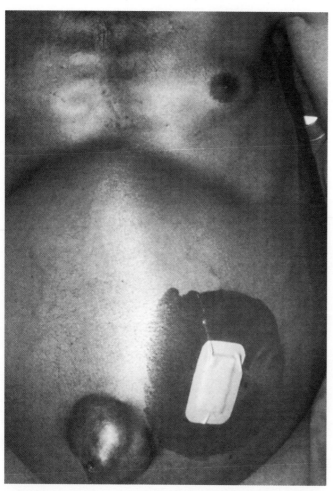

Fig. 12.6 Ascites with an everted umbilicus and venous distention in a patient with cirrhosis.

a combination of altered sodium and electrolyte balance, low plasma protein levels, hyperaldosteronism and local increases in hydrostatic pressure due to portal hypertension. Ascites in patients with hepatobiliary disease may also be secondary to advanced malignancy with hepatic and peritoneal deposits, so called 'malignant ascites'.

EXAMINATION OF THE LIVER

The liver is examined by a combination of palpation and percussion from above and below to delineate its borders. Dullness to percussion of the upper border extends as far as the fifth intercostal space. Auscultation is also important as a venous hum may be heard with portal hypertension and a bruit in association with hepatocellular carcinomas.

Enlargement of the liver occurs in a number of pathological states, although a tongue like extension from the right lobe, Riedel's lobe, which is of no pathological significance, may be mistaken for a tumor. Causes of hepatomegaly are listed in Table 12.1. A lobe may undergo hypertrophy and hence become palpable in an otherwise atrophied diseased liver, which is impalpable. Reduction in liver size is also important since this may occur in cirrhosis and certain types of hepatitis.

Consistency is also relevant and may aid in identifying the cause of hepatomegaly. For example a hard 'knobbly liver' often represents the presence of metastases whilst smooth enlargement may be due to cirrhosis.

Table 12.1 Causes of hepatomegaly

Variant anatomy:
Reidel's lobe
low lying diaphragm

Inflammatory:
hepatitis
abscesses—amebic and pyogenic
Schistosomiasis
cirrhosis—early
sarcoid

Biliary obstruction—especially extrahepatic

Metabolic:
amyloid
fatty liver
glycogen storage disease

Hematological:
leukemias
lymphomas
myloproliferative disorders
sickle cell disease
porphyrias

Tumors:
primary—benign and malignant
secondaries

Cardiovascular:
cardiac failure
hepatic vein obstruction

Table 12.2 Causes of splenomegaly

Infection:
acute—viral, bacterial
chronic—tuberculosis, brucellosis
parasitic—malaria, schistosomiasis

Hematological:
leukemias
hemolytic anemias
hemaglobinopathies

Portal hypertension—especially extrahepatic

Neoplastic:
lymphomas
myeloproliferative disorders
secondary deposits

Inflammatory:
rheumatoid
systemic lupus
amyloidosis

EXAMINATION OF THE SPLEEN

Examination of the spleen should commence in the right iliac fossa and proceed towards the left subcostal region since this is the direction in which splenomegaly occurs. Rotation of the patient by 45° to the right may aid palpation since the spleen then falls onto the examining right hand. During this maneuver the left hand should support the rib cage and relax the skin and abdominal musculature by drawing these down and to the right. Percussion may be useful and if ascites is present the spleen may become ballotable. If the spleen is sufficiently enlarged the notch on its anterior border may become palpable. Causes of splenomegaly are listed in Table 12.2.

GALLBLADDER SIGNS

Tenderness and guarding in the right hypochondrium exacerbated by inspiration (Murphy's sign) suggests cholecystitis. If the gallbladder is palpable in the presence of obstructive jaundice this suggests malignant obstruction of the biliary tree (Couvoisier's law) which is commonly due to carcinoma in the head of pancreas. Failure to palpate the gallbladder does not, however, exclude malignant disease.

Conversely it is possible for obstructive jaundice and a palpable gallbladder to be due to a stone impacted in Hartman's pouch leading to a mucocele or empyema with a stone obstructing the common bile duct.

Gallbladder distention and signs of sepsis, in the presence of gallstones, may indicate the formation of an empyema or mucocele of the gallbladder. In such instances initial treatment may consist of percutaneous aspiration and drainage with a delayed cholecystectomy whether laparoscopic or open. A gallbladder which is intermittently palpable suggests the presence of a periampullary carcinoma.

CLINICAL FEATURES OF PORTAL HYPERTENSION

Portal hypertension is due to either intrahepatic or extrahepatic portal venous obstruction. Intrahepatic portal hypertension is usually associated with hepatomegaly and may also be accompanied by splenomegaly and ascites. Dilated abdominal wall veins may also be found secondary to porto-systemic anastamosis, giving rise to a 'Caput medusae' (vide supra). The more common clinical site of porto-systemic anastamosis is at the gastro-esophageal junction leading to esophageal varices and therefore any evidence of upper gastrointestinal blood loss, whether hematemesis or melena, should be investigated with urgent endoscopy (Ch. 95). Rarely these patients may develop hemorrhoidal varices around the anus due again to porto-systemic anastamosis.

Extrahepatic portal hypertension is usually due to portal vein thrombosis and as such it is important to identify whether there has been a history of neonatal infection around the umbilicus, major intra abdominal sepsis, pancreatic cancer or a blood disorder which might lead to hypercoagulability. These patients almost invariably have splenomegaly (often associated with pancytopenia). In such cases the liver is normal, but ascites may be present.

CLINICAL FEATURES OF ALCOHOLIC LIVER DISEASE

The symptoms and signs of alcoholic liver disease may be directly related to alcoholism or to secondary hepatocellular dysfunction. Such patients commonly suffer repeated falls whilst inebriated and as such may have signs of trauma and bruising. Multiple 'old' rib fractures are common findings on chest X-ray and are related to such behaviour. Alcoholic neuropathy may also be present (as described above), especially given the malnourished state of many such patients.

Acute alcoholic hepatitis usually occurs after a bout of drinking and may be associated with liver tenderness, jaundice, pyrexia and a leucocytosis.

Advanced alcoholic liver disease may be associated with the other manifestations of hepatic impairment e.g. portal hypertension, ascites, hepatomegaly and ultimately liver failure.

CLINICAL FEATURES OF OTHER TYPES OF LIVER DISEASE

PRIMARY BILIARY CIRRHOSIS

Primary biliary cirrhosis (PBC), or chronic non-suppurative destructive cholangitis, usually affects middle aged women. Asymptomatic individuals may be diagnosed during routine examination where they are found to have hepatomegaly, autoantibodies or elevated plasma alkaline phosphatase. The earliest symptom is usually pruritis prior to jaundice developing, by which time the patients have developed hepatomegaly. Later on the patients develop jaundice, hepatosplenomegaly, xanthelasma (especially in the palms and around the eyes), vitiligo and arthritis. It is not uncommon to find PBC in association with connective tissue diseases.

ULCERATIVE COLITIS AND CROHN'S DISEASE

Both ulcerative colitis and Crohn's disease are associated with hepatobiliary disorders especially primary sclerosing cholangitis (Ch. 48). It is therefore important to include a detailed gastrointestinal systems review and investigation in any patient with unexplained liver disease.

INVESTIGATIONS OF HEPATOBILIARY DISEASE

LABORATORY INVESTIGATIONS

The routine liver function tests performed are not true measures of liver function but are in reality markers of liver disease. Although some diseases have characteristic altered patterns of liver function tests, there is a great deal of overlap between conditions. The majority of bilirubin in the plasma is unconjugated and a knowledge of the ratio of unconjugated to conjugated is only useful in congenital disorders of bilirubin metabolism and in hemolytic states. The

Table 12.3 Laboratory investigations in hepatopancreatobiliary disease

Hematological tests:
full blood count, erythrocyte sedimentation rate, reticulocyte count, haptoglobulin levels, Coomb's test

Liver function tests:
Conjugated and unconjugated bilirubin levels, aspartate amino transferase (AST), alanine aminotransferase (ALT), gamma glutamyl transferase, alkaline phosphatase

Proteins:
Albumin, globulin, prothrombin time

Immunological and serological tests:
mitochondrial antibodies
smooth muscle and antinuclear antibody
immunoglobulins
hepatitis B surface antigens (HBsAg)
IgM antibody to hepatitis A
hepatitis C antibodies
cytomegalovirus antibodies
EB virus antibody
leptospiral agglutinins
fasciola complement fixation test
amebic complement fixation test
hydatid complement fixation test
Wasserman reaction and other serological tests for syphillis

Tumor markers:
carcinoembryonic antigen (CEA)
alpha fetoprotein
CA 19-9

Alpha-1-antitrypsin levels
Serum amylase

Plasma ceroplasmin levels
Iron and iron binding capacity
Spot blood alcohol
Urine: urobilinogen, hemosiderin
Stools: ova and parasites

changes in the liver enzymes in conjunction with the bilirubin level may help to distinguish between intrahepatic cholestatic jaundice and extrahepatic obstruction (Ch. 21).

In addition to the 'liver function tests' other blood tests that can be performed in relation to hepatobiliary disease include: hematological studies, plasma proteins, immunological and serological assays and specific disease markers (summarised in Table 12.3). The indications for each test vary depending upon the clinical scenario and include certain disease specific investigations such as; anti-mitochondrial antibody which is specific for PBC, antibodies to hepatitis A, B and more recently C and ceroplasmin levels in Wilson's disease.

Markers of malignant disease vary in their clinical usefulness. Alpha-fetoprotein is a useful marker of hepatocellular carcinoma, whilst carcinoembryonic antigen is only of moderate sensitivity for following up patients with colorectal cancer. The marker CA 19-9 a carbohydrate antigen has been assessed in relation to pancreatic cancer. Unfortunately its lack of both organ and disease specificity has limited its role to follow up for tumor recurrence in patients whose levels fall after resection.

IMAGING

The following is a summary of imaging techniques currently in use and their indications in the management of hepatobiliary disease. A more detailed description of the indications and use of each modality can be found in subsequent chapters.

PLAIN ABDOMINAL AND CHEST X-RAYS

Some gallstones are calcified and therefore appear on abdominal X-ray, with calcification in the pancreas suggesting chronic pancreatitis. Air in the biliary tree in conjunction with small bowel obstruction suggests a gallstone ileus (Ch. 50).

The presence of lung metastases and/or pleural effusions is of importance in staging malignant disease and may identify a primary tumor. Old rib fractures are seen in patients with alcohol abuse and pathological fractures in patients with disseminated malignant disease.

TRANSABDOMINAL ULTRASOUND (Ch. 13)

Percutaneous ultrasound (US) remains one of the most widely used imaging modalities especially in the jaundiced patient. It is inexpensive, non-invasive and quick to perform, although it is operator dependent and suffers from image degradation due to body fat and intervening bowel gas.

It plays a pivotal role in the management of the jaundiced patient. US is able to identify the presence of and level of extrahepatic biliary obstruction in over 95% of patients (Taylor and Rosenfeld 1977, Lindsell 1990). The cause of obstruction may also be identified e.g. the presence of gallstones in the gallbladder, stones in the common bile duct or enlargement of the pancreatic head suggestive of pancreatic carcinoma. Defining the level of the obstruction is less accurate than identifying the presence of dilatation, but has been reported to be between 80 to 95% in experienced units, with small lesions in the distal bile duct, which is often obscured by bowel gas, the most difficult to define (Malini and Sabel 1977, Lindsell 1990).

Ultrasound also plays a role in the diagnosis of hepatocellular causes of deranged liver function. The echopattern from the liver may suggest underlying hepatic disease, with cirrhosis and chronic active hepatitis usually producing a bright, tightly packed echo pattern. Colorectal liver metastases are usually echogenic, whilst multiple liver metastases produce an irregular echo pattern (Lamb and Taylor 1982).

Many patients with liver disease will have normal echo patterns and those who are jaundiced without dilated ducts will usually require a liver biopsy to obtain a diagnosis.

LAPAROSCOPIC (INCLUDING INTRAOPERATIVE ULTRASOUND) AND ENDOSCOPIC ULTRASOUND (Chs 13 & 24)

Intraoperative ultrasound (IOUS) has the advantage over percutaneous US of being in direct contact with the intra-abdominal tissues and hence producing a more accurate image. It has been shown to be of use in hepatic surgery in identifying impalpable lesions not picked up on routine imaging, delineating lesions in relation to hepatic vascular structures and guiding the surgeon during resection. Similarly in pancreatic disease IOUS helps to determine resectability especially in regard to the peripancreatic vessels. Laparoscopic IOUS probes are now available and have been shown to be of use especially with regard to picking up unidentified hepatic tumors and in the assessment of resectability of pancreatic tumors.

Endoscopic ultrasound involves the use of a specially designed echoendoscope and uses similar principles to IOUS. An echoendoscope is attached to the distal end of the endoscope and allows visualization of adjacent tissues from within the lumen of the stomach and duodenum. This technique has been shown to be highly accurate in the diagnosis of both pancreatic and periampullary tumors, but is less sensitive in discriminating whether the lesion is benign or malignant. It is also useful in the staging of malignant pancreatic and periampullary tumors especially with regard to vascular invasion.

ISOTOPE SCANNING (Ch. 14)

^{99m}Technitium sulfur colloid when injected intravenously is selectively taken up by the reticuloendothelial cells of the liver and spleen. It is able to demonstrate hepatic tumors both primary and secondary, although its main uses are in advanced cirrhosis and alcoholic hepatitis. In advanced cirrhosis there is poor uptake by the liver and is mostly taken up by the spleen and bone marrow, whilst in alcohol hepatitis there is almost no uptake by the liver.

^{99m}Tc-HIDA scanning uses an imino-diacetic acid derivative, which when injected intravenously is taken up by the liver and excreted into the biliary system outlining the bile ducts, even in the presence of a moderate elevation bilirubin levels. This has been used in the diagnosis of acute cholecystitis, hepatitis due to biliary atresia in the neonatal period, in the assessment of biliary-enteric anastamosis and to demonstrate external and internal biliary fistulae.

ENDOSCOPIC RETROGRADE CHOLANGIOPANCREATOGRAPHY (ERCP) (Chs 17 & 28)

This technique is now widely used in the imaging and management of pancreatobiliary pathology. In particular it plays a key role in the management of the jaundiced patient with dilated ducts on US. ERCP demonstrates the level and cause of obstruction, permits biopsies to be taken for tissue diagnosis and provides the opportunity for therapeutic intervention. Given the increased use of laparoscopic cholecystectomy ERCP may also be used to exclude the presence of ductal stones in selected patients preoperatively.

ERCP is also helpful in the diagnosis of pancreatic pathology, not only in delineating the pancreatic ducts, but also in obtaining brushings for cytological diagnosis.

PERCUTANEOUS TRANSHEPATIC CHOLANGIOGRAM (PTC) (Ch. 17)

This technique is used in jaundiced patients with a dilated bile duct in whom ERCP is not possible and therefore provides the only route of access to the biliary tree. Needles are introduced percutaneously, under US guidance, into the intrahepatic bile ducts. Contrast may then be injected or a guidewire passed to allow stenting, or passed into the duodenum and grasped by the endoscope in a combined procedure. Up to 99% of patients with dilated bile ducts and 82% with normal or sclerosed ducts are sucessfully cannulated using this technique, although there is a higher incidence of bile leakage and bleeding compared to ERCP (Felluci and Wittenberg 1977, McPherson et al 1984).

COMPUTED TOMOGRAPHY (CT) (Ch. 15)

This investigation allows imaging of the liver, bile ducts, gallbladder and pancreas. It is particularly useful in identifying small lesions in the liver and pancreas and plays a key role in staging hepatopancreaticobiliary malignancy. With the advent of spiral CT scanning further improvements in imaging over previous CT has led to greater diagnostic accuracy, especially with regard to liver metastases and pancreatic tumors.

CT combined with angioportography (CTAP) allows further differentiation of even smaller hepatic tumors up to several mm in size, but does require cannulation of the major mesenteric arteries.

MAGNETIC RESONANCE IMAGING (INCLUDING MAGNETIC RESONANCE CHOLANGIOPANCREATOGRAPHY) (Ch.16)

Standard magnetic resonance imaging (MRI) is proving to be increasingly useful in the investigation of hepatobiliary disease, especially in diagnosing and staging malignant disease. Alterations in the weighting of the image leads to prominence of the ductal system in the biliary tree and pancreas, known as magnetic resonance cholangiopancreatography (MRCP). MRCP has an advantage over ERCP in being non-interventional and does not require contrast injection, although, unlike ERCP, it is purely diagnostic. This technique may eventually supersede ERCP in non-jaundiced patients in whom imaging of the biliary system, rather than intervention or biopsy, is required.

CHOLECYSTOGRAPHY

This investigation is of little value and cannot be used if the patient is jaundiced. In the non-jaundiced patient this technique may demonstrate gallstones in the gallbladder and occasionally the bile ducts. Non-opacification of the gallbladder in the absence of jaundice, chronic diarrhea or malabsorption indicates gallbladder pathology. The possible mechanisms for this picture are either a non-functioning gallbladder or a stone impacted in Hartman's pouch or cystic duct. Oral cholecystography is unable to predict the need for cholecystectomy, even if the gallbladder fails to opacify.

INTRAVENOUS CHOLANGIOGRAPHY

This technique involves the intravenous injection of an iodine-containing contrast medium, which binds to plasma proteins and is excreted by the liver. The bile ducts are then opacified, along with the gallbladder if the cystic duct is patent. This investigation is now rarely performed as it has been superseded by other techniques which are more accurate in the jaundiced and non-jaundiced state (Osnes et al 1978). Even if performed successfully the diagnostic yield is still low (Blumgart et al 1974).

Some centers have returned to intravenous cholangiography in an attempt to pick up bile duct stones and identify anomalous anatomy in patients about to undergo laparoscopic cholecystectomy, in order to avoid peroperative cholangiography.

OPERATIVE AND POST-OPERATIVE T-TUBE CHOLANGIOGRAPHY (Ch. 22)

The incidence of operative cholangiography has fallen since the advent of laparoscopic cholecystectomy and the adoption of a policy of selective preoperative ERCP in many centers. Traditionally operative cholangiography was performed during cholecystectomy to exclude the presence of stones in the common bile duct. Some groups are now performing laparoscopic cholangiography during cholecystectomy for this reason and also in an effort to reduce the incidence of bile duct injury, especially if the anatomy is unclear (Ch. 38).

It may also be used during laparotomy in patients in whom the cause of their jaundice is not apparent, although this is now unusual given the current expertise in ERCP available in most units.

ANGIOGRAPHY

There are a number of different types of angiography available, each with their own specific indications and uses.

Selective visceral angiography has been used in regard to pancreatic cancer, to assess resectability and to detect any coexisting vascular anomalies, which might affect the surgical procedure. With improved CT techniques such investigations have to a large extent been superseded and are no longer routine practice in many units.

Hepatic artery angiography has been used during the evaluation of hepatic tumors to exclude the presence of other lesions prior to resection and also to identify any variant vascular anatomy. Liver abcess and cysts can also be diagnosed by this technique if other investigations have failed to provide a definitive answer. Again improved CT technology has reduced the need for angiography in this field.

Hepatic artery angiography is still performed prior to insertion of hepatic arterial catheters for regional chemotherapy of hepatic tumors and chemoembolization is still performed via this route for certain endocrine tumors.

Angiography may be combined with CT (CTAP) to improve the diagnosis of small hepatic tumors.

Splenoportography is useful if shunt surgery is considered for esophageal varices, especially to determine the patency of the portal vein. However with greater use of sclerotherapy and other techniques for the control of acute variceal hemorrage the need for this investigation has reduced.

Inferior venacavography is occasionally performed prior to hepatic resection to delineate the vascular anatomy and to determine whether the inferior vena cava is compressed or invaded.

LAPAROSCOPY (Ch. 20)

Laparoscopic staging is now routine practice in many units prior to resection of both pancreatic and hepatic tumors, particularly given the low sensitivity of CT for the detection of peritoneal metastases.

Occasionally laparoscopy is used if liver biopsy has to be performed under direct vision. Laparoscopic cholangiography is also feasible as discussed above and is being increasingly utilized.

PERCUTANEOUS NEEDLE BIOPSY (Ch.19)

Liver biopsy is sometimes indicated in patients without dilated bile ducts in order to determine the etiology of the underlying disease. Liver biopsies may also be necessary in order to determine the nature of hepatic lesions which are indeterminate on conventional imaging.

Fine needle aspiration or core cuts of pancreatic lesions are not commonly used, especially in potentially resectable lesions, due to the risk of malignant needle track seeding.

REFERENCES

Blumgart L H, Salmon P R, Cotton P B 1974 Endoscopic retrograde cholangiopancreatography in the diagnosis of the patient with jaundice. Surgery, Gynaecology and Obstetrics 138: 565–570

Felluci J T, Wittenburg J 1977 Refinements in Chiba needle transhepatic cholangiography. American Journal of Roentgenology 129: 11–16

Lamb G, Taylor I 1982 An assessment of ultrasound scanning in the recognition of colorectal liver metastases. Annals of the Royal College of Surgeons 64: 391–393

Lindsell D R M 1990 Ultrasound imaging of pancreas and biliary tract. Lancet i: 390–394

Malini S, Sabel J 1977 Ultrasonography in obstructive jaundice. Radiology 123: 429–433

McPherson G A D, Benjamin I S, Hodgson H J F, Bowley N B, Allison D J and Blumgart L H 1984 Pre-operative percutaneous transhepatic biliary drainage: the results of a controlled trial. British Journal of Surgery 71: 371–375

Osnes M, Larsen S, Lowe P 1978 Comparison of endoscopic retrograde and intravenous cholangiography in diagnosis of biliary calculi. Lancet ii: 230

Taylor K J, Rosenfield A T 1977 Greyscale ultrasonography in the differential diagnosis of jaundice. Archives of Surgery 112: 820–825

Ultrasound of the liver and biliary tract

D.O. COSGROVE, M.J.K. BLOMLEY, R.J. ECKERSLEY

INTRODUCTION

Ultrasound is a tomographic imaging technique that is capable of providing anatomical and functional information with high resolution and great flexibility at low cost. Structural detail down to around a millimeter, e.g. for intrahepatic ducts, is available without the requirement for administration of contrast agents (Fig. 13.1). The high intrinsic contrast is produced by the tissues' structure at a submillimeter level, and is chiefly attributable to the differences in rigidity and density between fluids, watery tissue, collagen fibers and fatty tissue. The tomograms are formed very rapidly, allowing real time imaging. The studies are therefore quick and interactive. Immediate viewing of changing situations is a characteristic feature of routine ultrasound; examples include the effects of respiration or palpation on the organ and the direct 'real-time' observation of the position of a biopsy needle (Das et al 1997, Duysburgh et al 1997). The tomograms can be taken in any plane, allowing optimal display of critical anatomy. Since many scanners are small and self-contained, they may be wheeled to the ward, theatre or recovery room, a major asset for the surgical patient. Minimal preparation, or none at all, is required so that the procedure is well tolerated, the only practical problem being abdominal tenderness that may make probe contact painful. Ionizing radiation hazards do not exist.

The flexibility of the technique has led to several specialized applications of ultrasound. Its interactiveness and display of soft tissues in real time make ultrasound an ideal technique for guiding biopsies and other interventional procedures (Pederson et al 1993, Holm & Skjoldbye 1996, Abbitt 1998, Smith 1999). It is possible to make the transducer small enough to be accommodated on an endoscope with the advantage that higher quality images are obtained because higher frequency ultrasound can be used (Fukuda et al 1991, Bezzi et al 1998). Endoscopic ultrasound is, of course, rather more invasive than transcutaneous, and only tissues with a few centimeters of the gut wall are accessible. The same is true of intravascular ultrasound. Small transducers suitable for use in the operating theatre (Herman 1996), similarly, offer the benefit of higher resolution as well as of guiding needle placement for biopsies or cannulation of small portal vein branches (Klotter et al 1986) (Ch. 24) while the development of transducers small enough to fit into standard laparoscopic instruments (Ch. 20) extends these advantages to minimally invasive surgery (Barbot et al 1997).

The availability of Doppler has greatly extended the role of ultrasound in the diagnosis and management of vascular pathology of the liver and is now an indispensable tool in hepatic imaging (Grant 1992, Bolondi et al 1998, Jeffrey & Ralls 1998) (Fig. 13.2). It is particularly helpful in liver

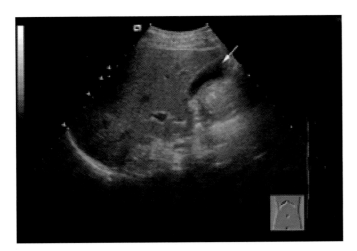

Fig. 13.1 Gray-scale scan. Modern scanners with high-resolution transducers give excellent resolution and high contrast as can be seen in this parasagittal section through a normal liver and gallbladder (arrow).

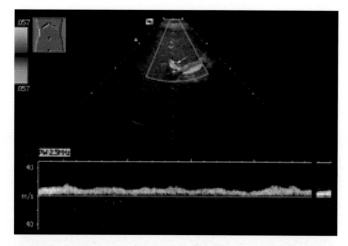

Fig. 13.2 Duplex Doppler of the portal vein. Using color Doppler (top portion) the spectral Doppler gate (arrow) has been placed over the vessel of interest, the portal vein. The trace in the lower portion is a normal spectral Doppler signal which shows the frequency shift as it changes with time (x-axis). Flow towards the transducer is depicted above the zero line and vice versa. The strength of the Doppler signal at each frequency is indicated by the brightness of the display, a measure of the amount of blood flowing at each velocity. If the angle between the Doppler beam and the flow direction is known (red line), the frequency shift can be converted to a velocity scale, as shown. The small variations in velocity are caused by transmitted cardiac and thoracic pressure changes.

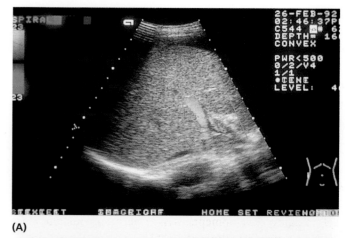

(A)

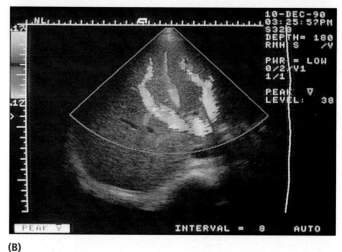

(B)

Fig. 13.3 Color Doppler of normal liver. The portal vein and hepatic artery are shown in tints of red in scans taken at the porta hepatis **(A)** while the interdigitating arrangement of the smaller portal vein branches (in red) with the hepatic veins (in blue) are well seen in a high transverse scan **(B)**.

transplants, both pre-operatively (to establish portal vein (PV) and caval patency) and postoperatively (for the portal vein and hepatic artery) and in the Budd–Chiari syndrome. In cirrhosis Doppler can establish the patency of the PV and of some types of shunts (others that are covered by gas-containing bowel are usually inaccessible). In pulsed Doppler, a sensitive gate is positioned over a region of interest, e.g. the PV, and the temporal pattern of flow analysed to display its velocity spectrum; volume flow can also be estimated though with less precision. With color Doppler, a vascular map is presented as an overlay on the gray scale scan (Foley 1992) to provide a form of angiogram that gives a non-invasive picture of vascular anatomy, for example, of the transplant hepatic artery (Fig 13.3). Though the flow information is crude (only mean velocity or, in power Doppler, the number of moving red cells, is presented) the anatomical information gained is an extremely valuable addition to imaging. Color and pulsed Doppler are complementary, the former providing images, the latter functional data on blood flow.

However, this description omits some important limitations to the uses of ultrasound. The variable quality of the images obtained is a problem. Slim patients give the best images because resolution deteriorates with depth; for this reason, ultrasound is particularly valuable in pediatrics.

Bone and gas are impenetrable and may also degrade the image quality of regions of interest lying close to them. In practical terms this is only an occasional problem for the liver because the intercostal spaces allow adequate access in almost all patients if the subcostal route is difficult to use. But for the pancreas and the lower end of the common bile duct, adequate imaging may be impossible in some 10 to 20% of cases, especially for hospitalized patients or those with ileus because of the larger amount of intestinal gas.

The small field of view of a real time ultrasound image makes the scan difficult to review and can also lead to difficulty in repeating the same tomogram for follow-up purposes. It makes explanation to referring physicians and surgeons difficult; understandably, they may find the more complete tomographic images of computed tomography (CT) or magnetic resonance imaging (MRI) more believable. However, the surgeon who can attend the actual scanning sessions will readily appreciate the completeness of the study and the added value of imaging in real time. The fact that the bony skeleton is not displayed, apart from causing difficulty in interpretation, poses a problem when it is necessary to compare ultrasound tomograms with CT or with radiographs.

The interactive nature of ultrasound renders it very operator dependent: a skilled and motivated operator can produce consistently good results but lack of experience and working without essential clinical information can severely devalue a study.

Many of these problems have been mitigated with recent technological developments. Tissue harmonic imaging, by selecting returning echoes at double the transmitted signals (these are generated as the ultrasound pulse propagates through the tissue, rather like the breaking of a wave as it approaches the shore), reduces the artefacts from heavily built patients and gives cleaner images (Fig. 13.4). Oral contrast agents displace upper intestinal gas and improve the display of retroperitoneal structures such as the lower end of the bile duct (Fig. 13.5), while the development of

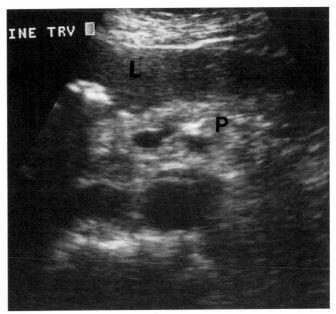

(A)

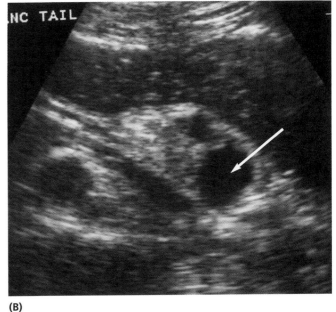

(B)

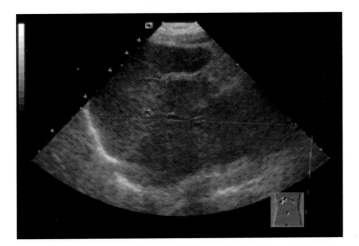

(A)

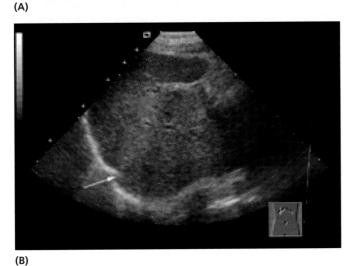

(B)

Fig. 13.4 Tissue harmonic imaging. In this new gray scale ultrasound mode the scanner's filters are set so that the transmitted frequency is half the received frequency—in this case 2 and 4 MHz. The resulting improvement in the clarity of the image (note the impression on the superior surface of the liver caused by a prominent diaphragmatic leaflet, arrow in **(B)**, compared with the conventional fundamental image **(A)** results from the improvement in beam profile.

Fig. 13.5 SonoRx improves ultrasound transmission. **(A)** Though the head and neck of the pancreas (P) are clearly visualized the body is obscured by gastric gas; after drinking SonoRx, a cellulose-simethicone agent, acoustic access was improved and a pseudocyst in the distal body of the pancreas could be seen (arrow in **(B)**). P, pancreas; L, liver. (Images courtesy of Dr Anna Lev-Toav, Thomas Jefferson Hospital, Philadelphia)

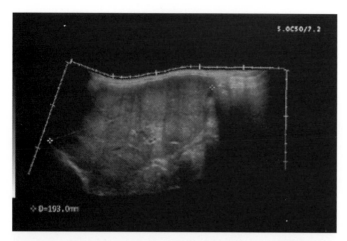

Fig. 13. 6 Extended field-of-view scan. Extended field of view scans (Sciescape, Siemens™) are useful when structures larger than can be accommodated on a single real-time image must be measured—in this case an enlarged liver measuring over 19 cm with multiple metastases (the rounded lesions) from a carcinoma of the stomach. They are also useful for communication, particularly for teaching and for demonstrating pathology to clinicians. They are made by the pattern recognition software in the scanner holding matching images from a real-time sweep and assembling them seamlessly.

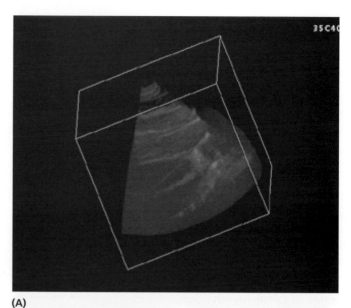

(A)

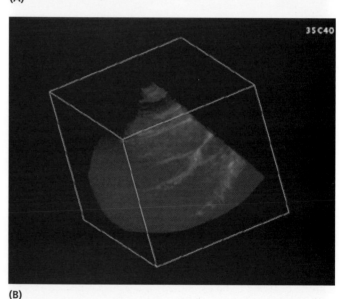

(B)

Fig. 13.7 Three dimensional reconstruction of flow to a liver metastasis. Following injection of a microbubble contrast agent, the vessels in the liver were enhanced so that they became whiter than the parenchyma and a three-dimensional data set was obtained by sweeping the transducer across the region containing a colo-rectal metastasis. In these two frames from a rotating loop, the vessels can be seen as sinuous lines surrounding the lesion; in the original stereoscopic movie the relationships were more clearly seen.

microbubble contrast agents for intravenous use not only rescues Doppler studies that would otherwise have been failures but also opens out important new diagnostic possibilities (see below). Application of sophisticated transducer technologies and of powerful computer systems has resulted in better image and particularly Doppler quality. An example of this is the availability of extended field of view images, obtained by cross-correlation pattern recognition techniques that allow much more complete body sections to be presented, partially at least, addressing the keyhole view limitation (Fig. 13.6). A further exploitation of this and of other registration techniques allow three dimensional data sets to be collected and rendered either for 3-D viewing or for reslicing to display otherwise unobtainable tomograms (Fig. 13.7).

It can be seen that ultrasound is continuing to develop rapidly and the process shows no sign of slowing down.

TECHNOLOGY

Ultrasound is a high frequency, mechanical vibration whereby alternate waves of compression and rarefaction travel through the tissue (McDicken 1991, Kremkau 1997). The waves are generated by piezo-electric crystals, shaped into a transducer which focuses the ultrasound waves into a beam. Commonly used frequencies are 5.0 or 3.5 mega-hertz (MHz); the corresponding wavelengths in tissue are 0.3 and 0.5 mm respectively and this sets theoretical limits to the spatial resolution that can be achieved.

The small proportion of the ultrasound that is absorbed by the tissue appears as heat. The remainder is reflected as the beam crosses between tissues of different acoustic properties (known as acoustic impedance, a complex of tissue density and rigidity). While both these components are familiar in that they are palpable in bulk, the ultrasound pulse responds to tissue structure in the sub-millimeter range. The smallest structure that can be resolved in practice depends on the contrast in reflectivity: well-defined structures such as ducts can be traced down to a millimeter or so in caliber but low contrast lesions such as liver metastases must be much larger, perhaps 5–10 mm in diameter.

The reflected portion of the sound beam that returns to the transducer is used to form the image. The depth (range) of a reflecting interface is calculated from the delay between the sending of the pulse and the detection of the returning echo, and its direction from the angle at which the transducer faces; this is the same 'pulse-echo' method used in Radar and Sonar. The velocity of ultrasound in different tissues is not quite constant but varies so little that the minor errors in calculating the depth of reflecting surfaces can be ignored.

The strength of the echoes is proportional to the change in acoustic impedance at the interface. At risk of oversimplifying a complex phenomenon, it may be said that impedance correlates with tissue rigidity. In the body this ranges from gases at the one extreme, through fluids and soft tissue, to bone and calcified tissue at the other. For soft tissues, the collagen content is usually the main contributor and this is found in a condensed form in fascia and in a diffuse form as the microskeleton of the parenchyma that surrounds blood vessels. It is probably the characteristic vascular pattern as reflected in the ultrasound image that lends tissue-specific textures to sonograms. Fatty tissue is strongly echogenic because of the abundant lipid/watery interfaces at cellular or lobular level.

Real-time scanners rapidly sweep the beam through the volume of tissue to be examined: the scan is repeated 20–30 times a second to give a moving image, as with a ciné film. The sweep may be angled from a point on the skin, so-called sector scanning, to form a triangular image. This method provides good access through small windows and so is particularly useful for intercostal scans of the liver. However, the triangular field of view gives a poor display of superficial structures and linear arrays are more convenient in this respect. Here the ultrasound beam is swept electronically along a block of piezo-electric material some 2 cm wide and 5–10 cm long. Curved linear arrays combine some of the advantages of the two geometries.

For Doppler, a different type of signal processing is used to assess the change in frequency in the returning echoes that occurs when the reflector is moving. For a given transducer frequency, the blood velocity is proportional to the Doppler shift with a correction for the beam-to-vessel angle, and the flow direction can also be provided. The

spectrum from a pulsed Doppler scanner is displayed as a chart of (blood) velocity against time, in which flow towards the transducer is shown above the zero line, and vice versa (Fig. 13.2). The amount of blood flowing at any particular volume is indicated by the degree of whitening of the trace. Simultaneous imaging and Doppler (known as 'duplex scanning', from their operation in two modes) is available on most systems, so that the Doppler-sensitive gate can be positioned precisely over the vessel of interest.

In color Doppler, similar processing is applied across the entire image (or a selected portion of it, since this minimizes the inevitable reduction in frame rate that occurs when Doppler is used) (Fig. 13.3). The color Doppler signals are shown as an overlay, conventionally coded in shades of red for flow towards, and blue for flow away from the transducer, though a variety of other color maps may be selected. Another way to display flow information depicts only the Doppler signal intensity as a power Doppler scan (Fig. 13.8). It has higher sensitivity than frequency-based color Doppler but lacks directional information and so is more useful for the small vessels, for example, in tumors, than for the portal vein where flow direction is clinically important. Inevitably the necessary circuitry is complex and therefore color Doppler is confined to 'high-end' scanners, but its value in picking out small flow abnormalities (e.g. occlusion of a hepatic artery) makes it essential for some important applications in the liver and elsewhere.

Ultrasound guidance of biopsy procedures is a valuable extension of the imaging process that makes use of its real-time interactiveness (Pederson & Pederson et al 1993). Ultrasound may be used simply for planning the biopsy by marking the skin site for a needle puncture; this is useful for

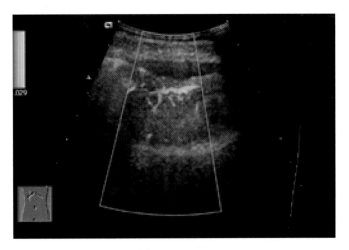

Fig. 13.8 Power Doppler scan. The abundant vasculature supplying this focal nodular hyperplasia are demonstrated as orange-red structures on this power Doppler study.

simple procedures such as paracentesis where the main value of ultrasound is to check that loops of bowel in the ascites will not be punctured. For biopsy guidance two general approaches in use are the freehand and needle-guided methods. The former is simpler in that any transducer can be used. The needle site and path are chosen and the needle (or its tip) is monitored continuously as it is advanced into the lesion. Keeping the needle path in view requires a high degree of hand/eye co-ordination and is not feasible for small or deep lesions where the needle guide approach is more reliable. For this, an attachment to the probe with a needle channel constrains the needle along a path that runs diagonally across the scan area; its line is indicated on screen and, once this has been positioned over the lesion, the needle should pass in the correct direction.

Using a fine (23 G, 0.7 mm OD) needle, cytological samples can be taken from almost any liver lesion with a very high degree of safety. In many units, even the obvious precaution of checking for a bleeding diathesis is dispensed with, and there are no restrictions against penetrating bowel loops, though the gall bladder and dilated bile ducts should be avoided.

If histological specimens are required (e.g. to differentiate between types of malignancy or for diffuse pathologies) a larger (16–18 G) cutting needle must be used. Automatic firing systems (e.g. the Biopty gun) make the procedure simple and reliable. Inevitably, there is an increased risk of bleeding and this is particularly high if a subcapsular metastasis is punctured. Bleeding tests and prolonged observation are required, though overnight admission is not always essential.

Ultrasound can also be used to guide placement of drainage catheters for abscesses (see Infective Conditions).

To make a scan the transducer is contacted to the skin using a coupling jell, and the examination consists of moving the probe gently across the surface of the abdomen. For the liver, subcostal views in transverse and longitudinal directions are convenient and access may be improved if the patient holds a deep breath. The gastro-esophageal junction can also be imaged in this way. If the upper abdomen is gassy, intercostal views give more limited access, but usually allow a full assessment while displacing the gas with an oral contrast agent (e.g. Oralex, or SonoRx, Bracco, Princeton, NJ) may be helpful (Fig. 13.5). Angled views can be useful, e.g. aligned along the common bile duct. No preparation is needed for liver scans but the gallbladder is easier to assess when distended, so a six-hour fast (clear fluids allowed) is useful but not obligatory.

For the lower common bile duct and the pancreas, transverse scans give the best anatomical display and usually these can be obtained without patient preparation. When overly-ing gas obstructs the ultrasound beam, scanning in the erect position can help by allowing bowel loops to drop away as well as by bringing the left lobe of the liver down over the pancreas, thus providing an 'acoustic window'. In difficult cases, access can be improved further by filling the stomach with water before scanning. Using these approaches, the head of the pancreas can be imaged adequately in over 75% of subjects and this can be improved by using an oral contrast agent (Harisinghani et al 1997). In patients with ileus (e.g. in acute pancreatitis) and the very obese, the image quality is usually poor—here CT is better able to provide a diagnosis. The spleen, together with the splenic vein, the tail of the pancreas and the left kidney, may be imaged in the coronal plane through left intercostal spaces or the left flank.

For Doppler the main constraint is the fact that flow at 90° to the beam gives no signal since there is no component of movement towards (or away from) the transducer. Thus, apparent absence of flow can be technical and is less reliable than the demonstration of flow (Parvey et al 1989). For quantitative velocity and volume flow measurements the beam-to-vessel angle must be measured—scanners are equipped with appropriate calculation packages to transform the Doppler shift into true linear velocity and to calculate the mean velocity from the spectrum of the velocities in the Doppler gate.

NORMAL FINDINGS

THE LIVER (see also Ch. 1)

A series of sagittal tomograms (Couinaud 1957, Lyons 1978, Wagner et al 1982, McGrath & Mills 1985) reveals the left lobe as an almond-shaped structure extending inferiorly from the fibrous portion of the diaphragm (Fig. 13.9) (Cosgrove & McCready 1982, Cosgrove 1993). Its inferior border is normally sharp. Its visceral surface is related to the aorta and the esophagogastric junction superiorly and to the stomach, lesser sac and body of the pancreas inferiorly. Moving to the right, segment 1 (caudate lobe) is detected superiorly where it overlies the inferior vena cava. The fissure for the ligamentum venosum, separating it from the left liver, is clearly seen and may pose an interpretative problem by partially shadowing the caudate itself. The ligamentum teres may be seen here and longitudinal sections further to the right reveal segment IV (the quadrate lobe) before the porta is encountered, where the portal vein and its left and right main branches predominate. Characteristic Doppler signals can be picked up from them, best demonstrated in intercostal scans (Fig. 13.2). Superiorly, the groove for the inferior vena cava is seen, though this and the hepatic veins are better displayed on transverse sections. Further to the right, the right liver (segments V–VIII) is visible up against the right hemidiaphragm. Its visceral surface contacts the right kidney, the hepatic flexure of colon and the duodenum, often with the gallbladder intervening. Again, the free edge of the liver has a sharp contour (Hollinshead 1982, Schneck 1983, Netter 1989).

Transverse sections high in the liver image the terminal inferior vena cava (IVC) as it penetrates the diaphragm to empty into the right atrium (Fig. 13.10). A little below this, the point of emptying of the hepatic veins is seen; usually the left and middle form a common trunk which joins the

inferior vena cava anteriorly. The right hepatic vein empties into the lateral part of the IVC, often a centimeter or so below. Simply by sliding the transducer inferiorly, the course of these major veins can be traced to define the sector to which structures belong. The smaller, inferior hepatic veins are sometimes also visualized on ultrasound and all can be demonstrated with Doppler (Fig. 13.11). The caudate lobe (segment I) and its process, lying in contact with the left liver, is often apparent in sections a little inferiorly. Segment VII may form a surprising appearance where its medial portion lies posterior to the IVC and partly enfolds it.

The ligamentum teres is well seen in cross section; though usually solid, a thread-like remnant of the umbilical

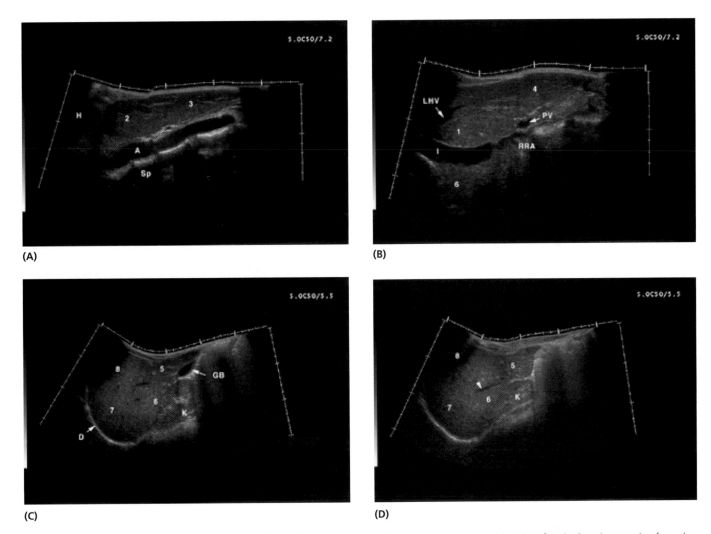

(A) (B)

(C) (D)

Fig. 13.9 Normal liver—sagittal sections. The liver's uniform stippled texture of mid-gray level is shown in this series of sagittal sections passing from the midline (**(A)**, **(B)**) to the right (**(C)**, **(D)**), together with the contiguous organs. Veins in the liver are seen as echo-free tubular structures; those with prominent walls are portal veins while the thin walls of the hepatic veins are not apparent. The Couinaud segments are numbered. In sagittal tomograms on ultrasound, the slices are displayed in the conventional orientation with the patient supine and viewed from the right, as in a clinical examination. Thus the patient's head is to the left of the image with the feet to the right and the anterior skin line is uppermost. The small scale divisions are 1 cm apart. (A, aorta; D, diaphragm; GB, gall bladder; H, heart; I, inferior vena cava; LHV, left hepatic vein; K, kidney; PV, portal vein; RRA, right renal artery; Sp, spine; arrowhead, right hepatic vein)

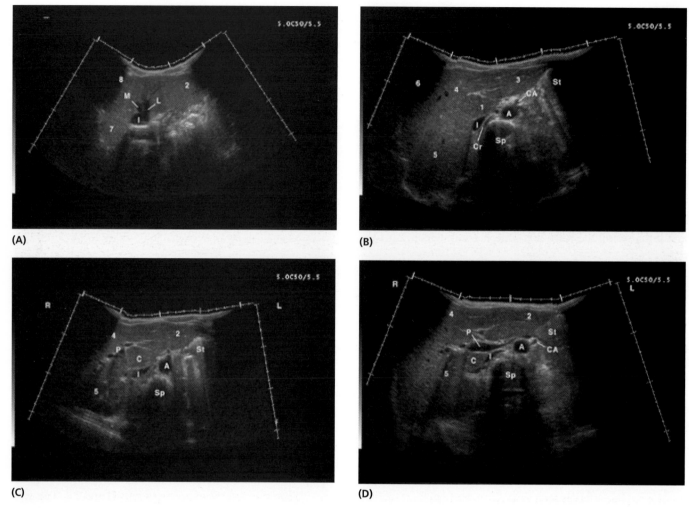

Fig. 13.10 Normal liver—transverse sections. **(A)** High transverse sections show the terminal portions of the hepatic veins, the left and middle usually forming a short common trunk before discharging into the inferior vena cava just below the diaphragm. The middle hepatic vein separates the left and right livers; the terminal branches of the portal veins that supply them can be discerned. A separate vein often drains segment VIII. Further inferiorly **(B–D)** the caudate lobe (segment I) and the portal vein are imaged. (A, aorta; C, caudate lobe; CA, celiac axis; Cr, crus; I, inferior vena cava; M, middle hepatic vein; L, left hepatic vein; P, portal vein; Sp, spine; St, stomach)

vein is normal. At this level the gallbladder is often visualized overlying the right kidney. The pancreas may be visualized here also.

The liver parenchyma appears as a stippled texture representing the interaction of the echoes from the liver lobules with the ultrasound beam. The texture therefore varies both with equipment parameters (especially the transducer) and with pathology. Distinguishing these influences at present is largely a matter of experience, though more quantitative methods are under development (so-called 'tissue characterization') (Cosgrove 1993).

The uniform liver texture is interrupted by vessels. The hepatic veins, with their thin walls, appear as branching, tubular 'defects' converging to the upper IVC. The portal tracts have strongly reflective walls due to the associated vessels and to the enveloping fat and fibrous tissue. The left

portal vein curves anteriorly from the main portal vein to supply the more anteriorly situated left liver. The right portal vein runs in about the same coronal plane as the porta, passing to the right before dividing into anterior and posterior branches. Within the liver the bile ducts and arterial branches are usually too small to be resolved on ultrasound though both are well seen at the porta (see below).

The liver vessels are well seen using color Doppler (Fig. 13.2). The hepatic veins appear as blue bands on color Doppler, because their flow is away from the transducer. On spectral Doppler their flow pattern is complex, being predominantly towards the IVC, but interrupted and usually reversed at each atrial systole (Fig. 13.11). This is because the IVC communicates directly into the right atrium, no valve intervening, so that in systole blood is ejected retrogradely into the cava and thence the hepatic veins. Usually

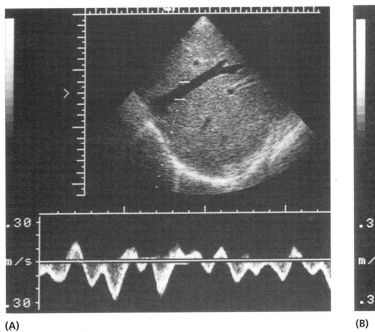

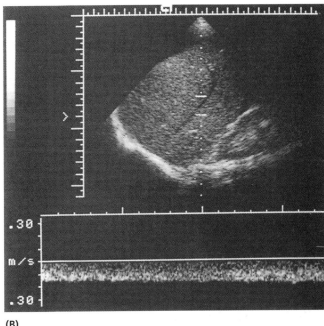

(A)

(B)

Fig. 13.11 Doppler of the hepatic veins. The normal hepatic veins show a fluctuating pattern since the flow in them is strongly affected by the pressure changes in the right atrium **(A)** Stiffening of the liver, as occurs in cirrhosis, prevents the retrograde inflow and the trace becomes monophasic **(B)** (Note the ascites in this case.)

the best approach for a Doppler study of the main portal vein is via a lower right intercostal space because in this position the blood flows directly towards the transducer and thus gives maximal signals. If the conventional color coding is used, normal hepatopetal flow is shown in red. The accompanying artery is seen as a narrow red line that is often discontinuous both spatially—because it is tortuous—and in time—because its flow is pulsatile. On spectral Doppler analysis the portal vein is seen to have continuous flow (perhaps with slight cardiac and respiratory modulation) with a peak velocity of some 15 cm/s in the fasting state increasing by as much as a factor of five in the absorptive state.

Also disturbing the homogeneous texture of the liver is the echogenic ligamentum teres passing from the free edge of the liver close to the midline, superiorly and to the right to end in the left portal vein. Superiorly the residual sinus venosus is represented by the limit of the echogenic line separating the caudate from the left liver. It passes superiorly to end at the IVC and contains the attachment of the lesser omentum whose fat accounts for the high reflectivity of this fissure. The fissure between the quadrate (segment IV) and the right liver can often also be visualized as an oblique band stretching from the origin of the right portal vein to the neck of the gallbladder (Fried et al 1984).

The liver capsule is seen as a smooth, fine echogenic line. It is not normally well marked though it is readily detected in ascites when the ultrasound beam is aligned at 90° across it.

The segmental anatomy of the liver (Ch. 1) is best appreciated in transverse sections. Superiorly the hepatic veins are easily demonstrated and provide obvious landmarks, with the middle hepatic vein (running from the gallbladder fossa), separating the left and right livers. The left hepatic vein runs in the plane between segments II and IV. The separation between segments III and IV is easily demonstrated a few centimeters inferiorly where the ligamentum teres is cut across. The falciform ligament itself cannot be defined except in the presence of ascites when it appears as a thin sheet attaching the anterior surface of the liver to the anterior abdominal wall. The fissure between segments IV and V is often clearly seen, though its oblique or near-coronal orientation may be surprising until it is remembered that segment IV lies anterior to segment V in the true anatomical orientation of the liver. The right hepatic vein, running in the coronal plane, separates the anterior segments V and VIII from the posterior segments VI and VII.

The interdigitating pattern of the portal vein branches, running into the centre of the segments, is most impressively demonstrated with color Doppler (Fig. 13.2). The division of the right portal vein into anterior and posterior sectoral branches is usually apparent and the division of the left portal vein may also be demonstrated.

The great variation in shape to which the liver is subject markedly affects its appearance on tomography. A Reidel extension of the right lobe is seen as a tongue lying over the right kidney: a useful practical application of ultrasound is the demonstration that an apparent right upper quadrant mass is actually a Reidel lobe. The diaphragmatic surface of the right liver is usually smooth, but prominent or hypertrophic diaphragmatic leaflets produce 'cough furrows' that may be seen on ultrasound as indentations, or, if the intervening parts of the liver catch the eye, as apparent lobulations that are easily mistaken for mass lesions.

The caudate lobe (segment I) is very variable in size and shape. Measured transversely to the deepest part of the fissure for the sinus venosus, it is usually half the width of the right liver and is less than half the AP thickness of the left lobe. These are exceeded in the hypertrophy of cirrhosis and in the Budd–Chiari syndrome. The caudate lobe may extend inferiorly as a tongue to below the level of the porta. It can then masquerade as precaval or pre-aortic lymphadenopathy or even be confused with a pancreatic mass.

The left lobe is very variable in size, occasionally being absent or replaced by a fibrous remnant. It has been suggested that this is due to an extension of the neonatal spasm of the umbilical vein into the left portal vein. This variation in size can also be demonstrated on ultrasound.

Due to the great variations in proportion of the liver, an estimation of its size cannot be made from any single tomogram (Fritsehy et al 1983, Niederau et al 1983). A complete series can be measured to determine the liver volume accurately; both CT and ultrasound are suitable for this time-consuming method, but the comparative ease with which the liver's margins can be traced on a CT scan makes this the preferred technique. However, 3-dimensional ultrasound techniques offer an alternative approach (Hughes et al 1996). Linear measurements, such as the span of the liver in the mid-clavicular line or its antero-posterior thickness at the left border of the spine, are easily made on ultrasound but are inaccurate as volume estimates, though useful for serial assessment.

THE BILIARY TREE

The filled gallbladder is usually a very obvious structure on sonography of the right upper quadrant because the echo-free bile shows up in strong contrast to the fine echogenic line of the wall (Fig. 13.12). Classically it is described as having a pear shape though in practice its shape is variable. Folds in the body or at the fundus are common and they can often be effaced by changing the patient's position or by continued filling. The position of the gallbladder is also very variable since it may possess its own mesentery and wander from its fossa on the visceral surface of the liver. However, the position of the neck of the gallbladder is relatively fixed below and just to the right of the porta; the fissure

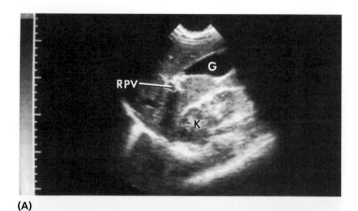

(A)

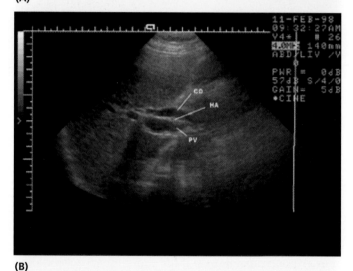

(B)

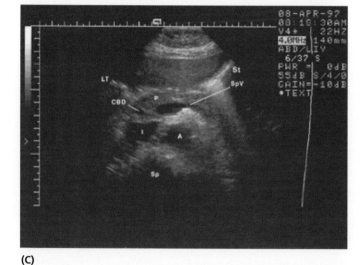

(C)

Fig. 13.12 The biliary tree. The pear-shape and thin wall of the filled gallbladder are seen in **(A)**. The upper portion of the bile duct is shown in the oblique tomogram **(B)** lying anterior to the right portal vein and right hepatic artery. It can be traced down to the level where it passes posterior to the first part of the duodenum: the retroduodenal portion is usually obscured by gas. The terminal portion can be detected again in the head of the pancreas **(C)**. (A, aorta; CBD, common bile duct; CD, common duct; G, gallbladder; HA, hepatic artery; I, inferior vena cava; K, kidney; LT, ligamentum teres; P, pancreas (neck); PV, portal vein; Sp, spine; SpV, splenic vein; St, stomach)

separating segment IV from the antero-lateral segment of segment V passes from the porta to the neck of the gall-bladder and is a useful landmark for its position when there is difficulty in identification such as a contracted or tumor-filled gallbladder. The initial portion of the cystic duct may be imaged as a tortuous tubular structure continuous with the neck of the gallbladder, but this is only possible when it is filled with bile. When empty, it produces strong echoes (due to the fibro-muscular wall) and there may be shadowing of deeper structures. This pattern is confusing since it simulates an impacted gallstone.

Identification of the biliary tree on ultrasound depends on its relationships with the portal vein. Starting high in the porta, portions can be identified lying anterior to the right portal vein; the best view is obtained in an oblique section approximately at right angles to the costal margin, either intercostally or subcostally (Fig. 13.12B). In this plane the right portal vein is cut across and so is seen as a ring; the duct is cut lengthways or obliquely and is seen as a tube lying anteriorly across the right portal vein. This portion of the duct probably represents the right hepatic duct. Where there is difficulty, Doppler can be helpful in distinguishing the duct from the hepatic artery. Traced inferiorly, it expands as it is joined sequentially by the left hepatic duct and the cystic duct forming the common hepatic and common bile ducts, respectively. Since the junctions themselves cannot usually be imaged, the imprecise term 'common duct' is often deliberately employed. Further inferiorly, the duct passes posterior to the first part of the duodenum and this portion may be difficult to image because of duodenal gas. It can be picked up again in the head of the pancreas; transverse sections are usually best for this, and allow its relationship to the pancreas and adjacent duodenum to be studied (Fig. 13.12C).

The lumen of the duct measures up to some 4 mm within the porta and some 7 mm inferiorly (common bile duct). A precise upper limit cannot be set because of the spread of the normal range, especially with age, though a useful rule is to allow 1 mm per decade of life. There is also some overlap with the size in minimal dilatation, these figures providing approximately 95% discrimination. The duct diameter on ultrasound is considerably smaller than that measured on contrast radiology. The smearing of strong echoes on ultra-sound serves to reduce the apparent lumen while tube magnification and choleretic or pressure effects on cholangiography enlarge it (Sauerbrei et al 1980). Observation of changes in caliber stimulated by a fatty meal may be useful in distinguishing large normal duct, which does not dilate further, from the obstructed duct, which dilates when an increase in bile secretion occurs (Hederstrom et al 1988).

ULTRASOUND IN LIVER PATHOLOGY

Ultrasound can be useful to the liver surgeon in both focal and diffuse disorders. It has applications in diagnosis, pre-operative evaluation and in postoperative assessment. Intraoperative uses are also important (Klotter et al 1986, Kawasaki et al 1996, Barbot et al 1997, Cheng et al 1998).

CYSTIC LESIONS (Chs 66 and 67)

Simple cysts are easily detected on ultrasound as well-defined, rounded, echo-free spaces which show accentuation of the distal echoes (because of the low attenuation of the cyst fluid) (Gaines & Sampson 1989). Their walls are smooth and thin. While ultrasound cannot differentiate between true congenital cysts and post-infective or post-traumatic cysts, complicated cysts (e.g. necrotic tumor, superinfection) are obviously different since they have internal echoes and irregular walls. Rarely cystic metastases, such as these from ovarian carcinoma, may appear as simple cysts ultrasonically; if this is a clinical consideration, serology for CA 19-9 may help in their discrimination (Horsmans et al 1996). Giant cysts so distort the local anatomy that even their organ of origin may be difficult to determine. Since vascular malformations can simulate simple cysts, a Doppler study is a useful precaution before 'cyst' puncture is attempted (Tanaka et al 1992) (Fig. 13.13).

Polycystic disease has a more complex appearance, with numerous cystic spaces which become compressed into polygonal forms where they are contiguous (Kuni et al 1978). The complex pattern and the marked increased through transmission of sound make complications difficult to assess: an abscess or tumor deposit in the affected region would probably be missed, though the vascularity (assessed with Doppler perhaps enhanced by microbubbles) may improve its performance. Generally, however, radiolabeled white cell scanning or CT is recommended.

INFECTIVE CONDITIONS

Because of its sensitivity to fluid spaces, ultrasound is highly reliable in the detection of liver abscess (Ch. 61) (Ralls et al 1979, Dewbury et al 1980, Seeto & Rockey 1996, N'Gbesso & Keita 1997). The typical pattern, with an irregular, shaggy margin and debris-containing fluid is easily recognized (Fig. 13.14). They usually have a hypervascular periphery (the 'inflammatory capsule') which can be viewed on color Doppler as a dramatic colored 'halo' around the abscess, particularly around pyogenic abscesses. However, it should be noted that abdominal ultrasound is rarely helpful

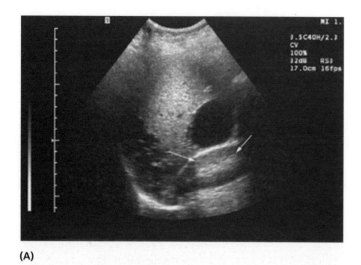

(A)

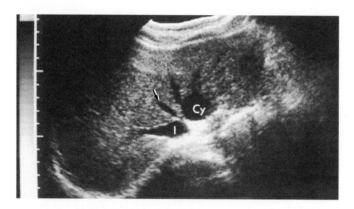

(B)

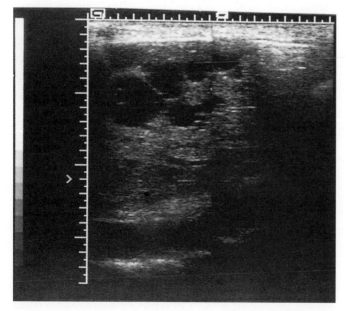

(C)

in the diagnosis of pyrexia of unknown origin unless there are localizing clues (de Kleijn et al 1997).

Ultrasound can be used to guide fine needle aspiration for culture and, if necessary, this may be performed at the patient's bedside using a portable scanner. Adequate sampling, both from the wall of the abscess as well as from the fluid region, and correct handling for culture (aerobic, anaerobic, TB, fungal) are important for successful diagnosis. In selected cases, a drain can be inserted under ultrasound control for definitive treatment. However insertion of a sufficiently large drain may be difficult under local anesthesia and, especially for abscesses lying high in the right lobe, the extrapleural route may be difficult to achieve. Similarly, for subphrenic collections a formal approach under general anesthetic is preferred unless the patient is too unwell to tolerate an anesthetic.

Abscesses do not always have the typical features. Early on, before a cavity has developed, they form an inflammatory mass (Dewbury et al 1980) which appears as a focal lesion, often poorly defined, with low or high level echoes. The changes may be very subtle, so that a negative ultrasound early in the course of a febrile illness does not exclude an abscess; a repeat ultrasound after a few days may show the typical changes as liquefaction supervenes. Eventually, an abscess cavity may shrink and disappear or it may leave a scar. In some cases a fluid space may persist indefinitely as a post-infective cyst (Ralls et al 1983).

Generally the different types of abscess are indistinguishable on ultrasound (Ralls et al 1979). However, ultrasound can often provide clues to the etiology of an abscess. For example, there may be features of cholecystitis, possibly with a pericholecystitic abscess. A mass in the right iliac fossa suggests an appendix abscess while a pelvic scan may demonstrate a tubo-ovarian abscess.

Fungal abscesses in immunosuppressed patients produce a characteristic appearance with multiple, echo-poor foci of a few millimeters diameter, each with a reflective central punctum that probably represents the artery into which the fungi have embolized (Pastakia et al 1988, Karthaus et al 1998).

Hydatid disease (*Echinococcus granulosus*) (Ch. 63) of the

Fig. 13.13 Liver cysts. Cysts show the distal echo enhancement that is the ultrasonic clue that they are fluid filled; in this example the enhancement falls over the right kidney (arrows in **(A)**). This benign cyst has the characteristic features of smooth walls and absent internal echoes. The hepatic vein that lies superior to it is seen in the transverse section **(B)** as the left and middle hepatic veins run to its right. This cyst involves segments II and IV. Note the separate vein (arrow) draining segment VIII. In polycystic disease the cysts have the same features though their contiguous surfaces tend to be flattened **(C)**. Assessment of the remaining liver may be difficult because the cysts disturb the acoustic texture of the unaffected liver. Cy = cyst; I = inferior vena cava).

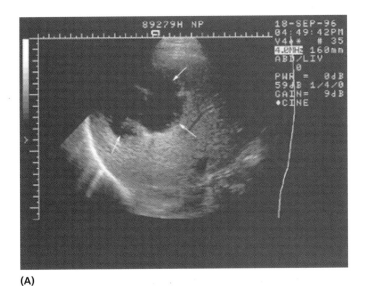

(A)

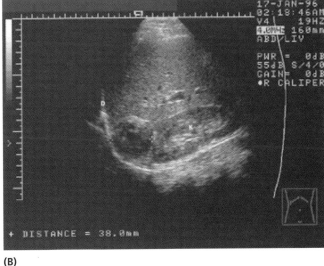

(B)

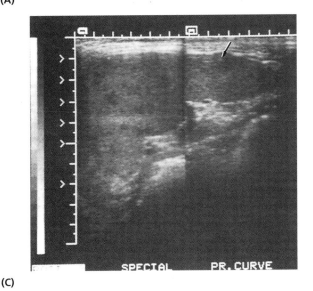

(C)

Fig. 13.14 Liver abscesses. The shaggy, thick walls of this fluid-filled lesion (arrows in **(A)**) are typical of an abscess, though a hematoma or a necrotic tumor deposit would be indistinguishable. This lesion lies in the right lobe of liver. A rounded cystic mass containing numerous smaller cysts is the typical pattern of a hydatid (calipers (D) in **(B)**). Daughter cysts are not always present and in this case the hydatid simulates a complex cyst. Fungal abscesses produce a characteristic pattern with multiple small echopoor foci, each often containing a small reflective punctum (arrow in **(C)**). Since they are small, they are best visualized with a high frequency ('small parts') transducer. D = calipers; K = kidney.

liver is readily detected on ultrasound as a cystic cavity, commonly in the right lobe and typically with a very well-defined thickened wall that represents the chitinous capsule (Abdel-Latif et al 1982, Hadidi 1983, Lewall & McCorkell 1985). The presence of daughter cysts (some 50% show this) gives a pathognomonic appearance of one or many cysts within the mother cyst (Beggs 1983). In the mature form the lesion is packed with polygonal cysts which may even show third generation daughters within them. In earlier cases, a careful search may be needed to demonstrate the separation of the inner germinal layer that represents the beginnings of daughter cyst formation and, in patients at risk, any apparently simple cyst must be considered suspicious. Hydatids often contain a sediment of debris, representing the shed scolices (hydatid sand) and they frequently calcify, detected on ultrasound as strong echoes. Superinfection with pyogenic organisms may occur; in that

event, the lesion has the same appearance as an abscess (el Hajjam et al 1996). There may be a marked increase in reflectivity as the lesions respond to antihelminthic treatment (Bezzi et al 1987). Palliative treatment by aspiration of the hydatid with instillation of a sclerosant has been successfully carried out in endemic rural areas (Saini et al 1983, Mueller et al 1985, Filice & Brunetti 1997).

Granulomas have been reported as producing a typical ultrasonic appearance with en echogenic focus surrounded by an echo-poor rim (Mills et al 1990). *Schistosoma mansonii* produces echogenic periportal thickening, the ultrasonic equivalent of pipe stem cirrhosis (Friis et al 1996).

TRAUMA

In liver trauma (Chs 68, 69) ultrasound is most useful in detecting hemoperitoneum; the extent of liver injury can

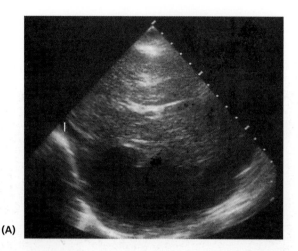

(A)

also be assessed but CT is more reliable here (Froelich et al 1982). Injured liver tissue gives low level echoes, together with a fluid space if there is an intrahepatic hematoma (Van Sonnenberg et al 1983). The ruptured liver surface may be detected as an irregularity of the capsule.

Blood in the peritoneum has the same echo-free appearance as ascites: the clinical background should suggest its true nature which is best confirmed by a directed tap, perhaps under ultrasound control. The fact that the scanner can be brought to the patient's bedside enhances the value of ultrasound in the evaluation of trauma but, if the chest or abdominal wall has been injured, the probe contact required for scanning may be difficult. It is impossible to scan through dressings; if these need to be removed, sterility can be maintained by covering the probe and using sterile contact jelly, as for biopsies. Similar considerations apply when scanning postoperative patients (Fig. 13.15).

TUMORS

Benign tumors of the liver (Ch. 72) usually form well-circumscribed masses with irregular internal echoes, but there is a wide range of appearances and some are difficult to distinguish from normal liver or from each other (De Carlis et al 1997). For example, focal nodular hyperplasia and estrogen adenomas have similar appearances (Rogers et al 1981, Di Stasi et al 1996, Sandler et al 1997). The Küpffer cells that are usually present in focal nodular hyperplasia phagocytose colloids (Casarella et al 1978) so that the lesions do not show as a defect on the isotope scan; the combination of a lesion apparent on ultrasound or CT and a normal isotope scan is characteristic of this condition and this pattern may be mirrored by the late liver-specific phase of some of the ultrasound contrast agents (see below). Biopsy of estrogen adenomas should be approached with caution because they are vascular—a feature that is obvious on color Doppler. The childhood adenomas found in type 1 glycogen-storage disease give multiple echogenic or echo-poor masses (Labrune et al 1997).

HEMANGIOMA

Hemangiomas are common and can be troublesome on ultrasound since they have a range of appearances that sometimes overlap those of more serious lesions, especially metastases. Ironically, the ease with which ultrasound can detect hemangiomas creates a management problem since further investigation is then required for a condition that is of no clinical importance (Gandolfi et al 1983). The pattern on ultrasound depends on whether the hemangioma is localized or diffuse, and on their structure. The common

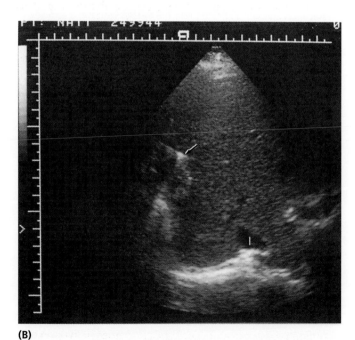

(B)

Fig. 13.15 Hematomas are poorly reflective when fresh ((**A**)—the consequence of a road traffic accident) and become more reflective as they mature. The eventual scar (transverse section (**B**)—the residue of a segmentectomy) is a strongly reflective line. (I, inferior vena cava)

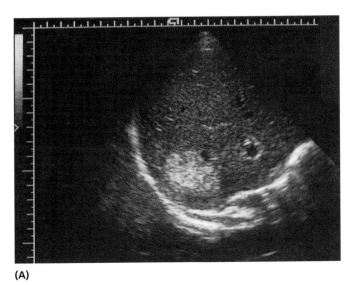

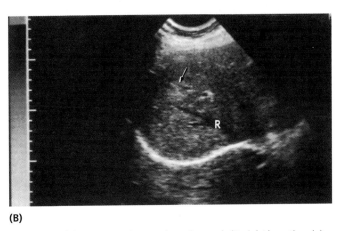

(A)

(B)

Fig. 13.16 Hemangioma. The strong echoes and clear margins of these lesions are typical of the common hemangioma (arrows). (R, right hepatic vein)

capillary type form highly echogenic rounded lesions, often lying in a subcapsular position (Bree et al 1983) (Fig. 13.16). While this typical pattern is reassuring, some 10% of hemangiomas are atypical in appearance, with an irregular echo texture and echo-poor regions that cannot be distinguished from malignancy. Doppler is of limited value: most cases give no signals, presumably because the flow is too slow to be detected, but sometimes venous (continuous) signals are obtained (Young et al 1998). However, pulsatile arterial signals are unusual and should be considered suspicious of malignancy (Wachsberg & Jilani 1999). Until the promise of microbubble contrast agent enhancement is clinically validated (Strunk et al 1998), correlative imaging with CT (Freeny et al 1979), MR (Mirowitz et al 1991) or angiography are required.

Cavernous hemangiomas are echo-poor unless there is thrombosis; this is the typical pattern of the pediatric hemangioma and the high flow within them gives striking color Doppler signals as well as causing dilation of both the hepatic artery and veins (Miller & Greenspan 1985, Stanley et al 1989). When there is thrombosis or calcification, regions with high-level echoes are also seen (Bruneton et al 1983). Ultrasound can be useful in assessing progress in the neonate presenting with high-output heart failure since repeat scans are easily performed.

PRIMARY LIVER TUMORS

Hepatoblastomas (Ch. 74) are often large and multiple; typically they are slightly more echogenic than the normal liver but with very poorly defined margins (Bottelli et al 1998). Vascular invasion, a common feature, can be demonstrated with color Doppler.

The focal form of hepatocellular carcinoma (Ch. 73) appears as a mass, rounded or lobular and often multiple, with high level echoes when small becoming heterogeneous with enlargement (Atomi et al 1984, Buscarini et al 1996, Ishiguchi et al 1996, Toyoda et al 1997) (Fig. 13.17). Necrotic or hemorrhagic regions are common. Invasion of hepatic veins or the portal vein can be demonstrated as echogenic foci within the vessels or as color voids on Doppler. Most hepatocellular carcinomas are vascular with vessels penetrating into the mass as well as lying around the periphery: they can be delineated with color Doppler (Ishiguchi et al 1996, Lencioni et al 1996a,b, Taylor et al 1997, Bolondi et al 1998, Kamalov et al 1998). Often they occur on the background of cirrhotic changes (see below) but, since most regenerating nodules are inapparent on ultrasound and have the same vascularity as the surrounding liver, any well-defined focus must be regarded as suspicious, especially if it is vascular. If excision of a hepatocellular carcinoma is proposed, ultrasound can provide useful information of the segmental distribution of the lesion but should be used in conjunction with other imaging techniques since each modality may detect lesions missed by the others. Intra-operative ultrasound is useful in confirming that there are not further occult lesions elsewhere in the liver.

Detection of the diffuse form of hepatocellular carcinoma is difficult for ultrasound since the alterations in liver texture may be subtle and indistinguishable from many other diffuse diseases such as cirrhosis and chronic active hepatitis. Cholangiocarcinomas pose the same problem.

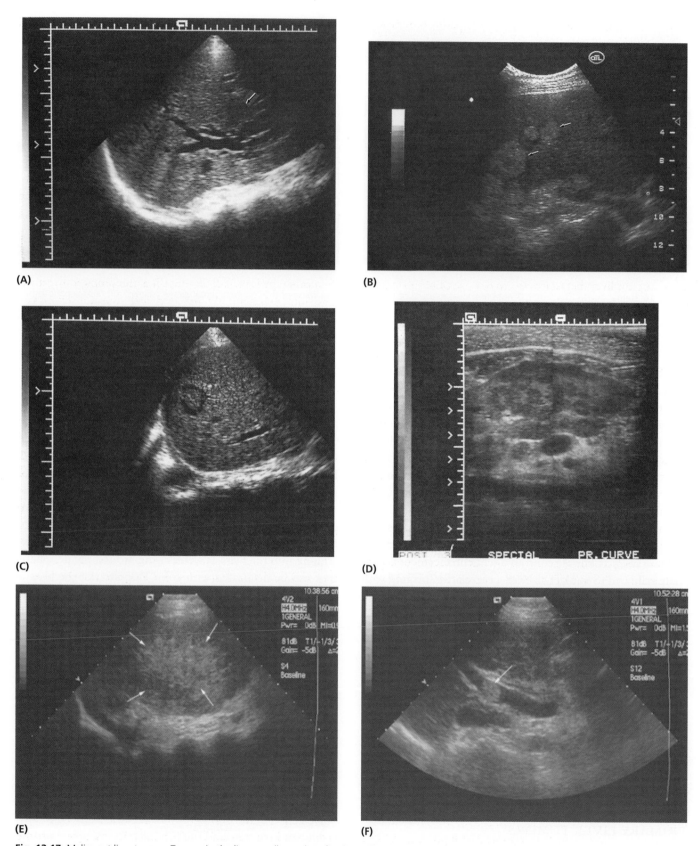

Fig. 13.17 Malignant liver tumors. Tumors in the liver usually produce focal masses, either echo-poor (arrow in **(A)**) or echogenic (arrows in **(B)**). They often have a concentric ring pattern **(C)** and may be multiple or so extensive **(D)** as to replace most of the liver's substance. The patterns in hepatocellular carcinoma are similar (arrows in **(E)**) an advanced HCC replacing the right lobe of liver and this tumor has a particular propensity to invade the liver's veins, in this case, the portal vein (arrow in **(F)**).

In populations at risk from primary hepatocellular carcinoma, ultrasound is used as a screening tool, being more readily available and quicker than CT and more sensitive than scintigraphy (Khakoo et al 1996) (Bottelli et al 1998) though screening has not yet been shown to improve survival (Larcos et al 1998). It may also prove useful in guiding local treatment by injection of alcohol directly into the lesion (Livraghi 1996) or by directing radio-frequency (RF) or laser interstitial therapy (Gillams et al 1997). Color Doppler, perhaps with microbubble enhancement, is proving useful in assessing the completeness of the ablation (Lagalla et al 1998).

METASTASES (Ch. 75)

Screening for liver metastases is a major use of ultrasound in many hospitals. Typically metastases appear as space occupying lesions, distorting the liver surface or internal anatomy) (Bruneton et al 1996, Carter et al 1996, Paley & Ros 1998) (Fig. 13.17). Like hepatocellular cancer, they may be echopoor or echogenic, while mixed patterns as well as fluid regions following necrosis also occur. Sometimes a clue to the origin may be obtained since echogenic lesions are typical of secondaries from urogenital and gastrointestinal tract tumors; they may also demonstrate the acoustic shadowing that indicates calcification and suggests a better prognosis (Easson et al 1996). For the most part, liver metastases do not show Doppler signals, neuroendocrine tumors being interesting exceptions.

Since metastases are almost exclusively supplied by the hepatic artery, one would expect a relative increase in the arterial supply to the liver and the change might be disproportionate to the size of the metastases because the responsible angiogenic factors seem to exert a general effect on the liver. Leen's group have reported interesting results in patients with cancer of the colon: using Doppler to measure the hepatic arterial and portal vein flow, they have demonstrated an increase in the relative hepatic artery flow (HA index = HA/HA + PV; normal ≤ 25%) in patients with liver metastases either diagnosed radiologically or at laparotomy—including some that were missed preoperatively (Leen et al 1996). In a few cases the index was raised but no metastases could be found—i.e. apparent false positives: intriguingly, some of these patients developed overt metastases on follow-up at 3 months, suggesting that they had, in fact, been understaged at surgery. Unfortunately, the technique has proved to be very demanding and attempts to reproduce it have been less successful (Oppo et al 1998); simpler methods using microbubble contrast agents are promising.

The limitations of ultrasound in the detection of metastases need to be born in mind (Scheibel 1982, Carter et al 1996). While false positives for metastases are rare (hemangioma mistaken for tumor being the only significant problem), false negatives occur in up to 15% of cases because some lesions are too small to be detected (< 1 cm) while others lie in portions of the liver that are difficult to scan (e.g. the anterior and extreme lateral portions). Others are missed despite being large and accessible because there is no contrast between these 'isoechoic' lesions and the liver parenchyma. CT often reveals these deposits; on the other hand, ultrasound readily detects others that are missed on CT. These considerations dictate the investigative policy in critical cases, i.e. where exclusion of metastases is essential to management, such as patients under consideration for excision of a presumed solitary deposit or where arduous chemotherapy is proposed. Since it is the simplest investigation, ultrasound should be used first, but CT employed when the ultrasound is negative, perhaps to be followed, in turn, by gadolinium-enhanced MRI (Bunk et al 1997).

Ultrasound can be used to monitor progress of metastases by serial assessment of their size. To be satisfactory, this requires the identification of an individual lesion that can be located and measured again at subsequent examinations.

An important development in liver surgery is the availability of intraoperative ultrasound scanning (Klotter et al 1986, Staren et al 1997, Cheng et al 1998, Kolecki & Schirmer 1998) (Chs 24 & 89). A small handheld probe that can be draped or gas sterilized and applied directly to the liver surface at laparotomy can demonstrate lesions far smaller than detectable by conventional ultrasound or by CT scanning. Bismuth has used intraoperative ultrasound as an extension to the inspection and palpation of the liver at laparotomy and found that it altered the surgical management in 22 out of 31 cases of cancer of the gastrointestinal tract (Bismuth 1982) and this has been confirmed (Klotter et al 1986, Herman 1996, Machi & Sigel 1996, Staren et al 1997) though less successful results have been reported from other centers (Leen et al 1996). Confirmation of the true nature of a lesion detected by ultrasound can be obtained by ultrasound guided biopsy and frozen section. If a solitary liver metastasis is discovered, it may be resected as a part of the radical excision of the primary while the demonstration of multiple metastases may dictate a limited, palliative resection of the primary. Similarly in hepatocellular cancer, intraoperative ultrasound can be used to confirm the extent of liver involvement (Makuuchi et al 1998). Ultrasound can be used to direct injection of a dye into the vessels feeding a tumor to stain the involved segment to guide the extent of the resection.

A novel approach to the remote ablation of abdominal

(and pelvic) masses uses a highly focused, high power ultrasound beam (ter Haar et al 1991). By heat coagulating the lesion, it has the potential of removing solitary liver tumors transcutaneously without damage to surrounding tissues and without using ionizing radiation, both of which would make it much easier to use than radiotherapy and simpler for the patient than conventional surgery or techniques using percutaneous alcohol injections or laser coagulation. The procedure would be planned in the same way as for radiotherapy but could also be continuously monitored using a conventional ultrasound scanner.

DIFFUSE LIVER DISEASES

Ultrasound is neither very sensitive nor specific in diffuse liver diseases. The changes seen may be divided into those affecting the liver uniformly and those showing patchy changes. Two main patterns can be identified, known as the 'bright' and the 'dark' liver patterns (Kurtz et al 1981, Joseph et al 1991, Caturelli et al 1996, Taylor & Ros 1998).

An overall increase in liver parenchymal echoes is the basic change in the bright liver (Fig. 13.18). The increase may be so marked as to be immediately obvious but, in less gross cases, comparison of the echo level with internal features is required (Dewbury et al 1980, Lonardo et al 1997). The renal cortex is normally only slightly less reflective than the liver; in the 'bright liver' the liver/kidney contrast is exaggerated so that the kidney appears relatively dark. Similarly, the normal contrast between the liver parenchyma and the reflective cuff around the portal vein branches is lost

when the liver is strongly reflective, so that the liver acquires a uniform appearance ('ground-glass pattern') with apparent loss of internal structure.

Fat and fibrous tissue are the common causes, fat probably being the predominant factor. Thus the bright pattern occurs in fatty change and in cirrhosis and also in hepatic fibrosis, lipid, glycogen and iron storage diseases. The finding is therefore non-specific but such a liver is always abnormal on biopsy (Sanford et al 1985, Needleman et al 1986, Saverymuttu et al 1986, Joseph et al 1991). However, ultrasound is not particularly sensitive to this group of disorders and the scan may look normal in milder cases (Gosink et al 1979). Conventional ultrasound cannot distinguish simple fatty change from non-alcoholic steato-hepatitis (NASH), though there is a possibility that microbubble techniques might achieve this (Laurin et al 1996).

In cirrhosis other changes may be detected, such as irregularity of the liver surface, hypertrophy of the caudate lobe (segment I) (Harbin et al 1980) and features of portal hypertension (Gaiani et al 1997) (Fig. 13.19). Generally regenerating nodules cause surprisingly change to the echo texture of the liver: macronodules are only occasionally demonstrable as masses with a reflectivity very similar to that of normal liver, while micronodules sometimes lend a granular texture to the liver though surface nodularity is readily demonstrated in the presence of ascites. Ultrasound is very sensitive to ascites, quantities down to 25 ml being detectable (Gefter et al 1982). Recanalization of the umbilical vein is readily demonstrated and varicosities at the splenic hilum and around the pancreas can be detected

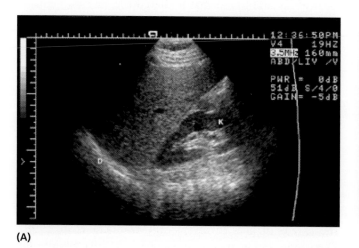

(A)

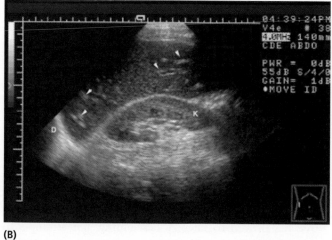

(B)

Fig. 13.18 Diffuse liver diseases. The even texture of the liver parenchyma in **(A)** is due to the increased echo levels of the 'bright liver' of this patient with fatty infiltration. The hepato-renal contrast is exaggerated. Cirrhosis and chronic hepatitis are other common causes. When the liver echo intensity is reduced **(B)**, the periportal echoes seem accentuated (arrowheads) and hepato-renal contrast is reversed. This 'dark liver' pattern is seen in acute hepatitis and congestive hepatomegaly. (D, diaphragm; K, kidney)

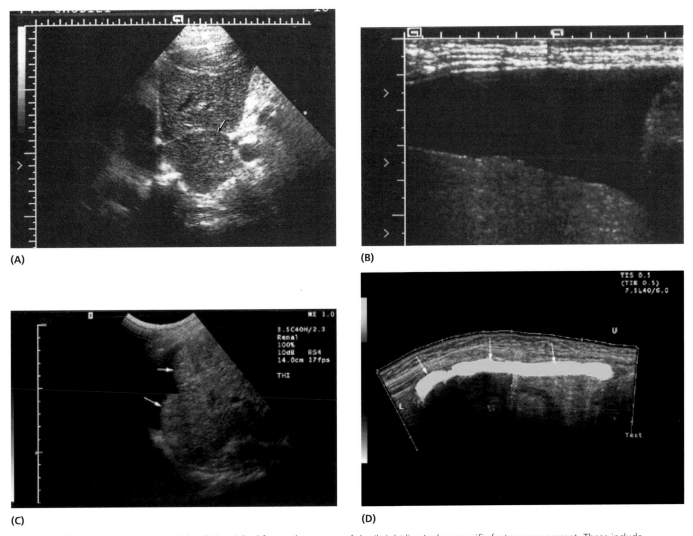

(A)

(B)

(C)

(D)

Fig. 13.19 Cirrhosis. Cirrhosis can only be distinguished from other causes of the 'bright liver' when specific features are present. These include enlargement of the caudate lobe (arrow in **(A)**), nodularity of the liver surface—best seen against the background of ascites (micronodular in **(B)**, macronodular in **(C)**), and signs of portal hypertension such as a reanalyzed umbilical vein (arrows in **(D)**) here seen extending down to umbilical level. However, sensitivity is low, the ultrasound examination being normal in some 50% of patients with cirrhosis. (L, liver; U, umbilicus)

(Juttner et al 1982). Varices at the esophago-gastric junction are best seen on endosonography (see below). The portal vein is often dilated above the normal of 13 mm diameter but this is not a useful index of pressure and failure to dilate after a meal seems to be more sensitive (Bolondi et al 1998). Screening studies for patients at risk of developing cirrhosis, such as those with hepatitis C, have been proposed (Izzo et al 1998).

Doppler is an essential supplement to imaging in cirrhosis and has proved useful in the evaluation and follow up of portal hypertension (Van Leeuwen 1990, Korner 1996, Bolondi et al 1998) (Fig. 13.20). Portal vein flow slows from its normal rate of more than 12 cm/s (in the fasting state) in portal hypertension and this seems to be more reliable than the caliber of the vein (Gaiani et al 1997, Iwao et al 1997). When there is recanalization of the umbilical vein,

normal or even increased Doppler shifts occur as the portal vein flow speeds up to feed the shunt; this can be confusing unless the presence of this type of porto-systemic shunt is recognized. Indices based on the ratio between portal vein and hepatic artery flow have been developed and attempts made to calculate true portal vein flow, though these are subject to a wide margin of error and so are disappointing as clinical tools (Dinc et al 1998).

Doppler is a very reliable method of demonstrating flow reversal in the portal veins while spectral Doppler reveals the sluggish to-and-fro pattern of 'balanced flow' when minor changes in the abdominal pressure with respiration determine whether flow is hepatopetal or hepatofugal (Fig. 13.21).

Ultrasound can also be useful in the follow-up assessment of porto-systemic shunts, depending on the anastomotic

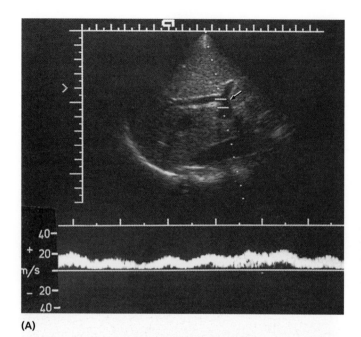

(A)

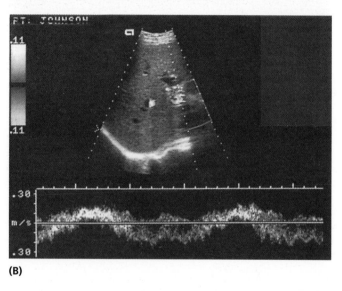

(B)

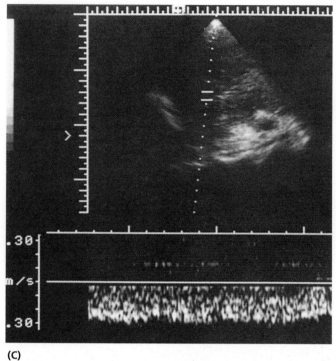

(C)

Fig. 13.20 Doppler of the portal vein. Normal flow in the portal vein gives a continuous signal above the baseline, indicating flow into the liver **(A)**. There may be slight phasic variations, corresponding to cardiac and respiratory pressure changes, as in this example. In the patient with portal hypertension in **(B)** there is 'balanced flow' that varies from hepatopetal to hepatofugal, depending on the abdomino-thoracic pressure gradient. The trace wanders across the zero-flow baseline. In a more severe case in **(C)** the hepatofugal flow is depicted as a trace consistently below the baseline. (In these duplex spectral images, the position of the Doppler-sensitive gate is indicated by the white bars on the scan in the upper portion [arrow in **(A)**] while the spectral trace itself shows flow velocity on the Y-axis [in cm or m/sec] with time [X-axis] in seconds. Flow towards the transducer is displayed above the line [+ in **(A)**] and flow away from it, below [– in **(A)**].)

site (Forsberg & Holmin 1983). Porto-caval and lieno-renal shunts are accessible but mesocaval shunts are usually obscured by overlying gut and portography is required. Transjugular intrahepatic porto-systemic shunt (TIPS) (Ch. 101) patency can be assessed with Doppler though stenoses have proved to be more difficult to evaluate (Skjoldbye et al 1998). Ultrasound does not usually provide sufficiently detailed anatomical information to plan TIPS procedures.

In the 'dark liver' (Kurtz et al 1980) the low intensity echoes from the liver parenchyma throw the periportal echoes into relief so that the texture shows accentuation of the vascular markings (Fig. 13.18) and the liver becomes less reflective than the kidney. This change is seen in inflammatory (Grumbach et al 1989) and congestive conditions where the increase in water content seems to be responsible. In a jaundiced patient, the finding of a dark liver with normal bile ducts suggests a cholestatic hepatitis. The dark pattern also occurs in lymphoreticular malignancies but ultrasound cannot distinguish between neoplastic and reactive lymphocytic infiltration.

In some diffuse liver diseases the process is patchy in its severity and so the ultrasound scan shows an irregular texture. Many infiltrative conditions fall into this category, the commonest examples being focal fatty change (Kissin et al 1986, Middleton 1989) and the irregular necrosis in paracetamol or alcohol toxicity. The scan appearances are confusingly similar to multiple metastases. Contrast enhanced studies or biopsy are generally required to establish the diagnosis.

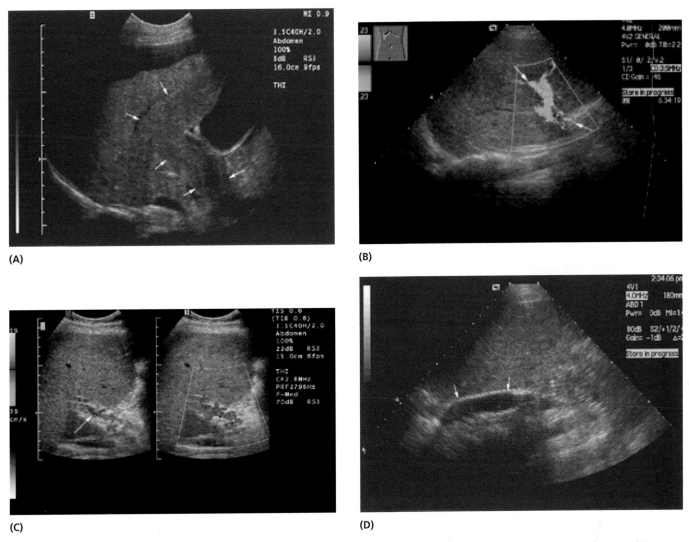

Fig. 13.21 Abnormalities of the portal venous system. A wide echogenic band (arrows in **(A)**) represents thrombus in a dilated portal vein, in this case the result of portal hypertension—note the ascites and knobby liver surface. Reversed flow in the portal vein is indicated by blue and green tints **(B)**; note also the enlarged artery (arrows) with hepatopetal flow (red and yellow tints). In **(C)** the portal vein is replaced by tortuous vascular channels (arrow in **(C)**). This is the appearance of 'cavernous transformation' of the portal vein. The gray scale study is shown on the left with the color Doppler on the right. A meso-caval shunt is imaged as an echogenic tubular structure (arrows in **(D)**) extending from the SMV to the upper IVC in this patient with portal vein thrombosis secondary to Budd–Chiari syndrome. With high resolution transducers the woven structure of the stent wall can be discerned. (SMV, superior mesenteric vein; IVC, inferior vena cava)

VASCULAR PROBLEMS

Portal vein thrombosis when acute can be difficult to detect on gray scale scanning because fresh thrombus is echo-poor, though it becomes more reflective as organization progresses (Fig. 13.21). A diagnostic trap is failure to appreciate that the portal vein can always be visualized as an echo-free structure—failure to do so suggests that it is filled with thrombus. Demonstrating flow on a Doppler study excludes occlusive thrombus (Miller & Greenspan 1985) but, because Doppler systems cannot demonstrate flow below a cut-off point (around 1 cm/s, depending on the

particular scanner), absence of Doppler signals does not necessarily mean thrombus: often in cases with minimal flow, to-and-fro signals can be obtained on provocation by breathing or abdominal pressure. Microbubble contrast agents have proved helpful in highlighting the weak signals that are typical of this situation. Often blood and tumor thrombus cannot be distinguished but if arterial flow is demonstrated within the thrombus on spectral Doppler, tumor is likely since only venous signals are found in blood thrombus (during recanalization). In 'cavernous transformation' of the portal vein, the chaotic pattern of the tangle of venous channels is striking on color Doppler though, if one channel predominates, this can be mistaken for a normal portal vein (Dinc et al 1998) and there is often hypertrophy of the hepatic artery in which flow is increased.

True abnormalities of the hepatic artery are rare, apart from complications of transplantation (see below), but the common normal variants are well shown with color Doppler (Lafortune & Patriquin 1999).

Flow in all three hepatic veins can normally be demonstrated with Doppler and the spectral trace shows a pulsatile pattern with transient reversed (hepatopetal) flow as blood is pushed back into the liver at atrial systole. This pulsatility is reduced or abolished if the liver loses its compliance and becomes stiff; flattening of the hepatic vein waveform is a sensitive but non-specific sign of diffuse liver pathology (Farrant & Meire 1997, Bolondi et al 1998).

In those patients with the Budd–Chiari syndrome (Ch. 105) who survive the acute crisis and are sent for investigation, one or two of the hepatic veins usually remain patent with intrahepatic shunts that drain the affected segments (Grant 1992, Noone et al 1996, Bjoro et al 1997, Mulholland et al 1997, Pande et al 1998). This produces the pathognomonic appearance of adjacent hepatic vein segments with opposite Doppler colors at the same time (Fig. 13.22). Thrombus may be demonstrated in the affected veins which appear thin and thready and there may be reverse flow in the portal vein. In the subacute phase, enlargement of the liver, especially segment I, is usually obvious as is the inevitable ascites. Where a caval web is the cause, this can sometimes be visualized but venography is more reliable.

While the arterio-venous shunts of Osler-Weber-Rendu syndrome are readily visualized on color Doppler, the smaller vascular lakes of peliosis are more difficult to delineate and appear on gray scale as a heterogeneous liver texture, a confusing appearance shared by numerous other conditions (Tateishi et al 1998).

LIVER TRANSPLANTATION (Chs 108, 112, 113, 114, 115, 116)

Ultrasound with Doppler is invaluable in the preoperative evaluation of the potential transplant recipient, in theater to establish satisfactory anastomoses (Cheng et al 1998) and in evaluating postoperative progress (Kok et al 1996, Pinna et al 1996, Seu et al 1996, Cook & Crofton 1997, Kok et al 1998, Leutloff et al 1998, Waldman et al 1998). Crucial to the preoperative evaluation is the demonstration that the portal vein is patent; this requires a careful Doppler assessment (preferably with color). If there is a delay before surgery, the portal vein should be re-examined because of the unstable state of portal vein flow in many of these patients. Suspected portal vein thrombus or cavernous transformation should be evaluated by angiography to help plan the anastomotic procedure. If the splenic vein and superior mesenteric vein are found to be patent, the surgeon may be able to remove the thrombus or, alternatively, interpose a vein graft between the intrahepatic portion of the portal vein and the splenic-superior mesenteric vein confluence. The IVC should also be assessed preoperatively since it is essential that there is a patent suprahepatic portion

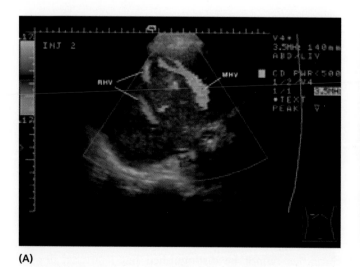

(A)

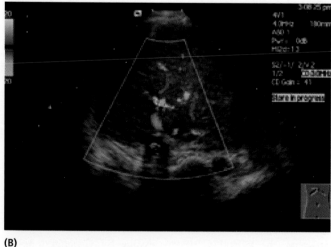

(B)

Fig. 13.22 Budd–Chiari syndrome. The pathognomonic pattern of flow in opposite directions in adjacent hepatic veins occurs in partial Budd–Chiari syndrome when one vein is spared in the thrombotic process (**(A)**, high transverse section). Blood flows retrogradely in the occluded vein, in this case the right, and empties via intrahepatic veno-venous shunts into the patent middle hepatic vein. (Because the signals were too weak to detect the flow patterns, this study was enhanced with a microbubble contrast agent.) In more severe cases, partial recanalization of the occluded portal veins produces a complex network of veins (**(B)**, high transverse section), the ultrasound equivalent of the angiographic 'bird's nest'. (MHV, middle hepatic vein; RHV, right hepatic vein.)

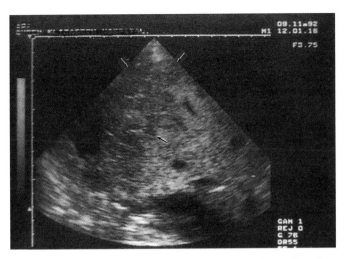

Fig. 13.23 Ischemic segments in a transplanted liver. Following hepatic artery occlusion, echopoor areas (arrows) may be seen in the periphery of the liver corresponding to necrotic tissue.

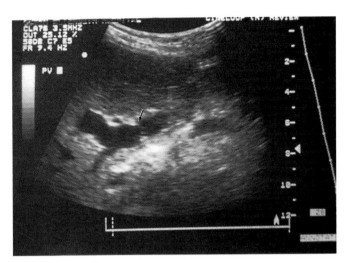

(A)

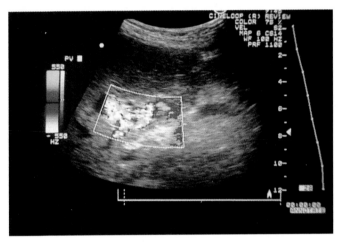

(B)

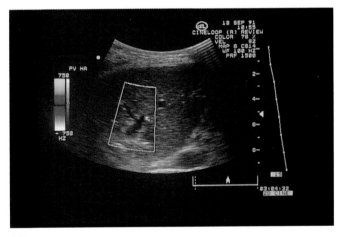

(C)

Fig. 13.24 Portal vein in the transplanted liver. Some degree of narrowing is usually seen at the anastomotic site (arrow in **(A)**) and the turbulent flow it causes makes for complicated color patterns on the Doppler study **(B)**. Since the patent portal vein is so readily demonstrated, occlusion can be diagnosed with confidence using color Doppler. In **(C)** the hepatic artery is demonstrated (colored dot) but no signals are obtained from the vein.

to receive the donor cava. Patency of the IVC below the liver is not as important and, indeed, this portion of the cava may be absent in some patients with biliary atresia. Ultrasound can detect other congenital abnormalities such as a preduodenal portal vein in these children. Unsuspected hepatocellular carcinoma should be sought in patients being transplanted for cirrhosis.

Cholangiocarcinoma, a risk in patients with primary sclerosing cholangitis, is difficult to detect on ultrasound because of its diffusely infiltrating margins though the new liver-specific microbubble methods promise to improve on this limitation (Tham et al 1996, Colli et al 1998). Where the transplant is being undertaken for malignancy, ultrasound should be used along with other imaging techniques to assess vascular invasion and extrahepatic extension of tumor. The search may be supplemented by an intraoperative ultrasound scan.

One of the most serious postoperative complications, hepatic artery occlusion (Ch. 115), can be assessed with a color Doppler study and routine assessments, perhaps daily, are recommended by some groups (Kok et al 1998) and this necessitates the availability of a sophisticated scanner in intensive care. Intravenous microbubble contrast agents simplify and speed this important and technically demanding study in sick patients (Schlief et al 1990). Peripheral areas of ischemia and local necrosis may be seen when there is branch occlusion (Cook & Crofton 1997) (Fig. 13.23). Since both hepatic artery and portal vein flow are normally in the same direction, their color Doppler signals can be confused so the spectral trace must be checked for pulsatile flow (Fig. 13.24). Other vascular complications that can be recognized include portal vein thrombosis. Baseline and frequent routine serial studies allow deterioration to be detected early (Kok & Slooff et al 1998). Unlike the changes in pulsatility that are seen in renal transplant rejection, liver rejection does not seem to alter the arterial waveform except perhaps in children (Griffith & John 1996, Kauffman et al 1997).

Collections are common in the early postoperative period. Diagnostic aspiration of these can be performed if clinically indicated using ultrasound guidance. Bile leaks can be confirmed by a T-tube cholangiograms and a pigtail drainage catheter can then be inserted under ultrasound guidance, traversing the liver if necessary.

MICROBUBBLE CONTRAST AGENTS

Unlike all other imaging technologies, ultrasound has lacked agents that can be administered to patients to improve or enhance the diagnostic information available: with the recent introduction of safe and effective agents that enhance the ultrasonic information, this has now changed. The most important are microbubbles, but some interesting attempts to improve imaging by other means include the use of gas absorbing and gas displacing oral fluids to improve access to the retroperitoneum, including the lower end of the bile duct. These agents consist of a suspension of chopped cellulose with simethicone (SonoRx, Bracco, Milan) and are well-tolerated despite the large volumes that have to be drunk. They seem to be more effective than a drink of plain water.

The field is a dynamic one, with many new agents being developed and new ways to exploit the opportunity (Cosgrove et al 1998, Dawson et al 1999).

History

When in the late 1960s Dr Charles Joiner noted transient 'clouds of echoes' in the left outflow tract whenever an injection was given into the left heart, the idea of an ultrasound contrast agent was born. Subsequent studies showed that the signals were produced by small bubbles formed at the catheter tip. Though effective as ultrasound enhancers, the short life and poor reproducibility of these hand-made bubbles limited their clinical use and so ways to improve them were investigated, culminating in the development of safe and stable microbubbles with a life of several minutes after intravenous injection. Levovist (Schering AG, Berlin) is the most widely studied and is now commercially available in many parts of the world (Calliada et al 1998). It is made of galactose formed as microcrystals that act as nucleation sites for air when mixed for injection. The survival of the microbubbles is improved by adding a trace of the surfac-

tant palmitic acid. Levovist increases the signal strength of blood by 10–20 dB, producing a degree of enhancement that can be detected on gray scale in the heart and in large vessels; in smaller vessels and especially in the microvasculature, the higher sensitivity of Doppler is required.

In these galactose-based agents the microbubbles are formed within the mixing vial. Optison (Malinckrodt, St Louis) is an example of a preformed microbubble or, more precisely, a microcapsule, which needs only agitation to resuspend the bubbles before injection. While air is the gas used in the early agents, there are advantages in using inert gases of larger molecular weight, chiefly because they diffuse more slowly and so confer a longer life in the blood; perfluoro gases are used in Optison and several newer agents while sulphur hexafluoride is used in SonoVue (Bracco, Milan).

Principles

The same mechanisms that determine the echogenicity of tissue interfaces apply to microbubbles: the echo intensity is proportional to the change in acoustic impedance as the sound beam crosses from blood to the gas in the bubbles. The impedance mismatch at such an interface is very high but, because of their small size and low concentration, they would be expected to be poorly reflective. The compressibility of gas compared to tissue is the key to their extraordinary efficacy: microbubbles resonate in sympathy with the ultrasound pressure waves and this makes them behave as though they are very much larger than their actual diameter (some $10^{14} \times$ larger) (de Jong et al 1991).

Obviously microbubbles must be made small enough to cross the capillary beds (≤ 7 μm) and, like any mechanical system, the critical frequency for resonance depends on their diameter. It is entirely coincidental that microbubbles in the 1–7 μm size range happen to resonate in the 2–15 MHz ultrasound frequencies that are used for clinical diagnosis. Because of their size, they do not diffuse across the endothelium (unlike the agents used for X-ray and MRI) and so they are essentially blood-pool markers with a distribution similar to those of labeled red cells. Some types of microbubbles, however, are taken up by the phagocytic cell systems and thus also target functioning liver and spleen tissue after the initial blood-pool phase, a feature of particular interest in liver diseases.

Clinical applications

The simplest use of microbubbles is to enable studies that were otherwise difficult or unreasonably time consuming; this 'rescue of a failed Doppler study' is the first widespread use. However, the blood-pool enhancement extends the role of Doppler into vascular beds that were previously beyond the sensitivity of ultrasound scanners, e.g. in tumors. Furthermore, the ability to track the passage of a microbubble bolus though a region of interest allows functional data similar to that available from dynamic isotope studies to be obtained but with better spatial resolution more cost effectively. Similar analyses can be performed with CT and MRI but at higher cost and, for CT, a radiation penalty.

The first clinical application is in enabling otherwise difficult vascular studies such as detecting the slow flow in a portal vein or TIPS shunt in a cirrhotic (Braunschweig et al 1996) (Fig. 13.25). In the microcirculation, flow in vessels down to perhaps 100 µm in diameter can be demonstrated under ideal situations, the limit being set by the overwhelming Doppler signals from the gross movement of surrounding tissues. This allows at least arterioles and venules to be picked up and shows regions of infarction or ischemia as color voids. Of wider interest is the improved display of the neovascularization of tumors: enhanced studies improve display of the tortuous and tangled pattern and can help differentiate benign from malignant lesions in the liver and elsewhere (Ernst et al 1996) (Fig. 13.26). Important examples are the lack of signal from hemangiomas and from regenerating nodules by comparison with metastases and hepatomas. While the main use is likely to be the differential diagnosis of masses, changes during treatment may be use-

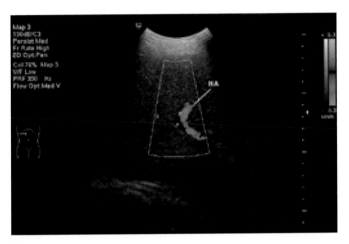

(A)

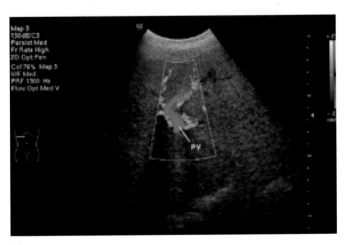

(B)

Fig. 13.25 Microbubble enhancement of the portal vein. In this patient with portal hypertension, Doppler signals from the hepatic artery were prominent but those from the portal vein could not be identified (**A**); after administration of a microbubble contrast agent (**B**), clear signals were obtained from the portal vein and their blue color indicates hepato-fugal flow (note the orientation of the color bar on the right of the images). (HA, hepatic artery; PV, portal vein)

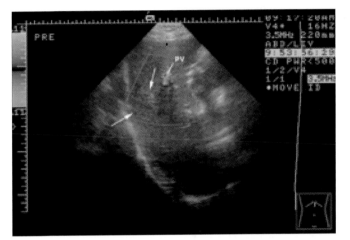

(A)

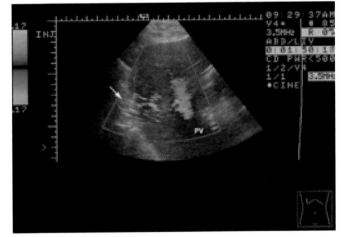

(B)

Fig. 13.26 Microbubble enhancement of a liver tumor. In this patient suspected of a renal cell carcinoma metastasis, only a vague alteration in liver texture (arrows in (**A**)) and no pathological Doppler signals could be seen; after administration of a microbubble contrast agent (**B**), the malignant neovasculature is revealed. (PV, portal vein)

ful indices of response or chemo-resistance and have been used to determine whether sufficient interstitial treatment by alcoholization or RF heating has been given (Lencioni et al 1997). With the development of specific blockers to angiogenesis factors, this application could become increasingly important.

Quantification of the wash-in and wash-out of microbubbles injected as a bolus allows transit-time curves to be generated, opening the way to functional studies analogous to dynamic isotope and CT techniques. Microbubbles are confined to the blood-pool markers, so that these measurements are complementary to those using diffusible agents such as iodinated X-ray contrast. There is every likelihood that physiological indices such as the mean transit time and true perfusion can be calculated and they can be presented as data for a region or point of interest or be displayed as functional images (Eckersley 1999).

An interesting way to use the dynamic properties of bolus injections of microbubbles is to track their appearance in the hepatic veins after a peripheral injection: normally the delays caused by passage through three capillary beds means that they start to appear in the hepatic veins after a delay of about 45 s. However, if there is arterio-venous shunting as occurs in cirrhosis and liver malignancy (Ho et al 1997), the arrival time is greatly shortened (Fig. 13.27). In early studies good discrimination between hepatitis and cirrhosis has been reported and metastases can be distinguished from hemangiomas which behave normally (Blomley et al 1998). This

simple technique could reduce the need for biopsies in chronic liver disease and may improve sensitivity to metastases (Albrecht et al 1999).

Some microbubbles target normal liver and, using special ultrasonic modes, can be used as markers to distinguish subtle focal lesions from functioning liver (Blomley et al 1998) (Fig. 13.28). In these so-called non-linear modes, the distinctive behavior of gas as it expands and contracts within the ultrasonic field is exploited to highlight their presence. While this approach is still experimental, initial results suggest that it improves the detection of metastases and that it improves specificity because many benign lesions such as regenerating nodules, focal nodular hyperplasia and, to a lesser extent, hemangiomas, show these signals.

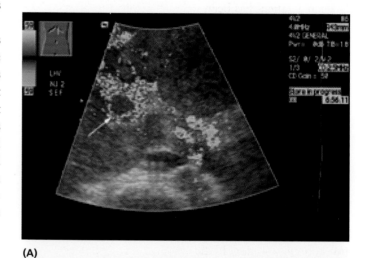

(A)

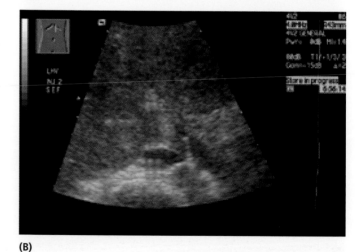

(B)

Fig. 13.27 Hepatic vein transit times. The changes in spectral Doppler signal strength in a hepatic vein after a peripheral intravenous injection of a bolus of a microbubble contrast agent is shown in this time-reflectivity chart. The arrival of contrast in the hepatic veins is normally late (> 40 s) because of the triple capillary beds they have to cross (controls). However, when shunting is present, as occurs in cirrhosis and liver malignancy, the contrast arrives much earlier (10–15 s in this series); this simple non-invasive test shows promise in the detection of cirrhosis and of liver malignancy.

Fig. 13.28 A liver-specific microbubble. This galactose-based agent (Levovist, Schering AG) pools in normal liver for some 30 min after it has cleared from the blood pool and it can be revealed using color Doppler at a high transmission level. Focal lesions are clearly revealed as color defects (arrow in **(A)**) unless, like FNH, they contain functioning liver tissue. This patient had multicentric hepatocellular carcinoma but the lesions were not visible on the gray scale scan taken at the identical location **(B)**.

ULTRASOUND IN DISEASES OF THE BILIARY TREE

THE BILE DUCTS

The exquisite sensitivity of ultrasound to dilatation of the bile ducts has made it the imaging technique of choice in the evaluation of jaundice problems (Barloon et al 1996) (Ch. 21). Dilated bile ducts are seen as tubules lying alongside the portal vein branches (Fig. 13.29). The pattern is characteristic and specific.

Ultrasound has proved to be thoroughly reliable in this application though, obviously, it displays anatomy and not duct pressure and therefore can be misleading in the rare cases where these do not correspond. An important instance is when a patient has been referred within a few days of the onset of obstruction, before dilatation has developed. The scan should be repeated in a few days if there is any remaining doubt as to the cause of the jaundice. Once dilated, the biliary tree may remain distended after relief of the obstruction. Thus the duct system may be prominent in patients with gallstone disease or after duct instrumentation at cholecystectomy. A ball-valve calculus can produce spectacular dilatation of the common bile duct without jaundice.

The level of obstruction can be defined by tracing the duct system down to the obstruction (Fig. 13.30). Obstruction at the porta gives dilatation of the ducts in one or both liver lobes but with a normal caliber common bile duct whereas it is dilated when obstructed at the lower end, the commonest site. If the lesion lies in the head of the pancreas, the pancreatic duct is also often dilated. Lesions in the retroduodenal portion of the duct may be more difficult to image because it is often shadowed here by duodenal gas. Nevertheless the level of obstruction can be predicted accurately in some 80% of cases.

Furthermore, ultrasound is often able to determine the etiology. The demonstration of stones in the common bile duct depends on their size and position. Larger stones (> 5 mm) are readily visualized unless excessive intestinal gas precludes adequate imaging (Dong & Chen 1987) (Fig. 13.30). Smaller stones may not cast an acoustic shadow (for this the stone must be large enough to block the ultrasound beam) and, since it is the shadow that draws attention to the stone, they are more difficult to detect. In addition, since smaller stones lodge further down the duct, they tend to lie closer to the duodenum where gas may degrade the image. Gas in the first part of the duodenum also obscures the retro-duodenal portion of the duct and even large stones in this position may be missed; the operator will know that the study was incomplete and recommend another investigation. The tell-tale shadowing is often missing, even with large stones, presumably of the crumbly, semi-solid variety (Dewbury & Smith 1984). They appear as intraductal soft tissue masses and may simulate tumors. A region of inflammation often develops around a stone impacted at the lower end of the common bile duct. This focal pancreatitis is indistinguishable from a tumor on ultrasound; guided fine-needle aspiration may be helpful.

Pancreatic tumors (Ch. 55) that cause jaundice are usually large enough to be detected as masses with irregular,

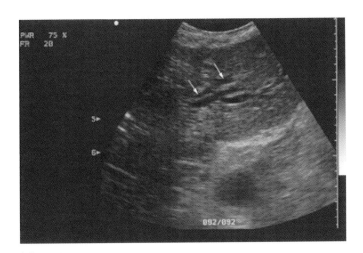

(A)

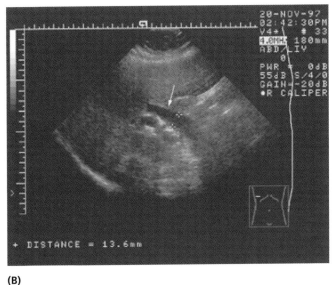

(B)

Fig. 13.29 Dilated bile ducts. Normally the intrahepatic bile ducts cannot be discerned on ultrasound but when dilated they appear as vessels lying parallel to the portal vein branches (arrows in **(A)**). The common duct, measured in the porta hepatis, should be less than 7 mm in diameter: in this example **(B)** it is dilated at 13.6 mm.

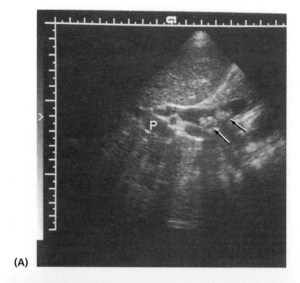

(A)

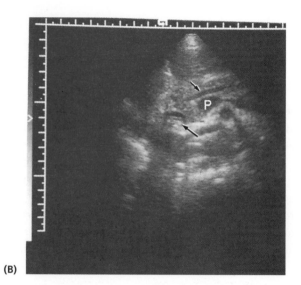

(B)

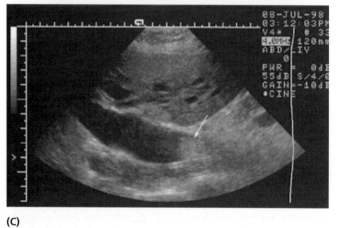

(C)

Fig. 13.30 Stones in the common bile duct. Several stones (arrows) are impacted in the lower end of the common bile duct in this patient with obstructive jaundice ((**A**) longitudinal section, (**B**) transverse section through the head of the pancreas). In this case they cast acoustic shadows which makes them easy to recognize; many duct stones do not shadow (arrow in (**C**)) and so are easily missed or confused with ductal or pancreatic tumors. Note the dilated pancreatic duct (short arrow in (**B**)). (P, portal vein)

predominantly low-level echoes (Barloon et al 1996). In some instances the changes may be recognized before the lesion has produced the mass effects of expansion and distortion of the pancreatic contour that are characteristic of more advanced tumors. On the other hand, ampullary carcinomas are too small to be detected though their presence may be inferred from the combination of dilated pancreatic and biliary ducts (the 'double duct sign'). Endoscopic ultrasound however is proving useful in this difficult problem (see below). Cholangiocarcinoma (Ch. 54) produces a soft tissue mass that may be demonstrated extending along the biliary tree though this is often difficult to recognize on ultrasound (Adam & Benjamin 1992) (Fig. 13.31). Strictures are almost impossible to demonstrate on ultrasound, the duct seeming to disappear at the site of narrowing with no characteristic features. Rarer causes that can also be imaged include choledochal cysts and ascaris worms.

Overall ultrasound is highly reliable in the detection of biliary tree dilatation and will usually indicate the level if not

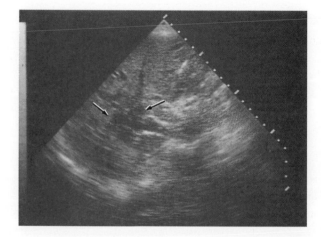

Fig. 13.31 Klatskin tumor. Cholangiocarcinomas arising in the porta are often difficult to demonstrate on ultrasound though the duct dilatation they cause is easily recognizable. In this case the tumor is seen as an ill-defined echo-poor region occupying the region of the porta (arrows). (See also Ch. 54.)

the precise site of obstruction. It is less good at determining the etiology though, in some cases the precise cause can be defined with confidence. Thus ultrasound should be the first imaging study for jaundiced patients. Where an obstructing stone is demonstrated, the study can provide all the information required for further management. When a pancreatic mass is demonstrated, fine-needle aspiration may be performed under ultrasound control to confirm malignancy. The demonstration of local extension (nodes, tumor in the splenic/portal vein) or liver metastases indicates that only palliative surgery or biliary stenting is appropriate. Where radical surgery is proposed, further investigation with CT and arteriography are required to evaluate local spread and vascular invasion more completely. In those cases of obstructive jaundice where no causative lesion is seen on ultrasound, further imaging is required; endoscopic ultrasound, endoscopic retrograde cholangiopancreatography (ERCP) or percutaneous transhepatic cholangiography (PTC) may be used.

The intra-operative applications of ultrasound for the biliary tree are promising (Klotter et al 1986, Machi & Sigel 1996, Catheline & Champault 1998, Silverstein et al 1998). As with its uses for hepatic surgery, a sterilized hand-held real-time probe is applied directly to the surface of the bile duct. Stones as small as a millimeter-or-so in diameter can be detected. The examination is simpler than an operative cholangiogram and should be performed first because air bubbles have a confusing appearance. The detection rate of the two techniques is identical but ultrasound gives fewer false positives so that unnecessary duct explorations can be avoided. However, ultrasound does not display the overall anatomy of the duct system so that variations and anomalies are not readily detectable.

Ultrasound is also valuable in post-operative evaluation. Chiefly this is directed to the biliary tree itself, but bilomas, hematomas and abscesses can be detected and aspirated (diagnostically or therapeutically) under ultrasound control. The speed and flexibility of ultrasound makes it the method of choice, especially for ill patients, because the scanner can be taken to the bedside. Evaluation of the biliary tree consists mainly in assessing its caliber; the duct system often does not return to completely normal dimensions but a second increase in caliber following the postoperative reduction suggests drainage failure as does dilatation after a fatty meal (Darweesh et al 1988). Prostheses and stents can be visualized on ultrasound (Fig. 13.32). An additional and often striking feature is the presence of gas in the biliary tree, including the gallbladder itself; it demonstrates that the anastomosis or stent is patent (Chu et al 1978) (Fig. 13.33).

Ultrasound may also be useful in other biliary disorders. Intrahepatic cholelithiasis produces echogenic foci accom-

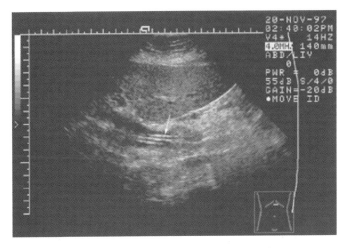

Fig. 13.32 Biliary stent. The typical parallel-lines pattern of a stent (arrow) is seen in this dilated common duct. While the position of such stents is readily demonstrated, ultrasound cannot assess their patency.

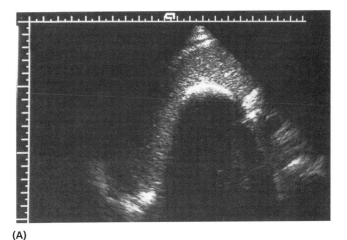

(A)

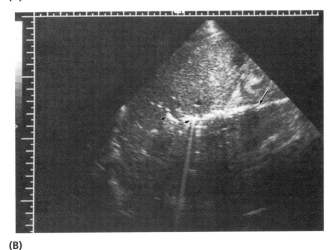

(B)

Fig. 13.33 Gas in the biliary tree. The gall bladder **(A)** returns very strong echoes with total distal shadowing in this patient with a biliary stent (arrow in **(B)**) that had been inserted to relieve obstruction from a carcinoma of the head of the pancreas. There is also gas in the bile ducts, seen as reflective foci, some with the 'comet tail' artifact (arrows in **(B)**) seen as a bright band distal to the gas pocket.

panied by shadowing in the distribution of the biliary tree (Lin et al 1989). However, since these stones are often small, they are easily missed on ultrasound so that cholangiography is a more reliable test. Intrahepatic stones can also be imaged intra-operatively. Intrahepatic stones are also a feature of Caroli's disease (Ch. 66) (Breysem et al 1998) and of sclerosing cholangitis. In the former the intrahepatic duct ectasia produces cystic spaces in the liver. In sclerosing cholangitis (Ch. 48) there is irregular dilatation of the ducts giving a beaded appearance on the ultrasound scan with the stones producing focal intense echoes accompanied by bands of acoustic shadowing. Complicating cholangiocarcinoma is difficult to detect on ultrasound before it becomes extensive.

Biliary atresia (Ch. 47) is best confirmed with biliary excretion isotope studies (Dick & Mowat 1986) but failure to demonstrate the common bile duct in a jaundiced baby is suspicious though not definitive because the small caliber of the normal duct sometimes makes demonstration difficult. In some cases cystic dilatation of residual biliary segments occurs, giving rise to a confusing appearance. Ultrasound can also demonstrate associated anomalies such as situs inversus and polysplenia and is useful in post-operative follow-up to check that the liver texture remains normal and to monitor for splenomegaly, an indicator of portal hypertension.

Choledochal cysts (Ch. 65) are mostly very obvious on ultrasound as a subhepatic cyst alongside the gallbladder; with careful scanning, its communication with the bile duct may be demonstrable (Meire & Farrant 1993). Some of the less common types of choledochal cyst (the fusiform and intrahepatic variants) are more difficult to recognize.

THE GALLBLADDER

Ultrasound is the simplest and most reliable method for demonstrating gallstones (Health and Policy Committee et al 1988). They appear as strongly reflective foci in the gallbladder and cast well-marked acoustic shadows (Fig. 13.34). Unless impacted, they move with changes in posture. The demonstration of all of these features is almost totally reliable down to stones of a millimeter or so in size. Confusion can occasionally be caused by polyps, especially when they are calcified. Difficulties arise when the gallbladder is contracted because stones may then simulate gas in a bowel loop; in this situation stones may be missed and occasionally duodenal gas has been misread as stones filling a contracted gallbladder. Since the gallbladder neck normally returns very strong echoes, a stone impacted here may be difficult to detect. Usually other stones are present in these cases and there may be additional features of cholecystitis.

Debris or sludge in gallbladder should not cause confusion since it does not shadow.

The limitations of ultrasound in stone detection, apart from very small stones, are the difficulty in estimating the size and number of stones and in detecting whether they are calcified (Simeone et al 1989). These are important considerations in the selection of cases for medical treatment of stones. Here X-ray cholecystography is preferred. Ultrasound can be used to guide lithotripsy (Mathieson et al 1989, Zhang et al 1997).

Ultrasound is reliable in the diagnosis of acute cholecystitis (Ch. 34) provided careful interpretation of the features is made (Dillon & Parkin 1980). Major signs are the demonstration of gallstones or of edema or gas in the gallbladder wall (Fig. 13.35). Edema produces thickening with an

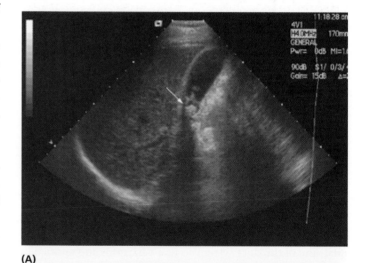

(A)

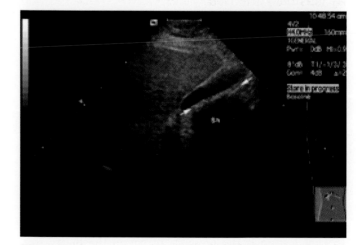

(B)

Fig. 13.34 Gallstones. Echogenic foci in the gallbladder with acoustic shadowing are the characteristic ultrasound appearances of gallstones, whether solitary **(A)** or multiple (between the arrows in **(B)**). Note the stone (arrow) in the neck of the gallbladder in **(A)**. (Sh, acoustic shadow)

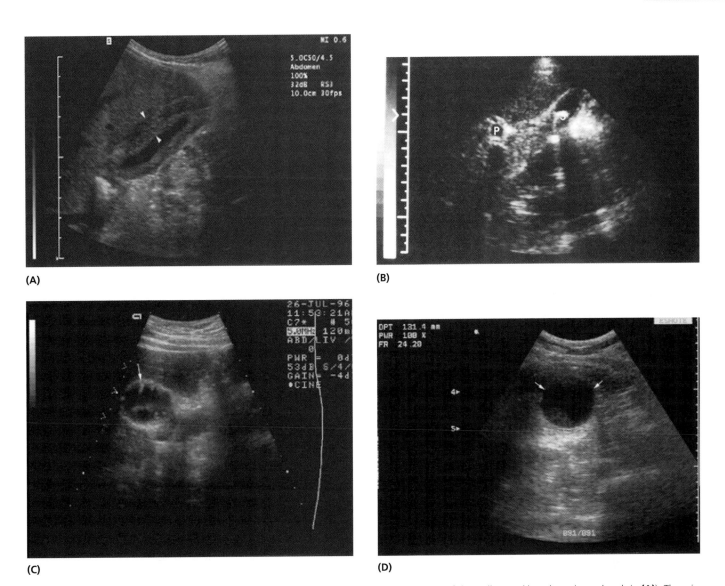

(A)

(B)

(C)

(D)

Fig. 13.35 Cholecystitis. Typical findings in acute cholecystitis are a thickening and lamination of the wall caused by edema (arrowheads in (A)). There is usually also local tenderness when the probe is pressed over the gallbladder (the ultrasound Murphy's sign). In chronic cholecystitis (B) the wall thickening is often less obvious and is uniformly echogenic. Adenomyomatosis has similar appearances to chronic cholecystitis though the wall thickening tends to be focal; in some cases a characteristic flare extending from echogenic foci in the wall (arrows in (C)) gives the so-called 'diamond ring' appearance. It is probably a form of reverberation artifact from the dilated sinuses within the wall. Mucocele of the gallbladder (arrow in (D)) is often an incidental finding; this patient presented with a right-sided mass that proved to be a grossly dilated gallbladder containing stones.

echo-poor band while gas is intensely echogenic. Non-visualization of the gallbladder is also a major sign. Simple wall-thickening is a minor sign as is local tenderness, a rounded shape or dilatation. Pericholecystitic fluid is also a minor sign. The demonstration of a major and a minor sign together gives an overall accuracy of over 90% and when the gallbladder is normal, ultrasound often indicates another cause for the symptoms. Acalculous cholecystitis is more difficult to diagnose with ultrasound because these generally ill patients have numerous other potential causes for gallbladder wall-thickening and often are unable to report whether the gallbladder is tender (Wiboltt & Jeffrey 1997).

In chronic cholecystitis the wall is also thickened but lacks the echo-poor halo and there is no local tenderness. The gall bladder fails to empty after a meal or CCK challenge (Hederstrom et al 1988). Stones are usually present.

Less common allied problems are also demonstrable on ultrasound. A mucocele appears as a large, sometimes enormous gallbladder which is non-tender and thin-walled (Fig. 13.35). The contents are usually echo-free, apart from stones, though debris may form. In adenomyomatosis there is gross wall-thickening, usually segmental in distribution and predominantly affecting the fundus (Rice et al 1981) (Fig. 13.35). When large, the Aschoff-Rokitansky sinuses can be visualized as 'intramural cysts' while calcifications give strongly echogenic foci in the wall, the combination being referred to as the 'diamond ring sign'. Cholecystography is more specific in this problem. The porcelain gallbladder has a striking appearance: the wall is replaced by a curvilinear band of intense echoes with shadowing (Kane et al 1984). The pattern is similar to that of gas in the gallbladder lumen but can be distinguished on a plain X-ray. Apparent thickening of the gallbladder wall is also encountered in a variety of unrelated conditions. It is a common feature of viral hepatitis, probably representing direct extension of the inflammatory process. It is also seen in most patients with ascites and in hypoalbuminemia.

Ascaris worms in the gallbladder and biliary tree have a characteristic appearance as parallel echogenic lines with a curved shape; if the parasite is alive, striking writhing movements are seen on real time (Ferreyra & Cerri 1998) (Ch. 62).

Adenomas of the gallbladder (Ch. 53) appear as polypoid increscences into the lumen (Carter et al 1978) (Fig. 13.36). They may have strong echoes and even cast acoustic shadows and so simulate stones but their position on the gallbladder wall remains fixed with changes in posture. Provided they are smaller than 5 mm in diameter, they may be ignored but larger polyps and those that are vascular on color Doppler need ultrasound follow up because of the risk that they may be malignant.

Carcinoma in the early stages is indistinguishable from adenoma or cholecystitis. More advanced cases are seen as a mass involving the gallbladder wall, sometimes filling the lumen and enveloping any associated stones and often extending into the porta to produce features of obstructive jaundice (Lampmann et al 1984) (Ch. 53). The abnormality is readily demonstrated by ultrasound though a specific diagnosis cannot always be made since chronic cholecystitis and adenomyomatosis can have similar appearances. Unfortunately, because of the late onset of symptoms with this tumor, improvements in imaging have not improved prognosis. The best chance of successful treatment is in those cases where the tumor is fortuitously detected at a stage when excision is still possible. Ultrasound offers the best prospect since it is so widely used for the gallbladder—ultrasonologists should have a low threshold for raising the possibility of gallbladder cancer whenever irregular thickening or focal masses are demonstrated, especially in the over-60s and even when no stones are present.

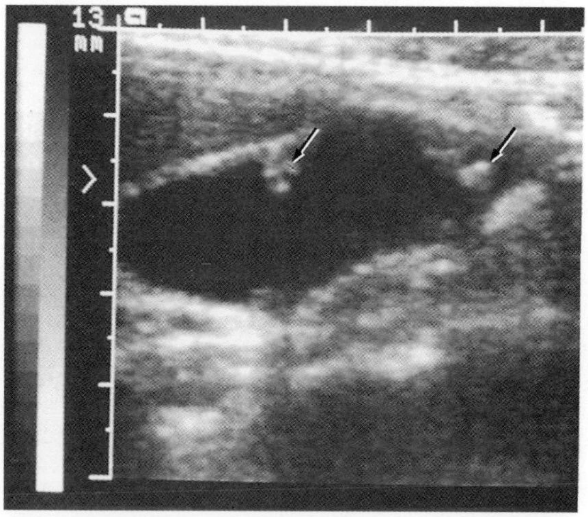

(A)

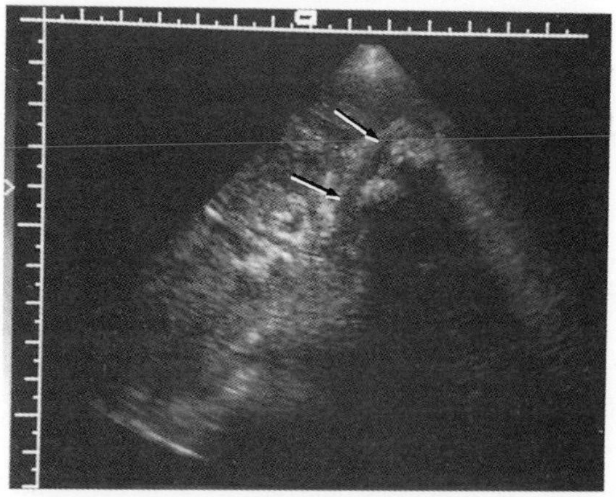

(B)

Fig. 13.36 Gallbladder tumors. Two gallbladder polyps are seen as small masses (arrows in (A)) attached to the gallbladder wall. Malignancy cannot be excluded but the small size and localized nature of these lesions are reassuring. Generalized thickening of the gallbladder wall (arrows in (B)) was due to a carcinoma that was inoperable because of spread to the porta with bile duct obstruction. Gallstones were present.

REFERENCES

Abbitt P L 1998 Ultrasonography. Update on liver technique. Radiologic Clinics of North America 36: 299–307

Abdel-Latif Z, Abdel-Wahab M F, El-Kady N M 1982 Evaluation of portal hypertension in cases of hepatosplenic schistosomiasis using ultrasound. Radiology 144: 216

Adam A, Benjamin I 1992 The staging of cholangiocarcinoma. Clinical Radiology 46: 299–303

Albrecht T A, Blomley M J K, Cosgrove D O et al 1999 Non-invasive diagnosis of hepatic cirrhosis by transit time analysis of an ultrasound contrast agent. Lancet 353: 1579–1583

Atomi Y, Inoue S, Kawano N, Morioki Y (eds) 1984 Hepatocellular carcinoma. Ultrasonic differential diagnosis of tumors. Igaku-Shoin

Barbot D J, Marks J H, Feld R I et al 1997 Improved staging of liver tumors using laparoscopic intraoperative ultrasound. Journal of Surgical Oncology 64: 63–67

Barloon T, Bergus G, Weissman A 1996 Diagnostic imaging to identify the cause of jaundice. American Family Physician 54: 556–562

Beggs I 1983 The radiological appearance of hydatid disease of the liver. Clinical Radiology 34: 555–563

Bezzi M, Silecchia G, De Leo A et al 1998 Laparoscopic and intraoperative ultrasound. European Journal of Radiology 27: S207–214

Bezzi M, Teggi A, De Rosa F et al 1987 Abdominal hydatid disease: US findings during medical treatment. Radiology 162: 91–95

Bismuth H 1982 Surgical anatomy and anatomical surgery of the liver. World Journal of Surgery 6: 3–9

Bjoro K, Blomhoff J P, Schrumpf E et al 1997 Hepatic vein thrombosis. Diagnostic and therapeutic difficulties. Tidsskrift for den Norske Laegeforening 117: 1274–1276

Blomley M, Albrecht T, Cosgrove D et al 1998 Stimulated acoustic emission in liver parenchyma with Levovist [letter]. Lancet 351: 568

Blomley M J, Albrecht T, Cosgrove D O et al 1998 Liver vascular transit time analyzed with dynamic hepatic venography with bolus injections of an US contrast agent: early experience in seven patients with metastases. Radiology 209: 862–6

Bolondi L, Gaiani S, Gebel M 1998 Portohepatic vascular pathology and liver disease: diagnosis and monitoring. European Journal of Ultrasound 7: S41–52

Bottelli R, Tibballs J, Hochhauser D et al 1998 Ultrasound screening for hepatocellular carcinoma (HCC) in cirrhosis: the evidence for an established clinical practice. Clinical Radiology 53: 713–716

Braunschweig R, Olif S, Oliff J 1996 Echo-enhanced liver and portal system ultrasound imaging with Levovist. Angiology 7 (suppl): 23–29

Bree R L, Schwabh R E, Neiman H L 1983 Solitary echogenic spot in the liver; is it diagnostic of a hemangioma? American Journal of Roentgenology 140: 41–44

Breysem L, Opdenakker G, Smet M et al 1998 Caroli's syndrome. Journal Belge De Radiologie 81: 1–2

Bruneton J N, Drouillard J, Fenart D et al 1983 Ultrasonography of hepatic cavernous haemangioma. British Journal of Radiology 56: 791–794

Bruneton J N, Raffaelli C, Balu-Maestro C et al 1996 Sonographic diagnosis of solitary solid liver nodules in cancer patients. European Radiology 6: 439–442

Bunk A, Stoelben E, Kohler T et al 1997 Value of color Doppler ultrasound in preoperative planning of the resection of liver tumors. Langenbecks Archiv Fur Chirurgie (suppl) Kongressband 114: 428–430

Buscarini L, Di Stasi M, Buscarini E et al 1996 Clinical presentation, diagnostic work-up and therapeutic choices in two consecutive series of patients with hepatocellular carcinoma. Oncology 53: 204–209

Calliada F, Campani R, Bottinelli O et al 1998 Ultrasound contrast agents: basic principles. European Journal of Radiology 27 (suppl) 2: S157–60

Carter R, Hemingway D, Cooke T G et al 1996 A prospective study of six methods for detection of hepatic colorectal metastases. Annals of the Royal College of Surgeons of England 78: 27–30

Carter S, Routledge J, Hirsch J 1978 Papillary adenoma of the gallbladder. Journal of Clinical Ultrasound 6: 433–435

Casarella W, Knowles D, Wolff M, Johnson P 1978 Focal nodular hyperplasia and liver cell adenoma. American Journal of Roentgenology 131: 393–402

Catheline J M, Champault G 1998 Laparoscopic ultrasound in abdominal surgery. Acta Chirurgica Belgica 98: 55–61

Caturelli E, Giacobbe A, Facciorusso D et al 1996 Percutaneous biopsy in diffuse liver disease: increasing diagnostic yield and decreasing complication rate by routine ultrasound assessment of puncture site. American Journal of Gastroenterology 91: 1318–1321

Cheng Y F, Huang T L, Chen C L et al 1998 Intraoperative Doppler ultrasound in liver transplantation. Clinical Transplantation 12: 292–299

Chu J, Husband J, Cosgrove D O, McCready V R M 1978 The B-scan appearance of gas in the biliary tree. British Journal of Radiology 51: 728–730

Colli A, Cocciolo M, Mumoli N et al 1998 Peripheral intrahepatic cholangiocarcinoma: ultrasound findings and differential diagnosis from hepatocellular carcinoma. European Journal of Ultrasound 7: 93–9

Cook G, Crofton M 1997 Hepatic artery thrombosis and infarction: evolution of the ultrasound appearances in liver transplant recipients. British Journal of Radiology 70: 248–251

Cosgrove D 1993 Liver anatomy and normal variations. In: Cosgrove D O, Meire H B, Dewbury K C (eds) Clinical Ultrasound. Churchill Livingstone, London

Cosgrove D, Blomley M, Jayaram V, Nihoyannopoulos P 1998 Echo-enhancing (contrast) agents. Ultrasound Quarterly 14: 66–75

Cosgrove D, McCready V R M 1982 Ultrasonic imaging, liver spleen and pancreas. Wiley, Chichester

Couinaud C 1957 Le Foie. Etude anatomiques et chirugicales. Masson, Paris

Darweesh R M A, Dodds W J, Hogan W J 1988 Fatty meal sonography for evaluating patients with suspected partial common duct obstruction. American Journal of Roentgenology 51: 63–68

Das D K, Tripathi R P, Kumar N et al 1997 Role of guided fine needle aspiration cytology in diagnosis and classification of liver malignancies. Tropical Gastroenterology 18: 101–106

Dawson P, Cosgrove D, Grainger R, (eds) 1999 Textbook of Contrast Media. Isis Medical Press

De Carlis L, Pirotta V, Rondinara G F et al 1997 Hepatic adenoma and focal nodular hyperplasia: diagnosis and criteria for treatment. Liver Transplantation Surgery 3: 160–165

de Jong N, Ten Cate F, Lancee C et al 1991 Principles and recent developments in ultrasound contrast agents. Ultrasonics 29: 324–330

de Kleijn E M, van Lier H J, van der Meer J W 1997 Fever of unknown origin (FUO). II. Diagnostic procedures in a prospective multicenter study of 167 patients. The Netherlands FUO Study Group. Medicine 76: 401–414

Dewbury K C, Clark B E 1980 The accuracy of ultrasound in the detection of cirrhosis of the liver. British Journal of Radiology 52: 945–950

Dewbury K C, Joseph A E A, Sadler G M et al 1980 Ultrasound in the diagnosis of early liver abscess. British Journal of Radiology 53: 1160–1167

Dewbury K C, Smith C L 1984 The misdiagnosis of common bile duct stones with ultrasound. British Journal of Radiology 56: 625–630

Di Stasi M, Caturelli E, De Sio I et al 1996 Natural history of focal nodular hyperplasia of the liver: an ultrasound study. Journal of Clinical Ultrasound 24: 345–350

Dick M, Mowat A P 1986 Biliary scintigraphy with DISIDA. A simpler way of showing bile duct patency in suspected biliary atresia. Archives of Diseases of Childhood 61: 191–195

Dillon E, Parkin G 1980 The role of upper abdominal ultrasonography in suspected acute cholecystitis. Clinical Radiology 31: 175–179

Dinc H, Sari A, Resit Gumele H, Cihanyurdu N et al 1998 Portal and splanchnic haemodynamics in patients with advanced post-hepatitic cirrhosis and in healthy adults. Assessment with duplex Doppler ultrasound. Acta Radiologica 39: 152–156

Dong B, Chen M 1987 Improved sonographic visualisation of choledocholithiasis. Journal of Clinical Ultrasound 15: 185–190

Duysburgh I, Michielsen P, Fierens H et al 1997 Fine needle trucut biopsy of focal liver lesions: a new technique. Digestive Diseases and Sciences 42: 2077–2081

Easson A M, Barron P T, Cripps C et al 1996 Calcification in colorectal hepatic metastases correlates with longer survival. Journal of Surgical Oncology 63: 221–225

Eckersley R 1999 Functional Imaging with ultrasound contrast agents. Ultrasound in Medicine and Biology (in press)

el Hajjam M, Essadki O, Chikhaoui N, Kadiri R 1996 Ultrasound signs of pseudoneoplastic forms of hepatic hydatid cysts. A prospective analysis of 50 cases. Annales De Radiologie 39: 172–181

Ernst H, Hahn E G, Balzer T et al 1996 Color doppler ultrasound of liver lesions: signal enhancement after intravenous injection of the ultrasound contrast agent Levovist. Journal of Clinical Ultrasound 24: 31–35

Farrant P, Meire H B 1997 Hepatic vein pulsatility assessment on spectral Doppler ultrasound. British Journal of Radiology 70: 829–832

Ferreyra N P, Cerri G G 1998 Ascariasis of the alimentary tract, liver, pancreas and biliary system: its diagnosis by ultrasonography. Hepato-Gastroenterology 45: 932–937

Filice C, Brunetti E 1997 Use of PAIR in human cystic echinococcosis. Acta Tropica 64: 95–107

Foley W D, Lawson T L 1992 Abdomen. In: Foley W D (ed) Color Doppler flow imaging. Andover Medical, Boston, Ch 3

Forsberg L, Holmin T 1983 Pulsed Doppler and B-mode ultrasound features of interposition meso-caval and porto-caval shunts. Acta Radiologica 24: 353–357

Freeny P C, Vimont T R, Barnett D C 1979 Cavernous hemangioma of the liver: ultrasonography, arteriography, and computed tomography. Radiology 132: 143–150

Fried A M, Kreel L, Cosgrove D O 1984 The hepatic interlobar fissure. American Journal of Roentgenology 143: 561–563

Friis H, Ndhlovu P, Kaondera K et al 1996 Ultrasonographic assessment of *Schistosoma mansoni* and *S. haematobium* morbidity in Zimbabwean schoolchildren. American Journal of Tropical Medicine and Hygiene 55: 290–294

Fritsehy P, Robotti G, Sehneekloth G et al 1983 Measurement of liver volume by ultrasound and computed tomography. Journal of Clinical Ultrasound 11: 299–303

Froelich J W, Simeone J F, McKusick K A et al 1982 Radionuclide imaging and ultrasound in liver/spleen trauma. Radiology 145: 457–461

Fukuda M, Hirata K, Mitani M et al 1991 Endoscopic sonography in gastroenterology. Hospimedica (Dec) 21–27

Gaiani S, Gramantieri L, Venturoli N et al 1997 What is the criterion for differentiating chronic hepatitis from compensated cirrhosis? A prospective study comparing ultrasonography and percutaneous liver biopsy. Journal of Hepatology 27: 979–985

Gaines P, Sampson M 1989 The prevalence and characterization of simple hepatic cysts by ultrasound examination. British Journal of Radiology 62: 335–367

Gandolfi L, Solmi L, Bolondi L et al 1983 The value of ultrasonography in the diagnosis of hepatic haemangiomas. European Journal of Radiology 3: 222–232

Gefter W B, Arger P H, Edell S I 1982 Sonographic patterns of ascites. Seminars in Ultrasound 2: 226–241

Gillams A, Brown S, Lees W 1997 Does interstitial laser therapy to hepatic metastases impact survival? Radiology 205: 200

Gosink B B, Lemon S K, Scheible W et al 1979 Accuracy of ultrasonography in diagnosis of hepatocellular disease. American Journal of Roentgenology 133: 19–25

Grant E 1992 Doppler imaging of the liver. Ultrasound Quarterly 10: 117–154

Griffith J F, John P R 1996 Imaging of biliary complications following paediatric liver transplantation. Pediatric Radiology 26: 388–394

Grumbach K, Coleman B G, Gal A A 1989 Hepatic and biliary tract abnormalities in patients with AIDS. Sonographic-pathologic correlation. Journal of Ultrasound Medicine 8: 247–254

Hadidi A 1983 Sonography of hepatic echinococcal cysts. Radiology 147: 913–927

Harbin W P, Robert N J, Ferrucci J 1980 Diagnosis of cirrhosis based on regional changes in hepatic morphology: radiological and pathological analysis. Radiology 135: 273–288

Harisinghani M, Saini S, Schima W et al 1997 Simethicone coated cellulose as an oral contrast agent for ultrasound of the upper abdomen. Clinical Radiology 52: 224–226

Health and Policy Committee, American College of Physicians 1988 How to study the gallbladder. Annals of Internal Medicine 109: 752–754

Hederstrom E, Forsberg L, Herlin P, Holmin T 1988 Fatty meal provocation monitored by ultrasonography. A method to diagnose ambiguous gallbladder disease. Acta Radiologica 29: 207–210

Herman K 1996 Intraoperative ultrasound in gastrointestinal cancer. An analysis of 272 operated patients. Hepato-Gastroenterology 43: 565–570

Ho S, Lau W Y, Leung W T et al 1997 Arteriovenous shunts in patients with hepatic tumors. Journal of Nuclear Medicine 38: 1201–1205

Hollinshead W 1982 Anatomy for surgeons: thorax, abdomen and pelvis. Harper and Row, New York

Holm H H, Skjoldbye B 1996 Interventional ultrasound. Ultrasound in Medicine and Biology 22: 773–789

Horsmans Y, Laka A, Gigot J F, Geubel A P 1996 Serum and cystic fluid CA 19–9 determinations as a diagnostic help in liver cysts of uncertain nature. Liver 16: 255–257

Hughes S W, D'Arcy T J, Maxwell D J et al 1996 Volume estimation from multiplanar 2D ultrasound images using a remote electromagnetic position and orientation sensor. Ultrasound in Medicine and Biology 22: 561–572

Ishiguchi T, Shimamoto K, Fukatsu H et al 1996 Radiologic diagnosis of hepatocellular carcinoma. Seminars in Surgical Oncology 12: 164–169

Iwao T, Toyonaga A, Oho K et al 1997 Value of Doppler ultrasound parameters of portal vein and hepatic artery in the diagnosis of cirrhosis and portal hypertension. American Journal of Gastroenterology 92: 1012–1027

Izzo F, Cremona F, Ruffolo F et al 1998 Outcome of 67 patients with hepatocellular cancer detected during screening of 1125 patients with chronic hepatitis. Annals of Surgery 227: 513–518

Jeffrey R B, Ralls P 1998 Color and Power Doppler Sonography. Lippincott-Raven, Philadelphia

Joseph A E A, Saverymuttu S H, Al-Sam S et al 1991 Comparison of liver histology with ultrasonogrupahy in assessing diffuse parenchymal liver disease. Clinical Radiology 43: 26–31

Juttner H-U, Jenney J M, Ralls P W et al 1982 Ultrasound demonstration of porto-syslemic collaterals in cirrhosis. Radiology 142: 459–466

Kamalov I R, Sandrikov V A, Gautier S V et al 1998 The significance of color velocity and spectral Doppler ultrasound in the differentiation of liver tumours. European Journal of Ultrasound 7: 101–108

Kane R, Jacobs R, Katz J 1984 Porcelain gallbladder: ultrasound and CT appearance. Radiology 152: 137–141

Karthaus M, Huebner G, Elser C et al 1998 Early detection of chronic disseminated Candida infection in leukemia patients with febrile neutropenia: value of computer-assisted serial ultrasound documentation. Annals of Hematology 77: 41–45

Kauffman W M, Heslop H E, Gronemeyer S A et al 1997 Hepatic arterial resistance index—an indicator of diffuse liver disease in children treated with bone marrow transplantation. Clinical Radiology 52: 903–906

Kawasaki S, Makuuchi M, Miyagawa S et al 1996 Extended lateral segmentectomy using intraoperative ultrasound to obtain a partial liver graft. American Journal of Surgery 171: 286–288

Khakoo S I, Grellier L F, Soni P N et al 1996 Etiology, screening, and treatment of hepatocellular carcinoma. Medical Clinics of North America 80: 1121–1145

Kissin C M, Bellamy E A, Cosgrove D O et al 1986 Focal sparing in fatty infiltration of the liver. British Journal of Radiology 59: 25–28

Klotter H, Ruckert K, Mentges B et al 1986 Intraoperative ultrasound study in surgery. Ultraschall Med 7: 224–230

Kok T, Slooff M J, Peeters P M et al 1996 Changes in portal hemodynamics and acute rejection in the first 2 weeks after orthotopic liver transplantation. A prospective Doppler ultrasound study. Investigative Radiology 31: 774–780

Kok T, Slooff M J, Thijn C J et al 1998 Routine Doppler ultrasound for the detection of clinically unsuspected vascular complications in the early postoperative phase after orthotopic liver transplantation. Transplant International 11: 272–276

Kolecki R, Schirmer B 1998 Intraoperative and laparoscopic ultrasound. Surgical Clinics of North America 78: 251–271

Korner T 1996 Diagnostic value of portal duplex ultrasound in liver cirrhosis. Ultraschall in Der Medizin 17: 79–84

Kremkau F 1997 Diagnostic ultrasound: principles and instruments. WB Saunders, Philadelphia

Kuni C C, Johnson N L, Holmes J H 1978 Polycystic liver disease. Journal of Clinical Ultrasound 6: 332–334

Kurtz A B, Dubbins P A, Rubin C S 1981 Echogenicity: analysis, significance, and masking. American Journal of Roentgenology 137: 471–475

Kurtz A L, Rubin C S, Cooper H S et al 1980 Ultrasound findings in hepatitis. Radiology 136: 717–725

Labrune P, Trioche P, Duvaltier I et al 1997 Hepatocellular adenomas in glycogen storage disease type I and III: a series of 43 patients and review of the literature. Journal of Pediatric Gastroenterology and Nutrition 24: 276–279

Lafortune M, Patriquin H 1999 The hepatic artery: studies using Doppler sonography. Ultrasound Quarterly 15: 9–26

Lagalla R, Caruso G, Finazzo M 1998 Monitoring treatment response with color and power Doppler. European Journal of Radiology 27 (suppl) 2: S149–156

Lampmann L, Meijer J G, Stroucken A 1984 Sonographic detection of early gallbladder cancer. Clin Med 53: 99–103

Larcos G, Sorokopud H, Berry G, Farrell G C 1998 Sonographic screening for hepatocellular carcinoma in patients with chronic hepatitis or cirrhosis: an evaluation. American Journal of Roentgenology 171: 433–435

Laurin J, Lindor K D, Crippin J S et al 1996 Ursodeoxycholic acid or clofibrate in the treatment of non-alcohol-induced steatohepatitis: a pilot study. Hepatology 23: 1464–1467

Leen E, Angerson W G, Cooke T G, McArdle C S 1996 Prognostic power of Doppler perfusion index in colorectal cancer. Correlation with survival. Annals of Surgery 223: 199–203

Leen E, Angerson W J, O'Gorman P et al 1996 Intraoperative ultrasound in colorectal cancer patients undergoing apparently curative surgery: correlation with two year follow-up. Clinical Radiology 51: 157–159

Lencioni R, Mascalchi M, Caramella D, Bartolozzi C 1996a Small hepatocellular carcinoma: differentiation from adenomatous hyperplasia with color Doppler US and dynamic Gd-DTPA-enhanced MR imaging. Abdominal Imaging 21: 41–48

Lencioni R, Pinto F, Armillotta N, Bartolozzi C 1996b Assessment of tumor vascularity in hepatocellular carcinoma: comparison of power Doppler US and color Doppler US. Radiology 201: 353–358

Lencioni R, Bartolozzi C, Ricci P et al 1997 Hepatocellular carcinoma: use of contrast enhanced color Doppler US to evaluate response to treatment with percutaneous ethanol injection. European Radiology 7: 792–794

Leutloff U C, Scharf J, Richter G M et al 1998 Use of the ultrasound contrast medium Levovist in after-care of liver transplant patients. Improved vascular imaging in color Doppler ultrasound. Radiologe 38: 399–404

Lewall D B, McCorkell S J 1985 Hepatic echinococcal cysts: sonographic appearance and classification. Radiology 155: 773–775

Lin H H, Changchien C S, Lin D Y 1989 Hepatic parenchymal calcifications—differentiation from intrahepatic stones. Journal of Clinical Ultrasound 7: 411–415

Livraghi T 1996 Physical and chemical locoregional therapy in liver metastasis. Annali Italiani Di Chirurgia 67: 799–804

Lonardo A, Bellini M, Tartoni P, Tondelli E 1997 The bright liver syndrome. Prevalence and determinants of a 'bright' liver echopattern. Italian Journal of Gastroenterology and Hepatology 29: 351–356

Lyons E 1978 A color atlas of sectional anatomy. Mosby, St Louis

Machi J, Sigel B 1996 Operative ultrasound in general surgery. American Journal of Surgery 172: 15–20

Makuuchi M, Kita Y, Takayama T 1998 Different strategies for treatment of hepatocellular carcinoma in the west and in the east. Japanese Journal of Cancer and Chemotherapy 25: 1137–1143

Mathieson J, So C B, Malone D E et al 1989 Accuracy of sonography for determining the number and size of gallbladder stones before and after lithotripsy. American Journal of Roentgenology 153: 977–980

McDicken W 1991 Diagnostic ultrasound, physical principles and use of instruments. Churchill Livingstone, Edinburgh

McGrath P, Mills P 1985 Atlas of Sectional Anatomy : Head, Neck and Trunk. Karger, Basel

Meire H B, Farrant P 1993 Paediatric biliary tree. In: Cosgrove D O, Meire H B and Dewbury K C (eds) Clinical Ultrasound. Churchill Livingstone, London

Middleton W D 1989 Sonography case of the day: focal hepatic fatty infiltration adjacent to falciform ligament. American Journal of Roentgenology 52: 1326–1327

Miller J H, Greenspan B S 1985 Integrated imaging of hepatic tumours in childhood. Radiology 154: 83–90

Mills P, Saverymuttu S, Fallowfield M et al 1990 Ultrasound in the diagnosis of granulomatous liver disease. Clin Radiol 41: 113–115

Mirowitz S A, Lee J K, Gutierrez E et al 1991 Dynamic gadolinium-enhanced rapid acquisition spin-echo MR imaging of the liver. Radiology 179: 371–376

Mueller P R, Dawson S L, Ferruci J T J, Nadi G L 1985 Hepatic echinococcal cyst: successful percutaneous drainage. Radiology 155: 627–628

Mulholland J P, Fong S M, Kafaghi F A, Fong W 1997 Budd–Chiari syndrome: diagnosis with ultrasound and nuclear medicine calcium colloid liver scan following non-diagnostic contrasted CT scan. Australasian Radiology 41: 53–56

N'Gbesso R D, Keita A K 1997 Ultrasonography of amebic liver abscesses. Proposal of a new classification. Journal De Radiologie 78: 569–576

Needleman L, Kurtz A B, Rifkin M et al 1986 Sonography of diffuse benign liver disease: accuracy of pattern recognition and grading. American Journal of Roentenology 146: 1011–1015

Netter F 1989 Atlas of Human Anatomy. Ciba collection of medical illustrations. Ciba-Geigy Corporation, Summit, New Jersey

Niederau C, Sonnenberg A, Muller J E, et al 1983 Sonographic measurements of the normal liver, spleen, pancreas and portal vein. Radiology 149: 537–540

Noone T C, Semelka R C, Woosley J T, Pisano E D 1996 Ultrasound and MR findings in acute Budd–Chiari syndrome with histopathologic correlation. Journal of Computer Assisted Tomography 20: 819–822

Oppo K, Leen E, Angerson W J et al 1998 Doppler perfusion index: an interobserver and intraobserver reproducibility study. Radiology 208: 453–457

Paley M R, Ros P R 1998 Hepatic metastases. Radiologic Clinics of North America 36: 349–363

Pande G K, Srinath C, Pal S, Reddy K S 1998 Hepatic venous outflow obstruction. Tropical Gastroenterology 19: 82–95

Parvey H R, Eisenberg R L, Giyanani V, Krebs C A 1989 Duplex sonography of the portal venous system: pitfalls and limitations. American Journal of Roentgenology 52: 765–770

Pastakia B, Shawker T H, Thaler M 1988 Hepatosplenic candidiasis: wheels within wheels. Radiology 166: 417–421

Pederson J, Pederson S T, Karstrup S 1993 Ultrasound guided biopsies. In: Cosgrove D O, Meire H B, Dewbury K (eds) Clinical Ultrasound. Churchill Livingstone, London

Pinna A D, Smith C V, Furukawa H et al 1996 Urgent revascularization of liver allografts after early hepatic artery thrombosis. Transplantation 62: 1584–1587

Ralls P, Meyers H I, Lapin S A et al 1979 Grey-scale ultrasonography of hepatic amoebic abscesses. Radiology 132: 125–137

Ralls P, Quinn M, Boswell W et al 1983 Patterns of resolution in successfully treated hepatic amoebic abscess: sonographic evaluation. Radiology 149: 541–543

Ralls P W, Meyers H I, Lapin S A, et al 1979 Grey-scale ultrasonography of hepatic amoebic abscesses. Radiology 132: 125–137

Rice J, Sauerbrie E, Semogas P 1981 The sonographic appearance of adenomyomatosis of the gall bladder. Journal of Clinical Ultrasound 9: 336–337

Rogers J V, Mack L A, Freenny P C 1981 Hepatic focal nodular hyperplasia: angiography; CT; sonography and scintigraphy. American Journal of Roentgenology 137: 983–991

Saini S, Mueller P, Ferruci J 1983 Percutaneous aspiration of hepatic cysts does not provide definitive therapy. American Journal of Roentgenology 41: 559–560

Sandler A, Rivlin L, Filler R et al 1997 Polycythemia secondary to focal nodular hyperplasia. Journal of Pediatric Surgery 32: 1386–1387

Sanford N L, Walsh P, Matis C et al 1985 Is ultrasonography useful in the assessment of diffuse parenchymal liver disease? Gastroenterology 89: 186–191

Sauerbrei E E, Cooperberg P L, Gordon P et al 1980 The discrepancy between radiographic and sonographic bile duct measurements. Radiology 137: 751–755

Saverymuttu S H, Joseph A E, Maxwell J D 1986 Ultrasound scanning in the detection of hepatic fibrosis and steatosis. British Medical Journal 292: 13–15

Scheibel W 1982 Diagnostic algorithm for liver masses. Seminars in Roentgenology 18: 84–97

Schlief R, Staks T, Mahler M et al 1990 Successful opacification of the left heart chambers on echocardiographic examinations after intravenous injection of a new saccharide-based contrast agent. Echocardiography 7: 61–64

Schneck C (ed) 1983 Tomographic anatomy. Clinics in Diagnostic Ultrasound. Churchill Livingstone, 11

Seeto R K, Rockey D C 1996 Pyogenic liver abscess. Changes in etiology, management, and outcome. Medicine 75: 99–113

Seu P, Imagawa D K, Olthoff K M et al 1996 A prospective study on the reliability and cost effectiveness of preoperative ultrasound screening of the 'marginal' liver donor. Transplantation 62: 129–130

Silverstein J C, Wavak E, Millikan K W 1998 A prospective experience with selective cholangiography. American Surgeon 64: 654–658

Simeone J F, Mueller P R, Ferrucci J T 1989 Non-surgical therapy of gallstones: implications for imaging. American Journal of Roentgenology 152: 11–17

Skjoldbye B, Wieslander S, Struckmann J et al 1998 Doppler ultrasound assessment of TIPS patency and function—the need for echo enhancers. Acta Radiologica 39: 675–679

Smith E H 1999 Hazards of fine-needle biopsy. Ultrasound Quarterly 15: 27–35

Stanley P, Gee G D, Miller J H 1989 Infantile hepatic hemangiomas, clinical features; radiologic investigations and treatment of 20 patients. Cancer 64: 936–949

Staren E D, Gambla M, Deziel D J et al 1997 Intraoperative ultrasound in the management of liver neoplasms. American Surgeon 63: 591–596

Strunk H, Stuckmann G, Frohlich E et al 1998 Native and signal-enhanced power Doppler sonography for characterization of liver lesions. Rontgenstrahlen Fortschritte 168: 344–351

Tanaka S, Kitamura T, Fujita M I H et al 1992 Intrahepatic venous and portal venous aneurysms examined by color Doppler flow imaging. Journal of Clinical Ultrasound 20: 89–98

Tateishi T, Machi J, Morioka W K 1998 Focal peliosis hepatis resembling metastatic liver tumor. Journal of Ultrasound in Medicine 17: 581–584

Taylor C R, Garcia-Tsao G, Henson B et al 1997 Doppler ultrasound in the evaluation of cirrhotic patients: the prevalence of intrahepatic arteriovenous shunting, and implications for diagnosis of hepatocellular carcinoma. Ultrasound in Medicine and Biology 23: 1155–1163

Taylor H M, Ros P R 1998 Hepatic imaging. An overview. Radiologic Clinics of North America 36: 237–245

ter Haar G, Rivens I, Chen L, Riddler S 1991 High intensity focused ultrasound for the treatment of rat tumours. Phys Med Biol 36: 1495–1501

Tham T C, Collins J S, Watson R G et al 1996 Diagnosis of common bile duct stones by intravenous cholangiography: prediction by ultrasound and liver function tests compared with endoscopic retrograde cholangiography. Gastrointestinal Endoscopy 44: 158–163

Toyoda H, Fukuda Y, Hayakawa T et al 1997 Changes in blood supply in small hepatocellular carcinoma: correlation of angiographic images and immunohistochemical findings. Journal of Hepatology 27: 654–660

Van Leeuwen M 1990 Doppler ultrasound in the evaluation of portal hypertension. Clinics in Diagnostic Ultrasound 26: 53–76

Van Sonnenberg E, Simeone J F, Mueller P R 1983 Sonographic appearance of hematoma in liver; spleen and kidney. Radiology 147: 507–512

Wachsberg R, Jilani M 1999 Duplex Doppler of small liver tumours: intralesional arterial flow does not exclude cavernous haemangioma. Clinical Radiology 54: 103–106

Wagner M, L L T 1982 Segmented anatomy. Macmillan, New York

Waldman D L, Lee D E, Bronsther O, Orloff M S 1998 Use of intraoperative ultrasonography during hepatic transplantation. Journal of Ultrasound in Medicine 17: 1–6

Wiboltt K S, Jeffrey R B, Jr 1997 Acalculous cholecystitis in patients undergoing bone marrow transplantation. European Journal of Surgery 163: 519–524

Young L K, Yang W T, Chan K W, Metreweli C 1998 Hepatic hemangioma: quantitative color power US angiography—facts and fallacies. Radiology 207: 51–57

Zhang W, Niu H O, Su Z X et al 1997 Intraoperative ultrasound-guided transhepatic lithotomy. A new alternative surgical procedure for the management of residual hepatic stones. Archives of Surgery 132: 300–303

Endoscopic ultrasound of the biliary tract

13b

P.D. STEVENS, C.J. LIGHTDALE

INTRODUCTION

The first endoscopic ultrasound (EUS) instruments were originally developed for pancreatic imaging, after the success of transrectal ultrasound for prostate imaging. Over the last 15 years, the applications of EUS have expanded to include the diagnosis and staging of primary gastrointestinal malignancies, the evaluation of pancreatic lesions, the evaluation of tumors and strictures of the bile duct, and the evaluation the bile duct and gallbladder for the presence of gallstones and/or biliary sludge. Extrahepatic biliary imaging with EUS has been possible because of the close apposition of the gastric antrum and duodenum with the porta-hepatis and the extrahepatic biliary tree. This juxtaposition creates an acoustical window through which a high-frequency ultrasound transducer, incorporated into an echoendoscope, can be maneuvered into position within the antrum and duodenum to produce clear images. Recently, ultrasound probes have been developed that can be placed into the bile ducts or gallbladder via either the transpapillary or percutaneous routes, and these may expand the usefulness of EUS for biliary diseases. The purpose of this chapter is to review the current instruments available for EUS and to discuss present and future applications of this technology to bile duct and gallbladder diseases.

INSTRUMENTS

ENDOSCOPE-BASED PROBES

Two types of echoendoscopes are available for the examination of the pancreas and biliary tree: those with mechanically rotating transducers (7.5 MHz, 12 MHz, and 20 MHz scanning frequencies) (Fig. 13.37) and those with an elec-tronic convex linear array (5 MHz and 7.5 MHz scanning frequencies) (Fig. 13.38). The chief advantage of the rotating transducer is the 360° tomographic image produced by the ultrasound beam sweeping perpendicular to the insertion shaft. The circumferential view obtained with this instrument makes orientation easier. This is particularly relevant when imaging the retroperitoneum through the duodenum, where a grasp of the anatomy is best obtained by relating organs and structures to major blood vessels (Snady 1992). The chief advantage of the electronic convex linear array transducers, where the ultrasound beam is directed parallel to the endoscope accessory channel, is that needles and other accessories passed through the channel of the endoscope can be placed into a target area under real-time endosonographic guidance. This facilitates directed tissue

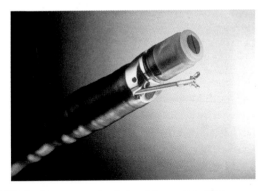

Fig. 13.37 The Olympus mechanical radial scanning video echoendoscope (GF-UM130, Olympus America, Melville, NY). The instrument produces a 360° tomographic image of structures within and adjacent to the wall of the GI tract. Accessories passed through the instrument channel can be used for all standard endoscopic applications such as mucosal biopsy and brushing. However, the transverse orientation of the ultrasound image plane does not allow real-time EUS-guided fine needle puncture.

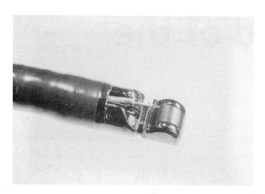

Fig. 13.38 The Olympus electronic curvilinear array echoendoscope (GF-UC30P, Olympus America, Melville, NY). The instrument produces images that are perpendicular to the instrument channel, allowing real-time EUS-guided fine needle puncture. The electronic transducer produces high-quality gray-scale images as well as color and duplex Doppler.

and fluid sampling or therapeutic injection. A second advantage of the convex linear array transducers is the availability of duplex and color Doppler, although the clinical value of these additional modalities for EUS exams has not been proved.

CATHETER-BASED PROBES

The availability of high frequency catheter-based ultrasound probes has made it possible to obtain ultrasound images from within the biliary tree. These mechanically-rotating high-frequency ultrasound probes, now equipped with transducer frequencies between 7.5 and 30 MHz, vary in width between 1.4 mm and 3.2 mm, and were first developed for use percutaneously (Engstrom & Wiechel 1990, Gerdes et al 1991). Recently, they have been increasingly used by endoscopists via the transpapillary route (Cushing et al 1993, Yasuda et al 1992, Gress et al 1995, Waxman 1995, Chak et al 1997). For the endoscopic approach, a sphincterotomy is sometimes necessary to facilitate the insertion of standard catheter-based instruments across the papilla without damaging the ultrasound transducer. However, wire-guided instruments are now available that allow efficient passage of these probes across the native papilla, through strictures, and into the intrahepatic biliary tree (Chak et al 1999). In addition, these probes can be placed via the transpapillary route through the cystic duct into the gallbladder (Uchida et al 1996) for high-frequency imaging of small mural lesions. Recently, specially designed catheter-based probes have been adapted for use with a system designed for 3-dimensional imaging of the bile duct (Kanemaki et al 1997), although clinical experience with this system is limited at present.

NORMAL ANATOMY

BILE DUCT

The normal bile duct can be imaged as a three layer structure: the inner hyperechoic layer represents the muscosa with a border echo, the middle hypoechoic layer represents the smooth muscle fibers and fibroelastic tissue, the outer hyperechoic layer represents the thin and loose connective tissue with a border echo (Mukai et al 1992). However, when imaging with an echoendoscope through the duodenum, the bile duct may appear as a single layer structure because of the thin second (muscular) layer. Occasionally, only two layers are imaged. In this situation, the inner hypoechoic layer represents both the mucosa and the muscular layer. When imaging with higher-frequency intraductal probes (Fig. 13.39) the three layer pattern is more consistent and has the same anatomic correlates as detailed above (Cushing et al 1993, Tamada et al 1998).

GALLBLADDER

The gallbladder wall typically appears as a three-layer structure both by echoendoscopic imaging and by intraluminal probe imaging (Morita et al 1988, Uchida et al 1996). The first layer is hyperechoic and represents the mucosa; the second layer is hypoechoic and represents the muscular layer,

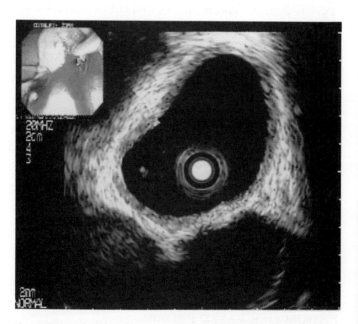

Fig. 13.39 An intraductal ultrasound (IDUS) image obtained with a 20 MHz catheter probe (Olympus UM 3R, Olympus America, Melville, NY) that has been placed within the bile duct under endoscopic and fluoroscopic guidance. The normal three-layer wall of this dilated bile duct is demonstrated. The endoscopic image is shown in a sub-screen located at the upper left corner of the figure.

the third layer represents the subserosal and serosal layers. Unfortunately, in some cases, the gallbladder may be positioned so that some or part of the wall is too far from the transducer for adequate imaging and thus may limit the usefulness of EUS for imaging this organ.

APPLICATIONS

BILE DUCT

Cancer detection

While there has been less information published concerning the role of endosonography for the detection and staging of bile duct cancers than there has been for esophageal, gastric, or pancreatic cancer, it does appear to have a role in these cancers, especially for smaller tumors. Primary bile duct cancers usually present with painless obstruction of the biliary tree and jaundice. While ultrasound and CT are reliable in establishing that the ductal system is obstructed and on what level, precise localization of tumors, especially if less than 2 cm, may be difficult.

The typical endosonography image of a bile duct tumor cancer shows a round or fusiform hypoechoic area arising from or surrounding the bile duct wall. While distal common bile duct tumors are usually easily imaged in a dilated duct, more proximal tumors may be difficult to detect due to limited penetration depth of the echoendoscope transducers. For the detection of small bile duct tumors, endosonography is as sensitive as endoscopic retrograde cholangiopancreatography (ERCP) and superior to ultrasound (US), computed tomography (CT) and angiography (Yasuda et al 1988, Sugiyama et al 1997a).

While EUS is highly sensitive for the detection of abnormalities of the bile duct, it has not yet been shown to be able to reliably distinguish benign from malignant thickening of the bile duct wall in cases of early lesions (Gress et al 1995, Tamada et al 1998a). In terms of ruling out malignant disease, however, the finding of a normal bile duct wall on EUS has a very high negative predictive value (Tamada et al 1998b).

Staging

Endosonographic staging of bile duct tumors is based on the TNM system (Anonymous 1999). The primary tumor is staged as follows: T1 tumors involve only the mucosa and or muscle layer; T2 tumors involve the perimuscular connective tissue, and T3 tumors involve adjacent structures including the liver, pancreas, duodenum, gallbladder, colon, stomach, and/or major blood vessels. Invasion is diagnosed when there is continuation of the hypoechoic tumor mass into adjacent structures. Regional lymph nodes are staged as follows: N0, no regional lymph nodes; N1, regional lymph nodes including celiac lymph nodes. In general, size criteria have not been used in the EUS studies of bile duct cancer staging, rather, lymph nodes with a hypoechoic texture and sharp boundaries, or those penetrated by the hypoechoic tumor mass are considered malignant. Lymph nodes with a hyperechoic pattern and indistinct boundaries are considered benign (Tio et al 1993, Qilian et al 1996).

Qilian et al (1996) evaluated the use of EUS for the preoperative assessment of 18 patients with extrahepatic bile duct tumors. The overall accuracy for T stage was 72%, for N stage 61%. In an earlier study, Mukai et al (1992) reported the accuracy of EUS for determining the T and N stage of CBD tumors in 16 patients. All 16 patients underwent resection. The extent of malignant invasion (T stage) was accurately diagnosed by EUS in 81% of patients. Over staging occurred in one patient due to inflammation around the common bile duct (CBD) and under staging occurred in two patients because of microscopic tumor invasion. The accuracy for lymph node staging was also 81%.

Tio et al, who reported their updated series of Klatskin tumors in 1993, have conducted the largest volume of work on EUS for staging of proximal bile duct cancers. They found that the overall accuracy of EUS for T stage was 86% and for N stage was 64% (Tio et al 1993). Although the accuracy of T staging is excellent, the accuracy for lymph nodes is less impressive. The problems with lymph node diagnosis should be largely addressed by EUS-guided fine needle aspiration biopsy, which has an overall accuracy of about 91% (Hoffman & Hawes 1995).

For determining resectability of bile duct cancer, portal venous invasion remains a key factor (Ch. 54). This particular aspect of staging was the subject of a recent comparative trial reported by Sugiyama et al (Sugiyama et al 1997). In their trial, EUS was prospectively compared to ultrasound, computed tomography, and angiography for the detection of portal venous system invasion in 19 bile duct cancers. All of the 19 lesions were resected, with or without portal venous resection, and underwent histopathologic staging. The authors of this study separated the degree of apparent involvement of the portal vein by tumor, as imaged by EUS, into 4 grades. In Grade 1, the tumor was away from the portal vein. In Grade 2, the tumor was in contact with the portal vein, but the echogenic interface was intact. In Grade 3, the tumor was contiguous with the portal vein and the echogenic interface was lost. In Grade 4, the tumor was seen in the vein or was occluding the vein. The authors defined EUS Grades 1 and 2 as negative for invasion, and EUS Grades 3 and 4 as positive for invasion. Using this system, they found that the accuracy for determining portal venous invasion was 93% for EUS, compared to 74% for US, 84% for CT, and 89% for angiography.

CATHETER-PROBE BASED INTRADUCTAL ULTRASOUND (IDUS)

The normal bile duct wall appears as a two- or three-layered structure on intraductal ultrasound and is similar to that seen with standard EUS (Cushing et al 1993, Tamada et al 1994, Furukawa et al 1992, Kuroiwa et al 1994, Tamada et al 1995). In contrast to EUS, IDUS is able to evaluate the proximal bile duct and surrounding structures at the hilum of the liver, including the portal vein, right hepatic artery, and contents of the hepatoduodenal ligament.

CANCER DETECTION AND STAGING WITH IDUS

The usefulness of IDUS for diagnostic imaging (Figs 13.39–13.41) is based on its ability to detect early lesions, to determine the maximal longitudinal extent of the bile duct cancer, and to determine the presence of extension into other organs or major blood vessels when this is not clear by other imaging methods (Fig. 13.40). Intraductal ultrasound has been shown to be useful in determining invasion into the portal vein, right hepatic artery, and pancreatic parenchyma (Kuroiwa et al 1994, Tamada et al 1995, Tamada et al 1996a, Tamada et al 1996b) with a diagnostic accuracy approaching 100%.

While IDUS alone cannot determine with a high degree of certainty whether any stricture is benign or malignant (Gress et al 1995), Tamada et al suggest that the IDUS findings can help direct management. If the IDUS of a stricture shows a wall-layer structure interrupted by a protruding tumor, one should perform prompt surgical exploration, even without tissue confirmation of a malignancy. If the IDUS shows a normal wall, further invasive testing is unnecessary. On the other hand, when the IDUS shows a lesion that leaves the wall layers undisturbed, direct biopsies should be obtained if possible, because only some of these will prove to be malignant (Tamada et al 1998b).

There are several important limitations of this technology. First, there is limited penetration depth with these high frequency probes, and certain structures are not well seen as a result, such as the main hepatic artery and the left hepatic artery. Also, because these probes cannot resolve the fibromuscular layer from the perimuscular connective tissue (both may appear as a single hypoechoic layer), differentiation between T1 and T2 cancers is not reliable (Tamada et al 1997). Another potential problem for IDUS is the influ-

ence of biliary drainage catheters on bile duct thickness. In one study (Tamada et al 1998a), it was demonstrated that bile duct wall thickness as measured by IDUS appears to be increased after placement of biliary drainage catheter. This could lead to an overestimation of the longitudinal (upstream or downstream) spread of disease. Further work

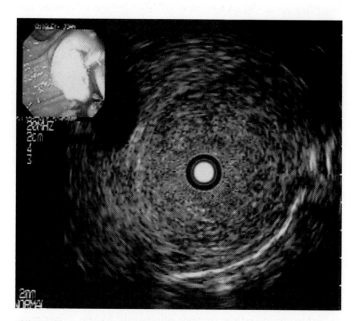

Fig. 13.40 An IDUS image of the distal portion of the bile duct shown in Figure 13.3. At this level, corresponding to a stricture on fluoroscopy, there is effacement of the wall layers and expansion of the wall by a hypoechoic process that extends into the surrounding pancreatic parenchyma.

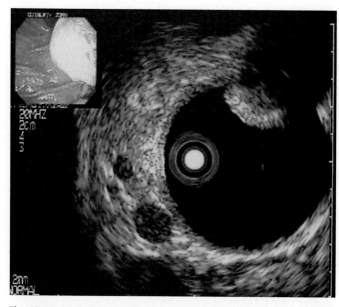

Fig. 13.41 An IDUS image of a common bile duct stone, which is seen in the upper right corner of the intraductal image as a curvilinear hyperechoic structure with a strong acoustic shadow.

is needed in this important area to try to distinguish patterns of malignant and benign thickening of the bile duct wall.

GALLBLADDER

Evaluation of polypoid lesions of the gallbladder

Sugiyama et al (Sugiyama et al 1999) evaluated the accuracy of EUS in diagnosing small (< 20 mm) polypoid lesions of the gallbladder. They retrospectively reviewed the preoperative EUS and transabdominal ultrasound in 65 patients who had undergone gallbladder resection for small polypoid lesions. The lesions resected were cholesterol polyp, $n = 40$; adenomyomatosis, $n = 9$; adenoma, $n = 4$; and adenocarcinoma, $n = 12$. They found that EUS showed a tiny echogenic spot or an aggregation of echogenic spots with or without echopenic areas in 95% of patients with cholesterol polyps, and multiple microcysts or comet tail artifacts in all adenomyomatosis cases. Adenomas and adenocarcinomas were not associated with the echogenic spots, microcysts, or artifacts. The authors concluded that a polypoid lesion (sessile or on a pedicle) without those features should be considered a neoplasm. Overall, EUS was superior to transabdominal ultrasound in differentiating the nature of the lesions (97% versus 71%).

Uchida et al reported the use of intraductal probes for evaluating gallbladder polypoid lesions in 4 patients, and was able to image the lesion of interest in three of the four patients (Uchida et al 1996). While this technique might improve image quality slightly over that obtained with endoscope-based EUS, it is not easy to insert the probe into the gallbladder and must be done with great care and over a guide-wire. The utility of this approach has not been proved, and further studies are awaited.

Gallbladder cancer staging

Mitake et al (1990) performed EUS in 39 patients before surgical resection for gallbladder carcinoma. They found that EUS accurately evaluated the depth of tumor infiltration with an overall T-stage accuracy of 79.5%. The N-stage accuracy was 89.7%. While there was some difficulty in distinguishing between T1 and T2 cancers, and in evaluating gallbladders with multiple gallstones, the authors concluded that endosonography is useful in the clinical staging of gallbladder carcinoma.

GALLBLADDER AND BILE DUCT STONES

When performing EUS, common bile duct stones are easily identified as curvilinear hyperechoic foci with strong acoustic shadowing by either standard or catheter-based EUS (Fig. 13.41). A number of studies have demonstrated the accuracy of EUS for common bile duct stones, even in small bile ducts harboring small distal stones (Norton & Alderson 1997, Sugiyama & Atomi 1997b, Palazzo et al 1995, 1996, Pratt et al 1996, Shim et al 1995, Amouyal et al 1994a, Edmundowicz et al 1992, Strohm et al 1984). In studies with over 50 patients, the sensitivity ranges from 84 to 100%, and the specificity ranges from 95 to 100%. Endoscopic ultrasound may also be useful for detecting small gallbladder stones missed on transabdominal imaging, especially those located in the neck of the gallbladder, where duodenal gas can obscure the image when scanning percutaneously.

Among the studies comparing EUS to ERCP for the detection of bile duct stones, most have used ERCP as the gold standard. However, when Prat et al compared the two procedures, they used endoscopic exploration of the bile duct with a balloon and basket as the gold standard. The procedures were similar in sensitivity (EUS 93%, ERC 89%), specificity (EUS 97%, ERC 100%), positive predictive value (EUS 98%, ERC 100%) and negative predictive value (EUS 88%, ERC 83%) (Pratt et al 1996).

Although EUS involves conscious sedation and requires the peroral introduction of an endoscope, the entire procedure can be performed efficiently in less that 15–20 minutes, and can be followed immediately by ERCP and stone extraction if needed (Edmundowicz et al 1992, Canto 1996).

Endoscopic ultrasound may prove most useful for evaluating patients who are at moderate risk of harboring bile duct stones and in whom a diagnostic ERCP might carry too great a risk of pancreatitis. Endoscopic ultrasound can be followed immediately by therapeutic ERCP during the same endoscopic session, if needed. Patients who might benefit from combined EUS/ERCP are those scheduled for laparoscopic cholecystectomy who are suspected of having common bile duct stones. In a recent preliminary report of a randomized clinical trial, we found that combined preoperative EUS/ERCP was equivalent to laparoscopic cholangiogram and transcystic common bile duct exploration for patients at a moderate risk for common bile duct stones in terms of overall success rate, length of hospital stay, and total hospital charges, but was associated with significantly shorter operating room times and fewer failed procedures (Shah et al 1999).

BILIARY SLUDGE

Biliary sludge, or microlithiasis, may be associated with biliary colic and acute cholecystitis and it may be responsible

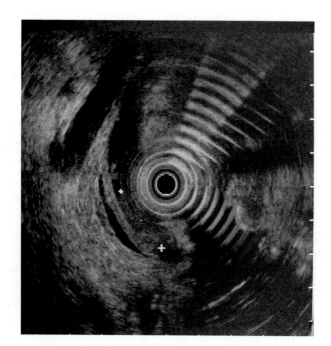

Fig. 13.42 An EUS image obtained with the mechanical radial scanning echoendoscope (Olympus GF-UM130) in a patient with idiopathic pancreatitis after standard imaging procedures. The cursor marks (+) are placed to show the layering biliary sludge partially occluding the bile duct just upstream of the papilla. The pancreatic duct is seen deep to the bile duct in the 7 to 9 o'clock position and the portal vein is seen deep to the bile duct in the 9 to 11 o'clock position.

for up to 60% of cases of idiopathic pancreatitis (Ros et al 1991, Lee et al 1992). There are reports that EUS can resolve very small concentrations of sludge in vitro (Stevens et al 1996) and that EUS is more sensitive than US in patients with idiopathic pancreatitis (Amouyal et al 1994b) (Fig 13.42). Dill et al (1995) reported that the detection of biliary sludge within the gallbladder by EUS predicts the response to cholecystectomy in patients with biliary-type pain from occult cholecystitis. If these studies are confirmed, EUS will come to occupy a pivotal role in the evaluation of patients with unexplained right upper quadrant pain or idiopathic pancreatitis.

SUMMARY

Endoscopic ultrasound is a minimally invasive imaging modality that provides high-resolution images of the extrahepatic biliary tree and the surrounding structures. It has been shown to be accurate for the detection and staging of bile duct and gallbladder cancers, and is especially useful for small tumors. Intraductal techniques, which are still in evolution, may provide even more information about the etiology and extent of biliary strictures and mural tumors. EUS has also been shown to be useful for the detection of biliary stones and sludge when transabdominal ultrasound is not diagnostic. In many cases, diagnostic endoscopic ultrasound can be followed immediately by therapeutic ERCP if needed. While the instruments and techniques for endosonography continue to improve, at present EUS can be considered a promising minimally invasive tool for evaluating the biliary tree.

REFERENCES

Amouyal P, Amouyal G, Levy P et al 1994a Diagnosis of choledocholithiasis by endoscopic ultrasonography [see comments]. Gastroenterology 106: 1062–1067

Amouyal G, Amouyal P, Levy P 1994b Value of endoscopic ultrasonography in the diagnosis of ideopathic acute pancreatitis. Gastroenterology 106: A283

Anonymous. American Joint Committee on Cancer. Annals of Surgery 1999

Canto M 1996 Endoscopic ultrasonography and gallstone disease. [Review] [43 refs]. Gastrointestinal Endoscopy 43: 37–43

Chak A, Canto M, Stevens P D et al 1997 Clinical applications of a new through-the-scope ultrasound probe: prospective comparison with an ultrasound endoscope. Gastrointestinal Endoscopy 45: 291–295

Chak A, Isenberg G, Kobayashi G, Wong R C K., Sivak M V J 2000 Prospective evaluation of over-the-wire catheter ultrasound probe. Gastrointestinal Endoscopy 51: 202–205

Cushing G L, Fitzgerald P J, Bommer W J et al 1993 Intraluminal ultrasonography during ERCP with high-frequency ultrasound catheters. Gastrointestinal Endoscopy 39: 432–435

Dill J E, Hill S, Callis J et al 1995 Combined endoscopic ultrasound and stimulated biliary drainage in cholecystitis and microlithiasis—diagnoses and outcomes. Endoscopy 27: 424–427

Edmundowicz S A, Aliperti G, Middleton W D 1992 Preliminary experience using endoscopic ultrasonography in the diagnosis of choledocholithiasis. Endoscopy 24: 774–778

Engstrom C F, Wiechel K L 1990 Endoluminal ultrasound of the bile ducts. Surgical Endoscopy 4: 187–190

Furukawa T, Naito Y, Tsukamoto Y, Mitake M, Yamada M, Ito A 1992 New technique using intraductal ultrasonography for the diagnosis of diseases of the pancreatobiliary system. Ultrasound Medicine 11: 607–612

Gerdes H, Botet J, Lightdale C J 1991 Percutaneous biliary endosonography in the evaluation of patients with recurrent obstructive jaundice. Gastrointestinal Endoscopy 37: 245

Gress F, Chen Y K, Sherman S et al 1995 Experience with a catheter-based ultrasound probe in the bile duct and pancreas. Endoscopy 27: 178–184

Hoffman B J, Hawes R H 1995 Endoscopic ultrasonography-guided puncture of the lymph nodes: First experience and clinical consequences. Gastrointestinal Endoscopy Clinics of North America. 5: 587–594

Kanemaki N, Nakazawa S, Inui K, Yoshino J, Yamao J, Okushima K 1997 Three-dimensional intraductal ultrasonography: preliminary results of a new technique for the diagnosis of diseases of the pancreatobiliary system. Endoscopy 29: 726–731

Kuroiwa M, Tsukamoto Y, Naitoh Y, Hirooka Y, Furukawa T, Katou T 1994 New technique using intraductal ultrasonography for the diagnosis of bile duct cancer. Ultrasound Medicine 13: 189–195

Lee S P, Nicholls J F, Park H Z 1992 Biliary sludge as a cause of acute pancreatitis. New England Journal of Medicine 326: 589–593

Mitake M, Nakazawa S, Naitoh Y et al 1990 Endoscopic ultrasonography in diagnosis of the extent of gallbladder carcinoma. Gastrointestinal Endoscopy 36: 562–566

Morita K, Nakazawa S, Kimoto E 1988 Gallbladder diseases. In: Kawai K (ed) Endoscopic Ultrasonography in Gastroenterology, 1st edn. Igaku-Shoin, Tokyo, p. 87–95

Mukai H, Nakajima M, Yasuda K, Mizuno S, Kawai K 1992 Evaluation of endoscopic ultrasonography in the pre-operative staging of carcinoma of the ampulla of Vater and common bile duct. Gastrointestinal Endoscopy 38: 676–683

Norton S A, Alderson D 1997 Prospective comparison of endoscopic ultrasonography and endoscopic retrograde cholangiopancreatography in the detection of bile duct stones. British Journal of Surgery 84: 1366–1369

Palazzo L, Girollet P P, Salmeron M et al 1995 Value of endoscopic ultrasonography in the diagnosis of common bile duct stones: comparison with surgical exploration and ERCP. Gastrointestinal Endoscopy 42: 225–231

Palazzo L, Levy P, Bernades P 1996 Usefulness of endoscopic ultrasonography in the diagnosis of choledocholithiasis. [Review] [51 refs]. Abdominal Imaging 21: 93–97

Prat F, Amouyal G, Amouyal P et al 1996 Prospective controlled study of endoscopic ultrasonography and endoscopic retrograde cholangiography in patients with suspected common-bile duct lithiasis [see comments]. Lancet 347: 75–79

Qilian Z, Weidong N, Lando Z, Jinyu L 1996 Endoscopic ultrasonography assessment in preoperative staging for carcinoma of ampulla of Vater and extrahepatic bile duct. Chinese Medical Journal 109: 622–625

Ros E, Navarro S, Bru C, Garcia-Puges, Valderrama R 1991 Occult microlithiasis in 'Idiopathic' acute pancreatitis: Prevention by cholecystectomy of ursodeoxycholic acid therapy. Gastroenterology 101: 1701–1709

Shah V H, Stevens P D, Memmo P et al 1999 Pre-operative EUS/ERCP vs. intraoperative cholangiography in patients with suspected CBD stones: A prospective randomized trial. Gastrointestinal Endoscopy 49: AB227

Shim C S, Joo J H, Park C W et al 1995 Effectiveness of endoscopic ultrasonography in the diagnosis of choledocholithiasis prior to laparoscopic cholecystectomy [see comments]. Endoscopy 27: 428–432

Snady H 1992 Endoscopic ultrasonography images of the normal retroperitoneum. Gastrointestinal Endoscopy Clinics of North America 2: 637–656

Stevens P D, Lightdale C J, Saha S A, Abedi M 1996 In-vitro comparison of endoscope-based vs. catheter-based endoscopic ultrasound for the detection of biliary sludge. Gastrointestinal Endoscopy 43: S57

Strohm W D, Kurtz W, Classen M 1984 Detection of biliary stones by means of endosonography. Scandinavian Journal of Gastroenterology (Suppl) 94: 60–64

Sugiyama M, Hagi H, Atomi Y, Saito M 1997a Diagnosis of portal venous invasion by pancreatobiliary carcinoma: value of endoscopic ultrasonography. Abdominal Imaging 22: 434–438

Sugiyama M, Atomi Y 1997b Endoscopic ultrasonography for diagnosing choledocholithiasis: a prospective comparative study with ultrasonography and computed tomography. Gastrointestinal Endoscopy 45: 143–146

Sugiyama H, Xie X Y, Atomi Y, Saito M 1999 Differential diagnosis of small polypoid lesions of the gallbladder: the value of endoscopic ultrasonography. Annals of Surgery 229: 498–504

Tamada K, Ido K, Ueno N, Ichiyama M, Tomiyama T, Kimura K 1994 Preoperative staging of extrahepatic bile duct cancer with intraductal ultrasonography (IDUS). American Journal of Gastroenterology 89: 239–246

Tamada K, Ido K, Ueno N et al 1995 Assessment of portal vein invasion by bile duct cancer using intraductal ultrasonography. Endoscopy 27: 573–578

Tamada K, Ido K, Ueno N, Ichiyama M, Tomiyama T, Nishizono T 1996a Assessment of the course and varications of the hepatic artery in bile duct cancer by intraductal ultrasonography. Gastrointestinal Endoscopy 44: 249–256

Tamada K, Ueno N, Ichiyama M et al 1996b Assessment of pancreatic parenchymal invasion by bile duct cancer using intraductal ultrasonography. Endoscopy 28: 492–496

Tamada K, Kanai N, Ueno N et al 1997 Limitations of intraductal ultrasonography in differentiating between bile duct cancer in stage T1 and stage T2: in-vitro and in-vivo studies. Endoscopy 29: 721–725

Tamada K, Tomiyama T, Ichiyama M et al 1998a Influence of biliary drainage catheter on bile duct wall thickness as measured by intraductal ultrasonography. Gastrointestinal Endoscopy 47: 28–32

Tamada K, Ueno N, Tomiyama T et al 1998b Characterization of biliary strictures using intraductal ultrasonography: comparison with percutaneous cholangioscopic biopsy. Gastrointestinal Endoscopy 47: 341–349

Tio T L, Reeders J W, Sie L H et al 1993 Endosonography in the clinical staging of Klatskin tumor. Endoscopy 25: 81–85

Uchida N, Ezaki T, Hirabayashi S et al 1996 Scanning of polypoid gallbladder lesions by ultrasonic microprobes using transpapillary catheterization. Endoscopy 28: 302–305

Waxman I 1995 Characterization of a malignant bile duct obstruction by intraductal ultrasonography [see comments]. American Journal of Gastroenterology 90: 1073–1075

Yasuda K, Mukai H, Nakajima M, Kawai K 1992 Clinical application of ultrasonic probes in the biliary and pancreatic duct. Endoscopy 24 Suppl 1: 370–375

Yasuda K, Nakajima M, Kawai K 1988 Diseases of the biliary tract and papilla of Vater. In: Kawai K (ed) Endoscopic ultrasonography in gastroenterology, 1st edn. Igaku-Shoin, Tokyo, p. 96–105

The role of nuclear medicine in the diagnosis and management of hepatobiliary disease

14

T. AKHURST, S.M. LARSON

INTRODUCTION

There has been a continual improvement in the care of patients with hepatobiliary disease. While much of this is due to innovative surgical technique and anesthesia, diagnostic imaging has also made major contributions to better care. Advances in crossectional imaging have led to significantly improved pre-surgical planning. Modern nuclear medicine contributes to pre-surgical diagnosis, with a vital role in the differential diagnosis of right upper quadrant pain as well as pre-surgical staging of malignant neoplasms involving liver.

Nuclear medicine should be regarded as the study of human pathophysiology, since the uptake of radiotracers used for nuclear imaging depend on either the function or molecular composition of normal or neoplastic tissues. Computed tomography (CT), ultrasound, magnetic resonance imaging (MRI), and plain X-ray excel at demonstrating anatomy. The addition of pathophysiologic information to high quality cross sectional imaging improves patient care by characterizing the processes that led to structural change. The power of nuclear medicine lies in its ability to perform dynamic studies to document physiologic processes quantitatively and/or to demonstrate the presence or absence of malignancy in normal sized structures.

The workhorse of nuclear medicine is currently the gamma camera that is capable of planar, tomographic and dynamic acquisitions. The availability of machines capable of acquiring positron emission data of the whole body is currently revolutionizing the practice of nuclear medicine particularly in the field of nuclear oncology. This is due to the improved physics of imaging of positron emitting radionuclides, and the fact that positron emitters are available for the most important biologic elements, i.e. carbon-11, fluorine-18, and oxygen-15. Since 1982 there has been an exponential rise in the number of papers reporting the utility of positron emission tomography in oncology (Fig. 14.1). In addition, new radiopharmaceuticals have been developed which offer more selective targeting to alterations in molecular structure of tissues. As one example among many, indium-111 octreotide targets tumors, which express somatostatin receptor. Since the last edition of this book was written there has been a major change in ability of nuclear medicine to contribute to management of the patient requiring hepatobiliary surgery and we will review these changes.

In particular, 2-fluoro-2-deoxy-D-glucose (FDG) positron emission tomography (PET) changes the management of patients with colorectal cancer metastatic to the liver and is a new and very exciting area of nuclear medicine practice. FDG PET is also being investigated in the management of other hepatobiliary malignancies. Hepatobiliary scintigraphy remains a powerful tool in the assessment of the functional status of the biliary tract and is the gold standard non-invasive test for the exclusion of cystic duct obstruction and by inference acute cholecystitis. General nuclear medicine imaging, using planar gamma camera imaging and Single Photon Emission Computed Tomography (SPECT) of a variety of technetium-99m and indium-111 labeled compounds continues to have an important role in the management of patients who have hepatobiliary disease both in terms of pre-operative assessment and post operative care.

POSITRON EMISSION TOMOGRAPHY (PET)

PHYSICS

Some elements undergo radioactive decay by emitting a positron from their nucleus (Table 14.1). A positron is a

PET Studies in Cancer

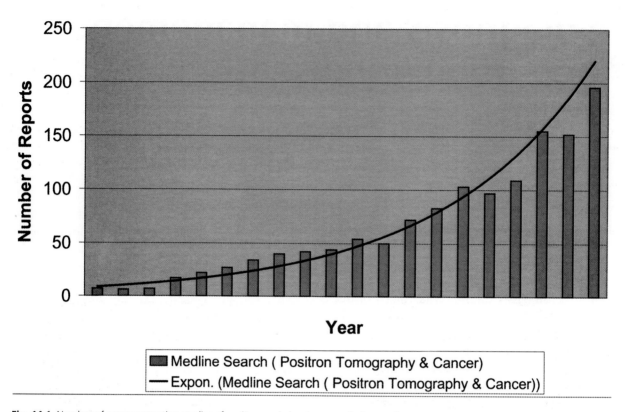

Fig. 14.1 Number of papers reporting studies of positron emission tomography in oncology.

Table 14.1 PET isotopes in clinical usage (Cho et al 1975).

Isotope	Maximal range (mm)	FWHM (mm)	Half-life (minutes)	Products/usage
^{18}F	2.6	0.22	110	FDG, F-MISO
^{11}C	4.2	0.28	20	Methionine, other aminoacids Colchicine
^{13}N	5.4	0.35	10	Ammonia
^{15}O	8.4	1.22	2	Water
^{82}Rb	17.1	2.6	1.3	Myocardial perfusion
^{86}Ga	9.0	1.35	68.3	Antibodies, peptides
^{124}I	10	8	6048 (4.2 days)	Antibodies, peptides

nuclear particle that has the same mass as an electron but has a positive charge. Once emitted, the positron moves through surrounding tissues for a millimeter or so, until eventually the positron combines with an electron in the environment and the rest mass of both particles is converted to two photons of energy (gamma rays) of 511 keV, which are emitted 180 degrees apart. It is these two photons which are detected by the PET camera.

CAMERA ISSUES

Dedicated PET systems

These machines are constructed using multiple rings of circularly arranged detectors comprising bismuth germanium oxide crystals (BGO) with associated collimators, or in some cases sodium iodide crystals (NaI). These cameras all work in coincidence, meaning that a true count is generated only when the two 511 keV gamma rays emitted during positron decay simultaneously strike a set of paired detectors (Fig. 14.2). These PET imaging devices have great 'sensitivity'; that is, a large amount of usable data is obtained from a given amount of activity injected into a patient so that the camera is able to detect small amounts of activity. The resolution of these machines is defined as the smallest distance between two sources of radiation whereby the imaging instrument is able to demonstrate two sources of radiation rather than one. This is currently around 5.0 mm for most clinical systems, and animal imaging devices are now available which have 2.0 mm (for fluorine-18) resolution. The first generations of machines were designed

to image only the brain, but in the last five years, whole body units have become available at major centers.

Gamma rays originating in the center of the body have to pass through tissue for a considerable distance in order to reach the detector, and if one or more of the paired annihilation photons are absorbed, that decay will not be recorded as a true count. Therefore a central source would be underrepresented if no attempt were made to correct for differing body tissue density and the depth of the origin of the gamma rays. One of the major advantages of PET imaging is that an accurate correction can be made for this process of 'attenuation' or loss of counts. Transmission data, collected using external rotating sources, is routinely acquired to

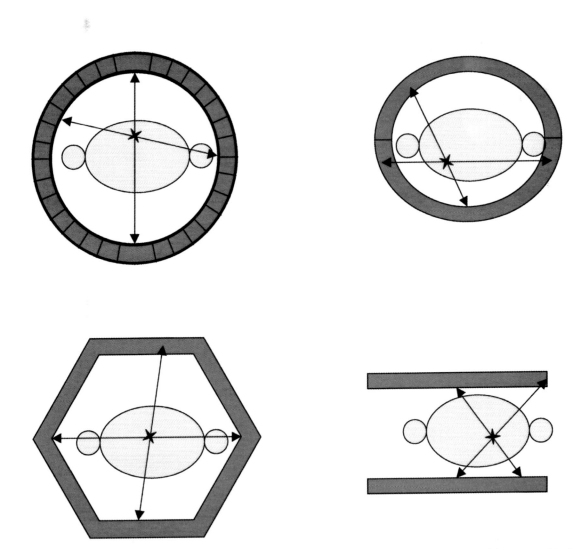

Fig. 14.2 This is a stylized representation of the (end on) geometry of types of cameras used for positron imaging in medicine arranged in decreasing detector performance. The top left image is of a dedicated BGO based system demonstrating one detector ring (of many) with a single crystal represented by one of the gray segments. The star represents the site of positron decay in the patient. Each arrowed line represents two photon pairs emitted as a result of positron decay. The top right image represents a dedicated curved NaI detector system. These systems usually have 6 large curved NaI crystals. The bottom left image is of a hexagonally arranged system with 6 large flat NaI crystals. The bottom right image is of a hybrid gamma camera system.

overcome the attenuation of activity originating in the center of the body. In this way the PET image becomes quantitative, so that the process of computerized data reconstruction ultimately generates a map of the three dimensional distribution of radioactivity. It is essential that attenuation be performed if there is to be good quality information obtained from areas like the porta hepatus, particularly if quantification of radioactivity content in the lesion is to be attempted.

Sodium iodide (NaI) based systems

The most rapid growth in the availability of positron imaging devices is in gamma camera based systems. At the time of writing, about 150 have been installed in the US. Conventional gamma cameras adapted for positron imaging use NaI crystal-based detector systems. These typically consist of two large rotating crystals with associated detectors the combination of which converts the gamma ray information into electrical signals enabling reconstruction and display. In positron imaging mode, the individual crystals and their associated detectors, are adapted to detect annihilation photons in coincidence. Attenuation correction methods have also been developed for these devices. These units are practical in that they can also image conventional single photon emitting radio-tracers using commonly available radiopharmaceuticals like technetium-99m (Tc-99m), when used in single photon imaging mode. However, the gamma camera based devices do not have the sensitivity or resolution of the dedicated PET systems.

CT/PET hybrid systems

Combination machines have been recently developed which comprise both a CT and a PET device in the same imaging gantry. The major advantage of this approach is the improvement in the speed of attenuation imaging. Also, near-perfect co-registration of structural and functional information is achieved. This promises near perfect anatomic localization of areas of functional changes.

BIOCHEMISTRY

2-Fluro-2-deoxy-D-glucose (FDG) PET

The commonest radiopharmaceutical in use in 1999 in PET imaging is FDG. This is a glucose analogue that crosses cell membranes sharing the glucose transporter molecules utilized by glucose. Like glucose it undergoes phosphorylation

by the enzyme hexokinase. The resulting molecule, FDG-6-phosphate, is polar and cannot cross cell membranes and is not a substrate for glucose-6-phosphate isomerase that converts glucose-6-phosphate to fructose-6-phosphate. FDG-6-phosphate is not a substrate for glucose-6-phosphatase in any tissue except the normal hepatocyte. The net effect of this is that there is a continuous accumulation and retention of FDG in cells (Fig. 14.3).

Warburg in 1930 reported that cancer cells show increased rates of glycolysis in comparison to normal cells. This discovery has stood the test of time and now underpins the utility of FDG-PET imaging in cancer. Glucose metabolism is the most efficient form of energy transfer and normal tissues all have characteristic glucose metabolic rates. The brain has a high rate of glucose metabolism, the lung and fat have low rates of glucose consumption. This means a clump of tumor cells are easier to detect in the lung or in fat than in the brain because the target to background ratio is high in these tissues. The liver has an intermediate glucose metabolic rate. Active inflammatory cells also exhibit an increased rate of glycolysis. This means that sites of active inflammation will exhibit increased FDG uptake, although in general the rate of glucose metabolism is less in inflammatory sites than most tumors. Sarcoidosis in particular can be quite FDG avid and may have similar patterns and degrees of uptake as some malignancies, such as lymphoma and small cell lung cancer. In such cases clinical judgement is called into play just as it is in the interpretation of opaque masses in the lung on CT scan.

The process of F-18 and FDG production and distribution is now routine and most major cities have intra-city distribution of unit doses as currently occurs for many other radiopharmaceuticals. It is likely that most tertiary hospitals will have some form of positron imaging capable camera in the very near future with many installing dedicated high end systems as clinicians realize the advantage of high resolution PET to their practices.

FDG-PET IMAGING IN THE MANAGEMENT OF PATIENTS WITH COLORECTAL CANCER METASTATIC TO THE LIVER

HISTORICAL REVIEW

The earliest human study of FDG PET in colorectal cancer was performed in 1982 by Yonekura et al. This study of large hepatic metastases in three patients with colorectal

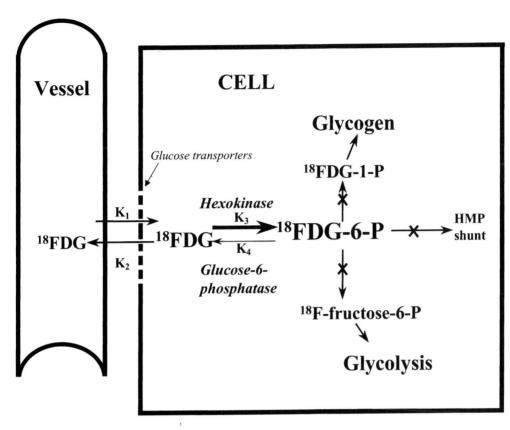

Fig. 14.3 This image illustrates the metabolic fate of F-18 FDG following injection. The curved object on the left represents the blood vessel, the gap, the extracellular space and the cell is on the right. Note the F-18 FDG is phosphorylated by hexokinase and thereafter effectively is not metabolized further.

cancer with FDG PET was successful and demonstrated that these tumors were highly glucose avid (Yonekura et al 1982) (Figs 14.3, 14.4 & 14.5). Numerous papers from multiple centers document that colorectal cancer is readily detected on FDG-PET scanning. Colorectal cancer is a common reason for referral of patients to have a FDG PET scan. For example, from Dec 1995 to Oct 1998, 411 scans were performed on patients with colorectal cancer at Memorial Sloan Kettering Cancer Center. The value of FDG PET in colorectal cancer patients is based on the consistently accelerated levels of glycolysis seen in colorectal cancer, which results in high FDG uptakes on PET scanning.

Resection of liver metastases is a procedure with a low peri-operative mortality and morbidity, with a 38% five-year survival rate (Fong et al 1997, D'Angelica et al 1997). This compares favorably with an untreated survival rate of 3% at 5 years without resection (Wagner et al 1984). Recurrent disease post resection is seen in about 65% of cases both in the liver (41%) as well as in the extra hepatic tissues (24%) (Nordlinger et al 1992). Recurrent disease in the liver post resection is potentially resectable and is associated with a

five year survival rate of 30% (Wanebo et al 1996a, Wanebo et al 1996b).

Staging

The role of preoperative imaging is to identify sites of disease in relation to the vascular anatomy of the liver as well as the exclusion of disease that renders the patient inoperable. Cross sectional imaging with CT, MRI and ultrasound are the method of choice in the elucidation of the vascular anatomy of the liver with nuclear medicine playing no direct role in this. A secondary role of preoperative imaging is in the demonstration of disease that renders the patient unresectable. In the best of centers, a significant number of patients who present for hepatic resection are found intraoperatively to have disease that if demonstrated initially would have led to a non-operative treatment plan (Jarnagin et al 1999). In a series reported by Scheele in 1995, the rates of resection with curative intent steadily increased between the years of 1960 and 1992 (Scheele et al 1995). There are a number of reasons for this, the first is more aggressive follow-up of patients leading to detection

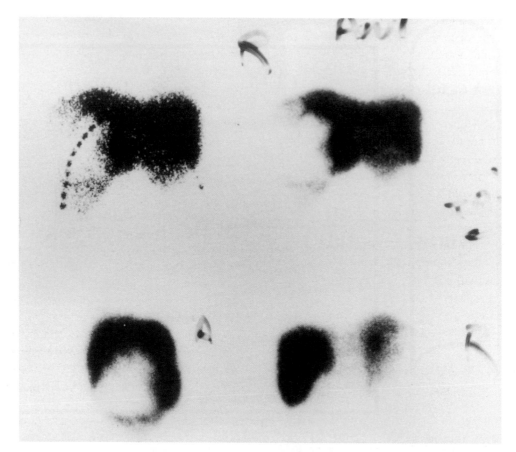

Fig. 14.4 This figure is of the first patient studied with F-18 FDG. This image is the Tc-99m sulfur colloid study demonstrating a large photopenic area in the right lobe of the liver. The black dots in the upper left panel are the markers over the lower border of the right ribs. The upper left panel is a short duration anterior marker view, the right upper panel is the formal anterior view, the lower left view is the right lateral view, the lower right panel is the posterior view, the spleen is seen on the left. (Yonekura et al 1982)

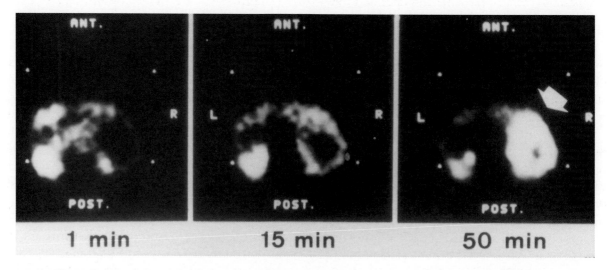

Fig. 14.5 This image is a transaxial slice of the same patient as Fig. 14.4 (viewed from above, so that the arrow in the right panel is pointing to the FDG avid metastasis). (Images 4 and 5 courtesy of Dr Samuel Yeh MD).

of disease at an earlier stage. A second reason is continued improvements in preoperative staging with more unresectable disease being found prior to surgery and finally improvements in operative technique as well as postoperative care.

The field of medical imaging is rapidly evolving with new approaches being developed, including new contrast agents, new machines with improved resolution and image display. It is very difficult to directly compare most of the studies in the literature as a variety of imaging techniques are reported each with their own gold standard. When there is a new technique with an increment in detection rate the initial reports published always report sensitivity rates of close to 100% as the new technique often becomes its own gold standard. There is always a trade off between sensitivity and specificity in any test with improvements in sensitivity being at the expense of specificity. Assessments of resectability are also difficult since surgeons vary in their judgement as to the limits of resection.

DETECTION OF LIVER METASTASES FROM COLORECTAL CANCER

Conventional imaging

In the detection of liver metastases that were confirmed with surgery, initial reports comparing MRI with Computed Tomographic Arterial Portography (CTAP) found the metastasis detection rate (sensitivity) was 94% (35 of 37) for CTAP and 78% (29 of 37) for high field strength MRI (Soyer et al 1993). Similar results have been reported with superparamagnetic iron oxide (SPIO)-enhanced MR combined with plain MR imaging versus CTAP (Strotzer et al 1997). The addition of SPIO-enhanced MR imaging at 1.5 T appears to increase the detection rates up to 99% of

lesions found pre-operatively but when compared to intraoperative ultrasound and post-resection pathology the detection rate fell to 56% (Hagspiel et al 1995). The high sensitivity of CTAP comes at a cost, as it is invasive, expensive and has a high false positive rate lowering the positive predictive value to levels around 79 (Lencioni et al 1998). A combined approach using CTAP as well as intraoperative ultrasound has been advocated by some and is a reasonable compromise where no other modalities are available.

FDG PET (Figs. 14.6–14.16)

The typical FDG-PET study is performed as a screening procedure with a scan performed of the whole body in an attempt to find as many sites of disease as possible. The typical FDG-PET study of the whole body takes 60–90 minutes depending on the machine used. The amount of time spent imaging the liver alone is between 10 and 20 minutes. If an acquisition of the liver was performed for an hour the accuracy of the PET will improve over the values reported in the literature. Nevertheless FDG PET imaging performs remarkably well with an extraordinarily good safety profile with no adverse effects reported in over 81 000 doses administered over a 4-year period in 22 centers (Silberstein, 1998).

DETECTION OF HEPATIC METASTASES (see Table 14.2)

A head to head retrospective comparison of CT versus FDG-PET clinical readings demonstrated an advantage of FDG PET over CT. The values reported were $n = 58$ with 23 with disease, FDG-PET sensitivity 95%, specificity 100% compared with CT 74% and 85% (Ogunbiyi et al 1997).

Table 14.2 FDG and the detection of hepatic disease

	Patients with disease	PET Sens.	PET Spec.	PET Acc.	CT Sens.	CT Spec.	CT Acc.	CTAP Sens.	CTAP Spec.	CTAP Acc.
Ogunbiyi et al 1997	23/58	95	100		74	85				
*Flamen et al 1999	45/103	99	100	99	93	95	94			
Lai et al 1996	27/34	89	67	85	100	14	82			
†Vitola et al 1996b	19/24	90	100	93	86	58	76	97	9	76
†Delbeke et al 1997	?/61	91	96	92	81	60	78	97	5	80
‡Schiepers et al 1995	34/80	94	100	98	85	98	93			
Valk et al 1998	57/118	95	100	97	84	95	90			

All studies used surgical findings, pathology and/or clinical follow-up of at least 1 year as the gold standard
* Equivocal lesions treated as negative
† Lesion by lesion analysis
‡ A combination of ultrasound and CT used as the comparative conventional tests

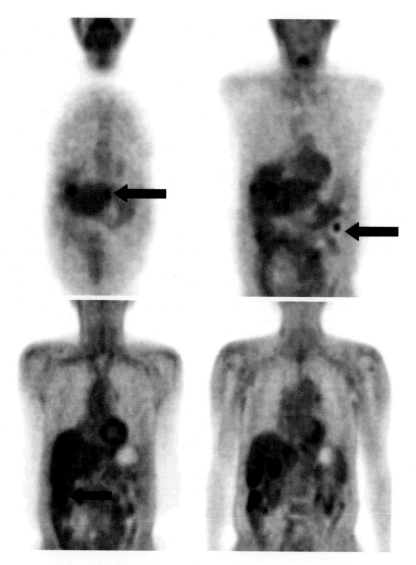

Fig. 14.6 This 74-year-old man with colorectal cancer synchronously metastatic to his liver was referred for assessment of FDG metabolism to assess for possible localized treatment to the liver. Increased FDG metabolism was seen in at least 8 sites within both lobes of the liver, consistent with multiple liver metastases. A further focus of abnormal FDG metabolism is seen in the left upper quadrant, consistent with an omental deposit as well as at the hepatic flexure, consistent with a probable anastomotic recurrence. A prior CT revealed liver disease only. As a result of this scan the patient underwent systemic chemotherapy.

The limitations of this study are its retrospective nature and the lack of information regarding the use of intravenous contrast, in addition the FDG-PET scans were read with knowledge of the CT while that converse may not have been true. A further report of 34 patients with colorectal cancer that was potentially resectable compared CT with contrast to FDG PET, this revealed FDG PET sensitivity 89%, specificity 67% compared with CT 100 and 14% giving overall accuracy FDG PET of 85% versus 82% for CT (Lai et al 1996). A further series of 24 patients of whom 19 had liver metastases compared CT, CTAP and FDG PET on a lesion by lesion basis. In terms of accuracy, FDG PET performed better than the radiological methods: 93% compared to 76% for both CT and CTAP. The reason the more sensitive CTAP performs worse than FDG PET is because the specificity of CTAP is only 9%. Similar findings were reported by a separate group; FDG-PET accuracy 92% compared to CTAP and CT accuracy of 80 and 78% respectively. The low specificity of CTAP (5%) again worked to the detriment of CTAP (Delbeke et al 1997).

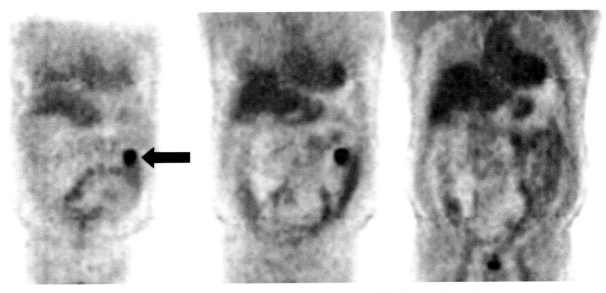

Fig. 14.7 This 49-year-old male with colon carcinoma was sent for evaluation of rising CEA following resection of his primary tumor. Two coronal views of the FDG-PET scan. Workup, including CT abdomen and pelvis was negative. At operation performed 6 weeks later a solitary metastasis was found in the jejunal mesentery, 4.5 × 4.0 × 2 cm in size. The arrow demonstrates the jejunal mesenteric metastasis.

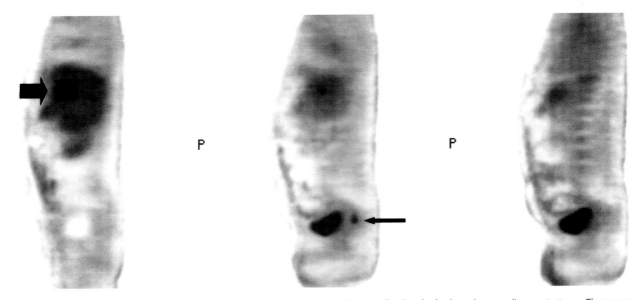

Fig. 14.8 This 66-year-old man underwent a low anterior resection in October 1996, at the time he had synchronous liver metastases. These were resected in November 1996. In December of 1996 he underwent 5FU-leukovorin chemotherapy for one year and pelvic radiotherapy. His CEA had been progressively rising, and he has been found to have liver metastasis. He was referred with a view to hepatic cryotherapy. The FDG-PET scan reveals a presacral pelvic recurrence (biopsy proven) (small arrow) as well as the known liver metastasis (large arrow).

DETECTION OF EXTRA-HEPATIC DISEASE

There has been a remarkable consistency in the rate that FDG PET alters the pre-operative stage of a patient following standard of care pre-operative diagnostic imaging (Table 14.3). In a wide variety of tumors, including colorectal cancer, about 30% of patients conventionally staged will have their treatment plans altered as a result of an FDG PET scan. A report of 34 patients with potentially resectable hepatic disease by Lai (Lai et al 1996), found retroperitoneal nodal metastases in six cases, pulmonary metastases in 3 cases and locoregional recurrences in two cases. One patient had unexpected disease in two sites leading to a total of ten of 34 patients (29%) in whom FDG PET had an influence on clinical management. The experience at MSKCC in the preoperative assessment of patients at high risk of recurrence following hepatic resection of colorectal cancer is very similar. We found nine of 40 cases (23%) had their management radically altered due to FDG PET findings of extensive unresectable disease, with another seven cases' management being influenced by the FDG PET findings confirming isolated, resectable, extra-hepatic disease giving a total of 40% patients in whom management was influenced. (Figs 14.6–14.14)

A real strength of FDG PET is therefore its ability to detect extra-hepatic disease and alter the surgical plan for the patient. Most if not all lesions detected with FDG PET are within the resolution of conventional imaging modalities and should theoretically be detectable but lesions are either not recognized as being abnormal ('missed') or appear normal. One reason why FDG PET performs so well is the accelerated glucose metabolism of the tumors makes the tumor stand out against the background of normal tissue, just as the light of a match is easily discerned, even at a

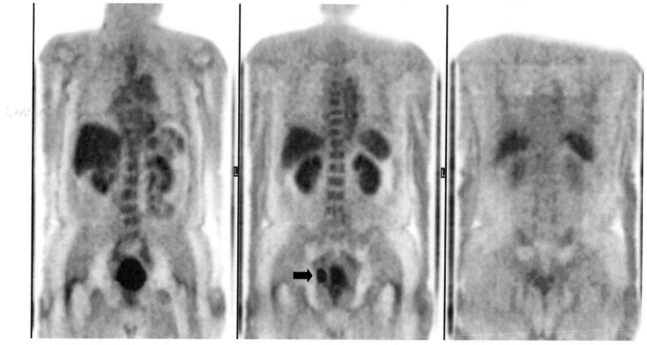

Fig. 14.9 This 57-year-old male was referred with a rising CEA. The patient underwent AP resection in 1996; he received 5FU-leukovorin in 10/97. An exploratory laparotomy in July 1998 was negative. The PET scan performed on 27th August 1998 showed an area in the posterior pelvis, beside the bladder (arrowed).

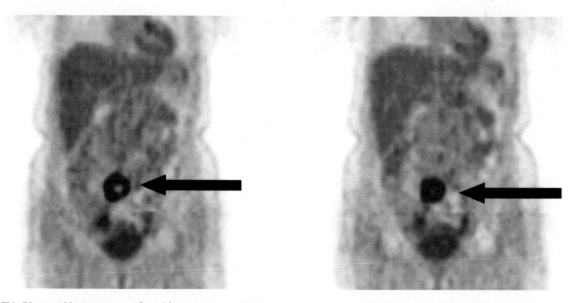

Fig. 14.10 This 59-year-old woman was referred for assessment of FDG metabolism in the setting of recurrent rectal cancer following surgery, radiation and chemotherapy. The scan reveals a large mass with partial necrosis within the peritoneum.

Table 14.3 The influence of FDG PET on patient management

	Number of patients considered for surgical resection	Percent in whom a change in management occurred as a result of FDG PET
Ogunbiyi et al 1997	23	43
Flamen et al 1999	37	11
Lai et al 1996	34	29
Vitola et al 1996b	24	25
*Delbeke et al 1997	61	28
†Schiepers et al 1995	76	26
Valk et al 1998	38	32

* All patients potential hepatic resection patients not reported separately
† Twenty-five unexpected lesions found in 20 patients

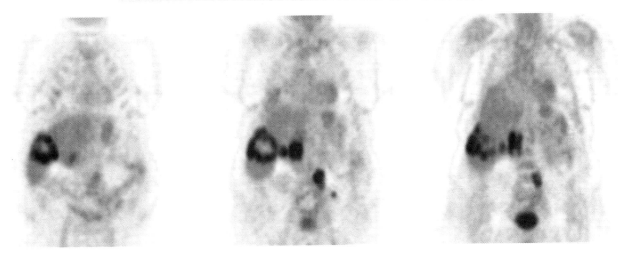

Fig. 14.11 This 74-year-old man presented in September 1997 with a T3N1 right colon ca invading his psoas muscle, he was treated with 5FU-leukovorin. The CT showed a caudate lesion, one lesion in segment 4 with questionable lesions elsewhere within the liver. The FDG-PET images demonstrate liver metastases with associated omental metastases.

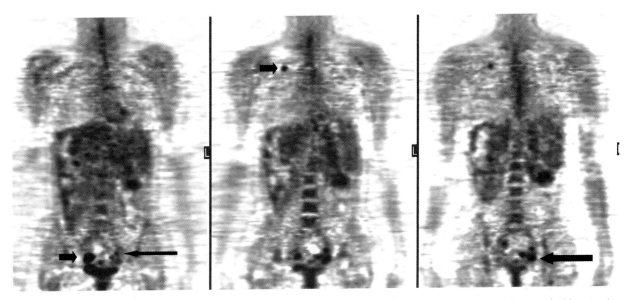

Fig. 14.12 This 31-year-old woman with colon cancer, status post-colon resection and right hepatectomy, recently treated with systemic and intra-arterial pump chemotherapy, with known pulmonary nodule, was referred for evaluation for possible resection of the right pulmonary nodule. The images demonstrate the right pulmonary nodule and pelvic recurrence of disease that was subsequently surgically confirmed. The liver reveals right lobe hypertrophy; the activity to the left of the liver is due to large bowel ptosed into the potential space left by the liver resection.

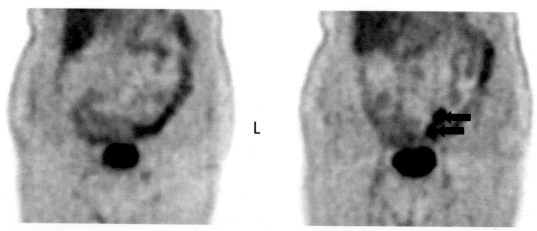

Fig. 14.13 Sixty-eight year-old woman with colon cancer, with a rising CEA with an equivocal CT for hepatic metastasis but no other disease. She has had no postoperative chemotherapy and feels well. The FDG-PET scan reveals two intraperitoneal lesions (arrowed) that were confirmed at operation.

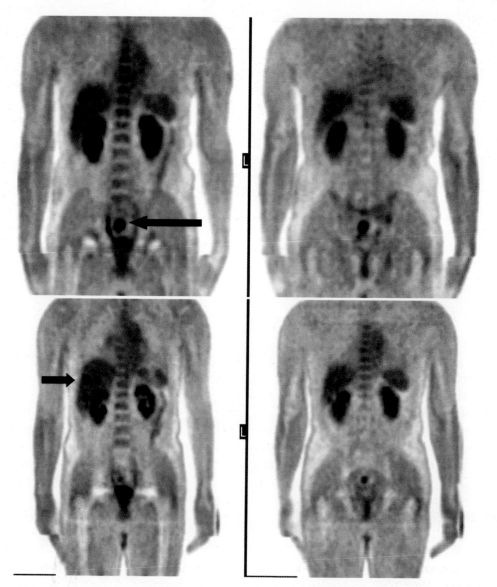

Fig. 14.14 This 59-year-old man with primary rectal cancer underwent two FDG-PET scans separated by chemotherapy with 5-fluorouracil and leukovorin and pelvic radiotherapy. The two top panels are the pre-treatment images and demonstrate the primary tumor with a local nodal metastasis in the top right panel and a liver metastasis seen lateral to the right kidney. The bottom panels demonstrate involution of the primary lesion but progression of the liver metastases.

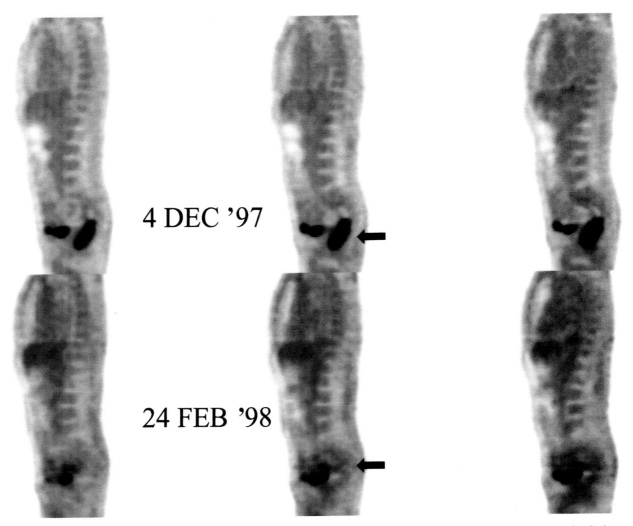

Fig. 14.15 This demonstrates the response of rectal cancer to the combination of chemotherapy with 5-fluorouracil and leukovorin and radiotherapy as a preoperative treatment.

distance, on a dark night. The effectiveness of FDG PET is its ability to demonstrate lesions mimicking a normal structure particularly intraperitoneal disease (Figs 14.7, 14.10, 14.12) that mimics unopacified loops of bowel as well as normal sized lymph nodes replaced by tumor. The influence of a finding of extra-hepatic disease depends on the approach to disease the treating clinician and the patient wish to undertake. Local pelvic recurrence if completely resectable should not necessarily stop a patient from undergoing hepatic resection. FDG PET is not a panacea however as an imaging study doesn't change the biology of a disease, and the fact that disease cannot be detected with FDG PET doesn't rule out micrometastatic disease. It is important in terms of informed consent that patients appreciate a workup including FDG PET doesn't rule out the later appearance of a distant metastasis.

EVALUATION OF PATIENTS POST-TREATMENT (Fig. 14.14, 14.15, 14.16)

There is a dearth of literature of the relative sensitivities of FDG PET and conventional imaging in the detection of recurrent intra-hepatic disease following liver surgery. There will be a group of patients post resection that will develop sub-phrenic abscesses that will be difficult to differentiate from recurrent tumor, however even in this situation FDG PET seems to perform well. In an initial report of seven patients who had previously undergone resection, PET correctly differentiated recurrent disease from post surgical change in all, CT misdiagnosed two of six with one false positive and one false negative with CTAP incorrect in three of five patients, all false positives (Vitola et al 1996b.

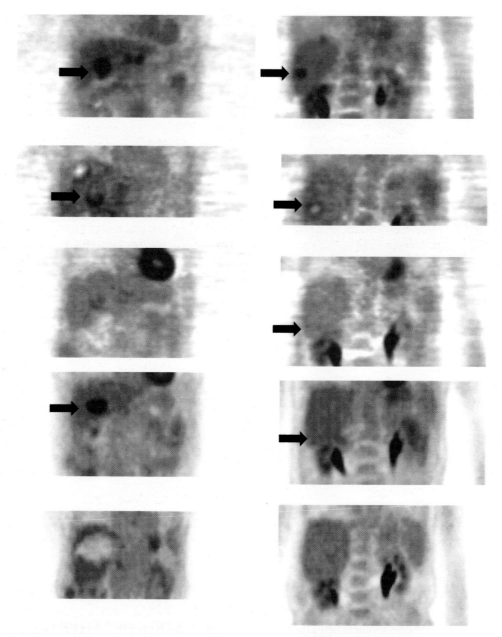

Fig. 14.16 This is a series of images performed on a 70-year-old patient with colorectal cancer metastatic to liver who underwent an FDG-PET study prior to intervention (first panel), immediately post cryotherapy (second panel), and while on hepatic artery pump therapy (third panel and fourth panel). The images show an incompletely cryotherapied lesion (arrowed) in the left column, which recurred, in comparison to an effectively cryotherapied lesion (arrowed) in the right column that did not recur. The bottom left panel reveals the resection cavity following resection of recurrence.

In the assessment of the effectiveness of chemoembolization FDG PET has been shown to be useful (Vitola et al 1996a), although an increment over CT and tumor markers has yet to be demonstrated.

Preliminary investigations suggest FDG PET performed within 24 hours post hepatic cryotherapy (Ch. 80) can predict sites of recurrent disease based on the pattern of FDG uptake (Akhurst et al 1999). This is a very exciting development as it helps clinicians identify those patients in whom cryotherapy has not been successful (Fig. 14.16). This is

particularly valuable as the early demonstration of potential treatment failure can assist in further treatment planning.

We have also been using FDG PET to follow patients who are being treated with hepatic artery infusaid pump therapy (Ch. 82). In both cases shown the information derived from the FDG PET scan would not have been obtainable from conventional imaging as the effects of cryotherapy persist on both CT and ultrasound leading to an inability to differentiate post treatment change from residual tumor.

In summary FDG PET alters pre-surgical staging in over 30% of cases that have had standard pre-operative testing. It appears to be at least as sensitive as conventional imaging in the detection of hepatic metastases, and more sensitive in the detection of extra-hepatic disease sites. FDG PET shows great promise in the evaluation of patients post treatment with particular reference to the detection of residual and recurrent disease (reflecting a failure of treatment and the biology of the disease respectively).

FDG PET IMAGING IN THE MANAGEMENT OF PATIENTS WITH HEPATOCELLULAR CARCINOMA (HCC)

DIAGNOSIS

In general the ease of lesion detection on imaging depends on the target to background ratio. The higher the target to background ratio, the easier it is to detect a lesion. A low grade lesion is likely to have a metabolic profile similar to the surrounding normal tissues. The liver is a homogeneous solid structure in terms of imaging. Therefore it is understandable that a lesion arising in liver from liver may be difficult to detect. This is in fact so with a number of reports demonstrating reduced efficiency of FDG PET in demonstrating HCC (Schroder et al 1998). A recent study aiming to evaluate FDG PET in the diagnosis of liver masses found all primary sarcomas and adenocarcinoma metastases and all cholangiocarcinomas had increased FDG uptake values but that seven of 23 patients with HCC had poor FDG uptake (Delbeke et al 1998). There is a sound pathophysiologic basis to this reduced efficacy as demonstrated by Torizuka et al in a study of HCC greater than 3 cm in size (Torizuka et al 1995). They demonstrated undifferentiated HCC had a pattern of continual FDG uptake shared by most solid tumors, whereas a moderately differentiated HCC demonstrated a pattern of uptake not dissimilar to the normal liver with an initial rise and then a slow fall. The difference in pattern was due to marked differences in the activity of transporters carrying glucose into the cell as well as hexokinase activity, but may also be due to a similarity between normal liver and HCC in terms of the rate of dephosphorylation of FDG-6 phosphate.

TREATMENT PLANNING AND ASSESSMENT OF PROGNOSIS

The survival rate of HCC patients seems to correlate with the degree of FDG uptake into the tumor with patients with low FDG uptake demonstrating a longer survival than those with high FDG uptake (Enomoto et al 1991). FDG uptake may correlate with the degree of expression of p53 (Schroder et al 1998), (Yoon et al 1998) a known factor in hepatocellular carcinogenesis (Hui et al 1998). In a similar fashion to other tumors FDG PET has been shown to be effective in monitoring Lipidol® chemoembolization (Torizuka et al 1994).

In summary FDG PET is of some value in the management of patients with HCC. The greatest utility will probably be in those cases in where the tumor is technically unresectable. In these cases a pretreatment scan will determine if FDG PET can detect the tumor and can then be used in therapeutic monitoring. If the primary is known to be FDG avid or tissue specimens demonstrate high levels of hexokinase activity, then a follow-up FDG scan may be useful in determining a site of recurrence or metastatic disease.

Cholangiocarcinoma

The detection of cholangiocarcinoma with endoscopic cholangiopancreatography (ERCP) in patients with primary sclerosing cholangitis can be difficult as the findings of the underlying disease may mimic those of tumor. Preliminary reports seem to indicate a potential role of FDG-PET imaging as they seem to be FDG avid (Keiding et al 1998, Delbeke et al 1998) although this may be limited to follow up assessment (Berr et al 1999).

Focal liver lesions

A focal liver lesion in a patient with a recent past history of colorectal cancer and a rising CEA will very likely be due to a metastasis, this in part explains the high success rates in detecting malignant disease reported by some groups (Delbeke et al 1998). In a separate group, FDG PET was not found to be useful in the characterization of liver masses in patients with chronic hepatitis C infection (Schroder et al 1998).

HEPATOBILIARY SCINTIGRAPHY

INTRODUCTION

Scintigraphic imaging of the hepatobiliary system aims to mimic the extraction of precursor of bile from the blood, the formation of bile and the excretion of bile into the bile ducts and gut. Iminodiacetic acid derivatives can be labeled with Tc-99m. These compounds are rapidly extracted from the circulation by hepatocytes and excreted into the biliary system without undergoing conjugation. The hepatic half-clearance time varies with the particular agent used

(Table 14.4) There is some renal excretion of iminodiacetic acid derivatives with proportionally increased renal excretion in hepatocellular dysfunction (Fig. 14.21).

Patient preparation is important in the performance and interpretation of hepatobiliary scintigraphy. Detailed clinical information is required for the proper interpretation of the studies. In order to image the gallbladder the patient should be fasting for between 2 and 24 hours. If a study is performed immediately post-prandially, the gallbladder will be contracted leading to non-visualization (Klingensmith et al 1981), with an over distended gallbladder leading to non-visualization in patients fasting for more than 24 hours (Larsen et al 1982).

NORMAL SCAN

A hepatobiliary study is usually acquired in a number of dynamic acquisitions, the immediate post-injection sequence is performed with rapid frame times (2–5 seconds duration) to assess perfusion (Fig. 14.17). The later images are acquired for a longer duration (2–5 minutes per frame)

Table 14.4 Iminodiacetic acid derivatives

Name	Liver half-clearance time (min)	Hepatic uptake %
m-Bromo-o-p trimethyl (Mebrofenin)	17	98
O-Diisopropyl (DISIDA)	19	88
O-Diethyl (EIDA)	37	82
O-Dimethyl (HIDA)	42	84
P-Isopropyl (PIPIDA)	59	85
P-n-Butyl (BIDA)	107	94

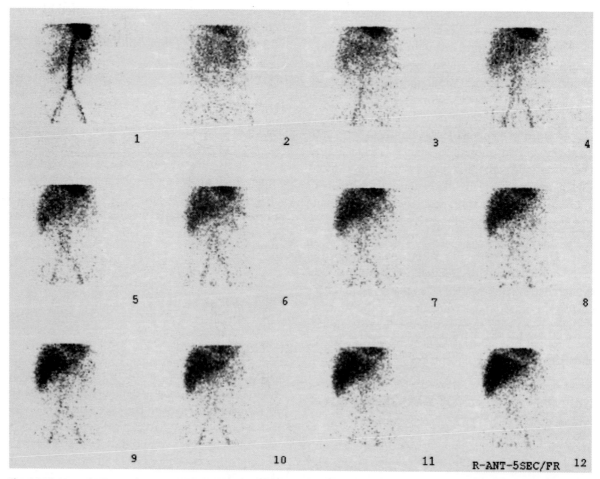

Fig. 14.17 Normal HIDA perfusion study demonstrating the biphasic influx of the tracer into the liver reflecting the dual blood supply of the liver. Note the relatively reduced uptake that coincides with the aortic activity.

to assess the uptake and excretory phase (Fig. 14.18). Right lateral and/or oblique images are often needed to distinguish gall bladder activity from underlying renal pelvis or duodenal activity (Fig. 14.19).

Following injection of the radiopharmaceutical (tracer) there is a biphasic influx of the tracer to the liver (Fig. 14.17). This reflects delivery of tracer from hepatic arterial and then portal circulation. The hepatocytes are efficient at extracting the tracer so there is rapid uptake of the tracer leading to hepatic uptake rapidly exceeding that of the cardiac blood pool. The hepatic activity reaches a peak at about 10 minutes post injection. The hepatocytes clear the tracer

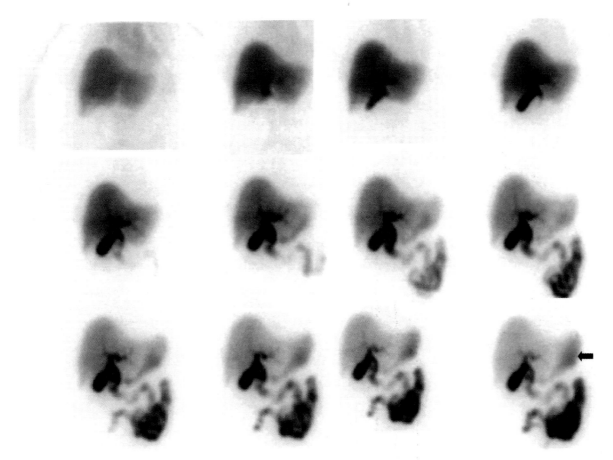

Fig. 14.18 Normal HIDA study demonstrating free passage of the tracer into the proximal bile ducts and gallbladder with subsequent free drainage into the gut. The images are acquired in the anterior projection 5 minutes apart for one hour. Note the reflux of bile into the stomach (arrowed) seen after 30 minutes and reaching a peak at 55 minutes.

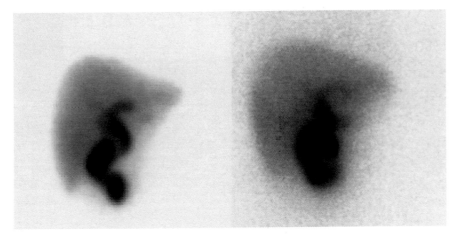

Fig. 14.19 This study demonstrates the benefit of a right anterior oblique view in separating the gallbladder and renal pelvis. Images acquired 60 minutes post injection.

into the biliary canuliculi and within 30 minutes the right and left hepatic ducts as well as the common hepatic duct can be seen (although such detail may not be seen in very small infants). The gallbladder is seen in 90% of normals within 30 minutes post injection with 100% being seen within 1 hour. The bowel is seen in 80% of normals within 60 minutes. The remaining 20% of patients eventually drain to the gut with delayed drainage either due to mild dehydration or mildly increased sphincter of Oddi dysfunction. In those patients who have had a cholecystectomy the gut can usually be seen by 20 minutes in most patients (Fig. 14.20) (Sostre et al 1992b). Bile reflux into the stomach can often be seen (Figs 14.18 and 14.22). If a patient has a contracted gallbladder as is often seen in chronic cholecystitis, the gallbladder filling may be delayed (Fig. 14.23).

AUGMENTED HEPATOBILIARY SCINTIGRAPHY

A number of drugs affect the function of the hepatobiliary tree and are used to improve the diagnostic efficacy of hepatobiliary scintigraphy. Phenobarbital is used to increase the production of bile in infants to improve the diagnostic accuracy of the test in cases of neonatal jaundice. Cholecystokinin (CCK) infusion leads to increased bile flow, contraction of the gallbladder and relaxation of the sphincter of Oddi, nitroglycerin relaxes (Staritz 1988) and morphine contracts the sphincter of Oddi (this effect is promptly relieved by CCK or naloxone) (Helm et al 1988, Patch et al 1991). The duration of rise of pancreatic CCK levels secreted in response to a fatty meal are much longer than the effects of infusion. A repeat dose of CCK given after a CCK infusion given as a premedication leads to an equivalent gallbladder ejection of bile. This means patients who have had a prolonged fast can have one injection to empty the gallbladder to enable subsequent filling and a later injection to assess gallbladder ejection fraction in the same sitting with no loss of diagnostic accuracy. (Sostre et al 1992a).

RIGHT UPPER QUADRANT PAIN

The differential diagnosis of right upper quadrant pain is beyond the scope of this chapter, but hepatobiliary scintigraphy has a role in the assessment of both acute and chronic

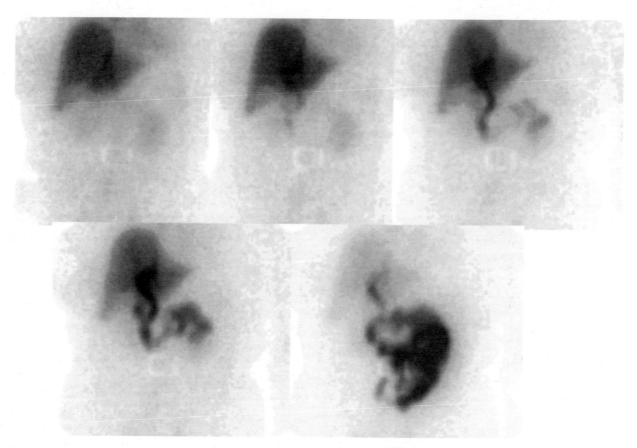

Fig. 14.20 This study demonstrates rapid transit into the gut post cholecystectomy; the intestines are seen 10 minutes post injection. Images acquired 2, 5, 10, 15 and 60 minutes post injection.

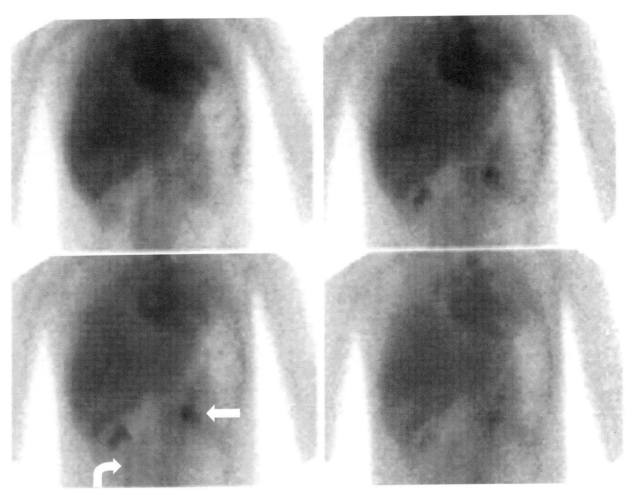

Fig. 14.21 This study demonstrates severe hepatocellular dysfunction with the kidneys exhibiting increased clearance of the tracer. Note the parallel reduction in activity in the cardiac blood pool and the liver. The two bright foci beneath the liver are due to activity in the pelvis of the right and left kidneys. The straight arrow is pointing to the left renal pelvis, the curved arrow points to the right ureter. Images acquired at 2, 15, 25 and 60 minutes post injection.

right upper quadrant pain. There has been a 30% increase in the number of cholecystectomies performed over the last 10 years. An even more interesting phenomenon is the change in the spread of indications, with rates of operations for biliary dyskinesia, acute acalculous cholecystitis and chronic acalculous cholecystitis increasing 348, 139, 138% respectively in the same time frame (Johanning & Gruenberg 1998). This study was a review of ICD-9 discharge codes and may be in part due to a reporting bias as these disease states become more widely appreciated but more probably due to the reduced morbidity of the laparoscopic operative procedure. It should be remembered that preoperative testing with biliary scintigraphy predicts those patients with acalculous biliary pain (Ch. 6) who are likely to benefit from cholecystectomy (Reed et al 1993, Goncalves et al 1998) and should be performed in this group (Barron & Rubio 1995). (See below.)

Cholecystitis

The diagnosis of acute cholecystitis is largely clinical, however ancillary tests are often performed to increase clinical confidence prior to surgery. The two competing imaging tests are ultrasound and hepatobiliary scintigraphy. The key finding on hepatobiliary imaging is non-visualization of the gallbladder (Fig 14.22). Sensitivity rates of over 96% have been consistently reported by many groups (Freitas et al 1982, Szlabick et al 1980, Suarez et al 1980, Velasco et al 1982). An additional finding of a hot rim around the gallbladder fossa is also strongly associated with a diagnosis of acute cholecystitis (Cawthon et al 1984) but is not 100% specific as had previously been thought (Oates et al 1996). The specificity of unaugmented hepatobiliary scintigraphy is lower however as prolonged fasting may lead to nonvisualization of the gallbladder. This has led to many investigators

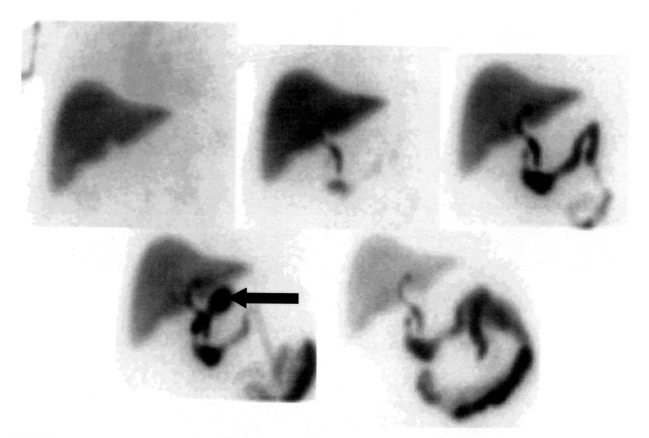

Fig. 14.22 This study reveals non-visualization of the gallbladder even after administration of morphine. Pathology revealed acute cholecystitis. (Images acquired 10, 30, 40 and 60 minutes post injection of tracer and 20 minutes post morphine). The 60-minute image reveals refluxed activity in the stomach (arrowed).

routinely using morphine augmentation (Choy et al 1984) and/or CCK pretreatment (Eikman et al 1975) to increase biliary tree pressure and demonstrate cystic duct patency. The addition of this step increases the specificity of hepatobiliary scintigraphy (Choy et al 1984, Fink-Bennett et al 1991a, Chen et al 1997, Cabana et al 1995) over and above delayed imaging (an example of which is shown in Fig. 14.19) (Kim et al 1993). Morphine augmented hepatobiliary scintigraphy in the detection of acute cholecystitis has sensitivity, specificity, positive and negative predictive values of 95, 99, 97, and 98%, respectively (Fink-Bennett et al 1991a). These figures compare favorably with ultrasound and it appears hepatobiliary scintigraphy is the diagnostic test of choice in the diagnosis of acute cholecystitis (Shea et al 1994).

Ultrasound relies on a combination of sonographic findings including the presence of stones, gallbladder-wall thickening, peri-gallbladder fluid, a positive Murphy's sign over the gallbladder fossa rather than demonstration of cystic duct obstruction itself (Lauritsen et al 1988, Dykes et al 1986, van Weelde et al 1986, Soiva et al 1986, Samuels et al 1983).

Chronic cholecystitis

In this group of patients the critical imaging finding is the presence of cholelithiasis and this is best demonstrated with ultrasound (Shea et al 1994). The majority of patients with chronic cholecystitis demonstrate cystic duct patency. Delayed filling of the gallbladder is associated with chronic cholecystitis but this is a non-specific finding as fasting may give the same appearance (Fig. 14.23). Ultrasound remains the diagnostic test of choice in the detection of chronic cholecystitis.

Chronic acalculous right upper quadrant pain

Chronic acalculous disorders of the biliary tree comprise acalculous cholecystitis, cystic duct syndrome, sphincter of Oddi dysfunction, and gallbladder dsykinesia.

Acalculous cholecystitis and the cystic duct syndrome

Cystic duct syndrome is defined as fibrotic narrowing of the cystic duct lumen by 60%, and/or kinking or adhesions of

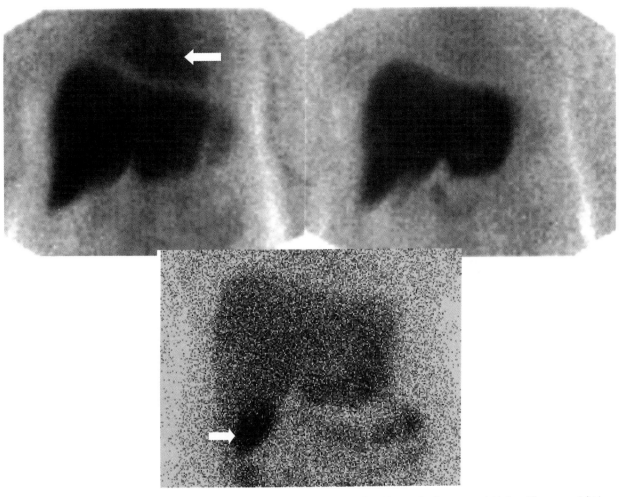

Fig. 14.23 Delayed gallbladder demonstration: the left-facing arrow outlines blood-pool activity at 10 minutes post injection. The upper right image demonstrates non-visualization of the gallbladder at 60 minutes post injection, the 4-hour image demonstrates the gallbladder (right facing arrow). Note the 6-hour half-life of Tc-99m and biologic clearance of the tracer leads to a reduction in counts acquired in time leading to a more 'grainy' image at 4 hours.

the duct seen at surgery. Chronic cholecystitis is defined pathologically as hypertrophy of the gallbladder wall (> 1.5–2 mm thick), the presence of Aschoff–Rokitansky sinuses, a mononuclear infiltrate, foamy macrophages, diffuse muscularis hypertrophy and yellow papillary nodules (Fink-Bennett et al 1991b). Using a standardized protocol of CCK infusion (0.2 ng/kg administered over 3 minutes) a normal range for the ejection of bile from the gallbladder has been established. Fink-Bennett et al studied this group in detail. Those patients with reduced gallbladder ejection fraction (GBEF) (< 35% ejected in the first 20 minutes post CCK infusion) were considered abnormal. Of those patients with an abnormal gall bladder ejection fraction, 108 of 115 (94%) had either cystic duct narrowing or chronic cholecystitis on pathology (with only one of 106 who had follow up reporting no amelioration of symptoms), and 69 of 78 (88%) who were medically managed have had continued symptoms suggestive of biliary colic. This suggests the find-

ing of reduced gallbladder ejection fraction in response to CCK is a strong indicator of the need for surgical intervention. Only seven (6%) of the 115 with histopathologic confirmation of disease had a gallbladder ejection fraction of > 35% being a false negative result. The negative predictive value of a normal gallbladder ejection fraction is 91% with 130 of 143 of those patients with improvement post-treatment for non-gallbladder pathology having a GBEF > 35% (Fink-Bennett et al 1991b).

The post cholecystectomy syndrome-Sphincter of Oddi dysfunction

A significant proportion of patients subjected to cholecystectomy will suffer continued pain post operatively (Ch. 43), many will be diagnosed as having irritable bowel syndrome, pancreatitis, gastritis, and esophagitis but about 6% have unexplained pain. Sphincter manometry is considered one of the main objective tests for the presence of sphincter of Oddi dysfunction (SOD) (Ch. 6).

The overall incidence of pancreatitis in patients undergoing ERCP manometry alone has been reported as being 9.3% with a 26% incidence if sphincterotomy is combined with manometry (Maldonado et al 1999). The high rate of this side-effect is acting as a continued stimulus to investigate non-invasive methods of diagnosing SOD. Augmented hepatobiliary scintigraphy is a promising method in the non-invasive diagnosis of SOD. The most common abnormal finding with hepatobiliary scintigraphy is an obstructive pattern of biliary drainage, but some patients who have no symptoms at the time of the examination will have a normal study. A variety of criteria for analysis have been developed using quantitative hepatobiliary scintigraphy (Roberts-Thomson et al 1986). Augmentation techniques include an improvement in biliary drainage following amyl nitrate therapy (Madacsy et al 1994) to exclude a fixed stenosis (that will not respond to drug therapy) and the development of an obstructive pattern with prostigmine-morphine administration (Madacsy et al 1995). Madacsy suggests only those with prostigmine-morphine induced obstruction should undergo manometry (Madacsy et al 1995).

BILIARY TRACT COMPLICATIONS FOLLOWING SURGERY (Figs 14.24–14.29)

The complication rates of laparoscopic cholecystectomy fall as the number of cases performed by a particular surgical group increases (Walker et al 1993). Hepatobiliary scintigraphy is a powerful, noninvasive tool in the detection of bile leak and iatrogenic biliary obstruction (Reichelt, 1978).

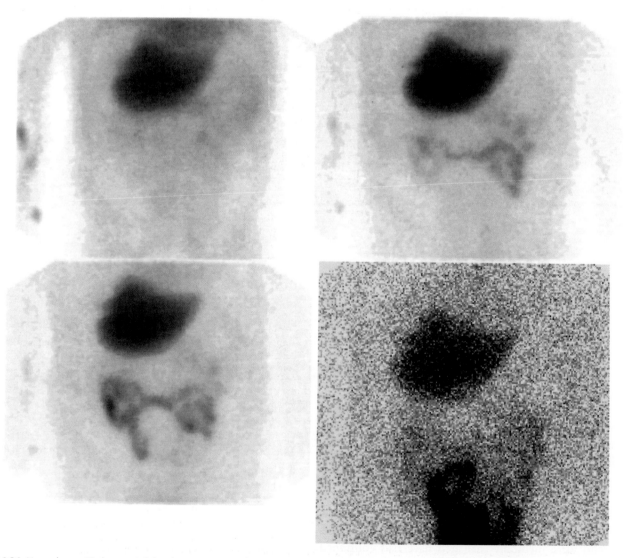

Fig. 14.24 Normal scan 12 days post right trisegmentectomy images acquired at 0, 30, 60 minutes and 3.5 hours post injection.

When there is a clinical suspicion of a bile duct injury post surgery (Ch. 49), hepatobiliary imaging should be one of the first tests considered. The degree of leak can be assessed and this can assist in the triaging of patients with bile leak towards conservative or operative repair. After bile drainage has been achieved a follow up scan can assist in the triaging of patients who require further intervention (Walker et al 1992).

Improved disease-free survival following hepatic resection of metastases has led to an increase in the complexity and aggressiveness of hepatic resection, including complex operations involving the biliary tree. Hepatobiliary scintigraphy can assess efficacy of biliary drainage following these complex procedures.

LIVER TRANSPLANTATION

The major role of hepatobiliary imaging in liver transplant patients is in the post-operative assessment of the presence or absence of bile duct injury (Ch. 115) (Mochizuki et al 1991). The noninvasive assessment of the integrity of a bile duct anastomosis is best performed by hepatobiliary scintigraphy, as conventional imaging cannot characterize the nature of ascitic fluid. Bile duct stenoses do occur and these are also well demonstrated with scintigraphy. Acute vascular rejection is an uncommon event in liver transplantation but scintigraphy is able to noninvasively assess perfusion (Williams et al 1985). Preservation injury or peri-transplantation infarction is demonstrable on scintigraphy and may give the clinician a feel for the expected level of function expected from the graft (Karademir et al 1994) but such information is unlikely to change post transplant treatment. Cholestasis and rejection are two common problems post transplantation and unfortunately the two overlap in terms of their scintigraphic appearance (Engeler et al 1992), this had led to many units not including scintigraphy in their post operative assessment. Attempts at further analyzing the information within the hepatobiliary scan in an attempt to

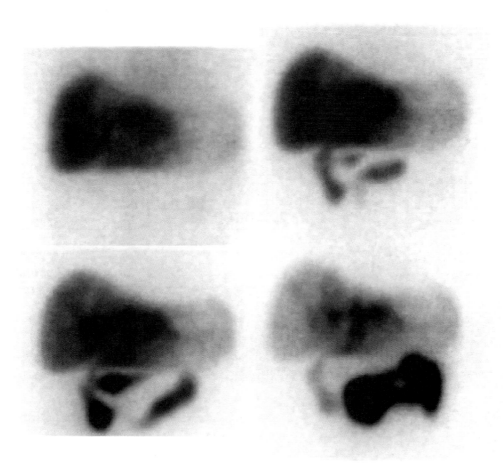

Fig. 14.25 This 47-year-old male with hypereosinophilic syndrome, status post right liver lobectomy for liver abscess is referred to rule out biliary obstruction and to evaluate the segmental drainage, 0, 10, 20 and 60 minutes post injection. The images demonstrate impaired drainage of the left ductal system with bile duct retention; ultrasound demonstrated bile duct stones. The patient required percutaneous drainage.

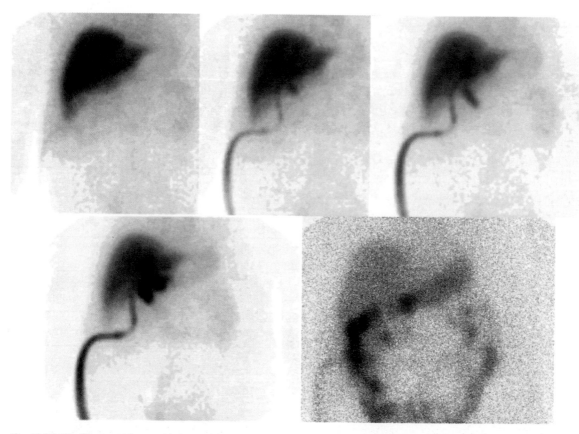

Fig. 14.26 This 70-year-old man with inoperable duodenal carcinoma had persistent bile drainage into the intraperitoneal drain tube inserted intra-operatively. The study reveals free passage of bile out of the drain tube with some drainage into the bowel. Images acquired 20, 30, 40 and 60 minutes and 3.5 hours post injection.

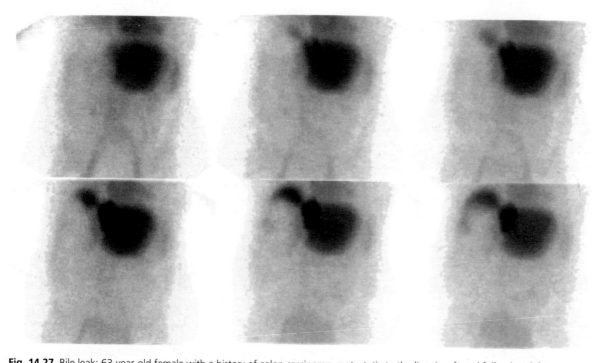

Fig. 14.27 Bile leak: 63-year-old female with a history of colon carcinoma, metastatic to the liver is referred following right trisegmentectomy for assessment of bile leak. The images demonstrate leakage from the anastomosis with tracking of the isotope into the right subphrenic space. The images presented are 10 minutes apart acquired over 1 hour.

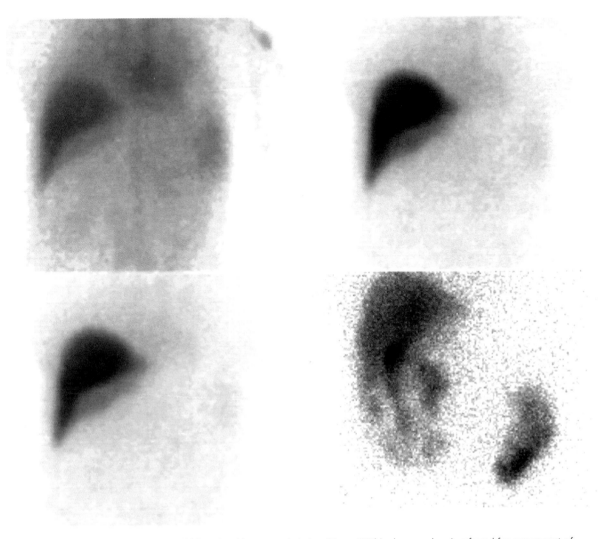

Fig. 14.28 Biliary obstruction: 40-year-old female with repeated cholangitis post Whipple procedure is referred for assessment of possible obstruction. Following this study an 8.5 French biliary drainage catheter was placed across a 1.5-cm high-grade bilio-enteric obstruction. Images 0, 30, 60 minutes and 3 hours post injection.

more accurately assess transplant viability have been promoted by some but have not become widely used (Brown et al 1988, Tagge et al 1987, Shah et al 1995). A normal study effectively excludes rejection or severe cholestasis but this information is unlikely to be additive to other simpler tests. Nuclear medicine studies are useful in the assessment of immunosuppressed patients with pyrexia of unknown origin.

HEPATOCELLULAR CARCINOMA

Hepatocellular carcinoma (HCC) has a variable pattern of uptake seen with hepatobiliary tracers. A poorly differentiated HCC appears as a cold lesion. A well-differentiated HCC typically exhibits retention of the tracer on delayed images performed 2–3 hours post injection (the normal liver having cleared). Therefore sequential studies can be

used to follow well-differentiated HCC if that was the course the clinician and patient wished to undertake. Focal nodular hyperplasia is the differential of focal retention of tracer, but an image at 5–10 minutes post injection should differentiate between FNH (iso-intense with normal liver) and HCC that usually is hypo-intense.

PEDIATRIC IMAGING

Neonatal jaundice

The task of the physician faced with a child who is jaundiced is to determine the etiology in order to determine whether intervention is required. The majority of cases of neonatal jaundice are due to physiologic jaundice of the newborn, breast milk jaundice and less commonly erythroblastosis

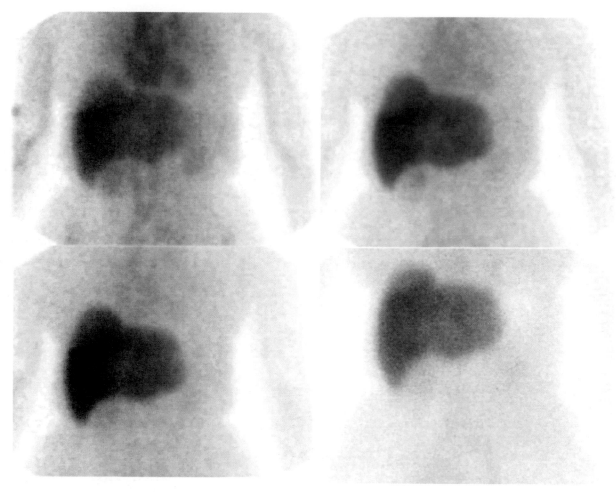

Fig. 14.29 Complete biliary obstruction. The images are immediately, 30, 60 minutes and 3 hours post-injection; note the lack of biliary excretion and the breast shadow over the right lobe of the liver.

fetalis. Idiopathic neonatal hepatitis is rare, as is biliary atresia (Ch. 47). Both of these conditions result in prolonged either mixed or conjugated hyperbilirubinemia (direct bilirubin of > 15%). Early diagnosis of biliary atresia is important because untreated biliary atresia leads to the development of cirrhosis and liver failure and an average untreated survival of 12 months (Emblem et al 1994). The differentiation of neonatal hepatitis and biliary atresia is difficult on clinical grounds and on occasion at liver biopsy (Manolaki et al 1983).

Biliary atresia

The differentiation of biliary atresia (Ch. 47) and neonatal hepatitis on histopathological grounds depends on the presence of ductal proliferation and portal fibrosis both of which may take some time to develop, and lead to reduced accuracy if the biopsy is performed too soon after birth.

The diagnosis of biliary atresia using hepatobiliary scintig-

raphy is primarily based on non-visualization of the gut at 24 hours but a secondary criteria of rapid uptake of the tracer into the liver without biliary excretion also suggests the presence of biliary atresia. Idiopathic neonatal hepatitis is characterized by impaired uptake of the tracer by the liver with slow hepatic clearance of the tracer that occurs in parallel to cardiac blood pool—due to renal excretion (this finding is mimicked by biliary atresia as cirrhosis develops leading to impaired hepatocyte extraction of the tracer). Therefore it is advisable to perform hepatobiliary imaging before 3 months of age to reduce the likelihood of the development of cirrhosis. Premedication with phenobarbital (5 mg/kg/day for 5 days) leads to increased bile flow and therefore improved specificity of the test as it reduces the number of cases where the gut is not visualized. The differential diagnosis of non-visualization of the gut at 24 hours is biliary atresia, bile plug syndrome, cystic fibrosis or severe hepatocellular dysfunction due to idiopathic neonatal hepatitis, total parenteral nutrition (Cooper et al 1985), infectious hepatitis, or septo-optic dysplasia (Kumura et al 1987). Bile plug syndrome is seen in dehydrated, septic infants. The characteristic scintigraphic features of this syndrome are excretion of the tracer into a dilated proximal biliary tract without gut excretion.

The diagnosis of biliary atresia on ultrasound is based on a number of ultrasonic features including inability to see a gallbladder, a hypoplastic gallbladder and no change in gallbladder size with food, and a new feature 'the triangular cord'. The triangular cord sign recently reported in a number of papers by a single group appears to have high sensitivity, specificity and accuracy (85 100 and 95% respectively) (Choi et al 1996, Park et al 1997, Choi et al 1998). The reported efficacy of DISIDA scanning (sensitivity 96%, specificity 35%, accuracy 56%) by this group is less than most other literature. A sensitivity rate of 85% of ultrasound utilizing this criteria alone however translates into 15% of infants with biliary atresia having a delayed surgical procedure so a combined approach would seem appropriate as the authors suggest. Ultrasound is a good initial test and is useful in ruling out the presence of a choledochal cyst, which may also present with neonatal jaundice. Hepatobiliary scintigraphy in such a case is useful if it demonstrates filling of the cyst with bile (Fig. 14.30).

Lin et al directly compared ultrasound with hepatobiliary scintigraphy with phenobarbital and cholestyramine premedication in a group of 66 patients with neonatal jaundice. The diagnostic sensitivity, specificity, and accuracy of scintigraphy in differentiating biliary atresia from other forms of neonatal jaundice of 100, 87.5, and 90.5%, respectively, compared to ultrasound results of 86.7, 77.1, and 79.4%, respectively (Lin et al 1997). Premedication with oral phenobarbital increases test accuracy by accelerating biliary excretion (Majd et al 1981a, Majd et al 1981b). Reduced specificity of hepatobiliary scintigraphy is seen if the child's birthweight is less than 2200 g (Spivak et al 1987).

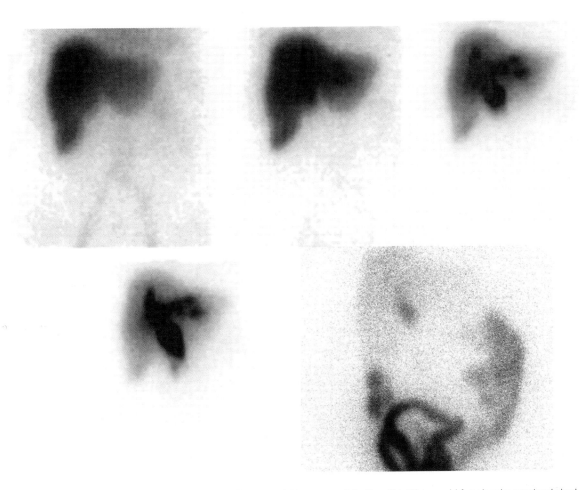

Fig. 14.30 Choledochal cyst: images 0, 20, 40, 60 minutes and 4 hours post injection. This 70-year-old female who previously had undergone a cholecystectomy was referred for assessment of a possible choledochal cyst. The study reveals a large bile-filled structure beneath the hepatic hilum consistent with a choledochal cyst.

SUMMARY

Hepatobiliary scintigraphy is the diagnostic test of choice in the diagnosis of cystic duct obstruction, predicts response to cholecystectomy in those patients with acalculous biliary pain, and plays a vital role in the assessment of patients with biliary tract injury and neonatal jaundice.

THE ROLE OF GENERAL NUCLEAR MEDICINE IN THE ASSESSMENT OF ADULTS WITH MALIGNANT DISEASE OF THE LIVER AND HEPATOBILIARY TREE

PREOPERATIVE ASSESSMENT

Cardiac preoperative risk assessment

In those cases where there is a significant risk of coronary disease, it is prudent to perform preoperative testing in attempt to risk stratify the patients prior to major surgery. Clinical groups who have been recommended to undergo preoperative testing include those patients with two or more of: diabetes, prior congestive cardiac failure, prior myocardial infarction, Canadian class I or II angina, poor functional capacity (< 4 mets on a treadmill exercise test) or where there is going to be a prolonged surgical procedure with large fluid shifts and/or blood loss (Leppo & Dahlberg 1998).

Pre-operative testing with myocardial perfusion scintigraphy with either thallium-201 (Tl-201) or ^{99m}Tc based perfusion agents is a powerful predictor of peri-operative events. The initial reports of thallium scintigraphy demonstrated a high positive predictive value of the test in the order of 20%, however the positive predictive value has slowly fallen over time (Leppo & Dahlberg 1998). In part this may be due to changes in scanning protocols (SPECT versus planar acquisition) or due to physicians over-reading the scans to avoid possible litigation, as the biology of the disease is unlikely to have changed significantly. A negative test remains highly predictive > 99% of a cardiac event-free peri-operative period.

SULFUR-COLLOID IMAGING

Historical background

Before high resolution CT, ultrasound, MRI were developed, the initial imaging investigation to evaluate potential hepatic involvement with tumor was colloidal scintigraphy. The initial work was done with radiolabeled gold but this was supplanted by technetium-99m labeled colloids. The colloids when injected undergo phagocytosis by reticuloendothelial cells that are found in liver, spleen and bone marrow.

In the normal patient, approximately 90% of the injected dose of Tc-99m sulfur colloid is taken up by the liver with the spleen and bone marrow each accounting for 5% (Fig. 32). Sulfur colloid imaging has been used in the assessment of diffuse parenchymal disease of the liver, with ratios of liver to spleen and bone marrow, 'the colloid shift', being used to assess the degree of hepatocellular dysfunction. The finding of a hypertrophied caudate lobe raises strong suspicions of the presence of Budd–Chiari syndrome (Ch. 105). The advent of high speed CT and color-doppler ultrasound has reduced the demand for liver spleen imaging for the establishment of this diagnosis.

DIAGNOSIS OF MALIGNANCY

The typical appearance of a malignant deposit is a focal defect on Tc-99m colloid imaging, as metastases do not contain the phagocytic cells necessary for uptake of the radiopharmaceutical (Fig. 14.4). The appearances of a 'cold spot' on colloid imaging are not specific as hepatic cysts, hemangioma, hepatic adenoma, all may appear cold as they do not contain Küpffer cells (Table 14.5).

A solid lesion identified on cross sectional imaging that is not accompanied by a photopenic defect on sulfur colloid imaging is likely to be focal nodular hyperplasia (Sandler et al 1980) or the rare hepatoblastoma usually only seen in children (Tanasescu et al 1991). Hepatic adenoma that take up sulfur colloid are quite rare (Low & Khangure 1990) and usually are gallium avid.

Table 14.5 Cold defects on Tc-99 sulfur colloid imaging

Lesion	Explanation
'Hepatic pseudotumor'	Hepatic regeneration or scar in cirrhotic patients may or may not be hot
Acute radiation injury	Radiosensitive reticuloendothelial cells
Extra-hepatic masses	Deformation of normal liver
Simple cysts	No target cells in lesion
Polycystic liver disease	No target cells in lesion
Hemangioma	No target cells in lesion
Adenoma	Usually cold rare cases with uptake present have been reported
Hamartoma	No target cells in lesion
Hydatid cyst	No target cells in lesion
Focal nodular hyperplasia	Variably hot or cold as may contain reticuloendothelial cells

Hot lesions on Tc-99m sulfur colloid imaging	
Budd–Chiari syndrome	Typically caudate lobe hypertrophy
Cirrhosis	
Hepatoma	
Hemangioma	
Hamartoma	
Abscess	
Focal nodular hyperplasia	

Dual tracer studies

The relative low specificity of sulfur-colloid imaging led to the development of a variety of dual tracer studies involving gallium-67 citrate (Ga-67) (Beihn et al 1974, Rovekamp et al 1983), Tc-99m-labeled red cells as well as indium-111-labeled white cells (Fawcett et al 1985) and more recently thallium-201 (Mochizuki et al 1994). The principle of the dual tracer studies was to use tracers of known physiologic processes to add specificity to the colloid findings. Thallium-201 acts as a potassium analogue when injected intravenously, and accumulates in viable cells. It has been used for many years for myocardial scintigraphy, and following serendipitous uptake in a tumor has been investigated as a tumor-seeking agent. Subtraction imaging with Tl-201 and Tc-99m labeled colloids have been used in the assessment of HCC (Mochizuki et al 1994). Ga-67 citrate is a non-specific tumor-seeking agent whose efficacy is probably related to shared metabolic pathways with iron. A lesion negative on colloidal imaging but positive on labeled white cell scan is suggestive of abscess, a lesion positive on Ga-67 and negative with colloid imaging is more likely to be a hepatocellular cancer (given the absence of fever and other signs of infection). Serial gallium studies can be a useful follow-up tool in patients post resection of HCC (Serafini et al 1988).

The improvements in the image achievable with ultrasound, CT and MRI as well as the limits of resolution 1.5–2 cm of the tracer techniques have led to the gradual replacement of colloid imaging with conventional radiological investigations. If there are contraindications to biopsy or equivocal lesions, combined tracer studies remain a useful non-invasive technique.

HEMANGIOMA (Fig. 14.31)

A hepatic hemangioma is almost always negative on sulfur-colloid imaging. If a lesion suspicious for a hemangioma can

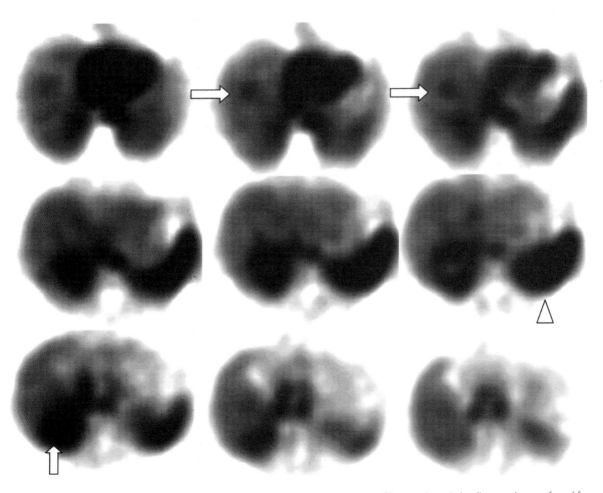

Fig. 14.31 This 52-year-old female with breast cancer was found to have lesions suggestive of hemangioma in her liver, and was referred for assessment. The images are sequential transaxial sections through the lower chest and upper abdomen. The study demonstrates the right and left ventricles in the top right image; the right facing arrows are pointing to a small hemangioma in the upper liver. The arrowhead is pointing to the spleen; the upward facing arrow is pointing to the larger hemangioma in the posterior right lobe of liver.

be identified as a cold spot with sulfur colloid, a red cell study can add weight to the diagnosis of hemangioma. A red cell study involves the labeling of the patient's red cells with Tc-99m using a stannous chloride chelate, which bonds the Tc-99m to the red cells (Royal et al 1981). As hemangiomas have an increased blood volume compared to normal tissues, they will appear as a hot spot on a blood pool scan and may even be visualized when other imaging modalities are negative (Krausz et al 1997). Lesions as low as 1.5–2 cm can be reliably detected with sensitivities of up to 89% (Guze & Hawkins 1989, Ziessman et al 1991, Siegel & Mazurek 1997). Hypervascular metastases do occur but are very rare (Ginsberg et al 1986, Swayne et al 1991, Farlow et al 1993, Shih et al 1996).

NEUROENDOCRINE RECEPTOR IMAGING

A large number of neuroendocrine tumors can be imaged using Indium-111 labeled octreotide, a somato-statin analogue, including carcinoids, gastrinomas, insulinomas, glucagonomas, medullary carcinoma of the thyroid, meningiomas, small cell lung cancer, and other tumors including non-Hodgkins lymphomas, Hodgkins (Krenning et al 1992). These agents can be used to characterize liver lesions in patients with the above underlying conditions. Uptake in the normal liver may obscure small lesions, so unless a lesion can be seen as a cold spot or a hot spot, there is limited diagnostic information in a scan showing homogeneous liver uptake of octreotide. The real advantage of somatostatin receptor imaging is in the demonstration of extra-hepatic metastases that may have not been demonstrated with the conventional imaging modalities, therefore altering the stage of the patient. The majority of patients with neuroendocrine tumors should have an octreotide scan prior to an attempted curative resection for metastatic disease (Fig. 14.32).

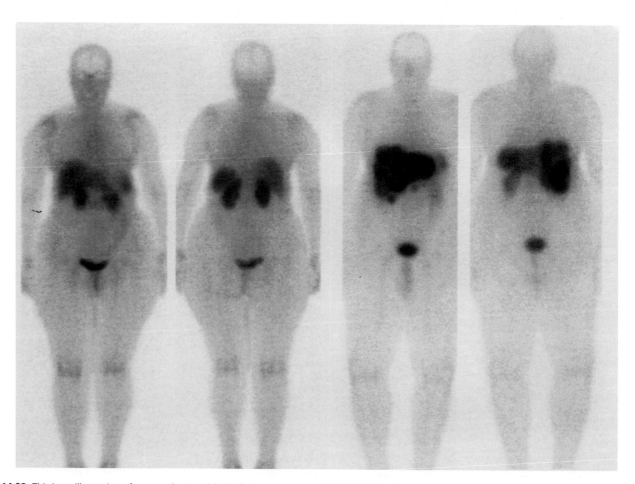

Fig. 14.32 This is an illustration of a normal octreotide study in a woman on the left with the images on the right being the case of interest. This 53-year-old man presented with confusion and was found to be hypoglycemic. Abdominal examination revealed hepatomegaly and a CT revealed metastases. FNA revealed small round cells suggestive of neuroendocrine origin. Note there is normally low-grade uptake of the tracer in the liver, spleen and kidneys. The images of the man on the right reveal extensive hepatic metastases and an epigastric mass.

HEPATIC ARTERIAL PERFUSION STUDIES
(Figs 14.33–14.39)

Technetium-99m macro-aggregated albumin (MAA)

This radiopharmaceutical is available in kit form, and is commonly used for pulmonary perfusion scintigraphy. A heating process makes an aggregate of the albumin. The end result of this process is a particle size of MAA 90% of which is between 10 and 90 µm in diameter. The net result is that this pharmaceutical when injected will embolize into the first capillary bed it meets and not pass on through the remainder of the circulation. This preparation has been used

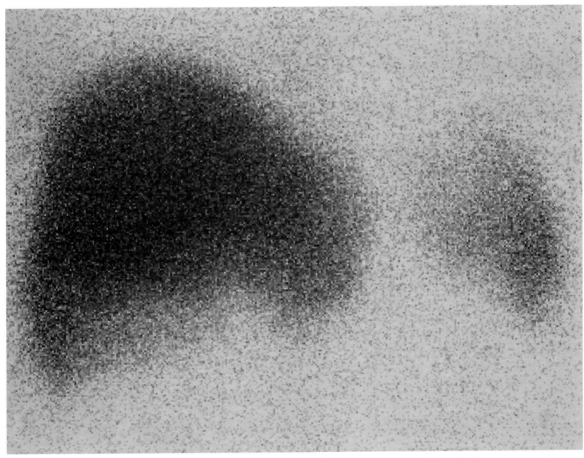

Fig. 14.33 Anterior delayed view of a normal liver and spleen scan after injection of Tc-99m sulphur colloid.

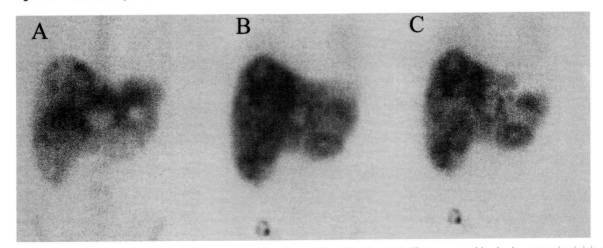

Fig. 14.34 The methodology of subtraction scintigraphy with Tc-99m sulfur colloid and Tc-99m MAA. The tracer requiring in vivo processing is injected first in a dose of 1 mCi (37 MBq). The second tracer MAA is injected through the hepatic catheter in a dose of 5 mCi (185 MBq). The left image **A** is the sulfur colloid image, the second **B** is the MAA image and the third **C** is the MAA minus the sulfur colloid image. Multiple hepatic metastases are seen demonstrating a hot rim of the MAA in the hypervascular rim of tumor. The activity in the right lower portion of the image is retained activity in the catheter.

to assess the perfusion of the liver by direct injection into the hepatic artery (Yang et al 1982). The addition of Tc-99m colloid imaging adds information regarding the relative perfusion of the liver via the hepatic artery as assessed by Tc-99m MAA and the intrahepatic distribution of the hepatic metastases as demonstrated by the Tc-99m colloid imaging (Ridge et al 1987) (Figs 14.35 & 14.36). Direct injection of chemotherapeutic agents into the hepatic has been shown to deliver ten times the concentration of 5-fluorouracil into liver metastases than that seen with the intravenous route (Hohenberger et al 1993).

The advent of intra-hepatic arterial drug therapy (Ch.

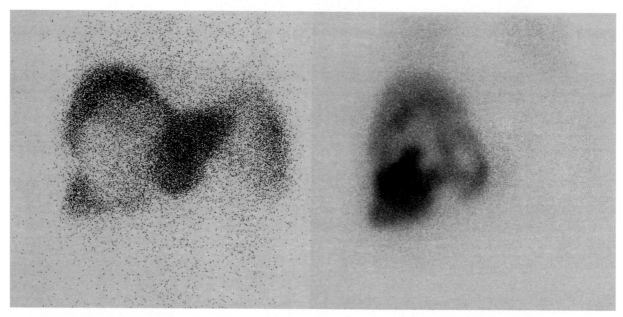

Fig. 14.35 Image of a patient with a lesion in the lower right liver, demonstrating reduced uptake of sulfur colloid (left panel) but relative hyperperfusion in the right panel taken after injection of the MAA intraarterially. This case demonstrates the principle of metastases being supplied by the hepatic artery rather than by the portal vein.

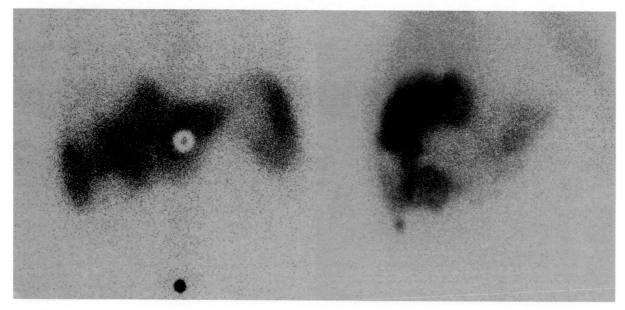

Fig. 14.36 Image of a patient with a lesion in the upper right liver, demonstrating reduced uptake of sulfur colloid (left panel) but relative hyperperfusion in the right panel taken after injection of the MAA intraarterially. This case demonstrates the principle of metastases being supplied by the hepatic artery rather than by the portal vein. The inferior black dot is an umbilical marker; the upper cold dot is an epigastric marker.

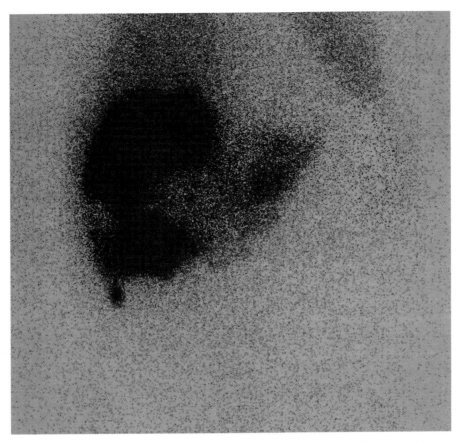

Fig.14.37 Same patient as Figure 14.35 with the contrast on the display 'wound up' demonstrating hepato-pulmonary shunting.

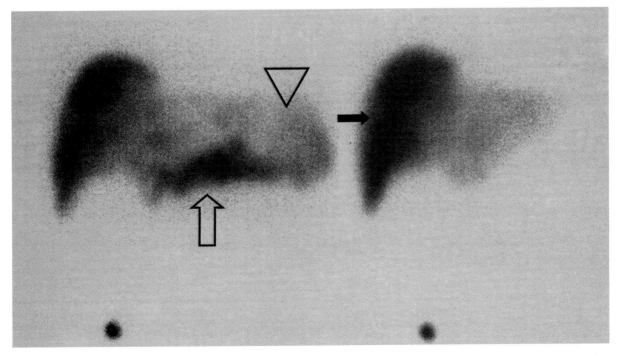

Fig. 14.38 This study demonstrates perfusion of the pancreas and spleen that was corrected with repositioning of the hepatic arterial catheter. The images to the right were acquired after the injection of Tc-99m MAA into the hepatic artery catheter and demonstrate aberrant perfusion of the pancreas, open arrow and the spleen (arrow-head). Following repositioning of the catheter the metastasis can be seen in the right lobe of the liver (solid arrow) with no extra-hepatic perfusion.

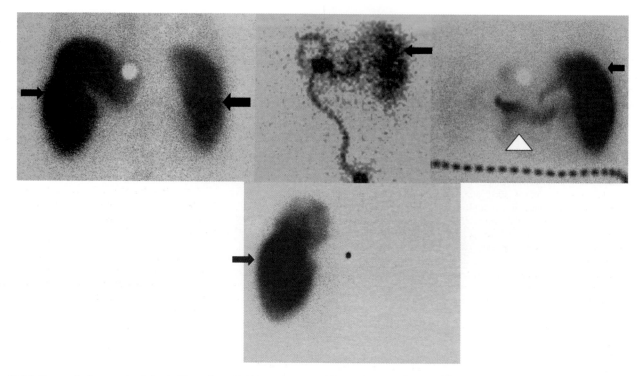

Fig. 14.39 Composite images: top left, Tc-99m sulfur colloid images; top middle, perfusion phase of hepatic pump study with Tc-99m MAA; top right, delayed pump study demonstrating perfusion of pancreas and spleen. The bottom panel demonstrates perfusion of the liver after repositioning of the arterial catheter.

82) has led to increasing use of combined Tc-99m MAA and Tc-99m colloid imaging to exclude extra-hepatic delivery of the radiopharmaceutical that may necessitate catheter revision (Habbe et al 1998). Inadvertent direct perfusion of the stomach, small gut or pancreas can lead to local chemotoxicity leading to localized inflammation, which is often symptomatic (Ottery et al 1986, Choplin et al 1983, Chuang et al 1981, Ku et al 1998) (Figs 14.38 & 14.39). In some cases the distribution of the tracer on scintigraphy has predicted the pattern of response of the metastases to the therapy (Borzutzky & Turbiner 1985), and is a useful adjunct in the assessment of response to therapy (Savolaine et al 1989). Hepatic artery scintigraphy has also been used to demonstrate the presence of arteriovenous shunting in hepatic tumors which can modify therapy in an attempt to limit pulmonary toxicity (Leung et al 1994) (Fig. 14.37).

Hepatic arterial therapy using radiopharmaceuticals

An adaptation of the chemotherapy approach has been made by a number of groups using therapeutic doses of unsealed radiotherapy. Hepatic delivery of beta particle emitting radiopharmaceuticals such as Yttrium-90 labeled microspheres has been associated with improved median survival and reductions in tumor markers in preliminary studies (Lau et al 1994).

SUMMARY

Nuclear medicine is a very diverse specialty. The tracer principle has been adapted to provide diagnostic information in both the preoperative and postoperative setting as well as towards the therapeutic administration of radiopharmaceuticals. Hepatobiliary scintigraphy has a vital role in the non-invasive assessment of patients with acute and chronic right upper quadrant pain as well as an integral role in the assessment of biliary dynamics in patients post biliary tract intervention. FDG PET is rapidly becoming a mainstream tool in the diagnosis of metastatic disease in patients with cancer and shows great promise in the assessment of response to treatment. The integration of FDG-PET information into treatment assessment is currently occurring and should lead to more appropriate management, as treatment algorithms become more refined over time. Other nuclear medicine techniques such as receptor imaging have a niche role to play in pre and postoperative assessment.

REFERENCES

Akhurst T, Larson S M, Macapinlac H, Fong Y, Kemeny N 1999 Flurodeoxyglucose (FDG) positron emission tomography (PET) immediately post hepatic cryotherapy predicts recurrence of tumor in the liver. Proceedings of the American Society of Clinical Oncology

Barron L G, Rubio P A 1995 Importance of accurate preoperative diagnosis and role of advanced laparoscopic cholecystectomy in relieving chronic acalculous cholecystitis. Journal of Laparoendoscopic Surgery 5: 357–361

Beihn R M, Damron J R, Hafner T 1974 Subtraction technique for the detection of subphrenic abscesses using 67Ga and 99mTc. Journal of Nuclear Medicine 15: 371–373

Berr F, Wiedmann M, Mossner J, Tannapfel A, Schmidt F 1999 Detection of cholangiocarcinoma in primary sclerosing cholangitis by positron emission tomography (letter). Hepatology 29: 611–613

Borzutzky C A, Turbiner E H 1985 The predictive value of hepatic artery perfusion scintigraphy. Journal of Nuclear Medicine 26: 1153–1156

Brown P H, Juni J E, Lieberman D A, Krishnamurthy G T 1988 Hepatocyte versus biliary disease: a distinction by deconvolutional analysis of technetium-99m IDA time-activity curves. Journal of Nuclear Medicine 29: 623–630

Cabana M D, Alavi A, Berlin J A, Shea J A, Kim C K, Williams S V 1995 Morphine-augmented hepatobiliary scintigraphy: a meta-analysis. Nuclear Medicine Communications 16: 1068–1071

Cawthon M A, Brown D M, Hartshorne M F, Karl R D Jr, Bauman J M, Howard W H D, Bunker S R 1984 Biliary scintigraphy. The 'hot rim' sign. Clinical Nuclear Medicine 9: 619–621

Chen C C, Holder L E, Maunoury C, Drachenberg C I 1997 Morphine augmentation increases gallbladder visualization in patients pretreated with cholecystokinin (see comments). Journal of Nuclear Medicine 38: 644–647

Cho Z H, Chan J K, Ericksson L, Singh M, Graham S, MacDonald N S, Yano Y 1975 Positron ranges obtained from biomedically important positron-emitting radionuclides. Journal of Nuclear Medicine 16: 1174–1176

Choi S O, Park W H, Lee H J, Woo S K 1996 'Triangular cord': a sonographic finding applicable in the diagnosis of biliary atresia. Journal of Pediatric Surgery 31: 363–6

Choi S O, Park W H, Lee H J 1998 Ultrasonographic 'triangular cord': the most definitive finding for noninvasive diagnosis of extrahepatic biliary atresia. European Journal of Pediatric Surgery 8: 12–16

Choplin R H, Gelfand D W, Hunt T H 1983 Gastric perforation from hepatic artery infusion chemotherapy. Gastrointestinal Radiology 8: 133–134

Choy D, Shi E C, McLean R G, Hoschl R, Murray I P, Ham J M 1984 Cholescintigraphy in acute cholecystitis: use of intravenous morphine. Radiology 151: 203–207

Chuang V P, Wallace S, Stroehlein J, Yap H Y, Patt Y Z 1981 Hepatic artery infusion chemotherapy: gastroduodenal complications. AJR. American Journal of Roentgenology 137: 347–350

Cooper A, Ross A J D, O'Neill J A Jr, Bishop H C, Templeton J M Jr, Ziegler M M 1985 Resolution of intractable cholestasis associated with total parenteral nutrition following biliary irrigation. Journal of Pediatric Surgery 20: 772–724

D'Angelica M, Brennan M F, Fortner J G, Cohen A M, Blumgart L H, Fong Y 1997 Ninety-six five-year survivors after liver resection for metastatic colorectal cancer. Journal of the American College of Surgeons 185: 554–559

Delbeke D, Vitola J V, Sandler M P, Arildsen R C, Powers T A, Wright J K Jr, Chapman W C, Pinson C W 1997 Staging recurrent metastatic colorectal carcinoma with PET. Journal of Nuclear Medicine 38: 1196–1201

Delbeke D, Martin W H, Sandler M P, Chapman W C, Wright J K Jr, Pinson C W 1998 Evaluation of benign vs malignant hepatic lesions with positron emission tomography. Archives of Surgery 133: 510–515; discussion 515–516

Dykes E H, Wilson N, Gray H W, McArdle C S 1986 The role of 99mTc HIDA cholescintigraphy in the diagnosis of acute gallbladder disease: comparison with oral cholecystography and ultrasonography. Scottish Medical Journal 31: 170–173

Eikman E A, Cameron J L, Colman M, Natarajan T K, Dugal P, Wagner H N Jr 1975 A test for patency of the cystic duct in acute cholecystitis. Annals of Internal Medicine 82: 318–322

Emblem R, Bentsen B, Stake G, Monclair T 1994 [Better results with early surgical intervention in biliary atresia. Icterus in infants older than 14 days should be investigated! (see comments)]. Tidsskr Nor Laegeforen 114: 1946–1947

Engeler C M, Kuni C C, Nakhleh R, Engeler C E, duCret R P, Boudreau R J 1992 Liver transplant rejection and cholestasis: comparison of technetium 99m-diisopropyl iminodiacetic acid hepatobiliary imaging with liver biopsy. European Journal of Nuclear Medicine 19: 865–870

Enomoto K, Fukunaga T, Okazumi S, Asano T, Kikuchi T, Yamamoto H, Nagashima T, Isono K, Itoh H, Imazeki K et al 1991 Can fluoro-deoxyglucose-positron emission tomography evaluate the functional differentiation of hepatocellular carcinoma. Kaku Igaku 28: 1353–6

Farlow D C, Little J M, Gruenewald S M, Antico V F, O'Neill P 1993 A case of metastatic malignancy masquerading as a hepatic hemangioma on labeled red blood cell scintigraphy (see comments). Journal of Nuclear Medicine 34: 1172–1174

Fawcett H D, Sayle B A, Winsett M Z 1985 Indium-111 chloride for detecting suspected hepatomas in patients with focal defects on technetium-99m sulfur colloid liver imaging. Clinical Nuclear Medicine 10: 410–412

Fink-Bennett D, Balon H, Robbins T, Tsai D 1991a Morphine-augmented cholescintigraphy: its efficacy in detecting acute cholecystitis (see comments). Journal of Nuclear Medicine 32: 1231–1233

Fink-Bennett D, DeRidder P, Kolozsi W Z, Gordon R, Jaros R 1991b Cholecystokinin cholescintigraphy: detection of abnormal gallbladder motor function in patients with chronic acalculous gallbladder disease. Journal of Nuclear Medicine 32: 1695–1699

Flamen P, Stroobant S, Van Cutsem E, Dupont P, Bormans G, De Vadder N, Penninckx F, Van Hoe L, Mortelmans L 1999 Additional value of whole-body positron emission tomography with fluorine-18-2-fluoro-2-deoxy-D-glucose in recurrent colorectal cancer. Journal of Clinical Oncology 17: 894–901

Fong Y, Cohen A M, Fortner J G, Enker W E, Turnbull A D, Coit D G, Marrero A M, Prasad M, Blumgart L H, Brennan M F 1997 Liver resection for colorectal metastases. Journal of Clinical Oncology 15: 938–946

Freitas J E, Mirkes S H, Fink-Bennett D M, Bree R L 1982 Suspected acute cholecystitis. Comparison of hepatobiliary scintigraphy versus ultrasonography. Clinical Nuclear Medicine 7: 364–367

Ginsberg F, Slavin J D Jr, Spencer R P 1986 Hepatic angiosarcoma: mimicking of angioma on three-phase technetium-99m red blood cell scintigraphy. Journal of Nuclear Medicine 27: 1861–3

Goncalves R M, Harris J A, Rivera D E 1998 Biliary dyskinesia: natural history and surgical results. American Surgeon 64: 493–497; discussion 497–498

Guze B H, Hawkins R A, 1989 Utility of the SPECT Tc-99m labeled RBC blood pool scan in the detection of hepatic hemangiomas. Clinical Nuclear Medicine 14: 817–818

Habbe T G, McCowan T C, Goertzen T C, Leveen R F, Culp W C, Tempero M A 1998 Complications and technical limitations of hepatic arterial infusion catheter placement for chemotherapy. Journal of Vascular and Interventional Radiology 9: 233–239

Hagspiel K D, Neidl K F, Eichenberger A C, Weder W, Marincek B 1995 Detection of liver metastases: comparison of superparamagnetic iron oxide-enhanced and unenhanced MR imaging at 1.5 T with dynamic CT, intraoperative US, and percutaneous. US Radiology 196: 471–478

Helm J F, Venu R P, Geenen J E, Hogan W J, Dodds W J, Toouli J, Arndorfer R C 1988 Effects of morphine on the human sphincter of Oddi. Gut 29: 1402–1407

Hohenberger P, Strauss L G, Lehner B, Frohmuller S, Dimitrakopoulou A, Schlag P 1993 Perfusion of colorectal liver metastases and uptake of fluorouracil assessed by H2(15O and [18F]uracil positron emission tomography (PET). European Journal of Cancer 29A: 1682–1686

Hui A M, Makuuchi M, Li X 1998 Cell cycle regulators and human hepatocarcinogenesis. Hepatogastroenterology 45: 1635–1642

Jarnagin W R, Fong Y, Ky A, Schwartz L H, Paty P B, Cohen A M, Blumgart L H 1999 Liver resection for metastatic colorectal cancer: assessing the risk of occult irresectable disease. Journal of the American College of Surgeons 188: 33–42

Johanning J M, Gruenberg J C 1998 The changing face of cholecystectomy American Surgeon 64: 643–647; discussion 647–648

Karademir S, Csete M E, Jurim O, Finstad T, Hawkins R, Bussuttil R W, Shaked A 1994 Role of 99mTc-labeled DISIDA scan in the assessment of marginal liver grafts after orthotopic transplantation. Clinical Transplantation 8: 54–58

Keiding S, Hansen S B, Rasmussen H H, Gee A, Kruse A, Roelsgaard K, Tage-Jensen U, Dahlerup J F 1998 Detection of cholangiocarcinoma in primary sclerosing cholangitis by positron emission tomography. Hepatology 28: 700–706

Kim C K, Tse K K, Juweid M, Mozley P D, Woda A, Alavi A 1993 Cholescintigraphy in the diagnosis of acute cholecystitis: morphine augmentation is superior to delayed imaging. Journal of Nuclear Medicine 34: 1866–1870

Klingensmith W C D, Spitzer V M, Fritzberg A R, Kuni C C 1981 The normal fasting and postprandial diisopropyl-IDA Tc 99m hepatobiliary study. Radiology 141: 771–776

Krausz Y, Levy M, Antebi E, Bar-Ziv J, Bocher M, Chisin R 1997 Liver hemangioma. A perioperative Tc–99m RBC SPECT correlation. Clinical Nuclear Medicine 22: 35–37

Krenning E P, Kwekkeboom D J, Reubi J C, Van Hagen P M, van Eijck C H, Oei H Y, Lamberts S W 1992 111In-octreotide scintigraphy in oncology. Metabolism 41: 83–86

Ku Y, Iwasaki T, Fukumoto T, Tominaga M, Muramatsu S, Kusunoki N, Sugimoto T, Suzuki Y, Kuroda Y, Saitoh Y 1998 Percutaneous isolated liver chemoperfusion for treatment of unresectable malignant liver tumors: technique, pharmacokinetics, clinical results. Recent Results in Cancer Research 147: 67–82

Kumura D, Miller J H, Sinatra F R 1987 Septo-optic dysplasia: recognition of causes of false-positive hepatobiliary scintigraphy in neonatal jaundice. Journal of Nuclear Medicine 28: 966–972

Lai D T, Fulham M, Stephen M S, Chu K M, Solomon M, Thompson J F, Sheldon D M, Storey D W 1996 The role of whole-body positron emission tomography with [18F]fluorodeoxyglucose in identifying operable colorectal cancer metastases to the liver. Archives of Surgery 131: 703–707

Larsen M J, Klingensmith W C D, Kuni C C 1982 Radionuclide hepatobiliary imaging: nonvisualization of the gallbladder secondary to prolonged fasting. Journal of Nuclear Medicine 23: 1003–1005

Lau W Y, Leung W T, Ho S, Leung N W, Chan M, Lin J, Metreweli C, Johnson P, Li A K 1994 Treatment of inoperable hepatocellular carcinoma with intrahepatic arterial yttrium-90 microspheres: a phase I and II study. British Journal of Cancer 70: 994–999

Lauritsen K B, Sommer W, Hahn L, Henriksen J H 1988 Cholescintigraphy and ultrasonography in patients suspected of having acute cholecystitis. Scandinavian Journal of Gastroenterology 23: 42–46

Lencioni R, Donati F, Cioni D, Paolicchi A, Cicorelli A, Bartolozzi C 1998 Detection of colorectal liver metastases: prospective comparison of unenhanced and ferumoxides-enhanced magnetic resonance imaging at 1.5 T, dual-phase spiral CT, and spiral CT during arterial portography. (In Process Citation) Magma 7: 76–87

Leppo J A, Dahlberg S T 1998 The question: to test or not to test in preoperative cardiac risk evaluation. Journal of Nuclear Cardiology 5: 332–342

Leung W T, Lau W Y, Ho S K, Chan M, Leung N W, Lin J, Metreweli C, Johnson P J, Li A K 1994 Measuring lung shunting in hepatocellular carcinoma with intrahepatic-arterial technetium-99m macroaggregated albumin. Journal of Nuclear Medicine 35: 70–73

Lin W Y, Lin C C, Changlai S P, Shen Y Y, Wang S J 1997 Comparison technetium of Tc-99m disofenin cholescintigraphy with ultrasonography in the differentiation of biliary atresia from other forms of neonatal jaundice. Pediatric Surgery International 12: 30–33

Low V, Khangure M S 1990 Hepatic adenoma and focal nodular hyperplasia: a diagnostic dilemma. Australasian Radiology 34: 124–130

Madacsy L, Velosy B, Lonovics J, Csernay L 1994 Differentiation between organic stenosis and functional dyskinesia of the sphincter of Oddi with amyl nitrite-augmented quantitative hepatobiliary scintigraphy. European Journal of Nuclear Medicine 21: 203–208

Madacsy L, Velosy B, Lonovics J, Csernay L 1995 Evaluation of results of the prostigmine-morphine test with quantitative hepatobiliary scintigraphy: a new method for the diagnosis of sphincter of Oddi dyskinesia. European Journal of Nuclear Medicine 22: 227–232

Majd M, Reba R C, Altman R P 1981a Effect of phenobarbital on 99mTc-IDA scintigraphy in the evaluation of neonatal jaundice. Seminars in Nuclear Medicine 11: 194–204

Majd M, Reba R C, Altman R P 1981b Hepatobiliary scintigraphy with 99mTc-PIPIDA in the evaluation of neonatal jaundice. Pediatrics 67: 140–145

Maldonado M E, Brady P G, Mamel J J, Robinson B 1999 Incidence of pancreatitis in patients undergoing sphincter of Oddi manometry (SOM). American Journal of Gastroenterology 94: 387–390

Manolaki A G, Larcher V F, Mowat A P, Barrett J J, Portmann B, Howard E R 1983 The prelaparotomy diagnosis of extrahepatic biliary atresia. Archives of Diseases in Childhood 58: 591–594

Mochizuki T, Tauxe W N, Dobkin J, Shah A N, Shanker R, Todo S, Starzl T E 1991 Detection of complications after liver transplantation by technetium-99m mebrofenin hepatobiliary scintigraphy. Annals of Nuclear Medicine 5: 103–107

Mochizuki T, Takechi T, Murase K, Tauxe W N, Bradfield H A, Tanada S, Hamamoto K 1994 Thallium-201/technetium-99m-phytate (colloid) subtraction imaging of hepatocellular carcinoma. Journal of Nuclear Medicine 35: 1134–1137

Nordlinger B, Jaeck D, Guiguet M, Vaillant J, Balladur P, Schaal J 1992 In: Nordlinger B, Jaeck D (Eds) Treatment of hepatic metastasesof colorectal cancer. Springer-Verlag, New York, p 129–146

Oates E, Selland D L, Chin C T, Achong D M 1996 Gallbladder nonvisualization with pericholecystic rim sign: morphine-augmentation optimizes diagnosis of acute cholecystitis. Journal of Nuclear Medicine 37: 267–269

Ogunbiyi O A, Flanagan F L, Dehdashti F, Siegel B A, Trask D D, Birnbaum E H, Fleshman J W, Read T E, Philpott G W, Kodner I J 1997 Detection of recurrent and metastatic colorectal cancer: comparison of positron emission tomography and computed tomography (see comments). Annals of Surgical Oncology 4: 613–620

Ottery F D, Scupham R K, Weese J L 1986 Chemical cholecystitis after intrahepatic chemotherapy. The case for prophylactic cholecystectomy during pump placement. Diseases of the Colon and Rectum 29: 187–190

Park W H, Choi S O, Lee H J, Kim S P, Zeon S K, Lee S L 1997 A new diagnostic approach to biliary atresia with emphasis on the ultrasonographic triangular cord sign: comparison of ultrasonography, hepatobiliary scintigraphy, and liver needle biopsy in the evaluation of infantile cholestasis. Journal of Pediatric Surgery 32: 1555–1559

Patch G G, Morton K A, Arias J M, Datz F L 1991 Naloxone reverses pattern of obstruction of the distal common bile duct induced by analgesic narcotics in hepatobiliary imaging. Journal of Nuclear Medicine 32: 1270–1272

Reed D N Jr, Fernandez M, Hicks R D 1993 Kinevac-assisted cholescintigraphy as an accurate predictor of chronic acalculus gallbladder disease and the likelihood of symptom relief with cholecystectomy. American Surgeon 59: 273–277

Reichelt H G 1978 Hepatobiliary sequential scintigraphy. Value of this nuclear-medicine-diagnostic technic in the pre- and postoperative stages following hepato-biliary-tract injuries. Chirurgica 49: 167–171

Ridge J A, Bading J R, Gelbard A S, Benua R S, Daly J M 1987 Perfusion of colorectal hepatic metastases. Relative distribution of flow from the hepatic artery and portal vein. Cancer 59: 1547–1553

Roberts-Thomson I C, Toouli J, Blanchett W, Lichtenstein M, Andrews J T 1986 Assessment of bile flow by radioscintigraphy in patients with biliary-type pain after cholecystectomy. Australia and New Zealand Journal of Medicine 16: 788–793

Rovekamp M H, van Royen E A, Folmer S C, van der Schoot J B 1983 Diagnosis of upper-abdominal infections by In-111 labeled leukocytes with Tc-99m colloid subtraction technique. Journal of Nuclear Medicine 24: 212–216

Royal H D, Israel O, Parker J A, Kolodny G M 1981 Scintigraphy of hepatic hemangiomas: the value of Tc-99m-labeled red blood cells: concise communication. Journal of Nuclear Medicine 22: 684–687

Samuels B I, Freitas J E, Bree R L, Schwab R E, Heller S T 1983 A comparison of radionuclide hepatobiliary imaging and real-time ultrasound for the detection of acute cholecystitis. Radiology 147: 207–210

Sandler M A, Petrocelli R D, Marks D S, Lopez R 1980 Ultrasonic features and radionuclide correlation in liver cell adenoma and focal nodular hyperplasia. Radiology 135: 393–397

Savolaine E R, Zeiss J, Schlembach P J, Skeel R T, McCann K, Merrick H W 1989 Role of scintigraphy in establishing optimal perfusion in hepatic arterial infusion pump chemotherapy. American Journal of Clinical Oncology 12: 68–74

Scheele J, Stang R, Altendorf-Hofmann A, Paul M 1995 Resection of colorectal liver metastases. World Journal of Surgery 19: 59–71

Schiepers C, Penninckx F, De Vadder N, Merckx E, Mortelmans L, Bormans G, Marchal G, Filez L, Aerts R 1995 Contribution of PET in the diagnosis of recurrent colorectal cancer: comparison with conventional imaging. European Journal of Surgical Oncology 21: 517–522

Schroder O, Trojan J, Zeuzem S, Baum R P 1998 Limited value of fluorine-18-fluorodeoxyglucose PET for the differential diagnosis of focal liver lesions in patients with chronic hepatitis C virus infection. Nuklearmedizin 37: 279–285

Serafini A N, Jeffers L J, Reddy K R, Heiba S, Schiff E R 1988 Early recognition of recurrent hepatocellular carcinoma utilizing gallium-67 citrate scintigraphy. Journal of Nuclear Medicine 29: 712–716

Shah A N, Dodson F, Fung J 1995 Role of nuclear medicine in liver transplantation. Seminars in Nuclear Medicine 25: 36–48

Shea J A, Berlin J A, Escarce J J, Clarke J R, Kinosian B P, Cabana M D, Tsai W W, Horangic N, Malet P F, Schwartz J S et al 1994 Revised estimates of diagnostic test sensitivity and specificity in suspected biliary tract disease (see comments). Archives of Internal Medicine 154: 2573–2581

Shih W J, Lee J K, Mitchell B 1996 False-positive results for hepatic hemangioma on Tc-99m RBC SPECT caused by a liver metastasis from small-cell lung carcinoma. Clinical Nuclear Medicine 21: 898–899

Siegel A, Mazurek R 1997 Early dynamic SPECT acquisition for the imaging of hepatic hemangiomas utilizing Tc-99m labeled red blood cells. Clinical Nuclear Medicine 22: 745–748

Silberstein E B 1998 Prevalence of adverse reactions to positron emitting radiopharmaceuticals in nuclear medicine. Pharmacopeia Committee of the Society of Nuclear Medicine. Journal of Nuclear Medicine 39: 2190–2192

Soiva M, Haveri M, Taavitsainen M, Suramo I 1986 The value of routine sonography in clinically suspected acute cholecystitis. Scandinavian Journal of Gastroenterology 21: 70–74

Sostre S, Canto M I, Kalloo A N 1992a Gallbladder response to a second dose of cholecystokinin during the same imaging study. European Journal of Nuclear Medicine 19: 964–965

Sostre S, Kalloo A N, Spiegler E J, Camargo E E, Wagner H N Jr 1992b A noninvasive test of sphincter of Oddi dysfunction in postcholecystectomy patients: the scintigraphic score (see comments). Journal of Nuclear Medicine 33: 1216–1222

Soyer P, Levesque M, Caudron C, Elias D, Zeitoun G, Roche A 1993 MRI of liver metastases from colorectal cancer vs. CT during arterial portography. Journal of Computer Assisted Tomography 17: 67–74

Spivak W, Sarkar S, Winter D, Glassman M, Donlon E, Tucker K J 1987 Diagnostic utility of hepatobiliary scintigraphy with 99mTc-DISIDA in neonatal cholestasis. Journal of Pediatrics 110: 855–861

Staritz M 1988 Pharmacology of the sphincter of Oddi. Endoscopy 20 (Suppl 1): 171–174

Strotzer M, Gmeinwieser J, Schmidt J, Fellner C, Seitz J, Albrich H, Zirngibl H, Feuerbach S 1997 Diagnosis of liver metastases from colorectal adenocarcinoma. Comparison of spiral-CTAP combined with intravenous contrast-enhanced spiral-CT and SPIO-enhanced MR combined with plain MR imaging. Acta Radiologica 38: 986–992

Suarez C A, Block F, Bernstein D, Serafini A, Rodman G Jr, Zeppa R 1980 The role of H.I.D.A./P.I.P.I.D.A. scanning in diagnosing cystic duct obstruction. Annals of Surgery 191: 391–396

Swayne L C, Diehl W L, Brown T D, Hunter N J 1991 False-positive hepatic blood pool scintigraphy in metastatic colon carcinoma. Clinical Nuclear Medicine 16: 630–632

Szlabick R E, Catto J A, Fink-Bennett D, Ventura V 1980 Hepatobiliary scanning in the diagnosis of acute cholecystitis. Archives of Surgery 115: 540–544

Tagge E P, Campbell D A Jr, Reichle R, Averill D R Jr, Merion R M, Dafoe D C, Turcotte J G, Juni J E 1987 Quantitative scintigraphy with deconvolutional analysis for the dynamic measurement of hepatic function. Journal of Surgical Research 42: 605–612

Tanasescu D E, Waxman A D, Hurvitz C 1991 Scintigraphic findings mimicking focal nodular hyperplasia in a case of hepatoblastoma. Clinical Nuclear Medicine 16: 236–238

Torizuka T, Tamaki N, Inokuma T, Magata Y, Yonekura Y, Tanaka A, Yamaoka Y, Yamamoto K, Konishi J 1994 Value of fluorine-18-FDG-PET to monitor hepatocellular carcinoma after interventional therapy. Journal of Nuclear Medicine 35: 1965–1969

Torizuka T, Tamaki N, Inokuma T, Magata Y, Sasayama S, Yonekura Y, Tanaka A, Yamaoka Y, Yamamoto K, Konishi J 1995 In vivo assessment of glucose metabolism in hepatocellular carcinoma with FDG-PET. Journal of Nuclear Medicine 36: 1811–1817

Valk P E, Abella-Columna E, Tesar R D, Pounds T R, Haseman M K, Myers R W 1998 Detection of recurrent colorectal cancer by FDG PET in patients with serum CEA elevation. Journal of Nuclear Medicine 39: 135P

van Weelde B J, Oudkerk M, Koch C W 1986 Ultrasonography of acute cholecystitis: clinical and histological correlation. Diagnostic Imaging Clinical Medicine 55: 190–195

Velasco J, Singh J, Ramanujam P, Friedberg M 1982 Hepatobiliary scanning in cholecystitis. European Journal of Nuclear Medicine 7: 11–13

Vitola J V, Delbeke D, Meranze S G, Mazer M J, Pinson C W 1996a Positron emission tomography with F-18-fluorodeoxyglucose to evaluate the results of hepatic chemoembolization (see comments). Cancer 78: 2216–2222

Vitola J V, Delbeke D, Sandler M P, Campbell M G, Powers T A, Wright J K, Chapman W C, Pinson C W 1996b Positron emission tomography to stage suspected metastatic colorectal carcinoma to the liver. American Journal of Surgery 171: 21–26

Wagner J S, Adson M A, Van Heerden J A, Adson M H, Ilstrup D M 1984 The natural history of hepatic metastases from colorectal cancer. A comparison with resective treatment. Annals of Surgery 199: 502–508

Walker A T, Shapiro A W, Brooks D C, Braver J M, Tumeh S S 1992 Bile duct disruption and biloma after laparoscopic cholecystectomy: imaging evaluation. AJR. American Journal of Roentgenology 158: 785–789

Walker A T, Brooks D C, Tumeh S S, Braver J M 1993 Bile duct disruption after laparoscopic cholecystectomy. Seminars in Ultrasound, CT and MR 14: 346–355

Wanebo H J, Chu Q D, Avradopoulos K A, Vezeridis M P 1996a Current perspectives on repeat hepatic resection for colorectal carcinoma: a review. Surgery 119: 361–371

Wanebo H J, Chu Q D, Vezeridis M P, Soderberg C 1996b Patient selection for hepatic resection of colorectal metastases. Archives of Surgery 131: 322–329

Warburg O 1931 The Metabolism of Tumors. Richard R. Smith, Inc: New York, p. 129–169.

Williams H C, Pope C F, Siskind B N, Lange R C, Flye M W 1985 Vascular thrombosis in acute hepatic allograft rejection: scintigraphic appearance. Journal of Nuclear Medicine 26: 478–481

Yang P J, Thrall J H, Ensminger W D, Niederhuber J E, Gyves J W, Tuscan M, Doan K, Cozzi E 1982 Perfusion scintigraphy (Tc-99m MAA) during surgery for placement of chemotherapy catheter in hepatic artery: concise communication. Journal of Nuclear Medicine 23: 1066–1069

Yonekura Y, Benua R S, Brill A B, Som P, Yeh S D, Kemeny N E, Fowler J S, MacGregor R R, Stamm R, Christman D R, Wolf A P 1982 Increased accumulation of 2-deoxy-2-[18F]Fluoro-D-glucose in liver metastases from colon carcinoma. Journal of Nuclear Medicine 23: 1133–1137

Yoon D S, Cheong J H, Park Y N, Kwon S W, Chi H S, Kim B R 1998 Cell proliferation index and the expression of p53 and Bcl-2 in tumorous and non-tumorous lesions of hepatocellular carcinoma and metastatic liver cancer. Yonsei Medical Journal 39: 424–429

Ziessman H A, Silverman P M, Patterson J, Harkness B, Fahey F H, Zeman R K, Keyes J W Jr 1991 Improved detection of small cavernous hemangiomas of the liver with high-resolution three-headed SPECT. Journal of Nuclear Medicine 32: 2086–2091

15

Computed tomography of the liver and biliary tract

M.E. RODDIE, A. ADAM

INTRODUCTION

In recent years the development of new technology has dramatically changed the imaging approach for hepatobiliary diseases. The clinician now has available computed tomography (CT), grey-scale and color-Doppler ultrasonography (Ch. 13) and magnetic resonance imaging (MRI) (Ch. 16). Despite competition from other imaging modalities, techniques for hepatobiliary CT continue to be refined and today CT remains the main imaging modality for studying the liver, including screening the liver for focal hepatic lesions, differentiating some benign masses from malignant ones, staging cancer patients prior to hepatic tumor resection and evaluating the biliary tree. The advantages of high-resolution images, short scan times and fast patient throughput have kept CT competitive with MRI which has more inherent tissue contrast and multiplanar capabilities. Compared with gray-scale ultrasonography CT is more accurate in the detection of focal hepatic lesions, is less operator-dependent and therefore more reproducible, and displays all of the upper abdominal anatomy, providing information about extrahepatic processes important in scan interpretation. Color-Doppler ultrasonography (Ch. 13) allows evaluation of the patency and flow characteristics of the hepatic and portal circulation but CT following administation of intravenous or intra-arterial contrast material provides excellent visualization of hepatic and portal vessels and provides information regarding the regional blood flow characteristics of focal lesions.

RECENT TECHNICAL ADVANCES

The development of helical (spiral) CT in the late 1980s has revolutionized the way CT of the body is performed.

Conventional 'step and shoot' CT requires that the patient take a separate breath for each individual slice performed, followed by an obligatory time to exhale, and take another breath. The shortest time in which the entire liver can be imaged using incremental CT is between 2 and 3 minutes. During helical CT (HCT), on the other hand, there is continuous tube rotation while the patient moves through the gantry and a volumetric data set is acquired within a single breath hold. The data can be reconstruced into standard axial images, or further manipulated to display 2-dimensional or 3-dimensional reconstructions of the area of interest. HCT has been made possible by the development of slip-ring technology and advances in radiographic tube heat dissipation (Kalender et al 1990) and the result has been a dramatic increase in scanning speed. An important advantage of HCT compared with conventional or incremental CT is the ability to reconstruct the data acquired on the initial scan at intervals as small as 1 mm. This significantly reduces partial volume artefact because, although the additional slice reconstructions remain the same thickness, the ability to shift the center of the slice can affect lesion conspicuity by placing the lesion directly within a reconstructed image, rather than between two contiguous reconstructed slices (Bluemke et al 1995). Another advantage of HCT compared with incremental CT is the absence of respiratory misregistration, which occcurs in conventional CT imaging when the patient takes different sized breaths between each image acquisition. This results in non-imaged areas of liver between consecutive scans, a problem that is eliminated with HCT, thus greatly enhancing diagnostic accuracy. Probably the most important advantage of HCT in the liver, however, is the reduced time required to image the entire liver (20–30 seconds) which allows imaging to be performed during the optimal phase (or phases) of hepatic enhancement following intravenous administration of contrast agent. It is now possible to image the liver in the hepatic arterial, portal venous and delayed phases of enhancement after intravenous contrast agent administration and this has improved the ability of the technique to both detect and characterize focal hepatic lesions.

HCT has recently undergone a further major advance with the development of a new class of multidetector-array scanners which utilize a substantially greater percentage of the X-rays emitted from the tube cathode, improving tube efficiency and permitting even faster scanning. This new generation of CT scanner is capable of imaging the entire liver in 7 seconds. Multidetector-array HCT also allows thinner collimation (2.5 mm) and the resultant improved resolution has been shown to increase the detection of small hepatic lesions by up to 46% (Weg et al 1998).

TECHNIQUE

As a result of the recent developments discussed above it will be appreciated that there is now a bewildering choice of protocols for CT of the liver but, as in the past, performance of an optimal CT study of the liver requires a thorough knowledge of the information the referring clinician hopes to gain from the examination. This allows the radiologist to tailor the scanning technique to the problem at hand. A variety of technical parameters can be chosen including slice thickness, table speed (pitch), image reconstruction interval and if contrast agent is to be given, its volume, rate and route of administration. The following paragraphs describe how to best use these various parameters with particular emphasis on focal lesion detection.

NON-CONTRAST CT

The easiest and simplest way to conduct a CT scan of the liver is to perform the study without administration of intravascular contrast medium. A slice thickness of 8–10 mm is selected with a pitch of 1.5. The attenuation value of the normal liver typically varies between 54 and 60 Hounsfield units (HU), which is approximately 8 HU greater than that of the spleen due to glycogen and iron stores in the liver. Hepatic neoplasms usually have a high water content resulting in relative hypoattenuation compared with liver parenchyma. The portal veins and bile ducts are also of lower attenuation than liver parenchyma, and a vessel running vertically through a section may mimic a small tumor, leading to errors in diagnosis. On unenhanced studies the attenuation difference between liver and tumor may be subtle and require viewing at very narrow window widths to allow focal lesion detection. Much higher lesion-

to-liver attenuation difference, however, can be achieved by the administration of intravenous contrast medium (Tidebrant et al 1990) and in the days when incremental contrast-enhanced CT of the liver was being performed (prior to the widespread availability of HCT) many centers abandoned the non-contrast component of the examination. This was due partly to pressure of time and partly because of the relatively low diagnostic benefit of non-contrast CT compared with intravenous contrast-enhanced CT. Non-contrast CT, however, is useful for detecting diffuse abnormalities such as hemochromatosis or fatty infiltration (Figs 15.1 & 15.2) where the attenuation of the liver is increased or decreased, respectively. Both these processes

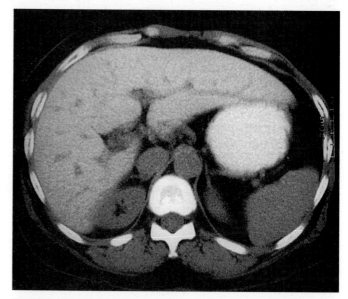

Fig. 15.1 Non-enhanced CT scan through the liver of a patient with hemochromatosis showing diffuse increased attenuation of the liver compared with the spleen.

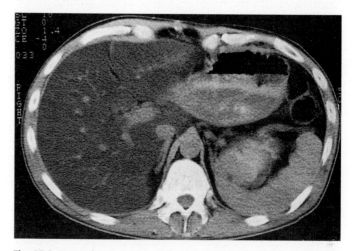

Fig. 15.2 Non-enhanced CT scan through the liver of a patient with fatty infiltration showing low attenuation of the hepatic parenchyma compared with the hepatic blood vessels and liver capsule.

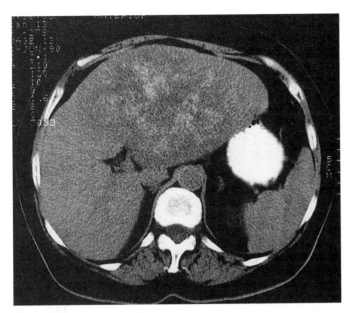

Fig. 15.3 Non-enhanced scan showing a large metastatic deposit in the left lobe of the liver from a primary colonic adenocarcinoma. Faint calcification is visible in the metastasis which would be masked following intravenous contrast medium enhancement.

may be obscured by the administration of intravascular contrast medium, which may also mask the presence of hemorrhage or faint calcification (Fig. 15.3). For this reason, and because the liver can now be scanned so rapidly, most centers perform a non-contrast examination prior to administration of an intravascular contrast agent. It is important, however, to remember that in some patients the clinical question may be answered by a non-contrast study alone. If, for example, a patient with a known primary tumor is shown to have numerous solid intrahepatic lesions, they are likely to represent metastases. The administration of intravenous contrast agent may make these lesions more conspicuous or even demonstrate a few additional lesions, but if a clinical management decision can be made on the non-contrast study alone, then there is no indication to perform any further imaging.

CONTRAST-ENHANCED HCT

In certain circumstances it is necessary to perform contrast-enhanced imaging of the liver, for example in patients with suspected hepatic metastases but a normal unenhanced CT, or those in whom hepatic resection is being considered. Contrast agent administration is essential in the characterization of an indeterminate lesion and certain patients, such as those with cirrhosis, should always have a contrast-enhanced scan unless there is a very strong contraindication to the administration of an intravenous contrast agent. The

aim of contrast-enhancement is to increase the conspicuity of hepatic lesions by increasing the lesion-to-liver attenuation difference. Slice thickness should be reduced to 5 mm if possible to maximize spatial resolution but the pitch can be maintained at 1.5. If this is not possible, it is better to increase the pitch to a level that will allow full coverage of the liver within a comfortable breath hold than to increase the slice thickness. It is accepted that intravenous contrast enhancement is best achieved by power-injection of a monophasic bolus of iodinated contrast agent (Birnbaum et al 1995) but the volume and rate of contrast agent injection varies from center to center.

The mean peak enhancement value of hepatic parenchyma increases when greater volumes of contrast agent are used (Chambers et al 1994a, 1994b). Increasing the injection rate does not, as was first thought, increase the level of maximum liver enhancement, but shortens the time to peak liver enhancement (Garcia et al 1996) which tends to occur approximately 25 s after the end of the bolus injection (Irie & Kusano 1996, Tublin et al 1999). There is considerable variation between the protocols used in different centers but volumes of 120–150 ml of contrast agent injected at 3 or 4 ml/s will result in satisfactory intravenous contrast-enhanced HCT of the liver.

The hepatic parenchyma obtains 75 to 80% of its blood supply from the portal venous system and only 20 to 25% from the hepatic artery. Most liver tumors, however, receive the majority of their blood supply from the hepatic arterial system (Honda et al 1992). During the first 20–30 seconds after the start of the contrast agent injection, the hepatic arterial phase, tumors may appear enhanced, depending on their vascularity, against a background of relatively unenhanced liver parenchyma. The arterial phase is short, lasting only 11–13 seconds (Kopka et al 1996) after which the large contrast load arriving via the portal venous system causes lesions to appear hypodense relative to brightly enhanced hepatic parenchyma. Commencing image acquisition at 20 s after the start of the contrast agent bolus will result in arterial (or arterial dominant) phase enhancement which is recognized by bright aortic and hepatic arterial enhancement, minimal hepatic parenchymal enhancement and early (patchy) splenic enhancement (Fig. 15.4A). The portal venous system is, as yet, unopacified (although opacification will tend to begin during the latter stage of arterial phase imaging) and no hepatic venous opacification is seen. Portal-phase imaging is performed during the period of peak hepatic enhancement. Image acquisition is commenced 60–70 s after the start of the injection and portal phase images are recognized by reduction in aortic enhancement, bright and uniform enhancement of the hepatic parenchyma, uniform splenic enhancement and opacifica-

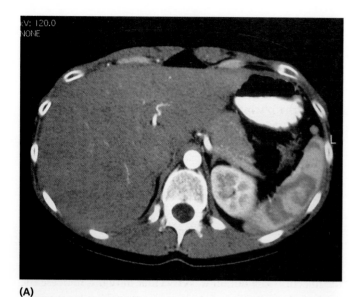

(A)

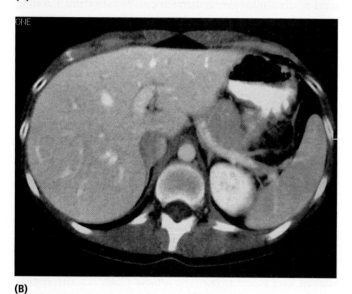

(B)

Fig. 15.4 Normal arterial and portal phases of hepatic enhancement following intravenous contrast agent administration. **(A)** Arterial phase shows bright aortic enhancement, minimal hepatic parenchymal enhancement and inhomogeneous splenic enhancement. **(B)** Portal phase shows intense hepatic parenchymal enhancement, uniform splenic enhancement and reduction in the aortic density.

Table 15.1 Vascularity of liver tumors

	Primary	Secondary
Hypervascular	Hepatocellular carcinoma	Renal cell carcinoma
	Focal nodular hyperplasia	Carcinoid
	Hepatic adenoma	Islet cell tumor
	Hemangioma	Thyroid carcinoma
		Adrenal carcinoma
		Leiomyosarcoma
		Choriocarcinoma
		Melanoma
Hypovascular	Cholangiocarcinoma	Pancreatic carcinoma
		Gallbladder carcinoma
		Esophageal carcinoma
		Gastric carcinoma
		Colonic carcinoma
		Bronchogenic carcinoma

These tumors may be obscured on the portal venous phase images because they may be enhanced to a similar degree to the surrounding liver parenchyma. They will be clearly identified, however, on the arterial phase images appearing hyperintense compared with unenhanced liver parenchyma. In this group of patients a dual-phase, contrast-enhanced scan should be performed with liver imaging in both the hepatic arterial and portal venous phases of enhancement. This type of scan is sometimes referred to as a 'triple phase' scan because, including the non-contrast phase, the liver is scanned three times in total. In evaluation of hepatocellular carcinoma (HCC) triple-phase HCT has been reported to detect additional nodules in 33% of patients (Oliver & Baron 1996) with tumors being seen only during hepatic arterial phase imaging in a significant number of cases (11%). In patients with hypervascular metastases the non-contrast component of the study has been shown to be as important as the hepatic arterial phase in lesion detection as some lesions are seen on only the non-contrast phase of the study (Oliver et al 1997, Paulson et al 1998).

If the imaging characteristics of a lesion on HCT suggest that it may be a benign cavernous hemangioma (see below) then delayed images may be performed through the lesion to record the characteristic 'in-filling' that occurs and takes up to 20 minutes in large lesions. A triple-phase HCT, however, will usually be so characteristic in cases of cavernous hemangioma that delayed scans are seldom required.

DELAYED CT

As described above, delayed HCT may be used in addition to a triple-phase study in cases of suspected hemangioma of the liver. The term 'delayed CT' was, however, originally used to describe a technique which was used prior to the

tion of the portal venous system and hepatic veins (Fig. 15.4B).

Most liver lesions are relatively hypovascular and will be most conspicuous (hypodense compared with liver parenchyma) during the portal phase of enhancement. A single-phase, contrast-enhanced scan performed during the portal phase of enhancement will be adequate to detect most focal lesions. There are, however, a group of lesions, both benign and malignant, which are relatively hypervascular because of an unusually rich arterial supply (Table 15.1).

introduction of HCT and involves a CT examination 4–6 h following administration of a double dose (up to 60 g) of iodinated contrast medium intravenously. The theory behind the technique is that iodinated contrast agents are primarily excreted by the kidneys but 1 to 2% of the administered dose is excreted by functioning hepatocytes (Bernardino et al 1986). The peak of extrarenal excretion of contrast agent occurs approximately 4 h after injection, when functioning hepatocytes will be hyperdense relative to non-excreting tissue such as spleen, muscle and blood vessels. Hepatic tumors (with the exception of focal nodular hyperplasia which contains some functioning hepatocytes) will be hypodense relative to hepatic parenchyma since they do not contain hepatocytes.

Despite improved sensitivity for detection of focal liver lesions demonstrated by several groups (Perkerson et al 1985, Phillips et al 1985, Bernardino et al 1986, Miller et al 1987), delayed CT never became widely used due to the inconvenience of the technique. Nevertheless, it is very occasionally used as an adjuvant imaging technique for clarification of subtle or questionable lesions seen during a routine CT study or CT arterial portography (see below).

CT ANGIOGRAPHY

An increasing number of patients are undergoing hepatic resection for either primary or secondary hepatic tumors, and preoperatively the surgeon needs to know the exact number, size and segmental location of each tumor nodule. Although more complex and invasive, the sensitivity of contrast-enhanced HCT of the liver can be improved by selectively delivering the contrast medium into either the portal vein or the hepatic artery, enabling lesions of only a few millimeters in diameter to be detected. The difference in blood supply between liver tumors and normal hepatic parenchyma (described above) which is exploited in dual-phase HCT results in an even greater lesion-to-liver attenuation difference when contrast medium is delivered selectively into one of the two vascular systems during HCT scan of the liver. CT angiography is performed by injecting contrast medium into either the hepatic artery directly or into the portal vein indirectly, via the superior mesenteric or splenic artery. As it is an invasive examination, the technique should be reserved for those patients who have been identified as having neoplastic lesions confined to one lobe and are being considered for partial hepatic resection.

To perform CT during hepatic arteriography (CTA), the tip of an angiographic catheter is placed into the proper hepatic artery. This minimizes the risk of contrast medium opacifying the portal system via the splenic artery. In the presence of replaced or accessory hepatic arteries, contrast administration can be administered selectively into the hepatic artery that perfuses the portion of the liver which will remain following a proposed hepatic resection, or multiple injections can be obtained. An injection of 70 ml of dilute (15 to 30%) iodinated contrast medium is delivered at a rate of 2 ml/s and thin-slice HCT through the entire liver commenced almost immediately; 3–5 s after initiating contrast administration (Chezmar et al 1993, Irie et al 1995, Takayasu et al 1995). Tumors will be hyperdense compared with the lower attenuation of the surrounding hepatic parenchyma. Hepatocellular carcinoma (HCC) tends to show homogeneous to heterogeneous enhancement whereas metastases usually demonstrate a ring enhancement pattern which is due to increased arterial perfusion in the surrounding liver parenchyma (Irie et al 1997). Hepatic arterial enhancement, however, can be very inhomogenous, particularly when hemodynamics are altered by the presence of hepatic tumors and/or cirrhosis.

Despite the fact that non-pathological areas of focal enhancement tend to occur peripherally (Kanematsu et al 1997a), CTA alone can be extremely difficult to interpret and, as a result, is not used commonly as a preoperative examination in the staging of focal liver disease. It may be of most value when combined with CT during arterial portography (CTAP), described below, when the enhancement characteristics at CTA may help characterize portal perfusion defects (Chezmar et al 1993, Kanematsu et al 1997b).

In CTAP the tip of the angiographic catheter is placed in the proximal superior mesenteric artery. A more distal placement is necessary if there is a replaced right hepatic artery, to avoid hepatic arterial opacification. Alternatively the catheter tip may be placed in the splenic artery. A total volume of 150 ml of a 60% iodinated contrast medium is administered at a rate of 3–5 ml/s and thin-slice HCT through the entire liver commenced within the period of peak hepatic enhancement, before systemic recirculation of the contrast material. A 30 s delay results in the best hepatic parenchymal and venous enhancement (Graf et al 1994). This delay allows time for the contrast medium to pass from the superior mesenteric artery through the mesenteric capillary bed into the portal venous and, eventually, the hepatic venous system. Liver tumors will be hypodense compared with the marked enhancement of the surrounding hepatic parenchyma (Fig. 15.5). Non-tumorous perfusion defects occur less frequently with CTAP than CTA and a number of factors including laminar flow in the portal vein, focal fatty infiltration or aberrant gastric venous drainage are thought to be responsible. Such 'pseudolesions' are well-described (Matsui et al 1994, Ohashi et al 1995, Kanematsu et al 1998) and tend to occur in typical locations such as the periportal region

(Fig. 15.6), around the gallbladder fossa and falciform ligament and adjacent to the right ribs. In difficult cases, however, delayed CT 4–6 hours later may be of great help in distinguishing true lesions from rounded perfusion defects (Fernandez & Bernardino 1990, McGrath et al 1993). CTAP has a slightly higher lesion detection rate compared with CTA. Several multimodality comparitive studies with operative correlation have shown that CTAP is the most sensitive pre-operative imaging modality for the detection of focal hepatic neoplasms with a reported sensitivity ranging from 81 to 91% (Nelson et al 1992, Paulson et al 1992, Bluemke & Fishman 1993, Graf et al 1994, Soyer et al 1994, Irie et al 1995, Lupetin et al 1996, McDermott et al 1996).

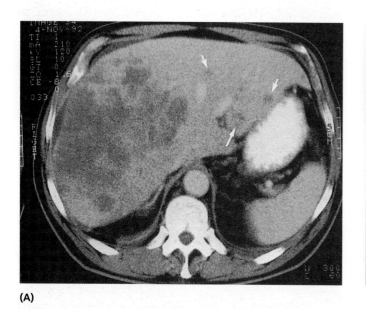
(A)

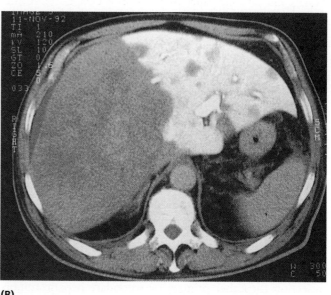
(B)

Fig. 15.5 CTAP in a patient with liver metastases being considered for hepatic resection. **(A)** Intravenous contrast-enhanced CT demonstrates numerous right sided metastases and three lesions in the left lobe (arrows). **(B)** CTAP at the same level demonstrates a straight line sign due to occlusion of the right portal vein and at least ten deposits in the left lobe.

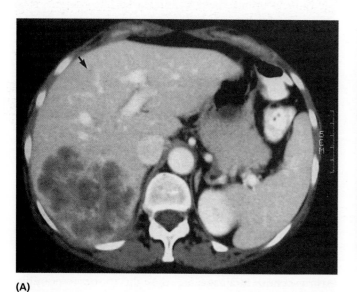
(A)

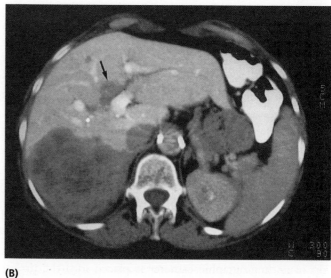
(B)

Fig. 15.6 Artefacts in CTAP. **(A)** Intravenous contrast-enhanced CT demonstrates a large right sided metastasis and a clear left lobe (the small arrowed lesion in the quadrate lobe was shown to be a simple cyst using ultrasonography). **(B)** CTAP at the same level shows a round periportal flow defect in the quadrate lobe (arrow). Note that the tumor in the right lobe appears larger with CTAP—this technique is more accurate in assessing tumor size.

LIPIODOL CT

This technique was developed primarily for the detection and treatment of hepatocellular carcinomas (Choi et al 1989a,b, Merine et al 1990) and involves administration of 2–10 ml of the iodized poppy seed oil Lipiodol, directly into the hepatic artery. There is selective and prolonged retention of iodized oil within highly vascular and abnormal hepatic tissue, especially HCC. This is due to a combination of trapping of Lipiodol within irregular and tortuous tumor vessels and slow clearance due to the absence of lymphatics and Küpffer's cells in HCC. Computed tomography scanning is performed 1–4 weeks later, when HCC appears hyperdense compared with hepatic parenchyma. The sensitivity and specificity of Lipiodol CT in the diagnosis of HCC has been reported to be as high as 97% and 77% respectively (Merine et al 1990, de Santis et al 1992, Lencioni et al 1997, Spreafico et al 1997). Limitations of the technique include the fact that poorly vascular, necrotic or fibrotic subtypes of HCC may not accumulate Lipiodol and there may be non-specific retention in normal parenchyma in the presence of focal inflammation or arterioportal shunts. Lipiodol is often mixed with lipophilic chemotherapeutic agents such as doxorubicin and mitomycin and embolic particles in an attempt to palliate the tumors or diminish their size prior to hepatic resection.

CT CHOLANGIOGRAPHY

Computed tomography following administration of intravenous cholangiographic contrast agents such as meglumine iodoxamate (Fig. 15.7) provides non-invasive opacification of the bile ducts and may be used for evaluation of congenital or acquired abnormalities of the biliary tree, ductal calculi and bile leaks. Pitfalls of this technique include lack of bile duct opacification in jaundiced patients and the fact that dense opacification of the ductal system may mask calculi or other subtle intraductal pathology. The facility to perform high-resolution CT with three dimensional reconstructions of the biliary tree has led to a resurgence of interest in the technique, and it has a role to play in conditions such as Caroli's disease (Fig. 15.8) where direct administration of contrast agent into the biliary tree, by percutaneous transhepatic cholangiography or endoscopic retrograde cholangiography, is undesirable (Stockberger et al 1994, Fleischmann et al 1996, Masui et al 1998). Computed tomography cholangiography is, however, relatively infrequently used due to the advances in magnetic resonance cholangiopancreatography (MRCP) which produces extremely high quality cholangiographic images without administration of a contrast agent or exposure to ionizing radiation.

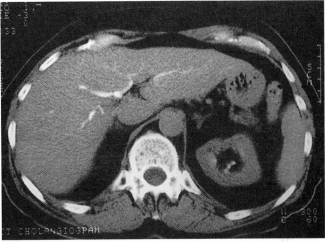

(A)

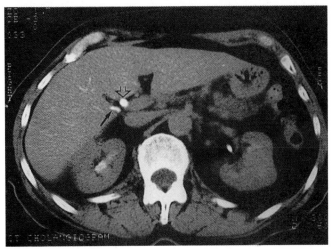

(B)

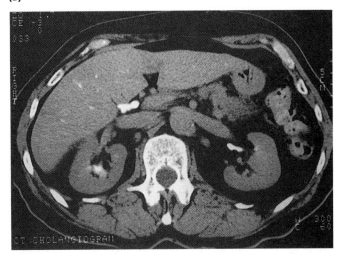

(C)

Fig. 15.7 CT performed after administration of intravenous cholangiographic agent showing normal variants of bile duct anatomy. **(A)** Contrast filling of non-dilated intrahepatic ducts. The confluence of the right anterior and left ductal systems is seen. **(B)** On a lower section, the right posterior sectoral duct (solid arrow) is seen separate to the common duct (open arrow). **(C)** At the level of the renal hila, the low insertion of the right posterior sectoral duct into the common duct is seen.

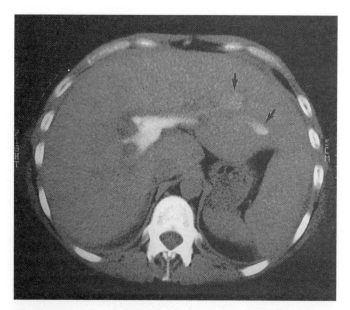

Fig. 15.8 CT following intravenous cholangiography in Caroli's disease showing pooling of contrast agent in large intrahepatic cystic spaces (arrows), proving that they are in communication with the biliary tree.

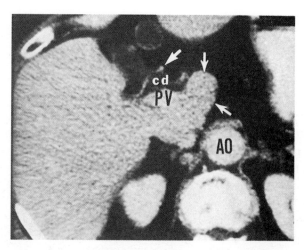

Fig. 15.9 Large papillary process of the caudate lobe (arrows) projects anteriorly and leftwards into the superior recess of the lesser sac. Note proper hepatic artery coursing anterior to the common hepatic duct (cd), which in turn lies on the right anterior surface of the portal vein (PV). AO, aorta.

ANATOMY (see also Ch. 1)

GROSS MORPHOLOGY

The liver is the largest organ in the abdomen and occupies most of the right upper quadrant. The right liver is generally larger than the left but there is considerable individual anatomic variation in size and shape, particularly of the left liver, which may remain entirely on the right of the abdomen or extend across the midline towards the left. The left liver consists of two lateral segments (segments II and III) and the medial segment (segment IV) (the quadrate lobe). Medially, the caudate lobe gives rise to the papillary process (Fig. 15.9), which protrudes to the left and anteriorly and invaginates the superior recess of the lesser sac. When large, the papillary process may be mistaken for an extrahepatic lymph node. In some cases the lateral segments may wrap around and appear contiguous with the spleen. The diaphragmatic surface of the liver is smoothly convex while the inferior or visceral surface is somewhat concave. The liver is covered in peritoneum with the exception of a portion of its posterior superior surface, where it is directly adherent to the diaphragm. This 'bare area' lies between the superior and inferior coronary ligaments which support the right lobe of the liver from the diaphragm. Due to the absence of a potential peritoneal space related to the bare area, any fluid seen posterior to the liver at this location must be either beneath the liver capsule or within the

pleural space. An important pitfall to be aware of when interpreting axial CT scans is that extrahepatic lesions arising from the right adrenal gland or perirenal region may mimic intrahepatic lesions arising from the right lobe of the liver (Fig. 15.10). The left lobe is supported from the diaphragm by the left coronary ligament, which becomes contiguous with the falciform ligament, anchoring the left lobe to the diaphragm and anterior abdominal wall. These ligaments are not normally seen on CT unless their margins are outlined by intraperitoneal fluid.

Three large fissures interrupt the surface of the liver and help define its segmentation. The interlobar fissure is an incomplete structure that defines the inferior margin of the separation between the right and the left liver. This fissure is generally difficult to identify on CT, but its position may be estimated as it is orientated in a vertical plane defined by the gallbladder fossa inferiorly (Fig. 15.11E) and the middle hepatic vein superiorly (Fig. 15.11B). The gallbladder, which is readily recognised on CT as an oval, water-dense structure, lies in the main interlobar fissure on the inferior surface of the liver (Fig. 15.11E).

Slightly to the right of midline, the anteroinferior portion of the diaphragmatic surface of the liver is notched by the fissure for the ligamentum teres or umbilical fissure which defines the inferior border between the medial and lateral segments of the left liver (Fig. 15.11D and E). The ligamentum teres passes through this fissure and is usually surrounded by a small amount of fat. When the ligamentum teres passes out of the liver ventrally, it is located in the free edge of the falciform ligament. The third fissure is present at the point of contact between the lateral segments of the left

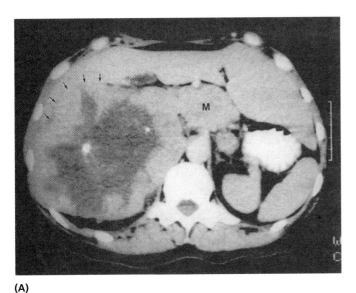

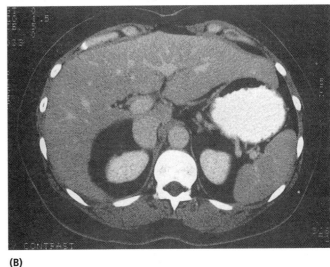

(A)

(B)

Fig. 15.10 Large right adrenal pheochromocytoma mimicking a right sided liver tumor. **(A)** Preoperative CT scan demonstrates a large tumor in the position of the right hepatic lobe. Careful inspection of the image reveals a thin plane between the tumor and the liver (arrows). The medial mass (M) proved to be a large lymph node mass. **(B)** Postoperative scan following removal of the adrenal tumor and lymph node mass confirms that the liver is normal.

hepatic lobe and the caudate lobe. This is the fissure for the ligamentum venosum (Fig. 15.11C and D), which is in continuity with the umbilical fissure. The former, however, has a right–left orientation on cross-sectional imaging, whereas the latter lies anteroposteriorly.

The mean density of hepatic parenchyma varies between 54 and 60 HU. Increased density may be seen in hemochromotosis, glycogen storage disease, Wilson's disease, β-thalassemia, sickle-cell disease and with certain drugs (amiodarone, cisplatin). A false appearance of inceased hepatic density may occur in anemia where the decreased attenuation of the blood pool gives the impression of increased hepatic density relative to the intrahepatic vessels. Decreased hepatic density is most frequently related to fatty infiltration of the liver, or occasionally secondary to hepatic edema.

SEGMENTAL ANATOMY

Many systems dividing the liver into segments have been described. A functional system, designed to correlate with surgical technique, has been described (Bismuth 1982). In this system, the three main hepatic veins divide the liver into four sectors, each of which is independent in that it receives a separate portal venous and hepatic arterial supply, and is drained by a separate bile duct (see Chs 1 & 83). The middle hepatic vein divides the liver into a right and left liver. The right liver is divided into two sectors by the right hepatic vein, and the left liver similarly by the left hepatic

vein. Since CT readily demonstrates the course of all three major hepatic veins on contrast-enhanced scans obtained near the diaphragm, the major hepatic sectors are easy to identify at this level (Fig. 15.11A and B). On scans obtained more caudally, the hepatic veins are difficult to differentiate from portal radicles, but a simple method to ensure better visualization of the hepatic veins is to tilt the gantry 20° caudally (Tidebrant et al 1991). The inferior boundary between the anterior and posterior sectors of the right lobe has to be estimated by extrapolating the line of the right hepatic vein on to lower sections. An imaginary line drawn between the inferior vena cava and the gallbladder, however, divides the right and left liver on caudal sections and corresponds to the line of the middle hepatic vein (Fig. 15.11E). The fissure for the ligamentum teres divides the medial and lateral segments of the left liver and corresponds to the line of the left hepatic vein (Fig. 15.11B, D and E). The anterior and posterior sectors of the right lobe are subdivided into inferior (V and VI) and superior (VIII and VII) segments. The right portal vein runs horizontally as it enters the right liver and this level demarcates the superior from the inferior segments (Fig. 15.11D).

VASCULAR ANATOMY

The portal vein originates at the junction of the splenic and superior mesenteric veins, immediately posterior to the neck of the pancreas. It then courses towards the right and cephalad as it enters the hepatoduodenal ligament. Within

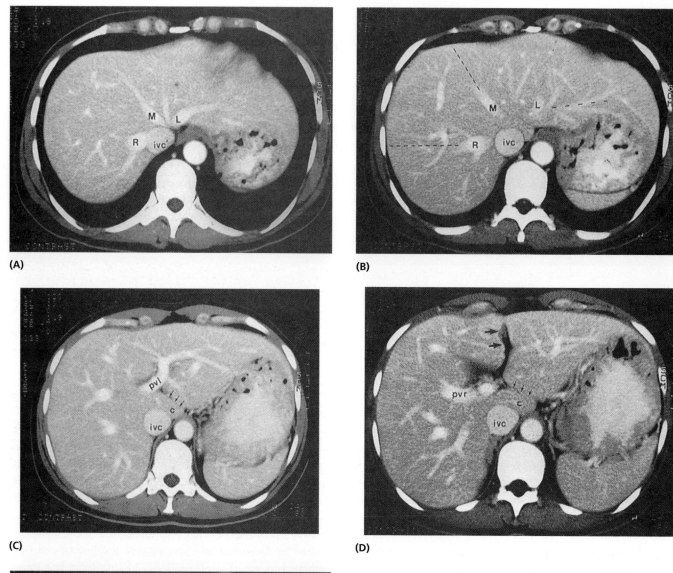

(A)

(B)

(C)

(D)

(E)

Fig. 15.11 Normal hepatic segmental and vascular anatomy on CT. **(A)** On cephalad sections the three hepatic veins are seen to enter the inferior vena cava. **(B)** The lines of the hepatic veins divide the liver into sectors. The right hepatic vein divides the right liver into an anterior and posterior sector; the middle hepatic vein separates the right from the left liver (and represents the line of the interlobar fissure); the left hepatic vein separates the segments of the left lobe (segments II and III). **(C)** Approaching the mid point of the liver the left portal vein is clearly seen. The fissure for the ligamentum venosum (arrows) divides the caudate lobe from the left lateral segments. **(D)** The next section demonstrates the horizontal portion of the right portal vein. The fissure for the ligamentum teres is now seen (large arrows) and this structure divides the lateral segments of the left liver from the quadrate lobe (segment IV). **(E)** On the last section the gall bladder has come into view and a line drawn along the axis of the gallbladder to the inferior vena cava represents the inferior extent of the interlobar fissure.

R, right hepatic vein; M, middle hepatic vein; L, left hepatic vein; ivc, inferior vena cava; c, caudate lobe; pvl, left portal vein; pvr, right portal vein; GB, gallbladder. (See also Ch. 1.)

this ligament, it runs a course parallel to the proper hepatic artery, which lies on its anteromedial surface, and the common bile duct which lies on its anterolateral surface. After entering the hepatic parenchyma, the portal vein branches in a predictable fashion to supply each portal sector. The branching patterns of the hepatic artery and bile ducts are identical with those of the portal vein.

A common normal variant which can be recognized on CT is an anomalous origin of the right hepatic artery, generally from the superior mesenteric artery. This vessel nearly always courses between the inferior vena cava and the portal vein to supply the right liver.

BILIARY ANATOMY (see Ch. 1)

The intrahepatic biliary tree branches in a fashion nearly identical to the portal system (Fig. 15.12). The left and right hepatic ducts form the common hepatic duct near the lateral margin of the main portal vein near its junction with the right portal vein. The common hepatic duct then continues inferiorly, towards the left and somewhat posteriorly, and maintains its anterolateral position with respect to the portal vein throughout its course within the hepatoduodenal ligament. It becomes retroperitoneal at the level of the head of the pancreas and occupies a position on the posterolateral surface of the pancreas until it joins the pancreatic duct immediately before entering the ampulla of Vater. The confluence of the right and left hepatic ducts is often seen lying anterior to the portal venous confluence. Visualization of the intrahepatic bile ducts with CT was originally considered to be evidence of biliary obstruction but, with newer scanners and thin collimation, peripheral bile ducts measuring 1–3 mm may be seen in normal subjects (Liddell et al 1990). The common duct, which measures 3–6 mm in cross-sectional diameter, is seen as a circular structure of near-water density posterolateral to the head of the pancreas on a postcontrast scan. The CT diagnosis of biliary obstruction is based on the demonstration of dilated intrahepatic or extrahepatic bile ducts. Dilated intrahepatic ducts appear on CT as linear branching or circular structure of near-water density enlarging as they approach the junction of the left and right hepatic ducts in the porta hepatis. The extrahepatic bile duct is considered unequivocally dilated if it is 9 mm or more in diameter (Fig. 15.13) and definitely normal if less than 7 mm. Although CT has proved to be accurate in establishing a diagnosis of biliary obstruction there is not always a direct correlation between the calibre of the biliary tree and the presence of clinically significant obstruction. In patients with significant dilation of the biliary tree in whom the obstruction is later relieved surgically or by spontaneous passage of a calculus, the bile

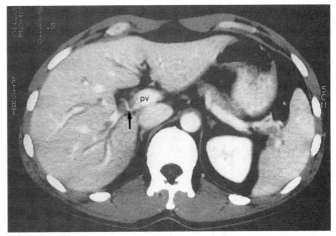

(A)

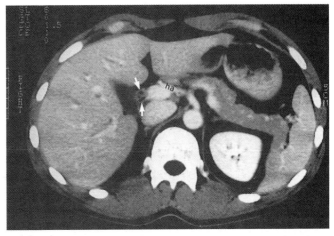

(B)

Fig. 15.12 Contrast-enhanced scan in a patient with a minimally dilated biliary system. **(A)** The intrahepatic bile ducts are seen as branching low-attenuation structures adjacent to the portal veins. At the porta hepatis the hepatic artery (arrow) is seen to pass between the main portal vein (pv) and the common hepatic duct. **(B)** A scan caudal to the porta hepatis demonstrates the common hepatic duct and the cystic duct running adjacent to each other in the hepatoduodenal ligament (arrows). The hepatic artery (ha) is in a more medial position.

duct may remain somewhat more dilated than normal for the remainder of the patient's life. In such patients, the CT findings may falsely suggest the presence of biliary obstruction. Likewise, a normal-calibre bile duct can be observed in the presence of a surgically correctable cause of jaundice. Intermittently obstructing calculi and subtle strictures of the extrahepatic duct may be present when the overall duct calibre is normal. In situations where there is discrepancy between clinical or biochemical evidence and the CT findings, MRCP or direct cholangiography by the percutaneous or endoscopic route should be performed to resolve the problem.

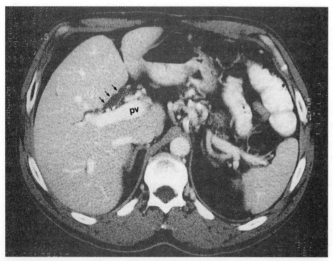

(A)

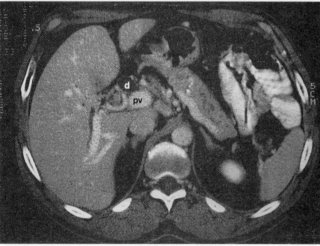

(B)

Fig. 15.13 (A) In a patient with dilated intra- and extrahepatic ducts the dilated confluence of right and left ducts (arrows) is seen lying anterior to the portal vein. **(B)** Below the porta hepatis the dilated common duct is seen lying anterolateral to the portal vein. pv, portal vein; d, common duct.

In addition to its ability to detect the presence or absence of biliary obstruction, CT is also able to predict the cause of obstruction in a majority of cases. While abrupt termination of the extrahepatic duct suggests a malignant process, smooth gradual tapering of bile ducts favors benign disease. The use of a negative oral contrast agent such as water will help in identification of small distal bile duct calculi.

PATHOLOGICAL PROCESSES

NEOPLASMS

The ability of CT to display precise anatomical information has made it a cornerstone in the evaluation of focal hepatic lesions. The ability of CT to characterize a hepatic mass, however, is limited to defining its size and location and displaying its response to contrast administration. No set of CT-derived criteria is capable of unequivocally distinguishing between a benign and a malignant lesion. It is, therefore, often necessary to perform a CT- or US-guided percutaneous biopsy to obtain tissue for histological examination.

MALIGNANT LESIONS

Hepatocellular carcinoma

Hepatocellular carcinoma, while not as prevalent in the West as it is in Africa and Asia, is still the most common primary hepatic tumor. It is a vascular neoplasm which may be solitary (30%), multifocal (65%) or may diffusely infiltrate the liver (5%). Complications include tumor invasion of the portal or hepatic veins, internal hemorrhage or rupture into the peritoneal cavity, biliary obstruction and metastatic spread.

On non-contrast CT, HCC appears as a solitary mass or multiple masses that are hypodense relative to normal hepatic parenchyma except in fatty livers where the tumor may appear hyperdense. Calcification is seen in less than 10% and fatty degeneration occurring within hepatocellular carcinoma has been reported (Itai et al 1981, Yoshikawa et al 1988, Freeny et al 1992). Following administration of intravenous contrast agent, HCC is normally hyperdense in the arterial phase due to its vascularity and hypo- or isodense compared with hepatic parenchyma in the portal venous phase. It is therefore not surprising that dual-phase scanning has been shown to detect a greater number of tumors than portal venous-phase imaging alone (Fig. 15.14). Imaging during the arterial phase has other advantages in that it can identify the early portal venous enhancement which is seen in the presence of arterioportal shunting and demonstrates enhancement of portal vein thrombus in cases where intravascular invasion has occurred (Fig. 15.15). Portal vein invasion is demonstrated in up to 44% of cases (Freeny et al 1992), and invasion of the inferior vena cava and hepatic veins also occurs (4 and 6%). Computed tomography findings of portal venous invasion by hepatocellular carcinoma include arterio-portal fistulae (Fig. 15.16), periportal streaks of high attenuation, or dilatation of the main portal vein or its major branches.

Encapsulated HCC is surrounded by a fibrous capsule and is characterized by a hypodense rim on the arterial-phase images (Fig. 15.17A). The capsule enhances on the portal phase images (Fig. 15.17B) and, if seen, indicates a well-differentiated, slow-growing tumor with a relatively

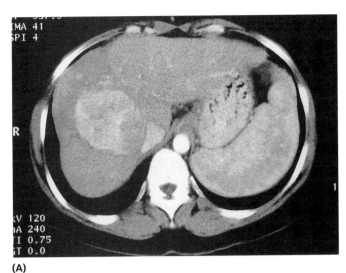

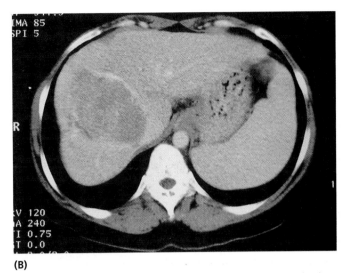

(A)   (B)

Fig. 15.14 Hepatocellular carcinoma **(A)** An arterial-phase image demonstrates a large brightly enhancing tumor abutting the inferior vena cava (IVC). A tiny daughter nodule is seen anteriorly. **(B)** A portal-phase image at the same level shows the HCC to be clearly visible but hypodense—the daughter nodule is no longer apparent.

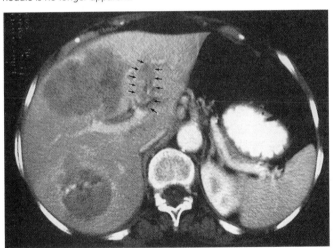

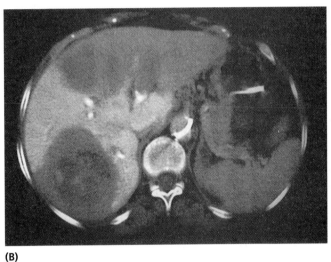

(A)   (B)

Fig. 15.15 Portal venous invasion by hepatocellular carcinoma. **(A)** Dynamic-bolus enhanced CT showing multifocal hepatocellular carcinoma. The proximal left portal vein appears amputated and more distally it is expanded by inhomogeneously enhancing soft tissue representing tumor thrombus (arrows). **(B)** These findings are confirmed by CTAP which demonstrates non-enhancement of the left liver (the straight line sign) due to left portal venous occlusion. The rounded edge of the tumor thrombus is clearly seen.

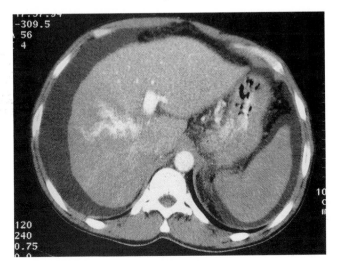

Fig. 15.16 Arterioportal shunting in association with a large right hepatocellular carcinoma. This section, caudal to the tumor, demonstrates peripheral streaks of high attenuation relating to the right portal vein.

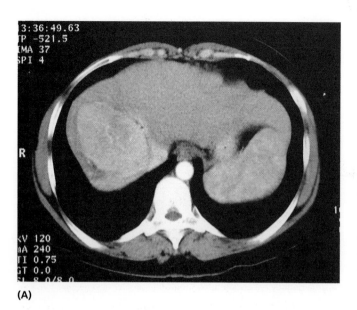
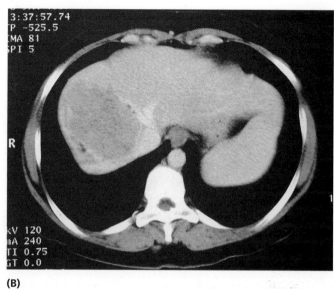

(A)   **(B)**

Fig. 15.17 Encapsulated HCC. **(A)** An arterial-phase image demonstrates a brightly enhancing HCC in the right liver surrounded by a hypodense rim. **(B)** The portal phase shows enhancement of the tumor capsule.

good prognosis (Ros et al 1990, Honda et al 1992). Fibrous septae forming a mosaic pattern within the tumor are also well seen on later scans and indicate a worse prognosis as they result from either tumor infiltration beyond the capsule or two or more separate tumors with a fibrous septum between them (LaLonde et al 1992). Computed tomographic arterial portography is an extremely effective imaging method for small tumors, with a detection rate of 95%. Computed tomography following injection of Lipiodol has also been reported to be an extremely sensitive method for detecting small hepatocellular carcinomas, detecting 93 to 96% of tumors. Extrahepatic metastatic disease from hepatocellular carcinoma is seen in up to 70% of cases. Nodes in the hepatoduodenal ligament are the commonest site of lymphatic spread; hematogenous metastases may be encountered in the lungs or adrenal glands.

Fibrolamellar hepatocellular carcinoma

This rare malignant tumor affects young adults without underlying hepatic cirrhosis. It is less aggressive than hepatocellular carcinoma and often has a good prognosis following tumor resection. Serum alpha-fetoprotein is usually normal but other markers may be elevated, such as vitamin B_{12} binding capacity, copper and copper binding proteins in malignant hepatocytes, and carcinoembryonic antigen. The tumor is composed of eosinophilic hepatocytes subdivided by laminated bands of stroma. It is usually a solitary, lobulated tumor which appears sharply demarcated from

surrounding hepatic parenchyma and often contains a central scar (Fig. 15.18). Central amorphous calcification is seen in up to 55% of cases (Brandt et al 1988, Soyer et al 1991) and is a major clue to the diagnosis on CT since calcification in untreated hepatocellular carcinoma is rare. Following intravenous contrast medium administration, variably intense enhancement occurs. There is no early enhancement of the central scar but this can occur on delayed images (Titelbaum et al 1988). Portal venous invasion can occur, but is much less frequent than with typical HCC.

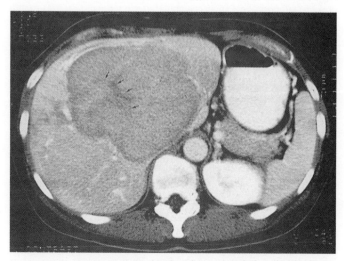

Fig. 15.18 Fibrolamellar hepatocellular carcinoma. The tumor has a smooth, well-circumscribed, lobulated outline and contains a central scar (arrows).

Angiosarcoma

Risk factors for angiosarcoma of the liver include hemochromatosis, radiotherapy, or exposure to compounds such as polyvinylchloride, arsenic, or Thorotrast. This last compound is a colloidal suspension containing 20% thorium dioxide by weight and was a widely used contrast agent from the late 1920s to the early 1950s. Following intravenous administration Thorotrast is deposited in the reticuloendothelial system of the liver and other organs where it is carcinogenic since it is an alpha-emitter with a biological half-life of 400 years and physical half-life of 1.4×10^{10} years. The mean latent period between Thorotrast administration and the subsequent development of malignancy is 29 years; most patients develop angiosarcoma, a malignant tumor of the reticuloendothelial system, but both hepatocellular carcinoma and cholangiocarcinoma have been described. Angiosarcoma is a vascular hepatic neoplasm that appears as an infiltrating, brightly enhancing mass on CT (Mahony et al 1982, Silverman et al 1983, Vasile et al 1983). High-attenuation thorium deposition may be seen in a patchy distribution in the liver, perihepatic lymph nodes and spleen. Histological 'cavernous' angiosarcoma may enhance in a similar way to hemangiomata, with the tumor becoming wholly or partly isodense with liver on delayed scanning (Itai & Teraoka 1989, White et al 1993).

Hepatic lymphoma

Primary lymphoma of the liver is a rare entity although the liver is a common secondary site of lymphomatous involvement, occurring at autopsy in 50% of patients with non-Hodgkin's lymphoma and 60% of patients with Hodgkin's disease. Less than 50 cases of primary hepatic lymphoma have been described, usually appearing as a large, multilobulated mass which enhances poorly following intravenous administration contrast medium (Osborne et al 1985, Sanders et al 1989). Central necrosis is frequently seen. Secondary lymphomatous involvement of the liver tends to be diffusely infiltrative or micronodular and CT may only show hepatomegaly with no evidence of focal lesions.

Hepatic metastases

The liver provides a fertile soil for metastases, not only due to its dual blood supply from both systemic and portal systems, but also because of humoral factors promoting cell growth and is second only to regional lymph nodes as a site of metastatic disease. Most hepatic metastases arise from primary tumors in the colon, breast, lung and pancreas. Peripheral sarcomas, melanoma, renal and thyroid malignancy and pelvic tumors are less common causes of hepatic metastases. Although metastases may be found anywhere in the liver, more lesions are found in the right liver compared with the left (Fink & Chaudhuri 1991). This may be because the right liver has more mass than the left but it has been hypothesized that tumor cells flow in a dependent laminar fashion in the portal vein and are therefore more likely to be directed to the right than the left.

The CT appearance of metastases is variable and depends on the size and vascularity of the tumor, the degree of necrosis and the CT technique used (see section on techniques above). Borders may be sharp, ill-defined or nodular. The shape may be round, ovoid or irregular. Attenuation is usually lower than that of surrounding hepatic parenchyma before non-contrast CT which on its own will detect only 50% of metastases (Paley & Ros 1998). Intravenous contrast agent enhancement increases the sensitivity to between 75 and 80%. Scanning during the appropriate phase of enhancement (arterial, portal, delayed) increases detection even further (see techniques section above). Peripheral ring enhancement occurs in all metastases but this is usually not appreciated in hypovascular metastases which appear of low attenuation compared with surrounding intensely enhancing hepatic parenchyma during portal phase scanning. Hypervascular metastases (see Table 15.1) may be obscured during the portal phase and are most clearly visualized during the arterial phase. Metastases from mucinous carcinomas tend to contain punctate or amorphous calcification (see Fig. 15.3). Cystic metastases are occasionally seen and can be distinguished from benign simple cysts since the former often contain mural nodules, fluid–fluid levels or septations. Differentiation of multiple hepatic metastases from multifocal hepatocellular carcinoma may be difficult but, generally, metastases present as multiple lesions of varying size scattered throughout the liver whereas, in hepatocellular carcinoma, the satellite lesions are usually small and relatively close to the primary mass. In addition, metastases rarely protrude prominently from the liver surface, a feature which is commonly seen with hepatocellular carcinoma.

Hepatic metastases missed on intravenous contrast-enhanced HCT are those that are relatively small, less than 1 cm in diameter and in patients who are potential candidates for surgical resection of metastases, CTAP is advised to best define the number and exact location of focal metastases. Computed tomographic arterial portography has a sensitivity ranging from 81 to 91% (see above) and in approximately 20% of patients there is an increase in the number of lesions detected by CTAP in comparison to intravenous contrast-enhanced hepatic CT. Computed tomographic arterial portography also gives a more accurate assessment of tumor size as lesions often appear smaller using intravenous contrast administration because the tumor edge becomes isodense with liver parenchyma (Fig. 15.6).

BENIGN TUMORS AND TUMOR-LIKE CONDITIONS

Cysts (Chs 66 and 67)

Hepatic cysts may be either congenital or acquired. Congenital cysts are more common than the acquired type, which are secondary to inflammation, trauma or parasitic disease. Small isolated congenital hepatic cysts are not uncommon and on CT are sharply defined, homogeneous areas of near-water attenuation, which do not enhance after administration of an intravenous contrast agent. Large cysts occur (Fig. 15.19) and can be multiseptated. Generally, the CT appearance of a simple cyst is so characteristic that no further evaluation is indicated. If the clinical history strongly suggests the possibility of a cystic neoplasm or abscess or if the CT appearance is atypical, ultrasonography should be performed followed by percutaneous needle aspiration of the lesion if appearances are confirmed to be atypical for a simple cyst.

Multiple hepatic cysts are usually associated with polycystic renal disease (Fig. 15.20), but may occur in the absence of renal cysts. Occasionally, patients may present with discomfort or biliary obstruction secondary to a large cyst. In such cases therapeutic aspiration and sclerosis of the cyst may be indicated.

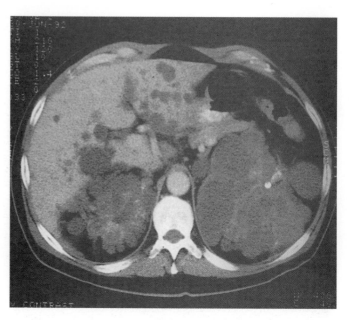

Fig. 15.20 Multiple simple hepatic cysts in a patient with polycystic kidneys.

Cavernous hemangioma

Hepatic cavernous hemangioma is a relatively common tumor, occurring in approximately 10% of the normal adult population. It occurs predominantly in females and is often located in the right liver. In 10% of patients, multiple hemangiomata are present. Cavernous hemangioma is the single tumor with so characteristic an enhancement pattern following intravenous contrast that its histology can be confidently predicted. Because of its extensive vascular compartment, intense globular peripheral enhancement occurs after a bolus of contrast is administered followed by slow diffusion from the periphery toward the center (Fig. 15.21). The enhancement is typically isodense with the aorta at all stages (Leslie et al 1995). In large lesions it may take up to 30 minutes for complete opacification to occur. CT features seen in cavernous hemangioma are listed in Table 15.2. Using the criteria shown, the positive predictive value of CT in the diagnosis of hemangioma was 100% in one series (Ashida et al 1987). With the exception of small tumors (less than 2 cm) which do not exhibit these typical enhancement patterns, the combination of the clinical and radiographic features are usually diagnostic of this entity. Giant hemangiomas (greater than 10 cm diameter) occur and typically contain a central low-attenuation stellate scar. If there is typical uniform centripetal enhancement the diagnosis of hemangioma can be made but large tumors may be complicated by extensive intralesional fibrosis resulting in an atypical enhancement pattern. In such cases, biopsy may be required for definitive diagnosis.

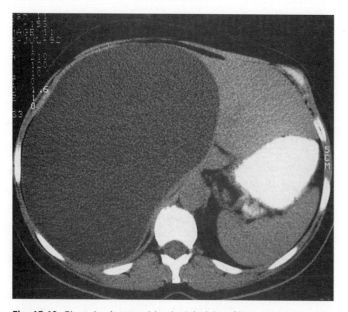

Fig. 15.19 Giant simple cyst arising in right lobe of liver. It is well-circumscribed and of homogeneous, near-water attenuation.

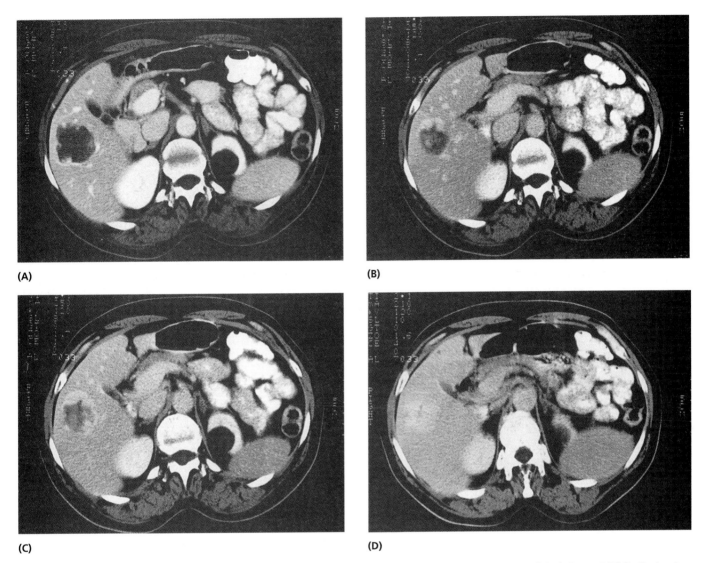

Fig. 15.21 Cavernous hemangioma of right liver showing **(A–C)** typical enhancement commencing at the periphery of the lesion and **(D)** finally showing complete opacification.

Table 15.2 CT features of hepatic cavernous hemangioma*

1. Low density lesion on unenhanced scan
2. Early peripheral contrast enhancement
3. Progressive opacification from the periphery to the center
4. A delay of at least 3 minutes before total opacification
5. Eventual isodense appearance with or without unopacified cleft

*Criteria for diagnosing cavernous hemangioma are 4 and 5 plus at least two of the remaining three.

Hepatocellular adenoma (Ch. 72)

These benign vascular tumors are composed of hepatocytes and demarcated by a fibrous capsule. They are found in young adult women in about 95% of cases. Recently, how-ever, there has been an increase in prevalence of this benign tumor, a fact which has been related to the widespread use of oral contraceptives.

Hepatocellular adenoma may present with spontaneous hemorrhage and may undergo malignant transformation. Hepatocellular adenoma is solitary in 80% and, on HCT, is typically a well-defined, encapsulated, low-attenuation mass because of the high lipid content of the hepatocytes within it. Areas that contain hemorrhage are hyperdense. Following contrast agent administration, transient periph-eral enhancement may be seen as a reflection of large subcapsular feeding vessels (Mathieu et al 1986). This enhancement may be missed unless arterial phase imaging is performed.

Focal nodular hyperplasia (Ch. 72)

Focal nodular hyperplasia (FNH) is composed of hepatocytes, bile ducts and Küpffer cells supported by a radiating fibrous stroma connected to a small central scar. A surrounding capsule is not seen. Focal nodular hyperplasia occurs primarily in young adult females but approximately 10 to 20% occur in men, and in 20% of patients are multifocal. Hemorrhage is rare unless lesions have undergone trauma. Focal nodular hyperplasia has no malignant potential. Unenhanced CT scans show a well-defined hypodense or isodense lesion. Only about 1% of FNH contain calcifications (Caseiro-Alves et al 1996). On contrast-enhanced HCT, FNH usually appears as a transiently homogeneously contrast-enhanced lesion (Fig. 15.22) that becomes isodense with hepatic parenchyma when portal haze or delayed scans are obtained (Welch et al 1985, Procacci et al 1992, Shamsi et al 1993). Contrast agent diffuses into the central scar and the scar may therefore be hyperdense relative to the rest of the lesion and to normal liver on delayed images.

Differentiation between hepatocellular adenoma and FNH may be impossible using CT alone. Focal nodular hyperplasia generally demonstrates uniform uptake on a technetium sulfur colloid scan but a small percentage of adenomas also demonstrate uniform isotope activity (Lubbers et al 1987). Fine needle aspiration cytology may differentiate between FNH and hepatocellular adenoma due to the presence of bile duct cells in the former (Ruschenburg & Droese 1989) but neither fine-needle aspiration biopsy nor wedge biopsy allows the pathologist to distinguish FNH and hepatocellular adenoma in all cases.

Regenerative hepatic nodules

Regenerative nodules are found in macronodular cirrhotic livers and represent islands of normal hepatic parenchyma containing bile ducts and Küpffer cells demarcated by the coarse fibrotic septa of the cirrhotic liver. It is thought that the natural progression of regenerative nodules is to low-grade dysplasia, high grade dysplasia and then to HCC but this may take many years and is not inevitable (Earls et al 1996). Regenerative nodules appear as isodense 'pseudo-masses', approximately 2 cm in diameter and enhance to the same degree as normal liver parenchyma following intravenous contrast agent administration. Evidence of arterial hypervascularity, shown by enhancement during the arterial phase, suggests that the nodule is dysplastic or contains foci of HCC (Lee et al 1997). Differentiation between metastases or hepatocellular carcinoma may be aided by Lipiodol CT since regenerating nodules, unlike tumors, tend not to retain the oily contrast agent, but definitive diagnosis often requires biopsy.

Peliosis hepatis

This is an unusual condition occurring in patients suffering from chronic debilitating diseases, such as tuberculosis or malignancy and in those receiving anabolic steroids. In this condition, multiple blood-filled cystic spaces occur within the liver, and generally range in size between a few millimeters and 1 cm. Some may be as large as 4–5 cm in diameter and there is danger of exsanguinating hemorrhage. Unenhanced CT displays multiple blood-dense irregular

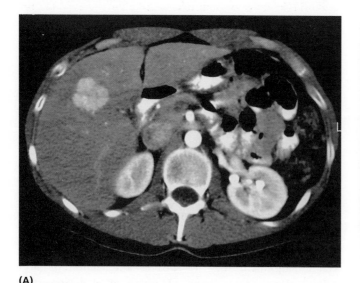

(A)

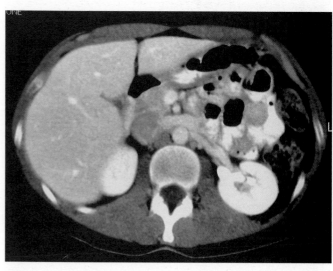

(B)

Fig. 15.22 Focal nodular hyperplasia **(A)** Arterial phase image demonstrates a well-circumscribed, brightly enhancing lesion in segment IV/V. **(B)** During the portal phase, the lesion is isodense with liver parenchyma and cannot be identified.

spaces which enhance following administration of contrast agent (Jamadar et al 1994). The condition may be complicated by hemorrhagic necrosis which may be mistaken for hepatic abscess (Vignaux et al 1999).

INFLAMMATORY DISEASE

Pyogenic abscess (Ch. 61)

Recent surgery, biliary disease, diverticulitis, Crohn's disease and alcoholism all predispose to pyogenic hepatic abscess. Due to the widespread use of broad-spectrum antibiotics the clinical presentation and CT appearance varies widely (Halvorsen et al 1984). Pyogenic hepatic abscesses may be classified as either microabscesses (less than 2 cm in size) or larger confluent lesions (macroabscesses). Microabscesses are well-defined, small, hypodense lesions on contrast-enhanced CT. They may be widely scattered or clustered with a tendency to coalesce (Jeffrey et al 1988). The relatively rare, diffuse, miliary pattern of pyogenic microabscesses is caused by staphylococcal infection in patients with generalized septicemia and the spleen is usually similarly affected. The cluster pattern, however, is associated with coliform bacteria and enteric organisms. This pattern is also seen in cholangitic abscesses related to biliary obstruction. Larger pyogenic abscesses range in appearance from unilocular cavities with smooth outer margins to highly complex and septated structures with internal debris and irregular contours. The majority of large pyogenic abscesses occur in the posterior portion of the right liver,

and on unenhanced CT appear as a well-defined mass of low attenuation. The attenuation value of the abscess cavity depends on the age of the abscess and becomes lower as the abscess matures. Gas bubbles may be seen if anaerobic bacteria are present. The periphery and any internal septae may enhance following contrast agent administration (Fig. 15.23). Patients with portal pyemia may have completely or incompletely occluding thrombi in the superior mesenteric or portal vein (Lim et al 1989) and CT evidence of appendicitis or diverticulitis.

Fungal abscesses

Fungal hepatic abscesses are generally disseminated microabscesses and occur in immunosuppressed patients. The most common fungal organism implicated is *Candida albicans*. Other fungi that cause microabscesses include cryptococcus, histoplasmosis, and mucormycosis. The sensitivity of CT in detecting hepatic fungal microabscesses is variable (Berlow et al 1984, Francis et al 1986, Pastakia 1988) and in a number of patients the abscesses are microscopic requiring core biopsy for diagnosis. With contrast enhanced CT, hepatic microabscesses appear as small, hypodense lesions ranging from several millimeters to 1.5 cm in size. Rarely, an actual target appearance may be identified with a small, high attenuation focus centrally surrounded by a low-attenuation zone.

Echinococcus (Ch. 63)

In endemic areas, involvement of the liver by hydatid disease is a common finding. *Echinococcus granulosus* presents with large single mass or multiple well-defined cystic lesions, which often contain internal 'daughter' cysts (Fig. 15.24A). Calcification in the wall of the large or internal cysts occurs in most patients. There is communication between the cysts and the biliary tree in approximately 25% of cases (Choli et al 1982) and frank rupture of cyst contents into the bile ducts occurs in 5 to 10%, accompanied by clinical features of cholangitis. *Echinococcus alveolaris* infection, by contrast, resembles both clinically and radiographically an infiltrating hepatic tumor (Fig. 15.24B) with irregular margins and heterogeneous density (Didier et al 1985).

Amebic abscess (Ch. 62)

The protozoan *Entamoeba histolytica* infects 10% of the world's population. Hepatic abscess is the most common extraintestinal complication of amebiasis and occurs in approximately 8.5% of all patients with amebic infection (Ralls 1998). On CT, amebic abscesses appear as well-

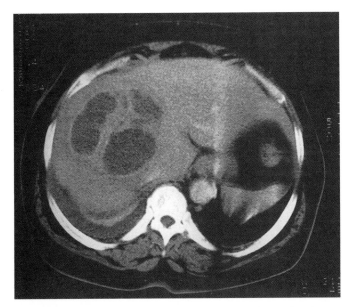

Fig. 15.23 Contrast-enhanced CT of a pyogenic liver abscess showing enhancement of the walls and internal septae. A sympathetic right-sided pleural effusion is seen.

defined masses of near-water attenuation with a thick enhancing rim (Fig. 15.25). One or more internal septations may be present. A feature of amebic liver abscess that may aid in distingishing it from other focal hepatic lesions is its tendency to extend beyond the surface of the liver (Radin et al 1988). The CT findings, however, are not specific and serological tests are necessary to confirm the diagnosis.

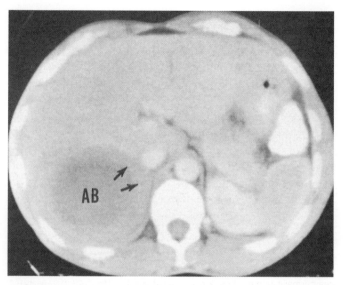

Fig. 15.25 Amebic abscess. A large abscess cavity (AB) is seen in the posterior segment of the right hepatic lobe. During intravenous infusion of contrast agent, a portion of the wall of the abscess cavity (arrows) is seen to enhance.

DIFFUSE HEPATOCELLULAR DISEASES

Fatty infiltration

Fatty infiltration, whether associated with cirrhosis or in a variety of other systemic disorders, including diabetes mellitus, cystic fibrosis, or malnourishment, results in a decrease in hepatic density. Mild degrees of fatty change may be subtle unless liver density is carefully compared to that of the spleen. The liver is normally 6–12 HU higher in attenuation than the spleen, and reversal of this relationship is the earliest CT indication of fatty infiltration. With more advanced changes, the hepatic parenchyma becomes less dense than intrahepatic vessels. In most instances, fatty infiltration is diffuse and uniform (Fig. 15.2), but non-uniform, focal distribution can also occur which can occasionally mimic a mass lesion. Fatty infiltration should be suspected, however, if blood vessels can be seen passing through the focal area in a normal pattern (Fig. 15.26).

Cirrhosis

Computed tomography is capable of demonstrating morphological changes associated with advanced hepatic cirrhosis. Typical CT features are a nodular hepatic outline (in macronodular cirrhosis) and relative atrophy of the right hepatic lobe and quadrate lobe with hypertrophy of the lateral segments of the left hepatic lobe and caudate lobe (Fig. 15.27). Comparative measurements of the transverse dimension of the caudate lobe in comparison to the

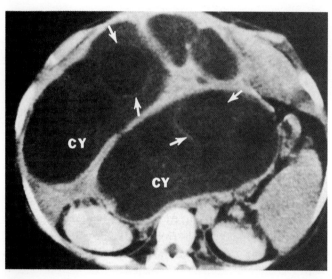

(A)

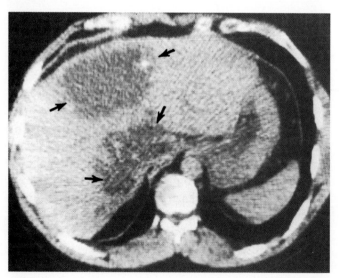

(B)

Fig. 15.24 Abscesses due to echinococcosis. **(A)** *E. granulosus* typically demonstrates multiple, well-circumscribed cysts (CY) in which smaller daughter cysts, some with peripheral calcification (arrows), are situated. **(B)** *E. alveolaris*, in contrast, typically involves the region of the porta hepatis and presents radiographically as low-attenuation areas with poorly-defined margins (arrows). These may be confused with metastases. (Part **A** courtesy of Dr MA Rudwan, Ibn Sina Hospital, Kuwait; part **B** courtesy of Dr M Cayle, Providence Hospital, Anchorage, Alaska.)

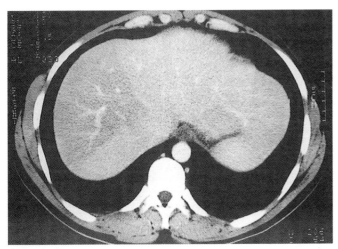

Fig. 15.26 Focal fatty infiltration. A wedge shaped area of low attenuation is visible in the right liver. The hepatic vessels pass through the area normally with no deviation, excluding the diagnosis of a mass lesion.

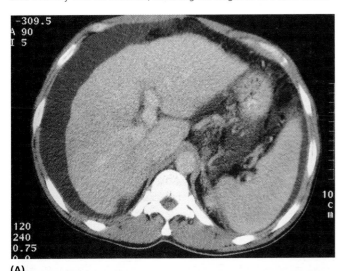

(A)

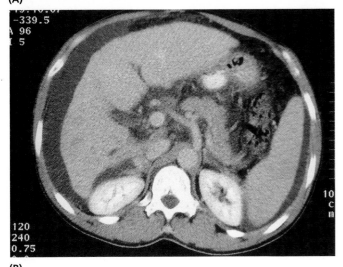

(B)

Fig. 15.27 Cirrhosis **(A)** The liver has an irregular outline. **(B)** The interlobar fissure (delineated by the gallbladder) is deviated towards the right as a result of atrophy of the right liver with hypertrophy of the left liver and the caudate lobe.

adjacent right lobe provides an index of right hepatic lobe shrinkage and is a relatively specific morphologic measurement of hepatic cirrhosis. A caudate-to-right-lobe ratio greater than 0.65 provides 96% confidence in the diagnosis of cirrhosis. Evidence of coexistent portal hypertension is provided by ascites, splenomegaly and portal-systemic varices.

Budd–Chiari syndrome (Ch. 105)

The Budd–Chiari syndrome is caused by chronic hepatic venous congestion due to obstruction to hepatic venous outflow. The CT appearance is characterized by hepatomegaly and ascites. The hepatic veins are either obliterated and therefore not seen or contain thrombus (Fig. 15.28A). Precontrast scans show decreased attenuation of hepatic parenchyma due to congestion and postcontrast scans demonstrate normal enhancement of the caudate lobe (which is hypertrophied in chronic cases) and patchy enhancement of the remainder of the liver (Fig. 15.28A) (Vogelzang et al 1987). Concomitant portal vein thrombosis is present in up to 20% of patients with the Budd–Chiari syndrome. A similar CT appearance of the liver, with patchy enhancement, is seen in patients with congestive heart failure but, unlike patients with true Budd–Chiari syndrome, these patients have patent and enlarged hepatic veins (Moulton et al 1988).

Hepatic infarction

Hepatic infarction is rare, and implies compromise to both the arterial and portal venous supply to a segment or lobe of the liver. CT findings include a well-defined, wedge-shaped area of low attenuation in segmental or subsegmental distribution, extending to the liver surface. After contrast administration, the affected zone is enhanced minimally; a peripheral, thin subcapsular rim often contains enhancing hepatic tissue. Gas formation within sterile infarcts (Fig. 15.29) is a recognized finding and does not necessarily imply superimposed infection. A late complication of hepatic infarction is formation of bile lakes in the affected segments due to disruption of biliary radicles.

HEPATIC TRAUMA (Chs 68 and 69)

Enhanced HCT is the imaging method of choice to evaluate hemodynamically stable patients with blunt hepatic trauma (Filicin 1991, Jeffrey & Olcott 1991). It can reliably diagnose and stage significant hepatic injuries and can aid the surgeon in deciding between early laparotomy or initial non-operative management. Preliminary non-contrast CT

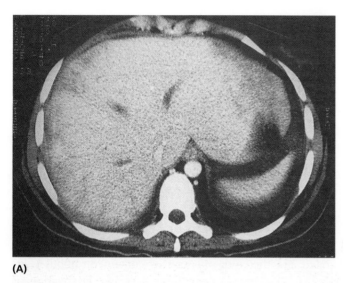

(A)

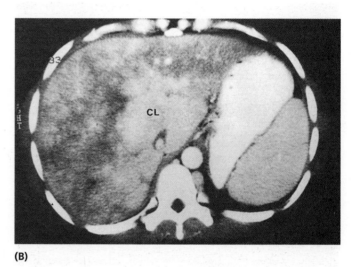

(B)

Fig. 15.28 The Budd–Chiari syndrome **(A)** A contrast-enhanced scan in a patient with acute hepatic venous thrombosis leading to the Budd–Chiari syndrome shows non-enhancement of the thrombosed hepatic veins. There is also patchy peripheral parenchymal enhancement. **(B)** In a patient with chronic Budd–Chiari syndrome due to a congenital stricture of the intrahepatic inferior vena cava there is enlargement of the caudate lobe (CL) and marked inhomogeneity of parenchymal enhancement. Splenomegaly is also seen.

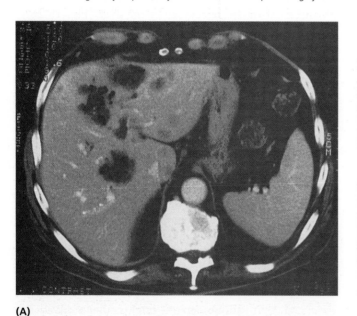

(A)

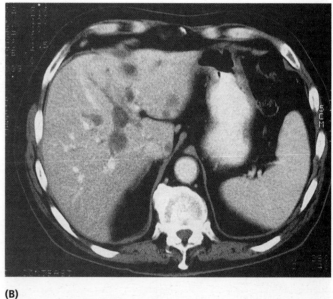

(B)

Fig. 15.29 Hepatic infarction **(A)** Multiple infarcted metastases following therapeutic hepatic embolization. The presence of gas within the infarcted areas does not necessarily imply superadded infection. **(B)** The patient was well and a follow-up scan, 3 weeks later, shows marked reduction in size of the infarcted areas with disappearance of the gas bubbles.

may demonstrate subtle parenchymal hematomas in some patients, but this does not warrant its routine use in all patients and although it may be useful for follow-up, non-enhanced CT often severely underestimates the extent of parenchymal injury.

The morphologic appearance of hepatic injuries may be specifically characterized with contrast-enhanced CT into parenchymal contusion, parenchymal laceration, parenchymal hematoma or subcapsular hematoma (Jeffrey & Olcott 1991). Hepatic contusions appear as ill-defined, low-atten-

uation lesions which do not disrupt major hepatic or portal venous vasculature. Hepatic lacerations appear as linear or branching low density lesions. Subcapsular hematomas have a characteristic lenticular configuration with scalloping of the peripheral aspect of the adjacent liver (Fig. 15.30). Hepatic parenchymal hematomas appear more rounded or oval in configuration. Both types of hematoma contain a central high-attenuation area of clot which decreases in density with time. More serious injuries include hepatic lobar destruction (Fig. 15.31) and major vascular injuries and the

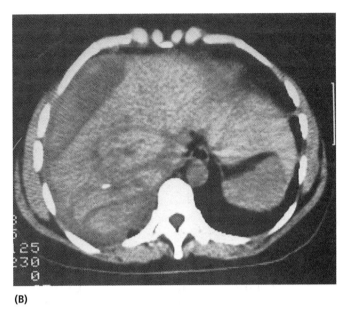

(A)

(B)

Fig. 15.30 Hepatic trauma **(A)** A patient who had been kicked by a horse demonstrated two large subcapsular collections related to the right lobe of the liver. The high attenuation areas within the subcapsular collections indicate that they represent recent hematomata. **(B)** The patient was hemodynamically stable and was therefore managed conservatively. A repeat scan, 1 week later, revealed no increase in size of the hematomata and a reduction in their attenuation suggesting that no new bleeding had occurred. The patient was discharged soon after, and the collections had completely resolved after 6 months.

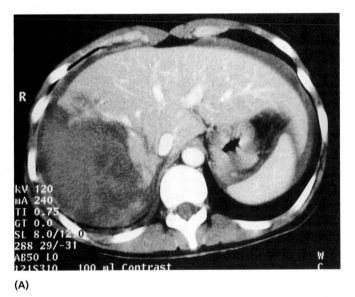

(A)

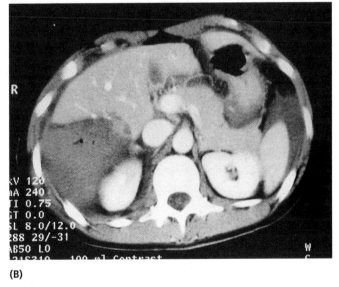

(B)

Fig. 15.31 Hepatic laceration. Scans performed after administration of intravenous contrast agent demonstrate: **(A)** a laceration through the right liver with devascularization of the posterior sector and **(B)** gas in the segment VI ducts due to bile duct injury.

importance of recognizing lacerations that involve major hepatic venous structures cannot be overemphasized. One of the most devastating hepatic injuries is avulsion of the confluence of the hepatic veins from the inferior vena cava.

Hepatic contusions typically resorb quickly and resolve within 5–7 days. The natural history on CT of other traumatic lesions is variable and depends on the degree of tissue necrosis and extent of bile leakage. The size of subcapsular hematomas may initially increase as a result of osmotic effects, and they may take months to resolve. Healing of parenchymal hematomas may similarly take months if a biloma develops. The presence within an area of hemorrhage of a discrete oval or round lesion which is isodense with adjacent major vascular structures should suggest an underlying arterial pseudoaneurysm. Similarly, rapid expansion of a hepatic injury, either pre- or postoperatively, may indicate the presence of an unrecognized arterial pseudoaneurysm.

LIVER TRANSPLANTATION (Chs. 108 and 115)

Computed tomography is useful for evaluating patients prior to liver transplantation and for following possible complications of the surgery. Computed tomography is not the examination of first choice in all cases and may need to be supplemented by other examinations such as arteriography and Doppler ultrasound (Nghiem 1998). A halo of decreased density surrounding the inferior vena cava and in the periportal region, thought to represent accumulation of lymphatic fluid, is seen early after transplantation. When this finding is seen peripherally there is an association with acute rejection but although this sign is fairly specific it is not very sensitive, limiting its use in the detection of transplant rejection. Lobar areas of inhomogeneous low attenuation are highly suggestive of partial or complete hepatic artery obstruction with ischemia. Other transplant complications such as bilomas, abscesses and hematomas are well seen on CT.

INTERVENTIONAL CT

In recent years, interventional radiology has assumed a major role in the diagnosis and management of hepatobiliary disease, often obviating the need for major surgical procedures. Following detection of pathology by an imaging technique it may be necessary to gain further diagnostic information by percutaneous fine needle aspiration or to perform a percutaneous drainage procedure. The choice of imaging modality includes CT, ultrasonography and fluoroscopy. Most liver lesions which can be adequately visualized with ultrasound should be biopsied using ultrasound guidance, as the procedure is simple, readily available (even

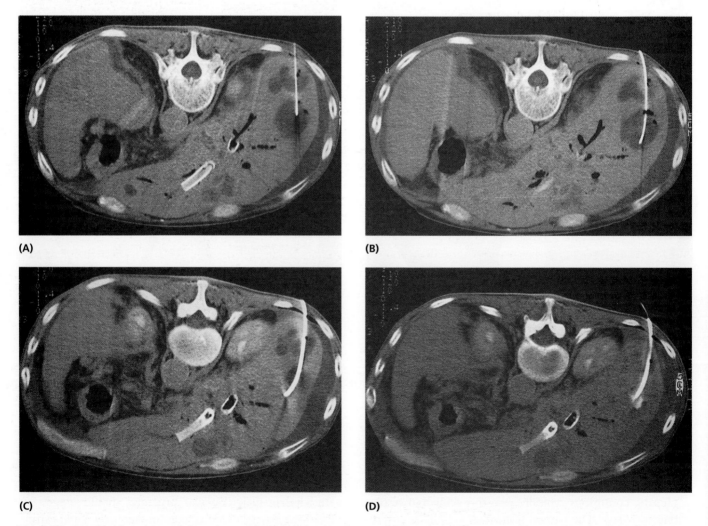

(A)   (B)   (C)   (D)

Fig. 15.32 CT-guided liver abscess drainage in a patient with cholangitic abscesses following tumor overgrowth of a metal stent inserted in the left and right hepatic ducts to palliate cholangiocarcinoma. **(A)** With the patient prone, a fine needle is inserted into the abscess cavity under CT guidance. **(B)** A guidewire is then placed into the cavity through the puncture needle. **(C)** A drainage catheter can then be inserted into the abscess. **(D)** The abscess is aspirated completely before the patient leaves the CT scanner.

at the patient's bedside) and involves no ionizing radiation. A certain number of lesions, however, will only clearly be seen with CT and for these lesions CT guided biopsy is necessary. Computed tomography guidance allows accurate needle placement in extremely small lesions but is not advised for lesions high in the right lobe of the liver as the needle path will cross lung or pleural space. This problem may be avoided by angling the CT gantry to avoid crossing the pleural space, but this will reduce the effective gantry diameter, leading to less working space for the operator, and is not entirely satisfactory. Drainage procedures are best performed using a combination of ultrasound and fluoroscopic guidance but in cases where the abscess cavity is poorly seen with US or where bile ducts are minimally or focally dilated, CT may be extremely useful to guide drainage (Fig. 15.32), to guide placement of the initial puncture needle into the lesion prior to transfer to the fluoroscopy suite, or to mark the best puncture site on the skin prior to the drainage procedure. Computed tomography fluoroscopy has recently been introduced into clinical practice making CT-guided intervention much more convenient and less time-consuming than before. With the addition of a monitor in the scanning room and a foot pedal, the operator is able to perform procedures using real-time, cross-sectional imaging (Froelich et al 1998).

THE BILIARY SYSTEM

The characteristics of biliary tract disease which can be assessed by CT are biliary dilatation, either focal or diffuse, and intrabiliary calcification. Since both of these primary characteristics can be assessed very well with ultrasound examination, CT is not used routinely as a screening examination for biliary disease. The major contribution of CT towards the understanding of biliary processes lies in its ability to depict the extrahepatic course of the biliary duct, and define those extrahepatic viscera adjacent to it. Information provided by CT is often critical in selecting an appropriate group of patients for surgical intervention to relieve obstructive jaundice. Minimal intrahepatic ductal dilatation may go undetected if intravenous contrast material is not used, and it is therefore mandatory to use intravenous contrast agent enhancement when evaluating the biliary tree. Oral contrast material is also helpful in defining portions of the extrahepatic biliary tree, particularly in the region of the head of the pancreas. If a calcified common duct stone is suspected, it may be helpful, although not absolutely necessary, to perform scans in the region of the ampulla of Vater prior to the administration of oral contrast, so that a small

calcified stone is not obscured. Helical computed tomography data can be post-processed to provide 2-dimensional images in the coronal or paracoronal plane (Fig. 15.33) which may make the level of obstruction more obvious than on the axial images.

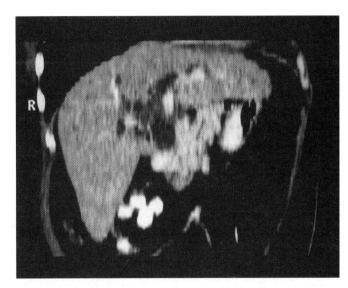

Fig. 15.33 Two-dimensional coronal oblique reconstruction of a contrast-enhanced HCT of the liver in a patient with a distal CBD cholangiocarcinoma. The low density bile ducts are dilated down to the level of the neck of the pancreas.

GALLSTONES

Computed tomography is inferior to US for detection of gallstones but may reveal unsuspected gallstones during studies performed for other reasons. Visualized gallstones are either calcified or of lower attenuation than the surrounding bile due to a high cholesterol content. Stones which are missed on CT are mixed cholesterol stones which are isodense with bile.

CHOLECYSTITIS

Computed tomography should not be used as a screening technique for the detection of acute cholecystitis. Occasionally, however, patients with cholecystitis will present with a confusing clinical picture and may undergo CT examination before the precise nature of the disease is clear. It is helpful, therefore, to recognize the appearance of cholecystitis on CT. Gallbladder distention, wall thickening and the presence of gallstones are often present in acute cholecystitis but are non-specific signs occurring in most patients with chronic cholecystitis. The presence of ill-defined pericholecystic lucency within the hepatic parenchyma adjacent to the gallbladder is suggestive of gallbladder inflammation (and not malignancy), as is soft tissue streakiness in the mesenteric and hepatoduodenal ligament fat (Fig. 15.34). Intramural edema within the gallbladder wall may be seen in acute cholecystitis and is a useful sign in an appropriate clinical setting but can also be seen in patients with ascites or hypoalbuminemia without gallbladder disease. The attenuation of the gallbladder bile is usually raised and extremely high attenuation of gallbladder contents can be seen in patients with hemorrhagic cholecystitis, a rare complication of cholelithias. Although many of the CT findings in uncomplicated acute cholecystitis are non-specific, CT is of great value when complications such as pericholecystic abscess, emphysematous cholecystitis or gallbladder perforation are present and can identify patients in need of emergency surgery. Gas in the gallbladder wall or lumen, which can be missed using ultrasonography, is particularly well seen using CT.

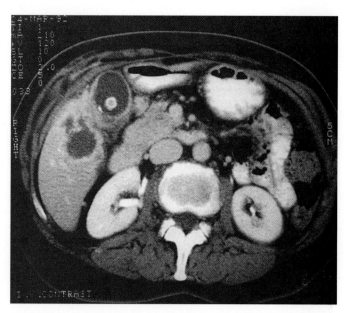

Fig. 15.35 Gallbladder carcinoma. CT demontrates irregular thickening of the posterolateral wall of the gallbladder with direct tumor extension into the adjacent liver. A calcified gallstone is seen within the gallbladder.

gallbladder. The latter is the most common appearance. Typical findings in advanced disease include direct liver, bowel or pancreas invasion, spread into the hepatoduodenal ligament, lymphadenopathy and hematogenous metastases.

Direct hepatoduodenal ligament invasion or hilar lymphadenopathy may produce biliary obstruction. Obstruction may also be caused by intraductal spread of the malignancy, which occurs in 4% of patients. Cholelithiasis is often present in patients with gallbladder cancer, and it may be difficult to distinguish between cholecystitis and carcinoma of the gallbladder. As mentioned above, the presence of a low-attenuation pericholecystic halo suggests benign disease, whereas the presence of irregular soft tissue lesions within the liver parenchyma adjacent to the gallbladder is a feature only of carcinoma.

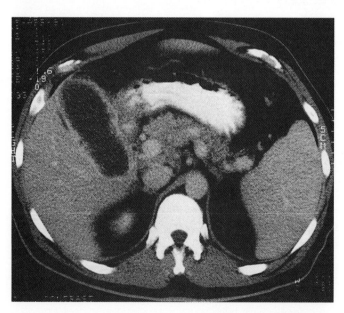

Fig. 15.34 Acute cholecystitis. CT demonstrates a distended, thick-walled gallbladder with pericholecystic fluid. No gallstones are seen.

GALLBLADDER CARCINOMA (Ch. 53)

Carcinoma of the gallbladder is the fifth most common gastrointestinal malignancy, but is extremely difficult to diagnose preoperatively. Small protruberences from the gallbladder wall into the lumen are common and are caused by adenomas, adenomyomas, cholesterosis and adherent stones. Carcinoma of the gallbladder tends to present as a much larger mass in a chronically diseased or porcelain gallbladder. Gallbladder carcinoma may appear as a polypoid intraluminal mass, focal or diffuse gallbladder-wall thickening (Fig. 15.35) or a large mass filling or engulfing the

CHOLEDOCHOLITHIASIS

The insensitivity of sonography in detecting choledocholithiasis has been well documented wth a reported detection rate in the range of 18 to 22%. CT has a much higher sensitivity with reported detection rates of up to 76% (Baron 1987). Meticulous attention must be paid to technique and, when a change in duct caliber is detected, thin collimation scans (3 to 5 mm) should be performed at close intervals through the transition area of the duct in order to detect the calculus. The only reliable indicators of choledocholithiasis are said to be the presence of dense intraluminal calcification or a 'target sign' within the duct. The latter refers to the appearance that results from a CT section being taken just above the midpoint of a stone within a dilated duct. A halo of bile is seen surrounding the higher density stone producing a targetlike appearance. Calcified stones lying within an obstructed duct present no challenge to the radiologist. Most errors in diagnosis are due to cholesterol stones, which may blend imperceptibly with the surrounding bile. Errors of diagnosis also occur in the presence of non-dilatation of the ductal system which occurs in about one third of patients with choledocholithiasis.

Intrahepatic calculi are rare in Western countries, most frequently occurring in association with iatrogenic bile duct strictures (Fig. 15.36). Computed tomography is of little value when stones are small and non-calcified and bile duct dilatation is minimal or absent. Intrahepatic choledocholithiasis may present a bizarre appearance, due to segmental or subsegmental biliary radicles filled with calculi. In Asian patients with recurrent pyogenic cholangitis who subsequently form bile pigment stones, the debris filling the biliary system is generally of higher attenuation than that of normal bile. Marked bile duct dilatation is present and often the larger intrahepatic ducts will be dilated without side branch dilatation. Eccentric and diffuse extrahepatic bile duct wall thickening is usually seen (Schulte et al 1990).

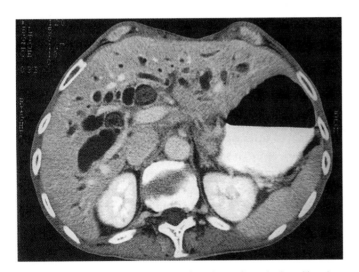

Fig. 15.36 Intrahepatic cholelithiasis. There is intrahepatic duct dilatation following recurrent anastomotic stricture formation at a hepaticojejunostomy. Several laminated, non-calcified calculi can be seen within the dilated ductal system.

MIRIZZI'S SYNDROME

Mirizzi's syndrome is an uncommon condition in which the common hepatic duct is obstructed due to stones impacted in or extruded from Hartman's pouch of the gallbladder or the cystic duct. Cholecystobiliary or cholecystoenteric fistulae are common complications. It is clinically important to recognize the diagnosis prior to surgery since failure to appreciate the extraluminal obstructing process will result in unrewarding exploration of the common duct and postoperative persistence of obstruction. The typical CT features of Mirizzi's syndrome are dilatation of the biliary system above the level of the neck of the gallbladder with a normal system below. Thin-section CT allows visualization of the cystic duct joining the common hepatic duct, and it is at this site where the gallstone causing Mirizzi's syndrome should be found. The gallstone may be impacted in a cystic duct or gallbladder neck and usually appears eccentrically located relative to the bile duct. An irregular cavity with surrounding edema and inflammation may be seen adjacent to the gallbladder neck. Since not all of the findings may be present on CT, direct cholangiography is recommended to document the nature of the obstruction and the presence or absence of a biliary fistula.

SCLEROSING CHOLANGITIS

Primary sclerosing cholagitis (Ch. 48) is an unusual entity consisting of progressive diffuse fibrosis of the biliary tree and is often seen in patients with pre-existing conditions such as ulcerative colitis or retroperitoneal fibrosis. Secondary sclerosing cholangitis is caused by previous biliary surgery, biliary stones, carcinoma or recurrent infection. Both may progress to produce cirrhosis and portal hypertension. Cholangiography is the accepted standard for the diagnosis of sclerosing cholangitis but characteristic finding may be seen using CT. The CT appearance is that of focal, discontinuous areas of minimal intrahepatic biliary dilatation without a mass lesion unless the disease is complicated by the development of cholangiocarcinoma. Thickening or nodularity of the bile duct wall may also be seen.

CYSTIC DISEASES OF THE BILIARY TREE

Several diseases may affect the biliary tree by causing cystic change (Chs 65 and 66). Caroli's disease causes marked segmental dilatation of intrahepatic bile ducts and is often associated with congenital hepatic fibrosis (Fig. 15.37). Computed tomography demonstrates multiple low-attenuation cystic lesions and may simulate polycystic liver disease. The diagnosis can be made by appreciating that the cysts are contiguous with the bile ducts and this can be aided by administration of an intravenous chlangiographic contrast agent (Fig. 15.38). The abnormally dilated bile ducts may surround the accompanying portal vein radicles and result in the appearance of a central dot within the center of the cystic masses (Choi et al 1990).

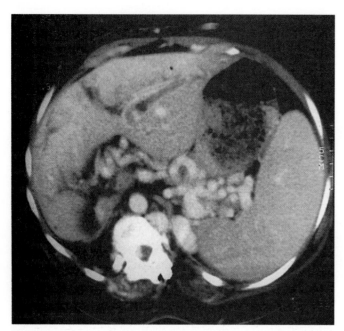

Fig. 15.37 Congenital hepatic fibrosis and Caroli's disease. There is right lobar atrophy, focal areas of intrahepatic duct dilatation and portal hypertension with gross splenomegaly and numerous venous collaterals.

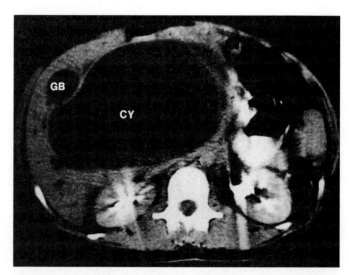

Fig. 15.39 Giant choledochal cyst (CY) displacing the gallbladder (GB) anteriorly.

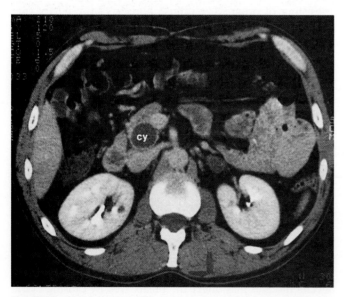

Fig. 15.38 Choledochal cyst. This patient has an entirely normal biliary tree apart from a 2 cm choledochal cyst in the distal common bile duct (cy).

Another entity is the choledochal cyst which represents focal dilatation of the common bile duct (Fig. 15.38). There may be associated proximal intrahepatic biliary dilatation but the common duct dilatation is usually disproportionately large for the degree of intrahepatic dilatation and may achieve giant size (Fig. 15.39). Chronic ulceration may occur within the dilated common duct leading to strictures or cholangiocarcinoma.

Herniation of the wall of the common bile duct into the duodenum results in a choledochocele, which is seen as a cystic mass contiguous with the common bile duct.

CHOLANGIOCARCINOMA (Ch. 54)

This is the most common primary malignancy of the bile ducts and is uncommon compared with hepatocellular carcinoma, but is an important cause of painless jaundice. In the majority of patients, the tumor arises centrally either at the junction of the left and right hepatic ducts, or more distally in the common hepatic and common bile duct. The remainder of cases arise in the intrahepatic ducts and may be difficult to distinguish from other intrahepatic neoplasms. Disparities between the degrees of biliary dilatation in the right and left lobes may occur despite the central location of the obstruction, with a tendency for the left system to dilate more than the right. Some patients may exhibit lobar atrophy, with dilated, crowded ducts, due to long-standing bile duct obstruction or concomitant portal venous obstruction (Fig. 15.40) (Ch. 3). Three types of tumor appearance are seen with CT. The infiltrating pattern is the most common, involving the bile duct wall and occluding the lumen. In such cases there is gross dilatation of the intrahepatic biliary tree in the absence of an obvious mass although careful attention to the wall of the duct at the site of obstruction will generally demonstrate diffuse mural thickening (Fig. 15.41). If seen, the tumor is ill-defined and enhances poorly during contrast-enhanced CT. Delayed CT often demonstrates tumor enhancement thought to be due to the retention of contrast agent in the tumors related to their high

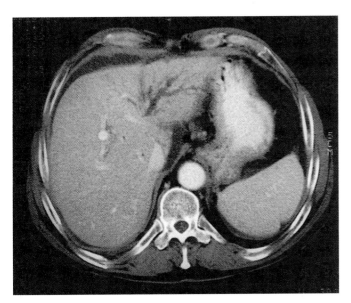

Fig. 15.40 Hilar cholangiocarcinoma causing left hepatic duct obstruction and left lobar atrophy with dilatation and crowding of the left sided ducts.

fibrous tissue content. The exophytic type of hilar cholangiocarcinoma, however, spreads more extensively into the surrounding hepatic parenchyma. The third type takes the form of a polypoid intraluminal mass which expands the duct and is usually clearly seen using CT. This type of cholangiocarcinoma is rare.

BILIARY CYSTADENOMA AND CYSTADENOCARCINOMA

Although these rare tumors arise from biliary tissue, they usually present as large intrahepatic lesions. They have a multilocular, cystic appearance and vary in size from 3.5 to 25 cm in diameter. The majority (85%) arise from intrahepatic ducts and may demonstrate fluid-fluid levels, mural nodules or septations. They are of higher density than simple cysts and may be confused with abscesses or cystic hepatic metastases.

METASTATIC DISEASE

Metastatic disease to the porta hepatis may manifest as biliary obstruction caused by an extrinsic mass effect on the common duct. This can be from direct invasion into the porta hepatis by gallbladder, pancreatic or gastric carcinoma or due to metastases to lymph nodes in the porta hepatis from lymphoma or other carcinomas. The CT appearance is similar to that of other masses obstructing the bile duct, with abrupt termination of the duct and surrounding soft tissue attenuation.

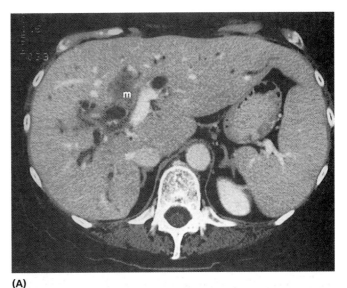

(A)

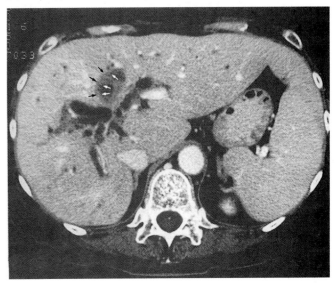

(B)

Fig. 15.41 Hilar cholangiocarcinoma. **(A)** At the level of the hilum there is an ill-defined, low attenuation mass (m) and intrahepatic duct dilatation. **(B)** On a more cranial section an area of ductal wall thickening can be seen (arrows).

REFERENCES

Ashida C, Fishman E K, Zerhouni E A, Herlong F H, Siegelman S S 1987 Computed tomography of hepatic cavernous hemangioma. Journal of Computer Assisted Tomography 11: 455–460

Baron R L 1987 Common bile duct stones: reassessment of criteria for CT diagnosis. Radiology 162: 419–424

Berlow M E, Spirit B A, Weil L 1984 CT follow-up of hepatic and splenic fungal microabscesses. Journal of Computer Assisted Tomography 8: 42

Bernardino M E, Erwin B C, Steinberg H V, Baumgartner B R, Torres W E, Gedgaudas-McClees R K 1986 Delayed hepatic CT scanning: increased confidence and improved detection of hepatic metastases. Radiology 159: 71–74

Birnbaum B A, Jacobs J E, Yin D 1995 Hepatic enhancement during helical CT: a comparison of moderate rate uniphasic and biphasic contrast injection protocols. American Journal of Roentgenology 165: 853–858

Bismuth H 1982 Surgical anatomy and anatomic surgery of the liver. World Journal of Surgery 6: 3–9

Bluemke D A, Fishman E K 1993 Spiral CT arterial portography of the liver. Radiology 186: 576–579

Bluemke D A, Soyer P A, Fishman E K 1995 Helical (spiral) CT of the liver. Radiologic Clinics of North America 33: 863–886

Brandt D J, Johnson C D, Stephens D H, Weiland L H 1988 Imaging of fibrolamellar carcinoma. American Journal of Roentgenology 151: 295–299

Caseiro-Alves F, Zins M, Mahfouz A E et al 1996 Calcification in focal nodular hyperplasia: a new problem for differentiation from fibrolamellar hepatocellular carcinoma. Radiology 198: 889–892

Chambers T P, Baron R L, Lush R M 1994a Hepatic CT enhancement. Part I. Alterations in the volume of contrast material within the same patients. Radiology 193: 513–517

Chambers T P, Baron R L, Lush R M 1994b Hepatic CT enhancement. Part II. Alterations in contrast material volume and rate of injection within the same patients. Radiology 193: 518–522

Chezmar J L, Bernardino M E, Kaufman S H, Nelson R C 1993 Combined CT arterial portography and CT hepatic angiography for evaluation of the hepatic resection candidate. Radiology 189: 407–410

Choi B I, Park J H, Kim B H, Han M C, Kim C W 1989a Small hepatocellular carcinoma: detection with sonography, computed tomography (CT), angiography and Lipiodol CT. British Journal of Radiology 62: 897–903

Choi B I, Lee J H, Han M C, Kim S H, Yi Y G, Kim C W 1989b Hilar cholangiocarcinoma: comparative study with sonography and CT. Radiology 172: 689–692

Choi B I, Yeon K M, Kim S H, Han M C 1990 Caroli disease: central dot sign in CT. Radiology 174: 161–163

Choli J D, Olaveni F J L, Casas T F, Zubieta S O 1982 CT in hepatic echinococcosis. American Journal of Roentgenology 139: 699–702

de Santis M, Romagnoli R, Cristani A et al 1992 MRI of small hepatocellular carcinoma: comparison with US, CT, DSA, and lipiodol-CT. Journal of Computer Assisted Tomography 16: 189–197

Didier D, Weiler S, Rohmer P et al 1985 Hepatic alveolar echinococcus: correlative US and CT study. Radiology 154: 179–186

Earls J P, Theise N D, Weinreb J C et al 1996 Dysplastic nodules and hepatocellular carcinoma: thin-section MR imaging of explanted cirrhotic livers with pathologic correlation. Radiology 201: 207–214

Fernandez M, Bernardino M E 1991 Hepatic pseudolesion: appearance of focal low attenuation in the medial segment of the left lobe at CT arterial portography. Radiology 181: 809–812

Filicin D V 1991 Diagnostic modalities in abdominal trauma. Surgical Clinics of North America 7: 241–256

Fink S, Chaudhury K 1991 Physiological considerations in imaging liver metastases from colorectal carcinoma. American Journal of Physiology 6: 150–160

Fleischmann D, Ringl H, Schofl R et al 1996 Three-dimensional spiral CT cholangiography in patients with suspected obstructive biliary disease: comparison with endoscopic retrograde cholangiography. Radiology 198: 861–868

Francis I R, Glazer G M, Amendola M A, Trenker SW 1986 Hepatic abscesses in the immunocompromised patient: role of CT in detection, diagnosis, management and follow-up. Gastrointestinal Radiology 11: 257–262

Freeny P C, Baron R L, Teefey S A 1992 Hepatocellular carcinoma: reduced frequency of typical findings with dynamic contrast-enhanced CT in a non-Asian population. Radiology 182: 143–148

Froelich J J, Saar B, Hoppe M et al 1998 Real-time CT-fluoroscopy for guidance of percutaneous drainage procedures. Journal of Vascular and Interventional Radiology 9: 735–740

Garcia P A, Bonaldi V M, Bret P M et al 1996 Effect of rate of contrast medium injection on hepatic enhancement at CT. Radiology 199: 185–189

Graf O, Dock W I, Lammer et al 1994 Determination of the optimal time window for liver scanning with CT during arterial portography. Radiology 190: 43–47

Halvorsen R A, Korobkin M, Foster W L Jr et al 1984 The variable CT appearance of hepatic abscesses. American Journal of Roentgenology 142: 941–946

Honda H, Matsura Y, Onitsuka H et al 1992 Differential diagnosis of hepatic tumors (hepatoma, hemangioma and metastasis) with CT: Value of two-phase incremental imaging. American Journal of Roentgenology 159: 735–740

Irie T, Kusano S 1996 Contrast-enhanced spiral CT of the liver: effect of injection time on time to peak hepatic enhancement. Journal of Computer Assisted Tomography 20: 633–637

Irie T, Takeshita K, Wada Y et al 1995 CT evaluation of hepatic tumors: comparison of CT with arterial portography, CT with infusion hepatic arteriography, and simultaneous use of both techniques. American Journal of Roentgenology 164: 1407–1412

Irie T, Tsushima Y, Terahata S, Hatsuse K, Kusano S 1997 Rim enhancement in colorectal metastases at CT during infusion hepatic arteriography. Does it represent liver parenchyma or live tumor cell zone? Acta Radiologica 38: 416–421

Itai Y, Teraoka T 1989 Angiosarcoma of the liver mimicking cavernous hemangioma on dynamic CT. Journal of Computer Assisted Tomography 13: 910–912

Itai Y, Furui S, Tasaka A 1981 Differential diagnosis of hepatic masses on CT, with particular reference to hepatocellular carcinoma. Journal of Computer Assisted Tomography 5: 834–842

Jamadar D A, D'Souza S P, Thomas E A, Giles T E 1994 Radiological appearances in peliosis hepatis. British Journal of Radiology 67: 102–104

Jeffrey R B Jr, Olcott E W 1991 Imaging of blunt hepatic trauma. Radiologic Clinics of North America 29: 1299–1310

Jeffrey R B Jr, Tolentino C S, Chang F C, Federle M P 1988 CT of pyogenic hepatic microabscesses: the cluster sign. American Journal of Roentgenology 151: 487–489

Kalender W A, Seissler W, Klotz E, Vock P 1990 Spiral volumetric CT with single-breath-hold technique, continuous transport, and continuous scanner rotation. Radiology 176: 181–183

Kanematsu M, Hoshi H, Imaeda T et al 1997a Nonpathological focal enhancements on spiral hepatic angiography. Abdominal Imaging 22: 55–59

Kanematsu M, Hoshi H, Imaeda T et al 1997b Detection and characterization of hepatic tumors: value of combined helical CT hepatic arteriography and CT during arterial portography. American Journal of Roentgenology 168: 1193–1198

Kanematsu M, Kondo H, Enya M, Yokoama R, Hoshi H 1998 Nondiseased portal perfusion defects adjacent to the right ribs shown on helical CT during arterial portography. American Journal of Roentgenology 171: 445–448

Kopka L, Rodenwaldt J, Fischer U, Mueller D W, Oestmann J W, Grabbe E 1996 Dual-phase helical CT of the liver: effects of bolus tracking and different volumes of contrast material. Radiology 201: 321–326

LaLonde L, Van Beers B, Jamart J, Pringot J 1992 Capsule and mosaic pattern of hepatocellular carcinoma: correlation between CT and MR imaging. Gastrointestinal Radiology 17: 241–244

Lee H M, Lu D S, Krasny R M, Busuttil R, Kadell B, Lucas J 1997 Hepatic lesion characterization in cirrhosis: significance of arterial hypervascularity on dual-phase helical CT. American Journal of Roentgenology 169: 125–130

Lencioni R, Pinto F, Armillotta N et al 1997 Intrahepatic metastatic nodules of hepatocellular carcinoma detected at Lipiodol CT: imaging-pathologic correlation. Abdominal Imaging 22: 253–258

Leslie D F, Johnson C D, Johnson C M et al 1995 Distinction between cavernous hemangioma of the liver and hepatic metastases on CT: value of contrast enhancement patterns. American Journal of Roentgenology 164: 625–629

Liddell R M, Baron R L, Ekstrom J E, Varnell R M, Shuman W P 1990 Normal intrahepatic bile ducts: CT depiction. Radiology 176: 633–635

Lim G M, Jeffrey R B Jr, Ralls P W, Marn C S 1989 Septic thrombosis of the portal vein: CT and clinical observations. Journal of Computer Assisted Tomography 13: 656–658

Lubbers P R, Ros P R, Goodman Z D, Ishak K G 1987 Accumulation of technetium–99m sulphur colloid by hepatocellular adenoma: scintigraphic-pathologic correlation. American Journal of Roentgenology 148: 1105–1108

Lupetin A R, Cammisa B A, Beckman I et al 1996 Spiral CT during arterial portography. Radiographics 16: 723–743

McDermott V G, Lawrance J A, Paulson E K et al 1996 CT during arterial portography: comparison of injection into the splenic versus mesenteric artery. Radiology 199: 627–631

McGrath F P, Malone D E, Dobranowski J, Stevenson G W 1993 CT portography and delayed high dose iodine CT. Clinical Radiology 47: 1–6

Mahoney B, Jeffrey R B, Federle M 1982 Spontaneous rupture of hepatic and splenic angiosarcoma demonstrated by CT. American Journal of Roentgenology 138: 965–966

Masui T, Takehara Y, Fujiwara T et al 1998 MR and CT cholangiography in evaluation of the biliary tract. Acta Radiologica 39: 557–563

Mathieu D, Bruneton J N, Drouillard J, Pointreau C C, Vasile N 1986 Hepatic adenomas and focal nodular hyperplasia: dynamic CT study. Radiology 160: 53–58

Matsui O, Takahashi S, Kadoya M et al 1994 Pseudolesion in segment IV of the liver at CT during arterial portography: correlation with aberrant gastric venous drainage. Radiology 193: 31–35

Merine D, Takayasu K, Wakao F 1990 Detection of hepatocellular carcinoma: comparison of CT during arterial portography with CT after intraarterial injection of iodized oil. Radiology 175: 707–710

Miller D L, Simmons J T, Chang R, et al 1987 Hepatic metastasis detection: comparison of three contrast enhancement methods. Radiology 165: 785–790

Moulton J S, Miller B L, Dodd G D III, Vu D N 1988 Passive hepatic congestion in heart failure: CT abnormalities. American Journal of Roentgenology 151: 939–942

Nelson R C, Thompson G H, Chezmar J L, Harned R K, Fernandez M P 1992 CT during arterial portography: diagnostic pitfalls. Radiographics 12: 705–718

Nghiem H 1998 Imaging of hepatic transplantation. Radiologic Clinics of North America 36: 429–443

Ohashi I, Ina H, Gomi N et al 1995 Hepatic pseudolesion in the left lobe around the falciform ligament at helical CT. Radiology 196: 245–249

Oliver J H, Baron R L 1996 Helical biphasic contrast-enhanced CT of the liver: technique, indications, interpretations and pitfalls. Radiology 201: 1–14

Oliver J H, Baron R L, Federle M P, Jones B C, Sheng R 1997 Hypervascular liver metastases: do unenhanced and hepatic arterial phase CT images affect tumor detection? Radiology 205: 709–715

Osborne B M, Butler J J, Guarda L A 1985 Primary lymphoma of the liver – ten cases and a review of the literature. Cancer 56: 2902–2910

Paley M R, Ros P R 1998 Hepatic metastases. Radiologic Clinics of North America 36: 349–363

Pastakia B, Shawker T H, Thaler M, O'Leary T, Pizzo P A 1988 Hepatosplenic candidiasis: wheels within wheels. Radiology 166: 417–421

Paulson E K, Baker M E, Hilleren D J et al 1992 CT arterial portography: causes of technical failure and variable liver enhancement. American Journal of Roentgenology 159: 745–749

Paulson E K, McDermott V G, Keogan M T et al 1998 Carcinoid metastases to the liver: role of triple-phase helical CT. Radiology 206: 143–150

Perkerson R B, Erwin B C, Baumgartner B R et al 1985 CT densities in delayed iodine hepatic scanning. Radiology 155: 445–446

Phillips V M, Erwin B C, Bernadino M E 1985 Delayed iodine scanning of the liver: a promising CT technique. Journal of Computer Assisted Tomography 9: 415–416

Procacci C, Fugazzola C, Cinquino, Mangiante G, Zonta L, Andreis I, Nicoli N, Pistolesi G 1992 Contribution of CT to characterization of focal nodular hyperplasia of the liver. Gastrointestinal Radiology 17: 63–73

Radin D R, Ralls P W, Colletti P M, Halls J M 1988 CT of amebic liver abscess. American Journal of Roentgenology 150: 1297–1301

Ralls P W 1998 Focal inflammatory disease of the liver. Radiologic Clinics of North America 36: 377–389

Ros P R, Murphy E J, Buck J L, Olmedilla G, Goodman Z 1990 Encapsulated hepatocellular carcinoma: radiological findings and pathological correlation. Gastrointestinal Radiology 15: 233–237

Ruschenburg I, Droese M 1989 Fine needle aspiration cytology of focal nodular hyperplasia of the liver. Acta Cytologica 33: 857–860

Sanders L M, Botet J F, Straus D J, Ryan J, Filippa D A, Newhouse J H 1989 CT of primary lymphoma of the liver. American Journal of Roentgenology 152: 973–976

Schulte S J, Baron R L, Teefey S A et al 1990 CT of the extrahepatic bile ducts: wall thickness and contrast enhancement in normal and abnormal ducts. American Journal of Roentgenology 154: 79–85

Shamsi K, De Schepper A, Degryse H, Deckers F 1993 Focal nodular hyperplasia of the liver: radiologic findings. Abdominal Imaging 18: 32–38

Silverman P M, Ram P C, Korobin M 1983 CT appearance of abdominal Thorotrast deposition and Thorotrast-induced angiosarcoma of the liver. Journal of Computer Assisted Tomography 7: 655–658

Soyer P, Roche A, Levesque M, Legmann P 1991 CT of fibrolamellar hepatocellular carcinoma. Journal of Computer Assisted Tomography 15: 533–538

Soyer P, Bluemke D A, Fishman E K 1994 CT during arterial portography for the preoperative evaluation of hepatic tumors: How, when, and why? American Journal of Roentgenology 163: 1325–1331

Spreafico C, Marchiano A, Mazzaferrro V et al 1997 Hepatocellular carcinoma in patients who undergo liver transplantation: sensitivity of CT with iodinated oil. Radiology 203: 457–460

Stockberger S M, Wass J L, Sherman S, Lehman G A, Kopecky K K 1994 Intravenous cholangiography with helical CT: comparison with endoscopic retrograde cholangiography. Radiology 192: 675–680

Takayasu K, Muramatsu Y, Furakuwa H et al 1995 Early hepatocellular carcinoma: appearance at CT during arterial portography and CT arteriography with pathologic correlation. Radiology 194: 101–105

Tidebrant G, Asztely M, Lukes P et al 1990 Comparison of non-enhanced, bolus enhanced and delayed scanning techniques in computed tomography of hepatic tumors. Acta Radiologica 31: 161–166

Tidebrant G, Lukes P, Tylen U, Wihed A 1991 Demonstration of hepatic veins by computed tomography using axial and angulated scanning. Acta Radiologica 31: 149–152

Titelbaum D S, Burke D R, Meranze S G, Saul S H 1988 Fibrolamellar carcinoma: pitfalls in non-operative diagnosis. Radiology 167: 25–30

Tublin M E, Tessler F N, Cheng S L, Peters T L, McGovern P C 1999 Effect of injection rate of contrast medium on pancreatic and helical CT. Radiology 210: 97–101

Vasile N, Lardé D, Zafrani E, Berard H, Mathieu D 1983 Hepatic angiosarcoma. Journal of Computer Assisted Tomography 7: 899–901

Vignaux O, Legmann P, de Pinieux G et al 1999 Hemorrhagic necrosis due to peliosis hepatis: imaging findings and pathological correlation. European Radiology 9: 454–456

Vogelzang R L, Anschuetz S L, Gore R M 1987 Budd–Chiari syndrome: CT observations. Radiology 163: 329

Weg N, Scheer M R, Gabor M P 1998 Liver lesions: improved detection with dual-detector-array CT and routine 2.5-mm thin collimation. Radiology 209: 417–426

Welch T J, Sheedy P F II, Johnson C M, Stephens D H, Charboneau J W, Brown M L, May G R, Adson M A, McGill D B 1985 Focal nodular hyperplasia and hepatic adenoma: comparison of angiography, CT, US and scintigraphy. Radiology 156: 593–595

White P G, Adams H, Smith P M 1993 The computed tomographic appearances of angiosarcoma of the liver. Clinical Radiology 48: 321–325

Yoshikawa J, Matsui O, Takashima T, Ida M, Takanaka T, Kawamura I, Kakuda K, Miyata S 1988 Fatty metamorphosis in hepatocellular carcinoma: radiologic features in 10 cases. American Journal of Roentgenology 151: 717–720.

Magnetic resonance imaging of the liver and biliary tract

16

L.H. SCHWARTZ AND D.R. DeCORATO

Magnetic resonance imaging (MRI) is a cross-sectional scanning technique, capable of obtaining images in any plane (Fig. 16.1). MRI utilizes magnetic fields and radio-frequency pulses to generate images with outstanding tissue contrast and excellent spatial resolution. The technique of magnetic resonance is not new and was, in fact, first described by Bloch (Bloch et al 1946) and Purcell (Purcell et al 1946) in the 1940s as a method for in vitro chemical analysis. Several decades later, Damadian (Damadian 1972) and Lauterbur (Lauterbur 1973) applied some of these basic principles to design a MRI technique capable of in vivo imaging. Today, MRI is used extensively as an imaging tool throughout the body to visualize and distinguish normal and pathologic tissue.

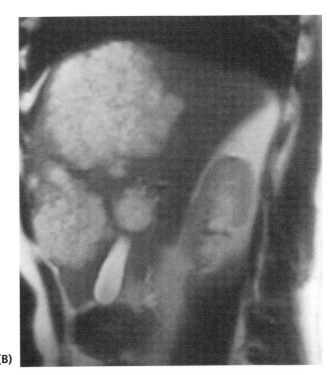

(B)

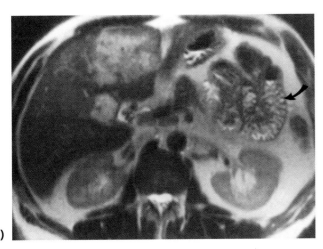

(A)

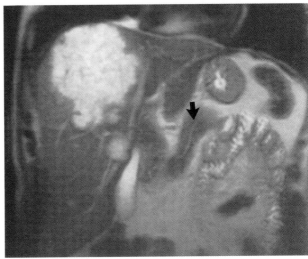

(C)

Fig. 16.1 Multiplanar T2-weighted images through the liver in a patient with multiple hepatic metastasis. **(A)** Axial image. **(B)** Sagittal image. **(C)** Coronal image. A variety of techniques can be used to obtain these images. Note fluid-containing structures including small bowel (curved arrow Fig. **A**), gallbladder, biliary tree and pancreatic duct (arrow Fig. **C**) are bright.

PRINCIPLES OF MRI

MRI is based upon the principles of nuclear magnetic resonance (NMR). Certain nuclei have a magnetic moment or spin. These nuclei when placed in a strong magnetic field react by trying to align themselves with the direction of the main magnetic field. A proton, for example, will align itself in one of two directions, either up or down. In addition, when placed in a magnetic field, the nuclei rotate or spin parallel to the magnetic field. The precise frequency of the nuclear spin is known as the Larmor frequency. The Larmor frequency depends upon the specific type nuclei imaged within the magnetic field, and the strength of the magnetic field. The most commonly imaged nucleus in clinical practice is the hydrogen nucleus (^{1}H), because of its great abundance in the human body. Other nuclei, which may be imaged by MRI, include phosphorus (^{31}P), sodium (^{23}Na) and carbon (^{13}C).

When nuclei are within the stable magnetic field, they are considered to be in equilibrium. There are almost an equal number of nuclei in the 'up' or 'down' alignment, and an equal number of transitions between the two states. Adding a momentary radiofrequency pulse at the precise frequency of the nuclear spin, or the Larmor frequency produces resonance (as in Magnetic *Resonance* Imaging). This radiofrequency pulse causes a change in the energy and a change in the transition state. The radiofrequency pulse is then turned off; the nuclei in the body return to the equilibrium state emitting a radiofrequency signal. The strength of this emitted signal, and the amount of time for the nucleus to return to the equilibrium state, determines the signal intensity of a tissue. The precise tissue signal intensity depends on several factors: longitudinal relaxation (T1), transverse relaxation (T2), proton density (nuclear spin) and flow.

The T1 value (longitudinal relaxation), or spin–lattice relaxation, is the time required for the rotating nuclei to return to the equilibrium state following the radiofrequency pulse. The initial energy absorbed by the nuclei is released and dissipated into the surrounding molecular environment or lattice. The precise T1 value is the time for the MRI signal to return to 63% of its maximum value. Most tissue T1 values vary between 200 and 800 ms. Tissue with a short T1 value will appear bright (hyperintense) on T1-weighted images by convention.

The T2 relaxation time (transverse relaxation or spin–spin relaxation) is a measure of the loss of signal in a plane perpendicular to the long axis of the magnetic field. This loss of signal is due to subtle inhomogeneities in the magnetic field because of the presence of spinning protons. The T2 value for a tissue is the time it takes for the signal to decrease to 63% of its equilibrium value. Most tissue T2 values vary between 50 and 200 ms. The T2 value can never be longer than the T1 value. By convention, tissues with a long T2 value will appear bright on T2-weighted images.

Fluid motion, such as from blood, plays a major role in the appearance of every MR image. In general, blood flow tends to produce spin dephasing, which will result in a loss of signal in a MR image. There are certain pulse sequences that are sensitive to flow and will produce images in which flow is high in signal. MR angiography (MRA) techniques utilize this principle to produce images in which flowing blood is bright and background tissue is relatively dark. This technique takes advantage of the fact that blood flow produces moving protons that will have a different signal from the static protons within the slice being imaged.

Improvements in MRI equipment and software used to control this machinery have resulted in decreasing the time needed to create an image. State of the art scanning equipment may create an image in less than one second. Additionally specialized surface coils (local antennas used to receive MR signal) are now used to obtain images with higher spatial resolution. There are fast techniques that can produce images with either T1-weighting or T2-weighting. Gradient recalled echo (GRE) techniques, for example can be applied to produce high quality T1-weighted images covering the entire liver with a total scan time of less than 20 seconds. This permits breathhold imaging and allows for the dynamic administration of certain contrast material with hepatic MR. New techniques utilizing a half-fourier technique (acquisition of slightly over 50% of the data and the computer reconstruction of the remaining data set) create sub-second T2-weighted images. Although rapid T2-weighting has previously been accomplished with techniques such as echo-planer imaging, the half-fourier techniques have significantly fewer artifacts. These new sub-second T2 sequences have several vendor specific trade names such as Single Shot Fast Spin Echo (SSFSE) or Half-fourier Acquisition Turbo Spin Echo (HASTE). Despite different nomenclature, these techniques produce similar highly effective results.

MRI SAFETY

MRI is safe for the majority of patients. There are however important considerations that both physicians and patients should be aware of. There are several contraindications to a MRI examination. Several of the absolute contraindications include: a cardiac pacing device, an implanted neurostimulator, an intracranial aneurysm clip of unknown composition and a metallic fragment in the globe of the eye. Relative contraindications for a MRI include: recent intravascular stent, filter and pregnancy. Depending on the location and composition of a particular stent or filter a variable time frame will exist before a MRI examination is obtainable. Pregnancy is a relative contraindication as there are no known long-term effects of MRI exams on the human fetus. It is prudent however to avoid scanning a pregnant patient prior to completion of organogenesis. These contraindications are not all-inclusive, and if questions arise about the safety of the patient, it is best to consult with the MRI specialist performing the exam.

MAGNETIC RESONANCE CHOLANGIOGRAPHY

MR cholangiography (MRC) or MR cholangiopancreatography (MRCP) is an imaging technique used to evaluate the biliary system. Heavily T2-weighted images are utilized to provide an overview of the biliary system and pancreatic duct. Excellent diagnostic quality images are obtainable, with high sensitivity and specificity for evaluation of biliary duct dilatation, strictures and intraductal abnormalities (Regan et al 1996, Becker et al 1997, Lomanto et al 1997, Mendler et al 1998). Cross-sectional images as well as projection images (Fig. 16.2) may be easily produced with current MRCP techniques. The projection images are similar to direct contrast-enhanced cholangiograms obtained with either endoscopic retrograde cholangiopancreatography

(ERCP) (Ch. 17) or percutaneous transhepatic cholangiography (PTC). The basic principal of MR cholangiopancreatography is to utilize T2-weighted images where stationary or slowly moving fluid, including bile, is high in signal intensity, and all the surrounding tissues including retroperitoneal fat and the solid visceral organs are lower in signal. There are varieties of MR specific techniques for obtaining cholangiographic images, including two- and three-dimensional sequences, breath hold or non-breath hold techniques, and respiratory gated techniques. MR

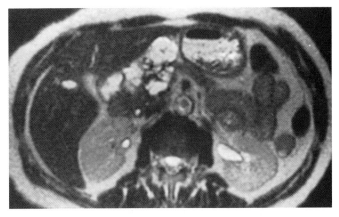

(B)

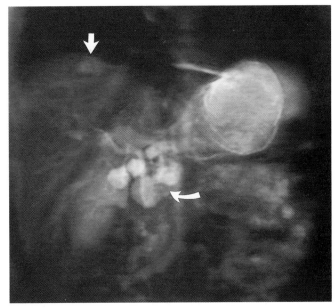

(C)

Fig. 16.2 Cross sectional images and projection image of the same patient. **(A)** Cross sectional coronal image obtained at a slice thickness of 4 mm. There is a focal mass (curved arrow) in the pancreas, which is hyperintense and is composed of multiple cysts. **(B)** Axial image through the pancreas also demonstrates the mass. **(C)** Projection image of the abdomen obtained at a slice thickness of 40 mm. The cystic mass within the pancreas (curved arrow) is easily identified. Fluid containing structures or lesions that act like fluids are seen easily with this technique. Note a small hemangioma at the hepatic dome (arrow).

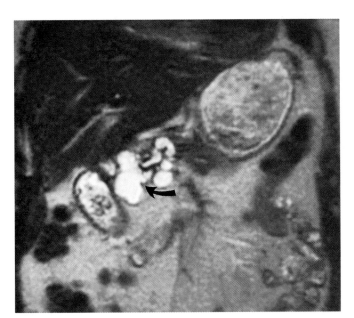

(A)

cholangiopancreatography will play a role in the future in imaging of benign disorders of the biliary and pancreatic system, as well as being part of a comprehensive imaging evaluation of malignancies of the biliary system. MRCP is noninvasive, thus eliminating the morbidity associated with ERCP. An additional advantage of MRCP includes visualization of the extrabiliary anatomy, thus allowing for exclusion or inclusion of alternative diagnosis.

MRI CONTRAST AGENTS

MRI contrast agents work by altering the T1 and T2 relaxation times of various tissue types. In the hepatobiliary system, MRI contrast agents can potentially improve the detection of liver lesions, as well as improve the characterization of focal liver abnormalities. MR contrast agents for hepatobiliary imaging are divided into two basic categories: intracellular and extracellular agents. The most commonly utilized contrast agents are the extracellular agents such as gadopentate dimeglumine (gadolinium (Gd)-DTPA). This agent is distributed within the intravascular compartment initially, and rapidly diffuses through the extravascular space, similar to the action of iodinated contrast agents in computed tomography. Agents such as gadolinium require fast MRI pulse sequences to preferentially enhance either tumor or normal tissue so that the difference between the two tissues will be great. Metastatic liver lesions for instance enhance irregularly predominately in the periphery of the lesion, and slowly, the central portion may or may not accumulate contrast material. Utilizing extracellular contrast agents such as gadolinium and dynamic fast scanning, one can differentiate hepatic hemangiomas from other tumors by their characteristic enhancement patterns. Hepatic hemangiomas fill in slowly (5–20 minutes) from the periphery with a nodular appearance. An advantage of gadolinium (over iodinated CT contrast) is the lack of renal toxicity even at high doses (Prince et al 1996). This fact has clinical implications in patients with decreased renal function or patients at risk for potential nephrotoxic effects of iodinated contrast agents.

A second type of hepatic contrast agent is categorized as intracellular agents. These agents are taken up either by hepatocytes or by the reticuloendothelial system. One of the hepatocyte specific agents is a T1 agent Mangafodipir trisodium (Mn-DPDP), which facilitates T1 relaxation in normal liver thus increasing conspicuity of lesions on T1-weighted images. Other agents, such as ferumoxides, are taken up primarily by the reticuloendothelial system in the liver and spleen. Ferumoxides (iron oxide based images) cause a decrease in normal hepatic parenchymal signal on T2-weighted images because of their iron content. Conspicuity of many hepatic lesions will be increased after administration of ferumoxides since the background normal hepatic parenchyma will decrease and the lesions will be relatively more hyperintense.

Newer T1 contrast agents are currently under investigation including gadolinium ethoxybenzyl DTPA (Gd-EOB-DTPA) and gadolinium benzyloxypropionictetra-acetate (Gd-BOPTA) (Giovagnoni & Paci 1996). These agents generate hepatic enhancement on T1-weighted images and are partially excreted via the biliary tree. Large clinical trials are currently under way to evaluate these newer hepatobiliary agents.

NORMAL HEPATIC APPEARANCE ON MRI

Hepatic MRI is a very sensitive technique to evaluate both diffuse and focal abnormalities. In normal hepatic parenchyma on T1-weighted images the liver is brighter (hyperintense) than the spleen. Depending on the specific technique chosen, the vessels may appear as dark (flow voids on spin echo technique) or may be bright (gradient echo technique). In T2-weighted images the spleen is relatively brighter than the liver (Fig. 16.3). Fluid is dark on T1-weighted images and bright on T2-weighted images due to both long T1 and T2 values. Although many hepatic lesions are low signal intensity on T1-weighted images, they may be variable on T2-weighted images depending on their water content.

DIFFUSE HEPATIC DISEASE

FATTY INFILTRATION OF THE LIVER

Fat may accumulate within hepatocytes due to a number of reasons, including alcohol abuse, and may be related to patients with diabetes or obesity. Fatty change may be diffuse, patchy or focal. The pattern of fatty infiltration is related to regional differences in perfusion. It is often difficult to distinguish fatty infiltration from focal hepatic lesions on computerized tomography (CT), because both will appear low in attenuation. Additionally, focal fatty sparing may appear similar to a vascular neoplasm on contrast enhanced CT. It is however easy to distinguish these entities on MRI because of different signal characteristics. On T1-weighted images, areas of fatty infiltration will appear bright because of the low T1 value of fat. The appearance on T2-weighted images depends upon the specific type of

T2-weighted sequence acquired. Conventional spin-echo T2-weighted sequences are relatively insensitive to the presence of fat (Wenke et al 1984). Areas of focal fatty infiltration may appear hyperintense to normal hepatic parenchyma on fast T2-weighted images due to the high signal intensity of fat on these sequences. Utilizing chemically selective fat suppression techniques, these areas of focal fatty infiltration will appear dark.

Chemical shift imaging is another technique that allows differentiation of the signals from fat and water protons. These chemical shift techniques are the most sensitive techniques for distinguishing fatty infiltration (Fig. 16.4)

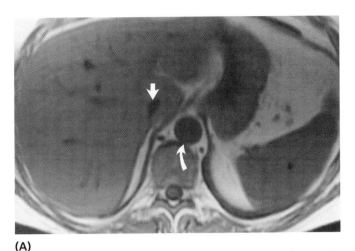

(A)

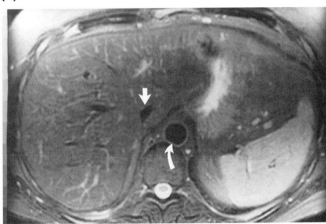

(B)

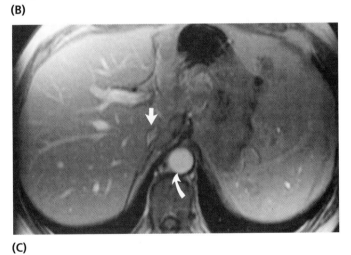

(C)

Fig. 16.3 Normal hepatic MRI. **(A)** T1-weighted spin echo image. The liver is brighter (hyperintense) relative to the signal of the spleen. Note that there are normal flow voids (dark areas in the visualized vessels) (arrow, intrahepatic portion of the inferior vena cava; curved arrow, aorta). **(B)** T2-weighted fast spin echo image. There has been reversal of the liver spleen contrast with the normal spleen now being brighter than the liver. Note once again the flow voids within the vessels (arrow, intrahepatic portion of the inferior vena cava; curved arrow, aorta). **(C)** Post contrast T1-weighted gradient echo image. There is normal enhancement in both the liver and spleen, with the parenchyma of both being about equal in this phase of the injection. Note that all the vessels (arrow, intrahepatic portion of the inferior vena cava; curved arrow, aorta) are bright due to the T1 shortening effect of gadolinium.

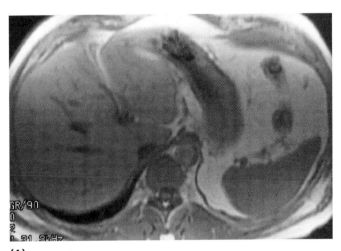

(A)

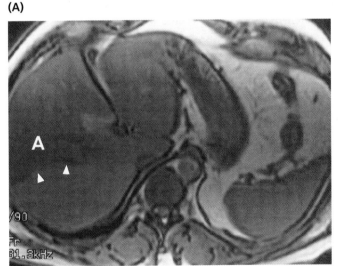

(B)

Fig. 16.4 Fatty infiltration of the liver. **(A)** T1-weighted in-phase gradient echo image (TE 4.2 demonstrates normal liver-spleen contrast. **(B)** T1-weighted out-of-phase image (TE 1.8) at the same level demonstrates a geographic area (A) that has lost signal (approached signal of the spleen). Arrowheads demarcate the transition to normal hepatic parenchyma. This area has normal vascularity coursing through it and no mass was present. This is the typical appearance of fatty infiltration on chemical shift imaging. Note on the out of phase images there is a black line (India ink effect) surrounding tissue interfaces.

(Mitchell et al 1991, Siegelman 1997). Chemical shift imaging techniques rely on the different resonant frequencies present in fat and water protons. Utilizing fast imaging techniques, the signal emanating from fat and water protons may be equal but opposite. Tissues, which have relatively equal quantities of fat and water, will appear dark because the signal from fat and water will cancel each other out. Areas of sparing will remain relatively hyperintense to the fatty infiltrated regions. Focal fatty infiltration should not enhance following gadolinium administration. The presence of a lesion with characteristic signal intensity findings on T1, T2 and gradient echo opposed phased imaging is diagnostic of fatty infiltration (Mitchell et al 1991, Kreft et al 1992). Any one of these sequences alone is not characteristic, as other lesions, including hepatocellular carcinoma and adenoma, may contain small quantities of fat within them.

IRON DEPOSITION DISEASE

Iron accumulation within the liver has two main etiologies: hemochromatosis and hemosiderosis. Hemochromatosis is characterized by abnormal intestinal absorption of iron. Iron accumulation is predominately in hepatocytes until late in the disease when there is 'spill-over' into the pancreatic parenchyma. The liver demonstrates abnormally low signal intensity when compared to spleen on T1-weighted sequences. Gradient echo sequences are the most sensitive sequence for detecting the presence of iron within the hepatic parenchyma. Primary or genetic hemochromatosis is important to diagnosis, as this entity may be unnoticed until late in the disease process. Long-term sequelae of this entity include fibrosis, cirrhosis and hepatocellular carcinoma, which may also be imaged with MRI. In addition, screening of family members is also important in primary hemochromatosis as it is an autosomal recessive trait. Hemochromatosis needs to be distinguished for the similar entity hemosiderosis. Hemosiderosis is not genetically linked and is associated with multiple blood transfusions, conversely it has a benign course. There is accumulation of hepatic iron in the reticuloendothelial system. MRI is excellent for identifying these entities, as iron changes the expected signal intensities of abdominal organs. In patients with hemochromatosis the normal liver–spleen pattern is reversed on T1-weighted images. In more advanced stages iron will also be deposited in the pancreatic parenchyma. Hemosiderosis affects the spleen and bone marrow early on in the disease process with the liver begin affected later. These distinguishing characteristics along with the patients history allow for correct differentiation between the two entities. Gradient echo imaging is very sensitive for the detection and characterization of these two processes (Rofsky & Fleishaker 1995) (Fig. 16.5).

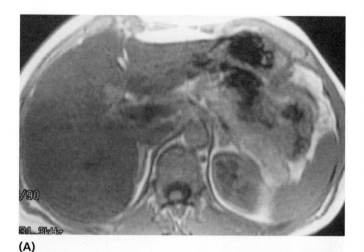

(A)

(B)

Fig. 16.5 Hemochromatosis. **(A)** T1-weighted in-phase gradient echo image (TE 4.2) demonstrates abnormal liver–spleen contrast. The liver is homogeneously darker than the spleen from preferential deposition of iron within the hepatic parenchyma. Note the difference from Figure 16.4. **(B)** T1-weighted out-of-phase gradient echo image (TE 1.8) demonstrates the liver spleen contrast returns to normal with the liver being brighter than spleen. This is opposite from Figure 16.4 and demonstrates early iron deposition disease within the liver.

FOCAL HEPATIC LESIONS

CYSTS

Cysts are common hepatic lesions, and may be simple (Ch. 66), or associated with polycystic disease of the kidney (Fig. 16.6). Small cysts (< 1 cm) may be difficult to characterize on CT due to volume averaging. The MRI criterion for a simple cyst is a lesion that is homogeneously low in signal intensity on T1-weighted images, and homogeneously bright on T2-weighted images. Lengthening the TE value on T2-weighted images allows for 'heavier T2-weighting'. Cysts maintain their high signal on these 'heavy' T2 images.

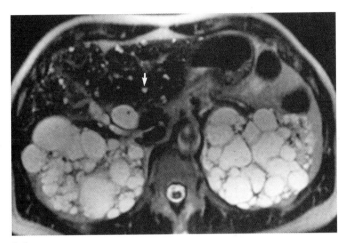

(A)

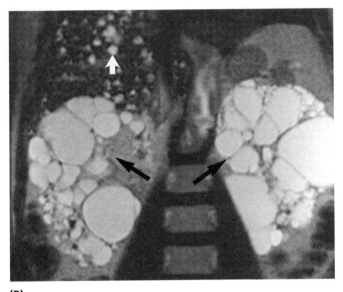

(B)

Fig. 16.6 Hepatic cysts associated with polycystic kidney disease. **(A)** Axial T2-weighted image at the level of kidneys, demonstrates bilaterally enlarged kidneys with multiple hyperintense cysts. Little normal renal parenchyma is present at this level. There are multiple small hepatic cysts as well (arrow). **(B)** Coronal T2-weighted images through the kidneys demonstrate similar findings of enlarged kidneys containing multiple cysts (black arrows) and small hepatic cysts are once again identified (white arrow).

A cyst should not enhance following Gd-DTPA administration. Hepatic cysts may also be associated with infectious etiologies such as echinococcal disease. Echinococcal cysts (Ch. 63) have a different MRI appearance, are usually multiloculated and complex, and may have components that enhance.

HEMANGIOMA

Hepatic hemangiomas (Ch. 72) are benign tumors of the liver and are found in up to 7.3% of autopsy specimens (Isak

& Rabin 1986, Birnbaum et al 1990). The vast majority of hemangiomas are found incidentally on other imaging studies, such as computerized tomography or ultrasound. MRI is ideal for characterizing hemangiomas, and is the preferred modality of choice. On T1-weighted images, hemangiomas are hypointense as compared with the surrounding hepatic parenchyma and have smooth, well-marginated borders and are frequently lobulated. Hemangiomas are hyperintense compared to normal liver on T2-weighted images and demonstrate a lobulated, well-demarcated border. Hemangiomas tend to retain their high signal on more heavily T2-weighted sequences. The presence of hyperintense peripheral nodular enhancement with either partial (especially when large) or complete filling in following gadolinium administration has been shown to be 100% specific, 84% sensitive and 95% accurate for the diagnosis of hemangioma (Fig. 16.7). (Whitney et al 1993, Mathieu et al 1997, Semelka & Sofka, 1997). Dynamic, fast MRI (following the administration of intravenous gadolinium) is useful for increasing the specificity of diagnosis of hepatic hemangioma and differentiating this lesion from others including metastases and hepatocellular carcinomas (Yoshida et al 1989). Larger hemangiomas tend to follow these criteria more frequently. Problems, however, arise with smaller hemangiomas that may 'flash-fill' and appear as hypervascular lesions. These smaller lesions (usually less than 1 cm) may be distinguished by their T2 characteristics (Outwater et al 1997). Hemangiomas may also be diagnosed after the administration of iron-based contrast agents (Harisinghani et al 1997).

FOCAL NODULAR HYPERPLASIA

Focal nodular hyperplasia (FNH) (Ch. 72) is another common benign tumor of the liver, though less frequent than hemangioma. Pathologically, FNH contains all the elements of normal liver, and may have a central fibrous scar, which is surrounded by hepatocytes and small bile ducts. FNH is the second most common benign tumor of the liver, and has been associated with oral contraceptive use (Christopherson et al 1977). Most FNH lesions are isointense or slightly hypointense compared to the normal liver parenchyma on T1-weighted images and are either isointense or minimally hyperintense on T2-weighted images (Fig. 16.8A and 16.8B). Frequently, FNH is visualized by displacement of the normal hepatic vasculature. Classic FNH has an early arterial peak enhancement with dynamic administration of intravenous contrast agent. A common feature of FNH is the presence of a central scar. Generally the central scar is hypointense on T1-weighted images and is hyperintense on T2-weighted images. The central scar

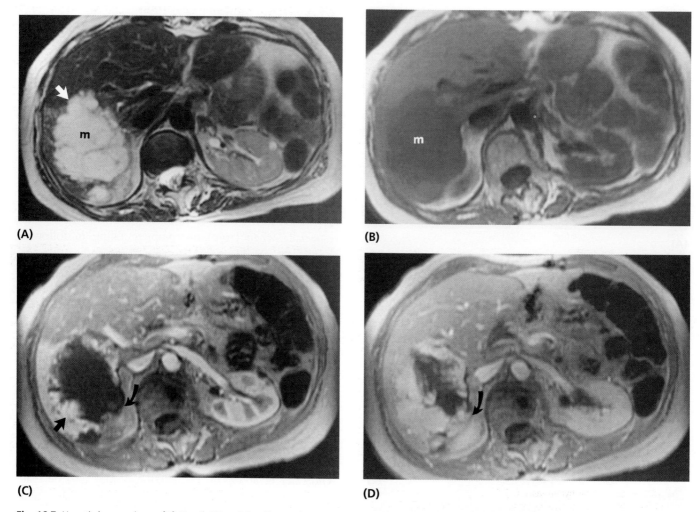

(A)

(B)

(C)

(D)

Fig. 16.7 Hepatic hemangioma. **(A)** Heavily T2-weighted image (TE 150) demonstrates a mass (m), which is hyperintense to hepatic parenchyma and contains some internal architecture. Note the lobulated well defined margins of this lesion (arrow). **(B)** Pre contrast T1-weighted gradient echo image at the same level demonstrates the mass (m) to be dark compared to background parenchyma. **(C)** T1-weighted GRE image during contrast administration demonstrates peripheral nodular or broken ring enhancement within this mass (arrow). Note the posterior medial aspect of this lesion fails to demonstrate enhancement during this phase of the contrast injection (curved arrow). **(D)** Delayed T1-weighted gradient echo sequence post contrast image demonstrates the lesion has partially filled in towards the central portion of the lesion. Note that the region identified in Figure 16.7C has filled in on delayed images (curved arrow). This constellation of findings is typical for hepatic hemangioma.

demonstrates contrast enhancement as well, but in a delayed fashion and with prolonged enhancement (Fig. 16.8C). Superparamagnetic iron oxide contrast agents will be taken up by FNH because they contain Kupffer cells. Many reports indicate that FNH will take up a significant percentage of superparamagnetic iron oxide particles after administration thus demonstrating signal loss post iron oxide agent (Grandin et al 1997). This is consistent with the experience of nuclear scanning with ^{99m}Tc–sulfur colloid. Therefore, lesions of FNH can be characterized with a high degree of specificity utilizing a variety of MRI techniques (Vilgrain et al 1992).

HEPATIC ADENOMA

Hepatic adenomas (Ch. 72) are also benign lesions associated with the use of oral contraceptives. They are commonly large, may cause upper abdominal pain and may rupture and bleed. Hepatocytes are present within adenomas; however, these lesions lack hepatic veins and bile ducts. In addition, there are only small numbers of reticuloendothelial cells if any present, therefore iron oxide scans demonstrate less uptake then FNH. Hemorrhage, which is one of the most common causes of pain, may be life threatening if it extends into the peritoneum. MRI tissue characterization of hepatic adenomas varies. Generally, hepatic adenomas are hyper-

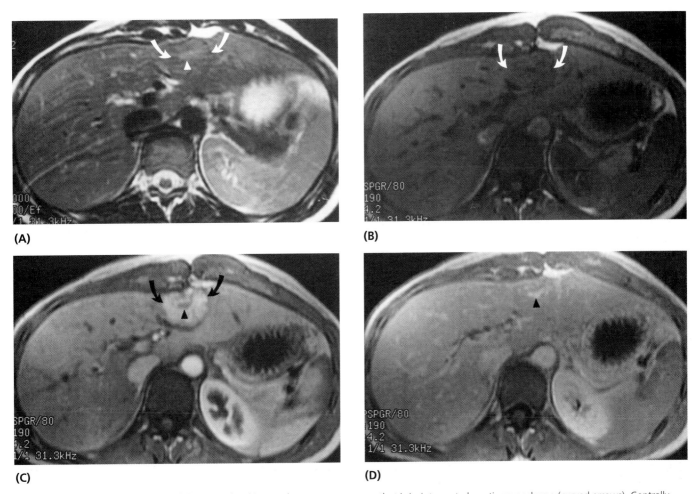

(A)

(B)

(C)

(D)

Fig. 16.8 Focal nodular hyperplasia. **(A)** T2-weighted image demonstrates a mass that is isointense to hepatic parenchyma (curved arrows). Centrally within this mass is a linear hyperintense focus (arrowhead). **(B)** Precontrast T1-weighted gradient echo image demonstrates the mass (curved arrows) to be mildly hypointense to liver. **(C)** Arterial dominant phase T1-weighted gradient echo sequence demonstrates the mass to enhance intensely with respect to hepatic parenchyma (curved arrows). The central focus, which was bright on the T2-weighted images, does not demonstrate enhancement on this phase of the injection (arrowhead). **(D)** Post-contrast equilibrium phase images demonstrate the mass to be isointense to background hepatic parenchyma. The central portion or scar demonstrates delayed enhancement (arrowhead), characteristic of FNH.

intense on T1-weighted images due to the presence of hemorrhage or fat. Infrequently, the T1-weighted images may demonstrate a low signal intensity pseudocapsule surrounding the adenoma, similar in appearance to hepatocellular carcinoma (Gabata et al 1990). A central scar may be seen within certain adenomas as well (Rummeny et al 1989). Adenomas are hypervascular lesions and demonstrate enhancement during the arterial dominant phase of the contrast injection. Small adenomas, without hemorrhage, may be difficult to differentiate from FNH (without a central scar) or well differentiated hepatocellular carcinoma.

HEPATIC ABSCESSES

Computed tomography is generally the modality of choice in the recent postoperative patient where there is a clinical

suspicion of a hepatic abscess (Ch. 61). Patients with a more atypical presentation may be a diagnostic dilemma. While some patients present with symptoms suggestive of abscesses, others do not. Patients with abscesses may be imaged with MRI. Abscesses are usually hyperintense on T2-weighted images with an irregular rim of intermediate signal intensity surrounding a hyperintense outer rim. Abscesses are generally hypointense on T1-weighted images unless they have hemorrhage or proteinacious debris within them. After administration of contrast material, the rim enhances while the central portion will not. The imaging findings may overlap somewhat with malignancies including gallbladder cancer.

HEPATIC METASTASES

The liver is the most common site for the hematogenous

spread of malignant neoplasms. Other hepatic lesions, including hemangiomas or fatty infiltration, may appear similar to metastases when imaged with CT or ultrasound. In addition, several types of lesions may coexist in the same patient, which may be challenging for the diagnostic radiologist. However, these lesions may be distinguished utilizing MRI. In general, metastases are of low signal intensity on T1-weighted images and are hyperintense on T2-weighted images. Metastases tend not to be as bright on T2-weighted images as hemangiomas or cysts. Metastases tend to have less well-defined borders than other benign lesions, and may have peripheral high signal intensity, which has been shown

to represent viable tumor (Fig. 16.9). During contrast administration metastases may demonstrate early peripheral rim enhancement. This peripheral rim washes out on delayed images, and actually appear hypointense on delayed images (Fig. 16.10). While this delayed hypointense rim is seen in the minority of cases it is 100% specific for the diagnosis of hepatic malignancy (Mahfouz et al 1994). Larger metastases tend to have a thick irregular rim of enhancement representing viable tumor with areas of central necrosis. MRI is the most sensitive noninvasive technique for evaluating patients for metastatic disease. It is less invasive and more cost-effective than CT arterial portography, and

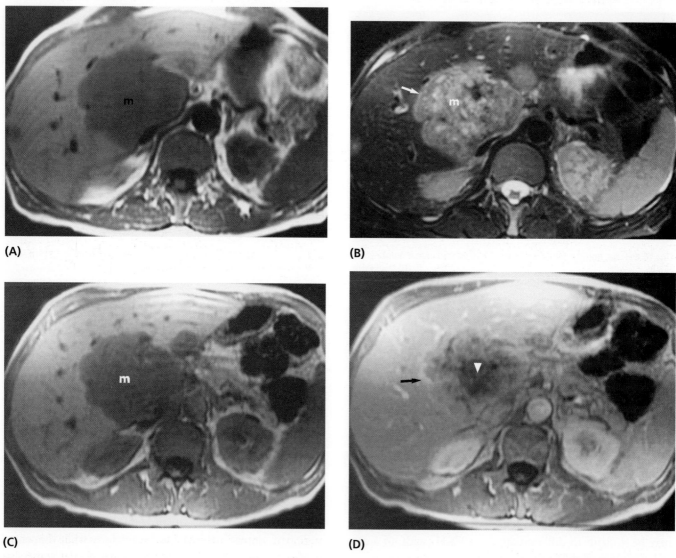

(A)　　　　**(B)**

(C)　　　　**(D)**

Fig. 16.9 Hepatic metastasis from colorectal carcinoma. **(A)** T1-weighted image demonstrates a large central low signal intensity metastasis (m) with several smaller lesions within the liver. **(B)** T2-weighted image demonstrates the mass (m) is brighter than background hepatic parenchyma. Note that the borders are somewhat ill-defined and there appears to be internal septations within this lesion. The periphery of the lesion is a rind of tissue which is mildly hyperintense to liver but darker than the central portion of the mass (arrow). **(C)** Pre-contrast enhanced T1-weighted gradient echo image demonstrates the large hepatic metastasis (m) in contrast to the normal hepatic parenchyma. **(D)** Pre-contrast enhanced T1-weighted gradient echo images fail to demonstrate the peripheral portion (black arrow) and internal septations have enhanced representing viable tumor, while the central necrotic portion (white arrowhead) fails to enhance. Note the distinct difference in appearance of that of the hemangioma (Figure 16.7).

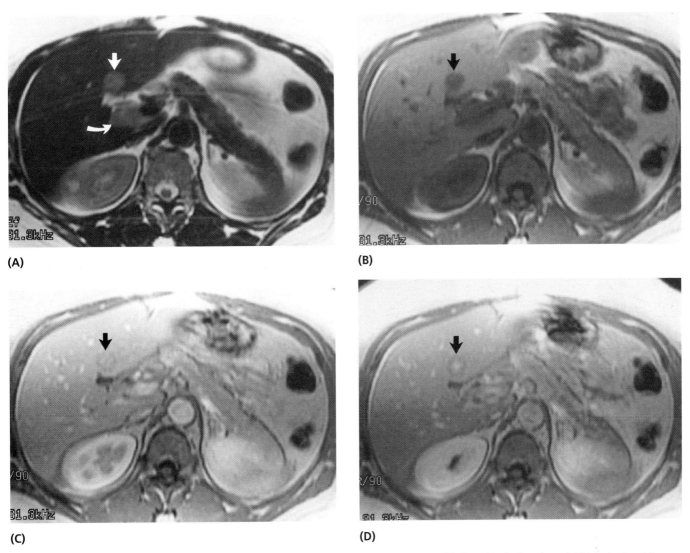

(A)

(B)

(C)

(D)

Fig. 16.10 Hepatic metastasis from breast carcinoma. **(A)** T2-weighted image demonstrates a small lesion with the liver (arrow). This lesion is mildly hyperintense. Note there is portal lymphadenopathy present as well (curved arrow). **(B)** Pre-contrast T1-weighted gradient echo image demonstrates a well-defined mass (arrow) that is hypointense to liver. **(C)** T1-weighted gradient echo image after the administration of contrast demonstrates the peripheral portion that enhanced irregularly during the arterial dominant phase (not shown) beginning to wash out suggesting an early target appearance (arrow). **(D)** Delayed post contrast gradient echo image demonstrates continued filling of the central portion of this lesion while the periphery has washed out (arrow).

therefore is an excellent screening tool for staging hepatic metastases for surgical resection. In addition, MR can also easily map out hepatic vasculature as well as image in multiple planes (e.g. coronal, sagittal or oblique) to allow for complete surgical planning.

HEPATOCELLULAR CARCINOMA

The diagnosis of hepatocellular carcinoma (Ch. 73) on CT and ultrasound is difficult due to its association with chronic liver disease. Chronic liver disease appears heterogeneous on CT and MRI (Fig. 16.11) and it is difficult to distinguish focal hepatic lesions in these patients. The heterogeneity is created by the presence of a nodular configuration. These nodules may represent regenerative nodules, dysplastic nodules or hepatocellular carcinoma. The advantage of MRI in the evaluation of hepatocellular carcinoma is that areas of carcinoma will demonstrate signal intensity changes relative to areas of cirrhotic hepatic parenchyma. Hepatocellular carcinoma generally is hypointense on T1-weighted images, and hyperintense on T2-weighted images, although the signal intensity can be variable on these sequences (Earls et al 1996, Kelekis et al 1998). Well-differentiated hepatocellular carcinoma, however, is hyperintense on T1-weighted images due to the presence of intracellular lipid (Ebra et al 1986) (Fig. 16.12). On T2-weighted images, large hepato-

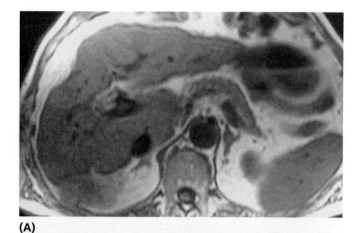

(A)

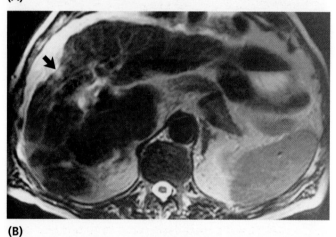

(B)

Fig. 16.11 Liver with cirrhotic configuration. **(A)** T1-weighted spin echo image at the level of the portal vein demonstrates hypertrophy of the left lobe and caudate, with atrophy of the right lobe of the liver. **(B)** T2-weighted image of the liver at the same level demonstrates mildly heterogeneous signal in the atrophied right lobe making exclusion of an underlying mass difficult. In addition note the focal hepatic scarring (arrow).

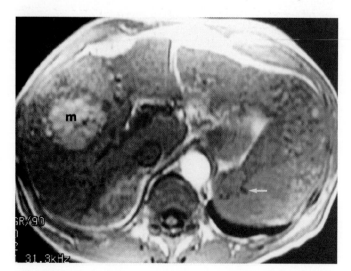

Fig. 16.12 Hepatocellular carcinoma containing intracellular lipids. T1-weighted in-phase gradient echo image demonstrates a mass (m) in the liver which is brighter than normal parenchyma. There are siderodic nodules diffusely present within the liver and also present in the spleen (gamma ghandi bodies) (arrow).

cellular carcinoma may have a 'mosaic' appearance produced by multiple centers of growth interspersed with areas of necrosis and regenerating liver tissue (Choi et al 1990, Lalonde et al 1992, Fujita et al 1997) (Fig. 16.13). The fibrolamellar type of hepatocellular carcinoma may have a central scar. These fibrous scars tend to be low in signal intensity on both the T1- and T2-weighted images. The presence of this fibrous scar, however, can not reliably distinguish between benign and malignant hepatic lesions since FNH may also have a central scar (Wilbur and Gyi, 1987). Gradient echo (bright blood technique) MRI and other flow-sensitive techniques are excellent for evaluating

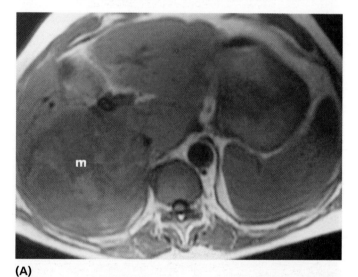

(A)

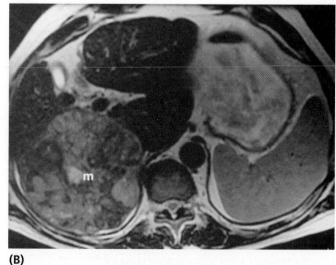

(B)

Fig. 16.13 Large hepatocellular carcinoma demonstrating the mosaic pattern. **(A)** T1-weighted image demonstrates a large heterogeneous mass (m) in the liver. Note the hypertrophied left hepatic lobe and caudate. **(B)** T2-weighted image also demonstrates the mass (m) to be heterogeneous with islands of tissue that are hyperintense with respect to other portions of the same mass. This pattern is known as the 'mosaic' pattern and can be seen in HCC especially when large.

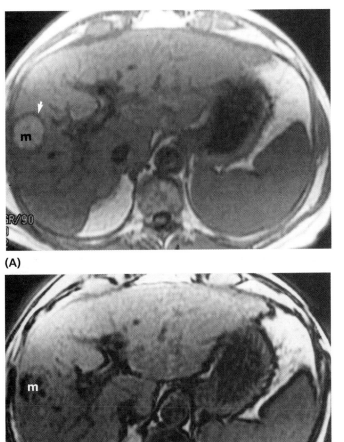

(A)

(B)

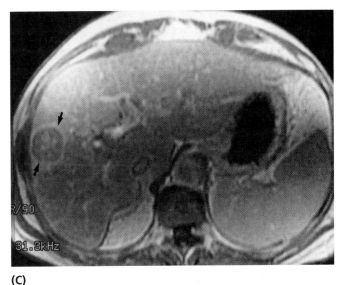

(C)

Fig. 16.14 Hepatocellular carcinoma with both intracellular lipid and capsular enhancement. **(A)** T1-weighted in-phase gradient echo image demonstrates a focal hyperintense mass (m). There is a dark rim around this mass making it appear encapsulated (arrow). **(B)** T1-weighted out-of-phase image demonstrates signal loss in this mass (m) representing intracellular lipid and water of approximately equal distribution. **(C)** Delayed post contrast image through the lesion demonstrates the 'capsule' around the lesion to have enhanced (arrows), the capsule did not enhance on the immediate post contrast images (not shown).

hepatic vascular tumor invasion. MRI is more sensitive than CT, sonography or angiography for detecting intrahepatic vascular invasion (Iton et al 1987). Contrast-enhanced MRI with Gd-DTPA demonstrates irregular and variable patterns of enhancement due to the vascular nature of the tumor. Most hepatocellular carcinomas are hypervascular in nature and demonstrate enhancement during the arterial dominant phase of the injection, in distinction to the other nodules seen in cirrhotic livers. These lesions tend to be isointense to the background liver parenchyma during the equilibrium phase of the examination. Although hepatocellular carcinomas are typically hypervascular lesions there has been a recent report of multiple dysplastic nodules presenting as hypervascular masses on both CT and MRI (Krinsky et al 1998). MRI is also excellent for identifying additional characteristics, which may aid in the diagnosis of hepatocellular carcinoma, including a capsule surrounding the lesion, which is low signal on the arterial dominant phase and enhances on delayed images (Fig. 16.14).

LESS COMMON HEPATIC TUMORS

LYMPHOMA

Non-Hodgkin lymphoma accounts for a vast majority of hepatic lymphoma. MRI demonstrates masses of varying size, which are generally low in signal intensity on T1-weighted images, and hyperintense on T2-weighted images. The degree of hyperintensity is not as great as with other focal benign hepatic lesions such as hemangiomas or cysts. This difference in signal intensity makes it relatively easy to determine the malignant nature of the lesion, but not the specific cause. The imaging characteristics of lymphoma overlap with other malignant hepatic lesions.

MESENCHYMAL TUMORS

Rarely, tumors of mesenchymal origin including angiosarcoma, leiomyosarcoma and fibrous histiocytoma may be present within the liver (Wunderbaldinger et al 1998). The MRI appearance of these tumors is nonspecific. Again, they are generally of low intensity on T1-weighted images and hyperintense on T2-weighted images.

EPITHELIOID HEMANGIOENDOTHELIOMA

Epithelioid hemangioendothelioma is a rare tumor of adults and should be distinguished from the infantile hemangio-endothelioma, which occurs in children. The prognosis is somewhat better than other parenchymal tumors such as sarcoma, though extrahepatic metastases do occur. Epithelioid hemangioendotheliomas are generally low in signal intensity on T1-weighted images and are hyper-intense on T2-weighted images, but not as hyperintense as hemangiomas. Following Gd-DTPA administration, there is an irregular nodular and concentric enhancement. Capsular retraction may also be seen with epithelioid hemangioendotheliomas helping to elucidate the diagnosis (Van Beers et al 1992).

BILIARY CYSTADENOMA AND BILIARY CYSTADENOCARCINOMAS

These lesions are rare tumors of the liver, which present as a predominately cystic mass containing septations (Fig. 16.15). These lesions may be low, intermediate or of increased signal on the T1-weighted images depending on the protein content within the mass. The lesions are usually hyperintense on T2-weighted sequences. The malignant variety may demonstrate nodular or irregular internal soft tissue; however distinction between the two is not always possible.

BILIARY TUMORS

GALLBLADDER CARCINOMA (Ch. 53)

Gallbladder carcinoma is well evaluated with MRI. This entity is best seen on T2-weighted images, as thickening of the gallbladder wall, generally adjacent to multiple gallstones.

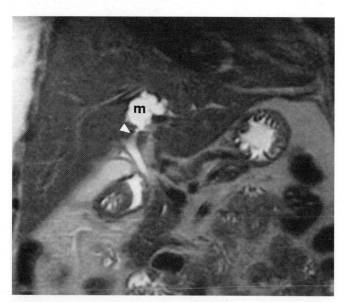

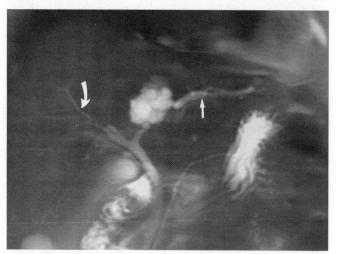

(A)

(B)

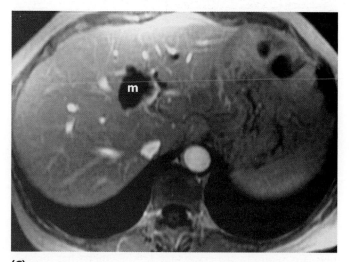

(C)

Fig. 16.15 Biliary cystadenoma. **(A)** Coronal T2-weighted image demonstrates a lobulated mass (m) in close proximity to the left hepatic duct (arrowhead). **(B)** Projection image in the coronal oblique plane demonstrates the well-defined hyperintense mass to be in continuity with a mildly dilated left sided biliary radical (arrow). Note the normal right sided biliary radical (curved arrow) well seen with this technique. **(C)** Post contrast T1-weighted gradient echo image demonstrates no enhancement within this mass (m).

Cholelithiasis is a predisposing condition. Evidence of liver invasion and spread to regional lymph nodes may also be identified with MRI. MRI is optimal for evaluation of these lesions due to its outstanding tissue contrast and ability to directly image in multiple planes (Demachi et al 1997, Yoshimitsu et al 1997).

BILE DUCT CANCER (Ch. 54)

Bile duct tumors are well seen on MRI. Central lesions (hilar cholangiocarcinomas) are generally associated with biliary dilatation, which is bright on T2-weighted images. The central tumors may be seen as areas of mildly hyperintense signal on T2-weighted images (Fig. 16.16), less so than the surrounding biliary dilatation. Peripheral or intrahepatic cholangiocarcinomas generally present as high signal intensity masses on T2-weighted images. They may appear similar to other malignant neoplasms of the liver but generally do not have capsules or areas of high signal intensity on the T1-weighted images as may be seen in hepatocellular carcinomas. Distinction of peripheral cholangiocarcinoma and confluent hepatic fibrosis is sometimes difficult; however late enhancement is seen in the malignant lesion.

BENIGN DISEASES OF THE BILIARY TRACT

CHOLELITHIASIS

Gallstones are easily identifiable on T2-weighted images as well as on MRCP sequences (Fig. 16.17). They usually appear as low signal intensity structures in a fluid filled gallbladder. MR is usually not the modality of choice in the evaluation of cholelithiasis, as ultrasound is highly sensitive and less expensive in uncomplicated cases. Choledocholithiasis,

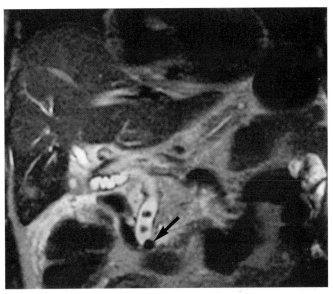

(A)

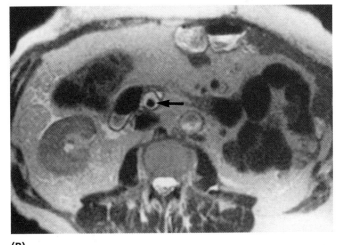

(B)

Fig. 16.17 Choledocholithiasis. **(A)** Coronal T2-weighted (SSFSE) image through the common duct, in a patient status post cholecystectomy, demonstrates multiple stones within the common bile duct. Note the distal stone impacted at the level of the ampulla (arrow). **(B)** Axial T2-weighted image with the same technique also demonstrates a stone, surrounded by bile, in the distal common bile duct (arrow).

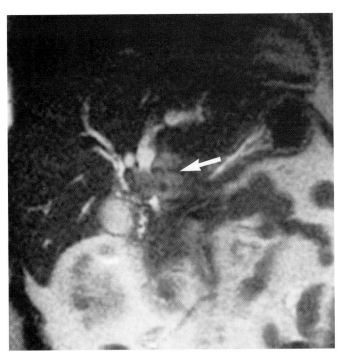

Fig. 16.16 Hilar cholangiocarcinoma. Oblique coronal T2-weighted image demonstrates dilatation of the intrahepatic biliary tree. A soft tissue mass (arrow) is present at the bifurcation of the common hepatic duct causing the ductal dilatation.

however, can be effectively and efficaciously imaged by MR (Dwerryhouse et al 1998, Musella et al 1998). Common duct stones are relatively uncommon in children (Rescorla, 1997) but are more common in elderly patients (Gonzalez et al 1997, Catheline et al 1998). Direct coronal T2-weighted imaging, readily available with MRI, easily identifies common duct stones. In addition if multiple stones are present in the common duct they too should be identifiable by MRI (Fig. 16.17). MRCP can also be obtained to evaluate if retained stones are present post cholecystectomy. If no stones are present on the MRCP this may negate the need for an ERCP.

CHOLEDOCHAL CYSTS

Choledochal cysts (Ch. 65) represent dilatation of the extrahepatic bile ducts. There may be associated intrahepatic biliary ductal dilatation as well. This entity is a relatively uncommon congenital anomaly, which usually presents before 10 years of age. The classic triad includes a palpable mass, abdominal pain and jaundice. Five types of cysts have been described (Todani et al 1977). Type I has been subdivided in A, B and C; in addition there are types II, III, IVA, IVB and V. MRI is well suited to not only diagnose this entity but also classify it. Not only can MR cholangiograms be generated to depict the normal and abnormal anatomy but also direct coronal imaging can be obtained for clearer evaluation.

POSTOPERATIVE BILIARY COMPLICATIONS

Complications from surgical procedures include bile leaks, abscess formation and biliary strictures (Chs 49 & 50). While utilizing other imaging modalities in the immediate postoperative setting to assess for bile leaks and abscesses may be prudent MR is uniquely suited for the assessment of the postoperative biliary tract. Bile duct injuries after surgery can be caused by a variety of reasons, but may lead to the same result – a stricture at the anastomotic site. MR using long echo train length imaging (MRCP technique) is uniquely suited for this problem. Surgical clips near the anastomosis may create streak artifacts during CT scanning. MR with its multiplaner capabilities, superior tissue contrast and the MRCP sequences' ability to minimize susceptibility due to multiple 180° refocusing pulses can allow for improved visualization of the region of the anastomosis and thus improve diagnostic confidence (Coakley et al 1998) (Fig. 16.18).

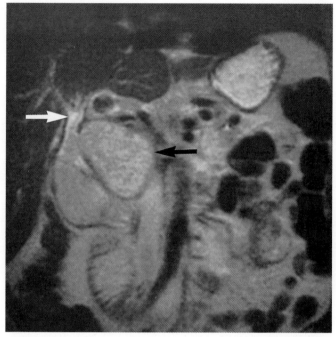

(A)

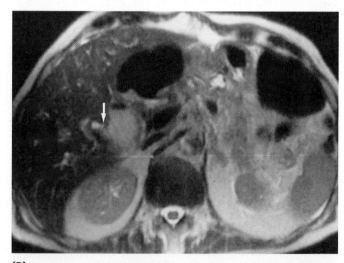

(B)

Fig. 16.18 Afferent loop syndrome. **(A)** Coronal T2-weighted sequence in a patient post pancreaticoduodenectomy for pancreatic carcinoma. The patient has a hepatojejunostomy with a patent anastomosis (white arrow). The afferent loop is markedly dilated (black arrow) in comparison to other loops of bowel. No mechanical obstruction was noted. **(B)** Axial T2-weighted image through the level of the anastomosis (arrow) demonstrates the site to be patent without evidence of a stricture. Again, the afferent loop is dilated.

REFERENCES

Becker C D, Grossholz M, Becker M, Mentha G, de Peyer R, Terrier F 1997 Choledocholithiasis and bile duct stenosis: diagnostic accuracy of MR cholangiopancreatography. Radiology 205: 523–30

Birnbaum B A, Weinreb J C, Megibow A J, Sanger J J, Lubat E, Kanamuller H, Noz M E, Bosniak M A 1990 Definitive diagnosis of hepatic hemangiomas: MR imaging versus Tc-99m-labeled red blood cell SPECT. Radiology 176: 95–101

Bloch F, Hansen W W, Packard H 1946 The nuclear induction experiment. Physical Review 70: 474–485

Catheline J M, Turner R, Rizk N, Barrat C, Buenos P, Champault G 1998 Evaluation of the biliary tree during laparoscoic cholecystectomy: laparoscopic ultrasound versus intraoperative cholanglography: a prospective study of 150 cases. Surgical Laparoscopy and Endoscopy 8:85–91

Choi B I, Lee G K, Kim S T et al 1990 Mosaic pattern of encapsulated hepatocellular carcinoma: correlation of magnetic resonance imaging and pathology. Gastrointestinal Radiology 15: 238–240

Christopherson W M, Mays E T, Barrows, G 1977 Clinicopathologic study of steroid-related liver tumors. American Journal of Surgical Pathology 1: 31–41

Coakley F V, Schwartz L H, Blumgart L H, Fong Y, Jarnagin W R, Panicek D M 1998 Complex postcholecystectomy biliary disorders: preliminary experience with evaluation by means of breath-hold MR cholanglography. Radiology 209: 141–6

Damadian, R 1972 Apparatus and method for detecting cancer in tissue. US Patent No 3789832

Demachi H, Matsui O, Hoshiba K, Kimura M, Miyata S, Kuroda Y, Konishi K, Tsuji M, Miwa A 1997 Dynamic MRI using a surface coil in chronic cholecystitis and gallbladder carcinoma: radiologic and histopathologic correlation. Journal of Computer Assisted Tomography 21: 643–51

Dwerryhouse S J, Brown E, Vipond M N 1998 Prospective evaluation of magnetic resonance cholanglography to detect common bile duct stones before laparoscopic cholecystectomy. British Journal of Surgery 85: 1364–6

Earls J P, Theise N D, Weinreb J C, DeCorato D R, Krinsky G A, Rofsky N M, Mizrachi H, Teperman L W 1996 Dysplastic nodules and hepatocellular carcinoma: thin-section MR imaging of explanted cirrhotic livers with pathologic correlation. Radiology 201: 207–14

Ebara M, Ohto M, Watanabe Y et al 1986 Diagnosis of small hepatocellular carcinoma: correlation of MR imaging and tumor histologic studies. Radiology 159: 371–377

Fujita T, Honjo K, Ito K, Matsumoto T, Matsunaga N, Hamm B 1997 High-resolution dynamic MR imaging of hepatocellular carcinoma with a phased-array body coil. Radiographics 17: 315–335

Gabata T, Matsui, O, Kadoya M et al 1990 MR imaging of hepatic adenoma. American Journal of Roentgenology 155: 1009–1011

Giovagnoni A, Paci E 1996 Liver. III: Gadolinium-based hepatobiliary contrast agents. (Gd-EOB-DTPA and Gd-BOPTA/Dimeg). Magnetic Resonance Imaging Clinics of North America 4: 61–72

Gonzalez J J, Sanz L, Grana J L, Bermejo G, Navarrete F, Martinez E 1997 Biliary lithiasis in the elderly patient: morbidity and mortality due to biliary surgery. Hepatogastroenterology 44: 1565–8

Gracy G R, Peters R L, Edmunson H A 1988 2nd series Atlas of tumor pathology

Grandin C B, Van Beers B E, Pauwels S, Demeure R, Jamart J, Pringot J 1997 Ferumoxides and Tc-99m sulfur colloid: comparison of the tumor-to-liver uptake in focal nodular hyperplasia. Journal of Magnetic Resonance Imaging 7: 125–9

Harisinghani M G, Saini S, Weissleder R, Halpern E F, Schima W, Rubin D L, Stillman A E, Sica G T, Small W C, Hahn P F 1997 Differentiation of liver hemangiomas from metastases and hepatocellular carcinoma at MR imaging enhanced with blood-pool contrast agent Code-7227. Radiology 202: 687–91

Ishak K G, Rabin L 1986 Benign tumors of the liver. Medical Clinics of North America 59: 995–1013

Itoh K, Nishimura K, Togashi K et al 1987 Hepatocellular carcinoma: MR imaging. Radiology 164: 21–25

Kelekis N L, Semelka R C, Worawattanakul S, de Lange E E, Ascher S M, Ahn I O, Reinhold C, Remer E M, Brown J J, Bis K G, Woosley J T, Mitchell D G 1998 Hepatocellular carcinoma in North America: a multiinstitutional study of appearance on T1-weighted, T2-weighted, and serial gadolinium-enhanced gradient-echo images. AJR. American Journal of Roentgenology 170: 1005–13

Kreft B P, Tanimoto A, Baba Y, Zhao L, Chen J, Middleton M S, Compton C C, Finn J P, Stark D D 1992 Diagnosis of fatty liver with MR imaging. Journal of Magnetic Resonance Imaging 2: 463–71

Krinsky G A, Theise N D, Rofsky N M, Mizrachi H, Tepperman L W, Weinreb J C 1998 Dysplastic nodules in cirrhotic liver: arterial phase enhancement at CT and MR imaging – a case report. Radiology 209: 461–4

Lalonde L, Van Beers B, Jamart J, Pringot, J 1992 Capsule and mosaic pattern of hepatocellular carcinoma: correlation between CT and MR imaging. Gastrointestinal Radiology 17: 241–4

Lauterbur P C 1973 Image formation by induced local interactions: examples employing nuclear magnetic resonance. Nature 242: 190–191

Lomanto D, Pavone P, Laghi A, Panebianco V, Mazzocchi P, Fiocca F, Lezoche E, Passariello R, Speranza V 1997 Magnetic resonance – cholangiopan-creatography in the diagnosis of biliopancreatic diseases. American Journal of Surgery 174: 33–8

Mahfouz A E, Hamm B, Wolf K J 1994 Peripheral washout: a sign of malignancy on dynamic gadolinium-enhanced MR images of focal liver lesions. Radiology 190: 49–52

Mathieu D, Vilgrain V, Mahfouz A E, Anglade M C, Vullierme M P, Denys A 1997 Benign liver tumors. Magnetic Resonance Imaging Clinics of North America 5: 255–88

Mendler M H, Bouillet P, Sautereau D, Chaumerliac P, Cessot F, Le Sidaner A, Pillegand B 1998 Value of MR cholanglography in the diagnosis of obstructive diseases of the biliary tree: a study of 58 cases. American Journal of Gastroenterology 93: 2482–90

Mitchell D G, Kim I, Chang T S, Vinitski S, Consigny P M, Saponaro S A, Ehrlich S M, Rifkin M D, Rubin R 1991 Fatty liver. Chemical shift phase-difference and suppression magnetic resonance imaging techniques in animals, phantoms, and humans. Investigative Radiology 26: 1041–52

Musella M, Barbalace G, Capparelli G, Carrano A, Castaldo P, Tamburrini O, Musella S 1998 Magnetic resonance imaging in evaluation of the common bile duct. British Journal of Surgery 85: 16–9

Outwater E K, Ito K, Siegelman E, Martin C E, Bhatia M, Mitchell D G 1997 Rapidly enhancing hepatic hemangiomas at MRI: distinction from malignancies with T2-weighted images. Journal of Magnetic Resonance Imaging 7: 1033–9

Prince M R, Arnoldus C, Frisoli J K 1996 Nephrotoxicity of high-dose gadolinium compared with iodinated contrast. Journal of Magnetic Resonance Imaging 6: 162–6

Purcell E M, Torrey H C, Pound R V 1946 Resonance absorption by nuclear magnetic moments in a solid. Physical Review 69: 37

Regan F, Smith D, Khazan R, Bohlman M, Schultze-Haakh H, Campion J, Magnuson T H 1996 MR cholangiography in biliary obstruction using half-Fourier acquisition. Journal of Computer Assisted Tomography 20: 627–32

Rescorla F J 1997 Cholelithiasis, cholecystitis, and common bile duct stones. Current Opinion in Pediatrics 9: 276–82

Rofsky N M, Fleishaker H 1995 CT and MRI of diffuse liver disease. Seminars in Ultrasound, CT and MR 16: 16–33

Rummeny E, Weissleder R, Sinomi S, Stark D D, Comptom C C, Hahn P F, Saini S, Wittenberg J, Ferrucci J T 1989 MR imaging of liver neoplasms. American Journal of Roentgenology 152: 493–499

Semelka R C, Sofka C M 1997 Hepatic hemangiomas. Magnetic Resonance Imaging Clinics of North America 5: 241–53

Siegelman E S 1997 MR imaging of diffuse liver disease. Hepatic fat ad iron. Magnetic Resonance Imaging Clinics of North America 5: 347–65

Todani T, Watanabe Y, Narusue M, Tabuchi K, Okajima K 1977 Congenital bile duct cysts: classification operative procedures, and review of thirty-seven cases including cancer arising from choledochal cyst. American Journal of Surgery 134: 263–9

Van Beers B, Roche A, Methieu D et al 1992 Epithelioid hemangloendothelioma of the liver. MR and CT findings. Journal of Computer Assisted Tomography 16: 420–424

Vilgrain V, Flejou J F, Arrive L, Belghiti J, Najmark D, Menu Y, Zins M, Vullierme M P, Nahum H 1992 Focal nodular hyperplasia of the liver: MR imaging and pathologic correlation in 37 patients. Radiology 184: 699–703

Wenker J C, Baker M K, Ellis J H et al 1984 Focal fatty infiltration of the liver: demonstration by magnetic resonance imaging. American Journal of Roentgenology 143: 573–574

Whitney W S, Herfkens R J, Jeffrey R B et al 1993 Dynamic breath-hold multiplanar spoiled gradient-recalled MR imaging with gadolinium enhancement for differentiating hepatic hemangiomas from malignancies at 1.5T. Radiology 189: 863–870

Wilbur A C, Gyi B 1987 Hepatocellular carinoma: MR appearance mimicking focal nodular hyperplasia. American Journal of Roentgenology 149: 721–722

Wunderbaldinger P, Turetschek K, Schima W, Harisinghani, M 1998 Primary malignant fibrous histiocytomas of the liver: CT and the findings. AJR. American Journal of Roentgenology 171: 900–1

Yoshida H, Itai Y, Ohtomo K et al 1989 Small hepatocellular carcinoma and the cavernous hemangioma: differentiation with dynamic FLASH MR imaging with Gd-DTPA. Radiology 171: 339–342

Yoshimitsu K, Honda H, Kaneko K, Kuroiwa T, Irie H, Ueki T, Chijiiwa K, Takenaka K, Masuda K 1997 Dynamic MRI of the gallbladder lesions: differentiation of benign from malignant. Journal of Magnetic Resonance Imaging 7: 696–701.

Direct cholangiography

17

R.C. KURTZ, R.N. GIBSON

INTRODUCTION

The most complete and detailed radiographic demonstration of the biliary system (cholangiography) is obtained when contrast medium is introduced directly into a bile duct (direct cholangiography). This can be performed preoperatively, intraoperatively, or via tubes placed in the biliary tract either surgically, radiologically or endoscopically. The non-operative techniques are percutaneous transhepatic cholangiography (PTC) and endoscopic retrograde cholangiopancreatography (ERCP).

PERCUTANEOUS TRANSHEPATIC CHOLANGIOGRAPHY

HISTORY

The first PTC is generally attributed to Huard and Do-Xun-Hop in 1937 (Wechsler & Wechsler 1975). Prior to this cholecysto-cholangiography had been performed by percutaneous puncture of the gallbladder in 1921 by Burckhardt and Muller. Later workers also used gallbladder puncture, either laparoscopically (Lee 1942, Keil & Landis 1951), or percutaneously. However, the risk of bile leakage and the limitations of the examination in the presence of cystic duct or common hepatic duct obstruction led to the abandonment of this technique in favour of percutaneous transhepatic puncture of intrahepatic bile ducts (Carter & Saypol 1952, Nurick et al 1953, Kidd 1956). Various techniques were developed using either an anterior, lateral or posterior puncture with a sheathed or unsheathed needle of up to 1.5 mm external diameter. However, the still significant risk of biliary peritonitis and hemorrhage meant that many patients underwent laparotomy immediately

following PTC (Seldinger 1966). The incidence of these complications has been substantially reduced by the popularization of the PTC technique developed at Chiba University (Ohto & Tsuchiya 1969, Okuda et al 1974) and at the same time the rate of duct opacification has significantly improved.

TECHNIQUE

The examination should be performed on a tilting fluoroscopic table as a sterile procedure, using local anesthesia and intravenous sedation. A clotting profile and platelet count should be near normal. Because of the high incidence of bacterial colonization of obstructed biliary systems (Keighley 1977) broad-spectrum antibiotics should be administered to provide adequate blood and tissue levels during the procedure; our current regimen is 4 g piperacillin and 0.5 g tazobactam intravenously just prior to the PTC. A 22 gauge (0.71 mm) flexible Chiba needle is inserted into the liver usually from the right side, just anterior to the mid-coronal plane and inferior to the visible lateral costophrenic recess. The needle is directed medially and slightly craniad (Fig.17.1A,B) avoiding puncture of the gallbladder and extrahepatic bile ducts. Successful entry of a duct is identified by aspiration of bile or on injection of contrast medium. Ultrasonographic guidance can also be used for duct puncture (Ohto et al 1980) and this is particularly useful if there is marked distortion of normal liver anatomy such as can occur following hepatic resection or in the presence of lobar atrophy. In an obstructed system as much bile as possible is aspirated and samples are sent for bacteriology and, when appropriate, cytology studies. Water-soluble contrast medium of 200–300 mg/ml iodine concentration is injected to fill as much of the intrahepatic and extrahepatic biliary system as possible without using undue pressure. Contrast medium has a higher specific gravity than bile and so, by tilting the fluo-

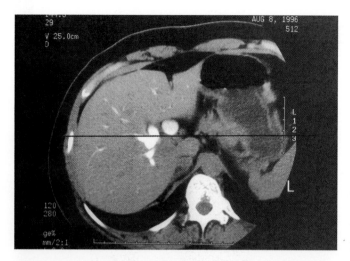

(A)

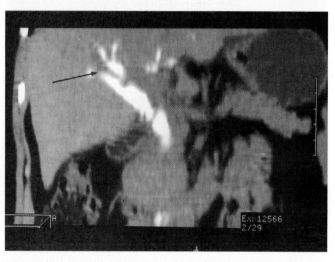

(B)

Fig. 17.1 Computed tomography scan following duct opacification with intravenous cholangiographic contrast medium. **(A)** Transverse scan and **(B)** coronal reconstruction through the optimal plane for needle entry, with the needle orientation shown (arrow).

roscopic table and rotating the patient, more of the biliary system can be opacified with a low pressure injection. Radiographs should be taken in multiple projections. In cases of near-complete duct obstruction delayed views may show more distal ducts and determine the length of the stricture or the presence of a second stricture. Delayed views can also be helpful for assessing the degree of obstruction produced by a partial stricture. After the procedure is completed, the patient should be observed closely for 24 hours as most complications will occur in this time period.

SUCCESS RATE AND ACCURACY OF PTC

The success rate of bile duct opacification depends on the presence of bile duct dilation and the number of needle passes made. With dilated ducts the opacification rate approaches 100% and at least a 95% success rate should be achieved even if the number of needle passes is limited to six (Jain et al 1977, Jaques et al 1980). If ducts are undilated the chance of success increases with the number of needle passes and in most series is between 60 and 80% (Fraser et al 1978, Jaques et al 1980, Harbin et al 1980). Surprisingly perhaps, no correlation has been shown to exist between the number of needle passes and the incidence of significant complications (Ariyama et al 1978, Harbin et al 1980), and the limiting factor to the number of passes made is usually patient discomfort. When duct opacification is achieved there may be duct obstruction without dilatation (Van Sonnenberg et al 1983). This occurs most often with choledocholithiasis and benign strictures. Secondary cholangitis tends to limit the distensibility of both intrahepatic and extrahepatic bile ducts (Benjamin 1982) and cirrhosis and liver metastases can have the same effect on intrahepatic ducts.

The level of duct obstruction will be accurately determined in all cases providing attention is paid to details of technique, in particular, the use of patient rotation and table tilt. The cause of obstruction is less accurately determined by PTC and although accuracy rates of over 90% are reported (Mueller et al 1982) there are patients in whom a specific diagnosis cannot be made on PTC grounds alone; indeed differentiation between benign and malignant stricturing is sometimes impossible. It is important to recognize this and take into account clinical features, other radiological findings and, preferably, histological or cytological evidence.

PITFALLS IN INTERPRETATION OF PTC

False localization of obstruction

Failure to inject adequate volumes of contrast or to position the patient appropriately can lead to false localization of the level of obstruction. This is a problem usually only with complete obstruction and may be recognized by the presence of a 'hazy' margin at the level of the apparent obstruction (Kittredge & Baer 1975) (Fig. 17.2).

Incomplete cholangiogram

Opacification of only the right-sided ducts is often mistaken for a complete cholangiogram leading to diagnosis of high common hepatic duct obstruction. This is recognizable by the absence of any left hepatic ducts, which should usually be visible overlying the spine. If the left ducts do not fill with further contrast injection in the left lateral decubitus position then a separate puncture and direct opacification of the left system should be performed, either from the right

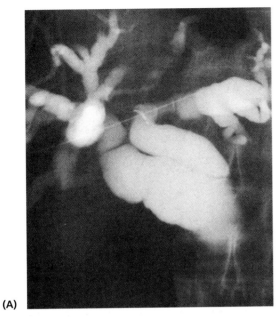

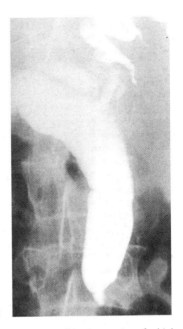

(A)

(B)

Fig. 17.2 Ampullary carcinoma. **(A)** With the patient supine, contrast pools proximally giving a false impression of a high bile duct obstruction The spurious nature of the level is suggested by the hazy inferior margin to the contast column. **(B)** With the patient semi-erect the contrast pools at the true point of obstruction, which is sharply defined.

side (Fig. 17.3) or via the epigastrium. Variations in duct anatomy can also cause some difficulty in interpretation and may result in incomplete cholangiogram if unrecognized. For example, the relatively common arrangement of a right

sectoral or segmental duct entering the left hepatic duct can be partially confusing in the presence of a hilar lesion.

Extraductal contrast injections

Contrast injected around a portal vein branch may mimic a dilated bile duct but should be recognizable by the central 'filling defect' which represents the portal vein. Opacification of hepatic lymphatics has no pathological significance in itself and the multiplicity of beaded channels should not be mistaken for narrow, irregular bile ducts. Extraductal contrast injections may obscure information and can compress bile ducts sufficiently to produce an artificial level of obstruction. Some contrast medium is frequently injected into a portal or hepatic vein branch and this is excreted by the kidney with resulting opacification of the renal pelvis or ureter. The latter should not be mistaken for a bile duct. Portal vein and hepatic vein branches are frequently visible on screening during the PTC but these are rarely visible on the radiographs. Extrahepatic injection of contrast is usually easily recognizable and tends to produce transient pain and sometimes local peritonitis.

COMPLICATIONS

Although the incidence of complications of PTC has fallen significantly since the introduction of the fine needle technique (Harbin et al 1980) major complications do

Fig. 17.3 Hilar cholangiocarcinoma involving first-order right and left hepatic ducts. Separate needle punctures were required to fill the right and left ducts.

Table 17.1 Complications reported with PTC

	No. of patients	Bile leakage	Sepsis	Hemorrhage	Miscellaneous	Deaths	Overall complication rate (%)
Ariyama (1983)	1149	2	0	0	0	0	0.2
Gibbons et al (1983)	123	6	3	0	1	0	9
Harbin et al (1980)	2005	29	28	7	5	4	3.6
Kreek & Balint (1980)	322	6	10	13	4	3	10.2
Kocher & Mousseau (1979)	94	0	2	–	–	0	2.1
Mueller et al (1980)	450	2	?	?	?	1	4.8
Michel & Adda (1980)	3472	62	24	7	17	4	6
Nagasue & Inokuchi (1979)	58	–	2	2	–	0	6.8
Ohto et al (1978)	1442	2	10	1	2	0	1.0
Total	9115	109 1.2%	151 1.7%	30 0.3%	59 0.7%	12 0.13%	4.1%

occasionally occur (Table 17.1). The commonest significant complications are bile leakage, sepsis and hemorrhage. The first two are almost unknown in the absence of ductal obstruction. Bile leakage is often asymptomatic but can result in peritonitis or subphrenic abscess (Harbin et al 1980). With routine antibiotic cover septic complications are usually minor in the form of transient fever but occasionally this is accompanied by hypotension and, rarely, endotoxic shock. Bacteremia and, more importantly, endotoxemia, occur via cholangiovenous reflux (Hultborn et al

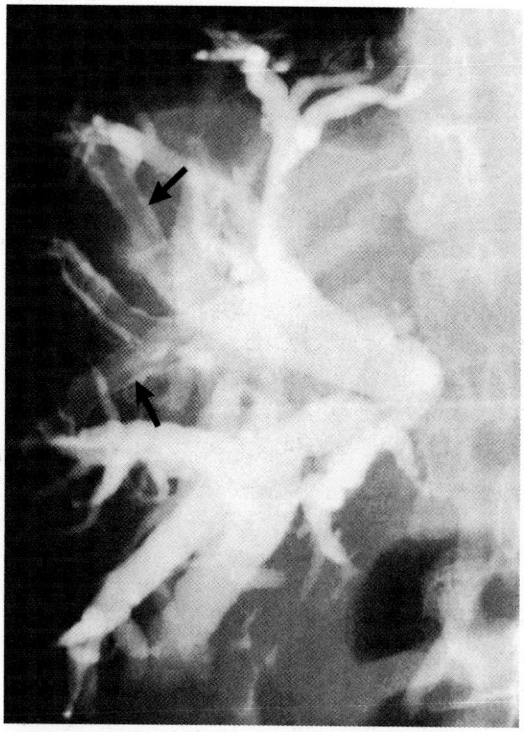

Fig. 17.4 Hemobilia indicated by cast-like filling defects (arrows) in several ducts.

1962) or biliary-venous fistulae created by the needle.

When major hemorrhage occurs it is usually either into the bile ducts (hemobilia) or intraperitoneal. Hemobilia may be recognized at the time of cholangiography by the presence of intraductal cast-like filling defects produced by blood clot (Fig. 17.4). Extensive clot should alert one to the possibility of continuing hemorrhage.

Arterioportal fistulae occurred in 3.8% of patients studied angiographically by Okuda (1978) following PTC. These most often are of no consequence but may be accompanied by significant bleeding which can be controlled by angiographic embolization (Sarr et al 1984), or may produce localized 'parenchymal' staining during hepatic arteriography which can mimic a small vascular tumor deposit. Small intrahepatic hematomas not uncommonly occur and produce discrete low attenuation areas on CT scanning (Tylen et al 1981) which should not be confused with tumor.

ENDOSCOPIC RETROGRADE CHOLANGIOPANCREATOGRAPHY

HISTORY

The procedure, endoscopic retrograde cholangiopancreatography (ERCP), was first reported in 1968 by McCune and colleagues and has remained an important diagnostic modality frequently used in the management of patients with hepatobiliary and pancreatic diseases (Oi et al 1970, Cotton et al 1972, Cotton 1977, Freeney 1988). Over the last 25 years, there has been continued progress in ERCP instrumentation. One major innovation was the development, in the late 1980s, of video or electronic endoscopy. Video endoscopy enables high-quality photographic and videotape documentation of important endoscopic findings, and has made the training of physicians in the technique of ERCP much easier. The endoscopic skills needed to perform ERCP are more difficult to learn than the standard procedures of upper endoscopy and colonoscopy, but there are now many endoscopists throughout the world who can easily, rapidly, and safely perform diagnostic ERCP. In fact, working with a cooperative patient and a well trained team, this procedure can often be completed in less than 15 min.

TECHNIQUE

Patient selection is important, as ERCP is commonly done in an outpatient setting. Patients should be alert and oriented and be able to give informed consent. In the rare situation when this is not possible, such as with an intubated patient on mechanical ventilation, consent is obtained from the next-of-kin. Patients with uncorrected shock, cardiac arrhythmias, profound neutropenia, or with a significant coagulopathy should not have an elective diagnostic test such as ERCP performed. Age is not a contraindication to ERCP as the procedure is safe even for selected patients in their 90s. While children less commonly have pancreatic and biliary disease, the standard technique is often all that is necessary, and instrumentation is the same except in children under 6 months old. General anesthesia is rarely needed for those over 11 or 12 years of age (Buckley & Connon 1990). ERCP has been shown to be a valuable adjunct in the evaluation of infantile cholestasis (Wilkinson et al 1991).

Patient comfort is maintained by the use of intravenous sedation under monitored control. We do not routinely use pharyngeal topical anesthetics. Drug combinations include narcotics, such as meperidine, droperidol, and the benzodiazepines midazalam or diazepam. Dosages are titrated for each patient with a total dose of meperidine generally ranging between 50 and 100 mg, droperidol between 2.5 and 5 mg, and midazalam between 2 and 10 mg. If excess duodenal motility is a problem, it is controlled by bolus injections of 0.2 mg–1 mg of intravenous glucagon. Oxygen is administered by nasal cannula to avoid the hypoxemia that has been described in up to 40% of patients undergoing ERCP (Woods et al 1989). The patient's EKG, blood pressure, oxygen saturation, and overall condition is continually monitored throughout the procedure by a dedicated nurse. Other personnel include the endoscopist, one or two endoscopy technicians, and an X-ray technician to help with fluoroscopy and film development. A radiologist is usually available to aid the endoscopist in the correct interpretation of unusual X-ray or fluoroscopic findings. Antibiotics are not routinely given for diagnostic procedures, but all ERCP equipment is chemically or gas sterilized.

A side-viewing duodenoscope is used to afford excellent visualization of the ampulla of Vater. In patients with a Billroth II type of gastrojejunostomy, a standard forward-viewing endoscope may be needed. An initial endoscopic evaluation of the stomach and duodenum is performed prior to cannulation of the ampulla. The pancreatic and biliary ducts are selectively cannulated and identified and a contrast agent such as diluted Renograffin-60 is injected into the desired duct under fluoroscopic control, with subsequent X-ray images of the duct anatomy. Material for pathological and cytological evaluation can be obtained from either the biliary or pancreatic duct system with a variety of dedicated endoscopic biopsy forceps and cytology brushes. Pathological and cytological material may also be obtained from the ampulla of Vater, duodenum, and stomach.

A skilled endoscopist can be expected to identify the ampulla of Vater in almost all patients with normal anatomy. If the ampulla is inside a duodenal diverticulum, or if the second portion of the duodenum is stenotic, compressed, or invaded by a pancreatic mass, identification of the ampulla may be very difficult. Once the ampulla is found, success rates for cannulating the common bile duct and pancreatic duct are well over 90% (Rosch 1985). When difficulty occurs in cannulation of the common bile duct, invasive maneuvers such as precut papillotomy can improve the success rate, but with an associated increase in the complication rate (Shakoor & Geenen 1992). In the patient with a Billroth II gastrojejunostomy, success rates for bile duct cannulation are much lower (Katon et al 1975, Osnes and Myren 1975).

Endoscopy and pancreatography during ERCP

The ability to perform endoscopy and pancreatography in addition to cholangiography, during ERCP affords a major advantage to this procedure. It is common for endoscopic examination of the stomach and duodenum to provide important diagnostic information helpful in management planning. Displacement of the antrum or pylorus or a stricture or narrowing of the second portion of the duodenum may indicate the presence of a pancreatic mass responsible for obstructive jaundice. The diagnosis can be confirmed by biopsies and cytologic specimens taken during the procedure from the infiltrated or ulcerated duodenal wall.

Duodenal diverticula are almost always located near the papilla in the descending duodenum. Large juxtapapillary diverticula are of clinical significance because they are often associated with choledocholithiasis. On inspection of the ampulla, anatomical variants should be looked for before attempting cannulation (Phillip et al 1974). On occasion, two orifices are found and this indicates separate biliary and pancreatic duct systems. The minor ampulla is located about 1–

2 cm above the major papilla. Impacted gallstones give rise to a characteristic distention or bulge of the papilla. Previous spontaneous passage of bile duct stones can be recognized by a fissured splitting of the papillary orifice. Previous surgical dilatation of the papilla or spontaneous gallstone perforation above the papilla also produce a characteristic appearance. Occasionally, a fistulous perforation in the roof of the papilla is found as a result of a false passage produced at surgical dilatation (Tanaka & Ikeda 1983). Biliary-enteric anastomoses appear as circular or slit-like openings.

The endoscopic diagnosis of ampullary carcinoma is not difficult, especially if the tumor is exophytic. However, the diagnosis becomes more difficult when the tumor is predominantly intramural. In such instances, the diagnosis is frequently confirmed by biopsy and cytology after endoscopic papillotomy allows the tumor to be exposed (Bourgeois et al 1984). In a series from the Medical College of Wisconsin, the correct diagnosis was made by endoscopic biopsy in 42 of 44 patients with ampullary neoplasia and in 16 of 18 patients with invasive ampullary cancer (Komoroski et al 1991).

Imaging the pancreatic duct can be an important adjunct to cholangiography during ERCP. Strictures, stones, and other obstructing lesions can be identified. With increasing age, there is progressive atrophy and fibrosis of the pancreas. The diameter of the main pancreatic duct increases with age as well. One study found no difference in pancreatic duct length between patients younger than 40 years when compared to those over 40. Duct diameter, throughout the pancreas however, was significantly greater in those older than 40 years (Anand et al 1989).

Anatomic variations such as pancreas divisum (Fig. 17.5) may also be identified on pancreatogram. This abnormality has been described in up to 7.5% of ERCPs and can be confirmed by cannulation of the main pancreatic duct through the orifice in the minor papilla (Bernard et al 1990).

COMPLICATIONS OF ERCP

The experience of the endoscopist is one of the most significant factors related to the development of ERCP complications (Bilbao et al 1976). Statistics on complication rates vary accordingly. Acute pancreatitis following ERCP occurs in < 7% of patients (Rosch 1981) and should be distinguished from transient asymptomatic hyperamylasemia which occurs in 40 to 75% of cases (Classen & Demling 1975). Asymptomatic hyperamylasemia disappears within 1–2 days, as does hypertrypsinemia (Phillip & Hagenmuller 1983) and elevations of serum lipase and elastase 1 levels (Okuno et al 1985). X-ray documentation of renal excretion of the contrast agent injected into the pancreatic duct

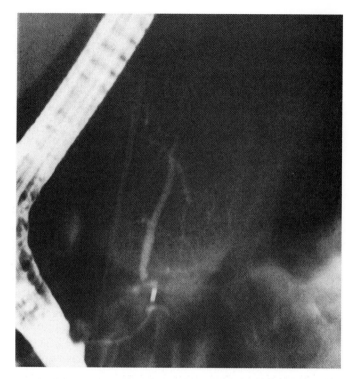

Fig. 17.5 Pancreas divisum. The cannula is in the major papillary orifice and contrast injection opacifies the proximal portion of the major pancreatic duct (Wirsung). Injection through the minor papillae will allow opacification of the duct of Santorini and the distal duct of Wirsung.

does not predict the development of acute pancreatitis (Hopper et al 1989). Necrotizing pancreatitis, a very serious complication, is observed in about 0.1% of pancreatograms. The recent use of nonionic contrast medium of low osmolarity has shown no advantage in preventing ERCP-related pancreatitis over the less expensive ionic contrast medium (Hannigan et al 1985). The risk of pancreatitis is reduced by careful and gentle injection of the contrast medium into the pancreatic duct, the avoidance of over distention or 'acinarization' of the pancreatic duct, and keeping repeated injection of the pancreatic duct to a minimum when encountering difficulty in filling the common bile duct. Prophylactic administration of somatostatin or its analog octreotide has not been shown to prevent pancreatitis during diagnostic or therapeutic ERCP (Borsch et al 1984, Sternlieb et al 1992). In addition, once pancreatitis has developed, the use of somatostatin does not improve its clinical course (Phillip et al 1985).

The most serious complication of ERCP is the development of post-procedure cholangitis. This occurs most commonly when there is a significant and high-grade bile duct obstruction. The most frequent bacterial pathogens are *Enterobacteria* spp. and *Pseudomonas aeruginosa* (Helm et al 1984). When an obstructed bile duct is identified on endoscopic cholangiogram, it is important to rapidly treat the obstruction by either nonsurgical or surgical means (Classen & Phillip 1982). While there are no studies that confirm the benefit of prophylactic antibiotics, it is reasonable to administer intravenous antibiotics which are preferentially excreted from the liver into the bile until adequate biliary drainage is achieved. One study looked at the prophylactic use of antibiotics in routine ERCPs (Sauter et al 1990). The authors found no difference in cholangitis rates when antibiotics were used, although the frequency of procedure-related bacteremia was significantly reduced. Antibiotics added to the injected radiographic contrast medium are of no benefit (Jandrzejewski et al 1980). Endoscopic instruments used in ERCP can be the source of serious infections (Earnshaw et al 1985). *Salmonella* spp. are the most common organisms transmitted by contaminated endoscopes (Axon 1991). For this reason, it is imperative to ensure that the endoscopic equipment used for ERCP is adequately disinfected or sterilized.

DIRECT CHOLANGIOGRAPHY AND PANCREATOGRAPHY BY PTC OR ERCP

BILIARY ANATOMY

The anatomy of the bile ducts is covered in Chapter 1. A knowledge of the common variations of ductal branching is essential for accurate interpretations of cholangiograms and these are shown in (Figs 17.6, 17.7). Segmental nomenclature is summarized in Table 17.2. In the right lobe the posterior segments lie more laterally than the anterior segments so that the most lateral ducts on a cholangiogram are usually

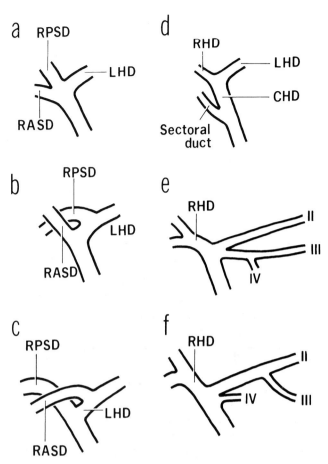

Fig. 17.7 Variations of perihilar ductal anatomy.

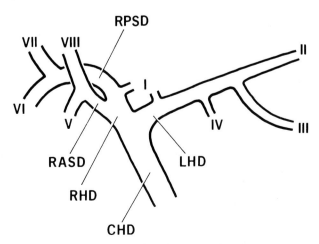

Fig. 17.6 Standard intrahepatic ductal anatomy. The segments are numbered according to Couinaud's description (see Table 17.2). RASD, right anterior sectoral duct; RPSD, right posterior sectoral duct; RHD, right hepatic duct; LHD, left hepatic duct; CHD, common hepatic duct.

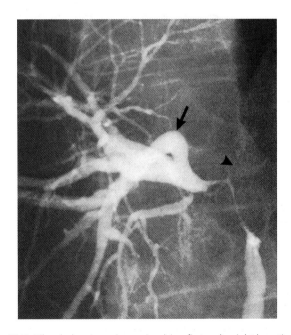

Fig. 17.8 Hilar cholangiocarcinoma involving first-order right hepatic duct, proximal common hepatic duct and faintly opacified left hepatic duct (arrowhead). Note the characteristic arched course of the right posterior sectoral duct (arrow).

segments VI inferiorly and VII superiorly. The posterior sectoral duct is often recognizable by an arched course close to the confluence (Figs 17.8, 17.9B). A right sectoral duct crosses to the left to join the left hepatic duct in 28% of cases according to Healey and Schroy (1953); in 22% this is the posterior sectoral duct (Figs 17.7b, 17.9B) and in 6% the anterior (Figs 17.7c, 17.9D). Occasionally a right sectoral or segmental duct, posterior more often than anterior, courses inferiorly and enters the common hepatic duct directly (Fig. 17.10) (Hand 1973). The confluence of the right and left ducts takes the form of a 'trifurcation' rather than a 'bifurcation' in 12% of cases according to Couinaud (1957) (Fig. 17.7a).

In the left lobe the superior and inferior lateral segment

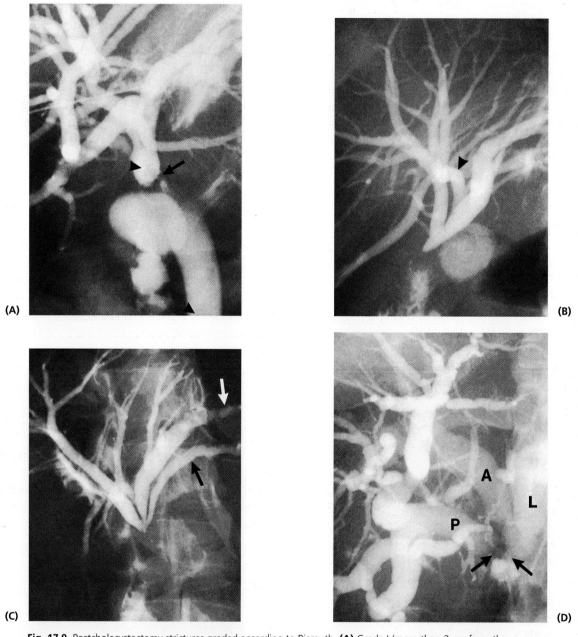

Fig. 17.9 Postcholecystectomy strictures graded according to Bismuth. **(A)** Grade I (more than 2 cm from the confluence of the right and left hepatic ducts)—calculi (arrowhead) lie above and below the stricture (arrow).
(B) Grade II (less than 2 cm from the confluence)—there has been a previous hepatojejunostomy; the right posterior sectoral duct (arrowhead) has an exaggerated arched course and enters the left hepatic duct as a normal variant.
(C) Grade III (the confluence is involved by stricture, but the right and left hepatic ducts are not completely separated)—ducts of segment II (white arrow) and segment II (black arrow) join the confluence independently as a normal variant.
(D) Grade IV (the right and left ducts are separated by the stricture)—the right anterior sectoral duct (A) is draining into the left hepatic duct (L) which is separated from the right posterior sectoral duct (P) by the stricture (arrows).

Table 17.2 Segmental nomenclature, after Couinard (1957) and Healey & Schroy (1953)

I	Caudate lobe
II	Left lateral superior segment
III	Left lateral inferior segment
IV	Left medial segment or quadrate lobe
V	Right anterior inferior segment
VI	Right posterior inferior segment
VII	Right posterior superior segment
VIII	Right anterior superior segment

ducts (segments II and III respectively) unite in the line of, or to the right of, the umbilical fissure in 92% of cases. In the latter instance the quadrate lobe (segment IV) may drain wholly or partially into the segment II duct. Rarely, segment II and III ducts join at or close to the confluence (Figs 17.7e, 17.9C) and segment IV drains directly into the common hepatic duct in 1% of cases (Fig. 17.7f) (Healey & Schroy 1953).

The caudate ducts are often difficult to identify. There are usually two or three ducts which drain most commonly into the right posterior sectoral duct, right hepatic duct or left hepatic duct (Healey & Schroy 1953). The recognizable caudate ducts are usually a few centimeters long and drain downwards or to the right.

The left hepatic duct (average length 17 mm) is considerably longer than the right (average length 9 mm) and has a longer extrahepatic course. The normal diameters of the

main bile ducts as measured at PTC are shown in Table 17.3. These figures are greater than the true duct dimensions because of some distention produced by direct cholangiography together with considerable magnification occurring on any fluoroscopic 'spot film.' The latter is of the order of 40% (Nichols & Burhenne 1984) and affects all structures in the image including calculi, tubes and strictures.

Table 17.3 Average duct diameters measured directly from 50 normal PTC examinations (Ohto et al 1978)

Duct	Diameter (mm)
Right hepatic	4.7
Left hepatic	5.2
Common hepatic	6.5
Common bile	7.6

The upper limits of normal for the diameter of the extra-hepatic bile ducts as measured by ERCP vary between 9 and 14 mm (Niederau et al 1984). Combined radiological and manometric studies (Poralla et al 1985) have shown that even in the absence of extrahepatic cholestasis the diameter of and the pressure difference in the bile ducts increases with advancing age. It should be noted that the diameter of the bile ducts as measured by ultrasonography is somewhat less than the measurements obtained during ERCP (Meier et al 1984, Niederau et al 1984). Anatomical abnormalities of the hepatobiliary system include cystic dilatations (Fig. 17.11) of the bile duct or of the intra-hepatic bile ducts (Caroli's disease). There is a wide variation in where the cystic duct joins the common hepatic duct. A low junction, with a correspondingly long cystic duct (Fig. 17.12), if not recognized, may result in difficulties. This is especially true when a cholecystojejunostomy is performed as a palliative biliary bypass for carcinoma of the head of the pancreas and either the jaundice is not relieved or recurs rapidly in the postoperative period.

INDICATIONS FOR DIRECT CHOLANGIOGRAPHY

Evaluation of the jaundiced patient is perhaps the most common and important indication for direct cholangiography. Noninvasive imaging procedures such as ultrasonography, CT scans or MRI should always be obtained first in the diagnostic work-up. When obstruction of the biliary system is demonstrated, PTC or ERC may then be performed to accurately identify the level of the obstruction and the probable cause. Frequently, the diagnostic cholan-

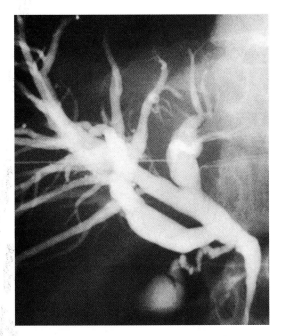

Fig. 17.10 Pancreatitis producing a typical incomplete long stricture of the common bile duct. The right posterior sectoral duct has a low entrance into the common hepatic duct, an uncommon but important normal variant.

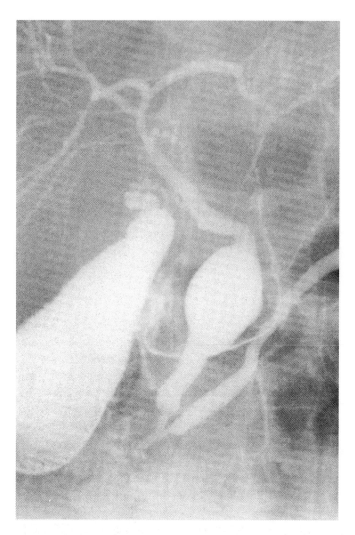

Fig. 17.11 Choledochal cyst.

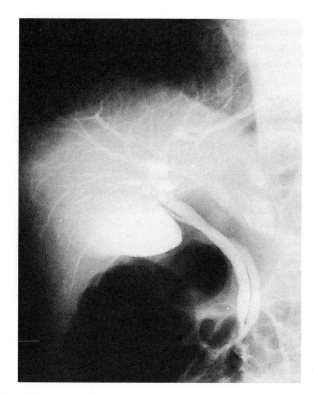

Fig. 17.12 Long cystic duct.

giogram will lead directly to a therapeutic procedure; endoscopic sphincterotomy, removal of bile duct gallstones, or placement of a biliary stent into the obstructed duct (Chs 28, 29).

Gallstone disease

Gallstone disease is the most frequent disorder affecting the biliary system. About 12% of the population in Western Europe and the United States have stones in the gallbladder. The incidence of gallstone disease is even higher, greater than 50%, in patients with portal hypertension and cirrhosis (Steinberg et al 1988). The majority of bile duct stones come from the gallbladder. It is estimated that 10 to 15% of patients undergoing cholecystectomy will have bile duct stones (Coelho et al 1984).

Direct cholangiography is the most accurate widely available imaging technique for the detection of ductal calculi. PTC will more reliably show intrahepatic calculi because of

generally better ductal filling while ERC is more appropriate for demonstrating common bile duct calculi. Either technique may fail to demonstrate small calculi if the concentration of the contrast medium is too high especially if there is significant ductal dilatation. Calculi can usually be differentiated from other causes of intraductal filling defects by using the features listed in Table 17.4. Occasionally an intraductal tumor will mimic an impacted calculus, e.g. at the lower end of the common bile duct. Common bile duct calculi may also be found in association with distal bile duct tumors.

In the United States, laparoscopic cholecystectomy is commonly performed in patients with gallbladder disease. ERC is often done preoperatively if the patient's history or liver chemistry profile is suggestive of common bile duct gallstones. In a large series of 1518 laparoscopic cholecystectomies performed in the southern United States (Meyers 1991), the incidence of undetected common bile duct gallstones was low at 2%. The authors attribute this to preoperative ERC in selected patients. Ductal calculi and benign strictures, including biliary-enteric anastomotic strictures, are frequently associated and if one is detected then the other should be carefully sought (Fig. 17.13). Intrahepatic duct stones (hepatolithiasis) are more commonly seen in the Far East. Most of these stones consist of calcium bilirubi-

Table 17.4 Intraductal filling defects and their differentiation

	Shape	Mobility	Constancy
Calculi	Rounded or *angulated**	If not impacted *fall** with repositioning	Usually on all films
Bubbles	*Round** unless filling duct	*Rise** on repositioning	Tend not to be on all films
Clot	Forms *casts** of ducts	Limited mobility	Usually absent or less prominent on early films
Intraductal tumour	Round, *irregular** or lobulated	*Immobile**	Should be on all films

* Main differentiating feature.

nate instead of the more common cholesterol gallstones seen in the West (Ohto et al 1984). In these patients, there is also an association between intrahepatic calculi and cholangiocarcinoma (Chen et al 1984) which may manifest itself on PTC as non-filling of a duct, stricture or an intraductal nodular filling defect.

Once the bile duct has been cannulated, it is possible to instil sufficient contrast medium to fill the entire biliary system, including the smallest intrahepatic branches. This ensures that all stones will be visualized (Fig. 17.14). The identification of bile duct stones is based on their characteristic shape and the lack of change of the image on several different radiographic views. The injection of air bubbles into the biliary system should be avoided since the bubbles may be mistaken for gallstones. Bubbles can usually be distinguished from stones by changing the position of the patient. When the patient is upright, the bubbles rise upwards in the bile duct, whereas stones generally sink. Smaller stones may only be identified in the initial stages of

the cholangiogram, when the contrast medium is first injected and the bile duct is only faintly filled. The small stones are often flushed upwards into the proximal biliary ducts with the contrast medium and they may no longer be visualized once the entire duct system is completely filled.

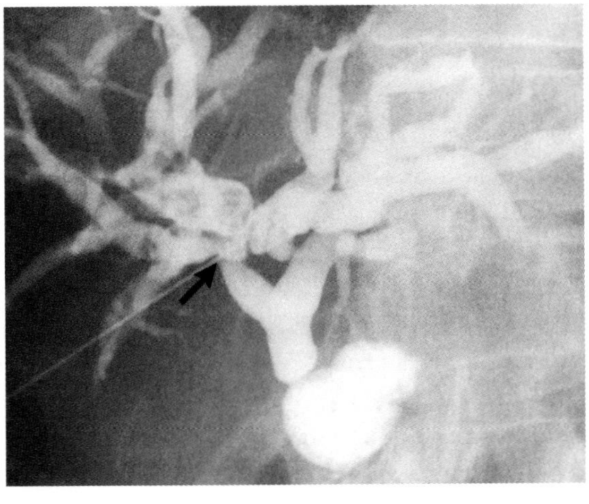

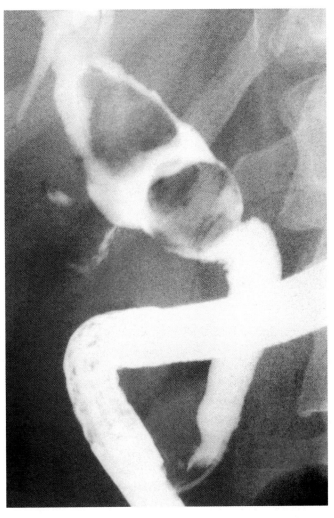

Fig. 17.13 Benign stricture of the right hepatic duct (arrow) with multiple ductal calculi proximal to it. The hepatojejunostomy is partially strictured.

Fig. 17.14 Choledocholithiasis.

For this reason, it is important to wait and observe the contrast emptying from the biliary system to aid in the detection of these small stones. In some patients, small stones will only be detected using a dilute solution of the contrast medium. Finding bile duct stones at the beginning of the ERC should not mislead the endoscopist into prematurely discontinuing the procedure. It is easy to overlook important additional findings, such as pancreatic or gallbladder cancers (Fig. 17.15) or biliary strictures. Recent studies have compared direct cholangiography with endoscopic ultrasound and MRCP to diagnose choledocholithiasis (Zidi et al 1999; de Ledinghen et al, 1999). MRCP seems to have a difficult time finding smaller bile duct gallstones (< 6 mm), but otherwise can be an effective non-invasive way to image the biliary system. EUS would also appear to be an important tool to aide in identification of those patients who require ERC before laparoscopic cholecystectomy.

It should be emphasized that neither PTC nor ERC are optimal modalities for assessment of the gallbladder, as neither technique consistently produces complete gallbladder opacification. The identification of gallbladder stones remains primarily in the domain of ultrasonography. Nevertheless, visualization of the gallbladder should not be omitted during the direct cholangiography. Identification of stones in the gallbladder requires the correct amount of gallbladder filling with contrast. Too little or too much contrast medium in the gallbladder may give rise to the incorrect diagnosis. Even if the gallbladder looks normal initially, an X-ray should always be taken while the gallbladder is emptying.

Mirizzi syndrome

Stones impacted in the infundibulum of the gallbladder (Fig. 17.16A,B), cystic duct, or cystic duct remnant may lead to compression and stricture of the common hepatic duct especially if the gallbladder infundibulum is inflamed. The duct becomes involved in the inflammatory and subsequent fibrotic processes. The result is biliary obstruction and jaundice This is the so-called Mirizzi syndrome (Fig. 17.16) (Koehler et al 1979). The affected segment of duct is usually 2–3 cm in length and is usually proximal although it may be distal if the cystic duct has a low insertion. On cholangiography there is partial or complete obstruction of the duct which may be visible adjacent to the stricture or, if a stone has eroded into the common hepatic duct, it may be seen as a filling defect (Fig. 17.17) or the resulting fistula may be opacified (Cruz et al 1983).

Awareness of this syndrome is very important as it must be distinguished from cholangiocarcinoma, gallbladder cancer, or metastatic tumors involving the porta hepatis.

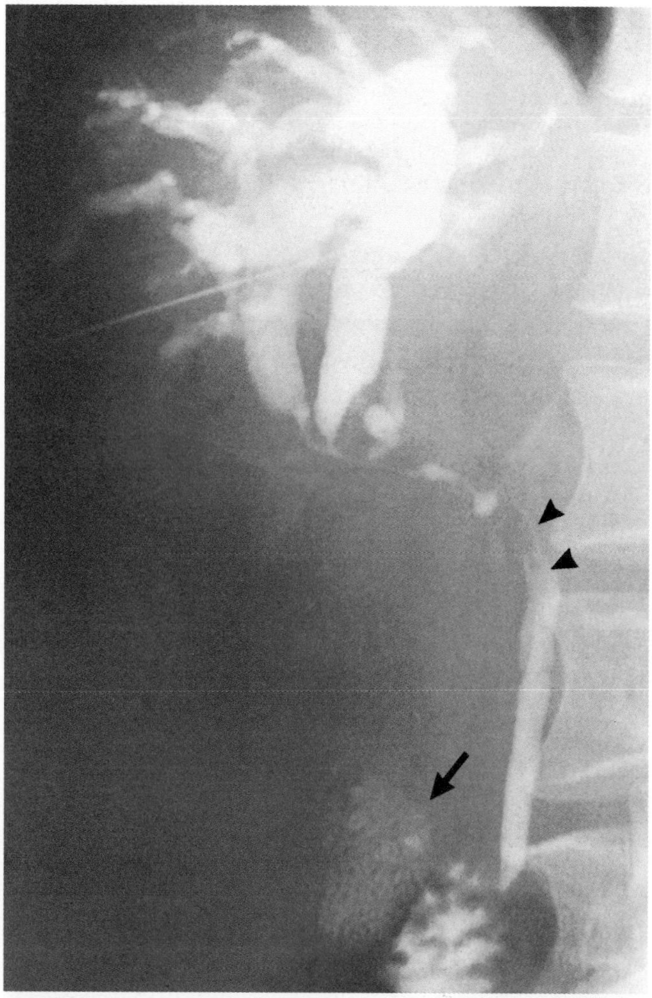

Fig. 17.15 Gallbladder carcinoma involving right third-order ducts and deviating upper common hepatic duct medially (arrowheads). There are multiple small calculi in the gallbladder fundus (arrow), which is separated from the strictured ducts by the tumor.

Post-cholecystectomy strictures (Ch. 49)

Iatrogenic injury to the extrahepatic bile ducts following cholecystectomy has been reported in < 1% of a selected group of patients (Femppel et al 1981). A large laparoscopic cholecystectomy series reported a similar incidence of bile duct injury (Meyers 1991). The location of the bile duct injury is somewhat dependent on the type of operation performed. Low bile duct strictures (Bismuth's type 1) almost always follow common bile duct exploration. High bile duct strictures (Bismuth type 2–4), are generally created during cholecystectomy (Moosa et al 1990), with the most common site at the hepatic duct junction with the cystic duct (Figs 17.18, 17.19). In most cases, the spindle-like nature

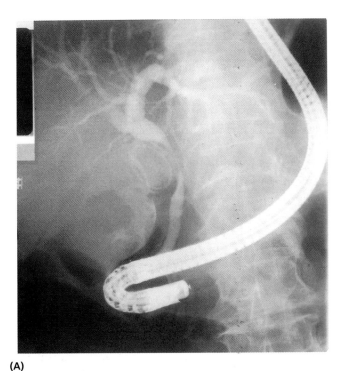

(A)

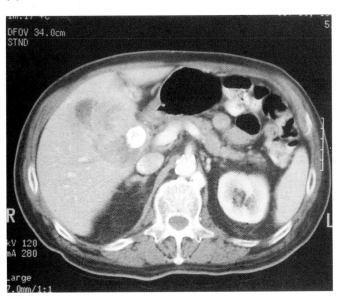

(B)

Fig. 17.16 Mirizzi syndrome. **(A)** ERCP demonstrates common hepatic duct stricture due to gallstone in the Hartman's pouch of the gallbladder. **(B)** CT scan shows the impacted stone. There is an associated gallbladder cancer.

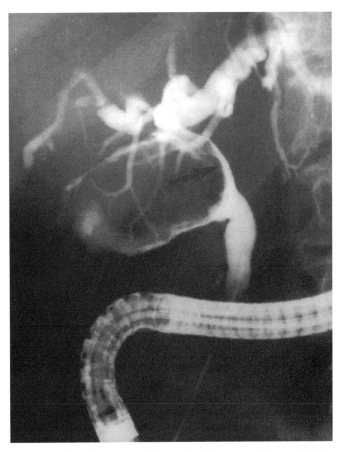

Fig. 17.17 Mirizzi syndrome. A large gallbladder calculus has eroded into the common hepatic duct (arrow) which is narrowed and deviated medially.

of the stricture points to the diagnosis. Associated segmental or lobar atrophy may result from either prolonged ductal obstruction or accompanying vascular injury (Blumgart et al 1984). Irregularity of duct caliber suggests secondary cholangitis. Single or multiple intrahepatic calculi may be seen, sometimes in association with additional strictures (Fig. 17.13). If there is a biliary fistula associated with bile duct injury then PTC or ERC may fail to delineate the damaged duct, particularly if it is a lobar or segmental duct. In this clinical setting the first approach should be to inject contrast directly into the fistulous tract and then proceed to PTC or ERC if necessary. In order to avoid bile duct injury during laparoscopic cholecystectomy, surgeons must not hesitate in converting to open cholecystectomy when laparoscopy does not permit good anatomical orientation (Hunter 1991).

Post-cholecystectomy syndrome (see also Ch. 43)

About 20% of cholecystectomy patients continue to have symptoms similar to those that led to their cholecystectomy. This symptom complex has been called the post-cholecystectomy syndrome. It may be caused by a number of different factors, including iatrogenic bile duct injury and subsequent stricture. These continued symptoms may also be caused by unrecognized esophagitis, peptic ulcer disease, irritable bowel syndrome, biliary dyskinesia, or papillary

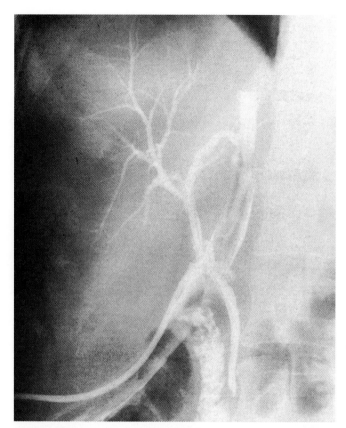

Fig. 17.18 T-tube following cholecystectomy. Late stricture subsequently developed (Fig. 17.19).

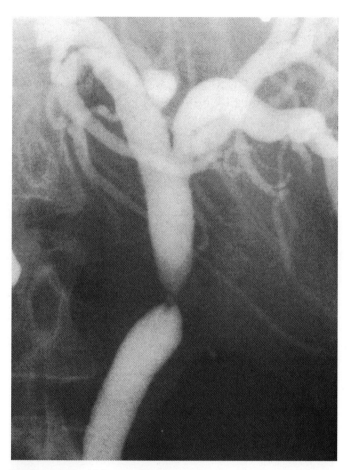

Fig. 17.19 Cicatricial stenosis of the common bile duct following cholecystectomy and biliary drainage via T-tube.

stenosis. If the pain lasts more than 6 months, there is clear evidence on noninvasive studies of partial bile duct obstruction, or there are abnormal liver function tests, ERCP should be performed (Ch. 6).

It has been suggested in the past that reproduction of the patient's pain on injection of contrast into the common bile duct during ERCP is correlated with sphincter-of-Oddi (SO) dysfunction. However, investigators at the University of Wisconsin found that only 6.7% of their patients with abnormal SO manometry had reproduction of their pain on common bile duct injection (Schmalz et al 1990). If there is delayed emptying of contrast from the common bile duct during ERCP, abnormal liver chemistries and abnormal SO manometry, endoscopic sphincterotomy may be beneficial (Geenen et al 1989) (Ch. 6). Postcholecystectomy syndrome symptoms may also result from a long cystic duct remnant left after cholecystectomy (Fig. 17.20). Stones will often form in the remnant and the remnant may fail to fill with contrast because of its occlusion by a stone. There is controversy about the pathological significance of this syndrome (Aaerimaa & Maekelae 1981, Grozinger 1984). Nevertheless, Daniels and colleagues (1980) report an incidence of about 5% in more than 4000 cholecystectomies,

with the belief that there was a causal connection with the symptoms in about one-third of the patients.

Pancreatic cancer (Ch. 55)

Approximately two-thirds of pancreatic cancers occur in the region of the ampulla of Vater and the head of the pancreas and accordingly, the bile duct is usually involved. ERCP is a sensitive and specific diagnostic test for pancreatic cancer. At Memorial Sloan-Kettering Cancer Center, ERCP had a sensitivity of 92% and a specificity of 97% in the evaluation of 116 patients. In 530 patients with pancreatic cancer, normal pancreatograms were seen in only 15 (2.5%) (Freeney 1988). Typical findings include complete occlusion or stenosis of the main pancreatic duct, narrowing or 'cut-off' of the intrapancreatic portion of the common bile duct, and the so-called 'double-duct' sign (Fig. 17.21), when there is stenosis or obstruction of both the main pancreatic duct and the common bile duct. Bile duct abnormalities are seen in about two-thirds of patients with carcinomas involving the

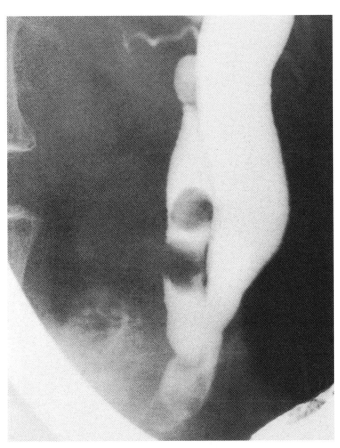

Fig. 17.20 'Cystic duct remnant syndrome'; stones in the cystic duct stump following cholecystectomy.

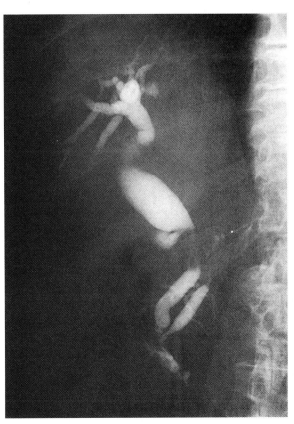

Fig. 17.21 Double duct sign (stenosis of the bile duct and pancreatic duct) in a case of pancreatic carcinoma.

head of the pancreas (Plumley et al 1982, Stolte 1984). In a small number of patients, differentiation from common bile duct narrowing due to pancreatitis may be difficult. Pancreatitis typically produces a longer, smooth, incomplete stricturing compared with carcinoma of either the pancreas or the lower common bile duct (Ariyama 1983) (Fig. 17.10). The course of the common bile duct above the obstruction is commonly rather horizontal (Fig. 17.22A) and this appears quite specific for pancreatic carcinoma (Freeny & Lawson 1982). Primary bile duct cancer of the intrapancreatic portion of the common bile duct may be indistinguishable from carcinoma of the head of the pancreas (Fig. 17.23). The pancreatic duct in these patients should be normal on ERCP. Endoscopic abnormalities such as a duodenal mass or ulcer, may be present and biopsy will document pancreatic cancer.

ERCP is an important tool when the patient's symptoms suggest pancreatic cancer, and the sonogram or CT scan are equivocal. Frick and colleagues (1982) described their experience in evaluating 26 patients with abdominal symptoms and indeterminate CT scans and found that ERCP aided the preoperative diagnosis in 25. In 140 patients (Ruddell et al 1983) with undiagnosed severe chronic abdominal pain, ERCP was abnormal in 18%. In approximately one-quarter of the patients, a diagnosis was made which included gallstones, peptic ulcer disease, pancreatic cancer, and chronic pancreatitis. ERCP may be difficult to interpret in the setting of chronic pancreatitis, and pancreatic cancers can be missed. Conversely, the finding on pancreatogram of a pancreas divisum may be misinterpreted as pancreatic cancer, especially if the CT scan shows enlargement of the pancreatic head as sometimes occurs in this congenital anomaly (Soulen et al 1989). While a recent study (Nix et al 1991) suggests that ERCP can help in determining tumor size and disease prognosis in carcinoma of the head of the pancreas, most clinicians do not use the technique in that way. Magnetic resonance cholangiopancreatography (MRCP) represents a new way to image the bile ducts and pancreatic duct. In a study comparing ERCP to MRCP in patients with pancreatic cancer done at MSKCC (Georgopoulos, 1999), MRCP was found to be a sensitive test for detecting the level of biliary ductal obstruction in patients with pancreatic cancer and the pancreatic mass. The results were comparable to ERCP. However, MRCP provided additional data regarding extent of disease that was not available from ERCP alone.

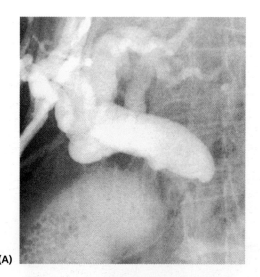

(A)

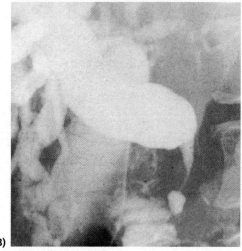

(B)

Fig. 17.22 Two of the common appearances of carcinoma of the pancreas. **(A)** Rounded obstruction with characteristic horizontal common bile duct. Note the coincidental stones in the distended gallbladder. **(B)** Tapered obstruction with slight shouldering. Compare this with pancreatitis (Fig. 17.10) where shouldering tends to be absent.

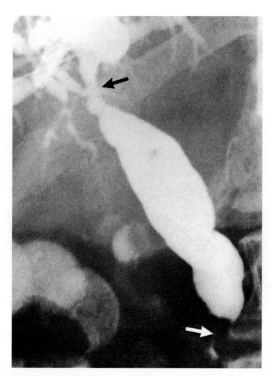

Fig. 17.23 Cholangiocarcinoma producing localized stricture of distal common bile duct (white arrow) indistinguishable from pancreatic cancer. Stricturing of the upper common hepatic duct (black arrow) is due to porta hepatis lymphadenopathy.

Mucin-producing pancreatic tumors have recently been described in Japan (Yamada et al 1991). These tumors typically occur within the pancreatic duct and produce large amounts of mucus which may be seen flowing from the papillary orifice on endoscopy. About half of these tumors will be benign, but even those which are malignant seem to have a better prognosis than the more common pancreatic adenocarcinoma.

Cholangiocarcinoma (Ch. 54)

Direct cholangiography is an important investigation for both diagnosis and preoperative evaluation of cholangiocarcinoma. In general PTC affords a better image of *hilar*

cholangiocarcinomas than does ERC. The extrahepatic ducts are involved more often proximally than distally with 53 to 68% of tumors occurring at or above the junction of the common hepatic duct and cystic duct (Warren et al 1972, Longmire et al 1973, Ohto et al 1978, Tompkins et al 1981). In a large series of 186 patients with bile duct cancers (Tompkins et al 1990), the majority (58%) occurred in the upper third of the bile duct system (at the level of the cystic duct junction or higher). The remainder diffusely involved the biliary duct system (7%) or involved the common bile duct either above the pancreas (17%) or the intrapancreatic portion of the bile duct (18%). By utilizing noninvasive imaging techniques, percutaneous cholangiography and ERC in the more recent years of this study, the investigators noted more than a 50% reduction in the time needed from the onset of symptoms to correct diagnosis and treatment.

Cholangiocarcinoma usually produces concentric stricturing (Figs 17.3, 17.8) which sometimes appears 'shouldered'; a polypoid appearance is very uncommon (Fig. 17.24). Mucin-producing cholangiocarcinoma can produce strand-like filling defects caused by the mucin which may also dilate the bile ducts distal to the tumor itself (Fig. 17.25). The length of stricture varies considerably but is usually at least 1 cm (Voyles et al 1983) in contrast to most

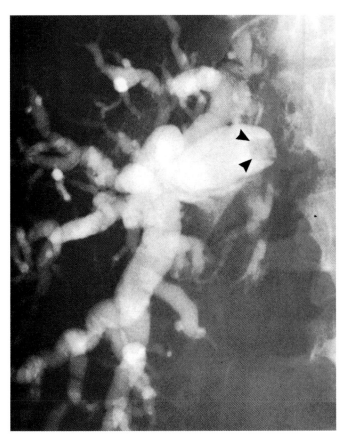

Fig. 17.24 Papillary hilar cholangiocarcinoma (arrowheads). Only the right ducts are opacified.

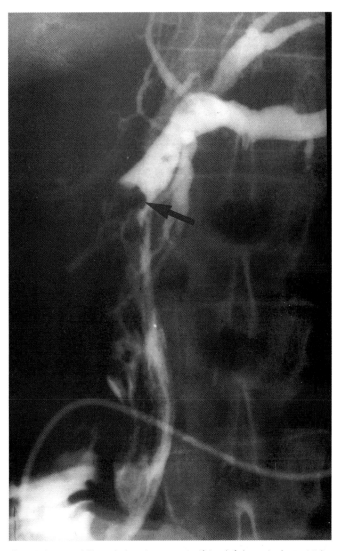

Fig. 17.25 Nasobiliary cholangiogram opacifying left hepatic ducts. Main left hepatic duct contains a small mucin-secreting papillary cholangiocarcinoma (arrow). The mucin results in expansion of the common bile duct below the tumor and the mucin appears as strand-like filling defects (courtesy Dr A Speer).

traumatic strictures. When complete obstruction involves the confluence of the right and left hepatic ducts separate punctures of the right and left ductal systems during PTC are necessary (Fig. 17.3). Stricturing may extend peripherally from the confluence on one or both sides to involve 2nd or 3rd order ducts. Frequently such extension is asymmetrical involving, e.g. second or third order ducts on one side but only the main duct (Fig. 17.26) on the other. Multiple strictures are occasionally seen either due to multifocal primary tumours or metastatic disease (Voyles et al 1983). When a focal stenotic lesion is identified on cholangiogram in a jaundiced patient, the presumptive diagnosis of a bile duct or Klatskin tumor is frequently made. Review of the final diagnosis in 98 consecutive patients with the preoperative diagnosis of a Klatskin tumor showed that 30 patients (31%) had a different final diagnosis (Wetter et al 1991). Of particular importance were five patients with a papillary type of bile duct cancer. Preoperative cholangiography in these five patients demonstrated extensive duct defects, which suggested unresectability, when in fact the resectability rate for these papillary tumors is often higher than the more common variety of bile duct carcinoma. When direct cholangiography is performed and the papillary bile duct

cancer involves the extrahepatic bile ducts, a 'golf-tee' appearance of the bile duct may be seen (Fig. 17.27).

In a significant number of cases lobar or segmental liver atrophy (Fig. 17.28) occurs in association with hilar cholangiocarcinoma due to either prolonged ductal obstruction or portal vein branch occlusion. Atrophy is indicated by crowding of ducts and has important implications when one is considering lobar resection or palliative biliary decompression by any technique.

ERC studies may point to the correct diagnosis in bile duct cancers (Fig. 17.29) and tissue specimens can be obtained by transampullary biopsy and cytology, but the yield is only 50 to 60% (Fig. 17.30) (Rustgi et al 1989, Foutch et al 1990, Kurzawinski et al 1992). The ability to obtain histological

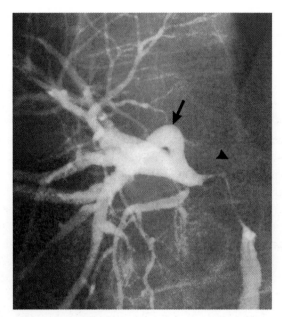

Fig. 17.26 Hilar cholangiocarcinoma involving first-order right hepatic duct, proximal common hepatic duct and faintly opacified left hepatic duct (arrowhead). Note the characteristic arched course of the right posterior sectoral duct (arrow).

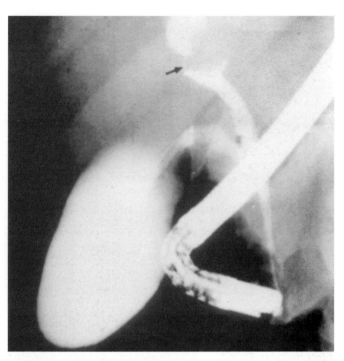

Fig. 17.27 'Golf-tee' appearance of a papillary bile duct cancer (arrowed) involving the common hepatic duct.

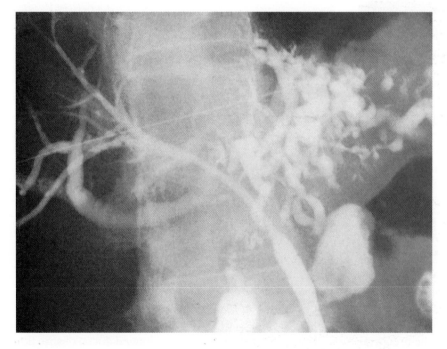

Fig. 17.28 Hilar cholangiocarcinoma with crowded left ducts indicating left-lobe atrophy. The right ducts are opacified via a percutaneous transhepatic drainage catheter.

confirmation by endoscopic means represents an important clinical tool which may help to avoid surgical exploration solely for a tissue diagnosis.

Primary sclerosing cholangitis (Ch. 48)

Sclerosing cholangitis usually produces cholangiographic changes in both the intra- and extrahepatic biliary tree (La

Russo et al 1984), although occasionally one part may be solely affected. Similar changes may be seen secondary to choledocholithiasis, post-cholecystectomy strictures, and sclerosing cholangitis may be indistinguishable from the diffuse form of cholangiocarcinoma. The detection of cholangiocarcinoma in a background of sclerosing cholangitis can be very difficult. Cholangiographic features suggesting cholangiocarcinoma include progressive focal stricturing,

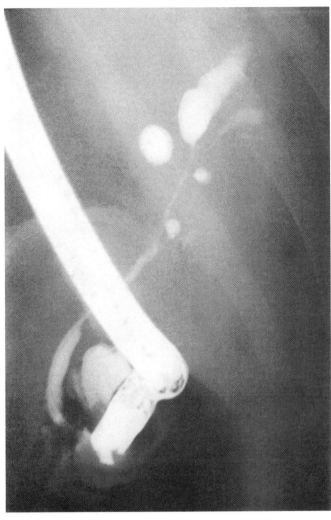

Fig. 17.29 Malignant stenosis of the common bile duct; bile duct carcinoma.

the presence of proximal uniform duct dilation, and nodular filling defects (Li-Yeng & Goldberg 1984). It has been suggested that by using these features together with careful sectional imaging techniques, most tumors can be detected (Campbell et al 1998). The two diseases often co-exist in patients with inflammatory bowel disease (Rohrmann et al 1978). The bile ducts in PSC are characterized by annular, concentric sclerosis which are usually multifocal and only rarely unifocal with duct dilation, usually of a mild degree, between strictures (Fig. 17.31). The larger bile ducts have irregularities of their walls called beading (Rogers et al 1972) (Fig. 17.32). Another characteristic sign is an absence of the smallest intrahepatic ducts leading to a reduction in the branching of the biliary tree or 'pruned-tree' appearance (Figs 17.32, 17.33). Parts of the biliary tree may be impossible to opacify (Li-Yeng & Goldberg 1984). While diverticular outpouchings of the extrahepatic ducts (Fig. 17.33) were at one time reported to be characteristic of PSC (La Russo et al 1984) they are no longer felt to be specific cholangiographic features (Gulliver et al 1991).

The diagnosis of PSC is being made more frequently and earlier in the disease course. Choledocholithiasis may also be part of the spectrum of PSC and may occur at the time of initial presentation or later in the course (Pokorny et al 1992). On ERCP, about 25% of patients with PSC will have pancreatic duct abnormalities (Lindstrom et al 1990). A study at the Mayo Clinic compared the course of PSC with the appearance of the cholangiogram (Craig et al 1991). Patients with high-grade intrahepatic strictures had

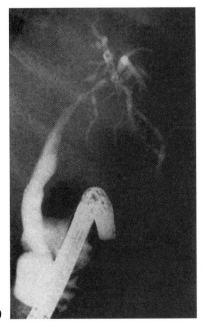

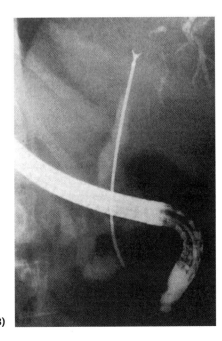

Fig. 17.30 Stenosis of the upper common bile duct. A biopsy forceps may be advanced under fluoroscopic control in the region of a suspected malignant stenosis.

(A)   **(B)**

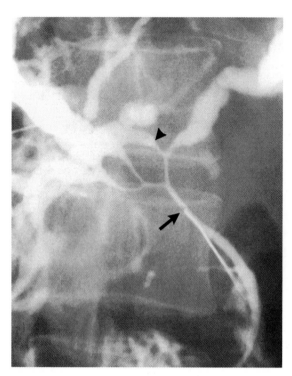

Fig. 17.31 Sclerosing cholangitis producing a stricture of the common hepatic duct extending into second-order ducts bilaterally. Differentiation from cholangiocarcinoma is aided by fine-needle aspiration cytology (arrow). Note the right posterior sectoral duct (arrowhead) entering the left hepatic duct.

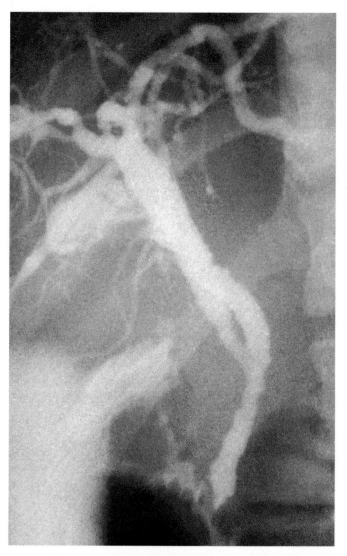

Fig. 17.32 Primary sclerosing cholangitis.

a 19% decrease in their 3-year survival when compared to patients with low-grade intrahepatic strictures. Diffuse involvement of the intrahepatic bile ducts with multiple strictures also predicted a lower 3-year survival rate. A large study of 126 patients at King's College Hospital in London showed that poor prognostic indicators of PSC included advanced histological stage, portal fibrosis, hepatosplenomegaly, portal hypertension, and cholestasis (Farrant et al 1991). It is also noteworthy that in 23% of patients in this series undergoing liver transplantation, cholangiocarcinoma was found.

In patients with ulcerative colitis, the incidence of PSC is about 1% (Mihas et al 1978). Conversely, in patients with PSC, ulcerative colitis is seen in about one-third of cases. Likewise, a combination of sclerosing cholangitis, chronic pancreatitis and Sjogren's syndrome appears to be a complex of symptoms with an autoimmune basis (Montefusco et al 1984).

Regional hepatic treatment by intra-arterial infusion (Ch. 82) of the chemotherapeutic agent FUDR in metastatic colorectal cancer, has been shown to produce a syndrome and cholangiographic picture that is similar to PSC

(Kemeny et al 1987). Decreasing or discontinuing the drug dosage may modify the course of this complication.

Secondary cholangitis

In contrast to primary sclerosing cholangitis, the cholangiogram in obstructive cholangitis is characterized by dilatation of the second and third order bile ducts. The appearance of irregularities in the bile duct walls, short stenoses and prestenotic dilatation of the intrahepatic bile ducts are reliable evidence of secondary cholangitis only if the clinical circumstances are taken into account.

A special type of secondary cholangitis is recurrent pyogenic cholangitis (RPC) (Cook et al 1954) (Ch. 64). This disease occurs predominantly in southeast Asia and is rarely

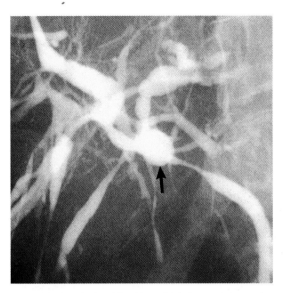

Fig. 17.33 Sclerosing cholangitis with multiple intra- and extra-hepatic segments of stricturing. A charteristic 'diverticulum' (arrow) overlies the confluence of the right and left hepatic ducts.

seen in Western countries. The infection and inflammation are restricted mainly to the biliary tree and this leads to bile duct strictures and the formation of bile duct stones. Gastrointestinal tract Gram-negative bacteria are usually involved. The common bile duct contains 80% of the stones (Lam et al 1978), while the remaining 20% of the stones are located in the intrahepatic bile ducts—these are predominantly bilirubin stones (Wong & Choi 1984). In the early stage of the disease, ERCP shows slight dilatation of the intrahepatic bile ducts with pronounced branching, 'arrowhead' formation, and abrupt termination of the duct (Lam et al 1978). The advanced stage of RPC is characterized by strictures of the intrahepatic bile ducts with proximal dilatation and stones. The radiological changes correlate well with the severity of the clinical picture. In addition, isolated, segmental or multiple cholangitic liver abscesses may occur. Abnormal pancreatic ducts are also found in up to 8% of the cases investigated.

Recently, cholangitis has been described in patients with AIDS. One form of this cholangitis is thought to be secondary to cryptosporidial infection of the bile ducts (McCarty et al 1989). The intrahepatic bile ducts are abnormal with an area of dilatation and focal strictures. Ultrasonography should be performed before ERC as it may be diagnostic and alleviate the need for the more invasive procedure. Other biliary tract abnormalities seen in AIDS patients include bile duct lymphomas, papillary stenosis, and a sclerosing cholangitis-like picture probably due to infection with cytomegalovirus (Schneiderman et al 1987, Cello 1989).

Cystic disease of the bile ducts (Ch. 66)

Direct cholangiography is useful in the diagnosis and preoperative assessment of this complex spectrum of diseases. The cholangiograms show cystic dilatations of bile ducts in one or more segments of the liver, which are frequently filled with multiple stones of various sizes (Kurtz et al 1980). Some endoscopists use the term, Caroli's syndrome, when stones are demonstrated in bile ducts which have undergone secondary dilatation. Intrahepatic cystic biliary dilatation may be demonstrated without associated extrahepatic duct dilatation, but is also seen in up to 44% of patients with choledochal cysts (Dayton et al 1983) (Fig. 17.34). Cholangiography may reveal evidence of complications including calculi, abscesses or cholangiocarcinoma, the latter having an incidence of 7% in Caroli's syndrome and 4% in choledochal cysts (Bloustein 1977). In patients with choledochal cysts ERCP may also demonstrate an abnormally proximal junction of the common bile duct with the pancreatic duct (Fig. 17.34), which is well documented and suggested to be an etiological factor (Kimura et al 1977).

Parasistic infestations (Chs. 62 and 63)

A proportion of hepatic hydatid cysts (5 to 10%) rupture into the bile ducts and this may simulate choledocholithiasis. The daughter cysts can cause biliary obstruction.

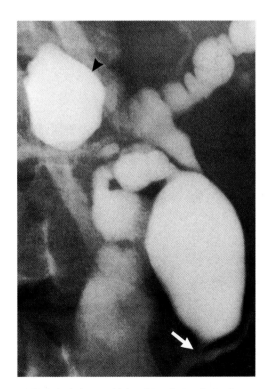

Fig. 17.34 Choledochal cyst with intrahepatic cyst formation (arrowhead). The common bile duct has an abnormally proximal junction with the pancreatic duct (arrow).

Calcified cysts are easy to recognize on X-ray. When the calcified cyst is not obvious, biliary strictures with obstruction may be noted on cholangiogram. The biliary ducts can show considerable irregularities in caliber and extensive displacement of the intrahepatic branches due to the mass effect of a large hydatid cyst (Cottone et al 1978, Ibrahim & Kawanishi 1981, Dyrszka & Sanghavi 1983).

Ascaris lumbricoides is a commonly seen helminth which has worldwide distribution. Its prevalence is 90% in some parts of Africa and the Far East. If the worm passes through the sphincter of Oddi it may cause acute pancreatitis or a cholestasis syndrome (Winters et al 1984). In the acute stage, the worm may occasionally be found and extracted from the ampulla, and it can be detected in the biliary tract by cholangiography.

Eating raw meat has been associated with *Clonorchis sinensis* infestation. The prevalence of this disease has been estimated to be as high as 60% of the general population of Hong Kong based on stool ova examinations. This worm can penetrate through the papilla into the bile ducts. In an ERCP study of 31 consecutive patients, the typical filamentous wavy or elliptical appearance of the worm in the bile ducts was felt to be pathognomonic (Leung et al 1989). Other common cholangiographic findings include widely dilated extrahepatic bile ducts which are filled with biliary sludge and stones and intrahepatic duct strictures that are predominantly found in the branches of the left hepatic duct (Yellin & Donovan 1981). The eggs of *Clonorchis sinensis* act as a nucleus for the development of the bile duct stones (Lam et al 1978). Naval et al (1984) reported successful endoscopic biliary lavage to eliminate the eggs.

Invasion of *Fasciola hepatica* into the biliary tract may also cause serious lesions and, in the chronic stage, can resemble the appearance of sclerosing cholangitis (Hauser & Bynum 1984). The appearance on ERCP is that of dilated bile ducts with unexplained sludge in the distal bile duct (Figs 17.35, 17.36).

Abscesses (Ch. 61)

Hepatic abscesses of any cause may communicate with the biliary tree and so be seen on cholangiography. Multiple hepatic abscesses are usually secondary to acute suppurative cholangitis in association with ductal obstruction, and appear as multiple small rounded cavities with slightly indistinct margins (Fig. 17.37). Such an appearance should lead to consideration of urgent biliary decompression, either surgically, percutaneously or endoscopically.

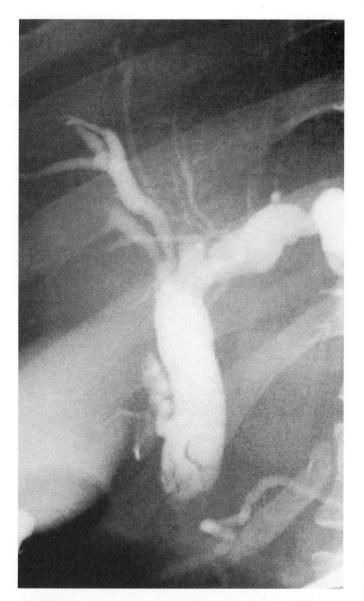

Fig. 17.35 Liver flukes in the distal bile duct presenting as 'biliary sludge'.

Intrahepatic trauma (Chs 68 and 70)

Damage to the hepatic parenchyma resulting from blunt abdominal injury (Fig. 17.38) may give rise to direct or indirect connections between the blood vessels and bile ducts . Depending on the existing pressure gradient, either blood enters the biliary tract (hemobilia) or bile enters the circulating blood (cholemia). Hemobilia may also occur after liver biopsy, percutaneous cholangiography, and percutaneously placed endobiliary stents. ERC is one method of diagnosing these complications, but angiography is more commonly performed after noninvasive imaging procedures.

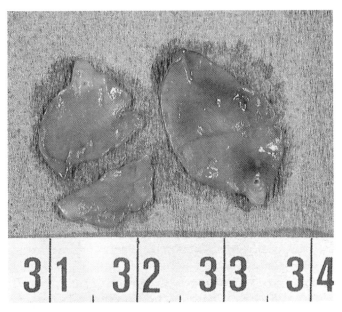

Fig. 17.36 Extracted liver flukes (same patient as Fig. 17.35).

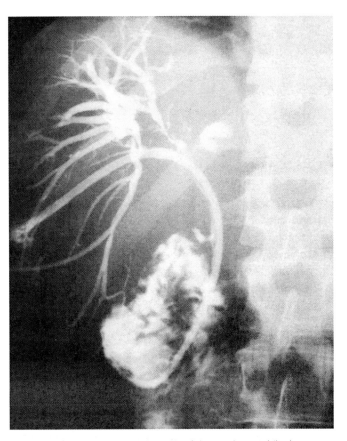

Fig. 17.38 Multiple traumatic stenoses of the intrahepatic bile ducts 2 years after liver rupture (motor vehicle accident).

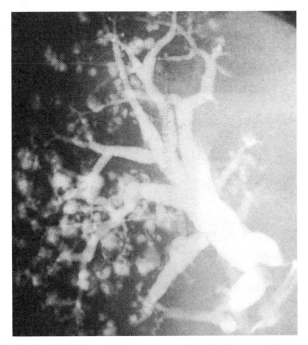

Fig. 17.37 Multiple hepatic abscesses associated with suppurative cholangitis in a patient with hilar duct obstruction.

biliary sludge in the form of casts, stones or debris. Ultrasonography was not as good as ERC in determining the cause of post-transplant cholestasis. Endoscopic sphincterotomy after diagnostic ERC was therapeutic.

Pancreatitis

The close anatomical relationship between the intrapancreatic portion of the common bile duct and the head of the pancreas is the reason for the frequent involvement of the bile duct in disorders of the pancreas. The clinical consequences are various degrees of cholestasis which may result in secondary cholangitis and stone formation.

In about 25% of patients with chronic pancreatitis the bile duct is involved. Bile duct involvement depends on the severity of the inflammation (Fig. 17.39). An analysis of 531 patients with chronic pancreatitis showed that over 60% had a significant bile duct stricture (Kasugai 1975). Signs of cholestasis occurred in 18.1% of the patients (Rosch et al 1981).

A long, smooth, and tapered stenosis of the bile duct

Liver transplantation

Orthotopic liver transplantation has become a relatively common procedure for the management of end-stage chronic liver disease. In a study of 178 liver transplant patients, 12 (7%), underwent post-transplant ERC for cholestasis, cholangitis, or persistent bile leaks (O'Connor et al 1991). The most common abnormality noted was

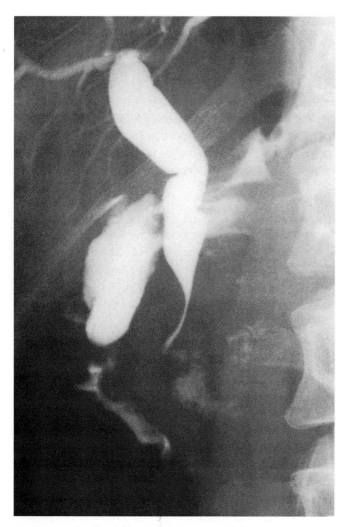

Fig. 17.39 Filiform stenosis caused by chronic pancreatitis.

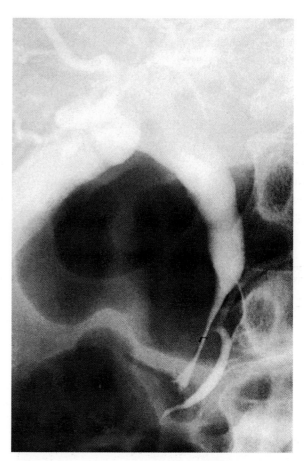

Fig. 17.40 Acute pancreatitis with pseudocyst in the head of the pancreas (verified on operation) leading to cholestasis.

characteristic of chronic pancreatitis is found in 27 to 58% of patients (Stolte et al 1984). Patients with bile duct strictures due to chronic pancreatitis may be observed without intervention if they do not develop cholangitis or stones, and cancer of the head of the pancreas can be comfortably excluded (Frey et al 1990).

Pancreatic pseudocyst, a worrying consequence of acute pancreatitis, may also cause symptoms of cholestasis due to compression of the bile duct (Fig. 17.40).

Pancreatography can be a potential source of serious infection when a large pancreatic pseudocyst is present, and ultrasonography or CT scans, not ERCP, should be used to diagnose and follow the course of patients with pseudocysts. ERCP, however, has been shown to be useful in the preoperative assessment of patients with pancreatic pseudocysts. In one series, ERCP findings altered the operative plan in over 50% of patients with pseudocysts (Nealon et al 1989).

ERCP has no role in acute pancreatitis, except in those patients where there is a possibility that the pancreatitis may be secondary to gallstone disease. In this event, ERCP is an important diagnostic option and will identify patients with biliary pancreatitis (Goodman et al 1985, Neoptolemos 1989). Diagnostic ERCP coupled with endoscopic sphincterotomy may be life-saving in this circumstance.

CONCLUSIONS

Direct cholangiography is an important option in the evaluation of patients with jaundice, unexplained abdominal pain, or equivocal imaging studies. Coupled with its therapeutic potential of biliary drainage and stone extraction, direct cholangiography will continue to help clinicians manage patients with hepatobiliary and pancreatic diseases. However, direct cholangiography should not be used only to determine the level of biliary obstruction, as it will rarely provide more important additional information than that obtained by a detailed transabdominal ultrasound examination (Gibson et al 1986). When direct cholangiography is indicated, the choice between PTC and ERC will be affected by the local availability and quality of the two services as well as by factors listed in Table 17.5. The authors' practice is to choose ERC if there is no intrahepatic bile duct dilatation on ultrasound, or if a low common bile duct obstruction is suspected. PTC is preferable if there is suspected high obstruction and intrahepatic duct dilatation or if there has been previous biliary-enteric anastomosis. Both examinations are sometimes necessary to determine the length of a stricture when biliary obstruction is complete.

Table 17.5 Comparison of PTC and ERC

	PTC	*ERC*
Advantages	Less expertise needed Less expensive equipment. Good duct filling above an obstruction	Visualization of stomach and duodenum. Biopsy of ampullary lesions possible. Simultaneous pancreatogram.
	Both may be followed by catheter or endoprosthesis insertion for biliary drainage	
Contraindications	Significant coagulopathy. Marked ascites*	Unfavorable anatomy. Pseudocyst.* Recent acute pancreatitis*
Success rates	98% – dilated ducts; 70% – undilated ducts†	Up to 90%‡
Major complications	4.1%	2–3%‡
Mortality	0.13%	0.1–0.2%‡

* Relative contraindications.
† Harbin et al (1980).
‡ Cotton (1977).

REFERENCES

Aaerimaa M, Maekelae P 1981 The cystic duct stump and the postcholecystectomy syndrome. An analysis of 54 patients subjected to ERCP. Annales Chirurgicae Gynaecologicae 70: 297–303

Anand B S, Vij J C, Mac H S, Chowdhury V, Kumar A 1989 Effect of aging on the pancreatic ducts: a study based on endoscopic retrograde pancreatography. Gastrointestinal Endoscopy 35: 210–231

Ariyama J 1983 Direct cholangiography. In: Herlinger H, Lunderquist A, Wallace S (eds) Clinical radiology of the liver. Marcel Dekker, New York, Ch 18, p 471

Ariyama J, Shirakabe H, Ohashi K, Roberts G M 1978 Experience with percutaneous transhepatic cholangiography using the Japanese needle. Gastrointestinal Radiology 2: 359–365

Axon A T 1991 Disinfection and endoscopy: summary and recommendations. Working party report to the World Congress of Gastroenterology, Sydney. Journal of Gastroenterology and Hepatology 6: 23–24

Benjamin I S 1982 The obstructed biliary tract. In: Blumgart L H (ed) The biliary tract. Churchill Livingstone, Edinburgh, Ch 10, p 157

Bernard J P, Sahel J, Giovannini M, Sarles H 1990 Pancreas divisum is a probable cause of acute pancreatitis: a report of 137 cases. Pancreas 5: 248–254

Bilbao M K, Dotter C T, Lee R G, Katon R M 1976 Complications of endoscopic retrograde cholangiopancreatography (ERCP). A study of 1000 cases. Gastroenterology 70: 314–320

Bloustein P A 1977 Association of carcinoma with congenital cystic conditions of the liver and bile ducts. American Journal of Gastroenterology 67: 40–46

Blumgart L H, Kelley C J, Benjamin I S 1984 Benign bile duct stricture following cholecystectomy: Critical factors in management. British Journal of Surgery 71: 836–843

Borsch G, Bergbauer M, Nebel W, Sebin G 1984 Der Einfluss von Somatostatin auf die Amylasespiegel und Pankreatitisrate nach ERCP. Medizinische Welt 35: 102–109

Bourgeois N, Dunham F, Verhest A, Cremer M 1984 Endoscopic biopsies of the papilla of Vater at the time of endoscopic sphincterotomy: difficulties in interpretation. Gastrointestinal Endoscopy 30: 163–166

Buckley A, Connon J J 1990 The role of ERCP in children and adolescents. Gastrointestinal Endoscopy 36: 369–372

Burckhardt H, Muller W 1921 Versuche ueber die Punkiton der Gallenblase und ihre Roentgendarstellung. Deutsche Zeitschrift fur Chirurgie 162: 168–197

Cameron J L, Pitt H A, Zinner M J, Kaufman S L, Coleman J A 1990 Management of proximal cholangiocarcinomas by surgical resection and radiotherapy. American Journal of Surgery 159: 91–98

Campbell W L, Ferris J V, Holbert B L, Thaete F L, Baron R L 1998 Biliary tract carcinoma complicating primary sclerosing cholangitis: evaluation with CT, cholangiography, US, and MR imaging. Radiology 207: 41–50

Carter R F, Saypol G M 1952 Transabdominal cholangiography. Journal of the American Medical Association 148: 253–255

Cattell R B, Braasch J W, Kahn F 1962 Polypoid epithelial tumours of the bile ducts. New England Journal of Medicine 266: 57–61

Cello J P 1989 Acquired immunodeficiency syndrome cholangiopathy: spectrum of disease. American Journal of Medicine 86: 539–546

Chen P H, Lo H W, Wang C S et al 1984 Cholangiocarcinoma in hepatolithiasis. Journal of Clinical Gastroenterology 6: 539–547

Classen M, Demling L 1975 Hazards of endoscopic retrograde cholangiopancreatography. Acta Hepatogastroenterologica 22: 1–3

Classen M, Phillip J 1982 Endoscopic retrograde cholangiopancreatography (ERCP) and endoscopic papillotomy (EPT). Seminars in Liver Disease 2: 67–74

Classen M, Phillip J, Wurbs D 1981 Fortschritte der direkten Cholangiographie und Cholangioskopie. In: Tittor W, Schwalbach G (eds) Leberdurch-blutung und Kreislauf. Thieme-Verlag, Stuttgart, p 158–161

Coelho J C, Buffara M, Pozzobon C E, Altenburg F L, Artigas G V 1984 Incidence of common bile duct stones in patients with acute and chronic cholecystitis. Surgery, Gynecology and Obstetrics 158: 76–81

Collier N A, Carr D, Hemingway A, Blumgart L H 1984 Preoperative diagnosis and its effect on the treatment of carcinoma of the gall bladder. Surgery, Gynecology and Obstetrics 159: 465–470

Cook J, Hou P C, Ho H C 1954 Recurrent pyogenic cholangitis. British Journal of Surgery 42: 188–203

Cotton P B 1977 Progress Report ERCP. Gut 18: 316–341

Cotton P B, Salmon P R, Blumgart L H et al 1972 Cannulation of the papilla of Vater via fiber-duodenoscope. Lancet 1: 53–58

Cottone M, Amuso M, Cotton P 1978 Endoscopic retrograde cholangiography in hepatic hydatid disease. British Journal of Surgery 66: 107

Couinaud C 1957 Le foie. Etudes anatomiques et chirurgicales. Masson, Paris

Craig D A, MacCarty R L, Wiesner R H, Grambsch P M, LaRusso N F 1991 Primary sclerosing cholangitis: value of cholangiography in determining prognosis. American Journal of Radiology 157: 959–964

Cruz F O, Barriga P, Tocornal J, Burhenne H J 1983 Radiology of the Mirizzi syndrome: Diagnostic importance of the transhepatic cholangiogram. Gastrointestinal Radiology 8: 249–253

Daniels C, Schmidt H D, Lenner V, Brunner H 1980 Langer Zystikusstumpf als Ursache der Restbeschwerden nach Cholezystektomie. Leber Magen Darm 10: 207–212

Danzi J T, Makipour H, Farmer R G 1976 Primary sclerosing cholangitis. American Journal of Gastroenterology 65: 109

Dayton M T, Longmire W P, Tompkins R K 1983 Caroli's disease: A premalignant condition? American Journal of Surgery 145: 41–48

De Ledinghen V, Lecesne R, Raymond J-M, Gense V, et al 1999 Diagnosis of choledocholithiasis: Eus or magnetic resonance cholangiography? A prospective controlled study. Gastrointestinal Endoscopy 49: 26–31

Dowdy G S, Olin W G, Shelton E L, Waldron G W 1962 Benign tumours of the extrahepatic bile ducts. Archives of Surgery 85: 503–513

Dyrszka H, Sanghavi B 1983 Hepatic hydatid disease: findings on endoscopic retrograde cholangiography. Gastrointestinal Endoscopy 29: 248–249

Earnshaw J J, Clark A W, Thom B T 1985 Outbreak of *Pseudomonas aeruginosa* following endoscopic retrograde cholangiopancreatography. Journal of Hospital Infection 6: 95–97

Farrant J M, Hayllar K M, Wilkinson M L, Karani J, Portmann B C, Westaby D 1991 Natural history and prognostic variables in primary sclerosing cholangitis. Gastroenterology 100: 1710–1717

Femppel J, Lux G, Rosch W 1981 Intraoperative Gallenwegslasionen. Medizinische Welt 32: 111–114

Foutch P G, Kerr D M, Harlan J R, Manne R K, Kummet T D, Sanowski R A 1990 Endoscopic retrograde wire-guided brush cytology for diagnosis of patients with malignant obstruction of the bile duct. American Journal of Gastroenterology 85: 791–795

Fraser G M, Cruikshank J G, Sumerling M D, Buist T A S 1978 Percutaneous transhepatic cholangiography with the Chiba needle. Clinical Radiology 29: 101–112

Freeney P C 1988 Radiology of the pancreas: Two decades of progress in imaging and intervention. American Journal of Radiology 150: 975–981

Freeny P C, Lawson T L 1982 Radiology of the Pancreas. Springer-Verlag, New York

Frey C F, Suzuki M, Isaji S 1990 Treatment of chronic pancreatitis complicated by obstruction of the common bile duct of duodenum. World Journal of Surgery 14: 59–69

Frick M P, Feinberg S B, Goodale R L 1982 The value of endoscopic retrograde cholangiopancreatography in patients with suspected carcinoma of the pancreas and indeterminant computed tomographic results. Surgery, Gynecology and Obstetrics 155: 177–182

Geenen J E, Hogan W J, Dodds W J, Toouli J, Venu R P 1989 The efficacy of endoscopic sphincterotomy after cholecystectomy in patients with sphincter-of-Oddi dysfunction. New England Journal of Medicine 320: 82–87

Georgopoulos S K, Schwartz L H, Jarnagin W R, Gerdes H, Breite I, Fong Y, Blumgart L H, Kurtz R C 1999 Comparison of magnetic resonance cholangiopancreatography (MRCP) and endoscopic retrograde cholangiopancreatography (ERCP) in malignant pancreaticobiliary obstruction. Archives of Surgery 134: 1002–1007

Gibbons C P, Griffiths G J, Cormack A 1983 The role of percutaneous transhepatic cholangiography and grey-scale ultrasound in the investigation and treatment of bile duct obstruction. British Journal of Surgery 70: 494–496

Gibson R N, Yeung E, Thompson J N et al 1986 Radiological evaluation of bile duct obstruction: level, cause and tumour resectability. Radiology 160: 43–47

Goodman A J, Neoptolemos J P, Carr-Locke D L, Finlay D B L, Fossard D P 1985 Detection of gall stones after acute pancreatitis. Gut 26: 125–132

Grozinger H H 1984 Zur Kritik des sog. Postcholezystektomie-syndromes. In: Demling L (ed) Klinische Gastroenterologie, Part II, p 378–386

Gulliver D J, Baker M E, Putnam W, Baillie J, Rice R, Cotton P B 1991 Bile duct diverticula and webs: nonspecific cholangiographic features of primary sclerosing cholangitis. American Journal of Roentgenology 157: 281–285

Hadjis N S, Blenkharn J I, Alexander N, Benjamin I S, Blumgart L H 1990 Outcome of radical surgery in hilar cholangiocarcinoma. Surgery 107: 597–604

Hadjis N S, Collier N A, Blumgart L H 1985 Malignant masquerade at the hilum of the liver. British Journal of Surgery 72: 659–661

Hand B H 1973 Anatomy and function of the extrahepatic biliary system. Clinics in Gastroenterology 2: 3–29

Hannigan B F, Keeling P W N, Stavin B, Thompson R P H 1985 Hyperamylasemia after ERCP with ionic and non-ionic contrast media. Gastrointestinal Endoscopy 31: 109–110

Harbin W P, Mueller P R, Ferrucci J T 1980 Transhepatic cholangiography. Complications and use patterns of the fine-needle technique. A multi-institution survey. Radiology 135: 15–22

Hauser S C, Bynum T E 1984 Abnormalities on ERCP in a case of human fascioliasis. Gastrointestinal Endoscopy 30: 80–81

Healey J E, Schroy P C 1953 Anatomy of the biliary ducts within the human liver. AMA Archives or Surgery 66: 599–616

Helm E B, Bauernfeind A, Frech K, Hagenmuller F 1984 Pseudomonas-Septikamie nach endoskopischen Eingriffen am Gallengangsystem. Deutsche Medizinische Wochenschrift 109: 698–701

Hopper K D, Wegert S J, Hallgren S E 1989 Renal excretion of endoscopic retrograde cholangiopancreatography injected contrast. A common phenomenon. Investigational Radiology 24: 394–396

Hossack K F, Herron J J 1972 Benign tumours of the common bile duct: report of a case and review of the literature. Australian and New Zealand Journal of Surgery 42: 22–26

Hultborn A, Jacobsson B, Rosengren B 1962 Cholangiovenous reflux during cholangiography. An experimental and clinical study. Acta Chirurgica Scandinavia 123: 111–124

Hunter J G 1991 Avoidance of bile duct injury during laparoscopic cholecystectomy. American Journal of Surgery 162: 71–76

Ibrahim M A H, Kawanishi H 1981 Endoscopic retrograde cholangiography in the evaluation of complicated echinococcus of the liver. Gastrointestinal Endoscopy 27: 20–22

Jain S, Long R G, Scott J, Dick R, Sherlock S 1977 Percutaneous transhepatic cholangiography using the 'Chiba' needle – 80 cases. British Journal of Radiology 50: 175–180

Jandrzejewski J W, McAnally T, Jones S R, Katon R M 1980 Antibiotic and ERCP: In vitro activity of aminoglycosides when added to iodinated contrast agents. Gastroenterology 78: 745–748

Jaques P F, Mauro M A, Scatliff J H 1980 The failed transhepatic cholangiogram. Radiology 134: 33–35

Kasugai T 1975 Recent advances in the endoscopic retrograde cholangiopancreatography. Digestion 13: 76

Katon R M, Bilbao M K, Parent J A, Smitz F W 1975 Endoscopic retrograde cholangio-pancreatography in patients with gastrectomy and gastrojejunostomy (Billroth II), a case for the forward look. Gastrointestinal Endoscopy 21: 164–165

Keighley M R B 1977 Micro-organisms in the bile. A preventable cause of sepsis after biliary surgery. Annals of the Royal College of Surgeons of England 59: 328–334

Keil P G, Landis S N 1951 Peritoneoscopic cholangiography. Archives of Internal Medicine 88: 36–41

Kemeny N, Daly J, Reichman B 1987 Intrahepatic or systemic infusion of fluorodeoxyuridine in patients with liver metastases from colorectal cancer. Annals of Internal Medicine 107: 459–465

Kidd H A 1956 Percutaneous transhepatic cholangiography. Archives of Surgery 72: 262–268

Kimura K, Ohto M, Ono T et al 1977 Congenital cystic dilation of the common bile duct: relationship to anomalous pancreaticobiliary ductal union. American Journal of Roentgenology 128: 571–577

Kittredge R D, Baer J W 1975 Percutaneous transhepatic cholangiography. Problems in interpretation. American Journal of Roentgenology 125: 35–46

Kocher F, Mousseau R 1979 Percutaneous transhepatic cholangiography with the Chiba needle. American Journal of Gastroenterology 71: 35–44

Koehler R E, Melson G L, Lee J K T, Long K 1979 Common hepatic duct obstruction by cystic duct stone: Mirizzi syndrome. American Journal of Roentgenology 132: 1007

Komoroski R A, Beggs B K, Geenan J E, Venu R P 1991 Assessment of ampulla of Vater pathology: an endoscopic approach. American Journal of Surgical Pathology 15: 1188–1196

Kreek M J, Balint J A 1980 'Skinny needle' cholangiography – results of a pilot study of a voluntary prospective method for gathering risk data on new procedures. Gastroenterology 78: 598–604

Kurtz W, Strohm W D, Leuschner U, Classen M 1980 Die kongenitale Dilatation der intrahepatischen Gallenwege (Caroli-Syndrom). Innere Medizin 7: 50–56

Kurzawinski T, Deery A, Dooley J, Dick R, Hobbs K, Davidson B 1992 A prospective controlled study comparing brush and bile exfoliative cytology for diagnosing bile duct strictures. Gut 33: 1675–1677

La Russo N F, Wiesner R H, Ludwig J, MacCarty R L 1984 Primary sclerosing cholangitis. New England Journal of Medicine 310: 899–903

Lam S K, Wong K P, Chan P K W, Ngan H, Ong G B 1978 Recurrent pyogenic cholangitis: A study by endoscopic retrograde cholangiography. Gastroenterology 74: 1196–1203

Lee W Y 1942 Evaluation of peritoneoscopy in intra-abdominal diagnosis. Review of Gastroenterology 9: 133–141

Leung J W C, Sung J Y, Chung S C S, Metreweli C 1989 Hepatic clonorchiasis—a study by endoscopic retrograde cholangiopancreatography. Gastrointestinal Endoscopy 35: 226–321

Lindstrom E, Bodemar G, Ryden B O, Ihse I 1990 Pancreatic ductal morphology and exocrine function in primary sclerosing cholangitis. Acta Chirurgica Scandinavica 156: 451–456

Li-Yeng C, Goldberg H I 1984 Sclerosing cholangitis: Broad spectrum of radiographic features. Gastrointestinal Radiology 9: 39–47

Longmire W P, McArthur M S, Bastounis E A, Hiatt J 1973 Carcinoma of the extrahepatic biliary tract. Annals of Surgery 178: 333–345

Matzen P, Malchow-Moller A, Lejerstofte J, Stage P, Juhl E 1982 Endoscopic retrograde cholangiopancreatography and transhepatic cholangiography in patients with suspected obstructive jaundice. Scandinavian Journal of Gastroenterology 17: 731–735

McCarty M, Choudhri A H, Helbert M, Crofton M E 1989 Radiological features of AIDS related cholangitis. Clinical Radiology 40: 582–585

McCune W S, Shorb P E, Moscowitz H 1968 Endoscopic cannulation of the ampulla of Vater: a preliminary report. Annals of Surgery 167: 752–756

Meier P, Ansel H, Silvis S, Vennes J 1984 Comparison of ultrasound and ERCP measurements of bile duct size. Gastroenterology 87: 615

Meyers W C 1991 A prospective analysis of 1518 laparoscopic cholecystectomies. New England Journal of Medicine 324: 1073–1078

Michel H, Adda M 1980 La cholangiographie transparietale laterale a l'aiguille fine. Gastroenterologie Clinique et Biologique 4: 137–143

Mihas A A, Murad T M, Hischowitz B I 1978 Sclerosing cholangitis associated with ulcerative colitis. American Journal of Gastroenterology 70: 614

Montefusco P P, Geiss A C, Bronzo R L, Randall S, Kahn E, McKinley M J 1984 Sclerosing cholangitis, chronic pancreatitis and Sjogren's syndrome: a syndrome complex. American Journal of Surgery 147: 822–826

Moosa A R, Mayer A D, Stabile B 1990 Iatrogenic injury to the bile duct: Who, how, where? Archives of Surgery 125: 1028–1031

Mueller P R, Harbin W P, Ferrucci J T, Wittenberg J, Van Sonnenberg E 1982 Fine needle cholangiography: reflections after 450 cases. American Journal of Roentgenology 136: 85–90

Nagasue N, Inokuchi K 1979 Diagnostic value of percutaneous transhepatic cholangiography judged by personal experience of 58 patients. Clinical Radiology 30: 451–455

Nakayama F, Wong J (eds) Intrahepatic calculi. Alan R Liss, New York, p 129–148

Naval F, Diner W C, Westbrook K C, Kumpuris D D, Uthman E O 1984 Endoscopic biliary lavage in a case of *Clonorchis sinensis*. Gastrointestinal Endoscopy 30: 292–294

Nealon W H, Townsend C M Jr, Thompson J C 1989 Preoperative ERCP in patients with pancreatic pseudocyst associated with resolving acute and chronic pancreatitis. Annals of Surgery 209: 532–538

Nebel O T 1975 Manometric evaluation of the papilla of Vater. Gastrointestinal Endoscopy 21: 126–128

Neoptolemos J P 1989 The theory of 'persisting' common bile duct stones in severe gallstone pancreatitis. Annals of the Royal College of Surgeons, England 71: 326–331

Nichols D M, Burhenne H J 1984 Magnification in cholangiography. American Journal of Roentgenology 141: 947–949

Niederau C, Sonnenberg A, Mueller J 1984 Comparison of the extrahepatic bile duct size measured by ultrasound and by different radiographic methods. Gastroenterology 87: 615–621

Nimura Y, Hayakawa N, Kamiya J, Kondo S, Shionoya S 1990 Hepatic segmentectomy with caudate lobe resection for bile duct carcinoma of the hepatic hilus. World Journal of Surgery 14: 535–544

Nix G A J J, Dubbelman C, Wilson J H P, Schutte H E, Jeekel J, Postema R R 1991 Prognostic implications of tumor diameter in carcinoma of the head of the pancreas. Cancer 67: 529–535

Nurick A W, Patey D H, Whiteside D G 1953 Percutaneous transhepatic cholangiography in the diagnosis of obstructive jaundice. British Journal of Surgery 41: 27–30

O'Connor H J, Vickers C R, Buckels J A et al 1991 Role of ERCP after orthotopic liver transplantation. Gut 32: 419–423

Ohto M, Karasawa E, Tsuchiya Y, Kimura K, Saisho H, Ono T, Okuda K 1980 Ultrasonically guided percutaneous contrast medium injection and aspiration biopsy using a real-time puncture transducer. Radiology 136: 171–176

Ohto M, Kimura K, Tsuchiya Y et al 1984 Diagnosis of hepatolithiasis. In: Okuda K, Ohto M, Ono T, Tsuchiya Y, Saisho H 1978 Cholangiography and pancreatography. Igaku-Shoin, Tokyo

Ohto M, Tsuchiya Y 1969 Non-surgically available percutaneous transhepatic cholangiography: technique and cases. Medicina, Tokyo 6: 735–739

Oi I, Kobayashi S, Kondo T 1970 Endoscopic pancreato-cholangiography. Endoscopy 2: 103–106

Okuda K, Musha H, Nakajima Y, Takayasu K, Suzuki Y, Morita M, Yamasaki T 1978 Frequency of intrahepatic arteriovenous fistula as a sequela t percutaneous needle puncture of the liver. Gastroenterology 74: 1204–1207

Okuda K, Tanikawa T, Emura T, Kuratomi S, Jinnouchi S, Urabe K et al 1974 Non-surgical, percutaneous transhepatic cholangiography-diagnostic significance in medical problems of the liver. American Journal of Digestive Diseases 19: 21–36

Okuno M, Himeno S, Kurakawa M et al 1985 Changes in serum levels of pancreatic isoamylase, lipase, trypsin, and elastase after endoscopic retrograde pancreatography. Hepatogastroenterology 32: 87–90

Osnes M, Myren J 1975 Endoscopic retrograde cholangiopancreatography (ERCP) in patients with Billroth II partial gastrectomies. Endoscopy 7: 225

Phillip J, Koch H, Classen M 1974 Variations and anomalies of the papilla of Vater, the pancreas and the biliary duct system. Endoscopy 6: 70–77

Phillip J, Usadel K H, Porro A, Hagenmuller F, Jessen K, Classen M 1985 Effekt von Somatostatin auf pankreatitische Komplikationen nach ERCP und Eingriffen an der Papilla Vateri. Fortschritte der Gastroenterologischen, Endoskopie 14: 124–129

Phillip J, Hagenmuller F 1983 Postoperative Syndrome an den Gallenwegen: das sog. Postcholezystektomie-Syndrome. In: Henning H (ed) Fortschritte der gastroenterologischen Endoskopie. Demeter Verlag, Grafelfing 12: 47–52

Plumley T F, Rohrmann C A, Freeny P C, Silverstein F E, Ball T J 1982 Double duct sign: Reassessed significance in ERCP. American Journal of Radiology 183: 31

Pokorny C S, McCaughan G W, Gallagher N D, Selby W S 1992 Sclerosing cholangitis and biliary tract calculi — Primary or secondary? Gut 33: 1376–1380

Poralla T, Staritz M, Manns M, Klose K, Honunel G, Meyer zum Buschenfelde K H 1985 Age and sex dependency of bile duct diameter and bile duct pressure—an ERC manometry study. Zeitschrift fur Gastroenterologie 23: 235–239

Rogers J V, Copeland A J, Schroder J S, Amerson J R 1972 Sclerosing cholangitis—roentgenographic features. South African Medical Journal 65: 587

Rohrmann C A, Ansel H J, Freeny P C et al 1978 Cholangiographic abnormalities in patients with inflammatory bowel disease. Radiology 127: 635–641

Rosch W 1981 Report on a symposium '10 years of ERCP': Diagnostic and therapeutic aspects. E.S.G.E. Newsletter 15: 7–9

Rosch W 1985 Endoskopische retrograde Gallenwegsdiagnostik (ERC). Krankenhausarzt 58: 27–34

Rosch W, Lux G, Riemann J F, Hoh L 1981 Chronische Pankreatitis und Nachbarorgane. Fortschritte der Medizin 99: 1118–1120

Ruddell W S J, Linott D J, Axon A T R 1983 The diagnostic yield of ERCP in the investigation of unexplained abdominal pain. British Journal of Surgery 70: 74–75

Rustgi A K, Kelsey P B, Guelrud P B, Saini S, Schapiro R H 1989 Malignant tumors of the bile ducts: Diagnosis by biopsy during endoscopic cannulation. Gastrointestinal Endoscopy 35: 248–251

Sarr M G, Kaufmann S L, Zuidema G D, Cameron J L 1984 Management of haemobilia associated with transhepatic biliary drainage catheters. Surgery 95: 603–607

Sauter G, Grabein B, Huber G, Mannes G A, Ruckdeschel G, Sauerbruch T 1990 Antibiotic prophylaxis of infectious complications with endoscopic retrograde cholangiopancreatography. A randomized controlled study. Endoscopy 22: 164–167

Schmalz M J, Geenen J E, Hogan W J, Dodds W J, Venu R P, Johnson G K 1990 Pain on common bile duct injection during ERCP: does it indicate sphincter of Oddi dysfunction? Gastrointestinal Endoscopy 36: 458–461

Schneiderman D J, Cella J P, Laing F C 1987 Papillary stenosis and sclerosing cholangitis in the acquired immunodeficiency syndrome. Annals of Internal Medicine 106: 546–549

Seifert E, Safrany L, Stender H St, Lesch P, Luska G, Misaki F 1974 Identification of bile duct tumors by means of endoscopic retrograde pancreato-cholangiography (ERCP). Endoscopy 6: 156

Seldinger S I 1966 Percutaneous transhepatic cholangiography. Acta Radiologica (suppl): 253

Severini A, Bellorni M, Cozzi G, Pizzetti P, Spinelli P 1981 Lymphomatous involvement of intrahepatic and extrahepatic biliary ducts. PTC and ERCP findings. Acta Radiologica Diagnosis 22: 159–163

Shakoor T, Geenen J E 1992 Pre-cut papillotomy. Gastrointestinal Endoscopy 38: 623–627

Soulen M C, Zerhouni E A, Fishman E K, Gayler B W, Milligan F, Siegelman S S 1989 Enlargement of the pancreatic head in patients with pancreas divisum. Clinical Imaging 13: 51–57

Steinberg H V, Beckett W W, Chezmar J L, Torres W E, Murphy F B, Bernardino M E 1988 Incidence of cholelithiasis among patients with cirrhosis and portal hypertension. Gastrointestinal Radiology 13: 347–350

Sternlieb J M, Aronchick C A, Retig J N et al 1992 A multicenter, randomized, controlled trial to evaluate the effect of prophylactic octreotide on ERCP-induced pancreatitis. American Journal of Gastroenterology 87: 1561–1566

Stolte M, Weiss W, Volkholz H, Rosch W 1984. A special form of segmental pancreatitis: 'Groove Pancreatitis'. Hepatogastroenterologica 29: 198–208

Tanaka M, Ikeda S 1983 Parapapillary choledochoduodenal fistula: an analysis of 83 consecutive patients diagnosed at ERCP. Gastrointestinal Endoscopy 29: 88–89

Thomas M J, Pellegrini C A, Way L W 1982 Usefulness of diagnostic tests for biliary obstruction. American Journal of Surgery 144: 102–108

Tompkins R K, Saunders K, Roslyn J J, Longmire W P 1990 Changing patterns in diagnosis and management of bile duct cancer. Annals of Surgery 211: 614–621

Tompkins R K, Thomas D, Wile A, Longmire W P 1981 Prognostic factors in bile duct carcinoma. Annals of Surgery 194: 447–457

Tylen U, Hoevels J, Nilsson U 1981 Computed tomography of iatrogenic hepatic lesions following percutaneous transhepatic cholangiography and portography. Journal of Computer Assisted Tomography 5: 15–18

Van Sonnenberg E, Ferrucci J T, Neff C C, Mueller P R, Simeone J F, Wittenberg J 1983 Biliary pressure: Manometric and perfusion studies at percutaneous cholangiography and percutaneous biliary drainage. Radiology 148: 41–50

Voyles C R, Bowley N J, Allison D J, Benjamin I S, Blumgart L H 1983 Carcinoma in choledochal cysts. Age-related incidence. Archives of Surgery 118: 986–988

Warren K W, Mountain J C, Loyd-Jones W 1972 Malignant tumours of the bile ducts. British Journal of Surgery 59: 501–505

Weismuller J, Gail K, Seifert E 1983 Maligner extrahepatischer Gallenwegsverschluss. Diagnostik und palliative Therapie. Deutsche Medizinische Woschenschrift 108: 203

Weschsler R L, Wechsler L 1975 The first application of transhepatic cholangiography to the localization of liver or biliary tract pathology: Hanoi, 1937. American Journal of Digestive Diseases 20: 699–700

Wetter L A, Ring E J, Pellegrini C A, Way L W 1991 Differential diagnosis of sclerosing cholangitis of the common hepatic duct (Klatskin tumors). American Journal of Surgery 161: 57–63

Wilkinson M L, Mieli-Vergani G, Ball C, Portmann B, Mowat A P 1991 Endoscopic retrograde cholangiopancreatography in infantile cholestasis. Archives of Diseases of Children 66: 121–123

Wilson C, Auld C D, Schlinkert R et al Hepatobiliary complications in chronic pancreatitis. Gut 30: 520–527

Winters C, Chobassian S J, Benjamin S B, Ferguson R K, Catran E L 1984 Endoscopic documentation of Ascaris-induced acute pancreatitis. Gastrointestinal Endoscopy 30: 83–84

Wong J, Choi T K 1984 Recurrent pyogenic cholangitis. In: Okuda K, Nakayama L, Wong J (eds) Intrahepatic calculi. Alan R Liss, New York, p 175–192

Woods S D, Chung S C, Leung J W, Chan A C, Li A K 1989 Hypoxia and tachycardia during endoscopic retrograde cholangiopancreatography: detection by pulse oximetry. Gastrointestinal Endoscopy 35: 523–525

Yamada M, Kozuka S, Yamao K, Nakazawa S, Naitoh Y 1991 Mucin-producing tumour of the pancreas. Cancer 68: 159–168

Yellin A E, Donovan A J 1981 Biliary lithiasis and helminthiasis. American Journal of Surgery 142: 128–135

Zidi S H, Prat F, Le Guen O, Rondeau Y, Rocher L, Fritsch J, Choury A D, Pelletier G 1999 Use of magnetic resonance cholangiography in the diagnosis of choledocholithiasis: prospective comparison with a reference imagining method. Gut 44: 118–122

Angiography

18

J.E. JACKSON, A.P. HEMINGWAY, D.J. ALLISON

INTRODUCTION

The medical and scientific significance of the ability to visualize structures angiographically was recognized from the earliest days of radiology. In January 1896, just two months after Roentgen had delivered his historic manuscript reporting the discovery of X-rays to the Physical Medical Society of Wurzburg, Haschek and Lindenthal produced a radiograph showing the injected vessels of an amputated hand (Haschek & Lindenthal 1896). During the next 2 decades detailed anatomical X-ray studies were obtained of the vascular system in animals and man by workers in both Europe and America, and it is astonishing to reflect on the fact that the first X-ray atlas of the arterial tree was published (in England) as long ago as 1920 (Orrin 1920). During the 1920s attention turned to obtaining arteriograms in vivo, and substances such as Lipiodol, strontium bromide, sodium iodide, thorotrast, and selectan were used in man to obtain peripheral arteriograms and venograms, aortic and pulmonary arteriograms and even cerebral arteriograms.

Portuguese workers such as Egas Moniz, Reynaldo dos Santos and Lopo de Carvalho were pre-eminent among the pioneers of human arteriography (Veiga-Pires & Grainger 1982), and the extent of their contribution has not been sufficiently acknowledged by many who have followed in their footsteps. The significance of the work they did was not lost on their contemporaries, however; when Moniz returned to Portugal after presenting his epoch-making paper entitled, 'Arterial encephalography, its importance in the localization of brain tumors' to the Academy of Medicine in Paris in 1928, he received a salutation from the combined professors of the Medicine Faculty at the railway station! (Goncalves 1982). Another pioneer in the field of arteriography was Forssmann who was particularly interested in techniques for visualizing the heart and pulmonary

vessels (Forssmann 1931). In 1928 after practising on a cadaver, he passed a catheter from his own antecubital vein into the right atrium, a procedure that not only paved the way for subsequent development in cardiac catheterization, but must also surely be remembered as one of the most courageous feats of self-experimentation in modern medicine.

In the early days of arteriography, vessel exposure by incision was required for vascular catheterization and, though this technique is still used in certain circumstances, percutaneous arterial puncture is the preferred method in most cases. Percutaneous puncture was used at first simply to introduce contrast medium directly through a needle into a vessel, but a major advance came with the introduction of percutaneous techniques for the introduction of catheters into blood vessels (Lindgren 1950, Peirce & Ramey 1953), and the 'percutaneous catheter replacement technique of Seldinger' (Seldinger 1953) introduced in 1953 soon became, and remains, the most widely used method of angiographic catheterization.

As vascular puncture and catheterization techniques developed, together with improvements in contrast media and catheters and the introduction of rapid film-changers, it became possible to obtain high-quality arteriograms of all the principal vascular beds in the body. Angiography rapidly occupied a vital place in diagnostic medicine and became not only an indispensable investigation in branches such as vascular surgery, cardiac surgery, neurosurgery and more recently gastrointestinal and hepatic surgery, but played no small part in influencing the actual direction of development of these and other specialities.

During the 1970s diagnostic arteriography, having reached its zenith, began a slow decline in importance as many of its roles were supplanted by less invasive and, for the most part, technically easier imaging techniques such as ultrasound (US), radionuclide studies, computerized tomography (CT) and, more recently, magnetic resonance imaging (MRI). This decline in the relative diagnostic value of the technique seems certain to continue, though its progress was considerably modified in the late 1980s by two factors. The first, *digital subtraction angiography* (DSA) is a technique which enables diagnostic images to be obtained using smaller quantities of contrast medium than was previously required and allows the electronic manipulation and review of data to be performed with great speed and facility. The second major factor influencing modern arteriographic practice was the introduction of the low-osmolality and non-ionic contrast media (Grainger 1997). These media do not give the sensation of intense heat or pain that conventional contrast agents induce when injected into vessels. They also cause less damage to the vascular endothelium and have fewer systemic toxic effects that the older agents.

Despite the improvements that these two advances have brought about in the comfort, speed, safety and diagnostic accuracy of arteriography, the current developments in ultrasound and, in particular, MRI make the demise of a large part (perhaps the majority) of current diagnostic work in arteriography seem inevitable.

It behoves all angiographers, wedded though they may be to the subspeciality, to accept with good grace and, indeed, encourage any developments that improve the safety and accuracy of diagnosis for the patient; it is both foolish and wrong to persist in using arteriographic techniques in clinical situations where equal or better diagnostic information can be obtained by less invasive techniques if these are readily available. In many areas of diagnosis, of course, arteriography still reigns supreme because of the outstanding resolution of its images and anatomical nature of its information display, and this will remain true for many years. The note of caution sounded above, however, will apply with increasing validity during the decade to come and arteriographers will have a crucial part to play in the critical evaluation of new techniques in comparison with the 'gold standard' of arteriography. One area where the future of arteriography does seem assured is in its therapeutic applications. Interventional vascular radiology, notably selective perfusion, angioplasty in all its forms, transjugular intrahepatic porto-systemic stent shunt (TIPS) insertion and embolization depend upon good angiographic technique for their success.

TECHNIQUE

The risks associated with modern angiography are extremely small. Angiography is still nevertheless an invasive proce-

dure and it should never be undertaken unless the radiologist is satisfied that the likely benefits justify the potential risks. An angiogram should never be done simply because it has been scheduled or 'routinely requested' by a clinical team; mistakes inevitably occur and the radiologist responsible for the procedure should be satisfied in every case that proper indications exist for the particular study requested. The angiographer should also be quite clear before starting as to what information is required from the procedure; this ensures that the correct studies and projections are obtained and allows rational decision-making during the procedure if something unexpected is shown or a problem arises.

PATIENT PREPARATION

Informed consent should be obtained for angiography. A doctor, preferably the responsible radiologist or a member of the radiology department, should see the patient before the procedure to explain what is to be done, check that no contraindications to the study exist, check the appropriate pulses and insure that adequate premedication is arranged. The groin should be shaved if a femoral approach is to be used. It has been the usual practice for patients to be on 'nil by mouth' for an appropriate period prior to the procedure to avoid the risk of aspiration during a possible contrast reaction or other serious accident. It is now the policy in many departments, however, only to stop solid foods and to permit free oral fluids unless general anesthesia or heavy premedication is being used. Whatever regimen is adopted adequate measures should be taken to avoid dehydration during the procedure and the recovery period.

CONTRAINDICATIONS

There are very few absolute contraindications to angiography but there are many factors which considerably increase the hazards of the technique. Always check that a patient is not *pregnant* before angiography as the radiation dose may be considerable. If angiography is essential in a pregnant patient, the dose to the fetus should be minimized by protection, field collimation and careful choice of filming sequences. Caution should be exercised in patients on *anticoagulant* therapy or with other *bleeding diatheses*, a point of particular relevance in patients with liver disorders. Arteriography should be avoided if possible in such cases; if it is essential then all possible steps should be taken to correct or improve the coagulation defect before and during the procedure if this is clinically acceptable. Other factors which increase the risk of bleeding from an arterial puncture site include systemic hypertension and disorders predisposing to increased fragility of the vessel wall such as Cushing's syndrome, prolonged steroid treatment and rare connective tissue disorders such as certain types of the *Ehlers–Danlos* syndrome. If angiography should prove to be necessary in patients with suspected or proven previous adverse reaction to iodinated contrast medium, appropriate steroid prophylaxis should be administered (Grainger 1997); alternatively carbon dioxide could be used (Kerns et al 1995, Yang et al 1995).

Arteriography can require larger doses of contrast medium than any other radiological procedure and particular care must be exercised in: infants, dehydrated or shocked patients, patients with serious cardiac or respiratory disease, patients in hepatic or renal failure and other patients with serious metabolic abnormalities.

ANESTHESIA

Most angiography is now performed under local anesthesia, though general anesthesia is necessary for babies and young children, confused, difficult or very nervous patients, and some complex interventional procedures. Although general anesthesia can be more pleasant for the patient than local anesthesia and reduces motion artefact on the radiographs, it nevertheless adds to the risks of angiography. This is not only because of the (small) risks inherent in general anesthesia, but also because it masks the patient's subjective symptoms and reactions. These may provide the radiologist with immediate warning of a mishap such as the subintimal injection of contrast medium or the inadvertent wedging of the catheter tip in a small artery, a warning which may well prevent more serious injury. A further point to remember is that many patients being investigated for 'surgical' liver disorders may well be operated on within a day or two of angiography and will then require another general anesthetic within a short period. When local anesthesia is to be used the patient should be sedated with a suitable premedication. This should contain an analgesic as most procedures cause some discomfort: it is not only kinder to the patient to make the study as painless as possible but it makes for appreciably better angiography. Premedication should be prescribed according to patient age and weight. Operators and clinicians must be aware of the sedative effects of the drugs administered and the potential for cardiorespiratory depression, a particular hazard in patients with advanced liver disease whose ability to metabolize certain compounds may be compromised. Patients must be carefully monitored. Pulse oximetry is advised for all patients and full resuscitation equipment, including drugs to reverse sedation and analgesia must be available at all times (Royal Colleges of Anaesthetists and Radiologists 1992).

It is also very important that the vascular puncture site is adequately anesthetized; 5–10 ml of 1–2% lignocaine should be infiltrated around the vein or artery; inadequate initial anesthesia not only causes patient discomfort but also predisposes to arterial spasm and restricts free catheter movement.

ARTERIAL PUNCTURE AND CATHETERIZATION

The majority of arterial studies are performed percutaneously via the femoral artery in the groin. The vessel is punctured using the Seldinger technique (Seldinger 1953) (Fig. 18.1). Occasionally it is necessary to use other routes of arterial access such as axillary or brachial artery puncture, or brachial artery cutdown. By manipulating the catheter under fluoroscopic control it is possible to insert the catheter selectively into various branches of the vascular system such as the renal artery, celiac axis and superior mesenteric artery. Different catheter shapes are available (Fig. 18.2) each of which is suitable for a particular maneuver or for catheterizing certain arterial branches. Superselective (subselective) catheterization of small subsidiary arteries

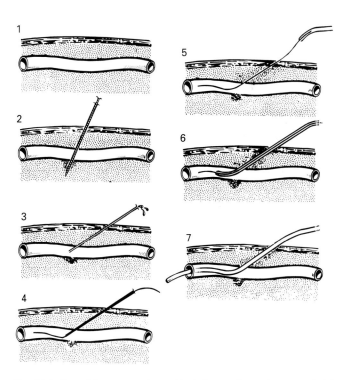

Fig. 18.1 One of the commonly used techniques of percutaneous arterial catheterization. The artery (1) is transfixed (2). The needle is partially withdrawn and re-angled (3). A guidewire is passed into the needle during free back-flow of blood (3, 4). The needle is removed and a catheter or introducer inserted over the wire (5, 6). When the catheter is safely within the arterial lumen the wire is withdrawn (7).

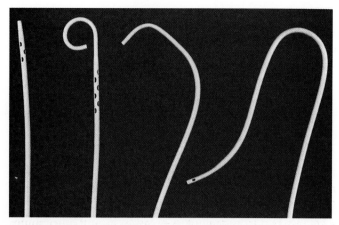

Fig. 18.2 Some of the many different available catheter shapes are illustrated. From left to right: straight 'flush,' 'pigtail,' 'cobra,' and 'sidewinder.' Note the side ports on some of the catheters.

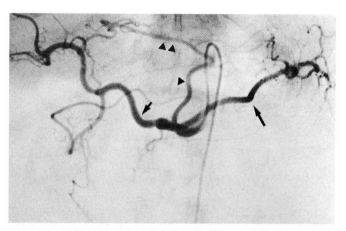

Fig. 18.3 Celiac axis arteriogram using a sidewinder catheter. The splenic (long arrow), left gastric (single arrowhead) and common hepatic arteries (short arrow) are well demonstrated. Note that the left gastric artery also gives rise to an accessory left hepatic artery (double arrowhead).

such as the pancreaticoduodenal arteries or intrahepatic branch vessels is routinely performed for embolization procedures (Ch. 77). Arteriographic anatomy is described in Chapter 1.

In the evaluation of liver disease it is necessary to inject selectively the celiac axis and the superior mesenteric artery.

The celiac axis

The celiac axis is the artery of the primitive foregut and through its three branches (left gastric, splenic and common hepatic) it supplies the stomach and upper duodenum, spleen, liver and pancreas (Fig. 18.3 and Fig. 18.4). The celiac stem arises from the front of the aorta at the level of L1; it can be catheterized with a femoral-visceral catheter, but a sidewinder catheter (Fig. 18.2) is preferred by the authors because it is less likely to be dislodged during a pump injection and can be further manipulated if necessary into the splenic or hepatic arteries in almost all patients. Super-selective studies of the left gastric, gastroduodenal, dorsal pancreatic and hepatic vessels (Fig. 18.5) can be obtained with appropriate catheters.

Oblique views are necessary for the complete demonstration of the duodenum and pancreas.

Using a digital subtraction technique (DSA), the celiac territory can normally be adequately opacified in the average

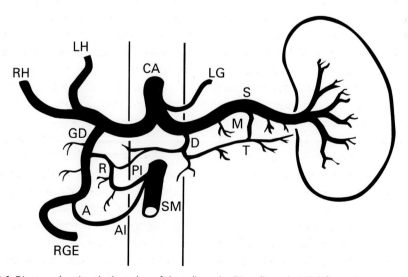

Fig. 18.4 Diagram showing the branches of the celiac axis. CA, celiac axis; LG, left gastric artery; S, splenic artery; M, arteria pancreatica magna; D, dorsal pancreatic artery; SM, superior mesenteric artery; T, transverse pancreatic artery; PI, posterior inferior pancreaticoduodenal artery; AI, anterior inferior pancreaticoduodenal artery; A, anterior superior pancreaticoduodenal artery; R, retroduodenal artery (posterior superior pancreaticoduodenal artery); GD, gastroduodenal artery; RH, right hepatic artery; LH, left hepatic artery; RGE, right gastroepiploic artery.

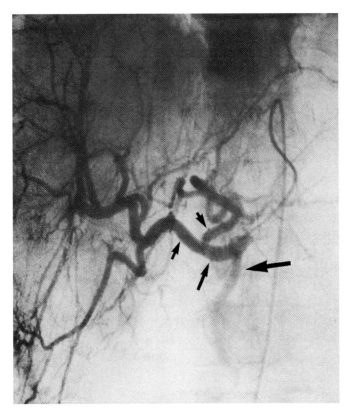

Fig. 18.5 Selective hepatic arteriogram. A sidewinder catheter has been positioned in the common hepatic artery with its tip just proximal to the origin of the gastroduodenal artery which is faintly opacified (large arrow). The proper hepatic artery (midsized arrow) divides into the right and left hepatic branches (short arrow).

adult by 25–40 ml contrast medium containing 250–350 mg iodine/ml delivered at 8–10 ml/s by a mechanical injector. Pump injections are often also necessary for splenic or common hepatic arteriograms, but hand injections suffice for superselective studies. One of the major disadvantages of DSA is that of movement artefact due to bowel peristalsis and patient respiration. The bowel should, therefore, be paralysed using an antimotility agent such as hyoscine (Buscopan) and each DSA acquisition is usually performed during suspended respiration. The radiographic filming sequence should extend sufficiently long to allow visualization for the portal venous system providing an *indirect splenoportogram* (see below). This occurs in 8–14 s after injection in most patients, but may take longer in the presence of splenomegaly or portal obstruction when venous images may be difficult to obtain due to the inability of the patients to hold their breath for a sufficient length of time. In such cases the angiogram is best performed with the patient breathing normally throughout; multiple images are obtained prior to the injection of contrast medium so that a suitable mark is available for each (or most) of the subsequent images. This technique is also useful in patients who are unable to hold their breath for even short periods of time.

Hepatic arteriography is usually performed for the assessment of liver tumors (primary or secondary) or hepatic arterial bleeding.

The hepatic vessels are best vizualized by selective catheterization and consistent success requires an experienced operator with a good knowledge of the variable vascular anatomy of the region. With conventional equipment, 15–20 ml of contrast medium (approximately 250–350 mg iodine/ml) injected by hand or with a pressure injector at a rate of 5–8 ml/s into the common hepatic artery provide an adequate demonstration of the vasculature. In many cases requiring hepatic angiography, more selective studies of individual vessels will be necessary and these will require proportionately smaller volumes of contrast medium.

The arterial and parenchymal phases of the study are usually of the greatest interest. Until the advent of DSA, the hepatic veins were only visualized in an arterial study if abnormal shunts were present (e.g. Osler–Weber–Rendu disease), but with the enhanced contrast resolution provided by digital studies the venous phase is now commonly seen in the absence of any known hepatic pathology (Fig. 18.6).

The portal vein is only shown on selective hepatic arteriography if flow reversal has taken place or, more commonly, if an arterioportal shunt exists. Such shunts are extremely important because they may be misdiagnosed as tumors or other causes of abnormal vascular staining. Opacified blood from the hepatic artery enters a radical of the portal vein and produces a cone-shaped segmental portal 'blush'. If this cone is at right angles to the X-ray beam its segmental nature will usually be obvious; if, on the other hand, it is in the line of the beam, only the round base of the cone will be visualized and it will look like a rounded lesion (Fig. 18.7).

An arterioportal fistula may be caused by any penetrating injury of the liver, and such lesions have become increasingly common owing to the increased use of percutaneous diagnostic and interventional techniques. It follows from this that if an abnormal vascular 'blush' is seen on hepatic arteriography in any patient who has previously undergone liver biopsy, percutaneous transhepatic, biliary drainage or any other percutaneous hepatic procedure, the possibility of an arterioportal fistula must be borne in mind. Such fistulae resolve spontaneously in the majority of cases; large or persistent lesions should be treated by selective arterial embolization as the shunting may increase progressively and result in portal hypertension.

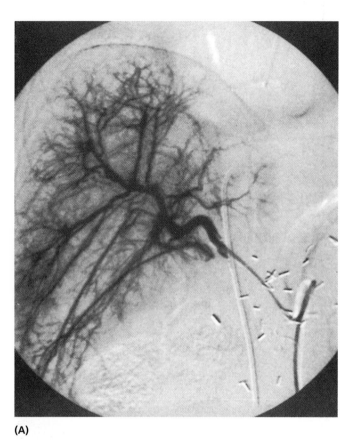

(A)

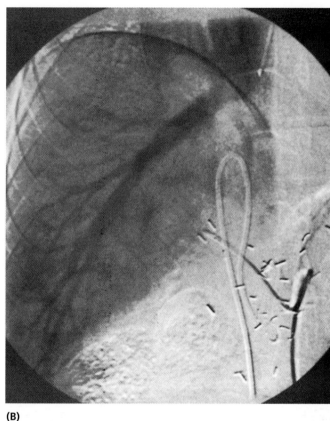

(B)

Fig. 18.6 Hepatic veins shown on DSA. **(A)** Hepatic arteriogram in a postoperative patient. **(B)** Late films showing the hepatic veins on DSA.

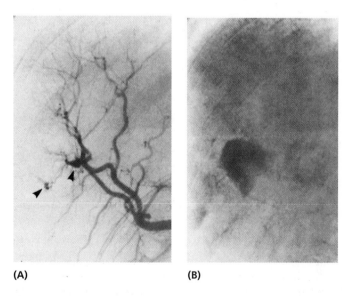

(A)   (B)

Fig. 18.7 Hepatic arteriogram in a patient who had undergone a PTC 2 days earlier. **(A)** Arterial phase (arrows point to a small arterioportal fistulae). **(B)** Capillary phase; dense 'blushes' due to portal venous staining.

The superior mesenteric artery

The superior mesenteric artery (SMA) supplies the bowel derived from the primitive mid-gut, from the mid-duodenum to the splenic flexure. It arises from the front of the aorta 1 cm below the celiac axis and is easily catheterized selectively in most individuals with a sidewinder or femoral-visceral catheter. Contrast medium (25–40 ml) containing approximately 250–350 mg iodine/ml, injected at 8–10 ml/s from an automatic injector (or by hand in some individuals) will opacify the SMA in the average adult (Figs 18.8A and 18.8B). It is important to continue filming up to 20 s after the contrast injection. This allows visualization of the superior mesenteric and portal veins. It is also of great importance to ensure that the presence of an accessory right hepatic artery (Ch. 1) is not missed by having the tip of the catheter too far into the stem of the SMA (Figs 18.8C and 18.8D).

Bowel movement should be inhibited using glucagon or Buscopan and it is again vital that respiratory movement is stopped during the acquisition of images—a noseclip is particularly useful in this respect as many patients simply continue to breath through their nose after closing their mouth! Alternatively a breathing technique, as discussed

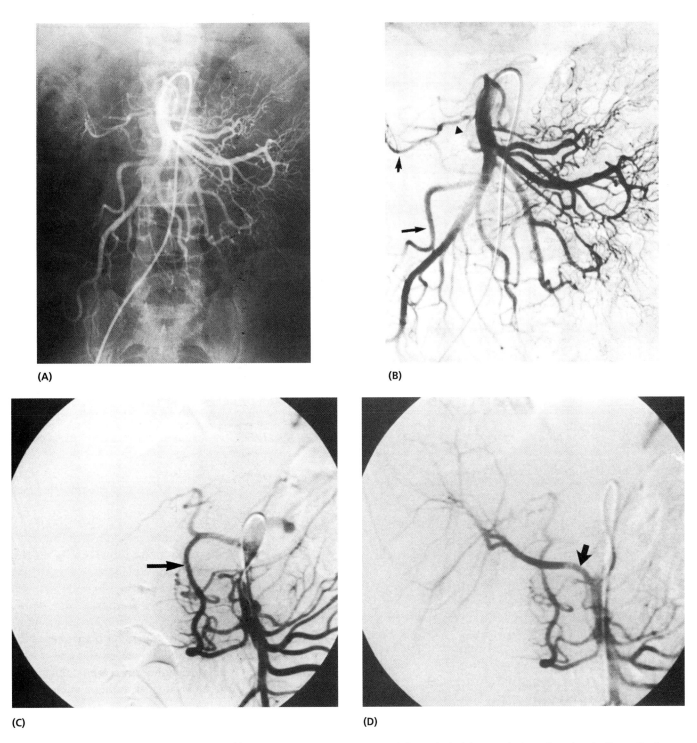

(A)

(B)

(C)

(D)

Fig. 18.8 (A,B) Superior mesenteric arteriogram. The upper branches on the patient's left supply the jejunum, the lower branches the ileum. On the right are the middle colic artery (arrowhead) the right colic artery (short arrow) and the ileocolic artery (long arrow). The continuation of the main arterial stem ultimately forms the left-hand limb of the ileocolic anastomotic loop. **(A)** The angiogram unsubtracted. **(B)** The subtraction point of the same study. **(C)** Superior mesenteric angiogram. The catheter is selectively inserted into the SMA. Following the injection of contrast medium there is filling of the SMA and retrograde filling of the celiac axis via the gastroduodenal artery (arrow). Note that there is no evidence of a right hepatic artery arising from the celiac axis. **(D)** Same patient as in **(C)**. The catheter has been withdrawn so that the tip lies nearer the orifice. When a further injection of contrast medium is made the accessory right hepatic arising from the SMA is now visualized (arrow).

above, may be used in those individuals who are unable to hold their breath satisfactorily.

VENOUS ACCESS

The venous system may be studied either directly by puncturing the vein under investigation with a needle or catheter and injecting contrast medium from an antegrade or retrograde approach, or indirectly by injecting the medium into the arterial system and imaging the venous return. In evaluation of hepatobiliary disease it is important to image both the systemic and portal venous systems. The detailed anatomy of these systems is discussed in Chapter 1.

Systemic venography

The hepatic veins are usually catheterized retrogradely; the catheter may be passed from an arm vein, a jugular vein or femoral vein into the hepatic venous system. It is frequently necessary to measure free and wedged hepatic venous pressures in the investigation of liver disease. Wedged hepatic venous pressure measurement requires that a catheter is impacted in a small branch of a hepatic vein. The catheter position is confirmed by the injection of contrast medium, and a dense stain is projected and there may be retrograde opacification of the portal vein, especially in those patients with portal hypertension. Reports have indicated (Casteneda-Zuniga et al 1978) that excess injection pressure may occasionally cause local hepatocellular damage.

Venography, with the catheter lying free in the hepatic veins, requires the injection of about 20–30 ml of contrast medium at a rate of 10–15 ml/s. Filling of the small hepatic venous radicles is assisted if the patient performs a Valsalva maneuver (Fig. 18.9).

Occasionally it is not possible to catheterize the hepatic veins retrogradely due to the presence of a stenosis or occlusion. In this situation direct transhepatic puncture of the hepatic veins can be performed (Fig. 18.10) and although this is rarely required as a diagnostic procedure it may prove very useful in Budd–Chiari syndrome in order to bypass a hepatic venous stenosis or occlusion and allow angioplasty and/or stent insertion (Griffith et al 1996).

The first in vivo *inferior venacavogram* was performed by Dos Santos (1935); he injected radio-opaque material via a saphenous vein cutdown. The technique has been greatly modified since then owing to the introduction of the Seldinger technique and developments in catheters, guidewires and imaging systems. The inferior vena cava can be approached antegradely from the femoral veins or retrogradely via the arm or neck veins. The technique employed depends on the indication and area of interest, but the most

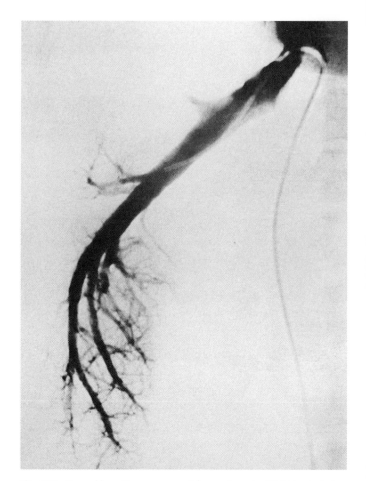

Fig. 18.9 Normal hepatic venogram. A femoral-cerebral III (sidewinder) catheter has been passed from the femoral vein into the inferior vena cava and hence the main right hepatic vein. Contrast medium has been injected into the hepatic vein while the patient performs a Valsalva maneuver. Small intrahepatic venous radicles can be seen.

commonly used approach is the one from the femoral vein. Puncture of the femoral vein has many similarities in technique to puncture of the femoral artery. The vein is not palpable however, to achieve a successful puncture, the operator relies on the fact that the vein is just medial to the artery. The procedure is usually performed under local anesthesia. It is useful to ask the patient to perform a Valsalva maneuver during the puncture as this temporarily distends the vein.

Once the catheter has been positioned satisfactorily then 20–40 ml of contrast medium is injected at a rate of 10–20 ml/s. Images are acquired at two films per second (Fig. 18.11) and the procedure is performed in the antero-posterior and lateral projections. In some cases (e.g. Budd–Chiari syndrome) it may be necessary to record pressure measurements.

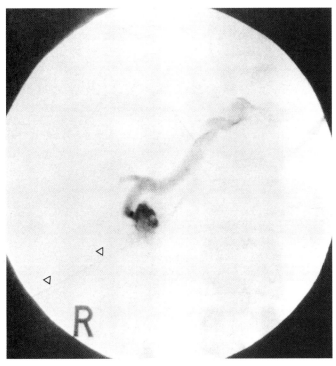

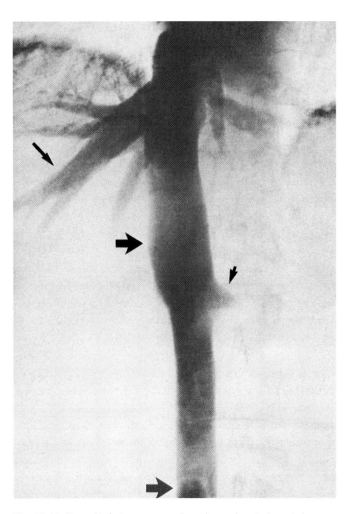

Fig. 18.10 Direct (hepatic) venogram. Retrograde right hepatic venography had been attempted but had failed. A Chiba needle (arrowheads) has been passed through the liver substance into a venous radicle. Contrast has been injected and a right hepatic vein has been opacified. A stenosis was demonstrated at the junction of the vein with the inferior vena cava.

Fig. 18.11 Normal inferior vena cava (broad arrow); anterioposterior projection. Contrast medium has been injected via the right femoral vein. The patient has performed a Valsalva maneuver during the contrast injection and reflux has occurred into the hepatic veins (long arrow) and the left renal vein (short arrow).

Portal venography

Visualization of the portal venous system may be helpful in the diagnosis of portal hypertension and is essential for its proper management. It may also be of great value in the evaluation of other liver disease and pancreatic disease (see below). The portal vein was first demonstrated by the direct injection of contrast medium into the main vein or one of its tributaries at laparotomy. This technique was devised by Blakemore and Lord (1945). In 1951, Abeatici and Campi demonstrated that contrast medium injected into the spleen flowed into the splenic and portal veins and, in the same year, Leger performed the first successful direct percutaneous splenoportogram in man. It was noted in the early 1950s that the portal vein was occasionally faintly visualized after injection of contrast medium into the aorta (Rigler et al 1953) and in 1958 Odman demonstrated the portal vein after injection of contrast medium into the celiac axis. In recent years developments in equipment (especially DSA), angiographic techniques and contrast agents have further improved the accuracy and safety of portography.

The portal venous system can be outlined in the following ways:

- Direct methods
  — percutaneous splenoportography
  — transjugular transhepatic portography
  — percutaneous transhepatic portography
  — perioperative mesenteric portography
  — transumbilical portography
  — transjugular portography
- Indirect methods
  — arterioportography
  — wedged hepatic venography.

The quality and wide availability of modern DSA systems has so improved the images available on indirect arterioportography that the direct methods are now used in only the most exceptional clinical circumstances.

Direct percutaneous splenoportography

This technique is now of historical interest only and will not be discussed further.

Transhepatic portography (Lunderquist & Ivancev 1997)

This technique was first described by Bierman et al (1952). Subsequent workers have modified the technique from the original simple needle puncture of an intra-hepatic portal venous radicle to sophisticated catheterization techniques. It is important that the procedure is not performed in patients with deranged blood coagulation. The portal vein is best punctured under ultrasound control. A catheter inserted transhepatically into the portal vein can be used for venography, venous sampling or embolization techniques. At the end of the procedure the catheter track can be embolized with absorbable gelatin sponge.

Complications (Lunderquist & Ivancev 1997). Complications of the procedure include: hemorrhage from the liver surface into the peritoneum or within the liver substance into the biliary system; fistula formation (arterioportal, arteriobiliary); portal vein thrombosis; biliary peritonitis; puncture of the gallbladder or colon (particularly in very sick patients who are unable to suspend respiration); pneumothorax; intrapleural bleed; pleural effusion; and biliary-pleural fistula.

Indications. The major indication for this technique nowadays is for the embolization of intrahepatic portal venous branches in order to induce liver hypertrophy in the non-embolized segments (Chs 54 & 87). Transhepatic cannulation of the portal vein may also be used for venous sampling procedures when a pancreatic hormone secreting tumor is suspected clinically, but cannot be localized by less invasive means (Allison 1980, Lunderquist & Ivancev 1997). Multiple samples are taken from the splenic, superior and inferior mesenteric veins, and also selectively from pancreatic veins. Simultaneous hepatic venous and arterial samples may also be obtained to assess whether or not functioning hepatic metastases are present and allow arteriovenous hormone gradients to be estimated. This technique has, however, been largely supplanted by that of arterial stimulation venous sampling (O'Shea et al 1996).

A transjugular, transhepatic approach to the portal vein is used for insertion of an intrahepatic portosystemic stent shunt (Ch. 101) for the treatment of variceal hemorrhage or ascites which is resistant to medical therapy. The other direct methods of portal venous opacification are largely obsolete due to improvements in imaging technology and indirect portography.

Indirect portography (arterioportography)

All the direct methods of opacifying the portal venous system are associated with a small but definite incidence of morbidity (Bron 1983). Indirect or arterioportography has not only the advantage of being less hazardous than many of the direct methods, but it can be combined with a study of the arterial system as well. It is also possible, by selective injections into the celiac axis (or splenic artery), superior mesenteric artery and inferior mesenteric artery, to opacify the splenic and mesenteric veins as well as the portal vein.

Technique. The splenic or superior mesenteric artery (or both) are selectively catheterized and films are exposed for up to 40 s following the injection of contrast medium, e.g. 30–40 ml at 7–10 ml/s (Figs 18.12, 18.13 and 18.14). Larger quantities of contrast medium may be required in patients with splenomegaly. The radiographs that are taken following the injection of contrast medium should be centered so that the lower esophagus is included on the film in order that varices are not missed. Oblique views may be needed to properly visualize the division into right and left intrahepatic portal branches.

Portal venous opacification may be improved by the intraarterial injection of a vasodilator (papaverine 15–30 mg or Tolazoline 30–50 mg) immediately before the angiogram. The dose of contrast medium injected should be increased when this technique is utilized.

Indications. The major indications for arterioportography are listed in Table 18.1. The portal vein may also be indirectly visualized by performing wedged hepatic venography and this may be usefully employed when performing a TIPS procedure in order to localize the right portal venous branches to aid in their transhepatic puncture. Iodinated contrast medium or carbon dioxide may be used (Sheppard et al 1998).

Table 18.1 Indications for arterioportography

Assessment of portal hypertension
Delineation and extent of varices
Evaluation of portosystemic shunts
Assessment of operability of hepatic biliary or pancreatic neoplasms
Assessment of feasibility of therapeutic hepatic arterial embolization

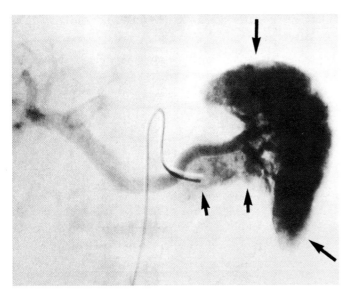

(A)

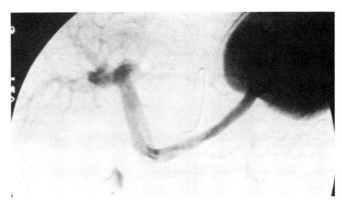

Fig. 18.13 Indirect splenoportogram using digital subtraction techniques. Diluted contrast medium (15 ml) was injected into the splenic artery.

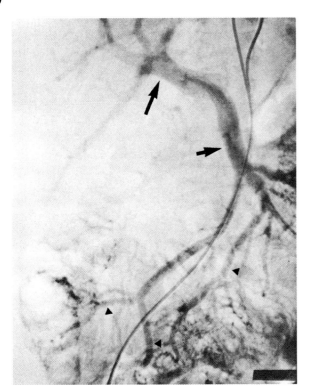

(B)

Fig. 18.12 (A) Indirect splenoportogram. A catheter has been placed selectively in the splenic artery. Contrast medium has been injected and films taken to 20 s. The spleen (long arrows) and tail of the pancreas (short arrows) are both opacified with contrast medium. The splenic vein, main portal vein and intrahepatic portal venous radicles are seen. **(B)** Superior mesenteric venogram. Late films have been taken following an injection of contrast medium into the superior mesenteric artery; the superior mesenteric vein (short arrow) and portal vein (long arrow) are demonstrated.

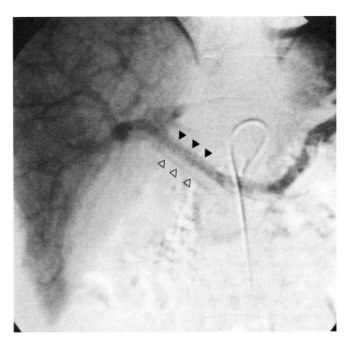

Fig. 18.14 Portal vein 'streaming.' A splenic arterial injection has opacified the splenic blood. In the portal vein the splenic blood (solid arrowheads) is seen outlining the upper axial portion of the vein, while unopacified blood from the superior mesenteric system is occupying the lower axial portion of the vessel (open arrowheads).

CT arterial portography (CTAP)

In patients with hepatic metastases who are being assessed for partial hepatectomy, CTAP should be considered (Matsui et al 1987, Seneterre et al 1996). This is presently the most sensitive technique for the demonstration of hepatic metastases and is therefore useful in those patients being considered on the basis of non-invasive imaging studies for hepatic resection. Magnetic resonance imaging scans using superparamagnetic iron oxide contrast media is the most sensitive non-invasive technique for detecting liver metastases (Blakeborough et al 1997) and should preferably be performed prior to CTAP to avoid an unnecessary invasive examination.

In CTAP, contrast medium is delivered selectively into the superior mesenteric artery (or less commonly the splenic artery) and a spiral CT scan is then performed through the liver during the portal venous phase of the study. Liver metastases, which derive their blood supply almost exclusively from the hepatic artery, are thus seen as areas of low attenuation within the surrounding enhanced normal liver parenchyma. Flow artefacts are relatively common and may cause some problems with interpretation as these tend to occur at certain well-recognized sites. Occasionally a second delayed spiral scan may be performed to aid in interpretation of the images.

AFTERCARE

When an arteriographic study is completed the catheter is withdrawn and firm manual pressure applied to the puncture site for 5–10 min. The radiologist should be absolutely satisfied that bleeding has stopped before the patient leaves the angiography suite. The wound site is then checked at regular intervals by the nursing staff who should also record pulse and blood pressure observations for a reasonable period following the procedure and check that distal pulses remain palpable. Pressure pads, sandbags and other accoutrements are generally a waste of time. It is much better to be able to see the puncture site than to cover it up. If bleeding does not stop from a puncture site, press for a longer period! Almost all postcatheterization bleeding can ultimately be controlled by local pressure unless the artery has been torn or there is a serious coagulation abnormality.

An adequate record of the procedure should be entered in the patient's case notes. This should include the date, the name of the operator, the names and doses of anesthetic agents, the volumes and concentrations of contrast medium and other drugs administered, preliminary findings, any complications during the procedure, the integrity or otherwise of the pulse peripheral to the puncture site at the end of the procedure, and the post-procedural nursing instructions. These notes are important not only for patient care but also as a medicolegal record, and they should be comprehensive and accurate.

COMPLICATIONS

Arteriography is extremely safe and although there are many possible complications (Table 18.2) most of these are rare (Allison & Jackson 1997).

Table 18.2 Complications of arteriography

1. *Complications related to contrast medium*
   Minor adverse reactions
   Major adverse reactions and death
   Local vascular changes (effects on blood cells, viscosity, vascular tone; results of extravasation, etc.)
   Systemic vascular changes (effects on blood volume, osmolality, etc.)
   Individual organ toxicity (heart, kidney, brain, etc.)

2. *Adverse reactions to local anesthetic or other drugs*

3. *Puncture site complications*
   Hemorrhage (external bleeding or hematoma)
   Intramural or perivascular injection of contrast medium
   Vascular thrombosis (dissection, local trauma)
   Peripheral embolization from puncture site
   Vascular stenosis or occlusion
   Aneurysm or pseudoaneurysm formation
   AV fistula
   Local sepsis
   Damage to nerves
   Damage to other local structures

4. *Catheter-related and general complications*
   Catheter thrombus embolism
   Air embolism
   Gauze embolism
   Dissection, perforation or rupture of vessels
   Organ ischemia or infarction secondary to spasm, dissection or embolism
   Interventional accidents
   Fracture and loss of guidewire or catheter fragments
   Knot formation in catheter
   Inadvertent injection of toxic material (e.g. skin cleansing lotion)
   Inadvertent overheparinization
   Vasovagal reaction

INDICATIONS

The indications for vascular studies in hepatobiliary disease can be divided into three broad groups: preoperative angiography, diagnostic angiography and therapeutic angiography.

PREOPERATIVE ANGIOGRAPHY

The indications for preoperative arteriography are relatively few due to the recent improvements in US, CT and MRI. Angiography was routinely used preoperatively to delineate vascular anatomy, to assess vascular involvement by the disease process and to determine venous patency but these are now well visualized in most individuals by non-invasive studies. It is important to detect the presence of any normal anatomical variants such as an accessory right hepatic artery (Figs 18.8C & 18.8D), or the entire hepatic artery arising from the SMA (replaced hepatic artery) and these anomalies will usually be visible on US, CT or MRI. Other common anomalies such as the presence of a left hepatic arterial supply arising from the left gastric artery may be more difficult to appreciate using these imaging modalities and if the detection of such a normal variant is important (as for example when performing a liver resection) then formal arteriography may be required.

Preoperative assessment is rarely necessary prior to the resection of hepatic neoplasms whether benign (Fig. 18.15) or malignant (Fig. 18.16) as their precise location

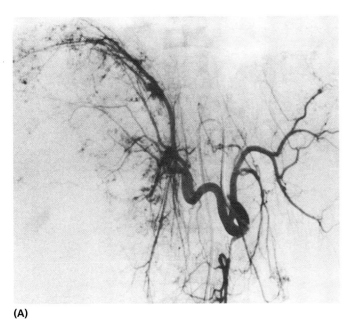

(A)

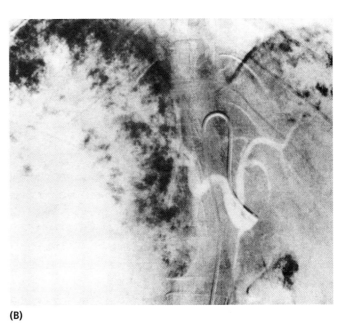

(B)

Fig. 18.15 Celiac axis arteriogram in a young woman shows the characteristic features of a massive benign hemangioma. There is filling of abnormal vascular lakes in the arterial phase **(A)** which retain contrast medium well into the venous phase **(B)** of the study.

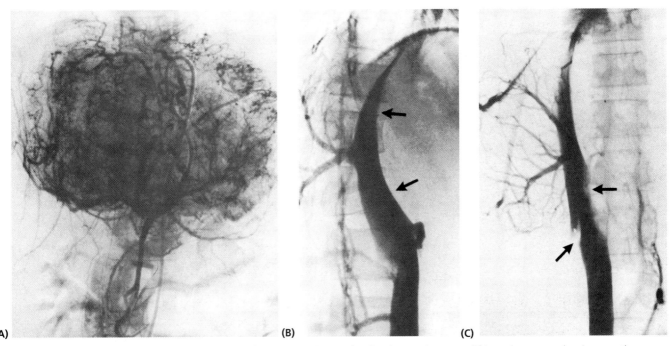

(A)   **(B)**   **(C)**

Fig. 18.16 Inferior vena caval compression by a heptoma. **(A)** Hepatic arteriogram showing the vascular tumor. **(B)** Lateral cavogram showing smooth posterior displacement and compression of cava (arrows). **(C)** Anteroposterior projection showing abnormal filling of the intrahepatic veins due to compression of the principal veins (note their extensive intercommunication). The filling defects in the caval contrast (arrows) are produced by the influx of unopacified blood from the renal veins. This study suggested the vena cava was compressed and displaced but not invaded and the liver tumor was successfully resected (see Ch. 83).

within the liver is best demonstrated on non-invasive cross-sectional images, especially MRI. The exception to this is the preoperative assessment of hilar cholangiocarcinoma (Ch. 54) where arterial and portal venous involvement may be better appreciated on conventional arteriography (Fig. 18.17); even with this tumor, however, MR angiography may soon replace DSA. The presence of a patent main portal vein and patent branch to the uninvolved part of the liver is important in determining resectability and this is usually well seen on US, CT and MRI as is involvement of the inferior vena cava and/or the hepatic veins (see Figs 18.16B & 18.16C). In a proportion of patients undergoing surgery for the repair of a benign biliary stricture secondary to previous surgery it may be important to determine whether or not the portal vein and/or hepatic artery were also damaged at the time of the biliary tract injury (Ch. 49) (Fig. 18.18).

The other group of patients who require preoperative vascular assessment are those with esophageal and/or gastric varices (Fig. 18.19). Prior to shunt surgery it may be necessary to determine caval, splenic, superior mesenteric and left renal vein patency; in the majority of individuals these are adequately assessed non-invasively but conventional arteriography may occasionally be necessary.

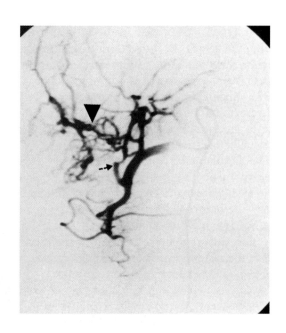

(A)

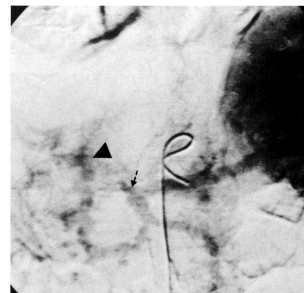

(B)

Fig. 18.18 (A) Selective hepatic arteriography in a woman who had undergone surgery for benign biliary disease, showing disruption of the normal right hepatic artery (arrow), with reconstitution via collateral vessels (arrowhead). **(B)** Indirect splenoportogram in same patient, showing disruption of the main portal vein (arrow) and cavernous transformation (arrowhead).

DIAGNOSTIC ANGIOGRAPHY

CONGENITAL LESIONS

Angiography does not play a major role in the diagnosis of congenital liver anomalies. The diagnosis of the major congenital lesions such as biliary atresia is made clinically and by other imaging modalities.

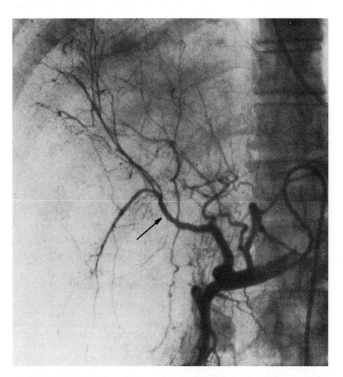

Fig. 18.17 Hepatic arteriogram in a case of cholangiocarcinoma. The tumor is arteriographically avascular but has produced a curved displacement of the right hepatic artery (arrow).

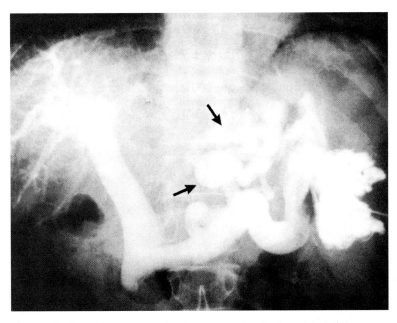

Fig. 18.19 Direct splenoportography. Contrast medium has been injected via a cannula into the splenic pulp. The splenic vein, portal and intrahepatic portal veins are visualized. Massive variceal dilatation of the left gastric vein is demonstrated (arrow). (Direct splenoportography as illustrated here is no longer used. See text.)

ACQUIRED LESIONS

Arteriography plays a considerably less important role than it once did in the diagnosis of intrahepatic neoplasms. It may still occasionally be useful, however, and the angiographic appearance of a number of benign and malignant hepatic tumors will therefore be discussed below.

Intrahepatic neoplasms

Benign tumors (Ch. 72) The most commonly encountered benign intrahepatic tumor is the hemangioma (Alfidi et al 1968, Pantoga 1968, Abrams et al 1969). This term is in fact a misnomer as these lesions are not tumors as the suffix '-oma' implies. They are more correctly termed vascular malformations, most being of a low-flow type; arteriovenous or arterio-portal shunting may, however, be seen in some lesions. Calcification is occasionally seen within these lesions on plain radiography or CT.

The characteristic angiographic appearances consist of abnormal vascular lakes around the periphery of larger lesions which fill in the arterial phase and which retain contrast medium within them well into the venous phase of the study (Fig. 18.15). Caution must be expressed, however, as other lesions including primary hepatocellular carcinomas and metastases can rarely produce an identical appearance. The lesions may be single, multiple, small or large. Depending on their position and size, giant lesions may cause displacement and/or compression of the portal veins

and inferior vena cava. Spontaneous hemorrhage may occur and if subcapsular this may prove fatal (Shearman & Finlayson 1982) although this is rare.

True hepatic hemangiomas occur in infants but are rare and are almost always associated with similar lesions involving the skin. When there is diffuse hepatic involvement massive arteriovenous shunting may result when these tumors pass through their proliferative phase. Angiographically there is massive hypertrophy of the hepatic artery with rapid arteriovenous shunting through numerous vascular hepatic tumors. Spontaneous involution of these lesions will occur in time if the child survives the often severe associated cardiac failure.

Adenomas These are uncommon tumors which are almost always associated with the contraceptive pill, anabolic steroids or abnormal carbohydrate metabolism such as familial diabetes mellitus, glycogen storage disease type 1a and galactosemia (International Working Party 1995). A decrease in size following withdrawal of the precipitating agent is useful for diagnosis. They may achieve a very large size prior to diagnosis and may rupture and bleed spontaneously. They are usually intensely vascular although they are occasionally partly or wholly avascular.

Focal nodular hyperplasia (FNH), which is multiple in about 20 to 30% of cases (Knowles & Wolff 1976, International Working Party 1995), may appear angiographically indistinguishable from an hepatic adenoma but the distinction is important (Casarella et al 1978), as the prognosis and management is different. The lesions are hypervascular (Fig. 18.20) and characteristically a dilated branch of the hepatic artery penetrates the lesion and at its center then divides into small radiating branches; there is a dense granular stain during the hepatogram phase (Casarella et al 1978).

Other benign tumors are rare. Hamartomas occur but the angiographic appearances are not specific and these lesions may undergo cystic degeneration.

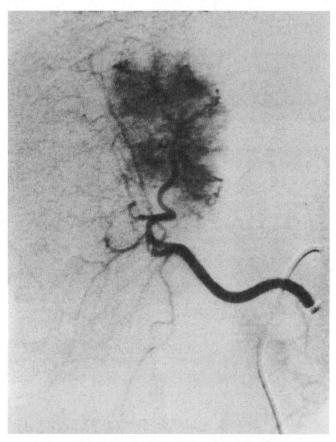

Fig. 18.20 Focal nodular hyperplasia. Selective hepatic arteriogram shows a highly vascular 'tumor,' the artery of supply dividing centrally to give a stellate pattern of vessels.

Primary malignant tumors Primary malignant tumors usually arise from the hepatic parenchyma (hepatocellular carcinoma), the biliary system (cholangiocarcinoma) or the vascular structures (angiosarcoma).

Hepatocellular carcinomas (Ch. 73) Approximately 80% of hepatocellular tumors occur in patients with pre-existing cirrhosis. They may be solitary but are frequently multifocal. They are characteristically hypervascular, showing a bizarre pathological circulation (Figs 18.21A & 18.21B) but occasionally relatively avascular lesions are encountered (Baum

1997). The tumors may reach enormous size and invade or obtain blood supply from adjacent structures such as the diaphragm (Fig. 18.21C) and kidney. The portal vein is frequently involved in the tumor process with frank invasion occurring in almost 50% of tumors. Portal venous invasion is usually associated with arterial to portal venous shunting which may be so massive as to cause reversal of portal venous flow. Angiographically the arterioportal shunting is usually obvious and when very prominent tumor thrombi may be visualized within the portal vein (Okuda et al 1975, Baum 1997).

Angiography plays a decreasing role in the assessment of resectability of hepatomas as their size and the extent of hepatic involvement are well delineated on cross-sectional imaging studies. Many tumors, however, are irresectable at diagnosis and these lesions may respond to chemoembolization or other ablative therapy.

The *fibrolamellar* variant of hepatoma is also usually hypervascular. These lesions are frequently solitary, very large at diagnosis and may appear on imaging to be quite clearly demarcated from the surrounding normal liver. As this type of tumor may respond favorably to resection, even when incomplete, adequate demonstration of its vascular supply and of the systemic and portal venous anatomy is essential (see Fig. 18.16) (Soreide et al 1985). Because they are often very large at presentation marked distortion of the portal and hepatic veins and the inferior vena cava may be present and this may be difficult to assess fully on cross-sectional imaging studies. In such cases preoperative angiography may be very useful.

Cholangiocarcinoma (Ch. 54) The major role of angiography in the assessment of cholangiocarcinoma is in the evaluation of resectability. The diagnosis is usually made by cholangiography, fine needle aspiration or brush cytology and non-invasive imaging. The tumors are typically hypovascular; a faint stain may be seen in the capillary phase, and they frequently cause arterial encasement and portal vein compression, occlusion or invasion (Fig. 18.22) (Walter et al 1976). In the assessment of resectability it is important to determine whether the changes are confined to the vascular supply to the right or left liver and to define the relationship of the vascular and biliary involvement (Soyer et al 1995, Thuluvath et al 1997). Portal venous involvement may occur in the absence of arterial changes and adequate views of both left and right systems should be obtained. Whilst angiography is still performed in most centers to assess the resectability of these tumors recent advances in MRI have meant that this modality may provide all the information required, not only in terms of arterial and portal venous encasement by the tumor but also of bile duct involvement by performing MR cholangiography.

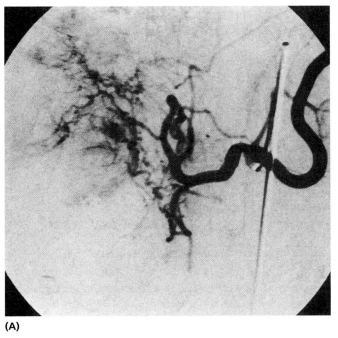

(A)

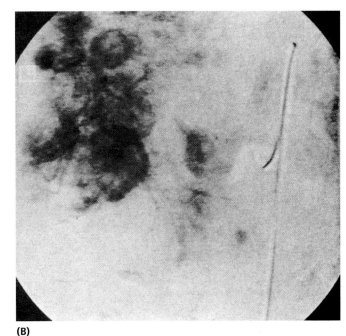

(B)

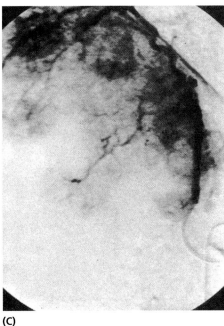

(C)

Fig. 18.21 Selective hepatic arteriography **(A)** shows evidence of a bizarre vascular pattern. In the venous phase **(B)** multiple vascular tumor nodules are seen within the liver parenchyma. The tumor is also being supplied by the phrenic artery **(C)**.

Angiosarcomas These are rare primary malignant tumors which may occur *de novo* but in 40% of cases their development has been linked to exposure to various substances, including vinyl chloride (Whelan et al 1976), thorotrast, arsenicals and radium (Lecker et al 1979). Angiographically the tumors characteristically show peripheral staining with central hypovascularity (Fig. 18.23).

Metastatic disease (Ch. 75) The commonest tumors to involve the liver parenchyma are metastases, their most frequent site of origin being the gastrointestinal tract, followed by the breast and genitourinary tract. Hepatic metastases are supplied almost exclusively by the hepatic artery. The vascularity of metastases is usually similar to that of the primary tumors, vascular primaries giving rise to vascular metastases and avascular primaries giving rise to relatively avascular deposits. The exception to this is a pancreatic tumor when the metastases may be more vascular than the primary (Baum 1997).

Hypervascular metastases frequently arise from neuroendocrine tumors (Fig. 18.24), colorectal primary tumors (Fig. 18.25), chorioncarcinomas, hypernephroma and

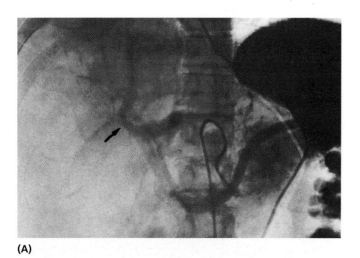

(A)

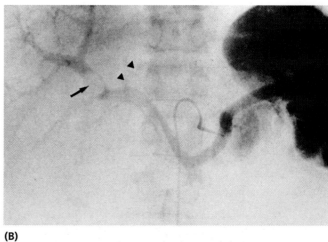

(B)

Fig. 18.22 **(A)** An indirect splenoportogram showing narrowing of the right portal vein due to encasement by tumor (arrow). **(B)** An indirect splenoportogram showing a filling defect in the right portal vein due to invasion of the vein by tumor (arrow). The left portal vein is occluded by tumor (arrowheads).

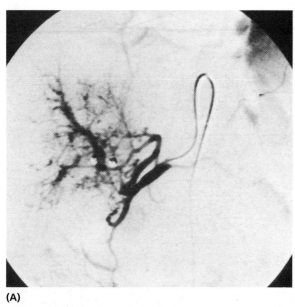

(A)

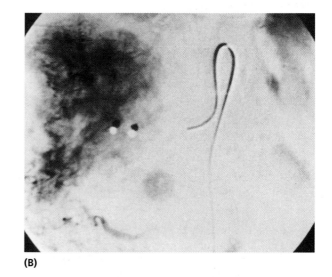

(B)

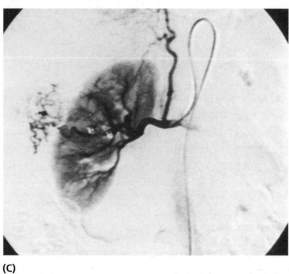

(C)

Fig. 18.23 Angiosarcoma. Arterial **(A)** and venous **(B)** phases from a hepatic arteriogram showing a highly vascular tumor. The two round, well defined opacities seen on both films represent artefacts caused by the presence of two Gianturco embolization coils. This tumor is also supplied by the renal artery **(C)**.

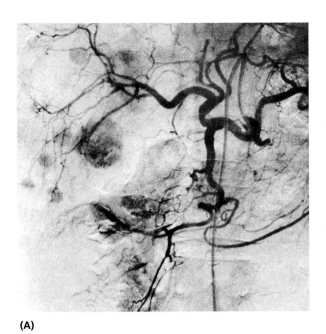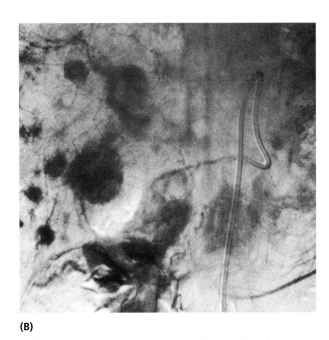

(A)   **(B)**

Fig. 18.24 Glucagonoma metastases. Selective hepatic arteriography shows multiple metastases throughout the liver substance in both the arterial **(A)** and capillary **(B)** phases.

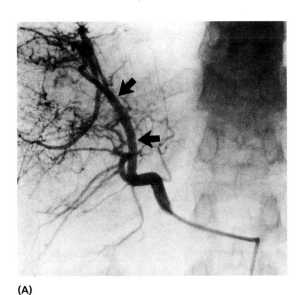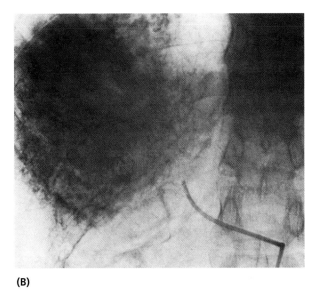

(A)   **(B)**

Fig. 18.25 Metastasis from a colorectal primary. Hepatic arteriography in a case of massive liver metastasis. **(A)** Arterial phase: the tumor deposit is displacing the hepatic artery (arrows). **(B)** Parenchymal phase: there is a dense 'blush' in the large tumor deposit.

leiomysosarcomas. Although angiography is a sensitive tool for diagnosing hypervascular lesions even when quite small, and may occasionally demonstrate tumors not seen on other modalities (Fig. 18.26), the diagnosis of metastatic disease is usually made on cross-sectional imaging studies; the number of lesions and extent of hepatic involvement is often well delineated on a contrast enhanced CT scan or MR scan. Angiography, therefore, has a limited role to play except as part of CT arterial portography (see above) or prior to embolization (Ch. 77).

Hypovascular metastases reveal themselves angiographically by causing displacement and distortion of vessels (arterial and portal venous) and negative filling defects in the hepatogram phase. They may be difficult to appreciate when small.

Extrahepatic neoplasms

Carcinoma of the gallbladder Carcinoma of the gallbladder (Abrams et al 1970, Collier et al 1984) (Ch. 53) may be

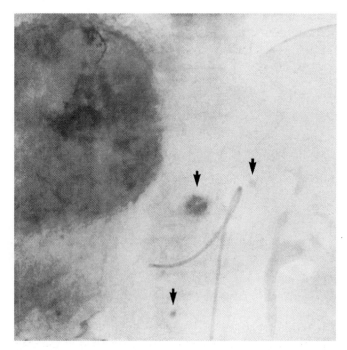

Fig. 18.26 Selective hepatic arteriography in a patient with metastatic tumor deposits in the liver. The large right lobe tumor was shown in CT, but the small deposits in the left lobe (arrows) were only demonstrated on this vascular study.

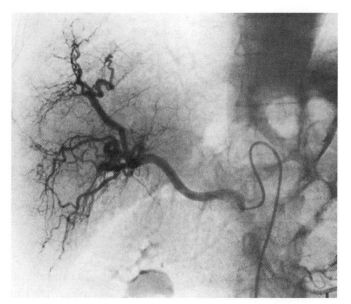

(A)

(B)

Fig. 18.27 Normal gallbladder 'blush'. Following selective hepatic arteriography the wall of the gallbladder is often visualized in the 'hepatogram' phase of the study.

found incidentally at cholecystectomy; alternatively, it may present as either a mass lesion or manifest the effects of spread into the liver, extrahepatic biliary system, stomach or duodenum. The gallbladder is supplied by the cystic artery, which usually arises from the right hepatic artery although it may occasionally arise from the left hepatic, celiac axis, common hepatic or gastroduodenal arteries (Ch. 1).

The outline of the normal gallbladder is not uncommonly seen on selective hepatic arteriography (Fig. 18.27). In the presence of malignancy the cystic artery may appear enlarged and encasement or occlusion of cystic artery branches has been reported (Abrams et al 1970). In the venous phase the wall of the gallbladder may be seen to be thickened and irregular. Neovascularity in the tumor is frequently detected. If the lesion is large, encasement and amputation of intrahepatic vessels can be seen secondary to invasion of liver substance by the tumor (Fig. 18.28).

Pancreatic neoplasia (Ch. 55) The diagnosis of pancreatic carcinoma is usually made clinically and by non-invasive imaging techniques. Whilst angiography was previously performed preoperatively in the majority of patients to assess resectability and to detect intrahepatic metastases, it now has a limited role because of the quality of images that are routinely obtained by CT and/or MRI. Encasement of the splenic and main portal veins and of the gastroduodenal

and/or the splenic arteries by the primary tumor are usually well visualized using these modalities. When some doubt exists angiography might still be useful.

Pancreatic neuroendocrine tumors present clinically with symptoms of excess hormone production, the hormone being produced by the primary tumor or the secondary deposits or both. Angiography may be very useful for the detection of small primary tumors of the pancreas, especially insulinomas and gastrinomas, and will often localize

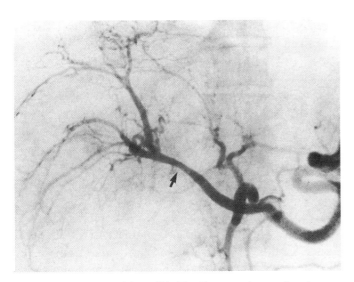

Fig. 18.28 Carcinoma of the gallbladder. The tumor has produced displacement and encasement (arrow) of the right hepatic artery.

Adrenal tumors Larger right-sided adrenal, hepatic and renal tumors can cause a serious diagnostic dilemma on cross-sectional imaging as their organ of origin may be difficult to determine. Angiography may be very useful in such cases as, although such lesions will often parasitize a vascular supply from adjacent organs, the principal feeding vessels usually arise from the organ of origin's normal arterial branches.

Cystic disease (Ch. 66)

The diagnosis and assessment of hepatic cystic disease is performed by US, CT and MRI. Angiography is not required in the evaluation of non-parasitic cysts; they may, however, be noted at the time of angiography performed for other reasons and will be seen as round avascular lesions with surrounding hypervascular rims due to compressed liver.

Hydatid cysts (Ch. 63) present as single or multiple intrahepatic lesions. Angiography is not performed in the diagnostic work-up of these patients and is rarely required prior to surgery. As with non-parasitic lesions the cysts may show rings of hypervascularity around an avascular center.

Vascular lesions

Primary venous disorders may involve the liver and show fairly characteristic appearances.

Peliosis hepatis Peliosis hepatis (Pliskin 1975) is a rare condition associated with the ingestion of anabolic steroids

lesions which have not been visualized using other modalities including US, CT and MRI (Fig. 18.29). Accurate localization may be improved by using the technique of arterial stimulation venous sampling in which calcium gluconate (for insulinomas) or secretin (for gastrinomas) is injected selectively in turn into the vessels supplying the pancreas and venous samples are obtained from the hepatic veins (O'Shea et al 1996). A rise in hormone level in the venous samples will occur after injection of the calcium gluconate or secretin into that vessel supplying the portion of pancreas containing the functioning tumor.

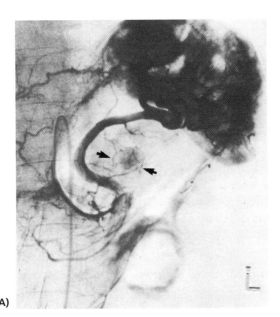

(A)

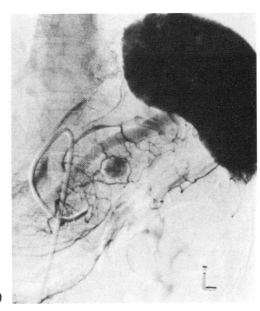

(B)

Fig. 18.29 Splenic arteriogram. Early **(A)** and late **(B)** radiographs showing the characteristic 'blush' of a pancreatic insulinoma (arrow).

and is also seen in patients with chronic debilitating diseases such as tuberculosis or malignancy. The characteristic angiographic changes in this disorder include areas of contrast accumulation of various sizes which persist through the venous phase. Although the lesions tend to respond to withdrawal of the causative agent, spontaneous rupture and intraperitoneal bleeding has been reported.

Polyarteritis nodosa This is a necrotizing vasculitis which characteristically involves small- and medium-sized arteries. In a significant proportion of cases this process leads to the formation of microaneurysms and these may rupture spontaneously. Arterial stenoses and/or occlusions may also occur. Angiography may be of value in establishing the diagnosis (Fig. 18.30). The renal and hepatic arterial trees should be examined; aneurysms occur in the liver in 40 to 60% of affected individuals and in the kidney in 80 to 100% (Travers et al 1979, Van Breda & Waltman 1984). From a technical point of view it is important to inject contrast selectively into the hepatic artery and to take films for at least 15 seconds. Similar appearances have been reported in patients suffering from drug abuse, in metastatic atrial myxoma and, rarely, in other collagen disease, such as systemic lupus erythematosus.

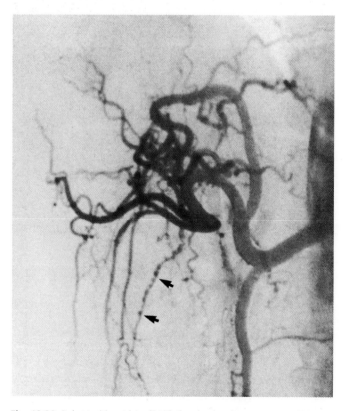

Fig. 18.30 Polyarteritis nodosa (PAN) the classic microaneurysms are seen in this hepatic arteriogram (arrows).

Aneurysms Aneurysms of the hepatic and splenic arteries and their branches may be atherosclerotic, traumatic, mycotic or inflammatory in nature; they have also been reported following intra-arterial cytotoxic agents (Forsberg et al 1978). They may be multiple and may attain a very large size. Large hepatic artery aneurysms may present with jaundice and/or an epigastric mass. Angiography is invaluable in detecting and accurately delineating these abnormalities and therapeutic embolization of the vessel of supply is frequently the most appropriate therapy.

Hereditary hemorrhagic telangiectasia (HHT) This condition (also known as Osler–Weber–Rendu disease) is a disease with an autosomal dominant mode of inheritance characterized by telangiectasia of the skin and mucous membranes. There may be associated arteriovenous malformations (AVMs) involving the hepatic or pulmonary circulations. Genetic linkage for this condition has been established on the long arm of chromosome 9 (Shovlin et al 1994, McDonald et al 1994) and the gene at this site has been identified as endoglin, an endothelial protein involved in the growth and function of blood vessels. Patients with this form of the disease (HHT Type 1) have an approximately 30% chance of developing pulmonary arteriovenous malformations but a very low risk of developing hepatic shunts. On the other hand, genetic linkage of HHT has also been established on chromsome 12 (Johnson et al 1995) and families with this form of the disease (HHT Type 2) are considerably less likely to develop pulmonary AVMs (only 3%) but are at greater risk of AVMs on the systemic side of the circulation notably within the liver. A further genotype (HHT Type 3) appears to be associated with an even greater risk of hepatic AVMs but the gene for this has not yet been identified. The typical appearances seen at angiography include multiple arteriovenous (hepatic artery to hepatic vein) fistulae (Fig. 18.31), usually involving the entire liver, and there is often rapid arteriovenous shunting with an elevated cardiac output. There may also be hepatic artery to portal vein and portal vein to hepatic vein communications.

Hepatic trauma

Angiography is generally reserved for those patients who show clinical or ongoing evidence of active hemorrhage especially if this occurs after satisfactory surgical packing of the liver. Hepatic vascular damage can be caused by either blunt or penetrating injury. (See Chs 68 & 69.)

Blunt trauma The commonest causes of blunt hepatic injuries are road traffic accidents and sports injuries (including horse riding, parachuting, skiing). Major liver injury has

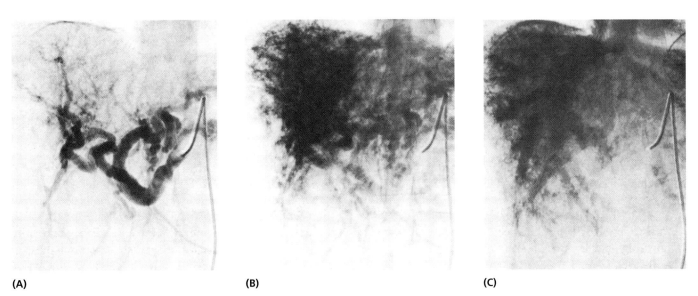

(A)   **(B)**   **(C)**

Fig. 18.31 Osler–Weber–Rendu disease. Selective hepatic arteriography, arterial **(A)**, capillary **(B)**, and venous **(C)** phases show abnormal vascularity, multiple small angiomas and hepatic artery to hepatic vein fistulae. Such dense opacification of the hepatic vein following injection of contrast into the hepatic artery is highly suggestive of pathology.

also occurred following external cardiac massage and in some areas of the world blast injury is an important cause. When angiography is performed following blunt trauma, several important points need to be considered. The operator needs to be aware if any arterial branches have not been filled, a finding suggestive of either transection or spasm; in this situation active bleeding may also be demonstrated in some cases. The hepatogram phase may show the lateral margin of the liver to be displaced medially by an extrahepatic or subcapsular hematoma (Fig. 18.32). It is also of great importance to determine portal vein patency and to take radiographs in the portogram phase as well as the arterial phase. Any area of the liver which appears avascular in both the arterial and portogram phases is non-viable and will usually require surgical intervention at some stage (usually earlier rather than later). Areas of hepatic infarction will, however, usually be more easily appreciated on CT.

Aneurysms of the hepatic artery and arterioportal fistulae may occur, often as late complications of injury (Ch. 69). These lesions may give rise to hemobilia (Ch. 70) which can be life-threatening (see below).

Penetrating injury Penetrating liver injury may be self-inflicted and violent injuries are usually due to stabbings, gunshot or shrapnel. Accidental injury such as may occur following road traffic accidents may be a mixture of blunt and penetrating trauma. The advent of more aggressive and invasive investigation of liver pathology has engendered its own complications. Biliary and hepatic surgery of all grades of complexity can also give rise to some specific vascular problems.

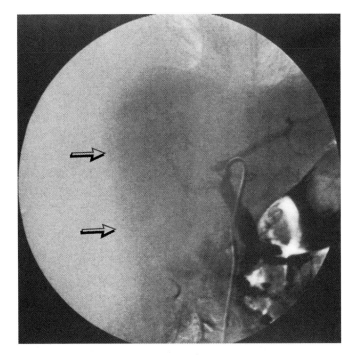

Fig. 18.32 Liver trauma. The late phase of a superior mesenteric arteriogram shows that the left portal vein is patent, the right portal vein is poorly seen and the liver is displaced medially (arrows) by a large hematoma.

The finding of *arterioportal fistulae* following penetrating injury such as stabbing, liver biopsy and percutaneous biliary drainage is not uncommon. Small fistulae will usually resolve spontaneously but larger lesions cause a rise in portal pressure and if left untreated may give rise to portal hypertension. These lesions can also involve the biliary tract and be associated with hemobilia; embolization is the treatment of first choice (Ch. 70). Intrahepatic arterial aneurysms are not infrequently seen following liver injury (Fig. 18.33) and may develop late when they are usually asymptomatic until they rupture causing life-threatening hemorrhage. Rupture usually occurs into either the peritoneal cavity or the biliary system. Transcatheter embolization is now the treatment of choice for many of these lesions, but consultation between surgeon and radiologist is important. It is important that the interventional radiologist occludes the aneurysm itself or isolates it completely from its vessel of origin and does not just block the feeding vessel proximally. The rich collateral network to the liver, and the rapid development of intrahepatic collaterals will in many instances render simple ligation or occlusion of the feeding vessel ineffectual. Surgical ligation of the main hepatic arterial trunk feeding such a lesion is often ineffective and

should be avoided if at all possible as it compromises interventional radiological therapy. The fact that injudicious surgical ligation may render embolization impossible should always be kept in mind.

Cirrhosis and portal hypertension

The diagnosis of cirrhosis and portal hypertension (see Section 13) is usually made by means other than angiography and the role of vascular studies in the investigation of portal hypertension is limited.

The etiology and classification of portal hypertension will not be discussed in this section. The angiographer should be acquainted with the general principles of investigation and management and the working diagnosis in each case, as this significantly affects the type of vascular study that should be performed.

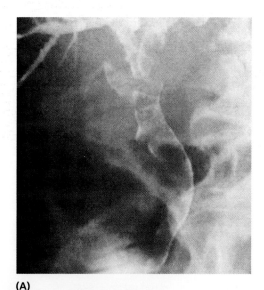

(A)

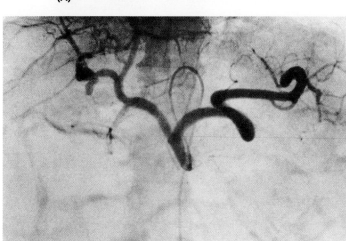

(B)

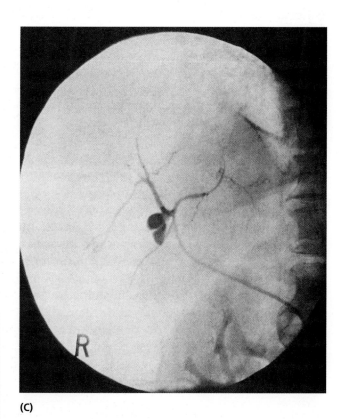

(C)

Fig. 18.33 Embolization of an intrahepatic aneurysm. The patient had undergone a difficult cholecystectomy three months earlier and now presented after recent jaundice and melena with active gastrointestinal bleeding. **(A)** A PTC shows the common bile duct to contain blood clot (filling defects). **(B)** A celiac arteriogram shows an aneurysm (presumably postsurgical) in the right hepatic artery. **(C)** A selective study shows detail of the aneurysm which is actively bleeding into the biliary tree. *continued*

Measurement of portal pressure The normal portal venous pressure ranges from 5 to 10 mmHg. Pressure may be measured by either direct or indirect means. Direct measurements are performed by catheterization of the portal venous system usually via a transjugular approach prior to the insertion of an intrahepatic porto-systemic stent. A percutaneous, transhepatic approach to the portal vein is less frequently utilized because of the increased morbidity and mortality associated with this technique and the measurement of splenic pulp pressure prior to direct splenoporto-

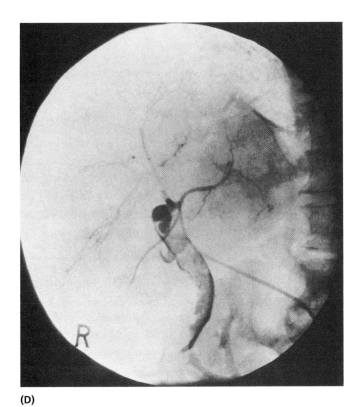

(D)

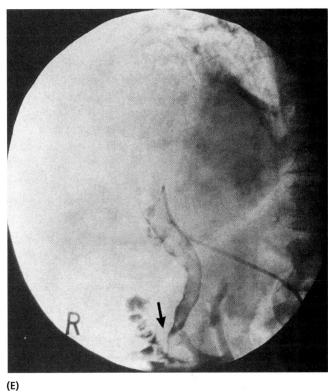

(E)

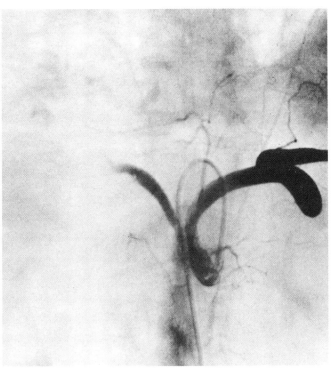

(F)

Fig. 18.33 *continued* **(D)**, **(E)** Note the contrast outlining the ampulla and duodenum (arrow) only 12 s after the arterial injection of contrast medium. **(F)** The hepatic artery has been embolized (arrow). The patient was discharged from hospital with no further treatment 1 week after the procedure.

graphy is of historical interest only. Indirect measurements of portal venous pressure are obtained by wedging a catheter into a peripheral hepatic vein; the reproducibility of these readings, which do not always give an accurate estimate of the pressure within the portal vein, is often poor.

Assessment of portal vein patency Cross sectional imaging techniques are now the most frequently used modalities for the assessment of portal venous patency and catheter angiography is infrequently required.

The portal vein may be compressed or invaded in its extrahepatic or intrahepatic course. Intrahepatic portal venous abnormalities may be due to cirrhosis where the necrosis and subsequent fibrosis and regeneration gradually impair circulation through the liver. Portal hypertension ensues, and varices may develop.

Schistosomiasis is in many countries the most common cause of hepatic fibrosis and portal hypertension. Tumors, either primary intrahepatic or metastatic, may compromise the intrahepatic portal veins. This abnormality may take the form of either direct invasion or compression and displacement of the vein. Portosystemic collateral vessels develop when the portal venous system is obstructed resulting in varices but they are usually unable to decompress the system completely.

The portal venous system may also be compressed or invaded in its extrahepatic course. Cavernous transforma-tion of the portal vein usually occurs as a result of neonatal umbilical vein infection, often associated with the use of umbilical vein cannulae. The extrahepatic portal vein is thrombosed and multiple tortuous collateral vessels develop around the thrombosed vessels and drain portal blood into the intrahepatic portal radicles (Fig. 18.34). Abdominal sepsis later in life may also cause portal vein thrombosis and give rise to cavernous transformation. Calcification may occur in the portal vein as a result of previous thrombosis. The extrahepatic portal vein may be compressed or invaded by tumors arising at or near the hilum of the liver.

Delineation of arterial anatomy It may be important to delineate accurately arterial anatomy, particularly if surgery is contemplated or if an arterioportal fistula is suspected. Arterial changes occur in cirrhosis where the intrahepatic vessels may show a characteristic corkscrew pattern. The liver may be noted to be small and, in the hepatogram phase, may be seen to be displaced from the lateral abdominal wall by ascites.

Demonstration of systemic venous anatomy and patency Hepatic vein occlusion, the Budd–Chiari syndrome, causes 'posthepatic' portal hypertension. The diagnosis is often made on ultrasound but angiography may be required especially if radiological recanalization is to be attempted (Griffith et al 1996). The appearances seen at selective

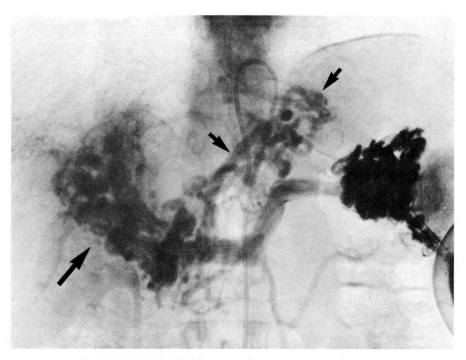

Fig. 18.34 A direct splenoportogram showing varices (short arrows) and cavernous transformation of the portal vein (long arrow). (Direct splenoportography is now seldom used.)

hepatic venography are characteristic, showing a spider's web pattern (Fig. 18.35). Prior to shunt surgery it is important to determine patency of both the inferior vena cava and left renal vein. Whilst this was previously performed angiographically, ultrasound, CT and/or MRI are now usually sufficient.

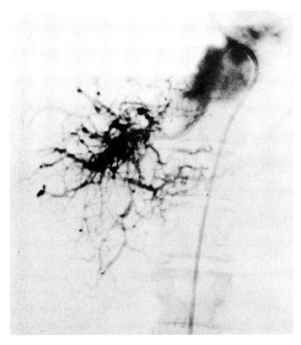

Fig. 18.35 Budd–Chiari syndrome. A catheter has been passed retrogradely into a right hepatic vein. An injection of a small volume (5 ml) of contrast medium has outlined an extensive fine network of collateral vessels. The 'spider-web' appearance is pathognomonic of the Budd–Chiari syndrome.

Visualization of portal venous collaterals If the main splenic or portal veins become occluded the many potential collateral routes of venous drainage may enlarge to partially decompress the system (Fig. 18.34). Gastric and esophageal varices are often well demonstrated on CT but their full extent may be best demonstrated by indirect splenoportography.

Transjugular intrahepatic porto-systemic stent shunt (Ch. 101) (Richter et al 1990) This technique involves the placement of a metallic stent between the hepatic and portal veins via a percutaneous, transjugular route and has proved very effective for the treatment of ongoing variceal hemorrhage, which has not responded to endoscopic sclerotherapy. Via a transjugular route the right or middle (less frequently the left) hepatic vein is catheterized with an angled catheter and through this the right branch of the portal vein is punctured transhepatically. Wedged hepatic venography may be useful in order to opacify indirectly the portal veins to aid their puncture as discussed above. The tract between the two veins is then dilated prior to the insertion of a metallic stent. The most severe immediate complication of the procedure is that of puncture of the liver capsule causing intraperitoneal hemorrhage but this is rare. Later complications include porto-systemic encephalopathy and shunt stenosis or occlusion.

Infection and infestation

Hepatic infection and infestation are usually diagnosed by clinical investigation and non-invasive radiological techniques, such as US and CT and angiography is practically never required. If performed for other reasons displacement of both arterial and venous structures may be seen. Abscesses are frequently avascular but may have a hypervascular ring (Nory et al 1974). Acute infection and abscess formation may produce arteriovenous shunting (Adler et al 1978) (Fig. 18.36). Multiple abscesses may be indistinguishable angiographically from metastatic disease.

Hydatid disease (Ch. 63) causes cystic change within the liver parenchyma. The cysts, which may reach a very large size, can cause marked displacement of arteries and displacement and compression of portal venous radicles.

Amebic abscesses (Ch. 62) occur within the liver; as with hydatid disease angiography is infrequently indicated and then usually in preoperative assessment and not primary diagnosis.

THERAPEUTIC ANGIOGRAPHY

It is possible, with experience, to place arterial catheters into superselective positions within the hepatic arterial tree. This capability may be employed for both infusion and embolization techniques. Angiographic techniques may also be used for the percutaneous placement of an intrahepatic, porto-systemic stent via a transhepatic route to treat variceal hemorrhage which has not responded to endoscopic sclerotherapy (see above).

INFUSION TECHNIQUES

The debate as to whether cytotoxic agents are more effective and cause less systemic side-effects if delivered selectively to the organ of interest will not be discussed here. Arterial catheters can be inserted into the hepatic artery either percutaneously or operatively for this purpose. This technique can cause permanent arterial damage (strictures,

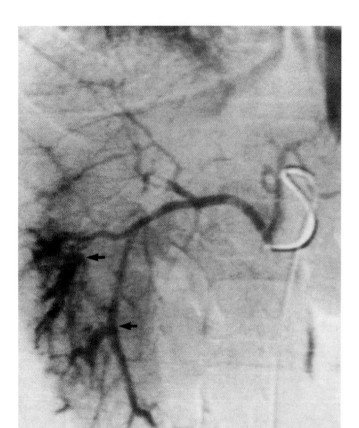

(A)

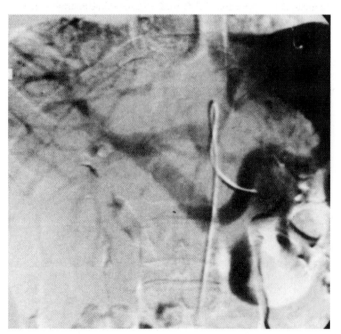

(B)

Fig. 18.36 Arteriovenous fistula in a patient with a liver abscess. **(A)** Hepatic arteriogram shows preferential filling of vessels in the lower part of the right lobe of the liver. Multiple small arterioportal fistulae are present (arrows). **(B)** An indirect splenoportogram shows that the portal vein segments in this area do not fill antegradely. The fistulae closed after treatment with antibiotics.

occlusions and aneurysms have all been reported) and catheter care requires close supervision.

EMBOLIZATION TECHNIQUES

Transcatheter therapeutic embolization may be used in the liver in the management of a wide variety of diseases. For further information on the types of embolic agents used and the potential hazards of the techniques the reader is referred to Chapter 77. It is worth stressing a few major guidelines at this point. Firstly, whatever the pathology, arterial embolization should generally not be performed in an area of the liver that does not have a portal venous supply because of the high likelihood of causing hepatic infarction. Secondly, it is important to observe a strict protocol with regard to patient preparation and antibiotic prophylaxis if complications are to be avoided. Thirdly, close post-procedural observation is required to manage the side effects (pain, fever) and complications (e.g. renal failure, abscess formation) that may occur. Finally, the angiographer should embolize as small an area of liver as possible, but must ensure that the desired therapeutic effect is achieved. The indications for hepatic arterial embolization are listed in Table 18.3.

Transhepatic (direct percutaneous or transjugular) embolization of gastric and oesophageal varices is less commonly employed since the success of TIPS has become evident for the acute management of variceal bleeding resistant to endoscopic sclerotherapy. Occasionally variceal embolization may be performed at the time of TIPS insertion although this is frequently not necessary.

REFERENCES

Abeatici S, Campi L 1951 Sur les possibilities de l'angiographie hepatique—la visualisation due systeme portal (recherches experimentales). Acta Radiologica (Stockholm) 36: 83–392

Abrams R M, Berenbaum E R, Santos J S, Lipson J 1969 Angiographic features of cavernous haemangioma of liver. Radiology 92: 308

Abrams R M, Meng C H, Firooznia H, Berenbaum E R, Epstein H Y 1970 Angiographic demonstration of carcinoma of the gallbladder. Radiology 94: 277–282

Adler J, Goodgold M, Mity H et al 1978 Arteriovenous shunts involving the liver. Radiology 129: 315–322

Alfidi R J, Rastogitt, Buonocore E, Brown C H 1986 Hepatic arteriography. Radiology 90: 1136–1142

Allison D J 1980 Therapeutic embolization and venous sampling. In: Taylor S (ed) Recent advances in surgery 10. Churchill Livingstone, Edinburgh, p 27–64

Allison D J, Jackson J E 1997 Angiography. In: Grainger RG, Allison DJ (eds). Diagnostic radiology. A textbook of radiological imaging. Churchill Livingstone, Edinburgh, ch 105

Anacker H, Deveris K, Linden G 1957 Leistungsfahigkeit und Grenzen der purkutanes Splenoportographie. Fortschritte auf dem Gebiete der Rontgenstrahlen 86: 411

Baum 1997 Hepatic arteriography. In: Baum S (ed). Abrams Angiography 4th edn. Little, Brown, Boston, ch 57

Bierman H R, Steinbach H L, White L P, Kelley K H 1952 Portal venipuncture: percutaneous transhepatic approach. Proceedings of the Society for Experimental Biology and Medicine 79: 550

Blakeborough A, Ward J, Wilson D et al 1997 Hepatic lesion detection at MR imaging: a comparative study with four sequences. Radiology 203: 759–765

Blakemore A H, Lord J W Jr 1945 Technique of using vitallium tubes in establishing portocaval shunts for portal hypertension. Annals of Surgery 122: 476

Bron K M 1983 Arterioportography. In: Abrams H L (ed) Angiography, 3rd edn. Little Brown, Boston, p 1605–1620

Casarella W J, Knowles D M, Wolff M, Johnson P M 1978 Focal nodular hyperplasia and liver cell adenoma: Radiologic and pathologic differentiation. American Journal of Roentgenology 131: 393–402

Casteneda-Zuniga W R, Jauregui H, Rysavy J A, Formanet A, Amplatz K 1978 Complications of wedge hepatic venography. Radiology 126: 53–56

Collier N A, Carr D H, Hemingway A P, Blumgart L H 1984 Preoperative diagnosis and its effect on the treatment of carcinoma of the gallbladder. Surgery, Gynecology and Obstetrics. 159: 465–470

Dos Santos R 1935 Phlebographie d'une veine cave inferieure suture. J Urol Med Chir 39: 586

Forsberg L, Hafstorm L, Lunderquist A, Sundquist K 1978 Arterial changes during treatment with intrahepatic arterial infusion of 5-fluorouracil. Radiology 126: 49–52

Forssmann W 1931 Ueber Kontrastdarstellung des Hohlen des levenden rechten Herzens under der Lungenschlagader. Munchen Med Mschr 78: 489–492

Goncalves A M 1982 Biography of Egas Moniz. Catalogo de exposicao intinerante da obra Egas Moniz e Reynaldo dos Santos. Publicacoes Ciencia e Vida Lda, Lisbon, p 77

Grainger R 1997 Intravascular contrast media. In: Grainger R, Allison DJ (eds) Diagnostic radiology. A textbook of radiological imaging. Churchill Livingstone, Edinburgh, ch 2

Griffith J F, Mahmoud A E, Cooper S, Elias E, West R J, Olliff S P 1996 Radiological intervention in Budd–Chiari syndrome: techniques and outcome in 18 patients. Clinical Radiology 51: 747–748

Hascheck E, Lindenthal O T 1896 A contribution to the practical use of the photography according to Roentgen. Wiener Klinische Wochenschrift 9: 63

Haskal ZJ 1997 Interventions in portal hypertension. In: Baum S, Pentecost MJ (eds). Abrams Angiography. Interventional Radiology. Little, Brown, Boston, ch 33

International Working Party 1995 Terminology of nodular hepatocellular lesions. Hepatology 22: 983–993

Johnson DW, Berg JN, Gallione CJ et al 1995 A second locus for hereditary haemorrhagic telangiectasia maps to chromosome 12. Genome Research 5: 21–28

Kerns S R, Hawkins I F Jr., Sabatelli F W et al 1995 Current status of carbon dioxide angiography. Radiologic Clinics of North America 33: 15–29

Knowles D M, Wolff M M 1976 Focal nodular hyperplasia of the liver: a clinicopathologic study and review of the literature. Human Pathology 7: 533–545

Lecker G Y, Doroshaw J H, Zwelling L A, Chabrie B A 1979 The clinical features of hepatic angiosarcoma: a report of four cases and review of the English literature. Medicine 58: 48–64

Lindgren E 1950 Percutaneous angiography of the vertebral artery. Acta Radiologica (Stockholm) 33: 389–404

Lunderquist A, Ivancev K 1997 Portal and pancreatic venography. In: Baum S (ed). Abrams Angiography 4th edn. Little, Brown, Boston, ch 56

Matsui O, Tokoshima T, Kayoda M et al 1987 Dynamic sequential computed tomography during arterial portography in the detection of hepatic neoplasms. Radiology 146: 721–727

McDonald M T, Papenberg K A, Ghosh S, et al 1994 Genetic linkage of hereditary haemorrhagic telangiectasia to markers on 9q. Nature Genetics 6: 197–204

Nory SB, Wallace S, Goldman AM, Ben-Menachen Y 1974 Pyogenic liver abscess. American Journal of Roentgenology 121: 388–395

Odman P 1958 Percutaneous selective angiography of the celiac artery. Acta Radiologica (Stockholm) (suppl 59): 1–168

Okuda K, Musha H, Yoshida T et al 1975 Demonstration of growing casts of hepatocellular carcinoma in the portal vein by celiac angiography: the thread and streak sign. Radiology 117: 303

Orrin H C 1920 The X-ray atlas of the systemic arteries of the body. Baillière, Tindall & Cox, London

O'Shea D, Rohrer-Theus A W, Lynn J A, Jackson J E, Bloom S R 1996 Localization of insulinoma by selective intraarterial calcium injection. Journal of Clinical Endocrinology and Metabolism 81: 1623–1627

Pantoga E 1968 Angiography in liver hemangioma. American Journal of Roentgenology 104: 874–879

Peirce E C, Ramey W P 1953 Renal arteriography: a report of a percutaneous method using the femoral artery approach and disposable catheter. Journal of Urology 69: 578–585

Pliskin M 1975 Peliosis hepatitis. Radiology 114: 29–30

Richter G M, Noeldge G, Palmaz J C et al 1990 Transjugular intrahepatic portocaval stent shunt: preliminary clinical results. Radiology 174: 1027–1030

Rigler L G, Olfelt P C, Krumbach R W 1953 Roentgen hepatography by injection of a contrast medium into the aorta. Radiology 60: 363

Royal Colleges of Anaesthetists and Radiologists 1992 Sedation and anesthesia in radiology. Report of a joint working party of the Royal Colleges of Anaesthetists and Radiologists

Seldinger S 1953 Catheter replacement of the needle in percutaneous arteriography. Acta Radiologica (Stockholm) 39: 368–376

Seneterre E, Taourel P, Bouvier Y et al 1996 Detection of hepatic metastases: Ferumoxides-enhanced MR imaging versus unenhanced MR imaging and CT during arterial portography. Radiology 200: 785–792

Shearman D J C, Finlayson N D C 1982 Diseases of the gastrointestinal tract and liver. Churchill Livingstone, Edinburgh, p. 681–701.

Sheppard D G, Moss J, Miller M 1998 Imaging of the portal vein during transjugular intrahepatic portosystemic shunt procedures: a comparison of carbon dioxide and iodinated contrast. Clinical Radiology 53: 448–450

Shovlin C L, Hughes J M B, Tuddenham E G D et al 1994 A gene for hereditary haemorrhagic telangiectasia maps to chromosome 9q3. Nature Genetics 6: 205–208

Soreide O, Czerniak A, Blumgart L H 1985 Large hepatocellular cancers; hepatic resection or liver transplantation? British Medical Journal 291: 853–857

Soyer P, Bluemke D A, Reichle R, Calhoun P S, Bliss D F, Scherrer A, Fishman E K 1995 Imaging of intrahepatic cholangiocarcinoma: 2. Hilar cholangiocarcinoma. American Journal of Roentgenology 165: 1433–1436

Thuluvath P J, Rai R, Venbrux A C, Yeo C J 1997 Cholangiocarcinoma: a review. Gastroenterologist 5: 306–315

Travers R L, Allison D J, Brettle R P, Hughes G R V 1979 Polyarteritis nodosa: a clinical and angiographic analysis of 17 cases. Seminars in Arthritis and Rheumatism 8: 184–198

Van Breda A, Waltman A 1984 Diagnostic hepatic angiography: mass and diffuse disease. In: Bernardino M E, Sones P J (eds) Hepatic radiography. Macmillan, New York, p 214–242

Veiga-Pires JA, Grainger RG 1982 Pioneers in angiography. MTP Press, Lancaster

Walter JF, Bookstein JJ, Bouffard EV 1976 Newer angiographic observations in cholangiocarcinoma. Radiology 118: 19–23

Whelan JG, Greech JL, Tamburro CH 1976 Angiographic and radionuclide characteristics of hepatic angiosarcoma found in vinyl chloride workers. Radiology 118: 549–557

Yang X, Manninen G, Soimakallio S et al 1995 Carbon dioxide in vascular imaging and intervention. Acta Radiologica 36: 330–337

Fine needle biopsy and aspiration cytology

19

O. SØREIDE, K. SØNDENAA

INTRODUCTION

Liver biopsy where tissue can be obtained for histological or cytological examination has been central to the investigation of liver diseases for many decades. The indications for biopsy have changed markedly over time. Contemporary imaging modalities (Ch. 21) allow a precise targeting and have facilitated the biopsy procedure. The availability of improved or new therapies, for instance a more aggressive approach to resection of liver and biliary tumors, may on the other hand reduce the need for a preoperative tissue proven diagnosis.

In surgical practice, the clinical problem is either that of a focal liver or biliary lesion or of a potential diffuse non-malignant parenchymal disease. The true nature of a newly diagnosed mass lesion must be ascertained, either during workup (vide infra) or by examination of a resection specimen. Biopsy of 'normal' liver is for surgeons only indicated if parenchymal liver disease such as liver cirrhosis which might affect treatment strategy, is suspected.

This chapter concentrates on percutaneous aspiration cytology (FNAC) and fine needle biopsy (FNB). Open surgical biopsies or laparoscopically-guided biopsy, and the use of liver biopsy in liver transplantation are discussed elsewhere (Chs 20, 54, 83, 111). An excellent review on liver biopsy from a physician's perspective is published by Desmet & Fevery (1995).

IMAGING AND PUNCTURE GUIDANCE

The pioneers of liver biopsy performed their aspirations without guidance of the needle. A blind (i.e. non-directed) biopsy so commonly used in the past is rarely if ever indicated in surgical patients although this is still common practice by medical gastroenterologists (Gilmore et al 1995). Such biopsy was soon replaced by percutaneous puncture in combination with some imaging technique. Initially, isotopic liver scan (Johansen & Svendsen 1978), angiography (Tylen et al 1976), fluoroscopy, for instance following percutaneous transhepatic cholangiography (PTC) or endoscopic retrograde cholangiopancreatography (ERCP) (Goldman et al 1977, Ho et al 1977, Gagnon et al 1991) were used for targeting. Puncture guided by these imaging techniques is, however, cumbersome and time-consuming (Ferrucci et al 1980) and they have now been replaced by ultrasound (US) imaging or puncture with computed (CT) or magnetic resonance (MR) guidance (vide infra).

'EXTERNAL' ULTRASONOGRAPHY (Ch. 13)

The modern high-resolution ultrasound (US) scanners allow real-time visualization of the target, the surrounding tissues, the needle and the needle track. US also allows multiple puncture directions; it is independent of organ function and no ionizing radiation is used. US provides a dynamic image—of importance when the target is small and moving—and the needle tip can be monitored during insertion. The method is convenient and the procedure rapid. Finally, the equipment is mobile and the patient can remain in bed during the procedure. The main disadvantages of US are related to its inability to penetrate gas and bone, so that intestinal gas may interfere with imaging of the abdominal organs, and the ribs may limit the accessibility of certain areas.

Three different methods of ultrasonographic guiding mechanisms are available (Holm et al 1985):

1. The freehand puncture, where the needle is introduced near to the transducer, and is visualized as it enters the soundfield.

2. Puncture through a puncture transducer which contains a needle canal which allows the needle to enter in the top of the soundfield, or guides the needle as it traverses the soundfield.
3. A steering attachment is added to the US transducer where the needle either enters the soundfield from the side in the same plane as the soundfield, or where the needle traverses the soundfield.

Jakobeit (1986) compared the freehand and transducer puncture techniques. There was no significant difference in accuracy between the two. Free-hand puncture is time-saving, allows a better visibility of the biopsy needle artifact and is more practicable.

Recently a new 'freehand' puncture technique has been developed. The ultrasound probe and the puncture needle are connected to a 'homing in' technology device, which initially was developed for warplane bombing. The lesion to be punctured is localized by US. The line that the needle will follow is shown real time on the US screen and can then be 'homed in' at the target. The advantage is that it is easy to use and allows selection of appropriate puncture sites.

ENDOSCOPIC ULTRASONOGRAPHY (EUS) (Ch. 13)

An extension of US as a puncture guide is that of endosonographically (EUS) guided biopsy. The first echoendoscopes had a mechanical radial scanning device, which mainly was used for diagnostic ultrasound. A needle could be seen to go through the ultrasound field of imaging, but could not be followed into the lesion to be biopsied.

The development of the curved array transducer endoscopes, or more recently the mechanical puncture scopes, allows the endoscopist to follow the needle all the way from exiting the echoendoscope to entering the lesion and facilitates either aspiration cytology or needle biopsy. Even a new automated spring-loaded biopsy device has been introduced (Binmoeller et al 1997). Needles are available in different lengths, which allow tissue sampling at some distance from the head of the echoendoscope.

Currently there are approximately 200 units of curved array echoendoscopes installed in Europe, but the number of advanced users trained in EUS guided biopsy is only around 20–25 (Vilmann 1998). There is a well-documented learning curve with this technique (Wiersema et al 1997). Common indications for EUS directed biopsy in hepatobiliary/pancreatic surgery are:

- Paraduodenal or pancreatic mass lesion(s)
- Celiac lymph node(s) enlargement in association with a

known upper GI-cancer or in a patient suspected of having cancer or lymphoma
- Intra-abdominal lymph node(s) masses in association with a known cancer or suspicion of cancer.

We will not present the results of endoscopic ultrasound guided fine needle aspiration here.

COMPUTER TOMOGRAPHY (CT) (Ch. 15)

CT is also a highly sensitive and specific guide for obtaining tissue.

With CT the radiologist has complete visualization of the entire field of study, and can therefore plan a safe route from skin to lesion. However, it is not possible to see the needle real-time, and the principles of stereotaxis must be applied. The steps as described by Lees (1998) are: determine and mark the desired entry point, calculate the depth and angle of needle placement, place the needle blind, check the needle position with one or more scans, and repeat until happy.

Pancreatic body and tail masses are often best approached by CT since visualization by US in such areas is limited. For areas visualized by both methods CT and US are equally effective in providing diagnostic material (Butler & Smith 1989, Brandt et al 1993). The choice of modality depends on personal preference, availability of CT scanning time, the expertise of the radiologist in CT and US and the cost.

MAGNETIC RESONANCE (MR) (Ch. 16)

MR-guided needle aspiration biopsy has also been described (Mueller et al 1986). With the new scanners MR offers the prospect of near real-time imaging for the biopsy procedure. MR-compatible needles, which reduce the image artifacts found with standard needles, have been developed although there are still major material compatibility problems. The main indication for MR-guided biopsy so far is hepatic lesions identified by MRI but not with noncontrast CT or US.

A recent extension is the 'open' MR machine (Signa SP; General Electrics) which allows the operator to work within the MR machine itself where he/she can view and puncture a lesion 'real-time' (Laerum et al 1998).

BIOPSY MODALITY

FINE OR COARSE NEEDLE?

Needles vary from small, skinny needles with a diameter of 19–23 gauge used primarily in aspiration cytology to larger core type needles that allow samples to be obtained for histopathologic studies. Biopsy specimen can also be sampled for cytogenetic and biochemistry studies.

The opportunity of obtaining morphologic diagnosis safely and rapidly by use of fine needle aspiration cytology (FNAC) is said to have been pioneered by Martin and Ellis (1930) at the Memorial Sloan Kettering Cancer Center in New York, although the first report on needle biopsy can be traced back to 1847 (Webb 1974). Frola (1935) from France also tried the fine needle aspiration technique and evaluated cytological smears. This technique did not receive much attention and seems to have been nearly forgotten until Lopes Cordozo (1954), Söderström (1966), Wasastjerna (1969) and Lundquist (1970a) published their extensive experience. The increased popularity of the method depends largely on the evolution of clinical cytology which allows the cytopathologist to provide a diagnosis based on the aspiration specimen which corresponds closely with that obtainable from histologic examination.

A fine needle has by definition an outer diameter of 1 mm (19 gauge) or less. It is a generally accepted fact that the complication rate increases with increasing diameter of the needle (Menghini 1970). The complication rate after abdominal biopsies of the liver using fine needles is extremely low (Table 19.6), and compares favorably with that following coarse needle liver biopsy (Perrault et al 1978).

Commonly we use a 19–22-gauge needle for aspiration cytology. Data from the literature suggest that a slightly thicker needle may increase the sensitivity. For instance, Andriole et al (1983) and Dickey and coworkers (1986) noted that increasing the caliber of the needle increased the sample size. Some authors argue that needles with specific tip design are more efficient and offer better material for evaluation by the cytopathologist. However, two well designed studies did not reveal any significant difference in tissue sampling among four different 22-gauge needles (Wittenberg et al 1982) or between a 22-gauge 300 angle-tipped Chiba and 22-gauge screw-tipped needles (Mindell & Korson 1990).

Fine needle biopsy (FNB) using cutting needles to obtain tissue fragments for histological examination was introduced by Menghini (1958). Such sampling has been facilitated by automatic spring-loaded sampling devices, so-called biopsy 'guns' (Lindgren 1982). Large series using such biopsy techniques have been published (Buscarini et al 1990, Elvin et al 1990, Jaeger et al 1990). Although a variety of needles are available (Andriole et al 1983), most reports are based on biopsies (so-called microhistology) using an 18-gauge cutting needle, i.e. a slightly thicker needle than that covered by the definition of a fine needle given above. Hopper et al (1993) have compared several needles and automated devices, and conclude that the 18-gauge needle is as effective as thicker needles, and that automated biopsy devices can provide more diagnostic specimens than manual or conventional needles in biopsy of cadaveric livers.

Needles, commercially available in varying lengths, are flexible and may bend as they are advanced through the abdominal wall. The fine needle can be stabilized by using an outer guide needle of larger diameter (10 cm long). This is first introduced through the superficial layers. This outer needle will not only ensure needle stability, but will also allow multiple passes of the fine needle without inconvenience to the patient.

Percutaneous coarse-needle biopsy is, in the author's opinion, contraindicated in liver, pancreatic and bile duct lesions. The difference in morbidity rates and the fact that an inconclusive FNB or FNAC can be repeated without adding any significant risk to the patient, lead to the conclusion that FNB and FNAC are superior to coarse liver biopsy techniques in the evaluation of focal liver lesions. Coarse liver biopsy should probably only be performed in patients where structural information is decisive, e.g. a biopsy of the non-tumorous liver in a patient with a focal liver lesion to exclude underlying cirrhosis or other significant parenchymal pathology. In such patients, FNB is probably a safer and better alternative. Percutaneous coarse needle biopsies of pancreatic or biliary tract lesions are not recommended.

FINE NEEDLE CYTOLOGY

ASPIRATION TECHNIQUE

The aspiration technique was pioneered by Franzèn et al (1960). When the ultrasonic examination has identified a puncture target, the optimum needle route is chosen. The fine needle is fitted to a disposable syringe, which is attached to an aspiration handle (Fig. 19.1). The outer supporting needle, if needed, is introduced and the fine needle is passed through it. When the tip of the fine needle is located within the lesion to be biopsied, the piston of the aspiration handle is retracted completely to apply full suction and the needle is moved back and forth to loosen cell clusters. With the needle still in the lesion, the negative pressure is equilibrated by slowly releasing the handle and the needle is withdrawn. The material in the needle is expelled onto glass slides. Expelling is facilitated by disconnecting the needle from the syringe, and filling of the syringe with air before expulsion of the needle contents.

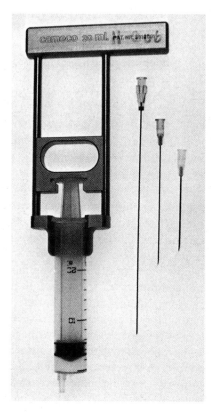

Fig. 19.1 Aspiration handle that permits a one-hand grip. The handle will fit a disposable 20-ml syringe.

Usually several passes of the needle will be performed in slightly different directions to ensure representative sampling. This is particularly important if the texture of the lesion is fibromatous or if there are necrotic areas in a tumor. Smith (1984) noted increased complication rates in proportion to the number of passes, but others disagree (Ferrucci et al 1980). Although Dickey et al (1986) demonstrated that there was no benefit in using two passes versus a single aspiration (of the pancreas), most investigators do several passes in order to secure representative sampling. Edoute et al (1991) showed that multiple repeated aspirations give a higher accuracy than a single aspiration (86% versus 57%). Repuncture also increases the accuracy (Evander et al 1978).

It is important though to standardize the aspiration technique. Kreula and coworkers (1989) have in an experimental study shown that there were differences in sample weights and cell count, including the amount of acellular material obtained by 3 groups of doctors who differed from each other in their technique and experience with FNAC. This difference disappeared when they all used a standardized technique based on moving the tip of the needle within the target at a standardized rate and with a set stroke amplitude.

Devices have been introduced to simplify FNAC. Hopper et al (1992) recently published a well-designed study comparing seven different techniques and devices for obtaining biopsy specimens using 22-gauge needles. None of the seven performed better in acquisition of the specimen with the exception that a nonaspiration, fine needle capillary biopsy technique provided less cellular material. While syringe holders may offer convenience and ease of use, they did not improve the quality of specimen obtained. On the other hand, Fagelman and Chess (1990) concluded that nonaspiration FNAC of the liver was as good as those from conventional aspiration technique.

Experience has shown that a fine-needle can traverse—without complication—stomach, bowel and urinary bladder to reach a mass lesion. Transpleural and transpulmonal puncture should, on the other hand, be avoided if possible. With a puncture through the liver, the edge should be avoided as it may be lacerated if the patient moves.

FNAC can be performed on an in- and outpatient basis without any special preparation. The skin and subcutaneous tissues can be anesthetized locally (rarely indicated), and diazepam may be given to an anxious patient.

PREPARATION OF THE SMEAR

The needle content is commonly expelled onto glass slides and spread immediately as shown in Fig. 19.2. Some authors also include a final rinse of the needle and syringe with saline solution. Such samples and fluid aspiration from cysts are spun down before being spread on slides, or mixed with 50% ethanol for centrifugation later.

The aspiration material is either fixed immediately or air dried. Wet fixation is either performed in 95% ethanol or by a commercially available spray fixative (standard in our hospital). This is followed by staining before cytomorphological evaluation. Some authors advocate that both wet and dry fixation should be done if sufficient material is obtained. Dry fixation can allow use of special stains such as immunocytochemical staining techniques.

There are, however, several methods of preparation including the smear technique, Millipore (R) filters, cytocentrifugation concentrations (cytospins) and cellblocks from the rinsed material. Experts often disagree on preparatory technique (for discussion, see Hajdu et al 1989). Although comparative studies are limited, one study would indicate that adding a rinse preparation to the smears increases the diagnostic rate (Axe et al 1986); smears that were interpreted as giving equivocal results, clearly showed a malignancy with a final rinse preparation. Others argue that the cellblock technique (inclusion cytology) is superior (Livraghi et al 1985).

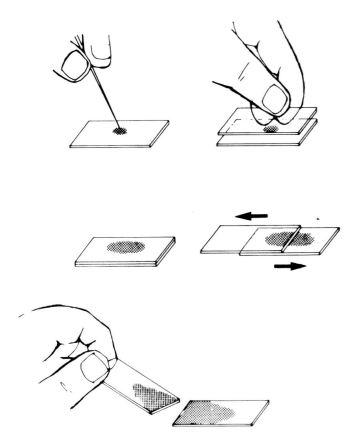

Fig. 19.2 Method of preparing aspiration biopsy smears. The needle content is expelled, and a second glass slide is put on top. The drop spreads between the slides which are then pulled in opposite directions, resulting in two specimens.

EXAMINATION OF CYTOLOGICAL OR HISTOLOGICAL SPECIMENS

The routine is to prepare FNAC and FNB specimens for conventional cytomorphologic or histologic evaluation. Specimens may also be used for immunohisto- or immunocytochemical studies; the presence of tumor-associated antigens may facilitate diagnosis. Molecular techniques may be used to evaluate oncogene products in cells or tissue. It is beyond the scope of this chapter to discuss such evaluation techniques in full. However, and as an example, Ki-ras gene mutations can be detected and used for diagnosing biliary strictures (Ito et al 1998, Watanabe et al 1994, Levi et al 1991), gallbladder lesions (Ajiki et al 1996) as well as in pancreatic tumors (Mora et al 1998, Shibata et al 1990, Tada et al 1991).

RESULTS

It is obvious from the literature that the results will vary widely according to whether the procedure was guided by some imaging technique, performed blindly, or by palpation. The results which follow refer only to US-, CT- or MR-guided biopsies, unless stated otherwise, as this reflects the current state of the technology.

The terminology in reported results also differs. To enable some comparison between different authors, the following terms will be used for evaluation of the results:

TP, true positive results; TN, true negative results; FP, false positive results; FN, false negative results. These figures form the basis for estimation of

$$\text{Sensivity} = \frac{TP}{TP + FN} \times 100\%$$

$$\text{Specificity} = \frac{TN}{TN + FP} \times 100\%$$

$$\text{Predictive value of a positive test} = \frac{TP}{TP + FP} \times 100\%$$
$$(PV_{pos})$$

$$\text{Predictive value of a negative test} = \frac{TN}{TN + FN} \times 100\%$$
$$(PV_{neg})$$

$$\text{Accuracy} = \frac{TP + TN}{TP + FP + TN + FN} \times 100\%$$

Not all authors report their results in this way, but the indices can often be calculated from published figures.

A general problem when reviewing the literature is that the selection of cases may influence the results (see below). Similarly, there seems to be no consensus of how to treat the nonrepresentative, equivocal or 'inconclusive' biopsies in analysis; the number of biopsy procedures, passes and sessions to establish the diagnosis are often not given. Lastly, the verification of the final diagnosis is often a problem, especially in patients with a negative 'result' and thought to have benign disease.

LIVER

Liver FNAC or FNB may be performed for either focal or diffuse disease. In this context only results from focal liver lesions will be given. FNAC of liver lesion(s) is done to answer the following questions:

1. What is the nature of a lesion, i.e. is it malignant or not?

2. If malignant, can the cellular or histologic characteristics indicate the site of origin?
3. Can cytology or biopsy identify benign liver lesions and differentiate between them?

Fine needle aspiration cytology

Table 19.1 gives a representative selection of papers, which indicates the usefulness of FNAC in diagnosing malignant liver lesions. The overall sensitivity varies from 67 to 100%, i.e. in those patients with malignant disease FNAC was positive for malignancy in 67 to 100%. The specificity was 99%, i.e. patients with benign disease had a benign cytological diagnosis in 99%. The predictive value of a positive (malignant) cytological test was 99%, whereas the predictive value of a negative cytology was only 71%. The interpretation of these figures is that *FNAC is a highly reliable test for malignant disease when positive. However, a negative (benign) cytology is of limited value in excluding hepatic malignancy because of many false negatives.* Further biopsies or other tests may be needed to establish the true nature of the lesion.

Table 19.1 also demonstrates that FNAC is useful for all types of focal liver lesion(s). This is not necessarily an argument for doing FNAC of all liver lesions (vide infra), but illustrates that if the FNAC is positive for malignancy this is highly unlikely to be false irrespective of the type of lesion. The relationship between size of lesion(s) and proportion in which a correct diagnosis was made has been studied by Reading et al (1988). They found correct diagnoses by

FNAC in 79% of lesions 1 cm or less in diameter, in 88% of those 1.1–2 cm, and in 98% of those 2.1–3 cm.

Many clinicians are worried about false positive cytology. These are exceedingly rare (Table 19.1). Analyses of the published series indicate that false-positives are due to sampling error or are based on aspiration material that often is scanty and probably should have been reported as 'not representative' (Ho et al 1981, Schwerk & Schmitz-Moormann 1981).

In contrast to other infradiaphragmatic organs, the liver may harbor a variety of malignant tumors. The cytological characteristics of aspirates from different liver lesions have been established (Eklund & Wasastjerna 1971, Wasastjerna 1979, Tao et al 1984). The trained cytologist is able to give a cytological diagnosis, which corresponds closely to the histology of the tumor (Jacobsen et al 1983, Droese et al 1984, Hajdu et al 1989, Fornari et al 1990, Edoute et al 1991). Others have been less successful and have been unable to differentiate primary from secondary tumors in 51 to 57% of patients (Sautereau et al 1987, Ohlsson et al 1999 in press). By establishing the histogenetic origin, the clinician can then direct further investigations, for instance, the gastrointestinal tract in the case of an adenocarcinoma.

Bile duct carcinomas, which make up 15 to 25% of primary carcinoma of the liver, are said to be often misdiagnosed as metastatic (Wasastjerna 1979), but data in the literature is difficult to evaluate. The features on imaging are nonspecific. It appears that FNB can give material for definitive diagnosis, but tissue typing accuracy is low (Berdah et

Table 19.1 Results of percutaneous FNAC in the diagnosis of malignant liver lesions

Author(s)	No. of patients	Type of lesion(s)	Sensitivity (%)	Specificity (%)	PVpos (%)	PVneg (%)
Montali et al 1982	108	M	92	100	100	70
Rosenblatt et al 1982	59	M	94	100	100	80
Jacobsen et al 1983	55	S	100	100	100	100
Pagani 1983	100	S	95	100	100	56
Schwerk et al 1983	130	S	92	93	98	77
Droese et al 1984	100	S	94	100	100	89
Whitlach et al 1984	86	M	87	100	100	76
Tatsuta et al 1984	41	M	94	96	94	96
Haubek 1985	380	S	91	100	100	65
Holm et al 1985	247	S	92	100	100	60
Bell et al 1986	197	S	67	100	100	45
Gebel et al 1986	854	M	88	100	–	
Servoll et al 1988	175	M	80	100	100	76
Butler & Smith 1989	40	S	98	100	100	88
Buscarini et al 1990	972	M	91	99	100	77
Fornari et al 1990	441	M	93	100	100	84
Edoute et al 1991	321	S	86	98	99	76
Ohlsson et al 1999	178	S	89	67	98	27

S, solid liver lesion(s); M, liver mass(es) of any type

al 1996; Colli et al 1998). There is some anecdotal experience suggesting that a combination of histology, histochemical and immunohistological examination may increase accuracy, in particular for the combined hepatocellular cholangiocarcinomas (Dusenbery 1997). Of 20 patients with a focal lesion of bile duct origin, 16 (80%) had a positive diagnosis of malignancy, but the histogenic nature of the lesions was not given (Montali et al 1982, Tatsuta et al 1984, Whitlach et al 1984, Haubek 1985).

Some clinicians have questioned the diagnostic accuracy of FNAC in hepatocellular carcinoma. However, several studies demonstrate that FNAC is accurate with a sensitivity rate of 80 to 95% and a specificity of 100% (Fornari et al 1990, Sbolli et al 1990, Hakim et al 1995). Bottles et al (1988) analyzed and characterized the different cytological features in the FNAC diagnosis of hepatocellular carcinoma. Others have shown that the cytologic patterns could be classified according to the World Health Organisation (WHO) histologic classification (Kung et al 1991).

A special problem is that of differentiating between a regenerative or hyperplastic hepatic nodule and a well-differentiated hepatocellular carcinoma, particularly in patients with cirrhosis (Hajdu et al 1989). The incidence of such nodules which appear as a focal mass lesion on imaging in patients with liver cirrhosis is around 10 to 20% (Ferrel et al 1992, Wada et al 1988). There are several problems related to terminology and prognostic importance; are they preneoplastic, borderline tumors or very early HCCs. (An International Working Party [1995] discussed the terminology.)

The final diagnosis of such nodules might be difficult to establish and five out of 54 nodules evolved to HCC during a median follow up of 35 months (Terasaki et al 1998). A correct diagnosis clearly depends on a skilled pathologist with competence to evaluate cytological or histological criteria commonly used to classify nonmalignant hepatocellular nodules (Terasaki et al 1998). In such patients an accurate diagnosis requires an abundant sample, and often a histological biopsy should be obtained.

Needle aspiration biopsy may occasionally be used as an additional staging procedure to distinguish tumor invasion in the portal vein from simple thrombus (Joly et al 1993, Dusenbery et al 1995).

The value of FNAC in the diagnosis of benign focal liver lesion(s) is difficult to establish. Numerous papers show that the cytological diagnoses in these patients have been nonspecific, i.e. that of no malignant tumor cells found. Solbiati et al (1985) performed FNAC in 33 patients with a liver hemangioma. The cytological diagnosis was based on the absence of malignant cells and the presence of capillary vessels in addition to blood and endothelial cells. A confident cytologic diagnosis was made in four (12%) and a probable diagnosis in another four (12%). Taavitsainen and coworkers (1990) in a study of 36 FNAC of liver hemangiomas were able to make a definitive diagnosis in seven (19%) and a scanty but indicative diagnosis in a further 14 patients (39%). Such results suggest that FNAC is unreliable in the diagnosis of hemangiomas, although a more recent study (Layfield et al 1998) concludes that fine needles aspirates from hemangioma were accurate in ten out of 11 cases. The fact that differentiation between benign lesions is essential for determining the type of treatment to be advocated, combined with the unreliability of cytology, suggests that the general picture of the usefulness of FNAC is less positive than that outlined for malignant tumors. Errors in diagnosis are particularly high in patients with lymphomas. FNAC rarely allows the subtyping of this malignancy, which is required for treatment (Welch et al 1989).

Simple liver cysts are a frequent finding in clinical practice. If the lesion exhibits the typical ultrasonographic or tomographic characteristics of a simple cyst, it is a general opinion that FNAC is unnecessary and unhelpful (Haubek 1985, Benhamou & Menu 1988). Most aspirates give acellular fluid. Some authors have warned against FNAC in patients with suspected hydatid disease of the liver although it appears that the procedure is safe and may contribute to the diagnosis (Stefaniak 1997, von Sinner et al 1995, Das et al 1995).

Reports on FNAC of hepatic adenoma, focal nodular hyperplasia (FNH) and fatty focal infiltration are limited. The hepatocytes of FNH are cytologically normal and are indistinguishable from those of normal liver, although they may contain excess glycogen (Knowles & Wolff 1976). Focal fatty infiltration may be more reliably diagnosed with CT (Yates & Streight 1986).

FNAC or histological fine needle biopsy (FNB)?

There is no agreement as to the superiority of cytology (FNAC) or microhistology (FNB) in the diagnosis of focal liver lesions. Table 19.2 gives a selection of the few comparative studies published. It is evident that neither method has clear advantages, and the retrieval rates and tissue typing accuracies are fairly similar. Recent data suggest that FNB is superior to FNAC in diagnosing benign lesions (Nyman et al 1995), but further studies are awaited. We know that cytology is inadequate in some patients, particularly in those with vascular lesions, in fibrotic, dense tumors, in lymphomas and endocrine lesions in whom subtyping is required and in well differentiated primary liver cancer.

Borzio and coworkers (1994) conclude, however, in a careful study that in patients with cirrhosis FNB is superior

Table 19.2 Comparison between cytology and fine needle histology in diagnosing liver mass lesion(s)

Author	No. of patients	Cytology	Sensitivity (%) Fine needle histology
Wittenberg et al 1982*	65	81	73
Sangalli et al 1989	112	74	82
Buscarini et al 1990	969	91	94
Hepatocellular carcinoma	389	90	93
Metastasis	504	93	94
Lymphoma	38	87	90
Edoute et al 1991	34	32	62
Rapaccini et al 1994	73	80	61
Nyman et al 1995	69	62	91

*Includes data published by Isler et al (1981)

to FNAC, particularly for small (< 3 cm) lesions. FNB is safe and its accuracy in diagnosing hepatocellular carcinoma is 85 to 90% patients with and without cirrhosis (Yu et al 1997, Huang et al 1996). Data suggest that the complications and death risk after FNB are of the same magnitude as after FNAC. The choice between the two biopsy modalities will therefore often depend on personal preference and the expertise of the pathologist. Further comparative studies are awaited.

In a recently published study Yu and coworkers (1998) have studied the diagnostic efficacy of FNB using an 18-gauge automated cutting needle in small (3 cm or less) focal hepatic lesions of different pathologies and different sizes (≤ 1 cm; > 1–2 cm; > 2–3 cm). The sensitivity for diagnosing malignancy was 96%, specificity 100%, positive and negative predictive values were 100% and 96% respectively; accuracy 98%. There was no difference related to tumor size.

Core needle biopsy of liver hemangioma using an 18–20 gauge needle with or without an automatic sampling device has also been used (Heilo and Stenwig 1997, Tung and Cronan 1993). It appears that FNB is accurate although Heilo and Stenwig (1997) report a fairly high false negative rate (15 out of 20). The procedure—even several passes—appears safe, in particular if some normal liver tissue is traversed before entering the hemangioma.

There are several commonly accepted principles, which should be noted during liver FNAC or FNB (Young 1992). Most will advocate that the needle should traverse some normal liver before entering the lesion to reduce the risk of post-biopsy hemorrhage. The risk of bleeding can be reduced by the plugged liver biopsy technique (Riley et al 1984, Zins et al 1992). Similarly, many are wary of needling vascular tumors, such as hemangiomas, hepatomas and endocrine metastasis lesions, although there seems to be no increased risk in such patients (Solbiati et al 1985, Croman

et al 1988). Caution should be exerted when taking a biopsy in a patient with an obstructive biliary tree due to the increased risk of bile leakage. Biopsies of hormone-producing tumors, e.g. carcinoids, can—although rare—lead to severe complications (Bissonette et al 1990).

Patients with uncorrectable coagulopathy may occasionally present a problem. Both the transjugular liver biopsy (cannot be used for puncturing of focal liver lesions) and the plugged liver biopsy techniques where the needle track is sealed with embolic material immediately after biopsy can be used. Ascites has also been considered a relative contraindication to biopsy. However, in a comparative study Murphy et al (1988) concluded that the risk from liver biopsies in the presence of ascites is not higher than biopsies done in its absence.

BILIARY TRACT

Percutaneous FNAC or FNA is one of many modalities in obtaining tissue from the biliary tract including the gallbladder. It is beyond the scope of this chapter to discuss and compare all sampling modalities. Kurzawinski et al (1993) has reviewed the diagnostic value of duodenal aspiration cytology, exfoliated cytology or bile brush cytology, endobiliary biopsy and aspiration FNAC. Later studies (de Paralta-Venturina et al 1996, Savader et al 1996) largely confirm the findings in this review. Others have provided data on endobiliary forceps biopsy during ERCP or PTC (Schoefl et al 1997, Pugliese et al 1995, Sugiyama et al 1996, Ponchon et al 1995).

The sensitivity of cytodiagnosis of extrahepatic biliary stricture can probably be increased by combining FNAC with bile cytology or other methods obtained at the time of percutaneous transhepatic cholangiography and/or brushing from the bile duct at ERCP (Desa et al 1991).

Extrahepatic bile duct

The literature on percutaneous FNAC of stricture of the extrahepatic bile duct is sparse, which may reflect the view taken by Longmire et al (1973) and many others, including us, that a tissue-confirmed diagnosis is not required when dealing with bile duct obstruction and cancer is suspected.

Table 19.3 gives the results in eight reports, although the papers published by Evander et al (1980) and Desa et al (1991) may contain some or all of the patients reported by the same groups in previous publications (Evander et al 1978, Dalton-Clark et al 1986). The reports indicate that PTC (percutaneous transhepatic cholangiography) and US were most commonly used for guidance.

Table 19.3 Results of percutaneous FNAC in the diagnosis of extrahepatic bile duct tumors

Author(s)	No. of patients	% Positive cytological diagnosis
Evander et al 1980	33	42
Chitwood et al 1982	12	67
Blumgart et al 1984	22	59*
Dalton-Clark et al 1986	18	87
Hall-Craggs & Lees 1986	32	57
Cohan et al 1986	13	92
Desa et al 1991	88	61*
Pelsang & Johlin 1997	5	80
Overall	223	62

*Both pre- and intraoperatively

Of FNAC performed in 223 patients, 62% proved to be positive for malignancy, i.e. a sensitivity of 62%. There is no information regarding the site of the tumors (proximal, mid-duct, distal or retroduodenal) in relationship to neither diagnostic accuracy, nor concerning the number of needle passes. Only one false-positive FNAC 'suspicious for malignancy' has been described in a patient with documented benign disease (Desa et al 1991). All authors point to the high frequency of false negatives and inadequate sample is common.

Gallbladder

Biopsy, particularly FNAC of gallbladder mass lesions is a well-established diagnostic method. The sensitivity of FNAC in diagnosing malignancy is around 60 to 70% (Das et al 1998; Akosa et al 1995, Shukla et al 1997, Zargar et al 1991). It also seems that FNAC is able to differentiate between adenocarcinoma and squamous cell and adenosquamous carcinoma (Das et al 1998).

Of note is, however, the fact that a gallbladder mass lesion has quite separate image characteristics; from a mass lesion almost filling the lumen, to an infiltrating mass or a polypoidal mass projecting into the lumen. There are no good data which show the efficacy of FNAC (or FNB) according to type of lesion although Wu and coworkers (1996) report the results of FNAC in 17 patients with gallbladder polyps of a size over 1 cm. From their data it is evident that FNAC of polypoid lesions fail to establish the diagnosis in many patients. Of interest though is the fact that all eight patients with cholesterol polyps were accurately diagnosed with FNAC.

PANCREAS

Aspiration cytology of the pancreas was pioneered by Christoffersen and Poll (1970), and percutaneous biopsies were first obtained by Oscarson et al in 1972.

Several series of percutaneous FNAC of pancreatic mass lesions have been published. Table 19.4 gives a representative selection with a total of 2975 patients. A positive cytology for malignancy (i.e. the sensitivity) has been obtained in around 76% of patients with verified cancer ranging from 58% to 94%. The frequency of false negatives is 15%, i.e. a negative cytology does not exclude malignancy.

The accuracy of FNAC of the pancreas seems to be independent of type of lesion, i.e. whether the aspirations were performed in patients with a malignant tumor only, or whether the biopsies were taken from any pancreatic mass lesion. This means that when malignant cells are demonstrated cancer is accurately diagnosed. Accuracy is higher with larger masses (> 3.0 cm, 92%; < or = 3 cm, 81%), and larger needle sizes (16–19 gauge, 92%; 20–22 gauge, 85%) (Brandt et al 1993).

The potential problem of false-positive cytology is also outlined in Table 19.4. Out of 1464 patients with benign disease, five (0.3%) biopsies were reported as showing malignant cells. In two of these (Holm et al 1985), the false-positives were due to misinterpretation of the specimen by the cytopathologist. Thus, false-positive biopsies are very rare in patients with benign pancreatic disease. Two false-positives were obtained from patients with chronic pancreatitis (Hancke et al 1984). We have also reported two false-positive intraoperative FNAC in a patient with chronic pancreatitis (Søreide et al 1985). In chronic pancreatitis both architectural and cytological changes may mimic carcinoma. We believe that most of these false-positives can be avoided by applying strict criteria for what constitutes a representative biopsy.

A specific problem for pancreatic FNAC seems to be the relatively high frequency of nonrepresentative specimens, also called 'insufficient material' or 'inconclusive' cytology by some authors. The figures range from 3.2% (Hancke 1981) to 44% (Søreide et al 1985) with an average between 10 and

Table 19.4 Results of percutaneous FNAC in the diagnosis of pancreatic mass lesion(s)

Author(s)	No. of patients	Type of lesion	Positive cytology (sensitivity) (%)	False positive(s)	False negative(s)*
Evander et al 1978	52	M	60	–	14/52 (27%)
Yamanaka & Kimura 1979	8	M + B	86	0/6	–
Hancke 1981	72	M + B	60	0/72	
Mitty et al 1981	53	M + B	86	0/10	8/53 (11%)
Hovdenak et al 1982	55	M + B	76	0/9	8/32 (25%)
Schwerk et al 1983	70	M + B	69	0/18	–
Hancke et al 1984	203	M + B	71	2/77 (2.6%)	30/126 (24%)
Bree et al 1984	32	M + B	86	0/11	3/22 (14%)
Holm et al 1985	190	M + B	72	2/73 (2.7%)	27/117 (23%)
Søreide et al 1985	61	M + B	58	0/24	2/22 (9%)
Lüning et al 1985	124	M + B	71	1/74 (1.4%)	8/44 (18%)
Dickey et al 1986	83	M + B	79	0/31	1/40 (3%)
Gebel et al 1986	322	M + B	69	0/214	9/89 (10%)
Hall-Craggs & Lees 1986	208	M	67	0/113	45/192 (23%)
Taavitsainen et al 1987	49	M	88	–	5/49 (10%)
Solmi et al 1987	43	M + B	90	0/13	0/42 (0%)
Ekberg et al 1988	79	M + B	86	0/10	10/69 (14%)
Kocjan et al 1989	62	M + B	86	0/41	5/31 (16%)
Glenthøj et al 1990	52	M + B	65	0/5	8/52 (15%)
DelMaschio et al 1991	81	M + B	94	0/27	0/52 (0%)
Brandt et al 1993	269	M + B	–	0/251	17/225 (8%)
Lerma et al 1996	109	M + B	73	0/109	19/69 (28%)
Linder et al 1997	334	M + B	69	0/64	0/270 (0%)
David et al 1998	364	M + B	98	0/212	–
Overall	2975		76	5/1464 (0.3%)	207/1423 (15%)

M, malignant tumors of the pancreas
M + B, malignant and benign pancreatic mass lesions
* Not including biopsies with nondiagnostic material

15%. The high figure in the latter series may reflect the strict criteria formulated by the cytologists for a representative specimen. The high frequency of nonrepresentative samples may not only reflect the relative inaccessibility of the pancreas but also imaging problems especially experienced with US.

Lastly, it must be emphasized that recognition of cells from an adenocarcinoma in FNAC of the pancreas does not necessarily mean that the tumor originates in this gland. Cyto- or histological examination alone cannot exclude origin in other or adjacent structures, e.g. intestines, stomach and distal bile duct or metastases to the pancreas. Similarly, experience seems to be insufficient to permit description of all variants of islet cell tumors. Cytologists state that extreme care is necessary in judging the biological behavior of such tumors on the basis of the cytological picture (Stormby 1979). A general impression is that cytology is not able to provide conclusive results in benign pancreatic conditions (Kocjan et al 1989, Di Stasi et al 1998).

FNAC OR HISTOLOGICAL FINE NEEDLE BIOPSY (FNB)?

As for the liver, there is no agreement as to the superiority of cytology or microhistology. Table 19.5 gives some com-parative studies published. It is evident that neither method has clear advantages and the choice between the two biopsy modalities will therefore often depend on institutional preferences.

In patients with unclear pancreatic lesions a full range of immunohistochemical stains is often required to establish a diagnosis. Therefore, the microhistology technique may be required and many authors argue that there are many advantages to the use of larger caliber automated cutting needles although all agree that there is a slight increase in risk. A particular problem is pancreatic cystic neoplasms. Recent data (Carlson et al 1998) suggest that needle aspiration and biopsy is helpful and can even differentiate between the mucinous cancer subtypes.

COMPLICATIONS AND RISKS

The relative safety of FNAC or FNB of intraabdominal organs has been studied in five large independent surveys (Livraghi et al 1983, Smith 1985, Weiss et al 1988, Fornari et al 1989, Smith 1991) and a summary of the results is given in Table 19.6. Smith (1991) in his review addressed

Table 19.5 Comparison between cytology and fine needle histology in diagnosing pancreatic cancer

Author	No. of patients	Sensitivity (%)	
		Cytology	Fine needle histology
Wirtenberg et al 1982*	41	78	46
Chagnon et al 1987	19	71	92
Vilgrain et al 1987	24	77	72
Glenthöj et al 1990	100	92	72
Solmi et al 1992	50	95	71
Frölich et al 1988	98	78	79
Lees 1998	n.a.	75	94
Di Stasi et al 1998	510	87	94

*Includes data published by Isler et al (1981)

the problems of bleeding and needle tract seeding specifically and an extract from his findings relevant to FNAC of the liver, biliary tree and pancreas will be presented.

The overall complication rate of FNAC in Smith's study (1985) was 0.16%. Livraghi et al (1983) reported an incidence of major complications of 0.05%, and an incidence of minor problems (mostly pain) of 0.5% (58/11 700). In comparison, Holm et al (1985) reported two complications following 2000 fine needle punctures of the abdomen giving a complication rate of 0.1%, Lundquist (1970b) had one complication in 2611 fine-needle liver biopsies (0.04%), Welch et al (1989) had 11 complications in 1000 biopsies (0.1%; only one required surgery) and Fornari et al (1989) reported a complication rate of 0.18%.

The potential hazards in percutaneous fine-needle cytology or biopsy of liver, biliary tract and pancreas are bleeding, bile leak, infection and tumor seeding or implantation in the needle tract (Table 19.6). Bleeding is the most common hazard, and may ultimately lead to death (Smith 1991). Of 27 patients dying after FNAC of the liver and pancreas, 17 deaths were caused by bleeding. Eleven of the 21 fatal liver biopsies occurred in patients with liver primary tumors often with chronic liver disease; nine in patients with liver metastases from various sites. Of the primary tumors, two were in patients with hemangioma and two were in individuals with angiosarcoma. An exceedingly rare complication is biliary-vascular fistula (Patel & Shapiro 1995).

As pointed out by Smith (1985) the frequency of bile leak (bile leak is not defined in any study) is probably over-inflated by inclusion of leaks following transhepatic cholangiography. If we look for the entity of 'bile peritonitis', only five cases have been reported (an incidence of 0.007%).

The infection group includes patients with generalized peritonitis after abscess puncturing, bacteremia, and patients with so-called generalized infections. The risk is small and only three deaths from sepsis have been found in the literature after puncture of the liver and pancreas (Smith 1991). It is apparent from the literature that both bacterial and parasitic abscesses can be punctured without any significant risk (Grönvall 1985, Smith 1985), and even hydatid cysts, often regarded as an absolute contraindication to biopsy, have been punctured without hazard to the patient. Others have reported complications such as pancreatitis, gastrointestinal tract bleeding—including biliary-vascular fistula and chylous ascites.

The risk of dying following fine needle biopsies (Table 19.6) varied from 0.006% to 0.02%. In four large institutional studies (Gebel et al 1986, Bret et al 1988, Weiss et al 1988, Nolsøe et al 1990) comprising 9392 biopsies, five

Table 19.6 Complication rates in abdominal FNAC

Complication	Livraghi et al 1983 (n = 11 700)	Smith 1985 (n = 63 108)	Weiss et al 1988 (n = 66 397)	Fornari et al 1989 (n = 10 766)	Smith 1991 (n = 16 381)
Bleeding	7 (0.06%)	27 (0.04%)	–	7 (0.07%)	–
Bile leak	2 (0.02%)	51 (0.08%)**	–	1 (0.009%)	–
Infection	3 (0.03%)*	16 (0.02%)	–	3 (0.03%)	–
Needle tract seeding	2 (0.02%)	3 (0.05%)	2 (0.003%)	1 (0.009%)	1 (0.005%)
Deaths	1 (0.008%)	4 (0.006%)	5 (0.008%)	2 (0.02%)	5 (0.03%)

* 12 patients with fever not included
** Probably inflated by inclusion of transhepatic cholangiography

deaths occurred giving a death rate of 0.05%. On the other hand, Drinkovic and Brkljacic (1996) had published two deaths—due to the bleeding from angiosarcoma and hepatocellular carcinoma in advanced cirrhosis among 1750 fine needle biopsies. Of 24 deaths after FNAC found in the literature (Smith 1991) four occurred after FNAC of the pancreas and 17 after liver FNAC. Cause of death was bleeding after biopsy of the liver and pancreatitis and sepsis after puncture of the pancreas.

Needle tract tumor seeding

The risk of needle tract tumor seeding or the potential spillage of tumor cells into the peritoneal cavity following biopsy of a malignant lesion has been used as an argument against biopsy. Experimental work (Ryd et al 1983) as well as clinical experience (Table 19.6) has indicated that the risk is very small. On the other hand, Ohlsson et al (1999 in press) have noted a 3% implantation rate after FNAC of liver tumors causing major local problems and death in four out of seven patients. As pointed out by these authors, overall estimates of the risk of needle tract seeding after FNAC are probably irrelevant. Untreated patients with advanced tumors have a short survival and the time for development of detectable implantation metastases will therefore be short. A better risk estimate is found in patients with radically resected liver tumors. *But as pointed out later (vide infra) biopsy should probably not be obtained in such patients.* Smith (1991) collected 23 cases of needle tract seeding. Eleven followed FNAC of pancreatic cancer, two after liver FNAC. It is unclear why seeding, although rare, appears to be more common after needling of a pancreatic carcinoma.

Little has been written or documented concerning the possibility that tumor cells can spread via the lymphatics or blood vessels in connection with aspiration biopsy of neoplastic lesions and thus result in metastatic growth. Experimentally, such dissemination occurs (Engzell et al 1971) but the clinical significance is difficult to evaluate.

In conclusion, the hazards of FNAC are small, and compare favorably with any invasive diagnostic modality used in clinical practice.

THE ROLE OF PERCUTANEOUS FNAC OR FNB IN PATIENTS WITH HEPATOBILIARY/PANCREATIC SURGICAL DISEASES—A PERSONAL VIEW

The results presented in this chapter may indicate that biopsy of liver, bile duct and pancreatic lesions is—with some reservations—a valuable diagnostic tool which can be performed safely in most patients. The problem with any collected review is that it provides general figures taken out of a clinical context, often in selected patients, and the authors will naturally give as good results as possible (i.e. the problem related to the number of procedures needed to establish the cytological diagnosis or publication bias). Often the result obtained from the biopsy procedure may only add marginal additional information or just confirm what the clinician knows (or should know) from the history or other clinical and laboratory results.

The authors' view is that biopsy of hepatobiliary-pancreatic lesions should not be done indiscriminately in any or all patients just because it is simple and safe. On the other hand, if it is included in a plan for management of specific problems (see below), biopsy can be accepted as an integrated and valuable investigation, which will prove to be highly cost-effective. The following personal recommendations for FNAC or FNB are briefly outlined.

LIVER

Simple cysts

These are frequent incidental findings and easy to diagnose, but infrequently symptomatic, and aspiration gives only clear fluid. If a typical appearance is found on imaging (US or CT), no fine-needle aspiration is required as FNAC is generally unhelpful (usually the cytological material is too sparse or completely missing and does not allow any diagnosis) and recurrence of the cyst(s) is a rule after emptying.

'Atypical' cysts

A cyst with irregular linings or margins and with an inhomogeneous content in an afebrile patient should be investigated and evaluated as a solid focal liver lesion (see below). If the patient is septicemic or presents with signs of an ongoing infection, immediate puncture of the lesion is advocated to obtain material for culture. In an area where hydatid disease is endemic, serological tests should be done and biopsy (FNAC) deferred.

Multiple solid liver lesions

The typical patient is one with a primary extrahepatic malignant lesion treated previously. FNAC or FNB should be performed in these patients early to establish the true nature of the disease and to avoid overinvestigation. In some patients the diagnosis of advanced malignant disease will be so obvious that biopsy will be of only academic interest and will add to the discomfort of the patient.

The problem of regenerative nodules or hyperplasia has been discussed. A differentiation between such lesions and a well differentiated hepatocellular carcinoma is difficult and often histology (FNB) is required.

A solid focal lesion

For the patient in whom a liver metastasis is suspected, and/or if he or she is unfit for surgery, biopsy should be performed early in the diagnostic process. Most other patients should be fully investigated before a decision whether FNAC or FNB is necessary. The reasons for this attitude are; a negative biopsy is unreliable and further investigations are often required; FNAC or FNB cannot identify the benign liver lesion and differentiate between them; and a primary malignant liver lesion should be resected whenever possible. *Thus, most patients in this group will eventually come to laparotomy irrespective of the cytological or histological findings. For the benign lesions where surgery is not indicated (i.e. most hemangiomas and FNH) the diagnosis will be established by CT, MR and/or angiography and rarely by addition of FNAC or FNB.*

In patients with suspected HCC who might be candidates for OLT (Orthotopic Liver Transplantation) biopsy should be avoided to remove the risk of recurrence in the needle track or cell spillage in the peritoneal cavity.

EXTRAHEPATIC BILE DUCTS AND PANCREAS

If US shows extrahepatic bile duct dilatation, a stenosis of the bile duct or a pancreatic tumor or mass *in combination with suspected liver metastases*, biopsy of the primary lesion and/or the metastases during the initial US examination is advocated. A positive cytology for malignancy of the liver mass(es) will thus obviate the need for more sophisticated and invasive tests in patients unfit for major pancreatic surgery.

Patients with a potentially resectable bile duct stricture or pancreatic mass should be investigated and prepared for surgery. FNAC or FNB is not required as part of the initial investigative strategy.

REFERENCES

Andriole I G, Haaga I R, Adams R B, Nunez C 1983 Biopsy needle characteristics assessed in the laboratory. Radiology 148: 659–662

Ajiki T, Fujimori T, Onoyama H, Yamamoto M, Kitazawa S, Maeda S, Saitoh Y 1996 K-ras gene mutation in gall bladder carcinomas and dysplasia. Gut 38: 426–429

Akosa A B, Barker F, Desa L, Benjamin I, Krausz T 1995 Cytologic diagnosis in the management of gallbladder carcinoma. Acta Cytologica 39: 494–498

Axe S R, Erozan Y S, Ermatinger S V 1986 Fine-needle aspiration of the liver. A comparison of smear and rinse preparations in the detection of cancer. American Journal of Clinical Pathology 86: 182–285

Bell D A, Carr C P, Szyfelbein W M 1986 Fine needle aspiration cytology of focal liver lesions. Results obtained with examination of both cytologic and histologic preparations. Acta Cytologica 30: 397–402

Benhamou J P, Menu Y 1988 Non parasitic cystic diseases of the liver and intrahepatic biliary tree. In: Blumgart L H (ed) Surgery of the liver and biliary tract. Churchill Livingstone, London, p 1013–1024

Berdah S V, Delpero J R, Garcia S, Hardwigsen J, Le Treut Y P 1996 A western surgical experience of peripheral cholangiocarcinoma. British Journal of Surgery 83: 1517–1521

Binmoeller K F, Jabusch H C, Seifert H, Soehendra N 1997 Endosonography-guided fine-needle biopsy of indurated pancreatic lesions using an automated biopsy device. Endoscopy 29: 384–388

Bissonette R T, Gibney R J, Barry B R, Buckley A R 1990 Fatal carcinoid crisis after percutaneous fine-needle biopsy of hepatic metastasis: case report and literature review. Radiology 174: 741–752

Blumgart L H, Benjamin I S, Hadjis N S, Beazley R 1984 Surgical approaches to cholangiocarcinoma at confluence of hepatic ducts. Lancet i: 66–69

Borzio M, Borzio F, Macchi R, Croce A M, Bruno S, Ferrari A, Servida E 1994 The evaluation of fine-needle procedures for the diagnosis of focal liver lesions in cirrhosis. Journal of Hepatology 20: 117–121

Bottles K, Cohen M B, Holly E A 1988 A step-wise logistic regression analysis of hepatocellular carcinoma; an aspiration biopsy study. Cancer 62: 558–563

Brandt K R, Charboneau J W, Stephens D H, Welch T J, Goellner J R 1993 CT- and US-guided biopsy of the pancreas. Radiology 187: 99–104

Bree R L, Jafri S Z H, Schwab R E, Farah I, Bernacki E G, Ellwood R A 1984 Abdominal fine needle aspiration biopsies with CT and ultrasound guidance; techniques, results and clinical implications. Computerized Radiology 8: 9–15

Bret P, Labadie M, Bretagnole M, Paliard P, Fond A, Valette P J 1988 Hepatocellular carcinoma: diagnosis by percutaneous fine needle biopsy. Gastrointestinal Radiology 13: 253–255

Buscarini L, Fornari F, Bolondi L et al 1990 Ultrasound-guided fine-needle biopsy of focal liver lesions: techniques, diagnostic accuracy and complications. A retrospective study of 2091 biopsies. Journal of Hepatology 11: 344–348

Butler J A, Smith C 1989 Fine-needle aspiration biopsy in the diagnosis of recurrent and metastatic intraabdominal malignancies. American Journal of Surgery 158: 589–592

Carlson S K, Johnson C D, Brandt K R, Batts K P, Salomao D R 1998 Pancreatic cystic neoplasms: the role and sensitivity of needle aspiration and biopsy. Abdominal Imaging 23: 387–393

Chagnon S, Coohand-Priallet B, Jacquenod P, Vilgrain N, Blery M 1987 Intéret de la cytoponction associée à la micro-biopsie dans les masses solides du pancréas. Journal de Radiologie 68: 733–736

Chitwood W R, Meyers W C, Heaston D K, Herskovic A M, McLeod M E, Jones R S 1982 Diagnosis and treatment of primary extrahepatic bile duct tumors. American Journal of Surgery 143: 99–105

Christoffersen P, Poll P 1970 Peroperative pancreas aspiration biopsies. Acta Pathologica Microbiologica et Immunologica Scandinavica (suppl 112): 28–32

Cohan R H, Illescas F F, Braun S D, Newman G E, Dunnick N R 1986 Fine needle aspiration biopsy in malignant obstructive jaundice. Gastrointestinal Radiology 11: 145–150

Colli A, Cocciolo M, Mumoli N, Cesarini L, Prisco A, Gaffuri I, Martinez E 1998 Peripheral intrahepatic cholangiocarcinoma: ultrasound findings and differential diagnosis from hepatocellular carcinoma. European Journal of Ultrasound 7: 93–99

Croman J J, Esparza A R, Dorfinan G S, Ridlen M S, Paolella L P 1988 Cavernous hemangioma of the liver: role of percutaneous biopsy. Radiology 166: 135–138

Dalton-Clarke H J, Pearse E, Krause T, McPherson G A D, Benjamin I S, Blumgart L H 1986 Fine needle aspiration cytology and exfoliative biliary cytology in the diagnosis of hilar cholangiocarcinoma. European Journal of Surgical Oncology 12: 143–145

Das D K, Bhambhani S, Pant C S 1995 Ultrasound guided fine-needle aspiration cytology: diagnosis of hydatid disease of the abdomen and thorax. Diagnostic Cytopathology 12: 173–176

Das D K, Tripathi R P, Bhambhani S, Chachra K L, Sodhani P, Malhotra V 1998 Ultrasound-guided fine-needle aspiration cytology diagnosis of gallbladder lesions: a study of 82 cases. Diagnostic Cytopathology 18: 258–264

David O, Green L, Reddy V, Kluskens L, Bitterman P, Attal H, Prinz R, Gattuso P 1998 Pancreatic masses: a multi-institutional study of 364 fine-needle aspiration biopsies with histopathologic correlation. Diagnostic Cytopathology 19: 423–427

DelMaschio A, Vanzulli A, Sironi S et al 1991 Pancreatic cancer versus chronic pancreatitis: diagnosis with CA 19-9 assessment, US, CT and CT-guided fine needle biopsy. Radiology 175: 95–99

Desa L A, Akosa A B, Lazzara S, Domizio P, Krausz T, Benjamin I S 1991 Cytodiagnosis in the management of extrahepatic biliary stricture. Gut 32: 1188–1191

Desmet V, Fevery J 1995 Liver Biopsy. Ballière's Clinical Gastroenterology 9: 811–828

Dickey J E, Haaga J R, Stellato T A, Schultz C L, Hau T 1986 Evaluation of computed tomography guided percutaneous biopsy of the pancreas. Surgery, Gynecology and Obstetrics 163: 497–503

Di Stasi M, Lencioni R, Solmi L, Magnolfi F, Caturelli E, De Sio I, Salmi A, Buscarini L 1998 Ultrasound-guided fine needle biopsy of pancreatic masses: results of a multicenter study. American Journal of Gastroenterology 93: 1329–1333

Drinkovic I, Brkljacic B 1996 Two cases of lethal complications following ultrasound-guided percutaneous fine-needle biopsy of the liver. Cardiovascular and Interventional Radiology 19: 360–363

Droese M, Altmannsberger M, Kehl A et al 1984 Ultrasound-guided percutaneous fine needle aspiration biopsy of abdominal and retroperitoneal masses. Accuracy of cytology in the diagnosis of malignancy, cytologic tumour typing and use of antibodies to intermediate filaments in selected cases. Acta Cytologica 28: 368–384

Dusenbery D 1997 Combined hepatocellular-cholangiocarcinoma. Cytologic findings in four cases. Acta Cytologica 41: 903–909

Dusenbery D, Dodd G D 3rd, Carr B I 1995 Percutaneous fine-needle aspiration of portal vein thrombi as a staging technique for hepatocellular carcinoma. Cytologic findings of 46 patients. Cancer 75: 2057–2062

Edoute Y, Tibon-Fisher D, Ben-Haim S, Malberger E 1991 Imaging-guided and non-imaging-guided fine needle aspiration of liver lesions: experience with 406 patients. Journal of Surgical Oncology 48: 246–251

Ekberg D, Bergenfeldt M, Aspelin P et al 1988 Reliability of ultrasound-guided fine-needle biopsy of pancreatic masses. Acta Radiologica 29 (Fasc 5): 535–539

Eklund P, Wasastjerna C 1971 Cytological identification of primary hepatic carcinoma cells. Acta Medica Scandinavica 189: 373–375

Elvin A, Andersson T, Scheibenpflug L, Lindgren P 1990 Biopsy of the pancreas with a biopsy gun. Radiology 176: 677–679

Engzell U, Esposti P L, Rubio C, Sigurdson Å, Zajicek J 1971 Investigation on tumour spread in connection with aspiration biopsy. Acta Radiologica 10: 385–398

Evander A, Ihse I, Lunderquist A, Tylén U, Åkerman M 1978 Percutaneous cytodiagnosis of carcinoma of the pancreas and bile duct. Annals of Surgery 188: 90–92

Evander A, Fredlund P, Hoevels J, Ihse I, Bengmark S 1980 Evaluation of aggressive surgery for carcinoma of the extrahepatic bile ducts. Annals of Surgery 191: 23–29

Fagelman D, Chess Q 1990 Nonaspiration fine-needle cytology of the liver: a new technique for obtaining diagnostic samples. American Journal of Roentgenology 155: 1217–1219

Ferrell L, Wright T, Lake J, Roberts J, Ascher N 1992 Incidence and diagnostic features of macroregenerative nodules vs. small hepatocellular carcinoma in the cirrhotic livers. Hepatology 16: 1372–1381

Ferrucci J T Jr, Wittenberg J, Mueller P R et al 1980 Diagnosis of abdominal malignancy by radiologic fine needle aspiration. American Journal of Roentgenology 134: 323–330

Fornari F, Civardi G, Cavanna L 1989 Complications of ultrasonically guided fine-needle abdominal biopsy: results of a multicenter Italian study and review of the literature. Scandinavian Journal of Gastroenterology 24: 949–955

Fornari F, Civardi G, Cavanna L et al 1990 Ultrasonically guided fine-needle aspiration biopsy: a highly diagnostic procedure for hepatic tumors. American Journal of Gastroenterology 85: 1009–1013

Fornari F, Filice C, Rapaccini G L, Caturelli E, Cavanna L, Civardi G, Di Stasi M, Buscarini E, Buscarini L 1994 Small (≤ 3 cm) hepatic lesions. Results of sonographically guided fine-needle biopsy in 385 patients. Digestive Diseases and Sciences 39: 2267–2275

Franzèn S, Giertz G, Zajicek J 1960 Cytological diagnosis of prostatic tumours by transrectal aspiration biopsy—a preliminary report. British Journal of Urology 32: 193–196

Frola E 1935 Etude clinique l'etat functionnel du foie par la punction hepatique. Presse Medical 43: 1198–1202

Frölich E, Wehrmann K, Seeliger H, Vierling P, Frühmorgen P 1988 Ultraschallgezielte Feinnadelzytologie und Feinnadelhistologie bei umschriebenen Pancreasprocessen. Leber, Magen Darm 18: 236–244

Gagnon P, Boustiere C, Ponchon T, Valette P-J, Genin G, Labadie M 1991 Percutaneous fine-needle aspiration cytologic study of main pancreatic duct stenosis under pancreatographic guidance. Cancer 67: 2395–2400

Gebel M, Horstkotte H, Köster C, Broakhorst R, Brandt M, Atay Z 1986 Ultraschallgezielte Feinnadelpunktion abdomineller Organe: Indikationen, Ergebnisse, Risiken. Ultraschall 7: 198–202

Gilmore I T, Burroughs A, Murray-Lyon I M, Williams R, Jenkins D, Hopkins A 1995 Indications, methods, and outcomes of percutaneous liver biopsy in England and Wales: an audit by the British Society of Gastroenterology and the Royal College of Physicians of London. Gut 36: 437–441

Glenthøj A, Sehested M, T'orp-Pedersen S 1990 Ultrasonically guided histological and cytological fine needle biopsies of the pancreas. Reliability and reproducibility of diagnosis. Gut 31: 930–933

Goldman M L, Naib Z M, Galambos J T et al 1977 Preoperative diagnosis of pancreatic carcinoma by percutaneous aspiration biopsy. Digestive Diseases and Sciences 22: 1076–1082

Grønvall S 1985 Diagnostic and therapeutic puncture of intraabdominal fluid collections. In: Holm H H, Kristensen J K (ed) Interventional ultrasound. Munksgaard, Copenhagen, p 154–159

Hajdu S I, Ehya H, Trable W J et al 1989 The value and limitations of aspiration cytology in the diagnosis of primary tumors. A symposium. Acta Cytologica 33: 741–790

Hakim J G, Kiire C F, Weinig M, Gudza I, Makunike R T, Muronda C, Siziya S 1995 Fine needle aspiration cytology in the diagnosis of hepatocellular carcinoma. Central African Journal of Medicine 41: 237–241

Hall-Craggs M A, Lees W R 1986 Fine needle aspiration biopsy: pancreatic and biliary tumors. American Journal of Roentgenology 147: 399–403

Hancke S 1981 Ultrasound in the diagnosis of pancreatic cancer. Scanning and percutaneous fine needle biopsy. Almquist and Wiksell, Stockholm

Hancke S, Holm H H, Koch F 1984 Ultrasound guided puncture of solid pancreatic mass lesions. Ultrasound in Medicine and Biology 19: 613–615

Haubek A 1985 Puncture of focal liver lesions. In: Holm H H, Kristensen J K (eds) 1985 Interventional ultrasound. Munksgaard, Copenhagen, p 43–53

Heilo A, Stenwig A E 1997 Liver hemangioma: US-guided 18-gauge core-needle biopsy. Radiology 204: 719–722

Ho C-S, McLaughlin M J, McHattie J D, Tao L-C 1977 Percutaneous fine needle aspiration biopsy of the pancreas following endoscopic retrograde cholangio-pancreatography. Radiology 125: 351–353

Ho C-S, McLoughlin M J, Tao L-C, Blendis L, Evans W K 1981 Guided percutaneous fine needle aspiration biopsy of the liver. Cancer 47: 1781–1785

Holm H H, Kristensen J K (eds) 1985 Interventional ultrasound. Munksgaard, Copenhagen

Holm H H, Torp-Pedersen S, Larsen T, Juul N 1985 Percutaneous fine needle biopsy. Clinics in Gastroenterology 14: 423–449

Hopper K D, Abendroth C S, Sturtz K W, Matthews Y L, Shirk S J 1992 Fine-needle aspiration biopsy for cytopathologic analysis: utility of syringe handles, automated guns, and the nonsuction method. Radiology 185: 819–824

Hopper K D, Abendroth C S, Sturtz K W, Matthews Y L, Shirk S J, Stevens L A 1993 Blinded comparison of biopsy needles and automated devices in vitro: 1. Biopsy of diffuse hepatic disease. American Journal of Roentengology 161: 1293–1297

Hovdenak N, Lees W R, Pereira J, Beilby J O W, Cotton P B 1982 Ultrasound-guided percutaneous fine-needle aspiration cytology in pancreatic cancer. British Medical Journal 285: 1183–1184

Huang G T, Sheu J C, Yang P M, Lee H S, Wang T H, Chen D S 1996 Ultrasound-guided cutting biopsy for the diagnosis of hepatocellular carcinoma—a study based on 420 patients. Journal of Hepatology 25: 334–338

International Working Party 1995. Terminology of nodular hepatocellular lesions. Hepatology 22: 983–993

Isler R J, Ferucci Jr, Wittenberg J et al 1981 Tissue core biopsy of abdominal tumors with a 22 gauge cutting needle. American Journal of Roentgenology 136: 725–728

Ito R, Tamura K, Ashida H, Nishiwaki M, Nishioka A, Yamamoto Y, Furuyama J I, Utsunomiya J 1998 Usefulness of K-ras gene mutation at codon 12 in bile for diagnosing biliary strictures. International Journal of Oncology 12: 1019–1023

Jackson J E, Adam A, Alison D J 1992 Transjugular and plugged liver biopsies. Baillière's Clinical Gastroenterology 6: 245–258

Jacobsen G K, Gammelgaard J, Fuglø M 1983 Coarse needle biopsy versus fine needle aspiration biopsy in the diagnosis of focal lesions of the liver. Ultrasonically guided needle biopsy in suspected hepatic malignancy. Acta Cytologica 27: 152–156

Jaeger H J, MacFie J, Mitchell C J, Couse N, Wai D 1990 Diagnosis of abdominal masses with percutaneous biopsy guided by ultrasound. British Medical Journal 301: 1188–1191

Jakobeit C 1986 Ultraschallgezielte Punktionsverfahren: Freihandpunktion versus Biopsieschallkopfpunktion. Erfahrungen aus 5 Jahren. Ultraschall 7: 290–292

Jennings P E, Coral A, Donald J J, Rode J, Lees W R 1989 Ultrasound-guided core biopsy. Lancet i: 1369–1371

Johansen P, Svendsen K 1978 Scan-guided fine-needle aspiration biopsy in malignant hepatic disease. Acta Cytologica 22: 292–296

Joly J-P, Delamarre J, Razafimahaeo A et al 1993 Occult hepatocellular carcinoma in cirrhosis: value of ultrasound guided biopsy of portal vein thrombus. Abdominal Imaging 18: 344–346

Knowles D M I I, Wolff M 1976 Focal nodular hyperplasia of the liver: a clinicopathologic study and review of the literature. Human Pathology 7: 533

Kocjan C, Rode J, Lees W R 1989 Percutaneous fine needle aspiration cytology of the pancreas: advantages and pitfalls. Journal of Clinical Pathology 42: 341–347

Kreula J, Bondestam S, Virkkunen P 1989 Sample size in fine needle aspiration biopsy. British Journal of Surgery 76: 1270–1272

Kung I T M, Chan S-K, Fung K-H 1991 Fine needle aspiration in hepatocellular carcinoma. Combined cytologic and histologic approach. Cancer 67: 673–680

Kurzawinksi T, Deery A, Davidson B R 1993 Diagnostic value of cytology for biliary strictures. British Journal of Surgery 80: 414–121

Laerum F, Borchgrevink H M, Fosse E, Faye-Lund P 1998 The new international centre—a multidisciplinary R & D clinic for interventional radiology and minimal access surgery. Computer Methods and Programs in Biomedicine 57: 29–34

Layfield L J, Mooney E E, Dodd L G 1998 Not by blood alone: diagnosis of hemangiomas by fine-needle aspiration. Diagnostic Cytopathology 19: 250–254

Lees W R 1998 Percutaneous Needle Aspiration and Cytology. In: The Pancreas, Beger H G, Warshaw A L, Büchler M W, Carr-Locke D L, Neoptolemos J P, Russel C, Sarr M G (eds) p 260–263

Lerma E, Musulen E, Cuatrecasas M, Martinez A, Montserrat E, Prat J 1996 Fine needle aspiration cytology in pancreatic pathology. Acta Cytologica 40: 683–686

Levi S, Urbano-Ispizua A, Gill R, Thomas D M, Gilbertson J, Foster C, Marshall C J 1991 Multiple K-ras codon 12 mutations in cholangiocarcinomas demonstrated with a sensitive polymerase chain reaction technique. Cancer Research 51: 3497–3502

Linder S, Blåsjö M, Sundelin P, von Rosen A 1997 Aspects of percutaneous fine-needle aspiration biopsy in the diagnosis of pancreatic carcinoma. American Journal of Surgery 174: 303–306

Lindgren R G 1982 Percutaneous needle biopsy: a new technique. Acta Radiologica (Diagnosis) 23: 633–656

Livraghi T, Damascelli B, Lombardi C, Spagoli I 1983 Risk in fine needle abdominal biopsy. Journal of Clinical Ultrasound 11: 77–79

Livraghi T, Pilotti S, Ravetto C, Sangalli G, Solbiati L 1985 Inclusion-cytology versus smear-cytology in fine needle abdominal biopsy. European Journal of Radiology 5: 111–114

Longmire W P, McArthur M, Basounis E, Hiatt J 1973 Carcinoma of the extrahepatic biliary tract. Annals of Surgery 1978: 333–345

Lopes Cordozo P 1954 Clinical cytology. Stafleu, Leiden

Lundquist A 1970a Fine needle aspiration biopsy for cytodiagnosis of malignant tumor of the liver. Acta Medica Scandinavica 188: 465–470

Lundquist A 1970b Liver biopsy with a needle of 0.7 mm outer diameter. Acta Medica Scandinavica 188: 471–474

Lüning M, Kursawe R, Schöpke W et al 1985 CT guided percutaneous fine-needle biopsy of the pancreas. European Journal of Radiology 5: 104–108

Martin H E, Ellis E B 1930 Biopsy by needle puncture and aspiration. Annals of Surgery 92: 169–181

Menghini G 1958 One-second needle biopsy of the liver. Gastroenterology 235: 190–199

Menghini G 1970 One-second biopsy of the liver—problems of its clinical application. New England Journal of Medicine 183: 582–584

Mindell H J, Korson R 1990 Comparison of 22-gauge Chiba and screw-tipped needles for cytologic diagnosis of malignancies in vitro tumor specimens. Radiology 176: 681–682

Mitty H A, Efremidis S C, Yeh H C 1981 Impact of fine-needle biopsy on management of patients with carcinoma of the pancreas. American Journal of Roentgenology 137: 1119–1121

Montali G, Solbiati L, Croce F, Ierace T, Ravietto C 1982 Fine-needle aspiration biopsy of liver focal lesions ultrasonically guided with a real-time probe. Report of 126 cases. British Journal of Radiology 55: 717–723

Mora J, Puig P, Boadas J, Urgell E, Montserrat E, Lerma E, Gonzalez-Sastre F, Lluis F, Farre A, Capella G 1998 K-ras gene mutations in the diagnosis of fine-needle aspirates of pancreatic masses: prospective study using two techniques with different detection limits. Clinica Chemica 44: 2243–2248

Mueller P R, Stark D D, Simeone J F 1986 MR-guided aspiration biopsy: needle design and clinical trials. Radiology 161: 605–609

Murphy F B, Basefield K P, Steinberg H V, Bernardino M E 1988 CT- or sonography-guided biopsy of the liver in the presence of ascites: frequency of complications. American Journal of Roentgenology 151: 485–486

Nolsøe C, Nielsen L, Torp-Pedersen S, Holm H H 1990 Major complications and deaths due to interventional ultrasonography: a review of 800 cases. Journal of Clinical Ultrasound 18: 179–184

Nyman R S, Cappelen-Smith J, Brismar J, von Sinner W N, Kagevi I 1995 Yield and complications in ultrasound-guided biopsy of abdominal lesions. Comparison of fine-needle aspiration biopsy and 1.2-mm needle core biopsy using an automated biopsy gun. Acta Radiologica 36: 485–490

Ohlsson B, Tranberg K-G, Nilsson J, Stenram U, Åkerman M 1999 Percutaneous fine needle aspiration cytology of the liver tumours—consequences for management and outcome. (Submitted)

Oscarson J, Stormby N, Sundgren R 1972 Selective angiography in fine-needle aspiration cytodiagnosis of gastric and pancreatic tumours. Acta Radiologica 12: 737–749

Pagani J J 1983 Biopsy of focal hepatic lesions. Comparison of 18 and 22 gauge needles. Radiology 147: 673–675

Patel R I, Shapiro M J 1995 Biliary venous fistula: an unusual complication of fine-needle aspiration biopsy of the liver. Journal of Vascular and Interventional Radiology 6: 953–956

Pelsang R E, Johlin F C 1997 A percutaneous biopsy technique for patients with suspected biliary or pancreatic cancer without a radiographic mass. Abdominal Imaging 22: 307–310

Peralta-Venturina M N de, Wong D K, Purslow M J, Kini S R 1996 Biliary tract cytology in specimens obtained by direct cholangiographic procedures: a study of 74 cases. Diagnostic Cytopathology 14: 334–348

Perrault J, McGill D B, Ott B J, Taylor W F 1978 Liver biopsy: complications in 1000 patients. Gastroenterology 74: 102–106

Ponchon T, Gagnon P, Berger F, Labadie M, Liaras A, Chavaillon A, Bory R 1995 Value of endobiliary brush cytology and biopsies for the diagnosis of malignant bile duct stenosis: results of a prospective study. Gastrointestional Endoscopy 42: 565–567

Pugliese V, Conio M, Nicolo G, Saccomanno S, Gatteschi B 1995 Endoscopic retrograde forceps biopsy and brush cytology of biliary structures: a prospective study. Gastrointestional Endoscopy 42: 520–526

Rapaccini G L, Pompili M, Caturelli E, Fursilli S, Trombino C, Gomes V, Squillante M M, Castelvetere M, Aliotta A, Grattagliano A et al 1994 Ultrasound-guided fine-needle biopsy of hepatocellular carcinoma: comparison between smear cytology and microhistology. American Journal of Gastroenterology 89: 898–902

Reading C C, Charboneau J W, James E M, Hurt M R 1988 Sonographically guided percutaneous biopsy of small (3 cm or less) masses. American Journal of Roentgenology 151: 189–192

Riley S A, Irving H C, Axon A T R, Ellis W R, Lintott D J, Losowsky M S 1984 Percutaneous liver biopsy with plugging of needle track: a safe method for use in patients with impaired coagulation. Lancet ii: 436

Rosenblatt R, Klutcher R, Moussouris H F, Schrieber K, Koss L G 1982 Sonographically guided fine-needle aspiration of liver lesions. Journal of the American Medical Association 248: 1639–1641

Ryd W, Hagmar B, Eriksson O 1983 Local tumour cell seeding by fine-needle aspiration biopsy: a semiquantitative study. Acta Pathologica Microbiologica et Immunologica Scandinavica 91(A): 17–21

Sangalli G, Livraghi T, Giordano F 1989 Fine needle biopsy of hepatocellular carcinoma: improvement in diagnosis by microhistology. Gastroenterology 96: 524–526

Sautereau D, Vive O, Cazer P Y et al 1987 Value of sonographically guided fine needle aspiration biopsy in evaluating the liver with sonographic abnormalities. Gastroenterology 93: 715–718

Savader S J, Prescott C A, Lund G B, Osterman F A 1996 Intraductal biliary biopsy: comparison of three techniques. Journal of Vascular and Interventional Radiology 7: 743–750

Sbolli G, Fornari F, Givardi G et al 1990 Role of ultrasound guided fine needle aspiration biopsy in the diagnosis of hepatocellular carcinoma. Gut 31: 1303–1305

Schoefl R, Haefner M, Wrba F, Pfeffel F, Stain C, Poetzi R, Gangl A 1997 Forceps biopsy and brush cytology during endoscopic retrograde cholangiopancreatography for the diagnosis of biliary stenoses. Scandinavian Journal of Gastroenterology 32: 363–368

Schwerk W B, Schmitz-Moormann P 1981 Ultrasonically guided fine-needle biopsies in neoplastic liver disease: cytohistological diagnosis and echo pattern of lesions. Cancer 48: 1469–1477

Schwerk W B, Dürr H K, Schmitz-Moormann P 1983 Ultrasound guided fine-needle biopsies in pancreatic and hepatic neoplasms. Gastrointestinal Radiology 8: 219–225

Servoll E, Viste A, Skaarland E et al 1988 Fine-needle aspiration cytology of focal liver lesions. Advantages and limitations. Acta Chirurgica Scandinavica 154: 61–63

Shibata D, Almoguera C, Forrester K, Dunitz J, Martin S E, Cosgrove M M, Perucho M, Arnheim N 1990 Detection of c-K-ras mutations in fine needle aspirates from human pancreatic adenocarcinomas. Cancer Research 50: 1279–1283

Shukla V K, Pandey M, Kumar M, Sood B P, Gupta A, Aryya N C, Shukla R C, Verma D N 1997 Ultrasound-guided fine needle aspiration cytology of malignant gallbladder masses. Acta Cytologica 41: 1654–1658

Smith E H 1984 The hazard of fine-needle aspiration biopsy. Ultrasound in Medicine and Biology 10: 629–634

Smith E H 1985 Fine needle aspiration biopsy: are there any risks? In: Holm H H, Kristensen J K (eds) Interventional ultrasound. Munksgard, Copenhagen, p 169–177

Smith E H 1991 Complications of percutaneous abdominal fine-needle biopsy. Radiology 178: 253–258

Söderström N 1966 Fine needle aspiration biopsy. Grune and Stratton, New York

Solbiati L, Livraghi T, De Pia L, Ierace T, Masciadri N, Ravetto C 1985 Fine-needle biopsy of hepatic hemangioma with sonographic guidance. American Journal of Roentgenology 144: 471

Solmi L, Gandolfi L, Muratori R, Leo P, Bacchini P 1987 Echo-guided fine-needle biopsy of pancreatic masses. The American Journal of Gastroenterology 82: 744–748

Solmi L, Muratori R, Bacchini P, Primerano A, Gandolfi L 1992 Comparison between echo-guided fine-needle aspiration cytology and microhistology in diagnosing pancreatic masses. Surgical Endoscopy 6: 222–224

Stefaniak J 1997 Fine needle aspiration biopsy in the differential diagnosis of the liver cystic echinococcosis. Acta Tropica 67: 107–111

Sugiyama M, Atomi Y, Wada N, Kuroda A, Muto T 1996 Endoscopic transpapillary bile duct biopsy without sphincterotomy for diagnosing biliary strictures: a prospective comparative study with bile and brush cytology. American Journal of Gastroenterology 91: 465–467

Søreide O, Skaarland E, Pedersen O M, Larssen T B, Arnesjø B 1985 Fine needle biopsy of the pancreas. Results of 204 biopsies in 190 patients. World Journal of Surgery 9: 960–965

Stormby N 1979 Pancreas. Monographs in Clinical Cytology 7: 194–211

Taavitsainen M, Koivuniemi A, Bondestam S, Kivisaari L, Tierala E 1987 Ultrasonically guided fine-needle aspiration biopsy in focal pancreatic lesions. Acta Radiologica 28 (Fasc. 5): 541–543

Taavitsainen M, Airaksinen T, Kreula J, Päivänsalo M 1990 Fine-needle aspiration biopsy of liver hemangioma. Acta Radiologica (Fasc. 1) 31: 69–71

Tada M, Omata M, Ohto M 1991 Clinical application of ras gene mutation for diagnosis of pancreatic adenocarcinoma. Gastroenterology 100: 233–238

Tao L C, Ho C S, McLaughlin J M, Evans W K, Donat E E 1984 Cytologic diagnosis of hepatocellular carcinoma by fine-needle aspiration biopsy. Cancer 53: 457–552

Tatsuta M, Yamamoto R, Kasugai H et al 1984 Cytohistologic diagnosis of neoplasms of the liver by ultrasonically guided fine-needle aspiration biopsy. Cancer 54: 1682–1686

Terasaki S, Kaneko S, Kobayashi K, Nonomura A, Nakanuma Y 1998 Liver, pancreas and biliary tract. Gastroenterology 115: 1216–1222

Torp-Pedersen S, Juul N, Vyberg M 1984 Histological sampling with a 23 gauge modified Manghini-needle. British Journal of Radiology 57: 151–154

Tung G A, Cronan J J 1993 Percutaneous needle biopsy of hepatic cavernous hemangioma. Journal of Clinical Gastroenterology 16: 117–122

Tylen U, Arnesjø B, Lindberg L G, Lunderquist A, Åkerman M 1976 Percutaneous biopsy of carcinoma of the pancreas guided by angiography. Surgery, Gynecology and Obstetrics 142: 737–739

Vilgrain V, Anagnostopoulos C, Chagnon S, Blèry M 1987 Etude de 90 ponctions à l'aiguille fine à visèe diagnostique de l'abdomen supèrieur sous controle èchographique. Apport de l'analyse cyto et histologique. Journal de Radiologie 68: 35–38

Villmann P 1998 Endoscopic ultrasound-guided fine-needle biopsy in Europe. Endoscopy 30: A161–A162

Vilmann P, Jacobsen G K, Henriksen F, Hancke S 1992 Endoscopic ultrasonography with guided fine needle aspiration biopsy in pancreatic disease. Gastrointestinal Endoscopy 38: 172–173

von Sinner W N, Nyman R, Linjawi T, Ali A M 1995 Fine needle aspiration biopsy of hydatid cysts. Acta Radiologica 36: 168–172

Wada K, Kondo F, Kondo Y 1988 Large regenerative nodules and dysplastic nodules in cirrhotic livers: a histopathologic study. Hepatology 8: 1684–1688

Wasastjerna C 1969 A cytochemical method for the study of bile canaliculi in fine needle aspirates of the liver. Acta Pathologica Microbiologica et Immunologica Scandinavica 77: 399–404

Wasastjerna C 1979 Liver. In: Zajicek J (ed) Aspiration biopsy cytology. Part 2: Cytology of infradiaphragmatic organs. S Karger, Basel, p 167–192

Watanabe M, Asaka M, Tanaka J, Kurosawa M, Kasai M, Miyazaki T 1994 Point mutations of K-ras gene codon 12 in biliary tract tumours. Gastroenterology 107: 1147–1153

Webb A J 1974 Through a glass darkly. (The development of needle aspiration biopsy). Bristol Medico-Chirurgical Journal 89: 59–68

Weiss H, Duntsch U, Weiss A 1988 Risiken der Feinnadelpunktion: Ergebnisse einer Unfrage in der BRD (DEGUM-Unfrage). Ultraschall Medizin 9: 121–127

Weiss H, Weiss A, Scholl A 1988 Todliche Komplikation einer Feinnadelbiopsie der Leber. Deutsche Medicinische Wochenschrifte 113: 139–142

Welch T J, Sheedy P F, Johnson C D, Johnson C M, Stephens D H 1989 CT-guided biopsy: prospective analysis of 1000 procedures. Radiology 171: 493–496

Whitlach S, Nunez C, Pitlik D A 1984 Fine needle aspiration biopsy of the liver. A study of 102 consecutive cases. Acta Cytologica 28: 719–725

Wiersema M J, Vilmann P, Giovannini M, Chang K J, Wiersema L M 1997 Endosonography-guided fine-needle biopsy: Diagnostic and complications assessment. Gastroenterology 112: 1087–1095

Wittenberg J, Mueller P R, Ferruci J T et al 1982 Percutaneous core biopsy of abdominal tumors using 22 gauge needles: Further observations. American Journal of Roentgenology 139: 75–80

Wu S S, Lin K C, Soon M S, Yeh K T 1996 Ultrasound-guided percutaneous transhepatic fine needle aspiration cytology study of gallbladder polypoid lesions. American Journal of Gastroenterology 91: 1591–1594

Yamanaka T, Kimura K 1979 Differential diagnosis of pancreatic mass lesions with percutaneous fine-needle aspiration biopsy under ultrasonic guidance. Digestive Diseases and Sciences 24: 694–699

Yates C K, Streight R 1986 Focal fatty infiltration of the liver simulating metastatic disease. Radiology 159: 83–84

Young E Y 1992 Percutaneous abdominal biopsy. Baillière's Clinical Gastroenterology 6: 219–244

Yu S C, Metreweli C, Lau W Y, Leung W T, Liew C T, Leung N W 1997 Safety of percutaneous biopsy of hepatocellular carcinoma with an 18 gauge automated needle. Clinical Radiology 52: 907–911

Yu S C, Lau W Y, Leung W T, Liew C T, Leung N W, Metreweli C 1998 Percutaneuous biopsy of small hepatic lesions using an 18 gauge automated needle. British Journal of Radiology 71: 621–624

Zargar S A, Khuroo M S, Mahajan R, Jan G M, Shah P 1991 US-guided fine-needle aspiration biopsy of gallbladder masses. Radiology 179: 275–278

Zins M, Vilgrain V, Gayno S et al 1992 US-guided percutaneous liver biopsy with plugging of the needle track: a prospective study in 72 high-risk patients. Radiology 184: 841–843

Zornoza J 1981 Percutaneous needle biopsy. Williams and Williams, Baltimore

Diagnostic laparoscopic techniques

20

C.H. WAKEFIELD, O.J. GARDEN

INTRODUCTION

Whilst the current impetus of minimally invasive surgery has been directed principally towards interventional laparoscopic procedures, the principles and technology of these procedures have evolved from the diagnostic techniques described nearly a century ago. The introduction of laparoscopic cholecystectomy in 1989 was a watershed in the development of minimal access surgery and brought with it an explosion of techniques and descriptions of a multitude of complex laparoscopic procedures. With these developments came the revival of diagnostic laparoscopy, for which there exists a definite role in the investigative algorithm of hepatobiliary disease. Diagnostic and staging laparoscopy is now therefore an established surgical procedure for the evaluation of gastrointestinal disease.

The first published report on laparoscopy by Jacobaeus, described 'the use of a cystoscope for the examination of the serosal cavities' in humans (Jacobaeus 1910). Meanwhile, at the Johns Hopkins University Medical School, Bernheim reported the first 'organoscopy' in the United States, in a patient of Halsted's with pancreatic cancer (Bernheim 1911). Kalk further pioneered the use of laparoscopy in the investigation of patients with liver disease and is credited with the design of the laparoscope upon which current designs are based (Kalk 1955). Ruddock (1934) was first to report on the usefulness of laparoscopy in liver and peritoneal disease, however the procedure was slow to gain popularity in the surgical community. It was the gynecologists who first recognized the usefulness of laparoscopy as both a diagnostic and therapeutic tool. The recognition of its efficacy and safety in their hands rekindled the interest of surgeons. Sugarbaker et al (1975) reported on the role of laparosocpy in the evaluation of abdominal pain and Cortesi et al (1979) utilized laparoscopy in the management of abdominal trauma. Hall et al (1980) is credited with one of the earliest reports on the use of laparoscopy in the assessment of the operability of intra-abdominal malignancies, particularly in the diagnostic challenge of the patient with jaundice and hepatomegaly. Despite the improvement in preoperative imaging modalities, the highly resolved and magnified views of the peritoneal cavity produced by modern optical systems at laparoscopy, allows the clinician to detect trace amounts of ascites and minute malignant serosal deposits. Armed with laparoscopic ultrasound, tissue parenchyma distant from the direct vision of the laparoscopist can be examined and biopsied safely for histological evaluation. Diagnostic laparoscopic techniques have increased the precision of diagnosis avoiding the committal to a potential nontherapeutic laparotomy. Some surgeons would regard diagnostic laparoscopy as a mandatory prelude to laparotomy, in the patient with suspected hepatobiliary and pancreatic malignancy, although this opinion is not universally held.

TECHNIQUES

The principles of laparoscopic procedures have remained the same since its first introduction. Namely the safe puncture of the peritoneum, followed by insufflation with gas to obtain an adequate pneumoperitoneum prior to insertion of a laparoscope. The careful systematic inspection of the peritoneum and insertion of further ports under direct vision is undertaken as indicated by initial laparoscopic findings.

PATIENT PREPARATION

Diagnostic laparoscopy may be performed either under local or general anesthesia. Examinations under local anesthetic should be carried out using the same sterile techniques as those under general anesthesia. The patient should be sedated and the facility for converting to general anesthesia and laparotomy should be immediately available. The authors routinely perform diagnostic laparoscopy under general anesthesia, since thorough examination of the peritoneal recesses is not possible under local anesthesia and sedation. Patients are requested to void urine prior to the induction of general anesthesia, as an empty bladder is advisable. Routine catheterization is not advocated since this is associated with an increased incidence of urinary tract infections (Ahktar et al 1985). Prophylactic antibiotics are not given, but we use subcutaneous heparin routinely at the time of induction for deep vein thrombosis prophylaxis. The patient is positioned supine on the operating table with normal pressure area precautions, the abdomen is fully prepared with antiseptic solution in case of recourse to full laparotomy and draped with sterile sheets as for any abdominal procedure.

The operating surgeon and assistants should be familiar with the workings and set up of the videophotographic equipment used, which prior to commencing the diagnostic procedure should be checked for correct function, picture quality, focus and color balance. Any ancillary equipment such as video recording, image capture, or ultrasonographic equipment should be tested for correct connection and interaction. The surgeon is reliant on the performance of these systems, therefore time taken in ensuring their proper functioning before embarking upon the procedure will allow the smooth and safe running of the diagnostic laparoscopy. Many recesses and organs are poorly visualized using end-viewing laparoscopes, such as the surface of the liver and pelvic recesses. These limited views may be improved by using an oblique (commonly 30°) viewing laparoscope, which may be rotated through a full 360° giving the surgeon greater flexibility and capabilities of viewing awkward areas within the abdominal cavity.

PRODUCTION OF PNEUMOPERITONEUM

The complications associated with diagnostic laparoscopy are related to the process of obtaining a pneumoperitoneum and to inadvertent instrumental injuries during laparoscopic examination. The majority of these complications are visceral or vascular puncture injuries caused by Veress needles and trocars. A recent meta-analysis has shown that open techniques of peritoneal access are significantly safer than percutaneous puncture in obtaining a pneumoperitoneum (Bonjer et al 1997). This meta-analysis reported on 489 335 laparoscopic procedures. The incidence of visceral injury using a closed technique was 0.083% compared with 0.048% for open cut-down. There were no reported vascular injuries with open techniques, whereas percutaneous puncture carried a vascular injury rate of 0.075%. Clearly

utilizing an open method of inserting ports is safer than a blind technique. In addition, it utilizes maneuvers which are familiar to surgeons who might not have had formal training in laparoscopic techniques and, in addition, open methods provide more rapid insufflation at lower overall financial cost.

Two open techniques are currently widely used, the first involves a direct cut-down onto the peritoneum through a small supraumbilical or infraumbilical incision and a purse string suture is placed around the fascia of the incised linea alba and peritoneum. The introduction of a modified port by Hasson has facilitated this procedure, there being two wings on the barrel of the port, in to which a blunt obturator fits. These wings allow the port to be held in position by sutures placed either side of the incision, thereby stabilizing the port and reducing the escape of gas around the barrel of the port. This technique can be used anywhere on the anterior abdominal, and is particularly appropriate in patients who have had previous surgery with possible adhesion formation (Hasson 1974). The authors use a second, more simple technique, which was first described by Fielding in 1992 (Paterson Brown 1994). The umbilicus is grasped using Kocher's forceps and everted. A small incision is made along the midline over the everted umbilicus where the skin is in close proximity to the underlying umbilical tube and peritoneum. Small retractors display the cylindrical umbilical tube which is incised longitudinally from its apex to the point where it fuses with the linea alba. Gentle blunt dissection with artery forceps through this plane permits safe entry into the peritoneal cavity. Thereafter a port without trocar or with a blunt trocar is inserted and gas insufflation commenced. Because of the improved efficacy and safety of the open cut-down technique, we currently do not use percutaneous puncture with a Veress needle to obtain pneumoperitoneum. Description of this closed and similar techniques may be found in other texts of laparoscopy.

INSUFFLATION OF GAS

Having inserted the 10 mm umbilical port, gas tubing is connected to the insufflating source. Early laparoscopists achieved pneumoperitoneum with room air introduced by the pumping action of a sterilized sphygmomanometer bulb. Some centers routinely use room air for insufflation, however reports of air embolism, pneumomediastinum and pneumopericardium prompted the search for alternative insufflating agents. Carbon dioxide is the most widely used agent, since it is non-combustible and therefore safe for use with electrocautery. It is readily absorbed and the risk of embolism is thereby reduced. Considerable volumes of carbon dioxide may be absorbed systemically during prolonged laparoscopic procedures and this may result in hypercapnia and acid-base disturbances which in turn may cause tachy-dysrythmias (Tan et al 1992). Carbon dioxide is too irritant to the peritoneal lining for laparoscopy to be undertaken under local anesthesia. Nitric oxide may be used for insufflation as an alternative and has additional analgesic properties. Electrocautery is however contraindicated with a nitric oxide pneumoperitoneum. Insufflation should be conducted under the control of a dedicated insufflating device; with an initial flow of gas at 1 liter per minute. The volume of gas introduced should be between 3 and 4 liters and an operating insufflation pressure well below 15 mmHg. When the intraabdominal pressure rises above 20 mmHg not only is the patient's ventilatory capacity reduced, but so is the pulse pressure and cardiac output as a consequence of diminished cardiac return. Even at lower pressures these changes may be sufficient to compromise patients with severe cardio-pulmonary disease (Wittgen et al 1991).

GENERAL LAPAROSCOPY OF THE PERITONEAL CAVITY

Following the development of an adequate pneumoperitoneum, the laparoscope is inserted and the omentum and viscera immediately adjacent to the umbilical port is examined for signs of trauma. In patients with liver disease and portal hypertension, distended periumbilical veins are prone to trauma and any bleeding at the port site should be viewed with suspicion and the source identified before proceeding further.

As for open laparotomy, diagnostic laparoscopy should follow a routine sequence. The pelvis and pelvic organs should be examined first. It is often necessary to insert additional ports, through which blunt probes and forceps may be passed to facilitate examination of other viscera. Such probes allow manipulation of viscera and the texture and fixity of structures can be determined in a limited way. An inspection of the abdominal cavity is performed and the parietal peritoneum carefully scrutinized. Attention is focused subsequently on the visceral peritoneum, the surfaces of the right and left lobes of the liver are examined and the anterior wall of the stomach, the lesser and greater omentum and spleen are all visualized in turn. If the greater omentum is turned upward and the colon retracted cranially, the root of the mesentry can be inspected, and the pancreatic head assessed through the mesocolon and duodenal curve. Atraumatic grasping forceps allow the surgeon to 'walk' along the small and large bowel. Some surgeons would routinely enter the lesser sac via the gastrocolic omentum, but this is unlikely to provide additional information except where the resectability of a tumor involving

the body of the pancreas is being assessed (Van Dijkum et al 1997). Conlon and his colleagues have advocated a trial dissection combined with lymph node sampling in patients with tumor of the pancreatic head (Conlon et al 1996).

EXAMINATION OF THE LIVER AND BILIARY TREE

The authors routinely use two 10 mm laparoscopic ports for examination of the liver and biliary tree. The first port is inserted at the umbilicus, and the second to the right in the midclavicular or anterior axillary line. Laparoscopic ultrasound is an integral part of our laparoscopic evaluation in hepatobiliary disease. At the outset of the examination the laparoscope is placed at the umbilicus and the laparoscopic ultrasound probe (a 10 mm diameter 7.5 MHz linear array probe) passed through the right lateral port (Fig. 20.1). These positions can be interchanged during the examination to allow different views and probe placements over the liver. In the initial part of the examination it is best to avoid displacement of the liver and structures at the porta hepatis, since the insufflation of gas in the subhepatic space may interfere with the quality of ultrasound images of the porta hepatis structures. All peritoneal and omental surfaces are scrutinized carefully, particularly along the falciform ligament and in the subdiaphragmatic recesses. The laparoscope is passed over both domes of the liver, noting its color, whether the surface is smooth or irregular and whether discrete lesions on the surface are visible. The liver edge and

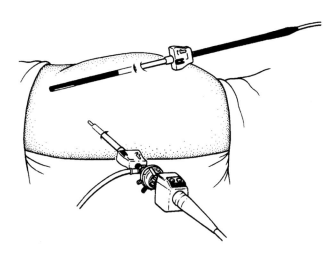

Fig. 20.1 The position of ports for laparoscopy and laparoscopic ultrasound evaluation of the liver. At the onset of the examination the laparoscope is placed through the umbilical port and the ultrasound probe at the right lateral port. These positions are later interchanged.

gallbladder should be inspected, noting the presence of adhesions around the gallbladder, its size and opalescence. Observations should be made on mesenteric vascularity and the size of the spleen, important features of portal hypertension and lymphomas. In the presence of portal hypertension, adhesions should by divided by coagulating cautery, since the presence of collateral vessels may produce troublesome bleeding if adhesions are inadvertently torn. At this point any ascitic fluid may be sampled by passing a sterile nasogastric tube through the second lateral port and aspirating into a catheter tip syringe. Instilling normal saline into the peritoneal cavity during the early part of the examination serves two purposes. It improves the acoustic coupling during laparoscopic contact ultrasonography; and by aspirating the saline at the end of the procedure, allows peritoneal cytology to be performed when only small volumes of peritoneal fluid are present.

The laparoscope is moved to the right lateral port and the ultrasound probe inserted at the umbilicus. Under laparoscopic vision the ultrasound probe is place in direct contact with the liver capsule of segment IV (quadrate lobe). From this position the portal vein and its bifurcation can be visualized and will act as a useful landmark upon which the remaining examination can be referenced. The probe is now placed over the right hemiliver in order to identify lesions within the liver parenchyma. Examination of the left lobe of the liver requires the surgeon to move the probe to the other side of the falciform ligament on to segments II and III. From segment IV, rotating the probe to the left brings the porta hepatis into view. The portal vein is separated from the vena cava by the caudate lobe (segment I), the common hepatic duct and hepatic artery lie anterior to the portal vein and the artery can be recognized by its pulsation. The segmental branches may be followed out as they run into the parenchyma of the left and right lobes of the liver. The middle hepatic vein runs from the antero-inferior aspect to the upper reaches of the liver, where it joins the cava at its confluence with the left hepatic vein. In order to identify the middle hepatic vein, the probe is placed over the junction of segments IV and V in the region of the gallbladder and advanced towards the vena cava (Fig. 20.2). Rotating the probe will bring the right or left hepatic veins into the image view. Further examination by lifting the undersurface of the liver allows direct inspection of the inferior surface with the laparoscope.

Appreciation of the vascular anatomy of the liver allows

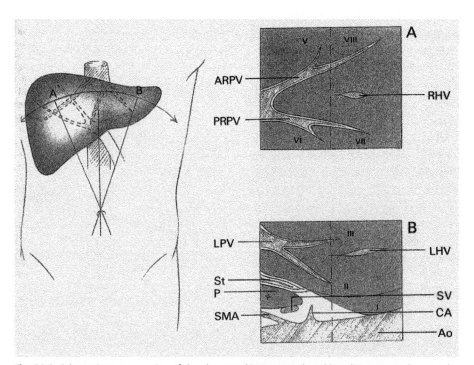

Fig. 20.2 Schematic representation of the ultrasound images produced by a linear array ultrasound probe placed through the umbilicus. **(A)** Oblique cross sectional scan of the right hemiliver. The anterior (ARPV) and posterior (PRPV) divisions of the right portal vein are displayed, the right hepatic vein passes in the plane between segments V and VIII anteriorly and segments VI and VII posteriorly. **(B)** Oblique sonogram of the left hemiliver, showing the left portal vein (LPV) and left hepatic vein (LHV). Structures lying posteriorly to the left lobe of the liver may be visualized. St, stomach; P, pancreas; SV, splenic vein; Ao, aorta; CA, celic axis; SMA, superior mesenteric artery.

the precise segmental location of lesions within the liver parenchyma to be determined, thus dictating the suitability and surgical approach to the lesion as well as identifying vascular involvement in the case of malignant disease of the liver. In order to examine the gallbladder, the ultrasound probe is best placed on the surface of segment IV, using the liver as an acoustic window; the size, wall thickness and the presence of calculi can be determined. As much of the biliary tree as possible should be examined through this window, after which the probe is moved directly onto the porta hepatis and drawn over the first part of the duodenum and head of the pancreas to allow the distal common bile duct to be examined. The duct can be traced along its intra pancreatic portion to the ampulla and the relationship to the vessels of any lesion arising from the common bile duct or pancreatic head can be assessed.

ACQUISITION OF MATERIAL FOR HISTOLOGY

Laparoscopically guided biopsies have the advantage over blind or radiologically guided biopsies, in that specific areas or lesions may be targeted without injury to adjacent structures. In addition, should there be bleeding following a biopsy, this can be controlled by direct tamponade by a probe or by diathermy. In this way the procedure of liver biopsy is considerably safer particularly in patients who are coagulopathic or have portal hypertension. Laparoscopic liver biopsy may be performed via a separate percutaneous puncture, and Tru-cut® biopsy needles are favored. Peritoneal or surface lesions on the liver may be sampled by pinch biopsies or excision using diathermy scissors and material from suspected lymph node metastases may be obtained using long fine needle aspiration. It is not our practice to routinely attempt laparoscopic needle biopsy in patients considered to have potentially resectable disease, because needle tract seeding to the parieties is a well documented phenomenon (Soreide 1990, John & Garden 1993). Surgeons undertaking laparoscopic assessment of intra-abdominal malignancy should be aware that tumor dissemination to port sites has been reported for hepatobiliary and other gastro-intestinal malignancies (van Dikjum et al 1996).

CONCLUSION OF LAPAROSCOPY

Once the examination is complete, instruments should be withdrawn under direct vision, following which auxiliary ports are removed and their insertion points inspected for bleeding from within the peritoneal cavity. The pneumoperitoneum is released and the final port and camera are removed. It is important to remove as much of the insufflating gas as possible, this minimizes postoperative pain and

lessens the potential for carbon dioxide absorption. Fascial defects of 10 mm or more should be closed and a J-shaped needle with absorbable suture material is preferred for the fascial layer. Following skin closure, the wounds should be infiltrated with local anesthetic to reduce the postoperative analgesic requirements.

COMPLICATIONS OF LAPAROSCOPY

The morbidity and mortality of diagnostic laparoscopic procedures is reported to be low. *These reports come from heterogenous patient groups and since they are retrospective, probably underestimate the true incidence.* Minor complications, defined as those which did not require immediate surgery or transfusion, occur in between 1 and 9% of laparoscopies (Kane & Kreis 1984). Major complications such as bowel perforations, lacerations of the spleen, hemorrhage and peritonitis occur with a frequency of 0.3 to 2.3%. The incidence of minor and major complications from a prospective series of patients undergoing laparoscopy for the assessment of gastrointestinal malignancies reported minor complication rates of 3% and major complications in 1% of procedures. The overall mortality reported in the literature ranges from zero to 0.49%, mainly from trocar injuries and cardiopulmonary complications (Nieveen van Dikjum 1998).

Port-site metastases following laparoscopic evaluation of malignant disease was first reported by Dobronte et al (1978). Since this first report, many similar cases have followed. There are a number of possible mechanisms which may account for this phenomenon, such as aerolization of tumor cells by insufflating gas, or by direct spread from handling by instruments. Port-site metastases after laparoscopy have only been reported in patients with advanced malignancy, having no influence on survival. The incidence is approximately 2% of staging laparoscopies, as of yet there is no concensus on means of prevention (van Dikjum 1998).

DIAGNOSTIC LAPAROSCOPIC ASSESSMENT IN CLINICAL PRACTICE

PRIMARY HEPATIC MALIGNANCY

Current radiological techniques are limited in their ability to detect small hepatic lesions of less than 1 cm diameter, particularly those situated superficially or on the liver capsule. In addition subtle parenchymal changes associated with liver disease such as cirrhosis are often not detected. Despite current radiologic imaging capabilities, up to 40% of patients with primary or metastatic hepatic malignancies have been found to have unresectable disease at the time of laparotomy (Soyer et al 1993). The role of laparoscopy in the diagnosis and management of hepatocellular carcinoma has been long established. Fornari et al (1988) reported on a series of 63 patients with focal liver lesions and compared the effectiveness of ultrasound guided needle biopsy with that of laparoscopically directed biopsy. Fine needle biopsy under ultrasound control showed a sensitivity of 75.6% with a rate of 84.1% in overall accuracy. Laparoscopy alone was associated with a sensitivity rate of 74.3% and an overall accuracy of 82.7%. The combination of the two procedures achieved an overall accuracy of 98.4% with a sensitivity of 97.5%. The authors commented that laparoscopy in addition to increasing the diagnostic accuracy of biopsy, also provided additional information to that of conventional imaging which could be of clinical relevance, particularly in the presence of cirrhosis (Fornari and others 1988). It is this additional information which provided early advocates of laparoscopy the advantage in surgical management of hepatocellular carcinoma. Jeffers et al (1988) studied 27 cases of presumptive hepatocellular carcinoma by means of laparoscopy and fine needle aspiration. In this study, fine needle aspirates provided positive and safe diagnoses of hepatocellular carcinoma in all the patients examined. The most significant finding from this cohort however was that from the laparoscopic findings, the entire cohort was

deemed unresectable on account of the presence of multifocal tumors, peritoneal spread and severe cirrhosis (Fig. 20.3). Thus in the assessment of hepatocellular carcinoma, laparoscopy is effective in obtaining representative tissue and thus providing a histological diagnosis. Moreover the additional information detected at laparoscopy provided means by which resectability could be accurately assessed, thus reducing the likelihood of performing an unnecessary exploratory laparotomy.

Subtle changes in liver morphology that might be detected at laparoscopy may also be of relevance. The appearance of yellow nodules on the surface of the liver has been shown to be a sensitive indicator of an underlying hepatocellular carcinoma. The presence too, of large complex regenerative nodules is closely associated with the occurrence of small subclinical hepatocellular carcinomas (Kameda & Shinji 1992). Cirrhotic patients with large complex regenerative nodules identified at laparoscopy have a cumulative hepatocellular carcinoma occurrence rate of 73% when followed over 3 years, whereas with similar patients in whom laparoscopy failed to detect such nodules, the cumulative rate of hepatocellular carcinoma was only 6% (Kameda and others 1997). In a prospective study of 442 patients examined by laparoscopy prior to treatment with interferon-α therapy for chronic type C hepatitis, specific laparoscopic findings before therapy were significantly associated with

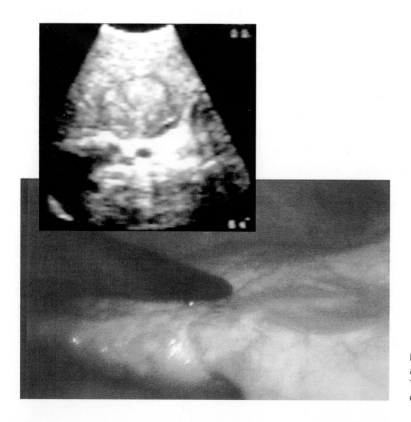

Fig. 20.3 A composite laparoscopic image of a cirrhotic liver and laparoscopic ultrasound picture of a typical hepatoma. These are generally hyperechoic lesions with a surrounding echolucent rim.

liver carcinogenesis. Hepatocellular carcinoma developed in 16 patients, but again only in those with irregular or nodular livers (Arase et al 1997).

The use of laparoscopy in the assessment of the patient with hepatocellular carcinoma will preclude approximately 50% of patients from subsequent laparotomy on the basis of unresectability (Babineau et al 1994). Laparoscopy is limited in that it is only able to provide information on the presence of obvious visible disease. This information can be supplemented by ultrasound images of tissues not directly accessible to laparoscopic examination. The information provided by intraoperative contact ultrasound has been shown to influence modifications to the surgical approach of patients under consideration for resection of primary and secondary liver tumors at open surgery (Bismuth et al 1987). It was inevitable that a combination of the two modalities of laparoscopy and contact ultrasonography would improve the assessment of the patient with intra-abdominal malignancy. Thus additional features such as deep parenchymal small multifocal lesions may be identified, as well as tumor thrombus formation in the portal vein and vascular involvement, findings which would render the patient unresectable and that would be concealed from routine laparoscopic examination. In a prospective study evaluating laparoscopy and laparoscopic ultrasonography in 91 patients intended for hepatic resection for hepatocellular carcinoma, 15 patients had evidence of unresectable disease using these combined modalities. Among the remaining 76 patients who underwent laparotomy, nine had exploration only and 67 underwent hepatic resection. Ultimately in this series, the combination of laparoscopy and laparoscopic ultrasound avoided an unnecessary exploratory laparotomy in 63% of patients (Lo et al 1998).

METASTATIC HEPATIC MALIGNANCY (see also Ch. 75)

Although metastases to the liver may arise from any primary tumor site, the hepatobiliary surgeon is mainly concerned with the management of those arising from a colorectal source. Up to 50% of patients with a diagnosis of colorectal carcinoma will develop metastases (Bengtsson et al 1981), the presence of which have profound implications on long-term survival. In a proportion of patients it is feasible to consider curative liver resection. Dynamic computed tomographic (CT) scanning, iodized oil-emulsion enhanced CT and computed tomographic arterioportography (CTAP) have all been evaluated in the assessment of hepatic metastatic disease. Overall sensitivity of these imaging techniques in detecting metastases range from 38 to 94%, but the sensitivity falls considerably with lesions

less than 1 cm in diameter (Tubiana et al 1992). Despite the sensitivity of CTAP, there is an associated high false-positive rate due to intrahepatic perfusion defects, which may occur in up to 40% of cases in some series (Soyer et al 1993). In our early experience of patients shown by radiological study to have resectable liver tumors (the majority metastatic) (John et al 1994), 46% of patients were demonstrated to have irresectable disease by laparoscopy as a consequence of extrahepatic spread, extensive bilobar disease and the presence of cirrhosis. The addition of laparoscopic ultrasound to the patient's assessment revealed liver tumors not detected by laparoscopy alone in a further 33%. In the cohort of 50 patients, 23 patients were precluded from resection by laparoscopy, and a further nine by laparoscopic ultrasound (due to the presence of bilobar diseases, hilar lymphadenopathy and vascular invasion). Two further patients originally thought to have malignant liver tumors, were found on laparoscopic ultrasound to have a regenerating liver nodule and a simple liver cyst. The combination of laparoscopy and laparoscopic ultrasound increased resectability to 98%, compared with a historical resectability rate of 58% before the introduction of these staging modalities. Clearly staging laparoscopy as a prelude to laparotomy reduces the physical and psychological morbidity of a non-therapeutic open surgical procedure (Fig. 20.4).

Whilst colorectal liver metastases may be the most frequently encountered, laparoscopy has been shown to be effective in the preoperative detection of liver deposits from esophageal, gastric (Shandall & Johnson 1985) pancreatic (Warshaw et al 1990), gallbladder (Dagnini et al 1984) and ovarian malignancies (Rosenhoff et al 1975). In the prospective evaluation of laparoscopy in the staging of gastro-oesophageal malignancy, Molloy et al 1995 detected hepatic metastases in 31% of biopsy proven carcinomas not detected by preoperative CT scanning. In the Netherlands there is an extensive experience in the efficacy of laparoscopy and laparoscopic ultrasound in the staging of gastrointestinal malignancy. In a recent review, 4% of patients with esophageal carcinoma were precluded from laparotomy by metastatic disease. Metastatic hepatic dissemination was identified in 21% of patients with primary liver tumors. Metastases or tumor ingrowth was detected in 43% of patients with proximal bile duct carcinomas at laparoscopy and laparoscopic ultrasound (van Dijkum et al 1999). Their experience is similar to our own with regard to the evaluation of pancreatic carcinoma (John et al 1995). Laparoscopy and laparoscopic ultrasound, as well as establishing resectability based on local and vascular invasion, lymph node and extrahepatic metastatic deposits, will identify liver metastases in 14 to

25% of patients assessed with pancreatic cancer (Fig. 20.5). Laparoscopy has principally been used for identifying metastases from intra-abdominal sources, however, some of the earliest reports of the role of laparoscopy in the staging of malignancy came from studies evaluating hepatic metastases from breast, bronchus and ovary (Lightdale 1992). Not only can metastases be identified, but an objective response to systemic therapies may be assessed, which may be particularly relevant in the restaging of ovarian cancer.

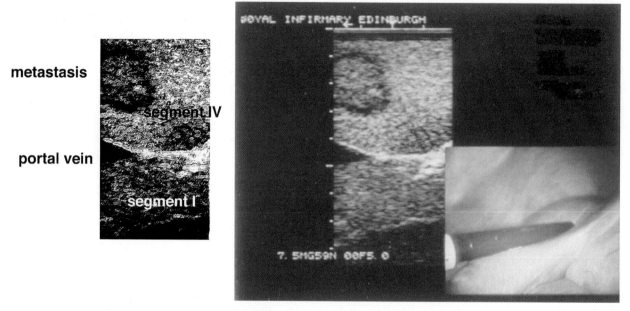

Fig. 20.4 An occult liver metastasis detected by laparoscopic ultrasound.

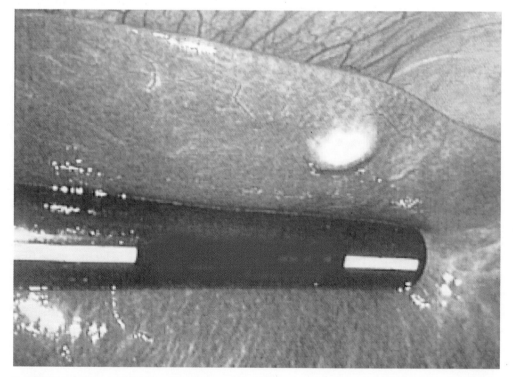

Fig. 20.5 The ultrasound probe may be used to manipulate structures, raising the left lobe of the liver reveals a small surface metastasis on the liver from a primary pancreatic carcinoma.

STAGING OF LYMPHOMAS

Hepatic involvement is frequently demonstrated in Hodgkin's and non-Hodgkin's lymphoma. Accurate staging of lymphoma at diagnosis determines the optimum therapeutic approach and allows an accurate estimation of prognosis. Data from the National Tumour Institute in Milan have shown an 80% accuracy in detecting hepatic involvement by laparoscopy (Lightdale 1982). However, it is unclear whether less invasive techniques such as CT scanning are sufficient in the assessment of the patient with lymphoma. A comparative trial of laparoscopy and laparoscopy-assisted liver biopsies with abdominal computed tomography, has been performed in the evaluation of patients who were diagnosed with having either Hodgkin's or non-Hodgkin's lymphoma (Sans et al 1998). The laparoscopic finding of white spots or nodules on the liver surface had 100% specificity in the diagnosis of lymphomatous liver involvement whereas hepatomegaly on both laparoscopy and computed tomography, had a low sensitivity and specificity for lymphoma affected liver. The use of laparoscopy in surgical staging of patients with lymphoma has the potential to decrease the morbidity and mortality of traditional staging laparotomy in these patients. All of the components of staging (liver biopsies, splenectomy, lymph node biopsies, and oophoropexy) can be performed laparoscopically (Johna & Lefor 1998). The splenectomy is completed after several liver biopsies have been obtained. Lymph nodes are then sampled from the celiac, portal, iliac, and periaortic regions. Lymph nodes identified as abnormal on pre-operative imaging studies are identified and excised. A histological classification may be made on the biopsy material obtained, thereby providing additional information to that obtained at staging radiology. This in turn may influence decisions on treatment schedules.

BENIGN LIVER DISEASE

Benign lesions of the liver are relatively common and it may be difficult to distinguish between these lesions and malignant tumor deposits within the liver. Accurate characterization of focal benign lesions may be achieved by a combination of transabdominal ultrasound and computed tomography. However these imaging techniques will not always produce a definitive diagnosis. The role of fine needle aspiration biopsy in the evaluation of focal liver lesions remains controversial, since biopsy may produce needle tract seeding in an unsuspected malignant lesion. It may also be difficult to distinguish between hepatocellular carcinoma and normal liver parenchyma from the histological analysis of biopsy material alone. The biopsy of other lesions such as hemangiomata, hemangioendotheliomas and ecchinococcal cysts are contraindicated. Laparoscopy may have a role in situations where a diagnosis can not be made with conventional radiologic imaging and where biopsy is best avoided (Fukuda et al 1992). Gross macroscopic features of a lesion may also avoid the necessity of a biopsy to obtain the diagnosis of a focal liver lesion. Additional information may be obtained by visualizing adjacent liver parenchyma and the chance of a sampling error is reduced with laparoscopically assisted liver biopsies.

The diagnosis of hepatic adenoma (Ch. 72) is usually made preoperatively, however laparoscopic evaluation may help in determining the nature of the lesion, and its location, as well as aiding in a targeted biopsy. Cuesta et al (1995) have reported on the laparoscopic resection of these tumors. This requires predissection localization and definition of the lesion by means of laparoscopy and laparoscopic ultrasonography. The importance of macroscopic appearances combined with histological findings is emphasized in the diagnosis of focal-nodular hyperplasia (FNH). The diagnosis is accepted only if different imaging techniques (CT, scintigraphy, magnetic resonance imaging) unequivocally demonstrate characteristic features (Marinone & Di Stasi 1997).

Occasionally a diagnosis of certainty requires laparoscopically guided biopsy of superficial lesions, with laparoscopic ultrasound being reserved for deep parenchymal lesions. The lesions are characterized by a bright hyperechoic center due to central fibrosis of the tumor, a subtle feature that may be missed by low-resolution transabdominal ultrasound. Although large symptomatic FNH nodules require surgical ablation, in the case of asymptomatic or small sized FNH nodules, these may best be managed by a programme of clinical observation with repeated US. The security of such a policy is entirely dependent on a correct diagnosis at the onset.

Intrahepatic cysts (Ch. 66) may be found in up to 10% of the normal population by routine scanning and are easily recognized by their ultrasound features alone. Cysts may be single or multiple and are generally smooth and spherical. Benign cysts are uniloculate, have a thin wall (Fig. 20.6), and can be differentiated from hydatid cysts on ultrasound appearances since the latter have fibrous and often calcified walls of greater echoicity. Small daughter cysts may be visualized embedded in the main cyst wall. Ultrasonography can identify the extent of the cyst, its nature and its relationship to major vessels and biliary radicals, and allow the surgeon to plan the procedure with greater precision than that previously afforded by conventional assessment. Laparoscopic ultrasonography has assumed great importance in this role, with the current trend towards the management of nonparasitic cysts by laparoscopic deroofing (Marvik et al 1993) (Ch. 83). Hemangiomas may appear as dense echoic areas in normal liver, but larger lesions may be difficult to distinguish from large tumors. It is these lesions which might inadvertently be subjected to fine needle aspiration biopsy (FNAB). In a report of ultrasound guided fine nee-

dle biopsy for the diagnosis of hepatic hemangiomas, giant lesions of greater than 5 cm diameter have been shown to bleed profusely when biopsied. The authors of this report recommended the use of laparoscopy to control the bleeding and to confirm the diagnosis (Caldironi et al 1998) (Fig. 20.7).

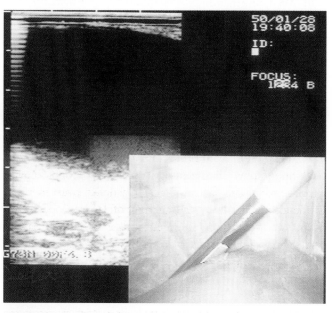

Fig. 20.6 A large benign intrahepatic cyst of the right hemiliver. There is no defined wall surrounding the fluid cyst which appears anechoic and is associated with posterior acoustic enhancement.

CHRONIC LIVER DISEASE

The mainstay of investigation for suspected liver disease is liver biochemistry, viral serology, autoimmune profiles and ultrasonography. However having undertaken a complete clinical evaluation, liver histology is frequently essential. Percutaneous liver biopsy (Ch. 19) is routinely employed to obtain liver tissue for histology, but has a relatively high complication rate (0.9 to 3.7%) and a mortality rate of between 0.01% and 0.12 (Piccinino et al 1986). Common causes of morbidity and mortality are from hemorrhage (0.02 to 0.2%), biliary peritonitis (0.02%) and perforation of the gallbladder or bowel (James & Lindor 1993). Because of the risks of blind biopsy and the potential for nonrepresentative biopsies by percutaneous means, nonsurgical gastroenterologists routinely employ laparoscopy and laparoscopic liver biopsy in the diagnosis of chronic liver disease (Haydon & Hayes 1997). Diagnostic laparoscopy with biopsy is as safe as percutaneous biopsy and is success-

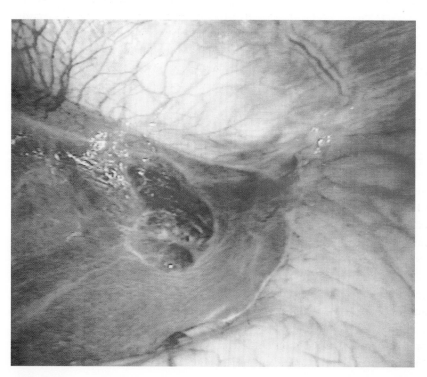

Fig. 20.7 A liver hemangioma. Diagnosis confirmed laparoscopically.

ful in greater than 95% of attempts made under local anesthesia. Since the biopsy can be directed at focal lesions, it is more specific in the evaluation of liver disease than percutaneous biopsy (Jalan et al 1995). Direct pressure or a heater probe can be applied to biopsy sites, reducing the incidence of hemorrhagic complications. It has been shown that the procedure may be performed safely in patients with platelets less than 80×10^6/ml and a prothrombine ratio (PTR) of greater than 1.3 (criteria that would normally contraindicate a blind biopsy). It is strongly recommended however that any reversible bleeding tendencies are corrected with blood products prior to undertaking the procedure.

An accurate assessment of the morphology of the surface of the liver is an important component in the management of chronic hepatitis. Progression to early cirrhosis in conditions such as chronic hepatitis C infection is associated with high failure rates in interferon-α treatment (Tsubota et al 1994). Cirrhosis may be localized and not detected by routine radiology and biopsy. The inflammatory changes in chronic active hepatitis is not a uniform process through the liver and variations in inflammatory severity at different liver sites may occur in 23.5% of cases (Poniachik et al 1996). Thus representative tissue samples are critical in assessing the true severity and activity of the disease prior to commencing treatment. It is also important in the context of potential liver transplantation to distinguishing between early cirrhosis and chronic hepatitis. Percutaneous biopsy for the diagnosis of liver cirrhosis, may produce a false-negative result, the rate of which is reported to be as high as 61% in some series. Comparative studies of laparoscopic findings with that of final histological diagnosis have shown that laparoscopy yields a sensitivity of 100% and a specificity of 97.9% in the diagnosis of cirrhosis (Jalan et al 1995). Fatty infiltration may be detected by the presence of yellow flecks on the liver surface and structural abnormalities in a cirrhotic liver, such as atrophy have been shown to be strongly associated with the presence of hepatocellular carcinoma (Kameda & Shinji 1992).

Laparoscopy plays an important part in the diagnostic evaluation of ascites. In a study of 129 patients with ascites of unknown origin, laparoscopic observation in combination with biopsy established the cause in 111 (86.0%) patients. Carcinomatosis peritonei was the most common cause in 78 cases (60.5%). Peritoneal biopsies revealed malignancy in 67 (adenocarcinoma 62, lymphoma 4, mesothelioma 1) and tuberculous peritonitis in 26 (20.2%). Cirrhosis was demonstrated in 7 (5.4%) and no gross abnormality was evident in 18 (14.0%) of cases. Most of the 18 patients without gross laparoscopic abnormality had underlying disease identified as a cause of ascites prior to evaluation and laparoscopy had been undertaken in these cases to exclude other processes that might have caused ascites (Chu et al 1994).

MALIGNANT DISEASE OF THE BILIARY TREE (see also Chs. 53 and 54)

Patients with cholangiocarcinoma often present with advanced disease, although it is recognized that resection is associated with prolongation of survival and provides the only chance for cure. In a retrospective review of patients with focal intrahepatic lesions detected by transabdominal ultrasound and subsequently histologically proven to represent cholangiocarcinoma, extrahepatic extension was found at operation in 46 of 52 patients (88.5%), while it was demonstrable by ultrasonography in only 16 (30.8%) (Wibulpolprasert & Dhiensiri 1992). Therefore, as with hepatic malignancies, laparoscopy may detect overt metastatic deposit. With the introduction of laparoscopic ultrasound an even greater detailed evaluation of the patient with a proximal bile duct obstruction is possible while careful preoperative study can be definitive (Ch. 54). Ultrasound examination in this situation may identify the level of obstruction of the biliary tree and demonstrate whether the primary or secondary biliary hepatic ducts are involved. Similarly vascular and lymph node involvement may be assessed, thereby determining resectability, and the need for liver resection. This information can be obtained without subjecting the patient to laparotomy and the potential morbidity and mortality of a trial dissection. Optimal treatment for the patient with unresectable disease however is currently still the subject of considerable debate and patients who have unresectable disease by radiologic or laparoscopic evaluation may be better served by nonsurgical internal biliary decompression (Ch. 58). Full laparoscopic assessment may allow this end-point to be achieved with the minimum of morbidity and with a lesser degree of surgical insult to the patient. In the event of a patient requiring a biliary bypass, such as a segment III cholangio-jejunostomy (Ch. 30), the identification of dilated ducts by ultrasonography identifies a ready target for the procedure. In addition the presence of left-lobe atrophy or involvement can be excluded. Laparoscopic ultrasound may have a role in alerting the surgeon to the presence of a gallbladder carcinoma at the time of laparoscopic cholecystectomy, or in cases where there is concern regarding the nature of the gallbladder pathology. Carcinoma of the gallbladder may be locally invasive of the liver parenchyma and the anatomical extent and presence of ductal or vascular involvement may be sonographically determined. The detection of a gallbladder carcinoma before an uninformed surgical intervention may avoid an inappropriate operation that compromises long-term survival (Dagnini et al 1984, Cuesta et al 1993).

BENIGN DISEASE OF THE BILIARY TREE

Whilst the diagnosis of gallstones will usually have been made preoperatively, laparoscopy and laparoscopic ultrasound may diagnose cholelithiasis in the evaluation of the biliary tree for presumed alternate pathology. In the patient with gallstones, the ultrasound examination may reveal a distended gallbladder filled with anechoic bile. The gallstone will invariably be situated posteriorly and will be seen as a crescentic hyperechoic image associated with posterior acoustic shadowing. The size of the stone(s) can be documented, and sludge or microcalculi will be seen as a layer of hyperechoic material settled on the posterior wall of the gallbladder. The gallbladder wall thickness may be assessed, and the signs of mural inflammation or edema recognized by loss of distinct echo-layers between mucosa and submucosa which are recognizable in the normal viscus. Cholesterosis may be distinguished from adenomatous polyps which do not typically cast an acoustic shadow (Fig. 20.8).

The appearance of common bile duct stones is identical to that of gallbladder calculi. Large duct calculi are obvious, but the presence of duct dilatation on laparoscopic ultrasonography should alert the surgeon to the possibility of the presence of small diameter (less than 5 mm) stones within the biliary tree. It is important to recognize that duct dilatation may occur in the absence of an obstructing calculus, and that choledocholithiasis may not cause duct dilatation. The supraduodenal portion of the common bile duct is more amenable to ultrasound examination and it may be difficult to define small calculi impacted in the distal duct, where duodenal gas may interfere with the image obtained. In the laparoscopic evaluation of patients with obstructive jaundice, tumors of the pancreas involving the lower bile duct must be distinguished from benign causes of biliary obstruction. The finding of an obliterated distal bile duct and pancreatic duct with proximal 'double duct' dilatation is highly suggestive of pancreatic or periampullary carcinoma (Ch. 17). Hypoechoicity of the pancreatic head is very often related to adenocarcinoma of the pancreas, whereas hyperechoicity is often caused by acute and chronic pancreatitis. Local complications of pancreatitis such as pseudocyst and abscess formation may be accurately evaluated by laparoscopy and laparoscopic ultrasound (John et al 1995).

The widespread enthusiasm for laparoscopic surgery has meant that fewer open cholecystectomies are being performed, with a concomitant move away from operative cholangiography. We and others have demonstrated that laparoscopic ultrasound is as accurate as intraoperative cholangiography in detecting common bile duct stones (Greig et al 1994) (Fig. 20.9). In addition ultrasonography

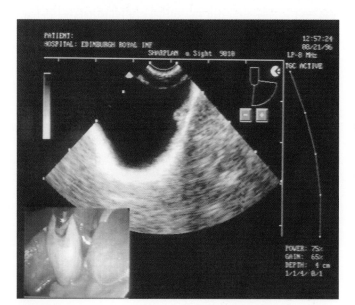

Fig. 20.8 Laparoscopic ultrasound demonstrating cholesterosis of the gallbladder.

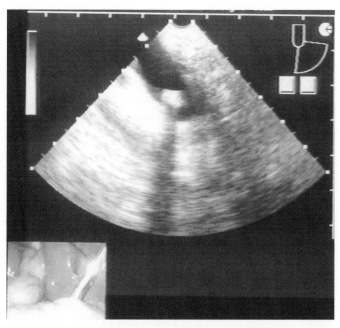

Fig. 20.9 A sector scanning ultrasound probe placed on the supraduodenal portion of the common bile duct. Choledocholithiasis is demonstrated, the gallstone is hyperechoic and produces a dense posterior shadow.

may be more sensitive in detecting micro-calculi in the biliary tree than conventional cholangiography. Operative ultrasonography has the benefit that, in experienced hands, it is quicker to perform than cholangiography and has the advantage of being able to image the intrahepatic biliary tree. There remains some debate regarding the role of contact ultrasonography to detect choledocholithiasis, however its usefulness in the detection of hepaticolithiasis is beyond question. The upper reaches of the biliary tree may not be reached by the instillation of contrast. Ultrasonography should detect even the smallest intrahepatic calculi, which will be hyperechoic in relation to the liver parenchyma. The associated segmental duct is often dilated, an important feature distinguishing air within the biliary tree as a cause of hyperechoic foci.

There have been reports of laparoscopic findings aiding the diagnosis of choledochal cysts at the time of laparoscopic cholecystectomy (Gibbs & Crist 1994), although there seems little logic in using laparoscopy to assess this condition. Prior to surgical intervention, the precise nature of a biliary stricture or focal lesion may be in doubt. Guided biopsies under laparoscopic or laparoscopic ultrasound control may allow accurate tissue determination of benign lesions such as bile duct adenoma, papillomas and granular cell tumors, whose presentation and radiological features may closely mimic malignant disease of the biliary tree.

CONCLUSIONS

Despite the improvements and availability of a range of imaging techniques, the preoperative assessment of benign and malignant hepatobiliary disease is frequently inconclusive. When a patient is being considered for curative resection underestimation of tumor stage can result in an unnecessary non-therapeutic laparotomy. In hepatobiliary and pancreatic malignancy, a non-operative intervention might be more appropriate. There is now compelling evidence that laparoscopy and laparoscopic ultrasound provide excellent evaluation of the extent of hepatobiliary disease. Laparoscopy and laparoscopic ultrasound may well replace conventional radiological investigations and in the hands of some allow selection of patients for operative treatment as a part of a rationalized staging protocol. Modern laparoscopic techniques can benefit the patient with malignant hepatobiliary disease, by reducing the number of investigative procedures and unnecessary laparotomies, thereby achieving prompt accurate diagnosis with minimal morbidity and mortality.

REFERENCES

Ahktar M S, Deere D M, Wright J T, MacRae K D 1985 Is bladder catheterisation really necessary before laparoscopy? British Journal of Obstetrics and Gynaecology 92: 1176–1178

Arase Y, Murashima N, Chayama K, Tsubota A, Koida I, Suzuki Y, Ikeda K, Saitoh S, Kobayashi M, Kumada H, Kobayashi M 1997 The superiority of laparoscopic examination in predicting hepatocellular carcinoma after inteferon therapy for chronic type C hepatitis. Digestive Endoscopy 9(1): 29–33

Babineau T J, Lewis W D, Jenkins R L, Bleday R, Steele Jr G D, Forse R A, Soper N J, Pitt H A, Way L W 1994 Role of staging laparoscopy in the treatment of hepatic malignancy. American Journal of Surgery 167(1): 151–155

Bengtsson G, Carlsson G, Hafstrom L, Jonsson P-E 1981 Natural history of patients with untreated liver metastases from colorectal cancer. American Journal of Surgery 141: 586–589

Bernheim B 1911 Organoscopy: cystoscopy of the abdominal cavity. Annals Surgery 53: 764–767

Bismuth H, Castaing D, Garden O J 1987 The use of operative ultrasound in surgery of primary liver tumors. World Journal of Surgery 11: 610–614

Bonjer H J, Hazebroek E J, Kazemier G, Giuffrida M C, Meijer W S, Lange J F 1997 Open versus closed establishment of pneumoperitoneum in laparoscopic surgery. British Journal of Surgery 84(5): 599–602

Caldironi M W, Mazzucco M, Aldinio M T, Paccagnella D, Zani S, Pontini F, De Bellis M E, Rebuffi A G, Costantin G 1998 The ultrasound (ultrasonographically guided) fine needle biopsy for the diagnosis of hepatic hemangiomas. Report on 114 cases. Minerva Chirurgica 53(6): 505–509

Chu C M, Lin S M, Peng S M, Wu C S, Liaw Y F 1994 The role of laparoscopy in the evaluation of ascites of unknown origin. Gastrointestinal Endoscopy 40(3): 285–289

Conlon K C, Dougherty E, Klimstra D S, Coit D G, Turnbull A D M, Brennan M F 1996 The value of minimal access surgery in the staging of patients with potentially resectable peripancreatic malignancy. Annals of Surgery 223: 134–140

Cortesi N, Zambarda E, Manenti A, Gigertinin G, Gotuzzo L, Malagoli M 1979 Laparoscopy in routine and emergency surgery: experience with 1720 cases. American Journal of Surgery 137: 647–649

Cuesta M A, Meijer S, Borgstein P J, Mulder L S, Sikkenk A C 1993 Laparoscopic ultrasonography for hepatobiliary and pancreatic malignancy. British Journal of Surgery 80(12): 1571–1574

Cuesta M A, Meijer S, Paul M A, De Brauw L M 1995 Limited laparoscopic liver resection of benign tumors guided by laparoscopic ultrasonography: Report of two cases. Surgical Laparoscopy and Endoscopy 5(5): 396–401

Dagnini G, Marin G, Patella M, Zotti S 1984 Laparoscopy in the diagnosis of primary carcinoma of the gallbladder: a study of 98 cases. Gastrointestinal Endoscopy 30: 289–291

Dobronte Z, Wittman T, Karacsony G 1978 Rapid development of malignant metastases in the abdominal wall after laparoscopy. Endoscopy 10: 127–130

Fornari F, Rapaccini G L, Cavanna L, Civardi G, Anti M, Fedeli G, Buscarini L 1988 Diagnosis of hepatic lesions: Ultrasonically guided fine needle biopsy or laparoscopy? Gastrointestinal Endoscopy 34(3): 231–234

Fukuda M, Hirata K, Mima S 1992 Preliminary evaluation of sonolaparoscopy in the diagnosis of liver diseases. Endoscopy 24(8): 701–708

Gibbs D H, Crist D 1994 Intraoperative diagnosis of choledochal cyst in preparation for laparoscopic cholecystectomy. Surgical Laparoscopy and Endoscopy 4(3): 225–229

Greig J D, John T J, Madhaven M, Garden O J 1994 Laparoscopic ultrasonography in the evaluation of the biliary tree during laparoscopic cholecystectomy. British Journal of Surgery 81: 1202–1206

Hall T J, Donaldson D R, Brennan T G 1980 The value of laparoscopy under local anesthesia in 250 medical and surgical patients. British Journal of Surgery 67: 751–753

Hasson H M 1974 Open laparoscopy: a report of 150 cases. Journal of Reproductive Medicine 12: 751–753

Haydon G H, Hayes P C 1997 Diagnostic laparoscopy by physicians: We should do it. QJM-Monthly Journal of the Association of Physicians 90(4): 297–304

Jacobaeus H C 1910 Uber die Moglichkeit die Zystoscope bei untersuchungen seroser Hohlungen anzuwenden. Munchener 57: 2090–2092

Jalan R, Harrison D J, Dillon J F, Elton R A, Finlayson N D C, Hayes P C 1995 Laparoscopy and histology in the diagnosis of chronic liver disease. QJM-Monthly Journal of the Association of Physicians 88(8): 559–564

James C H, Lindor K D 1993 Outcome of patients admitted with complications after outpatient liver biopsies. Annals of Internal Medicine 118: 96–98

Jeffers L, Spieglman G, Reddy R, Dubow R, Nadji M, Ganjei P, Schiff E R 1988 Laparoscopically directed fine needle aspiration for the diagnosis of hepatocellular carcinoma: A safe and accurate technique. Gastrointestinal Endoscopy 34(3): 235–237

John T G, Garden O J 1993 Needle track seeding of primary and secondary liver carcinoma after percutaneous liver biopsy. HPB Surgery 6: 199–204

John T G, Greig J D, Crosbie J L, Miles W F A, Garden O J 1994 Superior staging of liver tumors with laparoscopy and laparoscopic ultrasound. Annals of Surgery 220(6): 711–719

John T G, Greig J D, Carter D C, Garden O J 1995 Carcinoma of the pancreatic head and periampullary region. Annals of Surgery 221(2): 156–164

Johna S, Lefor A T 1998 Laparoscopic evaluation of lymphoma. Seminars in Surgical Oncology 15(3): 176–182

Kalk H 1955 Indikationsstellung und Gefahrenmoment bei der Laparaskopie. Deutsche Medizinische Wochenshrift 61: 1831–1833

Kameda Y, Shinji Y 1992 Early detection of hepatocellular carcinoma by laparoscopy: Yellow nodules as diagnostic indicators. Gastrointestinal Endoscopy 38(5): 554–559

Kameda Y, Asakawa H, Shimomura S, Shinji Y 1997 Laparoscopic prediction of hepatocellular carcinoma in cirrhosis patients. Journal of Gastroenterology and Hepatology 12(8): 576–581

Kane M G, Kreis G J 1984 Complications of diagnostic laparoscopy in Dallas: a 7 year prospective study. Gastrointestinal Endoscopy 30: 237–240

Lightdale C J 1982 Clinical applications of laparoscopy in patients with malignant neoplasms. Gastrointestinal Endoscopy 28: 99–102

Lightdale C J 1992 Laparoscopy for cancer staging. Endoscopy 24(8): 682–686

Lo C M, Lai E C S, Liu C L, Fan S T, Wong J 1998 Laparoscopy and laparoscopic ultrasonography avoid exploratory laparotomy in patients with hepatocellular carcinoma. Annals of Surgery 227(4): 527–532

Marinone M G, Di Stasi M 1997 Focal nodular hyperplasia: Value and limits of various imaging techniques. Giornale Italiano Di Ultrasonologia 8(1): 14–26

Marvik R, Myrvold H E, Johnsen G, Roysland P 1993 Laparoscopic ultrasonography and treatment of hepatic cysts. Surgical Laparoscopy and Endoscopy 3(3): 172–174

Molloy R G, McCourtney J S, Anderson J R 1995 Laparoscopy in the management of patients with cancer of the gastric cardia and oesophagus. British Journal of Surgery 82: 352–354

Paterson Brown S 1994 Principles, technique and complications of laparoscopy. Principles and practice of surgical laparoscopy. W B Saunders, London, p 44

Piccinino F, Sagnelli E, Pasquale G, Giusti G 1986 Complications following percutaneous liver biopsy. A multicenter retrospective study of 68 276 biopsies. Journal of Hepatology 2: 165–173

Poniachik J, Bernstein D E, Reddy K R, Jeffers L J, Coelho-Little M E, Civantos F, Schiff E R 1996 The role of laparoscopy in the diagnosis of cirrhosis. Gastrointestinal Endoscopy 43(6): 568–571

Rosenhoff S H, Young R C, Anderson T C et al 1975 Peritoneoscopy: a valuable staging tool in ovarian carcinoma. Annals of Internal Medicine 83: 37–41

Ruddock J C 1934 Peritoneoscopy. Western Medical Journal 42: 392–405

Sans M, Andreu V, Bordas J M, Llach J, Lopez-Guillermo A, Cervantes F, Bruguera M, Mondelo F, Montserrat E, Teres J, Rodes J 1998 Usefulness of laparoscopy with liver biopsy in the assessment of liver involvement at diagnosis of Hodgkin's and non-Hodgkin's lymphomas. Gastrointestinal Endoscopy 47(5): 391–395

Shandall A, Johnson C 1985 Laparoscopy or scanning in oesophageal and gastric carcinoma. British Journal of Surgery 72: 449–451

Soreide O 1990 Percutaneous aspiration cytology. Surgery of the Liver and Biliary Tract. Churchill Livingstone, New York, p 327–335

Soyer P, Lacheheb D, Levesque M 1993 False-positive CT portography: correlation with pathologic findings. American Journal of Roentgenology 285–289

Sugarbaker P H, Sanders J H, Bloom B S, Wilson R E 1975 Preoperative laparoscopy in the diagnosis of acute abdominal pain. Lancet 1: 422–445

Tan P L, Lee T L, Tweed W A 1992 Carbon dioxide absorption and gas exchange during pelvic laparoscopy. Canadian Journal of Anaesthesia 39: 677–681

Tsubota A, Chayama K, Ikeda K 1994 Factors predictive of response to interferon-α therapy in hepatitis C infection. Hepatology 19: 1088–1094

Tubiana J M, Deutsch J P, Taboury J, Martin B 1992 Imaging of hepatic metastases: diagnosis and resectability. Treatment of Hepatic Metastases of Colorectal Cancer. Springer-Verlag, Paris, p 55–69

van Dijkum Nieveen E J M, Wit L Th, de Obertop H, Gouma D J 1996 Port site metastases following diagnostic laparoscopy. British Journal of Surgery 83: 1793–1794

van Dijkum Nieveen E J M, De Wit L T, Van Delden O M, Rauws E A J, Van Lanschot J J B, Obertop H, Gouma D J 1997 The efficacy of laparoscopic staging in patients with upper gastrointestinal tumors. Cancer 79(7): 1315–1319

van Dikjum Nieveen E J S 1998 Diagnostic laparoscopy for staging gastrointestinal malignancies. Amsterdam: Astra Medica p 20–21

van Dikjum Nieveen E J M, Wit L Th, de Delden O M, van Kruyt P M, Lanschot J J B, van Rauws E A J, Obertop H, Gouma D J 1999 Staging laparoscopy and laparoscopic ultrasonography in over 400 patients with upper gastrointestinal carcinoma. British Journal of Surgery 85: in press

Warshaw A L, Gu Z, Wittenberg J, Waltman A C 1990 Preoperative staging and resectability of pancreatic cancer. Archives of Surgery 125: 230–233

Wibulpolprasert B, Dhiensiri T 1992 Peripheral cholangiocarcinoma: Sonographic evaluation. Journal of Clinical Ultrasound 20(5): 303–314

Wittgen C M, Andrus C H, Fitzgerald S D, Baudenistel L J, Dahms T E, Kaminski D L 1991 Analysis of the hemodynamic and ventilatory effects of laparoscopic cholecystectomy. Archives of Surgery 126: 928–932

21

Assessment of diagnostic techniques for liver masses and biliary obstruction

R.P. DeMATTEO, Y. FONG

INTRODUCTION

The hepatobiliary specialist frequently encounters liver masses and biliary obstruction. The diagnostic approach to these problems begins with the patient history and physical examination. Laboratory tests may provide additional information. However, it is the technological advances in radiologic imaging which have dramatically improved the ability to detect, characterize, and diagnose hepatic and biliary pathology. In particular, hepatobiliary neoplasms can now be identified at earlier stages when they are more amenable to therapy, especially curative resection. There are three goals in the evaluation of a patient. The first is to determine the diagnosis. The second objective is to stage the disease. To this end, radiologic investigation is used to define the extent of intrahepatic disease, the underlying state of the liver, and the presence of concomitant extrahepatic disease. The third purpose is to delineate the relationship of the disease to the vasculature and biliary ducts and identify anatomical variations in order to plan an operative approach for surgical resection or palliative ablative therapy when indicated.

Multiple preoperative tests are sometimes necessary to ascertain details that are not easily obtained even during laparotomy. The available array of diagnostic tests includes duplex ultrasound, nuclear scintigraphy, computed tomography, magnetic resonance imaging, angiography, direct cholangiography, liver biopsy, laparoscopy, intraoperative ultrasound, and laparotomy (Section 2). There is no one dominant imaging modality and different tests often provide complementary information. In selecting a diagnostic examination, one must balance the cost, availability, accuracy, resolution, invasiveness, and safety of the test (Bennett & Bova 1990, Moskal et al 1995, Saini 1997). While the diagnostic approach must be tailored to the history and

physical findings of a particular patient, there are general guidelines in the evaluation of liver masses and biliary obstruction that will be covered in this review.

LIVER MASSES

A hepatic mass may be discovered (1) in the assessment of other intra-abdominal disease with, for example, ultrasound or computed tomography, (2) in the evaluation of abdominal symptoms, or (3) in screening for metastatic disease. Benign hepatic tumors, which exist in over 20% of the population, must be distinguished from malignant ones (Karhunen 1986). A proper evaluation begins with the patient history. Symptoms are often absent or are nonspecific such as fever, weight loss, or abdominal pain. The patient should be questioned about previous cancer, hepatitis, alcohol intake, blood transfusion, oral contraceptive or steroid use, toxin exposure, foreign travel, genetic liver disorders, and inflammatory bowel disease. Physical examination (Ch. 12) should focus on the presence of jaundice, abdominal masses, nutritional status, adenopathy, and rectal examination. Signs of chronic liver disease such as gynecomastia, testicular atrophy, palmar wasting, and ascites should be sought. Hepatomegaly, splenomegaly, or spider nevi suggest the possibility of portal hypertension. Laboratory tests should include a hepatitis panel, liver function tests, complete blood count and platelets, prothrombin time, albumin, and serum alpha-fetoprotein and CEA levels. In particular, emphasis should be placed upon establishing the presence of cirrhosis or chronic hepatitis during the clinical assessment.

Only after a careful history and physical examination (Ch. 12) should radiologic imaging ensue. In the evaluation of a hepatic mass, the first consideration is whether the lesion is

Table 21.1 Differential of liver masses

Solid		Cystic	
Benign	Malignant	Benign	Malignant
Hemangioma	Metastasis	Simple cyst	Metastasis
FNH	Hepatocellular carcinoma	Abscess	Cystadenocarcinoma
Hepatic adenoma	Cholangiocarcinoma	Cystadenoma	
Fatty infiltration		Hydatid cyst	
Regenerative nodule		Amebic cyst	

solid or cystic, which is readily determined with computed tomography or ultrasound (Table 21.1).

SOLID LIVER MASSES

Triple phase helical computed tomography (CT) (Ch. 15), with precontrast, arterial phase, and portal phase images, is the preferred test for the assessment of solid liver masses (Jacobs & Birnbaum 1995, Oliver & Baron 1996, Saini 1997, van Leeuwen et al 1996). Liver images are captured during a single breath hold thereby limiting respiratory artifact, decreasing the required volume of contrast, and increasing the sensitivity for detection of small tumors. CT provides extensive anatomic detail of a lesion and its blood flow characteristics and surveys for the presence of extrahepatic disease. Precontrast CT scanning is often neglected but is essential for the evaluation of hypervascular liver tumors, steatosis, calcification, and hemorrhage. The ability to obtain arterial phase images allows for improved detection of hypervascular liver tumors because they are supplied predominantly by the hepatic artery (Hollett et al 1995, Itai & Matsui 1997). Meanwhile, the portal phase following contrast infusion facilitates the identification of hypovascular lesions that appear hypodense in comparison to the enhanced liver parenchyma. Delayed CT images obtained 4–6 hours later are inconvenient to obtain but may be even more sensitive in lesion detection. By that time, the liver parenchyma becomes hyperdense since 1 to 2% of contrast is excreted by hepatocytes while most neoplasms (except focal nodular hyperplasia) are hypodense (Bernardino et al 1986).

If the CT findings are nondiagnostic or CT is contraindicated because the patient has a severe allergy to iodinated contrast, then magnetic resonance imaging (MR) (Ch. 16) is performed. MR may provide better tissue characterization but the detection of subcentimeter nodules remains problematic. Numerous sequence protocols have been developed (Schnall 1995). Nearly all liver masses are hypointense on T1 images and 90% are hyperintense on T2

images (Wittenberg et al 1988). Contrast MR scanning is usually performed with the nonspecific extracellular contrast agent gadopentate dimeglumine (Gd-DTPA) though several agents that are specific for hepatocytes or reticuloendothelial cells are now in use (Ferrucci 1994, Hahn & Saini 1998, Van Beers et al 1997). MR during arterial portography with gadolinium has similar sensitivity and specificity to CT during arterial portography (CTAP) (Soyer et al 1994a).

Helical CT during arterial portography (Ch. 15) is a highly sensitive means of detecting liver masses (Soyer et al 1994b). It has an overall sensitivity of 72% in identifying primary malignant neoplasms with a sensitivity of 100% for lesions greater than 4 cm, 67% for masses between 2.1 and 4 cm, and 25% for masses less than 2 cm in size (Soto et al 1996a). It is limited by hepatofugal portal venous flow that may accompany cirrhosis. The 15% false positive rate that is encountered with benign tumors, regenerative nodules, and perfusion defects may be minimized by comparison to delayed (4 to 6 hours) images (Nazarian et al 1994, Soyer et al 1993, Soyer et al 1994b).

Although ultrasound (US) (Ch. 13) is highly sensitive in detecting solid hepatic masses, the appearance of any solid lesion is not sufficiently specific to render a definitive diagnosis. The distinction between a small hepatocellular carcinoma and a regenerating nodule in a cirrhotic liver is especially troublesome. Nevertheless, US is the most commonly used screening modality for hepatic neoplasms in the world. In addition, it does have a valuable role in monitoring the liver in patients who have had a previous liver resection or a history of an extrahepatic cancer. Intraoperative ultrasound (IOUS) (Chs 24, 89) is an invaluable tool for performing biopsy, cryotherapy, and ethanol injection, as well as defining vascular and biliary anatomy at the time of hepatic resection. IOUS can be used to stage a patient during laparoscopy (Ch. 83) and it has been reported to alter operative management in 10 to 48% of patients (Bismuth et al 1987, Castaing et al 1986, Ravikumar 1996, Rifkin et al 1987).

Angiography (Ch. 18) demonstrates the number of hepatic lesions, hepatic artery anatomy, vessel encasement, and vascular invasion. In patients with multifocal hypervascular tumors such as hepatocellular carcinoma, angiography may reveal small tumors that are not visible by other modalities. However, angiography is a highly invasive procedure that carries the risks of contrast toxicity and arterial injury. It has largely been replaced by other tests and is now reserved for the most difficult diagnostic dilemmas.

Although percutaneous biopsy (Ch. 19) is commonly endorsed by many clinicians, it is seldom indicated due to the associated risk of hemorrhage and the potential for tumor dissemination that may jeopardize a curative resection. Percutaneous biopsy is appropriate when a tumor is unresectable for anatomic or medical reasons. It is also performed when the diagnosis is equivocal or underlying parenchymal disease is suspected and the biopsy results may alter patient management. Biopsy may be carried out via US, CT, or laparoscopy.

HEMANGIOMA (Ch. 72)

Cavernous hemangiomas are the most common benign tumor of the liver. They exist in about 7% of the population and are multiple in 10% of cases (Ishak & Rabin 1975). They occur more frequently in women and tend to be located in the right lobe of the liver. Most hemangiomas are found incidentally though large ones may produce symptoms due to mass effect, thrombosis, or rupture. Rarely, they cause thrombocytopenia through platelet sequestration (Kasabach-Merritt syndrome). A central scar, calcification, or hemorrhage may be present. Ultrasound is not generally helpful in the diagnosis of a hemangioma since its appearance is nonspecific. Hemangiomas are well-circumscribed, round, homogeneous, and hyperechoic on US and their sluggish blood flow limits color flow Doppler examination (Nelson & Chezmar 1990).

Hemangiomas have a nonspecific appearance on noncontrast CT and appear as hypodense, well-defined, and homogeneous lesions. After contrast administration, peripheral nodular enhancement is seen in 67 to 88% of hemangiomas (Gaa et al 1991). Subsequently, centripetal filling develops within 15 minutes. This type of enhancement is virtually diagnostic as only 1 of 63 other hepatic neoplasms in one study and 2 of 34 other types of lesions in another report were found to have a similar pattern (Freeny & Marks 1986, Quinn & Benjamin 1992). Globular filling also distinguishes hemangiomas from hypervascular metastases that tend to fill uniformly and transiently (Leslie et al 1995). CT is less accurate in distinguishing both small (< 2 cm) hemangiomas that may fill rapidly and resemble a tumor as well as giant cavernous hemangiomas, which often have altered enhancement due to central fibrosis.

MR is 84 to 95% accurate in diagnosing hemangiomas and is the best test for lesions smaller than 2 cm and those that have atypical features on CT (Mitchell et al 1994). Hemangiomas have low attenuation on T1-weighted images but are uniformly very hyperintense on T2 images producing the characteristic 'light bulb' sign. Gadolinium administration reveals classic centripetal filling (similar to that seen on CT) in 50% of lesions less than 1.5 cm, 65% of those measuring 1.5–5 cm, but only 6% of those greater than 5 cm (Semelka et al 1994). In another study of 154 hemangiomas, all were hyperintense on T2 imaging and three patterns of contrast enhancement were observed (Semelka et al 1994). Early, uniform enhancement was seen in 35 of 81 lesions less than 1.5 cm. Peripheral enhancement with centripetal filling occurred in 75 of 154 lesions and peripheral filling alone existed in 44 of 154 hemangiomas and 16 of 17 large lesions. Hemangiomas usually retain contrast for over 10 minutes and are distinguished from hypervascular metastases that have rim enhancement with peripheral washout (Hamm et al 1990).

Technetium 99m labeled red blood cell scans are quite sensitive for diagnosing hemangiomas and are occasionally necessary when the diagnosis is uncertain (Birnbaum et al 1990). In combination with single photon emission computed tomography (SPECT), nuclear scintigraphy (Ch. 14) is highly accurate especially for lesions greater than 2 cm. Initially, there is no uptake of radionuclide but then pooling is seen on delayed images at 30–60 minutes (Birnbaum et al 1990). In general, red blood cell scans have been replaced by MR which provides additional diagnostic information. Angiography is rarely required to diagnose a hemangioma. Arteriography shows homogeneous, early peripheral filling with prolonged pooling resulting in a characteristic 'cotton wool' appearance around the normal caliber vessels that supply the neoplasm.

If a hemangioma is suspected, contrast CT and contrast MR provide the best means of diagnosis. Tagged red blood cell scan and, on occasion, arteriography are required for indeterminate lesions with atypical enhancement patterns. Biopsy is not generally recommended due to the risk of hemorrhage though others have reported it to have minimal complications (Heilo & Stenwig 1997).

FOCAL NODULAR HYPERPLASIA (Ch. 72)

Focal nodular hyperplasia (FNH) occurs mostly in women from 30 to 60 years of age. Patients are typically asymptomatic but some may have abdominal pain. FNH contains hepatocytes, bile ductules, and Kupffer cells and lacks a capsule. FNH is multiple in up to 20% of cases. There is no risk of hemorrhage or malignant transformation but FNH must be distinguished from other lesions that require treatment. Ultrasound is not helpful in diagnosing FNH since its appearance is usually hyperechoic or isoechoic but nondiagnostic. Duplex US may detect high peripheral blood flow.

On noncontrast CT, FNH is hypodense or isodense and homogeneous in nature. With contrast, it is seen to have early enhancement but becomes isodense on late portal phase images (Welch et al 1985) (Fig. 21.1). The central scar, if present, is hypodense at first and hyperdense on delayed images. A central scar is detectable in 60% of lesions by CT (Cherqui et al 1995). However, in one study, only 2 of 12 patients with FNH had 'typical' features on triphasic helical CT (Choi & Freeny 1998). Sulfur colloid scan, MR,

or biopsy was required for diagnosis in the other patients. Calcification is rarely present in FNH and was detected in only 5 of 357 lesions (Caseiro-Alves et al 1996). Dynamic CT can be used to distinguish FNH from adenoma as the latter usually has foci of hemorrhage (Mathieu et al 1986).

MR is the best overall test for FNH with a sensitivity of 70% and specificity of 98% (Cherqui et al 1995, Lee et al 1991). T1-weighted images usually show the lesion to be uniformly isointense with a hypointense scar (Fig. 21.2). On T2-weighted images, the lesion is usually iso- to slightly hyperintense with a hyperdense central scar as opposed to the hypodense scar of fibrolamellar carcinoma (Fig. 21.2). MR detects a central scar in 49 to 78% of lesions (Cherqui et al 1995, Lee et al 1991). Gadolinium administration yields an early intense lesion with a hypodense scar followed by a late isodense lesion with a hyperdense scar (Mahfouz et al 1993).

Nuclear scintigraphy (Ch. 14) and arteriography are less commonly utilized in the diagnosis of focal nodular hyperplasia. FNH is identified on technetium 99m-labeled sulfur colloid scan since its Kupffer cells take up sulfur colloid. Normal or increased uptake is seen in 70% of cases while most other lesions (except regenerative nodules and fatty change) are usually seen as cold defects (Welch et al 1985). One group also reported that hepatic adenomas take up sulfur colloid in 23% of cases (Lubbers et al 1987). The value

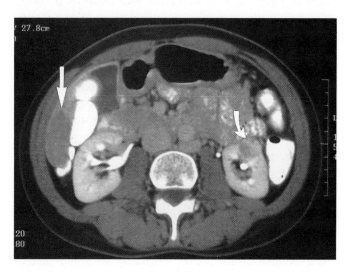

Fig. 21.1 Contrast CT of an FNH. CT with intravenous contrast in patient 1 who has a left renal cancer (curved arrow) demonstrates a 4 cm mass (arrow) in segment VI that is slightly hyperdense. The lesion was minimally hyperechoic on ultrasound (not shown).

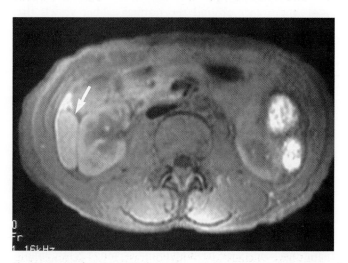

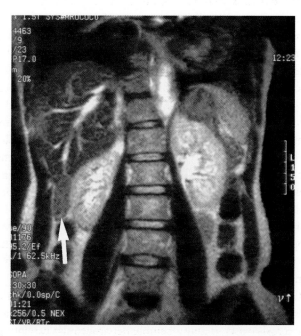

Fig. 21.2 MR of an FNH. MR shows the mass in patient 1 to be isointense (arrow) on cross-sectional T1-weighted images (left) and slightly hyperintense on T2 coronal (right) images and these findings are consistent with an adenoma or FNH. The lack of ducts or vessels makes it unlikely to be a Reidel's lobe. To exclude the possibility of a renal metastasis, a CT guided biopsy was performed which revealed benign hepatic tissue suggesting an FNH, which the lesion proved to be at the time of nephrectomy.

of nuclear scanning is limited in lesions less than 2 cm in size. Arteriography is occasionally required to make the diagnosis of FNH. In 90% of cases, it has a central vessel with radiating branches supplying the periphery that appear like the spokes of a wheel (Rogers et al 1981, Welch et al 1985). The lesion is hypervascular with AV shunts and early capillary filling and centrifugal enhancement. The scar is hypovascular.

When an FNH is suspected contrast CT and dynamic MR are the preferred tests. However, the appearance of FNH may be nondiagnostic with these modalities. The presence of a central scar is helpful but not pathognomonic since one may also be found in hemangioma, hepatic adenoma, and hepatocellular carcinoma (Rummeny et al 1989). *If the diagnosis remains uncertain, then sulfur colloid scan or angiography may be required.* Occasionally, biopsy is necessary.

HEPATIC ADENOMA (Ch. 72)

Hepatic adenoma usually occurs in young women as a solitary mass. It is associated with the use of oral contraceptive (or with anabolic steroids in men). Patients often have pain or discomfort. Hepatic adenoma does carry a risk of hemorrhage and malignant transformation (Foster & Berman 1994). The CT appearance of an adenoma is nonspecific and variable. Hepatic adenomas usually have low attenuation on noncontrast scans. With contrast, early and transient enhancement is seen followed by isodensity and then hypodensity on late films (Mathieu et al 1986). Adenomas often have areas of hemorrhage, fibrosis, or necrosis that gives them a heterogeneous appearance. MR typically shows a heterogeneous, hyperintense mass on T1 images due to glycogen and fat content or hemorrhage and the T2-weighted images are also hyperintense (Chung et al 1995, Paulson et al 1994). Gadolinium enhancement demonstrates an early and brief blush after which the lesion becomes isointense (Paulson et al 1994). MR is often necessary to distinguish hepatic adenomas from hemangiomas. Angiography outlines a predominantly hypervascular mass with areas of hypovascularity due to hemorrhage or necrosis (Welch et al 1985). The blood supply is typically peripheral and the surrounding arteries are enlarged. The US appearance of hepatic adenoma is nonspecific.

CT and MR are the initial diagnostic tests for hepatic adenoma but imaging is often inconclusive. When hemorrhage or necrosis exists, it may resemble hepatocellular carcinoma. Without these features, it is often difficult to distinguish an adenoma from a well-differentiated hepatocellular carcinoma. The age and gender of a patient and a history of oral

contraceptive use help to make a presumptive diagnosis. *In young women, the differential diagnosis includes focal nodular hyperplasia and sulfur colloid scintigraphy may help distinguish the two entities (vide supra).* Occasionally, biopsy may be necessary. For symptomatic lesions, hepatic resection can be performed without a preoperative histologic diagnosis.

HEPATOCELLULAR CARCINOMA (Ch. 73)

Hepatocellular carcinoma (HCC) is the most common visceral cancer in the world with an annual incidence of one million cases. In Western nations, it is usually a sequela of alcoholic cirrhosis. It is associated with hepatitis B and C infection, anabolic steroid or estrogen use, alpha-1 antitrypsin deficiency, Wilson's disease, hemochromatosis, and aflatoxin or Thorotrast exposure. Clinically, the onset is often insidious with the development of fatigue, weight loss, right upper quadrant pain, and ascites. However, some patients present with tumor rupture and intraperitoneal hemorrhage. Paraneoplastic syndromes such as hypoglycemia, feminization, or polycythemia may be present. Serum alpha-fetoprotein is elevated in over 90% of patients. Hepatocellular carcinoma tends to grow by expanding and displacing normal surrounding structures ('pusher'), projecting from the edge of the liver ('hanger'), or diffusely infiltrating the liver parenchyma (Ch. 83). HCC has a propensity to invade and grow within blood vessels and bile ducts. It invades the portal vein in up to 57 to 62% of patients but involves the hepatic vein and inferior vena cava less frequently (Mathieu et al 1984, The Liver Cancer Study Group of Japan 1990) (Fig. 21.3). Multifocal liver tumors and extrahepatic disease are present in two-thirds of patients (Fig. 21.4).

Detection of cirrhosis is important in evaluating a patient with suspected HCC. While the CT appearance of cirrhosis is variable and nonspecific, several signs may be suggestive (Brown et al 1997a, Torres et al 1986). A small right liver lobe with an enlarged caudate and left lateral segment is typical. In fact, a ratio of the diameter of the caudate to that of the right lobe of 0.65 or greater (normal is 0.3) marks cirrhosis 96% of the time (Harbin et al 1980). Furthermore, liver surface nodularity, ascites, varices, and splenomegaly may also be seen.

Noncontrast CT scans are essential in the evaluation of hepatocellular carcinoma as they reveal the tumor to have low attenuation with irregular margins. Less than 10% of lesions have calcification. With contrast, HCC demonstrates heterogeneous and bright enhancement in the arterial phase and then becomes hypodense on later images. The hepatic arterial phase is the most sensitive for HCC detection

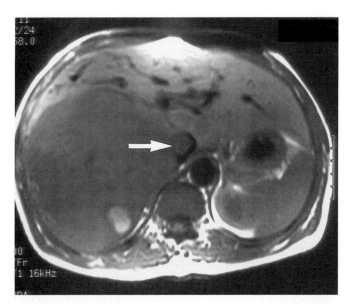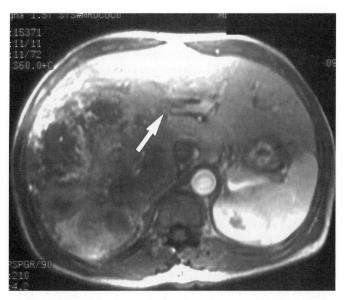

Fig. 21.3 MR of a hepatocellular carcinoma. T-1 weighted imaging (left) of patient 2 who has right upper quadrant pain and an AFP of 29 000 shows a large right-sided mass extending into segment I and IV. Note the tumor extension into the inferior vena cava (arrow). With contrast (right), tumor invasion into the portal vein is apparent (arrow).

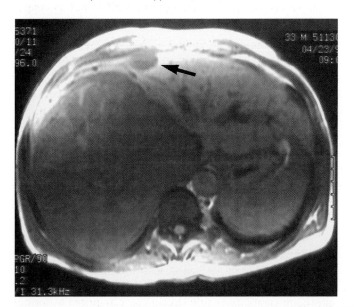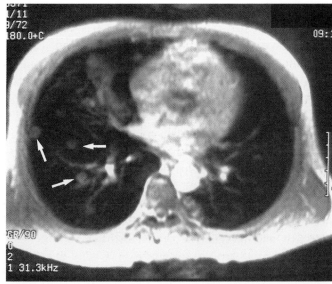

Fig. 21.4 MR of a hepatocellular carcinoma. A characteristic finding in HCC is the presence of a daughter nodule (left, arrow) and this was found in patient 2. Lung metastases (right, arrows) are also common as shown here on MR of the chest in this patient.

(Baron et al 1996). CT scanning has a sensitivity of only 56% in early, small HCCA and MR may be more accurate (Takayasu et al 1995). Early HCC is typically isointense prior to, early after, and late after contrast administration and the lesions that can be detected are seen as hypodense masses on late enhanced scans. In patients with HCC, segmental or lobar atrophy indicates occlusion of the bile duct or portal vein. Portal vein occlusion may be due to thrombosis from external compression or tumor invasion. Invasion of the portal vein by HCC (but not portal vein

thrombosis) results in vessel expansion and enhancement of the tumor thrombus during the hepatic arterial phase. The hepatic arterial phase may also demonstrate arterioportal shunting (Baron et al 1996). The presence of adenopathy, adrenal metastases, and lung metastases should be assessed. Detection of HCC is slightly more difficult in the presence of cirrhosis. CT has a sensitivity of 68% and specificity of 81% in detecting HCC in cirrhotics (Miller et al 1994).

The MR appearance of HCC is variable but it usually has slightly low attenuation on T1-weighted sequences and hyperintensity on T2-weighted images (Itoh et al 1987). Heterogeneous arterial phase enhancement is seen after contrast administration (Kelekis et al 1998). A mosaic pattern may be seen on T2 imaging. Areas of necrosis and fatty change are hyperintense on T2. A pseudocapsule may often be seen which has low signal on both T1 and T2 images. Small (< 1.5 cm) tumors are usually isointense on both T1 and T2 images and demonstrate homogeneous enhancement. MR with gadolinium is more sensitive than helical CT in detecting small HCC in patients with cirrhosis or chronic hepatitis. In a prospective study of 50 patients, MR had an overall sensitivity of 89% for lesions less than 3 cm and 85% for lesions less than 2 cm compared to a sensitivity of 64 and 52%, respectively, for CT (Yamashita et al 1996). With MR (and CT), it may be difficult to distinguish HCC from metastases which usually have peripheral enhancement. Differentiation from regenerative or dysplastic nodules may be cumbersome but is best carried out with MR (Mergo & Ros 1998). Regenerative nodules are usually mildly hypointense on T2 which distinguishes them from HCC. When HCC develops in a nodule, the T2 signal becomes intermediate in intensity (Mitchell et al 1991). Dysplastic nodules are slightly hyperintense on T1 and hypointense on T2 (Nagasue et al 1988). Contrast MR angiography may demonstrate portal vein invasion and portosystemic collaterals.

Computed tomography arterial portography (CTAP) is slightly more sensitive than helical CT in detecting HCC and in one study it identified 96 lesions in 23 patients versus 87 seen on CT (Kanematsu et al 1997a). In another report, 90% of HCC tumors were detected with CTAP (Ichikawa et al 1996). Helical CTAP offers no advantage over conventional CTAP in detecting HCC but is more sensitive than dynamic MR (Kanematsu et al 1997b, Soyer et al 1994c). The use of CTAP may be limited in the presence of cirrhosis as portal flow is slow or often reversed. As MR technology improves, there will be fewer indications for the invasive and expensive modality of CTAP in the diagnosis of HCC.

Angiography is useful when the diagnosis of HCC remains in question, when multifocal disease is suspected, and when information on vessel invasion is otherwise unsatisfactory. Angiography reveals the hypervascularity of HCC. It is most helpful in diagnosing small multifocal tumors. Blushing with irregular pooling occurs in the capillary phase. Neovascularity with a chaotic pattern of vessels of irregular caliber, arterioportal shunting, and vein invasion are typical features. The tumor often displaces the peripheral arterial feeding vessels. MR angiography and US may also be used to assess portal vein, hepatic artery, hepatic vein, and vena cava involvement.

On duplex ultrasonography (Ch. 13), HCC has variable echogenicity but is often hypoechoic. Without the demonstration of vascular invasion, though, the diagnosis is not certain. Duplex US is accurate in determining portal vein invasion and is comparable to CT portography in this regard (Bach et al 1996). In addition, it can be used to evaluate the confluence of the hepatic veins with equal accuracy to MR (Hann et al 1998). Sonography is severely limited by the presence of cirrhosis because regenerating nodules may resemble tumor. US does allow assessment of the direction of blood flow within the portal vein and thus provides important prognostic information by grading the degree of portal hypertension. Furthermore, ultrasound remains the most commonly utilized screening test for hepatocellular cancer in patients with cirrhosis because of its wide availability and low cost. IOUS is valuable to detect occult nodules and define anatomical relationships during partial hepatectomy.

CT and MR are the best modalities for diagnosing HCC. US is widely used as a screening test for HCC but its images are nonspecific although it may reveal vascular invasion. Positron emission tomography scanning is poor for detecting HCC and in one study, only 13 of 23 patients had increased [18]fluorodeoxyglucose (FDG) uptake (Delbeke et al 1998). Angiography is sometimes needed to discern vascular invasion or detect a small tumor. A liver mass in the presence of cirrhosis, portal vein invasion, or an elevated alpha-fetoprotein (AFP) (> 500 ng/ml) is presumed to be HCC until proved otherwise and the patient should undergo CT or MR for staging. The presence of venous invasion or an elevated AFP is particularly suggestive of HCC and may obviate the need for a tissue diagnosis if resection is planned. The existence of underlying cirrhosis confounds the detection of HCC. Difficulty also exists in recognizing early (< 1 cm) hepatocellular carcinoma that is the most amenable to therapy. Imaging assists in determining the resectability of a hepatocellular carcinoma by identifying the presence of extensive intrahepatic disease, vascular involvement, advanced cirrhosis, and extrahepatic metastases. Biopsy should be performed only if resection is contraindicated or if the diagnosis is unclear.

FIBROLAMELLAR HCC (Chs 71, 73)

The fibrolamellar variant of hepatocellular carcinoma (FLL) affects younger patients between 20 and 40 years old and has an equal sex distribution. These patients do not have underlying hepatic parenchymal disease and have normal alpha-fetoprotein levels. The lesion is well-circumscribed and sometimes contains a central scar. While it is generally thought that FLL has a better prognosis than HCC, the outcome is similar in the absence of cirrhosis or when matched for stage (Nagorney et al 1985, Ringe et al 1991). Up to 55% of tumors contain calcium which is often distributed in a stellate pattern unlike in FNH (Brandt et al 1988). Fibrolamellar HCC may be hard to distinguish from FNH or adenoma.

MR is the best diagnostic test for fibrolamellar HCC. It has a low attenuation on T1-weighted images. A heterogeneous high T2 signal is seen with a hypodense scar if one is present (recall that the scar of FNH is hyperdense). Heterogeneous enhancement occurs with gadolinium administration (Itoh et al 1987). CT demonstrates a solitary, well-circumscribed mass that is isodense or slightly hypodense with a central hypodense scar. With contrast, the tumor is isodense or hyperdense. FLL is hypervascular on angiography. The US appearance is nonspecific.

INTRAHEPATIC CHOLANGIOCARCINOMA

Intrahepatic (peripheral) cholangiocarcinoma is an uncommon tumor. It is associated with primary sclerosing cholangitis, biliary atresia, hepatolithiasis, and liver fluke infestation but most patients do not have pre-existent liver disease. Tumors that arise in the periphery of the liver become manifest later than central tumors that tend to produce jaundice. Cholangiocarcinoma invades the portal vein in 32% and the hepatic vein in 14% of patients (The Liver Cancer Study Group of Japan 1990).

Intrahepatic cholangiocarcinoma has nonspecific radiologic features and it is often mistaken for a metastasis or HCC. An intrahepatic mass in the setting of dilated biliary ducts should raise a suspicion of HCC or cholangiocarcinoma. The CT appearance is that of a hypodense mass with minimal enhancement. Some tumors have calcification. A common feature is that 74% have mild to moderate hyperintensity that is often confined to the periphery on delayed images post contrast (Lacomis et al 1997). The presence of intrahepatic metastases should be sought. On MR, the tumor is hypodense on T1 images and mildly to moderately hyperintense on T2 images (Hamrick-Turner et al 1992, Rummeny et al 1989). A scar, if present, is hyperdense on T2-weighted scans. Enhancement is peripheral initially and then progressively concentric (Soyer et al 1995). US reveals a hyperechoic, hypovascular mass with nonspecific features. Angiography is not useful for diagnosis as intrahepatic cholangiocarcinoma is hypovascular.

LIVER METASTASES (Ch. 75)

In the United States, metastatic liver tumors are 20 times more common than primary hepatic malignancies.

Metastases from neoplasms of the colon, breast, lung, pancreas, and stomach are encountered most frequently. Hepatic metastases are usually multiple and the diagnosis of metastatic disease should always be considered when there is a history of cancer. However, in patients with previous cancer, lesions less than 1 cm proved to be metastases only 11.6% of the time (Schwartz et al 1999). Metastases from the colon, pancreas, and ovary may be cystic and mistaken for simple cysts. Mucinous colorectal tumors as well as stomach, pancreas, breast, and ovarian metastases may be calcified (Bessot et al 1998). Diffuse metastases that occur with melanoma, lung, lymphoma, and breast cancer are especially difficult to detect. Metastases that tend to be vascular include neuroendocrine tumors (islet cell, thyroid, carcinoid, melanoma, and pheochromocytoma), renal cell carcinoma, breast cancer, and sarcoma. Meanwhile, tumors originating from the colon, stomach, lung, pancreas, esophagus, gallbladder, and bladder are usually hypovascular. In particular, characterization of colorectal metastases is essential to select those who are resectable since hepatic resection results in 5-year survival rates of 22 to 45% (Fong et al 1996). Resection has also proven to be useful for other metastatic tumors (Harrison et al 1997).

CT represents the most commonly performed test for the evaluation of liver metastases (Fig. 21.5). It has a sensitivity of 91% for detecting hepatic metastases greater than 1 cm which is comparable to the sensitivity of CTAP (Kuszyk et al 1996). However, helical CT has a sensitivity of only 56% for lesions less than 1 cm (Kuszyk et al 1996). Most metastases have low attenuation on noncontrast CT. With contrast, they have a variable appearance and some have peripheral rim enhancement. Hypervascular metastases may only be visible on noncontrast scans since they often become isodense after contrast infusion (Bressler et al 1987). Multiple hepatic metastases from the same primary tumor generally tend to have a similar appearance (Kruskal & Kane 1996).

CT during arterial portography (Ch. 15) represents the gold standard for assessing the number and distribution of hepatic metastases (Fig. 21.5). It is the most sensitive preoperative test for detecting small lesions, especially those less than 2 cm, and can detect colorectal liver metastases with greater than 90% sensitivity (Matsui et al 1987, Moran et al 1995, Nelson et al 1989, Soyer et al 1994a,b,c). CTAP assists surgical planning as it provides better definition of the relationship of a lesion to the vasculature and defines the arterial anatomy if hepatic artery pump placement is planned. The false negative rate is 9% in detecting colorectal metastases (Soyer et al 1992).

Liver metastases are dark on MR T1-weighted images with the exception of melanoma which is exceptionally

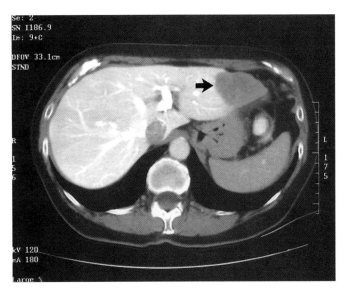

Fig. 21.5 Contrast helical CT and CT during arterial portography of a colorectal liver metastasis. Contrast helical CT (left) in patient 3 who has a history of colorectal adenocarcinoma shows a lesion in the left lateral segment (arrow). Note the origin of the segment III and IV vessels. The lesion is better appreciated on CT during arterial portography (right, arrow) which did not reveal any other intrahepatic masses.

bright. T2 images show moderate hyperintensity but can be very bright if the tumor is vascular or necrotic. With gadolinium, the entire mass or just its periphery may enhance transiently. Characteristic features on MR include a heterogeneous signal with an irregular border, a central increased signal with an outer area of lower density termed a target lesion, or a mass with a hyperintense rim called a halo (Lewis & Chezmar 1997). Peripheral washout of contrast is often seen on delayed images and can help distinguish a metastasis from a hemangioma (Mahfouz et al 1994). However, dynamic gadolinium offers no advantage over unenhanced MR in detecting liver metastases (Hamm et al 1997). MR is better than CT in detecting diffuse liver metastases.

Metastatic tumors to the liver have variable ultrasound appearance with respect to size, echogenicity, borders, texture, and blood flow though they frequently appear as hyperechoic lesions. Nevertheless, US is the most frequently used screening modality worldwide. Some lesions have the appearance of a halo (Wernecke et al 1992). Intraoperative ultrasound (Chs 24, 89) may be the best test for detecting small metastases (Bismuth et al 1987). It can detect occult colorectal metastases not apparent by CT or US and has an overall sensitivity of 96% compared to 91% sensitivity of CT during arterial portography (Soyer et al 1992). Laparoscopy is useful in the recognition of occult hepatic metastases as well as extrahepatic disease not detected by cross-sectional imaging (Babineau et al 1994, Jarnagin et al 1999, John TG et al 1994) (Ch. 83).

Angiography has little role in the diagnosis of hepatic metastases. However, because the hepatic artery is the primary blood supply to liver metastases, it is useful in determining the number and distribution of lesions. Angiography demonstrates neovascularization and sometimes arteriovenous shunts. Lesions may be hypervascular or hypovascular as outlined above. Hypovascular metastases are seen to displace normal vessels.

Nuclear scintigraphy has been applied to the diagnosis of metastatic liver tumors. Radiolabeled monoclonal antibodies are theoretically attractive for imaging colorectal metastases but have not yet proven to have clinical utility. Radioimmune imaging has a high false positive rate and is inferior to conventional CT (Doerr et al 1991). Positron emission tomography (PET) (Ch. 14) utilizing [18]fluorodeoxyglucose is under investigation for the detection of hepatic metastases and the presence of occult extrahepatic disease (Vitola et al 1996). Preliminary reports indicate that PET detects colorectal liver metastases with 90% sensitivity (Findlay et al 1996, Okazumi et al 1992) (Fig. 21.6). Further investigation is warranted to determine the clinical value and application of PET.

Helical CT is the best initial test for liver metastases. CT has similar sensitivity to MR but is better in detecting extrahepatic disease. Helical CT may be used as the sole preoperative test but it is our practice to also employ CT portography, MR, or ultrasound to determine the exact number of hepatic metastases and to plan resection. Helical CTAP is the most accurate test for determining the extent of metastatic liver disease. Intraoperative ultrasound is utilized to detect occult intrahepatic metastases during hepatic

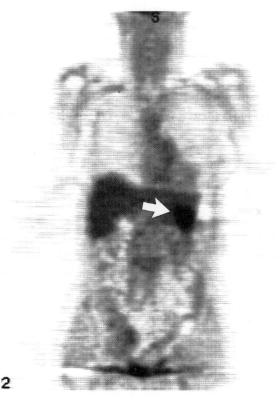
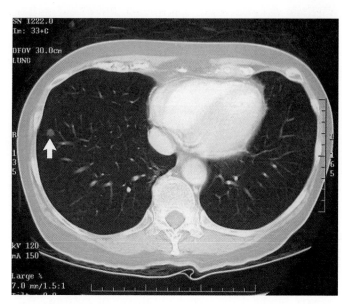

Fig. 21.6 PET scan and chest CT in metastatic colorectal cancer. Whole body PET scan (left) of patient 3 indicates that there is no extrahepatic disease and there is just one liver metastasis (arrow) as shown on the CT and CTAP. A preoperative CXR of patient 3 demonstrated a subcentimeter mass in the right lower lobe of the lung which was found to be an isolated nodule on CT (right, arrow) and proved to be a lung metastasis at thoracoscopic resection prior to hepatectomy.

resection. If surgery is indicated given the origin of the tumor and its intrahepatic location, then an extent of disease workup is performed to exclude concomitant extra-hepatic disease (Fong et al 1997, Harrison et al 1997) (Fig. 21.6). For instances where surgery is not indicated, percuta-neous biopsy should be performed to confirm the diagnosis.

PSEUDOTUMORS

Pseudotumors encompass a variety of lesions that can mimic the appearance of a hepatic neoplasm and include fatty change and, rarely, inflammatory pseudotumor (Fukuya et al 1994, Yates & Streight 1986). Hepatic lipid accumula-tion can arise from alcohol use, cirrhosis, malnutrition, steroids, obesity, diabetes mellitus, total parenteral nutri-tion, or chemotherapy. Fatty change may occur in a seg-mental or lobar distribution and be focal or multifocal. It is often adjacent to the falciform ligament or gallbladder fossa. Focal areas of normal parenchyma in an otherwise fatty liver may also resemble tumor. A key distinguishing feature of fatty change is that there is no mass effect or distortion of surrounding vessels. MR is the optimal method of diagnos-

ing fatty liver. It has a high signal on T1-weighted images that becomes hypointense with out of phase sequences. Fatty change is also often appreciated on unenhanced CT as areas of hypoattenuation (Jacobs et al 1998). It may con-found the detection of other neoplasms as hypointense lesions may appear isodense in the background of fatty change. Sulfur colloid uptake is normal and may support the diagnosis. Ultrasound is nonspecific and shows a hyper-echoic area.

CYSTIC MASSES (Ch. 66)

The diagnosis of a hepatic cystic lesion is usually suggested by a combination of patient history, clinical examination, and radiologic imaging. A simple cyst must be distinguished from an atypical cyst that contains internal septae or is associated with a mass. An atypical cyst may represent an abscess, cystic metastasis, cystadenoma, or cystadenocarci-noma and requires further evaluation. Ultrasound is the best initial test for cystic lesions of the liver.

SIMPLE CYST

Simple cysts occur in 10% of the population and are usually incidental. They are typically solitary and unilocular. They are readily diagnosed by ultrasound and are seen as homogeneous, well-demarcated, thin-walled structures that are anechoic and possess through transmission of sound waves with posterior enhancement. Additional tests are usually unnecessary. CT shows a discrete, homogeneous, and nonenhancing lesion with an attenuation similar to that of water or gallbladder fluid. Small cysts (< 2 cm) may be difficult to discern due to partial volume averaging. With MR, cysts are hypodense on T1 images, very hyperintense on T2 images, and they do not enhance with gadolinium. MR is only needed for complicated cysts that are hemorrhagic or infected. Other radiologic tests are generally not informative. Hepatic cysts are multiple in polycystic kidney disease and when hepatic resection is contemplated for this disorder, a brain CT should also be performed to rule out the presence of a coexistent cerebral aneurysm.

HYDATID CYST (Ch. 63)

Hydatid liver cysts occur from infestation with the parasite *Echinococcus granulosus*. Patients are often asymptomatic and the clinical course is latent. Some will develop right upper quadrant pain or jaundice. Otherwise, the disease may become manifest after a cyst complication such as infection, intrabiliary rupture, or extrahepatic rupture with anaphylaxis. *Hydatid cysts have characteristic radiologic features and ultrasound is the best diagnostic test* (Beggs 1983). Internal daughter cysts are present in half of cases. CT scan frequently shows rim calcification of the cyst wall. The diagnosis may be confirmed with a serum antibody test.

ABSCESS (Ch. 61)

Pyogenic hepatic abscess is usually a complication of cholangitis or intra-abdominal infection such as diverticulitis or appendicitis. An abscess arising from portal vein bacteremia usually develops in the right lobe of the liver while those of biliary origin are usually multiple and bilateral. Patients may have right upper quadrant pain or fever. Hepatic abscess may be unsuspected in an asymptomatic individual without an obvious contributory history. Abscesses may be multifocal or multilocular. Most fungal abscesses are due to *Candida albicans* and typically there are microabscesses scattered throughout the liver. US and CT have greater than 90% accuracy in detecting a hepatic abscess but may not differentiate an abscess from a cystic or necrotic metastasis (Kuligowska et al 1982). The ultrasound appearance is variable but classically reveals a hypoechoic, round lesion with internal echo scattering. CT reveals a thick wall, septae, air, or fluid that is denser than water (Mathieu et al 1985). Peripheral capsular enhancement is seen with contrast. The double target sign is seen in 30% of lesions with dynamic CT in which a hypodense center is surrounded by a hyperdense ring with an outer hypodense zone (Mathieu et al 1985). MR is rarely necessary to make the diagnosis. Abscesses have a low T1 signal 60% of the time and a hyperintense T2 signal in 72% of instances. All abscesses enhance with 86% showing rim enhancement (Mendez et al 1994). Percutaneous aspiration confirms the diagnosis of hepatic pyogenic abscess.

Amebic abscesses (Ch. 62) result from the protozoan *Entamoeba histolytica*. Patients present with fever and right upper quadrant pain. Amebic abscesses are round with fine internal echoes. They are usually single, located in the right lobe, and may be exophytic. They cannot be distinguished reliably from pyogenic abscesses by US or CT (Ralls et al 1987a). On MR imaging, there is a homogeneous low T1 signal and a heterogeneous hyperdense T2 signal (Elizondo et al 1987, Ralls et al 1987b). The diagnosis may be confirmed with serology.

BILIARY CYSTIC NEOPLASMS

Bilary cystic neoplasms are rare and tend to occur in middle-aged females. Biliary cystadenoma is thought to be a premalignant lesion. CT and MR demonstrate the presence of septae. Biliary cystadenocarcinoma may be difficult to discern but it usually has nodularity, wall hemorrhage, or hemorrhagic fluid in addition to septae (Buetow et al 1995). The MR appearance is variable and depends on the nature of the cystic fluid. Both cystadenoma and cystadenocarcinoma must be distinguished from hydatid cyst and abscess. US is particularly useful to detect irregularities in the wall and lining of a cyst.

BILIARY OBSTRUCTION

The evaluation of biliary obstruction begins with a careful history and physical examination (Ch. 12). Jaundice is the hallmark of biliary obstruction (Ch. 7). The patient should be questioned regarding pruritus, fever, weight loss, and the color of their feces and urine. A prior history of pancreatitis, ulcerative colitis, hepatitis, or cholangitis should be determined. Intermittent jaundice suggests stone-related disease, ampullary carcinoma, or papillary cholangiocarcinoma. Prior biliary surgery suggests the possibility of a stricture or a retained stone. Late jaundice following a pancreaticoduodenectomy should raise the suspicion of recurrent disease, technical anastomotic failure, or an iatrogenic stricture if radiation was administered. There are numerous exceptions to the dictum that jaundice without pain belies cancer while jaundice with intermittent pain signifies benign disease. Medical causes of jaundice include viral hepatitis, cirrhosis, alcohol intake, hemolysis, impaired uptake or conjugation of bilirubin, and the use of certain medications.

In addition to jaundice, other physical findings of biliary obstruction may include lymphadenopathy, evidence of nutritional deprivation, and the signs of cirrhosis or portal hypertension like ascites and splenomegaly. A palpable, nontender gallbladder in a jaundiced patient suggests malignant biliary obstruction by Courvoisier's law. Cirrhosis may be the result of intrinsic liver disease or secondary to biliary obstruction. Pertinent laboratory tests include CBC, platelet count, liver enzymes, bilirubin, and alkaline phosphatase. An elevated alkaline phosphatase may sometimes be the only indicator of obstruction. Other tests should include a hepatitis panel, renal function studies, and nutritional parameters.

Obstructive jaundice may be distinguished from medical disorders through the patient's history, physical examination, and ultrasound imaging to look for the presence of dilated biliary ducts. However, bile duct obstruction without dilatation may occur when there is a recent obstruction, a chronic low grade obstruction, an intermittent obstruction, or with primary sclerosing cholangitis (Ch. 7). A suspicion of obstruction should prompt cholangiography even when the ducts are of normal caliber. Conversely, some patients without obstruction may have dilated ducts especially if there was a previous obstruction. At times, a percutaneous liver biopsy is necessary to exclude hepatic disease as the cause of jaundice.

There are a number of pathologic processes that cause biliary obstruction. The differential includes choledocholithiasis, biliary stricture, cholangitis, choledochal cyst,

cholangiocarcinoma, gallbladder cancer, periampullary neoplasm, and metastases or lymphoma in the porta hepatis. The primary goal of diagnostic evaluation is to determine the level of biliary obstruction (i.e. proximal or distal) (Table 21.2). This may be readily discerned based on the pattern of ductal dilatation. The second goal is to ascertain the cause of the obstruction.

US (Ch. 13) is the initial test of choice in biliary obstruction. It is relatively inexpensive, widely available, and noninvasive. It can determine the level of biliary dilatation in 92% of cases and the cause in 71% of patients (Laing et al 1986). US may be limited in the distal biliary tree by overlying bowel gas. The upper limits of normal for the diameter of the common bile duct and common hepatic duct are 8 and 6 mm, respectively. CT is 95% accurate in determining the level and cause of an obstruction (Pedrosa et al 1981).

Direct cholangiography (Ch. 17) (via percutaneous transhepatic cholangiography (PTC) or endoscopic retrograde cholangiopancreatography (ERCP)) provides the most anatomic detail of the biliary tree and enables inspection for filling defects, stenoses, occlusions, masses, and dilatation (Blumgart et al 1974). ERCP is generally preferred for distal bile duct obstruction while PTC is performed for proximal pathology. With PTC, the biliary system can be cannulated in nearly all those with dilated ducts and in greater than 80% of those with normal ducts. PTC and ERCP are complementary tests and choosing between them is subject to their availability and local expertise. In a prospective, randomized study, they had similar accuracy in diagnosing jaundice (Elias et al 1976). Direct cholangiography may suggest segmental or lobar biliary obstruction when the intrahepatic ducts are crowded, dilated, and tortuous. In contrast, the intrahepatic ducts are crowded but of normal caliber in the presence of portal vein obstruction. Segmental or lobar atrophy (Ch. 3) of the liver from portal vein or duct obstruction is best visualized with CT. The gallbladder is not reliably visualized by direct cholangiography and is better examined with ultrasound.

Table 21.2 Differential of biliary obstruction

Proximal obstruction		Distal obstruction	
Biliary origin	*Extrinsic etiology*	*Biliary origin*	*Extrinsic etiology*
Cholangiocarcinoma	Hepatic neoplasm	Cholangiocarcinoma	Periampullary neoplasm
Choledocholithiasis	Extrahepatic mass	Choledocholithiasis	Pancreatitis
Gallbladder cancer	Lymphadenopathy	Choledochal cyst	Pancreatic cyst
Biliary stricture		Biliary stricture	
Malignant masquerade			
Mirizzi's syndrome			
Sclerosing cholangitis			
Caroli's disease			

MR cholangiography (MRCP) (Ch. 16) is a promising new tool that provides detail of the liver parenchyma, biliary tree, pancreas, and vasculature and identifies anatomic variants (Taourel et al 1996). MRCP exploits the property that stationary fluids, like bile and pancreatic juice, have higher T2 values than surrounding tissues (Schwartz et al 1998, Soto et al 1996a). It is noninvasive and averts the risk of pancreatitis, bleeding, perforation, and biliary sepsis associated with direct cholangiography. It can be employed when there is a contraindication to PTC or ERCP, a therapeutic intervention is not likely to be required, after failure of ERCP or PTC, or when there is a previous biliary-enteric or Billroth II anastomosis (Barish & Soto 1997, Soto et al 1996b). MRCP has a 95% sensitivity for detecting obstruction though it is inaccurate in assessing the grade of obstruction (Guibaud et al 1995, Morimoto et al 1992). Similarly, strictures cannot be well-characterized due to signal dropout. It has equal accuracy as ERCP in determining the level of obstruction and whether it is due to a neoplastic process (Lee et al 1997, Soto et al 1997). *Unlike PTC or ERCP, MRCP enables the biliary tree to be visualized above and below a complete obstruction (Vrachliotis et al 1997). Although it has already replaced direct cholangiography in many clinical circumstances, PTC and ERCP remain the tests of choice when therapeutic intervention such as biliary stent placement is necessary (Brown et al 1997b).*

CHOLEDOCHOLITHIASIS (Section 5)

Patients with choledocholithiasis may be asymptomatic or present with jaundice, cholangitis, or pancreatitis. *Direct cholangiography (Ch. 17) is the gold standard in detecting common duct stones which appear as filling defects.* Magnetic resonance cholangiopancreatography is also highly accurate and is comparable to ERCP in detecting choledocholithiasis (Becker et al 1997, Chan et al 1996). Magnetic resonance cholangiopancreatography has a sensitivity of 88 to 92% and a specificity of 91 to 98% in detecting choledocholithiasis (Becker et al 1997, Guibaud et al 1995, Reinhold C et al 1998). While US has a sensitivity of greater than 95% for detecting gallstones, it is not reliable in visualizing cystic duct stones due to sound wave distortion from the valves of Heister and has only a 56% sensitivity and 68% specificity in demonstrating choledocholithiasis (Tobin et al 1986). Meanwhile, CT has a sensitivity of 79% and a specificity of 100% for gallstones and a 75 to 88% sensitivity for choledocholithiasis and a specificity of 97% in detecting common duct stones (Barakos et al 1987, Neitlich et al 1997). Intraductal stones frequently appear as a target sign on CT. In those suspected of having cholangitis due to choledocholithiasis, evaluation should begin with US to define the level of obstruction. Patients that do not respond to resuscitation and antibiotics need emergent drainage by means of ERCP, PTC, or operation.

BILIARY STRICTURE (Chs 49, 54)

Long, smooth tapered strictures are usually the result of a benign process. The most frequent etiology of biliary stricture is iatrogenic injury following cholecystectomy or, less frequently, other right upper quadrant surgery. After cholecystectomy, the stricture is usually located in the common hepatic duct. The patient should be questioned about hemorrhage or fluid collection after their operation and current symptoms of fever or cholangitis. Additional causes of biliary stricture include pancreatitis, radiation, inflammation due to stone disease, and primary sclerosing cholangitis. Strictures from malignant disease tend to produce an abrupt change in the caliber of the bile duct. A proximal duct stricture may indicate the presence of a cholangiocarcinoma or a malignant masquerade such as a localized form of sclerosing cholangitis. An intrahepatic tumor causing extrinsic compression of the duct must be excluded. A mid bile duct stricture is caused by gallbladder cancer, cholangiocarcinoma, or Mirizzi's syndrome. A shrunken gallbladder with a stone should raise the suspicion of Mirizzi's syndrome which may harbor a cancer. Low ductal strictures are seen with periampullary neoplasms, pancreatitis, and cholelithiasis. In the presence of a distal stricture, the possibility of a choledochal–duodenal fistula should be kept in mind. As already stated, PTC is useful for proximal ductal disease while ERCP is preferred to examine the distal duct. Magnetic resonance cholangiopancreatography provides nearly the same information as direct cholangiography in the evaluation of a stricture.

PRIMARY SCLEROSING CHOLANGITIS (Ch. 48)

Primary sclerosing cholangitis is a progressive fibrosis of the biliary tree of unknown etiology. It is found in one-third of patients with ulcerative colitis. It occurs in men 2–3 times more commonly. Patients are initially asymptomatic though may have an elevated alkaline phosphatase. Progression to secondary biliary cirrhosis may ensue. *The diagnosis of primary sclerosing cholangitis is best made by ERCP.* The typical pattern is that of alternating short strictures (especially at duct bifurcations) and focal dilatation of the biliary ducts producing a string of beads sign. There is pruning of the intrahepatic ducts with absence of the smaller branches. The disease may occur anywhere along the biliary tract. In one study of 86 patients, all had intrahepatic disease, all but one had extrahepatic involvement, and 20% had intrahepatic disease with only proximal extrahepatic disease (MacCarty et al 1983). The possibility of cholangiocarcinoma must always be entertained in patients with primary sclerosing cholangitis 5 to 8% will develop it (Farrant et al 1991).

CHOLEDOCHAL CYST (Ch. 65)

The most common type of choledochal cyst is a solitary, fusiform dilatation of the extrahepatic bile duct. The classic presentation of jaundice, pain, and a mass is seen in one third of patients. Many other patients are asymptomatic. Choledochal cysts tend to manifest in childhood and usually involve the lower bile duct (Guibaud et al 1995). Magnetic resonance cholangiopancreatography has been shown to provide comparable information to direct cholangiography (Matos et al 1998). Caroli's disease is a congenital cystic dilatation of the intrahepatic ducts. It may be diagnosed with CT, US, PTC, or ERCP.

CHOLANGIOCARCINOMA (Ch. 54)

Patients with cholangiocarcinoma typically are discovered as a result of obstructive jaundice. The papillary variant of cholangiocarcinoma often produces intermittent jaundice. Ultrasound is the preferred initial test (Fig. 21.7). It detects hilar tumors and predicts the extent of bile duct involvement in 87% of patients (Hann et al 1996, Hann et al 1997). US demonstrates a heterogeneous mass with irregular margins that is slightly hyperechoic due to fibrotic tissue. *Duplex ultrasound may be as accurate in determining the extent of disease and vascular involvement* as the more invasive and expensive modalities of angiography and portography (Hann et al 1996, Looser et al 1992). In fact, US is as accurate as CTAP in determining portal vein involvement in a variety of tumors (Bach et al 1996, Hann et al 1997).

Cholangiography is an integral component in the evaluation of cholangiocarcinoma. *Magnetic resonance cholangiopancreatography may be the single best test.* It may be used to determine resectability through visualization of tumor extension along the biliary tract (Fig. 21.8), intrahepatic metastases, vascular involvement, and nodal metastases. Direct cholangiography has the advantage that specimens for bacterial culture and cytology may be obtained. PTC is preferred for proximal lesions. ERCP is used in distal tumors and a pancreatogram may be necessary when the diagnosis is unclear (Fig. 21.7). Both tests may be necessary when there is a complete obstruction (Soyer et al 1995).

CT is the best test for appreciating segmental or lobar atrophy and hyperplasia (Ch. 3). Lobar atrophy is an indication of ipsilateral portal vein obstruction or long-term biliary obstruction alone or a combination of both. In one

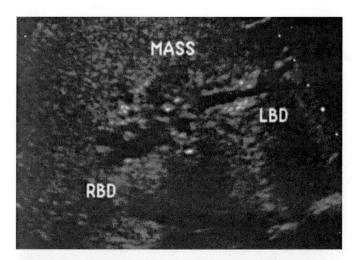

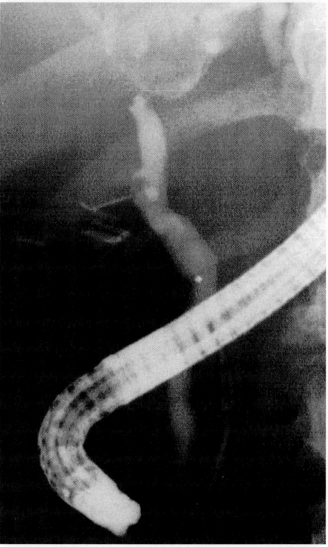

Fig. 21.7 Ultrasound and ERCP of a Klatskin tumor. Patient 5 presented with jaundice and by US (top) a mass was identified at the confluence of the left bile duct (LBD) and right bile duct (RBD) with slight extension into the right duct. The portal vein was patent but slightly compressed. ERCP (bottom) shows irregularity at the confluence and obstruction of the right hepatic duct.

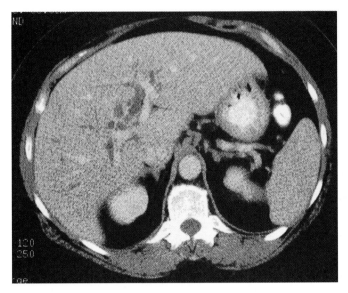 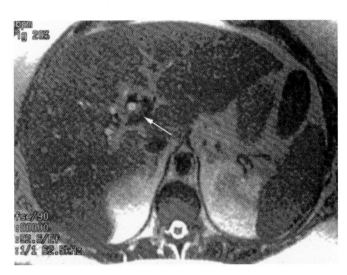

Fig. 21.8 CT and MR of a Klatskin tumor. CT (left) of patient 5 shows bilateral ductal dilatation but fails to identify a mass. MR (right) demonstrates a hilar mass (arrow). Note the presence of a metallic stent in the bile duct that was placed prior to surgical evaluation. Tumor clearance was obtained with a right trisegmentectomy and bile duct resection and the left duct was reconstructed with a Roux-en-Y loop of jejunum.

study of 30 patients with hepatic atrophy, 80% had concomitant biliary and portal vein involvement. Lobar atrophy accompanied by contralateral portal vein involvement precludes resection and the patient should undergo percutaneous drainage. The patient without liver atrophy can undergo exploration for resection or bypass. CT often cannot demonstrate an actual mass and only ductal dilatation is appreciated. CT is poor at determining portal vein involvement, arterial encasement, the nature of the lesion, and the exact level of proximal tumor extension (Feydy et al 1999). Helical CT has only 60% accuracy in determining resectability and an underestimation of the proximal extent of disease accounts for unresectability in most of the tumors that were thought to be resectable (Tillich et al 1998).

Angiography is not helpful in the diagnosis of cholangiocarcinoma and it is used primarily to identify vascular invasion. Angiography reveals the mass to be generally hypovascular without neovascularization though the periphery of the mass may stain initially (Soulen 1995). Arterial and portal vein compression, encasement, or invasion may be revealed. MR angiography (MRA) may someday supplant many of the applications of conventional angiography but at present it is relatively underdeveloped in abdominal imaging (Muller & Edelman 1995).

The diagnosis of small cholangiocarcinomas may be quite difficult. These are also the most important tumors to detect since these patients may undergo curative resection (Burke et al 1998). *When a radiologist experienced in ultrasonography is available, a combination of MRCP and duplex US is sufficient for diagnosis and preoperative staging.* CT may be used instead of MRCP but direct cholangiography may be required. Percutaneous biopsy is not routinely performed and clinical suspicion is adequate to proceed to exploration. Radiologic imaging of cholangiocarcinoma is essential in selecting patients for resection or palliation. Vascular involvement, local extension, liver metastases, liver segment atrophy, and the extent of intraductal disease determine resectability. A tumor is considered unresectable if it involves the secondary ducts bilaterally, the contralateral bile duct or vessels, common hepatic artery, or the portal vein in an extensive manner (Stain et al 1992).

GALLBLADDER CANCER (Ch. 53)

Most gallbladder cancers are discovered incidentally at the time of laparoscopy, laparotomy, or at pathologic examination of a resected gallbladder. Early gallbladder carcinoma is especially difficult to diagnose and requires a high index of suspicion. A shrunken gallbladder with a stone should raise the suspicion of Mirizzi's syndrome that may be associated with a gallbladder cancer in one third of cases. Gallbladder polyps greater than 1 cm in size should be suspected of harboring a cancer (Koga et al 1988). Gallbladder cancer tends to spread by direct extension (into the pancreas, liver, duodenum, or porta), through the lymphatics, into the biliary tree, via the peritoneum, or through the blood to the liver.

Ultrasound may show gallbladder wall-thickening, stones, a gallbladder mass, or ductal dilatation (Soyer et al 1997). Biliary obstruction usually occurs in the mid to proximal extrahepatic duct (Fig. 21.9). Ultrasound is accurate in

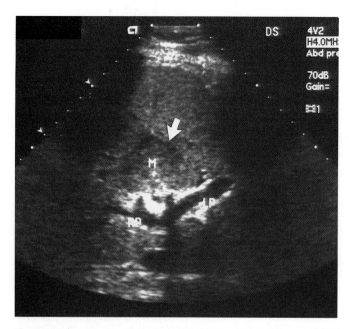 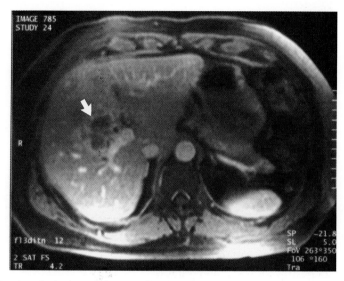

Fig. 21.9 Ultrasound and MR of a gallbladder carcinoma. Ultrasound (left) of patient 6 who has painless jaundice reveals a mass (arrow) just anterior to the portal confluence. The mass is seen in segment V on MR T1-weighted imaging with contrast (right, arrow). Note the left-sided intrahepatic biliary ductal dilatation.

the evaluation of the gallbladder mass and its extent of local spread but does not detect lymph node or peritoneal metastases (Bach et al 1998). Gallbladder cancer usually appears hypoechoic and hypovascular and stones are present in 80% of cases. Gallbladder wall thickening is defined as greater than or equal to 3 mm and is a nonspecific finding since it is also seen in cholecystitis, hepatitis, hepatic congestion, adenomyomatosis, and hypoalbuminemia (Wegener et al 1987).

As is the case with cholangiocarcinoma, MR with MRCP is the test of choice as it allows noninvasive visualization of the ductal system and further definition of the local spread of the tumor into the liver, porta hepatis, and adjacent organs (Fig. 21.9). It is superior to ultrasound in visualizing portal, retropancreatic, and aortocaval lymph nodes. Magnetic resonance cholangiopancreatography (as well as ERCP) may show a mid common bile duct stricture, a gallbladder irregularity, polyp, sludge, stone, filling defect, mass, or gallstones. Gadolinium enables examination of the vasculature. Overall, MRCP may determine resectability and guide the appropriate operative strategy. It is superior to direct cholangiography which often does not visualize the gallbladder. PTC may also be used to delineate the ductal anatomy and, in addition, it may provide access for palliative stenting (Ch. 29). It must be emphasized that patients should not be prematurely stented and denied surgical evaluation for resection.

The CT findings of gallbladder cancer are often nonspecific. An intraluminal mass, asymmetric gallbladder wall thickening, or a mass replacing the gallbladder may be seen. There may be dilated ducts, liver metastases, enlarged nodes, or a calcified (porcelain) gallbladder (Berk et al 1973). CT has a sensitivity of only 60% in detecting gallbladder carcinoma versus 82% of US (Chijiiwa et al 1991).

When a gallbladder cancer is discovered preoperatively, an *MRCP and US serve to diagnose and stage the patient.* CT may be employed instead of MRCP and then cholangiography may also be necessary. Angiography is rarely needed and only yields information on portal vein or hepatic artery involvement. Resectability is determined as with cholangiocarcinoma. A gallbladder cancer is unresectable if it involves the secondary ducts bilaterally, the contralateral bile duct or vessels, the common hepatic artery, or the portal vein in an extensive manner. Liver metastases (but not direct invasion) and lymph node metastases beyond the porta hepatis preclude resection.

PERIAMPULLARY NEOPLASMS (Ch. 55)

Distal bile duct obstruction may be the result of a biliary stricture, pancreatitis, pseudocyst, or a periampullary neoplasm. The latter includes cholangiocarcinoma, pancreatic adenocarcinoma, duodenal adenocarcinoma, ampullary adenocarcinoma, and, less frequently, lymphoma or metastases. It may be difficult to distinguish whether prominence of the head of the pancreas represents an adenocarcinoma or pancreatitis. A cystic lesion may result from a pseudocyst or a cystic tumor. Whether the patient has a benign or malignant process may be distinguished if there is a history of gallstones or alcohol use but the diagnosis cannot be definite even with a negative percutaneous or endoscopic biopsy. We do not routinely perform percutaneous or intraoperative biopsy except in unresectable disease. It is important to advise the patient of the possibility of having benign pathology when planning surgical resection such as pancreaticoduodenectomy.

Ultrasound demonstrates the distal nature of the obstruction and is often the initial test. Helical CT is the best overall test for assessing periampullary lesions and determining resectability (Nghiem & Freeny 1994, Strotzer et al 1997). It reveals a low attenuating mass, pancreatic ductal dilatation, bile duct dilatation, tumor extent, metastases, adenopathy, and vascular invasion. Pancreatic adenocarcinoma does not usually enhance or contain calcium in contrast to neuroendocrine tumors. CT has an accuracy of about 70% for resectability but is 91 to 100% accurate when the patient is deemed unresectable (Bluemke et al 1995, Diehl et al 1998, Freeny et al 1993). Thin cut (5 mm) CT is 88% correct in predicting resectability (Fuhrman et al 1994). CT is not accurate in detecting liver and peritoneal metastases, local extension, or adenopathy and 24% that are thought to be resectable on preoperative imaging will have occult metastasis at the time of laparoscopy (Conlon et al 1996, Fernandez-del Castillo et al 1995). In a report of 189 patients, CT had similar accuracy (73%), sensitivity (77%), and specificity (50%) as noncontrast MR in determining resectability (Megibow et al 1995). In a comparison of helical CT to dynamic MR, there was no difference (Ichikawa et al 1997). Helical CT is equivalent to endoscopic ultrasound in staging pancreatic tumors (Legmann et al 1998). Helical CT is equivalent to angiography in detecting arterial invasion (Kaneko et al 1997).

Direct cholangiography is not as useful as it is with proximal duct tumors. ERCP is indicated for lesions that are equivocal by CT and when preoperative biliary drainage is desired. In 376 patients, ERCP had a sensitivity of 94% and a specificity of 97% for pancreatic cancer (Freeny & Ball 1981). Irregular stenosis or abrupt termination of the duct raises the suspicion of malignancy. The 'double duct sign,' in which both the common bile duct and pancreatic ducts are dilated, occurs in 27% of patients at ERCP (Freeny et al 1976, Freeny & Ball 1981).

On MR, periampullary neoplasms are generally hypodense on T1, hyperdense on T2, and hypodense with gadolinium (Mitchell et al 1992). In 20 cases of pancreaticobiliary duct obstruction from neoplastic causes, MRCP identified the site of obstruction in 86% (Schwartz et al 1998). Overall though, MRCP is inferior to ERCP in the distal duct and consequently it is reserved for equivocal cases. MRA is comparable to angiography in demonstrating portal vein invasion (McFarland et al 1996). In a comparison of EUS, dynamic CT, and MR in 49 patients with pancreatic tumors, MR had a sensitivity of 83% and a specificity of 100% (Muller et al 1994). Its sensitivity fell to 67% in lesions smaller than 3 cm.

Helical CT is the best test to assess periampullary neoplasms and determine vessel involvement (Chs 55, 56). US is sometimes also performed to evaluate vessel involvement. On occasion, MRCP is needed to define the mass. ERCP is not typically required and routine preoperative biliary drainage with a stent should be avoided as it is associated with a higher incidence of postoperative infectious complications (Heslin et al 1998).

SUMMARY

Liver masses and biliary obstruction are frequent clinical scenarios. Often, a careful history, physical examination, and laboratory data suggest a differential pathologic diagnosis. A number of imaging modalities are available to confirm or refute a particular diagnosis. Radiologic evaluation also enables the staging of a patient's disease. In addition, it provides the anatomical relationship of a lesion to the biliary tree and vasculature making it instrumental in planning surgical intervention or palliative ablative therapies.

REFERENCES

Babineau T J, Lewis W D, Jenkins R L, Bleday R, Steele G D J, Forse R A 1994 Role of staging laparoscopy in the treatment of hepatic malignancy. American Journal of Surgery 167: 151–154

Bach A M, Hann L E, Brown K T, Getrajdman G I, Herman S K et al 1996 Portal vein evaluation with US: comparison to angiography combined with CT arterial portography. Radiology 201: 149–154

Bach A M, Loring L A, Hann L E, Illescas F F, Fong Y, Blumgart L H 1998 Gallbladder cancer: can ultrasonography evaluate extent of disease? Journal of Ultrasound in Medicine 17: 303–309

Barakos J A, Ralls P W, Lapin S A et al 1987 Cholelithiasis: Evaluation with CT. Radiology 162: 415–418

Barish M A, Soto J A 1997 MR cholangiopancreatography: techniques and clinical applications. American Journal of Roentgenology 169: 1295–1303

Baron R L, Oliver J H, Dodd G D, Nalesnik M, Holbert B L, Carr B 1996 Hepatocellular carcinoma: evaluation with biphasic, contrast-enhanced, helical CT. Radiology 199: 505–511

Becker C D, Grossholz M, Becker M, Mentha G et al 1997 Choledocholithiasis and bile duct stenosis: diagnostic accuracy of MR cholangiopancreatography. Radiology 205: 523–530

Beggs I 1983 The radiological appearances of hydatid disease of the liver. Clinical Radiology 34: 555–563

Bennett W F, Bova J G 1990 Review of hepatic imaging and a problem-oriented approach to liver masses. Hepatology 12: 761–775

Berk R N, Armbuster T G, Saltzstein S L 1973 Carcinoma in the porcelain gallbladder. Radiology 106: 29–31

Bernardino M E, Erwin B C, Steinberg H V, Baumgartner B R, Torres W E, Gedgaudas-McClees R K 1986 Delayed hepatic CT scanning: increased confidence and improved detection of hepatic metastases. Radiology 159: 71–74

Bessot M, Duprez A, Paley M R, Ros P R 1998 Hepatic calcification. Radiologic Clinics of North America 36: 391–398

Birnbaum B A, Weinreb J C, Megibow A J et al 1990 Definitive diagnosis of hepatic hemangiomas: MR imaging versus Tc-99m-labeled red blood cell SPECT. Radiology 176: 95–101

Bismuth H, Castaing D, Garden O J 1987 The use of operative ultrasound in surgery of primary liver tumors. World Journal of Surgery 11: 610–614

Bluemke D A, Cameron J L, Hruban R H et al 1995 Potentially resectable pancreatic adenocarcinoma: Spiral CT assessment with surgical and pathologic correlation. Radiology 197: 381–385

Blumgart L H, Salmon P R, Cotton P B 1974 Endoscopy and retrograde choledochopancreatography in the diagnosis of the patient with jaundice. Surgery Gynecology Obstetrics 138: 565–570

Brandt D J, Johnson C D, Stephens D H, Weiland L H 1988 Imaging of fibrolamellar hepatocellular carcinoma. American Journal of Roentgenology 151: 295–299

Bressler E L, Alpern M B, Glazer G M, Francis I R, Ensminger W D 1987 Hypervascular hepatic metastases: CT evaluation. Radiology 162: 49–51

Brown J J, Naylor M J, Yagan N 1997a Imaging of hepatic cirrhosis. Radiology 202: 1–16

Brown K T, Kemeny N, Berger M F et al 1997b Obstructive jaundice in patients receiving hepatic artery infusional chemotherapy: etiology, treatment implications, and complications after transhepatic biliary drainage. Journal of Vascular and Interventional Radiology 8: 229–234

Buetow P C, Buck J L, Pantongrag-Brown L et al 1995 Biliary cystadenoma and cystadenocarcinoma: Clinical imaging pathologic correlation with emphasis on the importance of ovarian stroma. Radiology 196: 805–810

Burke E C, Jarnagin W R, Hochwald S N, Pisters P W T, Fong Y, Blumgart L H 1998 Hilar cholangiocarcinoma: Patterns of spread, the importance of hepatic resection for curative operation, and a presurgical clinical staging system. Annals of Surgery 228: 385–394

Caseiro-Alves F, Zins M, Mahfouz A-E et al 1996 Calcification in focal nodular hyperplasia: a new problem for differentiation from fibrolamellar hepatocellular carcinoma. Radiology 198: 889–892

Castaing D, Emond J, Kunstlinger F, Bismuth H 1986 Utility of operative ultrasound in the surgical management of liver tumors. Annals of Surgery 204: 600–605

Chan Y L, Chan A C, Lam W W et al 1996 Choledocholithiasis: comparison of MR cholangiography and endoscopic retrograde cholangiography. Radiology 200: 85–89

Cherqui D, Rahmouni A, Charlotte F et al 1995 Management of focal nodular hyperplasia and hepatocellular adenoma in young women: a series of 41 patients with clinical, radiological, and pathological correlations. Hepatology 22: 1674–1681

Chijiiwa K, Sumiyoshi K, Nakayama F 1991 Impact of recent advances in hepatobiliary imaging techniques on the preoperative diagnosis of carcinoma of the gallbladder. World Journal of Surgery 15: 322–327

Choi C S, Freeny P C 1998 Triphasic helical CT of hepatic focal nodular hyperplasia: incidence of atypical findings. American Journal of Roentgenology 170: 391–395

Chung K Y, Mayo-Smith W W, Saini S, Rahmouni A, Golli M, Mathieu D 1995 Hepatocellular adenoma: MR imaging features with pathologic correlation. American Journal of Roentgenology 165: 303–308

Conlon K C, Dougherty E, Klimstra D S, Coit D G, Turnbull A D, Brennan M F 1996 The value of minimal access surgery in the staging of patients with potentially resectable peripancreatic malignancy. Annals of Surgery 223: 134–140

Delbeke D, Martin W H, Sandler M P, Chapman W C, Wright J K J, Pinson C W 1998 Evaluation of benign vs malignant hepatic lesions with positron emission tomography. Archives of Surgery 133: 510–515

Diehl S J, Lehmann KJ, Sadick M, Lachmann R, Georgi M 1998 Pancreatic cancer: Value of dual-phase helical CT in assessing resectability. Radiology 206: 373–378

Doerr R J, Abdel-Nabi H, Krag D, Mitchell E 1991 Radiolabeled antibody imaging in the management of colorectal cancer. Results of a multicenter clinical study. Annals of Surgery 214: 118–124

Elias E, Hamlyn A N, Jain S et al 1976 A randomized trial of percutaneous transhepatic cholangiography with the Chiba needle versus endoscopic retrograde cholangiography for bile duct visualization in jaundice. Gastroenterology 71: 439–443

Elizondo G, Weissleder R, Stark D D, Todd L E, Compton C et al 1987 Amebic liver abscess: diagnosis and treatment evaluation with MR imaging. Radiology 165: 795–800

Farrant J M, Hayllar K M, Wilkinson M L et al 1991 Natural history and prognostic variables in primary sclerosing cholangitis. Gastroenterology 100: 1710–1717

Fernandez-del Castillo C, Rattner D W, Warshaw A L 1995 Further experience with laparoscopy and peritoneal cytology in the staging of pancreatic cancer. British Journal of Surgery 82: 1127–1129

Ferrucci J T 1994 Liver tumor imaging. Current concepts. Radiologic Clinics of North America 32: 39–54

Feydy A, Vilgrain V, Denys A et al 1999 Helical CT assessment in hilar cholangiocarcinoma: Correlation with surgical and pathologic findings. American Journal of Roentgenology 172: 73–77

Findlay M, Young H, Cunningham D et al 1996 Noninvasive monitoring of tumor metabolism using fluorodeoxyglucose and positron emission tomography in colorectal cancer liver metastases: correlation with tumor response to fluorouracil. Journal of Clinical Oncology 14: 700–708

Fong Y, Cohen A M, Fortner J G et al 1997 Liver resection for colorectal metastases. Journal of Clinical Oncology 15: 938–946

Fong Y, Kemeny N, Paty P, Blumgart L H, Cohen A M 1996 Treatment of colorectal cancer: hepatic metastasis. Seminars in Surgical Oncology 12: 219–252

Foster J, Berman M 1994 The malignant transformation of liver cell adenomas. Archives of Surgery 129: 712–717

Freeny P C, Traverso L W, Ryan J A 1993 Diagnosis and staging of pancreatic adenocarcinoma with dynamic computed tomography. American Journal of Surgery 165: 600–606

Freeny P C, Ball T J 1981 Endoscopic retrograde cholangiopancreatography (ERCP) and percutaneous transhepatic cholangiography (PTC) in the evaluation of suspected pancreatic carcinoma: diagnostic limitations and contemporary roles. Cancer 47: 1666–1678

Freeny P C, Bilbao M K, Katon R M 1976 'Blind' evaluation of endoscopic retrograde cholangiopancreatography (ERCP) in the diagnosis of pancreatic carcinoma: the 'double duct' and other signs. Radiology 119: 271–274

Freeny P C, Marks W M 1986 Patterns of contrast enhancement of benign and malignant hepatic neoplasms during bolus dynamic and delayed CT. Radiology 160: 613–618

Fuhrman G M, Charnsangavej C, Abbruzzese J L et al 1994 Thin-section contrast-enhanced computed tomography accurately predicts the resectability of malignant pancreas neoplasms. American Journal of Surgery 167: 104–111

Fukuya T, Honda H, Matsumata T et al 1994 Diagnosis of inflammatory pseudotumor of the liver: value of CT. American Journal of Roentgenology 163: 1087–1091

Gaa J, Saini S , Ferrucci J T 1991 Perfusion characteristics of hepatic cavernous hemangioma using intravenous CT angiography (IVCTA). European Journal of Radiology 12: 228–233

Guibaud L, Bret P M, Reinhold C, Atri M, Barkun A N 1995 Bile duct obstruction and choledocholithiasis: diagnosis with MR cholangiography. Radiology 197: 109–115

Hahn P F, Saini S 1998 Liver-specific MR imaging contrast agents. Radiologic Clinics of North America 36: 287–297

Hamm B, Fischer E, Taupitz M 1990 Differentiation of hepatic hemangiomas from metastases by dynamic contrast-enhanced MR imaging. Journal of Computer Assisted Tomography 14: 205–216

Hamm B, Mahfouz A E, Taupitz M et al 1997 Liver metastases: improved detection with dynamic gadolinium-enhanced MR imaging? Radiology 202: 677–682

Hamrick-Turner J, Abbitt P L, Ros P R 1992 Intrahepatic cholangiocarcinoma: MR appearance. American Journal of Roentgenology 158: 77–79

Hann L E, Fong Y, Shriver C D et al 1996 Malignant hepatic hilar tumors: can ultrasonography be used as an alternative to angiography with CT arterial portography for determination of resectability? Journal of Ultrasound Medicine 15: 37–45

Hann L E, Greatrex K V, Bach A M, Fong Y, Blumgart L H 1997 Cholangiocarcinoma at the hepatic hilus: sonographic findings. American Journal of Roentgenology 168: 985–989

Hann L E, Schwartz L H, Panicek D M, Bach A M, Fong Y, Blumgart L H 1998 Tumor involvement in hepatic veins: comparison of MR imaging and US for preoperative assessment. Radiology 206: 651–656

Harbin W P, Robert N J, Ferrucci J T J 1980 Diagnosis of cirrhosis based on regional changes in hepatic morphology: a radiological and pathological analysis. Radiology 135: 273–283

Harrison L E, Brennan M F, Newman E et al 1997 Hepatic resection for noncolorectal, nonneuroendocrine metastases: a fifteen-year experience with ninety-six patients. Surgery 121: 625–632

Heilo A, Stenwig A E 1997 Liver hemangioma: US-guided 18-gauge core-needle biopsy. Radiology 204: 719–722

Heslin M J, Brooks A D, Hochwald S N, Harrison L E, Blumgart L H, Brennan M F 1998 Preoperative biliary stenting is associated with increased complications after pancreaticoduodenectomy. Archives of Surgery 133: 149–154

Hollett M D, Jeffrey R B J, Nino-Murcia M, Jorgensen M J, Harris D P 1995 Dual-phase helical CT of the liver: value of arterial phase scans in the detection of small (< or = 1.5 cm) malignant hepatic neoplasms. American Journal of Roentgenology 164: 879–884

Ichikawa T, Haradome H, Hachiya J et al 1997 Pancreatic ductal adenocarcinoma: Preoperative assessment with helical CT versus dynamic MR imaging. Radiology 202: 655–662

Ichikawa T, Ohtomo K, Takahashi S 1996 Hepatocellular carcinoma: Detection with double-phase helical CT during arterial portography. Radiology 198: 284–287

Ishak K, Rabin L 1975 Benign tumors of the liver Medical Clinics of North America 59: 995–1013

Itai Y, Matsui O 1997 Blood flow and liver imaging. Radiology 202: 306–314

Itoh K, Nishimura K, Togashi K 1987 Hepatocellular carcinoma MR imaging. Radiology 164: 21–25

Jacobs J E, Birnbaum B A 1995 Computed tomography imaging of focal hepatic lesions. Seminars in Roentgenology 30: 308–323

Jacobs J E, Birnbaum B A, Shapiro M A et al 1998 Diagnostic criteria for fatty infiltration of the liver on contrast-enhanced helical CT. American Journal of Roentgenology 171: 659–664

Jarnagin W R, Bodniewicz J, Dougherty E, Conlon K, Blumgart L H, Fong Y 1999 A prospective analysis of staging laparoscopy in patients with primary and secondary hepatobiliary malignancies (submitted)

John T G, Greig J D, Crosbie J L, Miles W F, Garden O J 1994 Superior staging of liver tumors with laparoscopy and laparoscopic ultrasound. Annalls of Surgery 220: 711–719

Kaneko K, Honda H, Hayashi T et al 1997 Helical CT evaluation of arterial invasion in pancreatic tumors: Comparison with angiography. Abdominal Imaging 22: 204–207

Kanematsu M, Hoshi H, Murakami T et al 1997a Detection of hepatocellular carcinoma in patients with cirrhosis: MR imaging versus angiographically assisted helical CT. American Journal of Roentgenology 169: 1507–1515

Kanematsu M, Oliver J H, Carr B, Baron R L 1997b Hepatocellular carcinoma: the role of helical biphasic contrast-enhanced CT versus CT during arterial portography. Radiology 205: 75–80

Karhunen P J 1986 Benign hepatic tumors and tumor like conditions in men. Journal of Clinical Pathology 39: 183–188

Kelekis N L, Semelka R C, Worawattanakul S et al 1998 Hepatocellular carcinoma in North America: A multiinstitutional study of appearance on T1 weighted, T2 weighted, and serial gadolinium enhanced gradient echo images. American Journal of Roentgenology 170: 1005–1013

Koga A, Watanabe K, Fukuyama T, Takiguchi S, Nakayama F 1988 Diagnosis and operative indications for polypoid lesions of the gallbladder. Archives of Surgery 123: 26–29

Kruskal J B, Kane R A 1996 Imaging of primary and metastatic liver tumors. Surgical Oncology Clinics of North America 5: 231–260

Kuligowska E, Connors S K, Shapiro J H 1982 Liver abscess: Sonography in diagnosis and treatment. American Journal of Roentgenology 138: 253–257

Kuszyk B S, Bluemke D A, Urban B A et al 1996 Portal-phase contrast-enhanced helical CT for the detection of malignant hepatic tumors: sensitivity based on comparison with intraoperative and pathologic findings. American Journal of Roentgenology 166: 91–95

Lacomis J M, Baron R L, Oliver J H, Nalesnik M A, Federle M P 1997 Cholangiocarcinoma: delayed CT contrast enhancement patterns. Radiology 203: 98–104

Laing F C, Jeffrey R B J, Wing V W, Nyberg D A 1986 Biliary dilatation: defining the level and cause by real-time US. Radiology 160: 39–42

Lee M G, Lee H J, Kim M H et al 1997 Extrahepatic biliary diseases: 3D MR cholangiopancreatography compared with endoscopic retrograde cholangiopancreatography. Radiology 202: 663–669

Lee M J, Saini S, Hamm B et al 1991 Focal nodular hyperplasia of the liver: MR findings in 35 proved cases. American Journal of Roentgenology 156: 317–320

Legmann P, Vignaux O, Dousset B et al 1998 Pancreatic tumors: Comparison of dual-phase helical CT and endoscopic sonography. American Journal of Roentgenology 170: 1315–1322

Leslie D F, Johnson C D, Johnson C M, Ilstrup D M, Harmsen W S 1995 Distinction between cavernous hemangiomas of the liver and hepatic metastases on CT: value of contrast enhancement patterns. American Journal of Roentgenology 164: 625–629

Lewis K H, Chezmar J L 1997 Hepatic metastases. Magnetic Resonance Imaging Clinics of North America 5: 319–330

Looser C, Stain S C, Baer H U, Triller J, Blumgart L H 1992 Staging of hilar cholangiocarcinoma by ultrasound and duplex sonography: a comparison with angiography and operative findings. British Journal of Radiology 65: 871–877

Lubbers P R, Ros P R, Goodman Z D, Ishak K G 1987 Accumulation of technetium-99m sulfur colloid by hepatocellular adenoma: scintigraphic-pathologic correlation. American Journal of Roentgenology 148: 1105–1108

MacCarty R L, LaRusso N F, Wiesner R H, Ludwig J 1983 Primary sclerosing cholangitis: findings on cholangiography and pancreatography. Radiology 149: 39–44

Mahfouz A E, Hamm B, Taupitz M, Wolf K J 1993 Hypervascular liver lesions: differentiation of focal nodular hyperplasia from malignant tumors with dynamic gadolinium-enhanced MR imaging. Radiology 186: 133–138

Mahfouz A E, Hamm B, Wolf K J 1994 Peripheral washout: a sign of malignancy on dynamic gadolinium-enhanced MR images of focal liver lesions. Radiology 190: 49–52

Mathieu D, Bruneton J N, Drouillard J, Pointreau C C, Vasile N 1986

Hepatic adenomas and focal nodular hyperplasia: dynamic CT study. Radiology 160: 53–58

Mathieu D, Grenier P, Larde D, Vasile N 1984 Portal vein involvement in hepatocellular carcinoma: dynamic CT features. Radiology 152: 127–132

Mathieu D, Vasile N, Fagniez P L, Segui S, Grably D, Larde D 1985 Dynamic CT features of hepatic abscesses. Radiology 154: 749–752

Matos C, Nicaise N, Deviere J et al 1998 Choledochal cysts: Comparison of findings at MR cholangiopancreatography and endoscopic retrograde cholangiopancreatography in eight patients. Radiology 209: 443–448

Matsui O, Takashima T, Kadoya M et al 1987 Liver metastases from colorectal cancers: detection with CT during arterial portography. Radiology 165: 65–69

McFarland E G, Kaufman J A, Saini S et al 1996 Preoperative staging of cancer of the pancreas: Value of MR angiography versus conventional angiography in detecting portal venous invasion. American Journal of Roentgenology 166: 37–43

Megibow A J, Zhou X H, Rotterdam H et al 1995 Pancreatic adenocarcinoma: CT versus MR imaging in the evaluation of resectability – Report of the Radiology Diagnostic Oncology Group. Radiology 195: 327–332

Mendez R J, Schiebler M L, Outwater E K, Kressel H Y 1994 Hepatic abscesses: MR imaging findings. Radiology 190: 431–436

Mergo P J, Ros P R 1998 Imaging of diffuse liver disease. Radiology Clinics of North America 36: 365–375

Miller W J, Baron R L, Dodd G D, Federle M P 1994 Malignancies in patients with cirrhosis: CT sensitivity and specificity in 200 consecutive transplant patients. Radiology 193: 645–650

Mitchell D G, Rubin R, Siegelman E S, Burk D L J, Rifkin M D 1991 Hepatocellular carcinoma within siderotic regenerative nodules: appearance as a nodule within a nodule on MR images. Radiology 178: 101–103

Mitchell D G, Saini S, Weinreb J et al 1994 Hepatic metastases and cavernous hemangiomas: distinction with standard- and triple-dose gadoteridol-enhanced MR imaging. Radiology 193: 49–57

Mitchell D G, Shapiro M, Schuricht A, Barbot D, Rosato F 1992 Pancreatic disease: findings on state-of-the-art MR images. American Journal of Roentgenology 159: 533–538

Moran B J, O'Rourke N, Plant G R, Rees M 1995 Computed tomographic portography in preoperative imaging of hepatic neoplasms British Journal of Surgery 82: 669–671

Morimoto K, Shimoi M, Shirakawa T et al 1992 Biliary obstruction: evaluation with three-dimensional MR cholangiography. Radiology 183: 578–580

Moskal T L, Charnsangavej C, Ellis L M 1995 Workup, diagnosis, and treatment of benign hepatic tumors. Cancer Bulletin 47: 385–391

Muller M F, Meyenberger C, Bertschinger P, Schaer R, Marincek B 1994 Pancreatic tumors: Evaluation with endoscopic US, CT, and MR imaging. Radiology 190: 745–751

Muller M F, Edelman R R 1995 Magnetic resonance angiography of the abdomen. Gastroenterology Clinical of North America 24: 435–456

Nagasue N, Yukaya H, Chang Y C, Kimura N, Ota N, Nakamura T 1988 Hepatocellular pseudotumour (regenerating nodule) in the cirrhotic liver mimicking hepatocellular carcinoma. British Journal of Surgery 75: 1124–1128

Nagorney D M, Adson M A, Weiland L H, Knight C D J, Smalley S R, Zinsmeister A R 1985 Fibrolamellar hepatoma. American Journal of Surgery 149: 113–119

Nazarian L N, Wechsler R J, Grady C K et al 1994 CT done 4–6 hr after CT arterial portography: Value in detecting hepatic tumors and differentiating from other hepatic perfusion defects. American Journal of Roentgenology 163: 851–855

Neitlich J D, Topazian M, Smith R C, Gupta A, Burrell M I, Rosenfield A T 1997 Detection of choledocholithiasis: Comparison of unenhanced helical CT and endoscopic retrograde cholangiopancreatography. Radiology 203: 753–757

Nelson R C, Chezmar J L 1990 Diagnostic approach to hepatic hemangiomas. Radiology 176: 11–13

Nelson R C, Chezmar J L, Sugarbaker P H, Bernardino M E 1989 Hepatic tumors: comparison of CT during arterial portography, delayed CT, and MR imaging for preoperative evaluation. Radiology 172: 27–34

Nghiem H V, Freeny P C 1994 Radiologic staging of pancreatic adenocarcinoma. Radiologic Clinics of North America 32: 71–79

Okazumi S, Isono K, Enomoto K et al 1992 Evaluation of liver tumors using fluorine-18–fluorodeoxyglucose PET: characterization of tumor and assessment of effect of treatment. Journal of Nuclear Medicine 33: 333–339

Oliver J H, Baron R L 1996 Helical biphasic contrast-enhanced CT of the liver: technique, indications, interpretation, and pitfalls. Radiology 201: 1–14

Paulson E K, McClellan J S, Washington K, Spritzer C E, Meyers W C, Baker M E 1994 Hepatic adenoma: MR characteristics and correlation with pathologic findings. American Journal of Roentgenology 163: 113–116

Pedrosa C S, Casanova R, Lezana A H, Fernandez M C 1981 Computed tomography in obstructive jaundice. Part II: The cause of obstruction. Radiology 139: 635–645

Quinn S F, Benjamin G G 1992 Hepatic cavernous hemangiomas: simple diagnostic sign with dynamic bolus CT. Radiology 182: 545–548

Ralls P W, Barnes P F, Radin D R, Colletti P, Halls J 1987a Sonographic features of amebic and pyogenic liver abscesses: A blinded comparison. American Journal of Roentgenology 149: 499–501

Ralls P W, Henley D S, Colletti P M et al 1987b Amebic liver abscess: MR imaging. Radiology 165: 801–804

Ravikumar T S 1996 Laparoscopic staging and intraoperative ultrasonography for liver tumor management. Surgical Oncology Clinics of North America 5: 271–282

Reinhold C, Taourel P, Bret P M et al 1998 Choledocholithiasis: Evaluation of MR cholangiography for diagnosis. Radiology 209: 435–442

Rifkin M D, Rosato F E, Branch H M et al 1987 Intraoperative ultrasound of the liver. An important adjunctive tool for decision making in the operating room. Annals of Surgery 205: 466–472

Ringe B, Pichlmayr R, Wittekind C, Tusch G 1991 Surgical treatment of hepatocellular carcinoma: experience with liver resection and transplantation in 198 patients. World Journal of Surgery 15: 270–285

Rogers J V, Mack L A, Freeny P C, Johnson M L, Sones P J 1981 Hepatic focal nodular hyperplasia: angiography, CT, sonography, and scintigraphy. American Journal of Roentgenology 137: 983–990

Rummeny E, Weissleder R, Sironi S et al 1989 Central scars in primary liver tumors: MR features, specificity, and pathologic correlation. Radiology 171: 323–326

Saini S 1997 Imaging of the hepatobiliary tract. New England Journal of Medicine 336: 1889–1894

Schnall M 1995 Magnetic resonance imaging of focal liver lesions. Seminars in Roentgenology 30: 347–361

Schwartz L H, Coakley F V, Sun Y, Blumgart L H, Fong Y, Panicek D M 1998 Neoplastic pancreaticobiliary duct obstruction: evaluation with breath-hold MR cholangiopancreatography. American Journal of Roentgenology 170: 1491–1495

Schwartz L H, Gandras E J, Colangelo S M, Ercolani M C, Panicek D M 1999 Prevalence and importance of small hepatic lesions found at CT in patients with cancer. Radiology 210: 71–74

Semelka R C, Brown E D, Ascher S M et al 1994 Hepatic hemangiomas: a multi-institutional study of appearance on T2-weighted and serial gadolinium-enhanced gradient-echo MR images. Radiology 192: 401–406

Soto J A, Barish M A, Ferrucci J T 1997 Magnetic resonance imaging of the bile ducts. Seminars in Roentgenology 32: 188–201

Soto J A, Barish M A, Yucel E K, Siegenberg D, Ferrucci J T, Chuttani R 1996a Magnetic resonance cholangiography: comparison with endoscopic retrograde cholangiopancreatography. Gastroenterology 110: 589–597

Soto J A, Yucel E K, Barish M A, Chuttani R, Ferrucci J T 1996b MR cholangiopancreatography after unsuccessful or incomplete ERCP. Radiology 199: 91–98

Soulen M C 1995 Angiographic evaluation of focal liver masses. Seminars in Roentgenology 30: 362–374

Soyer P, Bleumke D A, Hruban R H, Sitzmann J V, Fishman E K 1994 Hepatic metastases from colorectal cancer: Detection and false-positive findings with helical CT during arterial portography. Radiology 193: 71–74

Soyer P, Bleumke D A, Reichle R et al 1995 Imaging of intrahepatic cholangiocarcinoma: 1. Peripheral cholangiocarcinoma. American Journal of Roentgenology 165: 1427–1431

Soyer P, Lacheheb D, Levesque M 1993 False-positive CT portography: Correlation with pathologic findings. American Journal of Roentgenology 160: 285–289

Soyer P, Bluemke D A, Fishman E K 1994a CT during arterial portography for the preoperative evaluation of hepatic tumors: how, when, and why? American Journal of Roentgenology 163: 1325–1331

Soyer P, Bluemke D A, Hruban R H, Sitzmann J V, Fishman E K 1994b Primary malignant neoplasms of the liver: Detection with helical CT during arterial portography. Radiology 192: 389–392

Soyer P, Bluemke D A, Reichle R et al 1995 Imaging of intrahepatic cholangiocarcinoma: 2. Hilar cholangiocarcinoma. American Journal of Roentgenology 165: 1433–1436

Soyer P, Gouhiri M, Boudiaf M et al 1997 Carcinoma of the gallbladder: imaging features with surgical correlation. American Journal of Roentgenology 169: 781–785

Soyer P, Laissy J P, Sibert A et al 1994c Focal hepatic masses: comparison of detection during arterial portography with MR imaging and CT. Radiology 190: 737–740

Soyer P, Levesque M, Elias D, Zeitoun G, Roche A 1992 Detection of liver metastases from colorectal cancer: comparison of intraoperative US and CT during arterial portography. Radiology 183: 541–544

Stain S C, Baer H U, Dennison A R, Blumgart L H 1992 Current management of hilar cholangiocarcinoma. Surgery, Gynecology and Obstetrics 175: 579–588

Strotzer M, Gmeinwieser J, Schmidt J et al 1997 Diagnosis of liver metastases from colorectal adenocarcinoma. Comparison of spiral-CTAP combined with intravenous contrast-enhanced spiral-CT and SPIO-enhanced MR combined with plain MR imaging. Acta Radiologica 38: 986–992

Takayasu K, Furukawa H, Wakao F et al 1995 CT diagnosis of early hepatocellular carcinoma: sensitivity, findings, and CT-pathologic correlation. American Journal of Roentgenology 164: 885–890

Taourel P, Bret P M, Reinhold C, Barkun A N, Atri M 1996 Anatomic variants of the biliary tree: diagnosis with MR cholangiopancreatography. Radiology 199: 521–527

The Liver Cancer Study Group of Japan 1990 Primary liver cancer in Japan: Clinicopathologic features and results of surgical treatment. Annals of Surgery 211: 277–287

Tillich M, Mischinger H J, Preisegger K H, Rabl H, Szolar D H 1998 Multiphasic helical CT in diagnosis and staging of hilar cholangiocarcinoma. American Journal of Roentgenology 171: 651–658

Tobin M V, Mendelson R M, Lamb G H, Gilmore I T 1986 Ultrasound diagnosis of bile duct calculi. British Medical Journal Clinical Research 293: 16–17

Torres W E, Whitmire L F, Gedgaudas-McClees K, Bernardino M E 1986 Computed tomography of hepatic morphologic changes in cirrhosis of the liver. Journal of Computer Assisted Tomography 10: 47–50

Van Beers B E, Gallez B, Pringot J 1997 Contrast-enhanced MR imaging of the liver. Radiology 203: 297–306

van Leeuwen M S, Noordzij J, Feldberg M A, Hennipman A H, Doornewaard H 1996 Focal liver lesions: characterization with triphasic spiral CT. Radiology 201: 327–336

Vitola J V, Delbeke D, Sandler M P et al 1996 Positron emission tomography to stage suspected metastatic colorectal carcinoma to the liver. American Journal of Surgery 171: 21–26

Vrachliotis T G, Shirkhoda A, Bis K G et al 1997 MR cholangio-pancreatography (MRCP). Critical Reviews in Diagnostic Imaging 38: 295–323

Wegener M, Borsch G, Schneider J, Wedmann B, Winter R, Zacharias J 1987 Gallbladder wall thickening: a frequent finding in various nonbiliary disorders – a prospective ultrasonographic study. Journal of Clinical Ultrasound 15: 307–312

Welch T J, Sheedy P F, Johnson C M et al 1985 Focal nodular hyperplasia and hepatic adenoma: comparison of angiography, CT, US, and scintigraphy. Radiology 156: 593–595

Wernecke K, Vassallo P, Bick U, Diederich S, Peters P E 1992 The distinction between benign and malignant liver tumors on sonography: value of a hypoechoic halo. American Journal of Roentgenology 159: 1005–1009

Wittenberg J, Stark D D, Forman B H et al 1988 Differentiation of hepatic metastases from hepatic hemangiomas and cysts by using MR imaging. American Journal of Roentgenology 151: 79–84

Yamashita Y, Mitsuzaki K, Yi T et al 1996 Small hepatocellular carcinoma in patients with chronic liver damage: prospective comparison of detection with dynamic MR imaging and helical CT of the whole liver. Radiology 200: 79–84

Yates C K, Streight R A 1986 Focal fatty infiltration of the liver simulating metastatic disease. Radiology 159: 83–84

Intraoperative radiology

22

T.A. BROUGHAN, R.E. HERMANN

There remains debate regarding the need for routine intra-operative cholangiography, which is now being compared to intraoperative (Birth et al 1998, Catheline et al 1998, Rothlin et al 1994, Siperstein et al 1999, Thompson et al 1998, Wu et al 1998, Soper 1998) and endoscopic ultrasound (Canto et al 1998, Montariol et al 1998, Sahai et al 1999), magnetic resonance cholangiography (Dwerryhouse et al 1998, Lomanto et al 1997, Mendler et al 1998) and helical CT scanning (Baron 1997, Prassopoulos et al 1998). Nevertheless, its simplicity and potential to demonstrate relevant surgical anatomy are advantages of the technique.

Operative cholangiography was introduced by Mirizzi (1932 & 1937) in Argentina, and was later recognized as an important addition to gallbladder, biliary, and hepatic surgery. There has however been disagreement as to whether selective use (Barkun et al 1993, Bogokowsky et al 1987, Braghetto et al 1998, Corder, et al 1992, Csendes et al 1998, Fiore et al 1997, Jones et al 1995, Huguier et al 1991, Mansberger et al 1988, Montariol et al 1995, Murison et al 1993, Silverstein et al 1998, Trondsen et al 1998, Wright & Wellwood 1998) or routine cholangiography (Bagnato et al 1991, Berci 1992, Berci 1998, Berci et al 1991, Corbitt & Cantwell 1991, Corbitt & Leonetti 1997, Flowers et al 1992, Hunter 1991, Khalili et al 1997, Koo & Traverso 1996, Kullman et al 1996, Vecchio et al 1998, Lezoche et al 1994 Rantis et al 1993, Rosenthal et al 1994, Sackier et al 1991, Shively et al 1990, Stuart et al 1998, Traverso et al 1994, Woods et al 1995, Woods et al 1994, Z'graggen et al 1998) is indicated.

Advocates of routine operative cholangiography have traditionally recognized its value in identifying the entire biliary system at operation so that unsuspected pathological findings are not missed (Figs 22.1 and 22.2). Routine cholangiography allows unsuspected bile duct stones to be found, surgically relevant anatomy to be identified, and earlier detection of bile duct injuries to be made.

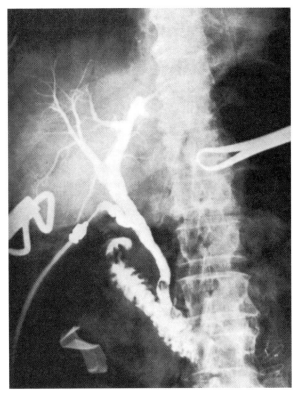

Fig. 22.1 Operative cholangiography showing a small stone in the non-dilated, distal, intrapancreatic bile duct, unsuspected by the surgeon.

Unsuspected stones, that is, stones found in the bile ducts on cholangiography that could not have been predicted pre-operatively by a relevant history or preoperative imaging (Koo & Traverso 1996, Stuart et al 1998, Traverso et al 1994) have been reported in 2.6 to 7.8% of cases at cholecystectomy (Flowers et al 1992, Vecchio et al 1998). Therefore using selective operative cholangiographic criteria, some 5% of patients will have retained bile duct stones after cholecystectomy. Thurston and McDougall (1976)

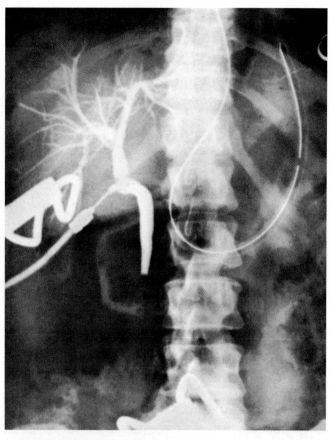

Fig. 22.2 Operative cholangiography showing an unsuspected distal bile duct obstruction due to a small stone. The patient had no prior history of jaundice or pancreatitis.

Before the advent of operative cholangiography, various preoperative and perioperative criteria were followed to determine the need for bile duct exploration (Glenn 1952, Bartlett & Waddell 1958, Saypol 1961). These included: (1) a palpable stone in the common bile duct; (2) a history of jaundice or cholangitis; (3) a thickened or dilated bile duct; (4) multiple small stones in the gallbladder or a single faceted stone; (5) a cystic duct larger than the stones in the gallbladder; (6) a past history of pancreatitis; and (7) a patient over 60 years of age with a long history of biliary disease. Various permutations of these criteria are still in use to determine the need for selective cholangiography at open cholecystectomy (Gregg 1988, Mansberger et al 1988, Lillemoe et al 1992). However, the use of these clinical criteria alone lead to a number of unnecessary common bile duct explorations. Thus Saypol (1961) and Appleman et al (1964) report that when clinical indications alone are used as a guide, biliary pathology is found in only 30 to 50% of the common bile ducts explored so that more than half of the patients are treated unnecessarily (Leichtling et al 1959). By contrast, when cystic duct cholangiography is performed routinely and used as the principal guide for the need to explore common bile duct, there are abnormal findings in the common bile duct in 90 to 95% of explorations (Pagana & Stahlgren 1980).

Unnecessary common bile duct explorations at cholecystectomy is potentially dangerous. McSherry & Glenn (1980) report a 0.5% mortality for cholecystectomy alone as compared with a 2.1% mortality for open cholecystectomy with common bile duct exploration. Glenn (1952) further relates the mortality for common bile duct exploration to the age of the patient; 1.5% for patients under 50 years of age and 9.6% for patients over 50 years of age. We have found that older patients have a higher incidence of common bile duct stones (Table 22.1) (Hermann 1983). Thus, it is particularly important to use operative cholangiography routinely when operating on older patients.

suggested that retained bile duct stones increase in size, perhaps over 10 years or more, and become symptomatic. There are few studies which document how often this occurs but Johnson and Hosking (1987) predict that 25 to 50% of retained stones will cause symptoms over time. It is known that bile duct stone can pass asymptomatically in at least 12% of patients (Acosta & Ledesma 1974, Kelly 1976) although Diehl et al (1997) report that gallstones smaller than 5 mm are more likely to cause gallstone pancreatitis, although this study has been debated. In an editorial, Cotton (1997) observes that in situations where T-tubes are left in place, small bile duct stones are often noted to pass asymptomatically in the first postoperative weeks and that the fragments of gallstones after extracorporeal lithotripsy most frequently pass asymptomatically. Routine operative cholangiography, especially with digital fluoroscopy, has a 0.017 to 2% false positive rate (Khalili et al 1997, Flowers et al 1992), a 0 to 0.3% false negative rate (Stuart et al 1998, Kullman et al 1996), and no reported injuries secondary to the procedure itself. It provides a reliable solution to the problem of the common bile duct stone.

Table 22.1 Incidence of bile duct stones at cholecystectomy

Age (years)	All patients/ patients with bile duct stones	Percentage
10–20	25/4	16
21–30	92/11	12
31–40	226/21	9
41–50	325/28	9
51–60	473/67	14
61–70	275/85	31
71–80	116/56	48
81–90	11/10	96
Total	1543/282	18

Bile duct injuries after laparoscopic cholecystectomy are 2–3 times more common than after open cholecystectomy (Berci 1992) and it has been questioned whether surgeons are properly informing patients of the risk of biliary injury and doing everything possible to minimize the risk (Berci 1998). Some surgeons feel that routine cholangiography decreases laparoscopic bile duct injuries (Bagnato et al 1991, Berci et al 1991, Corbitt & Cantwell 1991, Corbitt & Leonetti 1997, Hunter 1991, Khalili et al 1997, Lezoche et al 1994, Rosenthal et al 1994, Sackier et al 1991, Traverso et al 1994) while others report the prime advantage to be improved detection of bile duct injuries. (Woods et al 1995, Z'graggen et al 1998).

Our experience and that of others (Corbitt & Cantwell 1991, Lezoche et al 1994) demonstrate an ability to cannulate the cystic duct in 97% of cases during cholecystectomy. Khalili et al (1997) reported on the use of routine cholangiography in 1207 laparoscopic cholecystectomy cases. The findings were: 1016 (84%) normal studies; 149 (12.3%) common bile duct stones; 23 (1.9%) biliary anomalies; 10 (0.8%) duodenal diverticula; 4 (0.3%) ductal strictures; 5 (0.4%) common bile duct diverticula. Five (0.4%) bile duct injuries were demonstrated, of which four were minor and cholangiography is thought to have prevented bile duct transection. Traverso et al (1994) reported on 624 laparoscopic cholecystectomies of which 535 (86%) successfully underwent operative cholangiography and 420 (78%) were reviewed by both a surgeon and a radiologist. Relevant findings were defined as filling defects, strictures, leaks and anomalous bile ducts. The entire biliary tract was visualized in 86% of the cases and the common hepatic duct confluence in 95%. Without routine cholangiography, 68 relevant findings would have been missed in these 420 cases, including 47 (10%) bile duct filling defects and 18 (4%) dissection-relevant anomalous bile ducts. In a study at 669 German hospitals (Rosenthal et al 1994) fewer bile duct injuries and a better detection rate (80%) at cholecystectomy in the 30 of 174 units practising routine operative cholangiography were reported. Multicenter reports from the US and from Switzerland document the advantage of routine cholangiography in detecting bile duct injury during cholecystectomy. Woods et al (1994, 1995) reported that 62% of bile duct injuries were identified at the time of cholecystectomy when using cholangiography versus only 37% when no cholangiography was performed. Z'graggen et al (1998) found that operative cholangiography detected 75% of bile duct injuries compared to 33% of injuries being recognized at the time of cholecystectomy without cholangiography. The detection of bile duct injury at the time of cholecystectomy allows not only a medicolegal advantage but also a technical advantage. The possibility of repairing a freshly injured duct without infection, fibrosis, and inflammation is well-appreciated by the biliary surgeon (Berci 1992, Rantis et al 1993).

Proponents of selective operative cholangiography cite the added time and expense resulting from subsequent endoscopic cholangiography and sphincterotomy in patients with false-positive results during routine cholangiography (Barkun et al 1993, Bogokowsky et al 1987, Braghetto et al 1998, Corder et al 1992, Csendes et al 1998, Fiore et al 1997, Jones et al 1995, Huguier et al 1991, Mansberger et al 1988, Montariol et al 1995, Murison et al 1993, Silverstein et al 1998, Trondsen et al 1998, Wright & Wellwood 1998). Indeed false positive cholangiography does potentially expose the patient to the 9.8% morbidity and 0.4% mortality of subsequent endoscopic sphincterotomy. Additionally, several authors do not believe operative cholangiography decreases the incidence or increases detection of bile duct injury (Barkun et al 1993, Jones et al 1995, Wright & Wellwood 1998). However, there is no reported case of bile duct injury or complication secondary to operative cholangiography. The extra-operative time for digital fluorocholangiography is short. Average cholangiography time ranges from 3 to 15 minutes (average 5.5 minutes) (Berci et al 1991, Lezoche et al 1994). The added cost of routine cholangiography is $299.50 (Flowers et al 1992) to $737.00 (Ladocsi et al 1997, Soper & Dunnegan 1992). Carroll et al (1998) reviewed 46 cases which came to litigation after bile duct injury during laparoscopic cholecystectomy and found the average award to be $214,000 (US). Thus the prevention of a single bile duct injury pays for a large number of cholangiographies (Shea et al 1996). Many formulae have been devised to determine which patients need selective cholangiography (Barkun et al 1993, Bogokowsky et al 1987, Corder et al 1992, Csendes et al 1998, Fiore et al 1997, Huguier et al 1991, Mansberger et al 1988, Trondsen et al 1998) including the use of a back-propagation neural network program (BrainMaker Professional; California Scientific Software, Nevada City, LA), (Golub et al 1998). Using selective cholangiography in 253 patients submitted to laparoscopic cholecystectomy, Braghetto et al (1998) found 96.8% of patients were free from symptoms and had normal liver function tests with at least a 4-year follow-up. Jaundice and/or abnormal tests appeared in 3.2% of patients, and retained stones could be demonstrated in 2.3%. Murison et al (1993) followed 285 patients who did not have routine cholangiography at open cholecystectomy and predicted that 12% should have had unsuspected retained stones. No patient developed a single symptomatic retained bile duct stone over a 3-year period. However, in a group of patients who had cholangiography, there was an 86% positive bile duct exploration rate, whereas in the selective group there was only a 44% positive rate. One might reason that all of the patients would have been better served if all had undergone mandatory cholangiography.

How the surgeon employs operative cholangiography depends on the use of pre- and postoperative endoscopic retrograde cholangiopancreatography (ERCP) and laparoscopic bile duct exploration. Stuart et al (1998) report the management plan and results of routine laparoscopic cholangiography in Fig. 22.3. Preoperative ERCP results in 80 to 85% of normal and unnecessary studies (Hunter & Soper 1992). Traverso et al (1994) were unable to use preoperative indicators of common duct stones to predict the need for selective cholangiography or preoperative ERCP. There is debate as to whether preoperative or postoperative

ERCP is preferable in the context of laparoscopic cholecystectomy (Rhodes et al 1998, Prat et al 1998). Davis et al (1997) report that endoscopists in academic institutions performed a significantly higher proportion of postoperative procedures than were performed in community hospitals. Our preference is to use postoperative ERCP after laparoscopic cholecystectomy unless common duct stones have been imaged preoperatively, the patient has cholangitis, the plan is to leave the gallbladder in situ, or the patient has severe, unrelenting gallstone pancreatitis all indicating the need for preoperative study.

Laparoscopic common bile duct exploration is more difficult to perform than laparoscopic cholecystectomy, and the extent of its use by the average biliary surgeon remains to be seen. However, if laparoscopic common bile duct explo-

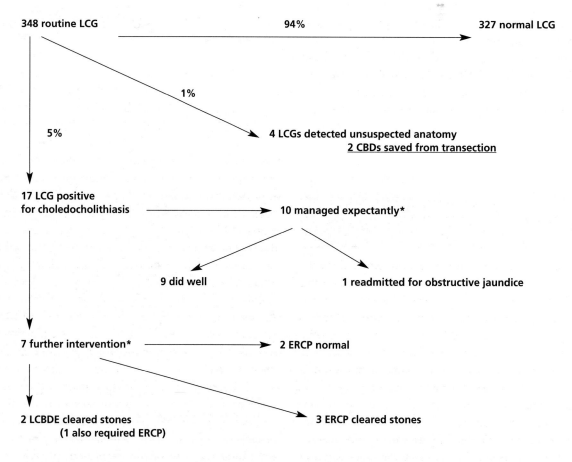

Fig. 22.3 Routine intraoperative laparoscopic cholangiography in 348 patients without preoperative evidence of choledocholithiasis. LCG, laparoscopic cholangiography; CBD, common bile duct; ERCP, endoscopic retrograde cholangiopancreatography; LCBDE, laparoscopic common bile duct exploration; *, at the discretion of the surgeon. (Adapted with permission from The American Journal of Surgery.)

ration is planned, operative cholangiography is a fundamental requirement and is preferable to laparoscopic ultrasound. The success rate of laparoscopic common bile duct exploration ranges from 68.8% (Berthou et al 1998) to 80% (Ferguson 1998). In a randomized trial comparing laparoscopic common bile duct exploration and postoperative ERCP both were found to be equally effective in clearing the bile duct of stones (Rhodes et al 1998). The patients having laparoscopic bile duct exploration had a significantly shorter hospital stay.

Endoscopic ultrasound has been proposed as an acceptable alternative to intraoperative cholangiography and preoperative ERCP (Canto et al 1998, Montariol et al 1998, Sahai et al 1999) but there is little evidence to strongly recommend it over other choices. *Intraoperative laparoscopic ultrasound* has had more surgical supporters (Birth et al 1998, Catheline et al 1998, Rothlin et al 1994, Siperstein et al 1999, Thompson et al 1998, Wu et al 1998, Soper 1998). Shorter examination time and lower cost are the suggested advantages of intraoperate ultrasound over operative cholangiography. There is doubt as to the cost advantage and, in addition, it is uncertain that laparoscopic ultrasound can match the potential fluorocholangiography has in identifying anomalous anatomy and bile duct injuries. Finally, reviewing the studies of bile duct repair (Woods et al 1994) and litigation (Carroll et al 1998) after laparoscopic cholecystectomy it is clear that not all surgeons can master the technique of cholangiography let alone laparoscopic ultrasound.

TECHNIOUES OF OPERATIVE CHOLANGIOGRAPHY

The instruments used are shown in Figure 22.4. Six techniques are used: (1) cystic duct cholangiography during laparoscopic cholecystectomy; (2) cystic duct cholangiography during open cholecystectomy; (3) cholecystocholangiography when the gallbladder is present and may be preserved; (4) common duct cholangiography when the gallbladder is absent, or when the common bile duct is dilated and appears to be the major site of disease; (5) transhepatic cholangiography when the anatomy of the extrahepatic bile duct is unclear or distorted from multiple previous operations on the bile ducts; and (6) post-exploration T-tube cholangiography performed after exploration of the common bile duct prior to terminating the operation. The techniques, indications, and advantages of these methods will be discussed individually.

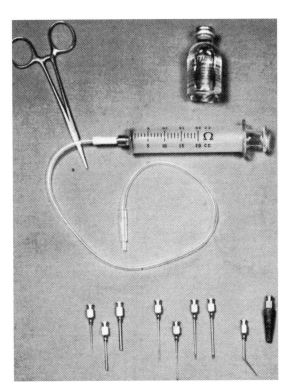

Fig. 22.4 Instruments used for operative cholangiography include a selection of blunt-tip needles, polyethylene tubing, a 20-ml syringe and a vial of contrast material (Renograffin-60).

LAPAROSCOPIC CYSTIC DUCT CHOLANGIOGRAPHY (see also Ch. 38)

Cholangiography is one of the most important aspects of laparoscopic operation on the gallbladder or bile ducts. Our approach is supported by Hugh et al (1997). The operation begins with dissection of the cystic duct. Our technique is illustrated (see also Ch. 38) from the beginning of the dissection. The visceral peritoneum along the right lateral-inferior side of the gallbladder is divided at the liver–gallbladder interface (Fig. 22.5). This is the 'safe side' of the gallbladder. By opening the visceral peritoneum in this area, the surgeon should be able to delineate the junction of the gallbladder and cystic duct. No duct is clipped or divided until the gallbladder–cystic duct junction is identified. Approximately 1 cm of cystic duct is dissected, providing adequate length to open the duct, insert a cholangiography catheter, and place two clips distal to the opening at the completion of cholangiography (Fig. 22.6). A large clip is placed on the base of the gallbladder (Fig. 22.7). Placing the clip at the base of the gallbladder provides maximum length of the cystic duct. No attempt is made to identify the proximal cystic duct and the junction of the cystic and common bile ducts. A small opening is made in the distal cystic duct (Fig. 22.8). The scissors are inserted into the opening, and the cystic duct is cut in order to provide an easy target for insertion of the cholangiography catheter (Fig. 22.9). The catheter can be used through any port, or a separate needle can be passed through the abdominal wall (Figs 22.10 and 22.11).

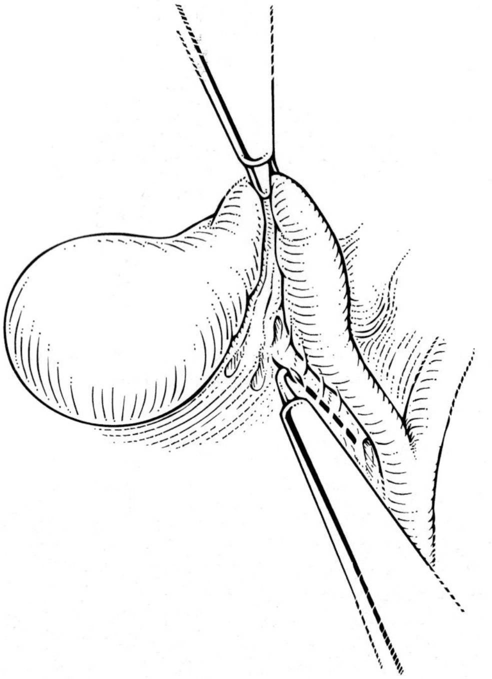

Digital fluoroscopy is particularly useful for laparoscopic cholangiography. It allows equipment on the operating field to be repositioned to provide an unobstructed view of the entire biliary system. Spot hard copy films are taken to document the findings (Fig. 22.12). Contrast medium is observed as it enters the duodenum through the sphincter of Oddi. Bruhn et al (1991) found that the results of routine operative cholangiography during laparoscopic cholecystectomy changed the course of operation in 10% of patients. For this reason, dissection of the cystic duct back to the common bile duct should not be attempted.

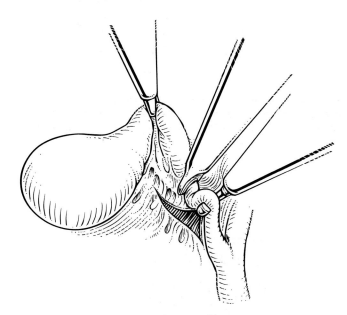

Fig. 22.5 Hook cautery is used to divide visceral peritoneum at the liver–gallbladder interface.

Fig. 22.7 A large clip is placed across the base of the gallbladder to prevent spillage of bile and/or gallstones when the cystic duct is opened.

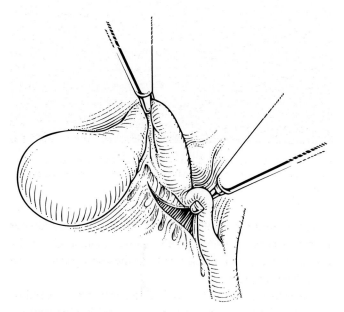

Fig. 22.6 The plane dissection has been established and dissection performed, allowing identification of the base of the gallbladder and the insertion of the cystic duct.

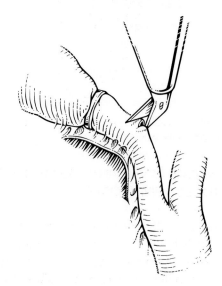

Fig. 22.8 A small opening in the cystic duct is made.

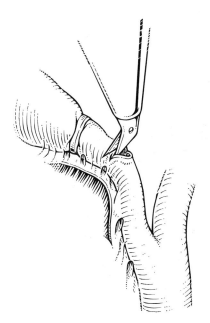

Fig. 22.9 The scissors enlarge this opening along the wall of the cystic duct which will be most accessible to the surgeon trying to thread a cholangiography catheter into the duct and through the valves of Heister.

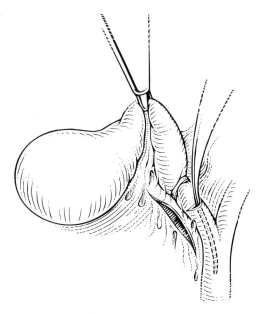

Fig. 22.11 The cholangiography catheter is threaded into the common bile duct, a step which minimizes leakage of contrast material from the unsecured opening in the cystic duct.

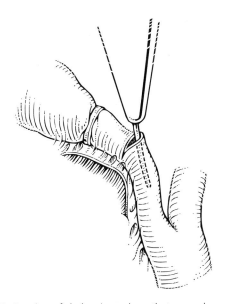

Fig. 22.10 A variety of cholangiography catheters can be used, depending on the surgeon's preference.

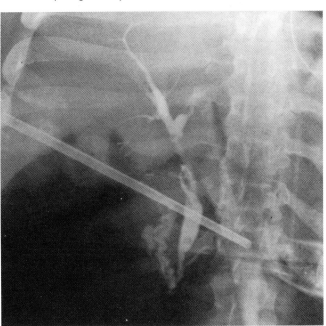

Fig. 22.12 A spot film taken during laparoscopic cholecystectomy showing an unsuspected common bile duct stone in a non-dilated bile duct.

CHOLANGIOGRAPHY VIA THE CYSTIC DUCT AT OPEN CHOLECYSTECTOMY

After the gallbladder is dissected from the liver bed, the cystic duct is identified. No attempt is made to dissect the cystic duct to its origin from the common duct. Any stones in the cystic duct are milked back into the gallbladder, and the neck of the gallbladder is ligated. Another ligature is placed around the distal cystic duct and left untied and later used to secure the catheter. Alternatively, cholangiography clamps or a clip can be used to hold the appropriate needle or catheter in place.

The instruments used in cholangiography are prepared by the surgical nurse; 15 ml of Renograffin-60 (iodine concentration of 29%) at room temperature is drawn into a 20 ml syringe attached to a short length of polyethylene tubing and a blunt 18 gauge needle. Care is taken to remove all air bubbles from the system. Room temperature contrast material should be used. The cystic duct is then opened, and the blunt 18 gauge needle attached to the syringe and tubing is inserted into the duct (Fig. 22.13). The distal ligature, clamp, or clip is secured around the duct and needle to keep them in place. Bile is gently aspirated into the tubing to confirm the position of the needle in the bile duct, and to aspirate any air from the system. The radiographic field is cleared of radiopaque material and equipment, but the retractor and drapes are not removed (retractors used during open operations on the biliary system are purposely placed so that they do not obstruct the radiographic visualization of the biliary system).

Renograffin-60 (15 ml) is used for the operative cholangiography (Figs 22.14 and 22.15). Approximately 3 ml is used for the initial injection, and a roentgenogram is taken. An additional 10–12 ml is used for the second injection, and a second roentgenogram is obtained. While awaiting development of the films, which takes approximately 10 minutes, the needle and tubing are removed from the cystic duct. Should a digital fluoroscope be available, fluorocholangiography is performed in a manner identical to the laparoscopic

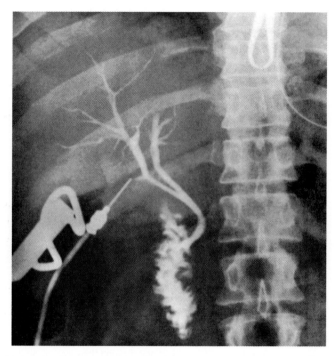

Fig. 22.14 Operative cholangiography showing a significant and dangerous anomaly of the biliary system; the cystic duct inserts into the main right hepatic duct.

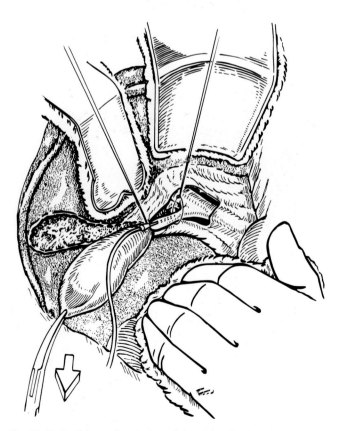

Fig. 22.13 Technique of cystic duct cholangiography.

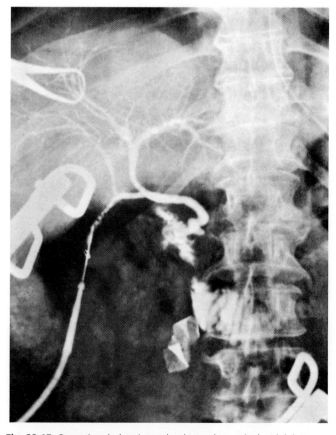

Fig. 22.15 Operative cholangiography shows the cystic duct joining a sectoral right hepatic duct.

situation. The cystic duct is ligated and divided, and the gallbladder removed.

Cystic duct cholangiography should be performed during cholecystectomy as a routine in all cases. This includes patients with acute (Fenton et al 1989) and chronic cholecystitis as well as those with jaundice or palpable stones in the common bile duct in whom a bile duct exploration is indicated.

CHOLECYSTOCHOLANGIOGRAPHY

Cholecystocholangiography is only possible when the cystic duct is patent. The surgeon may wish to preserve the gallbladder or cannot easily access the cystic duct due to inflammation or neoplasm. Indications for this technique include the adult patient with biliary tract obstruction in whom it is desirable to determine the level of obstruction or the baby with neonatal jaundice explored for the possibility of biliary atresia. A cholecystocholangiography may display the presence or absence of bile ducts.

The technique requires the placement of a purse-string suture at the fundus of the gallbladder. A 15–18 gauge needle is used to puncture the gallbladder through the purse-string suture, and the gallbladder is emptied of bile (Fig. 22.16).

Approximately 15–20 ml of Renograffin-60 is instilled into the gallbladder, the needle and syringe are withdrawn, and the purse-string suture is tied. With traction on the purse-string suture, the surgeon then squeezes the contrast material out of the gallbladder and into the biliary system. Two cholangiographs are obtained or fluorocholangiography is performed.

This technique provides visualization of the biliary system and demonstrates anatomy, but is less accurate than cystic duct cholangiography in the identification of small stones or other subtle pathology. It is important to express as much of the contrast medium out of the gallbladder as possible prior to obtaining the cholangiography. Retention of a large amount of contrast material in the gallbladder may obscure detail if the contrast-filled gallbladder overlies any segment of the biliary system.

COMMON DUCT CHOLANGIOGRAPHY

An operative cholangiography may be obtained directly through the wall of the common bile duct if the gallbladder has been removed previously, or if the common bile duct is dilated and appears to be the primary site of disease. A small 21 or 23 gauge needle, such as a scalp vein butterfly needle, attached to a segment of tubing and a 20 ml syringe is inserted into the common bile duct. Occasionally, bending the needle slightly aids insertion into the duct (Fig 22.17).

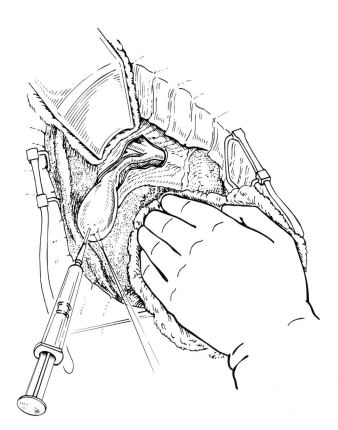

Fig. 22.16 Technique of cholecystocholangiography.

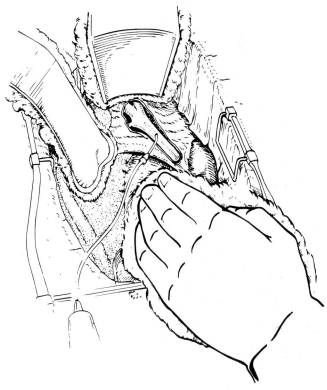

Fig. 22.17 Technique of common duct cholangiography.

Bile is aspirated to be certain of needle placement and to remove any air in the system. After removal of air bubbles, 10–15 ml of contrast material is gently introduced into the bile duct. Two radiographs are taken, one after the installation of approximately 3–4 ml, and the second after the instillation of the remainder of the contrast material. Alternatively fluorocholangiography is performed.

We obtain bile duct cholangiography prior to exploration of the common bile duct for stones if satisfactory preoperative direct cholangiography is not available. This pre-exploration cholangiography helps to define the location and number of stones in the bile ducts (Figs 22.18 and 22.19). When a satisfactory preoperative percutaneous transhepatic cholangiography or endoscopic retrograde cholangiography has been performed, we proceed directly to a common bile duct exploration.

TRANSHEPATIC CHOLANGIOGRAPHY

In the patient who has had multiple previous operations, especially when the anatomy or location of the bile duct is

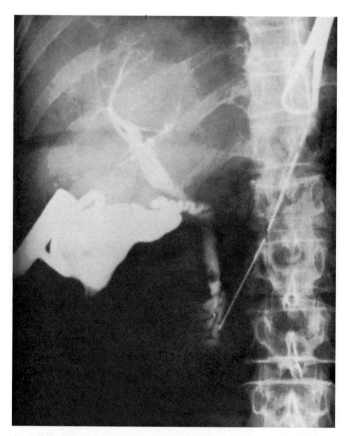

Fig. 22.19 Cholecystocholangiography showing a solitary stone in the non-dilated common bile duct.

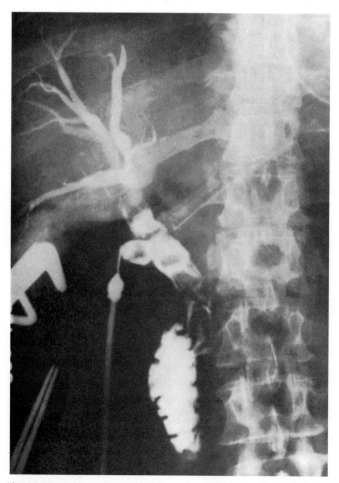

Fig. 22.18 Common duct cholangiography shows multiple stones in the common bile duct.

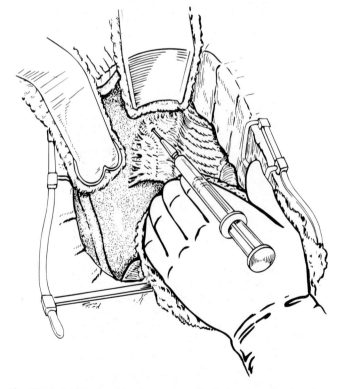

Fig. 22.20 Artist's drawing of a transhepatic cholangiography, inserting the needle into the hilar area of the liver. The extrahepatic anatomy is scarred from multiple previous operations to correct a bile duct stricture.

unclear to the surgeon, a direct needle puncture of the intrahepatic bile ducts is an option (Fig. 22.20). An example is the patient with a recurrent stricture of the bile duct who has had multiple previous operations. Ideally, preoperative percutaneous transhepatic cholangiography is performed to identify the stricture and dilated proximal bile ducts. In spite of this information, however, it may be diffi-

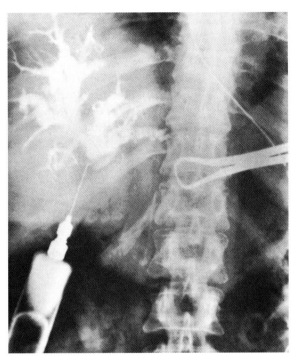

Fig. 22.21 Transhepatic cholangiography performed to identify and locate an obstructed bile duct (stricture).

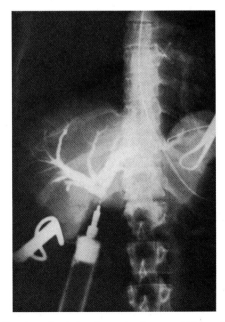

Fig. 22.22 Transhepatic cholangiography shows a stricture of the bile duct .

cult to find the biliary system at operation. At this time, a direct needle puncture of the liver may be performed to opacify the intrahepatic bile ducts.

A 21-gauge needle, directly attached to a 20 ml syringe, is used. After aspiration of bile, approximately 10 ml of contrast material are injected. The major value of this technique is the opacification of the intrahepatic biliary system (Figs 22.21 and 22.22). This method may also be used in the definition of intrahepatic ductal anatomy during surgery for hilar cholangiocarcinoma.

POSTEXPLORATION T-TUBE CHOLANGIOGRAPHY

After exploration of the common bile duct, a T-tube is usually placed in the bile duct to provide access to the biliary system for postexploration cholangiography and stone retrieval. An 18-Fr T-tube is employed in most patients so that postoperative extraction of any retained stones through the matured T-tube tract is possible (see Chs 41, 45).

Completion, postexploration cholangiography should be obtained while the patient is under anesthesia and before the abdominal incision is closed. If any stones have been overlooked, their identification allows removal before the operative procedure is terminated. Cholangiography also helps ensure that the T-tube has been properly placed and positioned. We perform T-tube cholangiography in all patients at 1 week following common bile duct exploration. A final T-tube cholangiograph may be obtained prior to hospital discharge. The T-tube is removed at follow-up 2–3 weeks later.

It has been shown in a number of surgical studies that T-tube cholangiography is more accurate than common bile duct exploration alone (Hicken & McAllister 1964, Mullen et al 1971, Way et al 1972, McCormick et al 1974, see Ch. 55). That is, stones have been identified on the postexploration T-tube cholangiography that were not seen by the surgeon during open common bile duct exploration (Fig. 22.23). Completion T-tube cholangiography reduces the likelihood of finding a residual stone on a later postoperative T-tube cholangiography, from 30 to 7% (Way et al 1972). Hicken & McAllister (1964) similarly showed that completion T-tube cholangiography reduced the incidence of residual bile duct stones from 11 to 4%. Excellent results have also been reported by LeQuesne and Bolton (1980). It is suggested that *operative choledochoscopy* can reduce the incidence of retained bile duct stones to 2% or less (Escat et al 1984) (vide infra).

Our technique of completion T-tube cholangiography is

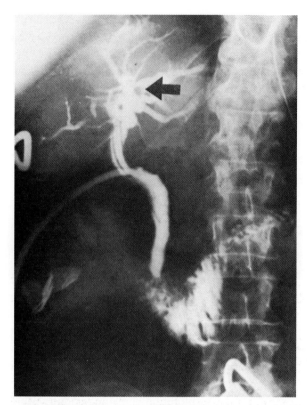

Fig. 22.23 Postexploration T-tube cholangiography identifies a residual stone in the intrahepatic bile ducts, missed during operative exploration of the bile duct.

to fill the right upper quadrant with saline solution. Saline is then used to irrigate and remove all of the air from the biliary system. A 20 ml syringe is attached directly to the T-tube. Two cholangiographs are obtained one after the instillation of approximately 5 ml of contrast medium and the second after the instillation of an additional 10 ml. Alternatively, fluorocholangiography is performed. The most common abnormal finding is sphincter spasm with no contrast material entering the duodenum. If the distal bile duct tapers smoothly, no stone deformity is seen, and the patient has had normal exploration of the distal bile duct, we disregard this spasm. If, however, there is any concern that there may be an organic obstruction, glucagon can be given intravenously. This will relax sphincter spasm, and permit a second injection. The best way to avoid these problems is to use fluorocholangiography, which will provide a dynamic view of the biliary system.

Other techniques of postexploratory cholangiography using a balloon catheter prior to insertion of the T-tube have been shown to be extremely effective (Myat et al 1973).

INTERPRETATION OF CHOLANGIOGRAPHY

Interpretation of intraoperative cholangiogram is extremely important and is usually and best performed by the surgeon. High-quality films must be obtained. It is important to position the patient in such a way that the common bile duct is to the right of and does not overlie the lumbar spine. For the most part, this can be accomplished simply by positioning the patient supine. An advantage of fluorocholangiography is the ability to move the C arm into any plane for added visualization. Undiluted contrast material is used, being careful not to inject too much of the agent initially and obscure small stones. The injection rate should be slow in order to avoid turbulence since a rapidly moving small stone may not be visible. The entire biliary system, including the intrahepatic and extrahepatic bile ducts and the flow of contrast material into the duodenum should be demonstrated. Extravasation of contrast may indicate bile duct injury. Some surgeons do not secure the cystic duct during laparoscopic fluorocholangiography, and extravasation is common. The total time involved in obtaining the cholangiography should be less than 10 minutes. It can be accomplished more rapidly using fluorocholangiography, and hard copy films should be made.

LeQuesne (1960) presented guidelines for the interpretation of cholangiography that are still important today. The normal duct should be no larger than 12 mm in size; contrast media must flow freely into the duodenum; at least one film should show the distal bile duct with its characteristic notch and the wider proximal duct; no filling defects should be present; and the hepatic ducts should be seen, but not overfilled. Visualization of the pancreatic duct is of no significance.

If high-quality cholangiography are not obtained, the value of the procedure is negated. Air bubbles, leakage of contrast material from the needle, over- or underpenetration, or other problems of technique lessen the value of intraoperative cholangiography (Hall et al 1973). These considerations imply that the surgeon, the nurse who prepares the equipment, and the radiology team all require frequent practice in performing intraoperative cholangiography. When operative cholangiography is performed routinely, optimal conditions for excellent cholangiography are obtained. When it is performed infrequently or selectively, a greater chance for poor-quality studies exists.

At one time, intraoperative cholangiography and intraoperative manometric studies of the biliary system were combined (Mallet-Guy 1952, Daniel 1972, McCarthy 1977, White & Bordley 1978) but are no longer thought to be of value.

Intraoperative choledochoscopy (see Ch. 23) is a valuable adjunct or alternative to intraoperative cholangiography (Schein et al 1963, Berci et al 1978, Keighley & Kappas 1980, King & String 1983, Escat et al 1984). We use it frequently to aid in stone detection and in the identification of bile duct changes seen on intraoperative cholangiography.

OPERATIVE FLUOROSCOPY AND CHOLANGIOGRAPHY

Berci et al (1978) have been strong advocates of operative fluoroscopy and cholangiography and report that the addition of fluoroscopy has reduced the incidence of retained stones to 1%. A portable high resolution digital-C arm with the capacity to take hard copy operative cholangiography is necessary; four to six films are obtained in addition to real-time fluoroscopy. Multiple views of the biliary system are possible by moving the C arm and changing the plane of projection. The average time for a study is no longer than 5 minutes. The rate and amount of contrast material injected can be optimized under real-time fluoroscopy. Fluoroscopy is also a valuable tool for analyzing and observing sphincter function. The sphincter may relax sporadically, and fluoroscopy is more likely to detect emptying of contrast medium into the duodenum.

Feeley and Peel (1982) have demonstrated a wide variation in biliary system volumes and emphasize the importance of observing early filling of the bile duct. The importance of early filling decreased as duct size increased. In 34 out of 41 patients whose bile ducts were filled by 2.9 ml or less of contrast material, the first film was the most important one diagnostically. Of 66 patients having ductal volumes greater than 10 ml, the first film was diagnostic in only seven.

RESULTS

We have now performed intraoperative cholangiography in more than 10 000 patients during the past 35 years. Our experience continues to be favorable. Routine use of the technique ensures that all patients are placed on an operating table equipped for intraoperative radiology, radiology technicians are available in the operating room, the nurses are prepared with instruments ready, and the surgical team gains daily experience with technique.

The complication rate for operative cholangiography should be nil. In our series there is not a single technique

related problem. More specifically, no instances of pancreatitis, cholangitis, or sepsis could be related to the procedure. In patients with a known allergy to iodinated contrast material, operative cholangiography has been safe, and no allergic reactions have been seen.

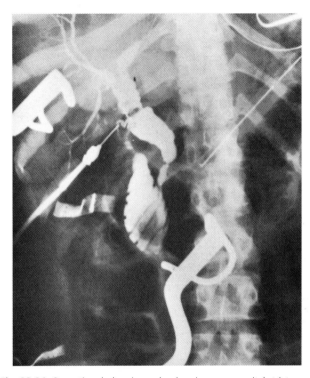

Fig. 22.24 Operative cholangiography showing a congenital stricture of the distal bile duct. Stones are present in the bile duct.

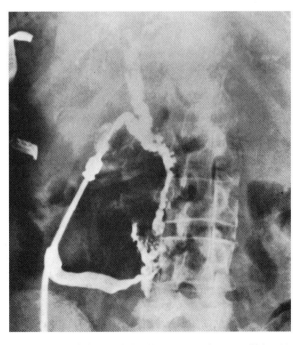

Fig. 22.25 Operative cholangiography showing sclerosing cholangitis, unsuspected preoperatively.

The overall incidence of unsuspected pathology, predominantly unsuspected stones in the bile duct, is 7% (Broughan & Hermann 1992). The pathology encountered, other than stones, included unsuspected strictures of the bile duct (Fig 22.24), inflammatory changes such as sclerosing cholangitis (Fig 22.25), congenital anomalies (Fig 22.26), and tumors of the biliary system (Fig 22.27). Intraoperative cholangiography proved to be the most valuable indication for exploration of the common duct. The incidence of false-positive cholangiography with resultant unnecessary bile duct exploration has been less than 2%. The incidence of false-negative cholangiography (difficult to ascertain) is about 2%. We believe the routine use of this procedure has

reduced the incidence of retained bile duct stones to less than 2% (Broughan et al 1985).

Operative cholangiography may suggest stenosis of the sphincter of Oddi, identify distal stones (Fig. 22.28), and contribute information of value as an indication for chole-

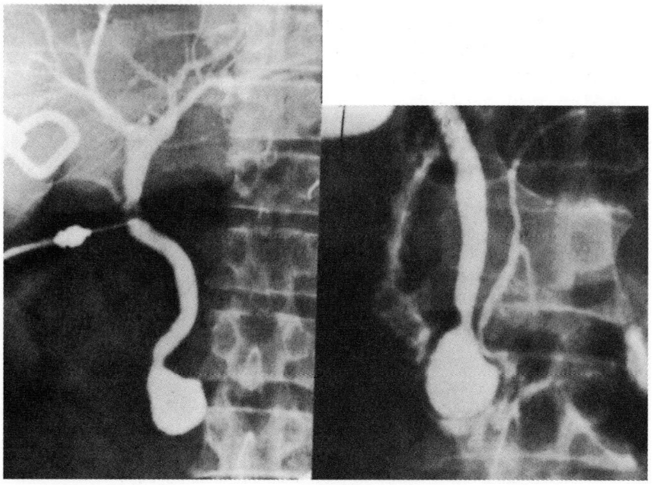

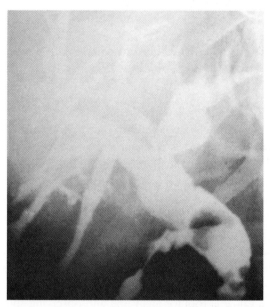

Fig. 22.28 Cystic duct cholangiography showing a dilated bile duct with multiple stones and moderate stenosis of the distal bile duct. Because of the distal duct stenosis, a choledochoduodenostomy was performed after common bile duct exploration.

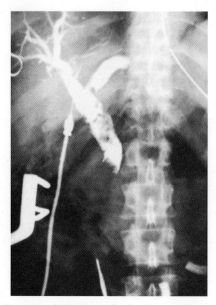

Fig. 22.26 Cystic duct cholangiography showing a choledochal cyst (choledochocele) of the distal bile duct, unsuspected by the surgeon.

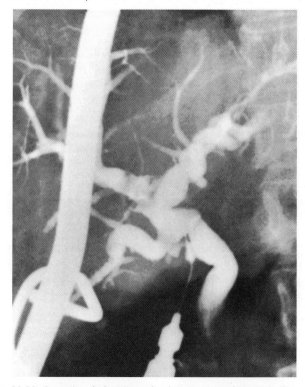

Fig. 22.27 Operative cholangiography showing an abrupt obstruction of the distal bile duct. A soft, villous tumor of the distal bile duct was found.

Fig. 22.29 Operative cholangiography showing several stones in the intrahepatic bile ducts.

dochoduodenostomy or choledochojejunostomy. Finally, in patients with intrahepatic duct changes or intrahepatic bile duct stones (Fig 22.29), operative cholangiography has led to the occasional transhepatic bile duct exploration or to liver resection for intrahepatic cystic dilation or stones.

REFERENCES

Acosta J M, Ledesma C L 1974 Gallstone migration as a cause of acute pancreatitis. New England Journal of Medicine 290(9): 484–487

Appleman R M, Priestley J T, Gage R P 1964 Cholelithiasis and choledocholithiasis: factors that influence relative incidence. Mayo Clinic Proceedings 39: 473–478

Bagnato V J, McGee G E, Hatten L E, et al 1991 Justification for routine cholangiography during laparoscopic cholecystectomy. Surgical Laparoscopy and Endoscopy 2: 89–93

Barkun J S, Fried G M, Barkun A N, et al 1993 Cholecystectomy without operative cholangiography. Annals of Surgery 218: 371–379

Baron R L 1997 Diagnosing choledocholithiasis: how far can we push helical CT? Radiology 203: 601–603

Bartlett M D, Waddell 1958 Indications for common duct exploration: evaluation in 1000 cases. New England Journal of Medicine 258: 164–167.

Berci G 1992 Biliary ductal anatomy and anomalies. Surgical Clinics of North America 72: 1069–1075

Berci G 1998 Complications of laparoscopic cholecystectomy. Surgical Endoscopy 12: 291–293

Berci G, Hamlin J A, Morgenstern L, Fisher D L 1978 Modern operative fluorocholangiography: utopia or overlooked entity? Gastrointestinal Radiology 3: 401–406

Berci G, Sackier J, Paz-Partlow M 1991 Routine or selected intraoperative cholangiography during laparoscopic cholecystectomy? American Journal of Surgery 161: 355–360

Berthou J C, Drouard F, Charbonneau P, et al 1998 Evaluation of laparoscopic management of common bile duct stones in 220 patients. Surgical Endoscopy 12: 16–22

Birth M, Ehlers K U, Delinikolas K, Weiser H F 1998 Prospective randomized comparison of laparoscopic ultrasonography using a flexible-tip ultrasound probe and intraoperative dynamic cholangiography during laparoscopic cholecystectomy. Surgical Endoscopy 12: 30–36

Bogokowsky H, Slutzki S, Zaidenstein L, et al 1987 Selective operative cholangiography. Surgery, Gynecology and Obstetrics 164: 124–126

Braghetto I, Debandi A, Korn O, Bastias J 1998 Long-term follow-up after laparoscopic cholecystectomy without routine intraoperative cholangiography. Surgical Laparoscopy & Endoscopy 8: 349–352

Broughan T A, Hermann R E 1992 Unpublished data

Broughan T A, Sivak M W, Hermann R E 1985 The management of retained and recurrent bile duct stones. Surgery 98: 746–750

Bruhn E W, Miller F J, Hunter J G 1991 Routine fluoroscopic cholangiography during laparoscopic cholecystectomy: an argument. Surgical Endoscopy 5: 111–115

Canto M I, Chak A, Stellato T, Sivak M V 1998 Endoscopic ultrasonography versus cholangiography for the diagnosis of choledocholithiasis. Gastrointestinal Endoscopy 47: 439–448

Carroll B J, Birth M, Phillips E H 1998 Common bile duct injuries during laparoscopic cholecystectomy that result in litigation. Surgical Endoscopy 12: 310–313

Catheline J M, Turner R, Rizk N, Barratt Christophe, Buenos P, and Champault G 1998 Evaluation of the biliary tree during laparoscopic cholecystectomy. Surgical Laparoscopy and Endoscopy 8: 85–91

Corbitt J D, Cantwell D V 1991 Laparoscopic cholecystectomy with operative cholangiogram. Surgical Laparoscopy and Endoscopy 1: 229–232

Corbitt J D, Leonetti L A 1997 One thousand and six consecutive laparoscopic intraoperative cholangiograms. Journal of Soc Laparoendosc Surg 1: 13–16

Corder A P, Scott S D, Johnson C D 1992 Place of routine operative cholangiography at cholecystectomy. British Journal of Surgery 79: 945–947

Cotton P B 1997 Comment. Do asymptomatic bile duct stones need to be removed? Gastrointestinal Endoscopy 46: 588–589

Csendes A, Burdiles P, Diaz JC et al 1998 Prevalence of common bile duct stones according to the increasing number of risk factors present: a prospective study employing routinely intraoperative cholangiography in 477 cases. Hepato-Gastroenterology 45: 1415–1421

Daniel O 1972 The value of radiomanometry in bile duct surgery. Annals of the Royal College of Surgeons of England 51: 357–372

Davis W, Cotton P B, Arias R, et al 1997 ERCP and sphincterotomy in the context of laparoscopic cholecystectomy: academic and community practice patterns and results. American Journal of Gastroenterology 92: 597–601

Diehl A K, Holleman D R, Chapman J B, et al 1997 Gallstone size and risk of pancreatitis. Archives of Internal Medicine 157: 1674–1678

Dwerryhouse SJ, Brown E, Vipond MN 1998 Prospective evaluation of magnetic resonance cholangiography to detect common bile duct stones before laparoscopic cholecystectomy. British Journal of Surgery 85: 1364–1366

Escat J, Glucksman DL, Maigne C, Fourtainer G, Fournier D, Vaislic C 1984 Choledochoscopy in surgery for choledocholithiasis: six-year experience in three hundred eighty consecutive patients. American Journal of Surgery 147: 670–671

Feeley M, Peel AL 1982 A critical assessment of fluoroscopy in preoperative cholangiography. Annals of the Royal College of Surgeons of England 64: 180–182

Fenton AH, Guyton DP, Evans DM 1989 The utility of intraoperative cholangiography with acute cholecystitis. American Surgeon 55: 392–395

Ferguson CM, 1998 Laparoscopic common bile duct exploration. Archives of Surgery 133: 448–451

Fiore NF, Ledniczky G, Wiebke E, et al 1997 An analysis of perioperative cholangiography in one thousand laparoscopic cholecystectomies. Surgery 122: 817–821

Flowers JL, Zucker KA, Graham SM, et al 1992 Laparoscopic cholangiography. Annals of Surgery 215: 209–216

Freeman ML, Nelson DB, Sherman S, et al 1996 Complications of endoscopic biliary sphincterotomy. New England Journal of Medicine 335: 909–918

Glenn F 1952 Common duct exploration for stones. Surgery, Gynecology and Obstetrics 95: 431–438

Golub R, Cantu R, Tan M 1998 The prediction of common bile duct stones using a neural network. Journal of the American College of Surgeons 187: 584–590

Gregg R O 1988 The case for selective cholangiography. American Journal of Surgery 155: 540–545

Hall R C, Sakiyalak P, Kim S K, Rogers L S, Webb W R 1973 Failure of operative cholangiography to prevent retained common duct stones. American Journal of Surgery 125: 51–63

Handy J E, Rose S C, Nieves A S, Johnson R L, Hunter J G, Miller F J 1991 Intraoperative cholangiography: use of portable fluoroscopy and transmitted images. Radiology 181: 105–107

Hayes M A, Goldenberg I S, Bishop C C 1958 The developmental basis for bile duct anomalies. Surgery, Gynecology and Obstetrics 107: 447–456

Hermann R E 1983 Common bile duct stone. In: Moody F G (ed) Advances in diagnosis and surgical treatment of biliary tract disease. Masson, New York, p 69–78

Hicken N F, McAllister A J 1964 Operative cholangiography as an aid in reducing the incidence of 'overlooked' common bile duct stones: a study of 1293 choledocholithotomies. Surgery 55: 753–758

Hugh T B, Kelly M D, Mekisic 1997 Rouviere's sulcus: a useful landmark in laparoscopic cholecystectomy. British Journal of Surgery 84: 1253–1254

Huguier M, Bornet P, Charpak Y, et al 1991 Selective contraindications based on multivariate analysis for operative cholangiography in biliary lithiasis. Surgery, Gynecology and Obstetrics 172: 470–474

Hunter JG 1991 Avoidance of bile duct injury during laparoscopic cholecystectomy. American Journal of Surgery 162: 71–76

Hunter J G, Soper N J 1992 Laparoscopic management of bile duct stones. Surgical Clinics of North America 72: 1077–1097

Isaacs J P, Daves M L 1960 Technique and evaluation of operative cholangiography. Surgery, Gynecology and Obstetrics 111: 103–112

Johnson A G, Hosking S W 1987 Appraisal of the management of bile duct stones. British Journal of Surgery 74: 555–560

Jones D B, Dunnegan D L, Soper N J 1995 Results of a change to routine fluorocholangiography during laparoscopic cholecystectomy. Surgery 118: 693–702

Keighley M R, Kappas A 1980 Evaluation of operative choledoscopy. Surgery, Gynecology and Obstetrics. 150: 357–359

Kelly T R 1976 Gallstone pancreatitis: pathophysiology. Surgery 80: 488–492

Khalili T M, Phillips E H, Berci G, et al 1997 Final score in laparoscopic cholecystectomy. Surgical Endoscopy 11: 1095–1098

King M L, String S T 1983 Extent of choledochoscopic utilization in common bile duct exploration. American Journal of Surgery 146: 322–324

Koo K P, Traverso L W 1996 Do preoperative indicators predict the presence of common bile duct stones during laparoscopic cholecystectomy? American Journal of Surgery 171: 495–499

Kullman E, Borch K, Lindstrom E, et al 1996 Management of bile duct stones in the era of laparoscopic cholecystectomy: appraisal of routine operative cholangiography and endoscopic treatment. European Journal of Surgery 162: 873–880

Ladocsi L T, Benitez L D, Filippone D R, et al 1997 Intraoperative cholangiography in laparoscopic cholecystectomy: a review of 734 consecutive cases. American Surgeon 63: 150–156

Leichtling J J, Rubin S, Breidenbach L 1959 The significance of in vivo measurement of the common bile duct. Surgery, Gynecology and Obstetrics 109: 773–777

LeQuesne L P 1960 Cholangiography. Proceedings of the Royal Society of Medicine 53: 852–855

LeQuesne L P, Bolton J P 1980 Choledocholithiasis incidence, diagnosis and operative procedures. In: Maingot R (ed) Abdominal operations, 7th edn. Appleton-Century-Crofts, New York, vol I, p 1055–1102

Lezoche E, Paganini A, Guerrieri M, et al 1994 Technique and results of routine dynamic cholangiography during 528 consecutive laparoscopic cholecystectomies. Surgical Endoscopy 8: 1443–1447

Lillemoe K D, Yeo C J, Talamini M A, Wang B H, Pitt H A, Gadacz T R 1992 Selective cholangiography: current role in laparoscopic cholecystectomy. Annals of Surgery 215(6): 669–676

Lomanto D, Pavone P, Laghi A, et al 1997 Magnetic resonance-cholangiopancreatography in the diagnosis of biliopancreatic diseases. American Journal of Surgery 174: 33–38

Mallet-Guy P 1952 Value of preoperative manometric and roentgenographic examination in the diagnosis of pathologic changes and functional disturbances of the biliary tract. Surgery, Gynecology and Obstetrics 94: 385–393

Mansberger J A, Davis J B, Scarborough C, et al 1988 Selective intraoperative cholangiography. American Surgeon 54: 31–33

McCarthy J D 1977 Radiomanometric guides to common bile duct exploration. American Journal of Surgery 134: 697–701

McCormick J S, Bremner D N, Thomson J W, McNair T J, Philp T 1974 The operative cholangiogram, its interpretation, accuracy and value in association with colecystectomy. Annals of Surgery 180: 902–906

McSherry C K, Glenn F 1980 The incidence and causes of death following surgery for nonmalignant biliary tract disease. Annals of Surgery 191: 271–275

Mendler M H, Bouillet P, Sautereau D, et al 1998 Value of MR cholangiography in the diagnosis of obstructive diseases of the biliary tree: a study of 58 cases. American Journal of Gastroenterology 93: 2482–2490

Mirizzi P L 1937 Operative cholangiography. Surgery, Gynecology and Obstetrics 65: 702–710

Mirizzi P L, La cholangiografia durante las operaciones de las vias biliares. 1932 Bol Soc Cir Buenos Aries 16: 1133–1135

Montariol T, Msika S, Charlier A, et al 1998 Diagnosis of asymptomatic common bile duct stones: preoperative endoscopic ultrasonography versus intraoperative cholangiography—a multicenter, prospective controlled study. Surgery 124: 6–13

Montariol T, Rey C, Charlier A, et al 1995 Preoperative evaluation of the probability of common bile duct stones. Journal of the American College of Surgeons 180: 293–296

Mullen J L, Rosato F E, Rosato E F, Miller W T, Sullivan M 1971 The diagnosis of choledocholithiasis. Surgery, Gynecology and Obstetrics 133: 774–778

Murison M S C, Gartell P C, McGinn F P 1993 Does selective perioperative cholangiography result in missed common bile duct stones? Journal of the Royal College of Surgeons of Edinburgh 38: 220–224

Myat Thu Ya, Robinson D, Gunn A A 1973 Preoperative cholangiography. British Journal of Surgery 60: 771–712

Pagana T J, Stahlgren L H 1980 Indications and accuracy of operative cholangiography. Archives of Surgery 115: 1214–1215

Prassopoulos P, Raptopoulos V, Chuttani R et al 1998 Development of virtual CT cholangiopancreatoscopy. Radiology 209: 570–574

Prat F, Amouyal G, Amouyal P, et al 1998 Laparoscopy versus endoscopy for bile-duct stones. Lancet 351: 984

Rantis P C, Greenlee H B, Pickleman J, et al 1993 Laparoscopic cholecystectomy bile duct injuries: more than meets the eye. American Surgeon 59: 533–540

Rhodes M, Sussman L, Cohen L, et al 1998 Laparoscopy versus endoscopy for bile-duct stones. Lancet 351: 984

Rhodes M, Sussman L, Coneh M P, et al 1998 Randomised trial of laparoscopic exploration of common bile duct versus postoperative endoscopic retrograde cholangiography for common bile duct stones. Lancet 351: 159–161

Rosenthal R J, Steigerwald S D, Imig R, et al 1994 Role of intraoperative cholangiography during endoscopic cholecystectomy. Surgical Laparoscopy and Endoscopy 4: 171–174

Rothlin M A, Schlumpf R, Lardiad'er Felix July 1994 Laparoscopic sonography: an alternative to routine intraoperative cholangiography? Archives of Surgery 129: 694–700

Sackier J M, Berci G, Phillips E, et al 1991 The role of cholangiography in laparoscopic cholecystectomy. Archives of Surgery 126: 1021–1026

Sahai A V, Mauldin P D, Marsi V et al 1999 Bile duct stones and laparoscopic cholecystectomy: a decision analysis to assess the roles of intraoperative cholangiography, EUS, and ERCP. Gastrointestinal Endoscopy 49: 334–343

Saypol G M 1961 Indications for choledochostomy in operations for cholelithiasis: analysis of 525 cases. Annals of Surgery 153: 567–574

Schein C J, Stern W Z, Hurwitt E S, Jacobson H G 1963 Cholangiography and biliary endoscopy as complementary methods of evaluation of the bile ducts. American Journal of Radiology 89: 864–874

Shea J A, Healey M J, Berlin J A, et al 1996 Annals of Surgery 224: 609–629

Shively E H, Wieman T J, Adams A L, et al 1990 Operative cholangiography. American Journal of Surgery 159: 380–384

Silverstein J C, Wavak E, Millikan K W 1998 A prospective experience with selective cholangiography. American Surgeon 64: 654–659

Siperstein A, Pearl J, Macho J, Hansen P, Gitomirski A, Rogers S 1999 Comparison of laparoscopic ultrasonography and fluorocholangiography in 300 patients undergoing laparoscopic cholecystectomy. Surgical Endoscopy 13: 113–117

Soper N J 1998 SSAT/SAGES Minimally invasive surgery symposium: advanced laparoscopic hepatobiliary surgery. Journal of Laparoendoscopic and Advanced Surgical Techniques 8: 169–183

Soper N J, Dunnegan D L 1992 Routine versus selective intra-operative cholangiography during laparoscopic cholecystectomy. World Journal of Surgery 16: 1133–1140

Stuart S A, Simpson T I G, Alvord L A, et al 1998 Routine intraoperative laparoscopic cholangiography. American Journal of Surgery 176: 632–637

Thompson D M, Arregui M E,Tetik C, Madden T, Wegener M 1998 A comparison of laparoscopic ultrasound with digital fluorocholangiography for detecting choledocholithiasis during laparoscopic cholecystectomy. Surgical Endoscopy 12: 929–932

Thurston O G, McDougall R M 1976 The effect of hepatic bile on retained common duct stones. Surgery, Gynecology and Obstetrics 143: 625–627

Traverso L W, Hauptmann E M, Lynge D C 1994 Routine intraoperative cholangiography and its contribution to the selective cholangiographer. American Journal of Surgery 167: 464–468

Trondsen E, Edwin B, Reiertsen O, Faerden A E, et al 1998 Prediction of common bile duct stones prior to cholecystectomy. Archives of Surgery 133: 162–166

Vecchio R, Macfadyen B V, Latteri S 1998 Laparoscopic cholecystectomy: an analysis on 114,005 cases of United States series. International Surgery 83: 215–219

Way L W, Admirand W H, Dunphy J E 1972 Bile duct injury during laparoscopic cholecystectomy without operative cholangiography. British Journal of Surgery 85: 191–194

Way L W, Admirand W H, Dunphy J E 1972 Management of choledocholithiasis. Annals of Surgery 176: 347–359

White T T, Bordley J I V 1978 One per cent incidence of recurrent gallstones six to eight years after manometric cholangiography. Annals of Surgery 188: 562–569

Woods M D, Traverso L W, Korzarek R A, et al 1994 Characteristics of biliary tract complications during laparoscopic cholecystectomy: A multi-institutional study. American Journal of Surgery 167: 27–33

Woods M S, Traverso L W, Kozarek R A, et al 1995 Biliary tract complications of laparoscopic cholecystectomy are detected more frequently with routine intraoperative cholangiography. Surgical Endoscopy 9: 1076–1080

Wright K D, Wellwood J M 1998 Bile duct injury during laparoscopic cholecystectomy without operative cholangiography. British Journal of Surgery 85: 191–194

Wu J S, Dunnegan D L, Soper N J 1998 Utility of intracorporeal ultrasonography for screening of the bile duct during laparoscopic cholecystectomy. Journal of Gastrointestinal Surgery 2: 50–60

Z'graggen K Z, Wehrli H, Metzger A, et al 1998 Complications of laparoscopic cholecystectomy in Switzerland. Surgical Endoscopy 12: 1303–1310

Choledochoscopy

23

G. BERCI

HISTORY

Seventy-five years ago, Bakes first recognized the fact that manipulation within a tubular organ, without direct vision is difficult and is accompanied by a high failure rate. He recommended an ear funnel with a mirror and a small electrical globe to allow inspection of the distal common bile duct (Bakes 1923). McIver (1941) suggested a cystoscope built in a right angle configuration with an electrical light bulb. He was unable to generate interest. In Europe, Wildegans popularized choledochoscopy by promoting an endoscope with a 60° angulation (Wildegans 1953). One of the major problems was the configuration of this instrument since manipulations were difficult in patients in whom the rib cage was near to the subcostal incision. The image was dim and optically substandard.

With the invention of the Hopkins-Rod lens system it was possible to design a small right-angled instrument (Fig. 23.1) with a better image quality and improved illumination. The first results were published 27 years ago (Shore et al 1971). It took many years until the concept and the instrument was accepted by the surgical community. The introduction of the flexible choledochoscope, (Yamakawa et al 1976) further facilitated endoscopy of the biliary tract (Fig. 23.2). Choledochoscopy introduced an important

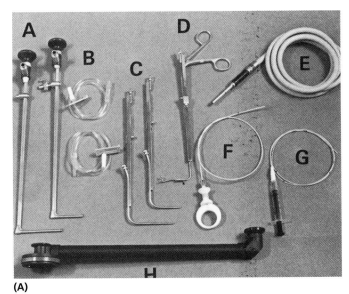

(A)

Fig. 23.1 (A) A Shorter and longer rigid choledochoscope: shorter horizontal length 40 mm; longer limb 60 mm. B Two venous extension tubes. C Instrument guide channel. D Biopsy forceps. E Fiber-optic light guide. F Dormia stone basket to be introduced through the instrument guide channel which is attached to the telescope. G A 4-French balloon catheter to be introduced to the same C instrument guide channel. H A teaching attachment which can be gas sterilized. **(B)** Instrument guide channel attached to the choledochoscope.

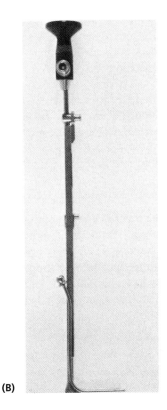

(B)

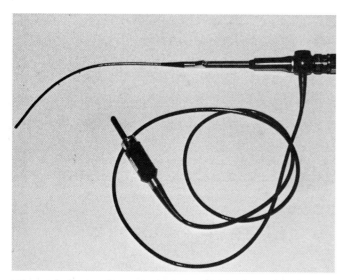

Fig. 23.2 Flexible choledochoscope with instrument channel (outer diameter 5 mm). This instrument is used mainly in the postoperative period for extraction of retained stones through the T-tube tract.

new parameter into biliary surgery, especially in the management of common bile duct stones and in the assessment and biopsy of tumors of the distal bile duct. Choledochoscopy is also of great help in the postoperative period to retrieve retained stones under visual control through the T-tube tract (Berci & Hamlin 1981).

RETAINED COMMON BILE DUCT STONES

Ever since Kehr (1913) published his unique textbook of biliary surgery, the problem of the retained common bile duct (CBD) stone has plagued patients and surgeons alike. The incidence of common bile duct stones is approximately 10 to 20% depending on the age of the patient. The real incidence of retained stone after duct exploration is not known but is reported as between 5 and 28% (Smith et al 1957, Hicken et al 1959, Schein et al 1966, Corlette et al 1978, Gartell & McGinn 1984, Cuschieri & Berci 1984, Berci & Hamlin 1984). Results depend on the accuracy of follow-up. It should be mandatory that all postoperative T-tube cholangiograms (if open cholecystectomy was performed) should be recorded in a hospital for a period of 5 years to allow an accurate reflection of the problem since the incidence may fluctuate from year to year. Following the introduction of endoscopic sphincterotomy (ES) for the treatment of common bile duct stones after open cholecystectomy it was clear that more stones are missed than surgeons are willing to believe. Laparoscopic cholecystectomy (LC) has resulted in a further and significant increase

in the need for endoscopic sphincterotomy (ES) which has a defined morbidity (10%) and mortality (0.5–1.0%) (Cotton et al 1991, Lambert et al 1991, Sherman et al 1991, Legorreta et al 1995, Fletcher 1997).

Endoscopic intraluminal inspection of the extrahepatic biliary system offers the most accurate method for the detection and removal of bile duct stones. During open cholecystectomy, some have attested to its value in reducing the number of missed stones to 0–3% (Griffin 1976, Finnis & Towntree 1977, Lennert 1980, Yap et al 1980, Reitsma 1981) whereas others have not supported these claims (Feliciano et al 1980, Rattner & Warshaw 1981). However, *all agree that if postexploratory choledochoscopy is employed after standard attempts of stone extraction further stones are recovered in 10 to 15% of cases* (Cuschieri & Berci 1984).

After the introduction of LC the experience of the open operative removal of CBD stones decreased significantly since, in many instances, patients undergo preoperative ES. If during preoperative investigation liver function tests shows abnormal values and endoscopic cholangiography (ERCP) is performed on this basis, up to 40 to 50% of studies will be negative and were thus never necessary (Stiegmann et al 1992, Fletcher 1997). However, if surgeons *routinely* perform fluorocholangiography the majority of preoperative ERCPs can be avoided. The exception to this rule is the high-risk case with severe comorbid conditions, cholangitis and/or jaundice. In these cases an endoscopic drainage or stone removal should be attempted.

TRAINING OF RESIDENTS AND TEAM EFFORT

The majority of surgical programs have structured training courses during which residents can practice choledochoscopy on an inanimate or animal model (Fig. 23.3). This is important since the removal of CBD stones laparoscopically requires a well-trained assistant. There is also need for dedicated scrub and circulating nurses to make sure that every accessory is in the room and that the choledochoscope is adequately prepared. The team concept means that every person involved in LCL, the surgeon, nursing and other operating room personnel be well acquainted with all the details of the operative and maintenance procedures (Fig. 23.4).

TECHNIQUE

Instrumentation (for open cholecystectomy)

The choledochoscope, the baskets (Fr. 2.7 or 3.0) and a vascular balloon (Fr. 4) as well as a guidewire and a flexible

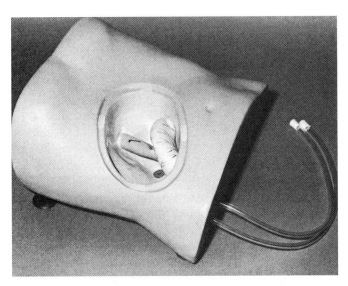

Fig. 23.3 Biliary model. The common bile duct and duodenum are pliable and simulate physiological conditions. During practice, irrigation can be used.

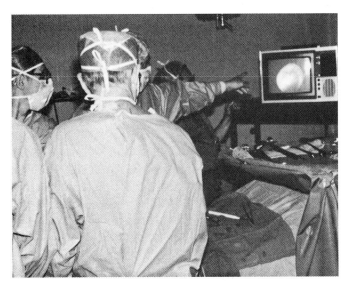

Fig. 23.4 The entire surgical team can follow the procedure. It is easy for the assistant to introduce stone retrieving instrument(s) and observe manipulations with the operator.

biopsy forceps should be kept together in one tray as a set on a separate table and be available in the room for each case (Fig. 23.3).

If the CBD has to be explored, the larger 5-mm flexible choledochoscope attached to a TV camera with a 2.0 mm instrument channel is preferred. It should be connected to a pressure irrigation system (150–200 mmHg) to provide a good stream through the instrument channel. The duodenum should be mobilized (Kocher maneuver) and kept on the stretch with the surgeon standing on the patient's left

introducing the choledochoscope through a 10-mm longitudinal incision in the CBD. If a yellowish or red disc is seen after the introduction of the instrument, the tip of the endoscope is in contact with the ductal wall. This can be corrected by a slow withdrawal or tilting of the tip of the choledochoscope until the tubal appearance of the distal duct or the sphincter is seen. Reversing the instrument allows recognition of the hilar branches of the duct. The best views are generally obtained on withdrawal of the instrument followed by slow advancement under direct visual control.

TELEVISION CHOLEDOCHOSCOPY

The majority of endoscopic procedures are performed with the aid of a television screen. Using this approach, the image is enlarged allowing observation of smaller details. The picture is seen with both eyes from a convenient distance (Fig. 23.4). The surgeon and the assistant can observe the image simultaneously and the maneuvers are carried out in a coordinated fashion (Berci et al 1985). The entire process can be recorded on videotape.

Cholangiography

Operative fluorocholangiography (OFC) (Ch. 22) does not exclude choledochoscopy. Both investigations are complimentary and should be employed. OFC can provide a valuable baseline of information to the surgeon *early in the course of the operation* in respect to unsuspected and/or suspected stones, the anatomy of the cystic and extrahepatic ductal system, the number and size of stones, locations of calculi and sphincter functions (Berci et al 1978). This information is important during open cholecystectomy and is essential during LC so as to allow the surgeon to determine whether the stone(s) can be retrieved laparoscopically (via et al cystic duct or CBD) or whether the conditions indicate the need for open surgery (Ch. 38). Not only is stone detection important during laparoscopic cholecystectomy but it is now clear that OFC can indicate biliary anomalies of surgical importance or reveal injuries to the biliary tree. Ductal injuries can never be completely eliminated but everything should be done to hold them to a minimum. OFC is of value in this endeavor (Cuschieri & Berci 1997).

Findings and operative maneuvers

The normal mucous membrane of the common bile duct is pale pink in appearance with a faint yellow tinge. There are usually several longitudinal folds present, which are flattened by the pressure of the irrigating fluid. A delicate submucosal vascular reticulum is usually visible. Approaching the ampulla the duct narrows, becomes funnel-shaped and curves towards the right posteriorly. The sphincter area itself has a characteristic appearance, which must be identified to ensure complete distal examination. The orifice is seen outlined against the darker background of the adjacent duodenal lumen. It usually appears stellate but may look somewhat fish-mouthed, pinpoint or patulous in nature. The mucosa and the papillary area are coarser and raised into folds and sometimes covered by fibrinous exudate. Failure to recognize the sphincter area precludes any diagnostic conclusions regarding the state of the distal duct. The bifurcation of the common hepatic duct is similar to the appearance of the main bifurcation of the bronchial tree seen at bronchoscopy. The right hepatic duct soon divides into its main sector or branches but the left hepatic duct has no major visible tributary. The mucosa of the hepatic ducts is paler than that of the distal duct. Anatomical variation of the ductal anatomy is common. In particular, a sectoral branch of the right hepatic duct may join the left hepatic duct and give the appearance of a trifurcation. The identification of the major hepatic ducts at the hilus is mandatory to the performance of a complete examination.

Cholangitis is a very common finding in patients with choledocholithiasis and can be of varying degrees. The appearance ranges from mucosal congestion and edema to a marked ulcerative cholangitis with fibrinous exudation. These inflammatory changes become more marked in the papillary regions. At times the examination of the sphincter area is obscured by an inflammatory exudate which has accumulated in this region. Removal of this debris by irrigation usually improves visualization. The changes are far less conspicuous in the proximal duct and in the hepatic ducts. The normal ampulla area is soft and pliable. If the area is observed for a minute or so, the opening and closing phases of the sphincter can be seen. Sphincter stenosis presents as a pinpoint opening which does not change in configuration but the appearance is unfortunately not diagnostic since a similar change can be caused by prolonged spasm due to frequent manipulation. IV administration of glucagon could be of help for better assessment of the sphincter area.

The continuous irrigation dilates the duct and with the mobilized stretched duodenum the distal CBD is better seen. The sphincter function can be observed and gentle advancement allows the characteristic appearance of the duodenum to be seen.

Gallstones are easily identified and may be free floating. Indeed they sometimes can pass spontaneously during irrigation on withdrawal of the endoscope. At times a stone can be found impacted in the orifice of the ampulla, partially imbedded in the ductal wall, or in a diverticulum of the distal duct. Multiple stones and biliary mud are frequently found behind the larger calculus. Repeated endoscopic examinations are necessary to ensure a stone-free duct. Multiple small calculi in a hepatic ductal branch are associated with biliary mud in a dilated duct, and in an elderly patient should cause the surgeon to consider a biliary enteric bypass. In the case of impacted intrahepatic stones it is important to manipulate under endoscopic control with precision so as to avoid perforation of the duct or hemobilia. A suitable attachment with forceps for removal of impacted stones is provided (Fig. 23.5).

In general terms, in the case of the floating stone, the basket or balloon (Fig. 23.6) should be advanced beyond the stone. The basket is then carefully opened and the position of the stone observed. The endoscope is tilted or moved together with the basket and this allows the stone to be entrapped. The endoscope and the basket with the entrapped stone are then withdrawn together.

The best opportunity to remove stones in a difficult situation is at the first attempt. Therefore, once the endoscope is in good position, it should not be withdrawn or moved. The position should be maintained and the assistant should advance the basket. Television choledochoscopy is essential for coordinated, fast, and efficient movements. If a stone is visualized, the irrigation should be decreased or stopped to avoid pushing the stone further in distally or in case of a hepatic calculus proximally. The operator should request the anesthesiologist to administer IV glucagon to relax the sphincter before choledochoscopy is started. Small calculi can be flushed into the duodenum, in some cases under visual control using warm saline. For larger calculi, the assistant advances the stone basket and with coordinated

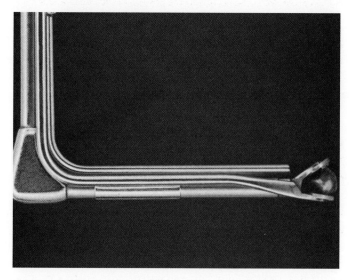

Fig. 23.5 For removal of impacted stones (distal duct) this attachable stone forceps can be of great help.

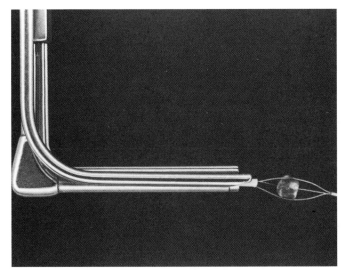

(A)

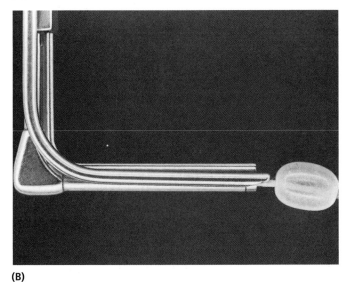

(B)

Fig. 23.6 (A) Dormia stone basket. The position of the basket and the stone can be easily observed and necessary movements carried out to entrap the calculus. **(B)** A 4-French balloon catheter. The balloon is passed beyond the stone. The endoscope with the stone is withdrawn (together) into the incision.

movements, the calculus is entrapped. Both instruments are withdrawn together. Completion cholangiography should confirm the existence of a stone-free duct.

Neoplasms of the biliary system (Chs 52 and 54) can be visualized and biopsied and specimens can also be obtained for cytological examination. Papillary tumors in particular protrude into the lumen of the biliary tract and are readily seen. Even though the biopsy specimens obtained are small, they are usually adequate for diagnosis. Extrinsic ductal obstruction due to neoplasm creates an appearance of complete occlusion of the ductal system through which the

instrument cannot be advanced. There may or may not be breaching of the mucosal integrity. Extrinsic compression of the distal common bile duct by an inflammatory mass is indistinguishable from a malignant lesion. Choledochoscopic examination in cases of papillary bile duct tumors, particularly lower bile duct tumors, is important and the whole biliary tree should be examined since multicentric tumors may be found in up to 7% of cases. Bile duct tumors may be unexpectedly encountered on exploration of the common bile duct for a stone, and it is important to remember this possibility.

LAPAROSCOPIC CBD STONE REMOVAL WITH THE CHOLEDOCHOSCOPE (see also Ch. 38)

Laparoscopic choledocholithotomy (LCL) is now an established procedure. By 1991 there were already reports that if fluorocholangiography and a choledochoscope were available, a common bile duct stone could be removed in one operative session (Berci 1991, Petelin 1991, Phillips & Carroll 1991). It is true that LCL requires more skill, but if a surgeon was able to learn laparoscopic cholecystectomy, he/she should be able to carry out biliary lithotomy.

The choledochoscope for laparoscopic choledocholithotomy (LCL)

A smaller diameter choledochoscope (2.8-mm flexible) is much easier to use during LCL than the standard choledochoscope (5-mm). It has a working channel of 1.2-mm through which irrigation and a French 2.7 mm basket can be advanced. The most recent version is the videoscope (Figs 23.7 & 23.8). The camera is built as an integral part of the grip. This system is ideal for LCL and has the advantage of allowing display of the choledochoscopic and abdominal images simultaneously (Fig. 23.9). In addition, a clear enlarged image is created (Fig. 23.10). During laparoscopic cholecystectomy, the cystic duct is defined and dissected. A small incision is made and a cholangiogram is performed. If it is positive, there are various techniques available to introduce the choledochoscope. If the duct lumen is larger than 3-mm, it can be introduced through a fourth trocar site. Another approach is an additional trocar, which penetrates the abdominal wall in the midline above the cystic duct area (Petelin 1991).

A guidewire with a soft tip should be available in case the instrument is difficult to introduce through the cystic duct incision. In this case the protruding guidewire which is advanced through the instrument channel into the cystic duct helps guide the choledochoscope. The instrument channel should be connected to a pressure bag with saline

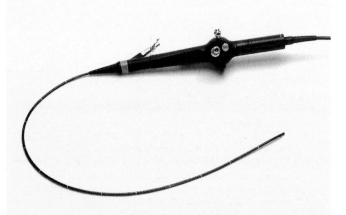

Fig. 23.7 The flexible video-choledochoscope. Outside diameter: 2.8 mm with a 1.2-mm instrument channel. Length: 55 cm. Bending the tip: 140°–140° on both sides. The miniature TV camera is a continuation of the grip and therefore it is more ergonomical during manipulation and more convenient. No focusing or attachments are necessary. The raster of the fiber structure is eliminated (Fig. 23.4) and a smooth enlarged image is seen.

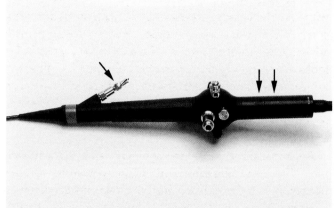

Fig. 23.8 Close up of Fig. 23.7. Single arrow—instrument channel for connecting irrigation or advancing a basket. Double arrow—miniature camera.

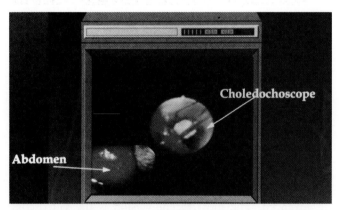

Fig. 23.9 Using two cameras and one 'twin video' control unit with a 'picture in picture' (PIP) modality, the operator can see the enlarged endoscopic image in the middle and the laparoscopic appearance of the choledochoscope in one corner simultaneously. In case of difficulty in advancing the choledochoscope, it is possible to see the instrument at the choledochotomy and rectify this by slowly withdrawing and repositioning the tip of the scope.

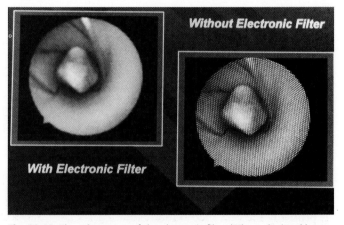

Fig. 23.10 The advantages of the electronic filter (EF) are depicted here. On the right is the normal appearance of the TV image of a fiberscope attached to a TV camera. The image displays the raster of the fiber structure. On the left is the same but shown this time with the inclusion of the EF. The image is smooth and detailed.

(150–200 mmHg) and infusion controlled by a stopcock. If a stone is easily visible, the infusion is decreased or even stopped; otherwise the stone will change position and be difficult to grasp. The basket is advanced by the assistant beyond the stone and is opened. By withdrawal and with coordinated movements the stone can be entrapped and extracted with the instruments.

If there is a small cystic duct, it can be dilated by introducing a guidewire followed by a balloon catheter (5-mm wide and 40-mm long, size French 7). The balloon is inflated to a predetermined atmospheric pressure dilating the cystic duct to 5-mm. It should be kept there for a few minutes then deflated. The balloon is then withdrawn over the guidewire and the choledochoscope is introduced over the guidewire.

If there is a stone located in the hepatic ductal system, it is very difficult to reverse the choledochoscope via the cystic duct approach. If it is impossible, laparoscopic or open choledochotomy should be considered.

If a large number of stones or larger sized calculi are found in a dilated duct, laparoscopic choledochotomy should be the next step. A 10-mm incision is made into the

CBD and the stones are recovered proximally and distally with the choledochoscope basket or balloon under visual control. If the duct shows some signs of cholangitis, it is advisable to insert a T-tube. However, if the duct lining looks clear, primary closure can be attempted but a cholangio-catheter should be introduced into the cystic duct. This not only acts as a decompressing drainage for 1–2 days but also allows postoperative cholangiography (Berci et al 1997).

An impacted stone in the sphincter area is fortunately rare. The usual alternatives are either to convert to open operation or to leave it for postoperative endoscopic management. However, if available, a laser transmitting flexible quartz bundle (200–500 microns) attached to a laser unit may be advanced through the choledochoscope instrument channel and the stone disintegrated under visual control. The prerequisite of this elegant method is the availability of lasers and special expertise of laser lithotripsy (Birkett 1992).

CONCLUSIONS

Familiarity and expertise with choledochoscopic techniques reduces the incidence of retained common bile duct stones considerably. The general surgeon should become familiar with laparoscopic choledocholithotomy.

While intraoperative cholangiography remains mandatory especially for early demonstration of anatomical anomalies and as an indication for duct exploration, choledochoscopy is probably the best method for exploring the duct and for ensuring complete clearance of stones (Berci 1998). While the overwhelming majority of cases of choledocholithiasis will, in the future, be managed endoscopically or laparoscopically, there will be a need to address the question of providing adequate training of surgical residents for those cases where open surgery is indicated.

REFERENCES

Bakes J 1923 Die Choledochopapilloskopie. Archiv fuer Klinische Chirurgie 126: 473–483

Berci G 1998 Laparoscopic cholecystectomy: Cholangiography. In: Scott-Connor C (ed) SAGES Manual: Fundamentals of Laparoscopy and GI Endoscopy. Springer, New York, Ch 13.3, p 143–162

Berci G 1991 Laparoscopic Surgery, Special Issue of Problems in General Surgery. Lippincott, Philadelphia p 2–18.

Berci G, Hamlin J A 1981 Retrieval of retained stones. In: Berci G, Hamlin J A (eds) Operative Biliary Radiology. Williams & Wilkins, Baltimore p 147–158

Berci G, Hamlin J A, Grundfest W 1984 Combined fluoro-endoscopic removal of retained stones. Archives of Surgery 118: 1395–1398.

Berci G, Shore J M, Morgenstern L, Hamlin J A 1978 Choledochoscopy and operative fluorocholangiography in the prevention of retained stones. World Journal of Surgery 2: 411–427

Berci G, Shulman A, Morgenstern L 1985 Television choledochoscopy. Surgical Gynecology and Obstetrics. 160: 176–7

Berci G, Petelin J B, Cuschieri A 1997 Laparoscopic ductal clearance. In: Berci G, Cuschieri A Bile Ducts and Bile Duct Stones. W B Saunders, Philadelphia, Chs 12, 13, 14

Birkett D H 1992 Biliary laser lithotripsy. Surgical Clinicics of North America 72: 641–654

Corlette M B, Achatzky S, Ackroyd F 1978 Operative cholangiography and overlooked stones. Archives of Surgery 113: 729–733

Cotton, P B, Lehman G, Vennes J, Geenen J E, Russell R C G, Meyers W C, Liguory C, Nickl N 1991 Endoscopic sphincterotomy complications and their management: An attempt at consensus. Gastrointestinal Endoscopy 37: 383–393

Cuschieri A, Berci G 1984 In: Common Bile Duct Exploration. Martinus-Nijhoff, Boston, p 54–61

Cuschieri A, Berci G 1984 Operative biliary endoscopy. In: Cuschieri A, Berci G, Common Bile Duct Exploration, Martinus Nijhoff, Boston. Ch 5, p 55–59

Cuschieri P, Berci G 1997 The role of fluorocholangiography during laparoscopic cholecystectomy. In: Berci G, Cuschieri P (eds). Bile Ducts and Ductal Stones. Saunders, Philadelphia, Ch 6L, p 33–44

Feliciano D V, Mattox K L, Jordan G L 1980 The value of choledochoscopy in exploration of the CBD. Annals of Surgery 191: 649–652

Finnis D, Towntree T 1977 Choledochoscopy in the exploration of the common bile duct. British Journal of Surgery 64: 661–664

Fletcher D 1997 Role of preoperative and postoperative ERCP. In: Berci G, Cuschieri A (eds), Bile Duct and Ductal Stones. Saunders, Philadelphia, Ch 6, p 33–43

Gartell P C, McGinn F P 1984 Choledochoscopy: are stones missed? A controlled study. British Journal of Surgery 71: 767–770

Griffin W T 1976 Choledochoscopy. American Journal of Surgery 132: 697–698

Hicken N F, McAllister J A, Walker G 1959 The problems of retained common duct stones. American Journal of Surgery 97: 173–183

Kehr H 1913 Praxis der Gallenweg Chirurgie. Lehman, Munich

Lambert M E, Betts C D, Hill J, Faragher E B, Martin D F, Tweedle D E F 1991 Endoscopic sphincterotomy: The Whole Truth. British Journal of Surgery 78: 473–476

Legorreta A P, Brooks R J, Staroscik R N, Yong X, Costantino G N, Zatz S L 1995 Increased ERCP rate following the introduction of laparoscopic cholecystectomy. Journal Laparoendo Surgery 5: 271–277

Lennert K 1980 Choledochoskopie. Springer, Heidelberg

McIver M A 1941 An instrument for visualizing the interior of the common bile duct at operation. Surgery 9: 112–114

Petelin J B 1991 Laparoscopic approach to common duct pathology. Surgical Laparoscopic Endoscopy 1: 33–41

Petelin J B 1996 Laparoscopic ductal stone clearance: Transcystic approach. In: Berci G, Cuschieri A (eds) Bile Ducts and Bile Duct Stones. WB Saunders, Philadelphia p 97–108

Phillips E, Carroll B J 1991 Problems in general surgery: new techniques for the treatment of common bile duct calculi encountered during laparoscopic cholecystectomy. Lippincott, Philadelphia 8: 387–395

Rattner D W, Warshaw A L 1981 Impact of choledochoscopy on the management of choledocholithiasis. Annals of Surgery 194: 76–79

Reitsma B J 1981 Common duct stones (Thesis). University of Limburg, Maastricht

Schein C J, Stern W Z, Jacobson H G 1966 Residual stones. In: Schein C J (ed) The Common Bile Duct. Thomas, Springfield, p 266–271

Sherman S, Ruffolo T A, Hawes R H, Lehman G A 1991 Complications of endoscopic sphincterotomy. Gastroenterology 101: 1068–1073

Shore J M, Morgenstern L, Berci G 1971 An improved rigid choledochoscope. American Journal of Surgery 122: 567–568

Smith S, Engel C, Averhook B, Longmire W P 1957 Problems of retained and recurrent common bile duct stones. Journal of American Medical Association 164: 231–236

Stiegmann G V, Goff J S, Mansour A, Pearlman N, Reveille R M, Norton L 1992 Precholecystectomy endoscopic cholangiography and stone removal is not superior to cholecystectomy, cholangiography and common duct exploration. American Journal of Surgery 163: 227–230

Traverso L W, Roush T S, Koo K 1995 Common bile duct stones—outcomes and costs. Surgical Endoscopy 9: 1242–1244

Wildegans H 1953 Grenzen der Cholangiographie und Aussichten der Endoskopie der tiefen Gallenwege. Med Klinik 48: 1270–1273

Yamakawa T 1976 An improved choledocho-fiberscope and non-surgical removal of retained biliary calculi under direct visual control. Gastrointestinal Endoscopy 22: 160–165

Yap P C, Atacador M, Yap A G, Yap R G 1980 Choledochoscopy as a complimentary procedure to operative cholangiography in biliary surgery. American Journal of Surgery 140: 648–650

Intraoperative ultrasound diagnostic aspects in liver surgery

24

A. MAZZIOTTI, G.L. GRAZI

Intraoperative ultrasonography (IOU) was introduced into clinical practice in the early 1980s. The development of small, easily sterilized, high frequency ultrasonographic probes has led to the intraoperative application of ultrasonography in liver, biliary, and pancreatic surgery. Liver surgery has become one of the most interesting and common applications of IOU. First investigated by the Japanese surgeons Makuuchi, Hasegawa and Yamasaki in 1981 (Makuuchi et al 1981), the technique has been progressively used to improve the diagnosis and management of liver lesions in many centers, including the East, Europe, and the USA (Nagasue et al 1984, Bismuth & Castaing 1985, Gunven et al 1985, Gozzetti et al 1986, Belghiti et al 1986, Olsen 1990, Solomon et al 1992, Gouillat et al 1992). In Europe, and more recently in the USA, the method has been accepted as an integral diagnostic and management modality in hepatobiliary clinics. In a survey by the World Association of Hepato-Pancreato-Biliary Surgery, 66 out of 67 European centers routinely employed IOU during hepatic surgery (Gozzetti et al 1994).

The aim of the investigation is to detect the presence or absence of liver lesions, to determine their location with regard to the adjacent vessels, and to provide an overall assessment of the extent of the disease. Using IOU, this information can be obtained immediately at the onset of the operation through an initial small incision, thereby avoiding unnecessary tissue dissection, traumatic surgical maneuvers, and the use of contrast medium at intraoperative radiology.

In this chapter the diagnostic use of intraoperative ultrasounds for hepatic surgery, specifically in the field of liver tumors, is explored and the experience gained over 15 years at the University of Bologna is reviewed.

INSTRUMENTATION AND THE TECHNIQUE OF EXPLORATION

The equipment employed for IOU is conventional ultrasonographic apparatus. It is best to limit the dimension of the machine in order to allow its accommodation in small operating rooms and to ensure that it is mobile and easily manageable. Adjustments of the 'gain' and of the 'gray scale', the freezing, taking of pictures, and other maneuvers are made by the operating room nurse and not by a specialized technician. It is advisable to have a screen big enough to allow the surgeon to see the images from 1 m away. The ultrasonographic probes must be small since they must be introduced into the abdominal cavity, often through a small incision. They must be easily sterilized and have a sufficient length of cord (about 2 m) to allow for ease of manipulation.

Linear array are the most commonly used probes in hepatic surgery (convex or sectorial probes are most commonly employed in pancreatic and biliary surgery). These probes have a T aspect with a field of view along the horizontal inferior bar of the T. The resulting images are rectangular with the superior part corresponding to the contact zone of the probe. Probes of this type can be hand-held by the surgeon and are maintained in contact with the hepatic surface, then passed along the anterior and lateral aspects of the liver (Ch. 89).

The width of the probe varies from 3 to 5 cm, with a maximum of 10 cm. The larger probes have a wide field of view and are very useful in allowing spatial topographic evaluation of lesions with respect to surrounding vascular structures. Such probes require a large subcostal access incision. Smaller 3 cm probes have a narrower field of view, with the disadvantage of providing a confined picture of the parenchyma and hence a more difficult assessment of the lesions. However, their use is mandatory in the case of a small laparotomy incision for initial exploration, a median laparotomy, or a lower midline incision. Such is the case for exploration of the liver prior to operation on other abdominal viscera; for example, the pancreas or colon.

The frequency of the ultrasound varies from 5 to 7.5 MHz and up to 10 MHz. Ultrasonographic resolution power depends on the frequency of ultrasound. As the frequency increases, the ultrasound loses energy across the tissue and the maximum depth of exploration is diminished. The 3.5 MHz probe has a more detailed depth of capacity but lower resolution (about 1 cm). High-resolution probes of 7.5 and 10 MHz have less depth of penetration but higher resolution. The 5 MHz probe is a good compromise between resolution power and depth of exploration (Franco et al 1990) and is the most useful for liver surgery.

The probe is placed directly on the liver surface which is methodically explored by the surgeon. It is necessary that the surgeon performing the study must also interpret the images because a radiologist will have difficulty interpreting the image, being ignorant of the position and direction of the probe. Furthermore, the studies are often repeated during the operation, for example in the evaluation of resection margins during liver tumor resection. It would be unduly time consuming for a radiologist to remain for many hours in the operating room. It is thus essential for the surgeon to learn the techniques of ultrasonography in order to be able to perform IOU in an expert manner.

The initial obstacle to the expansion of intraoperative ultrasound was the difficulty surgeons had in gaining experience with ultrasound images and learning how to scan the liver correctly. The two-dimensional images provided by ultrasonography must be considered in spatial content, along the 'gain', contrast, and the 'gray scale'. This coordination can only be performed by a surgeon who has gained familiarity with the technique. For this reason, those who wish to start using IOU should spend a period in a center where the technique is used routinely. The assistance of an expert sonographer in the early stages is also of considerable help.

Liver lesions situated in the superficial area of the liver are more difficult to detect than those lying deeply. In fact, immediately below the probe, for a depth of a few millimeters, there exists an artefactual zone (the 'bang effect') which conceals the area below the Glisson's capsule. To avoid this it is possible to place a water barrier between the probe and the liver surface (for example, the finger of a surgical glove filled with saline solution) in order to distance the probe from the surface and allow better identification of surface lesions. Occasionally, a Doppler probe can measure vessel flow. A rare application of IOU is verification of the patency of portosystemic anastomoses or arterial anastomoses during liver transplantation, especially in cases where a difficult arterial reconstruction is carried out. Recently, with the development of laparoscopic surgery, special probes have been developed which will enable initial exploration of the liver laparoscopically and prior to open laparotomy (Ch. 20). Special probes are available for use in the detection of bile duct but this use of IOU has not gained wide acceptance.

THE ULTRASOUND TECHNIQUE FOR HEPATIC EXPLORATION

Using a 3-cm probe, preliminary exploration can be carried out through a small laparotomy incision. However, this must be sufficiently large to allow the entry of the surgeon's hand. No preliminary division of the ligaments of the liver is required. Thus, in operations on colorectal tumors, a median laparotomy incision can be used. The hand is then passed upward from below to allow exploration of the liver. Systematic exploration of the liver should include a full examination of both lobes, the portal branches to each segment of the liver, and the course of the main hepatic veins from their origins to the confluence at the vena cava. The latter is of particular importance. It is also necessary to observe any anatomical anomalies, such as the presence of accessory hepatic veins. The presence of such veins can be useful during mobilization of the liver and in operations that involve the right posterior sector of the liver. Indeed, in some patients drainage of the posterior segment of the right liver can be carried by accessory hepatic veins (Makuuchi 1987) (Ch. 83).

Exploration of the right posterior sector of the liver can be carried out without division of the triangular ligaments, provided that the probe is moved obliquely to include in the field of vision the most posterior portion of the parenchyma. Ultrasound may be repeated during hepatic resection to verify the plane of parenchymal transection with respect to the limits of a tumor, in order to ensure sufficient resection margins. The importance of providing sufficient resection margins of at least 1 cm has been emphasized repeatedly in the literature (Hughes et al 1986, Ekberg et al 1987, Gozzetti & Mazziotti 1989), both in the management of metastatic disease and in primary hepatocellular carcinoma. It has been suggested that tumor margins less than 1 cm in width are associated with significantly higher recurrence rates after hepatectomy or segmentectomy (Gozzetti et al 1992).

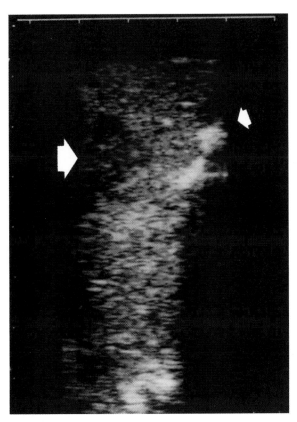

Fig. 24.1 Echo-assisted 'liver resection' for small hepatocellular carcinoma. The tumor (large arrow) is hypoechoic. The gauze (small arrow) situated in the resection plane is well visualized, as is the hyperechoic band. The limit between the tumor and the resection margin is 2 cm.

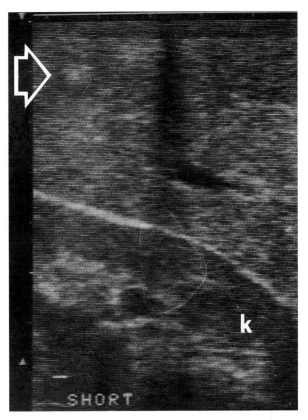

Fig 24.2 Small (8 mm) occult hyperechoic metastasis surrounded by an hypoechoic halo, discovered during IOU examination (k, kidney).

The correct plane of dissection is often difficult to evaluate in the course of liver resection, especially in the cirrhotic patient. Using IOU it is much easier to identify the distance from the tumor margin. To achieve this it is helpful to place at the resection margin an echogenic material such as surgical clamp or a piece of gauze; this allows identification of the direction of the resection plane and secures a distance from the lesion (Fig. 24.1).

DIAGNOSIS OF INTRAHEPATIC LESIONS

Lesions of about 1 cm in diameter are the limit of conventional preoperative radiological imaging techniques, as such lesions can easily escape definition during surgical exploration of the liver especially when they are deeply located in the parenchyma. This is particularly true in the presence of cirrhosis of the liver. The higher resolution capability of IOU probes allows the detection of lesions as small as 4–5 mm (Fig. 24.2). Several reports in the literature confirm the supe-

rior sensitivity of IOU for small lesions in normal or cirrhotic liver (Gunven et al 1985, Makuuchi 1987, Clarke et al 1989).

A study was conducted by the authors of 54 patients undergoing surgery for either primary liver tumors (28 were cirrhotics) or for metastatic lesions. All the patients underwent angiography, computed tomography (CT) scan, and ultrasound performed by the same surgeon perioperatively using 3.5 MHz probes. IOU proved to have greater diagnostic accuracy, especially for small lesions. Only two lesions about 1 cm in size located immediately beneath the liver surface in cirrhotics, and two lesions in the non-cirrhotic group escaped intraoperative ultrasonographic detection.

It should be emphasized that a high percentage of the lesions found in cirrhotic livers were not palpable during surgery. The sensitivity (the number of lesions detected compared with the total number of lesions) at the time of the preoperative studies and at IOU are shown in Table 24.1. The CT scan detected only half of the lesions less than 2 cm in size, and angiography rarely demonstrated minute lesions except for highly vascularized, small, hepatocellular carcinoma. Preoperative ultrasonography was also limited in detecting lesions less than 1 cm, particularly for lesions in

Table 24.1 Sensitivity of different diagnostic techniques in the diagnosis of liver neoplasms

	Lesion size (cm)	CT (%)	Angiography (%)	Preoperative US (%)	Intraoperative US (%)
Non-cirrhotic liver	< 1	50.0	16.6	50.0	66.6
	1–3	54.5	36.3	72.7	100
	> 3	92.5	88.8	96.2	100
Cirrhotic liver	< 1	0.0	20.0	20.0	60.0
	1–3	42.1	57.8	73.6	100
	> 3	80.0	80.0	100	100
Total		64.1	62.8	79.4	94.8

CT, computed tomography; US, ultrasonography

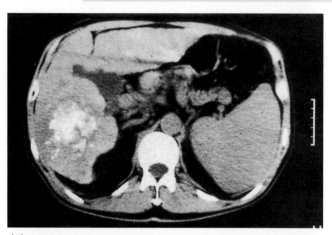

(A)

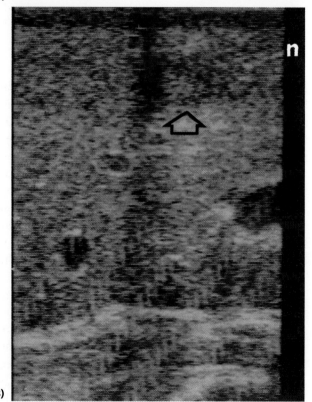

(B)

Fig. 24.3 (A) Hepatocellular carcinoma in cirrhosis in the right liver lobe; neither preoperative ultrasound nor CT scan (lipiodol contrast medium) shows other intrahepatic lesions. **(B)** Intraoperative ultrasonography shows a small (6 mm) secondary lesion in the left lobe (arrow).

the blind areas of the abdominal ultrasound, such as the posterior sector of the right liver and the most superficial part of the left lobes (Gozzetti et al 1989). More recently, the authors have studied 22 cirrhotic patients using angiography with lipiodol injection followed by a CT scan some 2–3 weeks later. Even using this technique, IOU revealed previously undetected lesions in three patients (Fig. 24.3).

DETECTION OF OCCULT LIVER METASTASES

The potential field for the detection of occult hepatic metastases using IOU during surgery for gastrointestinal neoplasms is evident when one considers that most patients operated on for these tumors do not routinely undergo exhaustive radiological imaging studies of the liver. Machi et al (1987) discovered unsuspected liver lesions in some 10% of patients submitted to operation for gastrointestinal tumors, and similar data have been reported by others (Bodrini et al 1987, Olsen 1990).

In the authors' experience of 110 patients operated on for gastrointestinal pancreatic cancer, additional information was obtained using IOU in eight patients. Illustration of such occult lesions are shown in Figs 24.4 and 24.5. Two such patients undergoing surgery for colorectal cancer had lesions smaller than 1 cm in diameter. In both these cases the lesions were removed by wedge resection at the time of colonic resection. Two lesions were of greater size (3 and 4 cm, respectively) and were located in segment VII of the right posterior sector. These were not revealed at preoperative ultrasonography. Neither of these lesions was palpable during surgery until the right triangular ligament was divided and the right liver mobilized. The other occult lesions were detected in patients with pancreatic carcinoma. In these patients, concomitant dilatation of the intrahepatic bile ducts may explain why these lesions were missed during preoperative ultrasonographic study and not recognized at subsequent surgical exploration. Discovery of these metastases contraindicated major pancreatic resection.

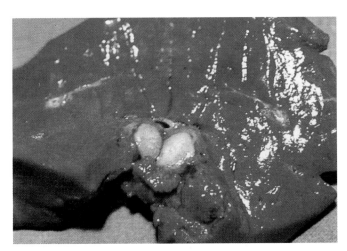

Fig. 24.4 Removal of small lesion in segment VI by wedge resection. This metastasis was seen only during intraoperative ultrasound (see Fig. 24. 5).

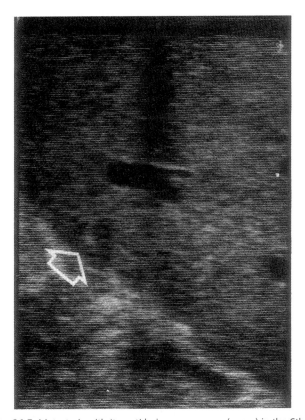

Fig. 24.5 Metastasis with 'target' lesion appearance (arrow) in the 6th segment in a patient operated on for carcinoma and removed by wedge resection (see Fig. 24.4).

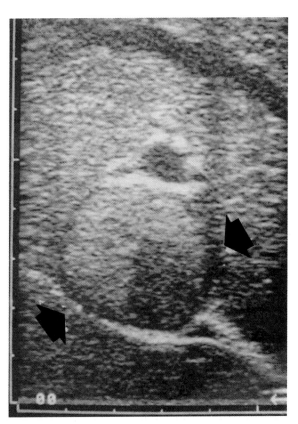

Fig. 24.6 A small (3 cm) isoechoic hepatocellular carcinoma in a cirrhotic patient. The tumor was not palpable within the liver parenchyma, and was resected by subsegmental resection. Note that the tumor is adjacent to a segmental portal branch.

SURGERY FOR HEPATOCELLULAR CARCINOMA IN CIRRHOTIC PATIENTS

Operation for primary hepatocellular cancer (HCC) in the cirrhotic patient is one of the more difficult problems in liver surgery (Chs 83 and 85). HCC is a common solid tumor of the liver the incidence of which appears to be significantly increasing in the East (Okuda et al 1987) and in Europe (Colombo et al 1991). The adoption of screening procedures (ultrasonography and measurement of serum alpha-fetoprotein) in patients with chronic hepatitis or cirrhosis has also resulted in an increasing number of patients being referred for surgical management. In this group, small, often single, symptom-free tumors are being detected at an early stage.

The experience of Eastern surgeons and recent data from European centers (Franco et al 1989, 1990, Gozzetti et al 1988, 1992) have demonstrated that the risks of resection in the cirrhotic liver are acceptable (Ch. 85) provided the residual liver function is carefully assessed and removal of tumor-free parenchyma is minimized. This implies the necessity for precise localization of the tumor and its relationship to the intrahepatic vasculature. Intraoperative ultrasonography is indispensable in this situation since it enables visualization of small tumors that usually escape detection at surgical exploration of the cirrhotic liver (Fig. 24.6). Nagasue et al (1984) have reported that approximately half the cancers in the cirrhotic livers less than 4 cm in size cannot be palpated. Sheu et al (1985) have reported that IOU decisively influenced surgical strategy in more than 30% of such patients submitted to surgery, and enabled limited resection in a significant number. The present authors' experience confirms these reports (Gozzetti et al 1988, 1989, Gandolfi et al 1992, Gouillat et al 1992).

Special techniques have been described for ultrasonographically guided hepatic resection in the cirrhotic patient. For small tumors the surrounding parenchyma to be excised can be tattooed (Gozzetti et al 1989) or mapped on the liver surface (Hasegawa et al 1988) so as to enable subsegmental resection. Makuuchi, Hasegawa, and Yamasaki have introduced the injection of methylene blue into the portal venous branch relative to the tumor, which allows visualization of the correct anatomical segment to be removed (Makuuchi et al 1985, Makuuchi 1987).

Bismuth et al (Bismuth & Castaing 1985, Bismuth et al 1987) have used a balloon catheter in the relevant segmental portal branch. The balloon is inflated to interrupt the blood flow and thus to allow a bloodless segmental resection to be performed. The present authors, however, conduct the resection using a meticulous technique of parenchymal division: in most of the cases the resection can be performed without any vascular control or limiting vascular clamping to the pedicle branches afferent to the hemiliver to be removed (Grazi et al 1997) while the Pringle maneuver, which is well tolerated in the cirrhotic liver (Gozzetti et al 1988, Mazziotti & Cavallari 1997), is performed more and more rarely. Another advantage of IOU is the detection of small satellite nodules or neoplastic thrombi in the small portal branches which may dictate a more extensive resection or contraindicate resection altogether (Gozzetti et al 1988, Mazziotti & Cavallari 1997).

Using the data from seven northern Italian centers, a retrospective multicentric study was done to evaluate the results of 256 hepatic resections in cirrhotic patients. IOU was performed in 186 of these patients and a significant correlation was found between improved results and the routine use of IOU. Thus, in centers where IOU was used routinely, better survival rates were observed (Gozzetti et al 1992). The explanation for these improved results may be found in the exclusion of patients with intrahepatic neoplastic spread and the improved resection margins obtained in the more experienced centres.

IOU DURING OPERATION FOR HEPATIC HYDATID DISEASE

The diagnosis of hydatid disease (Ch. 63) is easily made using routine preoperative ultrasonography or at CT scan-

ning. The classical picture of multiple cysts with calcified walls containing daughter cysts is characteristic. The diagnosis can, however, sometimes be in doubt. This is particularly true in the rare cases of cysts with dense and dishomogenous content, cysts without evident daughter cysts, or cyst membranes (Fig. 24.7). In these patients IOU can be of value since it may make evident the presence of proliferating membrane surrounding the liquid-filled cavity.

The importance of IOU in hydatid surgery lies in the possibility of evaluating the cyst wall in relationship to hepatic vascular anatomy. The vessels are distorted and displaced by the gradual growth of the cyst, which disturbs the normal intrahepatic vascular relationship. Display of the vessels is important in formulating a correct surgical approach.

Today there is an increasing preference for more radical surgery, such as total or subtotal pericystectomy. In an attempt to lower the recurrence rate and the postsurgical complications of abscess or biliary fistula, which may result from draining the cyst or marsupialization of the cavity (Magistrelli et al 1991), IOU is of special value. It is especially useful in the performance of total or subtotal pericystectomy since it clearly demonstrates the site of the pericystic membrane in relation to the hepatic venous and Glissonian pedicles, as well as the relationship to the retrohepatic vena cava. An example of such echo-guided pericystectomy is shown in Figures 24.8 and 24.9.

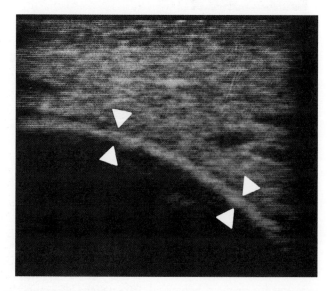

Fig. 24.7 Intraoperative ultrasound scan reveals a regular, highly echoic band clearly distinct from the surrounding liver parenchyma. This is the proliferating cyst membrane.

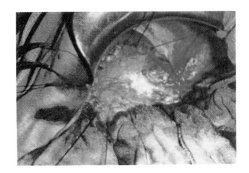

Fig. 24.8 The cyst in Fig. 24.9 was removed under intraoperative ultrasound guidance taking the resection up to the limit of the intrahepatic vessels. (Reproduced with permission from Gozzetti et al 1989).

IOU IN LIVING RELATED LIVER TRANSPLANTATION

The use of IOU has clearly emerged as of value in the field of living related liver transplantation (Ch. 14). In recent years, this procedure has met with increasing success due to the scarcity of cadaveric organ donors, in particular for pediatric recipients. It consists of two different steps: the first is the removal of a defined portion of liver from the donor using a conventional hepatic resection; the second is the implant of the graft in the recipient. One of the crucial aspects in the donor liver resection is to maintain the integrity of the vascular structures of the graft, but also not to damage the remaining vein of the recipient. The number of abnormalities already founded at the confluence of the hepatic veins is high. The use of IOU is thus of particular help in the detection of the anatomy of the liver to be

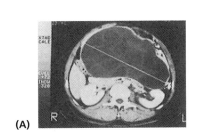

(A)

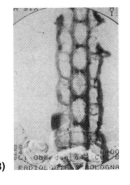

(B)

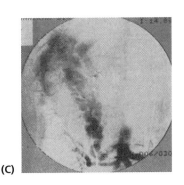

(C)

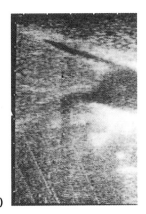

(D)

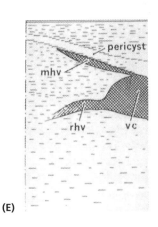

(E)

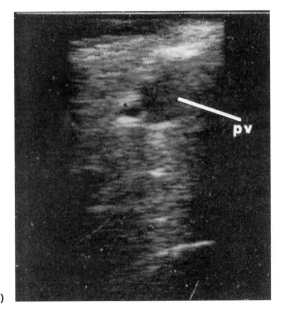

(F)

Fig. 24.9 (A) CT liver scan in a patient with a large hydatid cyst. **(B)** Inferior vena cavography. Obvious signs of compression (or thrombosis) of the lower vena cava. **(C)** Superior mesenteric arteriogram (venous phase). The portal vein fails to opacify and there are numerous collateral vessels. **(D), (E), (F)** After draining the cyst the image from inside the cavity shows a patent vena cava (vc), middle hepatic vein (mhv), and right hepatic vein (rhv), and a portal vein (pv) which are closely related to the pericystic membrane. (Reproduced with permission from Gozzetti et al 1989).

removed (Fig. 24.10), in the definition of the resection plane and to guide the surgeon during the division of the parenchyma (Kasai et al 1992).

The disposition of the hepatic vein tributaries around the juncture of the major hepatic veins with the inferior vena cava can be delineated before starting liver resection, using IOU. The left medial (umbilical) vein draining the left part of the medial segment can be recognized close to the confluence of the middle and left hepatic veins. This tributary can join the left hepatic vein in the majority of cases, but sometimes the middle hepatic vein (Kawasaki et al 1996).

THE IMPACT OF IOU ON SURGICAL STRATEGY

Although there are a large number of publications that favorably underline the sensitivity of IOU in relation to diagnosis, it is much more difficult to evaluate critically how its use influences surgical strategy or changes the surgeon's final decision as to the type of operation performed.

With regard to the detection of hepatic metastases prior to radical surgery for gastrointestinal tumors, IOU may have a decisive impact. Thus, in the presence of a pancreatic carcinoma, detection of hepatic metastases will change a decision to proceed with pancreaticoduodenectomy and allow the surgeon to carry out biliary bypass alone. In the performance of radical colonic surgery, detection of metastases may allow immediate treatment of such lesions or aid in planning future hepatic resection.

With regard to the performance of hepatic resection in the non-cirrhotic liver, the supplementary information supplied by IOU is limited—this is reported to be somewhere in the range 5 to 28% (Castaing et al 1986, Brower et al 1989, Gozzetti et al 1989, Boutkan et al 1992, Gouillat et al 1992), and has essentially been of the form to allow an extension of the excision to be performed, recognition of vascular infiltration, or the unmasking of multiple lesions. On the other hand, in hepatocellular cancer in the cirrhotic liver, IOU has considerable importance and allows additional information to be obtained which often alters the surgical decision. The examination may allow limited excision of small non-palpable tumors, or supply information which clearly indicates more extensive surgery (Nagasue et al 1984, Sheu et al 1985, Castaing et al 1986, Gozzetti et al 1989, Gouillat et al 1992).

Furthermore, IOU can be also of great help to guide the surgeon during cryoablation of hepatic lesions (Rozycki 1998) (Ch. 80). Under the guidance of the probe it is in fact possible to correctly place the cryosurgical applicator

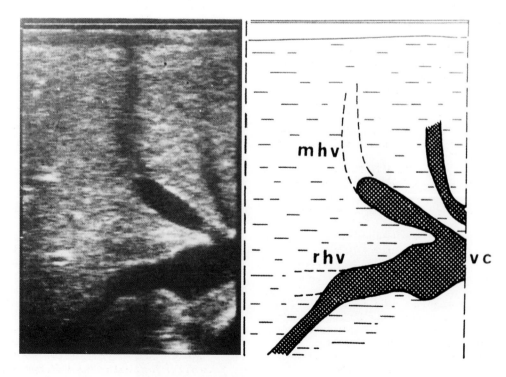

Fig. 24.10 Intraoperative ultrasonography revealed vessels anatomy during liver resection for living related liver transplantation; mhv, middle hepatic vein; rhv, right hepatic vein; vc, vena cava.

into the center of the lesion to be treated and to clearly detect the echogenic changes occurring during the performance of this procedure.

In hepatic surgery there should be great emphasis on the precision of correct preoperative indications and diagnostic protocols to be followed. For the majority of cases, relevant preoperative studies permit informed assessment in most cases. IOU can give supplementary information of particular importance in the cirrhotic liver, or when the intrahepatic anatomy is distorted by previous operations or by compression due to tumor. IOU is simple, rapid to perform, and easy to learn and is recommended for routine use during hepatic resection (Mazziotti & Cavallari 1997).

REFERENCES

Belghiti J, Cardi F, Men Y et al 1986 Surgical treatment of hepatocellular carcinoma on cirrhosis. Value of preoperative ultrasonography. Gastroenterology and Clinical Biology 10: 224–247

Bismuth H, Castaing D 1985 Echographie péropératoire du foie et des voies biliaires. Flammarion, Paris

Bismuth H, Castaing D, Garden O J 1987 The use of operative ultrasound in surgery of primary liver tumors. World Journal of Surgery 11: 610–614

Bodrini G, De Faetano A M, Giovannini I et al 1987 The systematic use of operative ultrasound for detection of liver metastases during colorectal surgery. World Journal of Surgery 11: 622–627

Boutkan H, Luth W, Meyer S, Cuesta M, Van Heuten E, Prevoo W 1992 The impact of intraoperative ultrasonography of the liver on the surgical strategy of patients with gastrointestinal malignancies and hepatic metastases. European Journal of Surgical Oncology 18: 342–346

Brower S T, Dumitrescu O, Rubinoff S et al 1989 Operative ultrasound establishes resectability of metastases by major hepatic resection. World Journal of Surgery 13: 649–657

Castaing D, Edmond J, Kustlinger F, Bismuth H 1986 Utility of operative ultrasound in the surgical management of liver tumors. Annals of Surgery 204: 600–605

Clarke M P, Kane R A, Steele G et al 1989 Prospective comparison of preoperative imaging and intraoperative ultrasonography in the detection of liver tumors. Surgery 106: 849–855

Colombo M, De Franchis R, Del Nino E et al 1991 Hepatocellular carcinoma in Italian patients with cirrhosis. New England Journal of Medicine 325: 675–680

Ekberg H, Tranberg K G, Anderson K et al 1987 Pattern of recurrence in liver resection of colorectal secondaries. World Journal of Surgery 11: 541–547

Franco D, Smadja C, Meakins J L, Berthoux L, Grange D 1989 The operative risk of elective hepatic resection for liver tumors: results of a series of one hundred consecutive hepatectomies in cirrhotic and non cirrhotic patients. Archives of Surgery 124: 1033–1037

Franco D, Capussotti C, Smadja C et al 1990 Resection of hepatocellular carcinoma. Results in 72 European patients with cirrhosis. Gastroenterology 98: 733–738

Gandolfi L, Mazziotti A, Caletti G, Bolondi L, Gozzetti G 1992 The role of gastroenterologist and digestive surgeons in ultrasonography. Italian Journal of Gastroenterology 24: 225–229

Gouillat C, Ben-Hayoun E, Detry L, Berard P 1992 Value of intraoperative ultrasonography in the surgical treatment of malignant tumors. Annales de Chirurgie, Paris 45: 534–539

Gozzetti G, Mazziotti A, Grazi GL 1994 HPB surgery: an independent speciality or a branch of digestive surgery? HPB Surgery 8: 111–113

Gozzetti G, Mazziotti A 1989 Expectations and possibilities of liver resections for metastases. In: Lygidakis N J, Tytgat G N J (eds). Hepatobiliary and pancreatic malignancies. Thieme Verlag, Stuttgart

Gozzetti G, Mazziotti A, Bolondi L et al 1986 Intraoperative ultrasonography in surgery for liver tumors. Surgery 99: 523–529

Gozzetti G, Mazziotti A, Cavallari A et al 1988 Clinical experience with liver resections for hepatocellular carcinoma in patient with cirrhosis. Surgery, Gynecology and Obstetrics 166: 503–510

Gozzetti G, Mazziotti A, Bolondi L, Barbara L 1989 Intraoperative ultrasonography in hepatobiliary and pancreatic surgery. Kluwer, Dordrecht

Gozzetti G, Belli L, Capussotti L et al 1992 Liver resection for hepatocellular carcinoma in cirrhotic patients. Italian Journal of Gastroenterology 24: 105–110

Grazi G L, Mazziotti A, Jovine E, et al 1997 Total vascular exclusion of the liver during hepatic surgery: selective use, extensive use or abuse. Archives of Surgery 132: 1104–1110

Gunven P, Makuuchi M, Hasegawa H et al 1985 Preoperative imaging of liver metastases. Comparison of angiography, CT scan and ultrasonography. Annals of Surgery 202: 573–579

Hasegawa H, Yamazaki S, Makuuchi M, Le Thai B 1988 Nouvelle technique d'hepatectomie utilisant l'echographie perop'ratoire et des aiguilles de repérage intra parenchymateuses. Technique du géometre. Journal de Chirurgie, Paris 125: 593–596

Hughes K S, Simon R, Soughrabodis et al 1986 Resection of the liver for colorectal carcinoma metastases: a multi institutional study of patterns of recurrence. Surgery 100: 278–284

Kasai H, Makuuchi M, Kawasaki S et al 1992 Intraoperative color Doppler ultrasonography for partial-liver transplantation from the living donor in pediatric patients. Transplantation 54: 173–176

Kawasaki S, Makuuchi M, Miyagawa S et al 1996 Extended lateral segmentectomy using intraoperative ultrasound to obtain a partial liver graft. American Journal of Surgery 171: 286–288

Machi J, Isamoto H, Yamashiti Y et al 1987 Intraoperative ultrasonography in screening for liver metastases from colorectal cancer: comparative accuracy with traditional procedures. Surgery 101: 678–684

Magistrelli P, Masetti R, Coppola R, Messia A, Nuzzo G, Picciocchi A 1991 Surgical treatment of hydatid diseases of the liver. A 20 year experience. Archives of Surgery 126: 518–523

Makuuchi M 1987 Abdominal intraoperative ultrasonography. Igaku Shoin, Tokyo

Makuuchi M, Hasegawa H, Yamasaki S 1981 Intraoperative ultrasonic examination for hepatectomy. Japanese Journal of Clinical Oncology 11: 367

Makuuchi M, Hasegawa H, Yamasaki S 1985 Ultrasonically guided subsegmentectomy. Surgery, Gynecology and Obstetrics 161: 346–350

Mazziotti A, Cavallari A. 1997 Techniques in liver surgery, Greenwich Medical Media, London

Nagasue N, Suchio S, Yakaya H 1984 Intraoperative ultrasonography for the surgical treatment of hepatic tumors. Acta Chirurgica Scandinavica 150: 311–316.

Okuda K, Fujimoto I, Hamai A, Urano Y 1987 Changing incidence of hepatocellular carcinoma in Japan. Cancer Research 47: 4967–4972

Olsen A K 1990 Intraoperative ultrasonography and the detection of liver metastases in patient with colorectal cancer. British Journal of Surgery 77: 998–999

Rozycki G S 1998 Surgeon-performed ultrasound: its use in clinical practice. Annals of Surgery 228: 16–28

Sheu J C, Leec S, Sung J L et al 1985 Intraoperative hepatic ultrasonography. An indispensable procedure in resection of small hepatocellular carcinoma. Surgery 97: 97–103

Solomon M J, Stephen M S, White G H, Eyers A A 1992 A new classification of hepatic territories using intraoperative ultrasound. American Journal of Surgery 163: 336–338

Pre- and postoperative care and anesthesia

25

The kidney and the liver: pre- and postoperative factors

N.G. MOSS, M.E.M. ALLISON

'Operations on patients with obstructive jaundice offer three avenues of danger, aside from the so-called accidents of surgery: (1) hemorrhage, (2) uremia, and (3) hepatic insufficiency.'

Walters & Parham 1922

HISTORICAL PERSPECTIVE

For almost 100 years surgeons have approached jaundiced patients with justifiable trepidation. Liver disease per se, and in particular obstructive jaundice, apparently predisposed the sufferer to innumerable postoperative complications, not least of which was death from uremia. The first clear description of this came from two German surgeons, Clairmont and von Haberer, in 1911, who described five previously healthy young women who died with renal failure shortly after cholecystectomy.

By 1938 the correlation had become so well recognized that Ayer could write 'fatal anuria has been observed frequently following operations on the biliary passages.' The cause of this problem exercised the minds of many investigators during the 1920s and 1930s. Definite abnormalities in renal structure and function were documented in clinical and experimental biliary tract obstruction (Wilbur 1934, Stewart & Cantarow 1935, Elsom 1937, Ayer 1938). Bile salts or other potential nephrotoxins originating in the obstructed liver were generally held responsible. Ravdin (1929) and later Shorr et al (1948) believed that specific vasodepressor substances were released from the obstructed liver which could result in profound postoperative shock. This is interesting today in the light of our understanding of endotoxemia (Ch. 9) and the vasodepressor effect of cholemia.

Lassen and Thomson expressed a different view in 1958

when they reported on 30 consecutive patients with obstructive jaundice and renal failure. Most were critically ill with pyrexia and hypotension before the onset of acute renal failure (ARF). It was unnecessary to evoke the presence of 'a mysterious nephrotoxic substance;' their patients had ARF due to shock.

The classic observations of Dawson (1964, 1968) on patients undergoing surgery for obstructive jaundice and on experimental animals reconciled these views. Postoperative ARF occurred more frequently in patients with obstructive jaundice than in nonjaundiced control patients undergoing surgery of comparable magnitude. He suggested that the presence of obstructive jaundice might 'render the kidney more sensitive to decreased blood flow—that is anoxia.'

The terms 'hepatorenal failure' and 'hepatorenal syndrome' are often used to describe any patient with jaundice and renal failure. Unfortunately, these expressions mean 'many things to many people' (Conn 1973) and their use can obscure proper consideration of underlying pathophysiological processes. Initially Helwig and Schutz (1932) used the expression 'hepatorenal failure' to refer to patients who were not necessarily jaundiced but who died with uremia after biliary tract surgery or acute liver injury. Today the phrase should only be used to describe patients with cirrhosis, salt and water retention and terminal renal failure, in whom there is no evidence of prerenal oliguria or established acute tubular necrosis (ATN) (Papper 1983).

Two aspects of liver and kidney function of relevance to the surgeon are considered in this chapter:

1. Obstructive jaundice and renal failure.
2. Chronic cirrhosis of the liver with ascites, sodium retention and renal failure, including the 'hepatorenal syndrome' (HRS).

OBSTRUCTIVE JAUNDICE AND RENAL FAILURE

The incidence of postoperative ARF in jaundiced patients undergoing surgery has apparently changed little in the past 30 years. In 1960 Williams et al reported that uremia occurred in 6% of 350 patients with obstructive jaundice after surgery and was the commonest cause of postoperative death. In Glasgow Royal Infirmary Renal Unit, an analysis of 251 patients treated for established ARF between 1959 and 1970 showed that in 12% renal failure was preceded by biliary tract surgery. 69% of these patients died (Kennedy et al 1973).

Today, despite improvements in anesthesia and perioperative care ARF after biliary tract surgery continues to be a significant problem, involving 6 to 18% of patients and associated with a high mortality rate (Pitt et al 1981, Blamey et al 1983, Armstrong et al 1984, Thompson et al 1987). Table 25.1 shows the fate of 114 patients after operation for liver, biliary tract or pancreatic disease, in a specialized unit in Glasgow Royal Infirmary during 1976. Before surgery 36 were jaundiced and one had renal failure; 78 were nonjaundiced and none of this group had renal failure. All were very ill, half of them having been referred from other hospitals because of complex hepatobiliary problems. Many of them had previously had biliary tract surgery and they were often infected and malnourished. Postoperative shock and ARF was significantly more common in the patients who were jaundiced before surgery and all of the patients who developed ARF died. The combination of liver disease, biliary tract surgery and renal failure is particularly sinister.

Table 25.1 Fate of 114 patients after surgery on liver/biliary tract/pancreas

Preoperative	Number	Postoperative	
		Shock/septicemia	Acute renal failure*
Jaundiced	36	13/36 (36%)	6/36 (17%**)
Nonjaundiced	78	15/78 (19%)	1/78 (1%)

*Mortality rate 100%
**Only one patient had preoperative renal impairment

THE PATHOPHYSIOLOGY OF ACUTE RENAL FAILURE

At a clinical level, the definition of ARF is reasonably clear. Incipient or potential acute renal failure is often seen in the critically ill patient in association with hypotension, hypovolemia and infection. These patients develop prerenal oliguria, which is a normal physiological response to acute hemorrhage, a fall in cardiac output, anesthesia, or surgery itself. Glomerular filtration rate (GFR) falls. There is a marked rise in the secretion of antidiuretic hormone (arginine vasopressin, AVP) and aldosterone, resulting in increased tubular reabsorption of salt and water. The patient with acute circulatory failure and prerenal oliguria thus produces a small volume of concentrated urine, with urine/plasma osmolality ratio greater than 1.05. Tubular reabsorption of urea also increases significantly and hence the plasma urea/creatinine ratio rises. Potential ARF is often reversible if appreciated and dealt with expeditiously (Luke et al 1970), otherwise *established* acute renal failure may rapidly ensue.

Established ARF should be defined simply as a rise in endogenous serum creatinine above normal in a patient with previously good renal function and which persists despite absence or correction of adverse hemodynamic or obstructive factors. Most patients are oliguric but a small number of nonoliguric or high output ARF problems also occur, probably more commonly than is generally recognized. Anderson et al (1977) observed that 54 out of 92 patients with progressive azotemia had urine volumes in excess of 600 ml per day. In 80% the urine volume exceeded 1 liter per day. The morbidity and mortality in this group was lower than in the oliguric patients.

This relatively simple clinical definition of ARF covers a multitude of complex pathophysiological events (Fig. 25.1). A wide variety of animal models have been studied, some of which have little obvious relevance to clinical practice. Two situations of particular interest for those involved with patients who have obstructive jaundice and renal failure are the effects of ischemia and of endotoxemia. Both models have been studied at four levels: whole animal, whole kidney, single nephron and single cell function. Both involve four mechanisms within the kidney itself: renal vasoconstriction, tubular obstruction, a fall in glomerular ultrafiltration coefficient and back leakage of filtrate across damaged tubular cells (Figs 25.1, 25.6). The relative importance of each depends on the precise precipitating cause and changes as the situation evolves.

Ischemic acute renal failure

Two mechanisms have been used to produce acute renal ischemia in experimental animals. Most commonly, the left renal artery is clamped for a varying period of time and then released. Less frequently the effect of systemic hypovolemia, produced by a period of hemorrhage followed by retransfusion, is studied.

As an example of the first situation a severe and reproducible (from rat to rat) model of ischemic ARF can be

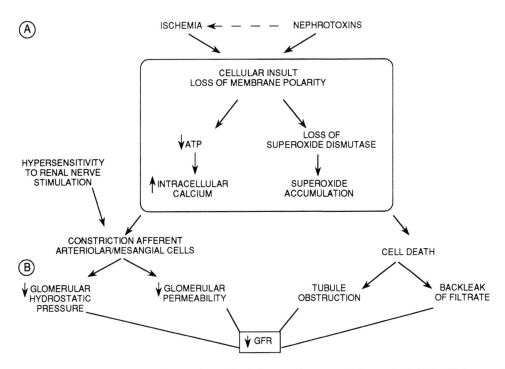

Fig. 25.1 Acute renal failure. **(A)** The onset is due to cellular insult resulting in intrarenal vasoconstriction and cell death. **(B)** Four mechanisms maintain the fall in GFR.

produced in the rat by cross clamping the left renal artery for 1 h. The presence of the contralateral kidney ensures the survival of the animal and allows sequential observations during recovery. In this model the course of renal failure can be divided into three phases: an initial phase, a maintenance phase and an early and late recovery phase. During the initial 24 h after release of the clamp there is a profound fall in urine flow rate, a reduction in GFR to less than 2% of control values and a fall in renal blood flow (RBF) to 20 to 50% of normal. The decrease in GFR, however, is due at this stage not to a fall in glomerular capillary hydrostatic pressure, which is within the normal range, but to tubular obstruction. Restoration of RBF to normal by volume expansion with isotonic sodium chloride does not improve the GFR.

Twenty-four hours later the renal failure is maintained because of a marked fall in glomerular capillary hydrostatic pressure and hence in single nephron filtration rate. This fall in glomerular capillary hydrostatic pressure is due to a marked increase in preglomerular vascular resistance. In addition, there is evidence of back leakage of glomerular filtrate across the damaged tubular epithelium.

Over the following 1–4 weeks recovery occurs in a biphasic manner. First there is regeneration and repair of tubular epithelium with a decrease in transtubular leakage and a loss of intratubular casts. Later there is progressive vasodilata-

tion, a rise in glomerular hydrostatic pressure and a return of GFR towards normal.

The duration of ischemia and the presence or absence of an untouched contralateral kidney is critical to the severity of renal failure. Prolonged ischemia, 2 h or more, leads to irreversible injury while 25 min or less results in only a mild form of renal failure. The degree of recovery of renal function is enhanced in a solitary ischemic kidney as compared to a kidney subjected to a similar episode in the presence of a normally functioning contralateral organ.

Renal ischemia produced by transient hypovolemia is of more relevance to those interested in clinical shock. This is usually produced by bleeding the animal to some predetermined blood pressure for a set period of time and then retransfusing the shed blood. During severe hemorrhagic hypotension there is patchy hypoperfusion of the renal cortex with a fall in RBF and a rise in renal vascular resistance. About 20% of the animals die during this period.

Retransfusion of shed blood in the survivors is followed by a 24-h period of diuresis with loss of urinary concentrating ability. Micropuncture studies have shown this to be due to a fall in reabsorption beyond the proximal convoluted tubule (Tanner & Selkurt 1970).

Very interesting changes take place in cell structure and function during and after ischemia. Studies of cell biology show that, on exposure to anoxia, all cells die in a similar fashion, be they renal tubular cells, cardiac myocytes or hepatocytes. Weinberg (1991) has recently reviewed these in detail (Fig. 25.1A).

Healthy proximal tubule cells are polarized in structural and functional terms, with distinct apical and basolateral membrane domains. Na/K ATPase is limited to the basolateral domain, separated from the apical brush border by a tight junction. Within 15 min of ischemia, half of these tight junctions are lost. Na/K ATPase thus redistributes to the apical membrane with resultant loss of sodium transporting ability (Molitoris 1992).

Early morphological changes involve the mitochondria which first lose their matrix granules, then become condensed and finally appear swollen. Blebs appear on the cell surface and the whole cell appears swollen. Up to this point recovery is still possible if the ischemic insult is removed. Continued anoxia, however, results in disruption of cellular membrane structures and death is inevitable. These structural abnormalities are associated with loss of calcium from the mitochondria into the cell cytoplasm and a significant rise in cytosolic ionized calcium. Membrane pumps are inhibited by the lack of ATP, since oxidative phosphorylation is quickly inhibited in the mitochondria by anoxia. Ion gradients are changed and the cell gains solute and water and hence appears swollen. Restoration of oxygen delivery brings another insult, namely the production of superoxide radicals (Paller et al 1984).

These changes have been described in some detail for two reasons. Firstly, it has been reported that bilirubin and bile salts also impair cellular metabolism and a number of membrane transport systems. Bilirubin can uncouple oxidative phosphorylation in isolated mitochondria, and changes in ultrastructure of glomerular endothelial cells have been described in rats with obstructive jaundice similar to those seen in anoxia (Figs 25.2, 25.3) (Allison et al 1978). Furthermore, Holt et al (1999) found that antioxidants partially reversed renal dysfunction in rats with bile duct obstruction. Thus, it should not be surprising that the changes in intracellular structure and function in cholemia resemble the effects of anoxia on cellular activities. An increased 'sensitivity' of these cells to anoxia might be expected.

Secondly, an understanding of the cellular effects of anoxia has led to the rational use of measures designed to attenuate these changes. Thus, the use of intravenous mannitol, a solute which penetrates cell membranes poorly and hence exerts an osmotic effect, has been shown to be of use clinically when given early during a period of anoxic insult. More recently calcium channel blocking drugs, such as verapamil, have been effective experimentally in animal models of ARF. Free radical scavengers such as superoxide dismu-

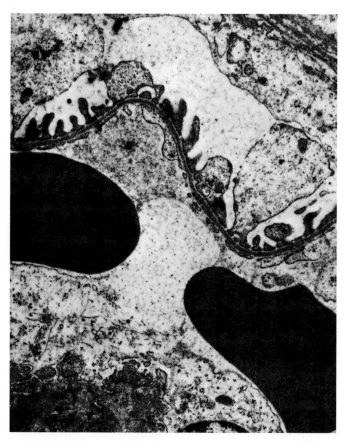

Fig. 25.2 Electron micrograph (original × 17 500) of glomerulus from sham operated control rat. The three layers of the basement membrane are clearly delineated and the epithelial and endothelial cells appear quite normal with no evidence of increased cytoplasmic activity. The normal fenestrated endothelial configuration is clearly visible, as are the epithelial foot processes. From Allison et al 1978.

tase and dimethylthiourea protect against renal failure during reflow after a 60-min period of warm ischemia in the rat (Paller et al 1984). As yet these substances await clinical trial but their use would be based on the results of careful studies of cell biology.

Endotoxin and acute renal failure

'Few, if any, biological substances have such varied effects on so many systems as does endotoxin.'

Nolan 1981

Endotoxins are lipopolysaccharide components of the outer cell membrane of Gram-negative bacteria which are normally present in the gut. They are released on the death of the cell and, if able to reach the circulation, have profound and disastrous effects on cell and organ function (Ch. 9).

The renal effects are summarized in Figure 25.4 (Wardle 1992).

Intense renal vasoconstriction occurs with profound damage to the endothelium and loss of its normal protective role against thrombosis. This may be due to a change in the balance between the production by the endothelial cells of prostacycline, a potent vasodilator and anti-platelet agent, and thromboxane, a most potent platelet aggregator and vasoconstrictor released by platelets. Administration of prostacycline or indomethacin, a prostaglandin synthetase inhibitor, can protect the rat with obstructive jaundice from renal fibrin deposition and death after intravenous endotoxin (Fletcher et al 1982). More importantly, endotoxin can induce excess nitric oxide production by endothelial and smooth muscle cells. This will render the vascular wall insensitive to the action of vasoconstrictors, resulting in profound systemic hypotension and circulatory collapse (Smith et al 1992).

In healthy subjects endotoxin is virtually absent from the peripheral circulation. In obstructive jaundice, however, endotoxemia, as detected by the limulus lysate assay, is found in 50–75% of patients in the preoperative period (Wardle 1975, Bailey 1976). Absence of bile salts, gut anoxia and decreased liver perfusion all contribute to the escape of endotoxin into the circulation. Patients with endotoxemia appear to be at particular risk of ARF. In rat studies Wardle and Wright (1970) showed that a single dose of intravenous endotoxin to an animal with obstructive jaundice produced ARF with intense intrarenal fibrin deposition. Increased endotoxin release in obstructive jaundice may thus lead to low grade disseminated intravascular coagulation. In particular, patients with increased fibrin degradation product levels (FDP) before operation have a poor prognosis (Allison et al 1979). 44% of patients with raised FDP levels died after operation compared with no deaths in those with normal levels of FDP. Renal failure was confined to those with increased levels of FDP.

WHY IS THE PATIENT WITH OBSTRUCTIVE JAUNDICE PARTICULARLY SUSCEPTIBLE TO ACUTE RENAL FAILURE?

Cholemia and liver damage per se are associated with adverse effects on renal structure and function, on circulatory homeostasis and on the integrity of the gastrointestinal barrier. It is scarcely surprising, therefore, that patients with obstructive jaundice have an increased risk of postoperative ARF.

Renal structure

There are well documented abnormalities in renal structure which 60 years ago investigators called 'cholemic nephro-

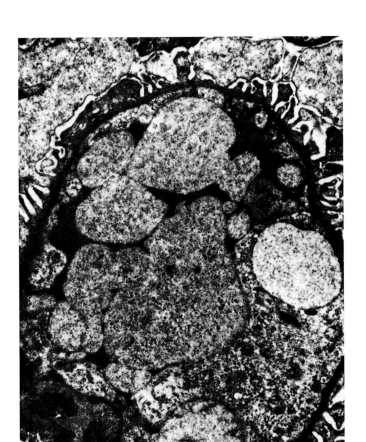

Fig. 25.3 Electron micrograph (original x 17 500) of a glomerulus from a rat with obstructive jaundice. There is an increase in activity of both epithelial and endothelial cells with marked endothelial cell swelling. The basement membrane appears muddy and the three layers are not clearly delineated. From Allison et al 1978.

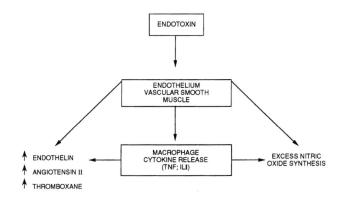

Fig. 25.4 Endotoxin and acute renal failure.

sis.' Light microscopy showed dilated tubules, lined by degenerating cells. Pigment casts were present in the distal convoluted tubule and collecting duct. The patients had albuminuria and there were cellular casts containing bile pigments in the urine.

Electron microscopic studies have confirmed that 'toxic' cellular degenerative changes occur, particularly in the middle segment of the proximal convoluted tubule. Within 12 h of bile duct obstruction in the rat there is an increase in pinocytotic organelles in the subapical cytoplasm of the proximal convoluted tubule cells, presumably due to increased active transport of bile acids. Rats fed a bile acid rich diet show similar changes. Significant changes in glomerular morphology are found in experimental animals with obstructive jaundice, similar to those seen in the human glomerulus in cirrhosis of the liver. Black granules appear in the basement membrane and subendothelial space, together with epithelial foot process fusion and considerable thickening of the basement membrane. We observed marked endothelial cell swelling with loss of the normal fenestrated appearance, a 'muddy' basement membrane and epithelial cell swelling with the presence of inclusion bodies in rats with obstructive jaundice (Figs 25.2, 25.3) (Allison et al 1978).

The mechanism of these changes in cell structure remains unknown despite extensive studies of the noxious effects of bilirubin and bile salts on the integrity of cells in vitro and in vivo. The constituents of bile are potentially nephrotoxic in a number of ways. Bile acids can inhibit ATPase activity, disrupt lysosomes, cause hemolysis and disrupt membranes. As discussed above, bilirubin can uncouple oxidative phosphorylation in mitochondria and decrease cell respiratory rate causing oxidative stress. Unfortunately, the relative toxicity of conjugated as compared to unconjugated bilirubin remains unclear.

Renal function

'The disturbance in renal function incident to jaundice may … become a matter which greatly influences the practical management of patients with biliary obstruction; hence its degree and course should be carefully assessed.'

Elsom 1937

There are numerous descriptions of impaired kidney function in association with obstructive jaundice per se, in the absence of any surgical insult. As many as 30% of patients with obstructive jaundice have been found to have a significant decrease in creatinine clearance before operation (McPherson et al 1982a). Preoperative acute renal failure has been found especially in the presence of cholangitis and sepsis (Sorenson et al 1971, Bismuth et al 1975).

We found an impairment in urinary concentrating ability in 24 patients with obstructive jaundice before surgery (Allison et al 1979). The mean GFR for the group as a whole was not different from controls. However, there was a small subgroup (5 of 24) in whom GFR was significantly reduced. After operation, three of these five subjects had significant renal failure.

In an important recent retrospective analysis aimed at defining the natural history of renal failure in obstructive jaundice Sitprija and colleagues in Thailand observed that renal impairment preceded operation in 64 out of 130 patients (49%) (Mairiang et al 1990). All patients had cholangiocarcinoma, none had been exposed to a known nephrotoxic agent, but all had been jaundiced for, on average, 40 days. Renal failure was nonoliguric in 80% and associated with severe jaundice, hypotension, hyponatremia and hypokalemia (Mairiang et al 1990).

More precise studies of renal function have been made in rats, dogs, rabbits and baboons. Unfortunately there is great variability in the effects of chronic bile duct ligation in different species making direct comparison difficult.

The general consensus of opinion can be summarized as follows (Better 1983): firstly, most investigators have found a fall in total RBF, particularly outer cortical blood flow. Indeed, medullary flow has been shown to rise and this has been used as an explanation for the fall in renal concentrating ability found in obstructive jaundice. This decrease in RBF could be due to an increased sensitivity of the renal vasculature to catecholamines, as shown both in vivo and in vitro (Bomzon & Kew 1983). As yet the factor or factors responsible for this remain speculative, but it would appear to involve stimulation of α adrenergic receptors and seems to be associated with the rise in the β lipoprotein fraction found in obstructive jaundice.

Secondly, in contrast to the significant decrease seen in RBF, whole kidney and superficial single nephron GFR are normal.

Thirdly, urinary concentrating ability is significantly decreased.

Finally, salt retention is rare in obstructive jaundice. Indeed, Alon et al (1982) have shown that the intrarenal infusion of diluted bile or bile acids, but not bilirubin, produces a diuresis and natriuresis in animals. Hence patients with obstructive jaundice may be especially vulnerable to salt and water depletion.

Circulatory homeostasis

Patients with obstructive jaundice seem more likely to develop hemorrhagic hypotension during surgery than nonjaundiced subjects. This decreased tolerance to even small volumes of blood loss can be demonstrated in the experimental animal. Thus a large and sometimes fatal fall in arterial blood pressure in the jaundiced rat could be precipitated by loss of only 10% of blood volume (Aarseth et al 1979). We found that 40% of rats with obstructive jaundice became hypotensive and died during routine surgery in preparation for kidney micropuncture studies (Allison et al 1978). The vasodepressor effects of cholemia per se have been extensively examined and are summarized in Figure 25.5 (Green et al 1984).

Theoretically, hypotension could result from a change in one or more of four primary factors: cardiac output, left ventricular performance, total plasma volume and its distribution between the splanchnic and systemic vascular beds and peripheral resistance. A significant fall in peripheral resistance and hence in arterial blood pressure is found when cholemia is produced either by ligation of the common bile duct or by diversion of the bile duct to the inferior vena cava. In addition, there is a redistribution of the total blood volume with trapping of blood in the splanchnic circulation in obstructive jaundice. Effective blood volume is thus reduced.

Cardiac output appears to be relatively unchanged in obstructive jaundice. Acute blood loss, however, results in a more marked fall in cardiac output with delayed recovery than that seen in control animals. The constituents of bile, in particular bile acids, have a cardiodepressor activity on left ventricular function. The precise factor or factors responsible for this remain speculative.

Integrity of the gastrointestinal barrier

The normal intestine and hepatobiliary system form a very efficient barrier against enteric pathogens, including endotoxins. Obstructive jaundice greatly reduces the efficacy of this barrier, putting the sufferer at increased risk of perioperative endotoxemia and multi-organ failure.

Bile salts, sodium taurocholate and deoxycholate act as surfactants and disrupt endotoxin, both in vitro and in vivo. In obstructive jaundice this important action of bile salts is lost, resulting in excessive endotoxin being absorbed into the portal blood system. This observation was first made in 1966 (Rudbach et al 1966) but only recently has its practical potential been appreciated and investigated (Bailey 1976, Evans et al 1982). However, no benefit in terms of systemic endotoxemia, renal function or mortality was found in a prospective, randomly allocated study of preoperative ursodeoxycholic acid in obstructive jaundice (Thompson et al 1986).

It is well recognized that liver disease is associated with a progressive decrease in the reticulo-endothelial phagocytic capacity of the Küpffer cell system. Approximately 50% of patients with obstructive jaundice can be shown to have a

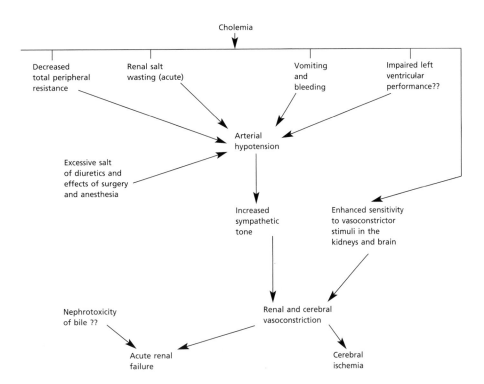

Fig. 25.5 Pathogenesis of arterial hypertension and renal failure in cholemia. From Green et al 1984.

decrease in the clearance of microaggregated iodinated human albumin (Drivas et al 1976) or of Tc-labelled sulphur colloid (Ingoldby 1983) indicating impaired reticulo-endothelial activity. These patients are especially at risk of developing postoperative endotoxemia. Tragically, endotoxins can themselves further suppress reticulo-endothelial cell activity and the function of hepatocytes, thus prolonging their active life. These changes have been attributed to a combination of the noxious metabolic effects of conjugated bilirubin, the detergent action of bile acids retained in the liver and to poor liver perfusion. Maintenance of normal liver blood flow therefore forms the third factor in the defense mechanisms of the gut and hepatobiliary tree. In all forms of surgery, good liver perfusion and freedom from hepatocellular anoxia are well recognized prerequisites for health. In 1946 it was shown that death from hemorrhagic shock in dogs could be prevented only if liver blood flow, and hence oxygen delivery, to the liver cells was maintained during bleeding (Frank et al 1946). Unfortunately, the effect of obstructive jaundice per se on liver blood flow in the human is unknown but in experimental animals liver blood flow has been shown to decrease at least in the early stages of biliary tract obstruction (Ch. 7). What is most important is that surgery and anesthesia can be associated with a significant fall in liver perfusion in the human (Gelman 1976).

There are two reasons why this might be especially important in patients with obstructive jaundice. The first is that liver anoxia could result in a further decrease in the clearance of endotoxin from portal blood. Secondly, the liver normally plays a crucial role in the removal of lactate from the extracellular fluid. Lactic acid, formed from pyruvate as the end product of anaerobic glycolysis in skeletal muscle, gut, brain, skin and red blood cells, is removed via gluconeogenesis in the liver (approximately 60%) and kidney (approximately 30%) (Park & Arieff 1981). Decreased lactate clearance is found in some types of liver disease and surgery or anesthesia will presumably further decrease clearance, resulting in profound metabolic acidosis.

WHICH PATIENTS ARE PARTICULARLY AT RISK?

Rapid identification of high-risk patients with obstructive jaundice is an essential prerequisite for good surgical management. Uncontrolled observations on small numbers of patients have suggested that the general risk factors for surgery such as advancing age, hypoalbuminemia, poor renal function, infection and weight loss are important (Allison et al 1979).

Statistical evaluation of risk factors measured in large numbers of patients undergoing biliary tract surgery have now been reported. Dixon et al (1983) studied 373 patients with obstructive jaundice and reported that a high plasma bilirubin (> 200 μmol/L), a low hematocrit and malignant disease were important independent risk factors for postoperative mortality. Both Pitt et al (1981) and Blamey et al (1983) found eight clinical and laboratory factors preoperatively which correlated significantly with postoperative mortality. Seven of the eight factors were common to both studies: malignant disease, age over 60 years, hematocrit less than 30%, albumin less than 30 g/L, white blood count greater than 10 000 per mm^3, hyperbilirubinemia and a raised serum alkaline phosphatase. A major difference between the two was in the statistical significance of a raised preoperative serum creatinine, which in the study of Pitt et al did not reach statistical significance. Blamey et al (1983) found it to be a factor of major prognostic importance. This is especially curious since renal failure was the commonest postoperative complication observed by Pitt et al (1981), accounting for 18% of total morbidity, and Bilbao et al (1998) and Lafayette et al (1997) have recently determined that renal dysfunction prior to orthotopic liver transplantation is strongly correlated with greater postoperative morbidity and mortality. This danger may be particularly acute in pediatric cases in which impaired renal function prior to surgery may exacerbate a predisposition in these patients for renal failure following liver transplantation (Bartosh et al 1997).

Linear discriminant analysis by Blamey et al (1983) further showed that serum creatinine and serum albumin in the week before surgery had independent significance in predicting mortality. Postoperative ARF occurred as a complication in 8% of their patients, especially when there was pre-existing renal impairment but also in association with hyperbilirubinemia, hypoalbuminemia, diabetes mellitus or malignancy.

McPherson et al (1982b) have suggested that measurement of antipyrine half-life might help in selecting high-risk patients with obstructive jaundice. This may well prove to be a useful measure of the hepatic deficit accompanying obstructive jaundice and of the rate of recovery, but further substantiation is required.

PREVENTION/AMELIORATION OF ACUTE POSTOPERATIVE RENAL FAILURE

Table 25.2 outlines the methods currently advised for the peroperative management of patients with obstructive jaundice.

Table 25.2 Preoperative management of patients with obstructive jaundice

General	Avoid prolonged hyperbilirubinemia
	Treat known infection, especially cholangitis
	Use aminoglycosides carefully
	Avoid prerenal failure
	Correct anemia, coagulation defects, hypoalbuminemia
	Avoid all NSAID*
Specific	IV saline and mannitol pre- and postoperatively
	Maintain good liver perfusion at surgery
No conclusive evidence for:	
Preoperative percutaneous biliary drainage	
Gut sterilization	
Polymyxin B	
Oral bile salts	

*Nonsteroidal anti-inflammatory drugs

Avoid delay

An impressive array of laboratory tests (Ch. 21) are available which enable prompt and precise diagnosis. Delay in investigation should not occur since it is recognized that the prognosis deteriorates as the depth and duration of the jaundice increases. Attention should be focused on sepsis and pre-existing renal impairment as the two most important associated problems, especially in the high risk group with raised serum creatinine concentration and a low serum albumin concentration.

Assess renal function

Renal function is best assessed simply by the measurement of serum creatinine concentration on 2 or 3 consecutive days. Hyperbilirubinemia and obstructive jaundice per se do not interfere with the measurement of creatinine by the Jaffe reaction (M. Smith, personal communication). Measurement of creatinine clearance, involving 24-h urine collections, is unnecessary and in any case usually notoriously inaccurate in clinical practice. Serum creatinine concentration should accurately reflect GFR in the absence of significant muscle breakdown. On the other hand, blood urea will not accurately reflect kidney function, since urea production is altered by liver disease and infection.

Treat infection

Infection of the biliary tree usually occurs in association with cholelithiasis or after previous biliary tract surgery (Ch. 8). About 10% of these patients develop ARF (Bismuth et al 1975). Our practise is to give all patients an aminoglycoside (e.g. netilimicin, 100 mg i.v.) just before any invasive pro-

cedure, together with metronidazole 1 g rectally. If the patient is pyrexial this is continued postoperatively. Peak and trough aminoglycoside levels should be monitored daily and the dose adjusted to keep peak levels between 5 and 10 mg/L and trough levels between 2 and 3 mg/L. In renal impairment aminoglycoside dosages must be greatly reduced and in those patients with a severe deficit in renal function who are dialysis dependent as little as 40 mg i.v. after each dialysis may be sufficient.

Correct prerenal deficits

Patients with obstructive jaundice are often elderly and malnourished. They tolerate anoxia, hypovolemia and hypotension poorly. Careful assessment of fluid balance should be made with measurement of central venous pressure before and for 2–3 days after surgery. The presence or absence of edema and serum albumin concentration should be noted. A serum albumin concentration less than 30 g/L in association with diminished skin turgor generally denotes significant volume depletion. Before any invasive procedure patients should have their volume defects corrected by the use of appropriate intravenous fluids. Plasma protein solution is useful to correct protein and salt deficiency. Concentrated albumin is available to increase albumin concentration to greater than 30 g/L when there is a danger of fluid overload. Hemoglobin should be 10 g/dL or greater.

All patients are empirically given vitamin K before surgery but a routine coagulation screen may detect other defects. The finding of diffuse intravascular coagulation carries an especially bad prognosis since it is generally associated with bacteremia and endotoxemia.

Avoid dangerous drugs

All nonsteroidal anti-inflammatory drugs (NSAID) should be stopped. They impair renal prostaglandin synthesis and can precipitate ARF especially in the elderly, hypovolemic and anoxic patient. Prostaglandins are required for the maintenance of intrarenal blood flow when this is threatened by hypovolemia and its associated increase in AVP (Yared et al 1985). In addition, NSAID can themselves produce acute interstitial nephritis and renal failure.

Mannitol and saline

Mannitol is a simple sugar, molecular weight 182. When given intravenously it is not metabolized but is freely filtered by the glomeruli into the tubular fluid where it acts as an osmotic diuretic. Intravenous mannitol in healthy individuals results in a profound diuresis and natriuresis.

The protective effect of mannitol in the ischemic kidney was first noted by Selkurt in 1945 and studied in more depth by Barry and Malloy in 1962 and by Eliahou in 1964. To date it remains the best substance available for the prophylaxis of ischemic ARF.

In the 1960s Dawson reasoned that since renal ischemia seemed particularly dangerous to patients with obstructive jaundice mannitol should be especially useful. He went on to demonstrate that this was indeed so. Patients with obstructive jaundice were given a constant infusion of 10% mannitol, equivalent to 50 g for 2 h before surgery. After surgery 10% mannitol infusion was continued to maintain a urine flow rate greater than 60 ml/h. He was thus able to prevent a postoperative fall in GFR.

There are four good theoretical reasons why mannitol could be effective. Firstly, it is an osmotic diuretic and by increasing tubule flow rate should flush out tubular casts and debris. Secondly, and the more importantly, it increases RBF even during hypotension. This is shown by the rise in partial pressure of oxygen found in the urine during mannitol infusion. Thirdly, it appears to prevent the endothelial cell swelling which occurs during ischemia, thus stopping the 'no reflow phenomenon' (Flores et al 1972). Finally, mannitol appears to be an effective hydroxyl radical scavenger. This is a fascinating observation in view of the recent recognition of the damaging effects of free radicals on cell function (Paller et al 1984).

Twenty years of clinical experience have established that renal function can be well maintained in patients with obstructive jaundice provided that adequate intravenous fluids and mannitol are given. Our practise is to give a bolus of 20 g (100 ml of 20% mannitol) 2 h before operation and again during anesthesia. All jaundiced patients are catheterized so that hourly urine volumes can be monitored. After operation 20 g mannitol is repeated if the urine flow rate falls to less than 50 ml/h on two successive occasions. Adequate intravenous saline must also be given because a marked natriuresis is seen during the two or three immediate postoperative days when mannitol is being used (Allison et al 1979). Indeed, a recent prospective, randomly allocated study on the role of mannitol has suggested that i.v. fluids are just as important. Mannitol per se did not improve postoperative renal function in jaundiced patients (Gubern et al 1988).

Injudicious overindulgence in mannitol might result in excessive intravascular volume expansion, hyponatremia and intracellular dehydration. During anuria 200 g mannitol given intravenously could theoretically expand the extracellular space by 2 L. One anuric patient given a total of 300 g mannitol over 24 h did become semicomatose with a serum sodium of only 96 mmol/L (Feldman et al 1971).

However, 20 g mannitol repeated up to five times over a 24-h period in a patient with some renal function is innocuous and should be used as the drug of first choice.

Anxiety over mannitol led to the use of the diuretics frusemide and ethacrynic acid to improve renal function in potential ARF. Even the most oliguric patient will respond to high dose loop diuretics with a few extra milliliters of urine, irrespective of the cause of their problem. Theoretically a rise in intratubular flow might help flush out casts and debris, as after mannitol. More importantly, loop diuretics, by inhibiting luminal sodium chloride transport will reduce the energy requirements of the cells of the thick ascending limb of Henle, perhaps helping them to resist hypoxia.

There is no convincing evidence, however, from clinical studies that loop diuretics per se, are of significant benefit. In particular, there are no studies devoted to jaundiced patients with renal failure. Attention to maintenance of intravascular volume and oxygen delivery should take precedence in the preoperative management of these patients.

Carcoana and Hines (1996) have recently reviewed the use of low dose dopamine infusion for the support of renal function and concluded that there is good evidence in its favour. For example, Henderson et al (1980) reported that dopamine infusion at a rate of 12 μg/kg body weight per min in the early stages of incipient ARF produced a rise in RBF and determined that it should be administered when hourly urine volumes are less than 50 ml/h on two successive occasions. Large inotropic doses of dopamine or dobutamine sometimes have to be used to sustain blood pressure but will have little beneficial effect on RBF.

PREOPERATIVE PERCUTANEOUS BILIARY DRAINAGE

It might seem logical to suppose that preoperative biliary decompression (Molnar & Stockum 1974) should improve the prospects for later definitive surgery especially in high-risk patients.

Initial results seemed favorable. The technique was described as being relatively safe, simple and, for the high risk patient, resulted in improved kidney function and better nutritional status.

Well-controlled clinical trials of external biliary drainage have failed to substantiate these claims (Hatfield et al 1982, McPherson et al 1984, Pitt et al 1985). Sepsis has proved to be a major problem when using external drainage although this can be overcome by careful attention to technique. The only objective improvement seems to be a significant fall in bilirubin. Although overall renal function in terms of creatinine clearance improved this was also seen in the control group treated by simple rehydration alone prior to definitive surgery. All these studies failed to demonstrate a decrease in mortality by the use of this technique. It is possible that preoperative internal biliary drainage may be more effective in preventing renal failure (Smith et al 1985) but this remains to be proven in a large trial.

THE MANAGEMENT OF ESTABLISHED ACUTE RENAL FAILURE

Preoperative ARF

A small number of patients with cholangitis, sepsis and obstructive jaundice will develop acute renal insufficiency (Bismuth et al 1975). The management of these patients is especially critical. They should be resuscitated with fluid replacement, correct antibiotics and, if necessary, dialysis before definitive surgery. The timing of the operation is determined by the evolution of the sepsis. Death from renal insufficiency may be prevented by adequate dialysis until postoperative renal recovery occurs.

Postoperative ARF

This is more difficult to manage since the patient has been the subject of a surgical insult and often has multiorgan failure. In general, such patients are best managed by a team of experts in an intensive care environment. Established ARF should always be considered to be potentially reversible since, should the patient survive the other problems, renal function will usually recover. The principles of management are quite simple: control fluid balance, control electrolytes, especially potassium, provide adequate calories and amino acids and watch closely for developing complications. No patient should be allowed to die of uremia, electrolyte imbalance or starvation. Dialysis can be carried out either by the use of an external semi-permeable membrane (hemodialysis) or across the peritoneal membrane. Peritoneal dialysis is often neither feasible nor desirable in a patient recovering from surgery for obstructive jaundice and will not be considered further.

Hemodialysis is generally carried out by the use of cellulosic-based membranes such as cupraphane. In classic hemodialysis substances with a molecular weight less than 1000 Daltons will pass across such a semipermeable membrane quite freely, diffusing from an area of high concentration to an area of low concentration. Thus urea and creatinine, present in the blood in high concentrations in uremia, will diffuse down a concentration gradient into the dialysate which bathes the membrane. The passage of water

occurs by convection, necessitating a relatively high transmembrane hydrostatic pressure gradient. Water removal by cellulosic-based membranes is thus limited and pressure dependent.

Recently exciting advances have been made in membrane technology. Highly permeable membranes, chiefly polysulphone and polyacrilonitrile membranes have appeared. They allow the free passage of substances up to a molecular weight of approximately 5000 Daltons. Considerable passage still occurs up to a molecular weight of 50 000 Daltons. They are very permeable to water and only a small transmembrane pressure gradient results in a large flux of water. The permeability characteristics of these membranes are therefore similar to those of the glomerular basement membrane complex and they have been termed the 'artificial glomerulus.' Such membranes can be used to produce a pure ultrafiltrate of plasma simply by the hydrostatic pressure of the arterial blood. This is known as hemofiltration. Up to 20 L of ultrafiltrate can be removed from the plasma over a 24-h period, thus keeping the concentration of blood urea etc. relatively constant. Replacement fluids must be given simultaneously to prevent loss of essential plasma electrolytes.

By combining simple ultrafiltration with dialysis (hemodiafiltration) one can use these membranes continuously to give smooth control of extracellular fluid composition over 3–6 weeks in patients with ARF. In addition, use of these membranes results in the removal of substances with molecular weights between 1000 and 5000 Daltons, an attribute of considerable theoretical interest to those involved in the management of patients with hepatic failure (Ch. 92).

RENAL FUNCTION IN CIRRHOSIS OF THE LIVER

'It is not the purpose of this article to review in its entirety the abundant literature ... but rather to attempt an appraisal and interpretation of some of the available information pertinent to Laennec's Cirrhosis of the Liver.'

Papper 1958

A vast multitude of clinical and experimental studies on the role of the kidney in cirrhosis of the liver have appeared over the past 100 years. Interested readers are referred to several excellent reviews (Papper 1958, Epstein 1983a, b, Papper 1983, Levensen et al 1983, Levinsky 1983, Gentilini et al 1990, Levy 1992, Davison 1996). The treatment of these conditions has recently been well reviewed by Epstein (1984).

Three aspects will be considered:

1. The nature of the renal problem in cirrhosis.
2. Renal failure in advanced cirrhosis.
3. Management of renal failure in cirrhosis.

1. RENAL STRUCTURE AND FUNCTION IN CIRRHOSIS

Renal structure

'The morbid alteration of the kidney, known to the name of Bright's disease, frequently accompanies cirrhosis, having been met with 15 times in 42 cases.'

Becquerel 1840

Despite this bold statement made over 100 years ago, attempts to correlate glomerular structure and function in cirrhosis of the liver have, until recently, been notoriously disappointing. For decades light microscopists examined autopsy material and considered degeneration of tubule cells to be the outstanding renal lesion. The recent introduction of electron microscopy and immunofluorescent techniques to examine renal biopsy material has yielded fascinating information. Significant glomerular abnormalities are present in over 95% of 116 renal biopsies examined by various authors (Eknoyan 1983). There is an increase in mesangial matrix, irregular thickening of the capillary basement membrane and occasionally pronounced glomerulosclerosis. Sakaguchi et al (1965) coined the term 'hepatic glomerulosclerosis' to describe these changes, since they were seen in a wide variety of liver diseases irrespective of the nature, duration or severity of the condition. Two distinct forms can be described. The first, a nonproliferative form, is associated with mesangial deposits of IgA. Patients usually do not have proteinuria. The second and more severe proliferative form shows both endothelial and epithelial cellular proliferation and intramembranous deposits of IgA. Patients often have pronounced proteinuria and hematuria. Hypocomplimentemia and cryoglobulinemia have been described in patients with cirrhosis.

Unfortunately, few studies have attempted to correlate these abnormalities in structure with functional changes. Indeed, Eknoyan (1983) in a recent review states that 'the glomerular lesions are accompanied by neither clinical manifestations nor biochemical abnormalities indicating renal dysfunction.' Detailed sequential studies correlating renal structure and function in cirrhosis of the liver are needed.

An interesting observation concerning the pathogenesis of renal failure in patients with liver disease has been made by histopathologists. Lecithin:cholesterol acyltransferase (LCAT) is an enzyme, made in the liver, which is responsible for the esterification of plasma cholesterol. Familial deficiency of the enzyme is associated with the appearance of unesterified cholesterol-rich lipoprotein in the plasma. A major problem for these sufferers is renal failure. Their glomeruli show deposition of cholesterol and phospholipids in the glomerular basement membrane, in the mesangium and significantly in the subendothelial space. These changes will develop within 5–6 months of the transplantation of a healthy kidney into a sufferer.

In 1978 Hovig et al found low plasma LCAT activity in patients with cirrhosis of the liver and renal failure. Theoretically, endothelial-cell swelling and damage due to these structures could result in a decreased ability of the cells to produce prostacycline or other cytoprotective vasoactive agents in response to stress. It should be remembered that endothelial cell swelling and damage is also a histological feature in animals with experimental biliary tract obstruction (Figs 25.2, 25.3).

Renal function

It is well established that cirrhosis of the liver is associated with a profound but variable degree of salt and water retention. Indeed, at times these patients can excrete urine which is almost free of sodium. Since this can occur when the glomerular filtration rate, and hence the filtered load of sodium, is normal or only slightly decreased, these patients must have a very significant rise in the tubular reabsorption of sodium. In 1977 Lopez-Novoa et al were able to confirm significant increased proximal reabsorption in the nephrons of rats with chronic cirrhosis by the use of kidney micropuncture techniques. The normal circadian rhythm for sodium excretion is changed, nocturnal sodium loss being increased in comparison to the reverse in normal subjects. In some patients the ability to excrete a water load is diminished, those with ascites and edema being particularly affected.

Recent studies (Naccarato et al 1981) have shown that increased tubular reabsorption of sodium can be found very early in the evolution of cirrhosis and pre-date the development of ascites. Levy and colleagues have described two phases in fluid retention. In the early or first phase (Unikowsky et al 1983) sodium retention may be the result of stimulation of a stretch receptor or a low pressure baroreceptor within the liver. Early intrahepatic hypertension would cause reflex stimulation of sympathetic nerves and increased tubular sodium reabsorption. This early first phase occurs before ascites formation and is associated with expansion of plasma volume. This is also associated with an attenuated renal response to atrial natriuretic factor which may contribute to salt retention (Levy 1997).

Later ascites develops, effective arterial blood volume decreases and plasma renin, aldosterone and estrogen concentrations rise. Increased tubular reabsorption of sodium continues and such patients are often unable to excrete a water load. They have dilutional hyponatremia.

Recent evidence points to an important contribution by endothelium derived relaxant factor (EDRF or NO) in the development of salt and water retention (reviewed by Martin et al 1998a). Constitutive NO production may be increased in cirrhosis (Bosch-Marce et al 1998) and inhibition of NO synthase prevents salt and water retention in cirrhotic rats (Martin et al 1998b). This effect appears to be a complex interaction in which increased renal perfusion pressure and a decreased tubular responsiveness to antidiuretic hormone (ADH) reverse the salt retaining state.

The precise pathophysiological mechanisms in ascites are still the subject of considerable research and have been discussed elsewhere (Ch. 94).

2. RENAL FAILURE IN ADVANCED CIRRHOSIS

Renal failure is distressingly common in cirrhosis of the liver, being found at some time in 50 to 75% of sufferers (Wilkinson et al 1975). Uremia has been described as the commonest extrahepatic cause of death in these patients (Clermont et al 1967). In many instances renal failure is due to prerenal deficits and/or ATN. In some, however, there is no obvious cause for renal failure and these patients are described as having 'the hepatorenal syndrome.' This has been defined by Papper (1983) as 'incompletely explained renal failure in patients with liver disease in the absence of clinical, laboratory or other known cause of renal failure.' Patients with HRS are often in the terminal stages of liver failure and the mortality rate is extremely high, although spontaneous recovery has been reported.

Table 25.3 contrasts the clinical and laboratory features of the three forms of renal failure which are found in cirrhosis of the liver. In both prerenal oliguria and in established ATN a clear precipitating event is usually obvious, with acute circulatory failure, infection or exposure to nephrotoxins. The patients need not necessarily have ascites. Prerenal oliguria is further characterized by a high urine/plasma osmolality ratio and a low urinary sodium excretion, indicating relatively intact tubular function. Replacement of measurement deficits with or without the addition of dopamine or mannitol is generally successful in correcting the oliguria, provided that the initiating events are under control. In established ATN, tubular function is lost, with a fall in the urine/plasma osmolality ratio to 1 or less and a high urinary sodium loss. Once tubular cell death has occurred volume expansion will not improve oliguria.

Table 25.3 Differential diagnosis of oliguria in cirrhosis

	Prerenal	ATN (established)	HRS
Clinical features	Associated with acute hypotension, hypovolemia, infection	Follows prerenal or nephrotoxins	Minor degree of salt/water depletion or hypotension, slow to develop
Urine sodium mmol/L	< 10	> 50	< 10 initially
Urine: plasma osmolality (no diuretics)	> 1.05	1 or less	> 1.05 initially
Response to volume expansion ± dopamine, mannitol	yes	no	no

These points have been covered in the first section of this chapter.

The HRS is therefore a clinical diagnosis of exclusion. Those at risk are generally in hospital, suffering from alcoholic cirrhosis with portal hypertension, are usually jaundiced and have moderate to severe ascites. They may be relatively hypotensive but not clinically shocked. Almost all have dilutional hyponatremia and the majority have hypoalbuminemia. Interestingly, a sense of false security may result from the presence of normal serum creatinine concentrations in these patients as measurement of GFR by insulin clearance has shown this to be significantly reduced in many patients with advanced cirrhosis and ascites (Papadakis & Arieff 1984). They conclude that HRS may represent only a slight deterioration in function in an already compromised kidney. Initially, tubular function is well maintained with a high urine/plasma osmolality ratio and a low urine sodium concentration. Unlike prerenal oliguria, however, volume expansion, whilst it may produce a very small and temporary improvement in renal function, has no long lasting beneficial effects.

Pathophysiology of HRS

Many factors present in cirrhosis of the liver may predispose the sufferer to both prerenal oliguria and HRS. Some of these, such as the noxious effects of cholemia and endotoxemia have already been discussed in the section on obstructive jaundice.

The hallmark of renal function in cirrhosis of the liver is vascular instability, with active cortical vasoconstriction. This was beautifully demonstrated in 1970 by Epstein et al using the [133]xenon washout technique and selective renal arteriography to study renal blood flow and its distribution in 15 patients with cirrhosis of the liver and differing renal function. In cirrhotic patients with renal failure there was marked variability and irregularity of xenon washout, in contrast to other patients without liver disease but with renal failure. Blood flow through the outer cortical compartment decreased in approximate proportion to the decrease in creatinine clearance.

The dynamics of forces normally governing glomerular ultrafiltration are now the subject of intense scrutiny. Each nephron's glomerular filtration rate is determined by the balance of hydrostatic and oncotic forces acting across the capillary bed together with the permeability and surface area of the capillary available for filtration, Kf (Fig. 25.6). High affinity glomerular receptors for vasoactive agents, such as angiotensin II, norepinephrine, endothelin, AVP, PGE_2, PGI_2, thromboxane A2, acetylcholine, bradykinin, histamine, dopamine and serotonin have been described (Dworkin & Brenner 1985). It is likely that a nice balance normally exists between intrinsic renal vascular tone, determined by AVP, prostaglandins and angiotensin II, and extrarenal vascular tone dependent on sympathetic nerves and cardiac output.

In cirrhosis of the liver, however, there may be a grave imbalance between renal vasoconstrictive mechanisms (e.g. AVP, angiotensin II, sympathetic nerve activity) and vasodilatory mechanisms (e.g. PGE_2, PGI_2, bradykinin). This is outlined in Figure 25.7. As a result there is variable renal cortical ischemia and loss of the protective mechanisms normally at work to maintain GFR in the face of systemic hypotension and hypovolemia. The evidence for this can be summarized as follows.

Firstly, immunoreactive circulating AVP is high in cirrhosis. This is due partly to an increased half-life but also to increased secretion due to a re-setting of normal osmoreceptor control. Exogenous AVP is a potent renal and systemic vasoconstrictor agent. Most important, AVP can also decrease GFR by decreasing glomerular capillary hydraulic permeability, Kf.

Secondly, renal PGE_2 production is increased in cirrhosis of the liver. This can be considered to be a compensatory adaptation to balance the renal vasoconstrictor effects of AVP and is linked to increased phospholipase A_2 (PLA_2) levels in cirrhosis (Niederberger et al 1998). In advanced cirrhosis, however, or after administration of NSAID, renal PGE_2 release decreases. These drugs can cause a significant fall in GFR and renal plasma flow in patients with alcoholic liver disease. There is also evidence that glomerular thromboxane release may be increased in HRS, causing a fall in Kf.

Thirdly, the renin–angiotensin system is activated in cir-

$$\mathrm{sng\,fr} = Kf\left(\bar{P}_{GC} - P_T\right) - \left(\bar{\Pi}_{GC} - \Pi_T\right)$$

Fig. 25.6 The factors determining the rate of ultrafiltration in a single glomerulus.
Sngfr: Single nephron glomerular filtration rate.
Kf: Glomerular capillary permeability, determined by local effective hydraulic permeability and the surface area available for filtration. Reduced by contraction of mesangial cells.
$\bar{P}_{GC}$: Mean hydraulic pressure within glomerular capillary, determined by efferent/afferent arteriolar constriction and systemic blood pressure.
P_T: Mean hydraulic pressure in Bowman's space.
$\bar{\pi}_{GC}$: Mean oncotic pressure within glomerular capillary, determined by plasma albumin concentration and glomerular filtration rate. Oncotic pressure rises exponentially with filtration.
π_T: Oncotic pressure within Bowman's space (negligible).

rhosis with ascites (Ibara et al 1998), with a marked rise in plasma renin levels. Indeed, these patients may be dependent on angiotensin II to maintain systemic blood pressure, administration of converting enzyme inhibitors resulting in profound hypotension. Unfortunately, angiotensin II can also cause renal afferent arteriolar vasoconstriction and a decrease in Kf, resulting in a fall in GFR.

Activation of the sympathetic nervous system may play an important role (DiBona & Sawin 1991). Animal studies have shown the existence of both a hepato-renal reflex and a splanchno-renal reflex which serve to decrease renal nerve activity in response to increased circulating volume or increased sodium intake. This mechanism may be defective in cirrhosis as Matsuda et al (1996) showed that the reflex inhibition in renal nerve activity that follows increased sodium intake is absent in dogs with bile duct ligation. This is consistent with observations of elevated plasma norepinephrine levels in patients with decompensated cirrhosis which correlate significantly with decreased RBF and sodium retention. In this case increased sympathetic nerve activity is believed to produce both renal vasoconstriction and an increase in sodium reabsorption from the proximal tubule (Moss et al 1992). The precise mechanisms for activation remain speculative, but could involve baroreceptors in the liver and portal vein.

Recently, attention has focused on the role of the endothelial cell as the source of two potent, but opposing, locally acting hormones, endothelin and nitric oxide. Patients with HRS have markedly elevated plasma endothelin 1 and 3 concentrations as compared to patients with acute or chronic renal failure or with liver disease alone (Moore et al 1992). When formed by glomerular endothelial cells these peptides bind to local specific receptors on mesangial cells. Mesangial contraction results in a fall in Kf and hence a fall in glomerular filtration rate.

On the other hand, the systemic hypotensive circulatory

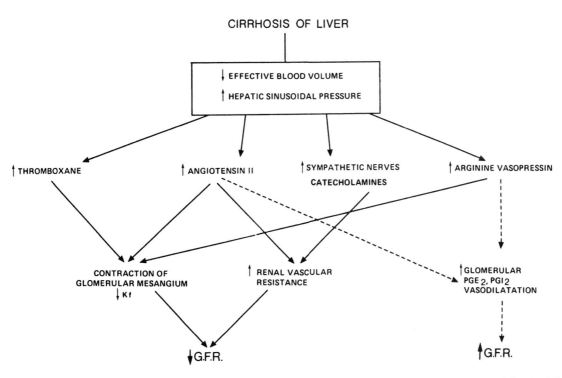

Fig. 25.7 Schematic representation of the possible intrarenal action of vasoactive hormones which might predispose to renal failure in cirrhosis of the liver. Endothelial cell damage (e.g. due to LCAT) may reduce ability to produce 'protective' vasodilatory PGE$_2$ and PGI$_2$.

changes of HRS may be due to prolonged production of nitric oxide–endothelial derived relaxing factor (Vallance & Moncada 1991). The induction of nitric oxide synthase by endotoxin has already been described (Fig. 25.4). Endotoxemia without sepsis has been reported in 92% of 39 cirrhotic patients by the use of a chromogenic Limulus assay (Bigatello et al 1987). The ability to block production and/or receptor activation of these powerful vasoactive substances may enable more specific treatment of HRS in the future.

3. MANAGEMENT OF RENAL FAILURE IN CIRRHOSIS OF THE LIVER (see also Ch. 92)

'The hepatorenal syndrome is one of the most frustrating diseases in medicine.'

Conn 1973

For those without access to liver transplantation the old addage that 'prevention is better than cure' certainly applies to renal failure in liver disease. All patients in hospital with cirrhosis of the liver should have renal function carefully monitored, especially when salt and water restriction or diuretics are in use, when gastrointestinal bleeding is likely or if surgery is proposed. Table 25.4 lists the basic requirements.

Renal failure in cirrhosis may be iatrogenic (Epstein 1984). For example, NSAID will prevent the intrarenal production of PGE$_2$ and PGI$_2$, vasoactive substances which play an essential protective role in normal glomerular hemodynamics and which are especially essential in cirrhosis of the liver. These drugs can cause renal impairment in liver disease (Boyer et al 1979, Zipser et al 1979). The hepatorenal syndrome begins insidiously and the surgeon cannot be too

Table 25.4 Prevention of renal failure in cirrhosis

Examine daily	weight
	tissue turgor
	ascites/edema
	blood pressure
	temperature
Measure	urine volume and osmolality
	sodium balance
	serum: creatinine, urea, sodium, potassium and albumin concentration
	hemoglobin/hematocrit
	liver function
Avoid	NSAIDs*
	nephrotoxins
	excessive weight loss (> 0.5 kg/day) due to diuretics, paracentesis or lactulose
	hypoalbuminemia
	infection

*Nonsteroidal anti-inflammatory drugs

obsessional in carefully examining the patient daily in terms of weight loss, presence or absence of edema, sodium balance and serum creatinine concentration. Large volume paracentesis to relieve aldorenal symptoms should always be accompanied by the simultaneous intravenous infusion of concentrated albumin to maintain or increase plasma volume and improve plasma albumin concentration. Re-infusion of concentrated ascitic fluid is also possible, although much less practical (see below).

In the first instance all patients with cirrhosis who develop oliguria should be considered to have either prerenal oliguria or established ATN (Table 25.3). Reversible volume depletion will respond to volume expansion with colloid, if albumin is low, or with saline. Patients with HRS given colloid will also respond favorably in the first instance but this is not sustained. A history of nephrotoxic drugs, severe infection or urinary obstruction would suggest ATN. Theoretically, these patients should recover once the aggravating factors have been corrected or removed. Hemodialysis support may be needed for 3–6 weeks while this occurs and should best be done using the more permeable polysulphone or polyacrilonitrile membranes and hemodiafiltration.

The outlook for patients with true HRS, however, is grim indeed; 'the overwhelming majority of patients with HRS die' (Epstein 1992). Essentially, improvement in renal function appears to be almost totally dependent on recovery of the liver and, indeed, kidney function in patients treated by liver transplantation returns to normal (Iwatsuki et al 1973). The advent of charcoal hemoperfusion, plasma exchange and the new permeable membranes for hemodiafiltration have led to reports of improvement in liver function in the short term with associated renal recovery. Such maneuvers may buy time to enable liver repair to occur and may occasionally be of benefit in the long term.

Somewhat in desperation an impressive array of 'specific medications' have been tried (Levenson et al 1983). While some are based on sound theoretical grounds, none have as yet been shown to be really effective in the long term. Vasopressor drugs such as dopamine and noradrenaline are without effect. Low-dose ornipressin (6 units/h) has been briefly reported as effective therapy for HRS (Lenz & Druml 1989). Infusion was associated with a pronounced increase in serum atrial natriuretic peptide concentration, a diuresis, natriuresis and increase in creatinine clearance during 2 h in six patients.

Since activation of the renin–angiotensin system may be involved in the diuretic 'resistance' of patients with cirrhosis and ascites, angiotensin converting enzyme therapy seemed logical. Unfortunately, systemic hypotensive effects have limited their usefulness. Recently Vliet et al (1992) reported that low-dose captopril (20 mg/day) was effective in restoring diuretic efficacy in four of eight cirrhotic patients without producing significant side effects.

Two maneuvers of particular interest to the surgeon are peritoneovenous shunting of ascitic fluid (Le Veen et al 1974) (PVS) (Ch. 94) and portacaval shunting. Both have been claimed to improve renal function in advanced cirrhosis and the HRS (Schroeder et al 1970, Wapnick et al 1977).

Role of peritoneovenous or portacaval shunting in improving renal function

Many patients with HRS have gross ascites. Increased intraabdominal pressure per se can be associated with a significant decrease in GFR and RPF (Bradley & Bradley 1947). The primary cause of anuria and renal failure is related to the level of abdominal pressure, pressures > 15 mmHg inducing oliguria and a fall in GFR. Acute renal failure has developed in patients in association with sudden rises in intra-abdominal pressure. However, in the 1950s it became recognized that repeated large volume paracentesis would result in hypovolemia, salt depletion and renal failure. This could be prevented by simultaneous intravenous reinfusion of the ascitic fluid. This maneuver was shown to produce a significant, but unfortunately transient, improvement in GFR and effective RPF with a diuresis and natriuresis. Kaiser et al (1962) claimed this technique to be of great value in the perioperative management of cirrhotic patients with ascites, conserving protein and maintaining renal function. More recently ultrafiltration of ascitic fluid using a polyacrilonitrile membrane with removal of salt and water before reinfusion was effective in preserving renal function in the short term (Parbhoo et al 1974). More recently Daimon et al (1998) reported on the successful treatment of ascites with the same procedure though no evidence of improved renal function was noted.

Recently Salerno (1992) has reinvestigated the whole problem. It was shown that, at intra-abdominal pressures in excess of 25 cm of water, the removal of 2 L of ascitic fluid over 15–30 min did not compromise overall renal function. Indeed, a significant rise in mean creatinine clearance was measured 2 h after the procedure.

Other studies demonstrated that intermittent large volume paracentesis can be safely carried out without immediate adverse effects on renal function. However, many advocate simultaneous albumin infusion (6 g/L of ascites drained) to reduce the risk of hypovolemia and renal failure. Careful comparative studies have shown that this procedure is successful in reducing ascites as effectively and more quickly than diuretics and salt restriction. Indeed, this is now suggested as initial therapy for ascites, diuretics being reserved for maintenance therapy (Kellerman & Linas 1990).

Recently synthetic plasma expanders (Dextran 70 and Hemaccel) have been compared with human albumin and found to be equally effective, at least in the short term (Salerno 1992). Indeed, simple isotonic saline, a solution without oncotic power may be equally effective in the short term.

Long-term observations of renal function and survival in cirrhotic patients subjected to either daily or weekly reinfusion treatments or managed by conventional diuretics and salt restriction are few. However, Clermont et al in 1967 could find no difference in the frequency of ultimate renal failure or survival between the two treatment groups.

The development by LeVeen et al in 1974 of a satisfactory valve first made possible long-term PVS of ascitic fluid. Subsequent modifications were made to prevent shunt occlusion (Denver shunt, Cordis-Hakim valve). Despite significant morbidity due to fever, diffuse intravascular coagulation and infection many thousands of these devices have now been implanted in ascitic patients. Significant improvement in nutritional and immunological well-being with reduction in ascitic fluid accumulation seems to occur in a significant proportion (Ch. 94).

The technique has also been widely advocated as an effective treatment for the HRS. Epstein (1982) has critically reviewed the evidence for this claim and found it lacking. Improvement in renal function with a diuresis and natriuresis is found for up to 2 weeks after shunt insertion. Simultaneously cardiac output increases, calculated peripheral resistance falls and both plasma renin activity and aldosterone concentration decrease (Schroeder et al 1979, Blendis et al 1979). In some patients these improvements have been noted for as long as up to 6 months after implanting the shunt (Greig et al 1981).

The evidence for improvement of renal function in HRS itself, however, is not good. Most investigators have claimed improvement in patients who undoubtedly had prerenal oliguria. Patients with true HRS have a dismal prognosis, irrespective of shunting (Linas et al 1986). Mean survival with medical treatment was only 4 days and 14 days in the surgical groups. The study of Schroeder et al (1979) is considered by Epstein to fulfill all the correct criteria for the diagnosis of HRS. They compared two techniques, either creation of a side-to-side portacaval shunt or a mesocaval shunt or insertion of a LeVeen shunt in 10 cachectic patients with massive ascites and oliguric renal failure. Interestingly, renal function improved and plasma renin activity fell to normal in seven of the 10 patients after either a portacaval shunt or a successful PVS. However, three of the five patients given a portacaval anastomosis died of liver failure post-operatively. The authors conclude 'that the efficacy of these procedures in prolonging the survival of patients with hepatorenal syndrome remains to be proven by controlled prospective study.'

REFERENCES

Aarseth S, Bergen A, Aarseth P 1979 Circulatory homeostasis in rats after bile duct ligation. Scandinavian Journal of Clinical Laboratory Investigation 39: 93–97

Allison M E M, Moss N G, Fraser M M 1978 Renal function in obstructive jaundice: a micropuncture study in rats. Clinical Science and Molecular Medicine 54: 649–659

Allison M E M, Prentice C R M, Kennedy A C, Blumgart L H 1979 Renal function and other factors in obstructive jaundice. British Journal of Surgery 66: 392–397

Alon U, Berant M, Mordechovitz D, Hashmonai M, Better O S 1982 Effect of isolated cholemia on systemic haemodynamics and kidney function in conscious dogs. Clinical Science 63: 59–64

Anderson R J, Linas S L, Berns A S 1977 Non-oliguric acute renal failure. New England Journal of Medicine 296: 1134–1138

Armstrong C P, Dixon J M, Taylor T V, Davies G C 1984 Surgical experience of deeply jaundiced patients with bile duct obstruction. British Journal of Surgery 71: 234–238

Ayer D 1938 Renal lesions associated with deep jaundice. Archives of Pathology 22: 26–41

Bailey M E 1976 Endotoxin bile salts and renal function in obstructive jaundice. British Journal of Surgery 63: 774–778

Barry K G, Malloy J P 1962 Oliguric renal failure. Evaluation and therapy by the intravenous infusion of mannitol. Journal of the American Medical Association 179: 510–513

Bartosh S M, Alonso E M, Whitington P F 1997 Renal outcomes in pediatric liver transplantation. Clinical Transplantation 11: 354–360

Better O S 1983 Bile duct ligation: an experimental model of renal dysfunction secondary to liver disease. In: Epstein M (ed) The kidney in liver disease. Elsevier Science, New York, pp 295–311

Bigatello L M, Broitman S A, Fattoril di Paoli M 1987 Endotoxemia encephalopathy and mortality in cirrhotic patients. American Journal of Gastroenterology 82: 11–15

Bilbao I, Charco R, Balsells J, Lazaro J L, Hidalgo E, Llopart L, Murio E, Margarit C 1998 Risk factors for acute renal failure requiring dialysis after liver transplantation. Clinical Transplantation 12: 123–129

Bismuth H, Kuntziger H, Corlette M B 1975 Cholangitis with acute renal failure. Annals of Surgery 181: 881–887

Blamey S L, Fearon K C H, Gilmour W H, Osborne D H, Carter D C 1983 Prediction of risk in biliary surgery. British Journal of Surgery 70: 535–538

Blendis L M, Greig P D, Langer B, Baigrie R S, Ruse J, Taylor B R 1979 The renal and haemodynamic effects of peritoneovenous shunt for intractable hepatic ascites. Gastroenterology 77: 250–257

Bomzon L, Kew M C 1983 Renal blood flow in experimental obstructive jaundice. In: Epstein M (ed.), The kidney in liver disease. Elsevier Science, New York, pp 313–326

Bosch-Marce M, Morales-Ruiz M, Jimenez W, Bordas N, Sole M, Ros J, Deulofeu R, Arroyo V, Rivera F, Rodes J 1998 Increased renal expression of nitric oxide synthase type III in cirrhotic rats with ascites. Hepatology 27: 1191–1199

Boyer T D, Zia P, Reynolds T B 1979 Effects of indomethacin and prostaglandin A1 on renal function and plasma renin activity in alcoholic liver disease. Gastroenterology 77: 215–222

Bradley S E, Bradley C P 1947 The effect of increased intra-abdominal pressure on renal function in man. European Journal of Clinical Investigation 26: 1010–1022

Carcoana O V, Hines R L 1996 Is renal dose dopamine protective or therapeutic? Yes. Critical Care Clinics 12: 677–685

Clairmont P, von Haberer H 1911 Ueber Aurie nach Gallensteinoperationen. Mitteilunger aus den Grenzgebieten der Medizen und Chirurgie 22: 159–172

Clermont R J, Vlahoevic Z R, Chalmers T C, Adham N F, Curtis G W, Morrison R S 1967 Intravenous therapy of massive ascites in patients with cirrhosis. II. Long term effects on survival and frequency of renal failure. Gastroenterology 53: 220–228

Conn H O 1973 A rational approach to the hepatorenal syndrome. Gastroenterology 65: 321–340

Daimon S, Yasuhara S, Saga T, Tokunaga S, Chikaki H, Dan K 1998 Efficacy of extracorporeal ultrafiltration of ascitic fluid as a treatment of refractory ascites. Nephrology, Dialysis, Transplantation 13: 2617–2623

Davison A M 1996 Hepatorenal failure. Nephrology, Dialysis, Transplantation 11 Suppl 8: 24–31

Dawson J L 1964 Jaundice and anoxic renal damage: the protective effect of mannitol. British Medical Journal 1: 810–811

Dawson J L 1968 Acute post-operative renal failure in obstructive jaundice. Annals of the Royal College of Surgeons of England 42: 163–181

DiBona G F, Sawin L L 1991 Role of renal nerves in sodium retention of cirrhosis and congestive heart failure. American Journal of Physiology 260: R298–R305

Dixon J M, Armstrong C P, Duffy S W, Davies G C 1983 Factors affecting morbidity and mortality after surgery for obstructive jaundice: a review of 373 patients. Gut 24: 845–852

Drivas G, James O, Wardle N 1976 Study of reticuloendothelial phagocytic capacity in patients with cholestases. British Medical Journal 1: 1568–1569

Dworkin L D, Brenner B M 1985 Biophysical basis of glomerular filtration. In: Geibisch G, Seldin DW (eds). The kidney: physiology and pathophysiology. Raven Press, New York, pp 397–426

Ecknoyan G 1983 Glomerular abnormalities in liver disease. In: Epstein M (ed) The kidney in liver disease. Elsevier Science, New York, pp 199–214

Eliahou H E 1964 Mannitol therapy in oliguria of acute onset. British Medical Journal 1: 807–809

Elsom K A 1937 Renal function in obstructive jaundice. Archives of Internal Medicine 60: 1028–1033

Epstein M 1982 Peritoneovenous shunt in the management of ascites and the hepatorenal syndrome. Gastroenterology 82: 790–799

Epstein M 1983a Pathogenesis of renal sodium handing in cirrhosis. A reappraisal. American Journal of Nephrology 3: 297–309.

Epstein M 1983b The renin-angiotensin system in liver disease. In: Epstein M (ed) The kidney in liver disease. Elsevier Science, New York, pp 353–375

Epstein M 1984 Therapy of renal disorder in liver disease. In: Suki WN, Massry SG (eds) Therapy of renal diseases and related disorders. Martinus Nijhoff, Dordrecht, pp 335–346

Epstein M 1992 The hepatorenal syndrome—new perspectives. New England Journal of Medicine 327: 1810–1811

Epstein M, Berk D P, Hollenberg N K 1970 Renal failure in the patient with cirrhosis. The role of active vasoconstriction. The American Journal of Medicine 49: 175–185

Evans H J R, Torrealba V, Hudd C, Knight M 1982 The effect of pre-operative bile salt administration on post-operative renal function in patients with obstructive jaundice. British Journal of Surgery 69: 706–708

Feldman B H, Kjellstrand C M, Fralby E E 1971 Mannitol intoxication. Journal of Urology 106: 622–623

Fletcher M S, Westwick J, Kakkar V V 1982 Endotoxin prostaglandins and renal fibrin deposition in obstructive jaundice. British Journal of Surgery 69: 625–629

Flores J, Dibona D R, Beck C H, Leaf A 1972 The role of cell swelling in ischemic renal damage and the protective effect of hypertonic solute. Journal of Clinical Investigation 51: 118–126

Frank H A, Seligman A M, Fine J 1946 Traumatic shock. XIII. The prevention of irreversibility in haemorrhagic shock by the viviperfusion of the liver. Journal of Clinical Investigation 25: 22–29

Gelman S I 1976 Disturbances in hepatic blood flow during anaesthesia and surgery. Archives of Surgery 111: 881–883

Gentilini P, Arias I M, Arroyo V, Schrier R W 1990 Liver diseases and renal complications. Raven Press, New York, pp 14–31

Green J, Beyar R, Bomzon L, Finberg J P M, Better O S 1984 Jaundice, the circulation and the kidney. Nephron 37: 145–152

Greig P D, Blendis L M, Langer B, Taylor B R, Colapinto R F 1981 Renal and haemodynamic effects of peritoneovenous shunt. II. Long-term effects. Gastroenterology 80: 119–125

Gubern J M, Sancho J J, Simo J, Sitges-Serra A 1988 A randomized trial on the effect of mannitol on post-operative renal function in patients with obstructive jaundice. Surgery 102: 39–44

Hatfield A R W, Terblanche J, Sataar S 1982 Pre-operative external biliary drainage in obstructive jaundice. Lancet ii: 896–899

Helwig F C, Schutz C B 1932 A liver kidney syndrome. Surgery, Gynecology and Obstetrics 55: 570–580

Henderson I S, Beattie T J, Kennedy A C 1980 Dopamine hydrochloride in oliguric states. Lancet ii: 827–828

Holt S, Marley R, Fernando B, Harry D, Anand R, Goodier D, Moore K 1999 Acute cholestasis-induced renal failure: effects of antioxidants and ligands for the thromboxane A2 receptor. Kidney International 55: 271–277

Hovig T, Blomhoff J P, Holme R, Faltmark A, Gjone E 1978 Plasma lipoprotein alterations and morphological changes with lipid deposition on the kidneys of patients with hepatorenal syndrome. Laboratory Investigation 38: 540–549

Ibarra F R, Galceran T, Oddo E, Arrizurieta E 1998 Changes in glomerular filtration rate and renal plasma flow in cirrhotic rats during converting enzyme inhibition. Renal Failure 20: 65–74

Ingoldby C 1983 Endotoxaemia and renal failure in obstructive jaundice. Thesis Dissertation, University of Cambridge.

Iwatsuki S, Popoutzer M M, Corman J L 1973 Recovery from 'hepatorenal syndrome' after orthotopic liver transplantation. New England Journal of Medicine 289: 1155–1159

Kaiser G C, Lempke R E, King R D, King H 1962 Intravenous infusion of ascitic fluid. Archives of Surgery 85: 83–91

Kellerman P S, Linas S L 1990 Large volume paracentesis in the treatment of ascites. Annals of Internal Medicine 112: 889–890

Kennedy A C, Burton J A, Luke R G 1973 Factors affecting prognosis in acute renal failure. Quarterly Journal of Medicine 42: 73–86

Lafayette R A, Pare G, Schmid C H, King A J, Rohrer R J, Nasraway S A 1997 Pretransplant renal dysfunction predicts poorer outcome in liver transplantation. Clinical Nephrology 48: 159–164

Lassen N A, Thomsen A C 1958 The pathogenesis of the hepatorenal syndrome. Acta Medica Scandinavica CLX: 165–171

Lenz K, Druml W V 1989 Ornipressin as a treatment of hepatorenal syndrome (HRS): effect on vasoactive hormones. Kidney International 35: 229

LeVeen H H, Christoudias G, Ip M, Luft R, Falk G, Grosberg S 1974 Peritoneovenous shunting for ascites. Annals of Surgery 180: 580–591

Levenson D J, Skorecki K L, Narins R G 1983 Acute renal failure associated with hepatobiliary disease. In: Bressner B M, Lazarus J M (eds) Acute renal failure. WB Saunders, Philadelphia, pp 467–498

Levinsky N G 1983 The hepatorenal syndrome. Medical Grand Rounds 2: 160–169

Levy M 1992 Hepatorenal syndrome. In: Geibisch G, Seldin DW (eds) The kidney: physiology and pathophysiology. Raven Press, New York, pp 3305–3326

Levy M 1997 Atrial natriuretic peptide: renal effects in cirrhosis of the liver. Seminars in Nephrology 17: 520–529

Linas S L, Schafer J W, Moore E E, Good J T 1986 Percutaneous shunt in the management of the hepatorenal syndrome. Kidney International 30: 736–740

Lopez-Novoa J, Rengel M A, Rodicio J L, Hernando L 1977 A micropuncture study of salt and water retention in chronic experimental cirrhosis. American Journal of Physiology 232: 315–318

Luke R G, Briggs J D, Allison M E M, Kennedy A C 1970 Factors determining the response to mannitol in acute renal failure. American Journal of Medical Science 259: 168–174

Mairiang P, Bhudhisawasdi V, Borirakchanyavat V, Sitprija V 1990 Acute renal failure in obstructive jaundice in cholangiocarcinoma. Archives of Internal Medicine 150: 2357–2360

Martin P Y, Gines P, Schrier R W 1998a Nitric oxide as a mediator of hemodynamic abnormalities and sodium and water retention in cirrhosis. New England Journal of Medicine 339: 533–541

Martin P Y, Ohara M, Gines P, Xu D L, St.John J, Niederberger M, Schrier R W 1998b Nitric oxide synthase (NOS) inhibition for one week improves renal sodium and water excretion in cirrhotic rats with ascites. Journal of Clinical Investigation 101: 235–242

Matsuda T, Morita H, Hosomi H, Okada M 1996 Response of renal nerve activity to high NaCl food intake in dogs with chronic bile duct ligation. Hepatology 23: 303–309

McPherson G A D, Benjamin I S, Boobis A R, Brodie M J, Hampden C, Blumgart L H 1982a Antipyrine elimination as a dynamic test of hepatic functional integrity in obstructive jaundice. Gut 23: 734–738

McPherson G A D, Benjamin I S, Habib N A, Bowley N B, Blumgart L H 1982b Percutaneous transhepatic drainage in obstructive jaundice. British Journal of Surgery 69: 261–264

McPherson G A D, Benjamin I S, Hodgson H J F, Bowley N B, Allison D J, Blumgart L H 1984 Pre-operative percutaneous transhepatic biliary drainage: the results of a controlled trial. British Journal of Surgery 71: 371–375

Molitoris B A, Dahl R, Geerdes A 1992 Cytoskeleton disruption and apical redistribution of proximal tubule Na(+)-K(+)-ATPase during ischemia. American Journal of Physiology 263: F488–495

Molnar W, Stockum A E 1974 Relief of obstructive jaundice through a transhepatic catheter—a new therapeutic method. American Journal of Roentgenology 122: 356–367

Moore K, Wendon J, Frazer M, Karani J, Williams R, Badr K 1992 Plasma endothelium immune activity in liver disease and the hepatorenal syndrome. New England Journal of Medicine 327: 1774–1778

Moss N G, Colindres R E, Gottschalk C W 1992 Neural control of renal function. In: Windhager E (ed) Handbook of Physiology, Section 8. Renal Physiology. Oxford University Press, New York, pp 1061–1128

Naccarato R, Messa P, D'Angelo A 1981 Renal handling of sodium and water in early chronic liver disease. Gastroenterology 81: 205–210

Niederberger M, Gines P, Martin P Y, St John J, Woytaszek P, Xu L, Tsai P, Nemenoff R A, Schrier R W 1998 Increased renal and vascular cytosolic phospholipase A2 activity in rats with cirrhosis and ascites. Hepatology 27: 42–47

Nolan J P 1981 Endotoxin reticuloendothelial function and liver injury. Hepatology 1: 458–465

Paller M S, Hoidal J R, Ferris T F 1984 Oxygen free radicals in ischemic acute renal failure in the rat. Journal of Clinical Investigation 74: 1156–1164

Papadakis M A, Arieff A T 1984 Hepatorenal syndrome: an expanded definition. Kidney International 25: 173

Papper S 1958 The role of the kidney in Laennec's cirrhosis of the liver. Medicine (Baltimore) 37: 299–316

Papper S 1983 Hepatorenal syndrome. In: Epstein M (ed), The kidney in liver disease. Elsevier Science Publishers, New York p 87–106

Parbhoo S P, Ajdukiewicz A, Sherlock S 1974 Treatment of ascites by continuous ultrafiltration and reinfusion of protein concentrate. Lancet 12: 949–952

Park R, Arieff A I 1981 Lactic acidosis: Current concepts. In: Shade P S (ed) Clinics in endocrinology and metabolism. W B Saunders, Philadelphia, pp 339

Pitt H A, Cameron J L, Postier R G, Gadacz T R 1981 Factors affecting mortality in biliary tract surgery. American Journal of Surgery 141: 66–72

Pitt H A, Gomes A S, Lois J F, Mann L L, Deutsch L S, Longmire W P 1985 Does pre-operative percutaneous biliary drainage reduce operative risk or increase hospital costs. Annals of Surgery 201: 545–553

Ravdin I S 1929 Vasodepressor substances in the liver after obstruction of the common duct. Archives of Surgery 18: 2191–2201

Rudbach J A, Anacker R L, Haskins W T, Johnson A G, Milner K C, Ribi E 1966 Physical aspects of reversible inactivation of endotoxin. Annals of New York Academy of Sciences 133: 629–643

Sakaguchi H, Dachs S, Grisham E, Paronetto F, Salomon M, Churg J 1965 Hepatic glomerulosclerosis. An electron microscopic study of renal biopsies in liver disease. Laboratory Investigation 14: 535–545

Salerno F 1992 Large volume paracentesis and volume reformation: can synthetic plasma expanders simply replace albumin? Journal of Hepatology 14: 143–145

Schroeder E T, Numann P J, Chamberlain B E 1970 Functional renal failure in cirrhosis. Recovery after portacaval shunt. Annals of Internal Medicine 72: 923–928

Schroeder E T, Anderson G H, Smulyan H 1979 Effects of portacaval or peritoneovenous shunt on renin in the hepatorenal syndrome. Kidney International 15: 54–61

Selkurt E E 1945 Changes in renal clearance following complete ischemia of the kidney. American Journal of Physiology 144: 395–404

Shorr E, Zweifach B W, Furchgott F 1948 Hepatorenal factors in circulatory homeostasis: III The influence of hormonal factors of hepatorenal origin on the vascular reaction to haemorrhage. Annals of the New York Academy of Science 49: 571–592

Smith R C, Pooley M, George C R P, Faithful G P 1985 Pre-operative percutaneous transhepatic internal drainage in obstructive jaundice: a randomised controlled trial examining renal function. Surgery 97: 641–647

Smith R E A, Radomski M W R, Moncada S 1992 Nitric oxide mediates the vascular action of cytokines in septic shock. European Journal of Clinical Investigation 438–439

Sorenson F H, Anderson J B, Ornsholt J, Skjoldborg H 1971 Acute renal failure complicating biliary tract disorders. Acta Chirurgica Scandinavica 137: 87–91

Stewart H L, Cantarow A 1935 Renal lesions following injection of sodium dehydrocholate in animals with and without biliary stasis. Archives of Pathology 20: 866–881

Tanner G A, Selkurt E E 1970 Kidney function in the squirrel monkey before and after haemorrhagic hypotension. American Journal of Physiology 219: 597–603

Thompson J N, Cohen J, Blenkharn J I, McConnell J S, Barr J, Blumgart L H 1986 A randomized clinical trial of oral ursodeoxycholic acid in obstructive jaundice. British Journal of Surgery 73: 634–636

Thompson J N, Edwards W H, Winearls C G, Blenkharn J I, Benjamin I S, Blumgart L H 1987 Renal impairment following biliary tract surgery. British Journal of Surgery 74: 843–847

Unikowsky B, Wexler M J, Levy M 1983 Dogs with experimental cirrhosis of the liver but without intrahepatic hypertension do not retain sodium or form ascites. Journal of Clinical Investigation 72: 1594–1604

Vallance P, Moncada S 1991 Hyperdynamic circulation in cirrhosis: a role for nitric oxide. Lancet 337: 776–778

Vliet V A A, Mackeng W H, Donkeraj M, Mevwissen S G M 1992 Efficacy of low dose captopril in addition to furosemide and splenoactine in patients with disseminated liver disease during blunted diuresis. Journal of Hepatology 15: 40–47

Walters W, Parham D 1922 Renal and hepatic insufficiency in obstructive jaundice. Surgery, Gynecology and Obstetrics 35: 605–609

Wapnick S, Grosberg S, Kinney M, LeVeen H H 1977 LeVeen continuous peritoneal–jugular shunt: Improvement in renal function in ascitic patients. Journal of the American Medical Association 237: 131–133

Wardle E N 1975 Endotoxaemia and the pathogenesis of acute renal failure. Quarterly Journal of Medicine 44: 389–398

Wardle E N 1992 Endotoxemia and acute renal failure. Care of the Critically Ill 8: 23–27

Wardle E N, Wright N A 1970 Endotoxin and acute renal failure associated with obstructive jaundice. British Medical Journal 4: 472–474

Weinberg J 1991 The cell biology of ischemic renal injury. Kidney International 39: 476–500

Wilbur O L 1934 The renal glomerulus in various forms of nephrosis. Archives of Pathology 18: 157–118

Wilkinson S P, Hirst D, Portman B, Williams R 1975 Pathogenesis of renal failure in cirrhosis and fulminant hepatic failure. Postgraduate Medical Journal 51: 503–505

Williams R D, Elliot D W, Zollinger R W 1960 The effect of hypotension in obstructive jaundice. Archives of Surgery 81: 335–340

Yared A, Kon V, Ichikawa I 1985 Mechanism of preservation of glomerular perfusion and filtration during acute extracellular volume depletion. Journal of Clinical Investigation 75: 1477–1487

Zipser R D, Hoefs J C, Speckart P F, Zia P K, Horton R 1979 Prostaglandins: modulation of renal function and pressor resistance in chronic liver disease. Journal of Clinical Endocrinology and Metabolism 48: 895–900

Pre- and postoperative nutrition in hepatobiliary surgery

26

M.L. BROWN, Y. FONG, W.S. HELTON

GOALS OF NUTRITIONAL SUPPORT IN HEPATOBILIARY SURGERY

The general objective of nutritional support in patients undergoing hepatobiliary surgery are the same as for any other patient undergoing operation, namely, to decrease postoperative morbidity and mortality. Nutritional intervention should attempt to maintain or restore immunity, support anabolism, and attenuate the catabolic response to injury. In addition, nutritional intervention should strive to restore specific hepatocellular functions, attenuate hepatocellular injury in response to ischemia and reperfusion and optimally support hepatocellular function and regeneration following transplantation or resection.

In addition to providing the basic components to correct protein calorie malnutrition, nutritional strategies have recently tried to identify and provide disease-specific nutrient requirements for individual organs, cells, and tissues. This new direction or application of nutritional science has been called nutritional pharmacology and is based on the observation that individual components of the immuno-inflammatory response to injury and infection can be influenced and manipulated by the timely administration of specific nutrients, in specific concentrations and by specific routes of feeding. Using the principles of nutritional pharmacology, clinicians and scientists have observed over the past few years that liver structure and function in both health and disease can be significantly influenced by nutritional means. This chapter will discuss the applications of nutrition in pre- and postoperative hepatobiliary surgery integrating recent developments with established practices.

ALTERATIONS IN LIVER METABOLISM THAT EFFECT NUTRITIONAL STATUS

The liver plays a critical role in metabolism and the assimilation of nutrients. It is central in the orchestration of protein and carbohydrate metabolism. Any defect or disease of the liver will result in significant metabolic derangements. Progression of liver dysfunction results not only in metabolic derangement from a decrease in the number of functioning hepatic cells but also in shunting of portal blood, which decreases the delivery of nutrients, growth factors and hormones to the remaining cells. Patients with advanced liver disease and cirrhosis also have increased circulating serum levels of growth hormone, glucagon, epinephrine and cortisol. The etiology of this altered hormonal pattern is not completely understood but is typical of a catabolic state and results in carbohydrate intolerance and muscle proteolysis (Eigler et al 1979, Sherwin et al 1974). It is further speculated that the catabolic profile of patients with cirrhosis and ascites may be due, in part, to a defective gastrointestinal mucosal barrier, which leads to the escape of endotoxin from the lumen of the bowel into the peritoneal cavity (Helton 1994). The transmigrated endotoxin stimulates peritoneal mononuclear phagocytic cells and Kupffer cells in the liver to release proinflammatory cytokines and mediators [interleukin-1 (IL-1), tumor necrosis factor (TNF), interleukin-6 (IL-6), eicosanoids, nitric oxide]. These mediators and cytokines modulate a number of metabolic functions of the liver including amino acid, protein, lipid, carbohydrate, and trace mineral metabolism (Andus et al 1991). The proinflammatory cytokines are produced by cells in the intestine and liver to mediate anabolic and catabolic functions, regulate hepatic blood flow, bile flow, liver regeneration, and the response to ischemia and reperfusion injury. Tumor necrosis factor is the proximal cytokine signal produced by hepatic Kupffer cells in response to endotoxin or ischemia-reperfusion. Tumor necrosis factor initiates a cascade of inflammatory events that are important in the pathogenesis of many types of surgically induced liver injury such as ischemia and reperfusion injury that occurs with liver resection and transplantation. Endotoxemia occurring in response to manipulation of the biliary tree in patients with biliary obstruction also stimulates the release of TNF, which is believed to mediate, in part, the increased organ failure associated with operating upon patients with biliary obstruction and infection (Wilkinson et al 1976, Nolan 1981).

Tumor necrosis factor and IL-6 cause a reprioritization of hepatic protein synthesis, a process involving accelerated production of acute-phase proteins at the expense of constitutive proteins. There is some indirect evidence that parenteral nutrition also weakens the intestinal barrier allowing endotoxin to escape from the gut where it then primes Kupffer cells for cytokine release in response to later infection (Fong et al 1989).

Increased skeletal muscle proteolysis and muscle wasting in advanced cirrhosis may be related, in part, to the fact that the cirrhotic liver does not respond appropriately to growth hormone because of low levels of growth hormone binding protein (GHBP) (Hattori et al 1992). Growth hormone normally binds to GHBP on hepatocytes and stimulates the production of insulin-like growth factor-1 (IGF-1), the principal mediator of growth hormone-induced protein synthesis and IGF-1 binding proteins. Patients with advanced cirrhosis therefore have low circulating plasma levels of IGF-1 and IGF-1 binding proteins (Hattori et al 1992, Poggi et al 1979). The net effect of this metabolic derangement is impaired glucose disposal by skeletal muscle and impaired skeletal muscle protein synthesis. Simultaneously, there is decreased protein synthesis by the diseased liver for the major secretory proteins such as albumin, and proteins in the coagulation cascade (Nachbauer & Fischer 1983). Due to the above alterations, the administration of recombinant IGF-1 but not growth hormone may enhance protein synthesis (Inaba et al 1994) and thus be an important adjunct to improving the nutritional state of patients with liver disease undergoing operation (Sato et al 1994).

Subclinical steatorrhea is common in patients with cirrhosis or obstructive jaundice and leads to fat soluble vitamin and trace element deficiencies (Gitlin & Heyman 1984). These deficits are under appreciated in the nutritional assessment of patients with hepatobiliary disease undergoing operation and should be corrected.

IDENTIFICATION OF PATIENTS AT RISK FOR POSTOPERATIVE COMPLICATIONS

To utilize nutrition support appropriately in a cost effective and clinically efficacious manner, it is necessary to identify which patients are at risk for nutritionally related complications and which will benefit from nutritional intervention. Malnutrition is recognized as an important predisposing factor in the morbidity and mortality of patients undergoing major abdominal surgery (Mullen et al 1979) (see Table 26.1). Up to 70% of patients with obstructive jaundice undergoing operation (Foschi et al 1986, Pitt et al 1981) and nearly all patients with advanced cirrhosis have significant malnutrition and are therefore at risk for postoperative complications. Infection is the most common complication in patients undergoing liver and biliary surgery and occurs in 22 to 40% of all patients (Foschi et al 1986, Pitt et al 1981, Dixon et al 1983, McPherson et al 1984, Smith et al 1985, Stimpson et al 1987). Furthermore, sepsis and sepsis-induced multiple organ failure are the most common causes of death in liver transplant recipients (Colonna et al 1988, Yokoyama et al 1989) and in patients with jaundice and cirrhosis undergoing abdominal operations (Pitt et al 1981, McPherson et al 1984, Armstrong et al 1984, Pitt et al 1985). Because the majority of patients with severe liver disease or jaundice are malnourished and since malnutrition leads to infection, nutritional intervention and repletion may decrease postoperative morbidity and mortality in patients undergoing hepatobiliary surgery.

Several prognostic scoring systems have been developed to identify malnourished patients at risk for developing postoperative complications (Buzby et al 1980). Although the use of such scoring systems allows prediction of postoperative complications in specific patient groups, their applicability in patients with significant liver disease or cirrhosis is not well established (Shronts 1988). Because conventional markers such as weight status and serum protein levels are altered and dependent on nonnutritional factors, one must

Table 26.1 Causes of malnutrition in cirrhosis

Poor dietary intake
Anorexia, nausea, alcohol abuse, dietary restrictions (protein, fat, sodium, fluid)

Malabsorption/maldigestion
Cholestasis, intraluminal bile deficiency, co-existing pancreatic exocrine insufficiency and fat malabsorption

Increased catabolism
Muscle proteolysis

Decreased protein synthesis
Decreased hepatocyte growth hormone receptor, decreased IGF-1 and IGF-BP, decreased hepatic transport proteins, fibrinogen, coagulation factors, lipoproteins

Drug therapy effects
Neomysin: villous atrophy, diarrhea, zinc deficiency
Lactulose: diarrhea, zinc deficiency
Diuretics: potassium, magnesium, zinc deficiency
Cholestyramine: diarrhea, fat-soluble vitamin deficiency.

also rely on other subjective measures. A dietary and medical history combined with physical examination is the most sensitive means of assessing nutritional risk in patients undergoing hepatobiliary surgery.

The evaluation of a patient's nutritional status should begin with an initial baseline evaluation and continue throughout the patient's course of treatment. A complete nutritional assessment includes the following: physical exam and clinical evaluation, assessment of muscle mass and strength, evaluation of serum albumin and c-reactive protein, vitamin and mineral deficits and determination of nutrient requirements (Shronts 1988) (Table 26.2). Historical questions should focus on the patient's nutritional intake, the degree and rate of weight loss over the past six months (Windsor 1993), use of alcohol, length of time with jaundice, and problems with diarrhea that may indicate fat malabsorption and steatorrhea. This assessment, although not clinically tested in prospective trials in patients undergoing liver surgery, is similar to the global nutritional assessment scale of Baker and Detsky (Baker et al 1982, Detsky et al 1987) and should provide a sensitive means of detecting patients at risk for nutritionally related problems following operation. Dixon (Dixon et al 1983), Pitt (Pitt et al 1981), and Halliday (Halliday et al 1988) identified

Table 26.2 Nutritional assessment

Clinical evaluation
Dietary and medical history
Physical activity
Weight loss over past 6 months

Physical exam
Body weight
Skin changes
Ascites?
Muscle mass and strength

Protein synthetic function
Albumin, transferrin
Prealbumin, protime
C-reactive protein

Vitamin, mineral, trace element deficits
Vitamins A, D, E, K, B6, niacin, folate, B_{12}
Thiamin, magnesium, potassium, zinc, iron, phosphorus

Table 26.3 Nutritional risk factors for postoperative complications in hepatobiliary surgery

Weight loss > 14% of lean body mass weight over previous 6 months
Serum albumin < 3.0 g/dl
Hct < 30%
Skin test alergy
< 25th percentile for mid-arm circumference and triceps skin fold
Total body potassium < 85% normal

From Pitt et al 1981, Halliday et al 1988, Harrison et al 1997

several nutritional risk factors in patients undergoing biliary tract surgery that were predictive of postoperative morbidity and mortality (Table 26.3). If these factors are identified in a patient being considered for an elective operation, preoperative nutritional repletion is probably indicated.

ANTIOXIDANT NUTRIENT DEPLETION IN THE PATHOGENESIS OF LIVER INJURY

Patients with liver disease, biliary obstruction, bacterial or viral infection and malnutrition have impaired antioxidant defenses coupled with increased oxidant stresses (Burra et al 1992, Bell et al 1992). Additional factors which deplete hepatic antioxidants include smoking, alcohol ingestion, general anesthesia and operation (Goode et al 1994, Bulger & Helton 1998). This likely contributes to increased risk for post operative infection and multiple organ dysfunction in this patient population. Data from animal studies suggest that a major pathophysiological event in hepatocellular injury is depletion of endogenous antioxidants (Burra et al 1992, Bell et al 1992) at the time of increased oxidative stress from infection (Sugino et al 1989, 1987), liver resection (Ouchi et al 1991), or transplantation (Serino et al 1990). Patients with chronic liver disease are at particularly high risk for having depleted stores of fat soluble vitamins. Patients with chronic liver disease have altered bile salt pools and enterohepatic circulation of bile salts, leading to impaired micelle formation which leads to malabsorption of fat and fat soluble vitamins (A, D, E, K). In fact, patients with advanced cirrhosis were found to have markedly depleted preoperative plasma levels of vitamin E, A and carotene which decreased even further following transplantation (Goode et al 1994). These low levels of antioxidants were associated with higher levels of lipid peroxide byproducts. Hence, patients with cirrhosis have lower antioxidant defenses, which compounds the insult of reperfusion injury by oxygen free radicals. Secondly, plasma levels of vitamin E decrease significantly in the first 48 hours after surgery or acute injury (Maderazo et al 1990, 1991). Low levels of vitamin E have also been previously reported in patients with varying levels of chronic liver damage (Goode et al 1994).

Obstructive jaundice is often associated with endotoxemia (Bailey 1976, Ding et al 1992) which leads to Kupffer cell production of oxygen radicals and nitric oxide which, in turn, inhibit protein synthesis (Curran et al 1990). Endotoxemia also reduces endogenous levels of the antioxidants glutathione, vitamin E and coenzyme Q (Marubayashi et al 1986). Studies in rodents demonstrate that supplemental vitamin E significantly attenuates liver ischemia reperfusion injury and hepatic lipid peroxidation (Sugino et al 1989). In vitro, physiological concentrations of vitamin E inhibit LPS-stimulated TNF secretion by Kupffer cells, suggesting that subnormal tissue or plasma levels of vitamin E may potentiate macrophage cytokine release (McClain et al 1994). Vitamin E has a variety of protective effects on the hepatobiliary system (Leo et al 1995). Vitamin E attenuates hepatocellular membrane lipid peroxidation and cellular damage following ischemia/reperfusion (Marubayashi et al 1986, Lee & Clemens 1992) and endotoxemia (Sugino et al 1989, Powell et al 1991). In rodents with bile duct obstruction, the concentrations of vitamin E and other antioxidants are reduced in liver tissue (Singh et al 1992, Sokol et al 1991). Large doses of enterally administered vitamin E inhibit the release of TNF in models of infection (Marubayashi et al 1989, Bulger et al 1997). Under these conditions, vitamin E supplementation improves survival following septic challenge (Yoshikawa 1984). These animal studies demonstrate a protective effect of vitamin E on liver function and survival during conditions commonly encountered in patients undergoing hepatobiliary surgery.

Vitamin C deficiency is evident in 50% of patients with alcoholic liver disease (Muller 1995) and is probably even lower in alcoholics who smoke. Vitamin C recycles reduced alpha-tocopherol and hence is intimately linked to vitamin E's ability to quench free radical mediated cellular damage (Sardesai 1995). The simultaneous administration of ascorbate and alpha tocopherol is more effective in inhibiting oxidation than either alone (Niki et al 1995). Ascorbate and vitamin E are located in different domains, with vitamin C acting as a first defense when the radicals are generated in the plasma, with vitamin E breaking the chain propagation at the cellular membrane level. The synergistic protective effects of vitamin C and E in preventing lipid peroxidation and cellular damage suggest that these vitamins should be administered together for maximal potential benefit (Bulger & Helton 1998).

The administration of fish oils or omega-3 fatty acids can also influence cytokine and prostanoid release by the intestine (Ogle et al 1995) and Kupffer cells of the liver (Bankey et al 1989, Billiar et al 1988). These observations demonstrate that hepatocellular function before and/or after hepatobiliary operations can be modulated by the administration of specific nutrients and vitamins (Marubayashi et al 1989, Helton 1994) and provide a potential opportunity whereby the hepatobiliary surgeon can influence patient outcome by nutritional means. While there are no clinical trials to date demonstrating that fish oil, omega three fatty acids or vitamin E supplemented diets improve the outcome of patients undergoing hepatobiliary operations, this is an area of nutritional support that should be studied in patients undergoing hepatobiliary operations.

SPECIFIC NUTRITIONAL PROBLEMS IN PATIENTS WITH HEPATOBILIARY DISEASES

Obstructive jaundice (see also Ch. 7)

Patients with significant jaundice often have anorexia and lose weight due to decreased oral intake. Approximately 45 to 70% of patients with obstructive jaundice present with malnutrition as judged by >10% weight loss, albumin < 3.0 g/dl, decreased triceps skin fold, and impaired delayed hypersensitivity reactivity (Foschi et al 1986). The primary nutritional deficit resulting from obstructive jaundice is malabsorption of fat and fat soluble vitamins. In addition, there is loss of trace minerals such as phosphate, calcium, magnesium and zinc due to salt formation from unabsorbed dietary fat (Shronts 1988). Patients with obstructive jaundice may suffer from ascites secondary to decreased serum albumin levels but rarely are the metabolism of carbohydrates and proteins altered (Flannigan et al 1985). Biliary sepsis in a patient with obstructive jaundice contributes to malnutrition by shifting protein synthesis from anabolic protein synthesis to acute phase protein synthesis (O'Neill et al 1997). This reprioritization of protein synthesis occurs as a result of endotoxin stimulated Kupffer cell production of tumor necrosis factor, interleukin-6, eicosanoids, nitric oxide, and other inflammatory mediators that directly inhibit protein synthesis (Curran et al 1990, Heinrick 1990). Because of these derangements, some have advocated biliary drainage prior to liver resection. Three randomized trials completed to date do not support such an approach (Hatfield et al 1982, McPherson et al 1984, Pitt et al 1985). In fact, in one of these trials, the preoperatively drained patients have increased morbidity due to increased incidence of infection. In our practice, therefore, we do not routinely perform biliary decompression preoperatively except in specific clinical scenarios: associated sepsis, renal failure, or severe malnutrition. To reverse the catabolic effects of chronic endotoxemia and restore hepatic protein synthesis, patients with biliary infection should be treated by biliary decompression for at least 4 weeks prior to major hepatobiliary surgery in order to allow hepatocytes to recover their protein synthetic capacity.

Cirrhosis and liver failure (see also Chs 92, 85)

The cirrhotic patient provides the clinician with a major challenge. Cirrhotics have multiple hormonal and metabolic alterations. Characteristics of cirrhotic patients include wasting symptoms: especially loss of fat and muscle mass, growth failure, glucose intolerance, hyperinsulinemia, insulin resistence, increased plasma glucagon and catecholamines, elevated serum free fatty acids, elevated glycerol, hypoproteinemia, hyperammonemia, hypophosphatemia and alterations in both plasma and cerebral spinal fluid amino acid profiles (Achord 1987, Petrides & de Fronzo 1989, Riggio et al 1984, Henriksen et al 1984). These hormonal and metabolic aberrations lead to altered metabolism of all three macronutrients (fat, protein and carbohydrate). The hormonal and metabolic changes seen in cirrhosis also lead to an increased skeletal muscle proteolysis for energy provision which leads to eventual muscle wasting. In addition, there is increased peripheral lipolysis with a decreased ability to utilize fat and carbohydrate which leads to hyperglycemia and hyperlipidemia (Katz 1986).

Compounding these metabolic alterations are issues that predispose cirrhotics to malnutrition. These include decreased dietary intake due to nausea, vomiting, and the common practice of imposing protein restriction in an effort to prevent encephalopathy. This practice of protein restriction is questionable in an already malnourished patient. Protein restriction exacerbates the problems inherently associated with malnutrition and prohibits the goal of liver regeneration. An alteration of plasma and cerebral spinal fluid amino acid profiles caused by catabolism, impaired hepatocellular function and portal shunting leads to decreased levels of branched chain amino acids (BCAA) (valine, leucine, isoleucine) and the preferred uptake into the brain of aromatic amino acids (phenylalanine, tyrosine, tryptophan). The increased uptake of aromatic amino acids is thought to alter the production of neurotransmitters resulting in encephalopathy. This theory led to the use of branched chain amino acids as dietary treatment for patients with liver disease. By correcting the serum amino acid profile by BCAA administration the hope is to reverse mental status changes and promote anabolism (Fischer et al 1976). In theory this practice sounds promising but unfortunately studies have been inconclusive with respect to the efficacy of BCAA and their use to prevent encephalopathy are not justified by clinical data (Naylor et al 1989).

Liver resection

Metabolic alterations occur in the regenerating liver following liver resection (Diehl 1991). Krebs cycle activity is depressed as is the redox state of the hepatic mitochondria with a switch from the utilization of glucose to fat as the preferred source of energy by way of beta oxidation (Nakatoni et al 1981). Because hyperglycemia and hyperinsulinemia suppress the release of fatty acids from adipose tissue and decrease ketone body production by the liver (Riou et al 1986) hypertonic glucose infusions and insulin administration should be avoided in the immediate (< 6 hours) postoperative period (Ozawa 1992). These observations indicate that selective administration of fat or ketone bodies shortly after liver resection or transplantation may be beneficial. In fact, in rodents, the provision of intravenous fat (30% of total nonprotein calories) (Nishiguchi et al 1991, Hamada 1993) or the ketone body monacetoacetate (Birkhahn et al 1989) immediately following liver resection accelerates liver regeneration. The administration of medium chain triglycerides following liver resection results in better hepatic energy charge and decreased lipid peroxidation when compared with the effects of intravenous glucose or long chain triglyceride infusions (Hamada 1993).

Sarac hypothesized that increasing fat oxidation preoperatively by way of fasting would improve liver function after extensive liver resection in rats. Rats subjected to 90% hepatectomy had improved survival to almost 100% when fasted 24 hours before operation and fed oral glucose immediately after operation (Sarac et al 1994). There was greater utilization of ketone bodies by the liver of fasted rats suggesting that the enzyme machinery for utilizing free fatty acids was induced by the previous fast. This study demonstrates that the surgeon can potentially manipulate the metabolic machinery of the liver preoperatively and subsequently provide the appropriate substrates by the appropriate route to optimize hepatocellular energetics and regeneration.

The regenerating liver has an increased demand for specific amino acids and provision of these in the diet accelerates regeneration. Immediately after liver resection there is an abrupt increase in the synthesis of the system A amino acid transporter (which transports alanine, serine, and methionine) but not of system N (glutamine, histidine, asparagine) or ASC (cysteine and others) (Fowler et al 1992). Increased system A activity is dependent on portal glucagon and insulin secretion as well as substrate amino acid supply (Dolais-Kitabgi et al 1981); system N and ASC are not similarly regulated (Fowler et al 1992). This fact supports the argument by many liver surgeons that enteral administration of glucose is the preferred route of feeding because of the effect on insulin release which is vital to the function of the regenerating liver (Ozawa 1992, Ozawa et al 1974).

Provision of adequate protein and calories is important to ensure adequate liver regeneration. Rats subjected to 50% of normal daily caloric intake for 1 week prior to and following liver resection had significantly impaired liver regeneration, even when administered exogenous IGF-I, compared with normally fed rats (Sato et al 1994). Specific types of protein supplemented diets such as a nucleoside-nucleotide-supplemented total parenteral nutrition (TPN) solution may improve protein synthesis following hepatectomy (Ogoshi et al 1989).

John et al reported that postoperative TPN (consisting of 45% fat calories) significantly impaired hepatic regeneration and albumin synthesis, caused cholestasis, and increased mortality when compared to the same diet administered by the enteral route after 70% hepatectomy in rats (John et al 1992). Mortality in rats fed TPN was 68%, 9% in those fed enterally, and 8% in those fed chow. This increased mortality in TPN fed rats could be due to increased bacterial translocation and (LPS) migration across the gut, which overwhelms the limited phagocyte capacity of the remnant Kupffer cell mass (van Leeuwen et al 1991) or excessive administration of intravenous glucose calories that adversely effects liver substrate metabolism (Ozawa 1992, Ozawa et al 1976). In fact, the same group of investigators subsequently demonstrated that the lethal consequences of parenteral nutrition after liver resection in rats could be ameliorated by decreasing the caloric and amino acid load (Delany et al 1994). This study suggested that the remnant liver has a limited capacity to metabolize intravenous glucose; a finding in keeping with Ozawa's contention that the liver slowly regains its ability to metabolize glucose after resection or transplantation (Ozawa 1992).

Transplantation (see also Section 14)

In the first 6 hours following liver transplantation, glucose utilization by the transplanted liver is impaired until the redox state of the mitochondria improves (Ozaki et al 1991). During this time, the liver preferentially uses fatty acid oxidation for ATP generation (Ozaki et al 1991, Takada et al 1993). After 6 hours, normally functioning liver allografts shift substrate utilization from fat to glucose, whereas failing livers continue to utilize fat. This shift in metabolism can be followed by measuring the plasma concentration of total ketone bodies and (AKBR) (Takada et al 1993). Based on these observations, Takada et al (1993) suggests that glucose should be administered in small quantities in the immediate postoperative period without insulin to avoid suppressing peripheral fat mobilization. Glucose infusion should be steadily increased as mitochondria respiration recovers and the Krebs cycle becomes active. When the redox state of mitochondria is sufficiently improved (e.g. AKBR > 0.7), amino acids and increased amounts of glucose can be administered.

The nutritional status of the donor liver may be one of the more important factors affecting posttransplant allograft function. Initially it was believed that liver allografts obtained from fasted subjects were more susceptible to anoxic liver injury due to an absence of glycogen as a source of glucose from glycolysis than livers obtained from subjects being administered glucose up to the time of liver donation (Bradford et al 1986). In addition, it was shown that livers from fasted animals had enhanced generation of oxygen radicals by Kupffer cells (Gasbarrini et al 1993). Subsequent work in animal liver transplant models (Palombo et al 1988, Astarcioglu et al 1991) and human liver donors (Cywes et al 1992) demonstrated that glucose administration to the donor increases liver glycogen and ATP content prior to cold preservation and attenuates liver injury following transplantation. However, more recent work by Southard and his colleagues demonstrates that the effects of fasting and feeding on liver allograft function after cold preservation and reperfusion are more complex. These investigators reported no relationship between hepatic glycogen content and post transplant function after cold preservation (Sumimoto et al 1993). In addition, Southard has shown that livers from fasted rats undergo two changes, one that sensitizes it to preservation/reperfusion injury (short-term fast (1–3 days)) and one that increases its tolerance to preservation injury (long-term fast (4 days)). Long-term fasting actually improves subsequent liver allograft function in the rat (Sumimoto et al 1993). The mechanisms for this protection are unclear but possibly related to the accumulation of metabolites within the liver that are readily used as a source of energy upon reperfusion or the fact that xanthine oxidase content is decreased (Rowe & Wingaarden 1996). The latter change may explain why livers from prolonged fasted rats generate less oxygen radicals after reperfusion.

Cancer

Hepatic cancer is commonly accompanied by progressive weight loss, anorexia and malnutrition. Patients with hepatocellular carcinoma usually have advanced cirrhosis and for that reason their malnutrition is often more pronounced. Inefficient energy utilization due to increased Cori-cycle activity (Holroyde & Reichard 1981) may be seen as well as other common occurrences with liver damage such as increased protein turnover rates with altered amino acid profiles, increased gluconeogenesis, and increased lipid oxidation (Holroyde & Reichard 1981, Young 1977, Waterhouse et al 1979). If jaundice is present, fat malabsorption will often occur in these patients. Profound malnourished patients with cirrhosis or chronic active hepatitis and hepatocellular carcinoma usually present in an advanced clinical stage such as Okuda class III. As a general rule, these patients should not undergo operation because of a prohibitive operative mortality (Okuda et al 1985).

NUTRITIONAL MANAGEMENT IN PATIENTS UNDERGOING HEPATOBILIARY OPERATIONS INCLUDING LIVER TRANSPLANTATION

The primary indication for nutritional support in any patient before and after a hepatobiliary operation is to decrease the incidence of postoperative complications by repleting nutrient deficits that occurred as a result of their anorexia, malabsorption and catabolic states. In addition, nutritional support strives to preserve protein synthesis, prevent hepatocellular dysfunction and injury, and provide a favorable environment for liver cell repair and regeneration. There are no data to support the routine use of nutrition support in well nourished patients undergoing hepatobiliary operations. In fact, the administration of parenteral nutrition to well-nourished patients undergoing operation is associated with a higher incidence of postoperative complications (Buzby 1991, Brennan et al 1994). Conversely, patients who are profoundly malnourished or deficient in specific vitamins probably benefit from pre- and post-operative nutritional support (Helton 1994, Halliday et al 1988, Buzby 1991).

There are several methods available to provide patients nutritional support. Most common and most physiologic is an oral diet tailored to the patient's specific needs. If the patient is unable to consume an oral diet or unable to meet their estimated caloric needs orally, a soft silastic nasogastric or nasoduodenal feeding tube should be placed. In the event that the patient is unable or unwilling to accept a nasoenteric feeding tube, then serious consideration should be given to placing a feeding jejunostomy or gastrostomy tube using the endoscopic or laparoscopic approach (Duh & Way 1993). Lastly, in the rare event that a patient can tolerate oral and/or enteral nutrients but can not meet his/her total nutritional needs by oral alone, combination diets utilizing partial enteral feeding or partial parenteral feeding are appropriate. Standard parenteral solutions usually are acceptable in these patients. Use of branched chain amino acid based solutions as stated earlier can not be justified at this time (McCullough & Tavill 1991). The increased infectious complications and costs associated with parenteral nutrition mandate that this route of feeding be used only when the enteral route is unavailable. Profoundly malnourished patients with malabsorption who develop diarrhea in response to enteral feeding can receive partial enteral nutrition with the balance of calories, protein, fat, trace elements and vitamins administered by the peripheral intravenous route (Benya et al 1990).

An enteral formula should be chosen based upon the patient's ability to digest and absorb nutrients. For most patients a standard enteral diet is sufficient. General guidelines for feeding are listed in Table 26.4 and are sufficient for the majority of patients. There are a few situations where modified special formulated diets may be of some benefit to the patient with hepatobiliary disease or pancreatic insufficiency. The theoretical potential of modulating the inflammatory and cytokine systems prior to operation by the administration of fish oils alone or in combination with antioxidants is a potential way of nutritionally improving patient outcomes but has not been studied to date.

Table 26.4 General guidelines for nutritional support

Oral route > enteral > picc line > TPN
Kcal: 30 kcal/kg/day
Nitrogen: 1.0–1.5 g/kg/day
Glucose: not to exceed 5 mg/kg/min
Fat calories: no more than 30% of total calories

Obstructive jaundice (see also Ch. 7)

If patients are profoundly malnourished and preoperative nutritional repletion is indicated, an argument can be made to reestablish bile flow by placing a biliary stent for decompression of the biliary tree prior to proceeding with a major operation. However, before undertaking this step each individual patient should be assessed for ability to tolerate fat and dietary recommendations based on this assessment. As a general rule, restoration of bile flow will improve absorption of fat and fat soluble vitamins. Foschi and colleagues reported a prospective randomized trial where patients with obstructive jaundice were randomized to biliary decompression followed by operation or biliary decompression combined with two weeks of alimentation followed by operation. Malnutrition was present in 70% of the patients. 85% of the patients receiving alimentation received at least partial enteral feeding. Patients receiving alimentation for 2 weeks had lower morbidity (17 versus 46%), mortality (3.5 versus 12.5%) and postoperative infection (14 versus 28%) compared to patients receiving only biliary decompression.

When bile flow is not re-established in patients with biliary obstruction who require nutritional support there is an impaired ability to tolerate fat in the diet. Such patients should ingest a low fat diet supplemented with water soluble forms of the fat soluble vitamins (e.g. Aquasol E®, ADEKS®). They should also receive supplements of calcium, phosphorus, and magnesium (Shronts 1988). Rather than struggle with the problems of inadequate oral intake in these anorectic patients, they are more easily and effectively repleted nutritionally by tube feedings because of the ability to administer more physiologic diets containing predigested protein (dipeptides and tripeptides) and a blend of medium chain triglycerides (MCTs) and long chain triglycerides (LCTs). These specialized diets help avoid diarrhea from fat maldigestion and malabsorption because the absorption of MCTs is not dependent on bile salts nor dependent on pancreatic lipase as are LCTs (Shopko et al 1991, McCullough et al 1989). Patients with obstructive jaundice require approximately 25–35 kcal/kg dry weight to maintain nitrogen balance (McCullough et al 1989). It is recommended that 25 to 40% of total calories be provided by fat as tolerated but this is unlikely without biliary decompression (McCullough et al 1989).

Cirrhosis and hepatic failure (see also Chs 92, 95)

The following discussion summarizes the essentials of nutritional management of the cirrhotic patient. For more detailed discussions, the interested reader is referred to other authors on this topic (Shronts 1988, McCullough & Tavill 1991, Nompleggi & Bonkovsky 1994).

Hospitalized patients with cirrhosis requiring operation have substantial morbidity and mortality (Rice et al 1997). Since malnutrition is a major problem in these patients aggressive nutritional support should be undertaken when operation is being contemplated or carried out. Prospective, randomized clinical trials have shown that hospitalized cirrhotics do not meet their nutritional needs with aggressive daily dietary counseling and have reduced hospital mortality and morbidity when fed via nasogastric or duodenal tubes (Cabre et al 1990). It is therefore recommended that all hospitalized cirrhotic patients undergoing emergency operation be fed via the enteral route unless otherwise contraindicated; use of parenteral nutrition in these patients is not indicated if the gastrointestinal track is functional.

Since the metabolic derangement of advanced liver disease affects all three macronutrients any dietary intervention needs to supplement all three. The caloric needs of patients with liver disease are increased (25–35 kcal/kg/day) particularly if they have ascites (McCullough & Tavill 1991). Protein needs depend on the patient's current nutritional status, ability to tolerate protein, and the presence or history of encephalopathy. In the nonencephalopathic patient 1–1.5 g protein/kg dry weight is recommended. If encephalopathy is present a thorough diet history should be taken to determine the tolerable amount of protein with recommendations to supply at least a minimum 0.5–0.7 g/kg dry weight per day. In a small number of patients with hepatic encephalopathy, the use of vegetable protein versus meat protein has been found to be beneficial

in some studies, though such use of vegetable protein (Shaw et al 1983) is not universally accepted.

Fluid and sodium restriction is often necessary depending on the severity of ascites and edema. A level of at least 2 g of sodium/day is recommended because lower levels are unpalatable and will usually decrease dietary intake further, thus exacerbating the patient's malnutrition. In cases of intractable ascites a 500–1000 mg sodium diet and 1.0–1.5 L of fluid has been recommended by some nutritional support experts (Shronts & Fish 1993). However, it is our opinion that treatment of massive ascites should rely more on aggressive diuretics rather than drastic limits on fluid intake. Cirrhotics and patients with hepatic failure commonly have micronutrient deficiencies (phosphate, magnesium, zinc) and these should be measured, monitored and aggressively repleted as necessary by the intravenous route (Shronts 1988).

Liver resection (see also Section 12)

The majority of patients in Western countries undergoing liver resection have no associated cirrhosis and therefore have no need for specialized nutritional support pre- or postoperatively. The majority can safely begin an oral diet on the first or second postoperative day and they are able to tolerate a full regular diet within 5 days. The malnourished patients being considered for elective liver resection should receive nutritional repletion pre- and postoperatively by the oral or enteral routes. In addition, patients undergoing extensive liver resection, particulary those with compromised preoperative hepatocellular function (e.g. steatosis, chronic viral hepatitis or cirrhosis) may benefit from specialized nutritional support. Based upon the physiology discussed previously, it is strongly recommended that patients not receive hypertonic glucose infusions in the immediate (less than 6 hours) postoperative periods since this can interfere with the liver's preferential use of fatty acids for energy and hepatic regeneration. If nutritional support is initiated within 24 or 48 hours after liver resection, it should be administered via the enteral route through a nasoduodenal or jejunal tube. Therefore, if the patient is profoundly malnourished preoperatively and the surgeon intends to administer postoperative nutrition, placement of a feeding jejunostomy tube at the time of operation should be considered.

Nutritional therapy can potentially attenuate damage to the residual liver in patients scheduled to undergo elective liver resection by preventing further reductions in endogenous antioxidants and repleting deficient antioxidant defenses. Patients at risk for depleted hepatic antioxidant defenses are those with a long history of obstructive jaundice, alcoholics, smokers, chronic biliary infection, and chronic active viral hepatitis (Bulger & Helton 1998, Helton 1994). Therefore, it is imperative that all patients stop smoking and cease ethanol ingestion a couple of weeks preoperatively in order to replete their intrinsic antioxidant defenses so as to avoid further oxidation stress and lipid peroxidation after operation. It can take up to 2 weeks of oral vitamin E supplementation to significantly increase vitamin E content in some tissues (Yau et al 1994). Therefore patients at risk for vitamin E deficits should receive supplements for 2 weeks preoperatively when possible.

A prospective randomized trial evaluated the effect of an antioxidant vitamin infusion (Omnibionta) which included 10 mg of alpha-tocopherol acetate, 2 mg of DL alpha tocopherol and 1 g of ascorbate in patients undergoing liver surgery (Cerwenka et al 1998). An antioxidant protective effect of Omnibionta was demonstrated by significantly less postischemic increases in transaminases and prothrombin time compared to patients not receiving the vitamin infusion. When taking into consideration the fact that vitamins are cheap, safe and readily available and that patients undergoing hepatobiliary operations are at risk for oxygen radical mediated injury, it is rational to administer vitamin E and C for several days preoperatively to patients at risk for postoperative complications.

To explore the hypothesis that the remnant liver following liver resection has limited capacity to metabolize glucose, Nishizaki and colleagues randomized patients after liver resection to receive peripheral glucose infusion (10 kcal/kg/day) or hypertonic glucose via central line for 7 days; both groups were allowed ad libitum food intake when tolerated. The average caloric intake of the two groups was 20 kcal/kg/day (peripheral dextrose) and 30 kcal/kg/day (hypertonic glucose) (Nishizaki et al 1996). There were no untoward effects from the hypertonic glucose infusion and patients in that group had improved prealbumin, decreased urinary 3-methylhistidine excretion and improved nitrogen balance as compared to the patients receiving peripheral glucose. The results of this study demonstrated that the remnant liver is not harmed by increased loads of glucose.

Haupt and colleagues investigated the effects of three separate parenteral diets on hepatocellular function in patients following segmental liver resection and did not find any adverse effects, even with a lipid-based diet providing 40% of total calories as fat (Haupt et al 1990). However, patients in this study were not profoundly malnourished and therefore a beneficial effect of TPN may not be expected or demonstrable. Shirabe and colleagues compared the effects of parenteral and early enteral nutrition in patients undergoing elective liver resection and reported that the group that received early enteral nutrition had improved postoperative immunologic function and decreased infectious complications compared to the parenteral group (8 versus 31% respectively) (Shirabe et al 1997).

Liver transplantation

Recent clinical and experimental observations demonstrate that nutrition plays an extremely important role in just about all aspects of the liver transplantation. The status of the donor, the function of the transplanted liver, the overall health of the recipient, the rejection process, the absorption and metabolism of immunosuppressive drugs, and a variety of metabolic pathways are influenced by nutrients and how they are administered. Clinical observations demonstrate that malnourished patients undergoing liver transplantation have significantly poorer outcome than well-nourished patients (Shaw et al 1985, Porayko et al 1991). Degree of malnutrition correlates significantly with days spent in the ICU, on a ventilator, and in the hospital as well as with mortality following transplantation (Pikul et al 1994). Furthermore, liver transplant recipients are predisposed to postoperative infectious complications not only because of severe preoperative protein calorie malnutrition but also because of the immunosuppressive drugs (O'Keefe et al 1980, 1981). Profoundly malnourished recipients have an incidence of infectious morbidity and 3-month mortality that is twice that of well-nourished patients undergoing liver transplant (Harrison et al 1997).

Several studies have investigated the effects of nutritional support in liver transplant patients (Harrison et al 1997, Hasse et al 1995, Chin et al 1990, Reilly et al 1990, Mehta et al 1995, Martin et al 1993, Wicks et al 1994). Based upon these studies, patients awaiting transplantation who are malnourished should receive aggressive nutritional counseling and support (Harrison et al 1997, Plauth et al 1997, Harrison et al 1993). Nutritional supplements including vitamins should be taken in an effort to attenuate further nutritional deficits and to replenish losses. Patients who ingest inadequate amounts of calories should be fed via a soft silastic nasogastric feeding tube. In contrast to what most people and physicians believe, these tubes are well-tolerated and can be used for months without much difficulty or patient discomfort.

Chin et al reported that children awaiting transplantation who were force fed via a nasogastric tube improved their nutritional status when receiving supplemental nutrition (Chin et al 1990) while those who were only encouraged to take supplements continued to deteriorate nutritionally while they were on the waiting list. In addition, aggressive nutritional support of pediatric patients awaiting liver transplantation improves clinical outcome following transplantation primarily by reducing the risk of infection (Charlton et al 1992).

Reilly prospectively studied the effects of three intravenous diets in hypoalbuminemic patients after liver transplanation. The three diets were a branched chain amino acid-based TPN solution, a standard TPN diet, and intravenous glucose (Reilly et al 1990). Both TPN diets provided 1.5 g protein/kg/day and 35 kcal/kg/day. Glucose was limited to 5 mg/kg/min and the balance of energy provided as 10% Intralipid. Patients in both TPN groups were extubated and discharged from the ICU a mean of 2.3 days earlier compared with patients receiving only glucose. In addition, overall hospital charges were estimated to be $21 000 less in the patients receiving either standard or branched chain TPN. Reilly concluded that malnourished patients undergoing transplantation can and should receive postoperative TPN.

A number of transplant centers subsequently demonstrated that liver transplant patients can be fed successfully and safely by a nasoduodenal or nasojejunal tube within hours after transplantation (Hasse et al 1995, Mehta et al 1995, Martin et al 1993, Wicks et al 1994). In three studies, early initiation of feeding (< 24 h) after operation was associated with a postoperative infection rate lower than expected (Hasse et al 1995, Mehta et al 1995, Martin et al 1993, Wicks et al 1994). In the prospective, randomized study reported by Hasse, the enterally fed patients had no viral infections in the first 2 postoperative weeks compared with 17% of patients fed intravenously ($P < 0.05$). Bacterial and overall infection rates were also decreased in the enterally fed group (14 versus 29% and 21 versus 41%, respectively) although the differences did not reach statistical significance. Mehta reported that post operative liver transplant patients fed immediately via the enteral route had decreased incidence of postoperative ileus (5 versus 28%, $P < 0.01$) and started on oral feedings much sooner (8 versus 12 days, $P = 0.07$) than patients fed intravenously (Mehta et al 1995). Based upon these studies, post operative nutritional support, if indicated for nutritional repletion or maintenance, should be administered via a nasoduodenal or jejunal tube.

Based upon the hypothesized benefits of increasing glycogen levels of the liver prior to cold preservation. The University of Toronto Liver Transplant Group carried out a prospective, randomized trail in which they treated the donor liver prior to procurement by a short-term intraportal glucose and insulin infusion (Cywes et al 1992). This study demonstrated that increasing liver glycogen content

decreased preservation and reperfusion injury compared to nontreated livers. The protective effect of glycogenation was not clinically apparent and only detected by differences in serum transaminase levels. Furthermore, the protective effects were predominantly evident in patients with prolonged warm ischemia times, suggesting that the extra glycogen provided substrate for anaerobic glycolysis as the liver warmed up prior to becoming reperfused.

Recent animal studies demonstrate that specific amino acids such as glycine and glutamate protect the liver from cold preservation injury (Marsh et al 1993, Southard et al 1990). The nutritional modulation of liver allografts is an area of active investigation by several labs and holds great promise for improving the outcome of patients undergoing liver transplantation in the future.

Cancer

A large number of liver cancer patients suffer from major metabolic alterations coupled with some degree of wasting. Therefore, each individual patient should be evaluated for current nutritional status and an individual nutritional plan devised to maintain and/or replete their nutritional status. This includes increased calorie and protein provision when necessary (up to 35 kcal/kg dry weight per day, up to 2.0 grams of protein/kg dry weight/day and micronutrient supplementation as needed (Fan et al 1994)). Dietary restrictions of any kind should be avoided if at all possible in these patients including sodium and fluid restrictions.

There are few well-conducted prospective randomized trials that have demonstrated any significant benefit from nutritional support for patients with cancer of the hepatobiliary tree undergoing operation. The best study published to date is by Fan and colleagues from Hong Kong who demonstrated the utility of pre- and postoperative TPN in patients undergoing elective liver resection for hepatocellular carcinoma. In this study the authors randomized 120 patients to one of two groups: standard oral diet preoperatively and intravenous dextrose postoperatively or TPN in addition to oral diet pre- and postoperatively. The perioperative nutritional therapy consisted of a solution enriched with 35% branched-chain amino acids, dextrose, and lipid emulsion (50% medium chain triglycerides) given intravenously for 14 days (7 days preoperatively for 12 hours a day and 7 days postoperatively continuously). The TPN diet provided 30 kcal/kg/day and 1.5 g of amino acid per kg of body weight per day. The TPN supplemented group of patients had a reduction in overall postoperative morbidity as compared with the control group (34 versus 55%) predominantly because of fewer septic complications (17 versus 37%). There was also less deterioration of liver function as measured by the change in the rate of clearance of indocyanine green and less ascites. Postoperative mortality in the perioperative TPN group was also 45% less than in the control group. Two important aspects of this study are that 90% of the patients had either cirrhosis or chronic active hepatitis and the average nutritional status of patients in both groups was adequate. The complication rates and deaths were not stratified according to the preoperative severity of malnutrition. Hence, it is unknown if the beneficial treatment effect of perioperative TPN was beneficial to all patients or specific for patients with malnutrition. Nevertheless, the general conclusion of this well-conducted study is that patients with cirrhosis and/or chronic active hepatitis with hepatocellular carcinoma undergoing liver resection appear to benefit from perioperative parenteral nutrition. Whether these clinical improvements in outcome observed by Fan from perioperative TPN could possibly be even greater if the enteral route of nutritional support is employed awaits future comparative trials, since this is the only major trial to demonstrate a benefit for TPN in the perioperative care of patients undergoing any major oncologic procedure, most clinicians have not yet begun to use TPN routinely in patients without major malnutrition. Most are awaiting further confirmatory data.

SUMMARY

Careful attention must be paid to the hepatobiliary patient's overall clinical condition, inadequacy of diet and degree of malnutrition to determine the appropriate level, if any, of nutrition support. Inappropriate therapy can result in further metabolic abnormalities and patient harm. There is increasing evidence that specific nutrients administered under specific conditions to selected patients can modulate metabolic events in the patient with hepatobiliary disease. Therefore, before prescribing nutritional therapy to the patient, a clinician or dietician with experience and expertise in liver metabolism should be consulted to evaluate the patient, provide recommendations for a diet and monitor the patient's course.

REFERENCES

Achord J 1987 Malnutrition and the role of nutritional support in alcoholic liver support. American Journal of Gastroenterology 82: 1

Andus T, Bauer J, Wolfgang G 1991 Effects of cytokines on the liver. Hepatology 13(2): 364–375

Armstrong C, Dixon J M, Taylor T V et al 1984 Surgical experience of deeply jaundiced patients with bile duct obstruction. British Journal of Surgery 74: 234–238

Astarcioglu I, Adam R, Gigou M et al 1991 High levels of glycogen in the donor liver improve survival after liver transplantation in rats. Transpl Proced 23(5): 2465–2466

Bailey M E 1976 Endotoxin, bile salts and renal function in obstructive jaundice. British Journal of Surgery 63: 774–778

Baker J, Detsky A S, Wesson D E et al 1982 Nutritional assessment: A comparison of clinical judgment and objective measurements. New England Journal of Medicine 306: 969–972

Bankey P, Billiar T R, Wang W Y et al 1989 Modulation of Kupffer cell membrane phospholipid function by n-3 polyunsaturated fatty acids. JSR 46: 439–444

Bell H, Bjorneboe A, Eidsvoll B et al 1992 Reduced concentration of hepatic alpha tocopherol in patients with alcoholic liver cirrhosis. Alcohol-Alcohol 27(1): 39–46

Benya R, Damle P, Mobarhan S 1990 Diarrhea complicating enteral feeding after liver transplantation. Nurt-Rev 48(3): 148–152

Billiar T, Bankey P E, Svingen B A et al 1988 Fatty acid intake and Kupffer cell function: fish oil alters eicosanoid and monokine production to endotoxin stimulation. Surgery 104: 343

Birkhahn R, Awad S, Klaunig J E et al 1989 Interaction of ketosis and liver regeneration in the rat. JSR 47: 427–432

Bradford B U, Marotto M, Lemasters J J et al 1986 New simple models to evaluate zone-specific damage due to hypoxia in the perfused rat liver: time course and effect of nutritional state. Journal of Pharmacology and Experimental Therapeutics 236: 262–268

Brennan M, Pisters P W, Posner M et al 1994 A prospective randomized trial of total parenteral nutrition after major pancreatic resection for malignancy. Annals of Surgery 220(4): 436–444

Bulger E, Helton W S, Clinton C M et al 1997 Enteral vitamin E supplementation inhibits the cytokine response to endotoxin. Archives of Surgery 132: 1337–1341

Bulger E, Helton W 1998 Nutrient antioxidants in gastrointestinal disease. Gastroenterology Clinics of North America 27(2): 403–419

Burra P et al 1992 Hepatic malondialdehyde and glutathione in end stage chronic liver disease. Hep 16(4 pt 2): 266A

Buzby G, Mullen J L, Matthews D C et al 1980 Prognostic nutritional index in gastrointestinal surgery. American Journal of Surgery 139: 160–167

Buzby G P 1991 Veterans Affairs total parenteral nutrition cooperative study group: perioperative total parenteral nutrition in surgical patients. New England Journal of Medicine 325: 525–532

Cabre E, Gonzales-Huix F, Abad-Lacruz A et al 1990 Effect of total enteral nutrition on the short-term outcome of severely malnourished cirrhotics. Gastroenterology 98: 715–720

Cerwenka H, Bacher H, Werkgartner G et al 1998 Antioxidant treatment during liver resection for alleviation of ischemia–reperfusion injury. Hepatogastroenterology 45(21): 777–782

Charlton C, Buchanan E, Holden C E et al 1992 Intensive enteral feeding in advanced cirrhosis: reversal of malnutrition without precipitation of hepatic encephalopathy. Archives of Disease in Childhood 67(5): 603–607

Chin S, Shepherd R W, Cleghorn G J et al 1990 Pre-operative nutritional support in children with end-stage liver disease accepted for liver transplantion: an approach to management. J Gastroenterol-Hepatol 5(5): 566–72

Colonna J, Winston D J, Brill J E et al 1988 Infectious complications in liver transplantation. Archives of Surgery 123: 360–364

Curran R, Billiar T et al 1990 Multiple cytokines are required to induce hepatocyte nitric oxide production and inhibit protein synthesis. Annals of Surgery 212: 460–471

Cywes R, Greig P D, Sanbria J R et al 1992 Effect of intraportal glucose infusion on hepatic glycogen content and degradation, and outcome of liver transplantation. Annals of Surgery 216: 235–247

Delany H, John J, Teh E L et al 1994 Contrasting effects of identical nutrients given parenterally or enterally after 70% hepatectomy. American Journal of Surgery 167: 135–144

Detsky A, Baker J P, O'RourkeK et al 1987 Predicting nutrition-associated complications for patients undergoing gastrointestinal surgery. J Parenteral and Enteral Nutrition 11: 440–446

Diehl A 1991 Nutrition, hormones, metabolism, and liver regeneration. Seminars in Liver Disease 11(4): 315–320

Ding J, Anderson R, Norgen L et al 1992 The influence of biliary obstruction and sepsis on reticuloendothelial function. European Journal of Surgery 158: 157–164

Dixon J, Armstrong C P, Duffy S W et al 1983 Factors affecting morbidity and mortality after surgery for obstructive jaundice: a review of 373 patients. Gut 24: 845–852

Dolais-Kitabgi J, Rey J F, Fehlmann M et al 1981 Effect of insulin and glucagon on amino acid transport in isolated hepatocytes after partial hepatectomy in the rat. Endocrin 109(868–875)

Duh Q, Way L 1993 Laparoscopic jejunostomy using T-fasteners as retractors and anchors. Archives of Surgery 128(1): 105–108

Eigler N, Sacca L, Sherwin R 1979 Synergistic interactions of physiologic increments of glucagon, epinephrine and cortisol in the dog. A model for stress induced hyperglycemia. Journal of Clinical Investigation 63: 114

Fan S, Lo C M, Lai E C et al 1994 Perioperative nutritional support in patients undergoing hepatectomy for hepatocellular carcinoma. New England Journal of Medicine 331: 1547–1552

Fischer J, Rosen H M, Ebeid A M et al 1976 The effect of normalization of plasma amino-acids on hepatic encephalopathy in man. Surgery 80: 77

Flannigan G et al 1985 Glucose and alanine metabolism in obstructive jaundice. Clin Nutr (suppl) 4: 26

Fong Y, Marano M A, Barber A et al 1989 Total parenteral nutrition and bowel rest modify the metabolic response to endotoxin in humans. Annals of Surgery 210(4): 449–457

Foschi D, Cavagna G, Callioni F et al 1986 Hyperalimentation of jaundiced patients on percutaneous transhepatic biliary drainage. British Journal of Surgery 73: 716

Fowler F, Banks R, Maillard M 1992 Characterization of sodium-dependent amino acid transport activity during liver regeneration. Hepatology 16: 1187–1194

Gasbarrini A, Caraceni P, Bernardi M 1993 Fasting enhances the anoxia/reoxygenation injury on freshly isolated rat hepatocytes. Hepatology 18(4): 125A

Gitlin N, Heyman M B 1984 Nutritional support in liver disease. Nutr Sup Serv 4(6): 14

Goode J et al 1994 Reperfusion injury, antioxidants and hemodynamics during orthotopic liver transplantation. Hepatology 19(2): 354–359

Greenburger M, Carley J, Schenker S et al 1977 Effect of vegetable and animal protein diets in chronic hepatic encephalopathy. Digestive Diseases and Sciences 22: 845–855

Halliday A, Benjamin I, Blumgart L 1988 Nutritional risk factors in major hepatobiliary surgery. J Parenteral and Enteral Nutrition 12(1): 43–48

Hamada H 1993 Effects of medium chain triglyceride administration on liver regeneration after partial hepatectomy in rats. Hokkaido-Igaku-Zasshi. 68(1): 96–109

Harrison J et al 1993 The effect of recipient nutrition on outcome in elective orthotopic liver transplantation (OLT) (abstract). Hepatology 18(4, pt 2): 333A

Harrison J, McKiernan J, Neuberger J. A prospective study on the effect of recipient nutritional status on outcome in liver transplantation. Transplant International 10(5): 369–374

Hasse J, Blue L S, Liepa G U et al 1995 Early enteral nutrition support in patients undergoing liver transplantation. JPEN 19(6): 437–443

Hatfield A R W, Terblanche J, Fataar S et al 1982 Preoperative external biliary drainage in obstructive jaundice. Lancet ii: 896–899

Hattori N, Kurahachi H, Ikekubo K et al 1992 Serum growth hormone-binding protein, insulin-like growth factor-I, and growth hormone in patients with liver cirrhosis. Metabolism 41(4): 377–381

Haupt W, Husemann B, Sailer D 1990 Postoperative parenteral nutrition following segmental liver resection—are fat emulsions a risk? Infusion 17(2): 94–98

Heinrich PC 1990 Interleukin-6 and the acute phase response. Biochemical Journal 265: 621–636

Helton W 1994 Nutritional issues in hepatobiliary surgery. Seminars in Liver Disease 14: 386–391

Henriksen J, Ring-Larsen H, Christensen N 1984 Sympathetic nervous activity in cirrhosis: a survey of plasma catecholamine studies. Journal of Hepatology a: 55

Holroyde C, Reichard A 1981 Carbohydrate metabolism in cancer cachexia. Cancer Treatment Report 65 (suppl): 55

Inaba T et al 1994 Insulin-like growth factor I improves organ nitrogen metabolism after surgery in rats with liver cirrhosis. J Parenteral and Enteral Nutrition 18(1): 23S

John J et al 1992 Seventy percent hepatectomy: comparative effects of parenteral and enteral nutrition on liver regeneration, morbidity, and mortality. Surg Forum 43: 124–125

Katz N ed. 1986 Metabolism of lipids. In: Thurman R, Kauffman F, Jungermann K (eds) Regulation of hepatic metabolism: intra- and intercellular compartmentalization. Plenum Press, New York 237–252

Lee S, Clemens M 1992 Effect of alpha-tocopherol on hepatic mixed function oxidases in hepatic ischemia/reperfusion. Hepatology 15(2): 276–81

Leo M, Ahmed S, Aleynik S I et al 1995 Carotenoids and tocopherols in various hepatobiliary conditions. J Hepatol 23: 550–556

McClain C et al 1994 Antioxidants depress monocyte/Kupffer cell tumor necrosis factor production. J Parenteral and Enteral Nutrition 18(1): 23S

McCullough A, Mullen K D, Smanik E J et al 1989 Nutritional therapy in liver disease. Gastroenterology Clinics of North America 18(3): 619–642

McCullough A, Tavill A 1991 Disordered energy and protein metabolism in liver disease. Seminars in Liver Disease 11(4): 265–277

McPherson G, Benjamin I S, Hodgson H J et al 1984a Preoperative percutaneous transhepatic biliary drainage; the results of a controlled trial. British Journal of Surgery 71: 371

McPherson G A D, Benjamin I S, Hodgson H J F, Bowley N B, Allison D J, Blumgart L H 1984b Preoperative percutaneous transhepatic biliary drainage: the results of a controlled trial. British Journal of Surgery 71: 371–375

Maderazo E, Woronick C L, Hickingbotham N et al 1990 Additional evidence of auto-oxidation as a possible mechanism of neutrophil locomotory dysfunction in blunt trauma. Critical Care Medicine 18: 141–147

Maderazo E, Woronick C L, Hickingbotham N et al 1991 A randomized trial of replacement antioxidant vitamin therapy for neutrophil locomotory dysfunction in blunt trauma. J Trauma 31(8): 1142–1150

Marsh D, Vreugdenhil P K, Mack V et al 1993 Glycine protects hepatocytes from injury caused by anoxia, cold ischemia and mitochondrial inhibitors, but not injury caused by calcium ionophores or oxidative stress. Hepatology 17(1): 91–98

Martin M et al. The benefit of early enteral feeding in patients undergoing liver transplantation (abstract). Hepatology 18(4 pt 2): p. 337A.

Marubayashi S, Dohi K, Ochi K et al 1986 Role of free radicals in ischemic rat liver cell injury: prevention of damage by alpha-tocopherol administration. Surgery 99: 184–92

Marubayashi S, Dohi K, Sugino K et al 1989 The protective effect of administered alpha-tocopherol against hepatic damage caused by ischemia-reperfusion or endotoxemia. Annals of the New York Academy of Sciences 570: 208–18

Mehta P, Alaka K J, Filo R S et al 1995 Nutritional support following liver transplantation: a comparison of jejunal versus parenteral routes. Clin Transplant, 5: 364–369

Mullen J L, Gertner M H, Buzby G P et al 1979 Implications of malnutrition in surgical patients. Archives of Surgery 114: 121–125

Muller M 1995 Malnutrition in cirrhosis. J Hepatol 23 (Suppl. 1): 31–35

Nachbauer C, Fischer S (eds) 1983 Nutritional support in hepatic failure. In: Fisher J Surgical Nutrition. Little, Brown and Co., Boston

Nakatoni T et al 1981 Changes in predominant energy substrate after hepatectomy. life sci 28: 257

Naylor C D, O'Rourke K, Detsky A S et al 1989 Parenteral nutrition with branched-chain amino acids in hepatic encephalopathy: a meta-analysis. Gastroenterology 97: 1033–1042

Niki E, Noguchi N, Tsuchihashi H et al 1995 Interaction among vitamin C, vitamin E, and beta carotene. American Journal of Clinical Nutrition 62 (suppl): 1322S–1326S

Nishiguchi Y, Sowa M, Birkhahn R 1991 Comparison of effects of long-chain and medium-chain triglyceride emulsions during hepatic regeneration in rats. Nutrition 7(1): 23–27

Nishizaki T, Takenaka K, Yanaga K et al 1996 Nutritional support after hepatic resection: a randomized prospective study. Hepatogastroenterology 43(9): 608–613

Nolan J 1981 Endotoxin, reticuloendothelial function, and liver injury. Hepatology 1: 458–465

Nompleggi D, Bonkovsky H 1994 Nutritional supplementation in chronic liver disease: an analytical review. Hepatology 19: 518–533

O'Keefe S, Abraham R R, Davis M et al 1981 Protein turnover in acute and chronic liver disease. Acta Chir Scand 507: 91–101

O'Keefe S, Williams R, Calne R 1980 Catabolic loss of body protein after human liver transplantation. Br Med J 2: 1107–1108

O'Neil S, Hunt J, Filkins J et al 1997 Obstructive jaundice in rats resulting in exaggerated hepatic production of tumor necrosis factor-alpha and systemic and tissue necrosis factor-alpha levels after endotoxin. Surgery 122(2): 281–287

Ogle C, Zuo L, Mao J X et al 1995 Differential expression of intestinal and splenic cytokines after parenteral nutrition. Archives of Surgery 130(12): 1301–1307

Ogoshi S, Mizobuchi S, Iwasa M et al 1989 Effect of a nucleoside-nucleotide mixture on protein metabolism in rats after seventy percent hepatectomy. Nut 5(3): 173–178

Okuda K, Ohtsuki T, Obabta H et al 1985 Natural history of hepatocellular cancer and prognosis in relation to treatment. Study of 850 patients. Cancer 56: 918–928

Ouchi K, Matsubara S, Muto T et al 1991 Hepatic resection under Pringle maneuver induces endotoxemia and lipoperoxidative attack in the jaundiced rat liver. Nippon-Shokakibyo-Gakkai-Zasshi 88(5): 1216–1220

Ozaki N et al 1991 Ketone body ratio as an indicator of early graft survival in clinical liver transplantation. Clin. Transplant 5: 48–54

Ozawa K, Ida T, Yamada T et al 1976 Significance of glucose tolerance as prognostic sign in hepatectomized patients. American Journal of Surgery 131: 541

Ozawa K 1992 Liver surgery approached through the mitochondria: the redox theory in evolution. Tokyo: Medical Tribune Inc. 96–100

Ozawa K, Yamada T, Honjo I 1974 Role of insulin as a portal factor in maintaining the viability of liver. Annals of Surgery 180: 716–719

Palombo P D et al 1988 Decreased loss of liver adenosine triphosphate during hypothermic preservation in rats pretreated with glucose: implications for organ donor management. Gastroenterology 95: 1043–1049

Petrides A, DeFronzo R 1989 Glucose and insulin metabolism in cirrhosis. Journal of Hepatology 8: 107

Pikul J, Sharpe M D, Lowndes R et al 1994 Degree of preoperative malnutrition is predictive of postoperative morbidity and mortality in liver transplant recipients. Transplantation 57: 469–472

Pitt H, Cameron J L, Postier R G et al 1981 Factors affecting mortality in biliary tract surgery. American Journal of Surgery 141: 66–71

Pitt H, Gomes A S, Lois J F et al 1985a Does percutaneous drainage reduce operative risk or increase hospital cost? Annalsof Surgery 201: 545–553

Pitt H A, Gomes A S, Lois J F, Mann L L, Duetsch L S, Longmire W P

1985b Does preoperative percutaneous biliary drainage reduce operative risk or increase hospital cost? Annals of Surgery 201: 545–553

Plauth M et al 1997 ESPEN guidelines for nutrition in liver disease and transplantation. Clin Nutr 16: 43–55

Poggi C, Marchand-Brustel Y, Zapt J 1979 Effects of binding of insulin-like growth factor-1 in the isolated soleus muscle of lean and obese mice: comparison with insulin. Endocrin 105: 723–730

Porayko M, Dicecco S, O'Keefe J 1991 Impact of malnutrition and its therapy on liver transplantation. Seminars in Liver Disease 11(4): 305–314

Powell R, Machiedo G W, Rush B F et al 1991 Effect of oxygen-free radical scavengers on survival in sepsis. American Journal of Surgery 57: 86–88

Reilly J, Mehta R, Teperman L et al 1990 Nutritional support after liver transplantation: a randomized prospective study. JPEN 14(4): 386–391

Rice H, O'Keefe G E, Helton W S et al 1997 Morbid prognostic features in chronic liver failure patients undergoing non-hepatic surgery. American Journal of Surgery 132(8): 880–884

Riggio O, Merli M, Cantafora A et al 1984 Total and individual free fatty acid concentration in liver cirrhosis. Metabolism 333: 646

Riou J, Beylot M, Laville M et al 1986 Antiketogenic effect of glucose per se in vivo in man and in vitro in isolated rat liver cells. Metabolism 35: 608–613

Rowe P, Wyngaarden J 1966 The mechanism of dietary alterations in rat hepatic xanthine oxidase levels. Journals of Biological Chemistry 241: 5571

Sarac T, Sax H C, Doerr R et al 1994 Preoperative fasting improves survival after 90% hepatectomy. Archives of Surgery 129: 729–733

Sardesai V 1995 Role of antioxidants in health maintenance. Nutr Clin Prac 10(1): 19–25

Sato N et al 1994 Insulin-like growth factor-I (IGF-1) in malnourished rats following major hepatectomy. J Parenteral and Enteral Nutrition 18(1): 25S

Serino F, Agnes S, Lippa S et al 1990 Coenzyme Q alpha tocopherol graft uptake and lipid peroxidation in human liver transplantation: evidence of energy metabolism protection in University of Wisconsin (UW) solution-preserved livers. Transplant-Proc 22(5): 2194–2197

Shaw B J, Wood R P, Gordon R D et al 1985 Influence of selected patient variables and operative blood loss on six-month survival following liver transplantation. Seminars in Liver Disease 5: 385–393

Shaw S, Worner T, Lieber C 1983 Comparison of animal and vegetable protein sources in the dietary management of hepatic encephalopathy. Am J Clin Nutr 38: 59–63

Sherwin R et al 1994 Hyperglucagonemia in Laennec's cirrhosis: The role of portal systemic shunting. New England Journal of Medicine 220–239

Shirabe K, Matsumata T, Shimada M et al 1997 A comparison of parenteral hyperalimentation and early enteral feeding regarding systemic immunity after major hepatic resection—the results of a randomized prospective study. Hepatogastroenterology 44(13): 205–209

Shronts E P 1988 Nutritional assessment of adults with end-stage hepatic failure. Nut Clin Practice 3(3): 113–119

Shronts E, Fish J 1993 Hepatic failure, in nutrition support dietetics core curriculum. In: Gottschlich M, Matarese L, Shronts E (eds) ASPEN. 311–326

Singh S, Shackleton G, Ah-Sing E et al 1992 Antioxidant defenses in the bile duct-ligated rat. Gastroenterology 103: 1625–1629

Smith R, Pooley M, George C R et al 1985 Preoperative percutaneous transhepatic internal drainage in obstructive jaundice: a randomized, controlled trial examining renal function. Surgery 97: 641–647

Snopko R, Gorny K, Sabesin S 1991 A fish oil diet does not provide hepatoprotection against galactosamine toxicity in rats. Gastro 100(4): A799

Sokol R, Devereaux M, Khandwala R 1991 Effect of dietary lipid and vitamin E on mitochondrial lipid peroxidation and hepatic injury in the bile duct-ligated rat. Journal of Lipid Research 32: 1349–1357

Southard J, van Gulik T M, Ametani M S et al 1990 Important components of the UW solution. Transplantation 49: 251–257

Stimpson R., Pellegrini C, Way L 1987 Factors affecting the morbidity of elective liver resection. American Journal of Surgery 153: 189–196

Sugino K, Dohi K, Yamada K et al 1987 The role of lipid peroxidation in endotoxin-induced hepatic damage and the protective effect of antioxidants. Surgery, 101: 746–752

Sugino K, Dohi K, Yamada K et al 1989 Changes in the levels of endogenous antioxidants in the liver of mice with experimental endotoxemia and the protective effects of antioxidants. Surgery Surgery (105): 200–206

Sumimoto R, Southard J, Belzer F 1993 Livers from fasted rats acquire resistance to warm and cold ischemia injury. Transplantation 55(4): 728–732

Takada Y, Ozawa K, Yamaoka Y et al 1993 Arterial ketone body ratio and glucose administration as an energy substrate in relation to changes in ketone body concentration after liver-related liver transplantation in children. Transplantation 55: 1314–1319

van-Leeuwen P, Hong R W, Rounds J D et al 1991 Hepatic failure and coma after liver resection is reversed by manipulation of gut contents: the role of endotoxin. Surgery 110(2): 169–175

Waterhouse C, Jeanprete N, Keilson J 1979 Gluconeogenesis from alanine in patients with progressive malignant disease. Cancer Research 39: 1968

Wicks C, Somasundaram S, Bjarnason I et al 1994 Comparison of enteral feeding and total parenteral nutrition after liver transplantation. Lancet 344: 837–840

Wilkinson S, Moodie H, Stamatakis J D et al 1976 Endotoxaemia and renal failure in cirrhosis and obstructive jaundice. British Medical Journal 2: 1415–1418

Windsor J 1993 Underweight patients and the risk of major surgery; symposium on perioperative care. World Journal of Surgery 17: 165

Yau T, Weisel R D, Mickle D A et al 1994 Vitamin E for coronary bypass operations. Journal of Thoracic and Cardiovascular Surgery 108(2): 302–10

Yokoyama I et al Endotoxemia and human liver transplantation. Transplantation Proceedings 21(5): 3833–3841

Yoshikawa T, Murakami M, Kondo M 1984 Endotoxin-induced disseminated intravascular coagulation in vitamin E deficient rats. Toxicology and Applied Pharmacology 74: 173–178

Young V 1977 Energy metabolism and requirements in the cancer patient. Cancer Research 37: 2336

Anesthesia and postoperative intensive care

27

J.A. MELENDEZ AND M. FISCHER

Anesthesia and operation on patients with major liver disease is a great challenge for the anesthesiologist and the surgeon. An increasing number of severely ill patients are being operated upon but with a significant peri- and postoperative mortality and morbidity. This is due to engagement of several vital organ functions in liver disease. A thorough understanding of the pathophysiology and pharmacology in liver disease and close monitoring of vital functions are crucial.

The anesthetic problems in connection with liver transplantation are dealt with elsewhere in this book (Ch. 107). This chapter mainly deals with the special anesthetic management of patients with liver disease undergoing hepatobiliary surgery. For a more detailed account of the progress of liver disease, changes in structure and liver function we refer to other chapters in this book. We have focused on anesthetic problems of special relevance for the joint (anesthetic and surgical) management of these patients. For detailed knowledge of anesthetic techniques, reference should be made to specialized texts (Brown 1988, Strunin & Thomson 1992).

PREOPERATIVE EVALUATION

With the advent of modern techniques, the anesthetic risk attributed to any surgical procedure is heavily dependent on the preoperative status of the patient. In hepatobiliary patients, the presence of preoperative pulmonary, cardiac and/or hepatic disease significantly augments the incidence of postoperative morbidity and mortality. The detailed evaluation of these major organ systems with a focus on corrective measures is combined with selected anesthetics, pharmacological agents and hemodynamic monitoring to provide optimal care. This approach significantly reduces perioperative complications.

Cardiac evaluation

Perioperative cardiac morbidity is one of the leading causes of perioperative death. The incidence of myocardial ischemia in patients suffering from coronary artery disease (CAD) may be as high as 74% (Mangano & Goldman 1995). This may occur up to 7 days following surgery. Myocardial infarctions occur in about 2% of patients with CAD with a resulting mortality in the range of 30 to 70%. Factors other than anginal syndrome that predispose to cardiac morbidity are shown in Table 27.1 (Goldman et al 1977). Preoperative evaluation should begin with an extensive history and physical examination, 12-lead EKG and, if

Table 27.1. Preoperative factors associated with postoperative life-threatening complications or fatal cardiac complications (modified from Goldman (1977), with permission of Massachusetts Medical Society, Boston)

History
  Age > 70 yrs
  Myocardial infarction in previous 6 months
Physical examination
  S_3 gallop or jugular venous distention
  Important aortic stenosis
Electrocardiogram
  Rhythm other than sinus or premature atrial contractions
  > 5 Premature ventricular contractions/min at any time
General Status
  $PO_2 < 60$ or $PCO_2 > 50$ mmHg
  $K < 3.0$ or $HCO_3 < 20$ meq/L
  BUN > 50 or creatinine > 3.0 mg/dL
  Abnormal SGOT
  Signs of chronic liver disease or patient bedridden
Operation
  Intraperitoneal, intrathoracic or aortic operation
  Emergency operation

necessary, proceed with radio-nucleotide stress test and echocardiography to clarify the extent of the ischemic disease. Drug therapy should be optimized in preparation for elective surgery. Unless contraindicated, there is compelling evidence to administer perioperative beta-blocker therapy in patients with CAD. Beta-blocker therapy has been demonstrated to reduce the incidence of perioperative ischemic events and myocardial infarction.

In the hepatobiliary patient population, cardiac assessment needs to stress the evaluation of myocontractile function. Cirrhotic cardiomyopathy classically occurs in men aged 30–55 years old who have been alcohol abusers for more than 10 years (Braunwald 1997). Putative mechanisms of damage are direct toxic effects of (1) ethanol and its metabolite acetaldehyde, (2) nutritional deficiencies particularly of thiamine (beri beri) and (3) additives in legitimate commercial products (cobalt in beer). Alcohol and acetaldehyde have been shown to decrease calcium binding and transport, myocardial lipid metabolism, myocardial synthesis, and myocardial ATPase activity. Two basic patterns of cardiac dysfunction have been demonstrated: left ventricular dilatation with impaired systolic function and left ventricular hypertrophy with diminished compliance and normal or increased contractile performance. Presenting manifestations range from insidious onset to catastrophic left sided cardiac failure. Anginal chest pain does not occur unless the patient has concomitant coronary artery disease or aortic stenosis.

Pulmonary evaluation

The nature and magnitude of the pre-existing respiratory conditions will determine the effect of a given standard anesthetic on respiratory function. Patients with poorly controlled respiratory disease are at higher risk for pneumonia and respiratory failure. Anesthesia will result in a decrease in mucus transfer and reductions of the functional residual capacity–closing capacity ratio (FRC:CC). In patients with emphysema, bronchitis and asthma, airway closure can occur with mild active expiration. In addition, inflammation and scarring can compromise bronchial structural integrity and further increase the risk of alveolar collapse. In patients with asthma or obstructive lung disease, high airway resistance favors deep slow respiration which may not be possible in patients with large abdominal incisions. Respiratory muscle abnormalities occur as a result of an abdominal surgical incision (Chuter et al 1990). Sub-costal incisions result in the largest change in respiratory patterns with a markedly decreased diaphragmatic excursion. Asthma and bronchospasm need to be resolved prior to an anesthetic. Patients may require pulmonary function tests and blood gas analy-

sis to establish the extent of disease and to optimize therapy. In severe cases, a course of preoperative antibiotics and corticosteroids is necessary to clear chronic bronchitis.

Hepatic evaluation

The operative outcome is clearly linked to severity of hepatic parenchymal disease and the extent of postoperative functional reduction. In patients with mild or well-compensated chronic hepatic disease, operative outcome is likely to be indistinguishable from the outcome in the general population. On the other hand, the unexpected diagnosis of viral hepatitis during emergency laparotomy carries a mortality of 9.5% (Aranha & Greenlee 1986). In some studies, the mortality in patients with acute viral or alcoholic hepatic failure approaches 100% (Greene 1981). Ideally, a measurement of metabolic liver function would provide the necessary predictive information. However, metabolic liver function tests (Ch. 2), such as the aminopyrine breath test and indocyanine green clearance, are not readily available for clinical use. Instead, metabolic capacity is usually estimated from other parameters and approximated by the Child's classification. Routine evaluation should include CBC, clotting factors, serum electrolytes, serum albumin, bilirubin and liver enzymes.

INTRAOPERATIVE MANAGEMENT

Surgical stimulation and manipulation of the liver markedly increases hepatic oxygen extraction ratio in connection with splanchnic vasoconstriction (Kainuma et al 1991; Whittle & Moncada 1998). There is a 16% drop in hepatic blood flow associated with anesthesia and mechanical ventilation (Gelman 1976). There is a further 10% decrease in liver blood flow with peripheral surgery and a 40% decrease with splanchnic surgery. This may be the direct effect of sympathetic control of the hepatic venous bed mediated through the hepatic innervation (Greenway et al 1986). PEEP decreases hepatic blood flow in step-wise manner. The response cannot be explained by a decrease in cardiac output alone; investigators postulate a vasoconstrictive response in the pre-portal vasculature. Intra-peritoneal insufflation and head-up tilt result in impairment of hepatic blood flow secondary to decreases in cardiac output (Berendes et al 1996b, Eleftheriadis et al 1996). The hepatic blood flow decrease caused by hypotensive spinal anesthesia is attenuated by ephedrine administration (Nakayama et al 1993). It is controversial whether catecholamines increase hepatic blood flow and oxygen supply. Dobutamine does not cause a significant increase in hepatic arterial blood flow (Kainuma et al 1992). However, total hepatic blood flow and portal venous blood flow are increased, resulting in an augmentation of hepatic oxygen delivery. The increase in hepatic oxygen delivery is countered by a rise in hepatic oxygen uptake with no overall improvement of hepatic oxygen supply-uptake ratio. Dopamine and norepinephrine increase hepatic venous oxygen saturation suggesting that the vasoactive treatment of patients in septic shock may not compromise splanchnic oxygenation (Ruokonen et al 1991, 1993). Hepatic portal flow does not decrease despite a 20 to 60% reduction in blood pressure as long as cardiac index is maintained during sodium nitroprusside hypotension (Chauvin et al 1985). A well-planned anesthetic will choose to maximize the relation between oxygen transport and oxygen utilization with the premise that reductions in systemic pressure are translated to reductions in hepatic blood flow. Anything resulting in reductions of systemic pressure and cardiac output—induced hypotension, hypovolemia and anesthetic overdoses—should be avoided.

Volatile anesthetics

Volatile anesthetics reduce hepatic blood flow in a dose-dependent fashion by effecting cardiac output and systemic pressure. Halothane, owing to its potent myocardial depression, produces the most decrease in hepatic blood flow. A study of 88 patients showed a 16% reduction in the estimated hepatic blood flow (EHBF), as measured by a colloidal gold technique. Surgical manipulation yields an additional decrease in EHBF. The reduction is more pronounced in patients undergoing partial gastrectomy (52%) or cholecystectomy than in patients undergoing herniorrhaphy or excision of a breast tumor (18%) (Garrison et al 1984, Gelman 1987). In the presence of halothane, the correlation of systemic arterial blood pressure and the hepatic blood flow indicates a loss of autoregulation (Altmayer et al 1991). In addition, halothane reduces oxygen delivery to a greater extent than it reduces systemic pressure. Animal studies point out that a 30% reduction in systolic pressure under halothane anesthesia leads to a 50% reduction in hepatic blood flow and a simultaneous increase in oxygen extraction.

The hepatotoxic effect of halothane has been widely studied. Fulminant hepatic failure is described in patients undergoing multiple halothane anesthetics. No safe exposure interval is demonstrated. The incidence 1:35 000 is linked to obesity, age, sex, level of enzyme induction, and genetic predisposition. Halothane-induced hepatic dysfunction has an unresolved etiology. Mechanisms suggested are based on metabolism, immunology, and hypoxia. The metabolic theory suggests that the P450 system of the liver, under hypoxic conditions, causes reductive metabolism of halothane rather than the usual oxidative pathway (Farrell et al 1985). The reductive metabolism causes production of various fluoride containing compounds. Yet, when the liver is directly challenged with these compounds hepatic dysfunction fails to occur. Other evidence suggests that halothane toxicity occurs during initial exposure rather than during metabolism. The suggestion that toxicity occurs prior to metabolism may involve hypoxia during anesthetic induction and not after reductive metabolism of halothane (Neuberger 1990). Hence, the origin of the hypoxic theory. The likelihood that hypoxia accounts for fulminant hepatic failure is not convincing. The strongest evidence lies with the immunologic theory. Hepatic damage is associated with multiple halothane exposures suggesting a possible sensitization (Hubbard et al 1988). Other signs of allergy are present such as eosinophilia and fever after the first exposure, and jaundice upon further exposure. Trifluroacetyl halide, a metabolic product of halothane, has been linked with a humoral response when bound to liver protein. There is also no reason to discount a cell mediated response. In some series, halothane antibodies have been demonstrated in up to 75% of patients. Hepatic necrosis may ensue with 10 to 80% mortality. Death occurs 1 to 2 weeks after the initiation of symptoms that include fever, and rash. In addition, a mild transaminase elevation after halothane exposure has been documented in close to 50% of cases. A significant increase in aminopyrine half-life has been shown to occur after halothane exposure not seen with other agents. This pattern should preclude the repeated use of halothane.

Enflurane hepatitis, if real, has an incidence well below 1:800 000 (Dykes 1984, Harper et al 1984). There is no documentation of antibodies or increase incidence with repeated anesthetics or cross-reactivity with halothane (Lewis et al 1983). Owing to its increased molecular stability and rapid egress from fatty tissues, enflurane does not undergo as extensive reductive metabolism as halothane (Masone et al 1982). The creation of free radicals and/or toxic products is almost completely eliminated. For equipotent doses, enflurane reduces hepatic blood flow to a lesser extent than halothane.

Isoflurane and desflurane undergo negligible hepatic metabolism (Elliot & Strunin 1993). As a result, isoflurane anesthetics are not accompanied by free radical formation. In 1987, the FDA concluded that there was no conclusive association between isoflurane exposure and postoperative hepatitis (Shingu et al 1983, Stoelting 1987). Isoflurane has been considered the agent of choice where preservation of splanchnic blood flow is required. Liver blood flow and the hepatic artery buffer response are maintained better in the presence of isoflurane than with any other volatile anesthetic agent (Berendes et al 1996a). Isoflurane preserves the hepatic blood flow buffer effect resulting in minimal change on total liver perfusion (Gelman et al 1983, Goldfarb et al 1990). In addition isoflurane is shown to attenuate the increases in hepatic oxygen consumption associated with surgery and liver manipulation. Desflurane is shown to have no deleterious effects on liver function and hepatocyte integrity. Desflurane anesthesia is associated with significantly greater gut blood flow than equipotent isoflurane. This difference cannot be explained by systemic hemodynamics alone. However, there is no difference in total hepatic flow between isoflurane and desflurane groups. This implies an intact hepatic artery buffer response with desflurane (O'Riordan et al 1997).

Sevoflurane appears to be similar to isoflurane and desflurane with a few exceptions. Indocyanine green clearance is better preserved during sevoflurane anesthesia than during halothane anesthesia. Sevoflurane appears similar to isoflurane in its effect on regional hepatic blood flow (Ebert et al 1995). However, in sevoflurane anesthetized beagles with ligation of the hepatic artery, the hepatic oxygen supply/uptake ratio, the hemoglobin oxygen saturation and oxygen partial pressure in hepatic venous blood are significantly lower than with halothane or isoflurane.

Nitrous oxide is extensively used in patients with hepatic disease (Lampe et al 1990, Khalil et al 1994). It is not shown to contribute to hepatic disease exacerbation. The sympathomimetic effects of nitrous oxide may increase hepatic metabolic requirements.

Intravenous anesthetics and muscle relaxants

Patients with hepatic disease often experience abnormal responses to drugs (Duvaldestin 1981). Although the most common cause of the unpredictability of the response is due to altered pharmacokinetics, changes in central nervous system effects have been described. The alterations of drug availability are dependent on changes in the drug plasma binding, volume of distribution, liver blood flow, drug metabolism, and the etiology and stage of liver dysfunction (Ghoneim & Korttila 1977, Prescott et al 1975). The expression of decreasing plasma proteins is an observed marker of chronic decline of liver anabolic capacity (Bond 1978); said reduction cuts down the number of drug binding sites and increases drug bio-availability. The decrease in plasma protein also yields ascites and peripheral edema increasing the volume of distribution of many drugs. The elimination of drugs with low extraction rate depends more on the metabolic capacity of the liver and less on the hepatic blood flow (Colli et al 1988). In patients with impaired liver function, such drugs will experience a prolonged length of

activity with no increase in peak levels. In contrast, the elimination of drugs with a high extraction rate depends on liver blood flow. Reductions in metabolic clearance will result in increases of peak drug level with minimal change in the elimination half-life. Protein binding, enzymatic induction, intrahepatic shunting and the effect of anesthetics on liver blood flow may affect the elimination of drugs with a high extraction rate. Chronic alcohol usage increases anesthetic requirements owing to the increase in drug metabolism (Couderc et al 1984).

The safety of barbiturate administration in patients with hepatic disease is well documented (Ghoneim & Pandya 1975, Pandele et al 1983). There are only rare reports of hepatitis following barbiturates (Black 1974). These are associated with fever, rash, eosinophilia, and an onset of symptoms within 5 weeks with several months of convalescence. The barbiturate-induced rise in cytochrome P450 reduction may increase toxic metabolites. The clearance of thiopental and methohexital is preserved in cirrhotics (Pandele et al 1983). The low serum albumin in decompensated cirrhotics results in the decrease in the volume of distribution and protein binding of drugs (Ghoneim & Pandya 1975). Consequently, free thiopental is increased in cirrhotics. The dosage should be reduced.

There are reports of hepatic injury ranging from cholestasis to centrilobular necrosis following prolonged usage of benzodiazepines. Benzodiazepines have a low hepatic clearance rate, hence have prolonged effects in patients with liver insufficiency. Adinazolam half-life is doubled in cirrhotics. The decrease in diazepam clearance in chronic liver disease correlates with serum albumin (Branch et al 1976, Branch 1987). Attention should be paid to active metabolites, which will further increase the duration of action. In compensated alcoholic cirrhotics, the metabolism rates of midazolam are similar to normals. Uncompensated cirrhotics may have prolonged pharmacological action. EEG response differences between cirrhotics and normals at similar drug concentrations suggest alterations in cerebral sensitivity. Dosages should be tailored appropriately (Hawkes et al 1973). Patients with hepatic encephalopathy may have increased endogenous benzodiazepines (Ferenci & Grimm 1990, Pomier-Layrargues et al 1994, Avallone et al 1998, Dasarathy & Mullen 1998).

Clinicians shy away from administering morphine to cirrhotics because of the profound effects seen with standard dosages. In poorly compensated liver disease, both synthetic and natural narcotics will exhibit accentuated central nervous system depression (Couderc et al 1984). Morphine is reported to have both unaltered and reduced clearance in cirrhotics (Patwardhan et al 1981, Hasselstrom et al 1990). In individuals with normal liver function, the clearance of morphine is dependent on hepatic blood flow (Park et al 1993). Although hepatic blood flow is reduced in cirrhotics, elimination of morphine is unchanged possibly as a result of extra-hepatic conjugation (Mazoit et al 1987). Hypo-albuminemia and hyperbilirubinemia decrease protein binding of morphine and yields more free drug for neurological effects. Alfentanyl has been shown to have a prolonged duration in patients with liver disease with a doubling of the elimination half-life (Bower et al 1992). The drop in clearance seems to be related to the etiology of liver disease. There is also a rise in the free alfentanyl fraction caused by the reduction of alpha-1-glycoprotein in cirrhotics (Belpaire & Bogaert 1991). H_2 blockers may further prolong the duration of action. Narcotics may be administered safely in reduced doses to well-compensated cirrhotics. Well-compensated cirrhotic patients do not experience a change in fentanyl elimination half-life, total plasma clearance and volume of distribution. Fentanyl has a high extraction ratio and hence, it is more dependent on hepatic blood flow and less on metabolic activity (Haberer et al 1982). Consistent with its minimal effect on cardiac output and systemic pressure, fentanyl has no effect on liver blood flow and oxygen deliver. In combination with isoflurane, fentanyl has the least effect on hepatic hemodynamics of any opiate, making it the narcotic of choice for anesthetics. Narcotics may cause biliary spasm, which can be relieved with glucagon or nalaxone.

There is not enough information about the effect of propofol on de-compensated cirrhotics. Protein binding is unchanged in cirrhotics (Kanto & Gepts 1989, Costela et al 1996). Although propofol is metabolized in the liver, pharmacokinetics are unchanged in uncomplicated cirrhotics (Servin et al 1990). Non-hepatic, possibly pulmonary metabolism of propofol has been documented during liver transplantation. Propofol causes reductions in systemic pressure, which may be translated to decreases in liver blood flow. When administered to well compensated cirrhotics, propofol has been well tolerated.

Etomidate is hydrolyzed by hepatic esterases to carboxylic acid. Terminal half-life is increased by 100% in cirrhotics. This is only important in prolonged infusions. Dosage should be decreased to prevent cumulative effect. The intermediate distribution phase is responsible for the short pharmacodynamic effect which is unchanged in cirrhotics (Carlos et al 1979). Although more common with prolonged infusions, etomidate may cause adrenal suppression, hence complicating the status of the de-compensated cirrhotic.

Ketamine is well tolerated in cirrhotics and has no hepato-toxic effects during short procedures (Abu et al 1988). Serum transaminase increase may result after prolonged continuous usage. The etiology is unknown. Ketamine does not alter portal or hepatic artery blood flow. It does decrease oxygen transport by increasing oxygen consumption of pre-portal organs. Increased intracranial pressure in comatose patients is a contraindication to its use.

There is an apparent resistance of patients with cirrhosis to muscle relaxants (Booij 1987, 1997). This is the result of an increase in the volume of distribution. Many muscle relaxants may also exhibit a prolonged duration of action caused by the decreased hepatic metabolic function. In essence, the initial dose of pancuronium or d-turbocurare required to achieve a specific degree of muscle relaxation is higher than expected (Duvaldestin et al 1978). This same dose has an unexpectedly prolonged duration of action (Abrams & Hornbein 1975). In patients with cirrhosis, the protein binding of turbocurare, pancuronium and vecuronium is similar to controls (Duvaldestin & Henzel 1982, Bencini et al 1986). Single dose vecuronium pharmacokinetics are not affected in patients with alcohol liver disease, however, large doses may behave like pancuronium (Hunter et al 1985, Arden et al 1988). Time to 50% twitch recovery is prolonged by 100% in cirrhotic patients receiving vecuronium (Arden et al 1988). Sustained usage of vecuronium in patients with cholestasis may lead to prolonged duration of action. Time to maximal neuromuscular blockade is unchanged for rocuronium (Bevan 1994, Khalil et al 1994). The reduced plasma clearance and the increased volume of distribution combine to increase the elimination half-life. There is no difference in the volume of distribution, plasma clearance and elimination half-life for doxacurium (Cook et al 1991).

Reductions in protein synthesis will result in decreased pseudocholinesterase activity. However, there is no clinically significant increase in succinylcholine activity. Mivacurium may be prolonged in patients with decreased pseudocholinesterase activity (Devlin et al 1993). Despite its increase in the volume of distribution, atracurium has an unchanged elimination half-life. Because atracurium is metabolized by Hoffman elimination, independent of liver and renal dysfunction, it may be considered the muscle relaxant of choice (Parker & Hunter 1989). There is also no change in laudanosine clearance, an atracurium metabolite. The drug has been shown to maintain its predictable dosage pattern in patients in extremis. Avoidance of large doses of any muscle relaxant is ideal.

There were no differences in a large number of indices of hepatic function and plasma composition prior to and during the second hour of a lidocaine infusion (Benowitz & Meister 1978, Davison et al 1982). This study suggests that a constant lidocaine concentration of about 6 µg/ml has no detrimental effect on hepatic function (Mets et al 1993,

1994). Amide linked local anesthetics are metabolized by the liver, hence caution should be used in patients with severe liver disease. There can be a substantial effect on local anesthetic pharmacokinetics (Endell et al 1983). The half-life of lidocaine may be increased by 300% (Aldrete et al 1970).

SPECIAL ANESTHETIC CONSIDERATIONS

Anesthesia for hepatectomy

Pre-resectional fluid loading is commonly practised in preparation for hepatic resection. This often results in a distended and tense vena cava. Inadvertently, the technique aimed at providing hemodynamic stability during episodes of uncontrolled bleeding, contributes to technical difficulties and handicaps the repair of venous injuries. Low central venous pressure anesthesia (LCVP) is designed to preclude vena caval distention and facilitate mobilization of the liver, and dissection of retrohepatic vena cava and major hepatic veins (Cunningham et al 1994, Melendez et al 1998). LCVP is performed in combination with surgical inflow and outflow control (Ch. 83). Neither the surgical nor the anesthetic components of the approach may be applied alone. This surgical-anesthetic technique compares very favorably with other techniques for major hepatic resection (Thompson et al 1983, Yanaga et al 1988, Delva et al 1989, Segawa et al 1993). Close cooperation between anesthesiologist and surgeon is necessary so that likely difficulties can be anticipated and appropriate measures taken.

A relationship between extent of intraoperative blood loss and morbidity has been demonstrated; blood loss in excess of 5 L is associated with prohibitive mortality (Yanaga et al 1988). LCVP minimizes hepatic venous bleeding during parenchymal transection and facilitates control of inadvertent venous injury. The blood loss resulting from a vascular injury is directly proportional to both the pressure gradient across the vessel wall and the fourth power of the radius of the injury. If the CVP is lowered from 15 mmHg to 3 mmHg, the blood loss through a vena caval injury will consequently fall by a factor greater than 5. Lowering CVP, not only lessens the pressure component of the equation, it minimizes the radial component of flow by reducing vessel distention (Fig. 27.1).

Fluid restriction is an important aspect of this technique. Preoperative overnight fluid replacement, a maneuver commonly performed prior to or immediately following the induction of general anesthesia, is withheld. Strict fluid restriction is practised until the liver resection is completed. Intermittently, small fluid boluses may be given to maintain hemodynamic stability. To guarantee the safety of patients,

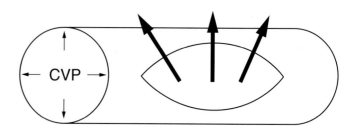

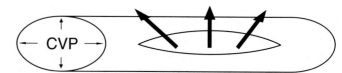

Fig. 27.1 Vena caval injury profile under various CVP conditions: (a) high CVP, (b) low CVP. Increased CVP leads to distention of vena cava with ensuing enlargement in diameter of injury and increase in the bleeding driving pressure.

appropriate cannulation is carried out and a high level of vigilance is maintained. Transfusion equipment such as the Woods Pump coupled to a Level 1 System is an important aid to emergency fluid resuscitation occasionally necessary with this anesthetic technique.

Intravascular hypovolemia is counteracted with 15° head-down tilt. By improving venous return, steep head-down tilt preserves hemodynamic stability and renal function. In animals, head-down tilt increases glomerular filtration rate (GFR), sodium excretion and urine output lasting up to 8 hours (McCombs et al 1996). Prolonged head-down tilt improves venous return and yields up to a 70% increase in plasma atrial natriuretic protein (ANP) (Hughson et al 1995, Terai et al 1995). Although some investigators report intraoperative oliguria during LCVP, there is no increase in the incidence of postoperative renal failure (Melendez et al 1998).

Anesthesia is maintained with a combination of isoflurane in O_2 and narcotics. Isoflurane provides vasodilatation with minimal myocardial depression (Schwinn and others 1990). Elimination of nitrogen from the anesthetic gas mixture is necessary to permit expiratory nitrogen monitoring for air emboli. Restriction of nitrous oxide in the gas mixture prevents the diffusion mediated increase in the size of circulating air pockets. In the majority of patients, fentanyl is the ideal narcotic to aid in the maintenance of anesthesia providing analgesia with minimal hypotension (Rosow et al 1982). However in a small group of patients, the anesthetic is supplemented with morphine in order to achieve the desired central venous pressure. Morphine reduces central venous pressure by inducing venous vasodilatation caused by histamine release and m_3 receptor activation (Rosow et al 1982, Stefano et al 1995, Grossman et al 1996). The combination of these anesthetics readily provides the favorable low central venous environment for hepatic resection. With this technique, intravenous nitroglycerin to lower CVP below 5 mmHg is rarely necessary.

The risk of intraoperative air emboli is likely to increase under LCVP-anesthesia. Transesophageal echocardiography can be used to monitor air emboli. The technology over-diagnoses clinically significant emboli. With surgical vigilance and rapid occlusion of open venous channels (Ch. 83), LCVP results in a very low incidence (0.4%) of clinically significant air emboli.

More complex LCVP management techniques have been described (Rees et al 1996). They employ epidural blockade and intravenous nitroglycerin. These patients may require intraoperative dopamine for systemic pressure support. The technique is cumbersome and adds an unnecessary level of complexity to an already challenging situation.

Anesthesia for vascular isolation

Prolonged inflow occlusion with or without hepatic vascular isolation is an alternative surgical approach for liver resection. Hepatic vascular isolation induces significant hemodynamic changes. The anesthetic management is therefore more complex, and many patients require pulmonary artery catheters during the procedure. Hepatic vascular isolation typically causes a decrease in venous return with a resulting decrease in cardiac index and increase in systemic vascular resistance. Mean arterial pressure is maintained by infusing large volumes of fluid to keep the central venous pressure high. Some patients require vasopressor support to maintain adequate perfusion during the cross clamping period. Most patients tolerate these hemodynamic changes reasonably well, although in some cases persistent hypotension and/or low

cardiac index demand that the procedure be abandoned. Several recent studies of hepatic vascular isolation are summarized in Table 27.2 (Delva et al 1989, Emre et al 1993, Hannoun et al 1993, Habib et al 1994, Emond et al 1995, Belghiti et al 1996, Melendez et al 1998). In these studies, blood loss and transfusion requirements were both greater than that reported by the authors using portal triad clamping with extrahepatic control of the hepatic veins. Thus hepatic vascular isolation is more complex and has not yielded better results than portal triad clamping and extrahepatic control of the hepatic veins (Cunningham et al 1994; Belghiti et al 1996).

Obstructive jaundice

Bile duct obstruction affects hepatic hemodynamics. Acute biliary obstruction is associated with an increase in liver blood flow but is decreased with chronic obstruction. Relief of long-term obstruction is not associated with a return to normal pressures and may even be associated with hemodynamic embarrassment and shock. The exact etiology of hemodynamic derangement in the face of biliary obstruction is not known but increased portal resistance is suggested as playing a role. Biliary sepsis may contribute to the exacerbation of the hemodynamic embarrassment. In these cases, aggressive hemodynamic monitoring may be lifesaving.

POSTOPERATIVE CARE

Due to surgical and anesthetic advance, and a better understanding of hepatic physiology, mortality and morbidity following hepatobiliary surgery has decreased (Melendez et al 1998, Ryan et al 1982) In fact, hepatobiliary surgery is increasingly common at major medical centers and postoperative recovery is becoming indistinguishable from that following other major abdominal surgery.

Table 27.2. Comparison of operative parameters between hepatic vascular isolation (HVI) and LCVP-aided hepatectomy (LCVP).

Author	Technique	Total cases	Major resections*	Blood loss (cc) Mean**	Median	Transfusions (units or cc)**
Delva et al, 1989[†]	HVI	35	35	–	–	8.0 ± 8.3
Emre et al 1993	HVI	16	13	1866 ± 1683	1325	–
Hannoun et al 1993	HVI	15	15	–	–	5.8 ± 4.7
Habib et al 1994	HVI	56	33	1651 ± 1748	1200	930 ± 750
Cunningham 1994	LCVP	100	69	1012 ± 964	1000	1.4 ± 2.1
Emond et al 1995	HVI	48	44	1255 ± 1291	–	1.9 ± 2.6
Belghiti et al 1996	HVI	24	24	1195 ± 1105	–	2.5 ± 3.4
Melendez et al 1998[†]	LCVP	496	357	849 ± 972	618	0.9 ± 1.8

*Major resections include all lobectomies and extended lobectomies. **Values are reported in mean ± S.D. [†]Denotes inclusion of cirrhotic patients in series

Immediate postoperative concerns

Some of the problems causing metabolic and functional changes after hepatobiliary surgery are common to all major intra-abdominal procedures (Aronsen et al 1969). Others are unique and require an in-depth understanding of liver physiology. Immediate postoperative concerns are bleeding, intravascular volume, renal function, and oxygenation. Anticipated respiratory compromise after upper abdominal surgery may preclude early extubation especially in combination with any baseline abnormality in gas exchange. Important laboratory tests are hematocrit, electrolytes, serum creatinine, blood urea nitrogen, PT/PTT, liver enzymes, chest roentgogram.

Unique postoperative concerns in the patient following hepatobiliary surgery include: phosphorus replacement, anesthetic elimination, drug metabolism, coagulation and postoperative pain control. Recent data suggest that hepatocellular regeneration may be critically dependent on cellular ATP stores (Greene 1981, Campbell et al 1990). Liver regeneration following partial hepatectomy involves rapid cell division as early as 24 to 72 hours after liver resection. Standard therapy for post hepatic resection should include the supplementation of intravenous fluids with KPO_4 (30–40 mmol/day). Particular attention must be paid to anesthetic elimination and residual drug effect, especially sedative, analgesic and neuromuscular blockers in those patients who have altered drug pharmacodynamics and pharmacokinetics. Postoperative pain management must be adapted to this population. Patient controlled analgesia (PCA) commonly employed for postoperative pain management should be employed without a basal narcotic infusion rate. After hepatic resection, patients experience an unpredictable reduction in the metabolism of narcotics. The half-life of coagulation factors is 6 hours so that coagulation factor deficiency is likely to evolve rapidly. Routine parental administration of vitamin K commonly corrects the coagulation abnormalities within 48 h. More rapid correction may be accomplished by fresh frozen plasma (FFP) but is rarely needed unless the prothrombin time (PT) is greater than 17 s.

Non-immediate complications

Identifying patients at high risk for complication is important for the hepatobiliary team. A recent study revealed that once postoperative hepatobiliary patients required admission to the intensive care unit mortality ranged from 37 to 79% regardless of admission diagnosis (Melendez et al 1998). A systematic pro-active approach that identifies early deviations from the norm is preferable to having to treat organ failure (Sesto et al 1987).

Jaundice

The diagnosis of postoperative jaundice is reflected in Table 27.3. The most common causes of elevated unconjugated hyperbilirubinemia are hematoma reabsorption and hemolysis of transfused blood. One should be suspicious of a bile duct injury at the time of surgery when faced with postoperative extrahepatic obstructive jaundice. Hemobilia, with temporary obstruction of the bile ducts by blood clots may occur. Hepatocellular injury is another possibility in the differential diagnosis of postoperative jaundice. Although it is tempting to attribute hepatocellular injury to the toxic effects of anesthetic agents, other etiologies causing a low flow state to the liver are more common, i.e. sepsis and low total hepatic blood flow. Infectious hepatitis may first manifest as jaundice in the postoperative period often related to intraoperative blood transfusions; in some cases, the responsible virus has no serologic marker. When all other factors are eliminated in the evaluation of postoperative jaundice, the diagnosis of anesthetic related hepatotoxicity might be entertained. The agent most commonly implicated is halothane. With newer less controversial volatile anesthetics, it is rarely seen today.

Ascites

Ascites manifests as a result of: (1) impaired albumin and protein synthesis, (2) increased hydrostatic pressure in hepatic sinusoids and splanchnic capillaries, (3) over-

Table 27.3. Differential diagnosis of postoperative jaundice (modified from Brown [1988] and Gelman [1992], with permission of F A Davis, J B Lippincott & W B Saunders, Philadelphia)

Increased bilirubin load	Biliary obstruction	Hepatocellular injury
Blood transfusion	Intrahepatic cholestasis	Hepatic hypoxemia
Hematoma	Drug induced	Exacerbated chronic hepatitis
Hemolytic anemia	Infection induced	Acute hepatitis: viral, alcoholic
Extracorporeal circulation hemolysis	Extrahepatic cholestasis	Gilbert's disease
	Bile duct injury	Sepsis
	Pancreatitis	Trauma
	Retained gallstones	Toxins, drugs

production of hepatic and splanchnic lymph leading to a transudation of lymph into the peritoneal space, (4) limited or reduced reabsorption of water and protein by peritoneal lymphatics, (5) sodium retention by the kidney secondary to hyperaldosteronism, increased sympathetic stimulation, alterations in metabolism of prostaglandins, and kinins and (6) impaired renal water excretion, partially due to increased concentrations of antidiuretic hormone (ADH). The decreased serum albumin, one to two weeks after hepatobiliary surgery, is clinically unimportant (Grundmann & Heistermann 1985). Even in the presence of severe hypoalbuminemia, albumin infusion is of no beneficial effect. The medical management of ascites emphasizes bed rest and sodium restriction. If a spontaneous diuresis does not occur, therapy is begun with the aldosterone antagonist spironolactone. Therefore, in patients with ascites electrolyte abnormalities (hyponatremia, hyperkalemia, hypochloremia, and hypokalemia) and contraction alkalosis, are commonly encountered as a result of both the primary process and medical therapy. If life-threatening complications such as cardiac or respiratory compromise occur, these patients require hemodynamic monitoring. Patients with ascites often respond to positive pressure ventilation as if hypovolemic although the physical findings are more consistent with hypervolemia. If ascites is refractory to medical management, paracentesis may be attempted.

Renal Failure (see also Ch. 25)

After hepatobiliary surgery, one may encounter rapidly progressive renal failure. The differential diagnosis includes acute tubular necrosis, pre-renal azotemia and hepatorenal syndrome. Hepatorenal syndrome is the development of otherwise unexplained renal failure in patients with advanced liver disease. In hepatorenal syndrome, urine sodium is typically < 10 meq/L with hyperosmolar urine, oliguria (< 400 ml/24 h), fractional excretion of sodium (FeNa$^+$) < 1, and urine creatinine to plasma creatinine ratio > 30:1. The pathophysiology of hepatorenal syndrome is based on the pooling of blood in splanchnic bed and decreasing plasma volume (Harleb et al 1997). The kidney perceives a decreased glomerular filtration rate; the resulting vasoconstriction shunts blood away from the renal cortex. Animal models with induced cirrhosis demonstrate an increased production of nitric oxide. Inhibition of nitric oxide synthesis benefits renal function in cirrhotic rats by increasing arterial pressure and increasing perfusion pressure. This improves systemic hemodynamics and down regulates baroreceptor tone. Cirrhotics show an increased synthesis of nitric oxide when compared to normals. Although further investigation in humans is required, hepa-

torenal syndrome may be reversed by inhibition of nitric oxide synthesis. In some cases, the precipitating event can be attributed to hemodynamic instability, nephrotoxic drugs, infection or overzealous diuresis and paracentesis. Although there is no specific treatment for hepatorenal syndrome, one should always assume that the primary pathophysiologic event is circulatory and invasive monitoring should be used to guide volume status. Dopamine (1–2.5 µg/kg/min) may help maintain urine output. Spontaneous recovery has been reported but the vast majority of patients die. Liver transplant may be indicated for the cirrhotic patient that develops hepatorenal syndrome.

Pulmonary care

Hepatopulmonary syndrome is defined as a triad of signs: (1) liver disease, (2) increased alveolar arterial gradients, and (3) evidence of intrapulmonary vascular resistance. Autopsy specimens of human and animal lung have shown pre-capillary pulmonary dilatations and direct arteriovenous communications. Such lesions have been documented in chronic cirrhotics, or after halothane-induced liver failure. Animal and limited human studies have shown the putative mechanism for pulmonary dilatation to be the endogenous circulating pulmonary vasodilator, nitric oxide. Increased nitric oxide concentrations have been measured in exhaled breath from cirrhotic patients prior to liver transplant and found to be significantly decreased post transplant. Hypoxemia requires oxygen supplementation and may progress to respiratory failure (Krowka & Cortese 1994).

Glucose metabolism

Glucose deprivation leads to hepatic glycogenolysis to provide glucose. After glycogen stores in the liver are exhausted (12 to 24 hours), the liver must synthesize glucose from other substrates (gluconeogenesis). The hormones insulin, glucagon and epinephrine are important modulators of these processes. On balance, the postoperative patient would seem to be prone to hypoglycemia secondary to diminished glycogen reserves, increased insulin levels and impaired gluconeogenesis; yet dangerous hypoglycemia is rare. Routine dextrose solutions should be ordered and glucose levels monitored.

Coagulation

Bleeding in the patient with liver disease is a complicated issue (Ch. 11) as hyper- and hypocoagulable states can exist. Portal hypertension induces splenomegaly and platelet sequestration leading to thrombocytopenia. Thrombocytopenia can result from alcohol related folate deficiency, and/or direct platelet toxicity. Profound thrombocytopenia can be seen in patients with aplastic anemia, secondary to hepatitis C. Liver transplant eliminates this state.

Cholestasis, which often accompanies cirrhosis, inhibits absorption and decreases hepatic vitamin K stores. The liver synthesizes vitamin K dependent factors II (prothrombin), VII, IX, X, protein S and protein C. Improvements in coagulation may be achieved with vitamin K 10 mg/day. If this fails to correct a prolonged international normalized ratio (INR) or PT after 2–3 days, Vitamin K administration should be stopped and additional causes sought. In addition to the Vitamin K dependent factors, the liver also synthesizes antithrombin III and factor I (fibrinogen). In this setting, fresh frozen plasma (FFP) may be administered at a dose 12 to 20 ml/kg (2–6 units) with the goal of decreasing the PT to within 3 seconds of control. If coagulopathy persists, dysfibrinogenemia should be entertained. The cirrhotic liver not only has decreased synthetic capacity but also decreased clearance of activated clotting factors, notably tissue plasminogen activator (tPA). The result is systemic fibrinolysis further inhibiting clot formation and continued bleeding. Decreased serum concentrations of protein S, protein C and antithrombin III result in hypercoagulable states. Deficiency of these factors can lead to disseminated intravascular coagulation (DIC). Although heparin is recommended for treatment of DIC, it should be used with caution in patients with cirrhotic liver disease as it may exacerbate bleeding as clotting factor supplies are exhausted.

The patient with liver disease failing to respond to standard corrective measures, may be given 1-deamino-8-D arginine vasopressin (DDAVP) at a dose of 0.3 µg/kg IV every 12–24 h depending on bleeding severity. DDAVP is a synthetic peptide that increases factor VIII concentrations and shortens PT. DDAVP may be used in concert with FFP.

Sepsis (see also Ch. 8)

Mortality after hepatic resection is often caused by abdominal sepsis (Bozzetti et al 1992). In one series, six of 14 deaths were the result of intra-abdominal sepsis (Melendez et al 1998). Biliary manipulation and placement of biliary stents, culture positive bile, retained gallstones, ascites, and blood loss may all predispose to abdominal sepsis. Other sources of sepsis include the respiratory and urinary systems. Upper abdominal incision, pleural effusion, COPD and poor pulmonary toilet may promote the development of pneumonia. Wound inspections and central line catheter changes should be routinely performed.

Gastrointestinal bleeding

Although the incidence of stress related gastric mucosal lesions is high, the actual incidence of bleeding ulcers is 5% with a mortality reported as high as 50%. Endoscopy allows identification of the bleeding site. Treatment is largely supportive with transfusions, antacids and H₂ blockers. Indeed, prophylactic therapy for prevention of stress ulceration should be considered in all patients following major hepatobiliary procedures.

One-third of cirrhotic patients have esophageal varices. The mortality rate associated with bleeding varices ranges from 15 to 40% with 60% dead at 5 years. Emergent supportive care with blood product transfusion should be instituted with an attempt at correcting coagulopathy. Emergency endoscopy should be pursued with variceal banding or sclerotherapy as indicated (Ch. 97). Acute control of bleeding can be gained with octreotide at 25–100 µg/min. If pharmacologic or endoscopic methods fail to control bleeding compression of the varices may be accomplished using a Sengstaken-Blakemore tube. Despite compression, re-bleeding occurs in 50% of patients. As complications may be severe (airway obstruction, aspiration, and/or perforation), compression should be used only as a temporary measure until patients can undergo transvenous intrahepatic portosystemic shunting (TIPS) (Ch. 101) or surgical portosystemic shunting (Ch. 100).

Encephalopathy

A sudden change in a patient's mental status or the onset of asterixis, a flapping tremor related to loss of extensor tone, should precipitate a search for cause and the start of therapy for hepatic encephalopathy (Gitlin 1998). Precipitating factors include GI bleeding, infection, drugs, diet or dehydration. The exact pathogenesis is unknown. Accumulation of endogenous ammonia is associated with the onset of encephalopathy and has been suggested as causative. Other contributory factors have been suggested: (1) changes in the blood–brain barrier permeability, (2) abnormal neurotransmitter balance, (3) altered cerebral metabolism, (4) impairment of neuronal Na⁺-K⁺ ATPase activity, and (5) increased endogenous benzodiazepines. Standard therapy is designed to reduce levels of ammonia and other potentially toxic metabolites. Short-term benefit from flumazenil administration has been reported (Ferenci et al 1989). Diet protein restriction and lactulose are still the gold standard.

REFERENCES

Abrams R E, Hornbein T F 1975 Inability to reverse pancuronium blockade in a patient with renal failure and hepatic disease. Anesthesiology 42(3): 362–4

Abu K A, Takrouri M, Toukan A, Abu K M, Amr S 1988 Ketamine hydrochloride as sole anesthetic for open liver biopsy. Middle East Journal of Anesthesiology 9(6): 537–43

Aldrete J A, Homatas J, Boyes R N, Starzl T E 1970 Effects of hepatectomy on the disappearance rate of lidocaine from blood in man and dog. Anesthesia and Analgesia 49(5): 687–90

Altmayer P, Grundmann U, Ziehmer M, Larsen R, Buch H P 1991 Cardiac output and liver blood flow in humans: effect of the volatile anesthetic halothane. Methods and Findings in Experimental and Clinical Pharmacology 13(10): 709–14

Aranha G V, Greenlee H B 1986 Intra-abdominal surgery in patients with advanced cirrhosis. Archives of Surgery 121: 774–8

Arden J R, Lynman D P, Castagnoli K P 1988 Vercuronium in alcoholic liver disease: a pharmacokinetic and pharmacodynamic analysis. Anesthesiology 68: 771

Aronsen K F, Ericsson B, Pihl B 1969 Metabolic changes following major hepatic resection. Annals of Surgery 169(1): 102–10

Avallone R, Zeneroli M L, Venturini I, Corsi L, Schreier P, Kleinschnitz M, Ferrarese C, Farina F, Baraldi C, Pecora N et al 1998 Endogenous benzodiazepine-like compounds and diazepam binding inhibitor in serum of patients with liver cirrhosis with and without overt encephalopathy [see comments]. Gut 42(6): 861–7

Belghiti J, Noun R, Zante E, Ballet T, Sauvanet A 1996 Portal triad clamping or hepatic vascular exclusion for major liver resection – A controlled study. Annals of Surgery 224: 155–61

Belpaire F M, Bogaert M G 1991 Binding of alfentanil to human alpha 1-acid glycoprotein, albumin and serum. International Journal of Clinical Pharmacology, Therapy and Toxicology 29(3): 96–102

Bencini A F, Scaf A H J, Sohn Y J 1986 Hepatobiliary disposition of vercuronium bromide in man. British Journal of Anaesthesia 58: 988–95

Benowitz N L, Meister W 1978 Clinical pharmacokinetics of lignocaine—Review. Clinical Pharmacokinetics 3(3): 177–201

Berendes E, Lippert G, Loick H M, Brussel T 1996a Effects of enflurane and isoflurane on splanchnic oxygenation in humans. Journal of Clinical Anesthesia 8(6): 456–68

Berendes E, Lippert G, Loick H M, Brussel T 1996b Effects of positive end-expiratory pressure ventilation on splanchnic oxygenation in humans. Journal of Cardiothoracic and Vascular Anesthesia 10(5): 598–602

Bevan D R 1994 Rocuronium bromide and organ function. European Journal of Anaesthesiology (suppl 9): 87–91

Black M 1974 Liver disease and drug therapy—Review. Medical Clinics of North America 58(5): 1051–7

Bond W S 1978 Clinical relevance of the effect of hepatic disease on drug disposition. American Journal of Hospital Pharmacy 35(4): 406–14

Booij L H 1987 Influence of renal and hepatic function on pharmacodynamics and pharmacokinetics of non-depolarizing muscle relaxants—Review. Scientific Edition Pharmaceutisch Weekblad 9(2): 56–60

Booij L H 1997 Neuromuscular transmission and its pharmacological blockade. Part 2: Pharmacology of neuromuscular blocking agents—Review. Pharmacy World and Science 19(1): 13–34

Bower S, Sear S, Roy R C, Carter R F 1992 Effects of different hepatic pathologies on disposition of alfentanil in anaesthetized patients. British Journal of Anaesthesia 68: 462–5

Bozzetti F, Gennari L, Regalia E, Bignami P, Montalto F, Mazzaferro V, Doci R 1992 Morbidity and mortality after surgical resection of liver tumors. Analysis of 229 cases. Hepatogastroenterology 39(3): 237–41

Branch R A 1987 Is there increased cerebral sensitivity to benzodiazepines in chronic liver disease? Hepatology 7(4): 773–6

Branch R A, Morgan R H, Read A E 1976 Intravenous administration of diazepam in patients with chronic liver disease. Gut 17: 975

Braunwald E (ed) 1997 Heart disease: a textbook of cardiovascular medicine. 5th edn. W B Saunders, Philadelphia, pp 1793–1799

Brown B R 1988 Postoperative jaundice. In Brown B R (ed) Anesthesia in hepatic and biliary tract disease. F A Davies, Philadelphia, pp 265–273

Campbell K A, Wu Y P, Chacko V P, Sitzmann J V 1990 In vivo ^{31}P NMR spectroscopic changes during liver regeneration. Journal of Surgical Research 49(3): 244–7

Carlos R, Calvo R, Erill S 1979 Plasma protein binding of etomidate in patients with renal failure or hepatic cirrhosis. Clinical Pharmacokinetics 4(2): 144–8

Chauvin M, Bonnet F, Montembault C, Lafay M, Curet P, Viars P 1985 Hepatic plasma flow during sodium nitroprusside-induced hypotension in humans. Anesthesiology 63(3): 287–93

Chuter T A, Weissman C, Mathews D M, Starker P M 1990 Diaphragmatic breathing maneuvers and movement of the diaphragm after cholecystectomy. Chest 97: 1110–4

Colli A, Buccino G, Cocciolo M, Parravicini R, Scaltrini G 1988 Disposition of a flow-limited drug (lidocaine) and a metabolic capacity-limited drug (theophylline) in liver cirrhosis. Clinical Pharmacology and Therapeutics 44(6): 642–9

Cook D R, Freeman J A, Lai A A, Robertson K A, Kang Y, Stiller R L, Aggarwal S, Abou-Donia M M, Welch R M 1991 Pharmacokinetics and pharmacodynamics of doxacurium in normal patients and in those with hepatic or renal failure. Anesthesia and Analgesia 72(2): 145–50

Costela J L, Jimenez R, Calvo R, Suarez E, Carlos R 1996 Serum protein binding of propofol in patients with renal failure or hepatic cirrhosis. Acta Anaesthesiologica Scandinavica 40(6): 741–5

Couderc E, Ferrier C, Haberer J P 1984 Thiopentone pharmacokinetics in patients with chronic alcoholism. British Journal of Anesthesia 56: 1393–7

Cunningham J D, Fong Y, Shriver C, Melendez J, Marx W L, Blumgart L H 1994 One hundred consecutive hepatic resections. Blood loss, transfusion, and operative technique. Archives of Surgery 129: 1050–6

Dasarathy S, Mullen K D 1998 Benzodiazepines in hepatic encephalopathy: sleeping with the enemy—comment. Gut 42(6): 764–5

Davison R, Parker M, Atkinson A J Jr 1982 Excessive serum lidocaine levels during maintenance infusions: mechanisms and prevention. American Heart Journal 104 (2 Pt 1): 203–8

Delva E, Camus Y, Nordlinger B, Hannoun L, Parc R, Deriaz H, Lienhart A, Huguet C 1989 Vascular occlusion for liver resections—operative management and tolerance to hepatic ischemia in 142 cases. Annals of Surgery 209: 211–8

Devlin J C, Head-Rapson A G, Parker C J, Hunter J M 1993 Pharmacodynamics of mivacurium chloride in patients with hepatic cirrhosis. British Journal of Anaesthesia 71(2): 227–31

Duvaldestin P 1981 Pharmacokinetics in intravenous anaesthetic practice. [Review]. Clinical Pharmacokinetics 6(1): 61–82

Duvaldestin P, Henzel D 1982. Binding of tubocurarine, fazadinium, pancuronium and Org NC 45 to serum proteins in normal man and in patients with cirrhosis. British Journal of Anaesthesia 54(5): 513–6

Duvaldestin P, Agoston S, Hanzel K 1978 Pancuronium pharmacokinetics in patients with liver cirrhosis. British Journal of Anaesthesia 50: 1131

Dykes MH 1984 Is enflurane hepatotoxic? Anesthesiology 61: 235–7

Ebert TJ, Harkin CP, Muzi M 1995 Cardiovascular responses to sevoflurane: a review. [Review]. Anesthesia and Analgesia 81 Supplement 6: S11–S22

Eleftheriadis E, Kotzampassi K, Botsios D, Tzartinoglou E, Farmakis H, Dadoukis J 1996 Splanchnic ischemia during laparoscopic cholecystectomy. Surgical Endoscopy 10(3): 324–6

Elliot R H, Strunin L 1993 Hepatotoxicity of volatile anaesthetics. Implications for halothane, enflurane, isoflurane, sevoflurane, and desflurane. British Journal of Anaesthesia 70: 339–48

Emre S, Schwartz M E, Katz E, Miller C M 1993 Liver resection under total vascular isolation—variations on the theme. Annals of Surgery 217: 15–9

Emond J, Wachs M E, Renz J F, Kelley S, Harris H, Roberts J P 1995 Total vascular occlusion for major hepatectomy in patients with abnormal liver parenchyma. Archives of Surgery 130: 824–31

Endell W, Oltmanns D, Pottage T 1983 Alteration of the kinetics of tocainide in combined hepatic and renal insufficiency. Methods and Findings in Experimental and Clinical Pharmacology 5(8): 589–90

Farrell G, Prendergast D, Murray M 1985 Halothane hepatitis. Determination of a constitutional susceptibility factor. New England Journal of Medicine 313: 1310–4

Ferenci P, Grimm G, Meryn S, Gangl A 1989 Successful long-term treatment of portal-systemic encephalopathy by the benzodiazepine antagonist flumazenil. Gastroenterology 96: 240–3

Ferenci P, Grimm G 1990 Benzodiazepine antagonist in the treatment of human hepatic encephalopathy. Advances in Experimental Medicine and Biology 272: 255–65

Garrison R N, Cryer H M, Howard D A, Polk H C 1984 Clarification of risk factors for abdominal surgery in patients with hepatic Cirrhosis. Annals of Surgery 199: 648–55

Gelman S 1976 Disturbances in hepatic blood flow during anesthesia and surgery. Archives of Surgery 111: 881–3

Gelman S 1987 General anesthesia and hepatic circulation. Canadian Journal of Physiology and Pharmacology 65: 1762–79

Gelman S 1992 Anesthesia and the liver. In: Barash P G, Cullen B F, Stoelting R K (eds) Clinical anesthesia, 2nd edn. J B Lippincott, Philadelphia, pp 1185–1214

Gelman S, Fowler K C, Smith K R 1983 Liver circulation and function during isoflurane anesthesia in dogs. Anesthesiology 59: A224

Ghoneim M M, Pandya H 1975 Plasma protein binding of thiopental in patients with impaired renal or hepatic function. Anesthesiology 42(5): 545–9

Ghoneim M M, Korttila K 1977 Pharmacokinetics of intravenous anaesthetics: implications for clinical use. Clinical Pharmacokinetics 2(5): 344–72

Gitlin N 1998 Hepatic encephalopathy. In: Zakim D, Boyer TD, editors. Hepatology A Textbook of Liver Disease. 3rd edn. WB Saunders, Philadelphia, pp 605–17

Goldfarb G, Debaene B, Ang E T, Roulot D, Jolis P, Lebrec D 1990 Hepatic blood flow in humans during isoflurane-N_2O and halothane-N_2O anesthesia. Anesthesia and Analgesia 71(4): 349–53

Goldman L, Caldera D L, Nussbaum S R, Southwick F S, Krogstad D, Murray B, Burke D S, O'Malley T A, Goroll A H, Caplan C H, Nolan J, Carabello B, Slater E E 1977 Multifactorial index of cardiac risk in noncardiac surgical procedures. New England Journal of Medicine 297: 845–50

Greene N M 1981 Anesthesia risk factors in patients with liver disease. Contemporary Anesthesia Practice 4: 87–109

Greenway C V, Dettman R, Burczynski F, Sitar DS 1986 Effects of circulating catecholamines on hepatic blood volume in anesthetized cats. American Journal of Physiology 250 (6 Pt 2): H992–H997

Grossman, M, Aboise A, Tangphao O, Blaschke T F, Hoffman B B 1996 Morphine-induced venodilation in humans. Clinical Pharmacological Therapy 60: 554–60

Grundmann R, Heistermann S 1985 Postoperative albumin infusion therapy based on colloid osmotic pressure. A prospectively randomized trial. Archives of Surgery 120(8): 911–5

Haberer J P, Shoeffler E, Coyderc E, Duvaldestin P 1982 Fentanyl pharmacokinetics in anaesthetised patients with cirrhosis. British Journal of Anaesthesia 54: 1267–70

Habib N, Zografos G, Dalla Serra G, Greco L, Bean A 1994 Liver resection with total vascular exclusion for malignant tumors. British Journal Surgery 81: 1181–4

Hannoun L, Borie D, Delva E, Jones D, Vaillant JC, Nordlinger B, Parc R 1993 Liver resection with normothermic ischaemia exceeding 1 h. British Journal Surgery 80: 1161–5

Harper M H, Johnson B H, Eger E I 1984 Celiac plexus block does not alter hepatic injury in rats. Anesthesia and Analgesia 63(5): 479–81

Hartleb M, Michielsen P P, Dziurkowska-Marek A 1997 The role of nitric oxide in portal hypertensive systemic and portal vascular pathology. Acta Gastroenterologica Belgica 60: 222–232

Hasselstrom J, Eriksson S, Persson A, Rane A, Svensson J O, Sawe J 1990 The metabolism and bioavailability of morphine in patients with severe liver cirrhosis. British Journal of Clinical Pharmacology 29(3): 289–97

Hawkes C H, Brunt P W, Prescott R J, Horn D B 1973 EEG-provocative tests in the diagnosis of hepatic encephalopathy. Electroencephalography and Clinical Neurophysiology 34(2): 163–9

Hubbard A K, Roth T P, Gandolfi A J 1988 Halothane hepatitis patients generate an antibody response towards a covalently bound metabolite of halothane. Anesthesiology 68: 791–6

Hughson R L, Maillet A, Gauquelin G, Arbeille P, Yamamoto Y, Gharib C 1995 Investigation of hormonal effects during 10-h head-down tilt on heart rate and blood pressure variability. Journal of Applied Physiology 78: 583–96

Hunter J M, Parker C J, Bell C F, Jones R S, Utting J E 1985 The use of different doses of vecuronium in patients with liver dysfunction. British Journal of Anaesthesia 57(8): 758–64

Kainuma M, Fujiwara Y, Kimura N, Shitaokoshi A, Nakashima K, Shimada 1991 Monitoring hepatic venous hemoglobin oxygen saturation in patients undergoing liver surgery. Anesthesiology 74(1): 49–52

Kainuma M, Kimura N, Nonami T, Kurokawa T, Ito T, Nakashima K, Shimada Y 1992 The effect of dobutamine on hepatic blood flow and oxygen supply–uptake ratio during enflurane nitrous oxide anesthesia in humans undergoing liver resection. Anesthesiology 77(3): 432–8

Kanto J, Gepts E 1989 Pharmacokinetic implications for the clinical use of propofol. Clinical Pharmacokinetics 17(5): 308–26

Khalil M, D'Honneur G, Duvaldestin P, Slavov V, De Hys C, Gomeni R 1994 Pharmacokinetics and pharmacodynamics of rocuronium in patients with cirrhosis. Anesthesiology 80(6): 1241–7

Krowka M J, Cortese D A 1994 Hepatopulmonary syndrome. Current concepts in diagnostic and therapeutic considerations. Chest 105: 1528–1537

Lampe G H, Wauk L Z, Whitendale P, Way W L, Murray W, Eger E I 1990 Nitrous oxide does not impair hepatic function in young or old surgical patients. Anesthesia and Analgesia 71: 606–9

Lewis J H, Zimmerman H J, Ishak K G, Mullick F G 1983 Enflurane hepatotoxicity. A clinicopathologic study of 242 Cases. Annals of Internal Medicine 98: 984–92

Mangano D T, Goldman L 1995 Preoperative assessment of patients with known or suspected coronary disease. New England Journal of Medicine 333: 1750–6

Masone R J, Goldfarb J P, Manzione N C, Biempica I 1982 Enflurane hepatitis. Journal of Clinical Gastroenterology 4: 541–5

Mazoit J, Sandouk P, Zetlaovi P 1987 Pharmacokinetics of unchanged morphine in normal and cirrhotic subjects. Anesthesia and Analgesia 66: 293–8

McCombs G B, Ott C E, Jackson B A 1996 Effects of thoracic volume expansion on cardiorenal function in the conscious rat. Aviation Space and Environmental Medicine 67: 1086–91

Melendez J A, Arslan V, Fischer M, Wuest D, Jarnagin W, Fong Y, Blumgart L 1998 Peri-operative outcome of major hepatic resections under low central venous pressure anesthesia—blood loss, blood transfusion and the risk of post-operative renal dysfunction. Journal of the American College of Surgeons 178: 620–25

Mets B, Hickman R, Neveling U, Emms M, Chalton D O 1993 Effect of lidocaine on in vivo hepatic function. Digestive Diseases and Sciences 38(12): 2163–9

Mets B, Hickman R, Chalton D 1994 Lidocaine extraction by the in vivo and isolated perfused pig liver. Journal of Hepatology 21(6): 1067–74

Nakayama M, Kanaya N, Fujita S, Namiki A 1993 Effects of ephedrine on indocyanine green clearance during spinal anesthesia: evaluation by the finger piece method. Anesthesia and Analgesia 77(5): 947–9

Neuberger J 1990 Halothane hepatitis. Incidence, predisposing factors and exposure guidelines. Drug Safety 5: 28–38

O'Riordan J, O'Beirne H A, Young Y, Bellamy M C 1997 Effects of desflurane and isoflurane on splanchnic microcirculation during major surgery. British Journal of Anaesthesia 78(1): 95–6

Pandele G, Chaux F, Salvadori C, Farinotti M, Duvaldestin P 1983 Thiopental pharmacokinetics in patients with cirrhosis. Anesthesiology 59(2): 123–6

Park G R, Saeid M, Manara A R, Atallah M M, Quinn K 1993 Morphine elimination and hepatic blood flow—a study in patients with portal hypertension. Middle East Journal of Anesthesiology 12(2): 101–11

Parker C J R, Hunter J M 1989 Pharmacokinetics of atracurium and laudanosine in patients with hepatic cirrhosis. British Journal of Anaesthesia 62: 177–83

Patwardhan R V, Johnson R F, Hoyumpa A J, Sheehan J J, Desmond P V, Wilkinson G R, Branch R A, Schenker S 1981 Normal metabolism of morphine in cirrhosis. Gastroenterology 81(6): 1006–11

Pomier-Layrargues G, Giguere J F, Lavoie J, Perney P, Gagnon S, D'Amour M, Wells J, Butterworth R F 1994 Flumazenil in cirrhotic patients in hepatic coma: a randomized double-blind placebo-controlled crossover trial [see comments]. Hepatology 19(1): 32–7

Prescott L F, Forrest J A, Adjepon-Yamoah K K, Finlayson N D 1975 Drug metabolism in liver disease. Review Journal of Clinical Pathology. (Suppl Royal College of Pathologists) 9: 62–5

Rees M, Plant G, Wells J, Bygrave S 1996 One hundred and fifty hepatic resections: evolution of technique towards bloodless surgery. British Journal of Surgery 83: 1526–9

Rosow C E, Moss J, Philbin D M, Savarese J J 1982 Histamine release during morphine and fentanyl anesthesia. Anesthesiology 56: 93–6

Ruokonen E, Takala J, Uusaro A 1991 Effect of vasoactive treatment on the relationship between mixed venous and regional oxygen saturation (see comments). Critical Care Medicine 19(11): 1365–9

Ruokonen E, Takala J, Kari A, Saxen H, Mertsola J, Hansen E J 1993 Regional blood flow and oxygen transport in septic shock (see comments). Critical Care Medicine 21(9): 1296–303

Ryan W H, Hummel B W, McClelland R N 1982 Reduction in the morbidity and mortality of major hepatic resection. Experience with 52 patients. American Journal of Surgery 144(6): 740–3

Schwinn D A, McIntyre R W, Reves J G 1990 Isoflurane-induced vasodilation: role of the adrenergic nervous system. Anesthesia and Analgesia 71: 451–9

Segawa T, Tsuchiya R, Furui J, Izawa K, Tsunoda T, Kanematsu T 1993 Operative results in 143 patients with hepatocellular carcinoma. World Journal of Surgery 17: 663–7

Servin F, Cockshott I D, Farinotti R, Haberer J P, Winckler C, Desmonts J M 1990 Pharmacokinetics of propofol infusions in patients with cirrhosis. British Journal of Anaesthesia 65(2): 177–83

Sesto M E, Vogt D P, Hermann R E 1987 Hepatic resection in 128 patients: a 24-year experience. Surgery 102(5): 846–51

Shingu K, Eger E I, Johnson B H, Lurz F W, Taber V 1983 Effects of halothane, isoflurane, enflurane, thiopental, and fentanyl on blood gas values in rats exposed to hypoxia. Anesthesia and Analgesia 62(2): 155–9

Stefano G B, Hartman A, Bilfinger T V, Magazine H I, Liu Y, Casares F, Goligorsky M S 1995 Presence of the m_3 opiate receptor in endothelial cells. Journal of Biological Chemistry 270: 30290–3

Stoelting R K 1987 Isoflurane and postoperative hepatic dysfunction. Canadian Journal of Anesthesiology 34: 223–6

Strunin L, Thomson S (eds) 1992 The liver and anaesthesia. Bailliere's Clinical Anaesthesiology 6(4): 697–956

Terai C, Anada H, Matsushima S, Shimizu S, Okada Y 1995 Effect of mild Trendelenburg on central hemodynamics and internal jugular vein velocity, cross-sectional area, and flow. American Journal of Emergency Medicine 13: 255–8

Thompson H H, Tompkins R K, Longmire W P, Jr 1983 Major hepatic resection: a 25 year experience. Surgery 197: 375–387

Whittle B J R, Moncada S 1998 Nitric oxide: The elusive mediator of the hyperdynamic circulation of cirrhosis. Hepatology 16(4): 1089–92

Yanaga K, Kanematsu T, Takenaka K, Matsumata T, Yoshida Y, Sugimachi K 1988. Hepatic resection for hepatocellular carcinoma in elderly patients. American Journal of Surgery 155: 238–41

Interventional radiology and endoscopic techniques. Biliary bypass and intubation

28

Interventional endoscopy (technical aspects)

K.F. BINMOELLER, N. SOEHENDRA

INTRODUCTION

The field of therapeutic biliary endoscopy has evolved rapidly since the first reports of endoscopic sphincterotomy in 1974 (Classen & Demling 1974, Kawai et al 1974). A spectrum of interventional procedures have gained widespread acceptance as therapeutic alternatives to operative management (Table 28.1). The minimally invasive nature inherent to endoscopic retrograde cholangiopancreatography (ERCP) coupled with its ability to be performed under conscious sedation resulted in its rapid dissemination around the world. Refinements in procedural technique and improvements in accessory equipment have improved results and safety. This chapter will focus upon these technical advances. The indications, contraindications, and complications of interventional biliary endoscopy are covered elsewhere (Chs 17, 40, 59) and therefore will not be directly addressed.

patients undergoing interventional ERCP, the sphincterotome can be used for both initial cannulation of the bile duct and subsequent sphincterotomy. Upwards bowing of the sphincterotome helps achieve the correct axis for selective cannulation of the bile duct (Fig. 28.1). If free cannulation of the bile duct fails, guidewire cannulation can be attempted by passing a guidewire through the sphincterotome. Hydrophilic guidewires with a special slippery coating are ideal for bile duct cannulation as they minimize trauma to the papilla and will more effectively seek out the path to the bile duct. The guidewire is extended several millimeters from the tip of the sphincterotome and the papillary orifice is cautiously probed with the wire until it slips into the bile duct (Fig. 28.2, top panel). Once deep cannulation is achieved, the sphincterotome can be advanced over the wire into the bile duct for sphincterotomy (Fig. 28.2, bottom panel). Using a double lumen sphincterotome, the wire can be left in the duct during sphincterotomy.

Table 28.1 Interventional endoscopy in biliary tract disease

Sphincterotomy
Stone extraction
Lithotripsy
    Mechanical
    Shock wave (electrohydraulic, laser)
    Chemical dissolution
Stent drainage
Balloon dilation
Sphincter of Oddi manometry
Photodynamic therapy
Papillectomy

CANNULATION

Selective cannulation of the bile duct is a prerequisite for sphincterotomy and interventional biliary procedures. For

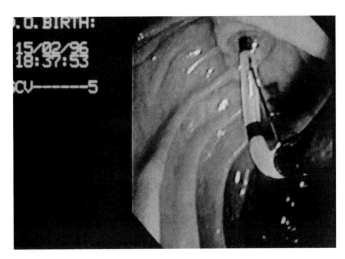

Fig. 28.1 Endoscopic view showing the use of a bowed sphincterotome for cannulation of the bile duct.

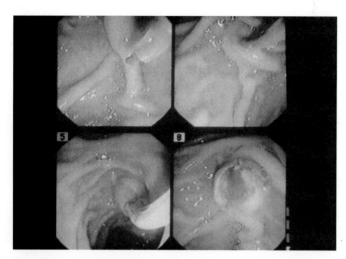

Fig. 28.2 Endoscopic views of bile duct cannulation using a guide wire (top panel) and sphincterotomy (bottom panel).

Precutting

Precutting is a useful technique to achieve selective bile duct cannulation when free- or wire-guided approaches fail. The objective of precutting is to incise the roof of the papilla to expose the underlying opening of the bile duct for selective cannulation. The widely used term 'precut papillotomy' is misleading since papillotomy has been used interchangeably with the term sphincterotomy. The term 'papillary roof incision' more accurately describes the procedure of precutting.

Precutting can be performed with either a needle-knife catheter (Fig. 28.3, top) or precut papillotome (Fig. 28.3, bottom). Most of the published experience has been with the needle-knife catheter (Huibregtse et al 1986a,b, Siegel et al 1989, Dowsett et al 1990, Tweedle & Martin 1991).

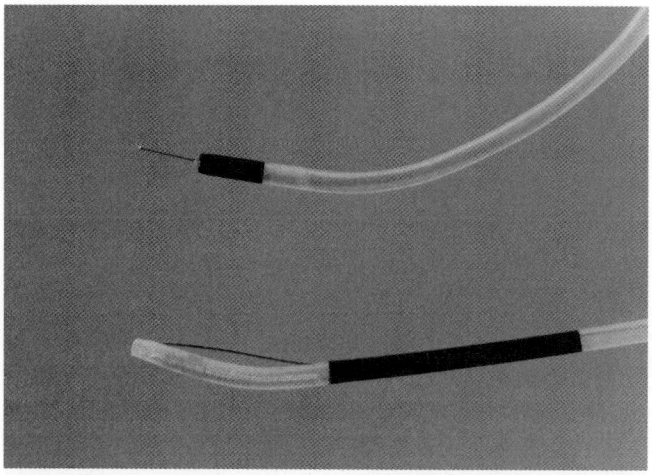

Fig. 28.3 Precut sphincterotomes. Above: Needle knife sphincterotome. Below: Precut sphincterotome. The cutting wire measures 10 mm and exists nearly directly at the tip of the sphincterotome.

This consists of a retractable bare diathermy wire which extends up to 5 mm from the tip of a catheter. The needle is inserted into the papillary orifice and the cut is directed upwards in the 11–12 o'clock direction. Caution must be taken not to incise too deeply, particularly at the papillary orifice, to avoid injury to the pancreatic duct. The ability to drill into the papilla with this instrument has been used by some to create a suprapapillary choledochoduodenal fistula (Osnes 1979, Schapira & Khawaja 1982, Kozarek & Sanowski 1983) This technique has been found to be particularly useful in patients with a papillary tumor. Another application is to free an impacted stone at the papilla. Here an incision is made directly into the most bulging portion of the papilla against the surface of the impacted stone (Binmoeller & Katon 1990, Leung et al 1990).

The precut papillotome resembles the conventional Erlangen-type sphincterotome, but has a shorter diathermy wire (15 mm) and practically no leading tip (Soehendra precut papillotome, Wilson Cook Inc) (Binmoeller et al 1996). The tip of the catheter is positioned at the papillary orifice and the incision is made by shifting the axis of the catheter to bring the wire in contact with the papillary roof (Fig. 28.4). After selective bile duct cannulation is achieved, a sphincterotomy can be immediately performed with the precut papillotome.

Precutting is not without risk. Two large multicenter studies identified precutting as a significant risk factor for post-sphincterotomy pancreatitis (Freeman et al 1996, Loperfido et al 1998), and there have been isolated reports of perforation. There is uniform agreement that precutting belongs strictly in the hands of the experienced biliary endoscopist and should be reserved for patients with a strong indication for sphincterotomy (Cotton 1989).

Rendez-vous procedure

If precutting fails, endoscopic biliary cannulation can be aided by a combined percutaneous and endoscopic approach ('rendez-vous' procedure). A guide wire is inserted via the percutaneous transhepatic route into the duodenum and subsequently grasped at the endoscopic end. The guide wire is then pulled through the working channel of the endoscope and serves as a guide rail to enable retrograde biliary cannulation, sphincterotomy and further endoscopic intervention (Kerlan et al 1984, Dowset et al 1989a,b, Hall et al 1990).

Juxtapapillary diverticula

Juxtapapillary duodenal diverticula, frequently found in elderly patients, alter the position and anatomical bound-

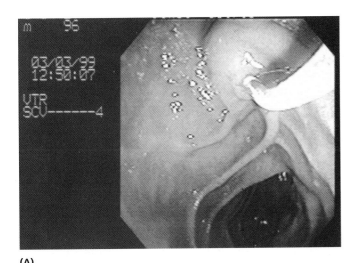

(A)

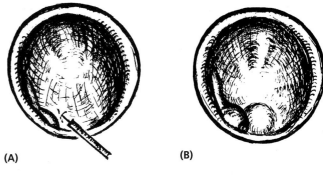

(A)   **(B)**

Fig. 28.5 Technique to improve accessibility of a papilla located on the inner surface of a diverticulum: **(A)** Using a standard injection catheter, 1–2 cc of saline is injected adjacent to the papilla on the diverticular side. **(B)** Raised submucosal tissue 'tilts' the papilla into view.

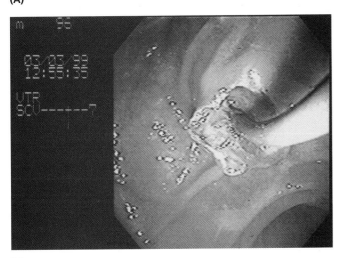

(B)

Fig. 28.4 Precutting technique. **(A)** Insertion of the tip of the precut sphincterotome in the papillary orifice followed by cephalad incision of the papillary roof at the 12 o'clock position with pure cutting current. **(B)** The incised roof retracts, exposing the underlying biliary duct orifice. The bile duct is selectively cannulated.

accessories (forceps and cannula) inserted together through the working channel to enable the endoscopist to simultaneously pull the papilla out of the diverticulum and cannulate the papilla has also been described.

Even with access to the papilla, deep cannulation of the bile duct adjacent to a large juxtapapillary diverticulum may be difficult, as the diverticulum will distort the course of the distal common bile duct. It is helpful to alter the direction of cannulation after entering the biliary orifice according to the anatomy of the diverticulum (Fig. 28.6). The direction of cannulation may actually be caudal rather than cranial. Use of a guide wire will tend to straighten the course of the duct and may facilitate deep cannulation.

aries of the papilla and displace the course of the bile duct, making cannulation more difficult (Vaira et al 1989). Accessing the papilla is a problem when the papilla is located within the diverticulum. Various ancillary maneuvers may improve access. Aspirating air from the diverticulum may help 'evert' the diverticulum, thereby bringing the papilla into a more favorable position for cannulation. Altering patient position and applying abdominal pressure may also be helpful. Failing these, a small depot of normal saline can be injected into the submucosal plane of the mucosa adjacent to the papilla. The injection should be made on the diverticular side of the papilla in an attempt to 'tilt' the papilla towards the endoscopist (Fig. 28.5). The use of two

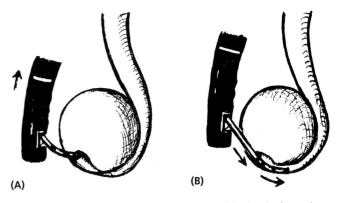

(A)   **(B)**

Fig. 28.6 Technique for deep cannulation of the bile duct in the setting of a large juxtapapillary diverticulum. **(A)** Slight withdrawal of the endoscope shifts the angle of cannulation more caudad. **(B)** The catheter is advanced while gradually straightening the cannulation angle.

Billroth-II gastrectomy

The patient who has undergone a Billroth-II gastrectomy poses a special challenge to the biliary endoscopist. Reaching the papilla is the first obstacle. If the afferent loop is long, the papilla may be beyond the reach of a duodenoscope. Intubation of the afferent loop with a forward-viewing pediatric colonoscope will usually enable access to the papilla. Cannulation of the Billroth-II papilla is the second obstacle. Because the endoscope approaches the papilla from below rather than above, the papillary anatomy in the Billroth-II patient will be reversed. The bile duct is cannulated by orienting the catheter downward at the 5–6 o'clock rather than the standard 11–12 o'clock position. It is helpful to use a new straight catheter, or even mold a downward bow into the catheter, to achieve this. Cannulation of the papilla is more difficult with a forward-viewing instrument owing to lack of an en-face view and the lack of an elevator (Fig. 28.7).

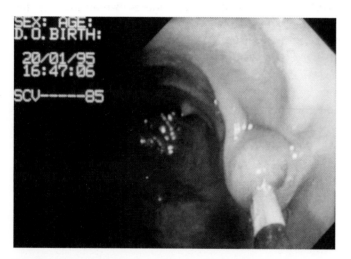

Fig. 28.7 Cannulation of the papilla using a forward-viewing pediatric colonoscope in a patient with Billroth-II anatomy. The bile duct is cannulated at the 5 o'clock position.

SPHINCTEROTOMY

Endoscopic sphincterotomy aims at opening the terminal part of the common bile duct by cutting the papilla and sphincter muscles. Although not always mandatory for interventional procedures, it greatly facilitates biliary access and manipulation.

The basic technique of sphincterotomy has changed little since its initial description nearly two decades ago. The standard sphincterotome (Erlangen 'pull-type' model) consists of a Teflon® catheter containing a cautery wire which is exposed for a variable length (20 to 30 mm) near the tip of the instrument. The leading tip distal to the wire ('nose') may be of variable length (5–15 mm). The preference of the authors is to use a sphincterotome with a shorter nose (5 mm) and shorter wire (20 mm), as this is easiest to manipulate in and around the biliary orifice.

Following deep bile duct cannulation, the sphincterotome is slowly retracted until approximately half of the wire length is exposed outside the papilla. The sphincterotome is slightly bowed so that the wire is in contact with the roof, but not excessively to avoid a 'zipper' incision. The incision is made by gently lifting the sphincterotome against the papillary roof using the elevator and up–down controls while applying short bursts of current. The power settings will vary according to the type of diathermy unit used. There is still debate as to whether blended or pure cutting current should be used. Theoretically, pure cutting current will be associated with less edema of the ampulla and may decrease the risk of pancreatitis, but the risk of postsphincterotomy hemorrhage might be greater. In a prospective randomized study the use of pure cut current was associated with a lower incidence of pancreatitis than with blended current sphincterotomy (Elta et al 1998). An insufficient number of patients were studied to comment on the relative risk of hemorrhage. If blended current is used, the cut should be monitored for excessive tissue blanching and edema, as this will increase the risk of pancreatitis.

The length of the sphincterotomy should be tailored to the indication. A small incision (up to 1 cm) will be adequate for stent insertion, whereas stone extraction usually requires a larger incision depending on the size of the stone to be extracted. The extent of the sphincterotomy will be limited by the size of the papilla and the length of the intraduodenal portion of the common bile duct. Particular caution is necessary when the papilla is small and the bile duct caliber is narrow. Although sphincterotomy in the presence of a juxtapapillary diverticula has not been found to be associated with higher complication rates (Vaira et al 1989), the risk of perforation is inherently greater. The incision should be performed in millimeter increments, paying close attention to the boundaries of the incision and the course of the intraduodenal segment of the bile duct.

In the Billroth-II patient, the standard Erlangen-type sphincterotome is unsuited for sphincterotomy due to the reversed anatomy of the papilla. Special sphincterotomes and techniques have been developed to accommodate this anatomical variation (Soehendra et al 1980, Shapira & Khawaja 1982, Osnes et al 1986, Ricci et al 1991). The Soehendra Billroth-II sphincterotome (Wilson-Cook) is most widely used, designed to produce an upside-down bow in the cutting wire so as to orientate the wire correctly within the bile duct. A new over-the-guide wire Billroth-II sphincterotome has been developed to enable sphincterotomy while leaving the guide wire in place (Wang et al 1996).

SPHINCTEROPLASTY

Balloon dilation of the sphincter using high-pressure hydrostatic balloons of 6- or 8-mm diameter has recently been used as an alternative to sphincterotomy (Mac Mathuna et al 1994, Bergman et al 1997). The theoretical advantage of this approach is the preservation of the sphincter function. Long-term complications after sphincterotomy such as cholangitis or papillary stenosis, however, have been found to be rare. The drawback of balloon dilation is a more limited size of the papillary opening that may limit the size of the stone that can be extracted using the balloon or basket catheter. Stones measuring > 8mm will often require mechanical lithotripsy to enable transpapillary extraction.

STONE EXTRACTION (see also Ch. 40)

Several series have shown that 85 to 90% of common bile duct stones can be effectively removed following endoscopic sphincterotomy combined with the Dormia basket or balloon catheter (Cotton & Vallon 1981, Geenen et al 1981). The choice of basket or balloon is largely dictated by stone size. The Dormia basket is sturdier and provides better traction for removal of a larger stone (> 0.5 cm). The balloon catheter occludes the lumen and is ideal for removing small stones or sludge.

Several technical points may increase the success rate of stone extraction. The sphincterotomy should be generous enough to enable extraction of the stone. The adequacy of the incision can be assessed by passing an inflated balloon catheter through the sphincterotomy opening. If multiple medium- or large-sized stones are present, it is important to remove stones individually, beginning with the lowermost stone, to avoid stone impaction. If a stone is mistakenly captured, it can be dislodged from the basket by pushing it upwards into the hepatic duct confluence where the basket will tend to fold over or advance into the hepatic duct, thereby releasing the stone. When extracting a stone, the direction of traction should be in the axis of the bile duct, which can be verified on fluoroscopy.

Intrahepatic stones pose a special challenge because they are difficult to access via the retrograde transpapillary route. These stones usually form above strictures and are tightly impacted. Use of a wire-guided basket may be helpful to gain access to these stones (Staritz et al 1990). Alternatively, a basket that can be introduced when endoscopic extraction fails has been reported (Binmoeller et al 1993a,b).

Intrahepatic stones can also be removed by the percutaneous transhepatic route (Burhenne 1980, Clouse et al 1986).

LITHOTRIPSY

Failure of standard stone extraction techniques is usually due to large stones (greater than 1.5 cm), multiple impacted stones, or stones proximal to a stricture. A variety of modalities are currently available to fragment these difficult stones prior to extraction. These include mechanical lithotripsy, intraductal shock wave lithotripsy, extracorporeal shock wave lithotripsy, and dissolution therapy. These modalities will be briefly discussed below.

Mechanical lithotripsy

Using mechanical lithotripsy, the stone is forcefully crushed in the arms of a Dormia basket after entrapment. This method is the simplest and most cost-effective of the lithotripsy techniques with success rates of 80 to 90% (Schneider et al 1988, Classen et al 1988, Siegel et al 1990a,b). There are two variations to the technique of mechanical lithotripsy: the non-endoscopic and through-the-endoscope methods. Using the non-endoscopic method, the stone is captured within a standard Dormia basket, the basket handle is cut off, and the endoscope is exchanged for the coil metal sheath. Using the through-the-endoscope method, a special basket contained within the metal sheath is inserted through the endoscope working channel (Fig. 28.8). Since the basket is part of a single unit lithotriptor device, this method presumes that the endoscopist anticipates the need for mechanical lithotripsy before an attempt is made to extract the stone. If stone extraction is attempted with a standard Dormia basket and the stone and basket become impacted in the bile duct, the endoscopist must use the non-endoscopic method to effect fragmentation.

Intraductal shock wave lithotripsy

Failure of mechanical lithotripsy is usually due to inability to capture the stone in the basket, which may occur if the stone is firmly impacted or very large. An alternative modality to achieve stone fragmentation is to use shock waves, which can be delivered intraductally or extracorporeally. Intraductal lithotripsy is performed using flexible probes that can be introduced into the bile duct. The shock waves are generated using electrohydraulic or laser technology (Liguory et al 1987, Leung & Chung 1989, Binmoeller et al 1993a,b, Kozarek et al 1988, Ell et al 1988, Cotton et al 1990, Ponchon et al 1991) and applied directly to the stone

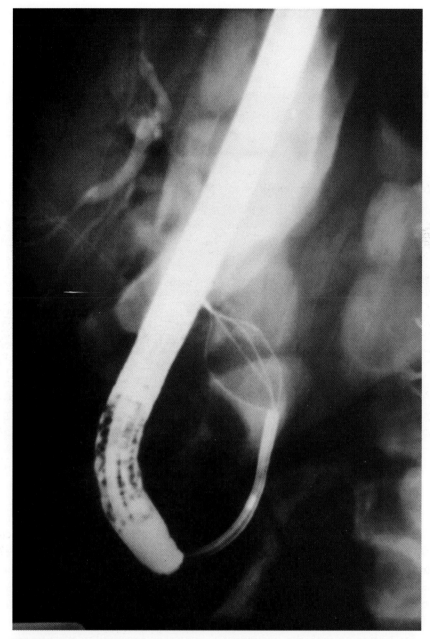

Fig. 28.8 Radiograph showing intraductal mechanical lithotripsy of a large stone using a through-the-endoscope lithotriptor device.

surface. Since shock waves can cause injury to the bile duct wall (Sievert & Silvis 1985, Harrison et al 1987, Thomas et al 1988, Bhatta et al 1990), intraductal lithotripsy is generally performed under cholangioscopic guidance using a cholangioscope that is inserted into the bile duct via the duodenoscope. The lithotripsy probe is inserted through the operating channel of the cholangioscope and shock waves are fired under visual guidance until adequate stone fragmentation is achieved (Fig. 28.9).

Extracorporeal shock wave lithotripsy

Extracorporeal shock wave lithotripsy (ESWL) has been shown to be an effective and safe method to fragment common bile duct and intrahepatic duct stones that defy endoscopic extraction. In a US multi-institution study stone fragmentation was achieved in 95% of patients, but 50% of patients required adjunctive treatments to achieve complete ductal clearance of stone fragments (Bland et al 1989).

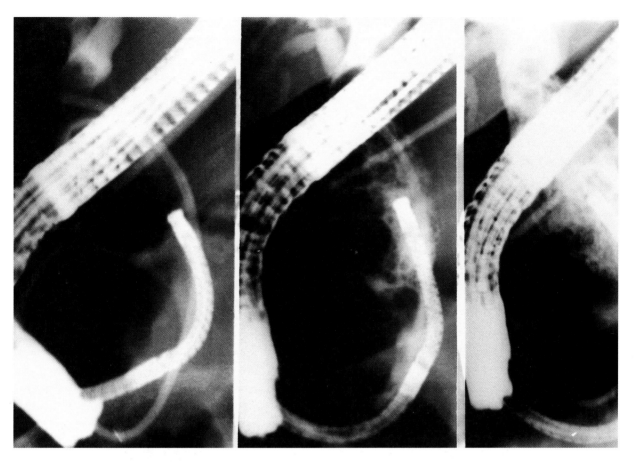

Fig. 28.9 Radiograph showing intraductal shock wave lithotripsy. The babyscope has been inserted into the bile duct and guides lithotripsy under direct cholangioscopic vision.

Extracorporeal shock wave lithotripsy was found in a prospective randomized study to be less effective than intra-ductal shock wave lithotripsy for the clearance of common bile duct stones (Neuhaus et al 1998). Although used in many countries for fragmentation of bile duct stones, ESWL is not approved in the US for this indication.

Chemical dissolution (Ch. 33)

Mono-octanoin and methyl-tert-butyl ether (MTBE) have been used to dissolve common bile duct stones via naso-biliary drainage catheters and T tubes (Allen et al 1985, Palmer & Hoffmann 1986). Despite encouraging initial reports, this approach has lost popularity due to the cumbersome, time-consuming technique and poor overall results (Dipadova et al 1986). This method is also not with-out hazard, particularly in patients who have undergone previous sphincterotomy and are thus prone to leakage of the solvent into the duodenum. The administration of ursodeoxychoic acid in combination with endoscopic stent placement was shown in one study to soften and decrease

the size of common bile stones, thereby facilitating endo-scopic extraction (Johnson et al 1993). This approach is appealing when high technology lithotripsy methods are not available.

BILIARY DILATION

Biliary dilation can be performed using push-type dilation catheters (bougies) or high-pressure hydrostatic balloons. The latter are commonly used to dilate benign biliary stric-tures, which may be caused by chronic pancreatitis, scleros-ing cholangitis, or operative injury (Foutch & Sivak 1985, Johnson et al 1991). The balloons are available in varying lengths and diameters. When inflated, the balloon applies radial dilating force. Strictures can be dilated in a graduated manner using balloons of increasing diameter (4–8 mm when inflated). The balloon is inflated with diluted contrast to the maximum atmospheric pressure allowable, and kept inflated until the stricture 'waist' disappears (generally 30–60 seconds of inflation). Balloon dilation is usually used in conjunction with stent placement to maintain the dilation effect (Davids et al 1992a,b). The duration of stenting required to achieve a permanent dilation effect is variable. Postoperative strictures may require up to 1 year of stenting (Smits et al 1996). The placement of multiple stents by adding a stent at 3-month intervals is one approach that may optimize the dilation effect.

Very tight strictures that do not permit passage of a bougie or balloon catheter can be opened with the Soehendra stent retriever device (Wilson Cook Medical) (van Someren et al 1996). The retriever device comes in diameters of 7, 8, 10, and 11.5 French. After placement of a guidewire across the stricture, the retriever device is coaxially inserted until it engages the stricture. Turning the shaft of the retriever clockwise, the screw-like tip of the instrument will bore a path through the stricture to enable dilation using a bougie or balloon catheter.

BILIARY STENTING

Endoscopic transpapillary stent placement is a well-standardized technique today and can be carried out with an overall success rate of over 90%. Stenting has become the treatment of choice for the palliative decompression of malignant biliary obstruction (Ch. 59) and is an accepted alternative to surgery for the treatment of benign biliary strictures although not all are in agreement as to the long-term efficacy (Ch. 49). Stenting has also been found to be an effective treatment for some postoperative biliary leaks (Binmoeller et al 1991, Davids et al 1992a,b) (Ch. 50).

Technique of stent placement

After diagnosing the type and site of obstruction with a diagnostic ERCP, a small sphincterotomy is often performed to facilitate insertion of further instruments. The stricture is then negotiated with a guide wire. The technical success has been enhanced in the last few years due to the availability of special hydrophilic wires which allow easier and less traumatic passage through strictures. Various maneuvers may facilitate the negotiation of a complicated biliary stricture. The angle of access to the stricture can be changed by adjusting the position of the guide catheter tip. An angulated guide wire tip may be helpful for negotiating eccentric strictures. For concentric strictures, an inflated balloon catheter inserted over the guide wire will center the guide wire in the lumen. Once the stricture is passed with a wire, a dilating catheter is coaxially inserted to dilate the stricture and obtain a complete cholangiogram. Cytology brushings can be obtained at this point to confirm malignant obstruction. A biliary stent (both plastic and expand-able metallic) is inserted using the Seldinger technique. Decompression of the obstructed biliary tree is typically indicated by a gush of dark stagnant bile into the duodenum.

Hilar strictures

Hilar strictures are often difficult to stent because they are further away from the endoscope and tend to be tortuous and sclerotic. For obstructing hilar cholangiocarcinoma (Klatskin tumors), the success rate of transpapillary stenting varies according to the level of obstruction. For Type I strictures (involvement of the common hepatic duct) the success rate is around 86%, but falls to 45% for Type II (involvement of both main hepatic ducts) and 15% for Type III strictures (involvement of secondary intrahepatic branches). There is controversy as to whether both lobes of the liver need to be drained when a bifurcation lesion obstructs both lobes. Although one early study that compared single and bilateral stent drainage for Type II and III malignant hilar obstruction did not show any difference in outcome (Polydorou et al 1989), two subsequent studies have shown bilateral drainage to be associated with a significantly lower complication rate and survival advantage (Deviere et al 1988, Chang et al 1998). As a rule, both lobes should be drained in Type II and III obstruction if contrast fills both hepatic ductal systems and fails to drain (Fig. 28.10). Some authors disagree with the use of endoscopic stenting for the management of hilar strictures emphasizing the change of curative resection for Type I strictures and the advantage of percutaneous transhepatic stenting for irresectable tumors (Chs 30, 54, 59).

Stent clogging

Stent clogging is a common problem which will necessitate a stent exchange. The mean duration of patency of plastic stents is approximately 5 months (Huibregtse et al 1986a,b). Exploring ways to prolong stent patency has been the subject of considerable research over the past years and continues to remain unsolved. Expandable metal stents, which can be inserted through the duodenoscope in a compressed state and expand to a diameter of up to 30 Fr, are less prone to clogging than plastic stents (Huibregtse et al 1989, Neuhaus et al 1991, Cremer et al 1990). Drawbacks of expandable stents are their high cost and difficulty removing these stents after placement. There have also been reports of technical difficulties with stent deployment (Bethge et al 1992). Although less prone to biliary sludge clogging, expandable stents may obstruct due to tumor ingrowth and overgrowth.

Replacement of a clogged plastic stent can be performed by either removing the clogged stent with a snare or forceps and inserting a new stent, or exchanging the stent over a guide wire using the Soehendra stent retriever (Fig. 28.11). The retriever consists of a 200 cm metal spiral catheter with a threaded tip that can be screwed into the end of the prosthesis (Soehendra et al 1990). The advantage of this method is that stent replacement can be performed without losing access to the stricture. This is particularly helpful when bilateral stent replacement is indicated.

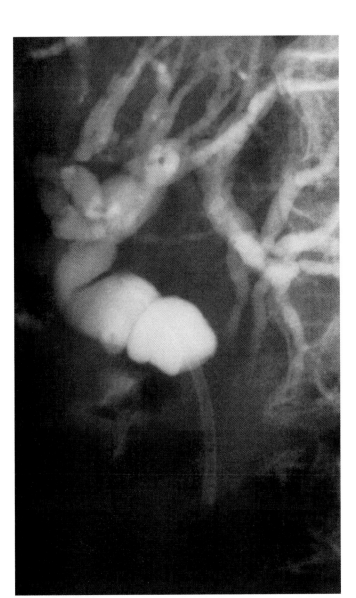

(A)

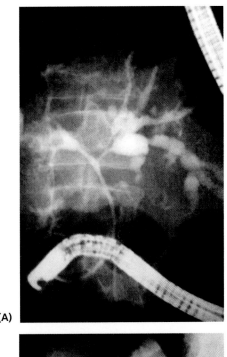

(A)

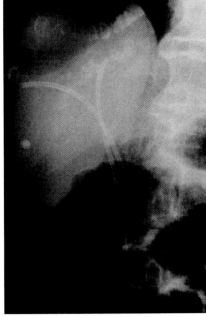

(B)

Fig. 28.10 **(A)** Radiograph showing endoscopic stent decompression of a malignant distal common bile duct stricture. **(B)** Endoscopic view of the biliary stent draining dark bile.

Fig. 28.11 Radiographs showing: **(A)** Type III malignant hilar obstruction upstream dilation of both the left and right hepatic ducts. **(B)** Placement of bilateral biliary stents for drainage of both lobes.

Endoprosthesis for stone impaction

Failure to clear the bile duct of stones after sphincterotomy places the patient at substantial risk for cholangitis and sepsis. Providing drainage is therefore mandatory. The placement of an endoprosthesis provides a temporizing measure to maintain biliary drainage and prevent stone impaction pending more definitive management (Cotton et al 1987, Foutch et al 1989, Soomers et al 1990). Stent placement may also be preferable to attempting stone extraction in the septic patient; clearance of the duct can be performed once the sepsis has settled and the patient's condition has stabilized. Stents should not be left in place as definite treatment or over an extended period of time, as late complications (mainly cholangitis) have been reported to occur in 40% of patients (Bergman et al 1995). The alternative of open surgical treatment of the problem should not be lost sight of (Ch. 39).

PHOTODYNAMIC THERAPY

Photodynamic therapy is a promising new therapy that may restore biliary drainage and improves quality of life in patients with nonresectable disseminated cholangiocarcinomas (Ortner et al 1998). Similar response has also been reported for patients experiencing obstructive jaundice from ampullary cancer, and the treatment may be applicable for pancreatic cancer as well. A photosensitizing cytotoxic agent is administered intravenously that is selectively taken up by tumor cells. Subsequent exposure to laser light of the proper wavelength activates the photsensitizing agent and results in tumor destruction. Application of laser light is performed under direct cholangioscopic view using thin laser fibers. Further study of this modality is necessary.

SPHINCTER OF ODDI MANOMETRY (SOM) (see also Ch. 6)

Sphincter of Oddi manometry is used in some centers to diagnose sphincter of Oddi dysfunction, of which papillary stenosis and sphincter dyskinesia are subtypes. Papillary stenosis is defined by an elevated basal sphincter pressure, and various manometric criteria are used to define sphincter dyskinesia. Postcholecystecomy pain is the dominant indication for SOM. The technique of SOM has become fairly standarized using special endoscopic manometry catheters that are introduced into the bile duct. Sphincterotomy has been shown to result in symptomatic improvement of biliary pain in patients documented to have sphincter of Oddi dysfunction (Geenen et al 1989). Endoscopic injection of botulinum toxin into the papilla of Vater is an alternative approach that has shown promising results and may predict which patients will respond best to endoscopic sphincterotomy (Wehrmann et al 1998).

PAPILLECTOMY

Benign adenomas of the papilla of Vater can be removed together with the papilla of Vater using a diathermic snare in an analogous manner to colon polypectomy (snare papillectomy) (Binmoeller et al 1993a,b, Bertoni et al 1997). The technique entails snaring of the papilla flush with the duodenal wall (Fig. 28.13). This is an alternative to local surgical resection if complete excision of the adenoma and papilla is achieved. It is critical that the excised tissue specimen is retrieved and submitted for complete histological evaluation. Surgical resection is indicated if the specimen shows malignancy or complete excision cannot be achieved endoscopically. Periodic endoscopic surveillance is mandatory to evaluate for adenoma recurrence. The technique of snare papillectomy has been used to facilitate cannulation of the bile duct in select cases where conventional cannulation techniques have failed (Farrell et al 1996).

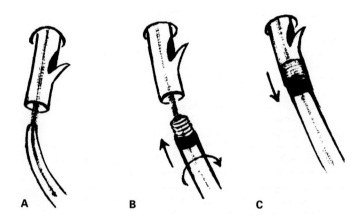

Fig. 28.12 Stent replacement using the Soehendra Retriever (Wilson-Cook Medical Inc). **(A)** A conventional 0.035 inch Teflon-coated guidewire is inserted through the prosthesis with the aid of an ERCP catheter. **(B)** The catheter is removed and the Retriever inserted over the wire until it abuts against the distal end of the prosthesis. The stent is rotated clockwise to screw the Retriever tip into the prosthesis. **(C)** The stent is removed over the indwelling guide-wire.

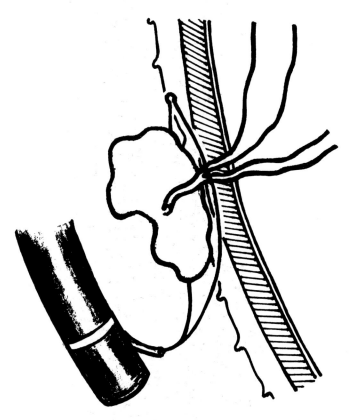

Fig. 28.13 Schematic diagram showing the technique of snare papillectomy of a benign villous adenoma. Note the plane of dissection to the level of the muscularis propria.

REFERENCES

Allen M J, Broody T J, Thistle J L, May G R, La Russo N F 1985 Cholelithiasis using methyl-tert-butyl-ether. Gastroenterology 88: 122–125

Bergman J J, Rauws E A, Tijssen J G, Tytgat G N, Huibregtse K 1995 Biliary endoprostheses in elderly patients with endoscopically irretrievable common bile duct stones: report on 117 patients. Gastrointestinal Endoscopy 42: 195–201

Bergman J J, Rauws E A, Fockens P, van Berkel A M, Bossuyt P M, Tijssen J G, Tytgat G N, Huibregtse K 1997 Randomised trial of endoscopic balloon dilation versus endoscopic sphincterotomy for removal of bileduct stones. Lancet 349: 1124–1129

Bertoni G, Sassatelli R, Nigrisoli E, Bedogni G 1997 Endoscopic snare papillectomy in patients with familial adenomatous polyposis and ampullary adenoma. Endoscopy 29: 685–688

Bethge N, Wagner H J, Knyrim K, Zimmermann H B, Starck E, Pausch J, Vakil N 1992 Technical failure of biliary metal stent deployment in a series of 116 applications. Endoscopy 24: 395–400

Bhatta K M, Rosen K J, Flotte T J, Dretler S P, Nishioka N S 1990 Effects of shielded and unshielded laser and electrohydraulic lithotripsy on rabbit bladder. Journal of Urology 143: 857–860

Binmoeller K F, Katon R M 1990 Needle knife papillotomy for an impacted common bile duct stone during pregnancy. Gastrointestinal Endoscopy 36: 607–609

Binmoeller K F, Katon R M, Shneidman R 1991 Endoscopic management of postoperative biliary leaks: Review of 77 cases and report of two cases with biloma formation. American Journal of Gastroenterology 86: 227–231

Binmoeller K F, Boaventura S, Ramsperger K, Soehendra N 1993a Endoscopic snare excision of benign adenomas of the papilla of Vater. Gastrointestinal Endoscopy 39: 127–131

Binmoeller K F, Bruckner M, Thonke F, Soehendra N 1993b Treatment of difficult bile duct stones using mechanical, electrohydraulic and extracorporeal shock wave lithotripsy. Endoscopy 25: 201–206

Binmoeller K F, Seifert, H, Gerke, H, Seitz U, Portis M, Soehendra N 1996 Papillary roof incision using the Erlangen-type pre-cut papillotome to achieve selective bile duct cannulation. Gastrointestinal Endoscopy 44: 689–695

Bland K I, Jones R S, Maher J W, Cotton P B, Pennell T C, Amerson J R, Munson J L, Berci G, Fuchs G J, Way L W et al 1989 Extracorporeal shock-wave lithotripsy of bile duct calculi. An interim report of the Dornier U.S. Bile Duct Lithotripsy Prospective Study. Annals of Surgery 209: 743–753

Burhenne H J 1980 Percutaneous extraction of retained biliary tract stones: 661 patients. American Journal of Roentgenology 149: 888–898

Chang W H, Kortan P, Haber G B 1998 Outcome in patients with bifurcation tumors who undergo unilateral versus bilateral hepatic duct drainage. Gastrointestinal Endoscopy 47: 354–362

Classen M 1987 Endoscopic papillotomy. In: Sivak M (ed) Gastroenterologic endoscopy. W B Saunders, Philadelphia: 631–651

Classen M, Demling L 1974 Endoskopische Sphincterotomie der Papilla Vateri und Steinextraktion aus dem ductus Choledochus. Deutsche Medizinische Wochenzeitschrift 99: 469–476

Classen M, Hagenmüller F, Knyrim K, Frimberger E 1988 Giant bile duct stones – non-surgical treatment. Endoscopy 20: 21–26

Clouse M E, Stokes K R, Lee R G L, Falchuk K R 1986 Bile duct stones: percutaneous transhepatic removal. Radiology 160: 525–529

Cotton P B 1989 Precut papillotomy—a risky technique for experts only (Editorial). Gastrointestinal Endoscopy 35: 578–579

Cotton P B, Vallon A G 1981 British experience with duodenoscopic sphincterotomy for removal of bile duct stones. British Journal of Surgery 68: 373–375

Cotton P B, Forbes A, Leung J W C, Dineen L 1987 Endoscopic stenting for long-term treatment of large bile duct stones: 2- to 5-year follow-up. Gastrointestinal Endoscopy 33: 411–412

Cotton P B, Kozarek R A, Schapiro R H, Nishioka N S, Kelsey P B, Ball T J, Putnam W S, Barkun A, Weinerth J 1990 Endoscopic laser lithotripsy of large bile duct stones. Gastroenterology 99: 1128–1133

Cremer M, Deviere J, Sugai B, Baize M 1990 Expandable biliary metal stents for malignancies: endoscopic insertion and diathermic cleaning for tumor ingrowth. Gastrointestinal Endoscopy 36: 451–457

Davids P H P, Rauws E A J, Coene P P L O, Tytgat G N J, Huibregtse K 1992a Endoscopic stenting for postoperative biliary strictures. Gastrointestinal Endoscopy 38: 12–18

Davids P H P, Rauws E A J, Tytgat G N J, Huibregtse K 1992b Postoperative bile leakage: endoscopic management. Gut 33: 1118–1122

Deviere J, Baize M, de Toeuf J, Cremer M 1988 Long-term follow-up of patients with hilar malignant stricture treated by endoscopic internal biliary drainage. Gastrointestinal Endoscopy 34: 95–101

Dipadova C, Dipadova F, Montorsi W, Tritapepe R 1986 Methyl tert butyl ether fails to dissolve retained radiolucent common bile duct stones. Gastroenterology 91: 1296–1300

Dowsett J F, Russell R C G, Hatfield A R W, Cotton P B, Williams S J, Speer A G, Houghton J, Lennon T, Macrae K 1989a Malignant obstructive jaundice: Prospective randomized trial of by-pass surgery versus endoscopic stenting. Gastroenterology 96: A128

Dowsett J F, Vaira D, Hatfield A R W, Cairns S R, Polydorou A, Frost R, Croker J, Cotton P B, Russell R C G, Mason R R 1989b Endoscopic biliary therapy using the combined percutaneous and endoscopic technique. Gastroenterology 96: 1180–1186

Dowsett J F, Polydorou A A, Vaira D, D'Anna L M, Ashraf M, Croker J, Salmon P R, Russell R C G, Hatfield A R W 1990 Needle knife papillotomy: how safe and how effective? Gut 31: 905–908

Ell C, Hochberger J, Müller D, Lux G, Demling L 1988 Laser lithotripsy for common bile duct stones. Gut 29: 746–751

Elta G H, Barnett J L, Wille R T, Brown K A, Chey W D, Scheiman J M 1998 Pure cut electrocautery current for sphincterotomy causes less post-procedure pancreatitis than blended current. Gastrointestinal Endoscopy 47: 149–153

Farrell R J, Khan M I, Noonan N, O'Byrne K, Keeling P W 1996 Endoscopic papillectomy: a novel approach to difficult cannulation. Gut 39: 36–38

Foutch P G, Sivak M V 1985 Therapeutic endoscopic balloon dilatation of the extrahepatic biliary ducts. American Journal of Gastroenterology 80: 575–579

Foutch P G, Harlan J, Sanowski R A 1989 Endoscopic placement of biliary stents for treatment of high risk geriatric patients with common duct stones. American Journal of Gastroenterology 84: 527–529

Freeman M L, Nelson D B, Sherman S, Haber G B, Herman M E, Dorsher P J, Moore J P, Fennerty M B, Ryan M E, Shaw M J, Lande J D, Pheley A M 1996 Complications of endoscopic biliary sphincterotomy. New England Journal of Medicine 335: 909–918

Geenen J E, Vennes J A, Silvis S E 1981 Resumé of a seminar on endoscopic retrograde sphincterotomy (ERS). Gastrointestinal Endoscopy 27: 31–38

Geenen J E, Hogan W J, Dodds W J, Toouli J, Venu R P 1989 The efficacy of endoscopic sphincterotomy after cholecystectomy in patients with sphincter-of-Oddi dysfunction. New England Journal of Medicine 320: 82–87

Hall R I, Denyer M E, Chapman A H 1990 Percutaneous-endoscopic placement of endoprostheses for relief of jaundice caused by inoperable bile duct strictures. Surgery 107: 224–247

Harrison J, Morris D L, Haynes J et al 1987 Electrohydraulic lithotripsy of gall stones in vitro and animal studies. Gut 28: 267–271

Huibregtse K, Katon R M, Tytgat G N J 1986a Precut papillotomy via fine-needle knife papillotome: a safe and effective technique. Gastrointestinal Endoscopy 32: 403–405

Huibregtse K, Katon, R M, Coene P P L, Tytgat G N J 1986b Endoscopic palliative treatment in pancreatic cancer. Gastrointestinal Endoscopy 32: 334–338

Huibregtse K, Cheng J, Coene P P L O, Fockens P, Tytgat G N J 1989 Endoscopic placement of expandable metal stents for biliary strictures—a preliminary report on experience with 33 patients. Endoscopy 21: 280–282

Johnson G K, Geenen J E, Venu R P, Schmalz M J, Hogan W J 1991 Endoscopic treatment of biliary tract strictures in sclerosing cholangitis: A larger series and recommendations for treatment. Gastrointestinal Endoscopy 37: 38–43

Johnson G K, Geenen J E, Venu R P, Schmalz M J, Hogan W J 1993 Treatment of non-extractable common bile duct stones with combination ursodeoxycholic acid plus endoprostheses. Gastrointestinal Endoscopy 39: 528–531

Kawai K, Akasaka Y, Murakami I, Tada M, Kohli Y, Nakajima M 1974 Endoscopic sphincterotomy of the ampulla of Vater. Gastrointestinal Endoscopy 20: 148–151

Kerlan R K, Ring E J, Pogancy A C, Jeffrey R B 1984 Biliary endoprosthesis-insertion using a combined peroral transhepatic method. Radiology 150: 828–830

Kozarek R A, Sanowski R A 1983 Endoscopic choledochoduodenostomy. Gastrointestinal Endoscopy 29: 119–121

Kozarek R A, Low D E, Ball T J 1988 Tunable dye laser lithotripsy: in vitro studies and in vivo treatment of choledocholithiasis. Gastrointestinal Endoscopy 5: 418–421

Leung J W C, Chung 1989 Electrohydraulic lithotripsy with peroral choledochoscopy. British Medical Journal 299: 595–598

Leung J W C, Banez V P, Chung S C S 1990 Precut (needle knife) papillotomy for impacted common bile duct stone at the ampulla. American Journal of Gastroenterology 85: 991–993

Liguory C L, Bonnel D, Canard J M, Cornud F, Dumont J L 1987 Intracorporeal electrohydraulic shock wave lithotripsy of common bile duct stones: preliminary results in 7 cases. Endoscopy 237–240

Loperfido S, Angelini G, Benedetti G, Chilovi F, Costan F, De Berardinis F, De Bernardin M, Ederle A, Fina P, Fratton A 1998 Major early complications from diagnostic and therapeutic ERCP: a prospective multicenter study. Gastrointestinal Endoscopy 48: 1–10

MacMathuna P, White P, Clarke E, Lennon J, Crowe J 1994 Endoscopic sphincteroplasty: a novel and safe alternative to papillotomy in the management of bile duct stones. Gut 35: 127–129

Neuhaus H, Hagenmüller F, Griebel M, Classen M 1991 Percutaneous cholangioscopic or transpapillary insertion in self-expanding biliary stents. Gastrointestinal Endoscopy 37: 31–37

Neuhaus H, Zillinger C, Born P, Ott R, Allescher H, Rosch T, Classen M 1998 Randomized study of intracorporeal laser lithotripsy versus extracorporeal shock-wave lithotripsy for difficult bile duct stones. Gastrointestinal Endoscopy 47: 327–334

Ortner M A, Liebetruth J, Schreiber S, Hanft M, Wruck U, Fusco V, Muller J M, Hortnagl H, Lochs H 1998 Photodynamic therapy of nonresectable cholangiocarcinoma. Gastroenterology 114: 536–542

Osnes M 1979 Endoscopic choledochoduodenostomy for common bile duct obstructions. Lancet 1: 1059–1060

Osnes M, Rosseland A R, Aabakken L 1986 Endoscopic retrograde cholangiography and endoscopic papillotomy in patients with a previous Billroth-II resection. Gut 27: 1193–1198

Palmer K R, Hoffmann A F 1986 Intraductal monooctanoin for the direct dissolution of bile duct stones: experience in 343 patients. Gut 27: 196–202

Polydorou A A, Chrisholm E M, Romanos A A, Dowsett J F, Cotton P B, Hatfield A R W, Russell R C G 1989 A comparison of right versus left hepatic duct endoprosthesis insertion in malignant hilar biliary obstruction. Endoscopy 21: 266–271

Ponchon T, Martin X, Barkun A, Mestas J L, Chavaillon A, Boustiere C 1990 Extracorporeal lithotripsy of bile duct stones using ultrasonography for localization. Gastroenterology 98: 726–732

Ponchon T, Gagnon P, Valette P J, Henry L, Chavaillon A, Thieulin F 1991 Pulsed dye laser lithotripsy of bile duct stones. Gastroenterology 100: 1730–1736

Ricci E, Bertoni G, Conigliaro R et al 1991 Endoscopic sphincterotomy in Billroth II patients: an improved method using a diathermic needle as a sphincterotome and a nasobiliary drain as a guide. Gastrointestinal Endoscopy 35: 47–50

Schapira L, Khawaja F I 1982 Endoscopic fistulosphincterotomy: an alternative method of sphincterotomy using a new sphincterotome. Endoscopy 14: 58–60

Schneider M U, Matek W, Bauer R, Domschke W 1988 Mechanical lithotripsy of bile duct stones in 209 patients—effect of technical advances. Endoscopy 20: 248–253

Shapira L, Khawaja F I 1982 Endoscopic fistulosphincterotomy: an alternative method of sphincterotomy using a new sphincterotome. Endoscopy 14: 58–60

Siegel J H, Ben-Zvi J S, Pullano W 1989 The needle knife: a valuable tool in diagnostic and therapeutic ERCP. Gastrointestinal Endoscopy 35: 499–503

Siegel J, Ben-Zvi J S, Pullano W 1990a Mechanical lithotripsy of common duct stones. Gastrointestinal Endoscopy 36: 351–356

Siegel J H, Ben-Zvi J S, Pullano W E 1990b Endoscopic electrohydraulic lithotripsy. Gastrointestinal Endoscopy 36: 134–136

Sievert C E, Silvis S E 1985 Evaluation of electrohydraulic lithotripsy on human gallstones. American Journal of Gastroenterology 80: 854

Smits M E, Rauws E A, van Gulik T M, Gouma D J, Tytgat G N, Huibregtse K 1996 Long-term results of endoscopic stenting and surgical drainage for biliary stricture due to chronic pancreatitis. British Journal of Surgery 83: 764–768

Soehendra N, Kempeneers I, Reynders-Frederix V 1980 Ein neues Papillotom für den Billroth-II Magen. Deutsche Medizinische Wochenzeitschrift 105: 362–363

Soehendra N, Maydeo A, Eckmann B, Bruckner M, Nam V C, Grimm H 1990 A new technique for replacing an obstructed biliary endoprosthesis. Endoscopy 22: 271–272

Soomers A J, Nagengast F M, Yap S H 1990 Endoscopic placement of biliary endoprostheses in patients with endoscopically unextractable common bile duct stones. Endoscopy 22: 24–26

Staritz M, Rambow A, Grosse A, Hurst A, Floth A, Mildenberger P, Goebel M, Junginger T, Hohenfellner R, Thelen M, et al 1990 Electromagnetically generated extracorporeal shockwaves for fragmentation of extra- and intrahepatic bile duct stones: indications, success and problems during a 15-month clinical experience. Gut 31: 222–225

Thomas S, Pensel J, Engelhardt R, Mezer W, Hofstetter A G 1988 The pulsed dye laser versus the Q switched Nd:YAG laser in laser-induced shock wave lithotripsy. Lasers in Surgery and Medicine 8: 363

Tweedle D E F, Martin D F 1991 Needle knife papillotomy for endoscopic sphincterotomy and cholangiography. Gastrointestinal Endoscopy 37: 518–521

Vaira D, Dowsett J F, Hatfield A R W, Cairns S R, Polydorou A A, Cotton P B, Salmon P R, Russell R C 1989 Duodenal diverticulum a risk factor for sphincterotomy? Gut 30: 578–579

van Someren R N, Benson M J, Glynn M J, Ashraf W, Swain C P 1996 A novel technique for dilating difficult malignant biliary strictures during therapeutic ERCP. Gastrointestinal Endoscopy 43: 495–498

Wang Y G, Binmoeller K F, Seifert H, Maydeo A, Soehendra N 1996 A new guide wire papillotome for patients with Billroth II gastrectomy. Endoscopy 28: 254–255

Wehrmann T, Seifert H, Seipp M, Lembcke B, Caspary W F 1998 Endoscopic injection of botulinum toxin for biliary sphincter of Oddi dysfunction 30: 702–707

29

Interventional radiologic techniques in the liver and biliary tract

K.T. BROWN, G.I. GETRAJDMAN

INTRODUCTION

As minimally invasive imaging guided techniques have become more sophisticated, and can be performed safely with smaller devices, the use of these techniques in the liver and biliary tract has become complementary to surgical methods. Procedures which can be performed safely include the simplest fine needle aspiration biopsy, to the most complicated biliary drainage procedures, or intervention for transjugular intrahepatic portosystemic shunt placement. With a basic understanding of both the anatomy and the physiology of the liver, the interventional radiologist is positioned to make valuable contributions to the hepatobiliary team. Many percutaneous methods of tumor ablation are currently being investigated. Because of the varied approach to hepatic tumor ablation, a full discussion of these techniques is beyond the scope of this chapter, and are covered separately in Chs 77, 78, 79 and 80.

LIVER BIOPSY (see also Ch. 19)

NON-TARGETED BIOPSY

Needle biopsy of the liver may be performed either to evaluate a diffuse hepatic abnormality, or to diagnose a specific lesion within the liver. Liver biopsy for diffuse disease has long been performed without imaging guidance, but rather with anatomic landmarks. On rare occasions anatomic landmarks may be unreliable, as in the case of patients who have undergone previous liver resection, or patients with very small high lying livers. Similarly, the presence of ascites may make an approach at the bedside difficult. In these situations imaging guidance may necessary to localize the liver. Following localization with either computed tomography

(CT) or ultrasound, an 18 to 15 g cutting needle is used in order to provide an adequate sample for analysis. Automated biopsy devices may be particularly useful in order to obtain samples free of crush artifact. Complications are primarily related to bleeding, and this procedure should be performed only when patients have normal or correctable coagulation studies.

TRANSJUGULAR BIOPSY

Patients with severe thrombocytopenia or coagulopathy being evaluated for diffuse liver disease are best biopsied with the transjugular technique. In the past the presence of ascites had also been considered a contraindication to percutaneous biopsy. In 1996, however, a study by Little et al (1996a) demonstrated no statistically significant difference in major or minor complications in patients with or without ascites undergoing percutaneous liver biopsy. In the absence of other risk factors (coagulopathy, uncooperative patient) these patients may undergo percutaneous biopsy. When transjugular biopsy is indicated it is best performed via puncture of either the internal or external jugular vein on the right side. For increased safety, ultrasound may be used to guide puncture of the internal jugular vein. Successful biopsy should be anticipated to result in diagnostic specimens in virtually all patients with use of semiautomated core cutting devices (Little et al 1996b).

IMAGING-GUIDED BIOPSY

Targeted needle biopsy is useful for the diagnosis of primary and secondary hepatic neoplasms. Ultrasound, CT, or even magnetic resonance imaging (MRI) may be used for guidance. Ultrasound is the fastest and least expensive, but requires more operator expertise. With regard to needles, studies have demonstrated that while per unit blood loss does not differ when comparing the amount of tissue recovered using 20 to 14 g needles, more tissue is obtained in fewer passes with larger needles (Plecha et al 1997). In reality, there is often little need for obtaining large volumes of tissue during targeted liver biopsy, particularly when diagnosing secondary neoplasms. This is in large part dependent on the available cytopathologic expertise, which varies from institution to institution. What the pathologist requires in order to arrive at a confident diagnosis must be taken into account when planning a biopsy. With proper specimen handling and preparation, fine needle aspiration (FNA) specimens may be used to diagnose a variety of hepatic lesions (Dodd et al 1997), although in some cases special stains may be necessary. The less blood present in the FNA samples the better, and it is sometimes useful to pre-rinse the aspiration syringe with heparin prior to obtaining a specimen. When entertaining the diagnosis of primary hepatocellular carcinoma (HCC) biopsy is not indicated when patients have a known risk factor (e.g. hepatitis B or C), obvious cirrhosis, and an elevated alpha-fetoprotein (> 500 ng/mL). When that is not the case, recognizing that the diagnosis of either a very well-differentiated or a very poorly differentiated HCC can be difficult on cytology alone, 18 g cutting needles are used for biopsy. Similar needles are used for performing biopsy when metastatic neuroendocrine tumor is suspected, to allow adequate material for special stains, and in cases where previous FNA has yielded an adequately cellular specimen, but where the diagnosis remains obscure. As with non-targeted percutaneous liver biopsy, complications are primarily related to bleeding, although in the case of lesions high in the liver near the dome of the liver pneumothorax may occur as well. Although deaths secondary to hemorrhage have been reported even following biopsy with 22 g needles (Drinkovic & Brkljacic 1996), with correction of coagulopathy, proper post-procedure observation, and the use of embolotherapy to treat post-procedure bleeding, major complications should occur very rarely if at all (see also Ch. 19).

TREATMENT OF HEPATIC CYSTS

Simple hepatic cysts (Ch. 67) are quite common, and typically occur as incidental findings on imaging studies obtained for other reasons. These cysts are lined with bile duct epithelium, but do not communicate with the biliary tree. On occasions they occur in the setting of polycystic disease (Ch. 66), with cysts present in the kidneys and pancreas as well. In the absence of symptoms these cysts require

no treatment. Symptoms usually consist of abdominal discomfort, or early satiety with or without weight loss. This may occur acutely when a patient bleeds into a pre-existing cyst. Infrequently a patient may present with jaundice or leg swelling related to cyst compression of either the bile duct or the inferior vena cava. Traditional therapy has typically been surgical, and many surgeons are currently electing to treat symptomatic cysts laparoscopically (Ch. 83). Before any therapy is undertaken it is important that the cyst be thoroughly imaged to assure that it meets all the criteria of a simple cyst. Wall-thickening, the presence of septations, or lack of enhanced through transmission on ultrasound should raise the question of a cystic metastasis, hydatid disease, or a cystadenoma.

Some patients are poor operative candidates, or would prefer to avoid the need for general anesthesia. Interventional techniques have been used to treat simple cysts, beginning with needle aspiration and catheter drainage. Although temporary symptomatic relief could be easily achieved, recurrence has been common. Attempts have been made to sclerose these cysts with a variety of agents including alcohol, tetracycline and formalin (Van Sonnenberg et al 1994) either at the time of drainage, or after a period of catheter drainage. More recently Tikkakoski et al (1996) described single-session treatment with alcohol, and Cellier et al (1998) with minocycline hydrochloride. Using alcohol, cysts are first emptied using a 5-F drainage catheter, and the absolute ethanol instilled and allowed to dwell for 20 minutes. During this time the patients are turned into various positions to distribute the ethanol. In some cases the procedure is repeated once or twice during the initial session, after which all the ethanol is aspirated and the catheter removed. Cellier et al (1998) removed only 25% of the cyst volume with a 22 g needle, and then injected 100–500 mg of minocycline hydrochloride, waited 5–10 minutes, and then removed the needle. Both authors found that patients with multiple cysts did less well than patients with solitary cysts. In addition, complete cyst regression was uncommon, although clinical success was achieved in 56 to 62% of patients.

HEPATIC ABSCESS DRAINAGE (see also Ch. 61)

Prior to the advent of sophisticated imaging studies the diagnosis of liver abscess was difficult, and mortality was high because of missed diagnosis. Radionuclide scanning with sulfur-colloid as well as gallium improved diagnosis of liver abscess, but advances in therapy awaited the development of cross-sectional imaging studies. In 1985 Gerzof et al reported the percutaneous treatment of pyogenic liver abscess using imaging guidance and, following the acceptance of this technique, mortality from this disorder dropped significantly. Liver abscess may occur in association with stone disease, bile duct obstruction, or related to ascending infection from sources such as appendicitis, or diverticulitis. Cryptogenic abscesses may be seen in diabetic patients, however at the time of diagnosis and treatment of a liver abscess a search should be made for the cause. When associated with ascending infection spread is via the portal venous system and pylephlebitis may occur. In this situation septic pylephlebitis may occur. The liver abscess and associated portal vein thrombosis may mimic the findings in primary hepatocellular cancer (Fig. 29.1A–C) The correct diagnosis may be suspected when the patient gives a history of fever or chills, the white blood cell count is elevated, and the patient appears ill. In addition, unlike patients with hepatocellular cancer, patients with pyogenic liver abscess usually do not exhibit findings of cirrhosis and portal hypertension. In many cases these can be successfully treated with antibiotics alone with complete resolution of the abscess (Fig. 29.1B), and cavernous transformation of the portal vein (Fig. 29.1C)

Uncomplicated pyogenic liver abscesses may be single or multiple, and may be unilocular, but frequently appear septated (Fig. 29.2A–D). It is frequently not possible to evacuate them completely at the time of catheter placement (Fig. 29.2B). Despite this fact, as well as a multi-loculated appearance (Fig. 29.2C), there is typically free communication between the locules, and most will resolve completely when treated with a single catheter (Fig. 29.2D), as well as appropriate antibiotics. It is not unusual to demonstrate communication with either the biliary tree or portal venous system when these catheters are injected with contrast (Fig. 29.2C). The treatment of liver abscess with antibiotics alone was reported by Herbert et al (1982) in 10 patients *following* diagnostic aspiration. In one of the earliest papers describing the successful treatment of

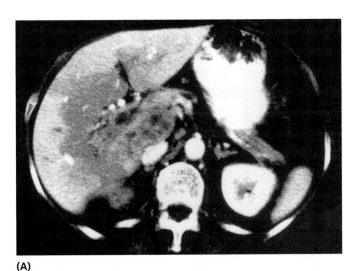

(A)

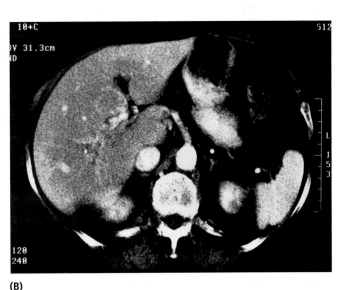

(B)

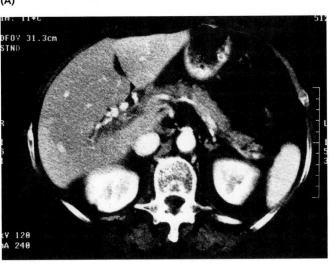

(C)

Fig. 29.1 Pylephlebitis. **(A)** CT scan demonstrating complex mass in the caudate lobe, and portal vein thrombosis. The unusual pattern of parenchymal liver enhancement with central low density is the characteristic pattern seen in patients with portal vein occlusion. **(B)** CT scan 1 month after treatment with antibiotics shows that the abscess in the caudate lobe has resolved. **(C)** Note the findings of cavernous transformation of the portal vein.

pyogenic liver abscess with catheter drainage, Gerzof et al (1985) suggested a dual role for aspiration alone: diagnostic, identifying the causative organism, and therapeutic in decompressing the abscess cavity. This decompression evacuates pus and accompanying endotoxins, relieving the

internal pressure and thereby ameliorating systemic toxicity and hematogenous dissemination. In addition, it is likely to allow for better entry of antibiotics into the wall of the abscess. This understanding has led some authors to advocate percutaneous needle aspiration (PNA) combined with antibiotic therapy, without placement of a drainage catheter. Giorgio et al (1995) described their experience with 115 patients treated with ultrasound-guided PNA and both intracavitary and systemic antibiotic therapy. Cure was achieved in 113 patients (98.3%), in 57 instances with only a single puncture. No recurrences were seen at 6–36 months follow-up. The use of PNA and antibiotics is simple and less expensive than catheter drainage. Giorgio et al (1995) believe it is also more acceptable to the patient.

(A)

(C)

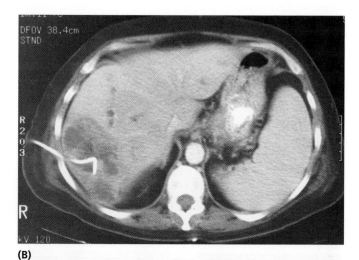

(B)

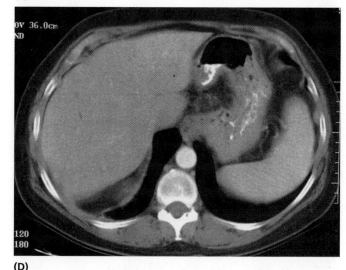

(D)

Fig. 29.2 Liver abscess. **(A)** CT scan demonstrating multiloculated abscess in right liver. **(B)** CT scan at the time of drainage catheter placement. **(C)** Contrast study via the drainage catheter demonstrates typical irregular loculated type appearance, as well as communication with biliary tree. **(D)** Follow-up CT scan 3 months after treatment of the hepatic abscess shows complete resolution.

Unfortunately, in the majority of cases more than one aspiration is necessary for complete treatment. Success rates of 70 to 98% of percutaneous therapies have been reported, with more recent studies (Miller et al 1997) all reporting success rates in the nineties. Given the mortality of 0 to 9% with percutaneous drainage, compared to a reported operative mortality of 12 to 26%, percutaneous therapy is now the treatment of choice (Miller et al 1997). Surgical intervention should be reserved for correctable causes, or for cases of failed percutaneous therapy. Whether indwelling catheter placement is necessary or not remains to be seen, although this is currently the most universally accepted method of therapy in the practice of most interventional radiologists.

AMEBIC ABSCESS (Ch. 62)

An appropriate travel history should raise the question of *Entamoeba histolytica*, which can be confirmed with serum hemagglutination studies. Amebic abscesses can virtually always be successfully treated with antibiotics alone (Ralls et al 1987) although aspiration may be useful to establish the diagnosis and exclude secondary concomitant bacterial infection. When aspiration is used for diagnosis the cavity should be aspirated as completely as possible. Assuming amebas are identified on microscopic examination, treatment with metronidazole alone is indicated.

ECHINOCOCCAL DISEASE (Ch. 63)

Echinococcal cysts have a characteristic multiloculated, or finely multiseptate appearance and rarely present with an acute illness. Serologic tests are often useful in establishing the diagnosis, in conjunction with the typical clinical and radiologic presentation. Although percutaneous aspiration had been considered contraindicated because of the risk of anaphylaxis, unintentional aspiration had been reported. Bret et al (1988) demonstrated the safety of aspiration and/or drainage of these cysts in 13 patients. None of the patients undergoing drainage were pre-medicated. If a catheter was placed for drainage, a scolicidal agent was injected into the cyst cavity following cystography. There were no complications or recurrences 6 months to 1 year after treatment. Khuroo et al (1991) treated 21 cysts in 12 patients under ultrasound guidance with percutaneous aspiration and instillation of hypertonic saline alone, re-aspirating the hypertonic saline after 20 minutes. All 21 cysts were successfully treated with only one mild atopic reaction.

TRAUMA

BILE DUCTS

Much of what we know about the role of the interventional radiologist in the management of traumatic injury to the bile ducts has been learned from patients who have experienced iatrogenic trauma, particularly following laparoscopic cholecystectomy (Boland et al 1996, Lund & Winick 1996, Lillemoe et al 1997). Similar principles would apply to the treatment of non-iatrogenic injuries. Patients with strictures who do not have a previous history of biliary surgery or significant right upper quadrant trauma should be investigated aggressively in an effort to establish that the stricture is indeed *not* malignant prior to treatment.

In general, small post-operative bile leaks typically heal spontaneously, assuming there is no outflow obstruction, and usually all that is required is drainage of any collection that may have formed (Ch. 50). Cystic duct leaks following cholecystectomy may respond best to endoscopic placement of a plastic biliary endoprosthesis. Major bile duct injuries consist of duct transection, laceration, and partial or complete ligation. These injuries are categorized according to the anatomic site of injury (Ch. 49). The length of duct available for surgical reconstruction, as well as the integrity of the hepatic duct confluence greatly influences treatment options. Most surgeons and radiologists agree that the best chance for a trouble free long-term outcome can be expected after primary surgical repair (Boland et al 1996, Lillemoe et al 1997). In a study by Lillimoe et al (1997) patients treated surgically demonstrated improved outcome compared to those treated with interventional techniques including drainage and balloon dilation. It is important to note, however, that all of the patients treated with interventional techniques had had previous surgical attempts at reconstruction. In the interventional group, patients who presented late and with low (Bismuth Type 1) (Ch. 48) injuries fared significantly better. Obviously these patients require a team approach. Those who are poor surgical candidates, have portal hypertension, or have had multiple previous attempts at surgical repair might be best treated with percutaneous drainage and balloon dilation (Ch. 49).

Mid to distal common bile duct strictures can be dilated with one balloon. Balloons should be sized slightly larger than the duct being dilated (usually 8–12 mm), and inflated to eliminate any 'waist'. When dilating strictures at the hilus (Fig. 29.3A–F), balloon dilation may require two or more catheters which may be used sequentially to dilate from side to side, and into the common hepatic duct, or across a bilioenteric anastamosis (Fig. 29.3B), or simultaneously.

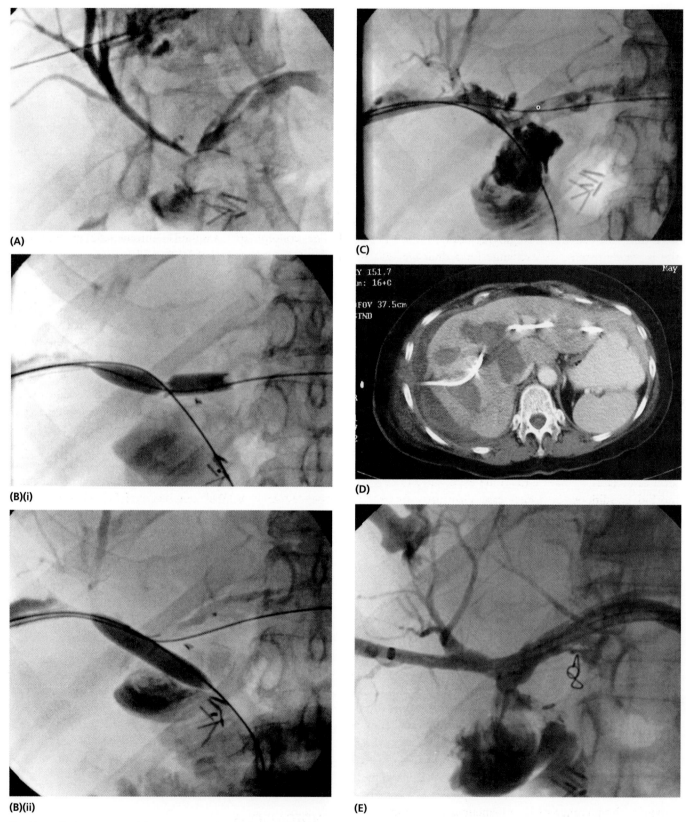

(A)

(B)(i)

(B)(ii)

(C)

(D)

(E)

Fig. 29.3 Bile duct stricture. **(A)** Note high-grade narrowing at the hepatobiliary anastomosis, involving the confluence of the right and left hepatic ducts. **(B)** Note 'waist' in balloon used to dilate from right hepatic duct to left hepatic duct (**Bi**), the waist has been eliminated on second balloon used to dilate across the bilioenteric anastomosis (**Bii**). **(C)** Note extravassation of contrast resulting from bile duct rupture following balloon dilatation. **(D)** CT scan from same patient demonstrating a significant intrahepatic hematomoa as well as a subcapsular hematoma. **(E)** Follow up cholangiogram 2 months later demonstrates the hepatic ductal confluence and hepatobiliary anastomosis to be widely patent.

When the simultaneous, or 'kissing balloon' technique is used, with one balloon placed from the right and one from the left, size should be adjusted appropriately. There is no evidence that prolonged inflation or multiple inflations enhance patency, and some believe this may promote ductal ischemia. Occasionally bile duct rupture occurs (Fig. 29.3C). We have seen a related arterial vascular injury (Fig. 29.3D) which required embolization. We have not found it necessary to treat the rupture with anything other than continued drainage, and have had good results (Fig. 29.3E) How long a catheter should be left in place following dilation is also controversial (Boland et al 1996). We leave a 10 or 12-F drainage catheter in place for 4 weeks, at which time we restudy the patient cholangiographically. If the stricture site is widely patent, we exchange for a drainage catheter above the treated area, and if the patient tolerates a clamping trial this catheter is removed within a week. If the follow-up cholangiogram demonstrates residual or recurrent narrowing, the site is re-dilated with a slightly larger balloon, followed by another 4-week observation period, a cholangiogram, and once again, a drainage catheter left above the dilated site and clamped. If the patient tolerates this 'capping trial', the catheter is removed. Patients who fail repeated dilations should be remanded either to continued catheter drainage or surgical treatment. We believe that self-expanding metallic stents should not be used to treat benign strictures unless the patients are extremely poor surgical candidates, or have limited life expectancy due to comorbid conditions, in which case Gianturco Rösch 'Z' stents (Cook, Bloomington, IN) should be used. This is because surgically treated patients have better outcomes, and once a metallic stent is placed it makes surgical repair more difficult.

VASCULAR INJURY (Chs 68, 69, 70)

Almost 15 years ago Sclafani demonstrated that angiographic methods could be used to control hemorrhage from injuries to the liver and spleen (Scalfani 1985). That this method is an effective alternative to surgery has been more recently shown by Hagiwara et al (1997). Fortunately, all but the most severe hepatic venous bleeding is self-limiting. Angiographic methods are suitable for treating hemorrhage secondary to blunt or penetrating trauma, including iatrogenic arterial injuries resulting from biliary interventions (Fig. 29.4A–C). Once the site of injury is established—either by the presence of pseudoaneurysm formation (Fig. 29.4B), extravasation (Fig. 29.5A), abrupt vessel cut-off, or spasm—the injured vessel(s) may be occluded with gelfoam and/or stainless steel coils (Figs 29.4 & 5). Should the use of small co-axial catheters be necessary, micro coils or polyvinyl alcohol (PVA) particles may be used. The dual blood supply to the liver, which allows the option of treating vascular tumors within the liver by embolizing the arterial blood supply, is also extremely tolerant of arterial occlusion for hemostasis, and this will not result in damage to the normal liver parenchyma.

TRANSJUGULAR INTRAHEPATIC PORTOSYSTEMIC SHUNTS (TIPS) (see also Ch. 101)

The concept of transjugular intrahepatic portosystemic shunts dates back to 1967, when Hannafee was performing diagnostic transjugular cholangiography, and on occasion punctured portal vein radicles (Hanafee & Weiner 1967). In 1969 Rosch et al explored the transjugular route as a means of visualizing the portal venous system as an alternative to many of the other more cumbersome methods available at that time, such as spleno-portography. Stimulated by Dotter's idea that the diagnostic catheter should be considered a therapeutic tool and a substitute for the surgeon's scalpel, the next step was the creation of an intrahepatic tract between the hepatic vein and portal vein that would serve as a portosystemic shunt. In 1969 Rosch et al created the first portosystemic shunt in dogs using co-axial catheters (Dotter technique) to dilate the intrahepatic tract (Rosch et al 1969, Rosch et al 1971). They discovered that without support the tract would close, and plastic tubing used to 'stent' the tract also thrombosed, or the tubing migrated. Balloon dilation (Burgener & Gutierrez 1979) and cryoprobes (Colapinto et al 1983) were then used, but intrahepatic tract patency remained problematic. In 1982 in the first human application, Colapinto used prolonged balloon inflation of up to 12 hours in an attempt to solve the tract patency problem (Colapinto et al 1982), but without success.

The technique remained dormant until the refinement of expandable metallic stents in the late 1980s. Richter et al (1989) published a landmark TIPS using Palmaz stents to maintain tract patency. The availability of WallStents (Schneider, Minneapolis, MN) has led to the rapid expansion of the procedure, which is now widely performed by interventional radiologists.

INDICATIONS

Creation of a TIPS is indicated for the treatment of recurrent variceal bleeding which is refractory to medical and/or endoscopic means. This is especially true for patients who

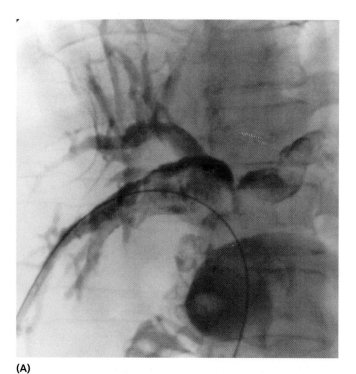

(A)

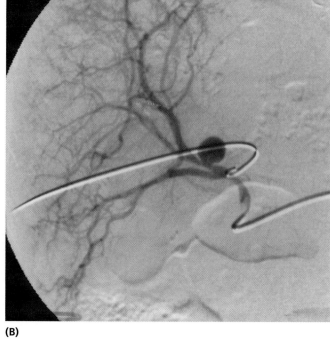

(B)

(C)

Fig. 29.4 Hemobilia. **(A)** Cholangiogram demonstrating an intraductal cast secondary to blood blot following biliary drainage of the right hepatic duct. **(B)** Pseudoaneurysm of the anterior sectoral division of the right hepatic artery. **(C)** Following stainless-steel coil embolization of the anterior sectoral branch of the right hepatic artery.

cases of Budd–Chiari syndrome (Seltzer et al 1993, Hastings et al 1996, Strunk et al 1997) (Ch. 105), particularly for patients with diffuse hepatic involvement.

CONTRAINDICATIONS

There are several contraindications to TIPS placement, both absolute and relative. Absolute contraindications include severe hepatic failure and severe right heart failure, which will both be exacerbated by shunt placement. In addition, in patients with markedly elevated right heart pressure, even reduction of the porto-systemic gradient to 12 mmHg or below may not be effective in decompressing varices because of the higher set point of the systemic pressures. Relative contraindications to TIPS include the presence of hepatocellular cancer or hepatic metastases, because of the increased risk of bleeding, or of polycystic changes within the liver. Chronic hepatic encephalopathy that has been controlled medically may worsen, although acute encephalopathy secondary to blood in the gastrointestinal tract may be improved. Thrombosis or cavernous transformation of the portal vein is a relative contraindication

are bleeding from gastric or peri-stomal varices, or patients with severe portal hypertensive gastropathy. It is an excellent technique to be used as a bridge to liver transplant, because when performed correctly it does *not* alter extrahepatic vascular anatomy. It is also indicated for the control of refractory ascites, as well as cirrhotic hydrothorax. The technique has also been applied to treatment of selected

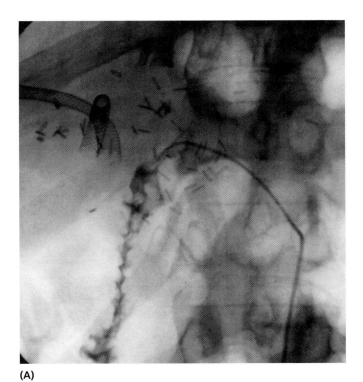

(A)

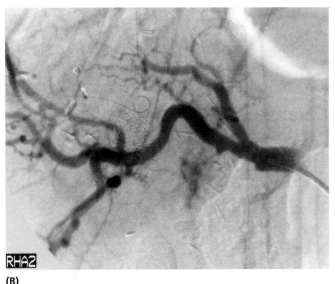

(B)

Fig. 29.5 Vascular trauma. **(A)** Patient with a history of bleeding duodenal ulcer initially treated with electrocautery, now with a re-bleed. Injection of contrast into a catheter in the right hepatic artery opacifies duodenum. **(B)** When catheter is pulled back and injected again, extravasation of contrast from the right hepatic artery is seen. **(C)** Unsubtracted angiogram following right hepatic artery occlusion with stainless-steel coils.

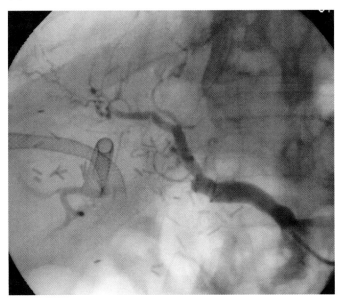

(C)

since it increases the difficulty of the procedure, and diminishes the chance of success. However, recanalization of the portal vein prior to performing a successful TIPS has been described (Rodosevich et al 1993).

TECHNIQUE

There are a variety of techniques and different systems available for performing a TIPS (Fig. 29.6A–D) After an upper endoscopy confirms esophageal varices, and excludes other sources of upper gastrointestinal bleeding, an ultrasound or CT scan is useful for demonstrating the anatomy, and confirming patency of the portal vein. Acutely bleeding patients should be stabilized. TIPS should not be attempted while the patient is undergoing aggressive resuscitative measures. After the administration of broad spectrum antibiotics, the procedure is performed under conscious sedation with anxiolytics and narcotics. Right internal jugular access is established, and a vascular sheath is placed. A selective catheter is advanced into one of the hepatic veins (Fig. 29.6A) and a wedged hepatic venogram performed with either contrast or CO_2. A steerable needle is then placed in the right hepatic vein, directed anteriorly, and used to puncture the right portal vein 2–3 cm from the main portal vein bifurcation, in an effort to remain intrahepatic. A guidewire is then advanced into the superior mesenteric vein or splenic vein, and used to place a catheter for pressure measurements and venography (Fig. 29.6B). The tract is pre-dilated with a balloon (Fig. 29.6C), and then an appropriately sized 10 or 12 mm WallStent is deployed and balloon dilated. Pressures are obtained, with the goal being a portal to IVC gradient of < 12 mmHg. If the gradient is higher then the stent may be dilated with a 12 mm balloon, if this does not result in a satisfactory pressure gradient, and collaterals fill persistently, then parallel stents should be considered. If the result is satisfactory (Fig. 29.6D) the procedure is concluded, and baseline ultrasound studies are performed the next day.

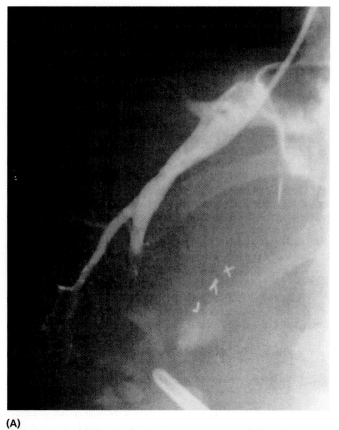

(A)

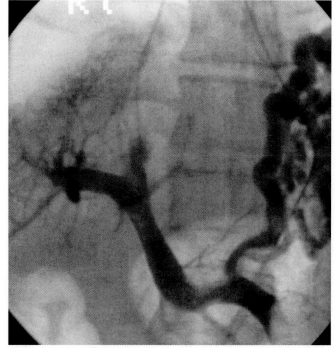

(B)

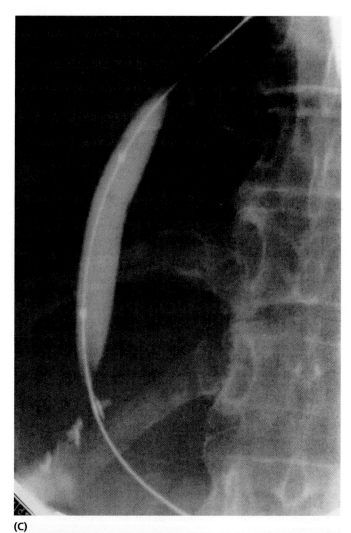

(C)

Fig. 29.6 TIPS. **(A)** Right hepatic venogram performed via a transjugular catheter. **(B)** Portogram demonstrates enlarged coronary vein with opacification of gastroesophageal varices. **(C)** Balloon dilatation of the transhepatic tract between right hepatic and right portal veins. **(D)** Post-TIPS placement. The dilated coronary vein and varices are no longer opacified.

(D)

RESULTS

In a review of 1750 patients at 9 institutions in the US and abroad (Barton et al 1995) the technical success rate was 97%. Failures were related to portal vein thrombosis, very hard livers, and massive ascites. The procedure controlled acute bleeding in 91% of patients. Re-bleeding increased in incidence with time with a 6% incidence at 3 months, 17% at 6 months, and 21% at one year. As is usually the case, Child class A patients fared better than Child class B, and Child class B better than Child class C. The procedure was successful in controlling ascites within 3 months in 65% of patients.

Complications include contrast induced ATN, allergic reactions to contrast, fever, hemobilia, and pulmonary edema. In addition, fatal outcomes were reported in 1.7% of patients caused by intraperitoneal, retroperitoneal and mediastinal hemorrhage, laceration of hepatic arteries, portal vein branches or the liver capsule, and right heart failure. The 30-day mortality was 11%, and was in general related to the patients' poor general underlying condition as manifested by hepatic failure, sepsis, ARDS, multi-organ failure and bleeding. The 5-year mortality was 32%, most commonly caused by progressive hepatic failure, again directly correlated with the patient's Child class.

The rate of encephalopathy was 20%, occurring most commonly in patients older than 60 with non-alcohol related liver disease, and with the use of larger stent sizes. Usually this side-effect is easily controlled medically, but in 5% of patients it was refractory to medical management. The incidence was somewhat higher in patients whose indication for TIPS was ascites.

Stenoses and occlusions occurred in 35 to 85% of stents. The wide range reflects differences in follow-up, with some centers using ultrasound and some venography. In addition, at some centers surveillance is carried out, in others patients were not studied unless and until they became symptomatic. The rate of stenosis is progressive during the first year, and increases more slowly thereafter, with 29% of stents affected at 6 months, 42% at 1 year, and 51% at 2 years. In asymptomatic patients surveillance demonstrates stenoses or occlusions in 39% of patients and in symptomatic patients in 92%. Only 25% of stent stenosis result in recurrent hemorrhage or ascites. With re-intervention, assisted patency of TIPS can be maintained in 95% of patients.

PORTAL VENOUS EMBOLIZATION

Branches of the portal vein may be embolized in order to induce ipsilateral atrophy and contralateral liver hyper-trophy in the preoperative management of some liver and biliary tumors (for details see Ch. 87).

BILE DUCTS AND GALLBLADDER

PERCUTANEOUS TRANSHEPATIC CHOLANGIOGRAPHY (PTC) (Ch. 17)

Direct percutaneous cholangiography today is utilized much less than in the past. Non-invasive methods of imaging the bile ducts, such as ultrasound and magnetic resonance cholangiopancreatography (MRCP) (Ch. 16) (Barish & Soto 1997) have almost eclipsed PTC in the diagnosis of biliary tract disease. It is our opinion that only in extremely unusual circumstances should transhepatic needle cholangiography be performed for diagnostic purposes alone, rather than in anticipation of a percutaneous intervention.

PERCUTANEOUS CHOLECYSTOSTOMY (Ch. 36)

Percutaneous cholecystostomy (PC) is indicated for patients with acute calculous cholecystitis who are too ill to undergo cholecystectomy, or as primary treatment for patients with acalculous cholecystitis. The diagnosis of acute acalculous cholecystitis can be difficult, however it usually occurs in elderly patients often being managed in intensive care units. The diagnosis should be suspected in this setting when there is no other explanation for fever and an elevated white blood cell in a patient with a distended tender gallbladder. Even patients with gas within the gallbladder wall can be treated with PC. The ease with which the procedure can be performed, and the low complication rate, allows PC to function as both a diagnostic test as well as a therapeutic method. A 56 to 80% clinical response to PC (Boland et al 1994) has been reported.

In the case of acalculous cholecystitis, initially thick, viscous, dark bile is aspirated from the distended gallbladder. As inflammation subsides and cystic duct patency is restored normal appearing bile begins to drain from the catheter. At that point a contrast study of the catheter can be performed to document patency of the common bile duct, and the PC catheter may be clamped. It is important not to remove the catheter until a tract to the skin has formed, in order to avoid intraperitoneal leakage of bile. Depending on the nutritional status of the patient and whether a transhepatic or transperitoneal approach was taken to the gallbladder, this typically occurs between the second and third week following the procedure (Hatjidakis et al 1998).

When gallstones are present the ultimate treatment will depend on the patient's underlying disease process, and age. In a patient with a long life expectancy PC may be a temporizing method performed during a period when the patient is critically ill, or recovering from a serious trauma. When the patient's condition improves, definitive treatment would consist of laparoscopic cholecystectomy. In a patient with limited life expectancy, either secondary to associated illness or advanced years, the stones may be removed from the gallbladder (or even the common bile duct) percutaneously prior to catheter removal, understanding that a diseased gallbladder will be left behind. Symptomatic calculous disease may be expected to recur in 20 to 50% of patients within 2–5 years (Gibney et al 1989).

Percutaneous cholecystostomy may also be performed as a means of relieving distal common bile duct obstruction in patients who are too ill to tolerate any other procedure, or in patients with minimal or no intrahepatic biliary ductal dilation. There is no question that PC is quicker, easier, and safer than percutaneous transhepatic drainage (PTD), and can even be performed at the bedside with ultrasound guidance. This makes it an ideal procedure for the septic patient with documented low bile duct obstruction. Patients without significant dilation of intrahepatic ducts can have a PC catheter placed which can be injected with contrast at a later time in order to opacify the intrahepatic ductal system, facilitating conventional transhepatic access to the biliary tree for common bile duct (CBD) stone removal, stent placement, brachytherapy, or stricture dilation.

RETAINED COMMON BILE DUCT CALCULI
(see also Ch. 41)

Retained common bile duct (CBD) stones may be successfully treated via a T-tube tract in the majority of patients, or even via a transhepatic approach (Fig. 29.7A–C). Stones are either extracted or crushed with baskets. A balloon dilatation of the sphincter (Fig. 29.7B) is performed to allow for passage of small fragments, typically with a 10 mm balloon. A survey of 39 institutions reported 5% morbidity and no mortality in 612 stone extraction procedures over 20 years ago (Burhenne 1976). Given the development of more sophisticated devices for minimally invasive procedures, including steerable catheters, cholangioscopes, and contact lithotripsy probes, the success rate for treatment of retained CBD stones is even greater, and these techniques and devices can be applied to the transhepatic removal of intrahepatic stones as well (Ch. 44).

The principal drawback to T-tube stone extraction is that 4–6 weeks is required for tract maturation. Endoscopic sphincterotomy and stone extraction (Ch. 40) may

be performed sooner, typically after 7–10 days with 90 to 95% success rate (O'Doherty et al 1986, Becker et al 1993). Complication rates vary between 4 to 19%, with a 0 to 2% mortality. In a review of the literature, Cotton (1990) suggested that the complication rates for endoscopic stone extraction when a T tube is in place may be lower than that reported after sphincterotomy in other patient groups. Despite this, he concluded that if an adequately sized and positioned T tube is present a percutaneous approach is probably safer, and should be performed unless the patient's condition dictates more immediate treatment.

PERCUTANEOUS TRANSHEPATIC BILIARY DRAINAGE (PTBD) (see also Chs. 7, 54, 58)

This procedure is indicated for relief of pruritis, cholangitis, or the lowering of serum bilirubin in order to permit the use of chemotherapeutic agents with biliary excretion routes. It may also be indicated as the initial step in the planned treatment of benign bile duct strictures or intrahepatic stones. *It is NOT indicated solely for the relief of jaundice or the treatment of dilated bile ducts.* Percutaneous transhepatic biliary drainage (PTBD) should be applied cautiously in truly asymptomatic patients, as it is a procedure associated with not insignificant complications, including bleeding, bile peritonitis, and sepsis. *In addition, patients with operable disease should be treated surgically.* A multidisciplinary consensus involving hepatobiliary surgeons, gastroenterologists, and interventional radiologists regarding the need for and proper technique of biliary drainage for a particular patient or clinical problem is important.

Pre-procedure evaluation

Pre-procedure evaluation should include a complete blood cell (CBC) with platelet count, prothrombin time (PT) partial thromboplastin time (PTT) and liver function tests. Although ultrasound is useful for confirming obstruction by demonstrating bile duct dilation, it is not as useful for planning PTBD, particularly if performed by an individual other than the one who will be performing the drainage procedure. The level of obstruction demonstrated on imaging studies should be used to triage patients to either percutaneous or endoscopic drainage. Patients found to have distal bile duct obstruction should be considered candidates for an endoscopic drainage procedure. We find ultrasound to be particularly useful for identifying the level and cause of obstruction (Gibson et al 1986), as well as evaluating portal vein patency (Hann et al 1997), but prefer CT scans for procedure planning. Findings such as

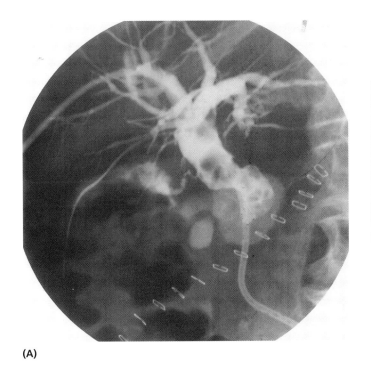

(A)

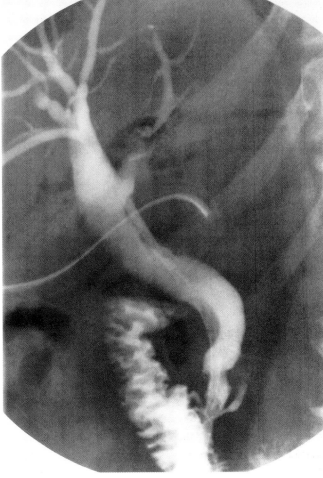

(C)

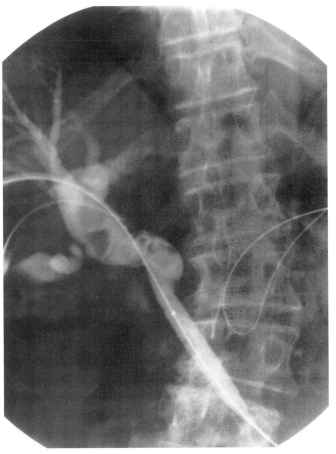

(B)

Fig. 29.7 Common bile duct calculi. **(A)** Note multiple angular filling defects in the common bile duct, representing stones. **(B)** Balloon inflated during dilatation of the sphincter at the ampulla of Vater. **(C)** Final study obtained after clearance of stones from common bile duct.

liver atrophy are readily identified on CT or ultrasound, but other anatomic considerations such as the presence of colonic interposition, location and extent of liver metastases or the sub-xyphoid extent of the left liver may be more easily appreciated on CT. Unlike ultrasound, CT renders a reproducible depiction of the liver in cross section, with easy identification of landmarks such as calcifications or surgical clips which may not be as evident on magnetic resonance imaging (MRI), but which may serve as useful flouroscopic landmarks. Translation of this information into a 3-dimensional mental image greatly facilitates the drainage procedure.

There is a high incidence of bacterbilia in patients undergoing drainage, particularly when there has been previous operation or instrumentation (Brody et al 1998), and

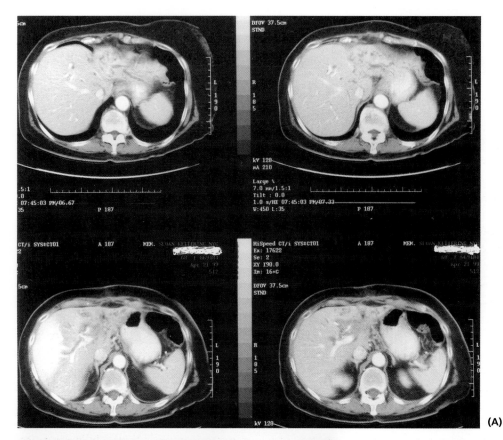

(A)

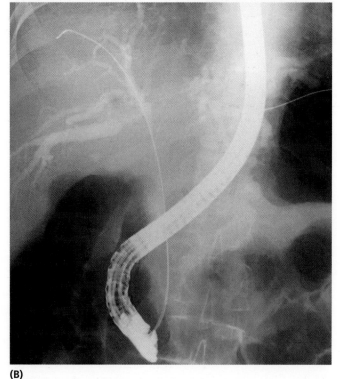

(B)

Fig. 29.8 Liver atrophy. **(A)** CT scan demonstrates small left liver, crowded bile ducts, and left portal vein occlusion, all classic imaging findings seen with lobar liver atrophy. **(B)** ERCP on the same patient shown in Fig. 29.9A demonstrating the typical cholangiographic findings of liver atrophy, with tortuous crowded bile ducts in the left liver. The right liver is not atrophic.

therefore prophylactic antibiotics are indicated. Ill patients may best be given broad spectrum agents that cover enterococci, streptococci, and both aerobic and anaerobic Gram-negative bacilli. Timentin® and Zosyn® provide excellent coverage in this regard. Patients with biliary sepsis may warrant the addition of an aminoglycoside for extended Gram-negative coverage. In addition, one may reduce the risk of nephrotoxicity, and take advantage of the post-antibiotic effect of aminoglycosides, by utilizing once-daily dosing (Lipsett 1996).

TECHNIQUE

The choice of a right- or left-sided transhepatic approach for PTBD should be made after careful evaluation of imaging findings. Particular attention should be paid to the presence of liver atrophy (Fig. 29.8A,B) and/or tumor involvement of the portal venous system. Drainage of an atrophic portion of the liver will do *nothing* to improve hepatic function or lower serum bilirubin. The only time it might be necessary to drain an atrophic section would be in the face of unrelenting biliary sepsis following drainage of the isolated functional liver parenchyma. In general, high biliary tract obstruction is more likely to result in isolation of the anterior and posterior sectoral ducts on the right side, and even extend to involve second order branches. Such isolation of ducts occurs later on the left. This is because the left hepatic duct is typically longer than the right. In addition, the right posterior sectoral duct joins the left hepatic duct rather than its anterior right counterpart in at least 20% of cases (Ch. 1). Thus, in high obstruction, in the absence of left portal vein compromise, a left approach may be preferred. Similarly, when ascites is present there is likely to be less of a problem with leaking ascites from an anterior left approach rather than a lateral right approach. Obviously, accessibility of the left liver relative to the xiphoid and stomach, and the location of metastatic deposits should be taken into consideration as well.

Once a decision has been made as to the best approach, an attempt should be made to puncture a peripheral bile duct. This will limit the risk of injuring a major vessel at or near the hilus and, importantly, provide for adequate side holes in the tube above the level of obstruction. This will ensure adequate drainage, as well as avoiding problems with hemobilia. It is also important to avoid puncturing the left ductal system from the right side, and vice versa, since this makes further catheter manipulations difficult. It is usually possible to place a multisidehole catheter across the obstructed area and into the doudenum at the time of initial drainage, allowing for drainage of bile into the bowel. In the presence of cholangitis, however, undue manipulation within the biliary tree is inadvisable, and we do not hesitate to leave an external drainage catheter and subsequently cross the obstruction later, after the patient has settled clinically. External catheters may also be necessary in the rare cases where the obstruction cannot be crossed at the time of initial drainage. In most patients, once the inflammatory component of the obstruction has resolved, and the bile ducts are not excessively dilated, conversion to an internal/external catheter, or placement of a biliary endoprosthesis is possible.

Patients with high bile duct obstruction frequently exhibit complete or near complete isolation of the right and left hepatic ducts. In some cases isolation extends to the sectoral or segmental level. This is more frequent on the right side as the right hepatic duct is short, and the anterior and posterior divisions become isolated. One drainage catheter only is placed at the initial encounter with the patient. It is necessary to have approximately 30% of the hepatic parenchyma drained and functional in order to alleviate jaundice. This is frequently accomplished with drainage of either the right or left liver. Pruritis is related to bile salt deposition within the skin, and usually responds immediately and dramatically to drainage of any part of the liver. If the serum bilirubin does not fall to an acceptable level, or if biliary sepsis is the dominant problem, it may be necessary to place more than one catheter. It may take up to

two weeks for the bilirubin level to plateau, particularly in long standing obstruction, so it is sometimes advisable to withhold final treatment decisions until the serum bilirubin has stabilized.

At the time of initial drainage of patients with malignant disease, thought should be given to the placement of an internal biliary endoprosthesis. Both plastic and metal endoprostheses are available, however data from many studies appear to support the cost effectiveness of metal stents (Lammer et al 1996). The metal stents most commonly used for malignant disease within the biliary tree are the Wallstent and the Strecker stent. These are non-removable, self-expanding, flexible, braided or woven stents, which can be placed through 7–10 French sheaths, but expand to diameters of 6–10 mm. This feature allows for placement at the time of initial biliary drainage in patients with mid to distal bile duct obstruction, where placement of additional drainage catheters is not going to be a consideration. It goes without saying that since these metallic stents are permanent they should not be used unless the patient has no possibility of curative resection. Hepatobiliary surgical resections are much more difficult once a metal stent has been placed.

Patients with high bile duct obstruction and isolated portions of the liver may require additional drainage procedures. It is best to wait until the patient shows a clinical response with decrease in serum bilirubin and resolution of sepsis before metal stent placement is considered. Although drainage catheters and endoprostheses *can* be placed through the interstices, or even sometimes alongside, an existing stent, it is much easier for the operator, and thus for the patient, if the stents are deployed simultaneously. In the case of isolation of the right and left hepatic ducts, this can be accomplished in one of two ways. From one transhepatic approach (Fig. 29.9A–C) a stent can be placed across to the contralateral side, while simultaneously deploying the second stent from the ipsilateral side into the distal common bile duct. Alternatively, when the patient has failed to respond to a single drainage, the contralateral side can be approached percutaneously (Fig. 29.10A–C), allowing for simultaneous placement of side-by-side stents across the obstruction at the ductal confluence and into the more distal common bile duct. We agree with Morgan & Adam (1996) that the latter approach is preferable in the event that it is necessary to re-intervene for subsequent stent occlusion. We do not agree with them on the issue of the need to always stent into the duodenum. For hilar lesions, although we are careful to 'overstent' (Lammer et al 1996) in an effort to avoid tumor overgrowth related occlusion, we only cross the ampulla if the stent will end within 2–3 cm and foster kinking and/or sphincter spasm. Unlike either of the authors mentioned above, we rarely pre- or post-dilate when placing WallStents, as the patients find balloon dilation to be quite painful, and satisfactory stent expansion is typically achieved within 24 hours (Figs. 29.9B and 29.10B) without the aid of balloons. There might be a role for balloon dilation if, following deployment, contrast material does not flow promptly across the stent, particularly at primary placement. Following stent deployment, the introducer system is removed, and a 4–5 French end hole catheter such as a Kumpe (Cook, Bloomington, IN) is left as a covering catheter. If dual access has been utilized, then two covering catheters are left. These catheters are used for follow-up cholangiography the next day (Fig. 29.9C and 29.10C), in order to ensure that there has not been asymmetric stent shortening or some other occurrence which would require placement of additional stents, or other intervention. In 95% of cases no other intervention is necessary.

BILE DUCT BIOPSY

Faced with inoperable, presumed malignant bile duct obstruction, a tissue diagnosis is often desirable prior to initiating brachytherapy, or sometimes simply in an effort to give meaningful prognostic information to the patient and

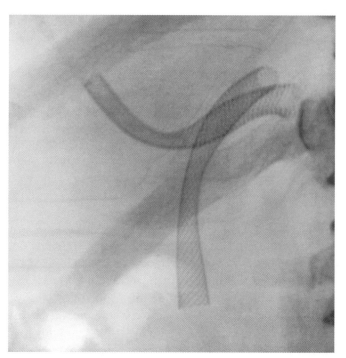

(B)

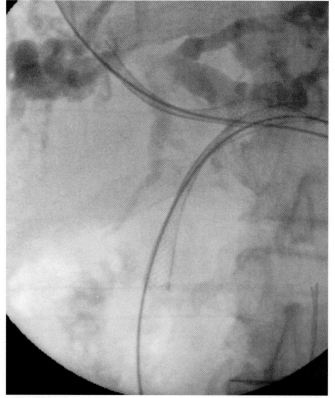

(A)

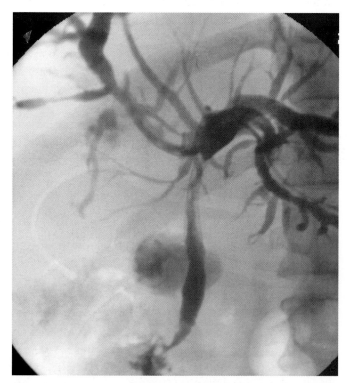

(C)

Fig. 29.9 Wallstents. **(A)** Patient with gallbladder cancer and hilar obstruction. Wallstents are simultaneously deployed from the left hepatic duct into the right hepatic duct, as well as from the left hepatic duct into the common bile duct. This was performed when cholangitis did not respond to drainage of the left side alone. **(B)** Wallstents 24 hours after placement nicely expanded without balloon dilatation.
(C) Cholangiogram demonstrating the stents to be well-positioned and widely patent.

family. A diagnosis can be arrived at in several ways. Bile cytology obtained at the time of initial drainage although not very sensitive has been found to be quite specific (Savader et al 1998), and there is virtually no disadvantage to sending a specimen. Alternatively, endoluminal biopsies can be obtained with brushes or forceps (Savader et al 1996). If these methods fail, we perform a cholangiographically guided percutaneous needle biopsy, which will frequently yield a diagnosis.

Brachytherapy

Brachytherapy involves the local delivery of radiation to a tumor, and can be used percutaneously to treat unresectable or recurrent cholangiocarcinoma (Ch. 54). We have also used this method to treat intraductal metastatic colorectal carcinoma. We first perform conventional biliary drainage, placing an internal/external catheter. After the bilirubin has normalized and any underlying infection subsided, a WallStent® (Schneider, Minneapolis, MN) is introduced to bridge the area of obstruction. A simulation catheter is positioned through the WallStent®, and photo spots obtained. After dosimetry is performed the radiation source is loaded within 24 hours, and remains in place for a predetermined time, dependent on dosimetry calculations. When therapy is complete, catheter and radiation source are removed at the bedside. This method is not only a means of local tumor therapy, but seems to prolong

WallStent® patency by decreasing the rate of tumor ingrowth (Eschelman et al 1996), at least when combined with external beam therapy.

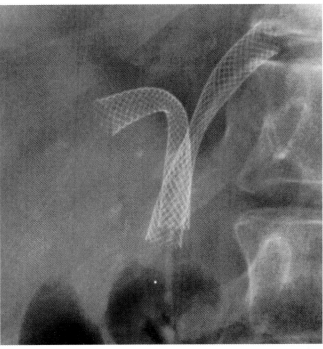

(B)

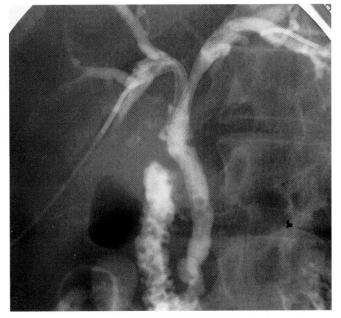

(C)

Fig. 29.10 Wallstents. **(A)** Patient with hilar obstruction secondary to cholangiocarcinoma. Bilirubin not low enough for chemotherapy after drainage of the right hepatic ducts underwent subsequent drainage of the left ducts and subsequent side-by-side Wallstent placement. **(B)** Without balloon dilatation after 24 hours the Wallstents are well expanded. **(C)** Cholangiography demonstrates the stents to be well-positioned and widely patent.

(A)

REFERENCES

Barish M A, Soto J A 1997 MR cholangiopancreatography: Techniques and clinical applications. Americal Journal of Roentgenology 169: 1295–1303

Barton R E, Rosch J, Saxon R et al 1995 TIPS: Short-and long-term results: A survey of 1750 patients. Seminars in Interventional Radiology 12(4): 364

Becker C D, Eigenmann T, Scheurer V, Halter F 1993 Comparison of percutaneous endoscopic retrograde removal of postoperatively retained bile duct stones. Cardiovascular Interventional Radiology 16: 144–149

Boland G W, Lee M J, Leung J, Mueller P R 1994 Percutaneous cholecystostomy in critically ill patients: early response and final outcome in 82 patients Americal Journal of Roentgenology 163: 339–342

Boland G W, Mueller P R, Lee M J 1996 Laparoscopic cholecystectomy with bile duct injury: Percutaneous management of biliary stricture and associated complications. Americal Journal of Roentgenology 166: 603–607

Bret P M, Fond A, Bretagnolle M et al 1988 Percutaneous aspiration and drainage of hydatid cysts in the liver. Radiology 168: 617–620

Brody L A, Brown K T, Getrajdman G I et al 1998 Clinical factors associated with positive bile cultures during primary percutaneous biliary drainage. Journal of Vascular and Interventional Radiology 9: 572–578

Burgener F A, Gutierrez O H 1979 Nonsurgical production of intrahepatic portosystemic venous shunts in portal hypertension with the double lumen balloon catheter. Rofo 130: 686–688

Burhenne H J 1976 Complications of non-operative extraction of retained common bile duct stones. American Journal of Surgery 131: 260–262

Cellier C, Cuenod C A, Deslandes P et al 1998 Symptomatic hepatic cysts: Treatment with single shot injection of minocycline hydrochloride. Radiology 206: 205–209

Colapinto R F, Stronell R D, Birch S J et al 1982 Creation of an intrahepatic portosystemic shunt with a Gruntzig balloon catheter. Canadian Medical Association Journal 126: 267–268

Colapinto R F, Stronell R D, Gildiner M et al 1983 Formation of intrahepatic portosystemic shunts using a balloon dilatation catheter: preliminary clinical experience. American Journal of Roentgenology 140: 709–714

Cotton P B 1990 Retained common bile duct stones: T-tube in place, percutaneous or endoscopic management? Gut 85: 1075–1088

Dodd L G, Mooney E E, Layfield L J, Nelson R C 1997 Fine-needle aspiration of the liver and pancreas: A cytology primer for radiologists. Radiology 203: 1–9

Drinkovic I, Brkljacic B 1996 Two cases of lethal complications following ultrasound-guided percutaneous fine-needle biopsy of the liver. Cardiovascular Interventional Radiology 19: 360–363

Eschelman D J, Shapiro M J, Bonn J et al 1996 Malignant biliary duct obstruction: Long-term experience with Gianturco stents and combined-modality radiation therapy. Radiology 200: 717–724

Gerzof S G, Johnson W C, Robbins A H, Nabseth D C 1985 Intrahepatic pyogenic abscesses: treatment by percutaneous drainage. American Journal of Surgery 149: 487–498

Gibney R G, Chow K, So C B et al 1989 Gallstone recurrence following cholecystolithotomy. Americal Journal of Roentgenology 153: 287–289

Gibson R N, Young E, Thompson J N et al 1986 Bile duct obstruction: Radiologic evaluation of level, cause, and tumor resectability. Radiology 160: 43–47

Giorgio A, Tarantino L, Marinielle N et al 1995 Pyogenic liver abscesses: 13 years of experience in percutaneous needle aspiration with US guidance. Radiology 195: 122–124

Hagiwara A, Yukioka T, Ohta S et al 1997 Nonsurgical management of patients with blunt hepatic injury: Efficacy of transcatheter arterial embolization. Americal Journal of Roentgenology 169: 1151–1156

Hanafee W, Weiner M 1967 Transjugular percutaneous cholangiography. Radiology 88: 35–39

Hann L E, Greatrex K V, Bach A M et al 1997 Cholangiocarcinoma at the hepatic hilus: Sonographic findings. Americal Journal of Roentgenology 168: 985–989

Hastings G S, O'Connor D K, Pais S O 1996 Transjugular intrahepatic portosystemic shunt placement as a bridge to liver transplantation in fulminant Budd–Chiari syndrome. Journal of Vascular and Interventional Radiology 7: 616

Hatjidakis A A, Karampekios S, Prassopoulos P et al 1998 Maturation of the tract after percutaneous cholecystostomy with regard to access route. Cardiovascular Interventional Radiology 21: 36–40

Herbert D A, Fogel D A, Rothman J et al 1982 Pyogenic liver abscesses: successful non-surgical therapy. Lancet 16: 134–136

Khuroo M S, Zargar S A, Mahajan R 1991 *Echinococcus granulosa* cysts in the liver: Management with percutaneous drainage. Radiology 180: 141–145

Lammer J, Winkelbauer F, Kontrus M, Thurner S 1996 Plastic versus metal biliary endoprostheses. Seminars of Interventional Radiology 13(3): 253–261

Lillemoe K D, Martin S A, Cameron J L et al 1997 Major bile duct injuries during laparoscopic cholecystectomy. Annals of Surgery 225(5): 459–471

Little A F, Ferris J V, Dodd III G D et al 1996a Image-guided percutaneous hepatic biopsy: Effect of ascites on the complication rate. Radiology 199: 79–83

Little A F, Zajko A B, Orons P D 1996b Transjugular liver biopsy: A prospective study in 43 patients with the Quick-Core biopsy needle. Journal of Vascular and Interventional Radiology 7: 127–131

Lipsett P A 1996 Preparation of the patient for biliary surgical or interventional procedures: Antibiotic prophylaxis. Seminars of Interventional Radiology 13(3): 201–206

Lund G B, Winick A B 1996 Complications from laparoscopic cholecystectomy and the role of interventional radiologic management. Seminars in Interventional Radiology 13(3): 263–275

Miller F J, Ahola D T, Brtezman P A, Fillmore D J 1997 Percutaneous management of hepatic abscess: A perspective by interventional radiologists. Journal of Vascular and Interventional Radiology 8: 241–247

Morgan R, Adam A 1996 Metallic stents in the treatment of patients with malignant biliary obstruction. Seminars in Interventional Radiology 13(3): 229–239

O'Doherty D P, Neoptolemos J P, Carr-Locke D L 1986 Endoscopic sphincterotomy for retained common bile duct stones in patients with T-tube in situ in the early post-operative period. British Journal of Surgery 73: 454–456

Plecha D M, Goodwin D W, Rowland D Y et al 1997 Liver biopsy: Effect of biopsy needle caliber on bleeding and tissue recovery. Radiology 204: 101–104

Ralls P W, Barnes P F, Johnson M B et al 1987 Medical treatment of hepatic amebic abscess: Rare need for percutaneous drainage. Radiology 165: 805–807

Richter G M, Palmaz J C, Nodge G et al 1989 The transjugular intrahepatic protosystemic stent-shunt (TIPSS): a new nonoperative, transjugular percutaneous procedure. Radiology 29: 406–411

Radosevich P M, Ring E J, LaBerge J M et al 1993 Transjugular intrahepatic portosystemic shunts in patients with portal vein occlusion. Radiology 4: 263–267

Rosch J, Hanafee W N, Snow H 1969 Transjugular portal venography and radiologic portacaval shunt: an experimental study. Radiology 92: 1112–1114

Rosch J, Hanafee W, Snow H et al 1971 Transjugular intrahepatic portocaval shunt. American Journal of Surgery 121: 588–592

Savader S J, Prescott C A, Lund G B, Osterman F A 1996 Intraductal biliary biopsy comparison of three techniques. Journal of Vascular and Interventional Radiology 7: 743–750

Savader S J, Lynch F C, Radvany M G et al 1998 Single specimen bile cytology: A prospective study of 80 patients with obstructive jaundice. Journal of Vascular and Interventional Radiology 9(5): 817–824

Sclafani S J R 1985 Angiographic control of intraperitoneal hemorrhage caused by injuries to the liver and spleen. Seminars in Interventional Radiology 2: 139–147

Seltzer M Y, Ring E J, LaBerge J M et al 1993 Treatment of Budd–Chiari syndrome with a transjugular intrahepatic portosystemic shunt. Journal of Vascular and Interventional Radiology 4: 263–267

Strunk H M, Textor J, Bronsing K A et al 1997 Acute Budd–Chiari syndrome: Treatment with transjugular intrahepatic portosystemic shunt. Cardiovascular Interventional Radiology 20: 311

Tikkakoski T, Makela J T, Leinonen S et al 1996 Treatment of symptomatic congenital hepatic cysts with single-session percutaneous drainage and ethanol sclerosis: Technique and outcome. Journal of Vascular and Interventional Radiology 7: 235–239

Van Sonnenberg E, Wroblicka J T, D'Agostino et al 1994 Symptomatic hepatic cysts: Percutaneous drainage and sclerosis. Radiology 190: 387–392

Biliary-enteric anastomosis

30

L.H. BLUMGART, W.R. JARNAGIN

HEPATICOJEJUNOSTOMY AND INTRAHEPATIC BILIARY-ENTERIC ANASTOMOSIS AND INTUBATION

Surgical relief of obstructive jaundice due to benign or malignant stricture of the hepatic ducts is best obtained by biliary-enteric anastomosis, usually to a Roux-en-Y loop of jejunum. It is often possible to form a hepaticojejunostomy between the common hepatic duct and the jejunum below or at the confluence of the major hepatic ducts. When this approach is rendered difficult because the right and left ducts converge within a deep hilus, or impossible because of tumor or dense adhesions involving a variable length of the hepatic ducts, adequate biliary drainage can only be obtained by intubation or biliary-enteric anastomosis to the right or left hepatic ducts or their intrahepatic branches.

The following description of techniques is based on an extensive experience, over three decades, of biliary reconstructions carried out at the hilus of the liver.

ANATOMY

The anatomical details of the extrahepatic biliary tree and adjacent hepatic arterial and portal venous structures are discussed in detail in Chapter 1 but some features are worthy of emphasis. The important ductal anomalies are nearly all related to the manner of confluence of the right and left hepatic ducts and of the cystic duct with the common hepatic duct and are so frequent that the surgeon must be acquainted with their range and should always expect the unusual.

The most common variation is an abnormal junction between the cystic duct and the main extrahepatic biliary channel. The cystic duct may join the common hepatic duct high and almost at the hilus of the liver. The right hepatic duct as such may be absent and the major ducts draining the anterior and posterior sectors of the right liver may join the left hepatic duct separately to form the common hepatic duct. In some cases the right anterior or right posterior sectoral duct may run a long extrahepatic course to join the common duct and the cystic duct may drain directly into such a duct. However, while these variations are common, there is almost always a consistent anatomy to the left hepatic duct and its branches.

The right hepatic duct has a short extrahepatic portion but the left hepatic duct *always* has an extrahepatic course (Fig. 30.1), the length of which at the base of the liver reflects the width of the quadrate lobe.

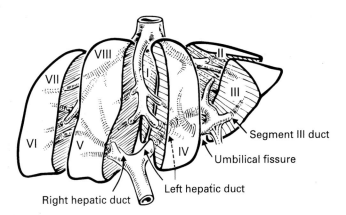

Fig. 30.1 Diagrammatic exploded view of the liver showing its segmental structure. Note that elements of the portal triad are distributed to the right and left liver on a segmental basis. The left hepatic duct always pursues an extrahepatic course beneath the base of the quadrate lobe (segment IV) in the groove separating the quadrate from the caudate lobe (segment I) (see Fig. 30.3). The ligamentum teres marks the umbilical fissure and runs to join the umbilical portion of the left branch of the portal vein. Each portal triad is composed of hepatic artery, left portal vein and biliary duct. Note particularly the distribution of the left portal triad in the umbilical fissure; major branches re-curve to the quadrate lobe medially and two major branches pursue a lateral course to segments II and III of the left lobe.

If the quadrate lobe has a broad, long base then the left hepatic duct has a longer rather transverse course whereas, if the quadrate lobe has a narrower more pyramidal base, the left hepatic duct has a shorter somewhat more oblique course. In the author's experience, these features may be predicted on the basis of cholangiographic appearance (Fig. 30.2).

The duct traverses to the left together with the left branch of the portal vein within a peritoneal reflection of the gastrohepatic ligament, fused with Glisson's capsule on the undersurface of the quadrate lobe (Fig. 30.3).

The left duct and left branch of the portal vein are joined by the left branch of the hepatic artery and enter the umbilical fissure of the liver within which division of vessels to and confluence of ducts from the left lobe (segments II and III) and the quadrate lobe (segment IV) occur. The left hepatic duct receives major tributaries from each of these segments, which converge in the umbilical fissure dorsocranial to the left portal vein. Hepatic ductal tributaries from the quadrate lobe (segment IV) and hepatic arterial and portal venous branches supplying it re-curve to segments IVA and IVB (Fig. 30.1).

The ligamentum teres in the lower edge of the falciform ligament traverses the umbilical fissure of the liver, which is usually, but not always, bridged in its lowermost part by a tongue of liver tissue joining the left lobe to the base of segment IV. The ligament joins the umbilical portion of the left portal vein as it curves anteriorly and caudally giving off branches to segments II and III of the left lobe and to segment IV (Fig. 30.1).

The techniques to be described rely on these anatomical features, anastomoses usually being carried out either at the hilus to the major right or left hepatic ducts or to the segment III duct of the left lobe.

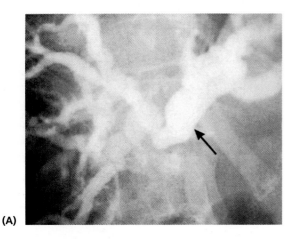

(A)

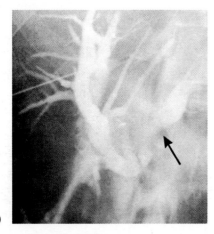

(B)

Fig. 30. 2 (A) Percutaneous transhepatic cholangiogram in a patient with a high benign bile duct stricture reveals a dilated intrahepatic ductal system with no evidence of the common hepatic bile duct. There is continuity at the confluence of the hepatic ducts. Note the transverse, rather horizontal course of the left hepatic duct (arrowed). It is predictable that this patient will have a rather broad-based quadrate lobe and that the left hepatic duct will be easily accessible. Repair was effected by means of an initial approach to the left hepatic duct after lowering of the hilar plate (see Figs 30.3 and 30.16) and subsequent hepaticojejunostomy. **(B)** Percutaneous transhepatic cholangiogram in a patient with benign postcholecystectomy bile duct stricture. Note the dilated intrahepatic ductal system. The stricture is at the confluence although there is continuity between the right and left ductal systems. There are two calculi in the right hepatic duct. The left hepatic duct (arrowed) pursues a vertical course and it is predictable that the quadrate lobe in this patient will have a narrow base and that dissection will be somewhat more difficult. Nevertheless, repair was effected after approaching the left duct and hilar area by initial dissection after lowering of the hilar plate and subsequent hepaticojejunostomy.

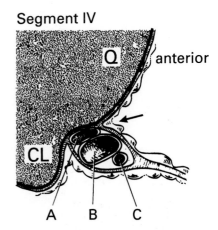

Fig. 30.3 Sagittal section showing in diagrammatic form the relationship of the quadrate (Q) and caudate (CL) lobe to the left portal triad, which is encased within a reflection of the lesser omentum which fuses with Glisson's capsule at the base of the quadrate lobe. The arrow indicates the point of incision for the dissection to lower the hilar plate (see also Fig. 30.18). A, left hepatic duct; B, left branch, portal vein. Note the left hepatic artery joins the left duct and left branch of the portal vein at the umbilical fissure.

TECHNIQUES

BASIC PRINCIPLES AND BILIARY INTUBATION

There are three critically important fundamentals in biliary-enteric anastomoses:

1. Identification of healthy bile duct mucosa proximal to the site of obstruction.
2. The preparation of a segment of the gastrointestinal tract, usually a Roux-en-Y loop of jejunum.
3. Direct mucosa-to-mucosa anastomosis between these two.

In selected cases, the anastomosis may be 'stented' by a transanastomotic tube passed either transhepatically, transjejunally or as a U-tube (Fig. 30.4), although the authors do not do this as a routine.

In selected cases where the anastomosis is technically quite difficult and stenosis is anticipated either due to recurrent malignancy or benign stricture, or in order to provide access for subsequent interventional radiological removal of intrahepatic stones, dilatation of strictures or introduction of brachytherapy catheters, the Roux-en-Y loop may be developed in such a way as to make its blind end subcutaneous (Fig. 30.5) (Kuvshinoff et al 1995, Barker & Winkler 1985, Schweizer et al 1991) (see also Ch. 101).

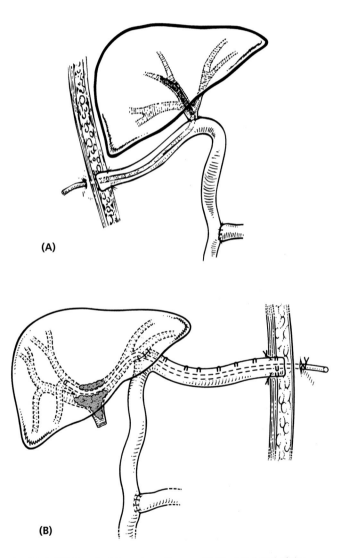

(A)

(B)

Fig. 30.5 (A) Hepaticojejunostomy Roux-en-Y. The blind end of the jejunal loop is kept deliberately long and brought to the abdominal wall. It is either delivered to the subcutaneous tissues or tacked to the peritoneum. The anastomosis is splinted with a transjejunal tube which is brought through the blind end of the jejunum and then through the abdominal wall. This tube track can be used as an avenue for subsequent interventional radiological or choledochoscopic maneuvers. **(B)** A similar anastomosis to the segment III duct. Note the clips on the jejunum and at the subcutaneous termination to guide the radiologist. In this case the loop is used to allow transtumoral intubation and subsequent radiotherapy.

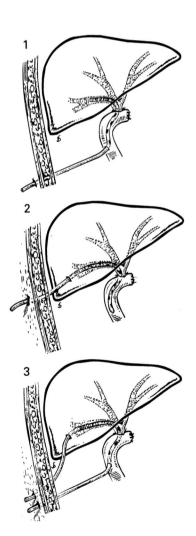

Fig. 30.4 A tube may be passed transjejunally (1), transhepatically (2) or as a U-tube (3).

If this technique is selected, the Roux loop must be made long enough to allow the blind end of the jejunum to reach the abdominal wall without tension. The hepaticojejunal anastomosis is made first and where this technique is selected we usually leave a silastic tube across the anastomosis and lead the tube transjejunally to emerge at the termination of the Roux loop.

It should be emphasized, however, that in the usual circumstance, where anastomosis is obtained between the mucosa of the bile duct and the jejunum, *there is usually no need for transanastomotic tubes and no evidence that intubation assists long term patency*. The authors now advocate a simple sutured anastomosis in the average case. Indeed, transanastomotic stents carry their own complications and these are thus obviated.

However, should direct anastomosis prove impossible at laparotomy, then intubation across the obstruction may be all that can be done. The passage of such tubes may be undertaken in a manner that allows the tube to traverse the obstructed ducts within the liver and the obstructing lesion and then drain into the common hepatic or common bile duct. However, the common bile duct may have been transected during dissection, hepaticojejunostomy to the bile duct below the lesion being necessary. The tube is then passed on below the obstructing lesion through the hepatic duct and on into the jejunum (vide infra). In some such cases the surgeon may elect to close the abdomen and proceed later with percutaneous transhepatic or endoscopic intubation. Adequate preoperative cholangiography will select most cases where intubation is a preferable approach and in whom laparotomy should not be performed.

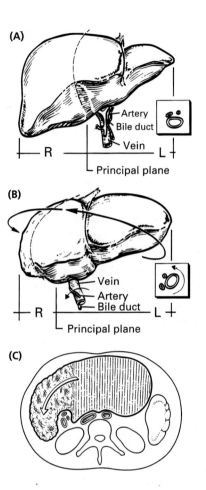

Fig. 30.6 Atrophy/hypertrophy complex. **(A)** The normal relationship of the right and left liver and of the hepatic artery, portal vein and common bile duct (see inset). **(B)** Gross atrophy of the right liver and hypertrophy of the left leads to rotation of the hilar structures so that the portal vein comes to lie relatively more anteriorly and the common bile duct is rotated posterolaterally (see inset). **(C)** Cross-section of the abdomen shows how this rotation carries the hilar structures posteriorly.

INCISIONS

Adequate exposure allowing full visualization is necessary for good biliary-enteric anastomosis. A right subcostal incision may be adequate but it is usually necessary to extend this incision as a bilateral subcostal (rooftop) incision in order to allow adequate exposure. If a bilateral subcostal incision is employed, the use of a broad-bladed ('gallows') retractor fixed to an overhead support and elevating the costal margin is valuable.

In cases of right lobe atrophy (Ch. 3), exposure is particularly difficult, the hilar structures being rotated posteriorly and to the right (Fig. 30.6) and the portal vein being encountered early during dissection. In such instances a thoracoabdominal incision through the right seventh interspace either electively but usually as an extension of a subcostal incision may prove to be essential (Bismuth 1982).

On opening the abdomen it is important to fully expose the liver and the supracolic compartment of the abdomen. *An important early step is division of the ligamentum teres and freeing of the falciform ligament from the abdominal wall back to the diaphragm.* If previous surgery has been carried out, adhesions are carefully taken down and there should be great care not to damage the bowel and particularly the colon. Indeed, preoperative bowel preparation is wise. Dissection of adhesions in the subhepatic area is best commenced from the right, mobilizing the colon from its adhesions to the undersurface of the liver and working medially so as to expose the area of the hilus. The duodenum will frequently be found adherent to the base of the liver; and the colon may be densely adherent to the scar of the gallbladder fossa.

BASIC ANASTOMOTIC TECHNIQUE

It is valuable to have an established routine for biliary-enteric anastomosis. Although some anastomoses are low and easily performed, a regular technique that allows anastomosis even in cases of high, difficult strictures should be developed.

The opened bile duct having been prepared, a *Roux-en-Y loop of jejunum 70 cm in length* is prepared and brought up preferably in a retrocolic fashion for side-to-side anastomosis. Should it be considered necessary to cross the anastomosis with a tube, this is inserted into the hepatic duct before commencement of the anastomosis. It is useful to fix the tube to the ductal wall using a single 4/0 catgut suture and this should be introduced in a mattress fashion across the lower duct wall and tied on the outside (Fig. 30.7). This fixation is important since it holds the tube in a predetermined position and avoids dislodgement during a difficult anastomosis. Side-to-side anastomosis is then performed using the technique described by Voyles and Blumgart (1982) and by Blumgart and Kelley (1984).

The anterior layer of sutures is placed first and prior to any attempt to place the posterior row. If more than one ductal orifice is visible at the hilus, these are best approximated with a row of sutures so that they can be treated as a single duct for anastomotic purposes (Fig. 30.8). If this cannot be done, then the *entire anterior row to all exposed ducts is inserted first so that the separated orifices can be treated as if single*. Attempts to complete one anastomosis and then another are difficult or impossible. These sutures (3/0 Vicryl [Ethicon, Edinburgh, UK] or other absorbable suture material) are serially introduced starting from the left and working to the right (Fig. 30.9).

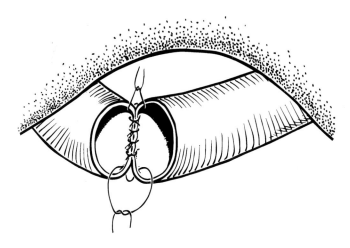

Fig. 30.8 Adjacent ductal orifices may be approximated prior to anastomosis.

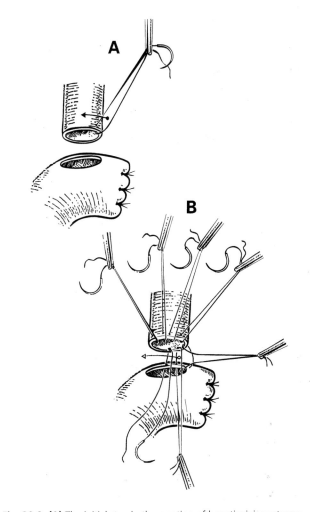

Fig. 30.9 (A) The initial step in the creation of hepaticojejunostomy Roux-en-Y. The anterior layer of suture (3/0 Vicryl) on the bile duct is inserted first, the sutures being passed from the inside out, commencing from the patient's left and working towards the right. The needles are retained and the sutures kept in order. **(B)** The anterior layer of sutures is elevated. This displays the posterior ductal wall and the posterior row of sutures is now placed, again from left to right.

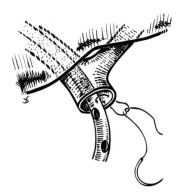

Fig. 30.7 Manner of fixation of trans-anastomotic tubes. Note the introduction of the absorbable suture in a mattress fashion across the ductal wall proximal to the future site of anastomosis. This secures the tube conveniently during anastomosis.

These maneuvers not only allow precise placement of the anterior row of sutures, which may be very difficult if the posterior layer is inserted first and tied, but also facilitate precise placement of the posterior layer (Fig. 30.9), which are likewise placed serially from left to right. The posterior layer of sutures is now tied (Fig. 30.10). The previously placed anterior row of sutures is now completed (Figs 30.11 and 30.12).

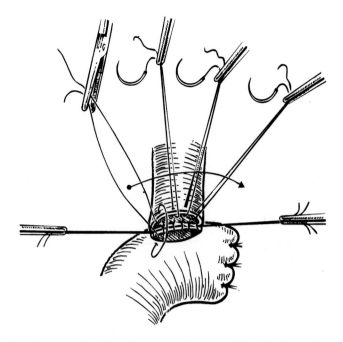

Fig. 30.11 Working from the patient's right toward the left, the needles of the anterior layer are now passed through the jejunal wall from the outside inwards (so as to allow subsequent tying of the knots within). The entire anterior row of sutures is completed in this way but not yet tied.

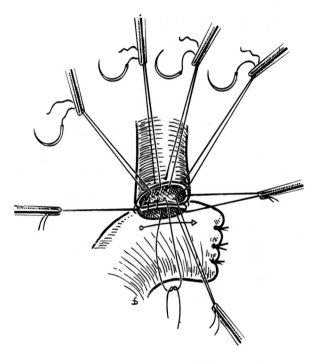

Fig. 30.10 The posterior sutures are now held taut and the jejunum is then 'railroaded' upwards into proximity with the bile duct. The posterior layer of sutures is now tied from right to left. Corner sutures are held. All other sutures are cut.

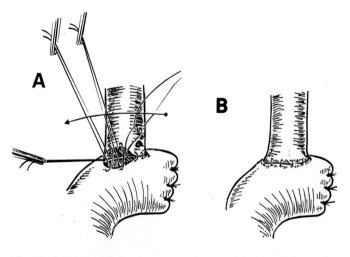

Fig. 30.12 (A) The left-hand stay suture is cut and the anterior layer of sutures is now completed, working from the patient's left to the right. **(B)** The completed anastomosis. Knots are all on the inside, thus approximating the mucosal surfaces of bile duct and jejunum accurately.

ALTERNATIVE ANASTOMOTIC TECHNIQUES

In some instances and, in particular, where the bile duct is large and there is some length of the common hepatic or common bile duct below the hilus, an alternative and quicker technique for anastomosis can be employed. This is particularly valuable in anastomosis of the biliary tract to the jejunum following pancreaticoduodenectomy (see Ch. 56) or as a method of anastomosis for palliative hepatico-jejunostomy for irresectable pancreatic cancer (vide infra).

The technique employs a running suture of 4.0 Vicryl or 4.0 P.D.S. and is depicted in Figs 30.13 A & B).

INTERPOSITION JEJUNAL LIMB

It has been suggested by some (Shamberger et al 1995, Bottger and Junginger 1992, Wheeler and Longmire 1978) but only rarely practiced by the authors that an interposition jejunal limb is more physiologically correct than the creation of a Roux-en-Y loop of jejunum. Such an inter-position limb (Fig. 30.14) allows bile to flow into the

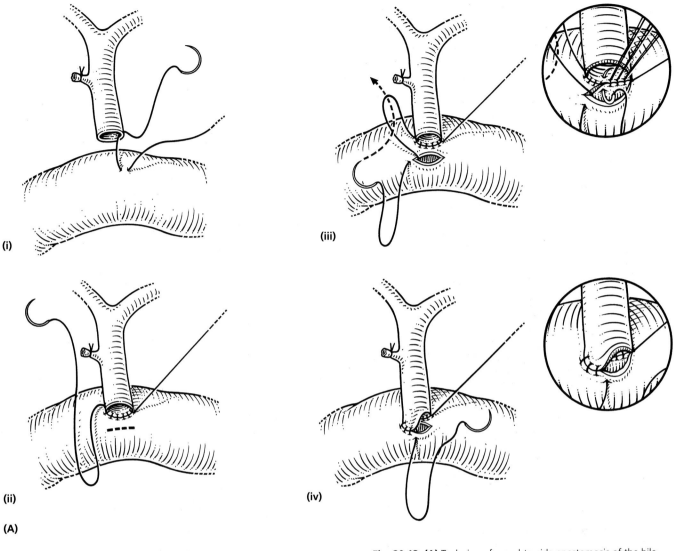

(i)

(ii)

(A)

(iii)

(iv)

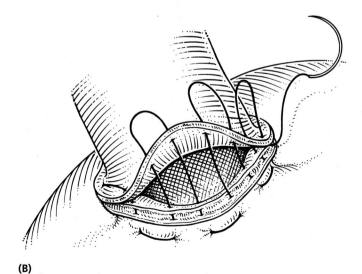

(B)

Fig. 30.13 (A) Technique for end-to-side anastomosis of the bile duct below the hilus to jejunum. **(i)** A 3.0 Vicryl suture is employed and the serosa of the jejunum is sutured to the full thickness of the bile duct. **(ii)** This suture is developed the posterior wall of the bile duct being attached to the jejunal serosa. The dotted line marks the point of incision in the jejunum, which is made after the posterior layer is attached. **(iii)** The suture is now developed either as a continuous or interrupted suture on the anterior layer. Note that the posterior layer of the jejunal mucosa is not sutured directly to the bile duct mucosa. However, several interrupted sutures may be inserted prior to completing the anterior layer so as to approximate the mucosae (inset). **(iv)** The anastomosis is completed. Inset shows the posterior layer with mucosal apposition. **(B)** Alternatively the jejunum may be opened and mucosa-to-mucosa anastomosis performed with a continuous PDS suture as illustrated (see also Ch. 56).

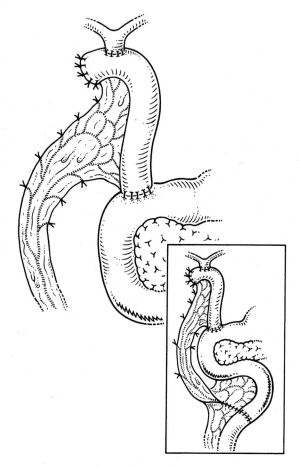

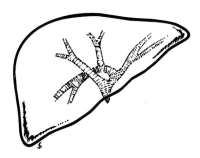

Fig. 30.15 Diagrammatic depiction of a high biliary stricture at the confluences of the bile ducts suggesting that the stricture and the left hepatic duct are intrahepatic structures. *This is an erroneous concept.*

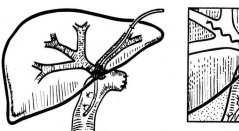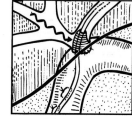

Fig. 30.16 Mucosal graft operation. The area of the stricture is dilated, exposing the biliary mucosa. A transhepatic tube is passed. A disc of seromuscular tissue is removed from a Roux loop and the tube is passed into the jejunum and fixed to the jejunal wall. The dome of jejunum so produced is pulled upwards into contact with the biliary mucosa. The inset illustrates how the dome of mucosa can obstruct a major hepatic duct (arrowed).

Fig. 30.14 A 15-cm segment of jejunum is isolated approximately 30 cm from the ligament of Treitz, the jejunum being reconstructed by end-to-end anastomosis. This limb must be isolated with care so as to carry with it a pedicle of the mesentery. The upper end of the limb is then sutured to the common hepatic duct and the lower to the commencement of the second part of the duodenum.

duodenum and may be free of the complication of late peptic ulceration, which occurs in some 10% of patients with a long-standing Roux-en-Y reconstruction.

MUCOSAL GRAFT OPERATION

A method for 'sutureless' anastomosis of the jejunum to the bile duct in high bile duct stricture, where exposure of biliary mucosa and consequently sutured hepaticojejunostomy are thought impossible was introduced by Smith (1969) and subsequently has been recommended (Smith 1981) as a standard repair for high biliary strictures (Smith 1969, Smith 1981). The authors do not employ this as a routine approach. Advocates of the mucosal graft operation (Knight & Smith 1982) tend to approach the scarred biliary hilus directly, the approach being dictated by an assumption that the stricture and the left hepatic duct are intrahepatic struc-

tures (Fig. 30.15). However, this is not so, the left hepatic duct being extrahepatic and accessible for direct anastomosis even in patients who have had several biliary operations.

The operation is carried out as indicated in Figure 30.16.

If there has been complete obstruction of the common hepatic duct and the right and left hepatic ducts are separated, these are sought and double grafts are inserted by means of two transhepatic tubes. It is important to emphasize that the ducts must be reasonably dilated for this approach to be feasible. Furthermore, the ducts intubated may not include the entire intrahepatic biliary ductal system.

HEPATICOJEJUNOSTOMY

The surgical approaches to be described can either: (1) display the *left hepatic ducts* by opening the umbilical fissure, elevating the base of the quadrate lobe and lowering the left hepatic ductal system from the undersurface of the quadrate lobe or, (2) expose the left hepatic ducts by dissection at the base of the ligamentum teres (ligamentum teres approach) (Blumgart & Kelley 1984).

Alternatively, if access to the left hepatic ducts is technically hazardous or impossible because of extensive tumor growth, it is possible to approach peripheral bile ducts in order to perform biliary-enteric bypass procedures (vide infra).

Hepaticojejunostomy can also be performed to the *right anterior or posterior sectoral hepatic ducts.*

APPROACH TO THE LEFT HEPATIC DUCT

At the hilum of the liver

Early division of the ligamentum teres and freeing of the falciform ligament from the diaphragm is important. A firm tie is placed on the divided ligamentum teres so that it may be elevated and used as a tractor. The liver is elevated so as to display its undersurface. Although often not necessary, the bridge of tissue (if present) connecting the left lobe of the liver to the quadrate lobe may now be divided by cutting it with diathermy (Fig. 30.17). Although not essential for approach to the left hepatic duct, this maneuver is useful in difficult cases. It exposes the umbilical fissure and allows considerably greater mobility and access for dissection at the base of the quadrate lobe.

The base of the quadrate lobe is now identified and dissection proceeded with in the plane between Glisson's

capsule and the peritoneal reflection encasing the left portal triad (Fig. 30.18). This dissection is deepened and the structures of the left portal triad are lowered from the inferior surface of the quadrate lobe and exposed for dissection (lowering of the hilar plate) (Fig. 30.19) (Hepp & Couinaud 1956, Bismuth 1982, Blumgart & Kelley 1984). Occasionally, an overhanging mass of the lower portion of the quadrate lobe may require excision in order to improve exposure. A thin-bladed curved retractor inserted from above, elevating the quadrate lobe, assists exposure.

If the right duct cannot be adequately exposed in this way, it is possible to obtain adequate exposure of the right hepatic duct by incising the liver parenchyma in the line of the gallbladder fossa. This hepatotomy (Blumgart 1980) together with the opening of the umbilical fissure described above allows elevation of the entire quadrate lobe (Bismuth 1982). Alternatively, the right portal pedicle can be delivered and the right anterior or, indeed, posterior sectoral ducts exposed (vide infra).

Stay sutures are placed in the left hepatic duct, which is then incised longitudinally. A Roux-en-Y loop of jejunum is

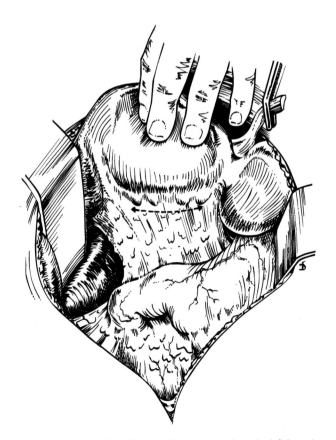

Fig. 30.18 The initial line of incision for an approach to the left hepatic duct by lowering of the hilar plate. The liver is elevated and the quadrate lobe retracted upwards. The incision is made at *precisely the point at which Glisson's capsule reflects to the lesser omentum.* (See also Fig. 30.3.)

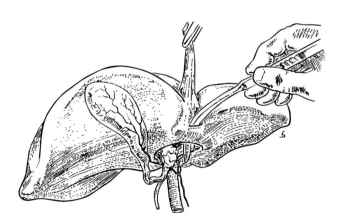

Fig. 30.17 The bridge of liver tissue frequently present between the base of the quadrate lobes (segment IV) and the left lobe of the liver can be divided. This is conveniently done by passing a curved director beneath it and cutting it with diathermy. Such division can be useful in aiding an approach to the left hepatic duct, particularly if the course of the duct is somewhat vertical and the base of the quadrate lobe short. The maneuver is always necessary (if the bridge of tissue is present) to allow dissection of the segment III duct. (See also Fig. 30.22).

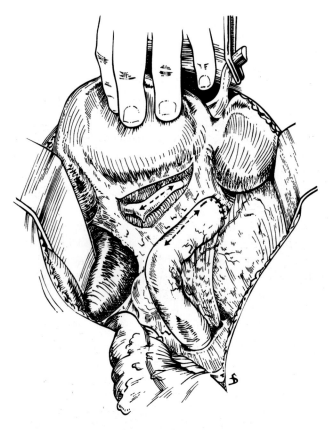

Fig. 30.19 The hilar plate (see Chapter 1) is lowered and the left hepatic duct exposed for dissection. The exposure is carried medially and to the right to expose the confluence and the right hepatic duct.

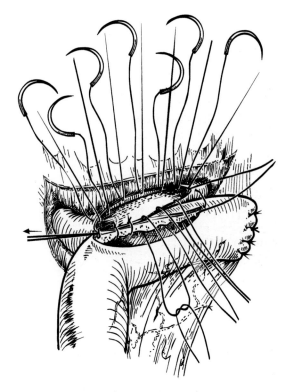

Fig. 30.20 The left hepatic duct and the jejunum are incised. The anastomosis is performed (see Figs. 30.8–30.12).

brought up. Should it be considered necessary to cross the anastomosis with a tubal splint, this is now inserted into the hepatic duct as described above. Side-to-side anastomosis is then performed by the technique illustrated in Figures 30.8–30.12. The Roux-en-Y loop of jejunum can be attached to Glisson's capsule at the point of reflection of the hilar plate with a few sutures (Figs 30.20 & 30.21)

Ligamentum teres (round ligament) segment III approach

While the vast majority of high benign strictures can be approached and dealt with as described above, it is occasionally difficult to expose the left hepatic duct beneath the quadrate lobe. This may be due to dense adhesions, bleeding or a large and overhanging quadrate lobe. On occasion the extrahepatic length of the left hepatic duct may be relatively short and oblique, making the approach to it difficult.

In carcinoma of the bile duct, a tumor extending into the left duct from the confluence area may preclude the use of the main left duct. *In any event, palliative anastomosis is best carried out at a reasonable distance from a malignant lesion.*

In such instances, repair can be effected by dissection of the left hepatic duct within the umbilical fissure (Soupalt & Couinaud 1957) and, while more often required and useful in malignant disease (Bismuth & Corlette 1956) and particularly in cancer of the hepatic duct confluence and gallbladder, the method is also useful in selected cases of benign stricture. *It is important to note that unilateral drainage of the left hepatic duct in the presence of a tumor which completely excludes the right liver and right hepatic ducts from the anastomosis is effective in the relief of jaundice provided the left lobe of the liver is not atrophic* (Baer et al 1994).

Careful preoperative assessment is mandatory. It is unwise to carry out percutaneous transhepatic drainage on the right side if it is not confidently expected that an endoprosthetic tube can be placed across an obstructing malignant lesion. In such instances, if surgical decompression of the left liver has been performed, the patient has a permanent biliary fistula on the right side unless suitable drainage of the right liver can be accomplished. Sometimes this situation can be met by anastomosis to the segment III duct and subsequent radiologic placement of an endoprosthesis from the right to left ductal systems utilizing the approach shown in Figure 30.5B. Such situations must be anticipated and, if there is an extensive lesion at the confluence involving the right ducts over a considerable length and any doubt

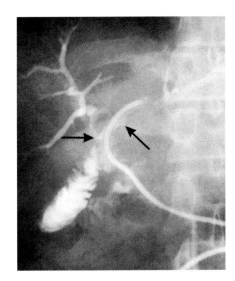

(A)

Fig. 30.21 (A) Cholangiogram obtained after injection of contrast medium across a transjejunal tube illustrates hepaticojejunostomy Roux-en-Y by the left approach in a patient with a high benign postcholecystectomy stricture. Note the anastomosis to the left duct and confluence area between the arrows. **(B)** Roux-en-Y hepaticojejunostomy has been completed and the Roux-en-Y loop is now sutured to the point of division of Glisson's capsule.

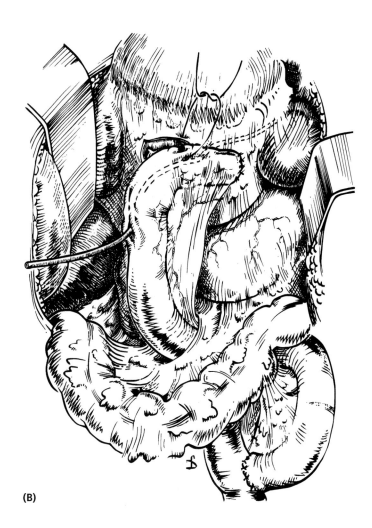

(B)

that a subsequent endoprosthesis can be introduced, percutaneous transhepatic intubation on the right is unwise. An immediate surgical approach to the segment III duct on the left is preferable, provided there is no atrophy of the left lobe of the liver.

Initially the ligamentum teres is elevated and the bridge of liver tissue joining segment IV to the left liver is divided as described above (Fig. 30.17). While the liver is then held up so that its inferior surface can be seen, the ligamentum teres is pulled downwards and dissected from the liver (Fig. 30.22).

An alternative and *preferable* method of exposure of the segment III duct is to open the liver to the left of the ligamentum teres and approach the duct from above. The liver is split just to the left of the ligamentum teres, and a small segment of liver tissue may be removed. In this manner, the duct may be exposed and opened without division of any of the portal venous supply to segment III (Fig. 30.23).

Side-to-side anastomosis to a loop of jejunum is then carried out by the techniques described above. An excellent anastomosis can be obtained (Fig. 30.24).

The procedure is not useful if there is left lobar atrophy and not necessary if the confluence and left hepatic duct is not involved by tumor and can be approached directly. In addition, the procedure may be difficult (a) in patients in whom longstanding obstruction has led to severe secondary biliary fibrosis rendering the liver substance rigid and difficult to maneuver, (b) if there is right liver atrophy and left liver hypertrophy, (c) after previous right hepatectomy.

Longmire procedure

An approach to the segment II duct of the left lobe of the liver, for use where approaches to the hilus were not possible, has been described. This procedure remains occasionally valuable but should not be employed when the left ductal system can be exposed below the quadrate lobe or within the umbilical fissure (see above). The Longmire approach (Longmire & Sandford 1948) involves removal of liver tissue with greater blood loss and often less effective biliary-enteric anastomosis than can be obtained by the other methods.

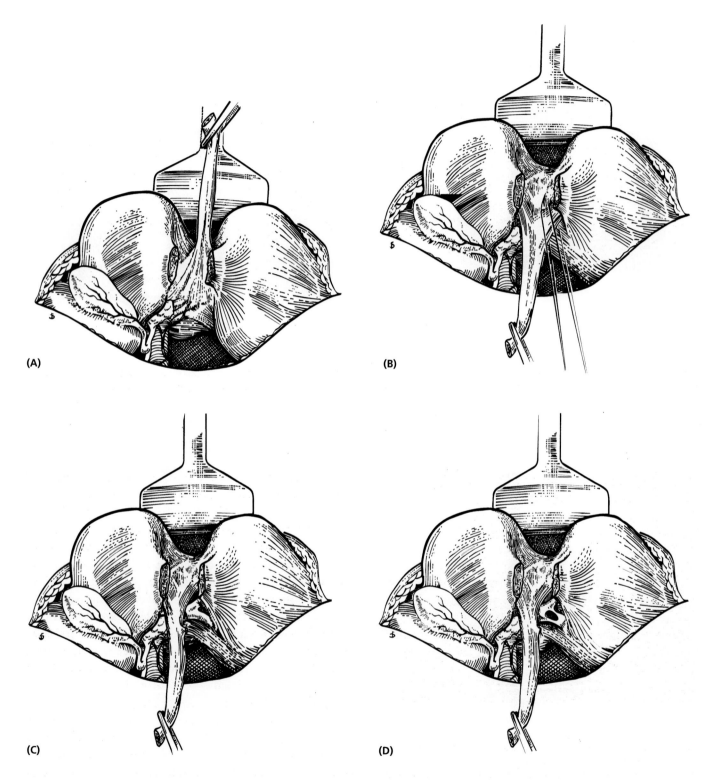

Fig. 30.22 **(A)** The liver is held up so that its inferior surface is seen. The bridge of liver between the quadrate lobe and the left lobe of the liver has been divided. The base of the ligamentum teres is seen. **(B)** The ligamentum teres is then pulled downwards. The peritoneum of its upper surface on the left side is incised and the extensions passing into the liver are exposed. The left of these extensions are divided between ligatures. These ligatures must be carefully passed using aneurysm needles. This part of the dissection is tedious and should be meticulously carried out since hemorrhage within the recess adjacent to the segment III duct can be difficult to control. **(C)** The segment III duct is exposed. **(D)** The duct is opened longitudinally for anastomosis which is carried out by the technique illustrated in Figures 30.8–30.11.

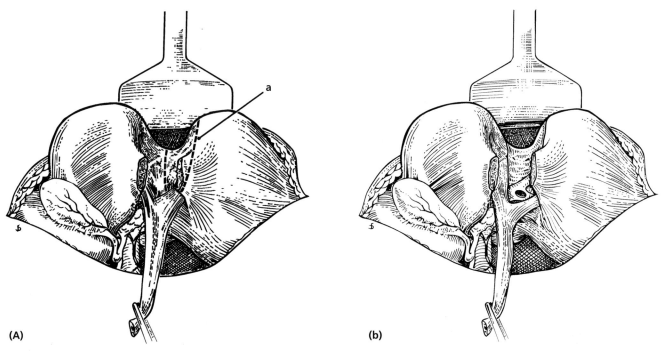

(A) **(b)**

Fig. 30.23 (A) The liver is split to the left of the ligamentum teres in the umbilical fissure. It may be necessary to remove a small wedge of liver tissue (a). **(B)** The segment III duct is exposed at the base of the liver split above and behind its accompanying vein and is ready for anastomosis.

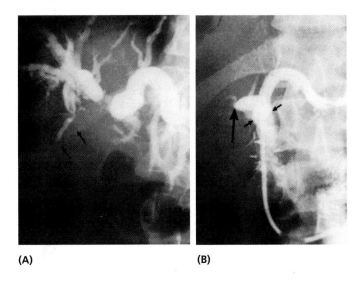

(A) **(B)**

Fig. 30.24 (A) Hilar obstruction of the biliary ductal system due to gallbladder carcinoma affecting branches of the segment V duct (arrows), causing complete obstruction at the confluence. The biliary ductal system was outlined by separate puncture of the right and left ductal system using a percutaneous transhepatic approach. **(B)** Transtubal cholangiography reveals that hepaticojejunostomy Roux-en-Y has been carried out to the segment III duct (between the small arrows). The large arrow indicates the area of the obstruction. The authors now omit the placement of a transjejunal/transanastomotic splint, this being unnecessary in the majority of cases. Excellent palliation was obtained in this patient for 20 months, advancing tumor within the liver then progressing to death.

The essence of the approach is the removal of a portion of the left lobe of the liver so as to expose the dilated intrahepatic ducts of segment II (and sometimes segment III). One of the great difficulties of the procedure is that the vessels of the portal triad run in close approximation with the ducts, so that some bleeding is inevitable and difficult to control without compromising the duct lumina. This is particularly so if the liver is fibrotic.

The operation is commenced by mobilizing the left lobe of the liver. The left triangular ligament is divided so allowing delivery of the left lobe forwards and into the wound. This maneuver itself may be difficult if the liver is tough and fibrous and if there is left lobe hypertrophy.

It is the authors' preference in the performance of this operation to apply a liver clamp to the left lobe just to the left of the ligamentum teres. The peripheral portion of the left lobe is then simply resected in order to reveal the exposed ducts and vessels. Slight release of the pressure of the clamp allows identification of the vessels, which can then be suture ligated.

This having been done, a Roux-en-Y loop of jejunum is prepared and brought up for anastomosis. Again, identification of a suitable size duct may be difficult. In such cases, the Roux loop may be opened over a considerable length and sutured to Glisson's capsule, although this is not easy.

Such suture may be carried out utilizing mattress sutures passed through the jejunal wall and through the exposed liver substance (Fig. 30.25).

Segment III hepaticojejunostomy

Occasionally, wedge excision of segment III (Fig. 30.26) allows exposure of the segment III duct with subsequent hepaticojejunostomy.

APPROACH TO THE RIGHT HEPATIC DUCTS

The right hepatic ductal system may be approached by excision of liver tissue on the right side, the procedure being similar to that described by Longmire for the left liver. The tip of segment V/VI of the right lobe is removed and hepaticojejunostomy carried out in a similar fashion to that described for the Longmire procedure above.

After removal of the gallbladder, incision at the base of the gallbladder fossa may expose the underlying segment V duct (Fig. 30.27), but the procedure is rarely applicable and not easy of execution.

Importantly, techniques have now been developed to expose the main right anterior sectoral duct for biliary enteric anastomosis. The pedicle to the right liver is exposed by excising the tissue anterior to it, the anterior sectoral pedicle is defined, and the relevant duct opened (Fig. 30.28). *This procedure is facilitated by delivery of the right pedicle as described for liver resection* (Launois & Jamieson 1992) (Ch. 83). If the entire right pedicle is to be delivered, it is necessary to first control the often multiple retrohepatic venous branches draining into the vena cava.

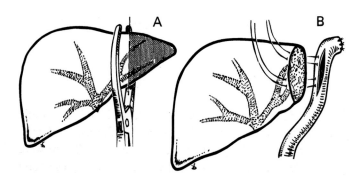

Fig. 30.25 (A) The Longmire operation. The left lobe of the liver is completely mobilized by division of the left triangular ligament. A clamp is applied across the mobilized lobe and this allows control of bleeding during removal of a portion of the left lobe so as to expose the segment II duct and occasionally the segment III duct. **(B)** Method of approximating the jejunal loop to the exposed liver surface. Alternatively, a tube can be passed into the biggest exposed duct and developed in a transjejunal fashion, a direct anastomosis being carried out between the jejunum and the exposed duct. The remainder of the jejunal loop is then approximated to the cut liver surface using the technique illustrated.

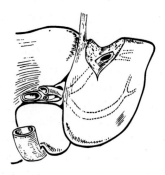

Fig. 30.26 Method of approach to the segment III duct. The left lobe of the liver is mobilized and a wedge of liver tissue involving segment III is removed anteriorly and medially. The segment III duct is thus exposed intrahepatically for anastomosis.

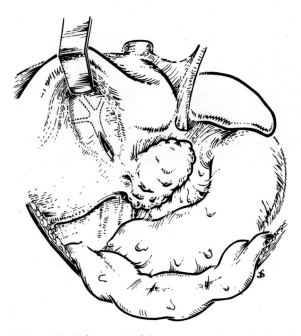

Fig. 30.27 Method of exposure of the segment V duct in the base of the gallbladder fossa (Ch. 2).

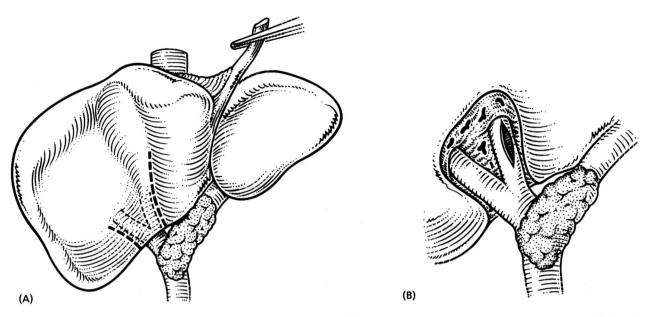

Fig. 30.28 **(A)** Exposure of the right hepatic pedicle. The liver is opened as indicated and liver tissue is cleared over a small distance. **(B)** The relevant duct (usually the anterior sectoral duct) is opened and anastomosis carried out.

RESULTS AND CONCLUSION

Roux-en-Y hepaticojejunostomy is the favored approach for the restoration of biliary-enteric continuity and good long-term results are reported (Bismuth et al 1978, Lane et al 1973, Pappalardo et al 1982, Chapman et al 1995). Despite some reports of stenosis at the anastomosis (Bowers 1964, Lane et al 1973, Leborgne et al 1974) there is no evidence that this problem is due to the use of the Roux loop rather than a consequence of the primary disease. In the past 30 years the authors have an extensive experience of Roux-en-Y· hepaticojejunostomy for benign and malignant disease (Chs 49, 54) and can confirm the efficacy and low operative mortality rate using this approach (Chapman et al 1995, Jarnagin et al 1998). Peptic ulceration can develop after this operation in some 7 to 13% of cases. For this reason some have suggested an interposed loop of jejunum between the bile ducts and the duodenum (Wheeler & Longmire 1978, Bottger & Junginger 1992, Shamberger et al 1995) (Fig. 30.14) but this approach has not been generally adopted, the advent of the histamine H_2 antagonists or pump inhibitors introduce a method of therapy for those who develop peptic ulceration. Indeed, these drugs could be used prophylactically for patients shown to have a high acid output preoperatively. Patients with proven duodenal ulceration should be considered for a definitive ulcer operation at the time of biliary repair.

We have recently reported the results of 55 biliary-enteric bypass operations over a 5-year period for cases of irresectable cancer of the extrahepatic biliary tree. There were 41 segment III bypasses and 14 bypasses to the right sectoral hepatic ducts. While initial good decompression and relief of symptoms was achieved in all patients, the long-term results were superior using the segment III duct, the one-year bypass patency being 80%. Moreover, segment III bypass for irresectable hilar cholangiocarcinoma was achieved with a tolerable morbidity and 0% mortality. On the other hand, bypass to the right sectoral hepatic ducts was associated with greater perioperative morbidity and mortality, and the long term results were not as good. Patients with gallbladder cancer, although effectively palliated, generally succumbed quickly as a result of rapid progression of the disease and are probably best treated with percutaneous biliary stenting (Jarnagin et al 1998) (Ch. 29).

Precise sutured hepaticojejunostomy can usually be carried out either after exposure of the left hepatic duct beneath the quadrate lobe by lowering of the hilar plate, or within the umbilical fissure by utilizing the ligamentum teres approach (Blumgart & Kelley 1984). The use of the mucosal graft procedure is rarely indicated. Left hepaticojejunostomy by the Longmire-Sandford operation or a similar right-sided intrahepatic hepaticojejunostomy are only indicated in special circumstances, usually in unilateral atrophy/hypertrophy of the liver or where both the hilus and umbilical fissure are compromised by tumor.

OPERATIVE INTUBATION OF THE BILIARY TRACT

The use of stents *placed at the time of operation* (Goetz 1951, Praderi 1961) has decreased markedly since the introduction of percutaneous transhepatic drainage methods and is likely to become obsolete. While some (Lillemoe & Cameron 1994) still use stenting regularly in a variety of situations, the authors very rarely use this approach.

Transhepatic biliary stents are claimed to have several advantages. The stent can be anchored at the skin precluding migration. Silastic stents allow healing of a biliary enteric anastomosis with a minimum of foreign body reaction. Since the stents exit through the liver and not through the biliary tree, the diameter can be large. The thickness of the wall of the stent prevents compression by tumor and, therefore, maintains patency of the biliary tree even with extensive local tumor growth. In malignant biliary strictures or sclerosing cholangitis, the stents may be left in place permanently with periodic changes to preclude obstruction of the side holes with biliary sludge. The stents can be easily replaced fluoroscopically on an outpatient basis by threading a guidewire through the stent, removing the old stent, and placing a new stent over the guidewire. It has been claimed that transhepatic stents assist the surgeon in identification of the left and right hepatic ducts at operation. By contrast, the authors have found no difficulty in locating the relevant ducts.

Disadvantages are that the stents protrude from the body and are a constant source of reminder to the patient of serious underlying disease, they can be very uncomfortable and inevitably lead to biliary tract infection and periodic attacks of cholangitis. Furthermore, in cases of malignancy, it is possible for tumor cells to migrate along the tube track and result in tumor seeding of peritoneum or even the skin.

INDICATIONS

BENIGN BILE DUCT STRICTURES

Benign bile duct strictures secondary to operative injury can be located anywhere along the extrahepatic biliary tree but are most commonly at or just below the hepatic duct bifurcation. Ideally, reconstruction is performed with a direct anastomosis of the bile duct to jejunal mucosa as described above. However, if at the time of surgery a perfect mucosa-to-mucosa anastomosis is not possible, hepaticojejunostomy may be carried out with an extension of the Roux-en-Y subcutaneously as described above (Fig. 30.5) or the mucosal

graft procedure may be employed. The tubes allow postoperative maneuvers as for example dilatation of stenoses or removal of intrahepatic stones. *We have had no need to carry out intubation or the mucosal graft procedure other than to allow radiological access for dilatation or intrahepatic stone extraction in over 200 consecutive repairs of benign bile duct stricture.*

PROXIMAL BILIARY TUMORS

A significant number of hilar tumors can be resected for potential cure (vide infra) (Ch. 54). Others are selected for operative bypass as described above or management by percutaneous drainage. The authors rarely employ operative stenting except to allow postoperative access for the introduction of postoperative radiotherapy (Fig. 30.5B). However, if operative placement of tubes is selected, the methods are as described below.

TECHNIQUE

The essentials of the technique are the initial introduction of percutaneously placed stents (Ch. 29), which are then used to 'railroad' transhepatic stents across the obstructing tumor or across anastomoses at the confluence of the hepatic ducts.

First the transhepatic catheters are passed and then are identified at operation and used to guide the operatively placed stents. After ultrasound or CT documentation of intrahepatic bile duct dilatation, the biliary anatomy is defined by percutaneous transhepatic cholangiography. The former is favored because it defines the extent of the proximal tumor involving the hepatic hilum, and permits the preoperative placement of percutaneous biliary catheters. For neoplasms involving the distal common hepatic duct and below, one right-sided percutaneous catheter is placed. For neoplasms involving the proximal common hepatic duct, or the bile duct confluence, both the right and left hepatic ducts are intubated with biliary catheters. If possible, these catheters are advanced through the neoplasm into the duodenum. If, at subsequent laparotomy, there is no evidence of disseminated tumor, the collapsed extrahepatic biliary tree is divided distally at the duodenum and the distal end oversewn. The proximal biliary segment is reflected cephalad and dissected off the portal vein (Ch. 54).

If the gallbladder is still in place, it is removed to allow access to the porta hepatis. Once the hepatic duct bifurcation is visualized, the surgeon palpates the transhepatic percutaneous catheters and the hepatic ducts above the tumor.

The dissection is continued up before dividing the right and left hepatic ducts. Bilateral silastic transhepatic stents are inserted. Both the right and left hepatic ducts are intubated and a bilateral hepaticojejunostomy is created to a Roux-en-Y jejunal loop. Two stents are generally required because the recurrence of tumor may obstruct the undrained hepatic lobe.

If the proximal bile duct tumor is not resectable because of extension into the portal vein or the hepatic parenchyma, the tumor is merely dilated and transhepatic stents inserted through the tumor. Hepaticojejunostomy can be performed to the common hepatic duct below the bifurcation, which is involved with tumor. For benign strictures, the stents are left in place temporarily. In proximal cholangiocarcinoma the stents are left in permanently. They are changed every four months on an outpatient basis to prevent occlusion of the side holes with sludge. External beam radiation therapy may be delivered following surgery, and in addition, the bilateral silastic stents can be used for the placement of an internal radiation source which can be placed in the area of the biliary resection to further boost the dose of radiation (Fig. 30.5B) (Kuvshinoff et al 1995).

U-TUBE TECHNIQUE

With this technique (Saypol & Kurian 1969, Terblanche et al 1972), a 16-Fr. Argyle nasogastric tube is inserted in a fashion similar to the silastic catheters; but the distal end, instead of being left free in a Roux-en-Y loop, is brought out through the common duct and subsequently through the abdominal wall to form a U. When the internal drainage is satisfactory, and the biliary leaks seal, the two ends of the U-tube are connected to form a circle. According to supporters, the advantage of this tube is easy replacement. However, this technique doubles the number of tubes coming out onto the patient's abdominal wall, and the silastic stents can now be changed just as easily using a guidewire. Furthermore, silastic is less reactive and may allow better anastomotic healing. While still used by many surgeons, the authors in a large experience of benign and malignant biliary strictures have not used this technique over the last fifteen years. Indeed, percutaneous transhepatic intubation has all but rendered operative intubational methods obsolete.

tion of the biliary tract in the periampullary region. Choledochoduodenostomy is infrequently used to relieve malignant obstruction (vide infra). These palliative procedures are directed at the relief of jaundice, itching, and vomiting. With the advent and development of interventional endoscopic intubational approaches for the relief of low biliary tract obstruction, the operation is seldom done electively in the older or infirm patients but may be elected as an option and performed in conjunction with gastrojejunostomy in patients in whom gastric outlet obstruction due to malignancy of the pancreatic head is a predominant at presentation. In addition, in younger patients judged to have a reasonable period of survival, elective hepatobiliary bypass may be performed in preference to endoscopic intubation, which is accompanied by necessity for frequent tube changes and a tendency to produce recurrent attacks of cholangitis.

Recent advances in diagnostic laparoscopic techniques have also resulted in a much higher resectability rate for those patients submitted to laparotomy for pancreatic malignancy and thus a decrease in the number of bypass procedures done as an alternative to resection at the time of laparotomy (Ch. 55).

Whereas the relief of jaundice may not prolong the patient's life (Sarr & Cameron 1982), this can at least improve the quality of life with well-being and appetite returning albeit temporarily. Surgical palliation of jaundice is achieved by anastomosis between the common hepatic duct or the gallbladder above and the stomach duodenum or jejunum below the obstructing tumor.

It is the authors' preference to remove the gallbladder if present and perform hepaticojejunostomy whenever possible since this allows direct relief of the obstructed biliary tree without the risk of compromising the cystic duct, which would render cholecystjejunostomy ineffective. Nevertheless, the relative merits of hepaticojejunostomy or cholecystjejunostomy are still under debate (Rappaport & Villalba 1990, Rosemurgy et al 1989, Singh & Reber 1989). Hepaticojejunostomy either end-to-side (described above) or side-to-side, yields reliable results. Others, however, prefer biliary-enteric bypass between the gallbladder and the proximal jejunum (Chs 55, 56).

CHOLECYSTDUODENOSTOMY—CHOLEDOCHOJEJUNOSTOMY AND CHOLEDOCHODUODENOSTOMY

In general, choledochoduodenostomy and choledochojejunostomy are performed for the relief of malignant obstruc-

CHOLECYSTJEJUNOSTOMY

INDICATIONS

The operation is suitable for patients with malignant obstruction of the low bile duct due to periampullary tumors and mainly pancreatic carcinoma. It is only suitable

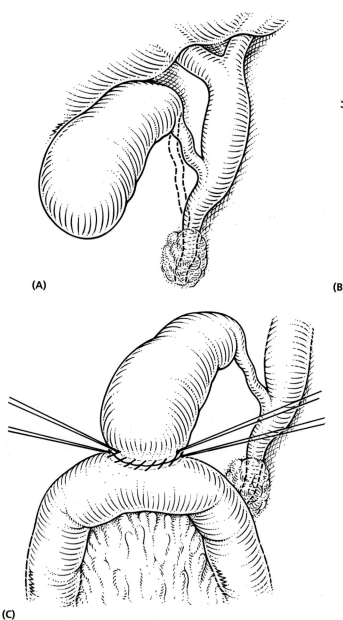

(A)

(B)

(C)

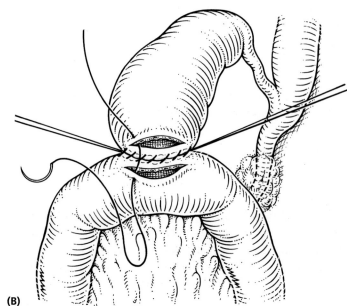

Fig. 30.29 (A)–(C) Technique of cholecystjejunostomy. (A) The cystic duct should join the common bile duct above the tumor. If it enters at the level of the tumor (dotted line) the procedure is contraindicated. **(B)** The posterior layer of the anastomosis is performed with a running suture between the opening at the fundus of the gallbladder and the jejunum. **(C)** The anterior layer of the side-to-side anastomosis is completed. (The authors do not employ an associated entero-enterostomy).

for patients in whom the cystic duct meets the common hepatic duct well above the tumor (Fig. 30.29). If indeed the cystic duct has a low junction with the common biliary channel and is already occluded by the tumor or close to the upper border of the tumor, then cholecystjejunostomy is an inappropriate operation.

Preoperative information as to this point should be available from cholangiographic studies or ascertained at operation. The authors never perform the procedure if opening of the gallbladder at the time of operation does not evidently relieve obstruction of the common bile duct or if there are multiple stones present in the gallbladder at the time of operation.

TECHNIQUE

The distended gallbladder is sutured either using interrupted sutures or a running 3-0 Vicryl suture to the first available loop of jejunum (Fig. 30.29).

This having been done, the gallbladder is opened and the content is sucked out. Bile is sent for culture. It is ascertained that the common hepatic duct has collapsed.

The jejunum is now opened opposite the gallbladder fenestration. The posterior and anterior layers are sutured with 3-0 Vicryl to complete the cholecystjejunostomy (Fig. 30.29).

HEPATICOJEJUNOSTOMY

It is the authors' preference to perform this operation as an end-to-side procedure. However, side-to-side hepatico-jejunostomy can be performed using techniques similar to those described for choledochoduodenostomy.

TECHNIQUE

The gallbladder, if present, is removed in a retrograde fashion.

The common bile duct well above the tumor is dissected, care being taken to avoid an accessory or replaced right hepatic artery if present. The duct is then divided and the lower end of the common bile duct is closed with a 3-0 Vicryl suture. The exposed common bile duct is now sutured into the jejunum using the techniques described above. In this situation, the authors employ the technique illustrated in Figure 30.13.

CHOLEDOCHODUODENOSTOMY

This operation is infrequently employed for the relief of malignant biliary tract obstruction although in selected cases, and particularly in those patients in whom the duodenum is mobile, it can give equally good results to hepatico-jejunostomy. If performed for malignant obstruction, it is the authors' preference to carry out end-to-side choledo-choduodenostomy utilizing precisely the same techniques as those illustrated in Figure 30.13.

It should be particularly noted that choledochoduo-denostomy, while infrequently employed for the relief of biliary tract obstruction in malignant disease, is *much more frequently used for the patient with biliary obstruction due to gallstones*. In the latter case, side-to-side choledochoduo-denostomy is preferable. Because this procedure is much more frequently performed for gallstone disease rather than for malignancy, it is described in detail in Chapter 45.

REFERENCES

Baer H U, Rhyner M, Stain S C, Glauser P W, Dennison A R, Maddern G J, Blumgart L H 1994 The effect of communication between the right and left liver on the outcome of surgical drainage for jaundice due to malignant obstruction at the hilus of the liver. HPB Surgery 8: 27–31

Barker E, Winkler M 1985 Permanent-access hepaticojejunostomy. British Journal of Surgery 71: 188–191

Bismuth H, Corlette M B 1956 Intrahepatic cholangiojejunostomy: an operation for biliary obstruction. Surgical Clinics of North America 36: 849–863

Bismuth H, Corlette MB 1975 Intrahepatic cholangioenteric anastomosis in carcinoma of the hilus of the liver. Surgery, Gynecology & Obstetrics 140: 170–178

Bismuth H, Franco D, Corlette M B, Hepp J 1978 Long-term results of Roux-en-Y hepaticojejunostomy. Surg Gyn Obstet 146: 161–167

Bismuth H 1982 Postoperative stricture of the bile duct. In: Blumgart LH (ed) The biliary tract. Churchill Livingstone, Edinburgh, p 209–218

Blumgart L H 1980 Hepatic resection. In: Taylor S (ed) Recent advances in surgery 10. Edinburgh: Churchill Livingstone, pp. 1–16

Blumgart LH, Kelley CJ 1984 Hepaticojejunostomy in benign and malignant high bile duct stricture: approaches to the left hepatic ducts. British Journal of Surgery 71: 257–261

Bottger T, Junginger T 1992 A small-bowel segment as a total extrahepatic bile duct replacement. Archives of Surgery 127: 1424–1428

Bowers R M 1964 Morbid conditions following choledochojejunostomy. Annals of Surgery 159: 424–427

Chapman W C, Blumgart L H, Benjamin IS 1995 Postcholecystectomy bile duct strictures: management and outcome in 130 patients. Archives of Surgery 130: 597–604

Goetz O 1951 Die tranchepatische Dauerdrainage bei der hoken gallanganstenose. Archives of Klinikum Chirurgie 270: 97

Hepp J, Couinaud C 1956 L'abord et l'utilisation du canal hepatique gauche dans le separation de la voie biliare principale. Presse Medicale 64: 947–948

Jarnagin W R, Burke E C, Powers C, Fong Y, Blumgart L H 1998 Intrahepatic biliary enteric bypass provides effective palliation in selected patients with malignant obstruction at the hepatic duct confluence. American Journal of Surgery 175: 453–460

Knight M, Smith Lord of Marlow 1982 Surgery of benign strictures of the extrahepatic bile ducts. In: Calne RY (ed) Liver Surgery, Piccin Medical Books, p 191–121

Kuvshinoff B W, Armstrong J G, Fong Y, Schupak K, Getradjman G, Heffernan N, Blumgart LH 1995 Palliation of irresectable hilar cholangiocarcinoma with biliary drainage and radiotherapy. British Journal of Surgery 82: 1522–1525

Lane C E, Sawyers J L, Riddell D H, Scott H W 1973 Long-term results of hepato-cholangiojejunostomy. Annals of Surgery 177: 714–722

Launois B, Jamieson G G 1992 The importance of Glisson's capsule and its sheath in the intrahepatic approach to resection of the liver. Surgery, Gynecology & Obstetrics 174: 7–10

Leborgne, Le Neel J C, Visset J et al 1974 Consideration sur un serie de 65 derivations bilio-jejunales pour lesion benignes de lavoie biliare principale. Annales Medicae, reims 11: 345–348

Lillemoe K D, Cameron J L 1994 Operative intubational techniques in biliary obstruction. In: Blumgart L H (ed) Surgery of the Liver and Biliary Tract, 2nd edn. Churchill Livingstone, London, p 1069–1078

Longmire W P, Sandford M C 1948 Intrahepatic cholangiojejunostomy with partial hepatectomy for biliary obstruction. Surgery 128: 330–347

McArthur M S, Longmire W P Jr 1971 Peptic ulcer disease after choledochojejunostomy. American Journal of Surgery 122: 155–158

Pappalardo G, Correnti S, Mobarhan S et al 1982 Long-term results of Roux-en-Y hepaticojejunostomy and hepaticoduodenostomy. Annals of Surgery 196: 149–152

Praderi RC 1961 Choledocostomia tranhepatico. Bolletino Societa (Uruguay) 32: 237

Rappaport M D, Villalba M 1990 A comparison of cholecysto- and choledochoenterostomy for obstructing pancreatic cancer. American Surgeon 56: 433–435

Rosemurgy A S, Burnett C M, Wasselle J A 1989 A comparison of choledochoenteric bypass and cholecystoenteric bypass in patients with biliary obstruction due to pancreatic cancer. American Surgeon 55: 55–60

Sarr M G, Cameron J L 1982 Surgical management of unresectable carcinoma of the pancreas. Surgery 91: 123–133

Saypol G M, Kurian G 1969 A technique of repair of stricture of the bile duct. Surgery, Gynecology & Obstetrics 51: 186–195

Schweizer W P, Matthews J B, Baer H U, Nudelmann L I, Triller J, Halter F, Gertsch P, Blumgart L H 1991 Combined surgical and interventional radiological approach for complex benign biliary tract obstruction. British Journal of Surgery 78: 559–563

Shamberger R C, Lund D P, Lillehei C W, Hendren W H 1995 Interposed jejunal segment with nipple valve to prevent reflux in biliary reconstruction. Journal of the American College of Surgeons 180: 10–15

Singh S M, Reber H A 1989 Surgical palliation for pancreatic cancer. Surgical Clinic of North America 69: 599–611

Smith R 1964 Hepaticojejunostomy with transhepatic intubation. British Journal of Surgery 51: 186–194

Smith R 1969 Strictures of the bile ducts. Proceedings of the Royal Society of Medicine 62: 131–137

Smith R 1981 Injuries of he bile ducts. In: Lord Smith of Marlow, Dame Sheila Sherlock (eds) Surgery of the gallbladder and bile ducts 2nd edn. London, Butterworths, Ch 19, p. 361

Soupault R, Couinaud C L 1957 Sur un procede nouveau de derivation biliaire intra-hepatique: les cholangio-jejunostomies gauches sans sacrifice hepatique. Presse Medicale 65: 1157–1159

Terblanche J, Saunders S J, Louw J H 1972 Prolonged palliation in carcinoma of the main hepatic duct junction. Surgery 71: 720–731

Voyles C R, Bowley N J, Allison D J, Benjamin I S, Blumgart L H 1983 Carcinoma of the proximal extrahepatic biliary tree radiologic assessment and therapeutic alternatives. Annals of Surgery 197: 188–194

Voyles C R, Blumgart L H 1982 A technique for the construction of high biliary-enteric anastomoses. Surgical Gynecology & Obstetrics 154: 885–887

Wheeler E S, Longmire W P Jr 1978 Repair of benign stricture of the common bile duct by jejunal interposition choledochoduodenostomy. Surgery, Gynecology & Obstetrics 146: 260–262

Gallstones and gallbladder

Gallstone formation

31

R. HERMON DOWLING

INTRODUCTION

The second (1988) edition of this book included a comprehensive review of gallstone formation and epidemiology. Much of the information in this chapter remains current today, and can be commended to the reader. Since then, however, there have been significant advances in this field particularly in our understanding of gallstone pathogenesis. Rather than attempting to re-write the entire chapter, the author has chosen to emphasize new developments in this area, which have emerged since the last edition.

The aim of this review is to focus on the genesis of cholecystolithiasis (gallbladder stones)—rather than on stones developing in the biliary tree (choledocholithiasis). The pathogenesis of gallbladder stones is quite different from that of stones forming in the biliary tract—as is the natural history of untreated stones in these two locations (Ch. 32). Moreover, the management of symptomatic choledocholithiasis is radically different from that of stones confined to the gallbladder.

Most investigators find that the natural history and surgical complications of gallstone disease are independent of gallstone type. In other words, in patients who develop specific symptoms, once the presence of the stones has been confirmed and the decision to operate taken, it does not matter if the stones consist predominantly of cholesterol, of bile pigments or of calcium salts. Despite this, the emphasis in this chapter is on the most common type of gallstone found in developed societies—the cholesterol-rich stone developing in the gallbladder.

There are several reasons for this decision. First, as noted above, cholesterol gallstones are by far the most common variety found in industrialized nations. Second, much more is known about the pathogenesis of cholesterol-rich stones than about the development of brown or black pigment stones. Third, in the past, medical (non-surgical) treatment of gallbladder stones was largely confined to the cholesterol-rich variety. In general, only cholesterol-rich stones could be dissolved using oral bile acid treatment or contact solvents, such as methyl tert butyl ether (MBTE) or ethyl propionate (Ch. 33). Today, the success of laparoscopic cholecystectomy means that the non-surgical approaches are seldom used. However, in the opinion of the author, there is still a limited role for oral bile acid treatment in selected patients who are at high risk for operation and/or anesthesia, or who wish to avoid a surgical operation.

CLASSIFICATION OF GALLSTONE TYPE AND COMPOSITION

During the past decade, there has been relatively little new work on gallstone classification and composition. Gallbladder stones are still classified as cholesterol stones, black pigment stones and brown pigment stones (Trotman & Soloway 1976, 1982, Soloway et al 1977).

BLACK PIGMENT STONES

Black pigment stones occur with increased frequency in patients with hemolysis (for any reason), and in those with hepatic cirrhosis (Bouchier 1969, Nicholas et al 1972, Duchmann et al 1997, De Olmo et al 1997, Benvegnu et al 1997, Maggi et al 1997, Conte et al 1999). They consist predominantly of polymerized bilirubin but may also contain calcium salts. Recent studies from Canada (Goresky et al 1995) have shown that, however efficient, the liver does not convert all the unconjugated bilirubin into bilirubin mono- and di-glucuronides: a small fraction of the unconjugated moiety escapes conjugation and 'spills' into bile. In situations where there is excessive hemolysis, or where hepatic function is impaired (as in cirrhosis), the fraction of bilirubin escaping conjugation in the liver increases. The resultant excess unconjugated bilirubin in bile is vulnerable to polymerization, and/or to co-precipitation with free ionized calcium. Indeed, Goresky et al (1995) showed that the pattern of bilirubin conjugates in bile is significantly different in gallstone patients from that in control subjects. The same conclusion was reached by Lesma et al from Italy (1997) who showed that in a subgroup of patients with cholesterol gallstones, there was more insoluble monoconjugated bilirubin in gallbladder bile, than normal.

If polymerization of unconjugated bilirubin and/or the co-precipitation of unconjugated bilirubin with free ionized calcium is indeed the basis of black pigment stones, the prevalence and incidence of non-cholesterol gallstones should not depend on the type of hemolysis. Most, but not all (Chawla et al 1997), recent evidence suggests that this is indeed the case. Thus Webb et al (1989) showed that in Jamaican children with homozygous sickle cell disease, approximately 50% had developed gallstones by the age of ten. Most of these stones were radio-opaque—suggesting that, in addition to polymerized bilirubin, the stones also contained calcium salts. The same group (Walker & Serjeant 1996) carried out a cohort study of sickle cell disease and detected sludge in seventeen which changed, with time, into discrete gallstones in 12 (71%)—which prompted the editorial suggestion that 'biliary sludge is a stone-in-waiting' (Werlin & Scott 1996). Certainly black pigment stones and sludge are common in sickle cell disease (Barrett-Connor 1968, Lachman et al 1979, Sarnaik et al 1980). The cation, calcium, co-precipitates with a number of anions in bile including bilirubinate, carbonate, phosphate and fatty acids (often described conveniently, but inaccurately, as 'palmitate').

BROWN PIGMENT STONES

Brown pigment stones are found more often in the biliary tree than in the gallbladder. Moreover in the Far East, these 'earthy' brown pigment stones occur more frequently than cholesterol-rich gallstones. This is usually attributed to bacterial infection, and occasionally to parasitic worms (*Ascaris lumbricoides*, *Clonorchis sinensis*, and even *Schistosoma japonicum*), in the biliary tree. The role of biliary parasites in the genesis of hepatolithiasis (intrahepatic stones) was the subject of a recent review (Leung & Yu 1997).

Since the previous edition of this book, several investigators (Ho et al 1995, 1996, Higashijima et al 1996) have revisited Maki's classical theory (1966) that brown pigment stones form in the biliary tree because of infection there.

Maki suggested that the bacterial enzyme, beta-glucuronidase, deconjugated the bilirubin mono- and di-glucuronides to yield unconjugated bilirubin, which then co-precipitated with calcium to form calcium bilirubinate. In turn, calcium bilirubinate combined with mucus glycoprotein, cellular debris, dead bacteria and amorphous material, to form typical 'earthy' brown pigment stones. Certainly, deconjugation of bilirubin, by incubation of sterile human gallbladder bile with beta-glucuronidase in vitro, accelerated the co-precipitation not only of bilirubin but also of cholesterol, fatty acids and glycoprotein (Higashijima et al 1996).

CHOLESTEROL-RICH GALLBLADDER STONES

Although the most common type of gallstone in Western society consists predominantly of cholesterol, in fact pure cholesterol gallstones are rare; most are mixed in composition—albeit still rich in cholesterol. The definition of 'cholesterol-rich' gallstones is somewhat arbitrary—ranging from more than 70% to more than 90% cholesterol by weight, on chemical analysis. By definition, therefore, 10 to 30% of these cholesterol-rich stones contain components other than cholesterol. Despite this, physical chemists and clinical investigators alike have repeatedly made the erroneous assumption that if one could understand and control cholesterol secretion and solubility in bile, it should be possible not only to understand how the stones form, but also to prevent them from forming in the first instance. This was also the basis for suggesting that once the cholesterol-rich stones have formed, it should be possible to dissolve them by rendering the bile unsaturated in cholesterol, with oral chenodeoxycholic acid (Danziger et al 1972a, Bell et al 1972).

As indicated above, the surgical management of patients with complicated gallstone disease is not influenced by gallstone composition: cholecystitis, biliary colic and gallstone-induced pancreatitis are likely to occur as frequently in patients with cholesterol, as in those with non-cholesterol, stones. However, since the pathogenesis of these various types of stones is radically different, if one wants to devise logical, scientifically-based strategies for their prevention, it would be an advantage if one could predict stone composition accurately and non-invasively. Furthermore, since oral bile acid treatment (with or without extracorporeal shock-wave lithotripsy (ESWL)) should be confined to patients with dissolvable stones, it is still sometimes important to be able to select patients with cholesterol-rich stones.

PREDICTION OF GALLSTONE TYPE

Before the advent of ultrasonography and computed tomographic (CT) scanning, the non-invasive prediction of gallstone type/composition relied on conventional radiology. In general, cholesterol gallstones are radiolucent by conventional radiography, while calcium containing stones are radio-opaque. It may be convenient for medical students to learn that 90% of gallstones are radiolucent while 90% of renal stones are radio-opaque. But even if one relies on traditional X-ray methods, this generalization is not correct. The results of epidemiological studies from Italy (GREPCO 1984) suggest that when gallbladder stones are detected by ultrasound screening and the patients then undergo cholecystography, approximately 30% of stones are radio-opaque. Similar results were reported by Plaisier et al (1994). They found that 26.3% of symptomatic patients with gallbladder stones had calcified stones—particularly if they had solitary (35%), rather than multiple (18%), stones. However, we now recognize that oral cholecystography is relatively insensitive in detecting the presence of small amounts of calcium, in vivo. CT scanning is much more sensitive.

Oral cholecystography (OCG) is seldom used today. Nonetheless during OCG, opacification of the gallbladder establishes that the cystic duct is patent (an essential requirement in patients being considered for oral bile acid treatment). Moreover, apart from giving us information about stone size and number, the lucency, buoyancy and contour of the stone(s) provide valuable clues about their composition. Indeed, Dolgin et al (1981) used discriminant analysis to refine the sensitivity of cholecystography in predicting gallstone composition.

Many groups (Rajagopal et al 1989, Brakel et al 1990, Walters et al 1992, Caroli et al 1992, Petroni et al 1995, Pereira et al 1997) have now shown that localized CT scanning of the gallbladder is by far the most sensitive method for predicting gallstone composition, in vivo. Thus, the maximum gallstone attenuation score, measured in Hounsfield units (HU), predicts gallstone composition. For example in one study, Rajagopal et al (1989) showed that the Hounsfield unit score, measured in vivo, correlated positively with both the total calcium ($r = 0.86$, $p < 0.0001$) and calcium carbonate ($r = 0.79$, $p < 0.001$), and negatively with the cholesterol ($r = -0.76$, $p < 0.001$), content of the stones measured in vitro. The HU score also predicted the rate of gallstone dissolution in vitro (Rajagopal et al 1989) and the dissolution response to oral bile acid treatment, in vivo (Rajagopal et al 1989, Caroli et al 1992, Petroni et al 1995, Pereira et al 1997). In order to obtain optimum gallstone dissolution response to oral bile acids, the maximum gallstone attenuation score before starting treatment should be less than 100 HU (Rajagopal et al 1989, Walters et al 1992) and preferably less than 75 HU (Pereira et al 1997). However, this conclusion was based on relatively small groups of patients and there was an imbalance in numbers between those with attenuation scores of > and < 75 HU. Thus 42 of 77 patients whose pre-treatment attenuation score was < 75 HU, became stone-free compared with only one of nine whose HU before starting oral bile acids was 75–100 HU.

When gallstones contain as little as 3% calcium salts by weight, they become radio-opaque (Rajagopal et al 1989). Moreover, Taylor and colleagues (1995) showed that as little as 3% calcium carbonate, by weight, could be detected by infrared spectroscopy of cholesterol-rich gallstones. However, radio-opacity of gallstones depends on the type of calcium salt present, and its distribution within the stone (Agarwal et al, 1993). Thus radio-opacity is usually due to the presence of calcium carbonate (and less frequently to calcium phosphate)— rather than to calcium bilirubinate or calcium fatty acid soaps. This is because the radius of the carbonate ion is small, and comparable in size to that of the calcium ion, while that of the bilirubinate and palmitate ions is relatively large. In other words, the large size of the bilirubin and fatty acid anions 'dilutes' the calcium and reduces the density of the radio-opaque material within the stones. Moreover, if the calcium salts are localized to one part of the gallstone, such as the center/nucleus or the rim/shell, the stone is more likely to appear radio-opaque than if the calcium salts are scattered diffusely throughout the stones.

CHOLESTEROL SOLUBILITY IN BILE

HISTORICAL ASPECTS

The cholesterol molecule has only one hydrophilic group in the 3-beta position. Therefore it is almost completely insoluble in water, and in aqueous media such as bile. Despite this, considerable quantities of cholesterol are 'carried' in normal bile as a clear, one-phase solution. In the past, it was assumed that the lipophilic cholesterol was solubilized in bile by the combined detergent action of bile acids and phospholipids. Indeed, in the 1950s, Isaksson and colleagues (1954) came close to defining the limits of cholesterol solubility in bile from the molar ratio of bile acids plus phospholipids:cholesterol, the so-called Isaksson ratio. They showed that the ratio was high in stone-free control subjects and low in gallstone carriers. However, there was considerable overlap between the two groups and this lack of sensitivity limited the value of measuring the Isaksson ratio.

Then in the 1960s, Small, Dervichian and colleagues (Small et al 1966, Bourges et al 1967a, 1967b) used classical physicochemical methods to characterize, more accurately, how cholesterol was solubilized by bile acids and phospholipids in water. They fixed the percentage of water at 90% (the proportion normally found in bile) and used triangular co-ordinates to prepare phase diagrams which defined the maximum solubility of cholesterol in model bile. This took the form of a curved boundary line which separated a one-phase micellar zone below from two or more phases, above. Subsequently, Admirand and Small (1968) applied these principles to humans and in a classic paper, showed that by measuring the relative molar concentrations of bile acids, phospholipids and cholesterol in native human bile (obtained by the needle puncture of the gallbladder at the time of cholecystectomy), it was possible to represent individual bile samples as single points on the triangular co-ordinate diagram. Furthermore, it was possible to distinguish between control subjects (whose bile composition fell within the one-phase micellar zone) and patients with gallstones (whose bile composition fell above the boundary line indicating that they all had supersaturated bile). Subsequently, many investigators studied duodenal bile (or, more correctly, bile-rich duodenal fluid) and again showed that it was possible to distinguish between unsaturated and supersaturated bile. Indeed, Thomas and Hofmann (1973) devised a polynomial equation to express individual bile results as saturation (SI) or lithogenic (LI) indices. Thus, an SI of 1.0 indicated a saturated solution: SIs of < 1.0 indicated unsaturated, while those of > 1.0 indicated supersaturated, bile.

For several reasons, we now know that there are limitations to this approach. First, many investigators were unable to reproduce Admirand and Small's original findings. In the hands of others (Holzbach et al 1973, Sedeghat & Grundy 1980, Busch et al 1990), many stone-free control subjects had supersaturated bile and there was a large degree of overlap in saturation indices between control subjects and gallstone patients (Muraca et al 1994). Second, as a result, the specificity of demonstrating supersaturated bile was low. The factor which distinguished best between stone-free controls and gallstone patients was not supersaturated bile but the nucleation time (Holan et al 1979)—that is, the time required for cholesterol micro-crystals to appear in bile, ex vivo (see below). Third, we now know that in dilute hepatic bile, cholesterol is not transported as micelles but rather as small phospholipid/cholesterol liposomes or vesicles (Somjen & Gilat 1983). In turn, there are unilamellar and multilamellar vesicles, although how these are defined depends on the methods used to detect them. These include gel permeation chromatography based on precise knowledge of the intermicellar bile acid concentration (Donovan et al 1991, 1998). Indeed, as discussed in the previous edition of this book, there may be multiple cholesterol transporters in bile including stacked lamellae (Somjen et al 1990, Corradini et al 1995)—although this is controversial (Cohen et al 1993).

QUANTITATIVE CHANGES: MEASUREMENT OF BILE LIPID SECRETION RATES

Despite the limitations of measuring cholesterol saturation indices in gallbladder bile, or in bile-rich duodenal fluid, the fashion for doing so remains current today. The presence of supersaturated bile is a pre-requisite for the development of gallstones: without it, they cannot form. However, measurement of the relative proportions of the three major lipids in bile provides only a 'snapshot' of bile composition at one point in time. Moreover, if the bile sample was supersaturated with cholesterol, there was no way of knowing whether the supersaturation was due to too much cholesterol, too few bile acids, too few phospholipids, or to some combined defect. However, by applying marker-corrected, duodenal secretion-perfusion techniques (Grundy & Metzger 1972a, Grundy et al 1972b, Adler et al 1974, Northfield & Hofmann 1975, Shaffer & Small 1977), it became possible to measure the hour-by-hour secretion rates of the three biliary lipids. These were difficult techniques for patients and investigators alike. They involved intubation of the duodenum with multi-lumen tubes which remained in situ for many hours. Nonetheless, the results obtained using these techniques were valuable. They showed that the bile could become supersaturated with cholesterol in multiple different ways. The principal defect is undoubtedly hypersecretion of cholesterol (Nilsell et al 1985)—particularly in the obese (Bennion & Grundy 1975, Mabee et al 1976, Shaffer & Small 1977, Reuben et al 1985) who are pre-disposed to develop cholesterol-rich gallstones. However, supersaturated bile may also result from hyposecretion of bile acids or phospholipids (or both). This may relate to the reduced bile acid pool size seen in gallstone patients (Vlahcevic et al 1970, 1972) although there is controversy about whether the small bile acid pool in these individuals, cycles with normal (Reuben et al 1985), or increased (Northfield & Hofmann 1975), frequency.

QUALITATIVE CHANGES

In addition to the quantitative changes in bile lipid composition and secretion discussed above, qualitative changes in bile acid, and phospholipid fatty acid, composition may also be important.

The individual bile acids vary considerably in their detergent properties, and therefore in their capacity to solubilize cholesterol in bile (and other lipids in the intestinal lumen). However, this must not be considered in isolation. In the context of gallstone formation, one is more concerned about the combined detergent action of bile acids plus phospholipids, in solubilizing biliary cholesterol. However, the balance between hydrophobic and hydrophilic bile acids may also influence the pattern of bile lipid secretion across the canalicular membrane. Certainly it is known that oral bile acid treatment with the hydrophilic bile acids, cheno- or urso-deoxycholic acids, reduces biliary cholesterol secretion and saturation (Nilsell et al 1983, von Bergmann et al 1984). Conversely, when the percentage of the hydrophobic bile acid, deoxycholic acid, increases in bile (as a result of a variety of maneuvers, see below), the moles % cholesterol and the saturation indices, also rise (Marcus & Heaton 1986, 1988). The proportion of deoxycholic acid (DCA) may also influence the luminal concentrations of pro-nucleators, such as immunoglobulin G (IgG) and mucus glycoprotein (Sanabria et al 1995). Although the evidence incriminating DCA in the pathogenesis of cholesterol gallstones is strong, it is largely indirect and somewhat controversial (Noshiro et al 1995, Jungst et al 1999).

If there is uncertainty about the role of hydrophobic bile acids, such as deoxycholic acid, in the pathogenesis of gallstones, there is even less information about the importance of phospholipid fatty acid composition. Nonetheless, the results of several studies (Cantafora et al 1981, Berr et al 1992, Angelico et al 1992, Hatsushika et al 1993) suggest that when the proportion of arachidonic acid-rich phospholipids increases, there are adverse effects on the partitioning of cholesterol between vesicles and micelles, and on cholesterol solubility in bile (Demel et al 1972).

In bile, the principal phospholipid is phosphatidyl choline. It has a phosphoryl choline head group and, in common with other phospholipids, two long-chain fatty acids. The first of these, in the substitution one (sn-1) position, is almost invariably a saturated fatty acid while the second, in the sn-2 position, is usually unsaturated. The double bonds make the unsaturated fats rigid and space-occupying. This is particularly true when the sn-2 fatty acid is arachidonic acid. When this occurs, there is preferential 'shunting' of the arachidonic acid-rich phospholipids from the vesicles to the micelles. As a result, the molar ratio of cholesterol: phospholipids in the vesicles increases. They then become vulnerable to fusion and aggregation (Afdhal et al 1995), with the formation of unstable multi-lamellar vesicles, from which cholesterol micro-crystals precipitate (Kibe et al 1984). However, the various cholesterol 'carriers' (vesicles, micelles, etc.) in bile reach an equilibrium (Noshiro et al 1992) and crystalline cholesterol probably precipitates from all the various carriers, and not just from aggregated, unstable, multi-lamellar vesicles—at least in animal models (Ahrendt et al 1994).

THE TRIPLE DEFECT IN CHOLESTEROL GALLSTONE FORMATION

SUPERSATURATION

Although supersaturation of bile with cholesterol (or other solutes) is a *sine qua non* for cholesterol gallstone formation, as indicated above, it is a non-specific finding: supersaturation is common in stone-free controls. However, measurement of the cholesterol micro-crystal nucleation time does discriminate well between stone formers and gallstone-free subjects (Holan et al 1979). In other words, although supersaturation of bile with cholesterol is an essential prerequisite for stone formation, supersaturation is only part of the story. The precipitation of micro-crystals of cholesterol usually requires some additional factor, known as the nucleation defect—an imbalance between promoters and inhibitors of micro-crystal precipitation.

NUCLEATION DEFECT

When a sample of fresh bile is filtered or centrifuged (rendering it a one-phase isotropic solution), maintained at 37°C in a dust-free, clean environment and examined daily under the microscope, the time at which cholesterol micro-crystals appear is defined as the nucleation time (measured in days). In stone-free individuals, the nucleation time is long (> 10–15 days) but in stone formers it is abnormally rapid (< 5, and often < 2–3, days). Given the fact that the gallbladder fills and empties several times each day, it is obvious that the 'residence time' of bile within the gallbladder is measured in hours, while the nucleation time in vitro is measured in days. Therefore, the value of the measurement is in comparative studies between individuals (or groups of individuals). Moreover, the technique for measuring nucleation time is crude and imprecise. For this reason, alternative terms, such as the cholesterol micro-crystal detection, observation or appearance time, have been proposed (Corradini et al 1995, Lipsett et al 1995) and alternative methods, such as cholesterol crystal growth assays (Busch et al 1990b, Teramen et al 1995, Janciauskiene et al 1998, Ringel et al 1998), developed.

Although an entire chapter could be devoted to the nucleation defect in cholesterol gallstone formation, for the non-expert, research into pro- and anti-nucleating factors has proved to be a difficult and confusing field. Suffice to say that a large number of pro-nucleating, and a much smaller number of anti-nucleating, factors has now been identified (Table 31.1). Most of the cholesterol crystal promoters and inhibitors are proteins and of these, mucin or mucus glyco-

Table 31.1 Partial list of putative pro- and anti-nucleating substances shown to promote or inhibit the nucleation/precipitation of cholesterol microcrystals in model and/or native human gallbladder bile (see also review by He et al 1999)

Pro-nucleators		Anti-nucleators	
ACon A Bound 130 kDa (later shown to be Aminopeptidase-N)	Groen et al 1990 Nunez et al 1995 Offner et al 1994 Rigotti et al 1993	Apolipoproteins A-I, A-II	Kibe et al 1984a Donovan et al 1987
Phosopholipase C Fibronectin	Pattinson et al 1991 Chijiiwa et al 1991	Apolipoprotein B	Ahmed et al 1994
'A low density particle'	De Bruijn 1996		
Acute phase proteins α-1-acid glycoprotein	Abei et al 1993	Lectin bound proteins	Busch et al 1995
Haptoglobin	Yamashita et al 1996	*Helix pomatia* bound protein (120 kDa with 63 kDa subunits)	Busch et al 1993
Immunoglobulin A (IgA) Immunoglobulin M (IgM) Immunoglobulin G (IgG)	Upadhya et al 1993 LaRusso 1984 Harvey et al 1991	Phospholipids	Jungst et al 1993 Ringel et al 1998
Serpins (serine proteinase inhibitors) in low concentrations α-1-antitrypsin and α-1-antichymotrypsin	Janciauskiene et al 1998 Zijlstra et al 1996	*Serpins* (serine proteinase inhibitors) in high concentrations α-1-antitrypsin and α-1-antichymotrypsin	Janciauskiene et al 1998
Mucin glycoproteins (Mucus)	Lee et al 1981a Levy et al 1984 Gallinger et al 1985 Smith et al 1986 Afdhal et al 1993 Shiffman et al 1993b		
Non-mucin glycoproteins 84 kDa	Lipsett et al 1995		
Con A Bound Glycoproteins 40,50,58,80,98,143 kDa	Teramen et al 1995		
Anionic Polypeptide Fraction (6.5 kDa): Calcium binding protein (14 kDa) (APF/CBP)	Lafont et al 1997	Anionic Polypeptide Fraction (in vitro)	Konikoff et al 1997
Deoxycholic acid (?indirect effect)	Hussaini et al 1995	Ursodeoxycholic acid	Jungst et al 1993 Tudyka et al 1994
Ionized Calcium (vesicle aggregation and fusion)	Teramen et al 1995	Fatty acid, bile acid Conjugates (FABACs)	Gilat et al 2000
Transferrin	Janciauskiene et al 1996		
Arachidonic acid-rich phospholipids	Konikoff et al 1994b		
Hydrophilic proteins (myoglobin, chymotrypsin)	Ahmed et al 1994		

protein (MGP) is particularly important as a pro-nucleator (Levy et al 1984, Afdhal et al 1993, Shiffman et al 1993b) even if there is considerable heterogeneity of biliary mucins in humans (Klinspoor et al, 1994). Mucin is encoded by mucin core polypeptide genes (the MUC genes) (Kim & Gun 1995) which may well be important in the pathogenesis of cholesterol gallstones (Offner et al 1996, Kano et al 1998). In some cases, proteins extracted from native bile have been added to model bile solutions, and shown to accelerate the precipitation of cholesterol micro-crystals from supersaturated solutions. However, critics claim that many of these pronucleating proteins are not relevant physiologically (Yamashita et al 1995, LaFont et al 1997). Nonetheless, the importance of identifying promoters and inhibitors of cholesterol micro-crystal nucleation/precipitation lies in the hope that if one could decrease the concentration of the promoters, or increase the concentration of the inhibitors, it should be possible to prevent this crucial stage in the development of gallstones.

GALLBLADDER STASIS

In theory, it would not matter if susceptible individuals developed supersaturated bile and/or abnormal nucleation —provided that an actively motile gallbladder contracted efficiently and expelled resultant micro-crystals, into the duodenum. However, we have known for many years that in patients with gallstone disease, on average there is impaired gallbladder emptying (Fisher et al 1982, Forgacs et al 1984a, Pomeranz & Shaffer 1985, Festi et al 1990, Howard et al 1991, Jazrawi et al 1995). Moreover, the results of studies in experimental animals and humans suggest that impaired gallbladder emptying in response to food (or other cholecystokinetic stimuli) antedates, and contributes to, cholesterol gallstone formation. Thus when prairie dogs or Richardson ground squirrels are fed a lithogenic diet which induces the formation of supersaturated bile, the animals showed evidence of gallbladder stasis *before* the micro-crystals or gallstones developed (Gurll et al 1977, Meyer et al 1978, Roslyn et al 1980, Doty et al 1983, Fridhandler et al 1983, Pellegrini et al 1986, Pauletzki et al 1995). Similarly, in a simple but important clinical study, van der Linden and colleagues (1974) measured gallbladder motor function in 21 individuals who initially were gallstone-free and, on the basis of the results, divided them into 'strong' and 'weak' contractors. He then followed the patients for 14 years and found stones in seven of the twelve weak contractors, but in only one of the strong contractors. Furthermore, impaired gallbladder emptying is an independent determinant of gallstone recurrence in patients whose stones were cleared with lithotripsy. Thus Pauletski et al (1996) showed that over a 3-year period, recurrent stones formed in 53% of patients who had an ejection fraction of < 60%, compared with only 13% of patients whose ejection fraction was equal to or > 60%. Many other investigators have studied gallbladder motor function and, on the basis of the results, divided the patients into strong and weak contractors (for review, see Portincasa et al 1995). Whether this retrospective splitting of the patients/subjects into two groups is justified or not, is debatable. In the opinion of the author, it is justifiable but only if there is a bi-modal distribution of data—as opposed to a spectrum of results, some of which are normal and overlap with control values.

There is also a long list of conditions in which gallbladder motor dysfunction, and a high prevalence of gallstones, co-exist. This includes pregnancy (Friedman et al 1966, Valdivieso et al 1983, Maringhini et al 1987, Braverman et al 1980, Bolondi et al 1985, Maringhini et al 1993, Hahm et al 1997, Van Bodegraven et al 1998), total parenteral nutrition (Messing et al 1983, Roslyn et al 1983, Cano et al 1986, Nakano et al 1992), somatostatinomas (Krejs 1986), chronic octreotide treatment (Dowling et al 1992, Redfern & Fortuner 1995, Newman et al 1995), high spinal cord injury (Apstein & Dalecki-Chipperfield 1987, Stone et al 1990, Ketover et al 1996, Tandon et al 1997), vagotomy (Sapala et al 1970, Tompkins et al 1972, Ihasz & Griffith 1981, Masclee et al 1990), gastrectomy (Inove et al 1992, Ikeda et al 1995, Chijiiwa et al 1996, Maselli et al 1996), obesity (Weinsier et al 1955, Palasciano et al 1992, Spirt et al 1995, Attili et al 1995, Misciagna et al 1996) and, more important, rapid weight loss—as a result of very low calorie (500–600 kcal/day) diets (Shiffman et al 1991, Marks et al 1996, Gebhard et al 1996, Vezina et al 1998), or gastric by-pass surgery (Shiffman et al 1993a, Sugerman et al 1995, 1998)—and even prolonged overnight fasting (Ortega et al 1997, Attili et al 1998).

ROLE OF MUCUS GLYCOPROTEIN

In susceptible experimental animals, gallstone formation can be induced by feeding the appropriate lithogenic diet. Given these controlled conditions, it is possible to examine the gallbladder carefully at regular intervals, before and during stone formation. When this is done, the gallbladder is found to synthesize and secrete excess mucus glycoprotein which forms a gel on the surface of the gallbladder mucosa. In the early stages of gallstone formation, all the crystals and micro-calculi are trapped in the surface gel (Smith 1987, Rege & Pyrstowsky 1998). Whether or not this phenomenon also happens in spontaneous *human* gallstone formation, is unknown. Nonetheless, crystal trapping by mucus glycoprotein gel is another component of stasis within the gallbladder.

Apart from the influence of mucus glycoprotein on the nucleation and trapping of cholesterol micro-crystals, mucin may also be involved as a cement substance by acting as an 'endoskeleton' for crystal agglomeration and growth. Many years ago, Bouchier et al (1965) showed that split gallstones could be stained for the presence of mucin. Later, Sutor and Wooley (1974) showed that after the crystalline component of gallstones had been dissolved, an opalescent sponge-like structure remained which was almost certainly a mucus glycoprotein skeleton. De la

Porte et al (de la Porte et al 1996) noted that the crystals of cholesterol-rich gallstones were arrayed on a mucin plus protein matrix. They suggested that the cholesterol crystals bound directly to the mucin. Similarly, Bogren et al (1995) found that there was an inorganic matrix in all human gallstones.

ROLE OF BACTERIA

Many years ago, Lord Moynihan suggested that 'A gallstone is a tombstone erected to the memory of the organism within it'. However most gallstones, and samples of gallbladder bile removed at surgery, proved to be sterile. As a result, Moynihan's aphorism fell into disrepute—until the advent of scanning electron microscopy and molecular techniques which revived the concept that bacteria might be important in the genesis of cholesterol (as opposed to pigment gallstones (Trotman and Soloway 1976, Soloway et al 1977, Trotman and Soloway 1982).

By scanning electron microscopy, several investigators have noted the presence of chains of cocci on the outer surface and in the interior of split gallstones, often nestling in the clefts between sheets of crystals (Wetter et al 1994). Recently, Swidsinski et al (1998) used the nested polymerase chain reaction (PCR), followed by cloning and sequencing of the PCR products, to look for bacteria DNA in gallstones. On routine bacteriological culture, only 9% of gallstones from 100 patients were positive although bacterial DNA was found in the stones from 82 of the remaining 91 patients (90%). Lee et al (1999) also studied bacterial DNA in different types of gallstones and found that most mixed cholesterol stones had bacterial DNA sequences whereas only one in seven (14%) pure cholesterol stone yielded a PCR product.

ROLE OF NON-CHOLESTEROL MATERIAL AT THE CORE OF CHOLESTEROL GALLSTONES

It has been known for many years that when human cholesterol-rich gallstones are split in two, the interior may display a radiating, spoke-like array of cholesterol crystals but in the center of the stone, there is often a non-cholesterol, pigment-rich core or nucleus which consists of calcium bilirubinate, calcium carbonate and mucin (Womack et al 1963, Kaufman et al 1994). This observation fuelled the speculation that the initiating event in the formation of cholesterol-rich stones is not the deposition of cholesterol crystals, but the precipitation of bile pigments and calcium salts.

It is beyond the scope of this chapter to review the factors governing the solubility and precipitation of bile pigments and calcium salts in patients who form non-cholesterol stones (or at least pigment/calcium salt cores in otherwise cholesterol-rich stones). Nonetheless, a few of the underlying principles are summarized here.

SOLUBILITY AND PRECIPITATION OF CALCIUM SALTS IN BILE

As indicated above, the most common calcium salt in gallstones is calcium carbonate. Calcium salts precipitate out of solution when the product of their cation concentration, times their anion concentration, exceeds the solubility product (or K'SP) of that salt. The K'SP for vaterite (one of the crystalline forms of calcium carbonate) has been determined in saline (Moore & Verine 1985) and this has been used as a 'gold standard' to work out a calcium carbonate saturation index (Knyrim et al 1989, 1992)—in much the same way that the biliary cholesterol saturation index was derived.

MEASUREMENT OF CALCIUM AND CARBONATE ION CONCENTRATIONS IN BILE

The [calcium ion] × [carbonate ion] product has been studied both in human (Marteau et al 1990, Gleeson et al 1992) and in animal bile. Biliary $[Ca^{++}]$ can be measured using a calcium-selective electrode but when free ionized calcium concentrations were compared in patients with calcified stones, with those from patients with cholesterol stones, there were no significant differences (Gleeson et al 1992). However, one group of investigators (Rudnicki et al 1992) did find that the ionized calcium in gallbladder bile was significantly higher in patients with gallstone disease, than in those without gallstones. In patients with radio-opaque (calcified) stones, the defect leading to calcium carbonate precipitation must lie with the anion. However, determination of the carbonate ion concentration is more difficult and less direct, than measurement of the calcium ion concentration. Nonetheless, the $[CO_3^{--}]$ can be derived, indirectly, by measuring pH and pCO_2 with a blood gas analyzer, and total CO_2 with a microgasometer—using a modification of the van Slyke method. The carbonate ion concentration $[CO_3^{--}]$ can then be derived from the Henderson–Hasselbalch equation and Henry's law, the ion product $[Ca^{++}] \times [CO_3^{--}]$, calculated, and the results related to the K'SP for $Ca\,CO_3$ (vaterite), in saline (Moore & Verine 1985).

THE $[Ca^{++}] \times [CO_3^{--}]$ PRODUCT: HEPATIC VERSUS GALLBLADDER BILE

Using this approach, several groups of investigators have measured the $[Ca^{++}] \times [CO_3^{--}]$ product in different situations (Knyrim et al 1989, Marteau et al 1990, Rudnicki et al 1992, Knyrim et al 1992, Gleeson et al 1992, 1995)—such as comparing hepatic bile versus gallbladder bile (Gleeson et al 1992) or in gallbladder bile from patients with radio-opaque, calcium-containing stones versus those with radiolucent, cholesterol gallstones (Andrews 1933, Harvey et al 1985, Marteau et al 1990, Gleeson et al 1992). When the cation $\times$ anion concentrations are compared in gallbladder and hepatic biles, there are obvious and significant differences between the two. Hepatic bile is almost invariably supersaturated with calcium carbonate and the mean $[Ca^{++}] \times [CO_3^{--}]$ product there, is high (around $4.7 \times 10^{-8}(mol/L)^2$). In contrast, normal gallbladder bile is usually unsaturated in calcium carbonate and its mean $[Ca^{++}] \times [CO_3^{--}]$ product is $1.9 \times 10^{-8}(mol/L)^2$. That being the case, one might expect that calcified gallstones would form in the biliary tree—rather than in the gallbladder. However, as for cholesterol cholelithiasis, supersaturation alone is not sufficient to explain stone formation. Additional factors, such as stagnation or stasis, seem to be equally important in the pathogenesis of calcium-containing stones, as they were for cholesterol-rich gallstones. Even though the solubility of calcium carbonate is precarious in the biliary tree, the flow rate of hepatic bile there is high, and presumably high enough to prevent calcium salt precipitation.

THE $[CA^{++}] \times [CO_3^{--}]$ PRODUCT IN BILE FROM PATIENTS WITH CALCIFIED VERSUS CHOLESTEROL STONES

In patients who form calcified gallstones, although the gallbladder bile is supersaturated with calcium carbonate, the cation concentration $[Ca^{++}]$, is normal. The factor responsible for the supersaturation is a high anion concentration $[CO_3^{--}]$. In turn, the explanation for the high carbonate ion concentration seems to be defective acid secretion by a diseased gallbladder mucosa (for review, see Plevris & Bouchier 1995). The normal gallbladder secretes hydrogen ions (and absorbs bicarbonate ions) which ensures that the biliary calcium carbonate remains in solution. However, in patients with calcium-containing radio-opaque gallstones, the impaired hydrogen ion secretion results in a raised pH within the gallbladder lumen. In turn, this is responsible for a low $[CO_2]$, a high $[CO_3^{--}]$ and, therefore, a high $[Ca^{++}] \times [CO_3^{--}]$ product in gallbladder bile (Gleeson et al 1992), which exceeds the K'SP for calcium carbonate in saline (and, presumably, in bile).

RECENT DEVELOPMENTS IN BILIARY CHOLESTEROL SUPERSATURATION

THE GENETIC CONTROL OF BILIARY CHOLESTEROL SECRETION

Hints that cholesterol secretion and saturation, and therefore the risk of cholesterol gallstone formation, might be under genetic control came from epidemiological studies which showed that the prevalence of gallstone disease was higher in the first degree relatives of index cases, than in matched controls (Danziger et al 1972b, van der Linden 1973, Gilat et al 1983, Pixley et al 1985, Jorgensen 1988, Kesaniemi et al 1989, Sarin et al 1995, Attili et al 1997, Miquel et al 1998). For example, Sarin et al (1995) found that in 39 of 105 index cases (37%), one or more family members had gallstones (positive index cases). Put another way, 51 of 330 first-degree relatives had gallstones (15.5%) compared with a prevalence of only 12 of 330 matched controls (3.6%)—a four and a half times increase in the relative risk. In the large Italian multicenter study (MICOL) of almost 30 000 individuals, Attili et al (1997) found that there was a significant association between a positive maternal family history, and the presence of gallstone disease in both men and women. There was also a significant link between a positive paternal family history and the presence of gallstone disease in women. Moreover in Chilean Amerindians and Hispanics (who have a high prevalence of gallstones), cholesterol lithogenic genes are found frequently (Miquel et al 1998). However, the most convincing evidence that bile lipid secretion is at least partly under genetic control, comes from two separate groups of studies in experimental animals.

TRANSGENIC ANIMALS

In the Netherlands, Smit and colleagues (1993) were studying the role of the multiple drug resistance (mdr) gene in oncology (Oude Elferink & Groen 1995a, Kuipers et al 1997). They developed a homozygous transgenic 'knock-out' model in which the mdr-2 gene was deleted (mdr 2 −/−). This gene encodes for a canalicular p-glycoprotein that functions as a 'flippase', flipping phosphatidylcholine from the inner to the outer hemi-leaflet of the canalicular membrane. When the gene encoding the mdr-2 p-glycoprotein is disrupted, the animal continues to secrete bile acids normally but phospholipid secretion into bile is absent while cholesterol secretion is minimal (Oude Elferink et al 1995b). These severe abnormalities of bile lipid secretion cause liver disease (Smit et al 1993, Mauad et al 1994, Oude Elferink et al 1995b) with bile duct proliferation and portal inflammation (Mauad et al 1994), are incompatible with life and animals often die a few days after birth. The corresponding gene in humans is called the MDR-3 gene and already two patients have been identified with a deficiency of this gene and an associated severe disruption of bile lipid secretion and hepatic function (Deleuze et al 1996, Jacquemin et al 1997).

Although dramatic, the relevance of these interesting observations to human gallstone disease is uncertain. However, they clearly establish that in animals, and perhaps also in man, bile lipid secretion can be influenced markedly by genes. (For reviews, see Oude Elferink & Groen 1995a, Kuipers et al 1997).

LITH GENES IN INBRED STRAINS OF MICE

In Boston, Carey and colleagues (Khanuja et al 1995, Wang et al 1997, Lammert et al 1999) have been studying inbred strains (C57/L; SWR; SWA; C57BL/6; C3H and SJL) of mice which are susceptible to cholesterol gallstone formation, when fed a lithogenic diet—one containing 15% dairy fat, 1% cholesterol and 0.5% cholic acid. These investigators compared strains of animals which had high, intermediate and low prevalence rates of stone formation and found a major gene, named Lith 1, which mapped to mouse chromosome 2. They showed that the hepatic activity of the rate-limiting enzyme for cholesterol synthesis, HMGCoA-reductase, was up- and down-regulated in response to changes in dietary cholesterol in the gallstone-resistant, but not in gallstone-susceptible, strains. They suggested that the genetic regulation of cholesterol homeostasis, via the rate-limiting enzyme in cholesterol synthesis, was pivotal in determining the severity of cholesterol hypersecretion, and therefore the lithogenicity of gallbladder bile and the risk of cholesterol gallstone formation.

The results of these studies are, at the same time, both compelling and fascinating. Nonetheless, their relevance to human gallstone disease is uncertain. In family studies where there is a high incidence and prevalence of gallstone disease in first degree relatives (Danziger et al 1972b, van der Linden 1973, Gilat et al 1983, Pixley et al 1985, Jorgensen 1988, Kesaniemi et al 1989, Sarin et al 1995, Attili et al 1997, Miquel et al 1998), it remains to be seen if molecular genetic studies can identify 'marker genes' responsible for abnormal bile lipid secretion and cholesterol-gallstone formation.

The molecular biology of the bile acid and bile lipid transporters has been studied extensively in recent years, as has the molecular control of hepatic bile acid and cholesterol synthesis. However, these are somewhat peripheral to the objectives of this chapter. They are, therefore, not discussed

further but for those readers who are interested, several excellent reviews on these topics can be recommended (Crawford et al 1995, Muller & Jansen 1998).

RECENT DEVELOPMENTS IN CHOLESTEROL MICRO-CRYSTAL NUCLEATION

IDENTIFICATION OF NEW PRO- AND ANTI-NUCLEATING FACTORS

Table 1 summarizes the ever-growing list of promoters ($n = 14$) and inhibitors ($n = 5$) of cholesterol crystal precipitation. As indicated above, most of these factors are proteins and the strongest evidence incriminates mucus glycoprotein (MGP) as a pro-nucleator (Lee et al 1981a, 1981b, LaMont et al 1984, Levy et al 1984, Gallinger et al 1985, Smith & LaMont 1985, Smith 1987). (Basic aspects of the role of mucus glycoproteins in the pathogenesis of gallstones were reviewed recently by Madrid et al 1997.)

Several recent studies have emphasized the role of non-mucin glycoproteins, as promoters of cholesterol crystal precipitation. These non-mucin glycoproteins can be isolated from bile by lectin affinity chromatography—using columns containing conconavalin A, *Helix pomatia* and even lentils! However, there is little agreement about the molecular size/weight of these candidate proteins. Thus Lipsett et al (1995) isolated an 84 kDa non-mucin pro-nucleating glycoprotein while Busch and colleagues (1995) identified 16, 28, 63 and 74 kDa anti-nucleating glycoproteins which inhibited crystal growth by 40 to 76%—apparently by binding to the cholesterol crystals. In contrast, Teramen et al (1995) isolated six different conconavalin A-bound glycoproteins (40, 50, 58, 80, 98 and 143 kDa), all of which either shortened the nucleation time, accelerated the growth of the cholesterol micro-crystals, or both.

The inhibitors of cholesterol crystal nucleation include the apolipoproteins A-I and A-II, and phospholipids. Thus, Jungst et al (1993) showed that the addition of micromolar amounts of synthetic or naturally occurring phosphatidyl-cholines to aliquots of gallbladder bile, increased the nucleation times from around 2 days to > 21 days.

THE ROLE OF ASPIRIN AND NONSTEROIDAL ANTI-INFLAMMATORY DRUGS (NSAIDS)

Since mucus glycoprotein (MGP) has been shown repeatedly to promote cholesterol crystal nucleation/precipitation (Lee et al 1981a, 1981b, LaMont et al 1984, Levy et al 1984, Gallinger et al 1985, Smith & LaMont 1985, Smith

1987), several investigators have studied the mechanisms controlling MGP synthesis and secretion, within the gall-bladder. Thus, Carey and Cahalane (1993) postulated that arachidonic acid, originating from the hydrolysis of biliary phospholipids, might act as a precursor for prostaglandin synthesis within the gallbladder wall. This postulate was supported by the results of recent studies from Japan (Shoda et al 1997) which showed that phospholipase A2 was increased in the gallbladder wall and in gallbladder bile, of patients with multiple cholesterol gallstones, and this was associated with increased prostaglandin E2 levels and increased free arachidonate. If this concept is correct, the use of cyclo-oxygenase inhibitors, such as aspirin or NSAIDs, might be expected to inhibit prostaglandin synthesis and, thereby, to reduce mucus glycoprotein synthesis and secretion. The evidence that it does so is controversial: it was reviewed in a recent editorial (Sterling & Shiffman 1998).

A group of gastroenterologists from Boston (Lee et al 1981a, LaMont et al 1983) showed that when prairie dogs are given a lithogenic diet, they develop supersaturated bile and gallstones. These and other authors (Freston et al 1969, Sahlin et al 1992) also showed that the lithogenic diet induces excess mucus glycoprotein synthesis and secretion *before* micro-crystal and stone formation. Furthermore, when the animals were given a lithogenic diet plus aspirin, the experimental gallstone formation was prevented (Lee et al 1981b). Similar results were seen with a novel leukotriene/5-lipoxygenase inhibitor (Kam et al 1996).

Later, Broomfield and colleagues (1988) showed that in high-dose (1300 mg per day), aspirin inhibited the micro-crystal, micro-stone and gallstone formation that would otherwise have occurred, in obese patients undergoing rapid weight loss (who are at increased risk of gallstone formation) (Shiffman et al 1991, Shiffman et al 1993, Sugerman et al 1995, Gebhard et al 1996, Marks et al 1996, Sugerman et al 1998, Vezina et al 1998). Ursodeoxycholic acid also reduces the nucleation time—in part by lowering biliary cholesterol secretion and saturation, and in part by inhibiting gallbladder mucin (Broomfield et al 1988, Shiffman et al 1993b).

On this basis, Hood and colleagues from the British–Belgian gallstone study group carried out a retrospective survey of NSAID consumption in 75 patients whose gallstones had been dissolved completely with oral bile acid treatment (Hood et al 1988). They compared gallstone recurrence rates in the 12 individuals who regularly took aspirin and/or NSAIDs, with those in the 63 patients who never (or only occasionally) took these drugs. The regular ingestion of the cyclo-oxygenase inhibitors completely prevented gallstone recurrence while in patients who never (or

only rarely) took NSAIDs, 20 of the 63 individuals developed recurrence stones ($p < 0.02$).

However, aspirin and NSAIDs have other effects on the gallbladder—including a stimulatory effect on gallbladder emptying (O'Donnell et al 1992; Das et al 1995). Thus, Das and colleagues (1995) showed that after 2 weeks aspirin treatment in doses of 350 or 1400 mg/day, the gallbladder ejection fraction improved. O'Donnell et al (1992) found similar results and suggested that the protective effect of NSAIDs against gallstone recurrence (Hood et al 1988) might be explained not by their influence on the mucus glycoproteins, but rather by their effect on gallbladder emptying.

Rhodes et al (1992) studied the effect of one 300 mg aspirin tablet/day for 7 days, on mucus glycoprotein synthesis by explants of freshly excised human gallbladders, 'harvested' at the time of cholecystectomy, and maintained in organ culture for 24 hours. There was a considerable scatter of the data for 3-H glucosamine (precursor) incorporation into the glycoprotein component of mucin, with some overlap in results between the untreated and treated groups. Nonetheless, the mean value in the aspirin-treated patients (1347 fmol/g wet weight) was approximately half that in the untreated disease controls (2008 fmol/g wet weight; $p < 0.005$). Similar results were reported by Sterling et al (1995). In morbidly obese individuals whose bile was examined at the time of gastric by-pass surgery, the concentration of mucus within the gallbladder was increased in those with stones, but decreased in those with stones and 'a history of chronic NSAID use'. Moreover, Marks et al (1996) showed that in obese patients taking very low calorie weight reduction diets, ibuprofen in a dose of 1600 mg/day for 12 weeks countered the adverse effects of the diet on biliary cholesterol saturation, microcrystal nucleation and growth, and gallbladder contraction.

Taken at face value, the results of these studies might suggest that treatment with cyclo-oxygenase inhibitors should prevent stone formation/recurrence in high-risk groups. However, this is not the whole story. When investigators from the Department of Surgery at Boston University (O'Leary et al 1991) and elsewhere (Myers et al 1989) tried to repeat the early studies of Lee (1981a) and LaMont (1983), they were unable to do so. It now seems that this model of gallstone disease is distinctly fickle. The vulnerability of these animals to develop diet-induced gallstones may depend on their sex, and even on the time of the year when the studies are carried out. This may also explain why Cohen et al (1991) found that aspirin did not prevent gallstone formation either in hamsters or in prairie dogs, given lithogenic diets. Moreover, several other groups have studied the effect of long-term aspirin and/or NSAID ingestion on the prevalence and incidence of human gallstone disease—again with negative results (Kurata et al 1991, Attili et al 1997, Pazzi et al 1998).

THE MORPHOLOGY OF CRYSTALLINE CHOLESTEROL PRECIPITATES

Since bile is an aqueous medium (containing approximately 90% water), it was assumed that when biliary cholesterol precipitated out of solution, it always did so as typical, triclinic crystals of cholesterol monohydrate—flat rhomboid-shaped crystals which often had a notch missing from one corner (Craven 1976, Loomis et al 1979). Indeed, it is this form of crystalline cholesterol which is readily identified in samples of gallbladder bile or bile-rich duodenal fluid, from patients with cholesterol gallstones. However, as a result of studies from the United States, Israel and the Netherlands (Konikoff et al 1992, 1994; Portincasa et al 1996a, van Erpecum et al 1996a), we now know that initially at least, cholesterol precipitates as anhydrous crystals of many different forms. These include arcs, needles, spirals or helical structures, tubules, ribbons, triangular or trapezoid, and asymmetrical or symmetrical monoclinic (hexagonal) crystals etc. The results of studies using model bile solutions suggest that the crystal morphology is influenced by the type of bile acid present (van Erpecum et al 1996a).

Since cholesterol precipitates preferentially as triclinic crystals, and this is the form recognized in native human bile, the clinical significance of identifying transient anhydrous forms of cholesterol crystals is doubtful. (For further information, see recent reviews (O'Leary 1995, Portincasa et al 1997a)).

RECENT DEVELOPMENTS IN GALLBLADDER STASIS

Several investigators have examined the influence of changes in the bile acid and lipid composition of gallbladder bile, on gallbladder motor function. Thus in an elegant series of experiments, Behar Chen and colleagues (Behar 1989, 1993, Yu 1995, Chen 1997a, 1997b, 1999) have shown that the contractile response of strips of freshly excised human gallbladder, and of isolated myocytes, is impaired in carriers of cholesterol gallstones, but not in those with pigment stones. The altered gallbladder motility seems to be associated with the presence of supersaturated bile within the gallbladder. The mystery of how the gallbladder wall can 'read' the composition of bile within the gallbladder lumen may be explained by lipid transport across the gallbladder mucosa (Jacyna et al 1987, Ross et al 1990, Ginanni Corradini et al 1998a, 1998b). Certainly the presence of supersaturated bile seems to influence the cholesterol content and the cholesterol:phospho-

lipid molar ratio in the sarcolemmal membrane of the myocytes (Chen et al 1997b, 1999). In turn, this seems to impair the relaxation of the muscle cells and the contractile response of the gallbladder.

Gallbladder filling and emptying are under complex neural and hormonal control. It has been known for many years that the principal hormonal stimulus to gallbladder emptying is cholecystokinin (CCK). However, other peptide hormones also influence gallbladder motor function. For example, Ortega Lopez and colleagues (1997b) showed that in response to a semi-liquid test meal, gallstone patients have basal (fasting) and postprandial hypersecretion of substance P, when compared to controls. They also have a 'moderate decrease' of neurotensin after the test meal. Motilin may also influence gallbladder motility—particularly in the interdigestive state—probably by influencing phase III migratory motor complexes (MMCs) originating in the gastric antrum and duodenum which, in turn, affect gallbladder filling and emptying. Moreover somatostatin, pancreatic polypeptide, neuropeptide Y, gastrin releasing peptide, vasoactive intestinal polypeptide (VIP), peptide YY and calcitonin-gene related peptide (CGRP) may also play minor roles: for review see O'Donnell & Fairclough (1993). Nonetheless, given the fact that CCK is the most important hormone in regulating postprandial gallbladder emptying, and that most investigators find impaired gallbladder emptying in gallstone patients, the obvious questions arise—

(i) is meal-stimulated CCK release from the intestine in gallstone patients any different from that in controls?
(ii) if so, is the contractile response of the end-organ (the gallbladder) normal in gallstone patients?

The answer to the first of these rhetorical questions is that fasting and post-prandial immuno-reactive CCK levels are indeed comparable in control subjects and gallstone patients (Forgacs et al 1984b, van Erpecum et al 1990, 1992, Pauletzi et al 1993). However, many investigators claim that in gallstone carriers, there are 'strong' and 'weak' contractors (van der Linden 1974, Stolk et al 1995, Sanger et al 1997, Schneider et al 1997) and in the weak-contractor subgroup, Schneider et al (1997) found that the CCK receptor structure of the gallbladder myocytes was altered—possibly secondary to changes in nitric oxide, although this was not confirmed by Nardone et al (1995).

Once again, cell and molecular biology techniques have been applied extensively to the basic physiology and biochemistry of gallbladder contraction. For example, the cholecystokinin receptors have been characterized in the muscle cells of the gallbladder. Furthermore, the second messenger cascade within the myocytes has been defined (Chen et al 1997b). In brief, the impaired gallbladder muscle relaxation, which characterizes cholesterol-gallstone disease, seems to be in the plasma membranes. There is lower cyclic AMP production and it involves steps before G-protein activation (protein kinase C translocation from cytosol to membranes (Yu et al 1995)). Based on studies in an animal model of cholesterol-gallstone disease (ground squirrels fed a 1% cholesterol diet for 28 days), Xu et al (Xu & Shaffer 1996a) reached similar conclusions: the defect in gallbladder contraction did not involve an intracellular signal transduction pathway—but rather the sarcolemmal membrane. Moreover, as noted above (Chen et al 1999), the increased cholesterol content and the abnormal cholesterol:phospholipid molar ratio in the myocyte membrane is associated with altered membrane fluidity (anisotropy) but this could be corrected by incubating the membranes with cholesterol-free liposomes for four hours.

In general, however, these studies are judged to be somewhat tangential to the main aims of this chapter. Therefore, they are not discussed further but once again, the reader is referred to some excellent reviews on this topic (O'Donnell & Fairclough 1993, Panataker et al 1995, Duane 1996, Portincasa et al 1997b).

'MODELS' OF HUMAN GALLSTONE DISEASE

HIGH SPINAL CORD INJURY

In 1987, Apstein and colleagues noted that the prevalence of gallbladder stones was greater than normal in patients with high spinal cord injury—a finding which has been confirmed by several other investigators (Ketover et al 1996, Tandon et al 1997, Moonka et al 1991). Thus Ketover et al (1996) showed, by ultrasound, that in patients with spinal cord injury, the minimum prevalence of gallstones was 21% while the maximum was 30%. However, the authors concluded that gallbladder stasis 'did not appear to be etiologic' (in gallstones forming secondary to spinal cord injury). Similarly, in a study from India, Tandon and colleagues (1997) concluded that although gallbladder sludge was common (nine out of 18) in patients with spinal lesions above the tenth neuronal segment (T10), it was rare (two out of 18) in those with lower lesions. The Indian authors also concluded that gallbladder 'contractility' was normal.

OBESITY AND RAPID WEIGHT LOSS

With very few exceptions, the results of all epidemiological studies carried out to date show that obesity and a high body mass index (BMI), are risk-factors for cholesterol gall-

stone disease (Weinsier et al 1955, Attili et al 1995, Spirt et al 1995; Misciagna et al 1996). In obesity, total body cholesterol synthesis is increased (Miettinen et al 1971, Nestel et al 1973) as is biliary cholesterol secretion (Bennion & Grundy 1975, Mabee et al 1976, Shaffer & Small 1977, Reuben et al 1985). Moreover, gallbladder motility is abnormal in the obese (Hendel et al 1998). More important than obesity per se, is the observation that sludge and stones develop rapidly in obese individuals undergoing rapid weight loss—either as a result of gastric stapling operations (gastric by-pass) or of very low calorie diets. Indeed, in a meta-analysis, Weinsier et al (1995) concluded that the risk of gallstone formation increased dramatically when the rate of body weight loss exceeded 1.5 kg per week. However, Festi et al (1998) suggested that even within the confines of very low calorie diets (< 580 kcal/day), it is possible to prevent gallstone formation simply by increasing the daily quota of dietary fat from 3.0 to 12.2 g per day. Thus, asymptomatic gallstones developed in six of 11 (54%) of subjects taking the 3.0 g fat, very low calorie diet but in none of 11 taking the 12.2 g fat, very low calorie diet per day—probably because the higher fat diet induced significantly greater gallbladder emptying. Similar results were reported by Gebhard et al (1996). They randomized obese subjects to one of two low calorie liquid diets: either 520 kcal/day with <2 g fat/day, or 900 kcal/day with 30 g fat/day (which included one 10 g fat meal) 'to stimulate maximal gallbladder emptying'. They confirmed (by ultrasound) that the 520 kcal diet resulted in poor gallbladder emptying (35%) compared with 'maximal' (66%) gallbladder emptying on the 900 kcal diet. Despite this difference, weight loss was comparable with both regimes. More important, gallstones formed in four of six subjects on the 520 kcal diet, but in none of seven on the 900 kcal diet. The authors suggested that the gallstone risk during rapid weight loss may be reduced by maintaining gallbladder emptying with a small amount of dietary fat.

This conclusion is supported by similar results in 70 moderately obese individuals given a 1200 kcal/day diet, which contained approximately 20 g fat/day (Heshka et al 1998). On this regime, they too lost weight but none developed new gallstones during the study period of 16 weeks. The evidence incriminating the fat restriction in the genesis of gallstones during weight loss in the obese is strong—despite the suggestion by Vezina et al from Canada (1998) that fat restriction is not the main culprit. However, this apparent conflict of opinion was based on a comparison of de novo gallstone formation in subjects taking 900 kcal/day liquid diets containing either 16 g fat ($n = 94$) or 30 g fat ($n = 178$) per day, for 13 weeks. The incidence of gallstone development (17.0% versus 11.2%, respectively) was not significantly different in the two dietary groups—perhaps because (according to Gebhard et al (1996)), an intake of 16 g fat/day is more than adequate to ensure maximal gallbladder emptying and, therefore, to prevent gallstone formation.

Studies by Broomfield et al (1988), Shiffman et al (1991, 1992, 1993) and Sugerman et al (1995, 1998) showed that new gallstones form in 23 to 35% of patients undergoing rapid weight loss, who received no prophylactic treatment. However, there was a dose-dependent protection from stone formation in those receiving oral ursodeoxycholic acid in different doses (300 mg, 600 mg and 1200 mg/day). The results of a recent large survey in 47 000 female nurses suggests that weight cycling (intentional weight loss followed by weight regain) was associated with an increased risk for cholecystectomy—presumably and hopefully only for symptomatic gallstone disease—in approximately 55% of the cohort patients (Syngal et al 1999).

TOTAL PARENTERAL NUTRITION (TPN)

It has been known for several years that in patients nourished exclusively by the parenteral route, there is a high incidence of sludge and stone formation within the gallbladder (Messing et al 1983, Roslyn et al 1983). The natural history of biliary sludge has been studied extensively by Lee and colleagues—both in experimental animals and in man (Pekow et al 1995, Ko & Lee 1999). They showed that echogenic, non-shadowing, mobile debris within the gallbladder (sludge) is often transient—as is commonly the case during pregnancy (Friedman et al 1966, Braverman et al 1980, Valdivieso et al 1983, Bolondi et al 1985, Maringhini et al 1987, Maringhini et al 1993, Hahm et al 1997, Van Bodegraven et al 1998)—but that sometimes it is a precursor of stone formation. Indeed, the Seattle group suggested that biliary sludge is not always innocent: occasionally it can induce biliary colic, cholecystitis and even pancreatitis (Pekow et al 1995).

The mechanism for the formation of sludge and stones during TPN is complex. First, the absence of food from the gut leads to stagnation of bile acids within the enterohepatic circulation. And, since the hepatic transport of bile acids represents one of the major driving forces for bile flow, this stagnation leads to relative cholestasis (Lirussi et al 1989). Second, the meal-stimulated neural and hormonal 'messages' from the intestine to the gallbladder are either absent or diminished during TPN, and this is associated with gallbladder motor dysfunction. Indeed this may be the principal mechanism for sludge and stone formation during parenteral nutrition. In the short-term (2 weeks), daily stimulation of gallbladder emptying with parenteral CCK prevented stone formation in patients receiving TPN (Sitzmann et al 1990). Sludge and stone formation also occur, with increased frequency, in patients requiring intensive care and this can be countered by parenteral treatment with the CCK analogue, caerulin (Hasse et al 1995).

CHRONIC OCTREOTIDE TREATMENT

Octreotide (OT) is a relatively long-acting analogue of native human somatostatin. It is used widely in the treatment of a number of disorders—including acromegaly, a condition characterized by increased circulating levels of growth hormone and insulin like growth factor-1 (IGF-1). Chronic OT treatment suppresses growth hormone and IGF-1 levels and is, therefore, an effective treatment for acromegaly. However, after 1–2 years OT treatment, 10–60% (mean 29%) of patients develop gallstones.

The inhibitory effect of octreotide on peptide hormone levels is not confined to growth hormone and IGF-1: OT also inhibits meal-stimulated CCK release from the intestine (Lembcke et al 1987, Ewins et al 1992, Stolk et al 1993). This is the principal, but not the sole, mechanism whereby OT markedly inhibits gallbladder emptying (Lembcke et al 1987, Ewins et al 1992, Stolk et al 1993, Hussaini et al 1996, Ho et al 1999). Initially, it was assumed that the resultant gallbladder stasis was the explanation for OT-induced iatrogenic gallstones. However, given the multiple pathogenetic mechanisms involved in spontaneous gallstone disease (unrelated to acromegaly or OT treatment), Hussaini et al (1994) were reluctant to accept that OT-induced 'paralysis' of the gallbladder was responsible for the iatrogenic stones (Shi et al 1993). They, therefore, studied the lipid and bile acid composition, and the physical chemistry, of fresh gallbladder bile from three groups of individuals:

(i) stone-free acromegalics untreated with OT (the closest available approximation to a control group)
(ii) acromegalic patients with OT-associated gallstones and
(iii) a disease control group of non-acromegalic patients with cholesterol-rich gallstones.

In the patients with OT-associated stones, the gallbladder bile was invariably supersaturated with cholesterol. Most of the excess biliary cholesterol was in the vesicular fraction and the molar ratio of cholesterol:phospholipids in the vesicles was high—predicting vulnerability to aggregation, fusion and rapid nucleation of cholesterol micro-crystals. Indeed, this is what Hussaini et al (1994) found. The nucleation time in the patients with OT-associated stones was abnormally short (< 5 days), and comparable to that in the non-acromegalic disease controls, while in the stone-free group it was always > 10 days. The authors also found changes in biliary bile acid composition. Thus the proportion of the hydrophobic bile acid, deoxycholic acid (DCA; % of total bile acids), was approximately 12% in the stone-free patients compared with 24% in the two groups of stone carriers.

In a small number of acromegalic patients, the gallbladder bile was sampled on two occasions—before and during OT treatment. In these paired studies, again the % of DCA in bile doubled as a result of the somatostatin analogue therapy—in the absence of induced gallstones. At the same time, the bile changed from being unsaturated in cholesterol before treatment, to being supersaturated during therapy.

This profile of abnormalities in bile-lipid composition and physical chemistry was comparable to that seen in conventional cholesterol-gallstone disease. However the changes were apparently due to the OT treatment and not to the presence of stones. Furthermore, they developed in days or weeks—in contrast to the months or years required for spontaneous gallstone formation (Small 1980, Mok et al 1986).

Mechanism for the increased proportion of DCA in bile during OT treatment

The results of previous studies in non-acromegalic patients (control subjects and patients with the irritable bowel syndrome) suggested that a single, $50 \mu g$ injection of octreotide markedly prolongs mouth-to-cecum transit time (MCTT) (Lembcke et al 1987, Ewins et al 1992, Fuessl et al 1987, Moller et al 1988, O'Donnell et al 1990, Hussaini et al 1996). However, there was little information about the effects of chronic OT treatment on oro-cecal transit in acromegalic patients, and none about the effects of the somatostatin analogue on colonic transit—of relevance since deoxycholic acid (see below) is formed mainly in the large bowel (DCA).

To study this, Hussaini and colleagues (1996) measured MCTT using the lactulose breath hydrogen technique (Bond & Levitt 1974), and large bowel transit time (LBTT) by recording the transit of radio-opaque markers through the intestine, by the Metcalf technique (Metcalf et al 1987). The authors confirmed that OT markedly prolongs oro-cecal transit both in control subjects and in acromegalic patients. More important (at least in the context of DCA metabolism), they also showed that LBTT was significantly longer in acromegalic patients untreated with OT, than in controls. However, it took the power of paired studies (Veysey et al 1999), when LBTT was measured in the same acromegalic patients before and during OT treatment, to

prove that the somatostatin analogue consistently, and significantly, increased colonic transit. At the same time, Veysey et al (1999) again measured the % DCA—but this time in fasting serum, rather than in bile—and as before, the OT treatment doubled the mean % DCA. The authors went on to show that there was a highly significant linear relationship between LBTT and the % DCA in serum—suggesting that the longer the colonic transit, the greater was the % DCA in serum (and, by inference, in bile).

In order to calculate the percentages of the individual bile acids in fasting serum (surrogate markers for the proportions of bile acids in bile), Veysey et al (1999) used the highly sensitive method of gas chromatography-mass spectrometry. This measured the serum acid profile at one point in time. In contrast, the relatively crude technique used to measure LBTT took 4 days. In an attempt to redress this imbalance, Veysey and colleagues (1997, 1998) used serum sampling and a stable isotope dilution technique (Stellaard et al 1986) to estimate the pool size and the 'synthesis'/formation rate of DCA, over the same 4–5 days required for measurement of LBTT. The investigators confirmed that not only the % DCA in fasting serum, but also the pool size and formation rate (input into the enterohepatic circulation) of DCA increased significantly during OT treatment. Moreover, again there were significant correlations between LBTT and both the pool size and formation rate of this hydrophobic bile acid.

Mechanism whereby prolongation of colonic transit increases the size of the DCA pool

In theory, slowing of transit through the colon could affect DCA metabolism in several different ways (Thomas et al 1997a, 2000). Thus, the prolonged LBTT could allow more time for anaerobic bacterial proliferation in the colon. If so, assuming that the enzyme specific activity (which approximates to the amount of enzyme per bacterium) remains unchanged, any increase in the numbers of anaerobic bacteria present in the colon should increase the total amount or mass of the deconjugating and 7α-dehydroxylating enzymes present there. Alternatively, the changes in colonic transit could be associated with increases in enzyme specific activities. In theory, either or both of these mechanisms could increase DCA formation.

Previous studies by El Oufir and colleagues (1996) showed that changes in colonic transit time markedly influence the intra-colonic pH, or the pH of the stools—apparently by influencing short chain fatty acid absorption from the colon. Thus, when colonic transit was prolonged pharmacologically (with drugs such as loperamide), the fecal pH rose and the concentration of butyrate (the principal short chain fatty acid in the colon) fell. Similar results were obtained by Lewis and Heaton (1997).

There are at least three ways by which changes in large bowel luminal pH could influence DCA metabolism (Thomas et al 1997b). First, changes in colonic luminal pH could influence the activity of the deconjugating and dehydroxylating enzyme systems—both of which have pH optima (Thomas et al 1997c). Second, the growth of colonic anaerobes in a controlled environment in vitro (using a 'Chemostat'), is also influenced by pH (Fadden & Owen 1992). Third, we know from the results of titration studies (Dowling & Small 1968, Small 1971, Roda et al 1983, Carey 1985) that unconjugated bile acids, such as DCA, have relatively high pKa values and are insoluble in acid environments—such as those found in the normal cecum (Bown et al 1974, Evans et al 1988, Fallingborg et al 1989) (because of short chain fatty acid metabolism there). For this reason, the unconjugated bile acids are likely to be insoluble, and therefore unavailable, for absorption from the colon. In other words, induced changes in colonic transit could influence DCA solubilization and bioavailability. Finally, prolongation of LBTT could simply allow more time for DCA absorption—presumably by passive non-ionic diffusion—from the colon.

The influence of colonic transit, quantitative anaerobic bacteriology, bile acid metabolizing enzymes and intra-colonic pH, on DCA metabolism

To study this, Thomas and colleagues (1997a, 2000) studied two groups of individuals: (i) 20 stone-free 'controls' and (ii) 20 patients with presumed cholesterol-rich gallstones. All 40 were undergoing clinically-indicated colonoscopy but were found, in retrospect, to have no large bowel pathology. In preparation for the colonoscopy, the patients took no oral purgation. Instead, the contents of the left colon were 'washed out' by an instant enema with the aim of leaving those in the right colon undisturbed. After examining the left colon endoscopically, the colonoscope was advanced proximal to the hepatic flexure and samples of cecal contents obtained by aspiration. Then quantitative anaerobic bacteriology (total and Gram positive anaerobic counts) was carried out, and bile acid metabolizing enzyme activities measured, in the cecal aspirates.

In all 40 individuals, LBTT was again measured using the Metcalf technique (Metcalf et al 1987); the pH profile of the intestinal tract was recorded by telemetry (Bown et al 1974, Evans et al 1988, Fallingborg et al 1989, Thomas et al 1997) and, as a marker of DCA metabolism, the % DCA in fasting serum was quantitated by GC-mass spectrometry (Setchell & Matsui 1983).

The results of these studies showed that the gallstone patients had significantly longer colonic transit times than did the stone-free controls. They also had significantly more total and Gram-positive anaerobes in their cecal contents. In addition, the specific activity (enzyme units/mg protein) of the rate-limiting enzyme pathway for the conversion of conjugated cholic acid into unconjugated DCA (7-α dehydroxylase), was also significantly increased in the gallstone patients. At the same time, Thomas et al (1997a) confirmed that the prolonged colonic transit was associated with significant increases in the luminal pH of both the proximal and distal colon (Thomas et al 1997a, 1997b, 2000). The 'bottom line', however, was the demonstration that the gallstone patients also had significant increases in the % DCA in fasting serum (and again by implication, in bile). The same group of authors carried out comparable studies in two groups of acromegalic patients—those untreated with OT and those taking long-term somatostatin therapy—with broadly similar results (Thomas et al 1998) to those described above.

Based on these findings, the authors concluded that prolongation of LBTT is likely to favor increased DCA formation, solubilization (and therefore bioavailability) and absorption. They also proposed that prolonged colonic transit is a feature not only of acromegalic patients treated with OT, but also of spontaneous gallstone disease.

THE ROLE OF THE INTESTINE IN THE PATHOGENESIS OF SPONTANEOUS CHOLESTEROL GALLSTONE DISEASE

Investigators from Bristol (Low-Beer & Pomare 1975, Marcus & Heaton 1986, 1988, Low-Beer 1998) have long suspected that changes in colonic bacteria and altered DCA metabolism are important in the genesis of 'conventional' cholesterol gallstones—unrelated to acromegaly or octreotide treatment. Indeed, the evidence linking changes in intestinal transit with the % DCA in bile, the DCA pool size, biliary cholesterol saturation and the formation of cholesterol-rich gallstones, was comprehensively summarized by them some years ago (Marcus & Heaton 1988). Moreover, the results of animal studies support the concept that slow intestinal transit contributes to cholesterol gallstone formation. Xu et al (1996b) showed that when ground squirrels are fed a 1% cholesterol diet, their aboral intestinal transit becomes significantly delayed, the % DCA in the bile acid pool doubles and the cholesterol saturation index increases.

The evidence that prolonged intestinal transit really is involved in the development of spontaneous gallstone disease is limited, but that which is available all points in the same direction. Thus, Heaton and colleagues (1993) compared whole gut transit time and fecal wet weight in normal weight women with gallstones (and no obvious risk factors for cholelithiasis) with those in matched controls. On average, the mean whole gut transit time was almost 20 hours longer in the gallstone patients than in the controls, whereas their average fecal weight was only half that of the stone-free individuals. To paraphrase their findings, the women with gallstones suffered from slow transit constipation. Moreover in Ladakh, a mountainous region in Northern India, Spathis et al (1997) found that gallstones were common in non-obese women whose stool characteristics 'implied' that they had slow intestinal transit or 'intestinal stasis'. If this implication is correct, one might expect to find that constipation would be risk factor for gallstone formation, or that the prevalence of gallstones would be high in individuals with constipation. There are few good data to prove or disprove this point but in southern Italy, Misciagna et al (1996) found that constipation (as shown by the use of laxatives) was positively associated with the incidence of gallstones. Watkins et al (1993) also showed that constipation was a risk factor for cholesterol gallstones.

Whether physical activity influences intestinal transit, and the frequency of bowel movements, is uncertain but in a survey of more than 45 000 men followed for an 8-year period, Lietzmann et al (1998) showed that increased physical activity was inversely related to the risk of symptomatic gallstone disease. Conversely, sedentary behavior (watching television for more than 40 hours/week) was positively related to the risk for symptomatic gallstone disease. Conceivably, prolongation of intestinal transit with ageing might also be important since oro-cecal transit times and the prevalence of gallstones both increase with increasing age (Pilotto et al 1995, Kratzer et al 1998).

Subsequently, a group of investigators from Japan and Sweden (Shoda et al 1995) measured a large number of variables, including small bowel transit time, the % DCA in bile and biliary cholesterol saturation, again comparing gallstone patients with matched controls. They too found that when compared to the controls, the gallstone carriers had significantly prolonged intestinal transit, increased proportions of DCA in bile and supersaturated bile. Similar results were obtained from Bologna in Italy by Azzaroli et al (1999) although they too measured small, and not large, bowel transit time. In association with the prolonged oro-cecal transit, they found that the mean proportion of DCA increased from 15% in the controls to 23% in the gallstone patients, while the mean cholesterol saturation index in bile increased from 0.7 to 1.2.

These results, taken together with those from the Guy's Hospital group (Thomas et al 1997a), strongly support the claim that, in addition to the 'guilty gallbladder' and the 'lithogenic liver', one should now add the 'indolent intestine' to the list of putative culprits in gallstone pathogenesis. Indeed, this concept was reviewed recently (Dowling et al 1997) and several other editorials and review articles on this subject, have appeared (Low-Beer 1998, Heaton 1999).

MISCELLANEOUS TOPICS

THE PATHOGENESIS OF BILIARY SLUDGE AND MICROLITHIASIS

The sensitivity of ultrasound in detecting the presence of individual calculi within the gallbladder is around 2 mm. However because of their collective bulk, when multiple particles coalesce (as is the case with biliary sludge) ultrasound can detect much smaller deposits—even if they often lack an acoustic shadow. Despite this, microlithiasis is defined as the presence of stones in the gallbladder measuring < 3 mm in diameter, that are undetectable by transabdominal ultrasound and oral cholecystography (Houssin et al 1983, Ros et al 1991). By microscopy, the bile of these patients often contains cholesterol monohydrate crystals, calcium bilirubinate granules and microspheroliths. A group of investigators from India (Lee & Nicholl 1986) measured biliary cholesterol saturation indices and microcrystal nucleation times in patients with microlithiasis, and compared the results with those in stone-free controls and in patients with radiolucent, presumed cholesterol-rich gallstones. They showed that the saturation indices were significantly higher, and the nucleation times significantly shorter, in the patients with microlithiasis than in the controls. Similar results were reported for patients with biliary sludge. Thus, Lee and Nicholls (1986) found that the bile lipid composition and biliary cholesterol saturation indices were comparable in patients with biliary sludge, to those in patients with gallstones. Taken together, the results of these studies suggest that the pathogenesis of biliary sludge and microlithiasis may well be similar to that of conventional gallstone disease. Indeed, it is quite possible that the increased sensitivity of the imaging techniques has simply unmasked cholesterol cholelithiasis at a very early stage.

IRON DEFICIENCY

Adult prairie dogs were fed high cholesterol, plus either iron-supplemented or iron-depleted diets. Those with iron-deficient diets had lower 7α-hydroxylase levels, higher saturation indices and more cholesterol crystals per high-powered field, than did those with iron supplemented diets (Johnston et al 1997).

APOLIPOPROTEIN E4

In 1993, Juvonen et al showed that the cholesterol content of gallstones was related to the serum apolipoprotein E phenotype. This apolipoprotein increases intestinal cholesterol absorption (Kesaniemi et al 1987), hepatic lipoprotein uptake and dietary fat clearance (Weintraub et al 1996). Therefore, Bertomeu et al (1996) designed a study to test the hypothesis that carriage of the apo-E4 isoform could promote cholesterol gallstone formation by increasing hepatic and biliary cholesterol concentrations. To study this, the authors assessed the apo-E phenotype in 160 subjects with, and 125 without, gallstones. They found that in those carrying the E4 isoform, the relative risk (odds ratio) of developing gallstones was 2.67 ($p < 0.006$). Indeed, they suggested that carriage of the apo-E4 isoform was a genetic risk factor for cholelithiasis in humans. Subsequently, Portincasa et al (1996b) showed that the apolipoprotein E4 genotype also influenced the risk of gallstone recurrence, after extracorporeal shock-wave lithotripsy.

The role of apo-E4 as a risk factor for cholesterol gallstone formation was the subject of a recent editorial (van Erpecum & Carey 1996b).

MICRONUTRIENT ANTIOXIDANTS: ROLE OF FREE RADICALS IN GALLSTONE FORMATION

Braganza and colleagues (1995) have suggested that an absolute or relative insufficiency of micronutrient antioxidants may mobilize 'ancillary hepatobiliary resources'—such as bilirubin, lactoferrin and mucin—to combat oxidative stress, thereby promoting gallstone formation 'inadvertently'. In support of this contention, the same group (Worthington et al 1997) carried out a pilot study of antioxidant intake, and based on food inventories over a 6-month period, found that the patients ingested significantly lower amounts of 10 out of a total of 16 antioxidants—particularly alpha tocopherol. Reactive oxygen metabolites are also believed to induce gallbladder inflammation and may promote cholesterol monohydrate crystal precipitation from supersaturated gallbladder bile (Sipos et al 1997).

REFERENCES

Abei M, Kawczak P, Nuutinen H et al 1993 Isolation and characterization of a cholesterol crystallisation promoter from human bile. Gastroenterology 104: 539–548

Adler R D, Metzger A L, Grundy S M 1974 Biliary lipid secretion before and after cholecystectomy in American Indians with cholesterol gallstones. Gastroenterology 66: 1212–1217

Admirand W H, Small D M 1968 The physico-chemical basis of cholesterol gallstone formation in man. Journal of Clinical Investigation 47: 1043–1052

Afdhal N H, Niu N, Gantz D, Small D, Smith B F 1993 Bovine gallbladder mucin accelerates cholesterol monohydrate crystal growth in model bile. Gastroenterology 104: 1515–1523

Afdhal N H, Niu N, Nunes D P et al 1995 Mucin-vesicle interactions in model bile: evidence for vesicle aggregation and fusion before cholesterol crystal formation. Hepatology 22: 856–865

Agarwal D K, Choudhuri G, Kumar J 1993 Chemical nature and distribution of calcium compounds in radiolucent gallstones. Scandinavian Journal of Gastroenterology 28: 613–616

Ahrendt S A, Fox-Talbot K, Kaufman H S et al 1994 Cholesterol nucleates rapidly from mixed micelles in the prairie dog. Biochim Biophys Acta 1211: 7–13

Andrews E A 1933 Detailed study of a series of gallbladder bile cases. Surgery, Gynecology and Obstetrics 57: 36–56

Angelico M, Corradini G S, Masella R et al 1992 Molecular composition of biliary phosphatidylcholines, as related to cholesterol saturation, transport and nucleation in human gallbladder bile. Journal of Hepatology 15: 59–66

Apstein M D, Dalecki-Chipperfield K 1987 Spinal cord injury is a risk factor for gallstone disease. Gastroenterology 92: 966–968

Attili A F, Pazzi P, Galeazzi R 1995 Prevalence of previously undiagnosed gallstones in a population with multiple risk factors. Digestive Diseases and Sciences 40: 1770–1774

Attili A F, Capocaccia L, Carulli N, Festi D et al 1997 Factors associated with gallstone disease in the MICOL experience. I. Hepatology 26: 809–818

Attili A F, Scafato E, Marchioli R et al 1998 Diet and gallstones in Italy: the cross-section MICOL results. Hepatology 27: 1492–1498

Azzaroli F, Mazzella G, Mazzeo C et al 1999 Sluggish small bowel motility is involved in determining increased biliary deoxycholic acid in cholesterol gallstone patients. American Journal of Gastroenterology 94: 2453–2459

Barrett-Connor E 1968 Cholelithiasis in sickle cell anemia. American Journal of Medicine 45: 889–898

Behar J, Lee K Y, Thompson W R, Biancani P. 1989 Gallbladder contraction in patients with pigment and cholesterol stones. Gastroenterology 97: 1479–1484

Behar J, Rhim B Y, Thompson W et al 1993 Inositol triphosphate retores impaired human gallbladder motility associated with cholesterol gallstones. Gastroenterology 104: 563–568

Bell G D, Whitney B, Dowling R H 1972 Gallstone dissolution in man using chenodeoxycholic acid. Lancet 2: 1213–1216

Bennion L J, Grundy S M. 1975 Effect of obesity and caloric intake on biliary lipid metabolism in man. Journal of Clinical Investigations 56: 996–1011

Benvegnu L, Noventa F, Chemello L et al 1997 Prevalence and incidence of cholecystolithiasis in cirrhosis and relation to the etiology of liver disease. Digestion 58: 293–298

Berr F, Schrieber E, Frick U 1992 Interrelationships of bile acid and phospholipid fatty acid species with cholesterol saturation of duodenal bile in health and gallstone disease. Hepatology 16: 71–81

Bertomeu A, Ros E, Zambon D et al 1996 Apolipoprotein E polymorphism and gallstones. Gastroenterology 111, 1603–1610

Bogren H G, Mutvei H, Renberg G. 1995. Scanning electron microscope studies of human gallstones after plasma etching. Ultrastruct. Pathology. 19: 447–453

Bolondi L, Gaini S, Testa A, Labo G 1985 Gall bladder sludge formation during prolonged fasting after gastrointestinal tract surgery. Gut 26: 734–738

Bond J H, Levitt M D 1974 Investigation of small bowel transit time in man utllizing pulmonary hydrogen measurements. Journal of Laboratory and Clinical Medicine. 85: 546–556

Bouchier I A D, Cooperband S R, El Kodsi B M. 1965 Mucous substances and viscosity of normal and pathological human bile. Gastroenterology 49: 343–353

Bouchier I A D 1969 Postmortem study of the frequency of gallstones in patients with cirrhosis of the liver. Gut 10: 705–710

Bourgés M, Small D M, Dervichian D G 1967a Biophysics of lipidic associations. II. The ternary systems: cholesterol-lecithin-water. Biochim. Biophys. Acta 137: 157–167

Bourgés M, Small D M, Dervichian D G 1967b Biophysics of lipid associations. III. The quarternary systems lecithin-bile salt-cholesterol-water. Biochim. Biophys. Acta 144: 189–201

Bown R L, Gibson J A, Sladen G E, Hicks B, Dawson A M. 1974 Effects of lactulose and other laxatives on ileal and colonic pH as measured by a radiotelemetry device. Gut 15: 999–1004

Braganza J, Worthington H V 1995 A radical view of gallstone aetiogenesis. Medical Hypotheses 45: 510–516

Brakel K, Lameris J S, Nijs H G T et al 1990 Predicting gallstone composition with CT: In vivo and in vitro analysis. Radiology 174: 337–341

Braverman D Z, Johnson M L, Kern F Jr 1980 Effects of pregnancy and contraceptive steroids on gallbladder function. New England Journal of Medicine 302: 362–364

Broomfield P H, Chopra R, Sheinbaum R C et al 1988 Effects of ursodeoxycholic acid and aspirin on the formation of lithogenic bile and gallstones during loss of weight. New England Journal of Medicine 319: 1567–1572

Busch N, Tokumo H, Holzbach R T 1990 A sensitive method for determination of cholesterol growth using model solutions of supersaturated bile. Journal of Lipid Research 31: 1903–1909

Busch N, Lammert F, Marschall H U, Matern S 1995 A new subgroup of lectin-bound biliary proteins binds to cholesterol crystals, modifies crystal morphology, and inhibits cholesterol crystallization. Journal of Clinical Investigation 96: 3009–3015

Cano N, Cicero F, Ranieri F et al 1986 Ultrasonographic study of gallbladder motility during total parenteral nutrition. Gastroenterology 91: 313–317

Cantafora A, Angelico M, DiBase A et al 1981 Structure of biliary phosphatidylcholine in cholesterol gallstone patients. Lipids 16: 589–592

Carey M C, Cahalane M J 1993 Whither biliary sludge? Gastroenterology, 95: 508–523

Carey M C 1985 Physical-chemical properties of bile acids and their salts. In Danielsson H, Sjovall J (Eds) Sterols and bile acids. Elsevier Science, p 345–403

Caroli A, Del Favero G, Di Mario F et al 1992 Computed tomography in predicting gall stone solubility: a prospective study. Gut 33: 698–700

Chawla Y, Sarkar B, Marwaha R K, Dilawari J B 1997 Multitransfused children with thalassemia major do not have gallstones. Tropical Gastroenterology 18: 107–108

Chen Q, de Petris G, Yu P, Amaral J, Biancani P, Behar J 1997a Different pathways mediate cholecystokinin actions in cholelithiasis. American Journal of Physiology 272: G838–G844

Chen Q, Amaral J, Oh S, Biancani P, Behar J. 1997b Gallbladder relaxation in patients with pigment and cholesterol stones. Gastroenterology 113: 930–937

Chen Q, Amaral J, Biancani P 1999 Excess membrane cholesterol alters human gallbladder muscle contractility and membrane fluidity. Gastroenterology 116: 678–685

Chijiiwa K, Koga A, Yamasaki T 1991 Fibronectin: a possible factor promoting cholesterol monohydrate crystallization in bile. Biochim Biophys Acta, 1086: 44–48

Chijiiwa K, Makino I, Kozaki N, Tanaka M 1996 Differences in gallbladder bile lithogenicity in patients after gastrectomy and colectomy. European Surgery Research 28: 1–7

Cohen D, Kaler E W, Carey M C 1993 Cholesterol carriers in human bile. Are 'Lamellae' involved? Hepatology 18: 1522

Cohen B I, Mosbach E H, Ayyad H et al 1991 Aspirin does not inhibit cholesterol cholelithiasis in two established animal models. Gastroenterology 101: 1109–1116

Conte D, Fraquelli M, Fornari F et al 1999 Close relation between cirrhosis and gallstones: cross-sectional and longitudinal survey. Archives of Internal Medicine 159: 49–52

Corradini S G, Arancia G, Calcabrini A et al 1995 Lamellar bodies coexist with vesicles and micelles in human gallbladder bile. Ursodeoxycholic acid prevents cholesterol crystal nucleation by increasing biliary lamellae. Journal of Hepatology 22: 642–657

Craven B M 1976 Crystal structure of cholesterol monohydrate. Nature 260: 727–729

Crawford J M, Moeckel G-M, Crawford A R et al 1995 Imaging biliary lipid secretion in the rat: ultrastructural evidence for vesiculation of the hepatocyte canalicular membrane. Journal of Lipid Research 36: 2147–2163

Danzinger R G, Hofmann A F, Thistle J L, Schoenfield L J 1972a Dissolution of gallstones by chenodeoxycholic acid. New England Journal of Medicine 286: 1–8

Danzinger R G, Gordon H, Schoenfield L J, Thistle J L 1972b Lithogenic bile in siblings of young women with cholelithiasis. Mayo Clinic Proceedings 47: 762–766

Das A, Baijal S S, Saraswat V A 1995 Effect of aspirin on gallbladder motility in patients with gallstone disease. A randomized, double-blind, placebo-controlled trial of two dosage schedules. Digestive Diseases and Sciences 40: 1782–1785

de la Porte P L, Domingo N, van Wijland M et al 1996 Distinct immuno-localization of mucin and other biliary proteins in human cholesterol gallstones. Journal of Hepatology 25: 339–348

DeBruijn M A C, Mok K S, Nibbering C P et al 1996 Characterization of the cholesterol crystallization-promoting low-density particle isolated from human bile. Gastroenterology 1996 110: 1936–1944

Deleuze J-F, Jacquemin E, Dubuisson C et al 1996 Defect of multidrug-resistance 3 gene expression in a subgroup of progressive familial intrahepatic cholestasis. Hepatology 23: 904–908

Demel R A, Guerta van Kessel W S M, van Deenan L L M 1972 The properties of polyunsaturated lecithin in monolayers and liposomes and the interactions of these lecithins with cholesterol. Biochimica et Biophysica Acta 266: 26–40

De Olmo J A, Garcia F, Serra M A et al 1997 Prevalence and incidence of gallstones in liver cirrhosis. Scandinavian Journal of Gastroenterology 32: 1061–1065

de Vree J M L, Jacquemin E, Sturm E et al 1999 Mutations in the MDR3 gene cause of progressive familial intrahepatic cholestasis. Proceedings of the National Academy 95: 282–287

Dolgin S M, Schwartz J S, Kressel H Y et al 1981 Identification of patients with cholesterol or pigment gallstones by discriminant analysis of radiographic features. New England Journal of Medicine, 304: 808–811

Donovan J M, Benedek GB, Carey M C 1987 Formation of mixed micelles and vesicles of human apolipoproteins A-I and A-II with synthetic and natural lecithins and the bile salt sodium taurocholate; quasi-elastic light scattering studies. Biochemistry 26: 8116–8125

Donovan J M, Timofeyeva N, Carey M C 1991 Influence of total lipid concentration, bile salt: lecithin ratio, and cholesterol content on inter-mixed micellar/vesicular (non-lecithin-associated) bile salt concentrations in model bile. Journal of Lipid Research 32: 1501–1512

Donovan J M, Jackson A A 1998 Accurate separation of biliary lipid aggregates requires the correct intermixed micellar/intervesicular bile salt concentration. Hepatology 27: 641–648

Doty J E, Pitt H A, Kuchenbecker S L, Den Besten L 1983a Impaired gallbladder emptying before gallstone formation in the prairie dog. Gastroenterology 85: 168–174

Doty J E, Pitt HA, Kuchenbecker S L 1983 Role of gallbladder mucus in the pathogenesis of cholesterol gallstones. American Journal of Surgery 145: 54–61

Dowling R H, Small D M 1968 The effect of pH on the solubility of varying mixtures of free and conjugated bile salts in solution. Gastroenterology 54: 1291 (abstr)

Dowling R H, Hussaini S H, Murphy G M, Besser G M, Wass J A H 1992 Gallstones during octreotide therapy. Metabolism: Clinical and Experimental 41: Suppl. 2, 22–33

Dowling R H, Veysey M J, Pereira S P et al 1997 Role of intestinal transit in the pathogenesis of gallbladder stones. Canadian Journal of Gastroenterology. 11: 57–64

Duane W C 1996 Something in the way she moves: gallbladder motility and gallstones. Gastroenterology 111: 823–825

Duchmann J C, Joly J P, Decrombecque C et al 1997 Cirrhosis: a new, but expected cause of biliary sludge. Alcoholism, Clinical and Experimental Research 21: 119–121

El Oufir L, Flourie B, Bruley des Varannes S et al 1996 Relations between transit time, fermentation products, and hydrogen consuming flora in healthy humans. Gut 38: 870–877

Evans D F, Pye G, Bramley R et al 1988 Measurement of gastrointestinal pH profiles in normal ambulant human subjects. Gut 29: 1035–1041

Ewins D L, Javaid A, Coskeran P B et al 1992 Assessment of gallbladder dynamics, cholecystokinin release and the development of gallstones during octreotide therapy for acromegaly. Quarterly Journal of Medicine 83: 295–306

Fadden K, Owen R W 1992 Faecal steroids and colorectal cancer: the effect of lactulose on faecal bacterial metabolism in a continuous culture model of the large intestine. European Journal of Cancer Prevention. 1: 13–27

Fallingborg J, Christensen L A, Ingeman-Nielson M et al 1989 pH profile and regional transit times of the normal gut measured by a radiotelemetry device. Alimentary Pharmacology and Therapeutics 3: 605–613

Festi D, Frabboni R, Bazzoli F et al 1990 Gallbladder motility in cholesterol gallstone disease. Gastroenterology 99: 1779–1785

Festi D, Colecchia A, Orsini M et al 1998 Gallbladder motility and gallstone formation in obese patients following very low calorie diets. Use it (fat) or lose it (well). International Journal of Obesity and Related Metabolic Disorders 22: 592–600

Fisher R S, Stelzer F, Rock E, Melmud L S 1982 Abnormal gallbladder emptying in patients with gallstones. Digestive Diseases and Sciences 27: 1019–1024

Forgacs I F, Maisey M N, Murphy G M, Dowling R H 1984a Influence of gallstones and ursodeoxycholic acid on gallbladder emptying. Gastroenterology 87: 299–307

Forgacs I C, Murphy G M, Dowling R H 1984b Gallbladder contraction and plasma immunoreactive CCK in gallbladder and intestinal disease. In: Paumgartner G, Stiehl A, Gerok W (Eds) Enterohepatic circulation of bile acids and sterol metabolism. MTP Press, Lancaster p 147–154

Freston J W, Bouchier I A D, Newman J 1969 Biliary mucus substances in dihydrocholesterol-induced cholelithiasis. Gastroenterology 57: 670–678

Fridhandler T M, Davison J S, Shaffer E A 1983 Defective gallbladder contractility in the ground squirrel and prairie dog during the early stage of cholesterol gallstone formation, Gastroenterology 85: 830–836

Friedman G, Kannel W, Dawber T 1966 The epidemiology of gallbladder disease: Observations in the Framingham Study. Journal of Chronic Diseases 19: 273–292

Fuessl H S, Carolan G, Williams G, Bloom S R 1987 Effect of a long-acting somatostatin analogue (SMS 201-995) on postprandial gastric emptying of 99mTc-tin colloid and mouth-to-caecum transit time in man. Digestion, 36: 101–107

Gallinger S, Taylor R D, Harvey P R C, Petrunka C N, Strasberg S M 1985 Effect of mucous glycoprotein on nucleation time of human bile. Gastroenterology 89: 648–658

Gebhard R L, Prigge W F, Ansel H J et al 1996 The role of gallbladder emptying in gallstone formation during diet-induced rapid weight loss. Hepatology 24: 544–548

Gilat T, Feldman C, Halpern Z, Dan M, Bar-Meir S 1983 An increased familial frequency of gallstones. Gastroenterology 84: 242–246

Gilat T, Somjen G, Mazur Y et al 2000 The prevention of cholesterol crystallization in bile using fatty acid bile acid conjugates. Gastroenterology 118: A714

Ginanni Corradini S, Yamashita G, Nuutinen H et al 1998a Human gallbladder mucosal function: effects on intraluminal fluid and lipid composition in health and disease. Digestive Diseases and Sciences. 43: 335–343

Ginanni Corradini S G, Ripani C, Guardia P D et al 1998b The human gallbladder increases cholesterol solubility in bile by differential lipid absorption: A study using a new in vitro model of isolated intra-arterially perfused gallbladder. Hepatology 28: 314–322

Gleeson D, Hood K A, Murphy G M, Dowling R H 1992 Calcium and carbonate ion concentrations in gallbladder and hepatic bile. Gastroenterology 102: 1707–1716

Gleeson D, Murphy G M, Dowling R H 1995 Effect of acute bile acid pool depletion on total and ionised calcium concentrations in human bile. European Journal of Clinical Investigations. 25: 225–234

Goresky C A, Gordon E R, Hinchey E J, Fried G M 1995 Bilirubin conjugate changes in the bile of gallbladders containing gallstones. Hepatology 21: 373–382

GREPCO (Rome Group for the Epidemiology and Prevention of Cholelithiasis) 1984 Prevalence of gallstone disease in an Italian adult female population. American Journal of Epidemiology 119: 796–805

Grundy S M, Metzger A L 1972a A physiological method for estimation of hepatic secretion of biliary lipids in man. Gastroenterology 62: 1200–1217

Grundy S M, Metzger A L, Adler R D 1972b. Mechanisms of lithogenic bile formation in American Indian women with cholesterol gallstones. Journal of Clinical Investigations. 51: 3026–3043

Gurll N J, Meyer P D, DenBesten L 1977. Effect of cholesterol crystals on gallbladder function in cholelithiasis. Surgical Forum 28: 412–413

Hahm J S, Park J Y, Song S C et al 1997 Gallbladder motility change in late pregnancy and after delivery. Korean Journal of Medicine 12: 16–20

Harvey P R C, Upadhya G A, Straberg S M 1991 Immunoglobulins as nucleating proteins in the gallbladder bile of patients with cholesterol gallstones. Journal of Biological Chemistry 266: 13996–14003

Harvey R C, Taylor D, Petrunka C N 1985 Quantitative analysis of major, minor and trace elements in gallbladder bile of patients with and without gallstones. Hepatology 5: 129–132

Hasse C, Nielke A, Nies C, Al-Bazaz B, Gotzen L, Rothmund M 1995 Influence of ceruletid on gallbladder contraction: a possible prophylaxis of acute acalculous cholecystitis in intensive care patients. Digestion 56: 389–394

Hatsushika S, Tazuma S, Kajiyama G 1993 Nucleation time and fatty acid composition of lecithin in human gallbladder bile. Scandinavian Journal of Gastroenterology 28: 131–136

He C, Fisher S, Kullak-Ublick G A et al 1999 Electrophoretic analysis of proteins in bile. Analytica Chimica Acta 383:185–203

Heaton K W, Emmett P M, Symes C L, Braddon F E M 1993 An explanation for gallstones in normal-weight women: slow intestinal transit. Lancet 341: 8–10

Heaton K W 1999 Gall bladder and bowel: the links multiply. Editorial commentary. Gut 35: 166

Hendel H W, Hojgaard L, Andersen T et al 1998 Fasting gallbladder volume and lithogenicity in relation to glucose tolerance, total and intra-abdominal fat masses in obese non-diabetic subjects. International Journal of Obesity and Related Metabolic Disorders 22: 294–302

Heshka S, Spitz A, Nunez C et al 1998 Obesity and risk of gallstone development on a 1200 kcal/d (5025 kJ/d) regular food diet. International Journal of Obesity and Related Metabolic Disorders 22: 282–284

Higashijima H, Ichimiya H, Nakano T et al 1996 Deconjugation of bilirubin accelerates coprecipitation of cholesterol, fatty acids, and mucin in human bile—in vitro study. Journal of Gastroenterology 31: 828–835

Ho K J, Lin X Z, Yu S C, Chen J S, Wu C Z 1995 Cholelithiasis in Taiwan. Gallstone characteristics, surgical incidence, bile lipid composition, and role of beta-glucuronidase. Digestive Diseases and Sciences, 40: 1963–1973

Ho K J 1996 Biliary electrolytes and enzymes in patients with and without gallstones. Digestive Diseases and Sciences, 41: 2409–2416

Ho K Y, Weissberger A J, Marbach P et al 1990 Therapeutic efficacy of the somatostatin analog SMS 201–995 (octreotide) in acromegaly. Annals of Internal Medicine 112: 173–181

Holan K R, Holzbach R T, Hermann R E et al 1979 Nucleation time; a key factor in the pathogenesis of cholesterol gallstone disease. Gastroenterology 77: 611–617

Hood K A, Gleeson D, Ruppin D C, Dowling R H and the British/Belgian Gallstone Study Group 1988 Prevention of gallstone recurrence by non-steroidal anti-inflammatory drugs. The Lancet, I: 1223–1225

Houssin D, Castaing D, Lemoine J et al 1983 Microlithiasis of the gallbladder. Surgery, Gynecology and Obstetrics 157: 20–24

Holzbach R T, Marsh M, Olszewski M, Holan K 1973 Cholesterol solubility in bile. Evidence that supersaturated bile is frequent in healthy man. Journal of Clinical Investigations. 52: 1467–1479

Howard P J, Murphy G M, Dowling R H 1991 Gall bladder emptying patterns in response to a normal meal in healthy subjects and patients with gall stones: ultrasound study. Gut 32: 1406–1411

Hussaini S H, Murphy G M, Kennedy C, Besser G M, Wass J A H, Dowling R H 1994 The role of bile composition and physical chemistry in the pathogenesis of octreotide-associated gallbladder stones. Gastroenterology 107: 1503–1513

Hussaini S H, Pereira S P, Murphy G M, Dowling R H 1995 Deoxycholic acid influences cholesterol transport and microcrystal nucleation time in gallbladder bile. Hepatology 22: 1735–1744

Hussaini S H, Pereira S P, Veysey M J et al 1996 The roles of gallbladder emptying and intestinal transit in the pathogenesis of octreotide induced gallbladder stones. Gut 38: 775–783

Ihasz M, Griffith C A 1981 Gallstones after vagotomy. American Journal of Surgery 141: 48–50

Ikeda Y, Shinchi K, Kono S, Tsuboi K, Sugimachi K 1995 Risk of gallstones following gastrectomy in Japanese men. Surgery Today, 25: 515–518

Inoee K, Fuchigami A, Higashide S et al 1992 Gallbladder sludge and stone formation in relation to contractile function and after gastrectomy. A prospective study. Annals of Surgery 215: 19–26

Isaksson B 1954 On the dissolving power of lecithin and bile salts for cholesterol in human bladder bile. Acta Soc. Med. Upsalien 59: 296–306

Jacyna M R, Ross P E, Bakar M A, Hopwood D, Bouchier I A D 1987 Characteristics of cholesterol absorption by human gallbladder: relevance to cholesterolosis. Journal of Clinical Pathology 40: 524–529

Janciauskiene S, Gerbord M-C, Lindgren S 1998 Effect of serpins on cholesterol crystallization in model bile. Journal of Hepatology 29: 541–549

Jazrawi R P, Pazzi P, Petroni M L et al 1995 Postprandial gallbladder motor function: refilling and turnover of bile in health and in cholelithiasis. Gastroenterology 109: 582–591

Johnston S M, Murray K P, Martin S A et al 1997 Iron deficiency enhances cholesterol gallstone formation. Surgery 122: 354–361

Jorgensen T 1988 Gallstones in a Danish population: familial occurrence and social factors. Journal of Biosocial Science 20: 111–120

Jungst D, Lang T, Huber P, et al 1993 Effect of phospholipids and bile acids on cholesterol nucleation time and vesicular/micellar cholesterol in gallbladder bile of patients with cholesterol stones. Journal of Lipid Research 34: 1457–1464

Jungst D, Muller I, Kullak-Ublick G A, Meyer G, Frim-Berger E, Fischer S 1999 Deoxycholic acid is not related to lithogenic factors in gallbladder bile. Journal of Laboratory and Clinical Medicine 133: 370–377

Juvonen T, Kervinen K, Kairaluoma M I et al 1993 Gallstone cholesterol content is related to apolipoprotein E polymorphism. Gastroenterology 104: 1806–1813

Kam D M, Webb P A, Sandman A et al 1996 A novel 5-lipoxygenase inhibitor prevents gallstone formation in a lithogenic prairie dog model. I American Surgery 62: 551–555

Kano M, Shoda J, Irimura T et al 1998 Effects of long-term ursodeoxycholic administration on expression levels of secretory low-molecular-weight phospholipases A2 and mucin genes in gallbladders and biliary composition in patients with multiple cholesterol stones. Hepatology 28: 302–313

Kaufman H S, Magnuson T H, Pitt H A 1994 The distribution of calcium salt precipitates in the core, periphery and shell of cholesterol, black pigment and brown pigment gallstones. Hepatology 19: 1124–1132.

Kesaniemi YA, Ehnholm C, Miettinen TA 1987 Intestinal cholesterol absorption efficiency in man is related to apoprotein E phenotype Journal of Clinical Investigations 80: 578–581

Kesaniemi Y A, Koskenvuo M, Vuoristo M, Miettinen T A 1989 Biliary lipid composition in monozygotic and dizygotic pairs of twins. Gut 30: 1750–1756

Ketover S R, Ansel H J, Goldish G, Roche B, Gebhard R L 1996 Gallstones in chronic spinal cord injury: is impaired gallbladder emptying a risk factor? Archives of Physical Medicine & Rehabilitation 77: 1136–1138

Khanuja B, Cheah Y C, Hunt M et al 1995 Lith 1, a major gene affecting cholesterol gallstone formation among inbred strains of mice. Proceedings of the National Academy of Sciences 92: 7729–7733

Kibe A, Holzbach R T, LaRusso N F, Mao S J 1984a Inhibition of cholesterol crystal formation by apolipoproteins in supersaturated model bile. Science 225: 514–516

Kibe A, Breuer A C, Holzbach R T 1984b Cholesterol nucleation in human bile by video-enhanced contrast-differential interference microscopy (VEM). The role of vesicles in metastable supersaturation. Gastroenterology 86: 1326 (abstr)

Kim Y S, Gun J R Jr 1995 Diversity of mucin genes, structure, function and expression. Gastroenterology 109: 999–1013

Klinspoor J H, van Wijland M J, Koeleman C A et al 1994 Heterogeneity of human biliary mucin: functional implications. Clin Chim Acta 86: 75–82

Knyrim K, Vakil N, Pfab R, Classen M 1989 Effect of intraduodenal bile acid administration on biliary secretion of ionised calcium and carbonate in man. Hepatology 10: 134–142

Knyrim K, Vakil N 1992 Bile composition, microspheroliths, antinucleating activity and gallstone calcification. Gastroenterology 103: 552–559

Ko C W, Lee S P 1999 Gallstone formation. Local factors. Gastroenterol Clinics of North America 28: 99–115

Konikoff F M, Chung D S, Donovan J M, Small D M, Carey M C 1992 Filamentous, helical and tubular microstructures during cholesterol crystallization from bile. Evidence that biliary cholesterol does not nucleate classic monohydrate plates. Journal of Clinical Investigations 90: 1156–1161

Konikoff F M, Carey M C 1994a Cholesterol crystallization from a dilute bile salt-rich model. Journal of Crystal Growth 144: 79–86

Konikoff F M, Cohen D E, Carey M C 1994b Phospholipid molecular species influence crystal habits and transition sequences of metastable intermediates during cholesterol crystallization from bile salt-rich model bile. Journal of Lipid Research 35: 60–70

Kono S, Shinchi K, Todoroki I et al 1995 Gallstone disease among Japanese men in relation to obesity, glucose intolerance, exercise, alcohol use and smoking. Scandinavian Journal of Gastroenterology 30: 1228

Kratzer W, Kächele V, Mason R A et al 1998 Gallstone prevalence in Germany. The Ulm gallbladder stone study. Digestive Diseases and Science 43, 1285–1291

Krejs G J, Orci L, Conlon J M et al 1979 Follow-up of a patient with Somatostatinoma syndrome biochemical, morphologic and clinical features. New England Journal of Medicine 301: 285–292

Kuipers F, Oude Elferink R P, Verkade J H, Groen A K 1997 Mechanism and (patho) physiological significance of biliary cholesterol secretion. Sub-cellular Biochem 28: 295–318

Kurata J H, Marks J, Abbey D 1991 One gram of aspirin per day does not reduce risk of hospitalization for gallstone disease. Digestive Diseases and Sciences 16: 1110–1115

Lachman B S, Lazerson J, Starshak R J et al 1979 The prevalence of cholelithiasis in sickle cell disease as diagnosed by ultrasound and cholecystography. Pediatrics 64: 601–603.

LaFont H, Domingo N, Groen A et al 1997 APF/CBP, the small, amphipathic, anionic protein(s) in bile and gallstones, consist of lipid-binding and calcium-binding forms. Hepatology 25: 1054–1063

Lammert F, Wang D Q, Paigen B, Carey M C 1999 Phenotypic characterization of lith genes that determine susceptibility to cholesterol cholelithiasis in inbred mice: integrated activities of hepatic lipid regulatory enzymes. Journal of Lipid Research 40: 2080–2090

LaMont T J, Turner B S, DiBenedetto D, Handin R, Schafrer A I 1983 Arachidonic acid stimulates mucin secretion in prairie dog gallbladder. American Journal of Physiology 245: G92–G98

LaMont J T, Smith B F, Moore J R L 1984 Role of gallbladder mucin in pathophysiology of gallstones. Hepatology 4: 51S–56S

LaRusso N F. Proteins in bile: how they get there and what they do.: American Journal of Physiology 1984; 247: G199–205

Lee D K, Tarr P I, Haigh W G, Lee S P 1999 Bacterial DNA in mixed cholesterol stones. American Journal of Gastroenterology 94: 3502–3506

Lee S P, LaMont J T, Carey M C 1981a Role of gallbladder mucus hypersecretion in the evolution of cholesterol gallstones. Studies in the prairie dog. Journal of Clinical Investigations 67: 1712–1723

Lee S P, Carey M C, LaMont T J 1981b Aspirin prevention of cholesterol gallstone formation in prairie dogs. Science 211: 1429–1430

Lee S P, Nicholls J 1986 Nature and composition of biliary sludge. Gastroenterology 90: 677–680

Leitzman M F, Giovannucci E L, Rum E B et al 1998 The relation of physical activity to risk for symptomatic gallstone disease in men. Annals of Internal Medicine 128: 417–425

Lembcke B, Creutzfeldt W, Schleser S et al 1987 Effect of somatostatin analogue Sandostatin (SMS 201-995) on gastrointestinal, pancreatic and biliary function, and hormone release in normal men. Digestion 36: 108–124

Lesma A, Monti D, Mezzabotta M et al 1997 Monoconjugated bilirubin as a possible factor in cholesterol gallstone pathogenesis. Minerva Chirurgica 52: 771–775

Leung J W, Yu A S 1997 Hepatolithiasis and biliary parasites. Baillières Clinical Gastroenterology 11: 681–706

Lewis S J, Heaton K W 1997 Increasing butyrate concentration in the distal colon by accelerating intestinal transit. Gut 41: 245–251

Levy P F, Smith B F, LaMont J T 1984 Human gallbladder mucin accelerates nucleation of cholesterol in artificial bile. Gastroenterology 87: 270–275

Lipsett P A, Fox-Talbot M K, Falconer S D et al 1995 Biliary nonmucin glycoproteins in patients with and without gallstones. Journal of Surgical Research 58: 386–390

Lirussi F, Vaja S, Murphy G M, Dowling R H 1989 Cholestasis of total parenteral nutrition: Bile acid and bile lipid metabolism in parenterally-nourished rats. Gastroenterology 96: 493–502

Loomis C, Shipley G, Small D M 1979 The phase behaviour of hydrated cholesterol. Journal Lipid Research 20: 525–535

Low-Beer T S, Pomare E W 1975 Can colonic bacterial metabolites predispose to cholesterol gallstones? British Journal of Medicine i: 438–440

Low-Beer T S 1998 How the colon begets gallstones. Lancet 351: 612–613

Mabee T M, Meyer P, DenBesten L, Mason E E 1976 The mechanism of increased gallstone formation in obese human subjects. Surgery 79: 460–468

Madrid J F, Hernández F, Ballesta J 1997 Characterization of glycoproteins in the epithelial cells of human and other mammalian gallbladder. A review. Microscopy Research and Technique 38: 616–630

Maggi A, Solenghi D, Panzeri A et al 1997 Prevalence and incidence of cholelithiasis in patients with liver cirrhosis. Italian Journal of Gastroenterology and Hepatology 29: 330–335

Maki T 1966 Pathogenesis of calcium bilirubinate gallstone: role of *E. coli*, beta-glucuronidase and coagulation by inorganic ions, polyelectrolytes and agitation. Annals of Surgery 164: 90–100

Marcus S N, Heaton K W 1986 Intestinal transit, deoxycholic acid and the cholesterol saturation of bile—three inter-related factors. Gut 27: 550–558

Marcus S N, Heaton K W 1988 Deoxycholic acid and the pathogenesis of gall stones. Gut 29: 522–533

Maringhini A, Marceno M P, Lanzarone F et al 1987 Sludge and stones in gallbladder after pregnancy. Prevalence and risk factors. Journal of Hepatology 5: 218–223

Maringhini A, Ciambra M, Bacelliere P et al 1993 Biliary sludge and gallstones in pregnancy: incidence, risk factors and natural history. Annals of Internal Medicine 119: 116–120

Marks J W, Bonorris G G, Schoenfield L J 1996 Effects of ursodiol or ibuprofen on contraction of gallbladder and bile among obese patients during weight loss. Digestive Diseases and Sciences 41: 242–249

Marteau C, Sastre B, Iconomidis N et al 1990 pH regulation in human gallbladder bile: study in patients with and without gallstones. Hepatology 11: 997–1002

Masclee A A M, Jansen J B M J, Driessen W M M et al 1990 Effect of truncal vagotomy on cholecystokinin release, gallbladder contraction and gallbladder sensitivity to cholecystokinin in humans. Gastroenterology 98: 1338–1344

Maselli M A, Pezzolla F, Piepoli A L et al 1996 Gallbladder motility in vitro in men with gallstones following Billroth II gastric resection. Neurogastro and Motility 8: 29–33

Mauad T H, van Nieubwkerk C M J, Dingemans K P et al 1994 Mice and homozygous disruption of the mdr2 P-glycoprotein gene: a novel animal model for studies of non-suppurative inflammatory cholangitis and hepatocarcinogenesis. American Journal of Pathology 145: 1237–1245

Messing B, Bories C, Kunstlinger F et al 1983 Does total parenteral nutrition induce gallbladder sludge formation and lithiasis? Gastroenterology 84: 1012–1019

Metcalf A M, Phillips S F, Zinsmeister A R, MacCarty R L, Beart R W, Wolff B G 1987 Simplified assessment of segmental colonic transit. Gastroenterology 92: 40–47

Meyer P D, Den Besten L, Gurll N J 1978 Effects of cholesterol gallstone induction on gallbladder function and bile salt pool size in the prairie dog model. I. Surgery 83: 599–604

Miettinen T A 1971 Cholesterol production in obesity. Circulation 44: 842–850

Miquel J F, Covarrubias C, Villaroel L et al 1998 Genetic epidemiology of cholesterol cholelithiasis among Chilean Hispanics, Amerindians and Maoris. Gastroenterology 115: 937–946

Misciagna G, Leoci C, Guerra V et al 1996 Epidemiology of cholelithiasis in southern Italy. Part II: Risk factors. European Journal of Gastroenterology and Hepatology 8: 585–593

Mok H Y, Druffel E R, Rampone W M et al 1986 Chronology of

cholelithiasis. Dating gallstones from atmospheric radiocarbon produced by nuclear bomb explosions. New England Journal of Medicine 314: 1075–1077

Møller N, Petrany G, Cassidy D et al 1988 Effects of the somatostatin analogue SMS 201-955 (Sandostatin) on mouth-to-caecum transit time and absorption of fat and carbohydrates in normal man. Clinical Science 75: 345–350

Moonka R, Stiens S A, Resnick W J et al 1999 The prevalence and natural history of gallstones in spinal cord injured patients. Journal of the American College of Surgery 189: 274–281

Moore E W, Verine J H. Pathogenesis of pancreatic and biliary CaCO₃ lithiasis: the solubility product (K'SP) of calcite determined with the Ca⁺⁺ electrode. Journal of Laboratory and Clinical Medicine 106: 611–618

Lord Moyniham 1964 in: Harding Rains A J 'Gallstone Causes and Treatment' London, Heinemann Medical Books, p. 31

Muller M, Jansen P L M 1998 The secretory function of the liver: new aspects of hepatobiliary transport. Journal of Hepatology 28: 344–354

Muraca M, Cianci V, Miconi L et al 1994 Ultrasound evaluation of gallbladder emptying with ceruletide: comparison to oral cholecystography with fatty meat. Abdominal Imaging 19: 253–258

Myers S I, Li Y F, Weisbrodt N W et al 1989 Endogenous gallbladder prostaglandin biosynthesis is not related to gallstone formation in the prairie dog fed a high-cholesterol diet. Surg Forum 40: 157–158

Nakano K, Chijiiwa K, Noshiro H et al 1992 Human gallbladder bile becomes lithogenic during short-term intravenous hyperalimentation. Journal of Surgical Research 53: 396–401

Nardone G, Ferber I A, Miller L J 1995 The integrity of the cholecystokinin receptor gene in gallbladder disease and obesity. Hepatology 22: 1751–1753

Nestel P J, Schreibman P H, Ahrens E H Jr 1973 Cholesterol metabolism in human obesity. Journal of Clinical Investigation 52: 2389–2397

Newman C B, Melmed S, Snyder P J et al 1995 Safety and efficacy of long-term octreotide therapy of acromegaly: results of a multicenter trial in 103 patients — a clinical research center study. Journal of Clinical Endocrinology and Metabolism 80: 2768–2775

Nicholas P, Rinaudo P A, Conn H O 1972 Increased incidence of cholelithiasis in Laennec's cirrhosis. Gastroenterology 63: 111–121

Nilsell K, Angelin B, Leijd B, Einarsson K 1983 Comparative effects of ursodeoxycholic acid and chenodeoxycholic acid on bile acid kinetics and biliary lipid secretion in humans. Gastroenterology 85: 1248–1256

Nilsell K, Angelin B, Liljeqvist L, Einarsson K 1985 Biliary lipid output and bile acid kinetics in cholesterol gallstone disease. Gastroenterology 89: 287–293

Northfield T C, Hofmann A F 1975 Biliary lipid output during three meals and an overnight fast. I. Relationship to bile acid pool size and cholesterol saturation of bile in gallstone and control subjects. Gut 16: 1–11

Noshiro H, Chijiiwa K, Hirota I 1992 Activity of cholesterol in human gallbladder bile in relation to nucleation of cholesterol monohydrate crystals. Clinica Chimica Acta 205: 167–169

Noshiro H, Chijiiwa K, Makino I, Nakano K, Hirota I 1995 Deoxycholic acid in gall bladder bile does not account for the shortened nucleation time in patients with cholesterol gall stones. Gut 36: 121–125

Nunez L, Amigo L, Mingrone G et al 1995 Biliary aminopeptidase-N and the cholesterol crystallisation defect in cholelithiasis. Gut 37: 422–426

O'Donnell L J D, Watson A J M, Cameron D, Farthing M J G 1990 Effect of octreotide on mouth-to-caecum transit time in healthy subjects and in the irritable bowel syndrome. Aliment. Pharmacology and Therapeutics 4: 177–182

O'Donnell L J D, Wilson P, Guest P et al 1992 Indomethacin and postprandial gallbladder emptying. Lancet 339: 269–271

O'Donnell L J D, Fairclough P D 1993 Gall stones and gall bladder motility. Gut 34: 440–443

Offner G D, Gong D, Afdhal N H 1994 Identification of a 130-kilodalton human biliary concanavalin A binding protein as aminopeptidase N. Gastroenterology 106: 755–763

Offner G D, Nunes D P, Zang F, McAnneny D B, Afdhal N H 1996 Alterations in gallbladder mucin gene expression in patients with cholesterol gallstones. Gastroenterology 110: A1282 (Abstr)

O'Leary D P, LaMorte W W, Scott T E et al 1991 Inhibition of prostaglandin synthesis fails to prevent gallbladder mucin hypersecretion in the cholesterol-fed prairie dog. Gastroenterology 101: 812–820

O'Leary D P 1995 Biliary cholesterol transport and the nucleation defect in cholesterol gallstone formation. Journal of Hepatology 22: 239–246

Ortega R M, Fernandez-Azuela M, Encinas-Sotillos A et al 1997 Differences in diet and food habits between patients with gallstones and controls. Journal of American College of Nutrition 16: 88–95

Ortega López D, Martínez S J, Borque M et al 1997 Study of the secretion of substance P, neurotensin and somatostatin in patients with cholelithiasis. Revista Espanola de Enfermedades Digestivas 89: 425–434

Oude Elferink R P, Groen A K 1995a The role of mdr2 P-glycoprotein in biliary lipid secretion. Cross-talk between cancer research and biliary physiology. Journal of Hepatology 23: 617–625

Oude Elferink R P, Ottenhoff O, van Wijland M, Smit J J, Schrinkel A H, Groen A K 1995b Regulation of biliary lipid secretion by mdr2 P-glycoprotein in the mouse. Journal of Clinical Investigations 95: 31–38

Palasciano G, Serio G, Portincasa P et al 1992 Gallbladder volume in adults, and relationship to age, sex, body mass index, and gallstones: a sonographic population study. American Journal of Gastroenterology 87: 493–497

Panataker R, Ozmen M M, Bailey I S, Johnson C D 1995 Gallbladder motility, gallstones, and the surgeon. Digestive Diseases and Science 40: 2323–2335

Pattinson N R, Willis K E 1991 Effect of phospholipase C on cholesterol solubilization in model bile. Gastroenterology 101: 1339–1344

Pauletzi J, Cicala M, Holl J et al 1993 Correlation between gallbladder fasting volume and postprandial emptying in patients with gallstones and healthy controls. Gut 34: 1443–1447

Pauletzki J G, Xu Q-W, Shaffer E A 1995 Inhibition of gallbladder emptying decreases cholesterol saturation in bile in the Richardson ground squirrel. Hepatology 22: 325–331

Pauletzki J, Althaus R, Holl J, Sackmann M, Paumgartner G 1996 Gallbladder emptying and gallstone formation: a prospective study on gallstone recurrence. Gastroenterology 111: 765–771

Pazzi P, Scagliarini R, Sighinolfi et al 1998 Nonsteroidal antiinflammatory drug use and gallstone disease prevalence: a case control study. American Journal of Gastroenterology 93: 1420–1424

Pekow C A, Weller R E, Schulte S J, Lee S P 1995 Dietary induction of cholesterol gallstones in owl monkey: preliminary findings in a new animal model. Laboratory Animal Science 45: 657–662

Pellegrini C A, Ryan T, Broderick W, Way L W 1986 Gallbladder filling and emptying during cholesterol gallstone formation in the prairie dog. Gastroenterology 90: 143–149

Pereira S P, Veysey M J, Kennedy C, Hussaini S H, Dowling R H 1997 Gallstone dissolution with oral bile acid therapy: importance of pre-treatment CT scanning and reasons for non-response. Digestive Diseases and Sciences 42: 1775–1782

Petroni M L, Jazrawi R P, Grundy A et al 1995 Prospective, multicenter study on value of computerized tomography (CT) in gallstone disease in predicting response to bile acid therapy. Digestive Diseases and Sciences 40: 1956–1962

Pilotto A, Fransceschi M, Del Favero G et al 1995 The effect of aging on oro-cecal transit time in normal subjects and patients with gallstone disease. Aging 7: 234–237

Pixley F, Wilson D, McPherson K et al 1985 Effect of vegetarianism on development of gall stones in women. British Medical Journal 291: 11–12

Plaisier P W, Brakel K, van der Hul R L et al 1994 Radiographic features of oral cholecystograms of 448 symptomatic gallstone patients: implications for non-surgical therapy. European Journal of Radiology 18: 57–60

Plevris J N, Bouchier I A D 1995 Defective acid base regulation by the gall bladder epithelium and its significance for gall stone formation. Gut 37: 127–131

Pomeranz I S, Shaffer E A 1985 Abnormal gallbladder emptying in a subgroup of patients with gallstones. Gastroenterology 88: 787–791

Portincasa P, Stolk M F J, van Erpecum K J et al 1995 Cholesterol gallstone formation in man and potential treatments of the gallbladder motility defect. Scandinavian Journal of Gastroenterology 30: (Suppl 212) 63–78

Portincasa P, van Erpecum K J, Jansen A et al 1996a Behavior of various cholesterol crystals in bile from patients with gallstones. Hepatology 23: 738–748

Portincasa P, van Erpecum K J, van de Meeberg P C et al 1996b Apolipoprotein E4 genotype and gallbladder motility influence speed of gallstone clearance and risk of recurrence after extracorporeal shock-wave lithotripsy. Hepatology 24: 580–587

Portincasa P, van Erpecum K J, van Berge Henegouwen G P 1997a Cholesterol crystallisation in bile. Gut 41: 138–141

Portincasa P, van de Meeberg P C, van Erpecum K J et al 1997b An update on the pathogenesis and treatment of cholesterol gallstones. Scandinavian Journal of Gastroenterology (Supplement) 223: 60–69

Rajagopal S U, Keightley A, Bills P, Walters J R F, Murphy G M, Dowling R H 1989 Predictive value of pre-treatment CT scanning vs conventional radiology in determining composition, dissolvability and fragmentability of gallbladder stones (GBS). Journal of Hepatology 9: S211 (Abstract)

Redfern J S, Fortuner W J II 1995 Octreotide-associated biliary tract dysfunction and gallstone formation: Patho-physiology and management. American Journal of Gastroenterology 90: 1042–1052

Rege R V, Pyrstowsky J B 1998 Inflammation and a thickened mucus layer in mice with cholesterol gallstones. Journal of Surgical Research 74: 81–85

Reuben A, Maton P N, Murphy G M, Dowling R H 1985 Bile lipid secretion in obese and non-obese individuals with and without gallstones. Clinical Science 69: 71–79

Ringel Y, Somjen G J, Konikoff F M, Rosenberg R, Michowitz M, Gilat T 1998 The effects of phospholipid molecular species on cholesterol crystallization in model biles: the influence of phospholipid head groups. Journal of Hepatology 28: 1008–1014

Rhodes M, Allen A, Dowling R H, Murphy G M, Lennard T W J 1992 Inhibition of human gall bladder mucus synthesis in patients underoing cholecystectomy. Gut 33: 1113–1117

Roda A, Hofmann A F, Mysels K J 1983 The influence of bile salt structure on self-association in aqueous solutions. Journal of Biological Chemistry 258: 6362–6370

Ros E, Navarro S, Bru C et al 1991 Occult microlithiasis in 'idiopathic' acute pancreatitis: prevention of relapses by cholecystectomy or ursodeoxycholic acid therapy. Gastroenterology 101: 1701–1709

Roslyn J, DenBesten L, Thompson J, Cohen K 1980 Chronic cholelithiasis and decreased bile salt pool size. Cause or effect? American Journal of Surgery 139: 119–124

Roslyn J J, Pitt H A, Mann L L et al 1983 Gallbladder disease in patients on long-term parenteral nutrition. Gastroenterology 84: 148–154

Ross P E, Butt A N, Gallacher C 1990 Cholesterol absorption by the gallbladder. Journal of Clinical Pathology 43: 572–575

Rudnicki M, Jorgensen T, Thode J 1992 Increased activity of ionized calcium in gallbladder bile and gallstone disease. Gut 33: 1404–1407

Sahlin P, Schneider H, Hanisch E et al 1992 Nonadrenergic noncholinergic regulation of gallstone containing and gallstone free human gallbladders. European Journal of Gastroenterology and Hepatology 4: 1019–1024

Sanabria J R, Upadhya A, Mullen B, Harvey P R C, Strasberg S M 1995 Effect of deoxycholate on immunoglobulin G concentration in bile: studies in humans and pigs. Hepatology 21: 215–222

Sänger P, Schneider H, Hanisch E et al 1997 Nonadrenergic noncholinergic regulation of gallstone containing and gallstone free human gallbladders. Zentralblatt fur Chir 122: 418–424

Sapala M A, Sapala J A, Soto A D et al 1970 Cholelithiasis following sub-total gastric with truncal vagotomy. Surgery, Gynecology and Obstetrics 71: 196–200

Sarin S K, Negi V S, Dewan R, Sasan S, Saraya A 1995 High familial prevalence of gallstones in the first-degree relatives of gallstone patients. Hepatology 22: 138–141

Sarnaik S, Slovis T L, Corbett D P et al 1980 Incidence of cholelithiasis in sickle cell anemia using the ultrasonic gray-scale technique. Journal of Pediatrics 96: 1005–1008

Schneider H S, Sanger P, Hanisch E 1997 In vitro effects of cholecystokinin fragments on human gallbladders. Evidence for an altered CCK-receptor structure in a subgroup of patients with gallstones. Journal of Hepatology 26: 1063–1068

Sedeghat A, Grundy S M 1980 Cholesterol crystals and the formation of cholesterol gallstones. New England Journal of Medicine 302: 1274–1277

Setchell K D R, Matsui A 1983 Serum bile acid analysis. Clinica Chimica Acta 127: 1–17

Shaffer E A, Small D M 1977 Biliary lipid secretion in cholesterol gallstone disease. The effect of cholecystectomy and obesity. Journal of Clinical Investigations 59: 828–840

Sharma B C, Agarwal D K, Dhiman R K et al 1998 Bile lithogenicity and gallbladder emptying in patients with microlithiasis: effect of bile acid therapy. Gastroenterology 115: 124–128

Shi Y F, Harris A G, Zhu X F et al 1993 Clinical and biochemical effects of the long-acting somatostatin analogue SMS 201-995 in ten patients. Journal of Clinical Endocrinology and Metabolism 76: 32–37

Shiffman M L, Sugerman H J, Kellum J M et al 1991 Gallstone formation and after rapid weight loss: a prospective study in patients undergoing gastric bypass surgery for treatment of marked obesity. American Journal of Gastroenterology 86: 1000–1005

Shiffman M L, Sugerman H J, Kellum J M, Moore E W 1992 Changes in gallbladder bile composition following gallstone formation and weight reduction. Gastroenterology 103: 214–221

Shiffman M L, Sugerman H J, Kellum J M et al 1993a Gallstones in patients with morbid obesity. Relationship to body weight, weight loss and gallbladder bile cholesterol solubility. International Journal of Obesity and Metabolic Disorders 17: 153–158

Shiffman M L, Shamburek R D, Schwartz C C et al 1993b Gallbladder mucin, arachidonic acid, and bile lipids in patients who develop gallstones during weight reduction. Gastroenterology 105: 1200–1208

Shoda J, He B-F, Tanaka N et al 1995 Increase of deoxycholate in supersaturated bile of patients with cholesterol gallstone disease and its correlation with de novo syntheses of cholesterol and bile acids in liver, gallbladder emptying, and small intestinal transit. Hepatology 21: 1291–1302

Shoda J, Ueda T, Ikegami T et al 1997 Increased biliary group II phospholipase A2 and altered gallbladder bile in patients with multiple cholesterol stones. Gastroenterology 112: 2036–2047

Sipos P, Gamal E M, Blazovics A et al 1997 Free radical reactions in the gallbladder. Acta Chir Hungarica 36: 329–330

Sitzmann J V, Pitt H A, Steinborn P A, Pasha Z R, Sanders R C 1990 Cholecystokinin prevents parenteral nutrition induced biliary sludge in humans. Surgery, Gynecology & Obstetrics 33: 4–9

Small D M, Bourges M C, Dervichian D G, 1966 Ternary and quaternary aqueous systems containing bile salt, lecithin, and cholesterol. Nature 211: 816–818

Small D M 1971 in: Nair P P, Kritchevsky D (Eds) The Bile Acids. Plenum Press, New York, p 249–256

Small D M 1980 Cholesterol nucleation and growth in gallstone formation. New England Journal of Medicine 302: 1305–1307

Smit J J, Schrinkel A H, Oude Elferink R P et al 1993 Homozygous disruption of the murine mdr2 P-glycoprotein gene leads to a complete absence of phospholipid from bile and to liver disease. Cell 75: 451–462

Smith B F, LaMont J T 1985 Identification of gallbladder mucin-bilirubin complex in human cholesterol gallstone matrix: Effects of reducing agents on in vitro dissolution of matrix and intact gallstones. Journal of Clinical Investigations 439–445

Smith B F 1987 Human gallbladder mucin binds biliary lipids and promotes cholesterol crystal nucleation in model bile. Journal of Lipid Research 28: 1088–1097

Soloway R D, Trotman B W, Ostrow J D 1977 Pigment gallstones. Progress in hepatology. Gastroenterology 72: 167–182

Somjen G J, Gilat T 1983 A non-micellar mode of cholesterol transport in human bile. FEBS Letters 156: 265

Somjen G J, Marikovsky Y, Wachel E et al 1990 Phospholipid lamellae are cholesterol carriers in human bile. Biochemica et Biophysica Acta 1042: 28–35

Spathis A, Heaton K W, Emmett P M et al 1997 Gallstones in a community free of obesity but prone to slow intestinal transit. European Journal of Gastroenterology and Hepatology 9: 201–206

Spirt B A, Graves L W, Weinstock R, Bartlett S J, Wadden T A 1995 Gallstone formation in obese women treated by a low-calorie diet. International Journal of Obesity and Related Metabolic Disorders 19: 593–595

Stellaard F, Paumgartner G, van Berge Henegouwen G P, van der Werf S D J 1986 Determination of deoxycholic acid pool size and input rate using [24-13C] deoxycholic acid and serum sampling. Journal of Lipid Research 27: 1222–1225

Sterling R K, Shiffman M L, Sugerman H J et al 1995 Effect of NSAIDs on gallbladder bile composition. Digestive Diseases and Sciences, 40: 2220–2226

Sterling R K, Shiffman M L 1998 Nonsteroidal antiinflammatory drugs and gallstone disease: will an aspirin a day keep the gallstones away? American Journal of Gastroenterology 93: 1405–1407

Stolk M F, van Erpecum K J, Renooij W et al 1995 Gallbladder emptying in vivo, bile composition, and nucleation of cholesterol crystals in patients with cholesterol gallstones. Gastroenterology 108: 1882–1888

Stolk M F J, van Erpecum K J, Koppeschaar H P F et al 1993 Postprandial gallbladder motility and hormone release during intermittent and continuous subcutaneous octreotide therapy in acromegaly. Gut 34: 808–813

Stone J M, Nino-Murcia M, Wolf V A, Perkash I et al 1990 Chronic gastrointestinal problems in spinal cord injury patients: a prospective analysis. American Journal of Gastroenterology 85: 1114–1119

Sugerman H J, Brewer W H, Shiffman M L et al 1995 A multicenter, placebo-controlled, randomized, double-blind, prospective trial of prophylactic ursodiol for the prevention of gallstone formation following gastric-bypass-induced rapid weight loss. American Journal of Surgery 169: 91–97

Sugerman H J, Londrey G L, Kellum J M et al 1989 Weight loss with vertical banded gastroplasty and Roux-Y gastric bypass for morbid obesity with selective versus random assignment. American Journal of Surgery 157: 93–102

Sutor D J, Wooley S E 1974 The organic matrix of gallstones. Gut 15: 487–491

Swidsinski A, Khilkin M, Pahlig H, Swidsinski S, Priem F 1998 Time dependent changes in the concentration and type of bacterial sequences found in cholesterol gallstones. Hepatology 27: 662–665

Syngal S, Coakley E H, Willett W C et al 1999 Long-term weight patterns and risk for cholecystectomy in women. Annals of Internal Medicine 130: 471–477

Tandon R K, Jain R K, Garg P K 1997 Increased incidence of biliary sludge and normal gall bladder contractility in patients with high spinal cord injury. Gut 41: 682–687

Taylor D R, Crowther R S, Cozart J C, Sharrock P, Wu J, Soloway R D 1995 Calcium carbonate in cholesterol gallstones: polymorphism, distribution, and hypotheses about pathogenesis. Hepatology 22: 488–496

Teramen K, Tazuma S, Ohya T, Kajiyama G 1995 Comparative effects on biliary concanavalin A-bound glycoproteins and calcium ion on cholesterol crystal nucleation and growth in model bile. Journal of Gastroenterology 30: 500–507

Thomas P J, Hofmann A F 1973 A simple calculation of the lithogenic index of bile: expressing lipid composition on rectangular co-ordinates. Gastroenterology 65: 698–700

Thomas L A, Veysey M J, Murphy G M, Dowling R H, King A, French G R 1997a Is cholelithiasis an intestinal disease? Gut 41 (Suppl 3): A2

Thomas L A, Bathgate T, Veysey M J et al 1997b Do changes in colonic luminal pH explain the increased proportions of serum and biliary deoxycholic acid seen in patients with cholesterol gallbladder stones (GBS)? Gut 41 (Suppl 3): A32

Thomas L A, King A, French G L, Murphy G M, Dowling R H 1997c Cholylglycine hydrolase and 7-alpha-dehydroxylase optimum assay conditions in vitro and caecal enzyme activities ex vivo. Clinica Chimica Acta 268: 61–72

Thomas L A, Bathgate T, Veysey M J et al 1998 Roles of colonic transit, bacteriology, bile acid metabolising enzymes and deoxycholic acid in the pathogenesis of gallstones and colorectal cancer in acromegalic patients before and during octreotide treatment. Gastroenterology 114: A546(abstract)

Thomas L A et al 2000 Prolonged colonic transit, increased bacterial enzymes and higher luminal pH enhance deoxycholic acid formation in cholesterol gallstone disease. Gastroenterology (in press)

Tompkins R K, Kraft A R, Zimmerman E et al 1972 Clinical and biochemical evidence of increased gallstone formation after complete vagotomy. Surgery 71: 196–200

Trotman B W, Soloway R D 1976 Pigment vs cholesterol cholelithiasis: Identification and quantification by infrared spectroscopy. Gastroenterology 72: 495–498

Trotman B W, Soloway R D 1982 Pigment gallstone disease: Summary of the National Institutes of Health – International Workshop. Hepatology 2: 879–884

Tudyka J, Wechsler J G, Kratzer W et al 1994 The effect of ursodeoxycholic acid on nucleation time in patients with solitary or multiple gallbladder stones. American Journal of Gastroenterology 89: 1206–1210

Valdivieso V, Covarrubias C, Siegal F, Cruz F 1983 Pregnancy and cholelithiasis: Pathogenesis and natural course of gallstones diagnosed in early puerperium. Hepatology 17: 1–4

Van Bodegraven A A, Bohmer C J, Manoliu R A et al 1998 Gallbladder contents and fasting gallbladder volumes during and after pregnancy. Scandinavian Journal of Gastroenterology 33: 993–997

van der Linden W 1973 Genetic factors in gallstone disease. Clinics in Gastroenterology 2: 603–614

van der Linden W 1974 Emptying of the human gallbladder and predisposition to gallstone formation. Tijdschr Gastro 17: 121–128

van Erpecum K J, van Berge Henegouwen G P, Stolk M F J et al 1990 Effects of ursodeoxycholic acid on gallbladder contraction and cholecystokinin release in gallstone patients and normal subjects. Gastroenterology 99: 836–842

van Erpecum K J, van Berge Henegouwen G P, Stolk M F J, Hopman W P M, Jansen J B M J, Lamers C B H W 1992 Fasting gallbladder volume, postprandial emptying and cholecystokinin release in gallstone patients and normal subjects. Journal of Hepatology 14: 194–202

van Erpecum K J, Portincasa P, Gadellaa M et al 1996a Effects of bile salt hydrophobicity on crystallization of cholesterol in model bile. European Journal of Clinical Investigations 26: 602–608

van Erpecum K J, Carey M C 1996b Apolipoprotein E4: another risk factor of cholesterol gallstone formation? Gastroenterology 111: 1764–1767

Veysey M J, Gathercole D J, Mallet A et al 1997 Large bowel transit time influences deoxycholic acid input rate and pool size—risk factors for octreotide-induced gallstones. Gastroenterology 112: A525 (Abstr)

Veysey M J, Mallett A, Jenkins P, Besser G M, Murphy G M, Dowling R H 1998 Deoxycholic (DCA) and cholic acid (CA) kinetics in acromegalic patients treated with octreotide (OT). Gut 42 (Suppl 1): A11

Veysey M J, Thomas L A, Mallet A I et al 1999 Prolonged large bowel transit increases serum deoxycholic acid: a risk factor for octreotide-induced gallstones. Gut 44: 675–681

Vezina W C, Grace D M, Hutton L C et al 1998 Similarity in gallstone formation from 900 kcal/day diets containing 16 g vs 30 g of daily fat: evidence that fat restriction is not the main culprit of cholelithiasis during rapid weight reduction. Digestive Diseases and Sciences 43: 554–561

Vlahcevic Z R, Bell C C Jr, Buhac I, Farrar J T, Swell L 1970 Diminished bile acid pool size in patients with gallstones. Gastroenterology 59: 165–173

Vlahcevic Z R, Bell C C Jr, Gregory D H, Buker G, Juttijudata P, Swell L 1972 Relationship of bile acid pool size to the formation of lithogenic bile in female Indians of the Southwest. Gastroenterology 62: 73–83

von Bergmann K, Epple-Gutsfeld M, Leiss O 1984 Differences in the effects of chenodeoxycholic and ursodeoxycholic acid on biliary lipid secretion and bile acid synthesis in patients with gallstones. Gastroenterology 87: 136–143

Walker T M, Serjeant G R 1996 Biliary sludge in sickle cell disease. Journal of Pediatrics 129: 443–445

Walters J R F, Hood K A, Gleeson D et al 1992 Combination therapy with oral ursodeoxycholic and chenodeoxycholic acids: pretreatment computed tomography of the gall bladder improves gall stone dissolution efficacy. Gut 33: 375–380

Wang D Q, Paigen B, Carey M C 1997 Phenotypic characterization of Lith-genes that determine susceptibility to cholesterol cholelithiasis in inbred mice: physical-chemistry of gallbladder bile. Journal of Lipid Research 38: 1395–1411

Watkins J L, Wiley T E, Layden T J 1993 Constipation: is it a risk factor for cholesterol gallstones? Hepatology 18: 457–458

Webb D H K, Darby J S, Dunn D T et al 1989 Gall stones in Jamaican children with homozygous sickle cell disease. Archives of Disease in Childhood 64: 693–696

Weinsier R L, Wilson L J, Lee J et al 1955. Medically safe rate of weight loss for the treatment of obesity: a guideline based on the risk of gallstone formation. America J. Medicine 98: 115–117

Weintraub M S, Eisenberg S, Breslow J L 1987 Dietary fat clearance in normal subjects is regulated by genetic variation in apolipoprotein E. Journal of Clinical Investigation 80: 1571–1577

Werlin S I, Scott J P 1996 Is biliary sludge a stone-in-waiting? Journal of Pediatrics 129: 321–322

Wetter L A, Hamadeh R M, Griffiss J McL et al 1994. Differences in outer membrane characteristics between gallstone-associated bacteria and normal bacteria. Lancet 343: 444–447

Wolpers C-H Personal communication

Womack N A, Zeppa R, Irvin G L III 1963 The anatomy of gallstones. Annals of Surgery 157: 670–686

Worthington H V, Hunt L P, McCloy R F et al 1997 A pilot study of antioxidant intake in patients with cholesterol gallstones. Nutrition 13: 118–127

Xu Q-W, Shaffer E A 1996a The potential site of impaired gallbladder contractility in an animal model of cholesterol gallstone disease. Gastroenterology 110: 251–257

Xu Q W, Scott R B, Tan D T, Shaffer E A 1996b Slow intestinal transit: a motor disorder contributing to cholesterol gallstone formation in the ground squirrel. Hepatology 23: 1664–1672

Yamashita G, Corradini S G, Secknus R et al 1995 Biliary haptoglobin, a potent promoter of cholesterol crystallization at physiological concentrations. Journal of Lipid Research 36: 1325–1333

Yamashita G, Secknus R, Chernosky A et al 1996 Comparison of haptoglobin and apoliprotein A-I on biliary lipid particles involved in cholesterol crystalization. Journal of Gastroenterology and Hepatology 11: 738–745

Yu P, Chen Q, Harnett K M, Amaral J, Biancani P, Behar J 1995 Direct G protein activation reverses impaired CCK signaling in human gallbladders with cholesterol stones. American Journal of Physiology 269: G659–G665

The natural history of gallstones and asymptomatic gallstones

32

J.N. VAUTHEY AND P.F. SALDINGER

INTRODUCTION

In 1992 it was estimated that 10 to 15% of the adult population in the United States had gallstones (which amounted to more than 20 million people) (NIH Consensus Statement, 1992). About one million patients are newly diagnosed annually and approximately 600 000 patients underwent cholecystectomy in 1991. Gallstones are the most common digestive disease leading to hospitalization with an estimated annual cost of $5 billion (NIH Consensus Statement, 1992). Considering these numbers and the limited financial resources in health care, it appears impossible to treat every patient diagnosed with gallstones by cholecystectomy. Knowledge of the natural history and risk factors in patients with asymptomatic gallstones is therefore essential. While it is generally accepted that asymptomatic patients should not undergo cholecystectomy there is still debate with respect to certain subgroups.

This chapter will highlight the current knowledge on incidence and natural history and analyze the management of gallstone disease in asymptomatic patients.

HISTORICAL NOTE

Gallstones have been described long before the era of modern abdominal surgery. Numerous calculi were found in the gallbladder of the mummy of a priestess of Amenen of the 21st Egyptian Dynasty (1500 BC) (Schwartz 1981). The Greek physician, Alexander Trallianus, described calculi within the hepatic radicles of a human liver (Glenn & Grafe 1966). By the 16th century, both Vesalius and Fallopius described gallstones found in the gallbladders of dissected human bodies (Schwartz 1981). These observations indi-cate a clear recognition of the phenomenon of cholelithiasis, however, pathogenesis and clinical significance of gallstones are seldom referred to. It was Langenbuch in the late 19th century (Langenbuch 1882) who widened the understanding of gallstone pathology and performed the first chole-cystectomy.

PREVALENCE

The population of certain parts of Italy has been studied extensively as to the prevalence of gallstones.

The Rome Group for the Epidemiology and Prevention of Cholelithiasis (GREPCO) found gallstones in 8% of Roman male civil servants between the age of 20 and 69 years. Less than 8% had a history of symptoms compatible with biliary colic (GREPCO 1988). The same group found a prevalence of as high as 25% in female civil servants in the 60–64 year age group. One-third reported at least one episode of biliary pain over a period of 5 years (GREPCO 1984).

As part of the Multicenter Italian Study on Cholelithiasis (MICOL) 29 739 study participants were examined by ultrasound and questionnaire with respect to the presence of gallstones and related symptoms (Attili et al 1995b). The prevalence of gallstones for women was 10.5% and 6.5% for men. This increased to 18.9 and 9.5% respectively when subjects who had already undergone cholecystectomy were added. A linear increase in prevalence was noted with age in both sexes. The vast majority of subjects with gallstones were asymptomatic (84.9% of women and 87.0% of men). This study confirms the high prevalence of gallstone disease and also shows that most patients are unaware of it. Similar numbers were found in a Scandinavian study (Muhrbeck & Ahlberg 1995).

Table 32.1 Prevalence of gallstones

Country	n	Gallstones %	Asymptomatic patients %
Italy (Attili et al 1995b)	29 739	18.9 (women) 9.5 (men)*	84.9 (women) 87.0 (men)
Sweden (Muhrbeck & Ahlberg 1995)	800	15	

* Including patients who had a cholecystectomy

The overall prevalence of gallstone disease in industrialized countries appears to be between 10 to 20% (Table 32.1) with an increase for female sex and age. The incidence is close to ten per 1000 subjects per year (Misciagna et al 1996, Angelico et al 1997).

NATURAL HISTORY OF GALLSTONES

The analysis of the natural history of gallstones started with a landmark study by Gracie and Ransohoff. They followed 123 Michigan University faculty members (110 men and 13 women) who had been found to have gallstones through routine screening for 15 years. At 5, 10 and 15 years of follow-up 10, 15 and 18% had become symptomatic. None of them had developed complications. The approximate rate at which the subjects developed biliary pain was 2% per year for the first 5 years with a subsequent decrease over time. Three patients in this study developed biliary complications, all of which were preceded by biliary pain. They concluded based on the results that prophylactic cholecystectomy for asymptomatic gallstones could not be recommended (Gracie and Ransohoff 1982).

Attili and colleagues also followed 151 subjects identified to have gallstones during the GREPCO study (GREPCO 1984) over a period of 10 years (Attili et al 1995a). Thirty-three subjects had symptoms while 118 were asymptomatic at the beginning of the study. The cumulative probability of developing biliary colic was 12% at 2 years, 17% at 4 years, and 26% at 10 years. The cumulative probability of developing complications after 10 years was 3% in the initially asymptomatic group and 7% in the symptomatic group. The authors conclude that the natural history of gallstone disease might not be as benign as previously thought.

In a Japanese study Wada and colleagues found one-third of 1850 patients with cholelithiasis to be symptomatic.

Twenty percent of the remaining 680 asymptomatic turned symptomatic over a median follow up of 13 years. Patients over the age of 70 were more likely to become symptomatic than patients under 70 (Wada and Imamura, 1993). McSherry followed 135 asymptomatic men and women with gallstones subscribers to the Health Insurance Plan of Greater New York. Ten percent developed symptoms and 7% required cholecystectomy over a median follow-up of 46 months (McSherry et al 1985).

A placebo group of 193 asymptomatic patients who were part of a chemical dissolution trial were followed for 24 months (Thistle et al 1984). Thirty-one percent of them developed biliary pain. This number is quite high but could be explained by intense surveillance. Also, the patients had to be asymptomatic for the 12 months preceding the trial and some patients might have been symptomatic prior to that. Similarly, Cucchiaro et al (1990) followed 125 asymptomatic patients for a period of 5 years. Fifteen patients developed symptoms during that time and two patients had to undergo emergency surgery for gallstone complications. Fifty-four patients died during that period because of malignancies, cardiovascular disease or renal insufficiency. None of the deaths was gallstone related.

Friedman et al (1989) followed 123 asymptomatic patients for up to 20 years. Six percent of the patients developed severe symptoms related to their gallstones during the first 5 years after diagnosis.

Death as the ultimate complication from gallstones is rare (Godrey et al 1984, Cucchiaro et al 1989). It usually occurs in the elderly as a consequence of biliary or postoperative complications.

Different study designs and outcome measures make it difficult to deduct a uniform natural history for gallstones. Most studies support that between 1 and 4% of patients with asymptomatic gallstones will develop biliary symptoms per year (Table 32.2). One can extrapolate that after 20 years two-thirds of patients will remain symptom free (Friedman 1993).

Table 32.2 Natural history of gallstones

Author	n	Number of years	Biliary pain %	Biliary complications %
Gracie 1982 (Gracie & Ransohoff 1982)	123	15	18	2
Attili 1995 (Attili et al 1995a)	118	10	26	3
Juhasz 1994 (Juhasz et al 1994)	110	6	22*	
Wada 1993 (Wada and Imamura 1993)	680	10 to 17	20	
McSherry 1985 (McSherry et al 1985)	135	4	17	0
Friedman 1989 (Friedman et al 1989)	123	5		6
Thistle 1984 (Thistle et al 1984)	193**	2	31	
Cucchiaro 1990 (Cucchiaro et al 1990)	125	5	12	2
Angelico 1997 (Angelico et al 1997)	426	10	38	

* Patients requiring cholecystectomy
** Asymptomatic for 12 months preceding the study

ASYMPTOMATIC GALLSTONES

The natural history of gallstone disease indicates that most patients with gallstones will not require treatment during the course of their life. A few investigators have tried to address options of prophylactic cholecystectomy versus expectant management in patients with asymptomatic gallstones.

Fendrick and colleagues compared laparoscopic cholecystectomy to expectant management in a cohort of men and women aged 30 to 50 years. Subjects in the non-operative group underwent cholecystectomy when symptoms developed. Outcome measure was gallstone-related deaths and gallstone related life-years lost for each age and gender cohort by strategy. They concluded from their analysis that prophylactic laparoscopic cholecystectomy was not justified in asymptomatic patients (Fendrick et al 1993).

Ransohoff and Gracie (1993) performed a similar study with a mathematical simulation model using data from the literature. They estimated lifetime risks for gallstone-related mortality and for life expectancy, for prophylactic cholecystectomy and expectant management. Their model confirmed that expectant management is most suitable for patients with asymptomatic gallstones while patients with symptomatic gallstones should undergo cholecystectomy.

The general recommendation for patients with asymptomatic gallstones is expectant management unless the patient is at increased risk for cancer or complications (American College of Physicians 1993, Mulvihill (vide infra) 1998).

RISK FACTORS FOR EARLY SYMPTOMS AND COMPLICATIONS

DIABETES MELLITUS

The incidence of gallstones in diabetics is probably not increased (Chapman et al 1996). It has been stated that diabetic patients have a higher incidence of gallstone disease and are particularly prone to biliary complications from their stones. This has led some authors to advocate prophylactic cholecystectomy in asymptomatic diabetic patients (Gibney 1990, Patino & Quintero 1998). However, diabetic patients do not have an increased morbidity or mortality from stone disease once other comorbidities such as cardiovascular disease and renal insufficiency are taken into account (Sandler et al 1986, Ransohoff et al 1987). Recent reports comparing patients with asymptomatic gallstones over time support this view, showing no difference in the incidence of symptoms, complications and mortality comparing diabetic to non-diabetic patients (Del Favero et al 1994). Friedman and colleagues used a decision analysis to compare expectant management to prophylactic cholecystectomy in asymptomatic diabetic patients. They showed that prophylactic surgery for silent gallstones in diabetic patients did not increase life expectancy or quality of life and may in fact reduce it (Friedman et al 1988).

There is no clear benefit to prophylactic cholecystectomy in diabetic patients with asymptomatic gallstones. At present, diabetic patients with gallstones should undergo cholecystectomy for the same indications as in the general population (Friedman et al 1988, Aucott et al 1993, Angelico et al 1997).

GENETIC

The incidence of gallstones varies markedly among world populations. The Pima Indians of the United States, especially females, have an unusually high incidence of gallstones (Sampliner et al 1970, Lowenfels et al 1985, 1989). Stones develop at a young age and complications requiring cholecystectomy occur in the majority of those who live for longer than 50 years. In contrast, the Masai of East Africa (Biss et al 1971) have a very low incidence of cholelithiasis. In populations of relative genetic homogeneity the incidence of cholelithiasis has an established familial relationship. Gilat et al (1983) studied prospectively the frequency of gallstones in 171 first-degree relatives of patients with proven gallstones compared with 200 matched controls. Gallstones were found in 22.8% of the female and 16.7% of the male family members (20.5% overall), as opposed to 10.3% of the female and 8.0% of the male controls (9.0% overall). Gallstone disease and gallbladder cancer are frequent among the Chilean population (Nervi et al 1988, Strom et al 1995). Miquel and colleagues compared the incidence of gallstones to the degree of racial admixture in Chilean Hispanics, Mapuche Indians and Maoris from the Easter Island (Miquel et al 1998). They concluded that cholesterol lithogenic genes are widely spread in Chilean Indians and Hispanics. Gallstones in populations at high risk develop at an earlier age, and data from numerous studies show that the risk of symptoms and/or complications (including gallbladder carcinoma) is cumulative. Indications for cholecystectomy can therefore be liberalized in these high-risk populations (Patino & Quintero, 1998).

GALLBLADDER CARCINOMA AND CALCIFIED GALLBLADDER

Over 70% of patients developing gallbladder carcinoma have gallstones (Piehler & Crichlow 1978) (Ch. 53). The risk of developing carcinoma is estimated to be 1% of calculous gallbladders 20 years after the initial diagnosis of gallstones, with the risk increased mainly in men (Maringhini et al 1987).

A higher incidence of carcinoma has been reported in patients with larger stones (Diehl, 1983, Lowenfels et al 1985, 1989). Because it would take at least 100 cholecystectomies to prevent one death from gallbladder carcinoma, most authors do not recommend prophylactic cholecystectomy in patients with asymptomatic gallstones as a measure of preventing the development of gallbladder cancer (Diehl & Beral 1981, Godrey et al 1984). The American Indian women and the Chilean Hispanic and Indian population with gallstones represent the only exceptions to this rule. Because of the early onset of gallstones in that population, there is an increased risk of gallbladder carcinoma and prophylactic cholecystectomy appears to be justified (Weiss et al 1984, Lowenfels et al 1985, 1989, Nervi et al 1988, Strom et al 1995).

Calcified or porcelain gallbladder is associated with carcinoma in 13–22% of patients (Berk et al 1973, Ashur et al 1978). The diagnosis should be suspected when ultrasonography shows an irregular echogenic density similar to that found in patients with stone-filled gallbladders. A plain abdominal X-ray confirms the diagnosis. Cholecystectomy is indicated in these cases even in the absence of symptoms.

OTHER RISK FACTORS

Pigment gallstones are reported in 58% of patients with homozygous sickle disease (Hb SS) and in 17% of patients with heterozygous types of hemoglobinopathies (Hb SC and Hb Sb) (Bond et al 1987). Two-thirds of patients with gallstones have symptoms although it is often difficult to distinguish between a sickle cell crisis and acute cholecystitis (Serafini et al 1987). Patients with other hemolytic anemias are also at risk for gallstone development many of whom will become symptomatic (Goldfarb et al 1990). Several arguments stand in favor of elective cholecystectomy in patients with hemolytic anemias. Biliary complications and vaso-occlusive crisis both present similarly (nausea, abdominal pain, fever, leucocytosis and cholestatic jaundice) and differentiation is not easy. The onset of gallstones at a young age in sickle-cell disease raises the lifetime risk of biliary complications. Elective cholecystectomy can be performed in a totally controlled situation. Cholecystectomy following the diagnosis of asymptomatic gallstones in patients with sickle-cell disease is therefore advisable (Stephens & Scott 1980, Ware et al 1988).

INCIDENTAL CHOLECYSTECTOMY

Sometimes, consideration is given to perform an incidental cholecystectomy in addition to the planned operation in patients with asymptomatic gallstones. The purpose would be to prevent postoperative cholecystitis or the later development of symptoms. Of course the addition of one procedure should bear no added risks for the patient. Several investigators have tried to address this question.

Several studies have confirmed a high incidence of biliary symptoms following laparotomy for unrelated conditions. Ouriel et al (1983) studied 11 patients with cholelithiasis who underwent repair of abdominal aortic aneurysms without cholecystectomy. Nine (82%) developed biliary symptoms, including four in the early postoperative period. String (1984) also reported symptoms from gallstones necessitating cholecystectomy in nine of 17 patients (53%) between 2 weeks and 108 months following major vascular abdominal procedures.

Thompson et al (1984) described 23 patients with cholelithiasis undergoing laparotomy without concomitant cholecystectomy. The same group found comparable results in a later study in which 16 patients (70%) developed symptoms within 6 months (Bragg and Thompson, 1989). Saade et al (1987) reported another 25 patients with incidental gallstones without cholecystectomy of whom 13 (52%) developed symptoms and 7 (30%) required cholecystectomy within 1 year of the initial operation.

It appears that these patients could have benefited from a concomitant cholecystectomy. It is of course paramount not to increase the morbidity. There are some reports of an increase in morbidity for this approach (McSherry & Glenn 1981, Thompson et al 1984, Saade et al 1987, Green et al 1990). The morbidity can be kept to a minimum by proper patient selection including general health, uncomplicated primary operation and proper exposure (Wolff 1995). Juhasz and colleagues studied patients with asymptomatic cholelithiasis who underwent operation for colorectal disease. One hundred and ninety-five (4%) had an incidental cholecystectomy while 110 (36%) did not (Juhasz et al 1994). There was no increase in operative morbidity in the cholecystectomy group. A total of 20 patients required cholecystectomy during a median follow up of 6 years. The cumulative probability of needing a cholecystectomy at 2 and 5 years after the initial surgery was 12 and 22%. The authors therefore recommend incidental cholecystectomy in patients with asymptomatic gallstones who undergo operation for colorectal diseases.

Simple cholecystectomy is now widely accepted as a concomitant procedure during the course of laparotomy for unrelated conditions. Its purpose is not only to prevent immediate postoperative biliary complications but also to reduce the risk of later biliary symptoms. If the gallstones are discovered preoperatively, as is most often the case, cholecystectomy should be discussed with the patient preoperatively. The discussion should emphasize the safety and the purpose of the procedure and not dismiss the possible complications—as with any additional surgical procedure. Clinical judgement and caution as to the appropriateness of the procedure remain paramount in each specific case of incidental cholecystectomy.

RECOMMENDATIONS

A careful analysis of hepatobiliary and systemic risk factors should precede any decision regarding cholecystectomy for asymptomatic gallstones. The procedure cannot be recommended for the vast majority of the population.

Because the risk factors for symptoms and possibly the complications of gallstones are cumulative (2% per year), prophylactic cholecystectomy may be considered in some populations with genetically determined early development of gallstones and risk for gallbladder cancer. Whether patients with a life expectancy of several decades should undergo prophylactic cholecystectomy is debatable (Patino & Quintero 1998). At this point there is no data to support it.

Cholecystectomy for asymptomatic gallstones is indicated in all patients with calcified gallbladder and in young patients with sickle-cell disease.

Diabetic patients should be evaluated for cholecystectomy with the same criteria as the general population; prophylactic cholecystectomy cannot be supported.

Provided that the exposure is adequate and there are no associated hepatobiliary risk factors (abnormal liver function tests, dilated bile ducts, cirrhosis, a shrunken or scarred gallbladder), incidental cholecystectomy can be carried out safely as part of another abdominal procedure.

REFERENCES

American College of Physicians 1993 Guidelines for the treatment of gallstones. Annals of Internal Medicine 119: 620–622

Angelico F, Del Ben M, Barbato A, Conti R, Urbinati G 1997 Ten-year incidence and natural history of gallstone disease in a rural population of women in central Italy. The Rome Group for the Epidemiology and Prevention of Cholelithiasis (GREPCO). Italian Journal of Gastroenterology and Hepatology 29: 249–254

Ashur H, Siegal B, Oland Y, Adam Y G 1978 Calcified gallbladder (porcelain gallbladder). Archives of Surgery 113: 594–596

Attili A F, De Santis A, Capri R, Repice A M, Maselli S. 1995a The natural history of gallstones: the GREPCO experience. The GREPCO Group. Hepatology 21: 655–660

Attili A F, Carulli N, Roda E, Barbara B, Capocaccia L, Menotti A, Okoliksanyi L, Ricci G, Capocaccia R, Festi D et al 1995b Epidemiology of gallstone disease in Italy: prevalence data of the Multicenter Italian Study on Cholelithiasis (M.I.COL.). American Journal of Epidemiology 141: 158–165

Aucott J N, Cooper G S, Bloom A D, Aron D C 1993 Management of gallstones in diabetic patients. Archives of Internal Medicine 153: 1053–1058

Berk R N, Armbuster T G, Saltzstein S L 1973 Carcinoma in the porcelain gallbladder. Radiology 106: 29–31

Biss K, Ho K J, Mikkelson B, Lewis L, Taylor C B 1971 Some unique biologic characteristics of the Masai of East Africa. New England Journal of Medicine 284: 694–699

Bond L R, Hatty S R, Horn M E, Dick M, Meire H B, Bellingham A J 1987 Gall stones in sickle cell disease in the United Kingdom. British Medical Journal (Clin Res Ed) 295: 234–236

Bragg L E, Thompson J S 1989 Concomitant cholecystectomy for asymptomatic cholelithiasis. Archives of Surgery 124: 460–462

Chapman B A, Wilson I R, Frampton C M, Chisholm R J, Stewart N R, Eagar,GM, Allan R B 1996 Prevalence of gallbladder disease in diabetes mellitus. Digestive Diseases & Sciences 41: 2222–2228

Cucchiaro G, Watters C R, Rossitch J C, Meyers W C 1989 Deaths from gallstones. Incidence and associated clinical factors. Annals of Surgery 209: 149–151

Cucchiaro G, Rossitch J C, Bowie J, Branum G D, Niotis M T, Watters C R, Meyers W C 1990 Clinical significance of ultrasonographically detected coincidental gallstones. Digestive Diseases and Sciences 35: 417–421

Del Favero G, Caroli A, Meggiato T, Volpi A, Scalon P, Puglisi A, Di Mario F 1994 Natural history of gallstones in non-insulin-dependent diabetes mellitus. A prospective 5-year follow-up. Digestive Diseases and Sciences 39: 1704–1707

Diehl A K 1983 Gallstone size and the risk of gallbladder cancer. JAMA 250: 2323–2326

Diehl A K, Beral V 1981 Cholecystectomy and changing mortality from gallbladder cancer. Lancet ii: 187–189

Fendrick A M, Gleeson S P, Cabana M D, Schwartz J S 1993 Asymptomatic gallstones revisited. Is there a role for laparoscopic cholecystectomy? Archives of Family Medicine 2: 959–968

Friedman G D 1993 Natural history of asymptomatic and symptomatic gallstones. American Journal of Surgery 165, 399–404

Friedman G D, Raviola C A, Fireman B 1989 Prognosis of gallstones with mild or no symptoms: 25 years of follow-up in a health maintenance organization. Journal of Clinical Epidemiol 42: 127–136

Friedman L S, Roberts M S, Brett A S, Marton K I 1988 Management of asymptomatic gallstones in the diabetic patient. A decision analysis. Annals of Internal Medicine 109: 913–919

Gibney E J 1990 Asymptomatic gallstones. British Journal of Surgery 77: 368–372

Gilat T, Feldman C, Halpern Z, Dan M, Bar-Meir S 1983 An increased familial frequency of gallstones. Gastroenterology 84: 242–246

Glenn F, Grafe W R Jr 1966 Historical events in biliary tract surgery. Archives of Surgery 93: 848–852

Godrey P J, Bates T, Harrison M, King M B, Padley N R 1984 Gall stones and mortality: a study of all gall stone related deaths in a single health district. Gut 25: 1029–1033

Goldfarb A, Grisaru D, Gimmon Z, Okon E, Lebensart P, Rachmilewitz E A 1990 High incidence of cholelithiasis in older patients with homozygous beta-thalassemia. Acta Haematologica 83: 120–122

Gracie W A, Ransohoff D F 1982 The natural history of silent gallstones: the innocent gallstone is not a myth. New England Journal of Medicine 307: 798–800

Green J D, Birkhead G, Hebert J, Li M, Vogt R L 1990 Increased morbidity in surgical patients undergoing secondary (incidental) cholecystectomy [see comments]. Annals of Surgery 211: 50–54

GREPCO 1984 Prevalence of gallstone disease in an Italian adult female population. Rome Group for the Epidemiology and Prevention of Cholelithiasis (GREPCO). American Journal of Epidemiology 119: 796–805

GREPCO 1988 The epidemiology of gallstone disease in Rome, Italy.

Part I. Prevalence data in men. The Rome Group for Epidemiology and Prevention of Cholelithiasis (GREPCO). Hepatology 8: 904–906

Juhasz E S, Wolff B G, Meagher A P, Kluiber R M, Weaver A L, van Heerden J A 1994 Incidental cholecystectomy during colorectal surgery. Annals of Surgery 219: 467–472

Langenbuch C 1882 Ein Fall von Exstirpation der Gallenblase wegen chronischer Cholelithiasis. Berliner Klinische Wochenschrift 48: 725–727

Lowenfels A B, Lindstrom C G, Conway M J, Hastings P R 1985 Gallstones and risk of gallbladder cancer. Journal of the National Cancer Institute 75: 77–80

Lowenfels A B, Walker A M, Althaus D P, Townsend G, Domellof L 1989 Gallstone growth, size, and risk of gallbladder cancer: an interracial study. International Journal of Epidemiology 18: 50–54

Maringhini A, Moreau J A, Melton L J, Hench V S, Zinsmeister A R, DiMagno E P 1987 Gallstones, gallbladder cancer, and other gastrointestinal malignancies. An epidemiologic study in Rochester, Minnesota. Annals of Internal Medicine 107: 30–35

McSherry C K, Ferstenberg H, Calhoun W F, Lahman E, Virshup M 1985 The natural history of diagnosed gallstone disease in symptomatic and asymptomatic patients. Annals of Surgery 202: 59–63

McSherry C K, Glenn F 1981 Biliary tract surgery concomitant with other intra-abdominal operations. Annals of Surgery 193: 169–175

Miquel J F, Covarrubias C, Villaroel L, Mingrone G, Greco A V, Puglielli L, Carvallo P, Marshall G, Del Pino G, Nervi F 1998 Genetic epidemiology of cholesterol cholelithiasis among Chilean Hispanics, Amerindians, and Maoris. Gastroenterology 115: 937–946

Misciagna G, Leoci C, Guerra V, Chiloiro M, Elba S, Petruzzi J, Mossa A, Noviello M R, Coviello A, Minutolo M C, Mangini V, Messa C, Cavallini A, De Michele G, Giorgio I 1996 Epidemiology of cholelithiasis in southern Italy. Part II: Risk factors. European Journal of Gastroenterology & Hepatology 8: 585–593

Muhrbeck O, Ahlberg J 1995 Prevalence of gallstone disease in a Swedish population. Scandinavian Journal of Gastroenterology 30: 1125–1128

Mulvihill S J 1998 Surgical management of gallstone disease and postoperative complications. In: Sleisenger M H, Fordtran J S (eds) Gastrointestinal Disease 6th edn. W B Saunders Company, Philadelphia, pp 973–984

Nervi F, Duarte I, Gomez G, Rodriguez G, Del Pino G, Ferrerio O, Covarrubias C, Valdivieso V, Torres M I, Urzua A 1988 Frequency of gallbladder cancer in Chile, a high-risk area. International Journal of Cancer 41: 657–660

NIH Consensus Statement 1992 Gallstones and laparoscopic cholecystectomy. NIH Consensus Statements 10: No. 3

Ouriel K, Ricotta J J, Adams J T, Deweese J A 1983 Management of cholelithiasis in patients with abdominal aortic aneurysm. Annals of Surgery 198: 717–719

Patino J F, Quintero G A 1998 Asymptomatic cholelithiasis revisited. World Journal of Surgery 22: 1119–1124

Piehler J M, Crichlow R W 1978 Primary carcinoma of the gallbladder. Surgery, Gynecology and Obstetrics 147: 929–942

Ransohoff D F, Gracie W A 1993 Treatment of gallstones. Annals of Internal Medicine 119: 606–619

Ransohoff D F, Miller G L, Forsythe S B, Hermann R E 1987 Outcome of acute cholecystitis in patients with diabetes mellitus. Annals of Internal Medicine 106: 829–832

Saade C, Bernard D, Morgan S, Tasse D, Rabbat A, Nadeau N 1987 Should cholecystectomy be done en passant for asymptomatic cholelithiasis? Canadian Journal of Surgery 30: 350–353

Sampliner R E, Bennett P H, Comess L J, Rose F A, Burch T A 1970 Gallbladder disease in Pima Indians. Demonstration of high prevalence and early onset by cholecystography. New England Journal of Medicine 283: 1358–1364

Sandler R S, Maule W F, Baltus M E 1986 Factors associated with postoperative complications in diabetics after biliary tract surgery. Gastroenterology 91: 157–162

Schwartz S I 1981 Sequence of stones. Contemporary Surgery 18: 9

Serafini A N, Spoliansky G, Sfakianakis G N, Montalvo B, Jensen W N 1987 Diagnostic studies in patients with sickle cell anemia and acute abdominal pain. Archives of Internal Medicine 147: 1061–1062

Stephens C G, Scott R B 1980 Cholelithiasis in sickle cell anemia: surgical or medical management. Archives of Internal Medicine 140: 648–651

String S T 1984 Cholelithiasis and aortic reconstruction. Journal of Vascular Surgery 1: 664–669

Strom B L, Soloway R D, Rios-Dalenz J L, Rodriguez-Martinez H A, West S L, Kinman J L, Polansky M, Berlin J A 1995 Risk factors for gallbladder cancer. An international collaborative case-control study. Cancer 76: 1747–1756

Thistle J L, Cleary P A, Lachin J M, Tyor M P, Hersh T 1984 The natural history of cholelithiasis: the National Cooperative Gallstone Study. Annals of Internal Medicine 101: 171–175

Thompson J S, Philben V J, Hodgson P E 1984 Operative management of incidental cholelithiasis. American Journal of Surgery 148: 821–824

Wada K, Imamura T 1993 Natural course of asymptomatic gallstone disease. Nippon Rinsho 51: 1737–1743

Ware R, Filston H C, Schultz W H, Kinney T R 1988 Elective cholecystectomy in children with sickle hemoglobinopathies. Successful outcome using a preoperative transfusion regimen. Annals of Surgery 208: 17–22

Weiss K M, Ferrell R E, Hanis C L, Styne P N 1984 Genetics and epidemiology of gallbladder disease in New World native peoples. American Journal of Human Genetics 36: 1259–1278

Wolff B G 1995 Current status of incidental surgery. Diseases of the Colon and Rectum 38: 435–441

33

Dissolution of gallstones

F. BAZZOLI, F. AZZAROLI, E. RODA

INTRODUCTION

This chapter will review existing knowledge of the currently available treatments for dissolving gallstones. Since the common goal of these methods is to render the patient gallstone-free without removing the gallbladder, they have been generally termed non-surgical methods. Both surgical and non-surgical methods should only be utilized for symptomatic gallstone patients (Ch. 32).

At the time of writing, only cholesterol gallstones can be dissolved in vivo while gallstones composed of bilirubinate and other inorganic components can only be treated surgically. An understanding of how cholesterol gallstones are formed (Ch. 31) is fundamental to an appreciation of the mechanism of gallstone dissolution by agents such as bile acids. Because the available cholelitholytic agents are effective only for cholesterol gallstones, their identification as such is essential to determine eligible patients.

Chenodeoxycholic acid (CDCA) was first reported to induce gallstone dissolution, but currently ursodeoxycholic acid (UDCA) is accepted as the bile acid (BA) of choice for the medical treatment of cholesterol gallstones. A combination of the two agents has, however, been proposed by some authors as most effective.

In addition, extracorporeal shock-wave lithotripsy (ESWL) is a new method to 'non-invasively' fragment gallstones in the gallbladder. In this case, however, oral BA dissolution treatment is also needed to completely free the gallbladder of the fragments resulting from lithotripsy treatment.

Contact dissolution by direct instillation into the gallbladder of a potent organic solvent, such as methyl tert butyl ether (MTBE), is highly effective in dissolving cholesterol gallstones, but this is an invasive method and should be reserved for carefully selected patients and only performed by experienced operators.

Post-dissolution gallstone recurrence is a problem of the non-surgical methods with most of the recurrences, however, being free of symptoms and most likely not needing further treatment.

HISTORICAL PERSPECTIVE

The idea of medically treating stones in the biliary tract is probably ascribed to JLW Thudichum who wrote in 1863 '... physicians became naturally anxious to discover some remedy by which these concretions in the biliary channels might be chemically dissolved' (Thudichum 1863).

The concept that the ratio of solute (cholesterol) to solvents (BA plus phospholipids) is altered in gallstone patients and that lowering this ratio, by administering bile salts, could possibly lead to gallstone dissolution, was first recognized by Dr AG Rewbridge in 1937. His hypothesis was confirmed 20 years later, by Johnston and Nakayama (1957) who indicated that the characteristics of the ideal solvent for gallstones are '(a) cholesterol must be readily soluble in it; (b) it must be possible to provide a continuous flow over the stones; (c) it must be non-toxic and (d) it must be possible to introduce it into the biliary tree over a sufficient time and in adequate concentrations to be effective.' In spite of this brilliant early foresight, it was not until 1972 that the Mayo group reported the first gallstone dissolution in man using CDCA (Danzinger et al 1972).

A few years later, in 1975, Makino reported gallstone dissolution by administering UDCA, a BA which had been used in Japan for decades as a cholagogue in various liver diseases (Bachrach & Hofmann, 1982a, 1982b).

During the last two decades, both CDCA and UDCA have been confirmed to be effective cholelitholytic agents. UDCA should be considered the BA of choice because of its freedom from side-effects.

More recently, the list of non-surgical methods for treating gallstones has been expanded by the introduction of novel methods such as ESWL and contact solvent dissolution.

NATURAL HISTORY OF GALLSTONES AND DEFINITION OF SYMPTOMS

Generally, therapeutic decisions largely depend on our knowledge of the natural history of a disease. Cholelithiasis is a disease with an increasing incidence but in a great majority of cases it is asymptomatic with little tendency to develop symptoms over time.

Biliary colic is the only specific biliary symptom, while symptoms such as postprandial bloating and fullness, epigastric discomfort and fat intolerance are not specific, being similarly present in patients with gallstones and those with functional dyspepsia or other gastrointestinal diseases (Glambek et al 1989, Jorgensen 1989, Schoenfield et al 1989).

Asymptomatic (Ch. 32) or silent stones are stones that have not caused specific biliary symptoms. Studies conducted in Italy (Sirmione 1987, GREPCO 1984 and MICOL 1995 studies) show only 13 to 25% of patients with gallstones visible at ultrasonography were symptomatic.

Based on available studies (Comfort et al 1948, Ralston & Smith 1965, Newman et al 1968, Gracie & Ransohoff 1982, McSherry et al 1985), the yearly incidence of biliary pain or complications in patients with silent stones varies from 0.5 to 4%. Epidemiological studies in Italy show a higher incidence of biliary pain in previously asymptomatic gallstone patients; these estimates (25.8% at 10 years), however, are still low (GREPCO 1995).

The recommendation that silent gallstones should not be treated (Gracie & Ransohoff 1982), still holds, particularly in relation to the absolute number of complications expected when prophylactic treatments are applied. However, as discussed below, medical treatment with a single course of UDCA appears to be totally safe and assures that at least a subset of patients with small radiolucent, floating stones, i.e. stones with a high dissolution probability, can be cured without risk. The concept of defining symptoms to derive treatment options also allows differentiation of severely symptomatic from mildly symptomatic gallstone patients.

PATHOGENESIS OF CHOLESTEROL GALLSTONES (see Ch. 31)

Several factors with varying degrees of importance lead to nucleation and crystallization of monohydrate cholesterol and eventually to stone formation.

The prerequisite in the pathogenesis of cholesterol gallstones is cholesterol supersaturation. Biliary cholesterol supersaturation is related to the presence of excess cholesterol to the relative concentration of the two detergent-like lipid solubilizers, phospholipids and BA. Any condition or disturbance which interferes with the secretion of the major biliary lipids (BA, cholesterol and phospholipids) into bile will possibly lead to cholesterol supersaturation and predisposition to gallstone formation. These factors are fully discussed in Chapter 31. Of particular interest in relation to stone dissolution are studies concerned with gallbladder motility. A defective gallbladder motility (Fisher et al 1982, Kishk et al 1987) is well recognized as the third condition/disturbance participating in gallstone formation. A reduced gallbladder emptying is present in about 30% of gallstone patients (Portincasa et al 1995).

The hypothesis that bile stasis must occur in gallstone patients to allow crystal aggregation and gallstone growth has gained support only recently, with the advent of cholescintigraphy (Shaffer et al 1980) and ultrasonography (Everson et al 1980), permitting systematic studies of gallbladder motility.

We have conducted a study (Festi et al 1990) on a large number of gallstone patients suitable for oral BA medical dissolution treatment (i.e. with small or medium sized radiolucent gallstones in a functioning gallbladder). In this study, gallstone patients showed significantly greater fasting and postprandial volumes and a decreased percentage of gallbladder emptying, but a similar absolute emptying rate compared to a group of matched controls.

In the same study, a group of patients who achieved gallstone dissolution with UDCA remained gallstone-free and untreated for at least 1 year, but showed persistence of the motor defect. The main conclusion of the study is that larger fasting volumes and not gallbladder contractility account for the defective gallbladder function in cholesterol gallstone patients. This suggests the existence of a defect of gallbladder tone rather than a defect of gallbladder contractile activity. This defect is likely to precede and, therefore, to promote gallstone formation since it persists after gallstone dissolution.

Furthermore, using simultaneously scintigraphy and ultrasonography for the evaluation of gallbladder motility Jazrawi et al (1995) have been able to demonstrate that the gallbladder motility defect is coupled with a reduced refilling and turnover of gallbladder bile determining a reduced washout of gallbladder contents including cholesterol crystals.

Minor contractions (30 to 40% of the basal volume) of the gallbladder occur physiologically in the interdigestive state, during the late phase II of MMC. Alterations of these contractions have been proposed as additional pathogenetic factors (Portincasa et al 1995).

DISSOLUTION THERAPY WITH ORAL BILE ACIDS

PHARMACOLOGY

Thus far only CDCA and UDCA have been proven to be capable of reducing biliary cholesterol saturation and to be effective agents for cholesterol gallstone dissolution.

Other BA, such as ursocholic acid, or other non-BA molecules, such as the new HMGCoA reductase inhibitors, simvastatin and pravastatin, have been shown to reduce biliary cholesterol saturation, but there is no convincing evidence of their ability to induce cholesterol gallstone dissolution.

The ability of CDCA and UDCA to dissolve cholesterol gallstones is presently well recognized (Bell et al 1972, Barbara et al 1976a, 1976b, Schoenfield & Lachin 1981, Bachrach & Hofmann 1982a, 1982b, Roda et al 1982, Fromm et al 1983a, Erlinger et al 1984). Both are BA occurring naturally in man: CDCA is a primary BA synthesized by the liver from cholesterol (Danielsson & Sjovall 1975). UDCA is present in man only in trace amounts (Salen et al 1974, Fromm et al 1976) and can be formed both in the intestine and in the liver from CDCA through the intermediate 7-ketolithocholic acid (Fromm et al 1983a, 1983b).

Most gallstones in man are of the cholesterol type (Miyake & Johnston 1968, Salen et al 1975, Barbara et al 1987) and cholesterol is solubilized in bile by BA and phospholipids (Admirand & Small 1968, Carey & Small 1978). The rationale for using oral BA to dissolve gallstones is, essentially, to reduce the ratio of cholesterol to BA plus phospholipids in bile (Bachrach & Hofmann 1982a, 1982b, Fromm 1984).

BA, and particularly CDCA and UDCA, have been considered to be a new class of therapeutic agents and since their bioavailability is related to concentrations in the enterohepatic and not in the systemic circulation, they have been named the first enterohepatic drugs (Hofmann 1990). After oral administration, they are rapidly absorbed in the intestine and, via the portal blood, reach the liver where they are conjugated with glycine or taurine and secreted into bile (Hofmann 1988). Most of the ingested CDCA and UDCA is likely to be absorbed in the upper intestine by passive diffusion (Hofmann 1988); absorption is then completed by an active transport mechanism in the terminal ileum. Extraction of portal blood BA by the liver is extremely rapid and efficient (Reichen & Paumgartner

1976), resulting in very low serum concentrations (Barbara et al 1976a, 1976b). The presence of high concentration in the enterohepatic circulation (liver, bile, intestine and portal blood) and low serum concentration is the main peculiarity of these enterohepatic drugs. On the other hand, this is crucial since not only bioavailability, but also their efficacy is related to biliary and not to serum concentration.

Bacterial biotransformation occurs in the intestine and lithocholic acid (LCA) is the main catalytic product of 7-dehydroxylating enzymes from both CDCA and UDCA (Fedorowsky et al 1979, Bazzoli et al 1982). In addition, considerable amounts of CDCA can be biotransformed to UDCA through oxidation in the intestine of CDCA to 7-ketolithocholic acid which can be absorbed and reach the liver. It can also be directly metabolized by intestinal bacteria: the enzymatic reduction of 7-ketolithocholic acid in the liver yields mainly CDCA and only small amounts of UDCA, while the action of intestinal bacterial flora will primarily induce the formation of UDCA (Fedorowski et al 1979, Bazzoli et al 1982, Fromm et al 1983a, 1983b). Both CDCA and UDCA are effective in lowering the biliary cholesterol saturation index. It was initially postulated that the administration of CDCA and UDCA would reduce the relative concentration of cholesterol by increasing BA secretion. This cannot be the mechanism, since there are other BA, such as cholic acid, which can increase BA secretion and enlarge BA pool size (Einarsson & Grundy 1980), but do not desaturate bile and dissolve gallstones (Thistle & Hofmann 1973).

It is presently accepted that the most important effect of orally ingested CDCA and UDCA is to depress the secretion of cholesterol into bile.

Although both CDCA and UDCA are effective in decreasing cholesterol saturation by decreasing biliary cholesterol secretion, they achieve this effect in different ways. Studies evaluating biliary lipid secretion after acute replacement of the preexisting BA pool with either one of the two cholelitholytic BA have shown that UDCA, but not CDCA, induces a rapid and significant decrease of cholesterol secretion (Sama et al 1982). UDCA is a hydrophilic BA with low detergency and low capacity of dissolving cholesterol in mixed micelles; the finding of an acute decrease of cholesterol secretion is consistent with the hypothesis that this is related to the limited ability of UDCA for solubilizing cholesterol and transporting it through the canalicular membrane (Carulli et al 1984).

Accordingly, CDCA, which is a less hydrophilic, good detergent and very good micelle-forming BA, is unable to acutely reduce cholesterol secretion into bile; however, after chronic feeding, this BA was also shown to induce a significant reduction of cholesterol secretion (Tint et al 1986). In this case, the effect has been related to a reduced synthesis of cholesterol. This is supported by the studies describing a reduction in HMGCoA reductase activity, the rate-limiting enzyme in the hepatic cholesterol synthesis, after chronic CDCA administration (Carulli et al 1980, Ahlberg et al 1981).

Other major effects of the two cholelitholytic agents on cholesterol and BA metabolism concern intestinal cholesterol absorption and hepatic BA synthesis. A reduced intestinal cholesterol absorption has been reported during UDCA, but not during CDCA administration (Ponz de Leon et al 1980b, Hardison & Grundy 1984). Although the mechanism by which UDCA decreases cholesterol absorption in the intestine has not been elucidated, this observation seems very important because it supports the finding that during CDCA administration, but not during UDCA administration, there might be increases in body cholesterol stores due to decreased biliary excretion. This different effect on cholesterol metabolism might be even more pronounced due to the inhibition of 7-hydroxylase, the rate limiting enzyme for conversion of cholesterol to BA during CDCA administration (Tint et al 1986).

In contrast, the administration of UDCA seems not to affect, or only moderately increase, hepatic BA synthesis (Tint et al 1986). In other words, during reduced biliary cholesterol excretion induced by either of these cholelitholytic agents cholesterol balance is maintained during UDCA via a combined reduction of cholesterol absorption and an increase of BA synthesis. During CDCA administration body cholesterol stores might be slightly increased, as suggested by the increased LDL plasma levels, reported in the National Cooperative Gallstone Study (NCGS) (Schoenfield & Lachin, 1981).

Furthermore, both CDCA and UDCA can modify cholesterol solubilization in bile: the first via micelle formation (Tint et al 1986) and the second by decreasing proteins with a pro-nucleating activity in bile (Van Erpecum et al 1996).

PATIENT SELECTION CRITERIA

Symptoms

Only symptomatic gallstones should be treated. The so-called mildly symptomatic gallstone patients, (presenting occasional and uncomplicated biliary pain) represent the optimal candidates for oral BA treatment. Significant improvement in the incidence of biliary colic in patients treated with CDCA (Lanzini & Northfield 1990) has been reported. Severely symptomatic gallstone patients with frequent and recurring biliary colic, particularly if associated with fever, jaundice or other signs suggesting complications, should not be considered for medical treatment.

However, in some selected cases UDCA, a safe agent free of side-effects may be used in asymptomatic patients with small and floating stones, a condition in which a high success rate is expected and in whom complications may be expected to occur more frequently (e.g. acute pancreatitis with small stones) (Ch. 35).

Gallstone composition

Successful dissolution depends primarily on stone composition; only cholesterol-rich gallstones, can be treated with oral BA while calcified and pigment stones will not benefit from reducing cholesterol saturation in bile.

Since most cholesterol-rich gallstones are radiolucent, oral cholecystography plus a plain film of the abdomen represent the most common method used to select patients for oral BA treatment. Unfortunately, 20 to 33% of calcified stones are not identified correctly by this method (Trotman et al 1977, Sarva et al 1981). CT scans to detect stone calcifications have been proposed as an alternative (Barakos et al 1987) but their use is still under debate (Simone et al 1989).

Since the cost-effectiveness of CT in selecting patients for nonsurgical treatment has yet to be established, one should also consider flotation of gallstones during oral cholecystography. This method, although not sensitive, is very specific, the density of a floating stone being very close to that of cholesterol monohydrate and it being accepted that floating stones are associated with an approximately 90% dissolution rate.

Gallbladder function

An absolute prerequisite for gallstone dissolution is good gallbladder function. Gallbladder function is presently assessed either by oral cholecystography, which shows a well opacified gallbladder, or by ultrasonography which documents at least 50% initial volume reduction after a test meal.

On the other hand, there are anecdotal reports of successful gallstone dissolution in patients with a non-visualized gallbladder and the observation in the NCGS of patients developing a nonfunctioning gallbladder during successful dissolution treatment (Schoenfield & Lachin 1981). Indeed, it has been stated that the recommendation not to accept patients with a non-visualizing gallbladder seems logical, albeit conservative (Hofmann 1990).

Exclusion criteria

While CDCA is still contraindicated in gallstone patients with liver disease, diarrhea and/or hypercholesterolemia, there are no absolute exclusion criteria for UDCA.

Although no proof of adverse effect has been provided, oral BA are not given to subjects with inflammatory disease and peptic ulcer or during pregnancy. As regards pregnancy, it should be noted that UDCA has been recently reported to be beneficial during pregnancy in the case of third trimester cholestasis by inducing a normalization of liver function tests without adverse effect on the fetus.

Efficacy and safety

In early and uncontrolled clinical studies of gallstone dissolution, a wide range of dissolution rates were reported, claiming up to 80% success rates. However, such high rates can only be expected in patients with very small, floating gallstones. The reasons for the wide variations in results include differences in dose and duration of therapy, selection criteria, expression of results and evaluation of efficacy (either as partial or complete dissolution).

The NCGS (Schoenfield & Lachin 1981), which evaluated the efficacy and safety of CDCA versus placebo, is the largest controlled study of oral BA dissolution therapy. This study, however, tested only fixed and suboptimal doses of CDCA, the low and high doses being 350 mg/day and 750 mg/day, respectively. Complete dissolution was achieved in 5.2 and 13.5% of the patients on low and high doses, respectively. Indirect evidence of the suboptimal dosages is seen in the higher (up to 36%) frequency of gallstone dissolution obtained in patients with less than ideal body weight, who received a higher dose/kg.

In the early 1980s, several controlled studies identified the optimal dosages of both CDCA and UDCA and comparatively evaluated safety and the main features of both cholelitholytic agents (Roda et al 1982, Fromm et al 1983a, 1983b, Erlinger et al 1984). In patients with radiolucent gallstones not larger than 20 mm in diameter in functioning gallbladders, one can reasonably expect a 40% gallstone dissolution rate after a treatment period ranging between 6 and 24 months. These results are obtained with CDCA at a dose of 12–15 mg/kg/day and with UDCA at a dose of 8–10 mg/kg/day.

Furthermore, dissolution with UDCA was, at least in one study (Roda et al 1982), significantly more rapid than with CDCA. In fact, about 75% of the total dissolutions induced by UDCA administration were achieved during the first 6 months of treatment while only 40% were obtained with CDCA in the same time period. Although a stone-size-dependent response to treatment has been reported in

several studies showing higher dissolution rates in patients with small multiple stones than in patients with a large, single stone (possibly because of the higher surface/volume ratio in the former group), there is evidence that this observation is not true for UDCA which, if administered at a particularly high dose, seems to induce a comparable response in patients with both large and small stones (Roda et al 1982). Kinetic analysis of gallstone dissolution during oral BA therapy seems to indicate a linear relationship between decrease in stone diameter and time, and suggests that gallstone dissolution in responsive patients averages a size decrease of 1–2 mm per month.

In addition to better efficacy, lower dosages, and the shorter treatment period required, the major advantage of UDCA over CDCA is the lack of side-effects. In fact, while the administration of UDCA is virtually free of any side-effects, the administration of CDCA induces diarrhea and hypertransaminasemia (Barbara et al 1976a, 1976b, Schoenfield & Lachin 1981, Bachrach & Hofmann 1982a, 1982b, Hofmann et al 1982, Roda et al 1982, Fromm et al 1983a, 1983b, Erlinger et al 1984). Diarrhea has been reported in about 40% of patients treated with therapeutic dosages (15 mg/kg/day) of CDCA. Although these side-effects are dose and time-related and tend to disappear after 1–6 months, either spontaneously or by decreasing the dosage, diarrhea is a major problem. In clinical trials, diarrhea has been the major cause of dropout, thus projecting low compliance in the general population of patients.

Hypertransaminasemia has been reported in about 15% of patients treated with 15 mg/kg/day of CDCA. It is also dose dependent; it appears during the first 2–3 months of treatment and tends to disappear in most cases after 5–9 months of treatment. It is not yet clear whether hypertransaminasemia reflects significant histological liver damage. Significant liver abnormalities have been reported in three patients in the NCGS (Schoenfield & Lachin 1981). However, in these patients a pretreatment liver biopsy had not been obtained and one cannot rule out the possibility of preexisting liver disease.

Calcification of gallstones during treatment is a major problem since the appearance of an opacified rim on the stone surface definitely precludes dissolution. It was initially postulated (Bateson et al 1981) that calcification was a side-effect of UDCA treatment due to the formation of calcium glycoursodeoxycholate and it was suggested that the administration of tauroursodeoxycholic acid could prevent it. However, in recent studies we have shown that gallstone calcification occurs during both CDCA and UDCA treatment (Frabboni et al 1985a). We have also evaluated gallstone calcification during tauroursodeoxycholic acid administration, which showed a rate quite similar to that of

CDCA and UDCA (Frabboni et al 1985b). Although no predictive factors were identified for gallstone calcification, we observed an increased frequency with advancing age. These results, together with the findings by others of calcification during placebo administration (Schoenfield & Lachin 1981), suggest that this phenomenon may simply be a part of the natural history of gallstone disease rather than a side-effect of oral BA treatment.

The combination of CDCA and UDCA has given results similar to those obtained with monotherapy (Jazrawi et al 1992) while Podda et al (1989) reported a faster dissolution at six months of the combination therapy compared to UDCA alone.

POSTDISSOLUTION GALLSTONE RECURRENCE

The major problem of nonsurgical treatment of cholesterol cholelithiasis is that after dissolution or fragmentation and cessation of oral BA administration, gallstones may recur. In fact, the defects leading to primary gallstone formation, development of supersaturated bile, nucleation defects and gallbladder motor dysfunction, are likely to persist after both dissolution and fragmentation.

In 1972, Danzinger and Hofmann published the first report on cholesterol gallstone dissolution with oral BA administration but 2 years later, the same authors documented that after discontinuance of CDCA therapy, bile promptly returns to the supersaturated state and gallstone recurrence follows.

However, apart from sporadic reports, it was not until the early 1980s that systematic data on gallstone recurrence were available (Ponz de Leon et al 1980a). A wide range of recurrence rates was reported, varying from 11% up to almost 100%. These widely divergent results were due to the different and mainly short follow-up periods, the relatively small number of cases and/or the different methods of statistical analyses adopted. For the same reasons, probably, no predictive factors for gallstone recurrence were initially identified.

Similarly, conflicting results were reported as to the effectiveness of postdissolution treatment, particularly with long-term, low-dose oral BA. In the NCGS (Marks & Lan 1984), continuous treatment with low dose CDCA (375 mg/day) did not significantly reduce the frequency of gallstone recurrence over a 3.5-year period as compared with the frequency observed in the placebo-treated patients. Regarding UDCA, in the British-Belgian Study (Hood et al 1993), no statistically significant difference was observed between placebo and treated subjects (UDCA 3 mg/kg/day) while a study from Spain showed no recurrence in nine subjects

given 300 mg of UDCA per day (Perez-Aguilar et al 1985). After five years of follow-up, Hood and coworkers (1993) reported that none of 12 regular users of nonsteroidal anti-inflammatory drugs (NSAIDs) had postdissolution gallstone recurrence. However, the role of NSAIDs in the prevention of gallstone recurrence is still debated (Adamek et al 1994, Tudyka 1996, Pazzi et al 1998).

We have recently completed a study (Villanova et al 1989) which aimed to evaluate the long-term (12-year follow-up) recurrence rate of gallstones after a large number of successful oral BA treatments, to identify predictive factors for gallstone recurrence and to assess the effectiveness of continuous treatment with low-dose UDCA in preventing recurrence.

In untreated subjects, the recurrence rate rose to 69% at the ninth year and then levelled off, the median time of recurrence being 5.9 years. This means that > 50% of the subjects who achieve dissolution with oral BA treatment are free of recurrence for 5 years and that about 30% are likely to remain stone-free and, therefore, can be judged to be definitely cured.

On the other hand, it has been observed that in other studies, gallstone recurrence is confined to the first 5 years after dissolution. In studies with relatively short follow-up periods the estimates at the tails of the survival curves must be interpreted with caution because the number of patients at risk is usually quite low at the end of the observation period (Richardson 1987).

In our study, although the maximum follow-up period was 12 years, the survival curves have been cut where the population at risk fell to less than five subjects or less than 10% of the initial population. Gallstone recurrence and previous dissolution were assessed with oral cholecystography (OCG) in the initial part of our study and later by real time ultrasonography. Since ultrasound has greater sensitivity, dissolution and consequently recurrence could have been slightly overestimated in the earlier part of the study.

The problem of assessing gallstone recurrence reflects the problem of assessing gallstone dissolution. With the advent of reliable ultrasonography it was realized that some cases of negative OCG were paralleled by a positive ultrasound, which detected smaller particles. This implies the possibility of an overestimation of gallstone dissolution and consequently of gallstone recurrence up to the period when ultrasound or ultrasound plus OCG have been adopted to assess both dissolution and recurrence.

In our study, the long-term administration of UDCA at the fixed dose of 300 mg/day significantly reduced the overall recurrence rate. This observation, however, was mainly due to the effect of postdissolution treatment on subjects less than 50 years of age. In these subjects, in fact, we observed a 16% recurrence rate at 5 years and no further increase later on, while almost 60% of the treated subjects over 50 years of age experienced recurrence in spite of post-dissolution treatment. The reason for this age-related difference is not apparent. Low compliance, decreased absorption of UDCA and increased biliary DCA in older subjects are possible explanations. It could also be hypothesized that in older subjects bile is more supersaturated than in the younger ones or that they develop tolerance to the cholelitholytic agent. On the other hand, nucleation defects and impaired gallbladder motor function could be more pronounced in older subjects, thus promoting gallstone recurrence.

Identifying groups of subjects who are more likely to develop gallstone recurrence after dissolution is important since this will allow planning of appropriate follow-up programs and of the need for prophylactic therapy.

In our study, possible factors affecting gallstone recurrence were investigated by examining recurrence rates in subgroups identified by the following variables: sex, age, body weight, serum cholesterol, serum triglycerides, pretreatment gallstone size, and number and type of BA taken during previous dissolution therapy.

The only factor predictive of gallstone recurrence we have been able to identify was pre-treatment gallstone number; the frequency of gallstone recurrence was, in fact, significantly higher in subjects who had multiple stones prior to dissolution treatment. This is probably the consequence of a much more rapid cholesterol nucleation time in patients with multiple compared to those with solitary stones (Shoda et al 1997). In subjects with pre-treatment solitary stones, a 10% recurrence rate at the sixth year, rising to 32% over time, was observed; this suggests that the great majority of these subjects are unlikely to reform gallstones even if post-dissolution treatment is not administered.

We also evaluated the frequency of biliary colic in post-dissolution patients (Bazzoli et al 1992). Prior to treatment for primary gallstone disease, 85% of our patients were symptomatic. After gallstone dissolution all patients became asymptomatic. Out of the 49 subjects who subsequently developed gallstone recurrence, only 12, that is 24.5%, had biliary colic while the great majority remained free of specific biliary symptoms. Subjects not developing recurrence also remained symptom free.

Finally, we evaluated the efficacy of retreatment with UDCA on recurring gallstones (Bazzoli et al 1990). UDCA was administered in subjects with gallstone recurrence at a dosage of 8–10 mg/kg/day and the dissolution of recurring gallstones was evaluated every 6 months by ultrasound. Gallstone redissolution was obtained in 50% of cases and the retreatment period was significantly shorter than the first course of oral BA treatment. The time lapsing between the initial dissolution and gallstone recurrence was significantly shorter in those subjects who eventually achieved gallstone dissolution with the second course of oral BA treatment. The redissolution rate was significantly higher in younger subjects and particularly in those less than 50 years of age.

To summarize: (a) Patients successfully treated with UDCA or CDCA are at high risk of reforming gallstones; nevertheless, more than 50% of those who achieve dissolution are likely to be free of recurrence for 5 years and more than 30% to remain stone-free and thus considered definitely cured; (b) the probability of recurrence is significantly higher in subjects with pretreatment multiple stones (gallstone recurrence is very unlikely in subjects with a pretreatment solitary stone—therefore, they do not require prophylactic postdissolution treatment); (c) postdissolution treatment with low dose UDCA prevents gallstone recurrence in subjects under 50 years old. Dosages higher than 300 mg/day UDCA may be necessary to prevent recurrence in older people. (d) Symptomatic patients successfully treated with oral BA therapy, although prone to gallstone recurrence, are unlikely to develop specific biliary symptoms again. Patients with asymptomatic gallstone recurrence have a natural history similar to that reported in patients with asymptomatic, untreated, primary gallstone disease and are most likely not to need any further treatment. (e) Retreatment of recurring gallstones with UDCA yields a 50% dissolution rate in a relatively short period of time and continuing treatment over 12 months does not improve the success rate. (f) Redissolution is more likely in those subjects with gallstones recurring soon after initial dissolution.

DISSOLUTION THERAPY WITH METHYL TERT-BUTYL ETHER (MTBE)

A recently developed method for the rapid dissolution of gallstones consists of the instillation of a potent organic solvent directly into the gallbladder via a percutaneous catheter. The local cholelytholitic agent presently accepted and available is MTBE. MTBE is a potent cholesterol solubilizing agent which has been proven to dissolve cholesterol gallstone in vitro (Allen et al 1985a) and not to damage gallbladder mucosa or other abdominal organs in vivo in animal models (McGahan et al 1988).

MTBE is an alkyl ether physically similar to diethyl ether but with a higher boiling point (about 55°C) thus allowing its infusion within the gallbladder at body temperature. Since its first proposal for the treatment of cholesterol gallstones in man (Allen et al 1985b), it has been found to be highly effective and relatively safe. The MTBE topical disso- lution treatment should be considered only for symptomatic cholesterol gallstone patients. As opposed to other nonsur- gical treatments, the number and size of gallstones are not limiting factors in selecting patients for MTBE. In fact, MTBE is indicated particularly when the patient is not eligible (because stones are too large or too many) for either oral cholelitholytic therapy or ESWL, or when biliary colic is severe and/or frequent and more urgent treatment is called for. Of course these latter conditions would also indicate cholecystectomy which should be performed unless the patient refuses operation or it is judged that the risk of operation is prohibitive. As indicated above, the cholesterol content of gallstones is inaccurately determined by oral cholecystography (Trotman et al 1975) and some authors have recently proposed the use of CT scanning for a better evaluation of the calcium content of gallstones (Barakos et al 1987, Baron et al 1989). Furthermore, CT scanning seems to produce optimal information for choosing the access route of the catheter into the gallbladder. On the other hand, a well-opacified gallbladder at oral cholecystog- raphy seems to be the best way to establish a patent cystic duct which is a necessary condition for the treatment.

Complications of gallstone disease and conditions such as coagulative disorders, anticoagulative treatments, preg- nancy, hepatic, pancreatic and biliary diseases in acute stages, are contraindications to MTBE treatment.

PROCEDURE

Since the introduction of MTBE treatment, several techni- cal aspects of catheter placement into the gallbladder have been developed in order to reduce the risk of intraperitoneal extravasation of both bile and MTBE (Bender & Williams 1988, Miller & Rose 1990, van Sonnenberg et al 1990).

The catheter should be placed into the gallbladder at its upper middle or proximal third via a transhepatic access site, generally along the mid axillary line. The interposition of an adequate area of liver parenchyma is also required in order to maintain the catheter in the correct position. The maneuver of gallbladder catheterization is performed under fluoroscopy and is initiated utilizing a fine needle (21- or 22-gauge) to enter the gallbladder. A guide-wire is then positioned on the needle, followed by several dilators increasing up to the appropriate caliber catheter size. Displacement of the catheter is best avoided by forming sev- eral loops within the gallbladder lumen and good position- ing is obtained when the pigtail, with its multiple holes, is as close as possible to the stones.

After correct catheter positioning, it is important to determine the correct infusion volume of MTBE which should be sufficient to completely cover the stones without overflow from the gallbladder into the duodenum.

A continuous flow of the solvent around the stone is then most important to obtain fast dissolution. This can be done manually by repeated infusion and aspiration of MTBE with a glass syringe or by using automatic pumps.

Ultrasound follow-up during MTBE infusion allows eval- uation of the progressive reduction in gallstone size and detection of potential side-effects, such as damage to the gallbladder wall, while fluoroscopic evaluation is needed to confirm appropriate catheter positioning and, if necessary, to permit catheter replacement.

When dissolution is obtained and the catheter is removed, the track is embodied to avoid bile leakage.

Alternatively, infusion of MTBE is possible via endo- scopic transpapillary catheterization of the gallbladder (Uchida et al 1994).

EFFICACY

Factors affecting dissolution are directly correlated with cholesterol content and inversely correlated with total stone volume.

With appropriate patient selection, reported dissolution rates are very high ranging from 80 to 96% (van Sonnenberg et al 1988, Thistle et al 1989, Leuschner et al 1990). A major problem in evaluating dissolution rates concerns the significance of small echoic images, described in about 30 to 70% of treated patients, after catheter removal (Leuschner et al 1987, McCullough et al 1990, Nelson et al 1990a). Since about 30 to 70% of this material can be dissolved by a 3–6 month oral BA treatment, it has been referred to as cholesterol microlithiasis (Thistle et al 1989, Leuschner et al 1990). In the remaining cases of unsuccessful oral BA treat- ment, the use of other solvents has been proposed to dis- solve noncholesterol debris (Nelson et al 1990b).

SIDE-EFFECTS

Possible treatment side-effects are related to both the pro- cedure of gallbladder catheterization and to MTBE as a chemical compound. Regarding catheterization, a compli- cation rate of less than 2% has been reported (gallbladder damage, hypotension and bradycardia, bile leakage and catheter dislodgement) (Thistle et al 1989, Hellstern et al 1990, Leuschner et al 1990).

Although the gallbladder mucosa is remarkably resistent to MTBE, it is destructive of the gastrointestinal mucosa, and erosive duodenitis has been reported. Nausea and vomiting are not uncommon with manual delivery but are prevented by the use of automatic pumps which control the infusion volume.

In a search for safer topical dissolution agents Hofmann et al (1997) have recently studied the safety and efficacy of ethyl propionate (EP). EP is an organic solvent less volatile and flammable than MTBE. Complete dissolution of gallstones was obtained in 4 out of 5 patients. Side-effects included pain at the site of instillation and one case of hypotension in a patient with severe cardiac disease. These results suggest that EP could be an acceptable alternative to MTBE in high risk patients.

APPLICABILITY

MTBE treatment is applicable with a high probability of success in selected cases of symptomatic cholesterol gallstones. The main advantages of this method are represented by the short duration of treatment, the possibility of treating gallstones independently of their number and size and low cost. Limiting factors are the necessity for an invasive gallbladder catheterization and potential MTBE toxicity.

A European survey in 21 clinics from six different countries of a total of 803 treated patients report a recurrence rate of 40% in solitary stones and 70% in multiple stones over a 5-year follow-up (Hellstern et al 1998).

EXTRACORPOREAL SHOCK WAVE LITHOTRIPSY AND ADJUVANT ORAL BILE ACID DISSOLUTION THERAPY

ESWL was first proposed by the Munich group for treatment of cholesterol gallstones (Sauerbruch et al 1986). Low-energy (electromagnetic) and high-energy lithotripters (electrohydraulic) can be used to generate shock waves to fragment gallstones.

Although theoretically ESWL should produce fragments sufficiently small to be expelled from the gallbladder, in practice fragmentation is often incomplete and total fragment clearance requires more than 6 months despite continuous adjuvant oral BA administration (Sackmann et al 1988). Laparoscopic cholecystectomy is probably the treatment of choice at present. Stone recurrence is a major drawback (Sackmann et al 1994).

A multicenter study in 1990 confirms the relevant role of adjuvant oral BA administration, which can double the success rate of lithotripsy (Schoenfield et al 1990). Some have reported that the two BA given together are better than monotherapy (Tudyka et al 1995), while others report the combination of CDCA and UDCA to be more effective than using UDCA alone (Sackmann et al 1990).

More recently, it has been reported that high-energy

ESWL does not necessitate adjuvant oral BA administration provided that fragments less than 3 mm in diameter are obtained with the treatment. However, administration of UDCA tends to improve short term efficacy of ESWL in patients with solitary stones. Furthermore, multiple sessions of ESWL are often required, implying high cost, and 10% of patients had significant complications (Sauter et al 1997).

ROLE OF NONSURGICAL TREATMENTS IN THE MANAGEMENT OF GALLSTONE DISEASE

Oral BA administration is most effective in dissolving newly-formed gallstones in selected patients with radiolucent, small to medium-sized stones in functioning gallbladders.

More recently, the advent of innovative treatments, such as ESWL, direct contact solvent dissolution and the availability of more early ultrasound diagnosis of gallstones have increased the available therapeutic approaches. After much debate (Gracie & Ransohoff 1985) it has been generally accepted that the prognosis of asymptomatic gallstone disease is generally benign (Ch. 32). Available evidence (Fitzpatrick et al 1977, Ransohoff et al 1983, Kottke et al 1984, Taroni et al 1987) shows that delaying treatment until biliary pain or complications occur (expectant management) is preferable to prophylactic cholecystectomy. Thus, the choice of therapy treatment applies only to symptomatic patients.

Since the choice of therapeutic treatment for gallstone disease depends not only on the presence of symptoms but also on the functional characteristics of the gallbladder and the physicochemical characteristics of the stone, we preliminarily evaluated the distribution of these characteristics in the general population of several small towns in northern Italy using data obtained from both transverse (prevalence) and longitudinal (incidence) studies.

The radiological findings in the 'prevalence' group showed that 52% of the cases had radiolucent and 15% radio-opaque stones, while in 26% of the subjects the gallbladder was not functioning. Therefore, 41% of the cases, those with radio-opaque stones and a non-functioning gallbladder, were only suitable for surgery.

Since there is general agreement not to treat asymptomatic patients, the radiological characteristics were evaluated only in symptomatic patients. These accounted for 12.5% of the general population and showed no significant differences in radiological findings.

Therefore, 45% of the cases were a priori suitable for surgery while 53% offered the choice of alternative therapeutic strategies. In the gallstone patients identified in studies of incidence there was a greater percentage of radiolucent stones (72% versus 52%) and a lower percentage of non-functioning gallbladders (88% versus 26%) as compared to 'prevalent' gallstones. The evaluation of symptomatic cases shows a percentage very similar to that present in the population of the 'prevalent' studies already analyzed (14% versus 12.5%), but with a different distribution since symptomatic patients all have radiolucent stones. It seems, therefore, that 'incident' stones, that is the more recent ones, have radiological and symptomatic characteristics that differ from those of 'prevalent' stones, that is, those of older formation. These differences are reflected in choice of treatment since surgery is not necessarily indicated in patients with 'recent' gallstones.

For a more realistic use of these epidemiological data, we evaluated the optimal choice of therapy for patients who were both aware of the disease and who had symptoms. Three hundred and forty-one patients in the 'prevalence' studies, 8.5% knew of the disease and had biliary symptoms. By evaluating the radiological characteristics of the stones and the gallbladder in these patients and applying agreed selection criteria (Paumgartner et al 1988), it was observed that 48% of the cases were suitable for operation; 28% for oral BA treatment; 21% for ESWL; and 3% for local treatment. Seventeen per cent of the cases were suitable for both oral BA therapy and ESWL.

For the 'incidence' group, the percentage of patients who were symptomatic and aware of the disease was 9%. The use of the same criteria showed that 25% of the cases were suitable for surgery and 75% for oral BA treatment.

Thus, depending on the differences in the radiological and symptomatic characteristics, newly-formed stones differ from 'older' ones as to the optimal choice of therapy. In fact, whereas old stones are suitable for all types of treatment, the recently-formed stones are generally best treated with oral BA.

REFERENCES

Abaurre R, Gordon S G, Mann J G et al 1969 The effects of ileal resection upon fasting bile salt pool size and composition. Gastroenterology 57: 679–688

Adamek H E, Buttmann A, Weber J et al 1994 Can aspirin prevent gallstone recurrence after successful extracorporeal shock-wave lithotripsy? Scandinavian Journal of Gastroenterology 29: 355–359

Admirand W, Small D M 1968 The physiochemical basis of cholesterol gallstone formation in man. Journal of Clinical Investigation 47: 1043–1052

Ahlberg J, Angelin B, Bjorkhem I et al 1979a Hepatic cholesterol metabolism in normo- and hyperlipidemic patients with cholesterol gallstones. Journal of Lipid Research 20: 107–115

Ahlberg J, Angelin B, Einarsson K et al 1979b Prevalence of gallbladder disease in hyperlipoproteinemia. American Journal of Digestive Disease 24: 459–464

Ahlberg J, Angelin B, Einarsson K et al 1980 Biliary lipid composition in normo and hyperlipoproteinemia. Gastroenterology 79: 90–94

Ahlberg J, Angelin B, Einarsson K 1981 Hepatic 3-hydroxy-3-methylglutaryl coenzyme A reductase activity and biliary lipid composition in man: relation to cholesterol gallstone disease and effects of cholic and chenodeoxycholic acid treatment. Journal of Lipid Research 22: 418–422

Allen M J, Borodi T J, Bugliosi T F et al 1985a Cholelitholisis using methyl tert-butyl ether. Gastroenterology 80: 122–125

Allen M J, Borodi T J, Bugliosi T F et al 1985b Rapid dissolution of gallstones by methyl tert-butyl ether. New England Journal of Medicine 312: 217–220

Azzaroli F, Mazzella G, De Vergori E et al 1997 Sluggish gallbladder and small bowel motility are associated with cholesterol gallstones. Gastroenterology 112: A499

Bachrach W H, Hofmann A F 1982a Ursodeoxycholic acid in the treatment of cholesterol cholelithiasis. Part I. Digestive Diseases and Sciences 27: 737–761

Bachrach W H, Hofmann A F 1982b Ursodeoxycholic acid in the treatment of cholesterol cholelithiasis. Part II. Digestive Diseases and Sciences 27: 833–856

Barakos J A, Ralles P W, Lapin S A 1987 Cholelithiasis: evaluation of CT. Radiology 162: 415–418

Barbara L, Roda E, Roda A et al 1976a Diurnal variation of serum bile acids in healthy subjects and hepatobiliary disease patients. Rendiconti di Gastroenterologia 8: 194–198

Barbara L, Roda E, Roda A et al 1976b The medical treatment of cholesterol gallstones: experience with chenodeoxycholic acid. Digestion 14: 209–214

Barbara L, Sama C, Morselli Labate A M et al 1987 A population study on the prevalence of gallstone disease: The Sirmione Study. Hepatology 7: 913–917

Baron R L, Kuypers S J, Lee S P 1989 In vitro dissolution of gallstones with MTBE: correlation with characteristics at CT and MR imaging. Radiology 173: 117–121

Bateson M C, Bouchier I A D, Trash D B et al 1981 Calcification of radiolucent gallstones during treatment with ursodeoxycholic acid. British Medical Journal 283: 645–646

Bazzoli F, Fromm H, Sarvsa R P et al 1982 Comparative formation of lithocholic acid from chenodeoxycholic acid and ursodeoxycholic acid in the colon. Gastroenterology 83: 753–757

Bazzoli F, Mazzella G, Villanova N et al 1987 Influence of age and sex on biliary lipid secretion in normal and gallstone subjects. Gastroenterology 92(5): Abstract 1719

Bazzoli F, Parini P, Villanova N et al 1990 Gallstone recurrence: efficacy and timing of re-treatment. Gastroenterology 98(5): Abstract 244

Bazzoli F, Mazzella G, Parini P et al 1991 Bile acid metabolism and enterohepatic dynamics in non-obese, normolipidemic patients with cholesterol gallstones. Gastroenterology 100(5): Abstract 309

Bazzoli F, Festi D, Zagari R M et al 1992 Gallstone recurrence and history of specific biliary symptoms during a long-term postdissolution follow-up. Gastroenterology 102(4): Abstract 302

Bell G D, Whitney B, Dowling R H 1972 Gallstone dissolution in man using chenodeoxycholic acid. Lancet ii: 1213–1216

Bender C E, Williams H I 1988 Technical aspects of percutaneous gallstone dissolution. Seminars in Interventional Radiology 5: 186–194

Bennion U, Grundy S M 1975 Effects of obesity and caloric intake on biliary lipid metabolism in man. Journal of Clinical Investigation 56: 996–1011

Berr F, Schreiber E, Frick U 1992 Interrelationships of bile acid and phospholipid fatty acid species with cholesterol saturation of duodenal bile in health and gallstone disease. Hepatology 16: 71–81

Bertomeu A, Ros E, Zambón D et al 1996 Apolipoprotein E polymorphism and gallstones. Gastroenterology 111: 1603–1610

Besancon F, Marche C, Barrett C 1970 Pharmacologie de la lithiase vesiculare. Effect preventif et curatif de diverses medications chez la soutis. Therapie 25: 463–485

Cahalane M J, Neubrand M W, Carey M C 1988 Physical-chemical pathogenesis of pigment gallstones. Hepatology 4: 519–569

Carey M C, Cahalane M J 1988a Enterohepatic circulation. In: Arias I M, Jakoby W B, Popper H, Schachter D, Shafritz D A (eds) The liver: biology and pathobiology. Raven Press, New York pp 573–616

Carey M C, Cahalane M J 1988b Whither biliary sludge? Gastroenterology 95: 508–523

Carey M C, Mazer M A 1984 Biliary lipid secretion in health and in cholesterol gallstone disease. Hepatology 4: 31S–37S

Carey M C, Small M D 1978 The physical chemistry of cholesterol solubility in bile: relationship to gallstone formation and dissolution in man. Journal of Clinical Investigations 61: 998–1026

Carulli N, Ponz De Leon M, Zironi F et al 1980 Hepatic cholesterol and bile acid metabolism in subjects with gallstones; comparative effects of short-term feeding of chenodeoxycholic and ursodeoxycholic acid. Journal of Lipid Research 21: 35–43

Carulli N, Loris P, Bertolotti M 1984 Effects of acute changes of bile acid pool composition on biliary lipid secretion. Journal of Clinical Investigation 74: 614–624

Comfort M W, Gray H K, Wilson J M 1948 The silent gallstone: a ten to twenty year follow-up study of 112 cases. Annals of Surgery 128: 913

Danielsson H, Sjovall I 1975 Bile acid metabolism. Annual Review of Biochemistry 44: 233–241

Danzinger R G, Hofmann A F, Schoenfield U, Thistle J L 1972 Dissolution of cholesterol gallstones by chenodeoxycholic acid. New England Journal of Medicine 286: 1–8

Doran J, Keighley M R B, Bell G D 1979 Rowacol: a possible treatment for cholesterol gallstones. Gut 20: 312–317

Dowling R H, Bell G D, White I 1972 Lithogenic bile in patients with ileal dysfunction. Gut 13: 415–420

Einarsson K, Hellstrom K, Kallner M 1975 Gallbladder disease in hyperlipoproteinemia. Lancet 1: 484–494

Einarsson K, Grundy S M 1980 Effects of feeding cholic acid and chenodeoxycholic acid on cholesterol absorption and hepatic secretion of biliary lipids in man. Journal of Lipid Research 21: 23–24

Einarsson K, Nilsell K, Leijd B et al 1985 Influence of age on secretion of cholesterol and synthesis of bile acids by the liver. New England Journal of Medicine 313: 277–282

Erlinger S, Le Go A, Husson J M et al 1984 Franco-Belgian cooperative study of ursodeoxycholic acid in the medical dissolution of gallstones: a double blind randomized, dose-response study and comparison with chenodeoxycholic acid. Hepatology 4: 308–314

Everson G, Braverman D, Johnson J et al 1980 A critical evaluation of real-time ultrasonography for the study of gallbladder volume and contraction. Gastroenterology 79: 40–46

Fedorowsky T, Salen G, Tint G S et al 1979 Transformation of chenodeoxycholic acid and ursodeoxycholic acid by human intestinal bacteria. Gastroenterology 77: 1068–1073

Festi D, Frabboni R, Bazzoli F et al 1990 Gallbladder motility in cholesterol gallstone disease; effect of ursodeoxycholic acid administration on gallstone dissolution. Gastroenterology 99: 1779–1785

Fisher R, Stelzer F, Rock E, Malmud L 1982 Abnormal gallbladder emptying in patients with gallstones. Digestive Diseases and Sciences 27: 1019–1024

Fitzpatrick G, Neutra R, Gilbert J P 1977 Cost-effectiveness of cholecystectomy for silent gallstones. In: Bunker J P, Barnes B A, Mosteller F (eds) Cost, risk and benefit of surgery. Oxford University Press, London pp 246

Frabboni R, Bazzoli F, Mazzella G et al 1985a Acquired gallstone calcification during cholelitholitic treatment with chenodeoxycholic, ursodeoxycholic and tauroursodeoxycholic acids. Hepatology 5 (No 5): Abstract 232

Frabboni R, Bazzoli F, Sapia C et al 1985b Acquired calcification of radiolucent gallstones during cholelitholitic treatment with bile acids. In: Barbara L, Dowling RH, Hofmann AF, Roda E (eds) Recent advances in bile acid research. Raven Press, New York pp 273–275

Fromm H 1984 Gallstone dissolution and the cholesterol-bile acid-lipoproteins axis. Proposition effects of ursodeoxycholic acids. Gastroenterology 87: 229–233

Fromm H, Erbler H C, Eschler A et al 1976 Alterations of bile acid metabolism during treatment with chenodeoxycholic acid. Studies of the role of the appearance of ursodeoxycholic acid in the dissolution of gallstones. Klinische Wochenschrift 54: 1125–1131

Fromm H, Roat I W, Gonzalez V et al 1983a Comparative efficacy and bile effects of ursodeoxycholic and chenodeoxycholic acids in dissolving gallstones. A double blind controlled study. Gastroenterology 85: 1257–1264

Fromm H, Sarva R P, Bazzoli F 1983b Formation of ursodeoxycholic acid in the human colon: studies of the role of 7-ketolithocholic acid as an intermediate. Journal of Lipid Research 24: 841–853

Glambek I, Arnesjo B, Soreide O 1989 Correlation between gallstones and abdominal symptoms in a random population. Results from a screening study. Scandinavian Journal of Gastroenterology 24: 277–281

Gracie W A, Ransohoff D F 1982 The natural history of silent gallstones. The New England Journal of Medicine 307: 798–800

Gracie W A, Ransohoff D F 1985 Natural history and expectant management of gallstone disease. In: Cohen S, Soloway RD (eds) Gallstones. Churchill Livingstone Press, New York pp 27–43

GREPCO 1984 Prevalence of gallstone disease in an Italian adult female population. American Journal of Epidemiology 118: 796–805

GREPCO 1995 The natural history of gallstones: the GREPCO experience. Hepatology 21: 656–660

Grundy S M, Duane W C, Adler R D et al 1974 Biliary lipid outputs in young women with cholesterol gallstones. Metabolism 23: 67–73

Hardison W G M, Grundy S M 1984 Effect of ursodeoxycholate and its tautine conjugate on bile acid synthesis and cholesterol absorption. Gastroenterology 87: 130–135

Heaton K W, Austad W I, Lack L et al 1968 Enterohepatic circulation of C14 labelled bile salts in disorders of the distal small bowel. Gastroenterology 55: 15–16

Heaton K W, Emmett P M, Symes C L et al 1993 An explanation for gallstones in normal-weight women: slow intestinal transit. Lancet 341: 8–10

Hellstern A, Leuschner M, Frenk K H et al 1990 Gallstone dissolution with methyl tert-butyl ether: how to avoid complications. Gut 31: 922–925

Hellstern A, Leuschner U, Benjaminov A et al 1998 Dissolution of gallbladder stones with methyl tert-butyl ether and stone recurrence. A european survey. Digestive Diseases and Sciences 43: 911

Hill G H, Mair W S J, Goligher J C 1975 Gallstones after ileostomy and ileal resection. Gut 16: 932–940

Hofmann A F 1988 Pathogenesis of cholesterol gallstones. Journal of Clinical Gastroenterology 10(Suppl 2): S1–11

Hofmann A F 1989 Overview of bile secretion. In: Schultz SG Handbook of physiology. The gastrointestinal system III. American Physiological Society, Bethesda pp 567–596

Hofmann A F 1990 Nonsurgical treatment of gallstone disease. Annual Reviews of Medicine 41: 401–415

Hofmann A F, Grundy S M, Lachin J M 1982 The National Cooperative Gallstone Study Group: pre-treatment biliary lipid composition in white patients with radiolucent gallstones in the National Cooperative Gallstone Study. Gastroenterology 83: 738–752

Hofmann A F, Amelsberg A, Esch O et al 1997 Successful topical dissolution of cholesterol gallbladder stones using ethyl propionate. Digestive Diseases and Sciences 42: 1274–1282

Holan K R, Holzbach T, Hermann R E et al 1979 Nucleation time: a key factor in the pathogenesis of cholesterol gallstone disease. Gastroenterology 77: 611–617

Holzbach R T, Marsh M, Olszewski M et al 1973 Cholesterol solubility in bile: evidence that supersaturated bile is frequent in healthy man. Journal of Clinical Investigations 52: 1467–1479

Hood K, Gleeson D, Ruppin D C and BBGSC 1993 Gallstone recurrence and its prevention: the British/Belgian Gallstone Study Group's (BBGSC) post-dissolution trial. Gut 34: 1277–1288

Jazrawi R P, Pigozzi M G, Galatola G et al 1992 Optimum bile acid treatment for rapid gallstone dissolution. Gut 33: 381–386

Jazrawi R P, Pazzi P, Petroni M L et al 1995 Postprandial gallbladder motor function: refilling and turnover of bile in health and in cholelithiasis. Gastroenterology 109: 582–591

Johnston C G, Nakayama F 1957 Solubility of cholesterol and gallstones in metabolic material. Archives of Surgery 75: 436–442

Jorgensen L T 1989 Abdominal symptoms and gallstone disease: an epidemiological investigation. Hepatology 9: 856–860

Juvonen T, Kervinen K, Kairaluoma et al 1993 Gallstone cholesterol content is related to apolipoprotein E polymorphism. Gastroenterology 104: 1806–1813

Kern F Jr 1994 Effects of dietary cholesterol on cholesterol and bile acid homeostasis in patients with cholesterol gallstones. Journal of Clinical Investigation 93: 1186–1194

Kesäniemi Y A, Ehnholm C, Miettinen T A 1987 Intestinal cholesterol absorption efficiency in man is related to apolipoprotein E phenotype. Journal of Clinical Investigation 80: 578–581

Khanuja B, Cheah Y-C, et al 1995 *Lith 1*, a major gene affecting cholesterol gallstone formation among inbred strains of mice. Proceedings of the National Academy of Sciences of the United States of America 92: 7729–7733

Kibe A, Holzbach R T, La Russo N F et al 1984 Inhibition of crystal formation by apolipoproteins A-I and A-II in model systems of supersaturated bile: implications for gallstone pathogenesis in man. Science 225: 514–516

Kimura T, Shimamaura M, Yamaguchi A et al 1981 Solubilization of cultured cell membrane by bile acids. Acta Hepatologica Japonica 22: 717

Kishk S M A, Darweesh R M A, Dodds W J 1987 Sonographic evaluation of resting gallbladder volume and postprandial emptying in patients with gallstones. American Journal of Roentgenology 148: 875–879

Kottke T E, Feldman R D, Albert D A 1984 The risk ratio is insufficient for clinical decision: the case of prophylactic cholecystectomy. Medical Decision Making 177: A1–A12

Lanzini A, Northfield T C 1990 Review article: bile acid therapy. Alimentary and Pharmacological Therapy 4: 1–24

Lee S P 1981 Hypersecretion of mucus glycoprotein by the gallbladder epithelium in experimental cholelithiasis. Pathology 134: 199–207

Leijd B 1980 Cholesterol and bile acid metabolism in obesity. Clinical Science 59: 203–206

Leuschner V, Rothe W, Klicic X et al 1987 Methyl tert-butyl ether treatment of cholesterol stones: toxicity and dissolution of stone debris. Gastroenterology 92: 1750

Leuschner V, Hellestern A, Fisher H et al 1990 Methyl tert-butyl ether for gallstone dissolution: clinical results. In: Paumgartner G, Stiehl A, Barbara L, Roda E (eds) Strategies for the prevention of hepatobiliary diseases. Kluwer Academic Publishers, Dordrecht pp 185–187

Mabee T M, Meyer P, DenBesten L et al 1976 The mechanism of increased gallstone formation in obese human subjects. Surgery 79: 460–468

Makino I, Shinozaki K, Yoshino K et al 1975 Dissolution of cholesterol gallstones by ursodeoxycholic acid. Japanese Journal of Gastroenterology 72: 690–702

Marcus S N, Heaton K W 1986 Intestinal transit, deoxycholic acid and the cholesterol saturation of bile—three inter-related factors. Gut 27: 550–558

Marcus S N, Heaton K W. 1988 Deoxycholic acid and the pathogenesis of gallstones. Gut 29: 522–533

Marks J W, Lan S O 1984 The Steering Committee and the National Cooperative Gallstone Study Group. Low dose chenodiol to prevent gallstone recurrence after dissolution therapy. Annals of Internal Medicine 100: 376–381

Marks JW, Conley DR, Capretta TL et al 1977 Gallstone prevalence and biliary lipid composition in inflammatory bowel disease. American Journal of Digestive Diseases 22: 1097–1100

Marks JW, Sue SO, Pearlman BJ et al 1981 Sulfation of lithocholate as a possible modifier of chenodeoxycholic acid-induced elevations of serum transaminase in patients with gallstones. Journal of Clinical Investigations 68: 1190–1197

Mazzella G, Bazzoli F, Villanova N et al 1990 Effect of gemfibrozil administration of biliary lipid secretion in hyperlipidemic patients. Scandinavian Journal of Gastroenterology 25: 1227–1234

Mazzella G, Bazzoli F, Festi D et al 1991 Comparative evaluation of chenodeoxycholic and ursodeoxycholic acids in obese patients. Effects on biliary lipid metabolism during weight maintenance and weight reduction. Gastroenterology 201: 490–496

McCullough J E, Stadheim L M, Reading C C et al 1990 Gallstone recurrence after methyl tert-butyl ether dissolution. Gastroenterology 98 (No. 5): Abstract 55

McGahan I P, Resluk H, Brock J M et al 1988 Dissolution of gallstones using methyl tert-butyl ether in an animal model. Investigative Radiology 23: 599–603

McSherry C K, Ferstenberg H, Calhoun W F et al 1985 The natural history of diagnosed gallstone disease in symptomatic and asymptomatic patients. Annals of Surgery 202: 59–63

M.I.COL. 1995 Epidemiology of gallstone disease in Italy: prevalence data of the multicenter Italian study on cholelithiasis. American Journal of Epidemiology 141: 158–165

Midvedt T, Norman A 1967 Bile acid transformation by microbial strains belonging to genera found in intestinal contents. Acta Pathologica Microbiologica Scandinavica 71: 629–635

Miettinen T A 1971 Cholesterol production in obesity. Circulation 44: 842–849

Miller F J, Rose S C 1990 Intervention for gallbladder disease. Cardiovascular Interventional Radiology 13: 264–271

Miquel J F, Núñez L, Amigo L et al 1998 Cholesterol saturation, not proteins or cholecystitis, is critical for crystal formation in human gallbladder bile. Gastroenterology 114: 1016–1023

Miyake M, Johnston C G 1968 Gallstones: ethnological studies. Digestion 1: 219–228

Nakayama F, Miyazaki K, Koga D 1980 Effect of chenodeoxycholic and ursodeoxycholic acids on isolated human hepatocytes. Gastroenterology 78: 1228–1233

Nelson P E, Moyer T, Thistle J L 1990a Gallstone dissolution in vitro with methyl tert-butyl ether: radiologic selection criteria. Gastroenterology 98: 1280–1283

Nelson P E, Moyer T P, Thistle J L 1990b Dissolution of calcium bilirubinate and calcium carbonate debris remaining after methyl tert-butyl ether dissolution of cholesterol gallstones. Gastroenterology 98: 1345–1350

Nestel P J, Schreibman P, Ahrens E H Jr 1973 Cholesterol metabolism in human obesity. Journal of Clinical Investigation 52: 2389–2397

Newman H F, Northup J D, Rosenblum M A 1968 Complications of cholelithiasis. American Journal of Gastroenterology 50: 476–496

Nilsell K, Angelin B, Liljeqvist L et al 1985 Biliary lipid output and bile acid kinetics in cholesterol gallstone disease. Evidence for an increased hepatic secretion of cholesterol in Swedish patients. Gastroenterology 89: 287–293

Northfield T C, Hofmann A F 1975 Biliary lipid output during three meals and on overnight fast. I. Relationship to bile acid pool size and cholesterol saturation on bile in gallstone and control subjects. Gut 16: 1–11

Noshiro H, Chijiiwa K, Makino I et al 1995 Deoxycholic acid in gall bladder bile does not account for the shortened nucleation time in patients with cholesterol gallstones. Gut 36: 121–125

Palmer R H 1967 The formation of bile acid sulfates: a new pathway of bile acid metabolism in humans. Proceedings of the National Academy of Sciences of the United States of America 58: 1047–1050

Pauletzki J, Althaus R, Holl J et al 1996 Gallbladder emptying and gallstone formation: a prospective study on gallstone recurrence. Gastroenterology 111: 765–771

Paumgartner G, Carr-Locke D L, Roda E et al 1988 Biliary stones: nonsurgical therapeutic approach. Gastroenterology International 1: 5–15

Pazzi P, Scagliarini R, Sighinolfi D et al 1998 Nonsteroidal antiinflammatory drug use and gallstone disease prevalence: a case-control study. American Journal of Gastroenterology 93: 1420–1424

Perez-Aguilar F, Breto M, Alfonso V 1985 Gallstone recurrence following cessation of dissolving treatment and during prophylactic administration of either low-dose chenodeoxycholic acid (CDCA) or medium-dose ursodeoxycholic acid (UDCA). Hepatology 1 (5): Abstract 253

Podda M, Zuin M, Battezzati PM et al 1989 Efficacy and safety of a combination of chenodeoxycholic acid and ursodeoxycholic acid for gallstone dissolution: a comparative study with ursodeoxycholate alone. Gastroenterology 96: 222–229

Ponz de Leon M, Carulli N, Lori R et al 1980a Medical treatment of gallstones with chenodeoxycholic acid (CDCA). Follow-up report at four years. Italian Journal of Gastroenterology 12: 17–22

Ponz de Leon M, Carulli N, Lori R et al 1980b Cholesterol absorption during bile acid feeding. Effect of ursodeoxycholic acid (UDCA) administration. Gastroenterology 78: 214–219

Portincasa P, Van Erpecum KJ, Stolk MFJK et al 1995 Role of gallbladder dysmotility in gallstone formation. In: Fromm H, Leuschner U (eds), Bile acids–Cholestasis–Gallstones. Advances in basic and clinical bile acid research. Kluwer Academic Publishers, Berlin pp 180–193

Portincasa P, van Erpecum KJ, van de Meeberg PC et al 1996 Apolipoprotein E4 and gallbladder motility influence speed of gallstone clearance and risk of recurrence after extracorporeal shock-wave lithotripsy. Hepatology 24: 580–587

Ralston DE, Smith LA 1965 The natural history of cholelithiasis: a 15 to 30-year follow-up of 116 patients. Minnesota Medicine 48: 327–332

Ransohoff DF, Gracie WA, Wollenson LB et al 1983 Prophylactic cholecystectomy or expectant management for silent gallstones: a decision analysis to assess survival. Annals of Internal Medicine 99: 199–204

Reichen J, Paumgartner G 1976 Uptake of bile acid by perfused rat liver. American Journal of Physiology 231: 734–742

Reuben A, Maton PN, Murphy GM et al 1985 Bile lipid secretion in obese and non-obese individuals with and without gallstones. Clinical Science 69: 71–79

Rewbridge AG 1937 The disappearance of gallstone shadows following the prolonged administration of bile salts. Surgery 1: 395–400

Richardson SC 1987 On the probability of gallstone recurrence. Journal of Hepatology 4: 390–392

Roda E, Mazzella G, Rods A et al 1980 Lithocholic acid metabolism before and after chenodeoxycholic acid therapy in gallstone patients. Italian Journal of Gastroenterology 72: 171–176

Roda E, Bazzoli F, Morselli Labate AM et al 1982 Ursodeoxycholic acid versus chenodeoxycholic acid as cholesterol gallstone dissolving agents: a comparative randomized study. Hepatology 2: 804–810

Roda E, Mazzella G, Bazzoli F 1989a Effect of ursodeoxycholic acid administration on biliary lipid secretion in primary biliary cirrhosis. Digestive Diseases and Sciences 34: 525–585

Roda E, Morselli Labate AM, Sama C et al 1989b Epidemiology of gallstone disease. In: Burhenne HJ (ed) Biliary lithotripsy. Year Book Medical Publishers, Chicago, pp 131–138

Sackmann M, Delius M, Sauerbruch T et al 1988 Shock-wave lithotripsy of gallbladder stones. The first 175 patients. New England Journal of Medicine 318: 393–397

Sackmann M, Pauletzki J, Aydemir U et al 1990 Monotherapy with ursodeoxycholic acid is as efficient as a combination of urso- and chenodeoxycholic acid for dissolution of gallstone fragments. Hepatology 12(4): Abstract 126

Sackmann M, Niller H, Klueppelberg U et al 1994 Gallstone recurrence after shock-wave therapy. Gastroenterology 106: 225–230

Salen G, Tint G S, Eliav B et al 1974 Increased formation of ursodeoxycholic acid in patients treated with chenodeoxycholic acid. Journal of Clinical Investigation 53: 612–621

Salen G, Nicolau G, Shefer S et al 1975 Hepatic cholesterol metabolism in patients with gallstones. Gastroenterology 69: 676–684

Sama C, La Russo N F, Lopez Del Pino V et al 1982 Effects of acute bile acid administration on biliary lipid secretion in healthy volunteers. Gastroenterology 82: 515–525

Sarva R F, Farivar S, Fromm H et al 1981 Study of the sensitivity and specificity of computerized tomography in the detection of calcified stones which appear radiolucent by conventional roentgenography. Gastrointestinal Radiology 6: 165–170

Sauerbruch T, Delius M, Paumgartner G 1986 Fragmentation of gallstones by extracorporeal shock waves. New England Journal of Medicine 314: 818–822

Sauter G, Kullak-Ublik G A, Schumacher R et al 1997 Safety and efficacy of repeated shockwave lithotripsy of gallstones with and without adjuvant bile acid therapy. Gastroenterology 112: 1603–1609

Schoenfield L J, Lachin J M 1981 The Steering Committee and the National Cooperative Gallstone Study Group. Chenodiol (chenodeoxycholic acid) for dissolution of gallstones: the National Cooperative Gallstone Study. Annals of Internal Medicine 95: 257–282

Schoenfield L J, Carulli N, Dowling R H et al 1989 Asymptomatic gallstones: definition and treatment. Gastroenterology International 2: 25–29

Schoenfield L J, Berci G, Carnoval R L et al 1990 The effect of ursodiol on the efficacy and safety of extracorporeal shock-wave lithotripsy of gallbladder stones. The Dornier National Biliary Lithotripsy Study. New England Journal of Medicine 323: 1239–1245

Schreibman P H, Dell R B 1975 Human adipocyte cholesterol concentration, localization, synthesis and turnover. Journal of Clinical Investigation 59: 986–993

Shaffer E A, Small D M 1977 Biliary lipid secretion in cholesterol gallstone disease. The effect of cholecystectomy and obesity. Journal of Clinical Investigation 59: 828–840

Shaffer E A, McOrmand P, Duggan H 1980 Quantitative cholescintigraphy: assessment of gallbladder filling and emptying and duodenogastric reflux. Gastroenterology 89: 899–906

Shaffner F, Javitt N B 1966 Morphologic changes in hamster liver during intrahepatic cholestasis induced by taurolithocholate. Laboratory Investigation 75: 1783–1792

Shoda J, Veda T, Ikegami T et al Increased biliary group II phospholipase A2 and altered gallbladder bile in patients with multiple cholesterol stones. Gastroenterology 112: 2036–2047

Simone J F, Mueller P R, Ferrucci J T 1989 Nonsurgical therapy of gallstones: implications for imaging. American Journal of Roentgenology 152: 11–17

Sirmione 1987 XX European symposium on calcified tissues. Italy, October 4–8. Including satellite workshop on molecular and cell biology and satellite workshop in biology and regulation of bone metabolism: clinical significance. Abstracts. Calcified tissue International 41(Suppl 2): 1–96

Small D M, Dowling R H, Redinger R N 1972 The enterohepatic circulation of bile salts. Archives of Internal Medicine 130: 552–573

Taroni F, Sama C, Roda E 1987 Cost-effectiveness analysis of alternative treatments for silent gallstones. In: Serio A, Oore F, Tondini A (eds)

Medical Information Europe '87. Participants Editions, Roma p 155–160

Thistle J U, Hofmann A F 1973 Efficacy and specificity of chenodeoxycholic acid therapy for dissolving gallstones. New England Journal of Medicine 289: 655–659

Thistle J U, May G R, Bender C E et al 1989 Dissolution of cholesterol gallbladder stones using methyl tert-butyl ether administered by percutaneous transhepatic catheter. New England Journal of Medicine 320: 633–639

Thomas L A, Bathgate T, Veysey M J et al 1997 Is cholelithiasis an intestinal disease? Gut 41 (Suppl 3): A2

Thudichum J L W 1863 A treatise on gallstones: their chemistry, pathology and treatment. John Churchill, London

Tint G S, Salen G, Shaffer S 1986 Effect of ursodeoxycholic acid and chenodeoxycholic acid on cholesterol and bile acid metabolism. Gastroenterology 91: 1007–1018

Trotman B W, Petrella E J, Soloway R D et al 1975 Evaluation of radiologic lucency or opaqueness as a means of identifying cholesterol or pigment stones. Gastroenterology 68: 1563–1568

Trotman B W, Morris T A, Sanchez H et al 1977 Pigment versus cholesterol cholelithiasis: identification and quantification by infrared spectrometry. Gastroenterology 72: 495–501

Tudyka J, Kratzer W, Kuhn K et al 1995 Combined bile acid therapy is more effective on biliary lipids and dissolution rates than monotherapy after gallstone lithotripsy. American Journal of Gastroenterology 90: 1942–1948

Tudyka J, Weschsler J G, Kratzer W et al 1996 Gallstone recurrence after successful dissolution therapy. Digestive Diseases and Sciences 42(2): 235–241

Uchida N, Nakatsu T, Hirabayashi S et al 1994 Direct dissolution of gallstones with methyl tert-butyl ether (MTBE) via endoscopic transpapillary catheterization in the gallbladder (ETCG). Journal of Gastroenterology 29: 486–494

Valdivieso V D, Palms R, Nervi F et al 1979 Secretion of biliary lipids in young Chilean women with cholesterol gallstones. Gut 20: 997–1000

Van Erpecum K J, Portincasa P, Eckhardt E et al 1996 Ursodeoxycholic acid reduces protein levels and their nucleation-promoting activity in gallbladder bile. Gastroenterology 110: 1225–1237

Van Erpecum K J, Van Berge-Henegouwen G P, Eckhardt E R M et al 1998 Cholesterol crystallization in human gallbladder bile: relation to gallstone number, bile composition, and apolipoprotein E4 isoform. Hepatology 27: 1508–1516

van Sonnenberg E, Casola G, Zakko S F et al 1988 Gallbladder and bile duct stones: percutaneous therapy with primary MTBE dissolution and mechanical methods. Radiology 169: 505–509

van Sonnenberg E, D'Agostino H B, Casola G et al 1990 Interventional radiology in the gallbladder: diagnosis, drainage, dissolution and management of stones. Radiology 174: 1–6

Vessey D A, Whitney J, Gollan J L 1983 The role of conjugation reactions in enhancing the biliary secretion of bile acids. Biochemical Journal 214: 923–927

Villanova N, Bazzoli F, Frabboni R 1987 Gallstone recurrence after successful oral bile acid treatment: a three year follow-up and evaluation of long-term post-dissolution treatment. Gastroenterology 92: Abstract 1708

Villanova N, Bazzoli F, Taroni F et al 1989 Gallstone recurrence after successful oral bile acid treatment. A 12-year follow-up study and evaluation of long-term post-dissolution treatment. Gastroenterology 97: 726–731

Vlahcevic Z R, Bell C C Jr, Buhac I et al 1970 Diminished bile acid pool size in patients with gallstones. Gastroenterology 59: 165–173

Weintraub M S, Eisenberg S, Breslow J L 1987 Dietary fat clearance in normal subjects is regulated by genetic variation in apolipoprotein E. Journal of Clinical Investigation 80: 1571–1577

Cholecystitis

34

A. CUSCHIERI

Gallstones are common throughout the Western world and are found in about 10% of the adult population. In both sexes, the prevalence increases with age and peaks between 50 and 65 years (Barbara et al 1987). Overall gallstones are twice as common in females than in males (Holzbach 1989). In some countries such as Sweden, Czekoslovakia and Chile, and in certain ethnic groups, for example the Pima Indians, the incidence of gallstones is even higher and may approach 50% (Sampliner et al 1970, Bouchier 1988). The vast majority of gallstones remain silent and several studies have shown that only 20 to 30% of patients with gallstones have symptoms (Ch. 32) (Gracie & Ransohoff 1982, Kern 1983). The probability of a patient with silent gallstones developing biliary-related pain is 1 to 2% and the risk of developing a complication such as empyema of the gallbladder and perforated acute cholecystitis is even less; approximately 0.1% per year (Gracie & Ransohoff 1982).

The high prevalence rates for gallstone disease, despite the low symptomatic/complication rates translate to cholecystectomy being one of the commonest operations performed world wide and the cholecystectomy rate has increased significantly by an average of 20% since the introduction of laparoscopic cholecystectomy (Lam et al 1996) and this increase has affected all age groups. The exact reasons for this increased cholecystectomy rate during the 1990s are not known, but the rise is undoubtedly related to perceptions on the part of patients, general practitioners and surgeons that laparoscopic cholecystectomy (LC) is a lesser procedure than the open equivalent intervention and is attended by less pain, quicker recovery and reduced risk of death. To a large extent, these perceptions have been confirmed by data from large retrospective series of LC for symptomatic gallstone disease.

The indications for surgery include a wide range of biliary symptoms categorized clinically as gallstone dyspepsia; biliary colic, chronic cholecystitis and these account for the majority. Between 10 and 30% of patients undergoing cholecystectomy present with acute cholecystitis. This is most commonly obstructive in nature. In a small percentage, usually but not always, in critically ill patients the acute inflammation of the gallbladder arises in the absence of gallstones although biliary sludge is often present – acute acalculous cholecystitis.

ACUTE CALCULOUS CHOLECYSTITIS

PATHOLOGY

This is the commonest form of the disease and accounts for 90 to 95% of cases. The attack develops when the cystic duct becomes obstructed by a gallstone impacting in Hartmann's pouch. Although bacterial infection of the stagnant bile seems an obvious mechanism for the development of acute cholecystitis, cultures of gallbladder bile taken during open cholecystectomy are positive in only 15 to 30% of cases and in only 3% of patients undergoing LC for the same disease (Den Hoed et al 1998). The predominant microorganisms isolated from the gallbladder bile in these patients are *Escherichia coli* (60%), *Klebsiella pneumoniae* (22%) and *Streptococcus faecalis* (18%). There appears to be no relation between positive gallbladder cultures and postoperative wound infections for both open and laparoscopic cholecystectomy but the overall incidence of wound infection is much higher after the open procedure (14% versus 5%) and serious wound infections after LC are very rare. Thus the small incisions used in laparoscopic gallbladder surgery may be less susceptible to infective complications.

These observations indicate that the initial inflammatory process following obstruction of the cystic duct is of a chemical nature with infection supervening in some patients during the later stages of the disease. It is believed that trauma, secondary to gallstone impaction, leads to mucosal damage through the release of phospholipases that convert lecithin (a mucosal protective factor against bile acids) to lysolecithin, a known mucosal toxin. Alternatively, the release of the prostaglandin precursor arachidonic acid by the action of phospholipase A on lecithin may mediate the inflammatory response by producing prostaglandins (Sjodahl & Tagesson 1983). With conservative treatment, the inflammation resolves in some 80% of patients as the rising tension in the gallbladder lumen from the outpouring of the inflammatory exudate lifts the walls of Hartmann's pouch off the impacting stone. When this disengages and drops into the gallbladder lumen, cystic duct drainage leads to resolution. This fortuitous sequence is not encountered in 20% of patients, usually elderly, in whom patchy gangrene and or perforation with a large inflammatory phlegmon or peritonitis supervene.

DIAGNOSIS

CLINICAL FEATURES

The clinical presentation depends on the severity of the underlying disease. Generally it is characterized by a sudden and severe pain, mainly in the right hypochondrium which may radiate to the right or inter-scapular region. Often there is a history of less severe antecedent episodes of 'biliary colic'. Nausea and vomiting are frequent features in the early stages. On examination the patient is usually febrile (37.5–38.5°C) with tenderness and rigidity in the right upper quadrant and a positive Murphy's sign (mid-inspiratory arrest) although this is much better elicited ultrasonically (vide infra).

Jaundice when present may be due to common duct stones, cholangitis, or partial compression of the common hepatic duct by inflammatory edema caused by impaction of a gallstone in Hartmann's pouch (Mirizzi syndrome Type 1). Up to one quarter of patients with established acute cholecystitis will have a palpable mass in the right upper quadrant caused by a pericholecystic phlegmon, abscess or empyema, less commonly and in the elderly, a gallbladder carcinoma.

Usually the diagnosis of acute cholecystitis is not difficult, but other common intra-abdominal conditions, e.g., perforated peptic ulcer, acute pancreatitis or a retrocecal appendicitis associated with a high cecum and viral hepatitis need to be considered in the individual case. Enterally transmitted non-A non-B viral hepatitis can simulate acute cholecystitis quite closely (Dogra et al 1995).

Laboratory tests are frequently nonspecific, their greatest value being to rule out other important conditions in the differential diagnosis, particularly acute pancreatitis. Most patients will have a neutrophil leucocytosis ($>10 \times 10^9/L$) together with some abnormality of the liver function profile. The levels of serum bilirubin and alkaline phosphatase do not invariably correlate with the presence of ductal calculi (Dumont 1976) but are suggestive and clinical jaundice warrants investigation with endoscopic retrograde cholangiography (ERC) or magnetic resonance cholangiopancreatography (MRCP). Other laboratory findings include raised transaminases and minor elevations of the serum amylase, below the diagnostic threshold for acute pancreatitis (Williamson 1990).

IMAGING TESTS

The yield from a plain abdominal X-ray is limited. Calcified gallstones will be detected in 10 to 20% of patients. Gas in the gallbladder lumen and pericholecystic tissues caused by emphysematous cholecystitis (vide infra) is only visible in advanced cases by plain abdominal radiographs. Absence of free air under the diaphragm is useful for excluding perforated ulcer.

Real-time ultrasonography and biliary scintiscanning form the mainstays in the confirmatory diagnosis of acute cholecystitis. Gray scale B-mode ultrasound is the most commonly used test since it is readily available, non-invasive, quick and easy to perform. Furthermore, it has the advantage of providing information about the liver, biliary tract and pancreas together with other sources of non-biliary right upper quadrant pain (Duncan & Stoddard 1992). The sonographic features include a positive Murphy's sign, calculi or sludge, a thickened gallbladder wall and pericholecystic edema (Fig. 34.1). Ultrasound examination is hampered by obesity and overlying bowel gas and is, of course, observer dependent. There is now good evidence from reported studies that the diagnostic accuracy of ultrasound for acute cholecystitis is considerably improved with color velocity imaging and especially with power Doppler when compared to gray-scale imaging (sensitivity = 95% versus 86%, accuracy = 99% versus 92%) (Uggowitzer et al 1997, Soyer et al 1998). However, the high susceptibility of power Doppler to motion artifacts requires expert adjustments of the technical parameters, and if anything, increases the observer dependency. The resistive index within the intramural vessels of the gallbladder that can now be measured by ultrasound techniques does not differentiate between inflamed and non-inflamed gallbladders.

Gallbladder scintiscanning using iminodiacetic acid derivatives (HIDA, PIPIDA scans) can be used to confirm a

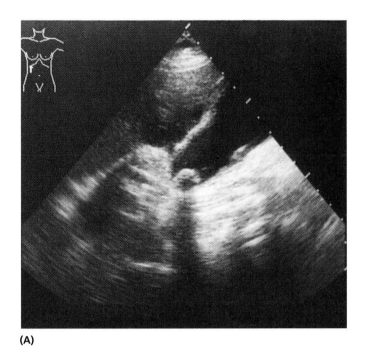
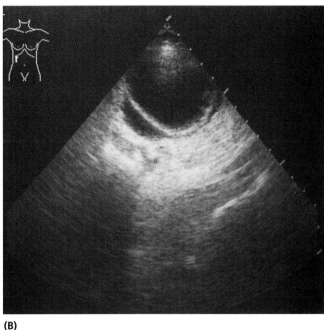

Fig. 34.1 (A) Ultrasound scan of an acutely inflamed gallbladder containing a stone impacted in Hartmann's pouch. **(B)** Acutely inflamed gallbladder wall with surrounding oedema.

nonfunctioning gallbladder (Fig. 34.2), and is regarded as the most accurate test of acute cholecystitis with a sensitivity of 97% and a specificity of 87% (Ralls et al 1982). A normal gallbladder scintiscan (Fig. 34.2A) is virtually 100% accurate in excluding acute cholecystitis (Cabellon et al 1984). The presence of pericholecystic uptake of the isotope is a valuable secondary sign in the diagnosis of acute cholecystitis and correlates with the presence of gangrenous cholecystitis or gallbladder perforation.

Intravenous cholangiography has been superseded by ultrasonography in the diagnosis of acute cholecystitis. CT scanning is useful in complicated cases but ill advised in the majority in view of the radiation dosage. Good diagnostic accuracy for acute cholecystitis has been reported with magnetic resonance imaging (Pu et al 1994).

INITIAL MANAGEMENT

This consists of intravenous fluid and electrolyte replacement, nasogastric suction, systemic antibiotics and parenteral analgesia. The patient is kept fasted to reduce the cholecystokinin release from the upper small bowel in order to minimize gallbladder stimulation. Although the inflammation is initially chemical and gallbladder bile cultures are negative in the majority of cases, most surgeons will choose to use systemic antibiotics because of the risk of progression

to an empyema and septic complications. Also, if surgery is performed, antibiotic prophylaxis will reduce the wound infection rate (Keighley 1977) although this has recently been questioned in patients undergoing LC (Den Hoed et al 1998). As the organisms cultured from gallbladder bile are predominantly Gram positive aerobes (*Escherichia coli, Klebsiella pneumoniae, Streptococcus faecalis*), a third generation cephalosporin is the antibiotic of choice. Anaerobes such as *Bacteroides fragilis* and *Clostridium perfringens* are associated with more severe, mixed infections particularly in the elderly. These require combination chemotherapy using metronidazole with an aminoglycoside and/or penicillin (Williamson 1990). The diagnosis of acute cholecystitis should be confirmed during this initial 12–24 hour period of stabilization by ultrasonography or gallbladder scintiscanning.

TIMING OF SURGERY

SEVERE PROGRESSIVE DISEASE

The timing of surgery is dictated by the severity of the attack. Table 34.1 summarizes the indications for emergency or urgent surgical intervention. Traditionally, such patients have been managed by laparotomy using a midline epigastric incision and the open approach is still favoured by many in critically ill elderly patients (Tokunaga et al 1997).

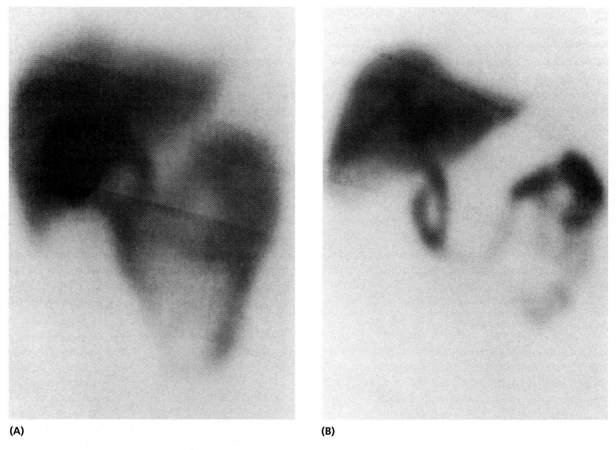

Fig 34.2 (A) HIDA scan showing filling of a normal gallbladder. **(B)** HIDA scan showing nonfilling of an acutely inflamed gallbladder.

Table 34.1 Indications for emergency or urgent intervention

- Deterioration in the patient's general condition or physical signs
- Evidence of generalized peritonitis
- Development of an inflammatory abdominal mass
- Gas in the gallbladder lumen or pericholecystic tissues
- Onset of intestinal obstruction

Hitherto, less than 10% of cases fell into this severe category (Mitchell & Morris 1982) but more recent reports from North America and Europe have highlighted an increasing proportion of acute severe cases requiring urgent surgical intervention (from 6 to 10% up to 25%). This has been attributed to (1) a decrease in the number of patients undergoing elective cholecystectomy though this has been reversed with the advent of LC, (2) an increasingly aged population, and (3) a rise in the actual incidence of acute complications of gallstone disease (Diettrich et al 1988, Reiss et al 1990).

ESTABLISHED NON-PROGRESSING DISEASE

These form the majority and the acute obstructive cholecystitis usually resolves with conservative treatment. There are two management options:

1. Early cholecystectomy carried out during the same hospital admission on the next available elective list
2. Interval cholecystectomy performed 6–8 weeks after resolution of the acute attack.

There have been at least six prospective randomized clinical trials comparing these two management options for open cholecystectomy (Van der Linden & Sunzel 1970, McArthur et al 1975, Jarvinen & Hastabacka 1980, Van der Linden & Edlund 1981, Norby et al 1983, Lathinen et al 1987). All have indicated clear benefit for early cholecystectomy. Essentially, early cholecystectomy benefits the patient by a reduction in the overall hospital stay and obviates the risk of recurrent bouts of acute cholecystitis requiring further hospital admissions. Fears that an early cholecystectomy is a more hazardous procedure have proved groundless, in particular the incidence of complications including missed common duct stones and mortality rates reported in these prospective trials have been similar to those after interval cholecystectomy. More recently, a randomized trial of early versus interval laparoscopic cholecystectomy for acute cholecystitis has demonstrated similar results. In particular there was no significant difference in the conversion rates (early 21% versus interval 24%), similar morbidity but a significantly ($p < 0.001$) shorter hospital stay, 7.6 versus 11.6 days, although the operating time was longer for the early group, i.e. 122 versus 106 min (Lai et al 1998). Similar benefits have been reported by another randomized trial comparing early versus interval LC for acute cholecystitis (Lo et al 1998). Thus early LC carries both medical and socioeconomic benefits over interval LC for acute cholecystitis.

An aggressive policy of early cholecystectomy is indicated in the elderly and diabetic patients unless they have co-morbid significant heart disease as these patients often have gangrenous disease (Tokunaga et al 1997, Tagle et al 1997).

SURGICAL TREATMENT

LAPAROSCOPIC VERSUS OPEN CHOLECYSTECTOMY

As with the elective situation, laparoscopic cholecystectomy offers significant advantages over open cholecystectomy for acute cholecystitis and early LC has rapidly become the treatment of choice for this condition. Aside from several retrospective reports indicative of reduced morbidity and hospital stay, the benefit of LC versus open cholecystectomy for acute cholecystitis has been confirmed by a prospective randomized clinical trial (Kiviluoto et al 1998). This study showed a significant reduction in the postoperative morbidity in the LC arm (only 3% minor complications versus 23% major complications and 19% minor complications in the open cholecystectomy group). In adopting LC as the routine option, it must be stressed that the need for conversion to open operation is encountered in 20–25% of cases. An early decision should be made to convert electively in the presence of obscured anatomy. This is far better than persistence with a difficult operation resulting in an enforced conversion because of the onset of an intraoperative complication. Patients requiring enforced conversion are at risk of severe postoperative complications (Lo et al 1997).

Thus the valid approach is a flexible one. The procedure starts with an exploratory laparoscopy to assess technical difficulty of the operation with particular reference to the structures in the triangle of Calot. A large distended gallbladder should be aspirated and lifted by a retractor rather than grasped. Large stones impacted in Hartmann's pouch that cannot be dislodged may prove problematic. The practical axiom is a simple one, i.e., if adequate exposure for a safe dissection cannot be obtained, the case should be converted. In some cases, a fundus first dissection of the gallbladder may be required (Wilson 1992).

INTRAOPERATIVE FLUOROCHOLANGIOGRAPHY

There is still considerable controversy on the need or otherwise for intraoperative cholangiography (Ch. 22) during cholecystectomy, and if anything, the debate has intensified since the introduction of LC. Some (author included) advocate it routinely, others selectively, and the majority have dispensed with this intraoperative investigation completely. Proponents of the selective policy cite the risks associated with negative common bile duct exploration associated with false negative cholangiograms (3%) and the potential for damage to the biliary tree by over manipulation as reasons against routine usage. Those in favor of routine cholangiography believe that its regular performance maintains the operator's technical expertise and ability to interpret results. In addition, the surgeon who has mastered laparoscopic fluorocholangiography can easily progress to trans-cystic extraction of ductal calculi. The case for routine fluorocholangiography is much stronger when cholecystectomy is performed for acute cholecystitis as these patients are more commonly jaundiced (by the inflammatory edema or by concomitant ductal calculi). The cholangiogram should outline the entire biliary tract (intra and extrahepatic). It ensures safe occlusion of the cystic duct stump without compromise of the common hepatic or common bile duct and differentiates stones from distortion caused by the inflammatory edema.

MINICHOLECYSTECTOMY

This implies performance of cholecystectomy through a small (5.0 cm wound) that should be placed in the midline and not in the right subcostal region (Dubois & Berthelot 1982, O'Dwyer et al 1990). Proponents recommend this technique for both elective cholecystectomy and for patients with acute cholecystitis (Baxter & O'Dwyer 1992). The procedure uses standard operating techniques with certain modifications such as the use of a headlight, a ring retractor, clip applicators and long instruments. The need to extend the incision is encountered in 15% of patients. A more recent modification has been described as 'cylindrical cholecystectomy' (Grau-Talens et al 1998). The operation is based on the introduction of a 3.8–5.0 mm cylinder that is 10.0 cm long which isolates the hepato-cystic region from the surrounding structures, and thus facilitates the intervention.

In general, minicholecystectomy is associated with a shorter hospital stay (3.5 days versus 8.5–11 days) as compared to patients undergoing cholecystectomy through an unrestricted incision (O'Dwyer et al 1990) and some have reported an earlier return to work after the procedure (Ledet 1990).

PARTIAL CHOLECYSTECTOMY

Many variations of this technique have been described involving a subtotal (fundus first) resection of the gallbladder but leaving the posterior wall attached to the hepatic bed (Bornman & Terblanche 1985). The same group has more recently reported this technique performed by the laparoscopic approach for patients with complicated acute cholecystitis or fibrosis (Michalowski et al 1998) and encountered one postoperative death (myocardial infarction) and 3 bile leaks in 29 patients. Thus suction drainage of the gallbladder bed is necessary after subtotal cholecystectomy (open or laparoscopic).

A modification using a 1.0 cm rim of Hartmann's pouch to buttress and occlude the internal opening of the cystic duct and leaving the structures of Calot's triangle undisturbed was described by Shein (1991) who reported favorably on the technique in 16 elderly/high risk patients. This author emphasizes its speed (mean operating time of 40 min), technical safety in obviating a difficult dissection of the liver bed and the practical advantage, in comparison to other conservative procedures, that leave the gallbladder in situ, of preventing gallstone formation.

CHOLECYSTOSTOMY

Cholecystostomy has frequently been criticized as an inferior operation because it is a temporizing procedure that palliates the patient's symptoms but leaves the patient at risk of development of further stones because the gallbladder is left in situ. Historical evidence suggests that approximately 50% of patients will develop further gallstones within 5 years of cholecystectomy (Hermann 1990). Despite these reservations, cholecystostomy still has a place in the management of those patients who are unfit for surgery because of co-morbid disease (ASA IV) or extreme old age in whom this simple quick procedure carried out surgically (open or

laparoscopic) or percutaneously under radiological or ultrasound control tides the patient over the critical illness in the short term, with the option of interval cholecystectomy if the patient's cardiorespiratory or general condition improves with medical treatment (Van Steenbergen et al 1990).

Open cholecystostomy can be performed through a small subcostal incision directly over the fundus of the gallbladder (localized by external ultrasound) under local or general anesthesia. After all accessible stones have been removed, a self-retaining tube drain is used to keep the gallbladder lumen decompressed and to allow a subsequent tube cholecystocholangiogram to assess whether there are any residual gallbladder stones (removed through the tract) or associated common duct stones (removed by endoscopic stone extraction). Although it has been generally assumed that these patients, if they survive long enough and their condition improves, will require definite surgery (Addison 1986), other reports suggest that adhesive obliteration of the gallbladder lumen provided it has been completely emptied of stones, may obviate the need for a subsequent cholecystectomy (Kaufmann et al 1990).

Percutaneous cholecystostomy (PC) under ultrasound or fluoroscopic guidance is an alternative to surgical or laparoscopic cholecystostomy that is favored by some and the reported results of recently published series have been good with an overall success rate of 95 to 98% and a mortality of 2 to 12% (England et al 1997; Hamy et al 1997). Response to this treatment defined as an improvement in clinical symptoms and signs or reduction in fever and WBC within 72 hours of PC is observed in 70 to 75%. The patients likely to respond are those with gallstones, symptoms and signs localized to the right upper quadrant and those with ultrasound radiological criteria of acute cholecystitis, especially pericholecystic fluid. The complications of PC (10%) include misplacement of the cholecystostomy catheter in the colon, exacerbation of sepsis and bile leakage. More recently ultrasound guided aspiration of the gallbladder without catheter drainage has been reported (Verbank et al 1998) in 27 critically ill patients (severe co-morbid disease) with acute cholecystitis with one death and improvement and survival in the rest.

ACUTE EMPHYSEMATOUS CHOLECYSTITIS

This has been regarded as a severe and fulminant form of acute cholecystitis caused by mixed infection of organisms, usually Coliform bacilli, Streptococci and gas-forming Clostridia. It is usually but not always acalculous. The condition has a peak incidence between the sixth and seventh decades, is three times more common in men than women and frequently affects diabetics (Mentzer et al 1975). Although the clinical picture is often identical to any other form of severe cholecystitis, a plain abdominal film may show gas bubbles in the gallbladder wall and pericholecystic tissues in the absence of an abnormal communication between the biliary system and the gastrointestinal tract. Gangrene, free perforation and generalized peritonitis are all common complications and dictate the need for emergency cholecystectomy as soon as the diagnosis is made (Williamson 1990).

More recent reports indicate that plain abdominal films are relatively insensitive and only diagnose severe disease. By contrast ultrasound examination and CT have a higher diagnostic yield, such that emphysematous cholecystitis is diagnosed more frequently nowadays because of the regular use of ultrasound in suspected acute hepato-biliary disease. This increased diagnostic frequency has uncovered a broad spectrum of disease ranging from mild to severe emphysematous cholecystitis (Gill et al 1997). Based on clinical assessment, emergency cholecystectomy (as opposed to early or interval) should be reserved for patients with severe disease.

ACUTE CHOLECYSTITIS IN AIDS PATIENTS

AIDS patients are susceptible to opportunistic gastrointestinal infections and this includes acute cholecystitis and cholangitis especially if their CD4 count is less than 200. The cholecystitis is acalculous in 52% of cases when the common infecting agents are Cryptosporidium and Cytomegalovirus. Less frequently, the infection is caused by fungus, yeast, *Mycobacterium tuberculosis* and *Mycobacterium avium cellulare*. The thirty-day mortality is 18%. In one report all the postoperative deaths ($n = 5$) occurred in 28 patients treated by open cholecystectomy whereas no deaths were encountered in 26 patients who underwent LC (Cacciarelli et al 1998). Postoperative mortality is related to a low CD4 count (< 200). Thus LC rather than open cholecystectomy should be the procedure of choice in AIDS patients especially if the CD4 count is below 200.

ACUTE ACALCULOUS CHOLECYSTITIS

PATIENT GROUPS

Acute acalculous cholecystitis (AAC) accounts for 5 to 14% of all cases of acute cholecystitis (Savoca et al 1990). It is a well recognized complication in patients who are critically injured following major trauma, burns, sepsis and major non-biliary surgery (including cardiac operations) who are

being nursed in intensive care units. AC has also been described as a complication of parenteral feeding (Petersen and Sheldon 1984) and is well documented in AIDS patients (Kavin et al 1986, Cacciarelli et al 1998). AAC occurs in 0.2% of surgical intensive care admissions and is associated with a high incidence of gangrene (60%). The mortality in this critically ill group is high and averages 40% (Kalliafas et al 1998).

However in one major report, over 70% of patients with AC did not fall into any of these categories but instead presented de novo as emergency admissions (Savoca et al 1990). Although the clinical presentation was indistinguishable from patients with acute calculus cholecystitis, the diagnosis was often missed by ultrasound evaluation. Over 70% of these patients had atherosclerotic cardiovascular disease, a risk factor that might explain the threefold preponderance in elderly male patients in this series (Savoca et al 1990). Although the morbidity rate following surgery was high (41%), there were no deaths. This indicates that the results of prompt surgery is this subgroup, 28% of whom had gangrenous cholecystitis, compare favourably to patients with acute calculous cholecystitis.

The impact of early diagnosis and prompt surgical intervention is also evident in those patients with major trauma in whom mortality rates of up to 75% have previously been reported (Glenn 1979). In one series (Cornwell et al 1989) the mortality rate over a 10-year period was reduced from 44 to 7% as a result of early diagnosis and prompt surgical intervention.

DIAGNOSTIC TESTS

Among the various tests used for ACC, morphine or cholecystokinin cholescintigraphy has the highest sensitivity (90 to 98%), followed by computed tomography (sensitivity of 67%) and ultrasonography (sensitivity of 29%); whereas the diagnosis was obtained in 97% of patients investigated by biliary scintiscanning. Morphine or cholecystokinin cholescintigraphy gives better results than the standard radionuclide investigation as it enables the assessment of the gallbladder ejection fraction reduction of which is essential for exclusion of ACC in these patients (Cacciarelli et al 1998).

MANAGEMENT

Outcome is dependent on the severity of the critical illness when present (Acute Physiology and Chronic Health II score), early diagnosis and emergency cholecystectomy. There are no comparative studies of LC versus open cholecystectomy for ACC.

CHOLECYSTITIS IN THE ELDERLY AND CHILDREN

THE ELDERLY

During this century there has been a gain in the life expectancy of 25 years in most Western countries (Piggot & Williams 1988). As a result, there has been an increasing population of elderly patients with gallstones that require surgical treatment. Operations for gallstones in the elderly have been associated with increased perioperative morbidity and mortality rates particularly if the common bile duct has been explored, when mortality rates as high as 30% have been reported (Vellacott & Powel 1979). Several factors are responsible for this poor outcome: (1) the clinical features at presentation may be nondescript and may lead to delay in diagnosis, (2) presence of co-morbid disease, e.g., cardiorespiratory, diabetes etc., (3) a significantly higher proportion of elderly patients present with life-threatening complications or severe cholecystitis. Thus in many series (Addison & Finan 1988, Irvin & Arnstein 1988) patients aged > 70 years have a 2–3 fold higher incidence of emergency presentation with jaundice, empyema, cholangitis, gangrene and perforation.

The poor outcome in the elderly group can be minimized by early diagnosis and prompt surgical intervention, appropriate antibiotic therapy and chemoprophylaxis against thromboembolic disease. These measures account for the improved survival (1.5 to 3% mortality after cholecystectomy) reported in some series (Irvin & Arnstein 1988, Tagle et al 1997). High mortality rates (10 to 20%) persist in the subgroup of elderly patients undergoing surgery for severe complicated disease and those who develop cardiorespiratory complications after surgery. In these patients percutaneous cholecystostomy may be a safer option in the absence of perforation, gangrene or peritonitis (Sugiyama et al 1998).

CHILDREN

Cholecystitis and choledocholithiasis are uncommon in children. Children with hereditary blood dyscrasias such as sickle cell disease or congenital spherocytosis are prone to pigment stone formation (Porkorny et al 1984). Gallstone disease has also been reported in children following ileal resection and following parenteral nutrition where a two-fold increase has been reported (Roslyn et al 1983, Bailey et al 1989).

COMPLICATIONS OF ACUTE CHOLECYSTITIS

Empyema of the gallbladder, gangrene, local or generalized peritonitis, pericholecystic abscess and cholecystoenteric fistula are the recognized specific complications. Severe disease with a high incidence of gangrene is encountered in the elderly, AIDS patients, those with emphysematous and acalculous cholecystitis, with gallbladder gangrene being common (up to 60%) in these high-risk groups. Postoperative complications include intra-abdominal bile/fluid blood collections, pulmonary collapse and consolidation, myocardial episodes especially in those with co-morbid ischaemic heart disease and bile duct injuries which may be higher after cholecystectomy in these patients.

THE FUTURE

The management of gallbladder disease including acute cholecystitis has been revolutionized with the introduction of LC (Ch. 38). It is now clear that LC can be undertaken for the vast majority of patients with acute cholecystitis without compromising the outcome. Indeed in some high-risk groups, the mortality may be reduced by LC. It is likely that in very critically ill patients, percutaneous ultrasound or fluoroscopy guided cholecystostomy may replace emergency cholecystectomy in the first instance. However, this simple procedure is not always successful in resolving the acute illness. Thus if this management option is adopted in the treatment of the critically ill patient, a time limit of 2 days should be set when surgery is undertaken as a salvage option. The relative merits of percutaneous radiologically guided cholecystostomy versus laparoscopic cholecystostomy should be compared within the context of a prospective randomized trial. The potential advantages of the laparoscopic approach include precise insertion of the drainage catheter into the gallbladder and the identification of pathology, e.g., gangrene, or perforation, that would require an immediate operation.

REFERENCES

Adamsen S, Hansen O H, Funch-Jensen P, Schulze S, Stage J G, Wara P 1997 Bile duct injury during laparoscopic cholecystectomy: a prospective nationwide series. Journal of the American College of Surgeons 184: 571–8

Addison N 1986 Iatrogenic bile duct stricture. British Journal of Surgery 73: 681–5

Addison N, Finan P J 1988 Urgent and early cholecystectomy for acute gallbladder disease. British Journal of Surgery 75: 141–3

Bailey P V, Connors R H, Tracey T F, et al 1989 Changing spectrum of cholelithiasis and cholecystitis in infants and children. American Journal of Surgery 158: 585–8

Barbara L, Sama C, Maria A et al 1987 A population study on the prevalence of gallstone disease: the Sirmione Study. Hepatology 7: 913–7

Baxter J N, O'Dwyer P J 1992 Laparoscopic or minilaparotomy cholecystectomy. British Medical Journal 304: 559–60

Bornman P C, Terblanche J 1985 Subtotal cholecystectomy for the difficult gallbladder in portal hypertension and cholecystitis. Surgery 98: 1–6

Bouchier I A D 1988 Gallstones: formation and epidemiology. In Blumgart L H (ed) Surgery of the Liver and Biliary Tract. Churchill Livingstone, London, p 503–16.

Cabellon S, Brown J M, Cavanaugh D G 1984 Accuracy of the hepatobiliary scan in acute cholecystitis. American Journal of Surgery 148: 607–8

Cacciarelli A G, Naddaf S Y, el-Zeftawy H A, Aziz M, Omar W S, Kimar M, Atay S, Abujudeh H, Gillooley J, Abdel-Dayem H M 1998 Acute cholecystitis in AIDS patients: correlation of Tc-99m hepatobiliary scintigraphy with histopathologic laboratory findings and CD4 counts. Clinical Nuclear Medicine 23: 226–8

Cornwell E E, Rodriguez A, Mirvis S E, Shorr R M 1989 Acute acalculous cholecystitis in critically ill injured patients Annals of Surgery 210: 52–55

Den-Hoed P T, Boelhouwer R U, Veen H F et al 1998 Infections and bacteriological data after laparoscopic and open gallbladder surgery. Journal of Hospital Infection 39: 27–37

Diettrich N A, Caioppo J C, Davies R P 1988 The vanishing elective cholecystectomy. Archives of Surgery 123: 810–4

Dogra R, Singh J, Sharma M P 1995 Enterically transmitted non-A, non-B hepatitis mimicking acute cholecystitis. American Journal of Gastroenterology 90: 764–6.

Dubois F, Berthelot B 1982 Cholecystomie par mini-laparotomie. Nouv Presse Med 11: 1139–42

Dumont A E 1976 Significance of hyperbilirubinaemia in acute cholecystitis. Surgical, Gynecogy and Obstetrics 142: 855–7

Duncan J L, Stoddard C J 1992 Acute inflammatory conditions of the alimentary tract. In: Gastrointestinal Emergencies. Gilmore I T, Shields R (eds) W B Saunders, London, pp 231–62

England R E, McDermott V G, Smith T P, Suhocki P V, Payne C S, Newman G E 1997 Percutaneous cholecystostomy: who responds? American Journal of Roentgenology 168: 1247–51

Gill K S, Chapman A H, Weston M J 1997 The changing face of emphysematous cholecystitis. British Journal of Radiology 70: 986–91

Glenn F 1979 Acute acalculous cholecystitis. Annals of Surgery 189: 458–65

Gracie W A, Ransohoff D F 1982 The natural history of silent gallstones: the innocent gallstone is not a myth. New England Journal of Medicine 307: 798–800

Grau-Talens E J, Garcia-Olives F, Ruperez-Arribas M P 1998 Transcylindrical cholecystectomy: new technique for minimally invasive cholecystectomy. World Journal of Surgery 22: 453–458

Hamy A, Visset J, Likholatinkov D, Lerat F, Gibaud H, Savigny B, Paineau J 1997 Percutaneous cholecystostomy for acute cholecystitis in critically ill. Surgery 121: 398–401

Herman R E 1990 Surgery for acute cholecystitis. Surgical Clinics of North America 70: 1263–75

Holzbach R T 1989 Pathogenesis and medical treatment of gallstones. In: Schlesinger M H, Fordtran J S (eds) Gastrointestinal Disease, 4th edn. W B Saunders, Philadelphia, p 1668–91

Irvin T T, Arnstein P M 1988 Management of symptomatic gallstones in the elderly. British Journal of Surgery 75: 1163–5

Jarvinen J H, Hastabacka J 1980 Early cholecystectomy for acute cholecystitis. A prospective randomised study. Annals of Surgery 191: 502–5

Kalliafas S, Ziegler D W, Flancbaum L, Choban P S 1998 Acute acalculous cholecystitis, risk factors, diagnosis and outcome. American Surgeon 64: 471–5

Kaufman M, Weissberg D, Schwartz I, Moses Y 1990 Cholecystostomy as a definitive operation. Surgery, Gynecology and Obstetrics 170: 533–7

Kavin H, Jonas R B, Chowdury L, Kabins S 1986 Acalculous cholecystitis

and cytomegalovirus infection in the acquired immunodeficiency syndrome. Annals of Internal Medicine 104: 53–4

Keighley M R B 1977 Micoorganisms in bile. A preventable cause of sepsis after biliary surgery. Annals of the Royal College Surgeons 59: 328–34

Kern F Jr 1983 Epidemiology and natural history of gallstones. Seminars in Liver Diseases 3: 87–96

Kiviluoto T, Siren J, Luukkonen P, Kivilaakso E 1998 Randomized trial of laparoscopic versus open cholecystectomy for acute and gangrenous cholecystitis. Lancet 351: 321–5

Lai P B, Kwong K H, Leung K L, Kwok S P, Chan A C, Chung S C, Lau W Y 1988 Randomized trial of early versus delayed laparoscopic cholecystectomy for acute cholecystitis. British Journal of Surgery 85: 764–7

Lam C M, Murray F E, Cuschieri A 1996 Increased cholecystectomy rate after the introduction of laparoscopic cholecystectomy in Scotland. Gut 38: 282–4

Lathinen J, Alhava E M, Aukes M 1987 Acute cholecystitis treated by early and delayed surgery. Scandinavian Journal of Gastroenterology 13: 673–8

Ledet W P 1990 Ambulatory cholecystectomy without disability. Archives of Surgery 125: 1434–5

Lo C M, Fan S T, Liu C L, Lai E C, Wong J 1997 Early decision for conversion of laparoscopic to open cholecystectomy for treatment of acute cholecystitis. American Journal of Surgery 173: 513–7

Lo C M, Liu C L, Fan S T, Lai E C, Wong J 1998 Prospective randomized study of early versus delayed laparoscopic cholecystitis. Annals of Surgery 227: 461–7

McArthur P, Cuschieri A, Sells R A, Shields R 1975 Controlled clinical trial comparing early versus interval cholecystectomy for acute cholecystitis. British Journal of Surgery 62: 850–2

Mentzer R M Jr, Golden G T, Chandler G T 1975 A comparative appraisal of emphysematous cholecystitis. American Journal of Surgery 120: 10–15

Michalowski K, Bornman P C, Krige J E, Gallagher P J, Terblanche J 1998 Laparoscopic subtotal cholecystectomy in patients with complicated acute cholecystitis or fibrosis. British Journal of Surgery 85: 904–906

Mitchell A Morris P J 1982 Trend in the management of acute cholecystitis. British Medical Journal 28: 427–30

Norby S, Herlin P, Holmin T, Sjodahl R, Tagesson C 1983 Early or delayed cholecystectomy in acute cholecystitis? A clinical trial. British Journal of Surgery 70: 163–5

O'Dwyer P J, Murphy J J, O'Higgins N J 1990 Cholecystectomy through a 5 cm incision. British Journal of Surgery 77: 1189–1190

Petersen S R, Sheldon G F 1984 Acute acalculous cholecystitis: a complication of hyperalimentation. Archives of Surgery 119: 1389–92

Piggot J P, Williams G B 1988 Cholecystectomy in the elderly. American Journal of Surgery 155: 408–10

Pokorny W J, Saleem M, O'Gorman R B et al 1984 Cholelithiasis and cholecystitis in childhood. American Journal of Surgery 148: 742–4

Pu Y, Yamamoto F, Igimi H, Shilpakar S K, Kojima T, Yamamoto S, Luo D 1994 A comparative study of usefulness of magnetic resonance imaging in the diagnosis of acute cholecystitis. Journal of Gastroenterology 29: 192–8

Ralls P W, Coletti P M, Halls J M et al 1982 prospective evaluation of 99m TC-IDA cholescintigraphy in the diagnosis of acute cholecystitis. Radiology 144: 369–71

Reiss R, Nudelman I, Gutman C, Deutsch A A 1990 Changing trends in surgery for acute cholecystitis. World Journal of Surgery 14: 567–71

Roslyn J J, Berquist W A, Pitt H A 1983 Increased risk of gallstones in children receiving total parenteral nutrition. Pediatrics 71: 784–9

Sampliner R E, Bennett P H, Commess L J et al 1970. Gallbladder disease in the Pima Indians. Demonstration of high prevalence and early onset using cholecystography. New England Journal of Medicine 283: 1358–64

Savoca P E, Longo W E, Zucker K A et al 1990 The increasing prevalence of acalculous cholecystitis in outpatients. Annals of Surgery 211: 433–7

Schein M 1991 Partial cholecystectomy in the treatment of acute cholecystitis in the compromised patient. Journal of the Royal College of Surgeons of Edinburgh 36: 295–7

Sjodahl R, Tagesson C 1983 On the development of primary acute cholecystitis. Scandinavian Journal of Gastroenterology 18: 577–79

Soyer P, Brouland J P, Boudiaf M, Kardache M, Pelage J P, Panis Y, Valleur P, Rymer R 1998 Color velocity imaging and power Doppler sonography of the gall bladder wall: a new look at sonographic diagnosis of acute cholecystitis. American Journal of Roentgenology 171: 183–8

Sugiyama M, Touhara M, Atomi Y 1998 Is percutaneous cholecystostomy the optimal treatment for acute cholecystitis in the very elderly? World Journal of Surgery 22: 459–63

Tagle F M, Lavergne J, Barkin J S, Unger S W 1997 Laparoscopic cholecystectomy in the elderly. Surgical Endoscopy 11: 636–8

Tokunaga Y, Nakayama N, Ishikawa Y, Nishitai R, Irie A, Kaganoi J, Ohsumi K, Higo T 1997 Surgical risks of acute cholecystitis in the elderly. Hepatogastroenterology 44: 671–6

Uggowitzer M, Kugler C, Schramyer G, Kammerhuber F, Groll R, Hausegger K A, Ratschek M, Quehenberger F 1997 Sonography of acute cholecystitis: comparison of color and power Doppler sonography in detecting a hypervascularized gallbladder wall. American Journal of Roentgentology 168: 707–12

Van der Linden W, Sunzel H 1970 Early versus delayed operations for acute cholecystitis. American Journal of Surgery 120: 7–13

Van der Linden W, Edlund G 1981 Early versus delayed cholecystectomy. The effect of a change of management. British Journal of Surgery 68: 753–7

Van Steenbergen W, Ponette E, Marchal G et al 1990 Percutaneous transhepatic cholecystostomy for acute complicated cholecystitis in elderly patients. American Journal of Gastroenterology 85: 1363–8

Vellacott K D, Powell P H 1979 Exploration of the common bile duct: a comparative study. British Journal of Surgery 66: 389–91

Verbank J, Ghillebert G, Rutgeerts L, Baert F, Goethals C, Schepekns H, Gelhof K, Surmont I 1998 Ultrasound-guided puncture of the gallbladder for acute cholecystitis. Acta Gastroenterologica Belgica 61: 151–2

Williamson R C N 1990 Acute cholecystitis: in Emergency Abdominal Surgery. Williamson R C N, Cooper M J (eds) Churchill Livingstone, Edinburgh, p 110–127

Wilson R G, Macintyre I M C, Nixon S J, Saunders J H et al 1992 Laparoscopic cholecystectomy as a safe effective treatment for severe acute cholecystitis. British Medical Journal 305: 394–6

Biliary acute pancreatitis

35

C.W. IMRIE

INTRODUCTION

The two most common etiological factors associated with acute pancreatitis are biliary disease and alcohol abuse. These two factors together account for over 80% of all patients with acute pancreatitis described in prospective studies of the disease. The major importance in identifying the presence of gallstones and biliary sludge/sand is almost 100% success rate in eliminating further attacks of pancreatitis when all calculi and similar material are removed. This efficient treatment contrasts markedly with the results in the treatment of alcohol abuse pancreatitis in which recurrent attacks are so common.

In European countries, most studies have found that approximately half of all patients with acute pancreatitis have gallstones. However, it has been reasonably claimed that, by sieving the feces to identify gallstones in the first bowel motions after the attack, the figure is actually around 60% (Mayer et al 1984). On this information a significant proportion of the co-called *idiopathic cases* are of biliary origin. Indeed, the idiopathic group which may comprise 20 to 25% of all cases in some prospective studies can be ascribed to biliary etiology when careful search is made for calculus and crystal material of less than 1–2 mm diameter. This is best done by examining biliary aspirate taken at endoscopic retrograde cholangiopancreatography (ERCP) (Neoptolemos et al 1988a, Ros et al 1991, Lee et al 1992). Thus the predominant cause of acute pancreatitis in most societies is biliary in origin with probably two-thirds of the idiopathic group consisting of patients with bile crystals, cholesterolosis or biliary sludge (Ros et al 1991). Exceptions to this are prospective studies from central areas of American and Scandinavian cities where alcohol is the predominant etiology (Ranson et al 1974, Kivilaakso et al 1981, Sainio et al 1995).

MECHANISM OF DISEASE

Although the classic paper by Opie (1901) illustrated the association between a small stone impacted at the ampulla of Vater and the presence of acute pancreatitis, it was not until 1974 that Acosta and Ledesma highlighted the frequent phenomenon of the transient migration of stones from the biliary tree, through the lower bile duct, and into the duodenum in patients with gallstone-associated pancreatitis. Other groups in the USA (Kelly 1976, Kelly & Swaney 1982), the UK (Mayer et al 1984) and Sweden (Elstrom 1978) have supported the evidence that transient migration of small gallstones is the hallmark of gallstone-associated acute pancreatitis. The task of fecal sieving to identify gallstones is not likely to prove popular unless a simple and reliable machine is designed to carry out this work which is unpleasant but very valuable in defining the etiology of pancreatitis.

A study from Manchester (Armstrong et al 1985) emphasized the importance of several features in the biliary and pancreatic duct systems which were specifically associated with gallstone pancreatitis (Fig. 35.1). The frequent finding of stones in the biliary tree not exceeding 3 mm in diameter in 90% of 59 patients with gallstone-associated pancreatitis, compared with less than 40% of 710 patients with gallstones and no pancreatitis, is important. In addition to patients with pancreatitis having *smaller stones*, they also harbor stones which are more numerous and associated with a larger diameter cystic duct (McMahon & Shefta 1980, Armstrong et al 1985). Furthermore, the *diameter of the common bile duct* (CBD) tends to be larger and pancreatic-duct reflux is seen much more frequently at operative cholangiography than in patients with biliary disease and no pancreatitis. Two other anatomical features were noted, the first of these being that the *interductal angle between the*

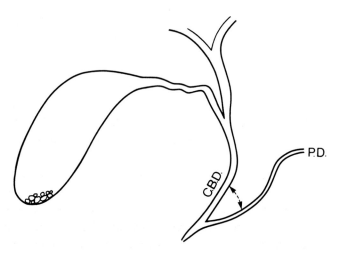

Fig. 35.1 Diagram illustrating features favoring gallstone pancreatitis (the arrows indicate the interductal angle). Larger angle; small stones; large cystic duct and long common channel (Armstrong et al 1985). CBD, common bile duct; PD, pancreatic duct.

lower CBD and pancreatic duct was larger in patients prone to pancreatitis. Secondly, the *common channel of the two ducts was at least 5 mm in length* in 73% of these patients, compared to less than 20% of those patients with gallstones and no pancreatitis (Armstrong et al 1985). There are, therefore, anatomical features which predispose to the presence of pancreatitis, but none of these fully explain the mechanism. The possible events at the lower end of the CBD, and pancreatic duct are represented in Fig. 35.2a where the hold-up of a stone or biliary sludge in the common channel may permit reflux of bile; a stone impacted in the exit of the pancreatic duct may facilitate reflux of pancreatic juice (Fig. 35.3); and a small irregular shaped stone stuck at the ampulla may cause pain and subsequent vomiting with duodenal juice potentially refluxing past the stone and into the pancreas.

In the situation of the *reflux of bile* initiating acute pancreatitis, it is known that bile lecithin and, in some circumstances, bile salts damage the mucosal barrier of the pancreatic duct and that potentiation by bacterial infection and drugs such as aspirin is also important. Pancreatic juice

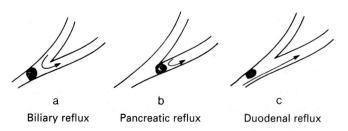

a	b	c
Biliary reflux	Pancreatic reflux	Duodenal reflux

Fig. 35.2 The various ways in which stone 'hold up' may facilitate reflux.

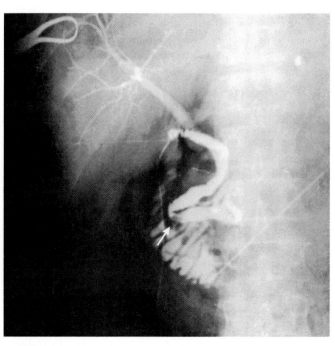

Fig. 35.3 Operative cholangiogram. Example of a gallstone impacted in the pancreatic duct (arrow) in a patient operated upon within 12 h of admission.

refluxing under pressure back up the duct system may well cause pain, but is relatively unlikely, on the basis of experimental studies, to initiate an attack of acute pancreatitis. The final situation depicted in Figure 35.2c would permit enterokinase in duodenal juice to be forced at high pressure along the pancreatic duct activating trypsinogen at the duct-cell interface and potentially initiating an attack of pancreatitis. It is even possible, when a stone is impacted at the ampulla, that a combination of bile reflux and duodenal reflux under pressure occurs simultaneously and initiates an attack of pancreatitis. Partial or complete obstruction of the pancreatic duct outflow, either within the common channel or at the duodenal orifice would possibly explain episodes of acute pancreatitis following operative or endoscopic instrumentation in this area. A similar mechanism may explain the acute pancreatitis which can occur if a long-limb surgical T-tube is allowed to pass through the lower CBD and on into the duodenum.

Of the many patients who suffer biliary-associated pancreatitis it is a relative rarity to find a stone truly impacted at the ampulla of Vater. Those surgeons or endoscopists who advocate immediate intervention (within 48 h of diagnosis) find many more stones in the lower CBD than those who advocate a longer delay before initiating active measures to eradicate stones. This supports the contention of Acosta that stones usually pass spontaneously into the duodenum (Acosta & Ledesma 1974).

It has frequently been shown that *very small stones*, or

even biliary sand may precipitate episodes of acute pancreatitis (Lee et al 1992). Some authors have suggested that even tiny biliary crystals or cholesterolosis might be responsible for initiating the disease. While it is probable that they represent an indicator of a stone former and that the main stone has passed, there is some evidence in the case of cholesterolosis from the histological study of almost 3800 gallbladders (Paricio et al 1990) that *cholesterolosis* on its own may be a primary determinant of acute pancreatitis caused by the passage of tiny cholesterol 'polyps'. In that study there was a documented attack of acute pancreatitis in 125 of 434 patients with gallbladders exhibiting cholesterolosis (29%). Subdividing those patients into 379 with cholesterolosis and gallstones, 98 (26%) had acute pancreatitis, while in the remaining 55 patients with cholesterolosis and no gallstones 27 (49%) had acute pancreatitis. This does not negate the view that cholesterolosis is a histological marker of the predisposition to the formation of small cholesterol gallstones, but certainly adds weight to the view that patients with cholesterol crystals (on analysis of bile) who have suffered acute pancreatitis would be eligible for laparoscopic or open cholecystectomy to remove the danger of further attacks.

Neoptolemos et al (1988a) were among the first to report on the use of polarizing microscopy to analyze bile obtained at ERCP in patients with 'idiopathic' pancreatitis. Of their 14 patients four were found on careful analysis to have small stones and five to have no stones but calcium bilirubinate crystals in their bile. Thus the majority of this small group had a biliary etiology and over one-third were found to have crystals indicating a persistent biochemical defect.

A much larger study (Ros et al 1991) showed that of 51 patients with a normal ultrasound scan following an attack of acute pancreatitis and no other identified etiology, 34 (67%) patients had cholesterol crystals, calcium bilirubinate granules or calcium carbonate microspheroliths on careful analysis. Gallstones were eventually identified in 35 patients, while in another 13 with cholesterol crystals treatment with ursodeoxycholate eliminated crystal formation and stopped further attacks of acute pancreatitis at a mean follow-up of 44 months.

It has also been contended that *biliary sludge* is an underestimated cause of so-called 'idiopathic acute pancreatitis' based on a study of 86 patients from two centers over an 8-year period from 1980 to 1988 (Lee et al 1992). The authors define biliary sludge as a suspension of cholesterol monohydrate crystals or calcium bilirubinate granules in bile, and is found predominantly, although not exclusively, in the gallbladder. Of their 86 patients, 31 were considered to have acute idiopathic acute pancreatitis. All had a sample of bile examined by polarizing microscopy, this bile being

obtained at ERCP in 15 patients, while in 16 bile was aspirated through a soft feeding tube placed beforehand into the duodenum after intravenous administration of 100 units of cholecystokinin. It is important to be aware that the bile samples were obtained during the convalescent phase of the disease varying intervals from 3 to 4 weeks after onset of acute pancreatitis. Of 31 patients no fewer than 23 (74%) were found to have cholesterol crystals, calcium bilirubinate granules or sludge. This biliary sludge was detected by ultrasound in 11 patients. In 10 patients the sludge had a predominant calcium bilirubinate content. To support further their contention of the importance of biliary sludge in the etiology of acute pancreatitis, patients who had effective treatment in the form of cholecystectomy or endoscopic sphincterotomy were subject to very few attacks of acute pancreatitis, while 11 patients who underwent neither of the above procedures suffered eight further attacks of acute pancreatitis.

It has therefore been shown that very small stones, or even biliary sand, may precipitate episodes of acute pancreatitis. Some authors have suggested that even tiny biliary crystals might initiate disease, although it is probable that they are an indicator of the stone former.

PREGNANCY AND ACUTE PANCREATITIS

It is worthy of note that the association between pregnancy and acute pancreatitis is usually gallstone related. In one study 90% of the pregnancy-associated cases of acute pancreatitis had gallstones present as the only identifiable explanation of their problem. Subsequent eradication of stones not only gave freedom from further attacks of pancreatitis beyond pregnancy but also during each subsequent pregnancy (McKay et al 1980).

BILIARY DYSKINESIA

Manometric studies at the sphincter of Oddi (Ch. 6) indicate that (occasionally) motility disorders of this area (found in patients with and without gallstones) may be implicated in the mechanism of acute pancreatitis (Toouli et al 1985). The preference by Toouli has been for open operative treatment to achieve a precise sphincterotomy of both bile duct and pancreatic duct where severe spasm has proven to be the most likely cause of recurrent acute pancreatitis.

Occasionally, acute pancreatitis may be associated with the presence of ampullary tumors, choledochal cysts or sclerosing cholangitis. In Asia, various worm infestations of the lower bile duct are well known to clinicians as a cause of acute pancreatitis.

It is important to remember that both biliary disease and

alcohol abuse are increasing in frequency in most Western societies. For this reason it is not unusual to find that 2 to 10% of patients will have both these etiological factors present (Trapnell & Duncan 1975, Imrie et al 1978a).

INVESTIGATION FOR THE PRESENCE OF STONES

Straight abdominal radiographs will reveal the presence of radio-opaque stones in 10 to 16% of patients; in the remaining 84 to 90% of cases other methods will be necessary. It has already been stated that fecal sieving has made the biggest single impact on defining the size of the idiopathic group of patients with acute pancreatitis (Acosta & Ledesma 1974, Kelly 1976, Mayer et al 1984). Ultrasound scanning (Ch. 12) has a very important role to play in the identification of gallstones which are often not well visualized by the more expensive computerized tomography (CT) scanner. Isotope scanning has been less helpful than in the patient with cholecystitis, and intravenous cholangiography is unreliable. Magnetic resonance (MR) scanning is now more frequently used. It is important to be aware that surgical clips may mimic the presence of stones with this modality. It must be remembered that although bowel gas can be troublesome there is little doubt that ultrasound has become a very important diagnostic modality in this disease (McKay et al 1982). In the situation where the ultrasound scan is equivocal, ERCP will provide the best indication of the presence or absence of stones (Fig. 35.4). It is particularly valuable in severe acute pancreatitis and has moved to a more prominent diagnostic role in recent years.

Liver function tests can differentiate between acute pancreatitis of biliary and alcohol origin (McMahon & Pickford 1979). Elevated levels of transferase (transaminase) enzymes, alkaline phosphatase and bilirubin are accurate indicators of the presence of gallstones (Blamey et al 1983). Elevations of transferase enzymes above 60 iu/L has been claimed to be as good as a whole group of liver function tests in identifying CBD stones (Neoptolemos et al 1984). Confirmation of the presence of CBD stones may be achieved by either careful ultrasound examination, MR scanning or ERCP. There continues to be a debate as to the exact place of both diagnostic and therapeutic ERCP in the management of biliary acute pancreatitis (Neoptolemos et al 1988, Fan et al 1993, Nowak et al 1993, Folsch et al 1997). Technical difficulties due to the presence of duodenal edema tend to increase the longer the delay in instituting ERCP such that it may be very difficult or impossible to identify the ampulla.

DISEASE SEVERITY

It frequently takes some time to identify the etiology in a particular episode of pancreatitis, and in the initial phases it is important to identify the severity of the attack. Those patients who do not have severe acute pancreatitis may be

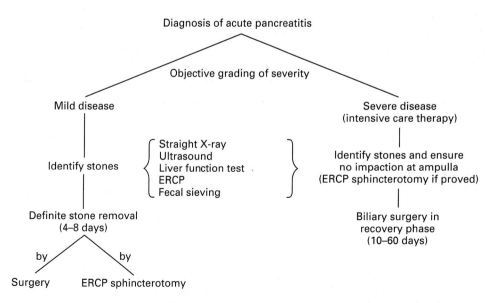

Fig. 35.4 Suggested optimum therapy in gallstone pancreatitis.

graded 'mild' or 'moderate', but it is important to identify the group at maximum risk of death and main complications. In order to achieve this, a number of grading systems have been devised. An initial system (Ranson et al 1974) was more relevant to patients with alcohol-associated disease. Indeed, Ranson subsequently introduced a modified grading system for the patient with biliary disease. This has complicated the system, since a dilemma exists as to which to utilize when the patient is initially admitted. This has not proved a problem with the *Glasgow grading system* which has been increasingly utilized in the UK and elsewhere (Imrie et al 1978, Osborne et al 1981, Wilson et al 1988). The system comprises eight factors; the presence of any three or more within 48 h of admission defines the patient as having severe disease (Table 35.1).

An extensive prospective study comparing three methods of assessment of prognosis in acute pancreatitis reveals that the Glasgow system (Table 35.1) is equally good for patients with either alcohol- or gallstone-related pancreatitis (Corfield et al 1985). The system is superior to clinical assessment alone and to peritoneal aspiration in grading patients with gallstone pancreatitis, but less good in grading the alcohol related group when compared with peritoneal aspiration. Indeed, initial clinical assessment and peritoneal aspiration/lavage approaches were found to be especially poor in assessing the severity of gallstone-related pancreatitis (Corfield et al 1985). Both identified less than 35% of such patients with a complicated outcome, while the *Glasgow grading system* was twice as accurate. In the clinical situation it is impossible to exclude the clinician's assessment, and combining this with the Glasgow assessment system is still useful in grading severity of disease in those with biliary-associated pancreatitis, while *APACHE II* is a more rapid, useful alternative system (Knaus et al 1984). The *APACHE II* system is also a little cumbersome, but has the advantage that it is in widespread use in the intensive-care situation, and also gives an objective monitor of progress beyond the first 2 days of illness (Larvin & McMahon 1989, Wilson et al 1990).

Obesity is an important adverse factor in outcome not only because of the increased amount of peri-pancreatic fat to be attacked by the disease process but by the increased risk of respiratory failure. Both a retrospective study in Cape Town (Funnell et al 1993) and a prospective study in Southampton (Johnson et al 1998) have shown that patients with a body mass index (BMI) in excess of 30 kg/m^2 are at significant additional risk. (Morbid obesity is usually defined if patients have a BMI in excess of 40 kg/m^2.) Indeed the prospective study indicated that organ failure was considerably more common in the overweight patients and suggested that the optimum marker of early severity of disease was a combination of *APACHE II* and obesity, the advantage being that much of this information is available soon after admission.

Contrast-enhanced CT scanning (CECT) gives an objective assessment of the disease state. Systems of grading the CT-scan information are based on the degree of pancreatic swelling, the amount of fluid in the peripancreatic tissue and the degree of non-perfusion of the pancreas (Balthazar et al 1990, London et al 1991, Sainio et al 1995). London et al (1991) used a CT-grading system which was not more accurate than the modified Glasgow scoring system. However, CECT does provide vital information for the surgeon about the dynamic changes in the size of the necrotic area and the presence of infection in or around the pancreas. Indeed this investigation is so important that all patients with severe illness should be moved to centers where there is a combination of clinical and radiological expertise to manage these patients effectively (Beger et al 1988, Bradley & Allen 1991, British Society of Gastroenterology 1998).

MR scanning is being increasingly utilized and ultimately may become as important as CECT scanning in the monitoring of these severely ill patients.

Organ failure is the most crucially important sign of severe disease and the development of scoring systems based on the systemic inflammatory response syndrome (SIRS) and other objective markers of respiratory renal and cardiac compromise are important. Patients who develop objective markers of organ failure are at highest risk but within this group clinical deterioration is the most important phenomenon as we cannot yet identify those who are going to improve and those who are going to deteriorate at a sufficiently early point.

SINGLE MARKERS OF SEVERITY OF DISEASE

There has been great interest in this area over the past 15 years but the only marker which is in clinical use is C-reactive protein. It has a similar drawback to the Ranson and Glasgow systems in that it requires 48 h to accurately identify the patients who have severe disease. The normal level of CRP is < 10 mg/l and patients who have elevations

Table 35.1 Glasgow system of prognostic factors*

WBC	> 15 000
P$_a$O$_2$	< 60 mmHg (8 kPa)
Glucose	> 10 mmol/L (excludes diabetics)
Urea	> 16 mmol/L (despite intravenous fluids)
Calcium	< 2.0 mmol/L
Albumin	< 32 g/l
LDH	> 600 international units/L
AST	> 200 international units/L

* The presence of any three or more of these factors within 48 h of admission indicates severe acute pancreatitis (Osborne et al 1981).

> 150 mg/l usually have clinically severe disease (Buchler et al 1986, Larvin & McMahon 1989, Wilson et al 1989, 1990, British Society of Gastroenterology 1998).

A considerable number of other markers have shown promise but have not yet been sufficiently proved in clinical practice to be recommended because the publications have invariably been based on batch analysis of frozen samples at a much later point than would provide useful clinical information. Most interest has been focussed on leukocyte elastase (PMN elastase), interleukin 6 (IL-6), procalcitonin (PCT) in blood measurements and the urinary measurement of trypsinogen activation peptide (TAP).

For the interested reader further information on PMN elastase (Dominguez Munoz et al 1991, Uhl et al 1991), interleukin-6 (Viedma et al 1992, Heath et al 1993), on procalcitonin, and on urinary TAP (Gudgeon et al 1990) are available.

THERAPY

In patients with *mild pancreatitis* (75%) it is usually sufficient simply to provide regular analgesia with pethidine (Demerol), intravenous fluids, nasogastric suction and hourly urine volume monitoring, the last two often being discontinued after 24 h. This contrasts with the problem of severe acute pancreatitis where multi-system organ failure is the major initial problem. At particular risk are the heart, lungs and kidneys. The hemodynamic upset closely mimics the problems encountered in septic shock with an elevation in cardiac index and a decrease in peripheral resistance (Bradley et al 1983, Beger et al 1986). The respiratory problem is the most frequent one encountered and occasionally necessitates ventilatory therapy. Humidified oxygen by face mask or nasal prongs is required for most of the patients in the severe group. Simple measures to combat the risk of renal insufficiency depend on the provision of high-volume intravenous fluid replacement due to the marked hypovolemia due to the combination of vomiting and the loss of intravascular fluid associated with the systemic inflammatory response syndrome. Such patients are best managed in a High Dependency or Intensive Care Unit where incipient renal failure may be managed by the use of various drugs before employing hemoperfusion or hemodialysis.

Other phenomena that tend to occur include hematological and biochemical abnormalities. Blood loss into and around the pancreas is rarely sufficient to necessitate transfusion, but the effect of hemodilution from the correction of hypovolemia requires careful monitoring.

Steady elevation of fibrinogen levels throughout the first week of illness rarely manifest in the full-blown syndrome of disseminated intravascular coagulation but rises in factor V and factor VIII are all part of the acute phase response.

In terms of biochemical upset the most frequent and important is a rapid and sustained loss of albumin from the intravascular space. High levels of albumin are found in the pleural effusion fluid as well as that which occurs in the peritoneal cavity. This is the major factor explaining hypocalcemia as correction for low levels of albumin usually indicate that the hypocalcemia is predominantly a protein bound phenomenon. Occasionally there may be justification for the infusion of calcium gluconate when true hypocalcemia is present but the parathyroid response is usually brisk resulting in the restoration of any depressed calcium levels within a short time (Imrie et al 1978b).

THE ROLE OF ANTIBIOTIC THERAPY

Since 1993 it has become increasingly customary for patients with severe acute pancreatitis to be managed with intravenous broad spectrum antibiotics utilizing either a third generation cephalosporin or imipenem. The use of these drugs has been based on studies of tissue penetration of antibiotics (Buchler et al 1989) and clinical studies using imipenem (Pederzoli et al 1993), cephalosporins (Luiten et al 1995, Sainio et al 1995, Delcenserie et al 1996). Other antibiotics have been studied in small numbers of patients (Schwarz et al 1997). The largest of these studies has been the one by Luiten et al whose main report on 102 patients concerned a controlled clinical trial of selective gut decontamination for the treatment of severe acute pancreatitis which combined an intravenous cephalosporin with the selective decontamination (Luiten et al 1995). The complex treatment of selective gut decontamination has not been generally accepted and the evidence for the use of intravenous antibiotics routinely is based on studies which are not large containing between 25 and 74 patients only. In terms of evidence based medicine the widespread use of such potent antibiotic has not been proved and there is increasing concern at the problem of fungal superinfection (Grewe et al 1999). Indeed our own group at Glasgow Royal Infirmary has abandoned the use of routine antibiotics except as a single shot cover for early ERCP intervention since more than half the patients with fungal superinfection have died (Eatock et al 2000). Despite these concerns about fungal superinfection a recent postal survey of current practice regarding antibiotics prophylaxis in the UK revealed that 89% of those involved in the treatment of severe acute pancreatitis used these antibiotics (Powell et al 1999).

The best current advice is probably to utilize a broad spectrum antibiotic with fluconazole but our own policy of withholding antibiotics except to cover coincident acute cholangitis may be the wiser policy in the initial phases of disease management.

EARLY INTERVENTIONAL ERCP (ENDOSCOPIC SPHINCTEROTOMY) (CH. 28)

Cholangitis complicating acute pancreatitis is a very serious entity and is an indication for early intervention. This is best performed by endoscopic sphincterotomy (Leese et al 1985, Neoptolemos et al 1987), although the alternative of surgical exploration with clearance of the CBD (and possible surgical sphincterotomy) is also possible. In a UK multicenter study of the management of severe acute pancreatitis, peritoneal lavage was found to be of no clear benefit (Mayer et al 1985), but a small number of patients who developed cholangitis ran a hazardous course, despite the initial attack being only moderately severe. Two of these patients died (Corfield et al 1985), and thus consideration of early endoscopic sphincterotomy is clearly important. Today there is a debate as to the place of early diagnostic and therapeutic ERCP with some advocating it in all patients with severe disease (Neoptolemos et al 1988b, Nowak et al 1993), while some recommend it for all patients (Fan et al 1993). A German multicenter study which acknowledged the place of ERCP sphincterotomy in those with acute pancreatitis and accompanying jaundice or cholangitis by excluding them from the study did not show any benefit at all for its application in other patients (Folsch et al 1997). The beneficial change in duct caliber and content from early ERCP sphincterotomy in appropriate patients is illustrated in Figure 35.5.

The surgical background to intervention in biliary acute pancreatitis was based on three different philosophies.

1. Immediate intervention originally advocated from Argentina (Acosta et al 1978) and later supported by a study from the United States (Stone et al 1981).

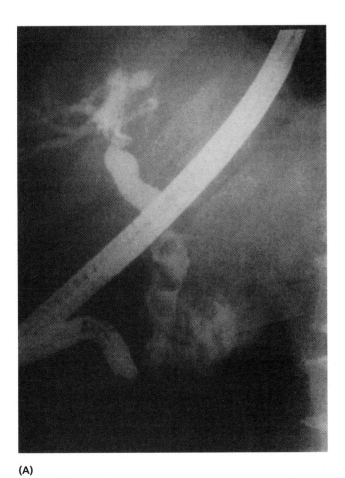

(A)

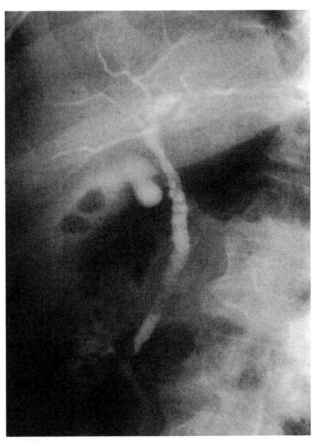

(B)

Fig. 35.5 (A) Dilated bile duct showing several stones in a patient with biliary-associated acute pancreatitis. The cystic duct is also blocked. **(B)** The same patient 3 weeks later with a non-dilated duct and the gallbladder now filling with two stones clearly illustrated within it.

2. Invervention between 2 and 7 days, allowing time for verification of the presence of gallstones (Ranson 1979, Osborne et al 1981, Tondelli et al 1982, Kelly and Wagner 1988).

3. Delayed intervention after resolution of the initial illness. This usually involved re-admission of the patient with the significant risk of a further attack of acute pancreatitis in the intervening period.

There were also those elderly and surgically unfit patients for whom little could be advocated prior to the ERCP approach. In this group therapeutic widening of the ampulla of Vater by sphincterotomy, with or without oral bile salt therapy in the form of ursodeoxycholate is the optimum therapy. The contentions about early endoscopic sphincterotomy can be very confusing to interpret as the results of the various studies are summarized in Tables 35.2–35.5. It is very important to be aware that in the multicenter German study (Folsch et al 1997) sphincterotomy was precluded from the active treatment group if stones were not shown to be present in the common bile duct at the time of the procedure. This had the effect that less than half the patients in the active treatment group had a therapeutic ERCP performed. The original paper (Neoptolemos et al 1988b) used a modified Glasgow scoring system to assess severity of disease found no benefit from early ERCP in those with mild acute pancreatitis while those with the severe form had significantly fewer complications and a lower mortality when sphincterotomy with duct clearance was employed. The reduction in mortality did not reach statistical significance because the number of patients was not sufficiently large. However, it was clear that no

obvious detrimental effect had stemmed from the intervention (Table 35.2). Studies from Poland (Nowak et al 1993) and from Hong Kong (Fan et al 1993) support the belief that this is the most appropriate approach to the initial management of all patients with acute pancreatitis of biliary origin (Tables 35.3 and 35.4). These studies represent persuasive evidence that this approach should be utilized, but the German data (Folsch et al 1997) with a higher incidence of complications in the treatment group has considerably slowed acceptance of this approach (Table 35.5). There were 22 centers involved in the German study and it took over 4 years to complete so that recruitment was slow and a large number of different operators carried out the procedures, compared to the other three studies in which very few experienced endoscopists were involved. In addition, the German study includes only 46 patients with proven severe acute pancreatitis compared to 53 in the original Leicester study (Neoptolemos et al 1988b, Table 35.2). A new international multicenter study is now proposed to try to answer some of the remaining questions regarding the place of early endoscopic sphincterotomy. It is proposed that the treatment group in this study all receive sphincterotomy and only patients with objective markers of severe disease qualify for inclusion.

NASO-ENTERAL FEEDING

After a period of more than 30 years during which absolute fasting combined with nasogastric suction, particularly in severe acute pancreatitis, was the norm many centers in Europe are now routinely using naso-enteral feeding. This

Table 35.2 Effect of early endoscopic sphincterotomy on the outcome of severe acute pancreatitis (Neoptolemos et al 1988b)

	No	No of complications	No of deaths
Endoscopic sphincterotomy within 72 h	25	6 (24%)	1
Conventional management	28	17 (61%)	5

Table 35.3 The effect of early endoscopic sphincterotomy on the outcome of all grades of biliary acute pancreatitis (AP) (Nowak et al 1993)

	No	No of recurrent AP	No of deaths
Endoscopic sphincterotomy within 24 h	178	0	3 (1.6%)
Conventional management	102	16	13 (12.7%)

Table 35.4 The effect of early sphincterotomy on the outcome of all grades of gallstone-associated acute pancreatitis (Fan et al 1993)

	No	No of complications	No of deaths
Endoscopic sphincterotomy within 24 h	64	10 (16%)	1
Conventional management	63	21 (33%)	5

Table 35.5 Active treatment including ERCP versus conventional therapy (Folsch et al 1997)

	No	Major complications	No of deaths
ERCP ± ES	126	38	14*
Conventional management	112	40	7

* 58 (46%) of the active treatment group had ES. Ten of the 14 patients in this group were reckoned to have died from biliary AP.

has been performed by a nasojejunal feeding tube placed early in the disease process in patients with clinically severe acute pancreatitis (Kalfarentzos et al 1997, Nakad et al 1998, Windsor et al 1998). Our own group in Glasgow has presented data on a pilot group of 26 patients with severe acute pancreatitis in whom nasogastric feeding through a fine bore tube was successfully performed in 22 (Eatock et al 2000). It was previously considered damaging to stimulate the pancreatic secretions but current evidence would suggest that even a slow rate of naso-enteral feeding may retard or reverse the adverse changes in gut permeability which occur very soon after onset of the attack of acute pancreatitis.

A similar study of 38 patient (Kalfarentzos et al 1977) had similar demographics in terms of age, etiology and objective markers of severity found that there was a significant reduction in major sepsis and cost of feeding when the naso-enteral approach was used. The period of time in Intensive Care and total hospital stay was not reduced. All patients had objective evidence of severe disease. On the other hand, Windsor et al (1998) studied 34 patients only 13 of whom had objective evidence of severe AP. These authors randomized 16 of the 34 patients to enteral feeding and 18 to intravenous feeding. In this small study there were fewer complications and deaths in the enterally fed group. Of special interest was the improvement in APACHE score and CRP in the first week in the patients in the enterally fed group as well as an enhancement of antioxidant capacity and a reduction in endotoxic response based on the levels of IgM anticore endotoxin antibodies. Confirmation of this study and the pilot studies by Nakad et al (1998) is still awaited.

In the Belgian study (Nakad et al 1998) there were 20 successful treatments of 21 patients at an average of 36 h following admission. A two lumen nasogastrojejunal tube was placed after endoscopic location of a jejunal guidewire. Interestingly antibiotics were withheld in the latter part of the study. Our own group found it possible to begin naso-enteral feeding via the stomach in 22 patients within 48 h of admission starting with a slow flow rate of 20 ml/h. We found it possible to increase this rate fairly quickly in almost all patients utilizing a commercially available low fat semi-elemental peptide feed (Nutricia). The feed was given at full strength at an initial slow rate increasing gradually to 100 ml/h. In only three patients was there a technical failure due to large nasogastric aspirate with the need to place the tube in the jejunum. Currently we are carrying out a randomized study comparing nasogastric with nasojejunal feeding.

At present enteral feeding has been used in a limited number of patients by four different groups of researchers but it does appear that a new approach to therapy is gaining ground quite quickly.

LATE COMPLICATIONS

In the most severe attacks of acute pancreatitis macroscopic areas of black necrosis may develop in the fatty tissue around the pancreas or, less commonly, in the gland itself. Surgical intervention may not be required if the necrotic tissue remains sterile, but infection is a prime indicator for intervention. In the very elderly or unfit this may be by means of percutaneously placed drains, but in all other patients surgical intervention is strongly advocated. The purpose of operation is to remove the infected necrotic tissue by blunt dissection utilizing the fingers and gentle traction with forceps. The CECT scan is an enormous advantage to the surgeon in planning this procedure. After the removal of necrotic issue, provided there is no troublesome venous ooze, postoperative lavage is a very useful method of treatment (Beger et al 1988). The best results involve continued lavage for a median time of around 3 weeks, and re-operation will be required in up to 25% of patients on account of continuing necrosis and/or infection (Beger et al 1988).

Where venous ooze is particularly troublesome, packing of the abdomen with large cotton packs enclosed in non-adherent paraffin gauze, or a similar method of applying local pressure is advocated. The optimum results with this approach and repeated changes of packs under general anesthesia have shown that over 85% of patients, even in this most severely affected of groups, may survive (Bradley & Allen 1991). *Whichever operative approach is chosen, it is crucial that the gallbladder is removed in all these patients since tiny stones may escape.*

PANCREATIC PSEUDOCYST

A pseudocyst is a collection of pancreatic juice enclosed by a wall of fibrous or granulation tissue, which arises as a consequence of acute pancreatitis, pancreatic trauma or chronic pancreatitis (Bradley 1993). Of all pseudocysts developing immediately after an attack of acute pancreatitis, approximately 50% will resolve spontaneously, provided patience is exercised and there is no clamant clinical problem. In the elderly and unfit percutaneously placed catheters may be of considerable value, but these may need to be left in place for up to 90 days. In fitter, younger patients who are symptomatic the synthetic analog of somatostatin, octreotide, may be used as a subcutaneous injection three times daily. This tends to be of more value in patients with chronic pancreatitis (Gullo & Barbara 1991). In our own experience, both percutaneous aspiration and catheter drainage have not been particularly valuable in patients with acute pseudocysts. We have previously shown that patients with gallstone-related pseudocysts have a higher mortality and morbidity (Table 35.6) than those with alcohol-related disease (Imrie et al 1988). We therefore advocate, when conservative means have failed, that internal drainage by anastomosis of the pseudocyst to the stomach (cystogastrostomy) or drainage into a Roux-en-Y loop, combined with cholecystectomy and duct clearance be performed. This may be achieved by minimally invasive laparoscopic or endoscopic approaches where the pseudocyst is adherent to the stomach or duodenum.

Table 35.6 Mortality of pseudocyst and etiology (data from a consecutive series of 88 patients).

Etiology	No	Deaths No	%
Alcohol	51	2	3.9
Gallstones	26	6	23.1
Trauma	6	1	16.6
Unknown	5	1	20.0
Total	88	10	11.4

REFERENCES

Acosta J M, Ledesma C L 1974 Gallstone migration as a cause of acute pancreatitis. New England Journal of Medicine 290: 484–487

Acosta J M, Rossi R, Galli O M R, Pellegrini C A, Skinner D B 1978 Early surgery for acute gallstone pancreatitis: evaluation of a systematic approach. Surgery 83: 367–380

Armstrong C P, Taylor T V, Jeacock J, Lucas S 1985 The biliary tract in patients with acute gallstone pancreatitis. British Journal of Surgery 72: 551–555

Balthazar E J, Ranson J H, Naidich D P, Megibow A J, Caccavale R, Cooper M 1985 Acute pancreatitis: prognosis value of CT. Radiology 156: 767–772

Balthazar E J, Robinson D L, Megibow A J, Ranson J H 1990 Acute pancreatitis: value of CT in establishing prognosis. Radiology 174: 331–336

Beger H G, Bittner R, Buchler M, Hess W, Schmitz J E 1986 Hemodynamic data patterns in patients with acute pancreatitis. Gastroenterology 90: 74–79

Beger H G, Buchler M, Bittner R, Block S, Nevalainen T, Roscher R 1988 Necrosectony and postoperative local lavage in necrotizing pancreatitis. British Journal of Surgery 75: 207–212

Blamey S L, Osborne D G, Gilmour W H, O'Neill J, Carter D C, Imrie C W 1983 The early identification of patients with gallstone associated pancreatitis using clinical and biochemical factors only. Annals of Surgery 198: 574–578

Bradley E L 1993 A clinically based classification system for acute pancreatitis. Archives of Surgery 128: 586–590

Bradley III E L, Allen K A 1991 Management of necrotizing pancreatitis: results of prospective longitudinal trial. American Journal of Surgery 161: 19–25

Bradley E L, Hall J R, Lutz J, Hammer L, Lattouf O 1983 Haemodynamic consequence of severe acute pancreatitis. Annals of Surgery 198: 130–133

British Society of Gastroenterology 1998 United Kingdom guidelines for the management of acute pancreatitis. Gut 42(suppl. 2): S1–S3

Buchler M, Malfertheiner P, Beger H G 1986 Correlation of imaging procedure, biochemical parameters and clinical stage in acute pancreatitis. In: Malfertheiner P, Ditschuneit H (eds). Diagnostic procedures in pancreatic disease. Springer-Verlag, Berlin, pp 122–129

Buchler M, Malfertheiner P, Freiss H et al 1989 The penetration of antibiotics into human pancreas. Infection 17: 20–25

Corfield A P, Cooper M J, Williamson R C N et al 1985 Prediction of severity in acute pancreatitis: Prospective comparison of three prognostic indices. Lancet ii: 403–407

Delcenserie R, Yzet T, Ducroix J P 1996 Prophylactic antibiotics in treatment of severe acute alcoholic pancreatitis. Pancreas 13: 198–201

Dominguez Munoz J E, Carballo F, Garcia M J et al 1991 Clinical usefulness of polymorphonuclear elastase in predicting the severity of acute pancreatitis: results of a multicentre study. British Journal of Surgery 78: 1230–1234

Elfstrom J 1978 The timing of cholecystectomy in patients with gallstone pancreatitis. Chirurgica Scandinavica 144: 487–490

Etoch F C, Brombacher G E, Steven A, Imrie C W, Carter C R 2000 Nasogastric feeding and severe acute pancreatitis may be practical and safe. International Journal of Pancreatology, in press.

Fan S T, Lai E C S, Mok F P T, Lo C-M, Zheng S-S, Wong J 1993 Early treatment of acute biliary pancreatitis by endoscopic papillotomy. The New England Journal of Medicine 4: 228–232

Folsch UR, Nitshe R, Ludtke R, Hilgers RA, Creutzfeldt W 1997 Early ERCP and papillotomy compared with conservative treatment for acute biliary pancreatitis. The German study group on acute biliary pancreatitis. New England Journal of Medicine 336:237–242

Funnell I C, Bornman P C, Weakley S P, Terblanche J, Marks I N 1993 Obesity: an important prognostic factor in acute pancreatitis. British Journal of Surgery 80: 484–486

Grewe M, Tsiotos G G, Luque de-Leon E, Sarr M G 1999 Fungal infection in acute necrotising pancreatitis. Journal of the American College of Surgery 188: 408–414

Gudgeon M, Heath D I, Hurley P et al 1990 Trypsinogen activation peptides assay in the early severity prediction of acute pancreatitis. Lancet 335: 4–8

Gullo L, Barbara L 1991 Treatment of pancreatic pseudocysts with octreotide. Lancet 338: 540–541

Heath D I, Cruikshank A, Gudgeon M, Jehanli A, Shenkin A, Imrie C W 1993 Role of interleukin-6 in mediating the acute phase protein and potential as an early means of severity assessment in acute pancreatitis. Gut 34: 41–45

Imrie C W, Benjamin I S, Ferguson J C et al 1978a A single centre double-blind trial of Trasylol therapy in primary acute pancreatitis. British Journal of Surgery 65: 337–341

Imrie C W, Beatstall G H, Allam B F, O'Neill J, Banjamin I S, McKay A J 1978b Parathyroid hormone and calcium homeostasis in acute pancreatitis. British Journal of Surgery 65: 717–720

Imrie C W, Buist L, Shearer M 1988 The importance of etiology in the outcome of pancreatic pseudocyst. American Journal of Surgery 156: 159–162

Kalfarentos F, Kehagias J, Mead N, Kokkinis K, Gogos C A 1997 Enteral nutrition is superior to parenteral nutrition in severe acute pancreatitis: results of a randomized prospective trial. British Journal of Surgery 84: 1665–1669

Kelly T R 1976 Gallstone pancreatitis: pathophysiology. Surgery 80: 488–492

Kelly T R, Swaney P E 1982 Gallstone pancreatitis: the second time around. Surgery 92: 571–574

Kelly T R, Wagner D S 1988 Gallstone pancreatitis: a prospective randomised trial of the timing of surgery. Surgery 104: 600–605

Kivilaakso E, Fraki O, Nikki P, Lempinen M 1981 Resection of the pancreas for acute fulminant pancreatitis. Surgery, Gynecology and Obstetrics 152: 493–498

Knaus W A, Wagner D P, Draper E A, Zimmerman J E 1984 APACHE-II final form and national validation results of a severity of disease classification system. Critical Care Medicine 12: 213

Larvin M, McMahon M J 1989 APACHE II score for assessment and monitoring of acute pancreatitis. Lancet ii: 201–205

Lee S P, Nicholls J F, Park H Z 1992 Biliary sludge as a cause of acute pancreatitis. New England Journal of Medicine 326: 589–593

Leese T, Neoptolemos J P, Carr-Locke D L 1985 Successes, failures, early complications and their management following endoscopic sphincterotomy: results in 394 consecutive patients from a single centre. British Journal of Surgery 72: 215–219

London N J M, Neoptolemos J P, Lavelle J, Bailey J, James D 1989 Serial computed tomography scanning in acute pancreatitis: a prospective study. Gut 30: 397–403

London N J M, Leese T, Lavelle J M et al 1991 Rapid bolus contrast-enhanced dynamic computed tomography in acute pancreatitis: a prospective study. British Journal of Surgery 78: 1452–1456

Luiten E J, Hop W C, Lange J F, Bruining H A 1995 Controlled clinical trial of selective decontamination for the treatment of severe acute pancreatitis. Annals of Surgery 222: 57–65

McKay A J, O'Neill J, Imrie C W 1980 Pancreatitis, pregnancy and gallstones. British Journal of Obstetrics and Gynaecology 87: 47–50

McKay A J, Imrie C W, O'Neill J, Duncan J G 1982 Is an early ultrasound scan of value in acute pancreatitis? British Journal of Surgery 69: 369–372

McMahon M J, Pickford I R 1979 Biochemical prediction of gallstones early in an attack of acute pancreatitis. Lancet ii: 541–543

McMahon M J, Shefta J R 1980 Physical characteristics of gallstones and the calibre of the cystic duct in patients with acute pancreatitis. British Journal of Surgery 67: 6–9

Mayer A D, McMahon M J, Benson E A, Axon A T R 1984 Operations upon the biliary tract in patients with acute pancreatitis: aims, indications and timing. Annals of the Royal College of Surgeons of England 66: 179–183

Mayer A D, McMahon M J, Corfield A P et al 1985 Controlled clinical trial of peritoneal lavage for the treatment of severe acute pancreatitis. New England Journal of Medicine 312: 399–404

Nakad A, Piessevaux H, Marot J C et al 1998 Is early nutrition in acute pancreatitis dangerous? About 20 patients fed by an endoscopically placed nasogastrojejunal tube. Pancreas 17: 187–193

Neoptolemos J P, Hall A W, Finlay D F, Berry J M, Carr-Locke D L, Fossard D P 1984 The urgent diagnosis of gallstones in acute pancreatitis: a prospective study of three methods. British Journal of Surgery 71: 230–233

Neoptolemos J P, Carr-Locke D L, Leese T, James D 1987 Acute cholangitis in association with acute pancreatitis: incidence, clinical features, outcome and the role of ERCP and endoscopic sphincterotomy. British Journal of Surgery 74: 1103–1106

Neoptolemos J P, Davidson B R, Winder A F, Vallance D 1988a The role of duodenal bile crystal analysis in the investigation of 'idiopathic' pancreatitis. British Journal of Surgery 75: 450–453

Neoptolemos J P, Carr-Locke D L, London N H, Bailey I A, James D, Fossard D P 1988b Controlled trial of urgent endoscopic retrograde cholangiopancreatography and endoscopic sphincterotomy versus conservative treatment for acute pancreatitis due to gallstones. Lancet ii: 979–983

Nowak A, Nowakowska-Dulawa E, Rybicka J 1990 Urgent endoscopic sphincterotomy versus conservative treatment in acute biliary pancreatitis—a prospective, controlled trial. 37: A5 (abstr)

Nowak A, Blaszcyska M, Nowaksja-Dulawa E, Marek T 1993 Endoscopic sphincterotomy in the therapy of acute biliary pancreatitis. In: Proceedings of the 2nd United European Gastroenterology Meeting

Opie E L 1901 The etiology of acute hemorrhagic pancreatitis. Bulletin of the Johns Hopkins Hospital 12: 182–188

Osborne D H, Imrie C W, Carter D C 1981 Biliary surgery in the same admission for gallstone-associated acute pancreatitis. British Journal of Surgery 68: 758–761

Paricio P P, Olmo D C, Franco E P, Gonzales A P, Gonzales L C, Lopez J B 1990 Gallbladder cholesterolosis: an aetiological factor in acute pancreatitis of uncertain origin. British Journal of Surgery 77: 735–737

Pederzoli P, Bassi C, Vesentini S, Campedelli A 1993 A randomized multicentre clinical trial of antibiotic prophylaxis of septic complications in acute necrotizing pancreatitis with impenem. Surgery, Gynecology and Obstetrics 176: 480–483

Powell J J, Campbell E, Johnson C D, Siriwardena A K 1999 Survey of antibiotic prophylaxis in acute pancreatitis in the UK and Ireland. British Journal of Surgery 86: 320–322

Ranson J H C 1979 The timing of biliary surgery in acute pancreatitis. Annals of Surgery 189: 654–663

Ranson J H C, Rifkind K M, Roses D F, Fink S D, Eng K, Spencer F C 1974 Prognostic signs and the role of operative management in acute pancreatitis. Surgery, Gynecology and Obstetrics 139: 69–81

Ros E, Navarro S, Bru C, Garcia-Puges A, Valderrama R 1991 Occult microlithiasis in 'idiopathic' acute pancreatitis: prevention of relapse by cholecystectomy or ursodeoxycholic acid therapy. Gastroenterology 101: 1701–1709

Sanio V, Kemppainen E, Puolakkainen P et al 1995 Early antibiotic treatment in acute necrotising pancreatitis. Lancet 346: 663–667

Schwarz M, Isenmann R, Mayer H, Beger H G 1997 Antibiotic use in necrotizing pancreatitis. Results of a controlled study. Dtsh Med Worchenschr 122: 356–361

Stone H H, Fabian T C, Dunlop W E 1981 Gallstone pancreatitis. Biliary tract pathology in relation to time of operation. Annals of Surgery 194: 305–312

Tondelli P, Stutz K, Harder F, Schupisser J-P, Allgower M 1982 Acute gallstone pacreatitis: best timing for biliary surgery. British Journal of Surgery 69: 709–710

Toouli J, DiFrancesco V, Saccone G, Kollias J, Schloithe A, Shanks N 1996 Division of the sphincter of Oddi for treatment of dysfunction associated with recurrent pancreatitis. British Journal of Surgery 83: 1205–1210

Trapnell J E, Duncan E H L 1975 Patterns of incidence in acute pancreatitis. British Medical Journal 2: 179–183

Uhl W, Buchler M, Malfertheiner P, Marini M, Beger H G 1991 PMN elastase in comparison with CRP, antiproteases, and LDH as indicators of necrosis in human acute pancreatitis. Pancreas 6: 253–259

Viedma J A, Perez-Mateo M, Dominguez J E, Carballo F 1992 Role of interleukin-6 in acute pancreatitis. Comparisons with C-reactive protein and phospholipase A. Gut 33: 1264–1267

Wilson C, Heads A, Shenkin A, Imrie C W 1989 C-reactive protein, antiproteases and complement factors as objective markers of severity in acute pancreatitis. British Journal of Surgery 76: 177–181

Wilson C, Heath D I, Imrie C W 1990 Prediction of outcome in acute pancreatitis: a comparative study of APACHE II, clinical assessment and multiple factor scoring systems. British Journal of Surgery 77: 1260–1264

Wilson C, Imrie C W, Carter D C 1988 Fatal acute pancreatitis. Gut 29: 782–788

Windsor A C, Kanwar S, Li A G et al 1998 Compared with parenteral nutrition, enteral feeding attenuates the acute phase response and improves disease severity in acute pancreatitis. Gut 42: 431–435

Percutaneous approaches to the treatment of gallbladder disease

36

C.D. BECKER

INTRODUCTION

Image-guided interventional techniques have been developed in order to provide minimally invasive treatment of gallbladder disease. Percutaneous, image-guided cholecystostomy is now an accepted method to decompress the acutely inflamed gallbladder if surgery is not indicated. A variety of methods aiming at elective, nonsurgical removal of gallbladder stones that were introduced in the early 1990s include extracorporeal shock-wave lithotripsy, contact dissolution of gallstones with methyl-tert-butyl-ether and percutaneous mechanical cholecystolithotomy. Due to the successful introduction of laparoscopic cholecystectomy (Ch. 38) surgical treatment of cholecystolithiasis has become less invasive and definitive treatment of cholecystolithiasis may now be accomplished with much shorter hospitalization. Since none of the existing nonsurgical techniques of gallstone removal can prevent recurrent gallstone formation, the indication to perform percutaneous gallstone removal without surgery is now limited. The current chapter gives an overview of image-guided treatment methods for gallbladder disease.

EXTRACORPOREAL SHOCK-WAVE LITHOTRIPSY

Extracorporeal shockwave lithotripsy (ESWL) of gallstones was developed in the 1980s as a noninvasive form of treatment in selected patients with symptomatic, uncomplicated cholecystolithiasis (Sauerbruch et al 1986, Sackmann et al 1991). ESWL is done with ultrasound guidance and requires no percutaneous cholecystostomy. The original investigators as well as the majority of subsequent investigators used

relatively strict selection criteria, including a normal gallbladder on ultrasound, opacification of the gallbladder on oral cholecystography, and a limited number (1–3) and size (0.5–3 cm) of the calculi. Cholestasis, pancreatitis, severe liver disease, hemorrhagic diathesis, abdominal aortic aneurysm, and pregnancy are considered contraindications. Most treatment protocols restrict ESWL treatment to calculi consisting of cholesterol, i.e., radiolucent or only faintly calcified calculi on plain radiography, and combine ESWL with adjuvant oral bile acid therapy (Ch. 33). Thus, there are usually two competing mechanisms leading to clearance of the gallbladder from fragments after ESWL: spontaneous passage of fragments through the cystic duct and fragment dissolution within the gallbladder by the adjuvant bile acids. ESWL alone may also lead to successful gallbladder clearance regardless of the composition of the calculi, but a high number of shockwaves and multiple treatment sessions are often needed to pulverize the calculi to a size of 2–3 mm so as to enable all of them to pass spontaneously (Rawat & Burhenne 1990, Fache et al 1990).

Three principles of shock-wave generators are available: spark-gap, piezoelectric and electromagnetic. All devices of the current generation use water cushions with coupling membranes for transmission of the shock-waves. Targeting is accomplished with real-time ultrasound (US). The mode of shock-wave treatment (i.e., the power settings and shock-wave numbers) may influence the result of ESWL considerably, but all three types of shock-wave generators allow effective gallstone fragmentation, and ESWL can be done successfully in an outpatient setting. Side effects of the treatment are minor, including cutaneous petechiae or, occasionally, hematuria. Approximately one third of patients develops at least one attack of biliary pain attributable to fragment passage; these episodes may occur any time between ESWL and complete gallbladder clearance. Mild transient biliary pancreatitis is observed in approximately 2%

of patients, cholestasis and acute cholecystitis are less frequent. The rate of fragment clearance after ESWL depends on the total stone volume and on the size of the largest remaining fragment. In the combination with adjuvant bile acids, ESWL may be considered successful if the remaining fragments are no larger than approximately 4 mm. This can usually be accomplished within 1–2 treatment sessions. On average, 70% of patients become stone-free within 1 year and 80% within 1.5 years after successful ESWL and adjuvant bile acid therapy (Ell et al 1990, Sackmann et al 1991, Becker et al 1992). If only patients with solitary gallstones up to 2 cm in diameter are treated, the stone clearance rate is 80 to 90% within 6–18 months (Sackmann et al 1991, Pauletzki et al 1994).

Over the past decade it has become clear that ESWL combined with oral bile acid treatment enables effective treatment of symptomatic patients who have a single, radiolucent gallstone in a functioning gallbladder (contraction more than 60% of the fasting volume). Advocates of ESWL treatment argue, therefore, that this group of patients should be offered ESWL because more than half of them can be cured definitively without general anesthesia, without any operation, and without any risk of bile duct injury and because failure of ESWL treatment does not preclude surgery at a later date (Sauerbruch 1997). On the other hand, it must be acknowledged that the problem of gallstone recurrence remains unsolved. Recent studies have shown that over two thirds of patients develop recurrence within 6 years, and it is argued that it may be preferable to perform laparoscopic cholecystectomy in the first place (Barkun et al 1997, Borch et al 1996, Cesmeli et al 1999, Go et al 1995).

PERCUTANEOUS CHOLECYSTOSTOMY FOR ACUTE CHOLECYSTITIS

Surgical cholecystostomy has long been used to provide external decompression of the acutely inflamed gallbladder in patients who are at high risk for operation or general anesthesia (e.g., sepsis, diabetes or severe cardiac, pulmonary, hepatic or renal failure). Percutaneous cholecystostomy (PC) was initially developed to provide a minimally invasive method of gallbladder decompression in elderly and very ill patients with acute acalculous or calculous cholecystitis or with gallbladder hydrops due to malignant disease (Elyaderani & Gabriele 1979, Pearse et al 1984). PC has also been employed to treat complications of cholecystitis, e.g., gallbladder perforation, empyema or pericholecystic abscesses or as an alternative to percutaneous transhepatic drainage of the bile ducts in obstructive jaundice. Most recently, PC has also been utilized to provide

access to the gallbladder for elective gallstone treatment with stone dissolution techniques, percutaneous cholecystolithotomy or other techniques.

The percutaneous access route to the gallbladder is usually determined with ultrasound (US) and based on the individual anatomical situation. Computed tomography (CT) can be used if ultrasound does not provide sufficient information. The transhepatic approach to the gallbladder has been favored by most authors because a puncture through the attached portion of the gallbladder should reduce the risk of bile leakage into the peritoneal cavity (Fig. 36.1). On the other hand, the area of attachment cannot be anticipated reliably with imaging techniques and the direct, transperitoneal route has also been used successfully (Vogelzang et al 1988). The acutely inflamed gallbladder is usually distended and immediately adjacent to the anterior

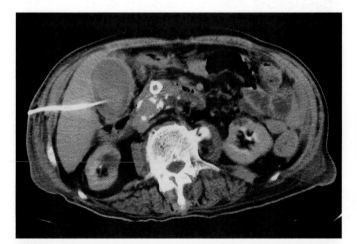

(A)

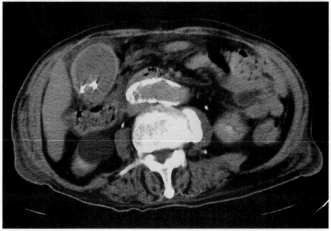

(B)

Fig. 36.1 CT-guided percutaneous cholecystostomy for acute acalculous cholecystitis in a patient with severe arteriosclerosis and ischemic heart disease. **(A)** shows the percutaneously placed drainage catheter and **(B)** the pigtail catheter in the gallbladder. The gallbladder wall is thickened and there is hyperdense sludge within the gallbladder.

abdominal wall, and the direct approach through the gall-bladder fundus avoids the trauma to the liver that may be associated with percutaneous gallstone removal at a later date. The use of a percutaneous removable anchor has recently been proposed in order to prevent the gallbladder wall from moving away from the trocar or from the catheter during exchange over a guide-wire (Cope et al 1990).

The initial gallbladder puncture is performed under local anesthesia. Prophylactic administration of atropine is advis-able in order to prevent vasovagal reactions (vanSonnenberg et al 1984). With portable US equipment, the PC proce-dure can be performed at the patients' bedside (e.g. in the intensive care unit). However, if there is doubt regarding a safe access route it may be preferable to combine US or CT with fluoroscopy (Fig. 36.2). Several suitable needle/ catheter or -guidewire systems are available, and the optimal method of catheter introduction is a matter of personal preference. Repeat punctures with introducer needles should always be avoided, because leakage of gallbladder content through the puncture channel may lead to internal decompression of the gallbladder into the peritoneal cavity and thus prevent further attempts to enter the gallbladder lumen. A catheter size of 6.5–7 Fr is usually sufficient to provide effective external gallbladder drainage; but 8 Fr or more may be necessary to drain gallbladder empyema or pericholecystic abscesses (vanSonnenberg et al 1991) (Fig. 36.3). If PC is done for acute cholecystitis, catheter manip-ulations should be kept to a minimum in order to avoid

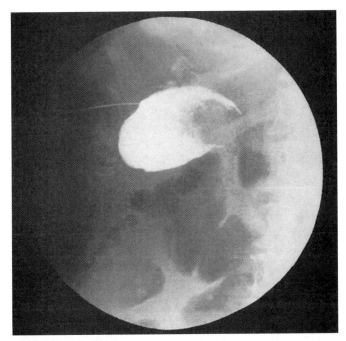

(A)

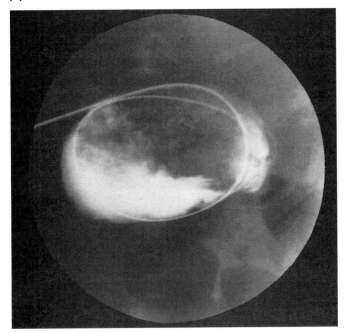

(B)

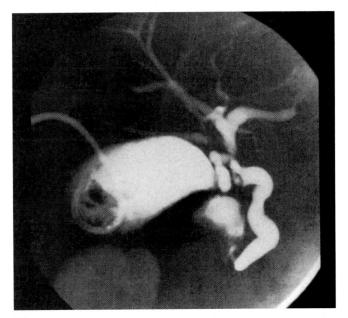

(C)

Fig. 36.2 Percutaneous-transhepatic cholecystostomy for acute acalculous hemorrhagic cholecystitis. Following an initial gallbladder puncture under ultrasound-guidance with a 22 gauge needle, the procedure was continued under fluoroscopic control. **(A)** Direct cholecystography demonstrated a large filling defect in the infundibulum of the gallbladder. **(B)** The 22 gauge access was converted to a larger caliber, and a guide-wire was introduced into the gallbladder. A 6.5-Fr self-retaining pigtail catheter was placed in the gallbladder lumen. There was no opacification of the cystic duct at the time of the initial procedure. **(C)** Repeat cholangiography was done 1 week after emergency cholecystostomy. The cystic duct was patent and there was unimpeded flow of contrast material into the duodenum. Most of the debris within the gallbladder had disappeared. The cholecystostomy catheter was removed 1 week after cholecystostomy; elective cholecystectomy was not required.

inadvertent perforation of the frail inflamed gallbladder wall or leakage of gallbladder contents alongside the catheter. To prevent inadvertent dislodgement of the catheter on the ward, it is preferable to use a self-retaining catheter.

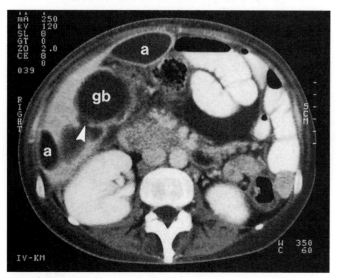

(A)

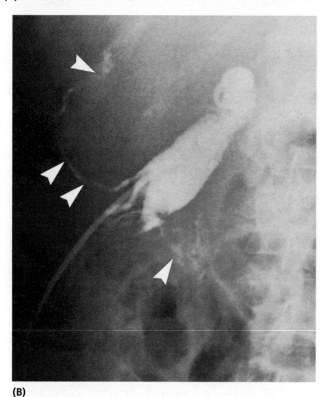

(B)

Fig. 36.3 Gallbladder empyema with perforation and pericholecystic abscess formation. **(A)** CT demonstrates a distended gallbladder (gb) with a perforated wall (arrow) and pericholecystic abscesses (a). **(B)** Using a subhepatic access under ultrasound guidance, a catheter was placed through the gallbladder fundus within the gallbladder lumen and drained pus. Injection of contrast material demonstrated the gallbladder lumen and at least 2 sites of perforation communicating with pericholecystic abscesses (arrows).

Diagnostic cholangiography through the cholecystostomy catheter may be obtained after a few days in order to assess the presence of gallstones and patency of the cystic duct. It is advisable to leave the cholecystostomy catheter in place for at least 7–10 days to let a tract develop and to avoid bile leakage into the peritoneal cavity.

While transient right upper quadrant pain is a relatively common side-effect of PC, serious procedure-related complications are uncommon. In a review of 252 percutaneous cholecystostomies reported in the English language literature, there were 4 cases of bile peritonitis and 1 death (0.3%); other procedure-related complications included vasovagal reaction or decrease in blood pressure, self-limited hemobilia and acute cholecystitis due to a stone being lodged in the cystic duct (Teplick 1989). In a recent series of 127 patients undergoing gallbladder puncture and cholecystostomy, the reported rate of minor and major complications was 3.9 and 8.7%, respectively. The 30-day mortality of that series was 3.1%, but all deaths were due to underlying diseases (vanSonnenberg et al 1992). Thus, in view of the severely compromised health of most patients undergoing the procedure, PC may be considered a safe procedure. The efficacy of PC is difficult to determine because the diagnosis of acute cholecystitis is often unreliable in patients with multiple concomitant medical and surgical problems (McGahan & Lindfors 1988, 1989). If the indication for percutaneous cholecystostomy is restricted to patients with clinical and/or imaging findings of acute cholecystitis a response rate of 90% may be expected (van Overhagen, 1996). However, if patients with unexplained abdominal sepsis are included, the response rate will of course be lower (McGahan & Lindfors 1989, Lee et al 1991, Boland et al 1994). Current experience thus indicates that PC is an effective temporizing measure in elderly or critically ill patients with acute cholecystitis and a safe alternative to emergency surgery. In patients with acute acalculous cholecystitis interval cholecystectomy is usually not necessary, and PC may, thus, be considered a definitive therapy (Vauthey et al 1992).

NONSURGICAL TECHNIQUES TO REMOVE GALLBLADDER STONES

PERCUTANEOUS GALLSTONE REMOVAL VIA CHOLECYSTOSTOMY

Percutaneous contact dissolution of gallbladder stones with methyl-tert-butyl-ether (see also Ch. 33)

Methyl-tert-butyl-ether (MTBE) is the most potent cholesterol solvent now available. Because of its boiling point of

55.2°C it remains liquid at body temperature and is therefore easier to handle than diaethyl ether. Direct instillation of MTBE through a small percutaneous cholecystostomy catheter has been successfully used to dissolve cholesterol stones of the gallbladder within hours (Allen 1985).

The selection criteria for MTBE therapy in the two largest studies reported to date included symptomatic, uncomplicated gallstone disease as well as normal hematologic and hepatic laboratory tests. Absence of calcifications of the gallstones is confirmed by plain computed tomography (CT) and patency of the cystic duct demonstrated by means of an oral cholecystogram to ascertain that non-cholesterol components and residual debris could pass spontaneously from the gallbladder to the intestine. There were no limitations regarding the number and size of gallstones (Thistle et al 1989, Hellstern et al 1990). The majority of treatments with MTBE have been performed on an elective basis in patients who had an increased risk of surgery or anesthesia because of coexisting medical conditions or who refused to undergo surgery for other reasons. However, MTBE has also been used to dissolve cholesterol calculi in patients who had undergone percutaneous cholecystostomy on an emergency basis (vanSonnenberg et al 1986, 1992). MTBE has even been used successfully in the presence of an occluded cystic duct (Mueller et al 1991).

The use of MTBE requires several precautions. Because of its unpleasant odour, its inflammability and its anesthetic effect, it must be used in a well-ventilated room. Catheters, syringes and stopcocks must be made of special materials, e.g., teflon, polyethylene, glass and metal, because several other synthetic materials become macerated by MTBE. Following percutaneous cholecystostomy as described earlier, a 5 Fr pigtail-catheter is positioned within the gallbladder under fluoroscopic control so as to provide close contact with the gallstones to be dissolved. The gallbladder 'overflow volume' is assessed by contrast injection into the gallbladder. A similar volume of MTBE (usually a few ml) is then instilled and aspirated in continuous cycles (Fig. 36.4). Depending on the stone volume, complete dissolution is usually accomplished during a hospitalization of 2–3 days with several hours of treatment each day. Automatic pumps have recently become available for MTBE treatment in order to reduce the relatively long operator time required for the procedure.

Minor side effects include nausea, vomiting or a burning sensation in the right upper abdomen which may be due to the drug itself, or to minor leakage of bile alongside the catheter or to catheter manipulations within the gallbladder. Serious complications such as major bile leakage, hemobilia or stone impaction in the cystic duct or common bile duct are uncommon. No deaths have been reported in the major

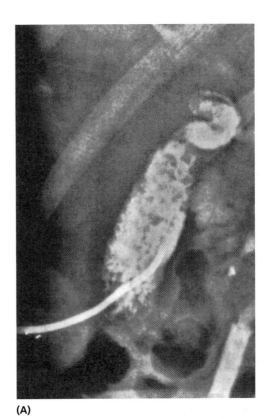

(A)

(B)

Fig. 36.4 Percutaneous dissolution of cholesterol gallstones with MTBE. **(A)** Direct cholangiography obtained through a cholecystostomy catheter demonstrated multiple small calculi in the gallbladder lumen. **(B)** After a few hours of MTBE dissolution treatment, the stone volume had diminished considerably.

series reported to date. The success rate of MTBE dissolution treatment has been reported to be 96% although residual debris was still visible on ultrasound in many patients at the time of discharge (Thistle et al 1989, Hellstern et al 1990, Thistle et al 1991). In the era of laparoscopic cholecystectomy, indications for MTBE dissolution treatment of gallbladder calculi may be considered extremely rare.

Percutaneous cholecystolithotomy

The term 'percutaneous cholecystolithotomy—(PCCL)' is used to describe a variety of technical modifications to remove gallbladder stones mechanically through a percutaneous access. Unlike MTBE dissolution treatment, PCCL can be done regardless of the size, number and composition of the calculi. A small, shrunken thick-walled gallbladder is generally considered a contraindication to all forms of PCCL. The common steps of all techniques of PCCL are: percutaneous access to the gallbladder by means of percutaneous cholecystostomy, immediate or sequential dilatation of the cholecystostomy tract to a relatively large size, introduction of instruments for gallstone fragmentation and removal and external drainage of the gallbladder after the procedure (Akiyama et al 1985, Kerlan et al 1985).

PCCL may be done through a transhepatic or through a transperitoneal access route. The size of the percutaneous tract which is needed for PCCL depends on the instruments used for stone fragmentation, ranging from 10 Fr to 30 Fr. Tract dilatation can be performed with fascial dilators of increasing diameters, with co-axial systems or with angioplasty balloon catheters. Regardless of the technique, the dilatation procedure is painful unless performed under heavy intravenous sedation or general anesthesia. The most important risks are hemorrhage if a transhepatic access is used and bile leakage and loss of access if a subhepatic transperitoneal route is chosen; these complications are less likely if tract dilatation and stone removal is done in multiple sessions. Instrumentation for stone removal is performed through a metal or teflon sheath. Smaller calculi can be removed with wire baskets (Cope et al 1990). Fragmentation of larger calculi may be done with electrohydraulic, ultrasonic or laser-mediated intracorporal lithotripsy (Burhenne et al 1975, Picus et al 1989, Bogan et al 1989, Gillams et al 1992). These techniques require direct contact between the lithotripsy probes and the calculi under endoscopic vision. A tract diameter of 18–30 Fr is necessary to introduce endoscopic devices with instrumentation channels. The 'rotary gallstone lithotrite' was specially designed for percutaneous gallstone lithotripsy and enables pulverization of gallbladder calculi in a manner similar to a household blender (Miller et al 1991a,b). The

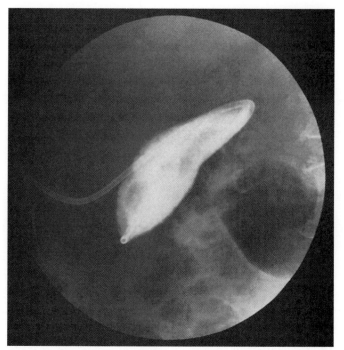

(A)

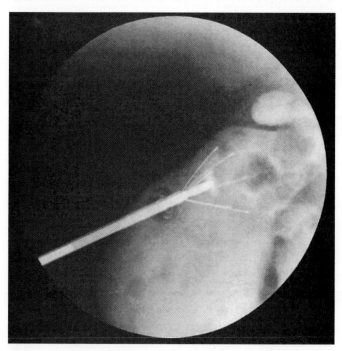

(B)

Fig. 36.5 Percutaneous cholecystolithotomy with the rotational 'lithotrite'. **(A)** Access to the gallbladder was established by means of percutaneous-transhepatic cholecystostomy using a right anterolateral entry into the gallbladder. The catheter entered the gallbladder wall in its distal half. There were multiple filling defects due to calculi. **(B)** Following dilatation of the percutaneous tract, the rotational lithotrite with its sheath has been introduced into the gallbladder lumen. The gallbladder was distended with dilute contrast material, and the calculi were well visualized. The struts around the propeller protected the gallbladder wall, while the calculi were attracted into the propeller by a vortex created within the gallbladder fluid.

device consists of a 6-pronged basket surrounding a 3 mm impeller. The impeller is mounted on a cable that rotates in a 7-Fr catheter and, driven by an electric motor, may rotate up to 30 000 rpm. This produces a strong fluid vortex pulling the stones automatically into the basket towards the impeller, and the stones are crushed into fragments mostly smaller than 2 mm within minutes (Miller et al 1991a,b). This technique can be performed under fluoroscopic vision and requires a percutaneous tract no larger than 10 Fr (Fig. 36.5). Because the device must be able to open freely within the gallbladder, the stone volume should not exceed 75% of the volume of the gallbladder.

The success rate of PCCL is 88% (Gillams et al 1992). Procedure-related complications occur in 15% and included subhepatic bile collections, cholangitis, gallbladder perforation with pericholecystitis and wound infections; most procedures are done on an elective basis. Although PCCL has been performed with local and intravenous anesthesia, the majority are done under general anesthesia (Picus et al 1989, Hruby et al 1989, Gillams et al 1992). Cannulation of the cystic duct with a guide-wire is usually feasible. This may even allow extraction of calculi from the common bile duct or cystic duct (Fache et al 1990).

In summary, PCCL may occasionally appear as a useful alternative to elective surgery in patients who have undergone percutaneous cholecystostomy on an emergency basis for acute calculous cholecystitis and in whom surgery remains contraindicated even after the inflammatory signs have settled. Although in the early 1990s elective PCCL was proposed to avoid cholecystectomy in patients with symptomatic but uncomplicated cholecystolithiasis this indication appears obsolete in the era of laparoscopic cholecystectomy.

Combined surgical and radiological intervention ('minicholecystostomy')

This procedure was described by Burhenne et al (1985) and included provision of both emergency decompression of the gallbladder and the possibility of percutaneous stone removal 7–10 days later without the need for tract dilatation (Burhenne & Stoller 1985). Following localization of the gallbladder by means of US, a small abdominal incision is made over the gallbladder fundus under local anesthesia and intravenous analgesia. To minimize the procedure, stone removal is not attempted immediately. A 24-Fr Foley catheter is placed into the gallbladder, and the fundus of the

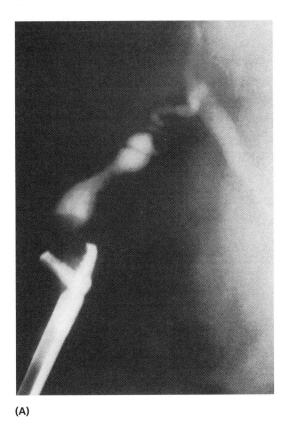

(A)

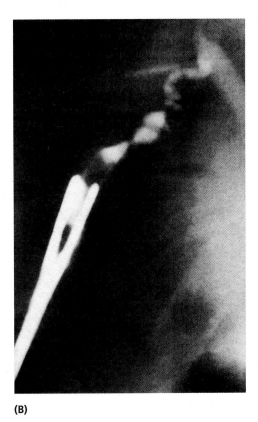

(B)

Fig. 36.6 Mechanical cholecystolithotripsy through a subhepatic surgical 'minicholecystostomy'. **(A)** Because the gallbladder fundus had been sutured to the anterior abdominal wall at the time of emergency cholecystostomy, percutaneous tract formation was not necessary and percutaneous gallstone removal was feasible 1 week later through a short, straight 24-Fr percutaneous tract. The Storz stone-crushing forceps was introduced into the gallbladder and a large calculus was fragmented. **(B)** The fragments were subsequently extracted with the Mazzariello-Caprini-forceps.

gallbladder is sutured to the combined peritoneum and posterior layer of the rectus sheath, thus creating a short, wide tract. Following one week of external gallbladder drainage, the gallstones can be removed under fluoroscopic control, usually without analgesia. Large stones can be fragmented with stone crushing forceps and removed mechanically with a variety of instruments (Fig. 36.6).

The 'minicholecystostomy' approach avoids the risks of hepatic hemorrhage, bile leakage and vasovagal reactions associated with dilatation of a percutaneous cholecystostomy tract and also facilitates repeated subhepatic access to the gallbladder. The success rate of stone removal was 97% for gallbladder stones, 86% for cystic duct stones and 63% for common bile duct stones; there were no serious complications and no deaths (Burhenne & Stoller 1985, Gibney et al 1987).

PERCUTANEOUS ABLATION OF THE GALLBLADDER

Despite successful gallstone removal, all the percutaneous techniques cannot provide definitive cure of gallstone disease since the functioning gallbladder remains in place. Although long-term follow-up regarding most of the newer treatment modalities is not yet available, gallstone recurrence must be expected to be common (Norrby & Schönebeck 1970, Gibney et al 1989, Villanova et al 1989). One must also consider that gallbladder-preserving treatment does not eliminate the risk of gallbladder carcinoma (So et al 1990).

Nonsurgical ablation of the gallbladder may be defined as fibrotic obliteration of the gallbladder lumen. Ideally, the gallbladder mucosa would be eradicated completely, because this would not only eliminate the possibility of gallstone recurrence, but also the long-term risk of gallbladder adenocarcinoma. Percutaneous gallbladder ablation was developed and tested experimentally and clinically in order to prevent gallstone recurrence by eliminating the functioning gallbladder through a cholecystostomy. A two-step approach was developed including preliminary obliteration of the cystic duct by means of bipolar RF electrocautery and subsequent sclerotherapy of the gallbladder. Concentrated ethanol and sodium-tetradecyl-sulfate were used for gallbladder sclerotherapy without toxic side effects. Histologic studies in preliminary animal experiments revealed necrosis of the gallbladder wall within 2 weeks and fibrotic obliteration of the gallbladder within 8 weeks (Becker et al 1988, 1989). The ablation procedure was then tested in a group of ten patients who, because of multiple medical risk factors,

had undergone cholecystostomy instead of cholecystectomy for acute gallbladder disease (Becker et al 1990). Although follow-up studies by ultrasound gave no evidence of mucocele formation or stone recurrence, small gallbladder lumina remained visible in all patients, indicating that mucosal ablation was still incomplete. Although occasional attempts at gallbladder ablation have been reported by other investigators (van Overhagen 1996), further technical improvement would be needed prior to wider clinical application.

SUMMARY

Percutaneous, image-guided cholecystostomy offers a minimally invasive treatment of acute cholecystitis in the high risk patient. In acalculous disease, PC alone is curative unless the gallbladder wall has already become necrotic in the course of gangrenous cholecystitis. In calculous disease, interval cholecystectomy is usually required although percutaneous gallstone removal through the cholecystostomy tract may, in some cases, be preferable.

The role for elective percutaneous gallstone removal by means of MTBE or PCCL has virtually disappeared because the hospitalization required for these procedures is similar to laparoscopic cholecystectomy and a definitive cure cannot be provided.

ESWL is a noninvasive outpatient procedure and may be considered as a useful treatment option in the small group of patients who fulfill the selection criteria. However, due to the relatively high recurrence rates observed in recent studies laparoscopic cholecystectomy appears to be the more effective treatment.

REFERENCES

Akiyama H, Nagusa Y, Fujita T et al 1985 A new method for nonsurgical cholecystolithotomy. Surgery, Gynecology and Obstetrics 161: 73–74

Allen M J, Borody T J, Bugliosi T F, May G R, La Russo N F, Thistle J L 1985 Cholelitholysis using methyl tertiary butyl ether. Gastroenterology 88: 122–125

Barkun AN, Barkun JS, Sampalis JS, Caro J, Fried GM, Meakins JL, Joseph L, Goresky CA 1997 McGill Gallstone Treatment Group. Costs and effectiveness of extracorporeal gallbladder stone shockwave lithotripsy versus laparoscopic cholecystectomy. A randomized clinical trial. International Journal of Technology Assessment in Health Care 13(4): 589–601

Becker C D, Quenville N F, Burhenne H J 1988 Long-term occlusion of the porcine cystic duct by endoluminal radiofrequency electrocoagulation. Radiology 167: 63–68

Becker C D, Quenville N F, Burhenne H J 1989 Gallbladder ablation through radiologic intervention: an experimental alternative to cholecystectomy. Radiology 171: 235–240

Becker C D, Fache J S, Malone D E, Stoller J L, Burhenne H J 1990 Ablation of the cystic duct and gallbladder: Clinical observations. Radiology 176: 687–690

Becker C D, Huber T, Glättli A, Renner E L, Gysi B, Seiler C 1992 Cholecystolithiasis: Three years experience with ultrasound-guided electromagnetic shock-wave lithotripsy. European Radiology 2: 478–482

Bogan M L, Hawes R H, Kopecky K K, et al 1989 Percutaneous cholecystolithotomy with endoscopic lithotripsy by using a pulsed-dye laser: Preliminary experience. Radiology 173: 481

Boland G W, Lee M J, Leung J, Mueller P R 1994 Percutaneous cholecystostomy in critically ill patients: Early response and final outcome in 82 patients. American Journal of Roentgenology 163: 339–342

Borch K, Jonsson K A, Lindstrom E, Carlsson P, Kullman E, Ihse I, Svanvik J 1996 Extracorporeal shock-wave lithotripsy of gallbladder stones: an alternative for the selected few. European Journal of Surgery 162(5): 379–84

Burhenne H J 1975 Electrohydrolytic fragmentation of retained common bile duct stones. Radiology 117: 721–722

Burhenne H J, Stoller J L 1985 Minicholecystostomy and radiologic stone extraction in high-risk cholelithiasis patients: Preliminary experience. American Journal of Surgery 149: 632–635

Burhenne H J, Becker C D, Malone D E, Rawat B, Fache J S 1989 Biliary lithotripsy: Early observations in 106 patients. Work in progress. Radiology 171: 363–367

Burhenne H J, 1989 Can the newer interventional procedures replace cholecystectomy for cholecystolithiasis? Radiology 170: 574

Cesmeli E, Elewaut A E, Kerre T, De Buyzere M, Afschrift M, Elewaut A 1999 Gallstone recurrence after successful shock wave therapy: the magnitude of the problem and the predictive factors. American Journal of Gastroenterology 94(2): 474–479

Cope C, Burke D R, Meranze S G 1990 Percutaneous extraction of gallstones in 20 patients. Radiology 176: 19

Ell C, Kerzel W, Schneider T et al 1990 Piezoelectric lithotripsy: Stone disintegration and follow-up results in patients with symptomatic gallbladder stones. Gastroenterology 99: 1439–1444

Elyaderani M, Gabriele O F 1979 Percutaneous cholecystostomy and cholangiography in patients with obstructive jaundice. Radiology 130: 601–602

Fache J S, Rawat B, Burhenne H 1990 Extracorporeal cholecystolithotripsy without oral chemolitholysis. Radiology 177: 719–721

Gibney R G, Fache J S, Becker C D et al 1987 Combined surgical and radiologic intervention for complicated cholelithiasis in high-risk patients. Radiology 165: 715–719

Gibney R G, Chow K, So C B, Rowley V A, Cooperberg P C, Burhenne H J 1989 Gallstone recurrence after cholecystolithotomy. American Journal of Roentgenology 153: 287–289

Gillams A, Curtis S C, Donald J, Russell C, Lees W 1992 Technical considerations in 113 percutaneous cholecystolithotomies. Radiology 183: 163–166

Glenn F 1981 Surgical management of acute cholecystitis in patients 65 years of age and older. Annals of Surgery 193: 56–58

Go P M, Stolk M F, Obertop H, Dirksen C, van der Elst D H, Ament A, van Erpecum K J, van Berge Henegouwen G P, Gouma D J 1995 Symptomatic gallbladder stones. Cost-effectiveness of treatment with extracorporeal shock-wave lithotripsy, conventional and laparoscopic cholecystectomy. Surgical Endoscopy 9(1): 37–41

Hellstern A, Leuschner M, Frenk H, Dillinger H W, Caspary W, Leuschner U 1990 Gall stone dissolution with methyl-tert-butyl ether: How to avoid complications. Gut 31: 922–925

Hruby W, Stackl W, Urbar M, Armbruster C, Manberger M 1989 Percutaneous endoscopic cholecystolithotripsy work in progress. Radiology 173: 477–479

Kerlan R K Jr, La Berge J M, Ring E J 1985 Percutaneous cholecystolithotomy: Preliminary experience. Radiology 157: 653–656

Lee M J, Saini S, Brink J, Zahn P F, Simeone J F, Morrison M C, Rattner D, Mueller P R 1991 Treatment of critically ill patients with sepsis of unknown cause: Value of percutaneous cholecystostomy. American Journal of Roentgenology 156: 1163–1166

McGahan J P, Lindfors K K 1988 Acute cholecystitis: Diagnostic accuracy of percutaneous aspiration of the gallbladder. Radiology 167: 669–671

McGahan J P, Lindfors K K 1989 Percutaneous cholecystostomy: an alternative to surgical cholecystostomy for acute cholecystitis? Radiology 173: 481–485

Miller F J, Rose S C, Buchi K N, Hunter J G, Nash J E, Kensey K R 1991 Percutaneous rotational contact biliary lithotripsy: Initial clinical results with the Kensey Nash lithotrite. Radiology 178: 781–785

Miller F J, Gordon R, Skolkin M, Cope S, Vogelzang R, Kopecky K 1991a Rotatory gallstone cholecystolithotripsy. Presented at the IV International Symposium on Biliary Stone Therapy, 2–4 October, Rochester, Minnesota, USA

Miller F J, Gordon R L, Cope C 1991b Rotary gallstone lithotripsy: Follow-up in 19 patients. In: Paumgartner G, Sauerbruch T, Sackmann M, Burhenne H J (eds) Lithotripsy and related techniques for gallstone treatment. Mosby Year Book, St. Louis, p 155–158

Mueller P R, Lee M J, Saini S, et al 1991 Percutaneous contact dissolution of gallstones: Complexity of radiologic care. Radiographics 11: 759–770

Norrby S, Schönebeck J 1970 Long-term results with cholecystolithotomy. Acta Chirurgica Scandinavica 136: 711–713

Pauletzki J, Sailer C, Kluppleberg U, von Ritter C, Neubrand M, Holl J, Sauerbruch T, Sackmann M, Paumgartner G 1994 Gallbladder emptying determines early gallstone clearance after shock wave lithotripsy. Gastroenterology 107: 1496–1502

Pearse D M, Hawkins, Shaver R, Vogel S 1984 Percutaneous cholecystostomy in acute cholecystitis and common bile duct obstruction. Radiology 152: 365–367

Picus D, Marx M V, Hicks M E, Lang E V, Edmundowicz S A 1989 Percutaneous cholecystolithotomy preliminary experience and technical considerations. Radiology 173: 487

Rawat B, Burhenne H J 1990 Extracorporeal shock-wave lithotripsy of calcified gallstones. Work in progress. Radiology 175: 667–670

Sackmann M, Ippisch E, Sauerbruch T, Holl J, Brendel W, Paumgartner G 1990 Early gallstone recurrence rate after successful shock-wave therapy. Gastroenterology 98: 392–396

Sackmann M, Pauletzki J, Sauerbruch T, Holl J, Schelling G, Paumgartner G 1991 The Munich Gallbladder Lithotripsy Study: Results of the first 5 years with 711 patients. Annals of Internal Medicine 114: 290–296

Sauerbruch T, Delius M, Paumgartner G, et al 1986 Fragmentation of gallstones by extracorporeal shock-waves. New England Journal of Medicine 314: 818–822

Sauerbruch T 1997 Extracorporeal shock wave lithotripsy. Digestion 58 (Suppl 1): 98–100

Skillings J C, Kumai C, Hinshaw J R. 1980 Cholecystostomy: A place in modern surgery? American Journal of Surgery 865–869

So D B, Gibney R G, Scudamore C H 1990 Carcinoma of the gallbladder: A risk associated with gallbladder preserving treatments for cholelithiasis. Radiology 174: 127

Teplick S K 1989 Diagnostic and therapeutic interventional gallbladder procedures. American Journal of Roentgenology 152: 913–916

Thistle JL, May GR, Bender CE et al 1989 Dissolution of cholesterol gallbladder stones by methyl-tert-butyl ether administered by percutaneous transhepatic catheter. New England Journal of Medicine 320: 633–639

Thistle J L 1991 Stone recurrence following MTBE dissolution. Presented at the IVth International Symposium on Biliary Stone Therapy. 2–4 October, Rochester, Minnesota, USA

vanSonnenberg E, Wing V W, Pollard J W, Casola G 1984 Life threatening vagal reactions associated with percutaneous cholecystostomy. Radiology 151: 377–380

vanSonnenberg E, Hofmann A F, Neoptolemus J, Wittich G R, Princenthal R A, Willson S W 1986 Gallstone dissolution with methyl-tert-butyl ether via percutaneous cholecystostomy: Success and caveats. American Journal of Roentgenology 146: 865–867

vanSonnenberg E, D'Agostino H B, Casola G 1991 Percutaneous treatment of gallbladder perforation and bile leakage. Radiology 178: 687–689

vanSonnenberg E, D'Agostino H, Goodacre B W, Sanchez R B, Casola G 1992 Percutaneous gallbladder puncture and cholecystostomy: Results, complications and caveats for safety. Radiology 183: 167–170

Vauthey J N, Martini M, Becker C D, Lerut J P, Gertsch P, Blumgart L H 1992 Percutaneous cholecystostomy for acute cholecystitis: Indications and limitations. Surgery, Gynecology and Obstetrics 176: 49–54

Villanova N, Bazzoli F, Taroni F et al 1989 Gallstone recurrence after successful oral bile acid treatment. A 12-year follow-up study and evaluation of long-term postdissolution treatment. Gastroenterology 97: 726–731

Vogelzang R L, Nemcek A A Jr 1988 Percutaneous cholecystostomy: diagnostic and therapeutic efficacy. Radiology 168: 29–34

The technique of cholecystectomy

The technique of cholecystectomy

37

P. GERTSCH

INTRODUCTION

Open cholecystectomy is increasingly performed only in the minority of cases where laparoscopic techniques do not allow a safe procedure. This might be recognized pre-operatively or during laparoscopy. In this situation, attempts at performing a laparoscopic operation might have obscured the anatomy by producing hematoma or even have resulted in an iatrogenic injury.

The revolutionary development of laparoscopic cholecystectomy has increased the trend, initiated earlier in open surgical techniques, of removing the gallbladder through smaller incisions (Dubois & Berthelot 1982, Moss 1986). Open cholecystectomy through a small incision has been compared with laparoscopic cholecystectomy and shown to give comparable results in terms of hospital stay and return to work in a prospective randomized study (Majeed et al 1996).

Basically two techniques are used to perform cholecystectomy: the retrograde technique, with initial dissection of the hilar structures of the gallbladder in Calot's triangle, and the anterograde or 'fundus down' technique where the gallbladder is first separated from the liver before the cystic duct and artery are transected. Retrograde cholecystectomy has been the technique used in most cases up to the advent of laparoscopic cholecystectomy, but the place of the anterograde technique is gaining in importance, since open cholecystectomy is now very frequently necessary in surgically difficult situations. In addition antegrade cholecystectomy has become routine for some authors using small incisions (Table 37.1).

INDICATIONS

The introduction of laparoscopic cholecystectomy has significantly influenced the treatment of patients with gallstones. This influence is detectable in both the outcome of cholecystectomy and the selection of patients. In a multivariate comparison of complications after laparoscopic and open cholecystectomy, the overall complication rate has been found distinctly lower after the laparoscopic approach (Jatzko et al 1995). An increase by 20 to 30% in the total number of cholecystectomies performed has been observed (Schweisinger & Diehl 1996), and this increase was restricted to patients with uncomplicated cholelithiasis and to those undergoing elective surgery (Shea et al 1998).

Table 37.1 Techniques of minilaparotomy cholecystectomy

Author and year	Muscle sparing incision	Standing side of surgeon	'Fundus down' technique	Special instruments
Pelissier 1990	Yes	Left	Yes	Front lamp
Tyagi et al 1994	Yes	Left	No	Laser, front lamp endoscopic instruments
McGinn et al 1995	No		Yes	No
Clezy 1996	Yes	Right	Yes	No
Majeed et al 1996	No		No	No
Assalia et al 1997			Yes	Front lamp

The decision to operate or not is based on the choice between operative risk and the danger of spontaneous progression of the disease. The lower complication rate of laparoscopic cholecystectomy compared to open cholecystectomy has not been sufficient to induce a detectable change in the well established indications for cholecystectomy. It is more likely that considerations such as postoperative discomfort, esthetic damage (abdominal scar), earlier return to work has made the procedure more acceptable to patients with minor symptoms.

Cholecystectomy is usually performed for symptomatic cholecystolithiasis and for related complications. Cholecystectomy for acalculous cholecystitis, adenomyomatosis or gallbladder carcinoma is less frequent. Asymptomatic cholecystolithiasis has been considered as an indication for cholecystectomy in diabetes or immunocompromised patients but this indication has remained controversial (Schweisinger & Diehl 1996).

There are two important areas where improvement in diagnosis is necessary. First, patients with right upper quadrant abdominal pain may have symptoms unrelated to the presence of stones in the gallbladder. Thus post-cholecystectomy pain, which has been observed in up to 30% of cases, may be the consequence of an operation performed for symptoms unrelated to the presence of gallstones (Ch. 43) (Bodvall & Overgaard 1967). Secondly and by contrast, patients with characteristic symptoms but with absence of stones in the gallbladder and who may be cured by a cholecystectomy have been identified (Lennard et al 1984, Rhodes et al 1988) and improvement in selection of cases for operation is necessary.

PREOPERATIVE ASSESSMENT

Some clinical features should alert the surgeon to possible operative difficulties. Repeated and prolonged attacks of biliary pain might be associated with chronic inflammation and dense adhesions or fibrous obliteration of Calot's triangle. Liver function tests should be performed systematically before cholecystectomy. Any abnormality (elevation of the serum bilirubin or alkaline phosphatase levels) requires serious attention, since the change may not be caused by the presence of stones in the bile duct, but may be an index of other extrahepatic biliary tract disease. Diagnoses such as the Mirizzi syndrome, tumor of the gallbladder or of the bile duct, choledochus cyst, sclerosing cholangitis are all possibilities. Although patients submitted to cholecystectomy will usually have undergone ultrasonography, more

detailed investigations should be performed if there is any doubt as to the integrity of the bile duct. Endoscopic retrograde cholangiography (Ch. 17) or MR cholangiography (Ch. 16) will usually allow identification of stones or other abnormalities.

Patients presenting with cirrhosis and portal hypertension, may also have symptoms unrelated to the presence of stones in the gallbladder. Cholecystectomy in this context represents a considerable risk of hemorrhage (Bornman & Terblanche 1985). Antibiotic prophylaxis is employed, a single dose being given at the time of anesthetic premedication.

Preoperative assessment may orientate the operation towards the laparoscopic or the open techniques. Apart from complicated cases where intraoperative difficulties can be anticipated, a suspicion of tumor of the gallbladder is a contraindication for the laparoscopic approach (Ch. 53). Port site recurrences have been reported in a significant number of cases. In a survey of 10 925 laparoscopic cholecystectomies, gallbladder carcinoma was observed in 37 cases. The port site recurrence rate of 14% was independent of the stage of the tumor but increased to 40% with intraoperative perforation of the gallbladder (Z'graggen et al 1998). Perforation of the gallbladder is frequent during laparoscopic cholecystectomy and may compromise the result of a subsequent curative operation.

THE OPERATION

A perfect knowledge of the anatomy of the bile ducts and of the possible variations (see Ch. 1) is necessary to perform safe cholecystecomy. Unidentified anatomical anomalies during operation often result in iatrogenic lesions of the bile duct. Therefore precise intraoperative identification of the anatomy is necessary before dividing or ligating any structure.

ANATOMY

The normal localization of the neck of the gallbladder and the cystic duct is between the peritoneal surfaces within the right anterior part of the hepatoduodenal ligament. The cystic artery runs transversely, forming with the cystic duct and bile duct the triangle described by Calot in 1891. The triangle of cholecystectomy (often misnamed as Calot's triangle) has for its upper limit not the cystic artery but the inferior surface of the liver (Rocko et al 1981). Dissection of this area should clearly demonstrate the anatomical structures and allow safe dissection (Fig. 37.1).

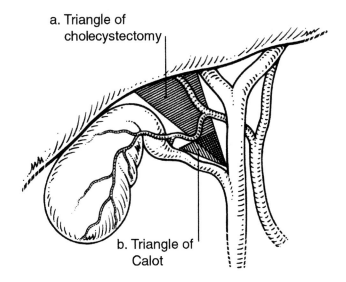

Fig. 37.1 (a) Triangle of cholecystectomy limited by the common hepatic duct and right hepatic duct, cystic duct and the liver. (b) Calot's triangle limited by the common hepatic duct, cystic duct and cystic artery.

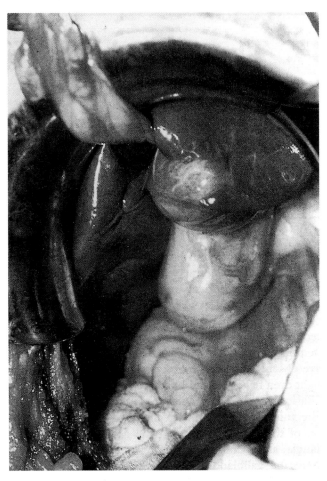

Fig. 37.2 Gallbladder located on the left side of the umbilical fissure and the ligament teres, attached to segment III of the liver.

A variety of abnormalities can alter the normal anatomy of the gallbladder. Bilobation and septa are usually not relevant. Duplication of the gallbladder is rare, and might be associated with one or two cystic ducts. Agenesis is extremely rare, and the apparent absence of a gallbladder is most frequently related to an intrahepatic location; in such cases, the infundibulum is usually extrahepatic. The gallbladder may be lying on the left side of a right-sided round ligament, being thus attached to the right lobe of the liver; in rarer instances the gallbladder has been observed attached to the left lobe of the liver, on the left side of the round ligament (Fig. 37.2) (Fujita et al 1998).

The junction between the cystic and common bile duct has many variations (Figs 37.3 & 37.4; see Ch. 1). The cystic duct may join the right side of the common bile duct after a parallel course, or it may be very short and almost non-existent. An apparently short cystic duct might, in reality, be a long duct fused and running parallel to the choledochus or it may be connected to the right hepatic duct. The cystic duct may also join the left side of the choledochus, having crossed it anteriorly or posteriorly. The cystic duct may on occasion be contracted as a result of a chronic inflammatory process such as seen in the Mirizzi syndrome.

An unappreciated abnormal confluence of the hepatic ducts probably represents the most important source of error leading to damage to the biliary tract during cholecystectomy. These variations may involve a direct hepatocystic ductal junction or a sectoral duct joining the choledochus just above or below the cystic duct. An abnormal confluence of the hepatic ducts has been reported in up to 43% of cases and a low junction with a right sectoral duct in 20% of cases (Fig. 37.4) (Couinaud 1957, Puente & Bannuva 1983, Champetrier et al 1989).

Abnormalities of the anatomy of the cystic artery are also frequent, and the right branch of the hepatic artery may inadvertently be transected if not identified. An origin of the right hepatic artery from the superior mesenteric artery results in passage of the vessel postero-laterally to the common bile duct and behind the cystic duct where it may be vulnerable (Ch. 1). Although the necessity to perform systematically an *intra-operative cholangiography* is still debated (Pernthaler 1990), the routine use of this procedure is advocated by most surgeons. Besides demonstrating unidentified stones or pathology in the intra- or extrahepatic bile ducts, intraoperative cholangiography provides a precise view of the anatomy of the biliary ductal system. This may help in avoiding operative errors resulting in biliary injury. Thus, a review of 78 post-cholecystectomy strictures has revealed that in only 29% of these was intra-operative cholangiography performed (Kelley & Blumgart 1985). Good technique is important and is detailed in Chapter 22.

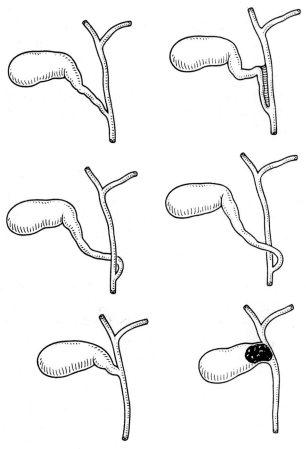

Fig. 37.3 Different modes of confluence of the cystic duct and common hepatic duct.

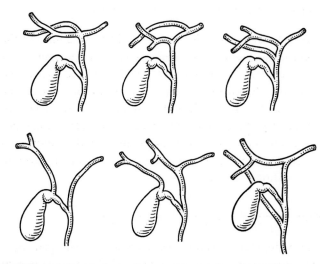

Fig. 37.4 Variations in the confluence of the extrahepatic bile ducts and cystic duct.

TECHNIQUE

Dissection must be performed close to the wall of the gall-bladder, particularly in the region of the infundibulum and cystic duct. The cystic artery may be identified and safely ligated only when its relation with the gallbladder has clearly been demonstrated.

The retrograde technique which involves initial dissection of the hilar structures of the gallbladder and of the chole-cystectomy triangle should be chosen when there is clear visualization of its anatomical limits. Whenever the features in this region are not perfectly clear as a result of acute or chronic inflammation, the anterograde or 'fundus down' technique is generally considered safer since initial dissection of the gallbladder from the fundus allows progressive demonstration of the anatomy down to the infundibulo-cystic junction. The basic principles of dissecting close to the gallbladder and demonstrating clearly any structure before ligature or section is performed must be respected.

THE INCISION

Different types of incisions may give access to the gallblad-der. The surgeon usually stands to the right of the patient. A right subcostal incision is usually performed and provides direct and good access. A midline incision also provides good exposure. Transrectal incisions have also been used.

The trend of 'minimally' invasive surgery has resulted in the description of shorter incisions which are justified only when access to perform a safe procedure is obtained, and when intra-operative assessment of the other intra-abdomi-nal structures is not necessary. In general few details have been given on the technical aspects of minilaparotomy cholecystectomies (Table 37.1). Ultrasonographic localiza-tion of the gallbladder may help to determine the site of inci-sion (Assalia et al 1997) whose size may vary between 2.5 and 10 cm having also been described as 'minimum neces-sary' and 'tailored to the individual patient' (Majeed et al 1996). The incision may be a small right subcostal incision or a right transverse incision, with section of the rectus muscle, thus corresponding to a classical but smaller incision.

Alternatively the small size of the incision may be exploited to reduce the trauma to the abdominal wall and the pain by muscle sparing approaches. Two important ele-ments have been taken into account in defining these inci-sions. Firstly, it is important that the incision gives good access more to the Calot's triangle (in the right paramedian region at the level of the 12th thoracic vertebra) than to the fundus of the gallbladder that can be mobilized by traction into the operative field. Secondly, an incision in the

'Minimal Stress Triangle' should result in less operative pain because the abdominal wall is less subject to tension and movements at this level during ventilatory and other movements (Tyagi et al 1994). The Minimal Stress Triangle is located in the subxiphoid area. It has for its base a horizontal line joining both the bilateral eighth chondrocostal cartilages and for vertex the xiphoid process. Calot's triangle lies within the boundaries of this triangle. The technique of microceliotomy described by Tyagi uses this approach with a 3 cm transverse skin incision located on the right of the midline at the level of the baseline of the Minimal Stress Triangle with corresponding vertical incision of the anterior and posterior rectus sheath 1 cm lateral to the linea alba for approximately 5 cm in length extending inferiorly from the xiphoid process. This incision involves lateral retraction of the rectus muscle and incision of the peritoneum through the falciform ligament. Pelissier (1990) described a 6 cm transverse incision in the epigastrium centered on the midline, 8 cm below the xiphoid process with transverse section of the linea alba extending slightly to the anterior sheath of both rectus muscles right and left; lateral retraction of the rectus muscles allowed limited incision of the posterior sheaths of both muscles. Section of the round ligament and retraction of the extremities upwards and downwards give direct access to Calot's triangle. Clezy (1996) described a horizontal incision at the same level but on the right side with incision of the anterior sheath of rectus muscle and, after simple medial retraction of the muscle, incision of the posterior sheath allowing access to Calot's triangle.

The advantages of performing a cholecystectomy through a minimal incision remain controversial. Prospective randomized studies showed on one side no clear advantage of small incision cholecystectomy over conventional cholecystectomy for elective operations (Schmitz et al 1997) but on the other less postoperative pain, shorter hospital stay and earlier return to full activities for emergency cholecystectomy (Assalia et al 1997).

EXPOSURE OF THE OPERATIVE FIELD AND INITIAL ASSESSMENT

The inferior aspect of the liver is normally accessible without dissection, but adhesions are often present and must be freed. Such adhesions may be dense and inflammatory, obscuring the anatomy of the region. Dissection should be performed close to the gallbladder, keeping in mind that a cholecystocolic or cholecystoduodenal fistula might be present. In this case, the fistula must be transected to expose the gallbladder. The opening in the colon or duodenum is subsequently sutured. If the gallbladder cannot be identified, one should suspect that it is scarred and contracted or that it is located within the liver. It might be safe in such a situation to identify first the distal bile duct and dissect it from below until the infundibulum of the gallbladder or cystic duct is encountered. Intraoperative ultrasound examination (see Ch. 13) may be useful.

Palpation of the intra-abdominal organs should be performed whenever possible, with special emphasis on the liver, hepatoduodenal ligament and pancreas. The gallbladder must be gently palpated and not emptied by compression even if stones are not detected because, first their presence has already been demonstrated by pre-operative investigations and, secondly, manual compression of the gallbladder may result in migration of small stones into the common bile duct.

PLACEMENT OF RETRACTORS AND EXPOSURE

A retractor should be placed in the upper right part of the wound, whatever the form of the incision. It can be held by an assistant, but it is usually better to have it fixed to the operating table as this not only spares a hand, but also provides steady, constant retraction.

Another retractor is necessary to rotate the inferior aspect of the liver cephalad and expose the infrahepatic region. A right-angle or Deever retractor is usually held by an assistant, who must take care not to tear the liver capsule. Abdominal pads will help to expose and isolate the operative field. The most important of these retractors is placed on the duodenum and transverse colon. A retractor, or the assistant's hand, by pulling downwards, provides a gentle traction on the hepatoduodenal ligament. Two other abdominal pads may be placed medially and laterally to isolate the infra-hepatic region.

EMPTYING OF THE GALLBLADDER

The dissection is usually eased by a slight distention of the gallbladder, and for this reason puncture of the gallbladder and aspiration of its content should not be performed systematically. Gross distention may, however, obscure the cholecystectomy triangle and grasping of a distended gallbladder with a forceps might be impossible. One should not hesitate in these circumstances to puncture the fundus and aspirate bile; bile culture is indicated, and is mandatory in cholecystitis or cholangitis.

RETROGRADE CHOLECYSTECTOMY

The peritoneum covering the hepatoduodenal ligament is incised anteriorly across the region of Hartmann's pouch; this incision is pursued posteriorly in the same way, giving easy access to the infundibulum of the gallbladder. A Duval or similar forceps is placed at the fundus of the gallbladder in the region of Hartmann's pouch (Fig. 37.5A) and dissection of the cholecystectomy triangle is commenced. It is important to keep close contact with the gallbladder and to demonstrate the junction between the gallbladder and the cystic duct. The lower limit of the triangle is the cystic duct and a ligature is passed around it but not tied. Slight tension produced by a clamp hanging on this ligature might prevent migration of stones from the gallbladder into the cystic duct. The cystic artery is normally above the cystic duct; it is important to dissect it towards the gallbladder to see its final distribution into the gallbladder wall (Fig. 37.5B). This is the best way to prevent ligature of an aberrant right hepatic artery. At this stage, the junction of the gallbladder infundibulum with the cystic duct and the distribution of the cystic artery into the gallbladder wall is clearly demonstrated. The cystic duct is palpated to detect stones which could, at this stage, be pushed back into the gallbladder (Fig. 37.6). The cystic artery can be ligated and transected (Fig. 37.7).

A ligature or a clamp is placed at the junction of the gallbladder and the cystic duct which is opened transversely 3 mm distally. A suitable canula for cholangiography is gently inserted into the cystic duct, taking care not to tear it (Fig. 37.8). If an obstacle is encountered, and if the presence of a stone has been excluded by palpation, a valve or tortuous cystic duct is probably the cause. It is useful in this event to insert the end of a long, fine clamp into the cystic duct and to dilate it gently. This usually allows easy subsequent placement of the canula.

A variety of canulae are described; the author prefers a

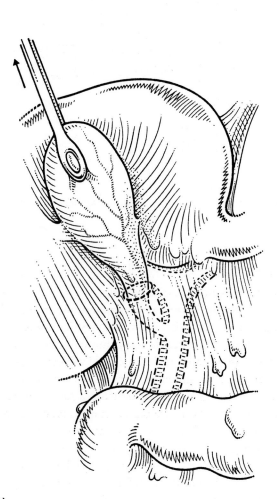

(A)

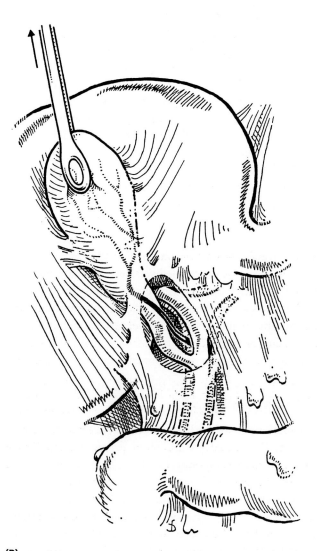

(B)

Fig. 37.5 The gallbladder is seized with a clamp and dissection of the cholecystectomy triangle started. The cystic artery is in its normal position, above the cystic duct.

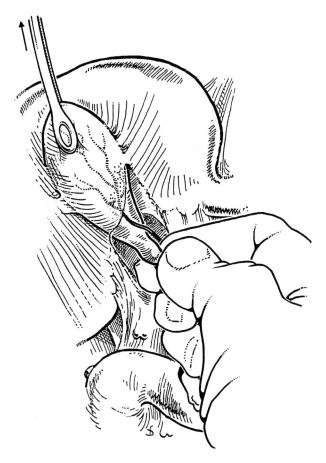

Fig. 37.6 Palpation reveals a stone in the cystic duct, which may be 'milked' back into the gallbladder.

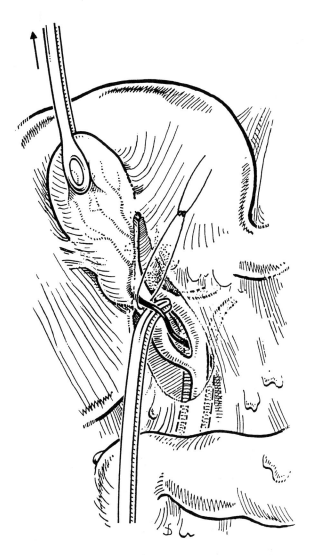

Fig. 37.7 The cystic artery is ligated close to the gallbladder wall.

transparent polyethylene catheter which allows easy identification and removal of air bubbles before insertion. This catheter is fixed by tying the ligature previously passed around the cystic duct. Cholangiography is performed using the technique of Bolton & Le Quesne (1980). All instruments and retractors are removed, and the patient is slightly rotated to the right (20 degrees) before contrast medium is injected. It is important to inject initially a small quantity (1–2 cc) of the contrast agent in order to be able to identify small stones in the bile duct. The ductal system of the biliary tract should be fully displayed, and fluoroscopy is valuable in this regard. Two or three films are taken. Whilst awaiting the cholangiograms, the cystic duct may be divided, leaving the catheter in place; the gallbladder is then dissected from its fossa either by sharp dissection or diathermy, with the help of gentle traction or, on occasions, finger dissection. The dissection should be kept close to the gallbladder, within the cystic plate (see Ch. 1), in order to avoid damage to the liver parenchyma, which may nevertheless occur in cases of chronic cholecystitis. In cases of acute cholecystitis with considerable edema, this plane is best found by sharp dissection using scissors.

There may occasionally be small bile ducts connecting the gallbladder to the intra-hepatic bile ducts. Transection of these is without consequence when the biliary tree is not obstructed. Hemostasis of the gallbladder fossa does not pose any problem. If available the argon beam coagulator is of value. However if the liver parenchyma has been lacerated, a gauze pack should be placed in the gallbladder bed and held in place with a retractor for at least 5 minutes. If the hemorrhage is not controlled, deep hemostatic sutures should be placed. Formal closure of the gallbladder bed is probably more harmful than useful in favoring postoperative local fluid collection.

The gallbladder should then be opened and checked for the presence of tumors. Inspection of stones may help to

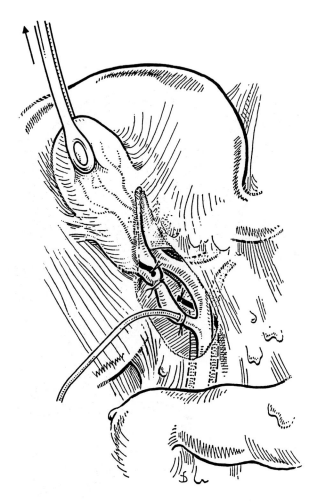

Fig. 37.8 The cystic duct is ligated at its junction with the gallbladder, and a catheter has been inserted for intra-operative cholangiography.

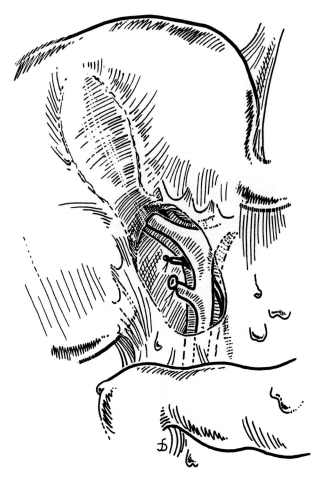

Fig. 37.9 The catheter is removed and the cystic duct suture ligated. The cholecystectomy is now complete.

interpret the cholangiograms, which are then assessed according to the criteria of Bolton & Le Quesne (1980). If there is any doubt as to the presence of stones or the normality of the bile duct, a further set of films should be obtained, especially if the initial cholangiograms were of poor quality.

The anatomy of the intra-hepatic bile ducts may be obscured by incomplete proximal filling because of early passage of contrast agent through the papilla. Low clamping of the hepatoduodenal ligament with an intestinal clamp may give better images if the cystic duct joins the hepatic duct above the clamp. A leak may be detected, and its origin should be identified. In most cases, it will originate from the gallbladder bed and may then be secured by a suture.

A small leak will be without consequence and will close spontaneously within a few days if there is no obstruction of the distal bile duct. The cholangiography catheter is then removed and the cystic duct suture-ligated, using resorbable suture material (Fig. 37.9). The insertion of a drain before closing the abdominal wall is controversial, and in most

cases is unnecessary. If a small bile leak is identified, insertion of a drain positioned close to the gallbladder bed will prevent collection of bile. Usually only 50 cc of hemoserous fluid will drain during the first 24 hours after which the drain may be removed; however, the drain should be retained if there is excessive oozing or leakage of bile.

ANTEROGRADE OR 'FUNDUS DOWN' CHOLECYSTECTOMY

An incision of the gallbladder serosa is performed 0.5 cm from the liver edge, and a plane is developed between the serosa and the gallbladder wall by sharp dissection, so as to allow entry to the cystic plate (see Ch. 1). The gallbladder is still vascularized via the cystic artery (Fig. 37.10). In the region of the infundibulum, the cystic artery is seen to enter the gallbladder wall (Fig. 37.11). After ligature and section of the cystic artery close to the gallbladder wall, the infundibulum is dissected free down to the junction with the cystic duct. This technique may cause migration of

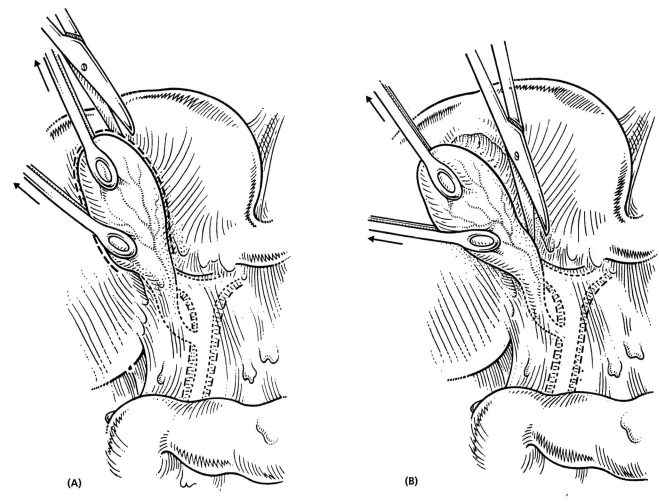

Fig. 37.10 (A) Anterograde of 'fundus down' cholecystectomy; the serosa of the gallbladder is incised 5 mm from the liver around the fundus. **(B)** A plane is developed between the serosa of the gallbladder and the gallbladder wall, and then between the liver and the gallbladder in the cystic plate, by sharp dissection.

stones from the gallbladder into the cystic duct but careful palpation could identify these stones after the cystic duct has been isolated. Not more than 0.5 to 1 cm of cystic duct should be dissected. Cholangiography and cystic duct ligature are performed in the same way as described for the retrograde technique.

CHOLECYSTECTOMY THROUGH SMALL INCISIONS

There is no fundamental difference with the above described techniques (Table 37.1). Some authors prefer operating from the left side of the patient. Smaller retractors are adequate and additional light (front lamp, light retractor, light suction) may be useful. Anterograde cholecystectomy is performed by some authors. The use of clips for

controlling the cystic artery and the cystic duct may be safer than awkward tying through a small incision.

PARTIAL CHOLECYSTECTOMY

Cholecystectomy may be hazardous when only the fundus of the gallbladder can be recognized and when the region of the infundibulum cannot be delineated because of fibrosis and inflammation obscuring the triangle of Calot (Fig. 37.12). It is then judicious to open the fundus and to introduce a finger into the gallbladder in order to guide the dissection (Fig. 37.13A). Impacted stones should be removed.

If no bile appears, the cystic duct is probably occluded by fibrosis and inflammation. A partial cholecystectomy is the safest procedure in this situation. The use of this technique has also been advocated in case of severe portal hypertension

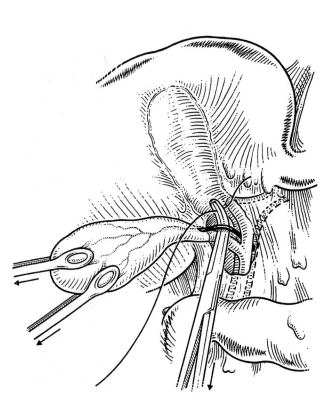

Fig. 37.11 As the anterograde dissection progresses towards the gallbladder neck, the cystic artery is identified, ligated and divided.

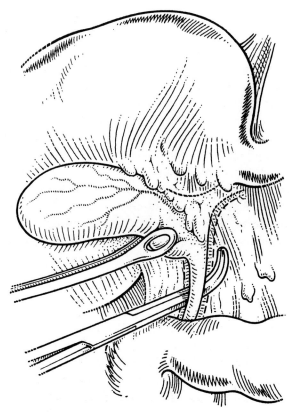

Fig. 37.12 The common hepatic duct can be mistaken for the cystic duct when the region of the infundibulum cannot be delineated because of fibrosis and inflammation.

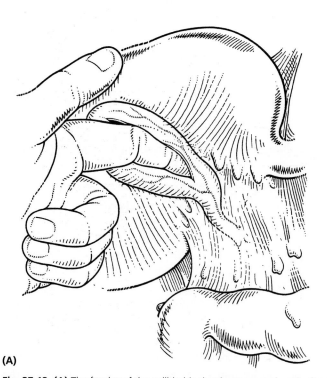

(A)

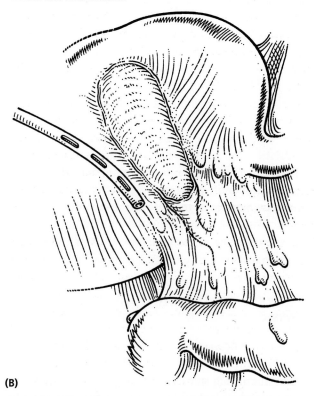

(B)

Fig. 37.13 (A) The fundus of the gallbladder has been opened, and a finger introduced into the gallbladder for palpation. **(B)** Partial cholecystectomy. The superficial part of the fundus and body of the gallbladder has been excised, leaving in place its attachment to the liver and the infundibulum. The remaining mucosa is removed by curettage and electrocoagulation and a drain placed near the infundibulum.

(Bornman & Terblanche 1985, Cottier et al 1991). The anterior visible wall of the gallbladder is excised, but the posterior wall in contact with the liver is left in place down to the region of the infundibulum. The mucosa is removed by curettage and electrocoagulation, and a drain is placed in the region of the infundibulum (Fig. 37.13B). No attempt at ligating the cystic duct should be made when the region is severely altered by inflammation. If a gush of bile appears when a big impacted stone is removed from the infundibulum, a cholecystocholedochal fistula is probably present (Mirizzi syndrome type II). It is then advisable to keep the opened distal part of the gallbladder intact to allow a cholecystoduodenostomy or a cholecystojejunostomy (Ch. 49). Attempted direct repair of the fistula is hazardous (Baer et al 1990).

INTRAOPERATIVE PROBLEMS

Intra-operative problems have been related to three main causes, namely dangerous surgery, dangerous anatomy and dangerous pathology (Johnston 1986; see Ch. 49). Insufficient preoperative assessment of a complicated situation is certainly another avoidable reason of intra-operative difficulties.

Dangerous surgery arises from inadequate or imprecise observation of the technical principles of cholecystectomy, insufficient experience, inadequate incision and exposure, or inadequate assistance (Smith 1979, Andren-Sandberg et al 1985). Some of the anatomical variations which have previously been mentioned are particularly dangerous and, in particular, a narrow common bile duct can be mistaken for the cystic duct (see Ch. 49).

Dangerous pathology includes chronic or acute inflammation which results in obscured anatomy and increased vascularity in the region of the cholecystectomy triangle (Fig. 37.12). Portal hypertension is associated with increased venous collateralization which makes the dissection hemorrhagic and dangerous. Partial cholecystectomy has been advocated in both situations (Bornman & Terblanche 1985, Cottier et al 1991).

Hemorrhage in the cholecystectomy triangle represents potential danger since attempts at hemostasis by placing clamps with obstructed and insufficient view may result in inadvertent clamping of the right or common hepatic artery, or of the bile duct (Fig. 37.14). In this situation, one should first attempt to control the hemorrhage by digital compression or by clamping the hepato-duodenal ligament (Fig. 37.15) in order to localize its precise origin.

Grasping the bleeding vessel should be done with precision so as to limit the risks of including another structure in the ligature. Cholangiography, even if already performed, may be repeated and carefully analyzed after hemostasis, as

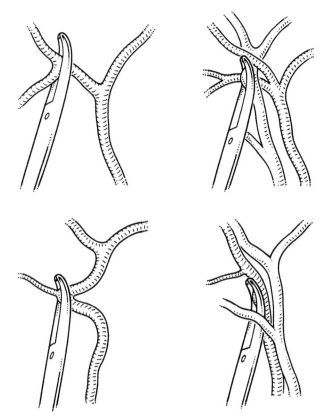

Fig. 37.14 Blind placement of clamps for hemostasis can result in lesions of the hepatic artery or bile duct.

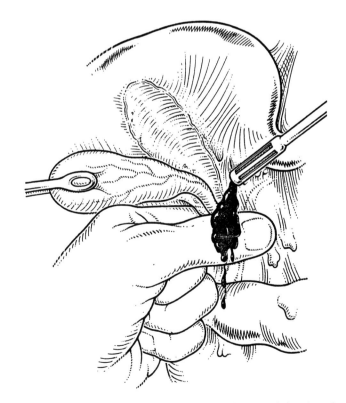

Fig. 37.15 Hemorrhage should first be controlled by manual clamping of the hepatoduodenal ligament until better view is obtained, making precise hemostasis possible.

it may reveal an iatrogenic lesion of the bile duct (leak, incomplete or complete occlusion).

Methods to deal with a fresh recognized iatrogenic lesion of the bile duct are discussed in Chapter 49.

REFERENCES

Andren-Sandberg A, Alinder G, Bengmark S 1985 Accidental lesions of the common bile duct at cholecystectomy. Pre and perioperative factors of importance. Annals of Surgery 201: 328–332

Assalia A, Kopelman D, Hashmonai M 1997 Emergency minilaparotomy cholecystectomy for acute cholecystitis: prospective randomized trial—implications for the laparoscopic era. World Journal of Surgery 21: 534–539

Baer H U, Natthews J B, Schweizer W P, Gertsch P, Blumgart L H 1990 Management of the Mirizzi syndrome and surgical implications of the cholecystocholedochal fistula. British Journal of Surgery 77: 743–745

Bodvall B, Overgaard B 1967 Computer analysis of postcholecystectomy biliary tract symptoms. Surgery, Gynecology & Obstetrics 124: 723–732

Bolton J P, Le Quesne L P 1980 Choledocholithiasis: Incidence, diagnosis and operative procedures. In: Maingot R Abdominal operation 9th edn. Appleton-Century-Crofts, New York, ch 66, p 1431–1450.

Bornman P C, Terblanche J 1985 Subtotal cholecystectomy: for difficult gallbladder in portal hypertension and cholecystitis. Surgery 98: 1–6

Champetrier J, Letoublon C, Arvieux C, Gerard P, Labrosse P A 1989 Les variations de division des voies biliaires extra-hepatiques: Signification et origine, conséquences chirurgicales. Journal de Chirurgie 126: 147–154

Clezy J K A 1996 Randomized trial of laparoscopic cholecystectomy and mini-cholecystectomy. Letter. British Journal of Surgery 83: 279

Cottier D J, McKay C, Anderson J R 1991 Subtotal cholecystectomy. British Journal of Surgery 78: 1326–1328

Couinaud C 1957 Le foie. Etudes anatomiques et chirurgicales. Vol 1. Masson, Paris

Dubois F, Berthelot B 1982 Cholecystectomie par mini-laparotomie. Nouvelle presse médicale 11: 1139–1141

Fujita N, Shirai Y, Kawaguschi H, Tsudaka K, Hatakeyama H 1998 Left-sided gallbladder on the basis of a right-sided round ligament. Hepatogastroenterology 45: 1482–1484.

Jatzko G R, Lisborg P H, Perti A M, Stettner H M 1995 Multivariate comparison of complications after laparoscopic cholecystectomy and open cholecystectomy. Annals of Surgery 221: 381–386

Johnston J W 1986 Iatrogenic bile duct stricture: an avoidable surgical hazard? British Journal of Surgery 73: 245–247

Kelly C J, Blumgart L H 1985 Per-operative cholangiography and post-cholecystectomy biliary stricture. Annals of the Royal College of Surgeons of England 67: 93–95

Lennard T W, Farndon J R, Taylor R M 1984 Acalculous biliary pain: diagnosis and selection for cholecystectomy using the cholecystokinin test for pain reproduction. British Journal of Surgery 71: 368–370

Majeed A W, Troy G, Smythe A, Reed M W R, Stoddard C J, Peacock J, Johnson A G 1996 Randomized, prospective, single-blind comparison of laparoscopic versus small-incision cholecystectomy. The Lancet 347: 989–994

McGinn F P, Miles A J G, Uglow M, Ozmen M, Terzi C, Humby M 1995 Randomized trial of laparoscopic cholecystectomy and mini cholecystectomy. British Journal of Surgery 82: 1374–1377

Moss G 1986 Discharge within 24 hours of elective cholecystectomy. Archives of Surgery 121: 1159–1161

Pelissier E P 1990 Une technique de cholecystectomie par minilaparotomie sans section musculaire. Annales de Chirurgie 44: 521–523

Pernthaler H, Sandbichler P, Schmied Th, Margreiter R 1990 Operative cholangiography in elective cholecystectomy. British Journal of Surgery 77: 399–400

Puente S G, Bannuva G C 1983 Radiological anatomy of the biliary tract: variations and congenital abnormalities. World Journal of Surgery 7: 271–276

Rhodes M, Lennard T W, Farndon J R, Taylor R M 1988 Cholecystokinin provocation test. Long-term follow-up after cholecystectomy. British Journal of Surgery 75: 951–953

Rocko J M, Swan K G, Di Gioia J M 1981 Callot's triangle revisited. Surgery, Gynecology & Obstetrics 153: 410–414

Schmitz R, Rhode V, Treckmann J, Shah S 1997 Randomized clinical trial of conventional cholecystectomy versus minicholecystectomy. British Journal of Surgery 84: 1683–1686

Schweisinger W H, Diehl A K 1996 Changing indications for laparoscopic cholecystectomy. Surgical Clinics of North America 76: 493–504

Shea J A, Berlin J A, Bachwich D R, Staroscik R N, Malet P F, McGuckin M, Schwartz J S, Escarce J J 1998 Indications for and outcomes of cholecystectomy. Annals of Surgery 227: 343–350

Smith R 1979 Obstruction of the bile duct. British Journal of Surgery 66: 69–79

Tyagi N S, Meredith M C, Lumb J C, Cacolac R G, Vanterpool C C, Rayls K R, Zerega W D, Silbergelit A 1994 A new minimally invasive technique for cholecystectomy. Annals of Surgery 220: 617–625

Z'graggen K, Birrer S, Maurer C A, Wehrli H, Klaiber C, Baer H U 1998 Incidence of port site recurrence after laparoscopic cholecystectomy for preoperatively unsuspected gallbladder carcinoma. Surgery 124: 831–838.

38

Laparoscopic cholecystectomy and choledocholithotomy

R.A. UNDERWOOD, N.J. SOPER

INTRODUCTION

First described in 1882 by Langenbuch, open cholecystectomy (OC) has been the primary treatment of gallstone disease for most of the past century (Beal 1984). However, the prevailing public perception of this operation as one that resulted in pain, disability, and a disfiguring scar engendered many attempts over the past two decades at nonoperative treatment of gallstones (Schoenfield & Lachin 1981, Schoenfield et al 1990). Despite successful removal or dissolution of gallstones with some of these techniques, each is limited by the persistence of a diseased gallbladder. In 1985, the first laparoscopically assisted cholecystectomy was performed by Mühe of Böblingen, Germany. Although meeting early skepticism from the academic surgical community, laparoscopic cholecystectomy was adopted rapidly around the world, and has subsequently been recognized as the new 'gold standard' for the treatment of gallstone disease (Soper et al 1992, 1994). By 1992, an estimated 80% of cholecystectomies in the United States were performed laparoscopically and an NIH Consensus Development Conference stated that laparoscopic cholecystectomy (LC) 'provides a safe and effective treatment for most patients with symptomatic gallstones. Indeed it appears to have become the procedure of choice for many of these patients' (Conference NC, 1992).

More than 600 000 cholecystectomies are performed annually in the United States, the majority of which are performed laparoscopically (Soper et al 1994). The advantages of LC over OC were immediately appreciated: earlier return of bowel function, less postoperative pain, improved cosmesis, shorter length of hospital stay, earlier return to full activity, and decreased overall cost (Barkun et al 1992, Bass et al 1993, McMahon et al 1994, Soper 1991, Soper et al 1992). There has been an increase in the rate of cholecystectomies subsequent to the introduction of LC accompanied by evidence of lower clinical thresholds for operative therapy of gallstones (Escarce et al 1995, Nenner et al 1994). Indeed, LC as a now mature mode of therapy has introduced the general surgical world to the revolutionary advantages and unique perspectives and concerns of minimal access surgery (Wu et al 1998). Based on our experience and that of others, this chapter will provide an overview of the operative technique and current status of laparoscopic cholecystectomy and laparoscopic management of common bile duct (CBD) stones.

HISTORY

The rapid acceptance of LC as the primary procedure for removal of the gallbladder has led general surgeons to embrace minimal access surgical techniques, yet closed cavity endoscopic techniques have been investigated since the early twentieth century with early proof of applicability established by gynecologists and urologists. Laparoscopy (from the Greek *laparo*, the flank, and *skopein*, to examine) was first performed in 1901 by George Kelling of Dresden, Germany, using room air filtered through sterile cotton for pneumoperitoneum and a Nitze cystoscope to view the abdominal cavity of a dog. Kelling named the procedure *Kölioskopie* and described it in a report published in *Münchener Medizinische Wochenschrift* in January 1902. Interestingly, as a correlate to current health care motivations, Kelling later reported that his use of the laparoscope had rapidly escalated in the postwar period secondary to the sparse economic resources in Germany. His reasons were basic—smaller incisions, more rapid recovery, and shorter, less costly hospital stays (Kelling 1923, Underwood 1997). Eight years later in the same publication, Jacobeus of

Stockholm, Sweden reported the first clinical application of laparoscopy and thoracoscopy, describing the laparoscopic diagnosis of intra-abdominal tuberculosis, cirrhosis, syphilis, and malignancy. Unlike Kelling, Jacobeus introduced a trocar for the cystoscope directly through the abdominal wall prior to establishing the pneumoperitoneum. Within a year, Jacobeus performed more than 100 procedures with only one major complication (bleeding) requiring open exploration (Jacobeus 1911). Over the next two decades, various gases were used to insufflate the abdomen and create a working space. The use of carbon dioxide (CO_2) for pneumoperitoneum was first recommended by Richard Zollikofer of Switzerland in 1924. As opposed to room air, CO_2 inhibits combustion and is rapidly absorbed postoperatively by the peritoneum. The primary mode for insufflation was the Veress needle which was introduced by Janos Veress of Hungary in 1938. This device incorporates a spring-loaded blunt obturator at its tip, which protects the internal viscera from the sharp needle tip once it has penetrated the fascia and peritoneum. This device was originally intended to produce therapeutic pneumothorax in patients with tuberculosis; however, it quickly found favor among laparoscopists and today is still used as the primary means to create the pneumoperitoneum for laparoscopy in many institutions (Veress 1938).

In 1929, the German hepatologist Kalk described a dual trocar laparoscopic technique for liver biopsy. He subsequently went on to develop many laparoscopic operating instruments. This expanded the role of laparoscopy from being strictly diagnostic to allowing therapeutic procedures (Kalk 1929). In 1933, a German general surgeon, Fervers, was the first to report laparoscopic lysis of abdominal adhesions for the diagnosis of bowel obstruction (Fervers 1933). However, laparoscopy remained in virtual obscurity until the 1960s when gynecologists such as Patrick Steptoe popularized laparoscopic tubal ligation (Steptoe 1967) which became accepted in England and caused a renewal of interest in laparoscopy worldwide. Meanwhile the German gynecologist and engineer Kurt Semm incorporated new aspects of fiber optics and used an automatic gas insufflator which allowed precisely controlled intra-abdominal pressure, greatly reducing the incidence of adverse effects of pneumoperitoneum such as hemodynamic or pulmonary compromise and hypercarbia. He championed what he termed 'endoscopic abdominal surgery' and developed many of the laparoscopic instruments still in use (Semm 1987).

In 1983, Lukichev and colleagues described laparoscopic cholecystostomy as treatment for acute cholecystitis (Lukichev et al 1983). However, resection of the diseased gallbladder using laparoscopic techniques was not performed until 1985 when the first laparoscopically assisted cholecystectomy was performed by Mühe of Böblingen, Germany. The missing link which brought laparoscopy into the mainstream of general surgery was the advent in 1985 of the charged coupled device (CCD) silicon chip solid state image sensor—i.e. the miniature video camera. Attaching a video camera to the laparoscope's eyepiece allowed all members of the operating team to view the operative field simultaneously and from the same orientation, as opposed to the now archaic single eyepiece viewing of the past. In 1987, a French surgeon in Lyon, Phillipe Mouret, performed the first video-laparoscopic cholecystectomy. In 1988 this new technique was introduced in the USA nearly simultaneously by McKernan and Saye in Marietta, Georgia, and Reddick and Olsen in Nashville, Tennessee (Reddick & Olsen 1989). Notably, these surgeons were in private practice in community-based hospital settings. During the years 1989–1991, it is estimated that some 20 000 American general surgeons received training in laparoscopic techniques. Laparoscopic cholecystectomy was quickly accepted as the new 'gold standard' technique to remove a diseased gallbladder. The resurgence of interest in the laparoscope initiated by laparoscopic cholecystectomy has led to near revolutionary change in the everyday practice of general surgery and the exponential development of newer applications such as laparoscopic antireflux procedures, appendectomy, adrenalectomy, inguinal herniorrhaphy, colon resection, and various intrathoracic videoscopic procedures.

INDICATIONS FOR CHOLECYSTECTOMY

There has been a documented increased frequency of cholecystectomy since the introduction of LC (Escarce et al 1995, Legorreta et al 1993, Nenner et al 1994, Steiner et al 1994). It is unclear whether patients simply are more willing to undergo a laparoscopic procedure rather than to endure biliary colic, or if the indications for cholecystectomy have become more liberal with the advent of LC.

The indications for LC are, and should be, the same as those for OC (Table 38.1). Patients generally have documented cholelithiasis and symptoms attributable to a diseased gallbladder. Biliary colic is typically a severe and episodic right upper abdominal or epigastric pain, often radiating to the back. Attacks frequently occur postprandially or awaken the patient from sleep. Patients with asymptomatic gallstones have less than a 20% chance of ever developing symptoms, and the risks associated with 'prophylactic' operation outweigh the potential benefit of surgery in most patients (Fendrick et al 1993, Ransohoff & Gracie 1993, Ransohoff et al 1983). However, prophylac-

Table 38.1 Indications for laparoscopic cholecystectomy

Symptomatic cholelithiasis
    Biliary colic
    Acute cholecystitis
Asymptomatic cholelithiasis
    Sickle cell disease
    Total parenteral nutrition
    Chronic immunosuppression
    No immediate access to health care facilities (e.g. missionaries, military personnel, peace corps workers, relief workers, etc.)
    Incidental cholecystectomy for patients undergoing laparoscopic procedure for other indications
Acalculous cholecystitis (Biliary dyskinesia)
Gallstone pancreatitis
Gallbladder polyps > 1 cm in diameter
Porcelain gallbladder

tic LC for asymptomatic cholelithiasis can be justified for certain individuals, such as those with sickle cell disease, requiring long-term total parental nutrition, or patients who are therapeutically immunosuppressed after solid organ transplantation. Patients with sickle cell disease often have hepatic or vaso-occlusive crises that can be difficult to differentiate from acute cholecystitis (Tagge et al 1994). In transplant patients, there is concern that immunosuppression will mask the signs and symptoms of inflammation until overwhelming infection has occurred (Hull et al 1994). Recommendations in the literature range from mandatory screening and treatment of biliary disease before transplantation (Girardet et al 1989), to prophylactic cholecystectomy 6 months post-transplantation (Boline et al 1991), to expectant management of all asymptomatic patients (Fendrick et al 1993, Steck et al 1991). Other possible indications for prophylactic LC include individuals who may not have access to modern health care facilities for an extended time period, such as missionaries and military personnel, and patients who are already undergoing laparoscopic abdominal surgery for other reasons (incidental LC).

Less commonly, individuals without gallstones but with typical biliary symptoms, i.e. acalculous cholecystitis or biliary dyskinesia, may also be considered for the procedure (Soper 1991). Other indications for LC include gallstone pancreatitis, gallbladder polyps greater than 1 cm in size.

In a patient with typical biliary colic, the only diagnostic study necessary prior to LC is an abdominal ultrasound revealing gallstones. Ultrasound demonstrates the size and number of stones, the thickness of the gallbladder wall, the presence or absence of pericholecystic fluid, and the diameter of the common bile duct (CBD) and other components of the biliary ductal system. Other non-biliary disorders

such as hepatic lesions or steatosis, masses in the pancreas, or renal tumors may also be diagnosed. When ultrasound is negative despite typical biliary symptoms, cholecystokinin-stimulated biliary scintigraphy demonstrating a low gallbladder ejection fraction with or without pain reproduction suggests acalculous cholecystitis (Soper 1993). If a patient with gallstones has atypical symptoms, however, a more extensive work-up including upper gastrointestinal contrast radiography or endoscopy, computerized tomography, or cardiac and pulmonary evaluation may be appropriate to rule out significant non-biliary disease processes.

CONTRAINDICATIONS

The number of absolute and relative contraindications to performing LC have decreased over the past 10 years as minimally invasive surgical equipment and skills have improved (Table 38.2). Absolute contraindications include the inability to tolerate general anesthesia or laparotomy, refractory coagulopathy, diffuse peritonitis with hemodynamic compromise, cholangitis, and potentially curable gallbladder cancer. Diffuse peritonitis with hemodynamic compromise represents a surgical urgency in which attempted LC is not prudent since the etiology is less than clear or secure. Standard open laparotomy allows rapid determination of the etiology and more expeditious management of the disorder. Suspicion of gallbladder malignancy (e.g. porcelain gallbladder) mandates that standard open resection be undertaken. This is due to persistent concerns with adequacy of resection and reports of port site metastases associated with the use of minimally invasive surgical techniques for the treatment of intra-abdominal malignancies.

Table 38.2 Contraindications to laparoscopic cholecystectomy

Absolute
    Unable to tolerate general anesthesia
    Refractory coagulopathy
    Suspicion of carcinoma
Relative
    Previous upper abdominal surgery
    Cholangitis
    Diffuse peritonitis
    Cirrhosis and/or portal hypertension
    Chronic obstructive pulmonary disease
    Cholecystenteric fistula
    Morbid obesity
    Pregnancy

Relative contraindications are dictated primarily by the surgeon's philosophy and experience. These include previous upper abdominal surgery with extensive adhesions, cirrhosis, portal hypertension, severe cardiopulmonary disease, morbid obesity, and pregnancy.

Intra-abdominal adhesions secondary to previous abdominal surgery can tether underlying viscera and consequently increase the risk of hollow organ injury during placement of laparoscopic trocars (Wolfe et al 1991). However, this risk can be reduced by using alternative initial access sites distant from the previous surgery and placement of initial trocars under direct vision using a direct cut-down technique on the peritoneum.

Cirrhosis results in a brittle, friable, heavy liver that may be difficult to retract in the cephalad direction, thereby limiting exposure of the porta hepatis and gallbladder. Cirrhosis may also be accompanied by decreased synthetic function of the liver resulting in coagulopathy and portal hypertension. Coagulopathies must be reversed prior to performance of LC. The ability to achieve effective hemostasis laparoscopically is significantly compromised compared with that of open exposure. Portal hypertension and aberrant portosystemic venous collateralization may lead to exsanguinating hemorrhage from small veins in the liver bed and porta hepatis, or large veins in the abdominal wall (such as a recanalized umbilical vein) at risk for laceration during trocar puncture. Laparoscopic cholecystectomy may be attempted with care in these patients by experienced surgeons, however, prompt conversion to an open procedure is recommended in the face of unusual bleeding, regardless of the stage of the operation (Soper 1993).

Pre-existing cardiac conditions mandate vigilant intraoperative observation for significant arrhythmias known to be associated with establishment of a CO_2 pneumoperitoneum including bradycardia and ventricular ectopy. Also, in patients with cardiac pacemakers, alternative energy sources such as bipolar electrosurgery or ultrasonic coagulation should be used due to known interference problems caused by monopolar electrosurgical devices.

Most patients undergoing LC exhibit mildly elevated arterial and alveolar carbon dioxide partial pressures (Pco_2) (Liu et al 1991). Chronic obstructive lung disease may predispose patients to CO_2 retention disproportionate to the measured end-tidal value during LC (Wittgen et al 1991). Obtaining preoperative pulmonary function tests and arterial blood gas determinations as well as maximizing pulmonary function by stopping smoking and bronchodilator therapy is prudent in these patients. An intraoperative arterial catheter should also be placed to allow frequent measurement of Pco_2 and pH. Hypercarbia may manifest as hypertension, tachycardia, or ventricular arrhythmias and should be addressed by immediate evacuation of the pneumoperitoneum and stabilization. Slow re-establishment of the pneumoperitoneum may be attempted, but the procedure should be terminated or converted to open if the hypercarbia recurs and is refractory to continued pneumoperitoneum.

Morbid obesity was initially a relative contraindication to LC primarily due to thickness of the abdominal panniculus relative to the length of early trocar and sheath designs making institution and maintenance of a pneumoperitoneum problematic if not impossible. Various instrument manufacturers have since developed longer port systems to obviate this problem. With pneumoperitoneum established, there is usually no additional risk with performance of LC in the obese patient unless the liver is diffusely infiltrated with fat making it more friable and prone to injury during forceful retraction or by inadvertent instrument contact with the hepatic capsule (Schirmer et al 1992). However, both retrospective and prospective studies have demonstrated modestly increased operative times with performance of minimally invasive procedures in obese patient group (Schirmer et al 1992, Underwood et al 1998). Today, LC is commonly performed in morbidly obese patients and appears to demonstrate the same advantages as in the non-obese patients and may offer advantages more specific to the obese patient such as decreased wound infections, incisional hernias, and thrombotic complications (Miles et al 1992, Talamini & Gadacz 1992). Indeed, rather than being contraindicated in the morbidly obese, LC may become the preferred mode of therapy for these patients.

Pregnancy is a controversial relative contraindication to LC due to the unknown effects of prolonged CO_2 pneumoperitoneum on the fetus. We have shown that LC can be performed safely during pregnancy but only with great care (Soper et al 1992). We limit this intervention to the second trimester of gestation after organogenesis is complete and prior to the uterine fundus reaching a size and height that encroaches on the operative field. Open insertion of the initial port or alternative location of the initial port in the right upper quadrant should be used to avoid injury to the gravid uterus and the insufflation pressure should be limited to less than 12 mmHg to avoid respiratory embarrassment and decreased vena caval return. Also, maternal hyperventilation with close monitoring of end-tidal CO_2 should be undertaken to prevent fetal acidosis. When visualization of the biliary tree is required, laparoscopic ultrasound is used in place of cholangiography in order to limit fetal radiation exposure. And finally, perioperative consultation with an experienced obstetrician is advisable, as is perioperative monitoring of the fetal heart.

ADVANTAGES AND DISADVANTAGES

The advantages of LC over other therapies for gallstone disease are multiple (Table 38.3). Unlike non-resective techniques for gallstone ablation, LC removes the diseased gallbladder along with its stones. Relative to traditional OC, postoperative pain and intestinal ileus are diminished with LC. The small size of the fascial incisions allows rapid return to heavy physical activities. The small incisions are also cosmetically more appealing than is the large incision used during traditional cholecystectomy. The patient can usually be discharged from the hospital either on the same day or the day following operation, and can return to full activity within a few days (Barkun et al 1992, Soper et al 1992). These factors lead to overall decreased cost of LC compared to its traditional open counterpart (Bass et al 1993).

There are, however, several potential disadvantages of LC (Table 38.3). As opposed to non-resective treatments for gallstones, patients must be acceptable candidates for general anesthesia and possible laparotomy. Three-dimensional depth perception is limited by the two-dimensional monocular image of the videoscope, and the operative field of view is usually directed by an individual other than the surgeon. It is more difficult to control significant hemorrhage using laparoscopic technology than in an open surgical field. There is also less tactile discrimination of structures using laparoscopic instruments as opposed to direct digital palpation during OC. CO_2 insufflation to create the pneumoperitoneum is associated with a number of potential risks, including reduction of vena caval flow and systemic hypercarbia with acidosis. Operative time is generally longer than for the traditional open operation, particularly during the early portion of the surgeon's experience. And finally, the videoscopic technology and minimal access instrumentation are costly, complex and continually evolving requiring the presence of appropriately trained support personnel.

Table 38.3 Advantages and disadvantages of laparoscopic cholecystectomy compared to open cholecystectomy

Advantages	Disadvantages
Less pain	Lack of depth perception
Smaller incisions	View controlled by camera operator
Better cosmesis	More difficult to control hemorrhage
Shorter hospitalization	Decreased tactile discrimination
Earlier return to full activity	Potential CO_2 insufflation complications
Decreased total costs	Adhesions/inflammation limit use
	Slight increase in bile duct injuries

INSTRUMENTATION

BASIC LAPAROSCOPY

High-intensity cold light transmitted via a flexible fiberoptic cable is necessary for adequate illumination of the abdominal cavity through the laparoscope. Most current laparoscopes transmit this light through a series of glass rods separated by small air spaces. This 'rod-lens' system, as introduced in 1960 by Hopkins in England, increased the optical efficiency relative to previous scopes by approximately 9-fold and allowed manufacture of smaller diameter scopes with larger viewing angles and brighter images (Fig. 38.1) (Cockett & Cockett 1998, Gow 1998, Jennings, 1998). Recently, true 'videoscopes' with video-chips located on the distal tip of the scope have been designed and marketed. Laparoscopes come in various sizes (2, 3, 5 and 10 mm diameter) and viewing angles (end-viewing 0° and oblique 30°, 40° or 50°). In general, smaller diameter laparoscopes have a smaller field of view and transmit less light than their larger counterparts. Although the end-viewing telescope is initially easier to use for the beginner, the oblique-view telescopes are valuable for 'looking around corners' (e.g. assessing the anterior abdominal wall or over the dome of the liver) and are generally preferred by experienced laparoscopists (Fig. 38.2). Flexible laparoscopes with variable deflection in two planes are also available, but have seen limited utilization.

For establishing pneumoperitoneum, a Veress needle can be used (Fig. 38.3). This device has an outer cutting needle of 2 mm diameter with an inner spring-loaded hollow blunt stylet with a side hole through its distal tip. When penetrating solid tissue such as the abdominal wall, the inner stylet is pushed back, allowing the cutting edges of the needle to be exposed. As soon as the sharp needle enters the abdominal cavity, the blunt stylet springs forward beyond the sharp end of the needle. This blunt tip then helps to prevent inadvertent injury to non-tethered abdominal viscera (Fig. 38.4).

An insufflator is required to deliver the appropriate gas through tubing connected to the Veress needle. The insufflator should be automatic and pressure triggered, with an upper limit set at 12–15 mmHg, since pressures higher than that can limit diaphragmatic excursion, reduce vena cava flow, and increase the possibility of gas embolism.

Laparoscopic trocars are available in various sizes (2–12 mm) and types (reusable versus disposable). Disposable trocars are always sharp, have more dependable gaskets to prevent gas leakage, may be radiolucent, and can incorporate a retractable 'safety shield' that covers the trocar point after abdominal entry to diminish the risk of trauma to internal viscera. However, these potential advantages are offset by greater expense.

It is mandatory that a set of laparotomy instruments be in the operating room to allow rapid laparotomy should a significant complication occur.

EQUIPMENT AND INSTRUMENTS FOR LAPAROSCOPIC CHOLECYSTECTOMY

Most surgeons utilize two video monitors, one on each side of the operating table to facilitate visualization by both surgeon and assistant. Forceps used to grasp the gallbladder without puncturing it should have handles with a ratchet mechanism apposing the jaws to reduce operator fatigue. Toothed grasping forceps may be useful when the gallbladder is markedly thickened and inflamed. Blunt dissection of the fibroareolar tissue overlying the infundibulum of the gallbladder is facilitated by fine-tipped dissecting forceps. Forceps with curved tips are useful for dissecting around tubular structures. Straight or curved scissors are used to cut

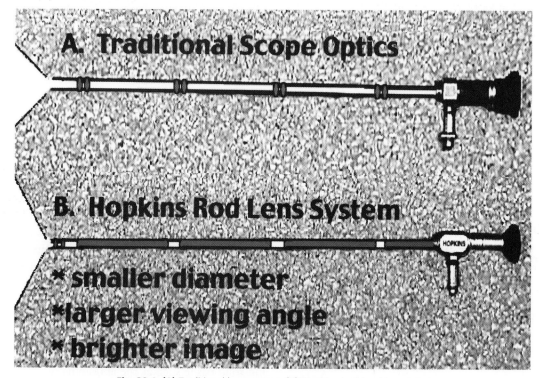

Fig. 38.1 (A) Traditional laparoscope; **(B)** Hopkins 'rod-lens' laparoscope.

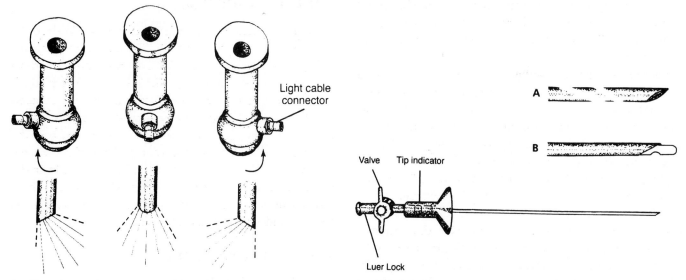

Fig. 38.2 Oblique-viewing laparoscope. (Reprinted with permission of Quality Medical Publishing.)

Fig. 38.3 Veress needle: **(A)** blunt core retracted; **(B)** blunt core extended. (Reprinted with permission of Quality Medical Publishing.)

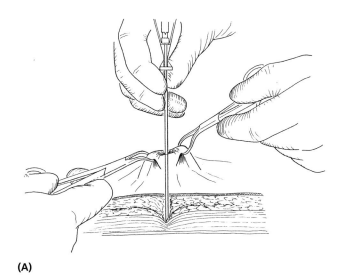

(A)

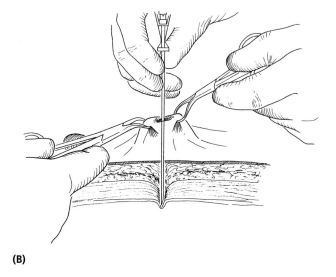

(B)

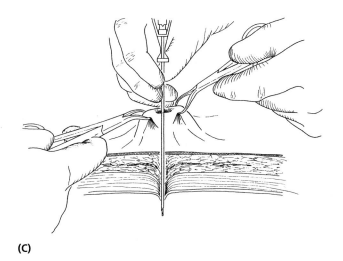

(C)

Fig. 38.4 Insertion of Veress needle. **(A)** Blunt tip retracts when encountering fascia; **(B)** Blunt tip springs forward when in preperitoneal space and then retracts again when peritoneum is encountered; **(C)** Blunt tip springs forward on entry into the abdominal cavity. (Reprinted with permission of Quality Medical Publishing.)

sutures and large structures, while microscissors with tips of 1–2 mm in length are useful for creating small cuts in the cystic ducts if an intraoperative cholangiogram is being performed.

Instruments that allow irrigation and aspiration of blood and bile are essential. Spatula-tipped or hook-tipped monopolar electrosurgical devices have become the most widely used dissecting tools, but other modalities such as ultrasonic coagulation and various forms of bipolar electrosurgical dissection may alternatively be employed. A clip applier is useful to control the cystic duct and artery. Equipment for intraoperative cholangiograms should be readily available. Various laparoscopic catheter systems have been developed and marketed with the common endpoint being placement of a 4- or 5-Fr catheter into the cystic duct with some form of fixation of the catheter allowing injection of radiographic contrast for visualizing the biliary tree.

OPERATING ROOM SET-UP

Using the 'American' technique, the surgeon stands to the left of the patient, the first assistant stands to the patient's right, and the laparoscopic video camera operator stands to the left of the surgeon (Fig. 38.5). In the 'French' technique, the patient's legs are abducted and the surgeon stands between the legs. The camera operator must always maintain the proper orientation of the camera and keep the operating instruments in the center of the video image. Following all instruments as they come into or exit from the operative field is a matter of surgeon preference. Sharp instruments should never be moved intracorporeally unless they are under direct videoscopic vision.

PATIENT PREPARATION

As with any abdominal operation, patients are fasted approximately 8 hours prior to the operation. Patients with

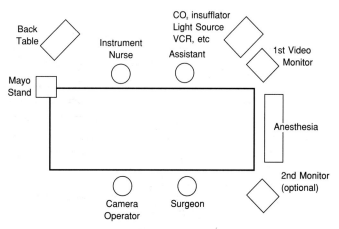

Fig. 38.5 Room set-up for LC.

no major comorbidity are admitted to the hospital on a same-day surgery basis. All patients are administered a single preoperative dose of intravenous broad-spectrum antibiotics. Sequential compression stockings are placed on both legs to avoid pooling of blood in the lower extremities by the reverse Trendelenburg position required for this operation. Following induction of general endotracheal anesthesia, an orogastric tube may be placed to decompress the stomach. The abdomen is shaved and prepared in standard sterile fashion with particular care taken to rid the umbilicus of all detritus.

OPERATIVE TECHNIQUE

PNEUMOPERITONEUM

A working space, generally provided by a pneumoperitoneum, is essential for the surgeon to view and to operate within the abdominal cavity. CO_2 has the advantage of being non-combustible and rapidly absorbed from the peritoneal cavity. It may, however, lead to hypercarbia in patients with significant cardiopulmonary disease (Fitzgerald et al 1992). Pneumoperitoneum can be established by either a closed or an open technique. In the closed technique, carbon dioxide is insufflated into the peritoneal cavity through a Veress needle, which is subsequently replaced with a laparoscopic port, placed blindly into the abdominal cavity. In the open technique, a laparoscopic port is inserted under direct vision into the peritoneal cavity via a small incision; only after ensuring definitive and safe peritoneal entry is the pneumoperitoneum established. There are advantages and disadvantages to both techniques. Surgeons performing LC should learn both and use them selectively.

For the closed technique, the surgeon should perform

various tests to ensure the safety of the needle insertion prior to insufflation. A syringe containing 5 ml of normal saline solution is attached to the end of the needle to aspirate and demonstrate the absence of blood, urine or enteric contents. If any one of the above is recovered, the needle should be removed and its position changed. If no fluid is aspirated, an assessment is made of the ease with which saline solution flows by gravity into the zero pressure abdominal cavity—the 'drop test'. This is done either by instilling a few drops of saline solution into the hub of the needle or by removing the barrel of the syringe. Manually elevating the abdominal wall near the needle site will decrease intra-abdominal pressure and enhance free flow; the fluid will flow much more slowly or not at all if the needle is in an extraperitoneal position.

Insufflator tubing is then connected to the Veress needle and carbon dioxide is insufflated at a low flow rate of ~1 L/min. The initial pressure of the abdomen is usually between 2 and 6 mmHg and should not increase appreciably during the early phase of insufflation. Asymmetric distention, a rapid rise in pressure with low insufflated volume, or an initial pressure above 10 mmHg suggest that the needle is not in the proper position. The abdomen should be serially percussed to confirm symmetric tympany associated with insufflation. The abdomen is then fully insufflated with the upper pressure limit set at 12–15 mmHg; this usually requires 3–6 L of CO_2, depending on the size of the abdominal cavity and degree of muscle relaxation. If intra-abdominal pressures exceed 20 mmHg, central venous pressures and blood pressures fall because of decreased venous return and diminished cardiac output (Chui et al 1993, Sharma et al 1997). Studies have also demonstrated direct negative effects on urine output relative to increased intra-abdominal pressures (McDougall et al 1996, 1997).

During the initial period of insufflation the patient must be closely monitored for signs of gas embolism (hypotension, decreased oxygen saturation, decreased end-tidal CO_2, 'mill-wheel' heart murmur), vagal reaction (hypotension and/or bradycardia), ventricular arrhythmias, and hypercarbia with acidosis. Most of these complications require immediate treatment by desufflating the CO_2 followed by gradual reestablishment of the pneumoperitoneum after the patient's condition has stabilized. Gas embolism results in an 'air-lock' right ventricular outflow obstruction with a dramatic fall in end-tidal CO_2 concentration. When suspected, this problem should be treated by placing the patient in a steep left decubitus Trendelenburg position followed by insertion of a central venous catheter to aspirate the carbon dioxide from the apex of the right ventricle (Chui et al 1993, Hanney et al 1995, Lantz et al 1994, Sharma et al 1997).

After the pneumoperitoneum is established, the Veress needle is replaced with a trocar/port through a periumbilical incision into which the laparoscope may be inserted. This port is inserted carefully while manually elevating the abdominal wall to avoid iatrogenic injury to intra-abdominal viscera or retroperitoneal structures.

Using the 'open' technique, the pneumoperitoneum is established similarly to an open diagnostic peritoneal lavage. A 1.5 cm skin incision is made in the infra- or supraumbilical skinfold. Dissection of the subcutaneous tissue is performed at the base of the umbilical raphé to reach the fascia rapidly, even in obese patients, as this is the thinnest part of the abdominal wall. Kocher clamps are then applied to both sides of the linea alba and a small vertical incision is made to gain access to the peritoneal cavity. A finger is placed into the wound to ensure that the free peritoneal cavity has been entered and to sweep away any adhesions that may be present. If a Hasson trocar (Weck & Co., Research Triangle Park, North Carolina, USA) is available, two sutures are placed on both sides of the fascial incision and are tied to the 'wings' of the wedge-tipped sheath after it is inserted into the peritoneal cavity under direct vision (Fig. 38.6). Alternatively, standard laparoscopic sheaths can be used after placing two concentric polypropylene purse-string stitches around the fascial incision (Figs 38.7 and 38.8). After removing the sheath at the conclusion of the procedure, the outer purse-string suture is removed and the inner one tied. Open insertion of the initial port takes a few minutes longer than its closed counterpart. However, extraction of the gallbladder at the conclusion of the operation is easier, thereby equalizing the time differential of the two access techniques. We currently primarily use the open insertion technique, as it may diminish the incidence of injury to intra-abdominal viscera and major retroperitoneal vascular structures.

PORT PLACEMENT AND EXPOSURE

Depending on the surgeon's preference, a 5 or 10 mm laparoscope is inserted into the abdomen through the umbilical port. The area immediately posterior to the umbilicus is initially viewed to ensure that there is no injury as a result of trocar insertion. Thorough intra-abdominal visual exploration is then performed. The pelvic viscera are examined for pathological abnormalities prior to evaluating the upper abdomen. The anterior surface of the intestines, the omentum and the stomach are also examined for disease. The patient is then placed in a reverse Trendelenburg position of 30° while rotating the table to the left by 15°. This maneuver allows the colon and duodenum to fall away from the liver edge. The falciform ligament and both lobes

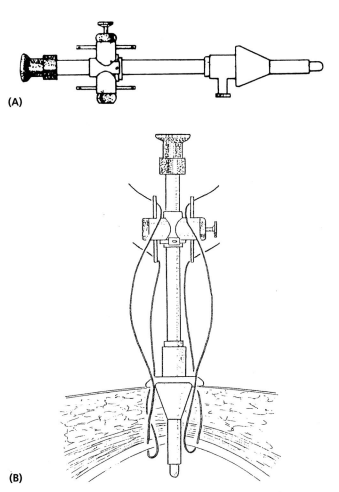

(A)

(B)

Fig. 38.6 (A) Reusable Hasson trocar/cannula. **(B)** Securing the Hasson cannula to the abdominal fascia. The fascial stay sutures are wound around the 'wings' of the cannula to secure it in place and seal the fasciotomy and peritoneotomy. (Reprinted with permission of Quality Medical Publishing.)

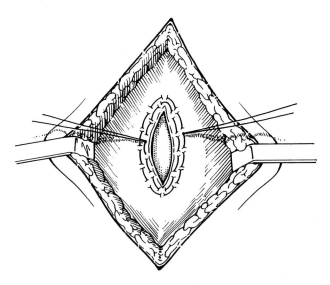

Fig. 38.7 Purse-string sutures around the fascial incision.

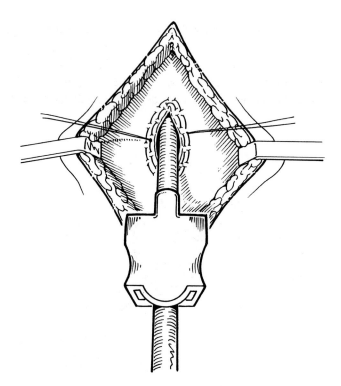

Fig. 38.8 Insertion of laparoscopic sheath under direct vision.

of the liver are examined closely for abnormalities. The gallbladder can usually be seen protruding beyond the edge of the liver.

Two small accessory subcostal ports are then placed under direct vision. The first 5 mm trocar is placed along the right anterior axillary line between the 12th rib and the iliac crest. A second 5 mm port is inserted in the right subcostal area in the midclavicular line. Grasping forceps are placed through these two ports to secure the gallbladder. The assistant manipulates the lateral grasping forceps, which are used to elevate the liver and to expose the fundus of the gallbladder. The surgeon uses a dissecting forceps to raise a serosal 'fold' of the most dependent portion of the fundus. The assistant's heavy grasping forceps are then locked onto this fold using either a spring or ratchet device. With these axillary grasping forceps, the fundus of the gallbladder is then pushed in a lateral and cephalad direction, rolling the entire right lobe of the liver cranially. This maneuver is complicated in patients with a fixed, cirrhotic liver or a heavy, friable liver due to fatty infiltration.

In patients with few adhesions to the gallbladder, pushing the fundus cephalad exposes the entire gallbladder, cystic duct and porta hepatis. Most patients, however, have adhesions between the gallbladder and the omentum, hepatic flexure and/or duodenum. These adhesions are generally avascular and may be lysed bluntly by grasping them with dissecting forceps at their site of attachment to the gall-

bladder wall and gently 'stripping' them down towards the infundibulum. After exposing the infundibulum, blunt grasping forceps placed through the midclavicular trocar are used to grasp and place traction on the neck of the gallbladder. The operative field is thereby established and the final working port is then inserted.

A final operating trocar/port is placed through an incision in the midline of the epigastrium. This trocar is usually inserted ~ 5 cm below the xiphoid process, but the precise position and angle depends on the location of the gallbladder as well as the size of the medial segment of the left lobe of the liver. When uncertain about the appropriate position for this trocar, a Veress needle may first be placed at the proposed site to ascertain whether its location and angle of insertion seen through the laparoscope are optimal. The trocar is inserted in a controlled fashion, angling its tip just to the right of the falciform ligament while aiming towards the gallbladder. Dissecting forceps are then inserted and directed towards the gallbladder neck. One should note that the orientation of the laparoscope is generally parallel to that of the cystic duct when the fundus is elevated, whereas the instruments placed through the other three ports enter the abdomen at right angles to this plane (Figs 38.9 and 38.10).

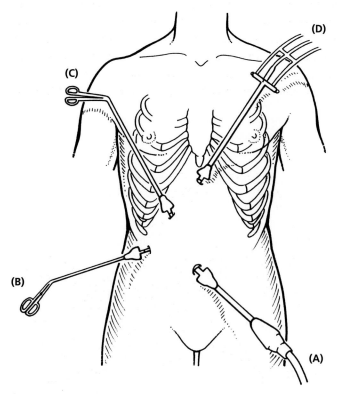

Fig. 38.9 Positions for insertion of the **(A)** initial and **(B–D)** accessory sheaths.

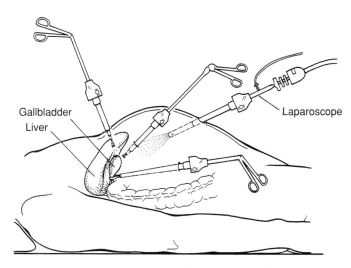

Fig. 38.10 Diagram of the abdomen after the creation of a pneumoperitoneum and the insertion of laparoscopic instruments.

DISSECTION

Two grasping instruments on the infundibulum exert traction on the gallbladder away from the common bile duct (CBD) in a superior and lateral direction. Fine-tipped dissecting forceps are used to dissect away the overlying fibroareolar structures from the infundibulum of the gallbladder. This is done with a blunt stripping action, always starting on the gallbladder and stripping the tissue towards the porta hepatis (Fig. 38.11). The dissection should begin on a 'known' structure, e.g. the gallbladder, rather than in an unknown area, to avoid damage to the underlying structures such as the bile duct or the hepatic artery.

It is important to clearly identify the structures forming the sides of Calot's triangle (i.e. cystic duct, cystic artery, and common hepatic duct)—the standard ventral aspect and its reverse (dorsal) aspect (Fig. 38.12). Distinction is here made with the hepatocystic triangle proper which is the ventral aspect of the area bounded by the gallbladder wall

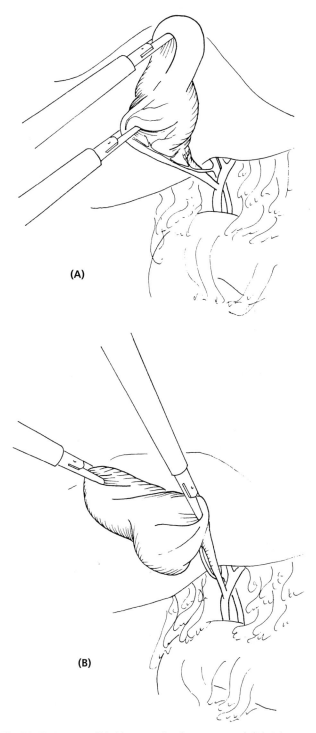

Fig. 38.12 Proper gallbladder retraction for exposure of: **(A)** Calot's triangle, **(B)** reverse Calot's triangle. (Reprinted with permission of Quality Medical Publishing.)

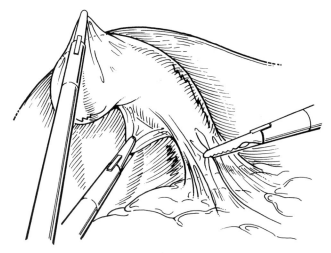

Fig. 38.11 The omentum and adhesions are bluntly divided by carefully pulling them away with atraumatic grasping forceps.

and cystic duct, the liver edge, and the common hepatic duct; the cystic artery (and hence Calot's triangle) lies within this space (Ch. 37). The hepatocystic triangle is maximally opened and converted into a trapezoid shape by retracting the infundibulum of the gallbladder inferiorly and laterally while maintaining the fundus under traction in a superior and medial direction. A lymph node usually lies adjacent to the cystic artery, and occasionally it is necessary to use a brief application of electrosurgical coagulation to obtain hemostasis as the lymph node is bluntly swept away. To expose the reverse of Calot's triangle, the infundibulum of the gallbladder is pulled in a superior and medial direction (Fig. 38.12). After clearing the structures from the apex of the triangle, the junction between the infundibulum and the origin of the proximal cystic duct can be clearly identified. The strands of peritoneal, lymphatic and neurovascular tissue are stripped away from the cystic duct to clear a segment from the surrounding tissue. Curved dissecting forceps are helpful in creating a 'window' around the posterior aspect of the cystic duct to skeletonize the duct itself. Alternatively, the tip of the hook cautery can be used to encircle and expose the duct. It is generally unnecessary and potentially harmful to dissect the cystic duct down to its junction with the CBD. The cystic artery is separated from the surrounding tissue by similar blunt dissection at this time. If the cystic artery crosses anterior to the duct, the artery may require dissection and division prior to approaching the cystic duct. The neck of the gallbladder is thus dissected away from its liver bed, leaving only two structures entering the gallbladder—the cystic duct and artery. No structure should be divided until the cystic duct and cystic artery are unequivocally identified. This is the 'critical view' of safety (Fig. 38.13) essential to prevent bile duct injury during LC (Strasberg et al 1995).

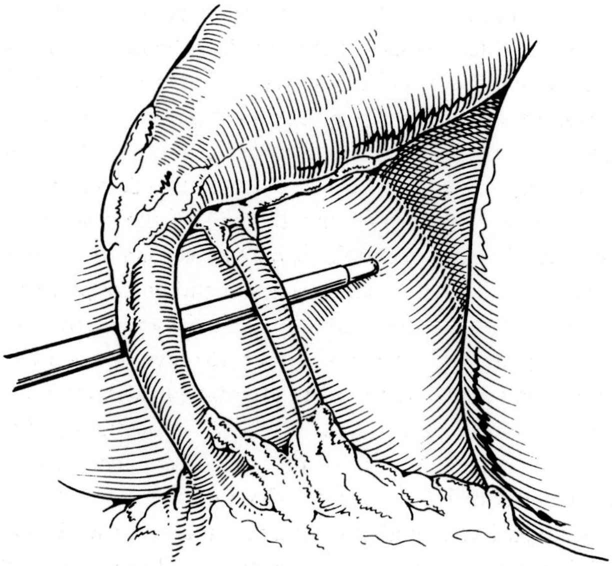

INTRAOPERATIVE EVALUATION FOR CHOLEDOCHOLITHIASIS

After initially dissecting the proximal cystic duct, the CBD should be imaged if there is any concern for choledocholithiasis or questions regarding the biliary anatomy. This can be achieved by radiographic intraoperative cholangiography (IOC) or intracorporeal laparoscopic ultrasonography (LUS) (see Ch. 22). Prior to either procedure, a clip is applied high on the cystic duct at its junction with the gallbladder to prevent stones migrating down the duct. To perform IOC, the anterolateral wall of the cystic duct is incised and dissecting forceps are used to gently compress the cystic duct systematically back towards the gallbladder, thereby 'milking' stones away from the CBD and out the ductotomy (Figs 38.14 and 38.15). A 4–5 Fr catheter is inserted into the duct through a hollow, 5 mm metal tube that has an appropriate gasket to prevent carbon dioxide leakage around the catheter itself. The cholangiography catheter is inserted into the cystic duct and a clip is applied loosely to secure the catheter in place (Fig. 38.16). If the introducer has grasping jaws, it can be used to secure the catheter into the duct (Fig. 38.17). Alternatively, catheters equipped with balloons proximal to the tip may be used for fixation. Cholangiography can be performed by either real-time fluoroscopy (dynamic IOC) or by obtaining two standard

Fig. 38.13 Critical view. Hepatocystic triangle is dissected free of all tissue except for the cystic duct and artery and the base of the liver bed is exposed. When this view is achieved, the two structures entering the gallbladder can only be the cystic duct and artery.

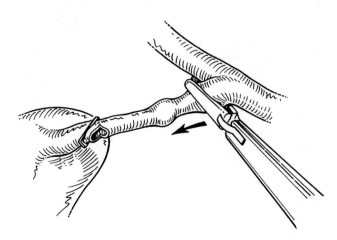

Fig. 38.14 After a clip is placed across the junction of the gallbladder with the cystic duct and a cystic ductotomy is made on the anterior side, the cystic duct is gently 'milked' back towards the ductotomy.

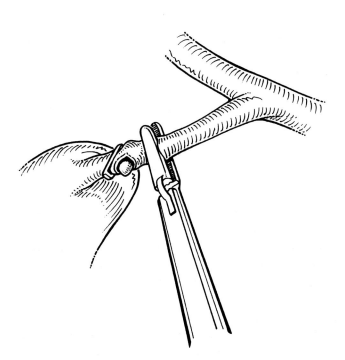

Fig. 38.15 A cystic duct stone is 'milked' out of the ductotomy.

radiographs (static IOC) after injecting 5 and 10 ml of water-soluble contrast medium (Figs 38.18 and 38.19). The films should be inspected for the following: (1) the length of cystic duct and location of its junction with the

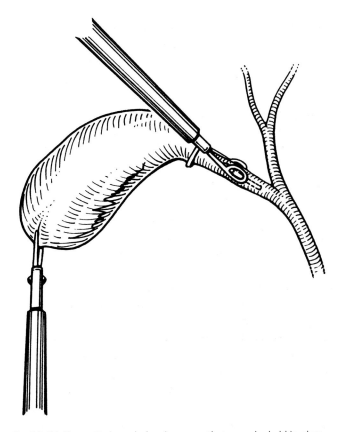

Fig. 38.17 Alternatively, a cholangiogram catheter can be held in place with a clamp.

CBD, (2) the size of the CBD, (3) the presence of intraluminal filling defects, (4) free flow of contrast into the duodenum, and (5) anatomy of the extrahepatic and intra-hepatic biliary tree. After the cholangiocatheter is removed, the cystic duct is doubly clipped below the ductotomy with care to avoid the wall of the CBD, and then divided. The posterior jaw of the clip applier must be visualized prior to applying each clip in order to avoid injuries to the sur-rounding structures. Great care should be taken so that the CBD is not 'tented up' into the clip. If the cystic duct is particularly large or friable, it may be preferable to replace one of the clips with a suture, either hand tied or preformed.

Evaluation of the CBD by LUS is an alternative to cholangiography. Several studies performed at open chole-cystectomy (OC) reported intracorporeal ultrasonography to be more accurate than operative cholangiography in assessing the CBD for stones (97–99% versus 89–94%) (Machie et al 1993a, 1993b, Orda et al 1994). However, few surgeons adopted ultrasound for this purpose. Recently, LUS has been used in several centers during LC and is gaining popularity (Jakimowicz 1993, John et al 1994, McIntyre et al 1994, Orda et al 1994, Steigmann et al 1994). With LUS, the transducer has a higher frequency

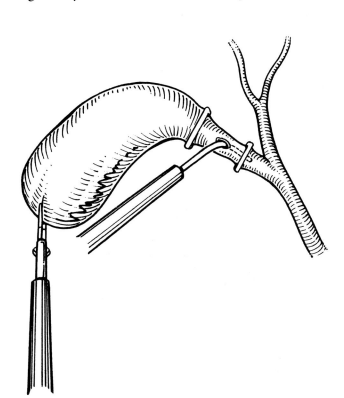

Fig. 38.16 Cystic duct cholangiography can be performed with a catheter clipped into place.

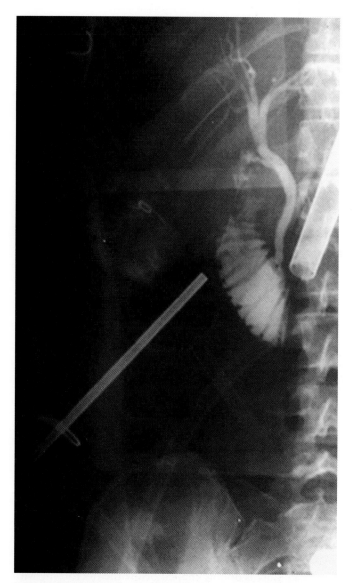

Fig. 38.18 Intraoperative cholangiogram showing absence of the bile duct calculus with free flow of contrast medium into the duodenum. (Reprinted from Blumgart LH & Fong Y (eds) Surgery of the Liver and Biliary Tract CD-ROM, 1997, Churchill-Livingstone.)

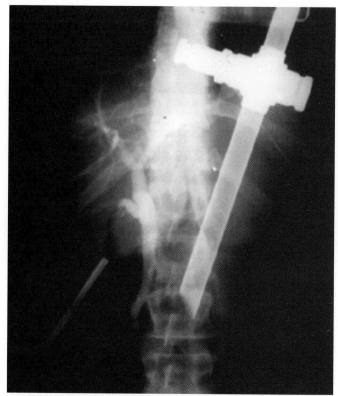

Fig. 38.19 Intraoperative cholangiogram showing a filling defect of the distal common bile duct. The defect has a characteristic 'meniscus' appearance, and there is no flow of contrast medium into the duodenum. (Reprinted from Blumgart LH & Fong Y (eds) Surgery of the Liver and Biliary Tract CD-ROM, 1997 Churchill-Livingstone.)

with improved resolution compared to that used with transabdominal ultrasonography. In experienced hands, LUS appears to be as accurate as cholangiography for demonstrating choledocholithiasis but can be performed more rapidly (Steigmann et al 1995). In a recent prospective multicenter trial with 209 LC patients, the time to perform LUS (7 ± 3 min) was significantly less than that of IOC (13 ± 6 min) (Steigmann et al 1995). The study showed that LUS was more sensitive for detecting stones but that IOC was better in delineating intrahepatic anatomy and defining anatomical anomalies of the ductal system. The authors concluded that the two methods of duct imaging

were complementary. Despite these promising data, more clinical experience will be necessary to establish the appropriate role of LUS for the detection of choledocholithiasis during LC (Soper 1997, Wu et al 1998).

COMPLETION OF CHOLECYSTECTOMY

Following clip ligation and division of the cystic duct, the cystic artery is dissected from the surrounding tissue for an adequate distance to permit placement of 3 clips. The surgeon must ascertain that the structure is indeed the cystic artery and not the right hepatic artery looping up onto the neck of the gallbladder or an accessory or replaced right hepatic artery (Ch. 1). After an appropriate length of cystic artery has been dissected free, it is clipped proximally and distally prior to its transection. Electrocautery should not be used for this division, as the current may be transmitted to the proximal clips leading to subsequent necrosis and hemorrhage. A common error is to dissect and divide the anterior branch of the cystic artery, mistaking it for the main cystic artery. This may result in hemorrhage from the posterior branch during dissection of the gallbladder fossa.

The ligated stumps of the cystic duct and the artery are then examined to ensure that there is no leakage of either bile or blood and that the clips are placed securely and compress the entire lumen of the structures without impinging on adjacent tissues. A suction-irrigation catheter is used to remove any debris or blood that has accumulated during the dissection. Separation of the gallbladder away from its hepatic bed is then initiated using an electrosurgical probe to coagulate small vessels and lymphatics. While maintaining cephalad traction on the fundus of the gallbladder with the axillary forceps, the midclavicular forceps pulls the neck of the gallbladder anterosuperiorly and then alternatively medially and laterally to expose and place the tissue connecting the gallbladder to the fossa under tension (Fig. 38.20). An electrocautery spatula or hook is used in a gentle sweeping motion with low-power (25–30 W) to coagulate and divide the tissue. Intermittent blunt dissection will facilitate exposure of the proper plane.

Dissection of the gallbladder fossa continues from the infundibulum to the fundus, progressively moving the midclavicular grasping forceps cephalad to allow maximal countertraction. The dissection proceeds until the gallbladder is attached by only a thin bridge of tissue. At this point, prior to completely detaching the gallbladder, the hepatic fossa and porta hepatis are once again inspected for hemostasis and bile leakage. Small bleeding points are coagulated and the right upper quadrant is liberally irrigated and then aspirated dry while checking for any residual bleeding or bile

leakage. The final attachments of the gallbladder are divided, and the liver edge is again examined for hemostasis.

After the cholecystectomy has been performed, the gallbladder must be removed from the abdominal cavity. If the stone burden is small, the gallbladder can be extracted at the subxiphoid port site. Usually, the gallbladder is most easily removed at the umbilical port site where there are no muscle layers anterior to the fascial plane. Also, if the fascial opening needs to be enlarged due to large or numerous stones, extension of the umbilical incision causes less postoperative pain and has better cosmesis than does enlarging the subxiphoid incision. The laparoscope is removed from the umbilical port and placed through the epigastric port. Large 'claw' grasping forceps are introduced through the umbilical port to grasp the infundibulum of the gallbladder. The forceps, trocar, and gallbladder neck are then retracted as a unit through the umbilical incision. The neck of the gallbladder is thus exteriorized through the anterior abdominal wall with the fundus remaining within the abdominal cavity.

If the gallbladder is not distended with bile or stones, it can be simply withdrawn with gentle traction. In most cases, however, a suction catheter introduced through an incision in the gallbladder neck is used to aspirate bile and small stones. Stone forceps can also be placed into the gallbladder to extract or crush calculi if necessary (Fig. 38.21).

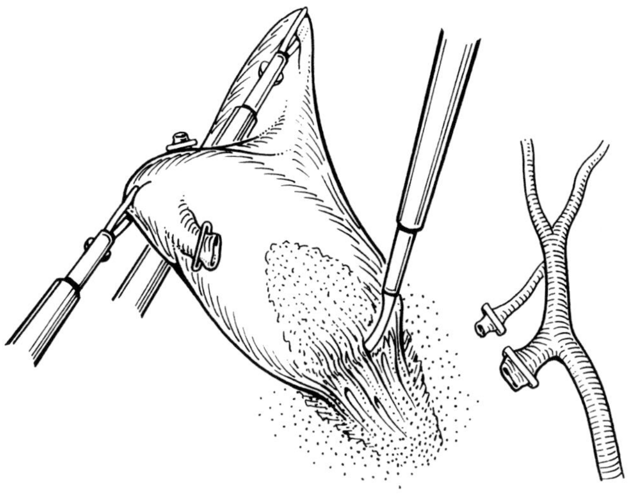

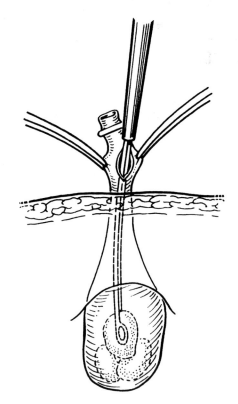

Fig. 38.20 Separation of the gallbladder from its bed by dissection with a blunt-tipped, thermal energy probe. The neck of the gallbladder is placed on traction in a superior direction, then twisted to the left and right to place tension on the junction between the gallbladder and hepatic fossa.

Fig. 38.21 Gallstones contained within the fundus may be crushed or removed after delivering the neck of the gallbladder through the umbilical incision.

Occasionally, the fascial incision must be extended to extract larger stones or thick-walled gallbladders. After the gallbladder is extracted, the operator's finger is used to occlude the port entry site. If any question concerning hemostasis or contamination of the right upper quadrant remains, the umbilical port can be replaced under direct vision and the upper part of the abdomen again copiously irrigated and aspirated. If not, all laparoscopic ports are now removed after allowing escape of the CO_2.

Each incision is infiltrated with bupivacaine for postoperative analgesia. The fascia of the umbilical incision is closed with one or two large absorbable sutures. Closure of the subxiphoid fascia is optional, as visceral herniation is unlikely to occur due to the oblique entry angle of the trocar into the abdominal cavity and its location anterior to the falciform ligament. The skin of the subxiphoid and umbilical incisions is closed with subcuticular absorbable sutures. The skin incisions at both 5 mm port sites can be closed with adhesive strips or skin closure adhesives. The orogastric tube is removed in the operating room, and the patient is transferred to the postanesthesia care unit.

INTRAOPERATIVE TREATMENT OF COMMON DUCT STONES

The reported incidence of CBD stones found during LC ranges from 3 to 10% (Barkun et al 1993, Frazee et al 1993). It is unclear whether uncomplicated choledocholithiasis requires treatment. Autopsy series have shown that many patients with silent gallbladder stones also harbor silent CBD stones (Crump 1931). Furthermore, smaller stones are known to pass through the ampulla of Vater, as demonstrated by stool analysis in patients with acute pancreatitis or acute biliary colic (Acosta & Ledesma 1974, Kelly 1980). However, in one study, the rate of symptoms or complications in patients with retained CBD stones following cholecystectomy was 94% with a mortality rate of 3% over 5 years (Hicken & McAllister 1964). It is not clear what stone size precludes passage nor which indicators will predict complications of cholangitis or pancreatitis if the stones are left in-situ. Therefore, it is generally recommended to treat choledocholithiasis when discovered intraoperatively; options include laparoscopic CBD management, open CBD exploration, and postoperative endoscopic or percutaneous transhepatic stone extraction. At the current state of evolving techniques and in the absence of prospective randomized trials guiding the management of patients with choledocholithiasis, the technical expertise of the particular local physicians is a major determining factor in CBD stone management.

Laparoscopic CBD exploration can take the form of accessing the CBD through the cystic duct (transcystic technique) or directly incising and opening the CBD with stone retrieval (laparoscopic choledochotomy). In the transcystic duct approach, stones smaller than 4 mm in size can often be flushed through the ampulla into the duodenum, a technique that is facilitated by pharmacologic relaxation of the sphincter of Oddi using sublingual nitroglycerine or intravenous glucagon. When these simple methods fail, a helical stone basket can be passed over a guidewire through the cystic duct and into the CBD to extract stones under fluoroscopic guidance (Fig. 38.22) (Hunter 1992). If attempts at transcystic basket extraction fail, the next step is to insert a 7–8 Fr choledochoscope to remove the stones under direct vision. If the CBD stone is larger than the lumen of the cystic duct, the cystic duct should first be balloon dilated to a maximum of 8 mm diameter, but never larger than the internal diameter of the CBD (Hunter & Soper 1992). The choledochoscope is then passed into the peritoneal cavity through the midaxillary port, utilizing a sheath to prevent damage to the scope by the port's valve. The choledochoscope is then inserted through the cystic duct into the CBD under direct vision. The lumen of the duct is optimally visualized by continuously infusing saline through the biopsy channel. Under visual guidance, the tip of a Segura-type stone basket is advanced beyond the stone and opened. As the basket is pulled backwards and rotated, the stone is ensnared (Fig. 38.23) (Jones & Soper 1996). A completion cholangiogram should always be performed to conclusively demonstrate clearance of the duct. Because of tissue edema secondary to ductal dilatation and manipulation, the cystic duct stump is ligated (rather than clipped) for added security. Successful extraction has been reported in 67 to 96% of patients thus treated in most series (Table 38.4) (Bagnato 1993, DePaula et al 1994, Dion et al 1994, Ferzli et al

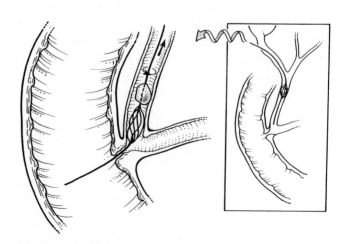

Fig. 38.22 Transcystic retrieval of common bile stones using a helical basket under fluoroscopy.

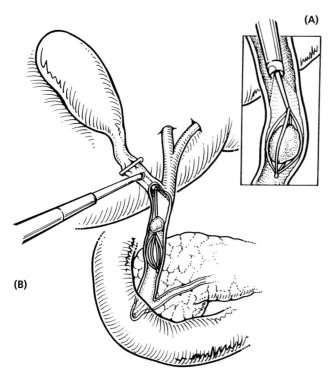

Fig. 38.23 Transcystic choledochoscopy. **(A)** The flexible choledochoscope is passed into the common bile duct through the cystic duct. Under direct vision the basket is advanced distal to the stone and opened. **(B)** As the basket is withdrawn through the working channel of the choledochoscope, the stone is ensnared. The basket, stone and choledochoscope are then removed as a unit.

1994, Franklin et al 1994, Hunter 1992, Petelin 1993b, Phillips et al 1994). Complications, such as infection and pancreatitis, have been reported in 5 to 10% of patients with a mortality rate of 1 to 2%. The duration of hospitalization following an uncomplicated transcystic duct stone extraction is the same as that for LC alone, averaging 1–2 days. The main advantage of the transcystic approach is that it avoids the need to incise the CBD with subsequent suture closure and placement of a T tube. Poor candidates for trans-cystic extraction techniques are those with large or multiple CBD stones, stones in the proximal ductal system, and those with small or tortuous cystic ducts.

Other novel transcystic approaches include balloon dilatation of the sphincter of Oddi and antegrade sphincterotomy. Carroll et al reported successful clearance of CBD stones in 17 of 20 patients (85%) by balloon dilatation; however, even in this small series, three patients (15%) experienced mild postoperative pancreatitis (Carroll et al 1993). This method should be avoided in patients with pre-existing pancreatitis, biliary dyskinesia, or anatomical sphincter anomalies. A sphincterotome may be inserted via the cystic duct and its tip placed just through the ampulla of Vater into the duodenum. A duodenoscope is passed transorally and used to allow proper positioning of the sphincterotome before applying current to perform a sphincterotomy. DePaula and associates have reported the performance of transcystic antegrade sphincterotomy at the time of LC in 22 patients, and all had successful stone clearance without complications; the procedure added only 17 minutes to the operation (DePaula et al 1993).

If the transcystic approach fails, we recommend direct incision of the CBD laparoscopically. Indications for laparoscopic choledochotomy are stones which are multiple, large or positioned within the proximal bile ducts in patients with a CBD diameter larger than 8–10 mm (Dion et al 1994, Phillips et al 1994). Stay sutures are usually placed on either side of the midline of the CBD wall to allow anterior traction on the duct. A longitudinal choledochotomy is made on the distal CBD, of adequate length to allow easy placement of a choledochoscope and removal of the largest stone. Stones are removed under endoscopic visualization and an appropriate sized T tube is placed in the duct. The ductotomy is closed with fine absorbable sutures using intracorporeal suturing techniques, and the T tube is exteriorized through the lateral port site. The patient is generally discharged 2–4 days postoperatively to return for a final T-tube cholangiogram and removal of the T tube at 14–21 days postoperatively. Retained stones demonstrated by T-tube cholangiography may be effectively removed percutaneously after allowing maturation of the T-tube tract. Percutaneous extraction is successful in more than 95% of patients with retained stones (Burhenne 1980). Overall,

Table 38.4 Techniques for treatment of choledocholithiasis

Method	Success rate (%)	Length of stay (days)	Return to work (days)
Transcystic duct extraction	70–95	1–2	7–10
Laparoscopic CBDE	85–100	4–7	14–30
Open CBDE	90–100	5–10	20–42
ERC/ES	85–95	2–3	7–14

CBDE, common bile duct exploration; ERC, endoscopic retrograde cholangiography; ES, endoscopic sphincterotomy laparoscopic choledochotomy is successful in more than 90% of patients with a minor morbidity rate of 5 to 10% and a mortality rate of 1 to 2% (Table 38.4). Complications of this technique include laceration of the CBD, bile leakage, sewn-in T tubes, and postoperative CBD strictures (Dion et al 1994). Many surgeons have not mastered laparoscopic suturing to the point where they feel comfortable closing the choledochotomy for fear of a resultant stricture. Nevertheless, advantages of the direct laparoscopic approach are that every portion of the ductal system can be accessed and stone size is unimportant. The alternative approach of open operation with exploration of the CBD with or without choledochoduodenostomy should not be forgotten in difficult cases (Chs 39, 42, 45).

The possibility of finding CBD stones and the means by which they can be treated must be discussed with the patient prior to operation in order to formulate a plan of therapy. Many surgeons routinely leave CBD stones in place during LC for planned postoperative endoscopic removal. Factors in favor of postoperative endoscopic therapy would include small non-obstructing duct stones, a patient with comorbidity making a prolonged operation risky, and a small CBD prone to postoperative stricture. In resorting to postoperative endoscopic retrograde cholangiography and sphincterotomy, the goals of minimally invasive surgery are maintained with a rapid return to full activity. However, relying on postoperative endoscopic sphincterotomy subjects the patient to an additional procedure with its associated morbidity, and possibly a second operation if endoscopic stone extraction fails. In experienced hands, endoscopic sphincterotomy has an overall failure rate for stone clearance of 5 to 10% (Cotton 1993). Leaving a transcystic catheter in the CBD at the time of LC may decrease the likelihood of failure by allowing a guidewire to be passed into the duodenum to facilitate cannulation of the CBD (Deslandres et al 1993). Certainly, one is more willing to submit a patient to postoperative endoscopic stone extraction when the endoscopic expertise is high, whereas an open CBD exploration (Ch. 45) should be strongly considered when only an inexperienced endoscopist is available in the local setting. Thus, the expertise of both laparoscopist and endoscopist remain critical determinants of the means by which CBD stones are managed (Cotton 1993).

POSTOPERATIVE CARE

Patients may be observed in the hospital overnight or be discharged later the same day. The patient is allowed clear liquids in the immediate postoperative period and is advanced to a regular diet as tolerated. Postoperative referred shoulder and neck pain may occur transiently due to diaphragmatic irritation. No activity restrictions are placed on the patient; functional status depends entirely on the degree of abdominal tenderness, which usually subsides by the second or third postoperative day. The patient may return to work as soon as the abdominal discomfort is tolerable, often within the first week.

Although LC was initially thought of as a procedure that could reduce a typical 5-day stay for an OC to 1–2 days, third-party payers in the USA have begun to push for discharge of the patient on the same day of surgery. The principal advantage is reduction of hospital costs. Nevertheless, not all patients are candidates for outpatient LC. In a recent prospective analysis of 506 consecutive LC cases, Saunders and associates argued that most complications, including those that are life-threatening, were not apparent by 8 hours postoperatively and only clinically detected 39% of the time at 24 hours following the procedure (Saunders et al 1995). Thus, they advocate great caution in selecting patients for outpatient LC. Patients who may benefit from an overnight stay include the elderly, those with significant co-morbid illnesses, those requiring substantial analgesia postoperatively, and cases in which complications have occurred. For same-day discharge, the patient should be healthy, reliable and sensible, have undergone an uncomplicated operation and have good home support. Written instructions are given to the patient and the family with detailed advice concerning signs of potential problems. Routine postoperative follow-up at 2–4 weeks is advised for all patients.

SPECIAL CONSIDERATIONS

CONVERSION TO OPEN OPERATION

Surgeons performing LC should not think of conversion to open operation as a complication, but rather mature judgment, and hence not hesitate to convert to a traditional OC if the anatomy is unclear, if complications arise, or there is failure to make reasonable progress in a timely manner (Table 38.5). It is 'better to open one too many than to open one too few', even if it means a longer hospital stay for the patient. Some complications requiring laparotomy are obvious, such as massive hemorrhage, bowel perforation, or major injury to the bile duct. Open laparotomy allows the additional tool of manual palpation and tactile sensation and should be performed when the anatomy cannot be delineated because of inflammation, adhesions or anomalies. Fistulae between the biliary system and bowel are rare,

Table 38.5 When to convert from open to laparoscopic cholecystectomy

Injury to major blood vessels, viscus or bile duct
Anatomy unclear
Failure to progress in a timely fashion
Pathology not amenable to minimal access surgical techniques
Choledocholithiasis untreatable by minimal access surgical techniques or postoperative endoscopic techniques
   Billroth II
   Previous failed ERCP
   Minimal endoscopic experience

ERCP, endoscopic retrograde cholangiopancreatography

but may require laparotomy for optimal management. The demonstration of potentially resectable gallbladder carcinoma (Ch. 53) also dictates an open exploration. Finally, CBD stones which cannot be removed laparoscopically and are unlikely to be extracted endoscopically (due to Billroth II anastomosis, previously failed endoscopic retrograde cholangiopancreatography (ERCP), or an inexperienced endoscopist) should be converted to open operation without hesitation.

ACUTE CHOLECYSTITIS

Acute cholecystitis (Ch. 34) may be treated by LC within the first 72 hours of presentation, after initiation of antibiotics and bowel rest, or allowed to 'cool down' and an elective LC performed 6–8 weeks following the acute attack (Soper 1991). Intervention during the early phase reveals an inflamed, thick-walled, tensely distended organ. To gain adequate traction on the gallbladder with the grasping forceps, it may be necessary to decompress the gallbladder by aspirating its contents with a large-gauge needle. As long as the inflammation is limited to the gallbladder, LC is usually technically feasible. However, if inflammation extends to the porta hepatis, great care must be taken in proceeding with the operation. The normally thin, minimally adherent tissue that invests the cystic duct and artery is markedly thickened and edematous and may not readily separate from these structures with the usual blunt dissection techniques. The duct wall also may be edematous, thus making its external diameter similar to the gallbladder neck and CBD. If the anatomy is unclear, cholangiography must be performed before clipping or dividing tissue. When acute inflammation has been present for several days or weeks before operation, the pericholecystic tissue planes may be obliterated by thick, 'woody' tissue that is difficult to dissect bluntly. The surgeon may therefore need to convert to OC if the minimal access approach is initially attempted during this subacute

phase. There is no harm in inserting the laparoscope and assessing the right upper quadrant. The decision to convert to an open operation is a matter of judgment, based on the existing anatomy, local conditions, and the surgeon's experience and confidence in his or her ability to complete the procedure using minimal access techniques.

Several authors have reported performing LC in the face of acute inflammation with success but with a higher conversion rate than for elective LC (Cooperman 1990, Hermann 1990, Rattner et al 1993, Reddick et al 1991, Unger et al 1991). Lo et al reported in their prospective study (1996) that despite longer operative times and postoperative stays for early LC in patients with acute cholecystitis (treatment within 5 days) versus delayed LC (initial conservative treatment followed by LC 3–4 months later), the advantage of early LC was the reduction in the total hospital stay, from 15 to 7 days. Rattner and associates retrospectively reviewed 20 patients who underwent attempted LC for acute cholecystitis and examined factors that were predictive of a successful procedure (Rattner et al 1993). Seven of the 20 patients (35%) required conversion to OC. The interval from admission to cholecystectomy in the successful cases was 0.6 days versus 5 days in the cases requiring conversion to OC. Converted cases also had a significantly higher white blood cell count, alkaline phosphatase levels and APACHE II scores compared to those undergoing successful LC. Ultrasonographic findings such as gallbladder distention, wall thickness and pericholecystic fluid did not correlate with the success of LC. In a recent prospective study of 105 patients randomized to early LC (within 24 hours of diagnosis of acute cholecystitis) versus delayed LC (6–8 weeks later), there was no significant difference in conversion rate (early 21% versus delayed 24%), postoperative analgesic requirement, or number of postoperative complications. The early group did have a longer operative time (123 min versus 107 min; $p = 0.04$), but total hospitalization was shorter (8 days versus 12 days; $p = 0.001$) (Lai et al 1998). It can be concluded that LC should be performed immediately after the diagnosis of acute cholecystitis. Delaying surgery allows inflammation to become more intense and neovascularized, thus increasing the technical difficulty of LC.

LARGE GALLSTONES

Extremely large gallstones (larger than 5 cm), although unusual, are difficult to manage during LC. The stone may completely fill the gallbladder, making it impossible to grasp the gallbladder wall and place it on adequate tension. Also, once the gallbladder has been excised, extracting the large calculus from the abdomen may necessitate enlarging the umbilical incision. The largest gallstone removed laparoscopically in our experience measured 8 × 5 cm, being essentially a cast of the gallbladder. Grasping forceps were used to push the gallbladder from side to side to maintain tension for dissection, and a ~4 cm incision was necessary for extraction. In such cases OC should be considered.

INTRAOPERATIVE GALLBLADDER PERFORATION

Perforation of the gallbladder with bile or stone leakage can be a nuisance but should not ordinarily require conversion to OC. Perforation may occur secondary to traction applied by the grasping forceps or because of electrosurgical thermal injury during removal of the gallbladder from its bed. In our experience, almost one-third of the patients have had intraoperative spillage of bile or stones (Jones et al 1995). Patients with a bile leak have not experienced an increased incidence of infection, prolongation of hospitalization or postoperative disability, nor adverse long-term complications (mean follow-up of 41 months in 250 consecutive LC patients). The only difference between those with and without bile leakage was that the operating time of patients with a gallbladder perforation was approximately 10 min longer, presumably due to the time spent cleaning up the operative field. When perforation does occur, the bile should be aspirated completely and irrigation used liberally. The hole in the gallbladder is best secured with a grasping instrument and then sutured or tied with an endoloop. The stones should be retrieved and removed. Gallbladder spillage, when treated in this manner, results in no adverse short- or long-term complications. Escaped stones composed primarily of cholesterol pose little threat of infection. However, pigment stones frequently harbor viable bacteria and may potentially lead to subsequent infectious complications if allowed to remain in the peritoneal cavity (Deziel et al 1993). The long-term complications of retained stones, either intra-abdominally with resultant abscess formation or intramurally with resultant port site abscess, have not been prospectively studied, but recent case reports and case series in the surgical literature document a clear potential for long-term infectious complications (Carlin et al 1995, Horton & Florence 1998, Parra-Davila et al 1998, Shocket 1995, Zamir et al 1999). The relative infrequency of these complications probably does not justify conversion to open operation in the face of spilled stones, but vigilance in avoidance of perforation, a careful search for escaped stones, and liberal use of a plastic retrieval bag for large and friable gallbladders is recommended (Zamir et al 1999).

ANATOMIC VARIATIONS

One of the most frequent anomalies is a right hepatic artery that loops up onto the infundibulum of the gallbladder. This may be misidentified as the cystic artery, leading to injury to the hepatic artery (Berci & Sackier 1994). The surgeon will also occasionally notice only a small cystic artery on the medial aspect of the gallbladder; when this occurs, one should be alert for a posterior branch leading onto the dorsal aspect of the gallbladder. If great care is not taken, brisk hemorrhage may occur.

A short cystic duct is seen frequently and may be draining into the right hepatic duct or a low entry right sectoral hepatic duct (2%), common hepatic duct (1%), or connect the infundibulum with the CBD by a duct of only a few millimeters in length in 5–6% of cases (Berci 1992, Reid et al 1986). During OC, this is relatively easy to recognize, especially if the cholecystectomy is performed in a 'fundus first' fashion. During LC, these ducts are in danger of being mistaken for a normal cystic duct and divided (Meyers et al 1996) (Fig. 38.24). In addition to anomalous biliary ducts, one may have accessory ducts either draining into the cystic duct or from the liver directly into the gallbladder ('ducts of Luschka'). Since the widespread use of LC, there has been an increased occurrence of bile leaks from so-called 'ducts of Luschka'. It is likely that many of these bile leaks are due to

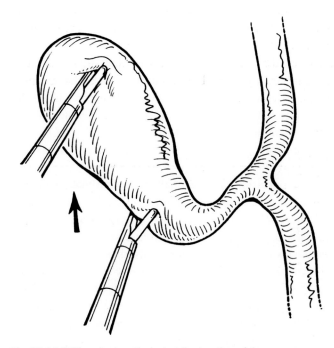

Fig. 38.24 With a short cystic duct at the junction of the common hepatic duct and the common bile duct, pulling the infundibulum can result in tenting of the common bile duct. This can mimic the appearance of the cystic duct.

dissection into the liver substance with injury to a normal, albeit superficial, intrahepatic biliary radicle.

If the liver is enlarged and heavy due to fatty infiltration or cirrhosis, it may be difficult, if not impossible, to expose the hepatocystic triangle. In cirrhosis, the firm enlarged liver is not only difficult to lift, but has a propensity to bleed when retracted. Furthermore, if there is associated portal hypertension, bleeding from small veins in the gallbladder bed, adherent omentum, or even trocar entry sites can make LC extremely difficult and dangerous.

COMPLICATIONS

Many complications related to laparoscopic removal of the gallbladder are similar to those occurring during traditional OC (Table 38.6). These complications include hemorrhage, bile duct injuries, bile leaks, retained stones, pancreatitis, wound infections, and incisional hernias. Other potential complications are pneumoperitoneum related (gas embolism, vagal reaction, ventricular arrhythmias, or hypercarbia with acidosis) and trocar related (injuries to the abdominal wall, intra-abdominal organ, or major blood vessels). The 'protective' shield on disposable trocars is not an insurance against perforation of intestine or major vessels, especially after previous abdominal operations. Regardless of the make of trocar, during its insertion one should never aim towards the spine or the location of the great vessels, and a hand is used as a 'brake' to prevent inadvertently introducing the trocar too far. Insertion of the initial trocar, especially when performed in a closed fashion, can cause iatrogenic injury to the bowel, bladder, aorta, iliac artery or vena cava (Cogliandolo et al 1998, Hanney et al 1995).

Table 38.6 Complications of laparoscopic cholecystectomy

Hemorrhage
Bile duct injury
Bile leak
Retained stones
Pancreatitis
Wound infection
Incisional hernia
Pneumoperitoneum related:
    CO_2 embolism
    Vaso-vagal reflex
    Cardiac arrhythmias
    Hypercarbic acidosis
Trocar related:
    Abdominal wall bleeding, hematoma
    Visceral injury
    Vascular injury

When a trocar injury to a major blood vessel is suspected, the patient must be opened immediately without removing the trocar until the involved blood vessel is isolated. In contrast, if the small-bore Veress needle enters a viscus or blood vessel, the operation can generally be completed and the patient monitored closely for signs of complications in the postoperative period.

The laparoscopic trocars may also lacerate blood vessels in the abdominal wall. Prior to removal, each trocar should be visualized from the peritoneal aspect using the laparoscope. If significant hemorrhage is seen, it can generally be controlled with cautery, intraoperative tamponade with a Foley catheter, or a through-and-through suture on each side of the trocar insertion site.

Most of the complications occur early in the surgeon's experience. For instance, in a recent multivariate regression analysis of 8839 LCs in which there were 15 bile duct injuries, the only significant factor associated with an adverse outcome was the surgeon's experience with the procedure (Moore & Bennett 1995). The regression model predicted that a surgeon had a 1.7% chance of a bile duct injury occurring in the first case and 0.17% chance of a bile duct injury in the 50th case.

Of all the potential complications, biliary injuries have received the most attention and are discussed at length elsewhere in this text (Ch. 49). Most series quote major bile duct injury rates of 0.30% or less during OC, whereas the incidence of bile duct injuries during LC is 0.40% or higher (Strasberg et al 1995). These injuries can cause major morbidity, prolonged hospitalization (Cates et al 1993), high cost and litigation (Asbun et al 1993). In addition to the surgeon's experience and aberrant anatomy, a number of reports mention chronic inflammation with dense scarring, operative bleeding obscuring the field, or fat in the portal area contributing to the biliary injuries (Adams et al 1993, Davidoff et al 1992, Moosa et al 1992, Soper et al 1993). The classic biliary injury, however, occurs when the CBD or a right hepatic duct is mistaken for the cystic duct and is divided between clips. Many surgeons attribute this misidentification to the direction of traction of the gallbladder, i.e. pulling the CBD and the cystic duct into alignment, thus making them appear to be one. Other contributing factors to misidentification are a short cystic duct, a large stone in Hartmann's pouch (making retraction and display of the cystic duct difficult), or tethering of the infundibulum to the CBD by acute or chronic inflammation (Figs 38.25 and 38.26). Constant awareness of these potential misidentifications and technical causes of biliary injuries is the best method of prevention. If a bile duct injury occurs, an immediate repair should be performed. When a bile duct injury is discovered in the postoperative period, a coordinated effort

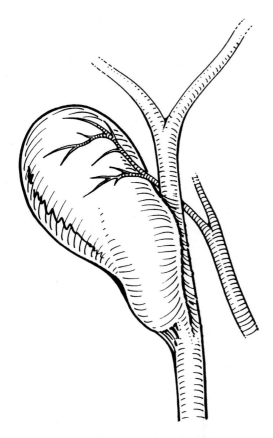

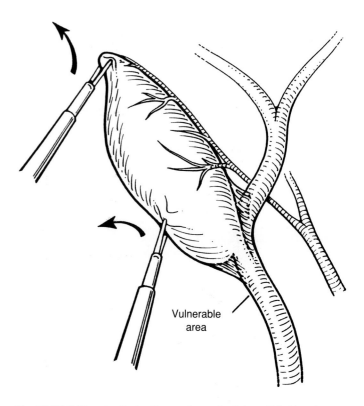

Vulnerable
area

Fig. 38.26 With excessive traction on the neck of the gallbladder, the common bile duct becomes tented and appears to be entering the gallbladder directly. The marked portion of the common bile duct is most vulnerable to injury during LC.

Fig. 38.25 Severe acute cholecystitis or long-standing chronic cholecystitis may result in the cystic duct and infundibulum of gallbladder becoming partially adherent or difficult to separate from the common bile duct itself (shaded area).

by radiologists, endoscopists and surgeons is necessary to optimize management (Strasberg et al 1995). There should be no hesitation in asking for the help of a surgeon experienced in biliary repair (Ch. 49).

RESULTS OF LAPAROSCOPIC CHOLECYSTECTOMY SERIES

AUTHORS' PERSONAL SERIES

Between November 1989 and January 1999, more than 4000 LCs were performed at Washington University's affiliated hospitals. Among the authors' personal series of >1200 LCs, there was a conversion rate of 2.1% and one perioperative death (0.1%) due to myocardial infarction at 1 week postoperatively. Significant postoperative complications occurred in 2.7%, including two minor duct injuries (0.2%). The mean operative time decreased from more than 100 minutes in the first 100 patients to 85 minutes in the most recent 100 patients. The postoperative course in most

patients was uneventful, with over 90% of patients discharged from the hospital within 24 hours of surgery, and only 10% required parental narcotics after leaving the recovery room. Similarly, the duration of disability was minimal, with the average postoperative interval to return to full activity being 10 days. These results compared favorably with those of traditional OC, in which the morbidity and mortality rates were similar but hospitalization for 3–5 days and return to work at 1 month after surgery were standard (Wu et al 1998).

OTHER REPORTED SERIES

Our data mirror those from most series of LC reported to date. There have been eight prospective, randomized trials comparing OC with LC and results have been mixed in demonstrating advantages of LC over OC in treating elective symptomatic cholelithiasis (Table 38.7). In the first study, 37 LC patients were compared to 25 patients undergoing minilaparotomy cholecystectomy (Barkun et al 1992). The mean hospital stay (including 1 preoperative day) was significantly shorter in the LC than the OC group (3 versus 4 days, respectively) as was the duration of convalescence (12

Table 38.7 Prospective randomized trials of open versus laparoscopic cholecystectomy

Study	Number of patients	Operating room time (min)	Complications (%)	Length of stay (days)	Return to work (days)
Barkun et al (1992)					
OC (minilap)	25	73	8.0	4*	20*
LC	37	86	2.7	3	12
Trondsen et al (1993)					
OC	35	50*	20	4*	34*
LC	35	100	17	3	11
Berggren et al (1994)					
OC	12	69*	—	3*	24*
LC	15	87	—	2	12
McMahon et al (1994)					
OC (minilap)	148	57*	20	4*	—
LC	151	71	17	2	—
McGinn et al (1995)					
OC (minilap)	155				
LC	155				
Majeed et al (1996)					
OC (minilap)	100	40*	xx	3	35
LC	100	65	xx	3	28
Squirrell et al (1998)					
OC (minilap)	100				
LC	100				
Kiviluoto et al (1998)					
OC	31	*	23*	6*	
LC	32		3	4	

*$p < 0.05$

versus 20 days, respectively). Use of narcotics throughout the first postoperative week was significantly greater in the OC group, but the duration of surgery was 12 minutes longer for LC than for OC (Barkun et al 1993).

The second study included 70 patients and also showed advantages of LC over OC in terms of length of hospital stay, postoperative opiate analgesia requirement, return to work, and time of convalescence (Trondsen et al 1993). Patients who underwent LC stayed in the hospital half the time of those who underwent OC (2 versus 4 days, respectively). The amount of pain as assessed by a visual analogue scale was significantly less in the LC group; the LC group also required less analgesics. Sick leave in the LC group was only one-third of that in the OC group (11 versus 34 days); full convalescence averaged 8 days in the LC group but 49 days in the OC group.

A third randomized trial of 27 patients also demonstrated advantages of LC over OC in regards to length of hospital stay, postoperative pain and convalescence (Berggren et al 1994). The mean duration of postoperative hospital stay was 2 days for LC and 3 days for OC. Patient-controlled opiate consumption in the first 12 h after operation was

similar in the two groups, but was significantly reduced thereafter in patients who underwent LC.

A fourth study prospectively randomized 299 patients to LC or minilaparotomy OC, and showed that LC resulted in shorter hospital stay and quicker return to normal activities (McMahon et al 1994a). The median postoperative hospital stay was 2 days shorter after LC. Laparoscopic patients returned to work in the home sooner and, at 1 week, had better physical and social functioning. Laparoscopic cholecystectomy was also associated with lower linear analogue pain scores, lower patient-controlled morphine consumption, a smaller reduction in postoperative pulmonary function, and better postoperative oxygen saturation (McMahon et al 1994b).

The fifth study prospectively randomized 310 patients to LC versus mini-laparotomy OC with 155 patients in each group. Conversion to large-incision cholecystectomy was significantly more common with LC (13% versus 4%) and complications were significantly more frequent with LC (9% versus 3%). When LC was successful, hospital stay was significantly shorter than for OC (2 versus 3 days respectively), but overall the hospital stay was not significantly different.

Postoperative analgesia requirements were reduced and return to normal activities and to work were faster after LC. There was no significant cost difference between the two procedures (McGinn et al 1995). Similarly, the sixth study prospectively randomized 200 patients in a single-blinded fashion (identical wound dressings were applied in both groups so that caregivers would be blinded to the type of operation) to LC versus mini-laparotomy OC. Laparoscopic cholecystectomy took significantly longer than small-incision cholecystectomy (median 65 min versus 40 min, $p < 0.001$). However, there was no significant difference in length of stay (median 3.0 for LC versus 3.0 for small-incision OC, $p = 0.74$), return to work (median 5.0 weeks versus 4.0 weeks; $p = 0.39$), and time to full activity (median 3.0 weeks versus 3.0 weeks; $p = 0.15$) (Majeed et al 1996). A follow-up to this study prospectively randomized 200 additional patients to LC or minilaparotomy OC. Postoperative pain, analgesic and antiemetic consumption, perceived health, and metabolic and respiratory responses were compared. Pain scores in both groups were low. Laparoscopic cholecystectomy, however, was associated with lower postoperative pain scores and analgesic requirements compared with small-incision OC, but the antiemetic requirements were greater after LC. The duration of hospital stay and the perceived health after operation were the same, and both procedures were associated with a similar reduction of respiratory function.

Twenty-four hours after operation the inflammatory (C-reactive protein, CRP) response to LC (22 ± 20 mg/L) was significantly lower than after small-incision OC (68 ± 30 mg/L), but the neuroendocrine (cortisol) response was similar (LC, 475 ± 335 nmol/L, compared with small-incision OC, 710 ± 410 nmol/L) (Squirrell et al 1998).

Most recently, a study of 63 patients prospectively randomized to LC versus OC for treatment of acute cholecystitis reported a LC to OC conversion rate of 16% and a significantly lower postoperative complication rate with LC (3% versus 23%) (Kiviluoto et al 1998). The postoperative hospital stay was significantly shorter in the LC than the OC group (4 versus 6 days) and the mean time to return to work was shorter in the LC group (14 versus 30 days).

Numerous clinical series of LC, either accrued prospectively or retrospectively, have also been reported (Table 38.8). Morbidity rates range from 1.5 to 8.6%, and bile duct injuries range from 0.2 to 0.7%. Mortality is rare after this procedure, and is usually attributed to unrelated events. The conversion rates from laparoscopic to open operation in most series range from 1.8 to 7.8% and generally is greater early in the surgeon's experience with the procedure.

As would be predicted for this excisional procedure, LC effectively treats gallstone disease. However, postcholecystectomy problems (Ch. 43) occur in some patients. Kane et al noted 89% of patients undergoing LC had preoperative

Table 38.8 Results of large series of LC

Study	Number of patients	Conversion (%)	Mortality (%)	Complications†	Bile duct injuries (%)
Deziel et al (1993)	77 604	—	0.04	2.0	0.6
Scott et al (1992)	12 397	4.3	0.08	4.0	0.4
Deveney (1993)	9597	—	0.04	2.5	0.3
Croce et al (1994)	6865	3.1	0.06	2.5	0.3
Orlando et al (1993)	4640	6.9	0.13	8.6	0.3
Schlumpf et al (1994)	3722	7.0	0.08	4.8	0.6
Collett et al (1993)	2955	4.8	0.20	3.4	0.6
SAGES (Airan et al 1992)	2671	4.6	0.15	—	0.2
Kane et al (1995)	2490	7.8	—	—	—
Litwin et al (1992)	2201	4.3	0.00	—	0.1
Kimura et al (1993)	1989	2.7	0.00	1.8	0.6
Larson et al (1992)	1983	4.5	0.10	2.1	0.3
Fullarton et al (1994)	1683	17.0	0.50	5.9	0.7
Newman et al (1995)	1525	2.2	0.26	4.1	0.0
Southern Surgeons Club (Meyers 1991)	1518	4.7	0.07	1.5	0.5
Cuschieri et al (1991)	1236	3.6	0.00	1.6	0.3
Brune et al (1994)	800	1.2	0.00	2.8	0.2
Perissat et al (1992)	777	5.5	0.10	3.3	0.4
Jatzko et al (1995)	740	5.4	0.14	1.9	—
Cappucino et al (1994)	563	4.8	0.00	6.9	0.3
Current series:					
Soper et al (1998)	1200	2.1	0.10	2.7	0.2

† Includes intraoperative and postoperative complications

biliary-type pain and only 10.6% of the patients had similar pain postoperatively (Kane et al 1995). Similarly, Ure et al found that the percentage of patients with biliary colic was reduced from 83% before LC to 6.4% after LC (Ure et al 1995). Fenster et al examined symptom relief in 225 patients undergoing LC followed postoperatively between 3 weeks and 3 months. They differentiated symptomatic gallstones from acalculous cholecystitis and discovered that 82% of patients with biliary colic and gallstones had complete relief of upper abdominal pain after the operation compared to only 52% of patients with acalculous cholecystitis (Fenster et al 1995). These data are comparable to the data for OC in which biliary-type pain persisted at follow-up (< 1 year) in 9 to 34% of patients with symptomatic gallstones (Bates et al 1991, Gilliland & Traverso 1990, Scriven et al 1993). In terms of cost-effectiveness, several studies have shown that LC is less expensive than the open procedure (Bass et al 1993, Fullarton et al 1994) while others have shown the contrary (McMahon et al 1994a).

CONCLUSIONS

Laparoscopic management of symptomatic gallstones has rapidly become the new standard for therapy throughout the world. Many patients can now undergo this operation in an ambulatory setting. Most common bile duct stones can be removed at the time of LC, either extracted through the cystic duct or by direct choledochotomy. Occasionally anatomical or physiological considerations will preclude the minimal access approach, and conversion to an open operation in such cases reflects sound judgment and should not be considered a complication.

REFERENCES

Acosta J M, Ledesma C L 1974 Gallstone migration as a cause of acute pancreatitis. New England Journal of Medicine 290: 484–487

Adams D B, Borowicz M R, Wootton F T I, Cunningham J T 1993 Bile duct complications after laparoscopic cholecystectomy. Surgical Endoscopy 7: 79–83

Airan M, Appel M, Berci G et al 1992 Retrospective and prospective multi-institutional laparoscopic cholecystectomy study organized by the Society of American Gastrointestinal Endoscopic Surgeons. Surgical Endoscopy 6: 169–176

Asbun H J, Rossi R L, Lowell J A, Munson J L 1993 Bile duct injury during laparoscopic cholecystectomy: mechanism of injury, prevention, and management. World Journal of Surgery 17: 547–552

Bagnato V J 1993 Laparoscopic choledochoscopy and choledocholithotomy. Surgical Laparoscopy and Endoscopy 3: 164–166

Barkun J S, Barkun A N, Sampalis J S et al 1992 Randomized controlled trial of laparoscopic versus mini-cholecystectomy. Lancet 340: 1116–1119

Barkun J S, Fried G M, Barkun A N et al 1993 Cholecystectomy without operative cholangiography. Implications for common bile duct injury and retained common bile duct stones. Annals of Surgery 218: 371–379

Bass E B, Pitt H A, Lillemoe K D 1993 Cost-effectiveness of laparoscopic cholecystectomy versus open cholecystectomy. American Journal of Surgery 165: 466–471

Bates T, Ebbs S R, Harrison M, A'Hern R P 1991 Influence of cholecystectomy on symptoms. British Journal of Surgery 78: 964–967

Beal J M 1984 Historical perspective of gallstone disease. Surg Gynecol Obstet 158: 181–189

Berci G 1992 Biliary ductal anatomy and anomalies; the role of intraoperative cholangiography during laparoscopic cholecystectomy. Surgical Clinics of North America 72: 1069–1077

Berci G, Sackier J M 1994 Laparoscopic cholecystectomy and laparoscopic choledocholithotomy. In: Blumgart LH (ed) Surgery of the Liver and Biliary Tract. Churchill Livingstone, Edinburgh, p 633–662

Berggren U, Gordh T, Grama D, Haglund U, Rastad J, Arvidsson D 1994 Laparoscopic versus open cholecystectomy: hospitalization, sick leave, analgesia and trauma responses. British Journal of Surgery 81: 1362–1365

Boline G, Clifford R, Yang H et al 1991 Cholecystectomy in the potential heart transplant patient. Journal of Heart and Lung Transplantation 10: 269–274

Brune I B, Scholenbenk, Omran S 1994 Complications after laparoscopic and conventional cholecystectomy: a comparative study. HPB Surgery 8: 19–25

Burhenne J 1980 Percutaneous extraction of retained biliary stones: 661 patients. American Journal of Roentgenology 134: 888–898

Cappucino H, Cargill S, Nguyen T 1994 Laparocopic cholecystectomy: 563 cases at a community teaching hospital and a review of 12,201 cases in the literature. Surgical Laparoscopy and Endoscopy 4(3): 213–221

Carlin C B, Kent R B, Laws H L 1995 Spilled gallstones—complications of abdominal wall abscesses. Surgical Endoscopy 9: 341–343

Carroll B, Phillips E, Chandra M, Fallas M 1993 Laparoscopic transcystic duct balloon dilatation of the sphincter of Oddi. Surgical Endoscopy 7: 514–517

Cates J, Tompkins R, Zinner M, Busuttil R, Kallman C, Roslyn J 1993 Biliary complications of laparoscopic cholecystectomy. American Surgeon 59: 243–247

Chui P T, Gin T, Oh T E et al 1993 Anaesthesia for laparoscopic general surgery. Anaesthesia and Intensive Care 21: 163–171

Cockett W S, Cockett A T 1998 The Hopkins rod-lens system and the Storz cold light illumination system. Urology 51: 1–2

Cogliandolo A, Monganaro T, Saitta F P et al 1998 Blind versus open approach to laparoscopic cholecystectomy: a randomized study. Surgical Laparoscopy and Endoscopy 8: 353–355

Collet D, Edye M, Perissat J 1993 Conversions and complications of laparoscopic cholecystectomy. Results of a survey conducted by the French Society of Endoscopic Surgery and Inververtional Radiology. Surgical Endoscopy 7: 334–338

Conference N C 1992 Gallstones and laparoscopic cholecystectomy. JAMA 269: 1018–1024

Cooperman A 1990 Laparoscopic cholecystectomy for severe acute, embedded, and gangrenous cholecystitis. Journal of Laparoendoscopic Surgery 1: 37–40

Cotton P 1993 Endoscopic retrograde cholangiopancreatography and laparoscopic cholecystectomy. American Journal of Surgery 165: 474–478

Croce E, Azzola M, Golia M, Russo R, Pompa C 1994 Laparocholecystectomy 6,865 cases from Italian institutions. Surgical Endoscopy 8(9): 1088–1089

Crump C 1931 The incidence of gallstones in gallbladder disease. Surgery Gynecology and Obstetrics 53: 447–455

Cuschieri A, Dobois F, Mouiel J et al 1991 The European experience with laparoscopic cholecystectomy. American Journal of Surgery 161: 383–388

Davidoff A, Pappas T, Murray E et al 1992 Mechanisms of major biliary injury during laparoscopic cholecystectomy. Annals of Surgery 215: 196–202

DePaula A, Hashiba K, Bafutto M 1994 Laparoscopic management of choledocholithiasis. Surgical Endoscopy 8: 1399–1403

DePaula A, Hashiba K, Bafutto M, Zago R, Machado M 1993 Laparoscopic antegrade sphincterotomy. Surgical Laparoscopy and Endoscopy 3: 157–160

Deslandres E, Gagner M, Pomp A et al 1993 Intraoperative endoscopic sphincterotomy for common bile duct stones during laparoscopic cholecystectomy. Gastrointestinal Endoscopy 39: 54–58

Deveney K E 1993 The early experience with laparoscopic cholecystectomy in Oregon. Archives or Surgery 128: 627–632

Deziel D, Millikan K, Economou S, Doolas A, Ko S, Airam M 1993 Complications of laparoscopic cholecystectomy: A national survey of 4,292 hospitals and an analysis of 77,604 cases. American Journal of Surgery 165: 9–14

Dion Y, Ratelle R, Morin J, Gravel D 1994 Common bile duct exploration: the place of laparoscopic choledochotomy. Surgical Laparoscopy and Endoscopy 4: 419–424

Escarce J, Chen W, Schwartz J 1995 Falling cholecystectomy thresholds since the introduction of laparoscopic cholecystectomy. JAMA 273: 1581–1585

Fendrick A, Gleeson S, Cabana M, Schwartz J 1993 Asymptomatic gallstones revisited. Is there a role for laparoscopic cholecystectomy? Archives of Family Medicine 2: 959–968

Fenster L, Lonborg R, Thirby R, Traverso L 1995 What symptoms does cholecystectomy cure? Insights fom an outcome measurement project and review of literature. American Journal of Surgery 169: 533–538

Fervers C 1933 Die Laparoskopie mit dem Cystoskop. Medizinsche Klinik 31: 1042–1045

Ferzli G, Massaad A, Kiel T, Worth M J 1994 The utility of laparoscopic common bile duct exploration in the treatment of choledocholithiasis. Surgical Endoscopy 8: 296–298

Fitzgerald S, Andrus C, Baudendistel L, Dahms T, Kaminski D 1992 Hypercarbia during carbon dioxide pneumoperitoneum. American Journal of Surgery 163: 186–190

Franklin M, Pharand D, Rosenthal D 1994 Laparoscopic common bile duct exploration. Surg Laparosc Endosc 4: 119–124

Frazee R, Roberts J, Symmonds R et al 1993 Combined laparoscopic and endoscopic management of cholelithiasis and choledocholithiasis. American Journal of Surgery 166: 702–705

Fullarton G, Darking K, Williams J, MacMillan R, Bell G 1994 Evaluation of the cost of laparoscopic and open cholecystectomy. British Journal of Surgery 81: 124–126

Fullarton G M, Bell G 1994 West of Scotland Laparoscopic Cholecystectomy Audit Group Prospective audit of the introduction of laparoscopic cholecystectomy in the west of Scotland. Gut 35: 1121–1126

Gilliland T, Traverso L 1990 Modern standards for comparison of cholecystectomy with alternative treatments for symptomatic gallstones with emphasis on long term relief of symptoms. Surgery Gynecology and Obstetrics 170: 39–44

Girardet R, Rosenbloom P, Deweese B et al 1989 Significance of asymptomatic biliary tract disease in heart tranplantation recipients. Journal of Heart Transplant 8: 391–399

Gow J G 1998 Harold Hopkins and optical systems for urology—an appreciation. Urology 52: 152–157

Hanney R M, All K M, Cregan P C et al 1995 Major vascular injury and laparoscopy. Australian and New Zealand Journal of Surgery 65: 533–535

Hermann R 1990 Surgery for acute and chronic cholecystitis. Surgical Clinics of North America 70: 1263–1275

Hicken N, McAllister A 1964 Operative cholangiography as an aid in reducing the incidence of 'overlooked' common bile duct stones. A study of 1,293 choledocholithotomies. Surgery 55: 753–758

Horton M, Florence M G 1998 Unusual abscess patterns following dropped gallstones during laparoscopic cholecystectomy. American Journal of Surgery 175: 375–379

Hull D, Bartus S, Perdrizet G, Schweizer R 1994 Management of cholelithiasis in heart and lung transplant patients: with review of laparoscopic cholecystectomy. Connecticut Medicine 58: 643–647

Hunter J 1992 Laparoscopic transcystic common bile duct exploration. American Journals of Surgery 163: 53–58

Hunter J, Soper N 1992 Laparoscopic management of common bile duct stones. Surgical Clinics of North America 72: 1077–1098

Jacobeus H 1911 Kurze Ubersicht uber meine Erfahrungen mit der Laparothorakoskopie. Muenchener Medizinische Wochenschrift 58: 2017–2019

Jakimowicz J 1993 Review: Intraoperative ultrasonography during minimal access surgery. Journal of the Royal College of Surgeons of Edinburgh 38: 231–238

Jatzko G T R, Lisborg P H, Perti A M, Stettner H M 1995 Multivariate comparison of complications after laparoscopic cholecystectomy and open cholecystectomy. Annals of Surgery 221(4): 381–386

Jennings C R 1998 Harold Hopkins. Archives of Otolaryngology Head and Neck Surgery 124: 1042

John T, Banting S, Pye S, Paterson-Brown S, Garden O 1994 Preliminary experience with intracorporeal laparoscopic ultrasonography using a sector scanning probe. A prospective comparison with intraoperative cholangiography in the detection of choledocholithiasis. Surgical Endoscopy 8: 1176–1180

Jones D, Dunnegan D, Soper N 1995 The influence of intraoperative gallbladder perforation on long-term outcome after laparoscopic cholecystectomy. Surgical Endoscopy 9: 977–980

Jones D, Soper N 1996 Advances in Surgery. Mosby YearBook, Chicago, pp 271–289

Kalk H 1929 Erfahrungen mit der laparoskopie. Zeitschrift für Klinische Medizin 111: 303–348

Kane R, Luie N, Borbas C et al 1995 The outcomes of elective laparoscopic and open cholecystectomy. Journal of the American College of Surgeons 180: 136–145

Kane R L, Luie N, Borbas C et al 1995 The outcomes of elective laparoscopic and open cholecystectomy. Journal of the American College of Surgery 180(2): 136–145

Kelling G 1923 Zur Colioskopie. Archiv für Klinical Chirurgie 1226: 226–229

Kelly T 1980 Gallstone pancreatitis: Pathophysiology. Surgery 80: 488–492

Kimura T, Kimura K, Suzuki K et al 1993 Laparoscopic cholecystectomy: The Japanese experience. Surgical Laparoscopy and Endoscopy 3: 194–198

Kiviluoto T, Siren J, Luukkonen P, Kivilaakso E 1998 Randomised trial of laparoscopic versus open cholecystectomy for acute and gangrenous cholecystitis. Lancet 351: 321–325

Lai P B S, Kwong K H, Leung K L, Kwok S P Y, Chan A C W, Chung S C S, Lau W Y 1998 Randomized trial of early versus delayed laparoscopic cholecystectomy for acute cholecystitis. British Journal of Surgery 85: 764–767

Lantz P E, Smith ?? 1994 Fatal carbon dioxide embolism complicating attempted laparoscopic cholecystectomy—case report and literature review. Journal of Forensic Sciences 39: 1468–1480

Larson G M, Vitale G C, Casey J et al 1992 Multipractice analysis of laparoscopic cholecystectomy in 1,983 patients. American Journal of Surgery 163: 221–226

Legorreta A, Silber J, Constantino G, Kobylinski R, Zatz S 1993 Increased cholecystectomy rate after introduction of laparoscopic cholecystectomy. JAMA 270: 1429–1432

Litwin D E M, Girotti M J, Poulin E C, Mamazz J, Nagy A G 1992

Laparoscopic cholecystectomy: Trans-Canada experience with 2201 cases. Canadian Journal of Surgery 35: 291–296

Liu S Y, Leighton T, Davis I, Klein S, Lippmann M, Bongard F 1991 Prospective analysis of cardiopulmonary responses to laparoscopic cholecystectomy. Journal of Laparoendoscopic Surgery 1: 241–246

Lo C, Liu C, Lai E, Fan S, Wong J 1996 Early versus delayed laparoscopic cholecystectomy for treatment of acute cholecystitis. Annals of Surgery 223: 37–42

Lukichev O, Filimonov M, Zybin I 1983 A method of laparoscopic choleyctostomy. Khirurugia 8: 125–127

Machi J, Sigel B, Zaren A et al 1993a Operative ultrasonography during hepatobiliary and pancreatic surgery. World Journal of Surgery 17: 640–646

Machi J, Sigel B, Zaren A, Kurahiji T, Yamashita Y 1993b Technique of ultrasound examination during laparoscopic cholecystectomy. Surgical Endoscopy 7: 545–549

Majeed A W, Troy G, Nicholl J P, Smythe A, Reed M W, Stoddard C J, Peacock J, Johnson A G 1996 Randomised, prospective, single-blind comparison of laparoscopic versus small-incision cholecystectomy. Lancet 347: 989–994

McDougall E M, Monk T G, Wolf J S Jr et al 1996 The effect of prolonged pneumoperitoneum on renal function in an animal model. Journal of the American College of Surgeons 182: 317–328

McDougall E M, Bennett H F, Monk T G et al 1997 Functional MR imaging of the porcine kidney: physiologic changes of prolonged pneumoperitoneum. J Soc Laparoendosc Surg 1: 29–35

McGinn F P, Miles A J, Uglow M et al 1995 Randomized trial of laparoscopic cholecystectomy and mini-cholecystectomy. British Journal of Surgery 82: 1374–1377

McIntyre R, Stiegmann G, Peralman N 1994 Update on laparoscopic ultrasonography. Endoscopic Surgery and Allied Technologies 2: 149–152

McMahon A, Russell I, Baxter J et al 1994a Laparoscopic versus minilaparoscopic cholecystectomy: A randomized trial. Lancet 343: 135–138

McMahon A, Russell I, Ramsay G et al 1994b Laparoscopic and minilaparotomy cholecystectomy: a randomized trial comparing postoperative pain and pulmonary function. Surgery 115: 533–539

Meyers W C, the Southern Surgeons Club 1991 A prospective analysis of 1518 laparoscopic cholecystectomies. New England Journal of Medicine 324: 1073–1078

Meyers W C, Peterseim D S, Pappas T N, Schauer P R, Eubanks S, Murray E, Suhocki P 1996 Low insertion of hepatic segmental duct VII–VIII is an important cause of major biliary injury or misdiagnosis. American Journal of Surgery 171: 187–191

Miles R H, Carballo R E, Prinz R A, McMahon M, Pulawski G, Olen R N, Dahlinghaus D L 1992 Laparoscopy: the preferred method of cholecystectomy in the morbidly obese. Surgery 112: 818–822

Moore M, Bennett C 1995 The learning curve for laparoscopic cholecystotomy. The Southern Surgeons Club. American Journal of Surgery 170: 55–59

Moosa A, Easter D, vanSonnenberg E et al 1992 Laparoscopic injuries to the bile duct. Annals of Surgery 215: 203–208

Morgenstern L, Wong L, Berci G 1992 1200 open cholecystectomies before the laparoscopic era: A standard for comparison. Archives of Surgery 127: 400–403

Nenner R, Imperato P, Rosenberg C, Ronberg E 1994 Increased cholecystectomy rates among medicare patients after the introduction of laparoscopic cholecystectomy. Journal of Community Health 19: 409–415

Newman C L, Wilson R A, Newman L 3rd et al 1995 1525 Laparoscopic cholecystectomy without biliary injury: a single institution's experience. American Surgeon 61(3): 226–228

Orda R, Sayfan J, Levy Y 1994 Routine laparoscopic ultrasonography in biliary surgery. Surgical Endoscopy 8: 1239–1242

Orda R, Sayfan J, Strauss S, Barr J, Oland J 1994 Intraoperative ultrasonography as a routine screening procedure in biliary surgery. Hepatogastroenterology 41: 61–64

Orlando R III, Russell J C, Lynch J, Mattie A 1993 The Connecticut Laparoscopic Cholecystectomy Registry Laparoscopic cholecystectomy. A statewide experience. Archives of Surgery 128: 494–499

Parra-Davila E, Munshi I A, Armstrong J H, Sleeman D, Levi J U 1998 Retroperitoneal abscess as a complication of retained gallstones following laparoscopic cholecystectomy. J Laparoendosc Adv Surg Tech A 8: 89–93

Perissat J, Collet D, Edye M, Magne E, Belliard R, Desplantez J 1992 Laparoscopic cholecystectomy: an analysis of 777 cases. Baillières Clinical Gastroenterology 6(4): 727–742

Petelin J 1993a Laparoscopic approach to common duct pathology. American Journal of Surgery 165: 487–491

Petelin J B 1993b Laparoscopic approach to common duct pathology. American Journal of Surgery 165: 487–491

Phillips E, Carroll B, Pearlstein A et al 1993 Laparoscopic choledochoscopy and extraction of common bile duct stones. World Journal of Surgery 17: 22–28

Phillips E, Rosenthal R, Carroll B, Fallas M 1994 Laparoscopic trans-cystic-duct common bile duct exploration. Surgical Endoscopy 8: 1389–1394

Ransohoff D, Gracie W 1993 Treatment of gallstones. Annals of Internal Medicine 119: 606–619

Ransohoff D, Gracie W, Wolfenson L, Neuhauser D 1983 Prophylactic cholecystectomy or expectant management for silent gallstones: a decision analysis to assess survival. Annals of Internal Medicine 99: 199–204

Rattner D, Ferguson C, Warshaw A 1993 Factors associated with successful laparoscopic cholecystectomy for acute cholecystitis. Annals of Surgery 217: 233–236

Reddick E, Olsen D 1989 Laparoscopic laser cholecystectomy: A comparison with mini-lap cholecystectomy. Surgical Endoscopy 3: 131–133

Reddick E, Olsen D, Spaw A et al 1991 Safe performance of difficult laparoscopic cholecystectomies. American Journal of Surgery 161: 377–381

Reid S, Cho S, Shaw C, Turner M 1986 Anomalous hepatic duct inserting into the cystic duct. AJR. American Journal of Roentgenology 147: 1181–1182

Saunders C, Leary B, Wolfe B 1995 Is outpatient laparoscopic cholecystectomy wise? Surgical Endoscopy 9: 1263–1268

Schirmer B D, Dix J, Edge S B, Hyser M J, Hanks J B, Aguilar M 1992 Laparoscopic cholecystectomy in the obese patient. Annals of Surgery 216: 146–152

Schlumpf R, Klotz H P, Wehrli H, Herzog U 1994 A nation's experience in laparoscopic cholecystectomy. Surgical Endoscopy 8: 35–41

Schoenfield I, Berci G, Carnovale R et al 1990 The effect of ursodiol on the efficacy and safety of extracorporeal shockwave lithotripsy of gallstones. New England Journal of Medicine 323: 1239–1245

Schoenfield I, Lachin J, The Steering Committee TNCGSG 1981 Chenodiol (chenodeoxycholic acid) for dissolution of gallstones: the national cooperative gallstone study. Annals of Internal Medicine 95: 257–282

Scott T R, Zucker K A, Bailey R W 1992 Laparoscopic cholecystectomy: a review of 12,397 patients. Surgical Laparoscopy and Endoscopy 2(3): 191–198

Scriven M, Burgess N, Edwards E, Morgan A, Bundred N, Lewis M 1993 Cholecystectomy: a study of patient satisfaction. Journal of the Royal College of Surgeons Edinburgh 38: 79–81

Semm K 1987 Operative Manual for Endoscopic Abdominal Surgery. Yearbook Medical Publishers, Chicago

Sharma K C, Kabinoff G, Ducheine Y et al 1997 Laparoscopic surgery and its potential for medical complications. Heart Lung 26: 52–64

Shocket E 1995 Abdominal abscess from gallstones spilled at laparoscopic cholecystectomy. Surgical Endoscopy 9: 344–347

Soper N 1991 Laparoscopic cholecystectomy. Current Problems in Surgery 28: 585–655

Soper N, Barteau J, Clayman R, Ashley S, Dunnegan D 1992 Laparoscopic versus standard open cholecystectomy: comparison of early results. Surgery Gynecology and Obstetrics 174: 114–118

Soper N, Hunter J, Petrie R 1992 Laparoscopic cholecystectomy during pregnancy. Surgical Endoscopy 6: 115–117

Soper N J, Stockmann P T, Dunnegan D L, Ashley S W 1992 Laparoscopic cholecystectomy: the new 'gold standard'? Archives of Surgery 127S: 917–921

Soper N, Flye M, Brunt L et al 1993 Diagnosis and management of biliary complications of laparoscopic cholecystectomy. American Journal of Surgery 165: 663–669

Soper N J 1993 Effect of nonbiliary problems on laparoscopic cholecystectomy. American Journal of Surgery 165: 522–526

Soper N J, Brunt L M, Kerbl K 1994 Laparoscopic general surgery. New England Journal of Medicine 330: 409–419

Soper N J 1997 The utility of ultrasonography for screening the common bile duct during laparoscopic cholecystectomy. J Laparoendosc Adv Surg Tech A 7: 271–276

Squirrell D M, Majeed A W, Troy G, Peacock J E, Nicholl J P, Johnson A G 1998 A randomized, prospective, blinded comparison of postoperative pain, metabolic response, and perceived health after laparoscopic and small incision cholecystectomy. Surgery 123: 485–495

Steck T, Castanfo-Nordin M, Keshavarzian A 1991 Prevalence and management of cholelithiasis in heart transplant patients. Journal of Heart and Lung Transplantation 10: 1024–1032

Steigmann G, McIntyre R, Pearlman N 1994 Laparoscopic intracorporeal ultrasound. An alternative to cholangiography? Surgical Endoscopy 8: 167–171

Steigmann G, Soper N, Filipi C, McIntyre R, Callery M, Cordova J 1995 Laparoscopic ultrasonography as compared with static or dynamic cholangiography at laparoscopic cholecystectomy. Surgical Endoscopy 9: 1269–1273

Steiner C, Bass E, Talamini M, Pitt H, Steinberg E 1994 Surgical rates and operative mortality for open and laparoscopic cholecystectomy in Maryland. New England Journal of Medicine 330: 403–408

Steptoe P 1967 Laparoscopy in Gynaecology. Livingstone Press, Edinburgh

Stoker M, Levielle R, McCann J et al 1991 Laparoscopic common bile duct exploration. Journal of Laparoendoscopic Surgery 1: 287–293

Strasberg S, Hertl N, Soper N 1995 An analysis of the problem of biliary injury during laparoscopic cholecystectomy. Journal of the American College of Surgeons 180: 101–125

Tagge E, Othersen H J, Jackson S et al 1994 Impact of laparoscopic cholecystectomy on the management of cholelithiasis in children with sickle cell disease. Journal of Pediatric Surgery 29: 209–212

Talamini M A, Gadacz T R 1992 Laparoscopic approach to cholecystectomy. Advances in Surgery 25: 1–20

Trondsen E, Reiertsen O, Andersen O, Kjaersgaard P 1993 Laparoscopic and open cholecystectomy: a prospective, randomized study. European Journal of Surgery 159: 217–221

Underwood R, Dunnegan D, Soper N 1998 Prospective, randomized trial of bipolar electrocautery versus ultrasonic coagulation for division of short gastric vessels during laparoscopic Nissen fundoplication. Surgical Endoscopy 12: 509

Underwood R A 1997 Chapter 1: The Laparoscopic Revolution. In: Jones D B, Wu J S, Soper N J (eds) Laparoscopic Surgery: Principals and Procedures. Quality Medical Publishing, Inc., St. Louis, p 3–8

Unger S, Edelman D, Scott J, Unger H 1991 Laparoscopic treatment of acute cholecystitis. Surgical Laparoscopy and Endoscopy 1: 14–16

Ure B, Troidl H, Spangenberger W et al 1995 Long term results after laparoscopic cholecystectomy. British Journal of Surgery 82: 267–270

Veress J 1938 Neues Instrument zur Ausführung von brust oder Bauchpunktionen. Deutsche Medizinische Wochenschrift 41: 1480–1481

Wittgen C M, Andrus C H, Fitzgerald S D, Baudendistel L J, Dahms T E, Kaminski D L 1991 Analysis of the hemodynamic and ventilatory effects of laparoscopic cholecystectomy. Archives of Surgery 126: 997–1000; discussion 1000–1001

Wolfe B M, Gardiner B N, Leary B F, Frey C F 1991 Endoscopic cholecystectomy. An analysis of complications. Archives of Surgery 126: 1192–1196

Wu J, Dunnegan D, Soper N 1998 The utility of intracorporeal ultrasonography for screening of the bile duct during laparoscopic cholecystectomy. Journal of Gastrointestinal Surgery 2: 50–59

Wu J S, Dunnegan D L, Luttmann D R, Soper N J 1998 The evolution and maturation of laparoscopic cholecystectomy in an academic practice. Journal of American College of Surgeons 186: 554–561

Zamir G, Lyass S, Pertsemlidis D, Katz B 1999 The fate of the dropped gallstones during laparoscopic cholecystectomy. Surgical Endoscopy 13: 68–70

39

Stones in the common bile duct – surgical approaches

R.M. GIRARD

The traditional approach in the treatment of symptomatic gallstones and choledocholithiasis has been open cholecystectomy and common bile duct exploration. Despite a long and successful history, few areas of surgical gastroenterology have seen, over the past two decades, so many changes as the management of common bile duct stones.

Recently, with the widespread acceptance of laparoscopic cholecystectomy for the treatment of symptomatic gallstones, the management of common bile duct stones has become even more controversial. Management options for choledocholithiasis have expanded and many procedures have challenged the place and preeminence of open choledochotomy. Alternative therapeutic options include precholecystectomy or postcholecystectomy endoscopic retrograde cholangiography and papillotomy with stone removal; laparoscopic common duct exploration; biliary lithotripsy and percutaneous transhepatic stone extraction.

In the era of open cholecystectomy, the common bile duct was explored in approximately 15% of all cholecystectomies and stones were removed in approximately 65% of these explorations. The incidence of concomitant choledocholithiasis varied between 8 and 20%. (Table 39.1). Open cholecystectomy with choledochotomy has been reported to have a mortality rate of less than 2% in many series (Bartlett & Waddel 1958, Ganey et al 1986, Pappas et al 1990, Schwab et al 1992, Moreaux 1995, Csendes et al 1998) and with the adjunct of routine postexploratory cholangiography and especially choledochoscopy an incidence of retained stones of less than 5% (Kappes et al 1982, Dayton et al 1984, DenBesten & Berci 1986).

ORIGIN OF CHOLEDOCHOLITHIASIS

It is generally accepted that the majority of common bile duct stones originally form in the gallbladder and later pass down through the cystic duct into the common bile duct; these stones are called secondary. Usually patients with choledocholithiasis also have gallstones but when they do not the gallbladder almost always shows chronic inflammatory change, suggesting that it previously contained stones.

Stones may also form primarily in the common bile duct and, when found in patients with congenital absence of the

Table 39.1 Incidence of choledocholithiasis in patients with gallstones

Reference	Total cases of gallstones	Exploration of common duct (%)	Exploration yielding stones (%)	Overall incidence of common duct stones (%)
McSherry & Glenn (1980)	8791	15.5	60	9.5
Hampson et al (1981)	2889	15	51	8
Doyle et al (1982)	4000	22	52.5	11.5
Lygidakis (1983)	3710	11.5	80	9.5
Coelho et al (1984)	908	21	72	15
Ganey et al (1986)	1024	26	36	9.5
DenBesten & Berci (1986)	983	24.5	81	20
Author's series	10 471	11	75	8
Total	32 776	15	63	9.5

gallbladder, provide an absolute proof of their origin; these stones are called primary. However, proving that a stone had its origin in the common duct in the presence of a gallbladder is difficult. The incidence of primary common duct stones is controversial and varies from 4% (Saharia et al 1977) to 56% (Madden 1973). Madden defined them as solitary ovoid, light brown in color, soft and easily crushable. More than 50% of primary stones in this study were noted at cholecystectomy and 21% of gallbladders contained no stones. However, Saharia et al (1977) classified patients as having primary stones if they met all the following criteria: (1) previous cholecystectomy with or without common duct exploration; (2) at least a 2 year asymptomatic period after initial biliary tract surgery; (3) presence of soft, friable, light-brown stones or sludge in the common duct; (4) absence of a long cystic duct or biliary stricture due to previous surgery.

CLINICAL FEATURES

The natural history of choledocholithiasis is unpredictable. Small stones may pass spontaneously into the duodenum without causing symptoms or they may temporarily obstruct the pancreatic duct, induce an episode of pancreatitis and then pass into the duodenum with relief of symptoms. Stones that do not pass spontaneously may reside in the bile duct for long, symptom-free periods and then suddenly precipitate an episode of jaundice or cholangitis. Choledocholithiasis may appear in any of the following five ways: without symptoms, biliary colic, jaundice, cholangitis or pancreatitis. The last four of these may appear in all possible combinations. Sometimes, common bile duct stones are an unanticipated finding during elective cholecystectomy for gallstones.

If stones obstruct the common duct and the bile becomes infected, acute cholangitis (Ch. 60) ensues. The classic triad of fever with chills, jaundice and pain leads to the suspicion of choledocholithiasis and, when associated with known cholelithiasis, the diagnosis is almost certain. When this triad is associated with hypotension and mental confusion, it confirms the presence of an acute obstructive suppurative cholangitis with impending bacteremic shock.

If a stone obstructs the common bile duct in the absence of infected bile, asymptomatic jaundice, often fluctuating, will ensue and in many patients there will be spontaneous complete resolution. This will happen if, as ductal dilatation develops, the stone floats back up the common bile duct and away from the narrow distal end as edema subsides; thus, it should not be assumed that the common duct is free

of stones when jaundice clears. However, occasionally jaundice is relieved because the stone indeed passes into the duodenum. Should incomplete obstruction persist for years before a definitive diagnosis is made and therapy instituted, secondary biliary cirrhosis with hepatic failure and portal hypertension may develop.

Pancreatitis (Ch. 35) is the second most frequent complication of choledocholithiasis whereas choledochoenteric fistula and common duct stricture are uncommon.

PREOPERATIVE DIAGNOSIS

In a multipractice analysis of 1983 patients undergoing laparoscopic cholecystectomy Larson et al (1992) noted a 3.8% incidence of common duct stones. This is consistent with another series (Csendes et al 1998) but considerably lower than that reported for open cholecystectomy (Table 39.1). This difference is probably due to a selection process. In an unselected group of patients, the incidence was 8.6% and rose to 12% with the addition of patients who had gallstone pancreatitis and were assumed to have passed a stone prior to endoscopic retrograde cholangiography (ERCP) (Miller et al 1995).

The preoperative evaluation of patients (those without jaundice) who are candidates for elective laparoscopic cholecystectomy should include a careful history and physical examination, serum chemistry evaluation (serum bilirubin, alkaline phosphatase, Y-glutamyl transferase, aspartate and alanine transaminases) and abdominal ultrasonography. The selection criteria include a common duct that measures less than 9 mm in diameter, normal liver function tests and no recent history of pancreatitis or jaundice. The application of these preoperative clinical, biochemical and ultrasonographic parameters has shown excellent negative predictive ability (Houdart et al 1995, Csendes et al 1998). Patients who do not exhibit any of these parameters preoperatively, have been shown to be free of duct calculi in 99% of the cases. Positive predictive ability has been less satisfactory and patients categorized as at-risk have been proven to have choledocholithiasis in 39% of cases (Houdart et al 1995). Therefore, it seems reasonable to avoid further diagnostic preoperative investigations and even routine intraoperative cholangiography in patients with absence of jaundice, normal liver function tests and ultrasonographic evidence of a normal biliary tree (common bile duct diameter under 9 mm) even in the presence of a recent acute cholecystitis.

On the other hand, investigation of the group at risk seems necessary to know to exclude common bile duct stones. If there is any suspicion that choledocholithiasis is present, preoperative magnetic resonance cholangiography (MRCP) or ERCP is performed. If no stone is found, laparoscopic cholecystectomy is performed. If bile duct stone is indeed present, preoperative endoscopic retrograde stone removal can then be performed. For the few non-jaundiced patients who may be candidates for elective open cholecystectomy, preoperative clinical indicators of chole-docholithiasis rather than expensive preoperative studies, should alert the surgeon to the need for accurate intra-operative assessment. The diagnosis of choledocholithiasis is usually made at operation by careful inspection, palpation and, importantly, operative cholangiography.

For patients with gallstones and concomitant jaundice, preoperative ERCP or MRCP should be performed to determine the presence or absence of obstruction and the nature of the obstructing lesion.

Similarly, if bile duct dilatation is clearly identified in a patient with gallstones, (common bile duct diameter above 9 mm) it is appropriate to perform a preoperative ERCP or MRCP or to carry out perioperative cholangiography.

COMMON BILE DUCT EXPLORATION AT CHOLECYSTECTOMY (Ch. 45)

The purpose of common bile duct exploration for choledo-cholithiasis is to detect and remove all stones within the bile duct system as safely as possible. However, this is not with-out risk. While open cholecystectomy alone may be per-formed with little morbidity, and a mortality of less than 0.5%, the addition of an exploration of the bile duct increases the morbidity, and mortality may rise by three to seven times (Table 39.2). Indeed, common bile duct explo-ration is the most important factor in influencing the mor-bidity and mortality of open cholecystectomy since the procedure is more often necessary in patients of advanced age and consequently with associated medical diseases. In addition, the longer duration of operation and the presence of jaundice, cholangitis or pancreatitis in patients with com-mon duct stones influence morbidity and mortality.

Thus, it is desirable that all those and only those patients with choledocholithiasis should have bile duct exploration at open cholecystectomy. Accurate diagnosis is therefore essential. In the past, many patients were selected for bile duct exploration on the basis of clinical and operative find-ings such as a previous history of jaundice or pancreatitis, a dilated common bile duct, a single faceted stone in the gall-bladder or multiple small gallstones. These are important observations which should alert the surgeon to the possibil-ity of choledocholithiasis, but the use of these criteria alone to predict the presence of common duct stones has led to negative choledochotomy in a high percentage of patients (Frazee & Van Heerden 1989). Clearly, the decision to explore the common bile duct must be based on the most accurate methods to confirm choledocholithiasis.

INDICATIONS FOR COMMON BILE DUCT EXPLORATION

Despite the fact that open choledochotomy is only occa-sionally necessary nowadays for the management of chole-docholithiasis, many current indications remain where it is still the management option of choice.

In several developing and less developed countries, elec-tive open cholecystectomies are still performed for many patients. Moreover, the availability of endoscopic retro-grade cholangiography and sphinctorotomy may be absent or scarce, so patients with acute or complicated gallstone disease are submitted directly to open cholecystectomy and common bile duct exploration if necessary. In these patients, the absolute indications for common duct explo-ration are: (1) palpable stones in the common bile duct; (2) jaundice with cholangitis; (3) a stone visualized at intra-operative cholangiography.

Palpation of the common bile duct is often underesti-mated but it is the most reliable indication for choledo-chotomy, having an accuracy of 98% if a stone is judged

Table 39.2 Mortality of biliary surgery for calculous diseases

Reference	Number of patients	Overall (%)	Cholecystectomy (%)	Cholecystectomy with CBDE (%)
Bartlett & Waddel (1958)	2243	1.1	0.6	1.8
DenBesten & Berci (1986)	983	1.6	0.6	4.4
Ganey et al (1986)	1024	0.5	0.4	0.7
McSherry (1989)	12 975	1.1	0.6	4.0
Pappas et al 1990	100	0	–	0
Author's series	10 471	0.45	0.3	1.6

palpable (Way et al 1972). Palpation should be performed from the liver hilum to the papilla after a Kocher maneuver. Obstructive jaundice with fever and chills is indicative of either cholangitis or acute cholecystitis. If patients with acute cholecystitis are excluded, this triad will be associated with choledocholithiasis in approximately 97% of the patients (Way et al 1972).

For the non-jaundiced patient, intraoperative cholangiography is, with palpation of stones, the most reliable determinant of the presence of choledocholithiasis and should be performed routinely at open cholecystectomy (Doyle et al 1982, Tompkins & Pitt 1982, Frazee & Van Heerden 1989). Its accuracy is between 85 and 98%. When technically satisfactory, the incidence of false-positive and false-negative examinations is 4 and 0.2%, respectively (Stark & Loughry 1980).

The main reasons to perform routine intraoperative cholangiography (Ch. 22) are: (1) exclusion from common bile duct exploration of patients who have clinical indications for choledochotomy, yet may not harbor stones at the time of surgery; (2) detection of unsuspected common duct stones in 3 to 7% of patients undergoing cholecystectomy (Tompkins & Pitt 1982); (3) pre-exploratory identification of the number and location of bile duct stones and their size; (4) visualization of the ampullary region and biliary anatomy. For these reasons, when technically possible, a cystic duct cholangiography should be performed on every patient prior to choledochotomy.

Specific diagnostic tests used preoperatively to demonstrate ductal stones should not be employed routinely in patients with proven gallstone but demonstration of choledocholithiasis by preoperative percutaneous or endoscopic cholangiography is a reliable indicator of common bile duct stones the accuracy rate for both being greater than 90%. However, the author considers that the presence of stones should be reconfirmed intraoperatively by cholangiography since stones may have passed into the duodenum in the interval between the performance of preoperative cholangiography and the time of surgery. Exploration of the common bile duct should be undertaken only when results from intraoperative cholangiography are unequivocally positive or when a stone is palpable within the common bile duct.

In developed countries where local endoscopic, radiologic or laparoscopic expertise may coexist in many hospitals, there are still occasional indications for open choledochotomy.

1. Patients with multiple common bile duct stones who are not candidates for ERCP or patients with stones which cannot be removed by endoscopic sphincterotomy.
2. Patients with gallstones and concomitant jaundice or acute suppurative cholangitis who cannot be managed by endoscopic sphincterotomy.
3. Patients in whom an open cholecystectomy is performed for different reasons such as suspicion of cancer or presence of a bilioenteric fistula or presence of Mirizzi syndrome, should have palpation of the common bile duct and operative cholangiography performed. If common bile duct stones are visualized, choledochotomy is mandatory.
4. Patients in whom, during laparoscopic cholecystectomy, there is finding by cholangiography of concomitant common bile duct stones and the surgeon decides that they cannot be removed intraoperatively at laparoscopy or postoperatively by endoscopic sphincterotomy.

TECHNICAL CONSIDERATIONS

Routine exploration of the common bile duct should be through a supraduodenal choledochotomy (Ch. 45) and the transduodenal route (Ch. 46) should be reserved for those patients in whom stones cannot be readily removed from above. Although impacted stones at the ampulla may be broken down and removed by a supraduodenal approach, they should probably be removed by means of a transduodenal sphincteroplasty since this is less traumatic in such circumstances.

The only reliable methods to confirm complete clearance of stone from the biliary tree are postexploratory choledochoscopy and cholangiography. The value of choledochoscopy has been confirmed by many authors (Nora et al 1977, Kappes et al 1982, Dayton et al 1984). Postexploratory cholangiography must also be used and should be obtained before closure of the abdomen, not only because it can locate occasional missed stones but also since it may reveal unsuspected disruption of the biliary ductal system. While often regarded as unreliable because of the failure of contrast material to enter the duodenum and the difficulty of eliminating air bubbles, postexploratory cholangiography can be carried out reliably with attention to detail. Myatt et al (1973) described a reliable technique which does not involve suture of the choledochotomy before postexploratory films are obtained. A small balloon catheter is introduced proximally and distally into the choledochus as the film is being taken after the introduction of the contrast material.

Postexploratory choledoscopy and cholangiography are mandatory in all patients following exploration of the common bile duct.

Following exploration, a T-tube (gauge at least 14 Fr) is left within the common bile duct so as to permit postoperative cholangiography and percutaneous extraction of retained stones (Ch. 41) if necessary.

In addition to routine postexploratory choledochoscopy and cholangiography, the selective use of biliary enteric drainage procedures is another method of decreasing the incidence of subsequently symptomatic retained stones. While the author does not recommend routine biliary enteric decompression at initial operation it should be carefully considered in patients with one or more of the following (see also Ch. 45):

1. Multiple duct stones, particularly in dilated ducts in elderly patients
2. One or several large stones within a dilated duct.

If these conditions pertain in an elderly or poor-risk patient, then choledochoduodenostomy may avoid reexploration. Other indications are:

3. Irretrievable intrahepatic stones
4. Proven ampullary stenosis
5. An impacted ampullary stone.

Choledochoduodenostomy and transduodenal sphincteroplasty both have their advocates. When the common duct is less than 1.5 cm in diameter in a young, low-risk patient with a solitary impacted ampullary stone, sphincteroplasty is preferable (Ch. 46). However, in elderly and high-risk patients with dilated ducts, choledochoduodenostomy is the procedure of choice (Schein & Gliedman 1981) (Ch. 45).

RESULTS OF CLINICAL EXPERIENCE

The author has reviewed the course of 1132 consecutive patients who underwent open cholecystectomy and concomitant bile duct exploration for presumed choledocholithiasis at the Maisonneuve-Rosemont Hospital in Montreal between 1971 and 1990. They constituted 10.8% of 10 471 patients who had cholecystectomy during this period and common duct stones were recovered in 850 (75%) patients (see Table 39.1). The age and sex distributions of the patients are shown in Table 39.3. The most reliable clinical indication of choledocholithiasis was jaundice associated with chills and fever (92%). The accuracy of preoperative intravenous cholangiography was 70%, while that of preoperative percutaneous or endoscopic cholangiography was 97%. Intraoperative findings that proved most reliable were palpation of common duct stones (96%) and positive cholangiography, which was 88% accurate in the demonstration of stones. The surgical procedures performed are shown in Table 39.4. It should be noted that 93% of the patients had only choledochotomy with stone extraction and T-tube drainage. The addition of a biliary enteric anastomosis was considered to be indicated in only 7% of the patients.

Table 39.3 Age and sex distribution of patients who had common duct exploration

Age (years)	Number of patients		
	Men	Women	Total
0–19	2	26	28
20–29	18	116	134
30–39	40	81	121
40–49	79	98	177
50–59	87	141	228
60–69	115	122	237
70–79	63	103	166
> 80	11	30	41
Total	415	717	1132

Table 39.4 Surgical procedures performed in addition to cholecystectomy

	Number of procedures	%
Choledochotomy with T-tube drainage	1050	92.8
Choledochotomy with transduodenal sphincteroplasty	45	4
Choledochotomy with choledochoduodenostomy	35	3
Hepaticojejunostomy	2	0.2

Postexploratory T-tube cholangiography was done intraoperatively in 906 patients. The examination was normal in 738 of these patients, and in 82, despite the absence of flow of contrast material into the duodenum, there was no filling defect and the appearances were accepted as indicating a stone-free duct. In 60 patients the examination revealed a stone, which was removed in 43 individuals, but in 17 patients the stones were abandoned within the ducts. Subsequent postoperative examination showed a missed stone in 26 cases. Operative choledochoscopy has been used since 1979 in more than 300 cases.

Of the 1132 patients, 18 died (1.6%). This mortality rate is significantly higher than the 0.3% mortality rate recorded for 9339 cholecystectomies without common bile duct exploration performed during the same period (Girard & Morin 1993). This confirms the increased risks associated with choledochotomy as reported by others (see Table 39.2). The mortality rate increases with age (Table 39.5) and was higher in patients with a positive duct exploration (1.9%) than in those with a negative exploration of the duct (0.7%). Of the 18 patients who died, 16 had either jaundice and/or acute pancreatitis at the time of surgery. The major cause of death was cardiac disease (six patients). Six other patients died of intraabdominal extrahepatic complications: three of a perforated duodenal ulcer, two from gastrointestinal bleeding and one from an abscess. Five patients

Table 39.5 Age-related mortality in common bile duct exploration

Age (years)	Number of patients	Number of deaths	Percentage
< 50	460	2	0.4
50–70	465	11	2.4
> 70	207	5	2.4
Total	1132	18	1.6

Table 39.6 Age-related morbidity in common bile duct exploration

Age (years)	Number of patients	Number of patients with complications	%
< 50	458	56	12
50–70	454	84	18.5
> 70	202	52	26
Total	1114	192	17

Table 39.7 Complications in patients with exploration of the common bile duct

Complication	Number of patients
Retained stone	61
Wound complication	38
Bile leakage	38
Pulmonary complication	31
Bile duct trauma	6
Intraabdominal abscess	4
Other	43

died of hepatobiliary complications: three from cholangitis with septic shock, one from hepatitis and one from a prolonged biliary fistula. The last patient died of pulmonary insufficiency.

It can be seen that most of the patients died from complications of associated diseases rather than from complications secondary to the choledochotomy itself. The causes of death are much more often related to the diseases for which the operation is performed and to medical conditions associated with age than to the specific performance of the choledochotomy.

The morbidity rate of 3.6% in 9337 cholecystectomies increased to 17% in patients with common bile duct exploration (Girard & Morin 1993). These results are in agreement with other studies that have reported increased morbidity in patients undergoing cholecystectomy with common bile duct exploration (Neoptolemos et al 1987). The incidence of complications was higher in positive than in negative explorations (19 versus 12%) and increased with age (Table 39.6). The most frequent complications were retained stones, bile leakage and wound complications (Table 39.7).

Retained stones were shown on postoperative T-tube cholangiography for 61 patients (5.4%). Nine (3.2%) of the 282 patients with negative choledochotomy had retained stones, whereas they were found in 52 (6.1%) of 850 patients with initial choledocholithotomy (positive exploration). Moreover, nine patients had residual or recurrent stones diagnosed 5 months to 8 years after the initial operation, giving an overall incidence of retained and recurrent stones of 6%.

Of the 61 patients with retained stones, spontaneous evacuation confirmed at T-tube cholangiography occurred in 12 individuals at intervals from 1 to 7 months after operation. Stones were successfully extracted in 28 patients via the T-tube tract and in two by endoscopic sphincterotomy, and nine patients underwent surgical choledocholithotomy 3 weeks to 6 months after the initial surgical operation. In 8 patients, a stone was abandoned in the bile duct, and two other patients were lost to follow-up.

COMMENTS

Open cholecystectomy with common bile duct exploration is a safe operation in young, healthy patients and has low mortality and morbidity rates. In the author's series, among 460 patients less than 50 years old who had an open cholecystectomy with common bile duct exploration, only two died (0.4%) (see Table 39.5) and the incidence of complications was 12% (see Table 39.6).

With advancing age, mortality and morbidity significantly increase (see Tables 39.5 and 39.6). Older patients, particularly those with obstructive jaundice and/or acute pancreatitis, are at a higher risk for complicated biliary tract disease necessitating choledochotomy. Moreover, other medical conditions often associated with advancing age also contribute to increased mortality and morbidity.

Before the introduction of laparoscopic cholecystectomy, it had been demonstrated that precholecystectomy endoscopic retrograde cholangiography with stone removal followed by open cholecystectomy was not superior to open cholecystectomy, operative cholangiography and common bile duct operation. In many studies, morbidity and mortality were similar and, in fact, the incidence of retained stones was lower with open choledochotomy (Neoptolemos et al 1987, Miller et al 1988, Stain et al 1991, Schwab et al 1992, Stiegmann et al 1992). Indeed, it was believed that routine precholecystectomy endoscopic retrograde cholangiography with stone removal was not worthwhile. However, since the introduction of laparoscopic cholecystectomy, preoperative ERCP has become, in many institutions, the standard approach for patients with suspected common bile duct stones. Numerous studies have confirmed the effectiveness of preoperative or postoperative endoscopic retrograde cholangiography ± sphincterotomy with stone removal for the management of stones in the common bile duct. (Frazee et al 1993, Duensing et al 1995, Miller et al 1995, Lorimer et al 1997).

Moreover, endoscopic retrograde cholangiography ± sphincterotomy with stone removal alone may be appropriate and is justified for common duct stones or their complications in elderly, debilitated, high-risk patients (Neoptolemos et al 1987). In these patients, the calculous gallbladder can be left in situ. Subsequent cholecystectomy for symptoms will be required in approximately 10% of the patients (Hill et al 1991). These patients are likely to die of underlying medical conditions before acute cholecystitis develops, but, should it do so, common duct exploration will not be required at the time of cholecystectomy, thus putting them in a lower-risk category.

The author agrees that the treatment of gallstones with choledocholithiasis in high-risk patients should be by endoscopic sphincterotomy alone. On the other hand, patients who are fit for cholecystectomy should not undergo only endoscopic sphincterotomy with common bile duct stone removal.

POSTCHOLECYSTECTOMY CHOLEDOCHOLITHIASIS

INCIDENCE

Although most initial operations for gallstone disease with or without demonstrated choledocholithiasis are curative, a small percentage of patients is found at some later date to have additional stones in the bile duct. About 1 to 2% of all patients who undergo cholecystectomy have stones left in the bile duct that require further intervention (Roslyn 1993). While retained or overlooked calculi following open cholecystectomy without common bile duct exploration are rare (Bergdahl & Holmlund 1976), their incidence following open cholecystectomy with concomitant common bile duct exploration has been reported to be less than 5% (Kappes et al 1982, Dayton et al 1984, Roslyn 1993) with a higher frequency following positive than in negative duct exploration. After a second operation on the biliary tract, a recurrence rate of approximately 20% has been reported (Way 1973, Saharia et al 1977), with even higher rates following subsequent reoperation (Allen et al 1981).

PREVENTION

Prevention of retained and recurrent bile duct stones is a very important goal and there is every reason to believe that most such stones can be prevented. Retained calculi are either knowingly left in the ductal system (abandoned stones) or inadvertently discovered on postoperative T-tube cholangiography, thus representing a failure in detection at the time of operation. Bergdahl & Holmlund (1976) reported that stones were retained in their patients for the following reasons:

1. Lodged inextricably in the intrahepatic duct (50%)
2. Overlooked because of technically inadequate postexploratory cholangiography (23%)
3. Not visualized despite good-quality postexploratory cholangiography (19%)
4. Misinterpreted as air bubbles on postexploratory cholangiography (8%).

The incidence of retained stones is almost certainly less if better techniques of postexploratory cholangiography and postexploratory choledochoscopy are used. The best treatment for retained and recurrent stones is undoubtedly: prevention through routine cystic duct cholangiography to discover the 3 to 7% common duct stones unsuspected at cholecystectomy; knowledge of when and how to explore the common bile duct; routine postexploratory choledochoscopy and cholangiography; and, finally, the selective use of adjunctive biliary enteric drainage procedures when indicated.

TREATMENT

Until 20 years ago, most retained and recurrent bile duct stones were treated operatively. However, over this period a variety of non-operative therapeutic alternatives have evolved and displaced operative management. These include:

1. Mechanical nonoperative extraction through the T-tube tract
2. Stone extraction after endoscopic sphincterotomy
3. Dissolution of stones by infusion of gallstone solvents into the T-tube
4. Biliary lithotripsy
5. Percutaneous transhepatic cholangiography and stone extraction.

The choice of management is determined by clinical presentation, the condition of the patient, availability of equipment, clinical expertise and the presence or absence of a T-tube. Today, the operative management of retained and recurrent bile duct stones is only resorted to if the non-operative procedures have failed.

RETAINED STONES IN THE PRESENCE OF A T-TUBE

With the advent of the laparoscopic biliary surgery, the use of the T-tube has become almost obsolete, eliminating methods for accessing the biliary tree postoperatively without an invasive procedure.

If a patient with a retained bile duct stone is in the immediate postoperative period and still has a T-tube in place, there are four management options: observation, mechanical extraction, endoscopic sphincterotomy or dissolution.

In the absence of biliary obstruction or infection, often no treatment is necessary for 4 to 6 weeks. During this period, 10 to 25% of retained stones found on postoperative cholangiography can be expected to pass spontaneously into the duodenum, and no further treatment will then be required. Occasionally, a radiological artefact (pseudo-calculus) strongly suggests the presence of a stone which is then not seen on repeated examinations.

If after 4 to 6 weeks the stone persists, active treatment should be instituted. In most patients, the choice of treatment lies between a radiological approach through the T-tube tract (Ch. 41) or early endoscopic retrograde sphincterotomy (Ch. 40). Because of its high success rate and low morbidity and mortality, nonoperative mechanical extraction through the T-tube tract is probably the treatment of choice in this situation. A success rate of 95% has been reported with a morbidity rate of only 4% (Mazzariello 1978). Burhenne (1980) reports no deaths in 661 patients. When complications do occur, they can be treated medically in most instances and only 0.2% have required surgery (Mazzariello 1978).

Endoscopic sphincterotomy has also been shown to be effective in the management of retained stones in the early postoperative period following exploration of the common bile duct with a T-tube still in place (O'Doherty et al 1986, Hammarström et al 1996). Although endoscopic sphincterotomy has the considerable advantage that it can be carried out as soon as retained stones are discovered, treatment may be unnecessary in some patients as stones may pass spontaneously. Moreover, the results of mechanical stone extraction through the T-tube tract are better than any reported for endoscopic sphincterotomy (Lambert et al 1988). Endoscopic sphincterotomy may be best employed when the patient is clinically unstable, when the T-tube is inappropriate in size and position or when mechanical extraction through the T-tube has failed.

Chemical dissolution is rarely indicated today and a sig-nificant role for this kind of management is difficult to support because better, safer and faster therapeutic alternatives exist. When endoscopic and interventional radiologic techniques fail to clear the stone from the common bile duct, chemical dissolution, as monotherapy or in conjunction with other non-surgical techniques could be indicated. Furthermore, if patients are at high surgical risk because of age or cardiopulmonary complications, and the hospital does not have the facility to perform extraction via a T-tube tract and endoscopic sphincterotomy, chemical lysis could be attempted.

Treatment of bile duct stones by extracorporeal shock-wave lithotripsy (Ch. 33) may occasionally play a role in the management of patients with retained common duct stones (Moody et al 1989). It is indicated in the management of stones that cannot be handled satisfactorily with percutaneous or endoscopic techniques. It may also, in certain circumstances, be a reasonable primary alternative for some patients.

If part or all of these techniques fail, however, operative management can be resorted to with the expectation of a very high success rate and comparable morbidity and mortality rates to endoscopic retrograde sphincterotomy (Girard & Legros 1981, Cameron 1989).

RETAINED OR RECURRENT STONES IN THE ABSENCE OF A T-TUBE

For the patient without a T-tube in place, endoscopic sphincterotomy is the procedure of choice and should be attempted first (Cameron 1989, Sivak 1989). Most reports of endoscopic sphincterotomy indicate a success rate in achieving overall clearance of stones from the common bile duct of more than 85% (Cotton 1984, Lambert et al 1991). Although early complication rates for endoscopic sphincterotomy is 5 to 10% with emergency surgery being required in 1 to 2% of cases, most complications can be managed conservatively (Cotton 1984, Escourrou et al 1984).

Hemorrhage, pancreatitis, cholangitis and perforation are the most frequent complications. Mortality is reported at usually between 0.5 and 2% (Sivak 1989, Lambert et al 1991). Long-term complication rate (mainly stenosis and/or new stones) is low (< 10%) and most of these complications can be managed endoscopically (Cotton 1984, Escourrou et al 1984, Sivak 1989, Hammarström et al 1996).

If for any reason there is a contraindication to endoscopic sphincterotomy, or if it fails, operative management is a reasonable alternative (Cameron 1989). It has been written many times that re-exploration of the common bile duct for a residual or recurrent stone is accomplished only with morbidity and mortality rates several times higher than those of the primary operation. However, it has been reported that reoperation for retained or recurrent stones can be performed with negligible operative mortality and morbidity (Girard & Legros 1981). This report, which included many series, showed that reoperation on the common bile duct for retained or recurrent stones is possible with a mortality rate of less than 2%. Miller et al (1988) reported 237 patients with common bile duct stones treated by common duct exploration or endoscopic sphincterotomy. Success was higher and mortality was lower for the operatively managed group. The complication rate was similar but the complications tended to be more serious and more apt to require surgery in the endoscopic sphincterotomy group. These studies demonstrate that the success, morbidity and mortality rates of surgery are comparable to those of endoscopic approaches and clearly suggest that operation should not be forgotten in the treatment of retained or recurrent bile duct stones.

When one is performing reoperation for retained bile duct stones, if they can be adequately and completely removed, the most appropriate surgical procedure is choledocholithotomy, choledochoscopy, placement of a T-tube and completion cholangiography. This procedure is adequate for the majority of patients at second operation, and there should be only a negligible recurrence rate of common bile duct stones if it was for a retained stone. The author's overall failure rate of 3% following choledochotomy for residual recurrent stone confirms this.

However, others have reported failure rates as high as 18 and 30% (Saharia et al 1977, Allen et al 1981). Because of this, Allen et al (1981) and Lygidakis (1982a) recommend a biliary enteric drainage procedure in all patients with previous choledocholithotomy. However, Tompkins and Pitt (1982) and Cameron (1989) emphasize that concomitant biliary drainage should not be carried out as mandatory in all patients with retained or recurrent stones. The author agrees with this, but biliary enteric drainage at reoperation should be carried out if any of the following occur:

1. Stricture of the distal bile duct or sphincter of Oddi
2. Marked dilatation of the duct (2 cm or more)
3. Multiple or primary bile duct stones
4. Inability to remove all stones from the duct
5. A third operation.

Either transduodenal sphincteroplasty (Ch. 46), choledochoduodenostomy (Ch. 45) or choledochojejunostomy are effective (Johnson & Harding Rains 1978, Jones 1978, Braasch et al 1980). Sphincteroplasty allows direct inspection of the papilla and extraction of an impacted stone but is not adequate to treat a long stricture of the distal duct. It is the treatment of choice in patients with a duct smaller than 1.5 cm in diameter to avoid possible stricture formation at the anastomosis but carries a greater risk of postoperative pancreatitis. Side-to-side or end-to-end choledochoduodenostomy, or end-to-side Roux-en-Y choledochojejunostomy are suitable for common ducts larger than 1.5 cm and offer better decompression of a very large duct. The mortality rate of choledochoduodenostomy is lower than that attending transduodenal sphincteroplasty, and it has been shown to be a safe and simple operation with low morbidity and mortality, especially in elderly patients (Schein & Gliedman 1981, Lygidakis 1982b). Occasionally, recurrent or primary stones are seen in patients with dilated ducts and a widely patent sphincter. In such cases, which have also been reported after endoscopic papillotomy, side-to-side choledochoduodenostomy or end-to-side Roux-en-Y choledochojejunostomy is necessary.

Treatment of bile duct stone by lithotripsy has been demonstrated (Ch. 33) and biliary lithotripsy may occasionally play a role in the management of patients with retained or recurrent common duct stones (Moody et al 1989).

RESULTS OF CLINICAL EXPERIENCE WITH REOPERATION

The course of all patients who had a reoperation for retained or recurrent choledocholithiasis at the Maisonneuve-Rosemont Hospital between 1969 and 1990 was reviewed. Eighty-five patients underwent a total of 88 operations: 85 were secondary operations and three patients needed a third operation. Common bile duct stones were confirmed in all patients before reoperation by either intravenous cholangiography, percutaneous cholangiography, endoscopic cholangiography or postoperative T-tube cholangiography. Seventy-three associated conditions which can be identified with increased operative risk were present in 44 patients (Table 39.8).

Table 39.8 Risk factors in 85 patients submitted to reoperation for retained or recurrent choledocholithiasis

Risk factor	Number of patients
Cardiac atherosclerosis	18
Septic cholangitis	15
Obesity	10
High blood pressure	8
Chronic pulmonary obstructive disease	7
Diabetes	5
Acute pancreatitis	5
Atrial fibrillation	3
Posthepatic cirrhosis	1
Chronic renal failure	1

There were 61 women and 24 men (age range 20 to 86 years, mean 57 years). Of the 88 reoperations, 43 were performed in patients over the age of 60 years. The initial biliary operations performed are shown in Table 39.9. The mean interval between the first and second operations was 81 months (range 1 month to 20 years) (Table 39.10) and the interval between the second and third operations in three patients was 2, 48 and 72 months.

There were three types of bile duct reoperation: choledocholithotomy with T-tube drainage (64 patients); choledocholithotomy with side-to-side choledochoduodenostomy (15 patients); choledocholithotomy with transduodenal

sphincteroplasty (six patients). Choledocholithotomy with T-tube drainage in one patient and choledocholithotomy with side-to-side choledochoduodenostomy in two patients were performed at a third operation. Choledochoscopy was used during the last 17 operations performed since 1979.

The average hospital stay was 9.3 days (range 5 to 24 days) and was approximately the same (9.7 days) for patients over 60 years of age. No patient died. There were only six minor complications and none of them necessitated urgent surgery (Table 39.11). In 43 reoperations performed in patients over 60 years of age, there were two complications (4.7%) (wound infection and pancreatic fistula). It is noteworthy that there was not a single complication in the last 17 operations. Two patients (3%) of the 64 who had choledocholithotomy with T-tube drainage developed recurrent bile duct stones 4 and 5 years after a second operation, and side-to-side choledochoduodenostomy was performed. To date, no patient has needed a fourth operation.

Taking the author's experience with that of other reported series, there have been 15 deaths among 920 patients submitted for reoperation for recurrent bile duct stones (Table 39.12). In one of these series (McSherry &

Table 39.9 Initial biliary operation performed

Type of operation	Number of patients
Cholecystectomy with operative cholangiography	8
Cholecystectomy without operative cholangiography	47
Cholecystectomy with choledocholithotomy	27
Cholecystectomy with choledocholithotomy and sphincterotomy	3

Table 39.10 Interval between first and second operation for retained or recurrent stones

Type of operation	Number of patients				Mean interval (months)
	Total	< 1 year	1–5 years	> 5 years	
Cholecystectomy with operative cholangiography	8	2	4	2	53
Cholecystectomy without operative cholangiography	47	10	12	25	98
Cholecystectomy with choledocholithotomy	27	13	7	7	46
Cholecystectomy with choledocholithotomy and sphincterotomy	3	0	0	3	152

Table 39.11 Complications of 88 common bile duct reoperations

Type	Number of complications
Lung atelectasis	2
Partial wound disruption	1
Stitch abscess	1
Wound infection	1
Pancreatic fistula	1
Total	6 (6.8%)

Table 39.12 Mortality rate of biliary reoperation for retained or recurrent bile duct stones

Reference	Number of operations	Mortality rate
Saharia et al (1977)	30	0
Jones (1978)	22	0
McSherry & Glenn (1980)	341	7 (2%)
Allen et al (1981)	47	1 (2%)
Choi et al (1982)	34	1 (3%)
Lygidakis (1982b)	116	2 (1.7%)
De Almeida et al (1984)	24	1 (4%)
Broughan et al (1985)	132	1 (0.8%)
DenBesten & Berci (1986)	86	2 (2.3%)
Author's series	88	0
Total	920	15 (1.6%)

Glenn 1980), 341 patients were reported in whom choledocholithotomy was carried out for retained or recurrent stones. Seven patients died after the procedure, resulting in a mortality of 2%. However, if three patients who were operated upon with cholangitis or pancreatitis were to be excluded, and only the elective procedure considered, only four patients will be found to have died (1%) after secondary choledocholithotomy.

These results show that the overall mortality rate for retained or recurrent stones is less than 2%, with most deaths occurring in elderly patients. This mortality rate is comparable to that of endoscopic sphincterotomy.

COMMENTS

Retained or recurrent bile duct stones can be managed safely with reoperation with little or no mortality, only minor morbidity and with a high success rate. It is effective and safe and should not be forgotten.

In a patient with a retained stone with a T-tube in place, extraction through the T-tube tract or endoscopic sphincterotomy should be attempted first. If available, chemical dissolution or biliary lithotripsy can be attempted. Otherwise, operative management is the alternative.

If a T-tube is not in place, endoscopic sphincterotomy should be attempted first. If there is any contraindication to sphincterotomy, or if it fails, operative management is a reasonable alternative, with the expectation of a very high success rate and comparable mortality and morbidity rates to sphincterotomy. Most patients will not require a biliary enteric drainage procedure. However, in selected patients, a drainage procedure will be required to prevent further problems.

CONCLUSION

Many options are now available for the management of common bile duct stones. Patients should be assessed by the gastroenterologist, radiologist and surgeon working in close relation. The choice between surgical and endoscopic removal of the stones should be made individually for each patient and multiple factors considered before making a decision. The traditional surgical management of patients with common duct stones has reached a high level of maturity and security even in elderly patients. The choice between open surgery, laparoscopic surgery and endoscopic sphincterotomy should take into account not only reported information and expertise but also the local availability and efficacy of the different methods.

The goal of surgeons performing open common bile duct exploration for calculous disease is to explore all and only all patients with choledocholithiasis, to detect and remove all stones within the bile ducts safely and to prevent retained and recurrent stones.

Before exploring a common duct, the surgeon must make an accurate diagnosis of choledocholithiasis which should be confirmed by preexploratory intraoperative cholangiography. The only reliable methods to confirm complete clearance of stones from the biliary tree at operation are postexploratory choledochoscopy and cholangiography, and these are mandatory procedures in all patients. Biliary enteric drainage procedures should be used selectively when indicated.

Patients with residual or recurrent bile duct stones should be managed depending on the general condition of the patient, available expertise and the presence or absence of a T-tube. The discovery of a retained or recurrent bile duct stone after biliary tract surgery is a signal for a thorough evaluation and subsequent decision.

REFERENCES

Allen B, Shapiro W, Way L W 1981 Management of recurrent and residual common duct stones. American Journal of Surgery 142: 41–47

Bartlett M K, Waddel W R 1958 Indications for common-duct exploration. Evaluation in 1000 cases. New England Journal of Medicine 258: 164–167

Bergdahl L, Holmlund D E W 1976 Retained bile duct stones. Acta Chirurgica Scandinavica 142: 145–149

Braasch J W, Fender H R, Boneval M M 1980 Refractory primary common bile duct stone disease. American Journal of Surgery 139: 526–530

Broughan T A, Sivak M V, Hermann R E 1985 The management of retained and recurrent bile duct stones. Surgery 98: 746–751

Burhenne H J 1980 Percutaneous extraction of retained biliary tract stones: 661 patients. American Journal of Roentgenology 134: 889–898

Cameron J L 1989 Retained and recurrent bile duct stones: operative management. American Journal of Surgery 158: 218–221

Choi T K, Lee N W, Wong J, Ong G B 1982 Extraperitoneal sphincteroplasty for residual stones. An update. Annals of Surgery 196: 26–29

Coelho J C U, Buffara M, Pozzobon C E et al 1984 Incidence of common bile duct stones in patients with acute and chronic cholecystitis. Surgery, Gynecology and Obstetrics 158: 76–80

Cotton P B 1984 Endoscopic management of bile duct stones (apples and oranges). Gut 25: 587–597

Csendes A, Burdiles P, Diaz J C 1998 Present role of classic open choledochotomy in the surgical treatment of patients with common bile duct stones. World Journal of Surgery 22: 1167–1170

Dayton M T, Conter R, Tompkins R K 1984 Incidence of complications with operative choledochoscopy. American Journal of Surgery 147: 139–145

De Almeida A M, Cruz A G, Aldeia F J 1984 Side-to-side choledochoduodenostomy in the management of choledocholithiasis and associated disease. Facts and fiction. American Journal of Surgery 147: 253–259

DenBesten L, Berci G 1986 The current status of biliary tract surgery: an international study of 1072 consecutive patients. World Journal of Surgery 10: 116–122

Doyle P J, Ward-McQuaid J N, McEwen-Smith A 1982 The value of routine peroperative cholangiography: a report of 4000 cholecystectomies. British Journal of Surgery 69: 617–619

Duensing R A, Williams R A, Collins J C et al 1995 Managing choledocholithiasis in the laparoscopic era. The American Journal of Surgery 170: 619–623

Escourrou J, Cordova J A, Lazorthes F et al 1984 Early and late complications after endoscopic sphincterotomy for biliary lithiasis with and without the gallbladder in situ. Gut 25: 598–602

Frazee R C, Van Heerden J A 1989 Cholecystectomy with concomitant exploration of the common bile duct. Surgery, Gynecology and Obstetrics 168: 513–516

Frazee R C, Roberts J, Symmonds R et al 1993 Combined laparoscopic and endoscopic management of cholelithiasis and choledocholithiasis. The American Journal of Surgery 166: 702–706

Ganey J B, Johnson P A, Prillaman P E, McSwain G R 1986 Cholecystectomy: clinical experience with a large series. American Journal of Surgery 151: 352–357

Girard R M, Legros G 1981 Retained and recurrent bile duct stones. Surgical or nonsurgical removal? Annals of Surgery 199: 21–27

Girard R M, Morin M 1993 Open cholecystectomy: its morbidity and mortality as a reference standard. Canadian Journal of Surgery 36: 75–80

Hammarström L E, Stridbeck H, Ihse I 1996 Long-term follow-up after endoscopic treatment of bile duct calculi in cholecystectomized patients. World Journal of Surgery 20: 272–276

Hampson L G, Fried G M, Stets J et al 1981 Common bile duct exploration: indications and results. Canadian Journal of Surgery 24: 455–457

Hill J, Martin D F, Tweedle D E F 1991 Risks of leaving the gallbladder in situ after endoscopic sphincterotomy for bile duct stones. British Journal of Surgery 78: 554–557

Houdart R, Perniceni T, Darne B et al 1995 Predicting common bile duct lithiasis: determination and prospective validation of a model predicting low risk. The American Journal of Surgery 170: 38–43

Johnson A G, Harding Rains A J 1978 Prevention and treatment of recurrent bile duct stones by choledochoduodenostomy. World Journal of Surgery 2: 487–496

Jones S A 1978 The prevention and treatment of recurrent bile duct stones by transduodenal sphincteroplasty. World Journal of Surgery 2: 473–485

Kappes S K, Adams M B, Wilson S D 1982 Intraoperative endoscopy. Mandatory for all common duct operations? Archives of Surgery 117: 603–607

Lambert M E, Martin D F, Tweedre D E F 1988 Endoscopic removal of retained stones after biliary surgery. British Journal of Surgery 75: 896–898

Lambert M E, Betts C D, Hill J et al 1991 Endoscopic sphincterotomy: the whole truth. British Journal of Surgery 78: 473–476

Larson G M, Vitale G C, Casey J et al 1992 Multipractice analysis of laparoscopic cholecystectomy in 1983 patients. The American Journal of Surgery 163: 221–226

Lorimer J W, Lauzon J, Fairfull-Smith R J et al 1997 Management of choledocholithiasis in the time of laparoscopic cholecystectomy. The American Journal of Surgery 174: 68–71

Lygidakis N J 1982a A prospective randomised study of recurrent choledocholithiasis. Surgery, Gynecology and Obstetrics 155: 679–684

Lygidakis N J 1982b Surgical approaches to postcholecystectomy choledocholithiasis. Archives of Surgery 117: 481–484

Lygidakis N J 1983 Incidence and significance of primary stones of the common bile duct in choledocholithiasis. Surgery, Gynecology and Obstetrics 157: 434–436

McSherry C K 1989 Cholecystectomy: the gold standard. American Journal of Surgery 158: 174–178

McSherry C K, Glenn F 1980 The incidence and causes of death following surgery for nonmalignant biliary tract disease. Annals of Surgery 191: 271–275

Madden J L 1973 Common duct stones: their origin and surgical management. Surgical Clinics of North America 53: 1095–1113

Mazzariello R M 1978 A fourteen-year experience with nonoperative instrument extraction of retained bile duct stones. World Journal of Surgery 2: 447–455

Miller J S, Ferguson C M 1990 Current management of choledocholithiasis. American Surgeon 56: 66–70

Miller B M, Kozarek R A, Ryan J A et al 1988 Surgical versus endoscopic management of common bile duct stones. Annals of Surgery 207: 135–141

Miller R E, Kimmelstiel F M, Winkler W P 1995 Management of common bile duct stones in the era of laparoscopic cholecystectomy. The American Journal of Surgery 169: 273–276

Moody F G, Amerson J R, Berci G et al 1989 Lithotripsy for bile duct stones. American Journal of Surgery 158: 241–247

Moreaux J 1995 Traditional surgical management of common bile duct stones: a prospective study during a 20-year experience. The American Journal of Surgery 169: 220–226

Myatt T Y, Robinson D, Gunn A A 1973 Peroperative cholangiography. British Journal of Surgery 60: 711–712

Neoptolemos J P, Davidson B R, Shaw D E et al 1987 Study of common bile duct exploration and endoscopic sphincterotomy in a consecutive series of 438 patients. British Journal of Surgery 74: 916–921

Nora P F, Berci G, Dorazio R et al 1977 Operative choledochoscopy. Results of a prospective study in several institutions. American Journal of Surgery 133: 105–110

O'Doherty D P, Neoptolemos J P, Carr-Locke D L 1986 Endoscopic sphincterotomy for retained common bile duct stones in patients with T-tube in situ in the early postoperative period. British Journal of Surgery 73: 454–456

Pappas T N, Slimane T B, Brooks D C 1990 100 consecutive common duct explorations without mortality. Annals of Surgery 211: 260–262

Roslyn J L 1993 Calculous biliary disease. In Greenfield L J (ed) Surgery: Scientific principles and practice. J B Lippincott, Philadelphia Ch 40: 936–953

Saharia P C, Zuidema G D, Cameron J L 1977 Primary common duct stones. Annals of Surgery 1985: 598–602

Schein C J, Gliedman M L 1981 Choledochoduodenostomy as an adjunct to choledocholithotomy. Surgery, Gynecology and Obstetrics 152: 797–804

Schwab G, Pointner R, Wetscher G et al 1992 Treatment of calculi of the common bile duct. Surgery, Gynecology and Obstetrics 175: 115–120

Sivak M V 1989 Endoscopic management of bile duct stones. American Journal of Surgery 158: 228–240

Stain S C, Cohen H, Tsuishoysha M, Donovan A J 1991 Choledocholithiasis. Endoscopic sphincterotomy or common bile duct exploration. Annals of Surgery 213: 627–634

Stark M E, Loughry W 1980 Routine operative cholangiography with cholecystectomy. Surgery, Gynecology and Obstetrics 151: 657–658

Stiegmann G V, Goff J S, Mansour A et al 1992 Precholecystectomy endoscopic cholangiography and stone removal is not superior to cholecystectomy, cholangiography and common duct exploration. The American Journal of Surgery 163: 227–230

Tompkins R K, Pitt H A 1982 Surgical management of benign lesions of the bile ducts. Current Problems in Surgery 19: 327–398

Way L W 1973 Retained common duct stones. Surgical Clinics of North America 53: 1139–1147

Way L W, Admirand W H, Dunphy J E 1972 Management of choledocholithiasis. Annals of Surgery 176: 347–359

Stones in the bile duct: endoscopic approaches

40

K. SOMNAY, D.L. CARR-LOCKE

INTRODUCTION

As endoscopic retrograde cholangiopancreatography (ERCP) transformed the diagnostic approach to suspected biliary disease and jaundice in the 1970s and 80s, so endoscopic sphincterotomy (ES), in the years since it was first performed in man (Kawai et al 1974, Classen & Demling 1974), has had a dramatic therapeutic impact on the management of biliary disease in general and the treatment of bile duct stones in particular. About 150 000 endoscopic biliary sphincterotomies are performed annually in the United States. It has undoubtedly influenced surgical decision-making, especially in the era of laparoscopic cholecystectomy, when bile duct stones are suspected and when ERCP and ES are readily available pre- or post-operatively. The introduction of ERCP and ES into the realm of bile duct stone management was at first resisted by the surgical community but their role became established once they were shown significantly to reduce the mortality rate in a range of situations (Cotton 1984). Though laparoscopic bile duct exploration (Ch. 38) is being performed in some centers, it requires considerable expertise and the position of laparoscopic bile duct stone retrieval in the treatment algorithm must await comparisons with peroral endoscopic management. A number of variable risk factors are present in all patients with biliary disease which, when combined together as clinical judgement, allow a decision to be made in favor of one or other mode of therapy. It is precise documentation of such factors and how they determine outcome from different treatments which needs to be examined carefully in relation to endoscopic approaches and their surgical alternatives. Recent studies show that ES for stones is safe even in younger patients with normal diameter bile ducts.

Interest in ERCP and ES as definitive therapy for bile duct stones has again grown enormously in the 1990s since the introduction of laparoscopic cholecystectomy. The views expressed in this chapter are based on an extensive personal ERCP experience and results derived from collected reports from recognized experts. Only peroral endoscopic techniques developed from ERCP will be considered here with no discussion of percutaneous choledochoscopy, nor per-laparoscopic biliary procedures except where these represent valid alternatives to endoscopic approaches.

INDICATIONS FOR ENDOSCOPIC THERAPY

Patients with bile duct stones present with a variety of clinical problems either alone or in combination e.g., cholestasis, pain, cholangitis, pancreatitis, or as asymptomatic demonstration on imaging or cholangiography. It has become increasingly acceptable to treat patients in all these categories endoscopically. Endoscopic sphincterotomy was initially considered justifiable only in elderly post-cholecystectomy patients with recurrent or retained bile duct stones who were at high risk of serious complications from open surgical bile duct exploration or re-exploration at a time when few endoscopy centers could offer the technique and criticisms by surgical experts were common (Blumgart & Wood 1978). The impressive successes of ES in this group, however, and an expansion of availability, together with a low level of complications and a strong patient preference, led many centers to widen their indications for the procedure to include younger and fitter post-cholecystectomy patients, and more recently, a range of patients in whom the gallbladder is still in situ but in whom bile duct stones give rise to the principal clinical problem. Much of this initially occurred in the absence of comparative trial data to aid decision-making and, indeed, there was such enthusiasm for ES that the establishment of randomized trials was difficult. Nevertheless, they were essential to settle arguments about relative morbidity and mortality risks as different groups of patients were likely to be treated empirically by endoscopic or surgical means and were not necessarily comparable (Cotton 1984).

The endoscopist is now faced with referral of a number of clearly defined groups of patients with confirmed or suspected bile duct stones for whom endoscopic management may be indicated:

- acute cholangitis irrespective of gallbladder status
- acute gallstone pancreatitis irrespective of gallbladder status
- obstructive jaundice
- post-cholecystectomy, stone(s) shown on intraoperative cholangiogram
- post-cholecystectomy, retained stone(s), early presentation
- post-cholecystectomy, late presentation
- gallbladder in situ, variable risk factors for surgery, possible need for subsequent cholecystectomy.

Many studies now show endoscopic therapy either as optimal in many of these settings or define its role in the treatment algorithm.

ENDOSCOPIC TECHNIQUES

The endoscopist now offering a service for the treatment of bile duct stones must have access to an appropriate endoscopy facility, high-quality image intensification and rapid film processing of permanent radiographs or digital storage. The team must be fully cognizant of all the basic procedures and lesser used techniques as well as potential complications and their management and must include medical, nursing and technical endoscopy staff together with radiography and patient transport personnel, all of whom allow the smooth running of an ERCP session and facilitate any decisions which must be made during an examination. It is essential for endoscopy staff to explain the nature of the procedure to the patient, outlining the purpose, benefits, advantages, alternatives, and possible hazards of the examination and therapy.

Endoscopic sphincterotomy immediately follows diagnostic ERCP which delineates the problem to be treated and allows accurate placement of instruments within the common bile duct (CBD). A vertical incision is made from the papillary orifice of the CBD in a cephalad direction along the intramural course of the CBD for a variable length (on average 10 to 15 mm) depending on local anatomy, the degree of CBD dilatation and the size of stone to be removed (Fig. 40.1). The incision is produced by the con-

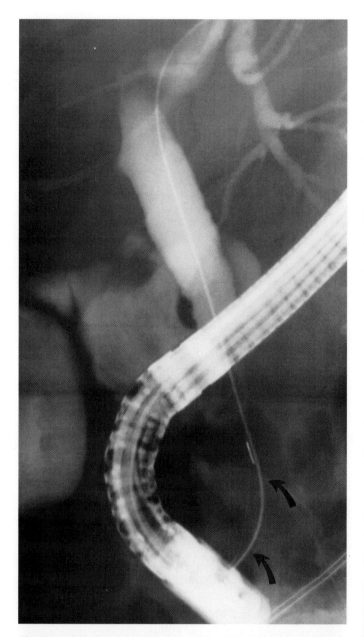

Fig. 40.1 ERCP showing cholangiography with dilated bile duct, a single duct stone just below the endoscope, a guidewire and sphincterotome in position during sphincterotomy (arrows).

trolled application of electrocautery delivered by a generator specifically made for endoscopic use which will not exceed 150 watts via a sphincterotome. It is fundamental to good ES technique that complete control of wire tension and electrocautery be maintained at all times whether or not the ES incision is made as a single continuous movement or in incremental steps. More recently developed 'smart' generators incorporate a pulsed generator (Erbe, Tubingen, Germany) with feedback-controlled power output and the potential for increased safety with regard to avoidance of 'zipper effect', pancreatitis and bleeding. Radiographic confirmation of correct sphincterotome placement is mandatory to avoid pancreatic trauma. Occasionally a 'pre-cut', more appropriately called 'access papillotomy' is needed to initiate ES when the standard instrument cannot be deeply inserted. More often cannulation is prevented by an impacted stone and the 'needle-knife' is more useful in this situation as the intramural CBD is usually grossly distended and easily incised to form a choledochoduodenal fistulotomy. In such situations the complication rate of using needle knife is comparable to standard sphincterotomy (Rabenstein et al 1997). Patients with Billroth II partial gastrectomy (Fig. 40.2) present special problems to the endoscopist and a number of methods have been described to obtain successful cannulation (Lin et al 1999) and when ES is required (Carr-Locke & Cotton 1985).

It is standard practice to attempt stone extraction from the bile duct immediately after ES as this decreases the likelihood of subsequent complications due to retained stones and removes the need for repeating the ERCP to check on ductal clearance at a later date. The two accessory instruments used most commonly for this are the Dormia type basket (Fig. 40.3) and the Fogarty-type balloon (Fig. 40.4) which are successful in clearing the bile duct in over 90% of attempts. It is also possible to extract stones without a preliminary ES either using a balloon dilator (Fig. 40.5) (Staritz 1983a) or after the lingual application of glyceryl

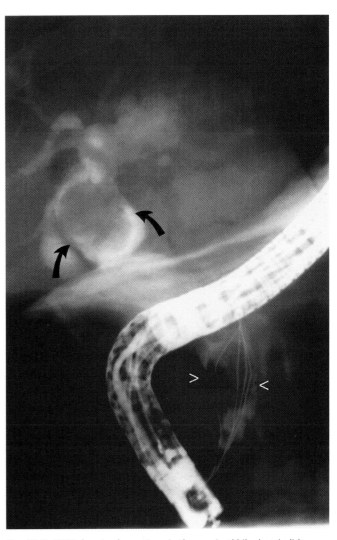

Fig. 40.3 ERCP showing large stone in the proximal bile duct (solid arrows) and basket extraction of a distal bile duct stone (white chevrons) following endoscopic sphincterotomy.

trinitrate to relax the sphincter of Oddi (Staritz et al 1985) and both techniques are highly successful for small stones. Randomized trials of balloon dilation of the papilla against ES have, however, shown a similar or worse morbidity, an increased need for lithotripsy and repeat examinations (Bergman et al 1998).

DIFFICULT STONES

Most experts would agree that the most difficult circumstances encountered during endoscopic stone removal are the result of technical difficulties with achieving deep biliary cannulation or performing ES. These are sometimes due to inaccessibility of the papilla and related to aberrant anatomy or unfavorable duodenal or papillary structures such as a periampullary diverticulum or prior surgery such as Billroth II or Roux-en-Y reconstruction. Adjuvant techniques with

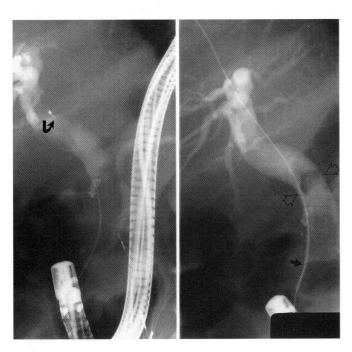

Fig. 40.2 ERCP in patient with Billroth 2 partial gastrectomy showing (left panel) insertion of a catheter (curved arrow) and placement of a guidewire (right panel), short biliary endoprosthesis (solid arrow) immediately prior to needle-knife sphincterotomy and demonstration of bile duct stones (open arrows).

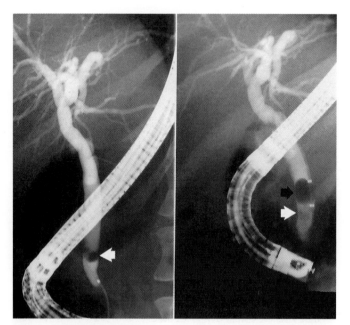

Fig. 40.4 ERCP showing (left panel) a non-dilated bile duct containing a single distal stone (white arrow) and (right panel) extraction balloon (black arrow) placed above the stone immediately prior to its removal following endoscopic sphincterotomy.

access papillotomy and combined percutaneous-endoscopic procedures will increase the success rates in these difficult circumstances (Dowsett et al 1989, Shakoor & Geenen 1992). The patient with a Billroth II partial gastrectomy poses a unique challenge with regard to selective bile duct cannulation for which techniques have been described. These include using straight catheters for selective CBD catheterization and cannulation with a guidewire (Lin et al 1999). The performance of ES is also difficult as the visualized anatomy is reversed. In difficult cases alternative techniques include needle-knife sphincterotomy with either a stent or naso-biliary drain used as a guide for cutting or use of specially designed reverse direction accessories.

Once ES has been successfully performed a variety of factors may hinder stone extraction including size, number, consistency, shape and location of stones, and ductal factors such as contour, diameter at the level of and distal to the stone(s), and the presence of co-existing pathology, such as stricture or tumor. Stones that appear larger than the endoscope on radiographic imaging (usually greater than 15 mm); a large number of stones; stones that are hard in consistency; stones that are square, 'piston' or faceted in shape that tightly fit the bile duct or that are packed against each other; intrahepatic stones or stones located proximal to a stricture or narrowed distal bile duct or in a sigmoid shaped duct are likely to be more difficult to extract and therefore may require adjuvant techniques to remove them. Techniques that have been developed to reduce stone size and facilitate

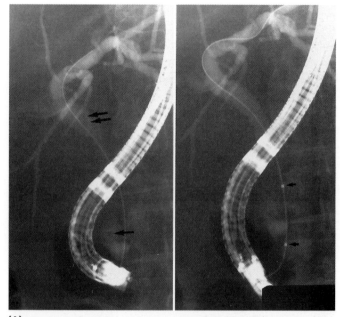

(A)

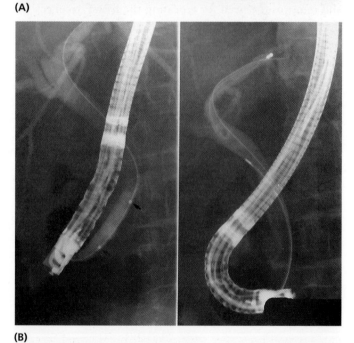

(B)

Fig. 40.5 ERCP series showing technique of balloon dilatation of the papilla for extraction of small stones. **(A)** Initial cholangiography (left panel) with demonstration of three small stones (long arrows) and placement of a guidewire and insertion of an 8-mm diameter dilating balloon (right panel) located between two radiopaque markers (small arrows). **(B)** Demonstrates inflation of the dilating balloon (left panel) followed by insertion of an extraction basket for stone removal (right panel).

endoscopic removal comprise mechanical lithotripsy, extracorporeal shock wave lithotripsy (ESWL), intracorporeal lithotripsy with laser or electrohydraulic probes and chemical contact dissolution therapy. Treatment options must be discussed jointly by endoscopist, surgeon, and interventional radiologist when difficulties are encountered (Fig. 40.6).

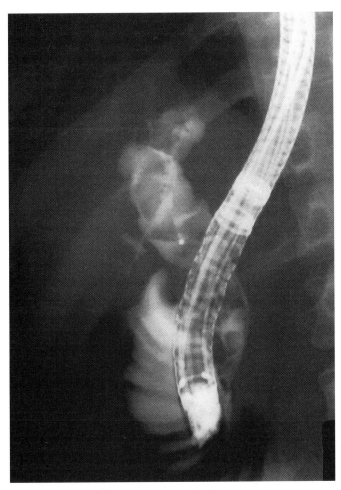

Fig. 40.6 ERCP demonstrating a dilated bile duct containing multiple faceted stones in a post-cholecystectomy patient positioned such that standard extraction techniques might be difficult.

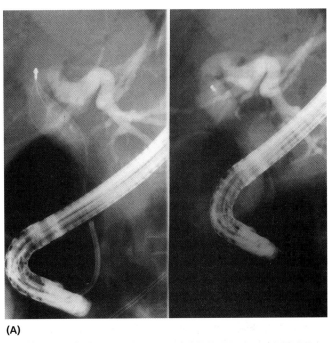

(A)

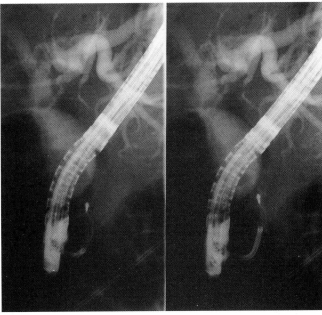

(B)

Fig. 40.7 ERCP sequence showing use of transendoscopic mechanical lithotripsy. **(A)** Shows positioning of the mechanical lithotripsy basket with its metallic sheath in the proximal bile duct (left panel) and its slow withdrawal towards the distally placed stone in order to entrap it (right panel). **(B)** Shows a process of lithotripsy following stone entrapment within the basket (left panel) as the basket wires cut through the stone (right panel) to produce stone fragmentation.

MECHANICAL LITHOTRIPSY

Removal of large common bile duct stones remains a challenge for the most skilled endoscopists. Mechanical lithotripsy (Staritz 1983b) has evolved and remains the best initial option for stones which cannot be removed by conventional techniques, as it can be applied safely and effectively during the initial endoscopic procedure. Standard retrieval baskets contained within a Teflon sheath may fail to crush large stones, as most exceed the breaking strength of the catheter. Mechanical lithotripters are modifications of standard Dormia baskets and possess great tensile strength (Fig. 40.7). The reinforced basket is opened in the bile duct and the stone entrapped within the braided wires. This can either be performed through the endoscope instrumentation channel or after the endoscope has been removed from the patient and a metal sheath extended over the inner Teflon catheter. The outer end is attached to a winding mechanism at the end of the metal sheath which when cranked, retracts the basket and captures the stone against the rigid distal end of the metal sheath leading to stone fracturing. The stone fragments can then be removed with the basket or a retrieval balloon. In experienced centers, this technique allows removal of more than 90% of difficult bile stones which are refractory to standard extraction techniques (Van Dam & Sivak 1993, Shaw et al 1993).

OTHER LITHOTRIPSY MODALITIES

Shockwave lithotripsy with extracorporeal (ESWL) and intracorporeal techniques (laser or electrohydraulic probes) are adjuncts to standard endoscopic management and mechanical lithotripsy in attempting bile duct clearance (Adamek et al 1996). The choice between these methods or surgery largely depends on availability and local expertise.

LASER LITHOTRIPSY

The first generation laser systems using continuous wave energy neodymium:yttrium aluminum garnet (Nd:YAG) devices were both ineffective in stone fragmentation and carried high risk for thermal bile duct injury (Ell et al 1988). Second generation devices which have gained acceptance are based on high-energy flashlamp pulsed-dye laser technology. The application of the laser pulse leads to rapid expansion and collapse of a plasma on the stone surface resulting in a mechanical shock wave. Initially, the only means to ensure laser-stone apposition was through the use of 'mother and baby' dual endoscope systems but, more recently, laser lithotripsy has been possible under fluoroscopic guidance with the use of devices that recognize the difference between stone and tissue (Cotton et al 1990, Neuhaus et al 1992, Ponchon et al 1991).

ELECTROHYDRAULIC LITHOTRIPSY (EHL)

Since its development during the 1950s in the USSR as a method to fragment rocks during mining, EHL has been adopted for medical use for the treatment of nephrolithiasis and, more recently, biliary tract calculi. The electrohydraulic probe consists of two co-axially isolated electrodes at the tip of a flexible catheter which is capable of delivering electric sparks in short rapid pulses leading to sudden expansion of the surrounding liquid environment, thereby generating pressure waves which result in stone fragmentation (Picus 1990). Stone contact with the electrode is achieved through the use of basket or balloon catheter systems (Siegal et al 1990) or under direct visual targeting (Fig. 40.8) through the working channel of a daughter endoscope (Hixon et al 1992), thus minimizing the risk of bile duct injury and perforation. Reports document complete stone clearance following multiple sessions in up to 86% of patients (Siegel et al 1990, Hixon et al 1992). Its main advantages over laser lithotripsy are its lower cost and increased portability.

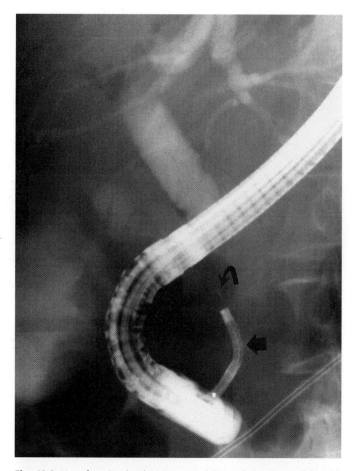

Fig. 40.8 Use of carrier duodenoscope and direct cholangioscope (broad arrow) inserted within the bile duct with protruding electrohydraulic lithotripsy probe (curved arrow) in close proximity to the stone to be fragmented (not visible).

EXTRACORPOREAL SHOCKWAVE LITHOTRIPSY (ESWL)

Extracorporeal shockwave lithotripsy (ESWL) with a variety of lithotripsy machines is now an accepted alternative to endoscopic fragmentation of difficult bile duct stones. In contrast to other techniques, direct contact with the stone is not necessary. Most centers have localized stones with fluoroscopic focusing during contrast perfusion of the bile duct through an endoscopically-placed nasobiliary catheter or percutaneous drain (Gordon et al 1991). Ponchon et al (1990) have reported ESWL success with an ultrasonographic localization system, although it was less effective when multiple stones were present. Several large series (Bland et al 1989, Sauerbruch & Stern 1989, Ponchon et al 1990, Weber et al 1992) indicate success rates for ESWL stone fragmentation of 53 to 91% and duct clearance in 58 to 86%. Minor complications are common, including hematuria, biliary pain, hemobilia, transient liver function test elevations, and cutaneous petechiae.

Overall, with the use of endoscopic techniques such as mechanical lithotripsy, electrohydraulic lithotripsy, laser lithotripsy and extracorporal shock-wave lithotripsy one report showed successful stone removal in 98% of 217 patients with only five patients requiring surgery (Schumacher et al 1998).

DISSOLUTION THERAPY

Contact chemical dissolution of stones has been attempted by perfusing the common bile duct with solvents administered via an indwelling nasobiliary tube, percutaneous transhepatic catheter, cholecystostomy tube or through an existing T tube. The initial results with these agents were disappointing due to incomplete stone dissolution and the potential for complications. A semi-synthetic vegetable oil, mono-ocatanoin, composed of 70% glycerol-1-mono-octanoate and 30% glycerol-1,2-dioctanoate was used experimentally for the dissolution of bile duct stones since 1977. Results collected from 222 clinicians treating 343 patients with bile duct stones between 1977 and 1983 reported a success rate for complete stone dissolution of only 25.6% and an additional partial success rate of 28% (Palmer & Hoffman 1986). Serious adverse effects leading to discontinuation of treatment occurred in 5% of patients, including hemorrhage from duodenal ulceration, acute pancreatitis, jaundice, pulmonary edema, acidosis, anaphylaxis, septicemia, and leukopenia, but no deaths were reported. The use of organic solvents such as the aliphatic ether, methyl-tert-butyl ether (MTBE) (Allen et al 1985), have also been disappointing with complete stone dissolution being achieved in only 30 to 45% and an unacceptable complication rate related to systemic absorption from spillover of solvent into the duodenum and intrahepatic bile ducts (Brandon et al 1988, Murray et al 1988, Neoptolemos et al 1990, Kaye et al 1990, Diaz et al 1992). Sophisticated computer-controlled two-way pump systems may reduce complications and improve efficacy but total success with cholesterol solvents for large CBD stones is less likely because these stones are primarily composed of bile pigments with small concentrations of cholesterol. Expectations of developing a solvent-chelating agent (EDTA) for pigment stones have not been realized. Therefore, due to its low efficacy and morbidity, contact dissolution therapy has not assumed an important role in patients with refractory CBD stones and newer agents with better methods for instillation are awaited.

ENDOPROSTHESIS PLACEMENT

In the few situations where stone extraction is incomplete or impossible because of stone size, local anatomy, bleed-

ing, or technical difficulty leading to incomplete ES, a nasobiliary tube (Fig. 40.9) or endoprosthesis (Fig. 40.10) should be inserted to provide biliary decompression and prevent stone impaction in the distal CBD. This serves as a temporizing therapy allowing for improvement in the patients' clinical condition until complete stone clearance is achieved either via additional endoscopic maneuvers or surgery. This is of paramount importance for those individuals with established cholangitis where the requirement for emergency surgery can be delayed into a semi-elective procedure. In those with uncertain duct clearance, a follow-up cholangiogram can be obtained via the nasobiliary tube without the need for repeat ERCP. Nasobiliary tubes are tolerated for periods of several days. The primary problem with tube placement has been accidental dislodgement and this led to the alternative therapy of temporary biliary endoprosthesis placement (Kiil et al 1989, Rustgi & Schapiro 1991). In the poor surgical risk patient, a proposed nonsurgical alternative was ES and long-term placement of a biliary endoprosthesis (Cotton et al 1987, Foutch et al 1989, Nordback 1989, Soomers et al 1990). Stent patency is not of major clinical importance in this situation, as the sphincterotomy typically provides an adequate conduit for bile flow around the prosthesis which then serves principally to prevent stone impaction. In three series totaling 53 elderly high-risk patients (Cotton et al

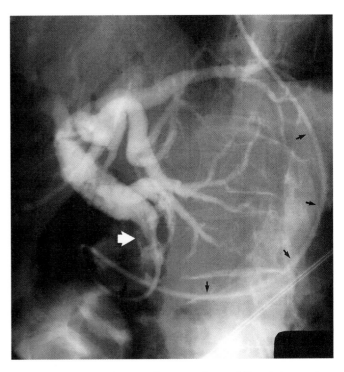

Fig. 40.9 Radiograph showing placement of a nasobiliary drainage tube (small arrows) for the initial treatment of severe cholangitis caused by a single bile duct stone (large arrow).

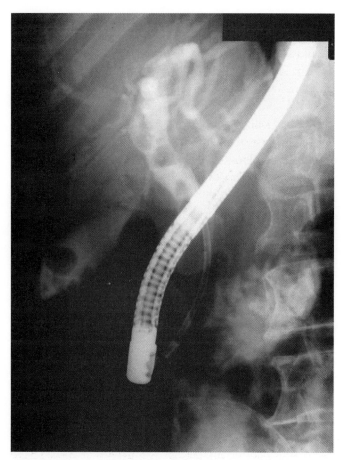

Fig. 40.10 ERCP showing placement of a 10-French diameter endoprosthesis for the temporary management of cholangitis caused by several bile duct stones.

RESULTS OF ENDOSCOPIC THERAPY

Successful endoscopic treatment of bile duct stones requires an adequate ES and this is now achieved in over 90% of attempts in most reported series, with noticeable improvement as experience increases (Blumgart & Wood 1978, Safrany 1978, Reiter et al 1978, Nakajima et al 1979, Siegel 1981, Geenen et al 1981, Cotton & Vallon 1981, Seifert et al 1982, Cotton 1984, Leese et al 1985a, Schumacher et al 1998). Although success rates for achieving ES are fairly uniform, rates for complete clearance of the CBD vary as not all endoscopists use extraction methods routinely and follow-up ERCP may be incomplete. Most experts would now expect to extract or confirm spontaneous passage of stones in at least 90% of successful sphincterotomies, making an overall successful therapeutic rate of over 85%. Failure to extract or pass stones may be due to size and/or number of stones within the duct or unfavorable duct diameter, usually in its retropancreatic segment. Stones up to 10 mm in diameter will not give rise to many problems but, in general, with increasing size above 15–20 mm chance of retention rises. Interpretation of success rates needs care as centers with greater expertise are more likely to be referred difficult cases who may be failures from attempts elsewhere and this will bias some results. Patient groups will also vary considerably from unit to unit and country to country reflecting different referral patterns, selection of patients and attitudes to endoscopic therapy.

Results from centers around the world (Cotton 1984, Safrany 1978, Reiter et al 1978, Nakajima et al 1979, Siegel 1981, Geenen et al 1981, Cotton & Vallon 1981, Seifert et al 1982, Leese et al 1985a, Schumacher et al 1998) with individual and collected series of from 430 to 7585 patients range from 78 to 98% for duct clearance with a median value of 88%. There does not appear to be any difference in technical success after ES in patients with and without gallbladders. In the past there was a predominance of elderly unfit cases with dilated bile ducts but, with time, younger patients with CBD stones and smaller ducts have been treated safely (Cotton et al 1998).

COMPLICATIONS OF ENDOSCOPIC THERAPY

Early complications of endoscopic sphincterotomy have been well-documented and, despite the disparate indications and selection of patients between centers, the incidence seems to be remarkably consistent at 8 to 10% (Cotton 1984, Safrany 1978, Reiter et al 1978, Nakajima et al 1979, Siegel 1981, Geenen et al 1981, Cotton & Vallon 1981, Seifert et al 1982, Leese et al 1985a, Freeman et al 1996, Vandervoort et al 1996).

1987, Foutch et al 1989, Soomers et al 1990), with up to 5 years follow-up, only three required surgery for biliary complications and four were operated on electively for treatment of stent occlusion or migration. An additional 16 patients had already died from nonbiliary causes. The addition of oral ursodeoxycholic acid to such patients has resulted in CBD stone disappearance, although additional studies are necessary to determine the true efficacy in this setting (Johnson et al 1991). More recent series (Bergman et al 1995, Maxton et al 1995) were not as enthusiastic for stenting as a long-term approach. Of 84 patients intentionally treated with permanent stents for endoscopically-irretrievable stones and followed for a mean of 3 years, 49 (58%) developed biliary complications and nine died as a result. However, most of the patients had a long, symptom-free interval before complications developed supporting stenting as effective short-term treatment. The high risk of long-term complications does not support the concept of permanent stent therapy except for those patients with severe comorbidity and a short life expectancy.

The expected higher complication rate during early experience of the technique is reflected in a personal series comparing the results of the first 394 procedures (Leese et al 1985a), which carried an overall morbidity of 10.4%, with a subsequent consecutive group of 300 sphincterotomies in which this rate fell to under 6%. The respective proportions of individual complications, however, remain similar in most reports with acute hemorrhage from the sphincterotomy site representing 2 to 2.9%, acute pancreatitis 1.5 to 5.4%, cholangitis 1 to 2.7% and retroperitoneal perforation 0.3 to 1%, with small numbers of other problems such as impacted basket, gallstone ileus and acute cholecystitis overall accounting for 1.1%. Emergency surgery is required in 1 to 2.5% of cases for bleeding, cholangitis, perforation and pancreatitis in descending order of frequency. There must be reservations about some figures, however, as definitions of hemorrhage, acute pancreatitis, cholangitis and perforation are often not given. We have always included any episode of overt bleeding (hematemesis and/or melena) and/or fall in hemoglobin of 2 g/dL or more following ES as significant hemorrhage although some have included only those requiring transfusion. Use of aspirin or related drugs in the usual doses does not seem to increase the incidence of hemorrhage (Nelson & Freeman 1994). Pancreatitis and cholangitis must depend on the presence of clinically recognizable syndromes rather than asymptomatic hyperamylasemia or transient elevation of temperature alone but these events may be under-reported. There does not appear to be an influence on significant complication rate or type by the initial presentation of the bile duct stone event (pain alone, jaundice alone, pancreatitis, a combination of these) except that cholangitis and cholecystitis are more likely post-ES if cholangitis pre-exists. Present evidence does not suggest that complications are more likely in older patients or after previous biliary surgery. A consensus conference provided a set of standards for defining complications and their severity (Cotton et al 1991).

Statistically significant risk factors for complications include difficulty in cannulation, precut sphincterotomy, suspected dysfunction of sphincter of Oddi, greater than two pancreatic cannulations, acinarization of the pancreas, failed biliary access or drainage, and the technical skill of the endoscopist, rather than to the age or general medical condition of the patient (Freeman et al 1996, Neoptolemos et al 1989, Vandevoort et al 1996).

Difficult duodenal diverticula, although sometimes rendering ERCP and ES technically more difficult, do not seem to add any further risk. In addition, many series do not include non-endoscopic complications occurring after ES, such as cardiovascular, cerebrovascular or respiratory events, and although surgery for the treatment of complications is

usually documented, that for failed endoscopic therapy is often not and these factors are important if comparative data from surgical reports are to be interpreted correctly.

MANAGEMENT OF COMPLICATIONS

The management of complications by centers performing ES will be well-standardized but many patients are referred from other hospitals and may be returned there shortly after the procedure where experience may be limited. Of all complications, hemorrhage requires surgical intervention most commonly (but only in a minority of cases) to control bleeding. The sphincterotomy is usually converted to a formal surgical sphincteroplasty which includes the likely bleeding artery. Immediate methods for hemostasis include balloon tamponade, direct bipolar electrocautery, injection or washing the area with 1:10 000 epinephrine solution, application of laser coagulation, superselective arterial catheterization and embolization, and infiltration with sclerosant (Grimm & Soehendra 1983). In the rare major arterial bleed, however, endoscopic view of the papillary area is often completely obscured by blood and further endoscopic therapy may not be possible.

Acute pancreatitis is managed along standard lines and, although many attacks will be mild and self-limiting, clinicians should not be complacent as some will be more severe and should therefore be graded and treated intensively as appropriate. There is no evidence that pre-ES or post-ES administration of Trasylol®, somatostatin or glucagon influences the incidence or severity of pancreatitis. Unlike hemorrhage, the onset of pancreatitis may be delayed for several hours and, rarely, 1 or 2 days. A multicenter, double-blind trial showed that Gabexate (ethyl-guanidine-hexanoloxy-dibenzoate-methyl-sodium sulfonate), a synthetic protease inhibitor reduced the extent of enzyme elevations, frequency of pancreatic pain and acute pancreatitis when used 30–90 minutes before and for 12 hours after ERCP (Cavallini et al 1996). Trials of platelet activating factor antagonists are in progress.

Cholangitis is almost completely confined to those patients in whom bile duct clearance has not been achieved and measures should be directed at providing adequate bile drainage, e.g. by nasobiliary catheter or endoprosthesis, as well as provision of parenteral antibiotics. Emergency surgery carries high risk when performed for cholangitis but will be indicated in those patients who do not improve within 24 hours.

Perforation may be asymptomatic and noticed only as retroperitoneal gas (Fig. 40.11) or extravasation of radiographic contrast but even in the symptomatic patient conservative treatment may be effective with spontaneous

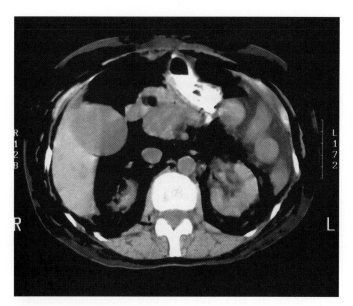

Fig. 40.11 Computed tomographic scan of the stomach with oral contrast showing extensive retroperitoneal, intraperitoneal and subcutaneous air caused by a perforation from endoscopic sphincterotomy. Patient made an uneventful recovery on conservative treatment.

resolution and avoidance of potentially difficult surgery. Occasionally this complication presents late after ES with a retroperitoneal collection of bile or pus pointing in the flank or inguinal region (Neoptolemos et al 1984a, Leese et al 1985a) and will require percutaneous or surgical drainage.

Gallstone ileus should be treated along standard surgical lines but its recognition needs to be emphasized as symptoms may be obscure in elderly patients and present many days after ES and stone release. Although rare complication of ES, the operation required to treat it may be considerably more straightforward than the biliary procedure which was avoided.

The impaction of an extraction basket now occurs rarely in experienced hands as many endoscopic maneuvres have been learned to prevent or save this situation. These include avoiding basket closure during initial attempts to extract a large stone to prevent impaling the basket wires in the stone surface, removal of the duodenoscope over an impacted basket catheter and reintroduction of it alongside the catheter to increase the ES incision, introduction of a second duodenoscope to enlarge the ES, passage of a sphincterotome along the same instrument channel as the impacted basket catheter when using large-channel (3.7 or 4.2 mm) endoscopes in order to enlarge the ES and conversion of the standard basket into a crushing type by replacement of the handle with a mechanical lithotripter.

MORTALITY

Mortality after ES has not been reported in a standardized way by different centers. Those deaths directly attributable to the procedure are fairly constant at 0.8 to 1.5% (Safrany 1978, Reiter et al 1978, Nakajima et al 1979, Siegel 1981, Geenen et al 1981, Cotton & Vallon 1981, Seifert et al 1982, Cotton 1984, Leese et al 1985a) with almost equal causation distributed between hemorrhage, pancreatitis, cholangitis and perforation with many deaths being postoperative. Deaths as a proportion of complications, however, range from 7 to 17% which presumably reflects the comprehensive reporting of all complications by some but only more severe ones by others. The accepted method of reporting surgical mortality within 1 month of the operation should be applied to ES results also. Treatment in this way (Leese et al 1985a) produced a mortality of 0.8% resulting from ES itself in 394 patients but an overall 3.3% within 1 month of ES. The additional deaths were due to a variety of vascular, respiratory, renal, infective and malignant conditions in a group whose mean age was 79 years. A further series of 59 elderly patients considered unfit for surgery (by surgeons) underwent ES (Neoptolemos et al 1984b) with only one death (1.7%).

LONG-TERM MORBIDITY

Long-term morbidity after ES in post-cholecystectomy patients, with follow-up information from 1 to 7 years after ES (Seifert et al 1982, Cotton 1984, Escourrou et al 1984, Rosch et al 1981, Hawes et al 1990) shows in excess of 90% of patients to be well on symptomatic review alone and about 8% with significant symptoms found to be due to recurrent stones (5%) and/or stenosis of the ES (3%) site on investigation. Radiological review of all patients after ES by plain abdominal radiograph for detecting pneumobilia, repeat ERCP, barium studies for duodenobiliary reflux, or radionuclide scanning does not seem justified outside clinical trials but a higher rate of asymptomatic stones and stenosis might be the result of such studies. The majority of these long-term complications are amenable to further endoscopic treatment. An air cholangiogram on plain radiography is present in half to two-thirds of patients after ES. Bile aspirated endoscopically long after ES (Gregg et al 1985, Hawes et al 1990) shows almost universal contamination with bowel organisms but the significance of this is unknown at present as there does not seem to be any long-term effect of this on liver function, bile flow or symptoms.

COMPLICATIONS, MORTALITY RATES AND LONG-TERM RESULTS OF BILE DUCT SURGERY

OPEN BILE DUCT EXPLORATION (Ch. 45)

Morbidity and mortality after open bile duct exploration have been well-documented (Kune 1972, Allen et al 1981, Way et al 1972, Glenn 1974, 1975, Vellacott & Powell 1979, McSherry & Glenn 1980, Pitt et al 1981, Girard & Legros 1981, Doyle et al 1982, Blamey et al 1983, Dixon et al 1983), with more recent interest in specific risk factors (Pitt et al 1981, Blamey et al 1983, Dixon et al 1983) allowing some prediction of likelihood of complications and perhaps the need for preoperative biliary drainage. Direct comparison with the endoscopic data is not scientifically accurate as it is clear that very different groups of patients are being treated by these modes of therapy. This highlights the concept of 'apples and oranges' succinctly stated by Cotton (1984) but mention must be given of published surgical figures to enable some clinical judgements to be made in the absence of randomized trials. It is immediately apparent that, unlike endoscopic therapy, surgical morbidity and mortality is very much determined by patient age, presence of other medical conditions (Glenn 1975, Vellacott & Powell 1979, McSherry & Glenn 1980), hemotologic and biochemical factors (Pitt et al 1981, Blamey et al 1983, Dixon et al 1983), and whether or not the operation is elective (Sullivan et al 1982, Houghton & Donaldson 1983) or an emergency (Boey & Way 1980, Thompson et al 1982). Mortality rates range from 1% in relatively fit younger patients to 28% in the unfit and elderly, and 12 to 14% in younger patients undergoing emergency surgery for cholangitis. These figures practically all refer to primary bile duct operations which should only be compared with results of ES when the gallbladder is in situ. Equivalent results for secondary bile duct explorations are less well recorded but mortality rates of up to 2% are possible for elective surgery (McSherry & Glenn 1980, Girard & Legros 1981). Consideration must also be given to biliary drainage operations which will avoid problems of stone retention but this may be at the expense of an increased postoperative morbidity and mortality. Average mortality rates of 1 to 5% for choledochoduodenostomy (CDD) and transduodenal sphincteroplasty (TDS) are reported (Capper 1961, Madden et al 1970, Stuart & Hoerr 1972, Jones 1978, Lygidakis 1981, Speranza et al 1982). A review of 246 such operations (Baker et al 1985) in which one of these drainage procedures was employed revealed a mortality of 5.4% for each of the two types of operations, with major morbidity of 12% for CDD and 21% for TDS.

LONG-TERM FOLLOW-UP OF SURGICALLY EXPLORED AND RE-EXPLORED BILE DUCTS

Long-term follow-up data after open bile duct exploration is surprisingly lacking. The wide variation in reported recurrent stone rates has been mentioned but morbidity and the need for further surgery has been found in 5% after 5 years (Larson et al 1966), 10% after 12 years (Peel et al 1975), and 21% after 6 to 11 years (Lygidakis 1983) when exploration without biliary drainage has been performed. Following CDD there may be no morbidity in a 6 to 11 year follow-up (Lygidakis 1983) with similar results for TDS (Degenshein 1964, Stuart & Hoerr 1972). Follow-up of 90% of the survivors of one series of 246 patients from 1 to 12 years postoperatively (mean 4.4 years) revealed that complications had been treated in 3% of the CDD group (mainly sump syndrome) and 6% of the TDS group (mainly cholangitis) with additional symptoms on interview in 8% of the CDD and 5% of the TDS groups.

LAPAROSCOPIC COMMON BILE DUCT EXPLORATION (LCBDE) (Ch. 38)

Laparoscopic common bile duct exploration (LCBDE) is now being performed increasingly in experienced tertiary referral centers (Rhodes et al 1995, Khoo et al 1996, Martin et al 1998). Ductal exploration may be accomplished through the cystic duct or directly through a choledochotomy. While the transcystic route is the least invasive and generally does not require any ductal manipulation or drainage procedure, choledochotomy requires either closure of the duct over a T tube or primary closure of the choledochotomy with or without a biliary stent placed in an antegrade fashion without need for a T tube (Rhodes et al 1995). In a recent randomized trial of LCBDE versus postoperative ERCP for CBD stones (Rhodes et al 1998), the clearance rates at the first intervention were the same (75%). With subsequent treatment, predominantly in the form of repeated ERCP, duct-clearance rates approached 100% in both groups. In a similar study sponsored by the European Association of Endoscopic Surgeons (Cuschieri et al 1996) patients were randomized to pre-operative ERCP followed by laparoscopic cholecystectomy or laparoscopic cholecystectomy with LCBDE. Duct clearance was similar in the two groups but they reported a shorter hospital stay for single stage surgical treatment. In a recent study (Tham et al 1997) we showed that therapeutic ERCP is safely performed as an outpatient procedure without need for hospitalization. This would need to be coupled with laparoscopic cholecystectomy requiring good co-ordination between surgeon and endoscopist to minimize hospital stay.

SPECIFIC CLINICAL PROBLEMS

POST-CHOLECYSTECTOMY WITH T TUBE IN SITU

Bile duct stones detected in the early postoperative period on T-tube cholangiography of less than 10 mm in diameter may pass spontaneously or with hydrostatic pressure from flushing or perfusing the T tube. However, the majority of these stones require additional mechanical manipulation. Increased morbidity, mortality and retained stone rate after secondary bile duct explorations has stimulated the development of alternative techniques including hydraulic T-tube irrigation with or without pharmacological relaxation of the sphincter of Oddi with glucagon or nitrates (Tritapepe et al 1988), T-tube infusion of cholesterol solvents (Tritapepe et al 1988), T-tube tract choledochoscopy and lithotripsy (Josephs & Birkett 1992) or percutaneous extraction of stones through a mature T-tube track. Results with this latter technique have ranged from 77 to 96% but multiple sessions are often required and the technique can be complicated by sepsis, biliary trauma, and biliary leakage in 4 to 8% of patients (Burhenne 1980, Mason 1980, Tritapepe et al 1988, Caprini 1988, Cotton 1990, Nussinson et al 1991). Delays of 4 to 6 weeks are required prior to manipulation to allow maturation of the T-tube track. Alternatively early ES can be safely and effectively applied after stone detection without the need for T-tube maturation allowing timely discharge from hospital. The results from eight endoscopic series totaling 337 patients indicate an overall endoscopic success rate of 90% with a morbidity of 7% and mortality of 0.6% (Soehendra et al 1981, Simpson et al 1985, O'Doherty et al 1986, Bickerstaff et al 1988, Lambert et al 1988, Danilewitz 1989, Tandon et al 1990, Nussinson et al 1991). The choice between these two techniques depends upon local expertise, as direct comparisons have not been made in controlled trials.

POST-CHOLECYSTECTOMY WITHOUT T-TUBE

The incidence of retained common bile duct stones remains at approximately 2 to 5% following conventional and laparoscopic cholecystectomy with an incidence as high as 5 to 15% following common duct exploration. Endoscopic sphincterotomy remains the treatment of choice for the elderly patient presenting days to years after cholecystectomy (Danilewitz 1989) as these individuals are at higher risk for further abdominal surgery (Cranley & Logan 1980, Sheridan et al 1987). Endoscopic sphincterotomy (ES) is also recommended for choledocholithiasis in the young, fit postcholecystectomy individuals even with normal diameter ducts (Cotton et al 1998).

PREGNANCY

Symptomatic choledocholithiasis during pregnancy poses a diagnostic and therapeutic challenge.

The frequency of choledocholithiasis in pregnancy requiring intervention may be as low as 1 in 1200. Traditionally intervention in these patients has been surgical. Although surgery has an overall low morbidity and mortality for the expectant mother, it carries with it a 4 to 6 week recovery period and a possibly increased risk of fetal loss.

Endoscopic treatment can be performed safely with a complication rate comparable to nonpregnant patients (Jamidar et al 1995). Certain precautions are necessary to minimize fetal exposure to radiation (Baillie et al 1990, Binmoeller & Caton 1990, Beck & Brodmekel 1991). During ERCP, the fetus is shielded with an abdominal lead apron, no radiographs are taken and dosimetry should be performed to estimate the amount of exposure to the fetus. These patients should undergo cholecystectomy upon completion of pregnancy to prevent recurrence.

SELECTED PATIENTS WITH GALLBLADDER IN SITU

In the elderly or in patients with significant co-morbidity, a deliberate decision is often made to leave the gallbladder in situ following ES and CBD stone removal. The short and long-term results and complications of ES in patients with gallbladders do not differ from those in the post cholecystectomy patient. These patients, in view of their shorter life expectancy, can be managed expectantly unless symptoms dictate otherwise. Careful follow-up for 5 to 10 years in patients with intact gallbladders indicates that approximately 10% will develop gallbladder symptoms or complications sufficient to warrant cholecystectomy and the majority occur in the first year (Escourrou et al 1984, Tanaka et al 1987, Davidson et al 1988, Rosseland & Solhaug 1984, Siegel et al 1988, Hill 1991). The risk for developing gallbladder symptoms is similar to that of patients with asymptomatic cholelithiasis (Gracie & Ransohoff 1982). Furthermore, the majority requiring cholecystectomy can be treated electively.

The risk for developing biliary symptoms appears to be dependent on the continuing presence of stones in the gallbladder. In two reports (Tanaka et al 1987, Siegel et al 1988), none of 155 patients with acalculous gallbladders at initial ES developed symptoms or complications that subsequently required cholecystectomy. In those with gallstones, there do not appear to be any reliable predictors to identify those patients with cholelithiasis who are likely to develop gallbladder complications following ES. Non filling of the gallbladder with radiographic contrast at ERCP (Worthley & Toouli 1988) or with radiotracer by nuclear scintigraphy (Holbrook et al 1991) may confer a higher likelihood for developing symptoms, although results from other series do not concur (Davidson et al 1988, Hill et al 1991). These results suggest that the low risk of subsequent gallbladder complications after ES and bile duct clearance, when patients are kept under supervision, outweighs the known higher mortality for cholecystectomy in the elderly and mitigates against routine cholecystectomy in this group. Few physicians would recommend this approach in the fit patient where the expectation for long-term survival and therefore development of symptoms necessitating cholecystectomy is greater. The risk of elective cholecystectomy is probably smaller than the risk of subsequently developing gallbladder symptoms in this group, and therefore elective cholecystectomy would seem most appropriate in this group.

The place of preoperative ES in young, good surgical risk patients with suspected choledocholithiasis has been examined to determine if preoperative ES confers an advantage in terms of morbidity, mortality and length of hospital stay compared with a conventional approach of open cholecystectomy, operative cholangiography, and CBD exploration. Two prospective, randomized controlled trials (Neoptolemos et al 1987, Stiegmann et al 1992) have addressed this question with the conclusion that no advantage is conferred by initial endoscopic bile duct clearance prior to cholecystectomy. High-risk surgical patients were excluded from these studies and both were conducted in the era of open cholecystectomy.

LAPAROSCOPIC CHOLECYSTECTOMY AND ERCP (see also Ch. 38)

Laparoscopic cholecystectomy has now replaced open cholecystectomy as the procedure of choice for gallbladder removal in the vast majority of individuals with symptomatic cholelithiasis. Optimal management of patients with suspected CBD stones varies according to the expertise available in a particular institution. Laparoscopic transcystic cholangiography (Sackier et al 1991, Flowers et al 1992) and choledochoscopy with stone extraction (Hunter 1992) or direct choledochotomy can be performed at the time of laparoscopic cholecystectomy, but the latter technique is only currently practiced at specialized surgical centers. Laparoscopic transcystic choledochoscopy is hindered by

the small size and tortuosity of the cystic duct making instrument passage and stone lithotripsy and removal potentially difficult. Thus a need for endoscopic management has evolved, with ERCP playing a central role in preoperative and postoperative CBD stone detection and removal. Initially, we and others (Cotton et al 1991) found it useful to stratify patients pre-operatively into low, intermediate and high likelihood for CBD stones (Table 40.1) based on established clinical and biochemical indicators including elevated function tests, a dilated CBD > 8 mm on ultrasound, and a history of jaundice or pancreatitis (Lacaine et al 1980, Del Santo et al 1985, Hauer-Jensen et al 1985). Some centers have advocated routine pre-operative or intra-operative cholangiography to document aberrant ductal anatomy and detect asymptomatic CBD stones. Aberrant ductal anatomy is however infrequently identified (Clair et al 1993) although it does contribute to operative ductal injury. Furthermore, in the absence of clinical or biochemical indicators ('low likelihood' category), CBD stones will be present in only 2 to 3% of individuals, a yield which would probably be offset by the risks of the ERCP itself (Neuhaus et al 1992). Small asymptomatic stones may be of minor clinical relevance as their natural history is not known and conceivably many, if not most, of these calculi would pass spontaneously without ever coming to clinical attention. We have favored selective cholangiography for patients only with risk factors for choledocholithiasis.

We have proposed three general strategies to manage these individuals with 'suspected' CBD stones. Algorithm 1 offers the advantage of complete surgical management at a single procedure without the need for additional postoperative stone extraction. The major disadvantage is the high rate of conversion to an open procedure which is not in

Table 40.1 Cholangiography stratification for 'risk' of choledocholithiasis

High likelihood (preoperative ERC)
Bilirubin > 2 mg% Alkaline phosphatase > 150 U/L Present/recent history of jaundice/pancreatitis Dilated CBD/stone on sonography
Intermediate likelihood (IOC) Bilirubin 1.5–2.0 mg% Alkaline phosphatase 110–150 U/L Transaminases > 2 × normal Remote jaundice/pancreatitis
Low likelihood (no ERC/IOC) Normal LFTs No ductal dilatation No jaundice/pancreatitis

keeping with the desire to maintain minimally an invasive approach to therapy. This strategy has not gained widespread acceptance, but would be a reasonable approach either in centers not capable of providing adequate endoscopic therapy or when techniques are achieved for performing laparoscopic CBDE. Algorithm 2 focuses on endoscopic cholangiography and stone clearance prior to performance of laparascopic cholecystectomy. This approach appears justified in the patient with a 'high likelihood' of a CBD stone in order to avoid prolonging the operative procedure with intraoperative cholangiography while maintaining the minimally invasive approach and reducing the need for conversion to an open CBD exploration for laparoscopic failures (Aliperti et al 1991, Neuhaus et al 1992, Boulay et al 1992). It is often possible to remove small stones (up to 3 mm in diameter) during ERCP through the intact papilla thereby sparing the patient the potential short- and long-term risks of ES (Staritz et al 1985, Ibuki et al 1992, Cotton 1993). Algorithm 3 utilizes laparoscopic transcystic cholangiography to detect CBD stones with postoperative ERCP to remove stones in these patients with positive cholangiograms. This strategy relies heavily on ERCP expertise, as failed stone removal will necessitate referral to a more experienced endoscopist or a second open operative procedure. The choice between these various strategies for the patient felt to be of 'intermediate likelihood' should be strongly influenced by the quality of the surgical and endoscopic therapy available.

At our institution in prospective series of 750 consecutive laparoscopic cholecystectomies (Table 40.2), preoperative endoscopic retrograde cholangiography ERCP (algorithm 2) was performed in 36 (4.8%) considered 'likely' to have CBD stones based on indicators of a total bilirubin >2 mg/dL, alkaline phosphatase > 150 U/L, a dilated CBD on ultrasound, or a recent history of jaundice or pancreatitis. Endoscopic retrograde cholangiography (ERC) was successful in 35 (97%) and 9 (25%) were positive. All stones were removed following sphincterotomy with only one complication of mild pancreatitis which delayed surgery by 3 days. Aberrant ductal anatomy was present in two, Mirrizzi's syndrome in one, and 23 were normal. Only one of nine patients with pancreatitis as the indicator for cholangiography had a CBD stone, questioning the utility of pancreatitis as a predictor of choledocholithiasis. We suggest performance of prelaparoscopic cholecystectomy ERCP 24–48 h prior to the planned surgery whenever logistically feasible to avoid the infrequent occurrence of stone migration from the gallbladder into the CBD during the ERCP–laparoscopy interval resulting in the possibility of a retained CBD stone. This sequence of events occurred early in our series in one patient who passed a stone from the gallbladder into the CBD during a 3-week interval between the pre-operative ERCP and laparoscopy. It has not recurred with subsequent performance of preoperative ERCP at the recommended 24–48 h interval. Selective intra-operative cholangiography (algorithm C) was performed in 45 (6%) felt to be of intermediate risk for CBD stones based on pre-operative indicators that included a total bilirubin elevation of 1.5–2.0 mg/dL, alkaline phosphatase of 110–150 U/L, transaminases > twice normal or a remote history of jaundice or pancreatitis. Only two (4.4%) of these studies were positive. Patients without pre-operative indicators (669 patients) considered 'low risk' did not undergo cholangiography and 11 (1.6%) have subsequently been found to have retained stones, all managed successfully by ERCP and ES. A more recent study by our group has shown an increased preoperative detection rate of bile duct stones with stricter criteria for selection (Tham et al 1997).

ACUTE CHOLANGITIS

Acute cholangitis due to bile duct stones was traditionally treated by initial supportive measures and parenteral antibiotics followed by early surgery if improvement was slow or absent. The mortality from emergency surgery can be as high as 12 to 16% with higher rates for elderly patients (Cotton 1984, Thompson et al 1982, Boey & Way 1980). In the 1980s we analyzed the results of treatment of 82 patients with severe acute cholangitis and bile duct stones admitted over a 7-year period during which ES was available (Leese et al 1985b). Mean age was 71 years (range 19 to 88), 87% were aged over 60 and 23% over 80 years. Overall 30-day mortality was 14.6% but varied considerably with different modes of therapy. Eleven received conservative treatment only. Of these, seven responded to antibiotics alone but four were moribund and died (36.4%) before any treatment could be instituted. Seventy-one underwent early biliary decompression surgically in 28 or endoscopically in

Table 40.2 ERCP in 750 laparoscopic cholecystectomies at Brigham & Women's Hospital 1990–1992

Preoperative ERCP	36 (4.8%)
Normal	23 (64%)
Stones	9 (25%)
Mirizzi's syndrome	1 (2.8%)
Aberrant anatomy	2 (5.6%)
Failed ERC	1 (2.8%)
Intraoperative cholangiography	45 (6.0%)
Successful	39 (87%)
Stones	2 (5.1%)
Not attempted	705 (94%)

ERCP, endoscopic retrograde cholangiopancreatography

43. Of the eleven who were post-cholecystectomy, four had early surgery with bilio-digestive bypass and two died within 30 days (50%) and seven had early ES with no mortality. Of the 60 with gallbladders, 24 were treated surgically (mean age 62 years) with a mortality of 16.7%, 13 had an ES followed by elective cholecystectomy (mean age 64 years) with no mortality and 23 had an ES with gallbladders in situ of whom six have died from unrelated causes, two have required surgery for empyema of the gallbladder at 19 days post-ES in one and recurrence of cholangitis at 5 months in the other. Complications after ES occurred in 10; hemorrhage in five, exacerbation of cholangitis in three, mild acute pancreatitis in one and gallstone ileus in one with only the latter requiring surgical intervention. Bile duct clearance was achieved in 40 out of 43 patients (93%). Of the three failures, one died without further therapy, one underwent surgery 4 weeks later and one remained asymptomatic having declined further treatment. Thus the 30-day mortality for patients treated by early surgery was 21.4% (six out of 28) and that for early ES irrespective of subsequent treatment was 4.7% (two out of 43). We concluded that patients not responding to standard initial therapy within 24 hours should be offered for endoscopic biliary decompression and bile duct clearance if this is locally available.

The only randomized trial of emergency endoscopic versus surgical management of severe calculous cholangitis (Lai et al 1992) showed a 3-fold difference in mortality (10% versus 32%, $P < 0.03$) in favor of ERCP.

GALLSTONE PANCREATITIS

Acute pancreatitis due to impaction of gallstones in the ampulla of Vater was first reported by Opie in 1901. From his observations was derived the 'obstructive theory' to explain the mechanism responsible for gallstone pancreatitis. Stone impaction in the common channel of the pancreatic and common bile ducts is postulated to result in obstruction of the two systems with resultant reflux of bile into the pancreatic duct (Moody et al 1993). In support of the (transient) obstructive theory, gallstones can be recovered from the feces of 85 to 95% of patients (Acosta & Ledesma 1974, Kelly 1980a,b), and the incidence of CBD stones is as high as 80% in those undergoing urgent operative or endoscopic intervention compared with a 5 to 30% incidence when the procedure is delayed (Acosta et al 1978, Ranson 1979, Kelly 1980a,b, Stone et al 1981). There are now well-established criteria e.g. Ranson, Imrie, Glasgow, and APACHE II) for assessing the severity of pancreatitis and thereby predict local adverse events of necrosis, hemorrhage, infection, and pseudocyst formation as well as systemic complications of adult respiratory distress syndrome,

disseminated intravascular coagulation, distant fat necrosis, and renal failure (Banks 1991). Stratifying the patients into severity of illness based on these criteria has been helpful in directing appropriate management. The majority of patients experience mild pancreatitis due to transient impaction of a stone in the ampulla followed by spontaneous migration into the duodenum. These individuals do well with conservative therapy alone and are unlikely to benefit from urgent intervention. In contrast, it has been proposed that the more severe cases of pancreatitis result from persistent stone impaction or choledocholithiasis with infected bile, offering the hope that early stone extraction by surgical or endoscopic techniques would halt progression of the acute event and also prevent the development of future attacks in the short term.

Early surgical therapy in cases of acute gallstone pancreatitis has been challenged due to the high operative morbidity and mortality. Results and conclusions from numerous series comparing early and late surgical therapy in gallstone pancreatitis are difficult to interpret. The mortality rates range from 2 to 67%, the studies are retrospective with frequent comparisons to historical controls, and stratification for severity of illness has not been utilized (Acosta et al 1978, Ranson 1979, Osborne et al 1981, Kim & Bosner 1988). In one series, Kelly and Wagner (1988) prospectively randomized 165 patients with gallstone pancreatitis to early or delayed surgery. In the group with severe pancreatitis they found 48% mortality following urgent operative intervention, compared with 11% mortality in patients in whom surgery was delayed for more than 48 hours for gallstones. In contrast, those patients with mild pancreatitis had mortalities of 3.3% and zero respectively. These results would favor avoidance of early operative intervention in the acute phase of biliary pancreatitis unless local complications from necrotizing disease dictate otherwise.

An endoscopic approach to gallstone pancreatitis offers the theoretical advantage of immediate relief of ampullary obstruction and ductal clearance without the risks of general anesthesia or the surgical procedure. There was initial reluctance to perform ERCP in patients with acute pancreatitis due to concerns that the procedure would exacerbate the illness and lead to death. Cotton and Safrany (1981) were the first to report ES in 11 patients with 'severe' gallstone pancreatitis. The procedure was performed within 24 hours of hospitalization and common duct stones were found in all patients with stone impaction at the ampulla in six individuals. Endoscopic removal of common duct stones resulted in 'prompt clinical and biochemical improvement' in ten of the 11 patients. Subsequent clinical studies supported the safety and efficacy of ERCP in the setting of acute biliary pancreatitis (Rosseland & Solhaug 1984, Neoptolemos et al

1984c, Shemesh et al 1990), but these reports were inconclusive due to methodological study flaws including non-randomization in patient selection, variation in timing of the procedure, and failure to stratify for severity of pancreatitis. The Leicester group (Neoptolemos et al 1986) were the first to perform a controlled study to evaluate the efficacy of ERCP in biliary pancreatitis. A group of 121 patients with suspected gallstone pancreatitis was randomized to urgent (within 72 hours of hospitalization) ERCP and ES if stones were present or conventional non-endoscopic management. Bile duct stones were found in 63% of the predicted severe group and only 26% of those with predicted mild attacks. Those with mild pancreatitis had favorable outcomes regardless of treatment strategy with a similar incidence of complications and no deaths. In the group of patients with 'severe' pancreatitis defined by modified Glasgow criteria, urgent ES significantly reduced the morbidity (local and systemic complications) from 61 to 24%, and length of hospitalization from 17 to 9.5 days) compared with conservatively managed patients. Mortality was lower in the ERCP group (4% versus 18%); but the difference did not reach statistical significance.

A second study published by the Hong Kong group (Fan et al 1993) prospectively randomized 195 consecutive patients with suspected gallstone pancreatitis to urgent (within 24 hours of hospital admission) ERCP with papillotomy or initial conservative treatment with selective ERCP only if the clinical condition deteriorated. In this region of the world, where biliary lithiasis is frequently responsible for acute pancreatitis, emergency ERCP resulted in a reduction in biliary sepsis from 12% in the conservatively-treated patients to zero in those undergoing endoscopic papillotomy and stone extraction. Overall, there were no significant differences in the incidences of either local (10.3% versus 12.2%) or systemic complications (10.3% versus 14.3%). However, in the subset of patients with 'severe' pancreatitis and common duct stones, urgent endoscopic sphincterotomy resulted in a decrease in the combined incidence of local and systemic complications to 21% and mortality rate to 5.3% compared with the conservatively-managed group where the rates were 68.8 and 25%, respectively.

A third randomized trial (Nowak et al 1998) had a very different design from the three preceding studies. All 280 patients with acute gallstone pancreatitis in the study underwent urgent duodenoscopy within 24 hours of onset of their disease, almost 25% were found to have impacted stones at the papilla and all were treated by immediate sphincterotomy. The remaining 205 patients were randomized to conventional treatment or sphincterotomy irrespective of the cholangiographic findings. In comparison to conventional treatment, the authors demonstrated a signifi-

cant advantage for patients treated endoscopically with respect to morbidity (17% versus 36%, $p < 0.001$) and mortality (2% versus 13%, $p < 0.001$). Both rates were also more strikingly reduced the earlier the endoscopic intervention was undertaken. As all patients seem to benefit irrespective of severity, the conclusion was that emergency ERCP and sphincterotomy was indicated in all patients with acute gallstone pancreatitis but further analysis of the data will be required when the full report is available.

A much criticized fourth recent randomized study from a large number of centers in Germany (Folsch et al 1997) set out to show that endoscopic intervention in gallstone pancreatitis in the absence of bile duct obstruction or low likelihood of bile duct obstruction would not show benefit and it succeeded but at the expense of an increased morbidity and mortality in the ERCP group not previously found in other trials.

These studies demonstrate that ERCP and endoscopic stone extraction can be safely performed in the setting of acute biliary pancreatitis. Furthermore, urgent ERCP and ES can be performed with good rationale in those patients with severe or progressive pancreatitis due to the resultant reduction in major local peripancreatic complications and the increasingly recognized coexistence of acute cholangitis potentially translating into a reduced mortality. Subsequent elective cholecystectomy should be considered although in the high-risk patient the gallbladder may be left in situ. In the patient with mild pancreatitis, no immediate intervention is advised. If later proven to have gallstones or microlithiasis (Targarona et al 1995, Lee et al 1992), elective laparoscopic cholecystectomy with preoperative ERCP or intra-operative cholangiography should be performed. In the post-cholecystectomy patient, endoscopic therapy is definitive. The role of endoscopic sphincterotomy in lieu of cholecystectomy for the high-risk patient with an intact gallbladder and gallstone pancreatitis in the absence of choledocholithiasis requires further evaluation (May & Shaffer 1991).

CONCLUSIONS

Endoscopic management of choledocholithiasis has matured in a very short time with wide acceptance as a respectable and highly effective therapy for choledocholithiasis. Endoscopic techniques are now well established and accessories have been developed to enhance success and safety. There would seem to be little argument against the use of ES in preference to surgery in the management of elderly high-risk patients with bile duct stones in the majority of clinical situations, irrespective of the presence or absence of the gallbladder and in all patients presenting with bile duct stones late after previous biliary surgery where the only alternative is further surgical intervention. The endoscopic removal of retained stones in the early postoperative period has been shown to be effective, carries a small risk of complications and allows early discharge from hospital. In addition, patients of all ages with acute cholangitis not responding to conventional therapy should be considered for endoscopic management before emergency surgery if this is logistically feasible. The case for ERCP and ES in the treatment of patients with severe gallstone-associated pancreatitis and fit patients with bile duct and gallbladder stones has been made in controlled trials. Integrated endoscopic therapy for biliary disease is now well advanced in those centers where surgical and endoscopic clinicians work closely together and where each provides the other with a suitable forum for critical evaluation of alternative therapeutic techniques. This has become increasingly manifest with the establishment of laparoscopic cholecystectomy with more complex laparoscopic manipulations of the bile ducts still evolving. As arguments and clinical practice come full circle, it is tempting to suggest the enthusiastic speculations of the early 1970s, that the surgeon should treat the gallbladder and the endoscopist the bile duct, may have come to pass three decades later.

REFERENCES

Acosta J M, Ledesma C I 1974 Gallstone migration as a cause of acute pancreatitis. New England Journal of Medicine 290: 484–487

Acosta J M, Rossi R, Galli O M R, Pellegrini C A, Skinner D B 1978 Early surgery for acute gallstone pancreatitis: evaluation of a systematic approach. Surgery 83: 367–370

Adamek H E, Maier M, Jakobs R, Wessbecher FR, Neuhauser T, Riemann J F 1996 Management of retained bile duct stones: a prospective open trial comparing extracorporeal and intracorporeal lithotripsy. Gastrointestinal Endoscopy 44: 40–47

Aliperti G, Edmundowicz S A, Soper N J, Ashley S W 1991 Combined endoscopic sphincterotomy and laparoscopic cholecystectomy in patients with choledocholithiasis and cholecystolithiasis. Annals of Internal Medicine 115: 783–785

Allen B, Shapiro H, Way LW 1981 Management of recurrent and residual common duct stones. American Journal of Surgery 142: 41–47

Allen M J, Borody T J, Bugliosi T F, May G R, Larusso N F, Thistle J L 1985 Rapid dissolution of gallstones by methyl-tert-butyl ether. New England Journal of Medicine 312: 217–220

Baker A R, Neoptolemos J P, Carr-Locke D L, Fossard D P 1985 Sump syndrome following choledochoduodenostomy and its endoscopic management. British Journal of Surgery 72: 433–435

Baillie J, Cairns S, Cotton P B 1990 Endoscopic management of choledocholithiasis during pregnancy. Surgery 171: 1–4

Banks P A 1991 Predictors of severity in acute pancreatitis. Pancreas S7–12

Beck G, Brodmekel G 1991 Choledocholithiasis in pregnancy: treatment by endoscopic sphincterotomy. Gastrointestinal Endoscopy 100: A 252

Bergman J J, Rauws E A, Tijssen J G, Tytgat G N, Huibregtse K 1995 Biliary endoprostheses in elderly patients with endoscopically irretrievable common bile duct stones: report on 117 patients. Gastrointestinal Endoscopy 42(3): 195–201

Bergman J J, Tytgat G N, Huibregtse K 1998 Endoscopic dilatation of the biliary sphincter for removal of bile duct stones: an overview of current indications and limitations. Scandinavian Journal of Gastroenterology (Suppl 225): 59–65

Bickerstaff K I, Berry A R, Chapman R W, Bitton J 1988 Early postoperative endoscopic sphincterotomy for retained biliary stones. Annals of the Royal College of Surgeons of England 70: 350–351

Binmoeller K F, Caton R M 1990 Needle knife papillotomy for impacted bile duct stone during pregnancy. Gastrointestinal Endoscopy 36: 607–609

Blamey S L, Fearon K C H, Gilmore W H, Osborn D H, Carter D C 1983 Prediction of risk in biliary surgery. British Journal of Surgery 70: 535–538

Bland K I, Jones R S, Maher J W et al 1989 Extracoporeal shock wave lithotripsy of bile duct calculi. Annals of Surgery 209: 743–755

Blumgart L H, Wood C B 1978 Letter on: Endoscopic treatment of biliary tract diseases. Lancet ii: 1249

Boey J H, Way L W 1980 Acute cholangitis. Annals of Surgery 190: 264–270

Boulay J, Schellenberg R, Brady P G 1992 Role of ERCP and therapeutic biliary endoscopy in association with laparosopic cholecystectomy. American Journal of Gastroenterolgy 1987: 837–842

Brandon J C, Teplick S K, Haskin P H et al 1998 Common bile duct calculi: Updated experience with dissolution with ethyl-tertiary-butyl-ether. Radiology 166: 665–667

Burhenne J H 1980 Percutaneous extraction of retained biliary tract stones. American Journal of Roentgenology 134: 888–898

Capper W M 1961 External choledochoduodenostomy, an evaluation of 125 cases. British Journal of Surgery 49: 292–300

Caprini J A 1988 Biliary stone extraction. American Journal of Surgery 54: 343–346

Carr-Locke D L, Cotton P B 1985 Endoscopic surgery: biliary tract and pancreas. British Medical Bulletin 42: 257–264

Cavallini G, Tittobello A, Frulloni L, Masci E, Mariana A, Di Francesco V 1996 Gabexate for the prevention of pancreatic damage related to endoscopic retrograde cholangiopancreatography. Gabexate in digestive endoscopy—Italian Group. New England Journal of Medicine 335(13): 919–23

Clair D G, Carr-Locke D L, Becker J M, Brooks D C 1993 Routine cholangiography is not warranted during laparoscopic cholecystectomy. Archives of Surgery 128: 551–555

Classen M, Demling L 1974 Endoscopische Sphinkterotomie der papilla Vater. Deutsche Medizinische Wochenschrift 99: 496–497

Cotton P B 1984 Endoscopic management of bile duct stones (apples and oranges). Gut 25: 587–597

Cotton P B 1990 Retained bile duct stones: T-tube in place percutaneous or endoscopic management? American Journal of Gastroenterology 85: 1075–1078

Cotton P B 1993 Removing duct stones without sphincterotomy. Gastrointetinal Endoscopy 39: 312

Cotton P B, Safrany L 1981 A preliminary report: urgent duodenoscopic sphincterotomy for acute gallstone pancreatitis. Surgery 89: 424–428

Cotton P B, Vallon A G 1981 British experience with duodenoscopic sphincterotomy for removal of bile duct stones. British Journal of Surgery 68: 373–375

Cotton P B, Burney P G J, Mason R R 1979 Transnasal bile duct catheterisation after endoscopic sphincterotomy. Gut 20: 285–287

Cotton P B, Forbes A, Leung J W C, Dineen L 1987 Endoscopic stenting for long term treatment of large bile duct stones: 2- to 5-year follow up. Gastrointestinal Endoscopy 33: 411–412

Cotton P, Cozarek R A, Schapiro R H et al 1990 Endoscopic laser lithotripsy of large bile duct stones. Gastroenterology 99: 1128–1133

Cotton P B, Lehman G, Vennes J, Russell R C, Meyers W C, Liguory C, Nickl N 1991a Endoscopic sphincterotomy complications and their management; an attempt at consensus. Gastrointestinal Endoscopy 37(3): 383–393

Cotton P B, Baillie J, Pappas T N, Meyers W S 1991b Laparosopic cholecystectomy and the biliary endoscopist. Journal of Gastrointestinal Endoscopy 37: 94–97

Cotton P B, Geenen J E, Sherman S, Cunningham J T, Howell D A, Carr-Locke D L, Nickl N J, Hawes R H, Lehman G A, Ferrari A, Slivka A, Lichtenstein D R, Baillie J, Jowell P S, Lail L M, Evangelou H, Bosco J J, Hanson B L, Hoffman B J, Rahaman S M, Male R 1998 Endoscopic sphincterotomy for stones by experts is safe, even in younger patients with normal ducts. Annals of Surgery 227(2): 201–43

Cranley B, Logan H 1980 Exploration of the common bile duct—the relevance of the clinical picture and the importance of pre-operative cholangiography. British Journal of Surgery 67: 869–872

Cuschieri A, Croce E, Faggioni A, Jakimowicz J, Lacy A, Lezoche E, Morino M, Ribeiro V M, Toouli J, Visa J, Wayand W 1996 EAES ductal stone study. Preliminary findings of multi-center prospective randomized trial comparing two-stage versus single-stage management. Surgical Endoscopy 10: 1130–1135

Danilewitz M D 1989 Early postoperative endoscopic sphincterotomy for retained common bile duct stones. Gastrointestinal Endoscopy 35: 298–299

Davidson B R, Neoptolemos J P, Carr-Locke D L 1988 Endoscopic sphincterotomy for common bile duct calculi in patients with gallbladder in situ considered unfit for surgery. Gut 29: 114–120

Degenshein G A 1964 Choledocho-duodenostomy; an 18-year study of 175 consecutive cases. Surgery 76: 316–324

Del Santo P, Kazarian K K, Rogers J F, Bevins P A, Hall J R 1985 Prediction of operative cholangiography in patients undergoing elective cholecystectomy with routine liver function chemistries. Surgery 98: 7–11

Diaz D, Bories P, Ampelas M, Larrey D, Michel H 1992 Methyl tert-butyl ether in the endoscopic treatment of common bile duct radiolucent stones in elderly patients with nasobiliary tube. Digestive Diseases Science 37: 97–100

Dixon J M, Armstrong C B, Duffy S W, Davies G C 1983 Factors affecting morbidity and mortality after surgery for obstructive jaundice; a review of 373 patients. Gut 24: 845–852

Dowsett J F, Vaira D, Hatfield R W et al 1989 Endoscopic biliary therapy using the combined percutaneous and endoscopic technique. Gastroenterology 96: 1180–1186

Doyle P J, Ward-McQuaid J N, McEwen-Smith A 1982 The value of routine per-operative cholangiography—a report of 4000 cholecystectomies. British Journal of Surgery 69: 617–619

Ell C, Lux G, Hochberger J, Muller D, Demling L 1988 Laser lithotripsy of common bile duct stones. Gut 29: 746–751

Escourrou J, Cordova J A, Lazorthes F, et al 1984 Early and late complications after endoscopic sphincterotomy for biliary lithiasis, with and without the gallbladder 'in situ.' Gut 25: 598–602

Fan S T, Lai E C S, Mok F P T, Lo C M, Zheng S S, Wong J 1993 Early treatment of acute biliary pancreatitis by endoscopic papillotomy. New England Journal of Medicine 328: 228–232

Flowers J L, Zucker K A, Graham S M, Scovill W A, Imbembo A L, Bailey R W 1992 Laparoscopic cholangiography: results and indications. Annals of Surgery 215: 209–216

Folsch U R, Nitsche R, Ludtke R, Hilgers R A, Creutzfeldt W 1997 Early ERCP and papillotomy compared with conservative treatment for acute biliary pancreatitis. The German Study Group on Acute Biliary Pancreatitis. New England Journal of Medicine 336: 237–242

Foutch H P G, Harlan J, Sanowski R A 1989 Endoscopic placement of biliary stents for the treatment of high risk geriatric patients with common duct stones. American Journal of Gastroenterology 84: 527–529

Freeman M L, Nelson D B, Sherman S, Haber G B, Herman M E, Dorsher P J, Moore J P, Fennerty M B, Ryan M E, Shaw M J, Lande J D, Pheley A M 1996 Complications of endoscopic biliary sphincterotomy. New England Journal of Medicine 335: 909–918

Geenen J E, Vennes J A, Silvis S E 1981 Resumé of a seminar on endoscopic retrograde sphincterotomy (ERS). Gastrointestinal Endoscopy 27: 31–38

Girard R M, Legros G 1981 Retained and recurrent bile duct stones: surgical or non-surgical removal? Annals of Surgery 193: 150–154

Glenn F 1974 Retained calculi within the biliary ductal system. Annals of Surgery 179: 528–539

Glenn F 1975 Trends in surgical treatment of calculus disease of the biliary tract. Surgery, Gynecology and Obstetrics 140: 877–884

Goodman A J, Neoptolemos J P, Carr-Locke D L, Finlay D B L, Fossard D P 1985 Detection of gallstones after acute pancreatitis. Gut 26: 125–132

Gordon S J, Stampfl D A, Grimm I S, Dahnert W, Goldberg B B, Taglienti G 1991 Successful shockwave lithotripsy of bile duct stones using ultrasound guidance. Digestive Diseases Science 36: 1102–1109

Gracie W, Ransohoff D 1982 The natural history of silent gallstones. New England Journal of Medicine 307: 798–800

Gregg J A, de Girolami P, Carr-Locke D L 1985 Effects of sphincteroplasty and endoscopic sphincterotomy on the bacteriologic characteristics of the common bile duct. American Journal of Surgery 149: 668–671

Grimm H, Soehendra N 1983 Unterspritzung zur Behandlung der Papillotomie-Blutung. Deutsche Medizinische Wochenschrift 108: 1512–1514

Hauer-Jensen M, Karesen R, Nygaard K et al 1985 Predictive ability of choledocholithiasis indicators. Annals of Surgery 202: 64–68

Hawes R H, Cotton P B, Vallon A G 1990 Follow-up 6 to 11 years after duodenoscopic sphincterotomy for stones in patients with prior cholecystectomy. Gastroenterology 98: 1008–1012

Hill J, Martin F, Tweeddle D E F 1991 Risk of leaving the gallbladder in situ after endoscopic sphincterotomy for bile duct stones. British Journal of Surgery 78: 554–557

Hixson L J, Fennerty M D, Jaffee P E, Pulju J H, Palley S L 1992 Peroral cholangioscopy with intracorporeal electrohydraulic lithotripsy for choledocholithiasis. American Journal of Gastroenterology 87: 296–299

Holbrook R F, Jacobson F L, Pezzuti R T, Howell D A 1991 Biliary patency imaging after endoscopic retrograde sphincterotomy with gallbladder in situ: Clinical impact of non visualization. Archives of Surgery 126: 738–742

Houghton P J W, Donaldson L A 1983 Elective biliary surgery—a safe procedure. Geriatric Medicine 13: 814–816

Hunter J G 1992 Laparoscopic transcystic common bile duct exploration. American Journal of Surgery 163: 53–56

Ibuki Y, Kudo M, Todo A 1992 Endoscopic retrograde extraction of common bile duct stones with drip infusion of isosorbide dinitrate. Gastrointestinal Endoscopy 38: 178–180

Ikeda S, Tanaka M, Itoh H, Kishikawa H, Nakayama F 1981 Emergency decompression of bile duct in acute obstructive suppurative cholangitis by duodenoscopic cannulation: a lifesaving procedure. World Journal of Surgery 5: 587–593

Jamidar P A, Beck G J, Hoffman B J, Lehman G A, Hawes R H, Agrawal R M, Ashok P S, Ravi T J, Cunningham J T, Troiano F et al 1995 Endoscopic retrograde cholangiopancreatography in pregnancy. American Journal of Gastroenterology 90: 1263–1267

Johnson G, Geenen J E, Venu R P, Schmalz M J, Hogan W J 1991 Treatment of non-extractable common bile duct stones with combination ursodeoxycholic acid (UDCA) plus endoprosthesis. Gastrointestinal Endoscopy 37: 253

Jones S A 1978 The prevention and treatment of recurrent bile duct stones by transduodenal sphincteroplasty. World Journal of Surgery 2: 473–485

Josephs L F, Birkett D H 1992 Laser lithotripsy for the management of retained stones. Archives of Surgery 127: 603–605

Kawai K, Akasaka Y, Murakami K, Tada M, Kohli Y, Nakajima M 1974 Endoscopic sphincterotomy of the ampulla of Vater. Gastrointestinal Endoscopy 20: 148–151

Kaye G L, Summerfield J A, McIntyre N, Dooley J S 1990 Methyl-tert-butyl ether dissolution therapy for common bile duct stones. Journal of Hepatology 10: 337–340

Kelly T R 1980a Gallstone pancreatitis: the timing of surgery. Surgery 88: 34–35

Kelly T R 1980b Gallstone pancreatitis: a prospective randomized trial of the timing of surgery. Surgery 104: 600–605

Kelly T R, Wagner D S 1988 Gallstone pancreatitis: a prospective randomized trial of the timing of surgery. Surgery 104: 600–605

Khoo D E, Walsh C J, Cox M R, Murphy C A, Motson R W 1996 Laparoscopic common bile duct exploration: evolution of a new technique. British Journal of Surgery 83: 341–346

Kiil J, Kruse A, Rokkjaer M 1989 Large bile duct stones treated by endoscopic biliary drainage. Surgery 105: 51–56

Kim U, Bosner B 1988 Timing of surgery for acute gallstone pancreatitis. American Journal of Surgery 156: 393–396

Kune G A 1972 Current practice of biliary surgery. Little Brown, Boston, p 221–223

Lacaine F, Corlette M B, Bismuth H 1980 Preoperative evaluation of the risk of common bile duct stones. Archives of Surgery 115: 1114–1116

Lai E C, Mok F P, Tan E S, Loc M, Fan S T, You K T, Wong J 1992 Endoscopic biliary drainage for severe acute cholangitis. New England Journal of Medicine 326: 1582–1586

Lambert M E, Martin D F, Tweedle D E F 1988 Endoscopic removal of retained stones after biliary surgery. British Journal of Surgery 75: 896–898

Larson R E, Hodgson J R, Priestly J T 1966 The early and long-term results of 500 consecutive explorations of the common duct. Surgery Gynecology and Obstetrics 122: 744–750

Lee S P, Nicholls J F, Park H Z 1992 Biliary sludge as a cause of acute pancreatitis. New England Journal of Medicine 326: 589–593

Leese T, Neoptolemos J P, Carr-Locke D L 1985a Successes, failures, early complications and their management following endoscopic sphincterotomy: results in 394 consecutive patients from a single centre. British Journal of Surgery 72: 215–219

Leese T, Neoptolemos J P, Baker A R, Carr-Locke D L 1985b Management of acute cholangitis and the impact of endoscopic sphincterotomy. Gut 26: A553

Lin L F, Siauw C P, Ho K S, Tung J C 1999 ERCP in post-Billroth II gastrectomy patients: emphasis on technique. The American Journal of Gastroenterology 94: 144–148

Livio M, Benigni A, Zoja C, Begnis R, Morelli C, Rossini M, Garattini S, Remuzzi G 1989 Differential inhibition by aspirin of platelet thromboxane and renal prostaglandins in the rat. Journal of Pharmacological Experimental Therapeutics 248: 334–341

Lygidakis N J 1981 Choledochoduodenostomy in calculus biliary tract disease. British Journal of Surgery 68: 762–765

Lygidakis N J 1983 Surgical approaches to recurrent choledocholithiasis. American Journal of Surgery 145: 633–639

Madden J L, Chun J Y, Kandalaft S, Parekh M 1970 Choledochoduodenostomy, an unjustly maligned surgical procedure? American Journal of Surgery 119: 45–54

McSherry C K, Glenn F 1980 The incidence and causes of death following surgery for non-malignant biliary tract disease. Annals of Surgery 191: 271–275

Martin L J, Bailey I S, Rhodes M, O'Rourke N, Nathanson L, Fielding G 1998 Towards T-tube free laparoscopic bile duct exploration: a methodologic evolution during 300 consecutive procedures. Annals of Surgery 228: 29–34

Mason R 1980 Percutaneous extraction of retained gallstones via the T-tube tract—British experience of 131 cases. Clinical Radiology 1: 497–499

Maxton D G, Tweedle D E, Martin D F 1995 Retained common bile duct stones after endoscopic sphincterotomy: temporary and longterm treatment with biliary stenting. Gut 36: 446–449

May G R, Shaffer E H 1991 Should elective endoscopic sphincterotomy replace cholecystectomy for the treatment of high-risk patients with gallstone pancreatitis? Journal of Clinical Gastroenterology 13: 125–128

May G R, Cotton P B, Edmunds S E, Chong W 1993 Removal of stones from the bile duct at ERCP without sphincterotomy. Gastrointestinal Endoscopy 39: 749–754

Moody F G, Senninger N, Runkel N 1993 Another challenge to the Opie myth. Gastroenterology 104: 927–931

Murray W R, Laferla G, Fullarton G M 1988 Choledocholithiasis—in vivo stone dissolution using methyl tertiary butyl ether (MTBE). Gut 29: 143–145

Nakajima M, Kizu M, Akasaka Y, Kawai K 1979 Five years experience of endoscopic sphincterotomy in Japan: a collective study from 25 centers. Endoscopy 2: 138–141

Nelson D B, Freeman M L 1994 Major hemorrhage from endoscopic sphincterotomy: risk factor analysis. Journal of Clinical Gastroenterology 19: 283–287

Neoptolemos J P, Harvey M H, Slater N D, Carr-Locke D L 1984a Abdominal wall staining and 'biliscrotum' after retroperitoneal perforation following endoscopic sphincterotomy. British Journal of Surgery 71: 684

Neoptolemos J P, Carr-Locke D L, Fraser I, Fossard D P 1984b The management of common bile duct calculi by endoscopic sphincterotomy in patients with gallbladders in situ. British Journal of Surgery 71: 69–71

Neoptolemos J P, Hall A W, Finlay D B, Berry J M, Carr-Locke D L, Fossard D P 1984c The urgent diagnosis of gallstones in acute pancreatitis: a prospective study of three methods. British Journal of Surgery 71: 230–233

Neoptolemos J P, London N, Slater N D, Carr-Locke D L, Fossard D P, Moossa A R 1986 A prospective study of ERCP and endoscopic sphincterotomy in the diagnosis and treatment of gallstone acute pancreatitis. A rational and safe approach to management. Archives of Surgery

Neoptolemos J P, Carr-Locke D L, Fossard D P 1987 Prospective randomized study of preoperative endoscopic sphincterotomy versus surgery alone for common bile duct stones. British Medical Journal 294: 470–474

Neoptolemos J P, Shaw D E, Carr-Locke D L 1989 A multivariate analysis of preoperative risk factors in patients with common bile duct stones. Implications for treatment. Annals of Surgery 209: 157–161

Neoptolemos J P, Hall C, O'Connor H J, Murray W R, Carr-Locke DL 1990 Methyl-tert-butyl-ether for treating bile duct stones: the British experience. British Journal of Surgery 77: 32–35

Neuhaus H, Feussner H, Ungeheuer A, Hoffmann W, Siewert J R, Classen M 1992 Prospective evaluation of the use of endoscopic retrograde cholangiography prior to laparoscopic cholecystectomy. Endoscopy 24: 745–749

Neuhaus H, Hoffmann W, Classen M 1992 Laser lithotripsy of pancreatic and biliary stones via 3.4 mm and 3.7 mm miniscopes: first clinical results. Endoscopy 24: 208–214

Nordback I 1989 Management of unextractable bile duct stones by endoscopic stenting. Annales Chirugiae et Gynaecologiae 78: 290–292

Nowak A, Marek T A, Nowakowska-Dulawa E, Rybicka J, Kaczor R 1998 Biliary pancreatitis needs endoscopic retrograde cholangiopancreatography wth endoscopic sphincterotomy for cure. Endoscopy 30: A256–259

Nussinson E, Cairns S R, Vaira D, Dowsett J F, Mason R R 1991 A 10-year single centre experience of percutaneous and endoscopic extraction of bile duct stones with T tube in situ. Gut 32: 1040–1043

O'Doherty D P, Neoptolemos J P, Carr-Locke D L 1986 Endoscopic sphincterotomy for retained common bile duct stones in patients with T-tube in situ in the early post-operative period. British Journal of Surgery 73: 454–456

Opie E L 1901 The etiology of acute hemorrhagic pancreatitis. Bulletin of the Johns Hopkins Hospital 12: 182–188

Osborne D H, Imrie C W, Carter D C 1981 Biliary surgery in the same admission for gallstone-associated pancreatitis. British Journal of Surgery 68: 758–761

Palmer K R, Hoffmann A F 1986 Intraductal mono-octanoin for the direct dissolution of bile duct stones: experience in 343 patients. Gut 27: 196–202

Peel A L G, Bourke J B, Hermon Taylor J et al 1975 How should the common bile duct be explored? Annals of the Royal College of Surgeons of England 56: 124–134

Picus D 1990 Intracorporeal biliary lithotripsy. Radiological Clinics of North America 28: 1241–1249

Pitt H A, Cameron J L, Postier R G, Gadacz T R 1981 Factors affecting mortality in biliary tract surgery. American Journal of Surgery 141: 66–72

Ponchon T, Gagnon P, Valette P J, Henry L, Chavaillon A, Thieulin F 1991 Pulsed dye laser lithotripsy of bile duct stones. Gastroenterology 100: 1730–1736

Ponchon T, Martin X, Barkun A, Mestas J L, Chavaillon A, Boustiere C 1990 Extracorporeal lithotripsy of bile duct stones using ultrasonography for stone localization. Gastroenterology 98: 726–732

Ranson J H C 1979 The timing of biliary surgery in acute pancreatitis. Annals of Surgery 189: 654–662

Rattner D W, Warshaw A L 1981 Impact of choledochoscopy in the management of choledocholithiasis. Annals of Surgery 194: 76–79

Reiter J J, Bayer H P, Mennicken C, Manegold B C 1978 Results of endoscopic papillotomy: A collective experience from nine endoscopic centers in West Germany. World Journal of Surgery 2: 505–511

Rhodes M, Nathanson L, O'Rourke N, Fielding G 1995 Laparoscopic exploration of the common bile duct: lessons learned from 129 consecutive cases. British Journal of Surgery 82: 666–668

Rhodes M, Sussman L, Cohen L, Lewis M P 1998 Randomised trial of laparoscopic exploration of common bile duct versus postoperative endoscopic retrograde cholangiography for common bile duct stones. Lancet 351(9097): 159–161

Rosch W, Riemann J F, Lux G, Lindner H G 1981 Long-term follow-up after endoscopic sphincterotomy. Endoscopy 13: 152–153

Rosseland A R, Solhaug J H 1984 Early or delayed endoscopic papillotomy (EPT) in gallstone pancreatitis. Annals of Surgery 199: 165–167

Rabenstein T, Ruppert T, Schneider H T, Hahn E G, Ell C 1997 Benefits and risks of needle-knife papillotomy. Gastrointestinal Endoscopy 46: 207–211

Rustgi A K, Schapiro R H 1991 Biliary stents for common bile duct stones. Gastrointestinal Endoscopy Clinics of North America 1: 79–91

Sackier J M, Berci G, Phillips E, Carroll B, Shapiro S, Pas-Parlow M 1991 The role of cholangiography in laparoscopic cholecystectomy. Archives of Surgery 126: 1021–1026

Safrany L 1978 Endoscopic treatment of biliary tract diseases. Lancet ii: 983–985

Sauerbruch T, Stern M 1989 Fragmentation of bile duct stones by extracorporeal shock waves. A new approach to biliary calculi after failure of routine endoscopic measures. Gastroenterology 96: 146–152

Schumacher B, Frieling T, Haussinger D, Niederau C 1998 Endoscopic treatment of symptomatic choledocholithiasis. Hepatogastroenterology 45: 672–676

Sees D W, Martin R R 1997 Comparison of preoperative endoscopic retrograde cholangiopancreatography and laparoscopic cholecystectomy with operative management of gallstone pancreatitis. American Journal of Surgery 174: 719–722

Seifert E, Gail K, Weismuller J 1982 Langzeitresultate nach endoskopischer Sphinkterotomie: follow-up-Studie asu 25 Zentren in der Bundesrepublik. Deutsche Medizinische Wochenschrift 107: 610–614

Shakoor T, Geenen J E 1992 Pre-cut papillotomy. Gastrointestinal Endoscopy 38: 623–627

Shemesh E, Czerniak A, Schneabaum S, Nass S 1990 Early endoscopic sphincterotomy in the management of acute gallstone pancreatitis in elderly patients. JAGS 38: 893–896

Sheridan W G, Williams H O L, Lewis M H 1987 Morbidity and mortality of common bile duct exploration. British Journal of Surgery 74: 1095–1099

Siegel J H 1981 Endoscopic papillotomy in the treatment of biliary tract disease: 258 procedures and results. Digestive Diseases and Sciences 26: 1057–1064

Siegel J H, Safrany L, Ben-Zvi J S et al 1988 Duodenoscopic sphincterotomy in patients with gallbladders in situ: reports of a series of 1272 patients. American Journal of Gastroenterology 83: 1255–1258

Siegel J, Ben-Zvi J, Pullano W 1990 Endoscopic electrohydraulic lithotripsy. Gastrointestinal Endoscopy 36: 134–136

Simpson C J, Gray G R, Gillespie G 1985 Early endoscopic sphincterotomy for retained common bile duct stones. Journal of the Royal College of Surgeons, Edinburgh 30: 288–289

Soehendra N, Kempeneers I, Eichfuss H P, Reynders-Frederix V 1981 Early postoperative endoscopy after biliary tract surgery. Endoscopy 13: 113–117

Soomers A J, Nagengast F M, Yap S H 1990 Endoscopic placement of biliary endoprostheses in patients with endoscopically unextractable common bile duct stones. Endoscopy 22: 24–26

Speranza V, Lezoche E, Minervina S, Carlei F, Basso N, Simi M 1982 Transduodenal papillostomy as a routine procedure in managing choledocholithiasis. Archives of Surgery 117: 875–878

Staritz M 1983a Endoscopic papillary dilatation. Endoscopy 15: 197–198

Staritz M 1983b Mechanical gallstone lithotripsy. Endoscopy 15: 316–318

Staritz M, Poarella T, Dormeyer H H, Meyer zum Buschenfelde K H 1985 Endoscopic removal of common bile duct stones through the intact papilla after medical sphincter dilation. Gastroenterology 88: 1807–1811

Stiegmann G V, Goff J S, Mansour A, Pearlman N, Reveille R M 1992 Precholecystectomy endoscopic cholangiography and stone removal is not superior to cholecystectomy, cholangiography, and common duct exploration. American Journal of Surgery 163: 227–230

Stone H H, Fabian T C, Dunlop W E 1981 Gallstone pancreatitis. Biliary tract pathology in relation to time of operations. Annals of Surgery 194: 305–312

Stuart M, Hoerr S O 1972 Late results of side to side choledocho-duodenostomy and of transduodenal sphincterotomy for benign disorders. American Journal of Surgery 123: 67–72

Sullivan D M, Ruffin-Hood T, Griffin W O 1982 Biliary tract surgery in the elderly. American Journal of Surgery 143: 218–220

Tanaka M, Ikeda S, Yoshimoto H, Matsumoto S 1987 The long-term fate of the gallbladder after endoscopic sphincterotomy. American Journal of Surgery 154: 505–509

Tandon R K, Nijhawan S, Arora A 1990 Management of retained common bile duct stones in patients with T-tube in situ: role of endoscopic sphincterotomy. American Journal of Gastroenterology 85: 1126–1131

Targarona E M, Balague C, Espert J J, Perez Ayuso R M, Ros E, Navarro S, Bordas J, Teres J, Trias M 1995 Laparoscopic treatment of acute biliary pancreatitis. International Surgery 80: 365–368

Tham T C, Vandervoort J, Wong R C, Lichtenstein D R, Van Dam J,

Ruymann F, Farraye F, Carr-Locke DL 1997 Therapeutic ERCP in outpatients. Gastrointestinal Endoscopy 45: 225–230

Thompson J E, Thompkins R K, Longmire W P 1982 Factors in management of acute cholangitis. Annals of Surgery 195: 137–145

Tritapepe R, di Padova C, di Padova F 1988 Non-invasive treatment for retained common bile duct stones in patients with T tube in situ: saline washout after intravenous ceruletide. British Journal of Surgery 75: 144–146

Vallon A G, Holton J M, Cotton P B 1986 Follow-up duodenoscopic sphincterotomy for recurrent duct stones (unpublished observations).

Van Dam J, Sivak M V 1993 Mechanical lithotripsy of large common bile duct stones. Cleveland Clinic Journal of Medicine 60: 38–42

Vandervoort J, Tham T C K, Wong R C K, Roston A D, Ferrari A P,

Slivka A, Musa A, Lichtenstein D R, Van Dam J, Ruymann F, Hughes M, Carr-Locke D L 1996 Prospective Analysis of Risk Factors for Pancreatitis after Diagnostic and Therapeutic ERCP. Gastrointestinal Endoscopy 43: 400

Vellacott K D, Powell P H 1979 Exploration of the common bile duct; a comparative study. British Journal of Surgery 66: 389–391

Way L W, Admirand W H, Dunphy J E 1972 Management of choledocholithiasis. Annals of Surgery 176: 347–359

Weber J, Adamek H E, Riemann J F 1992 Extracorporeal piezoelectric lithotripsy for retained bile duct stones. Endoscopy 24: 239–243

Worthley C S, Toouli J 1988 Gallbladder non-filling: an indication for cholecystectomy after endoscopic sphincterotomy. British Journal of Surgery 75: 796–798

Interventional radiology in the management of bile duct stones

41

L. MACHAN, C.D. BECKER

GENERAL CONSIDERATIONS

Radiology of the biliary tract owes its beginnings to contributions from surgery with the original description of transhepatic gallbladder puncture in 1921 (Burckhardt & Mueller 1921), cholecystography in 1923 (Cole 1960), and postsurgical cholangiography in 1924 (Cotte 1925). The specialties of radiology and surgery have had a close and important relationship ever since in the diagnosis of biliary disease, and later in therapy. Biliary interventional radiology (see also Ch. 29) expanded rapidly after description of non-operative retained biliary stone extraction in 1973 (Mazzariello 1973, Burhenne 1973). While the number of biliary interventions for stone disease has declined somewhat in the past few years because of improvements in endoscopic and laparoscopic techniques, biliary interventional radiology retains an important place in specific aspects of biliary stone disease.

EQUIPMENT AND RADIATION PROTECTION

A modern fluoroscopic unit with spot film capabilities, preferably digital, is required for radiology of the biliary tract. Small retained stones of 2 mm or less are better seen with radiographic than with fluoroscopic imaging. The roentgen-ray tube should be under the couch in order to decrease scatter to the radiologist, and the radiologist should have access to radiation shielding including a waist-high lead barrier, mobile radiation shield, and a lead shield or apron with a window which can be draped over the patient, leaving the area of interest free. Sterile gloves impregnated with a radiation dose reducing substance are recommended. The radiologist's fingers should never be in the primary beam, collimation should be to the smallest possible field, and magnification or imaging in an oblique projection should be kept to a minimum. Periodic patient skin exposure measurements should be obtained to augment and incite continuous re-evaluation of technique.

The equipment for instrumentation of the biliary tract via postoperative tracts or percutaneous transhepatic access includes standard angiographic guide-wires and catheters. A steerable catheter (Boston Scientific Corporation, Natick, MA) described by Burhenne in 1973 revolutionized the catheterization of T-tube tracts and still can be used in patients with tortuous anatomy, but its use has largely been supplanted by an extensive array of purpose designed, easily steerable, low profile devices. The devices used depend on radiologist choice but should be steerable and accommodate passage of baskets (Fig. 41.1) and biopsy forceps.

Percutaneous choledochoscopy (Fig. 41.2) has greatly facilitated the treatment of biliary stones by allowing direct visualization, enabling differentiation of stones from other ductal filling defects, and easy targeting of stones for fracture, retrieval, or dislodgement when impacted or situated in diverticula (Picus 1995). Most are 5 mm in diameter (15 Fr) with 6-Fr working channels. Smaller scopes are more flexible and can be inserted through smaller tracts, but have decreased torque control and field of view, and as they have smaller working channels, accommodate the use of smaller instruments.

INTERVENTIONAL ACCESS ROUTES

Access to the biliary tract for interventional procedures is gained via postoperative sinus tracts from a T tube or cholecystostomy tube, via surgically created Roux loops, or percutaneously through the liver.

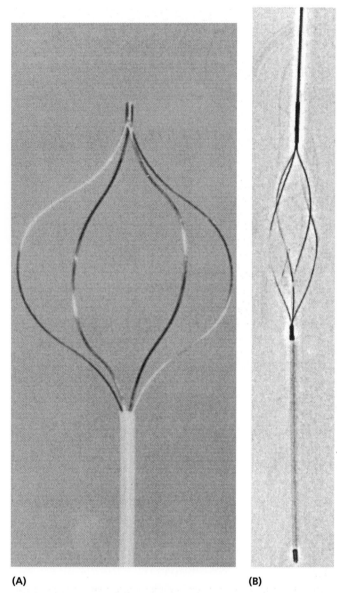

(A)   **(B)**

Fig. 41.1 Biliary stone baskets. **(A)** Standard 4 wire basket. **(B)** Four wire basket with a leading guidewire. This is particularly useful when the stone must be advanced into the duodenum.

T-TUBE TRACT

Instrumentation of a T-tube tract is an easy technical proce-dure and has implications for surgical T-tube placement. If T-tube insertion into the extrahepatic biliary tree is neces-sary, the calibre of the long arm of the rubber T tube should be at least 14 Fr (Fig. 41.3). If the common duct is small in caliber, the short arms of the T tube should be trimmed appropriately. Ideally, the T tube should connect at a 90° angle with the common bile duct, be as straight as possible, and exit through a stab wound in the right flank in the ante-rior axillary line. This will create the shortest possible tract

and allow access to the biliary tree both proximal and distal to the T-tube insertion site. Anterior T-tube placement through surgical incisions makes radiological instrumenta-tion considerably more difficult and the operator's hands are often in the field of radiation.

A T-tube cholangiogram should be obtained in the immediate postoperative period. This should be in the radiology department as high resolution spot radiographs in multiple obliquities are needed to ascertain the diagnosis and differentiate choledocholithiasis from a blood clot or tumor (Fig. 41.4).

If the postoperative T-tube cholangiogram demonstrates retained biliary stones, the patient is usally discharged as the T tube should be left in place for at least a total of 5 weeks to permit formation of a fibrous tract. This permits access to the bile ducts for stone extraction. A T-tube tract with a tube of less than 14 Fr may require more than a 5-week interval for tract formation, particularly if the patient is obese or on immunosuppressants. Fibrous reaction in adipose tissue occurs more slowly.

Radiological stone extraction is performed in the ambula-tory patient as a routine outpatient procedure using intra-venous sedation and local anesthetic. Admission to hospital is only required in complicated cases.

TRANSHEPATIC ROUTE

A percutaneous transhepatic approach to the biliary tract for stone removal may occasionally be used if a postoperative drainage tract is not available, when surgical or endoscopic stone removal is contraindicated or not possible (Fig. 41.5), or when the patient has calculi in intrahepatic ducts proximal to a biliary duct stricture e.g. segmental chol-angiohepatitis (Fig. 41.6). This is a further development of percutaneous transhepatic cholangiography (Dotter et al 1979). The technique is analogous to the biliary drainage procedures but carries a higher complication rate than instrumentation through a T-tube tract. The stone may be advanced into the duodenum (Fig. 41.7), or less ideally fragmented with an intracorporeal lithotripter or stone bas-ket (Fig. 41.8) in the bile duct, and the fragments are then expelled from the duct into the duodenum. Only as a last resort should transhepatic stone extraction be attempted as hepatic injury can occur during transhepatic stone extrac-tion.

CHOLECYSTOSTOMY TRACT

Similar to the use of the postoperative T-tube tract, radio-logical instrumentation through a cholecystostomy is feasi-

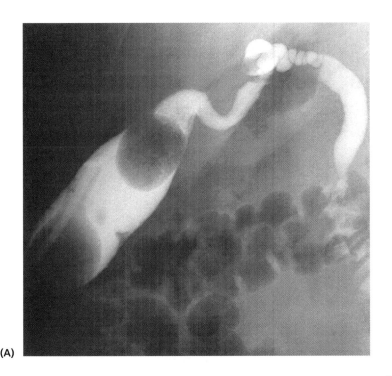

(A)

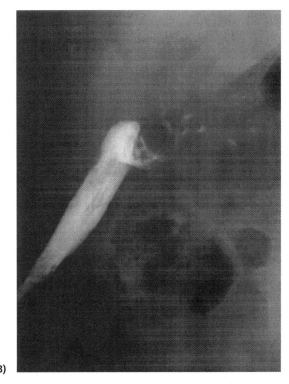

(B)

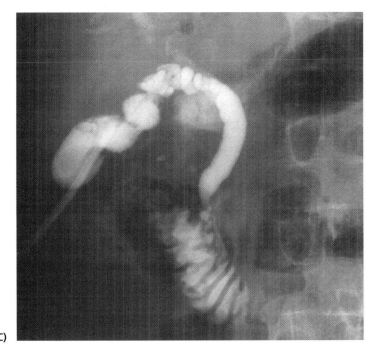

(C)

Fig. 41.2 Removal of stone via cholecystostomy. Debilitated 69-year-old man with acute cholecystitis. **(A)** Cholecystogram obtained via a Foley catheter in the gallbladder fundus one week after surgical minicholecystostomy demonstrating a large gallbladder calculus and a small calculus in the cystic duct. **(B)** After extrahydrolic lithotripsy, the gallbladder stone is fragmented. Fragments occlude the cystic duct. **(C)** After removal of fragments using choledochoscopic and fluoroscopic guidance, contrast drains freely through the cystic duct. The choledochoscope is seen in the gallbladder.

ble in order to gain access to the gallbladder or common duct for stone removal (Fig. 41.3). Access for this purpose can be achieved percutaneously with or without fixation of the gallbladder to the abdominal wall using a T fastener (Cope 1991) but the authors prefer surgical chole-cystostomy in high-risk patients with cholelithiasis. The gallbladder fundus is sutured to the peritoneum behind the rectus sheath. This permits radiological instrumentation for gallstone removal 1 week after operation.

JEJUNOSTOMY

The presence of a jejunostomy facilitates radiological intervention for stone removal in patients with intrahepatic

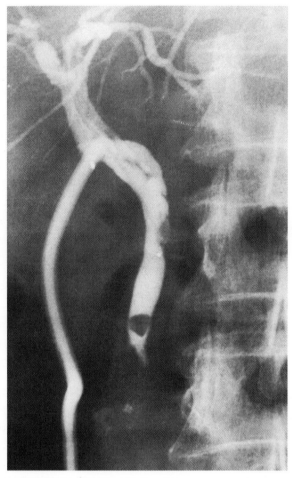

(A)

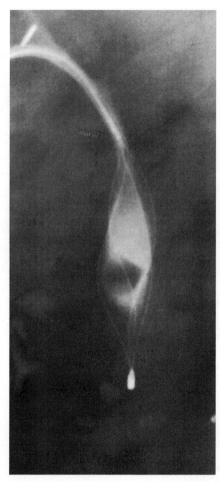

(B)

Fig. 41.3 (A) Retained distal common bile duct stone on T-tube cholangiography one week after operation. Note that the T tube is inserted in the common hepatic bile duct above the confluence of the cystic duct. **(B)** The retained common duct stone is ensnared in a wire basket before extraction. This stone measured 5 mm in diameter and was extracted intact through the sinus tract of a 14-Fr T tube.

stones proximal to a hepaticojejunostomy. The blind limb of the hepaticojejunostomy is sutured subcutaneously, and a radio-opaque clip is strategically placed to allow easy percutaneous localization, thus serving as an access port for repeated percutaneous intervention (McPherson 1998) (Ch. 30). This approach is ideal in patients who require repeated intrahepatic stone removal and stricture dilatation such as patients with Caroli's disease and recurrent pyogenic cholangitis who are not good candidates for endoscopic stone removal.

EXTRACTION OF STONES FROM THE BILE DUCTS

Despite improved preoperative and operative cholangiography, bile duct stones retained after operation can still be an exasperating problem. Perioperative endoscopic retrograde cholangiopancreatography (ERCP) and improved operative cholangiography have reduced the number of retained stones, but the incidence of false-negative completion cholangiograms is approximately 5% after common duct exploration. The additional use of intraoperative choledochoscopy can reduce this figure.

The problem is not new. More than 70 years ago, William Halstead, who performed one of the earliest operations on the gallbladder, stated that a simple, reliable method was needed to determine accurately the presence of stones in the common bile duct. Dr Halstead, 20 years later, was himself to die of complications after the removal of a retained common duct stone (Longmire et al 1979).

TECHNIQUE

Radiological intervention for retained stone removal is usually done in the ambulatory patient 5 weeks after cholecystectomy and common duct exploration. The T tube is removed and a

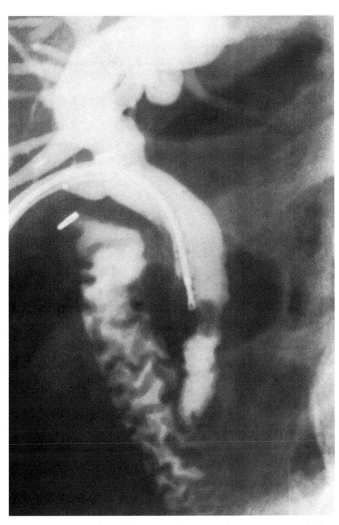

Fig. 41.4 Patient referred for retained common duct stone removal. The filling defect was immobile on instrumentation. Tissue was obtained using a flexible biopsy wire. Histopathological diagnosis reviewed cholangiocarcinoma of the common bile duct.

steerable catheter is introduced through the fibrous tract into the common duct (Fig. 41.9). A stone extraction basket is then maneuvered in its covering sheath or catheter in a closed position alongside the stone and opened behind it. The retained material is ensnared with the basket under fluoroscopic vision during cholangiography. The stones are then extracted through the sinus tract. The tract of a 14-Fr T tube will permit extraction of the intact stone if it measures 6 or 7 mm in diameter. Larger stones require fragmentation before the fragments are extracted. The radiologist must allow for a 30% magnification factor when measuring stones on cholangiograms. This magnification factor is larger in the distal common duct and less for intrahepatic stones.

Once engaged, the stone is best extracted in a continuous pulling motion without forcefully closing the basket on the stone. Even small stones will remain in the basket tip during continuous extraction through the duct system and sinus tract. Hesitant withdrawal, however, may permit small stones to fall outside the basket. Closure of the stone basket after the stone has been engaged often results in fragmentation or disengagement of the stone.

Small stones and fragments of about 3 mm in size and smaller frequently pass spontaneously through the ampulla. If the short arm of the T tube prevents retained small stones in the common hepatic duct from moving distally, the T tube should be exchanged for a straight tube early in the postoperative period to permit spontaneous passage of small stones. Small stones and fragments of 1 or 2 mm in size are difficult to identify on the fluoroscopic screen. Intermittent spot films are then indicated to assess stone location.

Large stones (over 6–8 mm in diameter) cannot be extracted intact through the sinus tract of a 14-Fr T tube (Fig. 41.10). Fragmentation is then required and is usually easily possible with a stone basket because large retained stones are almost always relatively soft. The stone is brought with the basket to the junction of the bile duct and the sinus tract, where strong resistance is felt. Increased and steady traction on the end of the basket wire is then applied over 1–2 minutes. A pulling force of no more than about 10 kg is necessary. The steady and increasing pull results in the stone being cut by the wire basket. No common duct injury has been experienced by the authors using this technique. Stones may also be fragmented by closing the basket within the duct. The open basket with the stone within it is pulled against the catheter tip. If the stone cannot be fragmented using a basket, it can be achieved by intracorporeal lithotripsy (Harris et al 1996) or by forceps (Mazzariello 1978).

Cystic duct remnant stones are very difficult or sometimes impossible to remove, particularly when the stone does not migrate from the cystic duct into the distal common duct with the patient in the erect position. A steerable catheter is then used in an attempt to mobilize the cystic duct stone by transmural pressure exerted on the common hepatic and cystic duct. If this is not successful, a combined choledochoscopic and fluoroscopic approach is attempted (Fig. 41.3).

Partially impacted stones in the distal end of the common duct are often difficult to engage in the wire basket since the basket must be opened beyond the papilla of Vater, there being insufficient space between the stone and the papilla. Impacted stones must therefore be moved to a more proximal position in the duct to permit satisfactory opening of the basket. This can be achieved through suction through a catheter, forcible contrast injection distal to the stone, or

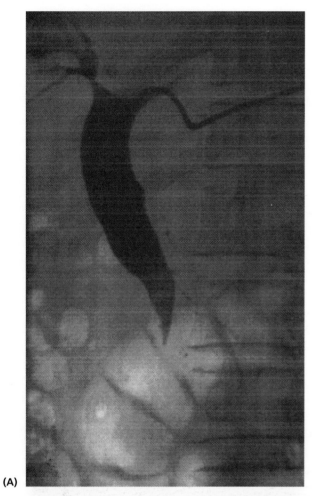

(A)

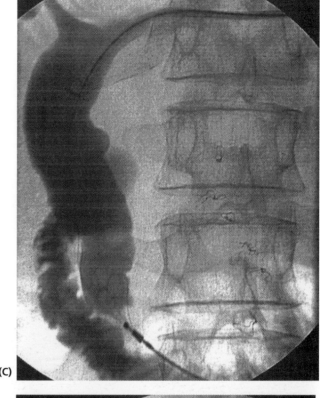

(C)

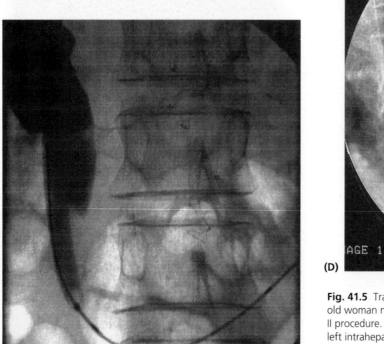

(B)

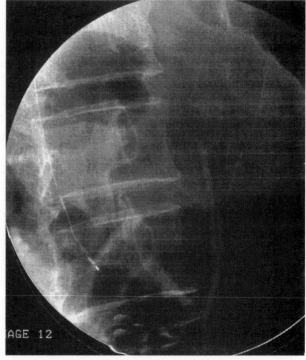

(D)

Fig. 41.5 Transhepatic stone removal and stricture therapy in a 67-year-old woman not a candidate for endoscopic treatment because of Billroth II procedure. **(A)** A smooth tapered occlusion at the ampulla is seen after left intrahepatic duct puncture. **(B)** Balloon dilatation of the stenosis. **(C)** The stones are basketed and advanced into the duodenum. **(D)** A papillotome was advanced through the transhepatic tract and a cut made at the 12 o'clock position. The patient remains well two and a half years after therapy.

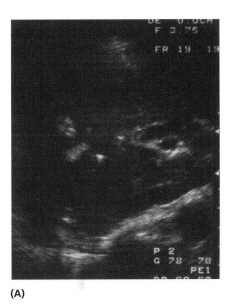

(A)

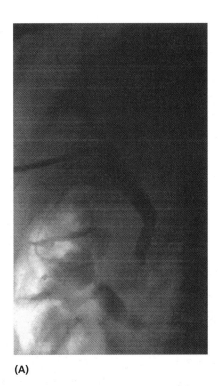

(A)

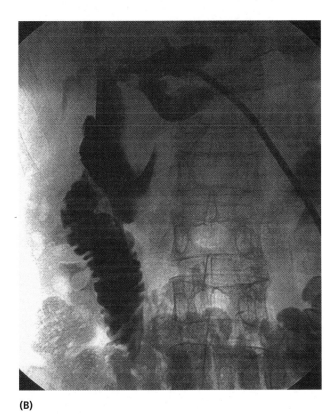

(B)

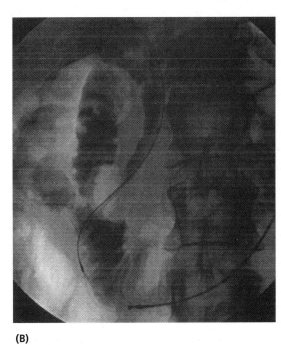

(B)

Fig. 41.6 Oriental cholangiohepatitis in a patient who is not a candidate for transplant. 54-year-old woman with recurrent episodes of septic biliary obstruction and chronic right lobe atrophy. **(A)** Hepatic ultrasound, sagittal projection. Echogenic material is seen in two radicals of the left-sided ductal system. These were punctured under ultrasound guidance. **(B)** Cholangiogram performed after left-sided intrahepatic duct puncture demonstrating a tight stenosis at the hilum and dilated deformed left-sided ducts which contained thick proteinaceous material. After balloon dilatation, the stricture was stented with an internal/external catheter for 3 months.

Fig. 41.7 Transhepatic advancement of common bile duct stone into duodenum. **(A)** An 8 mm calculus is seen in the distal CBD after right-sided puncture. **(B)** After capturing the stone (using a basket with a leading guidewire) the stone is deposited in the duodenum by opening the basket.

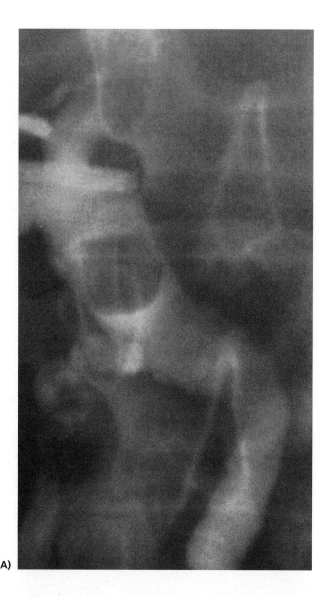

(A)

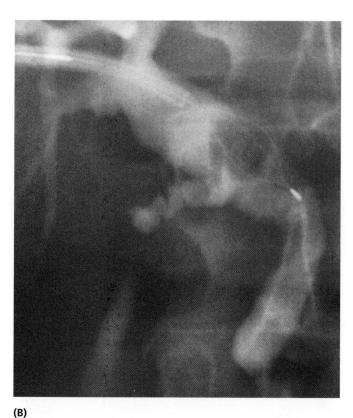

(B)

Fig. 41.8 **(A)** Transhepatic cholangiogram with a steerable catheter in the common hepatic duct demonstrating a large common hepatic duct stone in a patient with a previous Billroth II gastrectomy and the gallbladder in situ. **(B)** The wire basket has been passed through the transhepatic catheter and positioned around the bile duct stone. Gentle closure resulted in fragmentation of the stone, and fragments passed readily into the duodenum.

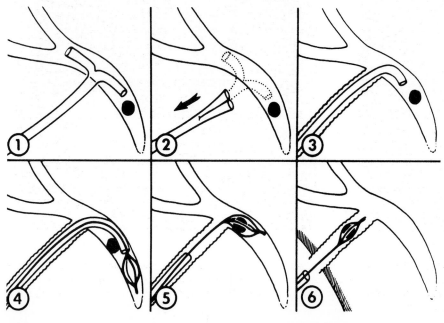

Fig. 41.9 Technical steps of retained common bile duct stone extraction with a T tube: (1) A cholangiogram shows location of the stone. (2) The T tube is extracted. (3) A steerable catheter is manipulated through the sinus tract into the common duct. (4) The tip of the steerable catheter is advanced beyond the stone and the wire stone basket is opened distally to the stone. (5) After partial withdrawal of the steerable catheter, the retained stone is ensnared in the open basket. (6) The stone is withdrawn through the sinus tract.

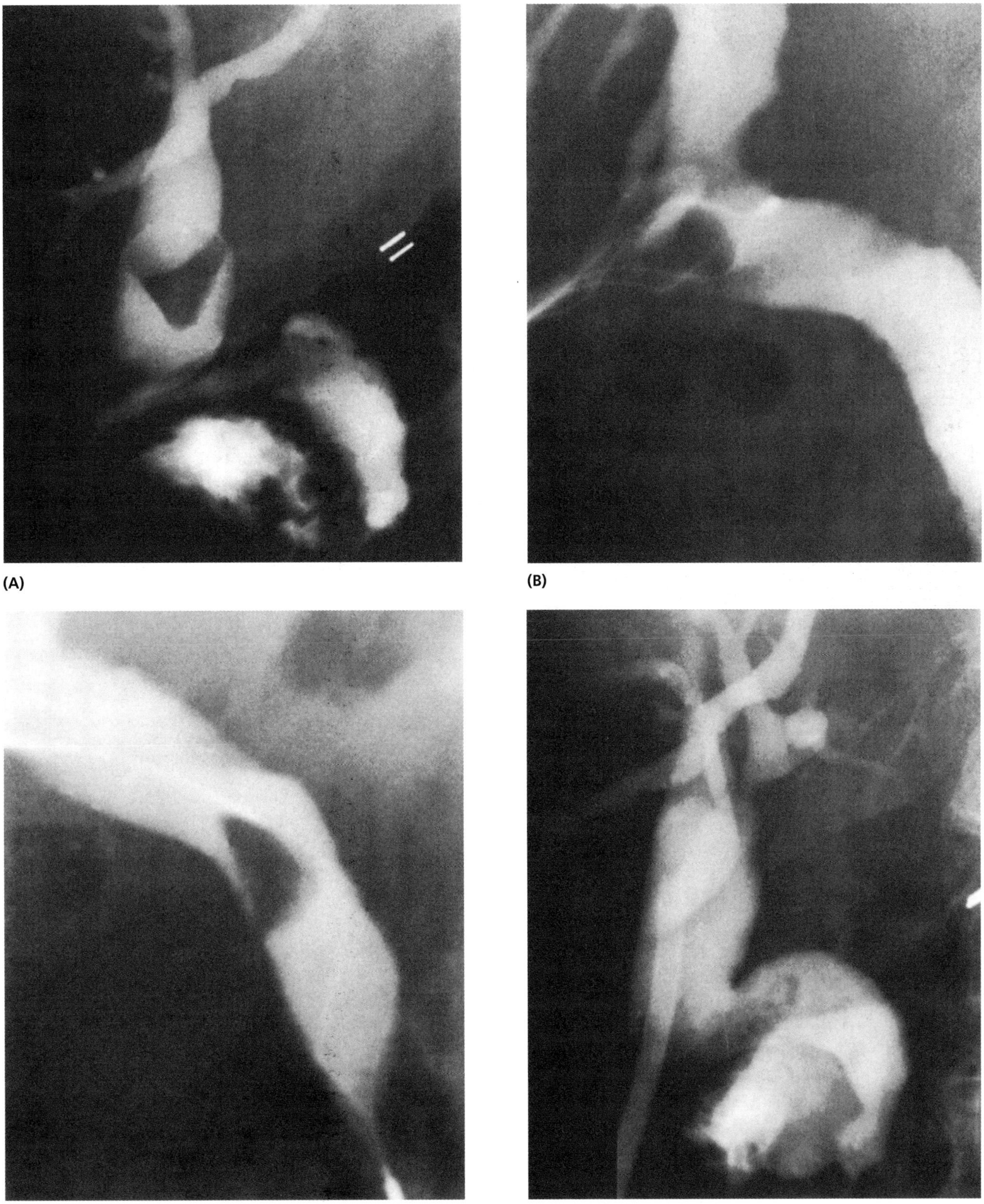

(A)

(B)

(C)

(D)

Fig. 41.10 (A) Large retained common hepatic duct stone. **(B)** The retained stone was fragmented at the junction of the bile duct and sinus tract. Note deformity of the wire basket due to traction. **(C)** Major fragments remaining are extracted. Note the straight cut margin of this fragment due to fragmentation with a wire basket. **(D)** The major fragments have been extracted. A few very small fragments remained, but passed spontaneously into the duodenum as confirmed on cholangiography 3 days later.

with a balloon catheter. This is distended with contrast material for exact visualization of size and position under the fluoroscope. The inflated balloon catheter is manipulated behind the stone and then eased centrally with a gentle pull. If the balloon is seen to wedge the stone sideways, no undue traction should be applied.

INTRAHEPATIC STONES

Biliary stones in intrahepatic radicles are often multiple and may be impacted (Fig. 41.11 and see also Fig. 41.15). As the steerable catheter cannot be passed alongside, the closed stone basket is moved beyond the stone for extraction. This is technically more demanding and represents a greater challenge than extraction of extrahepatic stones.

Intrahepatic stones, however, may move spontaneously into an extrahepatic location if the T tube is exchanged. It is often the case that the short arm of a T tube lying within the common hepatic duct or in one hepatic radicle prevents distal migration of stone. The T tube is extracted and exchanged for a straight catheter and the patient is then recalled after 1 or 2 weeks of ambulation.

Use of a Fogarty balloon is often required if intrahepatic stones are impacted. The balloon is inflated with contrast medium for fluoroscopic identification and gentle traction is applied. Overdistention of the balloon may lead to extravasation. Manipulation and extraction of intrahepatic stones, however, is more readily accomplished under postoperative fluoroscopy than during surgery.

Radiological intervention for intrahepatic biliary stones usually requires multiple sessions. A catheter is introduced through the sinus tract into the common duct in order to maintain access between sessions (Choi et al 1992).

RESULTS

The success rate of radiological percutaneous stone removal through the T-tube tract with the basket technique is 88 to 97% (Burhenne 1976, Geisinger et al 1989) and 95.3% using rigid forceps (Mazzariello 1978). Reasons for failure include stone impaction, stones situated in an inaccessible cystic duct remnant, a too small or too tortuous T-tube tract, inability to fragment a large stone or inadvertent injury to the sinus tract. Large calculi can usually be fragmented mechanically with the basket prior to extraction; adjuvant methods to deal with large and impacted calculi include intracorporeal and extracorporeal lithotripsy, and the use of balloon catheters (Harris et al 1996, Bean & Daughtry 1985, Meranze et al 1986, Burhenne 1975). Burhenne reported 2314 patients

with an overall success rate of 96%. About one-half of the patients in whom there was failure to remove all stones had intrahepatic stones. Other causes in his experience were inability to catheterize the sinus tract of a small T tube, inability to recatheterize the tract on a return visit, or impacted distal common duct stone. Cystic duct remnant stones are sometimes impossible to remove, particularly when the stone does not migrate from the cystic duct into the distal common duct with the patient in the erect position. The steerable catheter is then used in an attempt to mobilize the cystic duct stone by transmural pressure exerted on the common hepatic and cystic ducts.

Technical success rates improve with experience. It probably takes at least 20 extraction procedures for a radiologist to become sufficiently experienced in the technique.

COMPLICATIONS

The commonest complications of percutaneous stone removal are transient fever and sinus tract perforation. These usually are without clinical sequelae. Perforation of the sinus tract may render recatheterization impossible and does result in stone extraction failure. Patients with perforation of the sinus tract are placed on broad spectrum antibiotics. If clinical signs and symptoms develop, they usually subside within 48 hours even when there is communication between the perforated sinus tract and the peritoneal cavity (Burhenne 1980). Subhepatic bile collections occurred in 0.3% in this series.

Serious complications, e.g. bile leaks, sepsis, and severe pancreatitis are much less frequent. In a survey of 39 institutions reporting a total of 612 stone extraction procedures, a morbidity of 5% and no mortality was recorded (Burhenne 1976). However, a review of the same procedure performed in 26 British hospitals showed a complication rate of 9.2%, including pancreatitis, fever and perforation of the sinus tract (Mason 1980). In his own series of 2314 patients, Burhenne reported no perforation of the biliary tract (as opposed to the sinus tract) and no mortality. The morbidity rate was 4.1%.

Geisinger et al (1989) reported a complication rate of 3% in 189 procedures, including two cases of pancreatitis (1%). Two deaths have been reported from percutaneous stone extraction (Polack et al 1977, Mazzariello 1978), both due to acute pancreatitis after difficult radiological manipulations.

Even though major complications are much lower in benign than malignant disease (Lee 1987), if transhepatic access is required for biliary stone extraction complications relevant to establishment of ductal access do occur. These include hemobilia, sepsis, pneumothorax, bilithorax, hemorrhage, peritonitis and subphrenic abcess.

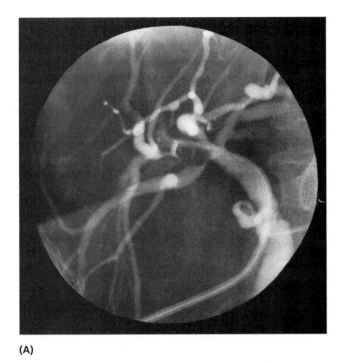

(A)

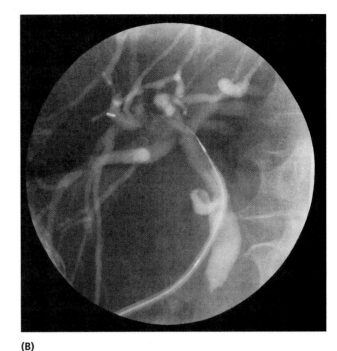

(B)

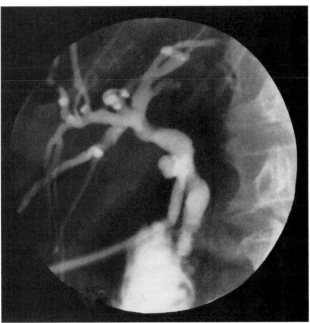

(C)

Fig. 41.11 Extraction of impacted intrahepatic calculi. **(A)** Direct cholangiography shows three impacted calculi in a right intrahepatic branch. **(B)** A small stone extraction basket has been maneuvered alongside and distal to the calculi and stone removal is being performed. **(C)** Completion cholangiogram showing no residual calculi and unimpeded passage of contrast material into the duodenum.

EXTRACTION OF GALLBLADDER STONES AND TRANSCHOLECYSTIC REMOVAL OF COMMON BILE DUCT STONES (Figs 41.12 and 41.13)

Radiological instrumentation through cholecystostomy tracts permits removal of stones from the gallbladder, the cystic duct and the common duct. This formerly difficult procedure now is easier as the invention of the hydrophilic guidewire greatly facilitates traversal of the cystic ducts. Large stones in the gallbladder are fragmented or removed with forceps or stone baskets. The same approach through the cholecystostomy tract may be used for removal of common bile duct stones. This usually requires use of a hydrophilic guidewire, dilatation of the cystic duct with an angioplasty balloon catheter, and

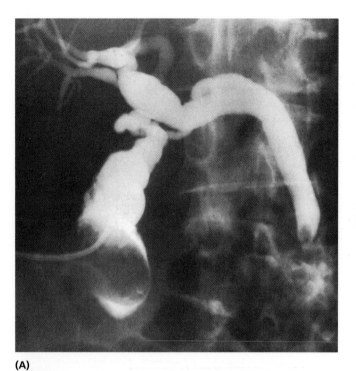

(A)

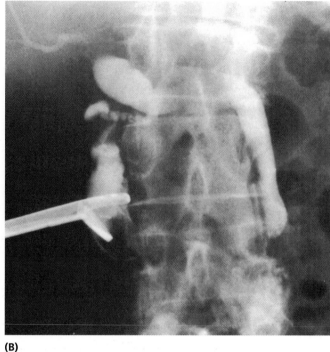

(B)

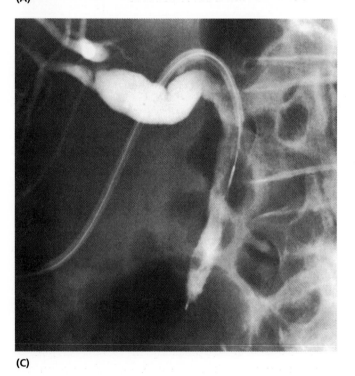

(C)

Fig. 41.12 **(A)** A solitary 4 × 6 cm gallbladder stone and a single distal common duct after cholecystostomy drainage for acute cholecystitis. **(B)** A Storz bladder stone crushing forceps was introduced through the cholecystostomy tract for fragmentation and complete removal of the gallbladder stone. **(C)** A steerable catheter was manipulated through the cystic duct and the distal common duct stone was engaged and removed through the cystic duct and gallbladder after balloon dilatation of the cystic duct. Following removal of all stones in multiple interventional sessions in this 93-year-old male, the cholecystostomy tube was removed and the gallbladder left in place.

advancement of the catheter for negotiation of the cystic duct. Stones are then basketed and advanced into the duodenum or retrieved through the cholecystostomy tract.

Cholecystostomy and subsequent radiologic stone removal is an alternative (Fig. 41.13) to cholecystectomy in high risk elderly individuals where cholecystectomy for acute cholecystitis carries a 9.8% operative death rate in patients over 65 years (Glenn 1981). This can be performed after surgical mini-cholecystostomy under local anesthetic followed by radiologic stone extraction (Gibney et al 1987) (Figs. 41.2 and 41.12) or after radiologically guided cholecystostomy (Cope 1991).

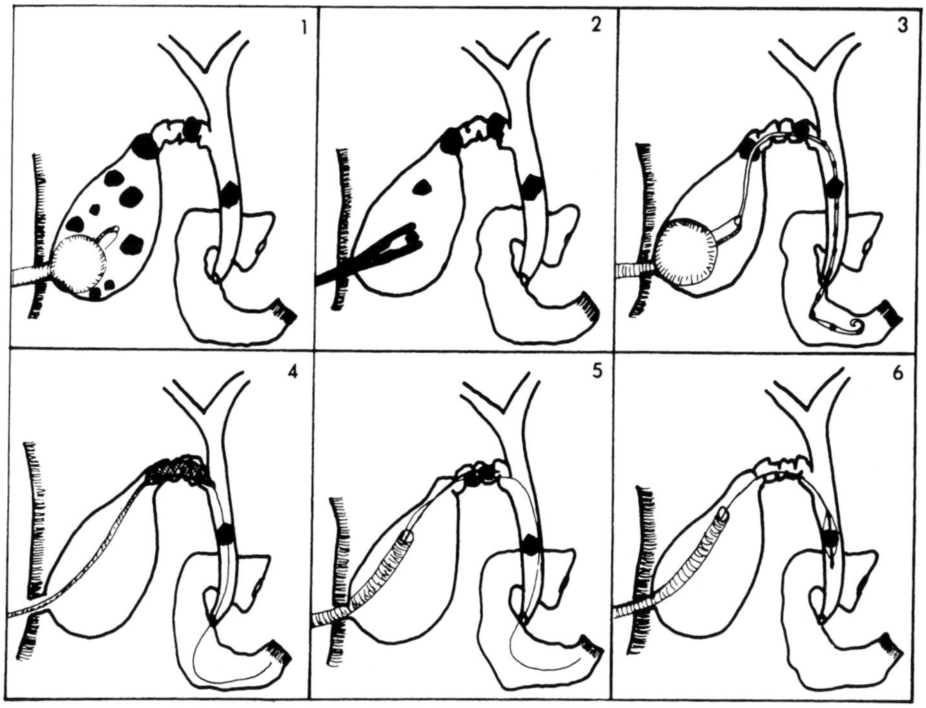

Fig. 41.13 Cholecystostomy intervention for cholelithiasis. (1) A balloon catheter is in place after mini-cholecystostomy with the gallbladder fundus sutured to the abdominal wall. Cholelithiasis affects gallbladder, cystic duct, and common duct. (2) 10 days after mini-cholecystostomy, stones are removed from the gallbladder with Mazzariello forceps under fluoroscopic control. (3) Drainage catheter with sideholes has been placed through the cystic and common ducts into the duodenum after manipulation with an 8-Fr steerable catheter and guidewire. The drainage catheter is placed through the 24-Fr cholecystostomy balloon catheter between procedures. (4) A guidewire is introduced through the drainage catheter into the duodenum and an angiographic balloon catheter is used for cystic duct dilatation. (5) Stones in the cystic duct are now retrieved into the gallbladder after inflation of the Fogarty balloon distal to the stone. A guidewire remains in place alongside the Fogarty balloon for access. (6) A final session involves catheter placement into the common duct followed by stone extraction basket positioning and extraction of the common duct stone through the cystic duct and gallbladder. The treatment is completed.

EXTRACTION OF STONES PROXIMAL TO STRICTURES

As opposed to malignant biliary strictures in which calculi are typically seen distal and virtually never proximal to the obstruction (Nichols & MacLeod 1998) intrahepatic stones are often situated above benign hepatic duct strictures. This is usually the case in recurrent pyogenic cholangitis and a complicating factor in Caroli's disease. Hepatic duct stones may also be present proximal to a stenosed hepatodochojejunostomy. Stone extraction in patients with benign biliary strictures cannot be accomplished without preceding stricture dilatation (Fig. 41.14).

Similar to percutaneous stone extraction, the subhepatic approach through postoperative drain tracts or via a jejunostomy is used to position angioplasty balloon catheters across the stricture for dilatation. Manual injection pressure usually suffices to obtain satisfactory stricture dilatation. If postoperative drain tracts are not available for instrumentation, percutaneous puncture of the dilated and stone-containing ducts is accomplished under ultrasonic or CT guidance. A guidewire is advanced through the stricture, followed by a dilatation balloon (Fig. 41.15). However, most strictures will recur without insertion of a plastic or metallic stent after dilatation. Removable metallic stents (Rey et al 1996) offer the advantages of metallic stents (larger diameter achieved through a smaller introducer size, lack of encrustation), without the disadvantage of the permanently implantable metallic stents, particularly tissue overgrowth (and may be especially useful in this application) (Fig. 41.16).

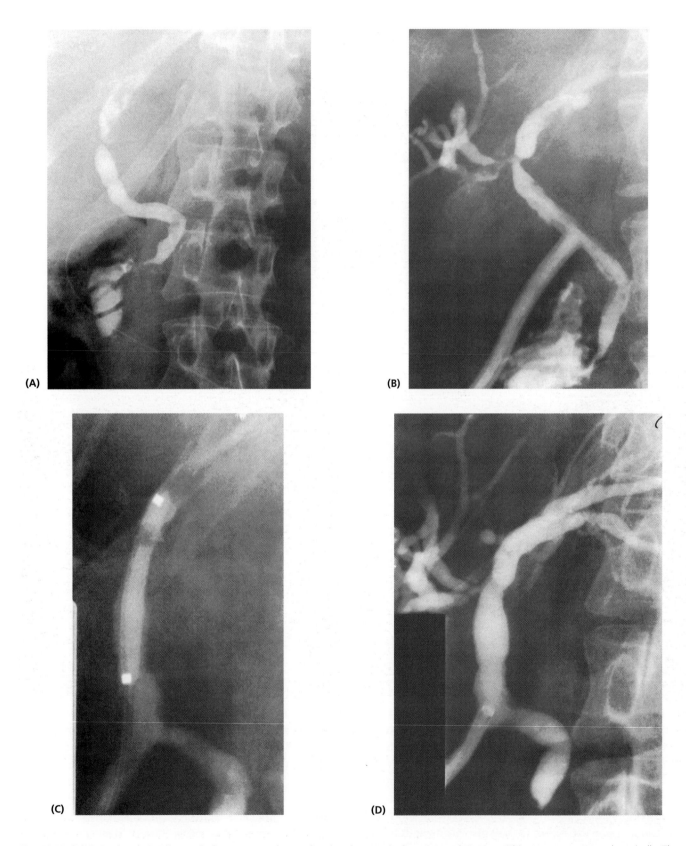

(A)

(B)

(C)

(D)

Fig. 41.14 (A) Operative cholangiogram before common duct exploration shows a single common duct stone. This stone was removed surgically. There is also a stricture at the porta hepatis with stones proximal to it in the distended left hepatic duct. **(B)** Five weeks after operation, the T tube is removed in the ambulatory patient. The cholangiogram shows multiple duct strictures at the porta hepatis. Percutaneous needle biopsy revealed inflammatory changes with no evidence of carcinoma. **(C)** Dilatation balloon placed in left hepatic duct for stricture dilatation. **(D)** The completion cholangiogram shows all stones to be removed. The left hepatic stricture has been dilated to a normal caliber. Right hepatic duct strictures remain.

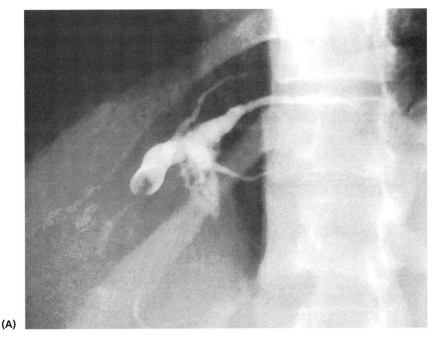

(A)

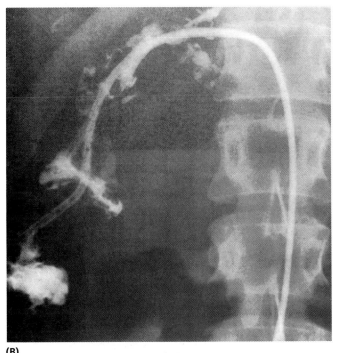

(B)

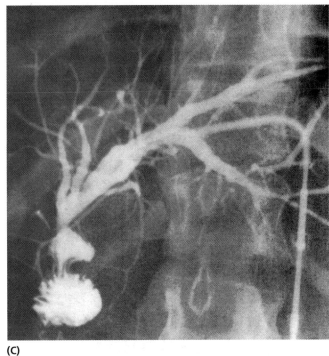

(C)

Fig. 41.15 (A) Deeply jaundiced patient 16 months after hepatodochojejunostomy shows an impacted intrahepatic stone in the left radical on subxiphoid transhepatic cholangiography. **(B)** An internal drainage catheter was placed over a guidewire after balloon dilatation of a stricture at the hepatodochojejunostomy anastamosis. Innumerable intrahepatic stones are now identified. **(C)** Cholangiography demonstrates that all stones were extracted or expelled and the anastamotic dilatation was maintained after three months of catheter stenting.

REPLACEMENT OF T TUBES

Postoperative drainage tubes often require replacement because of obstruction or inadvertent extraction. Restoration of tube patency may be accomplished by passing a guidewire through the obstructed tube, but obstruction of draining tubes by sediment is a recurrent problem and tube exchange over a guidewire is preferable. T tubes made especially for percutaneous reinsertion over a guidewire after interventional procedures are commercially available (Cook Inc., Bloomington, IN) (Fig. 41.17).

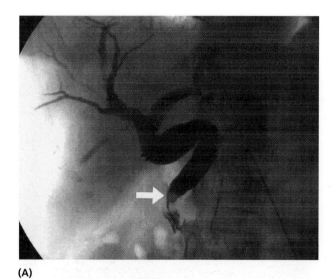

(A)

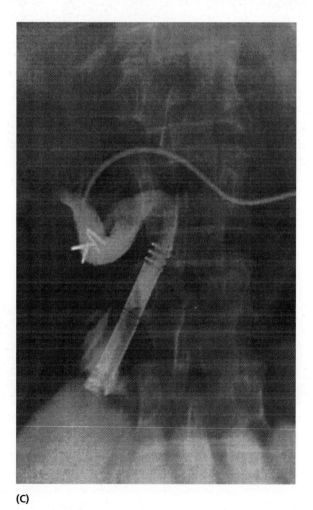

(C)

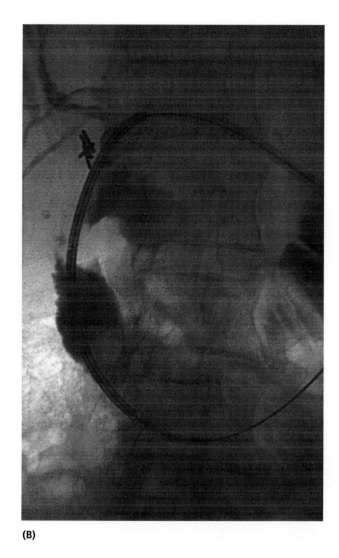

(B)

Fig. 41.16 Use of temporary metallic stent in patient with ampullary stenosis recurrent x 3 after sphincterotomy. **(A)** Transhepatic cholangiogram demonstrates a stone above ampullary stenosis. **(B)** After advancement of the stone into the duodenum a temporary nitinol stent is advanced across the sphincter. **(C)** After expansion of the stent excellent drainage was achieved. (*Continued*)

LITHOTRIPSY

A variety of techniques are available to deal with those calculi that cannot be removed or fragmented by means of the standard basket technique. Intra and extracorporeal lithotripsy have proven to be useful tools in certain situations (Bean & Daughtry 1985, Burhenne et al 1975, Harris et al 1996). In the rare situation that stones that are impacted or situated in inaccessible anatomical areas, e.g. in

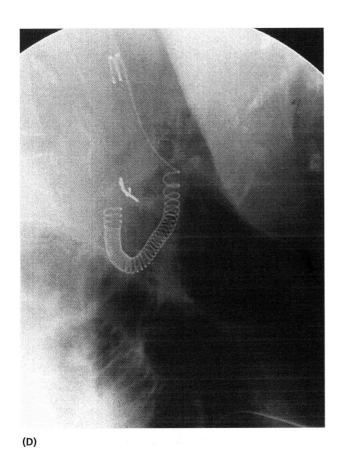

(D)

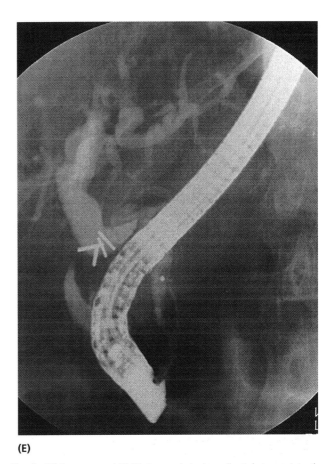

(E)

Fig. 41.16 (*Continued*) **(D)** The stent is removed by snaring one end and unravelling it. **(E)** Post removal ERCP demonstrated excellent drainage into the duodenum. The patient remains well 2 years later.

a cystic duct remnant or distal to bile duct strictures, they can be fragmented with extracorporeal shock wave lithotripsy (Becker et al 1993). Because larger fragments do not usually pass spontaneously through the papilla, additional interventional maneuvers are necessary in many cases. Therefore, shock wave lithotripsy is usually an adjunctive treatment to other interventional techniques rather than a single treatment modality.

Intracorporeal lithotripsy can be done with electrohydraulic, ultrasonic, or laser energy and clearance of stone burden in 94 to 96% of patients (Burton et al 1993, Harris et al 1996) is typical. Unlike extracorporeal shock waves, intracorporeal lithotripsy requires direct contact between the probe and the calculi. This is greatly enhanced by the use of the choledochoscope. Fragments are removed mechanically after lithotripsy. The lithotripsy catheter can be introduced through the T-tube tract or transhepatically (Lear et al 1984).

THE ROLE OF RADIOLOGICAL INTERVENTIONS IN RELATION TO OTHER TECHNIQUES FOR BILIARY STONE REMOVAL

In the 1970s and 80s it was appropriate that non-operative stone extraction techniques replaced reoperation for retained stones, as the latter procedure carries a higher mortality and morbidity than the initial operative procedure. Now laparoscopic cholecystectomy (Ch. 38) is the treatment of choice for uncomplicated cholecystolithiasis. Endoscopic sphincterotomy and stone removal has become the procedure of choice for patients having associated biliary ductal calculi (Ch. 40). In addition, operative cholangiography and choledochotomy are technically more difficult and thus these procedures are not commonly practiced. Therefore T-tube placement is performed much less com-

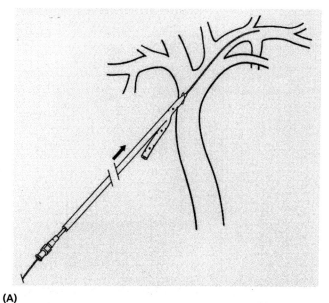

(A)

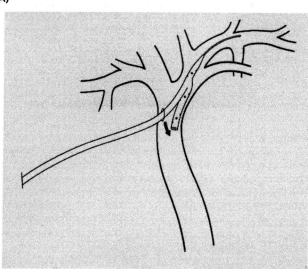

(B)

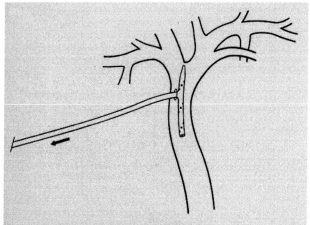

(C)

Fig. 41.17 Percutaneous T tube replacement. **(A)** T tube is advanced over a guidewire. **(B)** The T tube is retracted so that the inferior limb extends distally. **(C)** Final position.

monly. These factors have resulted in a marked decrease in the number of percutaneous fluoroscopically guided biliary procedures. The major role of fluoroscopically guided percutaneous interventions for biliary calculi is in those patients not amenable to surgical, endoscopic, or extracorporeal shock wave therapy (Sherman et al 1990). Endoscopic techniques are less effective for stones which are larger than 1.5 cm, impacted, associated with strictures, or peripheral to the central right and left main ducts (Sivak 1989). It is reasonable to favor a primary percutaneous radiologic approach if a T tube is in position and of appropriate size and position (Cotton 1990, Becker 1993). In other patients, and depending upon the resources in the specific hospital, removal of intrahepatic stones, fragmentation of large stones in bile ducts, and stricture dilatation may be performed more easily percutaneously. Percutaneous transhepatic removal of biliary stones should be reserved for cases where endoscopic sphincterotomy or surgery are contraindicated, not possible, or more likely to cause morbidity in that individual patient. In patients who require sphincterotomy, but for whom endoscopic access is not possible, fluoroscopically guided sphincterotomy can be performed (Angelini et al 1997) (Fig. 41.5).

Radiologically guided percutaneous biliary tract procedures require clinical judgement, manual skill, and responsibility to the patient before, during and after the procedure. Although their application has declined in number, they require close cooperation between the surgeon, endoscopist, and radiologist to evaluate results, treat complications, and especially to set indications to ensure that each individual patient receives the optimal therapy relevant to their specific circumstance.

REFERENCES

Angelini G, Mansueto G, Giacomin D et al 1997 Percutaneous transhepatic sphincterotomy of the major papilla and stone extraction without endoscopic control. Cardiovascular Interventional Radiology 20: 213

Bean WJ, Daughtry JD 1985 Ultrasonic lithotripsy of retained common bile duct stones. American Journal of Roentgenology 144: 1275–1276

Becker CD, Eigenmann F, Scheurer U, Halter F 1993 Comparison of percutaneous and endoscopic retrograde removal of postoperatively retained bile duct stones. Cardiovascular Interventional Radiology 16: 144–149

Burckhardt H, Mueller W 1921 Veruche uber die Paunktion der Gallenblase und ihre Rontgendarstellung. Deutche Zeitschrift fur Chirurgie 162: 168–197

Burhenne HJ 1973 Nonoperative retained biliary tract stone extraction: a new roentgenologic technique. American Journal Roentgenology 117: 338–399

Burhenne HJ 1975 Electrohydrolytic fragmentation of retained common duct stones. Radiology 177: 721–722

Burhenne JH 1976 Complications of nonoperative extraction of retained common duct stones. American Journal of Surgery 131: 260–262

Burhenne HJ 1980 Percutaneous extraction of retained biliary tract stones: 661 patients. American Journal of Roentgenology 134: 888–898

Burton KE, Picus D, Hicks ME et al 1993 Fragmentation of biliary calculi in 71 patients by use of intracorporeal electrohydraulic lithotripsy. Journal of Vascular and Interventional Radiology 4: 251–256

Choi BI, Han JK, Han MC 1992 Percutaneous removal of retained intrahepatic stones utilizing combination of techniques with emphasis of preshaped angulation catheter: review of 170 patients. European Radiology 2: 199–203

Cole WH 1960 The story of cholecystography. American Journal of Surgery 99: 206–222

Cope C 1991 Percutaneous cholecystolithotomy. Seminars in Roentgenology 26: 245

Cotte G 1925 Sur l'exploration des voies biliares au lipiodal en cas de fistule. Bulletin et Memories de la Societe nationale de Chirurgie 23: 759–764

Cotton PB 1990 Retained bile duct stones: T tube in place, percutaneous or endoscopic management? American Journal of Gastroenterology 85: 1075–1078

Dotter CT, Bilbao MK, Katon RM 1979 Percutaneous transhepatic gallstone removal by needle tract. Radiology 133: 242–243

Geisinger M, Owens DB, Meaney JF 1989 Radiologic methods of bile duct stone extraction. American Journal of Surgery 158: 222–227

Gibney RG, Fache JS, Becker CD et al 1987 Combined surgical radiologic intervention for complicated cholelithiasis in high-risk patients. Radiology 165: 715–719

Glenn F 1981 Surgical management of acute cholecystitis in patients 65 years of age and older. Annals of Surgery 193: 56–59

Harris VJ, Sherman S, Trerotola SO, Snidow JJ, Johnson MS, Lehman GA 1996 Complex biliary stones: tratment with a small choledochoscope and laser lithotripsy. Radiology 199: 71–77

Lear JL, Ring EA, Macoviak JA, Baum S 1984 Percutaneous transhepatic electrohydraulic lithotripsy. Radiology 150: 589

Lee CN, Ho CS 1987 Complications of percutaneous biliary drainage: benign vs malignant disease. American Journal of Roentgenology 148: 1207

Longmire WP Jr, Goldstein LI, Sample WF, Kadell B, Tompkins RK 1979 The treatment of retained gallstones. Western Journal of Medicine 130: 422–434

McPherson SJ, Gibson RN, Collier NA, Speer TG, Sherson ND 1998 Percutaneous transjejunal biliary intervention: 10 year experience with access via Roux-en-Y loops. Radiology 206: 665–672

Mason R 1980 Percutaneous extraction of retained gallstones via the T tube track: British experience of 131 cases. Clinical Radiology 31: 497–499

Mazzariello R 1973 Review of 220 cases of residual biliary tract calculi treated without reoperation: an eight year study. Surgery 73: 299–306

Mazzariello R 1978 A 14-year experience with nonoperative instrument extraction of retained bile duct stones. World Journal of Surgery 2: 447–455

Meranze SG, Stein EJ, Burke DR, Hartz WH, McLean GK 1986 Removal of retained common bile duct stones with angiographic occlusion balloons. Americal Journal of Roentgenology 146: 383–385

Nichols DM, MacLeod AJM 1998 Choledocholithiasis associated with malignant biliary obstruction – significance and management. Clinical Radiology 53: 49–52

Picus D 1995 Percutaneous biliary endoscopy. Journal of Vascular and Interventional Radiology 6: 303–310

Polack EP, Fainsinger MH, Bonnano SV 1977 A death following complications of roentgenologic nonoperative manipulation of common bile duct calculi. Radiology 123: 585–586

Rey JF, Duforest D, Marek TA 1996 Biliary stenting with self expandable Nitinol spring stent. Endoscopy 28: 58

Sherman S, Hawes RH, Lehman GA 1990 Management of bile duct stones. Seminars in Liver Disease 10: 205–221

Sivak MV 1989 Endoscopic management of bile duct stones. American Journal of Surgery 158: 228–240

42

Cholecystolithiasis and stones in the common bile duct: which approach, when?

A.G. JOHNSON, A.W. MAJEED

THE PROBLEM

Biliary surgeons now have a bewildering array of techniques for the diagnosis and treatment of gallstones. Yet there are large question marks over the appropriate use and relative cost effectiveness of each. While severe complications of gallstones may dominate our thinking, millions of people have gallstones and most are unaware of them. In Scandinavia, the risk of developing stones between the ages of 30 and 70 is 18% for men and 24% for women (Jensen & Jørgensen 1991), and it has been calculated that about a fifth of these will eventually proceed to surgery (Muhrbeck 1995). What, then, are the indications for elective chole-cystectomy? The ease and safety of abdominal ultrasound is revealing gallstones in patients with vague and mild symptoms, and doctors and patients alike are faced with the question: 'Are the gallstones causing the symptoms?', and 'What, indeed, are the symptoms of gallstones?'.

ELECTIVE CHOLECYSTECTOMY

There is considerable disagreement about indications for elective cholecystectomy. Scott and Black (1992) presented the case notes of over 200 patients who had undergone cholecystectomy to a panel of nine mixed specialists and a panel of nine surgeons, and asked whether they thought the cholecystectomy had been appropriate. Table 42.1 gives the result. Since the advent of laparoscopic cholecystectomy, the operation rate throughout the world has increased by between 20 and 70% (Bernard & Hartman 1993, Cohen et al 1996, Lothian Surgical Audit 1995), this in itself demon-strates the variability in the threshold for treatment.

Elective cholecystectomy may be performed for three reasons:

1. To treat symptoms
2. To prevent future symptoms
3. To prevent complications.

1. If the aim of operation is to treat symptoms, then the patient needs to be assured that the symptoms will be relieved by operation. Unfortunately, that cannot be guaranteed (Ch. 43), especially if the symptoms are those of reflux and flatulent dyspepsia, rather than pain (Johnson 1971). Indeed, cholecystectomy can make gastro (duodeno) esophageal reflux worse and can exacer-bate the diarrhea of irritable bowel syndrome. Long-term epidemiological studies from Denmark (Jørgensen, personal communication) found that pain in the right upper quadrant that is severe and precipitated by fatty food is the best predictor of gallstones in women, while in men, night time pain was the most accurate predictive symp-tom. Attempts at reproducing the pain with cholecys-tokinin or other stimuli have not been consistently predictive in the presence or in the absence of stones (Smythe et al 1998). Surgeons therefore have to make a clinical judgment about whether the stones are causing the symptoms and given the diffiulties, they would be most unwise to offer a guarantee of relief from symp-toms. Indeed, it is probably best to document that out-come cannot be guaranteed. Detailed symptom analysis of patients undergoing both lithotripsy and surgery show that persistent pain occurs most often in females with high scores for symptoms such as emotion, sleep and

Table 42.1 Appropriateness of cholecystectomy

	Mixed specialists (%)	Surgeons (%)
Appropriate	41	52
Inappropriate	30	2
Could not agree	29	44
TOTAL	100	98*

* 2% were agreed to be equivocal.

energy disturbances (Ahmed et al 1996). Patients with severe well-defined attacks of pain have usually the best symptomatic outcomes after cholecystectomy. These patients can usually remember the number of attacks and exactly when they occurred.

2. Studies in Italy (GREPCO 1988, Barbara et al 1987) and in Denmark (Jørgensen, personal communication) have found that long periods can elapse before patients with silent stones develop symptoms (see also Ch. 32). In the Danish study, patients were not told they had gallstones and were followed up for 11 years. In detailed analysis of lithotripsy for gallstones (Ahmed et al 1996) symptomatic stones became asymptomatic by being fragmented by extracorporal lithotripsy even when the fragments did not clear; thus the correlation between the existence of stones and symptoms is very unpredictable. In general, patients who are asymptomatic and who reside within a reasonable distance of adequate surgical care, may be treated expectantly. However, there are situations where prophylactic removal may be justified, e.g. in a patient who has perhaps developed symptomatic stones during one pregnancy and is planning a further pregnancy, or in patients who may intend to travel or live in a place with inadequate medical facilities.

3. Italian follow-up studies have shown that asymptomatic stones have a chance of causing complications of about 0.3% per year of follow up, and if they were symptomatic at presentation, 0.6% per year. The Danish study showed a complication rate of about 1% per year overall. Mortality from gallstones has also declined over the years and a Swedish study showed a steady decline through the period 1951 to 1996 (Persson 1998) (Fig. 42.1) and in surveys from the 1980s, 2.9 per 100 000 died of gallstone-related disease. The risk of dying from gallstones before the age of 65 is negligible, and after the age of 90, gallstones are insignificant compared with other causes of death. There

have been a few studies which have attempted to follow symptomatic patients who did not have operation. The overall conclusion is that the risk of developing a complication seems to be related to the severity of the initial presentation, and these patients should be treated accordingly. Asymptomatic or mildly symptomatic patients should *not* have a cholecystectomy to prevent complications unless there is a severe risk should the complication occur (e.g. in immuno-suppressed patients). Whether patients who have diabetes should undergo prophylactic cholecystectomy is not clear.

Cancer of the gallbladder

Gallbladder cancer (Ch. 53) is nearly always accompanied by gall stones, but this is a rare cancer while gallstones are very common and a causal relationship is difficult to establish. Gallbladder cancer is unusual before the age of 60 in men and 55 in women, but a calcified ('porcelain') gallbladder is a risk factor.

SUMMARY OF INDICATIONS FOR ELECTIVE CHOLECYSTECTOMY

1. Patients with severe or frequent well defined attacks of 'gallbladder' pain.
2. Patients who have had a complication e.g. acute cholecystitis or pancreatitis (if extra risk factors for anesthetic are not present) and the gallbladder is not shriveled and fibrosed especially in elderly patients.
3. Asymptomatic patients of any age with a calcified gallbladder if at low risk from operation.
4. Patients who are immuno-suppressed or in whom a complication would be particularly dangerous.

The presence of gallstones in itself is not an indication for cholecystectomy.

WHICH TECHNIQUES?

Operative techniques must be compared on the basis of at least six criteria (Table 42.2).

Safety must not be compromised for cosmesis and if a procedure is much more expensive, it must also show commensurate advantages. Costs can be calculated from the

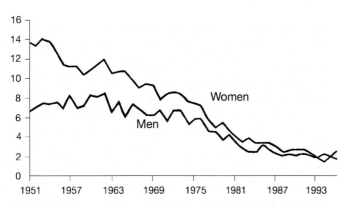

Fig. 42.1 Trends in annual mortality from gallstones per 100 000 of the population in Sweden (Persson G 1998).

Table 42.2 Criteria for comparing operative techniques	
Safety	Time off activity and work
Operating time	Cosmetic appearance
Post-operative hospital stay	Cost

point of view of the institution (National Health Service, or private insurers) on the one hand, and of patients and society (in terms of loss of income and productivity) on the other. When considering an operation as common as cholecystectomy, even a small extra cost for each operation can have a huge impact on the overall health budget.

There are many variables: for example, some surgeons naturally operate faster than others without compromising safety. Length of stay in hospital depends on patients' and carers' attitudes and social conditions at home; and return to work is influenced by the family doctor's views and whether the patient is self employed or receives full pay while off sick. Laparoscopic cholecystectomy has been credited with many perceived advantages but the only way to obtain meaningful data is to do prospective randomized trials with the same surgeons doing both operations on the same population of patients. In addition, well-documented analysis of trends in large populations gives further information about the impact of a change in surgical approach on delivery of healthcare (Cohen et al 1996, Fletcher 1995).

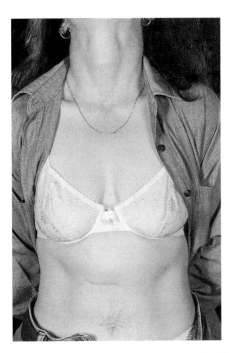

Fig. 42.2a Photograph of recent 'mini' cholecystectomy incision.

SAFETY

Unfortunately, accurate and complete prospective data on bile duct injuries before and after the introduction of laparoscopic surgery is not available. Estimates range from a two-fold increase in Holland (Gouma & Go 1994), a three-fold increase in Canada (Johnson 1971) and a five-fold increase in the USA (Strasberg et al 1995). It is doubtful if the 'learning curve' accounts for it. The operative mortality is, again, difficult to assess as the increase in the cholecystectomy rate after the introduction of laparoscopic cholecystectomy (from 20 to 70%) often involves younger, fitter patients. Many audits are voluntary and tend to be from those centers where the results are good.

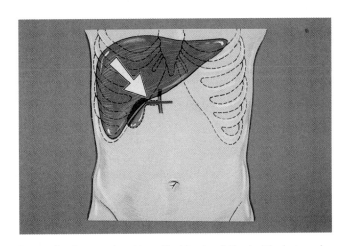

Fig. 42.2b Diagram of position of incision in relation to bile ducts and gallbladder.

SMALL INCISION (MINI) CHOLECYSTECTOMY

This is a much misunderstood operation because surgeons are still obsessed with the surface marking of the *fundus* of the gallbladder, whereas it is a clear view of the cystic duct/common bile duct junction that is essential for a safe cholecystectomy. A transverse incision is made high up in the epigastrium (sub-xiphoid) over the right rectus muscle (Fig. 42.2). The rectus can be cut transversely or split longitudinally. Only small retractors are needed, and unlike the traditional open operation, hands are not inserted into the wound but the operation is conducted with instruments. This incision allows a direct, vertically downward view of

Calot's triangle and bile duct and relative obesity of the patient does not affect vision and the operative space. A small incision over the *fundus* of the gallbladder in a moderately obese patient can make the operation extremely difficult. A high mini-incision combines the direct approach and speed of the open operation with the minimal access trauma of the laparoscopic approach without the other problems associated with the pneumoperitoneum. It is being done safely with a postoperative stay of less than 12 hours (Seale & Ledet 1999). Large incisions were used in the past, mainly because surgeons needed to do a full diagnostic laparotomy in the absence of ultrasound and other preoperative imaging, and also because muscle relaxation with anesthesia was not nearly so good.

OPERATING TIME, LENGTH OF STAY AND COSTS

There have been three (McMahon et al 1994, McGinn et al 1995, Majeed et al 1996) randomized controlled trials of laparoscopic versus mini cholecystectomy, with over 50 patients in each group. All have shown a shorter operating time for mini cholecystectomy and two showed slightly longer postoperative stay. When patients and carers were 'blinded' to which operation had been done, there was no difference. Trials which assessed time back to work found no difference, but the in-hospital cost of laparoscopic cholecystectomy was £400 more per operation which was almost entirely due to the longer theater time and increased cost of instruments (even using only a few disposables). Both laparoscopic and mini cholecystectomy are now being done with a hospital stay of 24 hours or less but the cost differences are likely to be maintained because they relate mainly to operating theater costs. Costings will vary in different health systems, e.g. the relative cost of theater time to ward time and the costs of disposable instruments in some systems are passed on to the insurer or patient. However, operating time is very variable and depends more on the pathology of the gallbladder and surrounding structures, rather than on the method of access. A Swedish study which compared the cost to patient and society, found that laparoscopic cholecystectomy cost an average £167 more in hospital than 'traditional' open cholecystectomy but a £200 saving is made on societal costs in favor of laparoscopic cholecystectomy (Berggren et al 1996). Fletcher (1995) found that the introduction of laparoscopic cholecystectomy led to a significant *increase* in the bed days occupied by patients with gallstones in Western Australia.

SPECIAL CASES

It is possible that laparoscopic cholecystectomy is technically easier in the very obese patient when the size of a small incision may have to be larger than normal. In the same way, patients who have had multiple upper abdominal operations with dense adhesions can make laparoscopic cholecystectomy more difficult and hazardous. The relative likelihood of having to explore the common bile duct may also influence choice (see below). For a patient for whom the cosmetic result is a major consideration, laparoscopic surgery has an advantage, but this must be balanced with the higher risk of bile duct injury, when obtaining informed consent from the patient.

PREDICTING THE 'DIFFICULT' CHOLECYSTECTOMY

It is very helpful in planning operating schedules to know beforehand if there is a high chance of a laparoscopic conversion, if the operation is likely to be lengthy or if a more experienced surgeon is required. A very thick walled gallbladder on ultrasound or an intra-hepatic gallbladder may predict a long and tedious procedure. It is also helpful to know about anatomical variations but, ironically, major common bile duct damage occurs in apparently easy and straightforward operations rather than difficult procedures. That is why it is strongly recommended that operative cholangiography should be done routinely and not just in difficult cases. The presence of common bile duct stones (see below) will alter the operative approach and its duration. A thin walled gallbladder in a thin patient is likely to herald a quick operation, but must not lead to complacency!

EMERGENCY CHOLECYSTECTOMY

There has always been a transatlantic difference in attitudes to the treatment of acute cholecystitis, with Americans recommending early operation and Europeans relying on conservative treatment followed by 'interval' cholecystectomy. This is largely due to the methods of payment and delivery of health care, rather than the difference in the pathology or natural history of the disease. More than 20 years ago, a prospective randomized trial had shown that open operation performed within 7 days of the start of the acute attack was quicker and safer than delayed operation at 2–3 months. Similarly, a recent randomized trial of early (less than 72 hours) versus delayed (8–12 weeks) laparoscopic cholecystectomy found a better outcome in those having early operation (Table 42.3) (Lo et al 1998). In the delayed group, 8 patients (20%) had to undergo urgent operation for spreading peritonitis and the laparoscopic conversion rate was actually higher in the delayed group (although other studies have shown a lower rate). In a small study comparing laparoscopic versus large incision open cholecystectomy for acute cholecystitis (Kiviluoto et al 1998) the

Table 42.3 Comparison of early (< 72 hours) and delayed laparoscopic operation for acute cholecystitis

	Acute	Delayed*
Hospital stay	6 days	11 days
Recuperation	12 days	19 days
Conversion	11%	23%
Complications	13%	29%

* 8 of 41 in the delayed group required urgent surgery for spreading peritonitis.

stay was shorter after laparoscopic cholecystectomy (4 versus 6 days). However, the groups were not comparable in that operative cholangiograms were only done in the open group, and most of the operations in the open group were done by junior surgeons, whereas the laparoscopic operations were performed by more experienced surgeons. A prospective study of a small incision (mini) cholecystectomy for acute cholecystitis has not yet been reported.

From the available evidence, acute cholecystectomy is a safe procedure and the total hospital stay and recovery period would be less than two-stage treatment. As with all laparoscopic operations the surgeon must be prepared to convert to open operation if there is any doubt about the anatomy, and operative cholangiography is an important method of confirming this.

STONES IN THE COMMON BILE DUCT (CBD)

As with stones in the gallbladder, CBD stones can be silent, painful or cause complications. If the patient presents with jaundice, it is essential to identify the cause and urgently relieve the jaundice to prevent liver failure. If there is a history which strongly suggests a stone in the common bile duct (painful jaundice) and ultrasonography shows gallbladder stones and a dilated common duct, further investigations to confirm or exclude CBD stones are essential, unless the decision is to proceed directly to surgery in the young, fit patient (see algorithm).

SILENT CBD STONES

If routine cholangiography (Ch. 22) is performed at operation, 8 to 10% of patients will be found to have incidental common bile duct stones even though the ducts are not dilated and the liver function tests are normal. These stones are usually small and their natural history is not known. There are two strongly opposing views on the management of these stones: (1) that they should all be removed because of the risk of acute pancreatitis or cholangitis—this view is often based on unfortunate anecdotal experiences; (2) that they can be ignored, because they probably pass spontaneously. Since the advent of laparoscopic cholecystectomy the proportion of patients having an operative cholangiogram has dropped significantly and, therefore, many stones are being left in the common bile duct with the surgeon blissfully unaware of their presence. Yet there does not seem to have been a large increase in post-cholecystectomy jaundice, cholangitis or pancreatitis (although this has not

been looked for prospectively). The only way to answer this question is a prospective randomized trial in which stones are identified at operative cholangiogram and half are removed by an appropriate technique and half are left alone and both groups are followed and the morbidity compared. The potential risk of acute pancreatitis in the group where stones are intentionally left would have to be taken into account when designing such a study.

IMAGING

Ultrasonography will show a dilated CBD and sometimes stones within it. Newer imaging techniques, particularly magnetic resonance cholangiopancreatography (MRCP) (Fig. 42.3) is non-invasive and gives excellent views of the stones in the common bile duct, but cannot be justified in every patient undergoing a cholecystectomy. It is probably most appropriate in patients with a dilated CBD on ultrasound and those with any past history of jaundice or abnormal liver function tests. There is a small group of patients with CBD stones (but no gallbladder stones) who are jaundiced at the time of presentation. They will need to be

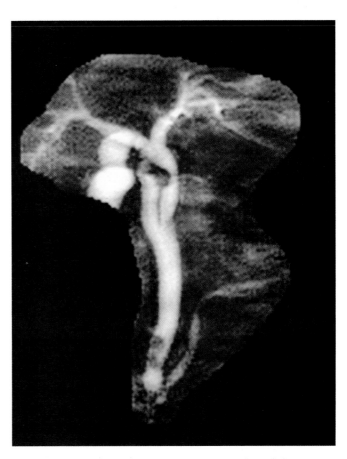

Fig. 42.3 Magnetic resonance scan of biliary system (MRCP) showing stones in common bile duct.

investigated to exclude other causes of jaundice (unless ultrasonography clearly demonstrates the CBD stones) and management will depend on their general fitness, the duration of jaundice and the degree of liver damage.

MANAGEMENT

In elderly unfit patients, endoscopic retrograde pancreatography (ERCP) and extraction of stones from the common bile duct will be the initial and probably the definitive treatment. In those who are fit for operation and for whom a cholecystectomy is also indicated (because of the risks of future complications if the gallbladder with its stones is left), the choice lies between operative exploration of the common bile duct and pre-operative or postoperative ERCP. A prospective randomized trial (Rhodes et al 1998) found that intention to treat by operative extraction at laparoscopic operation was more cost effective than postoperative ERCP as a separate procedure and this was confirmed in a non-randomized study (Liberman et al 1996). However, 28 out of 40 patients had stones < 9 mm and in 23 of these they were extracted through the cystic duct (the rest by postoperative ERCP). Five of the 12 who had larger stones were not cleared by laparoscopic choledochotomy.

Postoperative extraction of stones carries some risk because it is not always possible to remove them and if the opportunity at the operation is not taken, some patients will have failed ERCP and require re-exploration. At laparoscopic operation, there is the option to convert to open cholecystectomy or, if the incision is already a mini one, to open the duct and even perform a choledocoduodenostomy if this is indicated (multiple stones and debris, primary duct stones, evidence of obstruction of the lower end of the duct or if the surgeon is not sure that the duct is completely clear). Choledochoduodenostomy (Ch. 45) is an easy procedure through a well placed incision because the duodenum and common bile duct lie closely adjacent to each other. If the patient is fit (even if elderly), cholecystectomy and removal of duct stones is a better option than pre-operative ERCP followed by cholecystectomy (Tham & Carr-Locke 1999) as it avoids added morbidity from the ERCP. Figure 42.4 shows the algorithm for patients with no suspicion of common bile duct stones and Fig. 42.5 the algorithm when stones in the common bile duct are suspected. In both cases, it is assumed there are stones in the gallbladder. The decision in individual patients will depend, to some extent, on the local expertise such as experience with exploring the common bile duct laparoscopically, success rate for ERCP extraction and experience with mini-cholecystectomy and duct exploration.

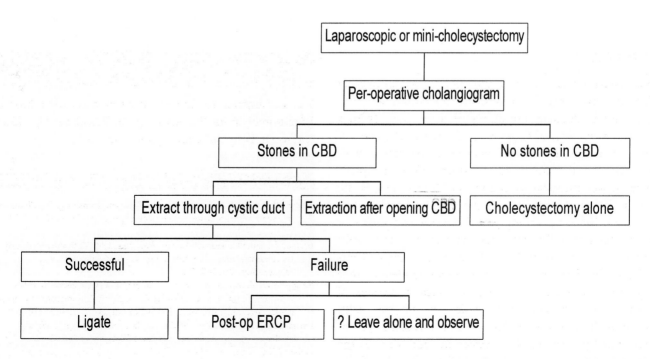

Fig. 42.4 Algorithm for the management of gallstone patients with no suspicion of stones in the common bile duct. It is assumed there are gallbladder stones. CBD, common bile duct; ERCP, endoscopic retrograde cholangiopancreatography.

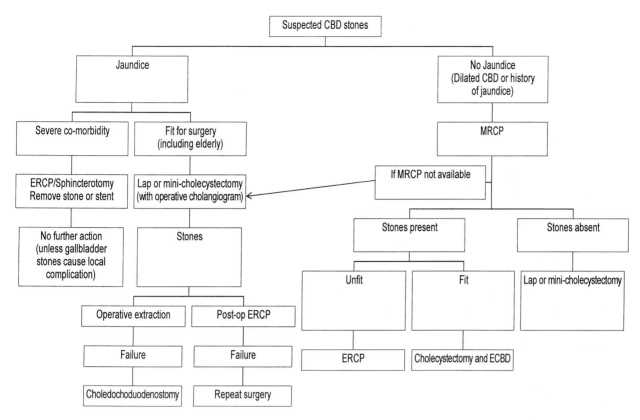

Fig. 42.5 Algorithm for the management of gallstone patients with suspected stones in the common bile duct. It is assumed there are gallbladder stones. CBD, common bile duct; ERCP, endoscopic retrograde cholangiopancreatography; MRCP, magnetic resonance cholangiopancreatography.

CONCLUSION

Cholecystectomy is a very safe and effective way of treating gallstones, but probably too many operations are performed for inadequate indications. In fit patients (with a low operative risk), a single procedure, i.e. cholecystectomy for acute cholecystitis and cholecystectomy with exploration of the common bile duct (open or laparoscopic) where there are common bile duct stones, is the safest and cheapest option with the shortest hospital stay. If a patient has longstanding jaundice, acute cholangitis or carries a high operative risk, then treating the acute problem with a procedure such as ERCP, that avoids an anesthetic, is the first priority. Management guidelines may need to be modified according to the local availability of imaging methods and endoscopic or surgical skills. Operation through a well placed 'mini' incision is just as effective as laparoscopic cholecystectomy and leads to the same rate of postoperative recovery. It also has the advantage that it may be significantly cheaper.

ACKNOWLEDGMENTS

We are grateful to Gunnar Persson and the Editor of Läkartidningen for Fig. 42.1, to Pat Elliott for Fig. 42.2b and to Dr Tony Blakeborough for Fig. 42.3.

REFERENCES

Ahmed R, Kohler B, Freeman J, et al 1996 Symptoms of gallstone disease five years after lithotripsy or cholecystectomy. GUT 39 (Suppl. 1): A43 (F172)

Barbara L, Sama C, Morselli Labate AM, et al 1987 A population study on the prevalence of gallstone disease: the Sirmione Study. Hepatology 7: 913–917

Berggren U, Zethraeus N, Avidsson D, Haglund U, Jonsson B 1996 Cost minimisation analysis of laparoscopic cholecystectomy vs. open cholecystectomy. American Journal of Surgery 172: 305–310

Bernard HR, Hartman TW 1993 Complications after laparoscopic cholecystectomy. American Journal of Surgery 165: 533–535

Cohen MM, Young W, Thériault M-E, et al 1996 Has laparoscopic cholecystectomy changed patterns of practice and patient outcome in Ontario? Canadian Medical Association Journal 154: 491–500

Fletcher D R 1995 Laparoscopic cholecystectomy: what national benefits have been achieved and at what cost? Medical Journal of Australia 163: 535–538

Gouma D J, Go P M N Y H 1994 Bile duct injury during laparoscopic and conventional cholecystectomy. Journal of the American Journal of Surgeons 178: 229–233

GREPCO 1988 The epidemiology of gallstone disease in Rome, Italy. Hepatology 8: 904–913

Jensen KH, Jørgensen T 1991 Incidence of gall stones in a Danish population. Gastroenterology 100: 790–794

Johnson AG 1971 Gallstones and flatulent dyspepsia: cause or coincidence? Postgraduate Medical Journal 47: 767–772

Jørgensen T. Personal Communication

Kiviluoto T, Siren J, Luukkonen P, Kivilaakso E 1998 Randomised trial of laparoscopic versus open cholecystectomy for acute and gangrenous cholecystitis. Lancet 351: 321–325

Liberman MA, Phillips EH, Carroll BJ, Fallas MJ, Rosenthal R, Hiatt J 1996 Cost-effective management of complicated choledocholithiasis: laparoscopic transcystic duct exploration or endoscopic sphincterotomy. Journal of the American Journal of Surgeons 182: 488–494

Lo C-M, Liu C-L, Fan S-T, Lai ECS, Wong J 1998 Prospective randomised study of early versus delayed laparoscopic cholecystectomy for acute cholecystitis. Annals of Surgery 227: 461–467

Lothian Surgical Audit 1995 Department of Surgery, Royal Infirmary, Edinburgh

Majeed A W, Troy G, Nicholl J P, et al 1996 Randomised, prospective, single blind comparison of laparoscopic v. small-incision cholecystectomy. Lancet 347: 989–994

McGinn F P, Miles A J G, Uglow M, et al 1995 Randomised trial of laparoscopic cholecystectomy and mini-cholecystectomy. British Journal of Surgery 82: 1374–1377

McMahon A J, Russell I T, Baxter J N, et al 1994 Laparoscopic v. mini-laparotomy cholecystectomy: A randomised trial. Lancet 343: 135–138

Muhrbeck O 1995 Gallstone disease in a Swedish population: An epidemiological investigation (dissertation). Karolinska Institutet, Danderyds Sjukhus, Stockholm

Persson G 1998 Vilka patienter behöver opereras för gallsten? Läkartidningen 95: 3530–3536

Rhodes M, Sussman L, Cohen L, Lewis MP 1998 Randomised trial of laparoscopic exploration of common bile duct versus postoperative endoscopic retrograde cholangiography for common bile duct stones. Lancet 351: 159–161

Scott EA, Black N 1992 Appropriateness of cholecystectomy. Annals of the Royal College of Surgeons 74 (suppl): 97–101

Seale AK, Ledet WP Jr 1999 Mini cholecystectomy: A safe, cost effective day surgery procedure. Archives of Surgery 134: 308–310

Smythe A, Majeed AW, Fitzhenry M, Johnson AG 1998 A requiem for the cholecystokinin provocation test. GUT 43: 571–574

Strasberg S M, Hertl M, Soper N J 1995 An analysis of the problem of biliary injury during laparoscopic cholecystectomy. Journal of the American Journal of Surgeons 180: 101–125

Tham TCK, Carr-Locke DL 1999 Endoscopic treatment of bile duct stones in elderly people. British Medical Journal 318: 617–618

Postcholecystectomy problems

43

I.J. BECKINGHAM, B.J. ROWLANDS

Cholecystectomy is the most commonly performed abdominal operation in most Western countries, with more than 50 000 cases per annum in the UK and 500 000 in the United States (Motson & Menzies 1997). The widespread adoption of laparoscopic cholecystectomy (LC) since 1990 has increased the number of gallbladders removed (Legoretta et al 1993, Orlando et al 1993, Steiner et al 1994) possibly because it is considered a less major procedure with less pain, reduced cardiopulmonary complications and faster recovery rates. Elderly and frail patients who previously were denied open surgery are undergoing the procedure laparoscopically and the threshold for offering patients gallbladder surgery seems to have been lowered (Steinle et al 1997, Wastell 1991). There are many conditions which masquerade as gall bladder disease preoperatively and, not surprisingly, many of these patients have persistent symptoms after cholecystectomy. Lowering the threshold for gallbladder removal in patients with vague abdominal pains and 'flatulent dyspepsia' is likely to result in a further increase in patients with postcholecystectomy pain. Performing cholecystectomy laparoscopically has brought new problems (e.g. port-site hernias and dropped stones) which may cause postcholecystectomy symptoms.

DEFINITIONS

The term 'postcholecystectomy syndrome' was widely used to describe biliary colic or dyspepsia (Bodvall 1973), or non-organic or functional (Primbam 1950, Schofield & MacLeod 1966) causes of pain following gallbladder removal. The term should be avoided as there is no single cause for these symptoms. In this chapter the term 'postcholecystectomy problems' refers to abdominal symptoms, new or recurrent, at any time after cholecystectomy, irrespective of their etiology. Symptoms fall into two main categories of postcholecystectomy pain (PCP) and post cholecystectomy diarrhea.

INCIDENCE OF POSTCHOLECYSTECTOMY SYMPTOMS

The long-term results of cholecystectomy were poorly documented until the late 1980s with previous data coming almost exclusively from retrospective questionnaires. The results of retrospective and prospective studies since 1987 are shown in Table 43.1. Older studies are not included as it is likely that a significant proportion of patients were operated on for a diagnosis other than cholelithiasis in the era before widespread availability of investigative techniques such as gastroscopy, ultrasound and endoscopic retrograde cholangiopancreatography (ERCP).

The wide range of satisfaction and symptom relief from these studies reflects the heterogeneous nature of the patients and studies and their origin from a mixture of general hospitals and tertiary referral centers. Other factors, often not outlined within the studies, must be taken into consideration when comparing results between centers. The following features may account for the wide variability in outcome, namely, the indication for surgery (biliary pain or flatulent dyspepsia); the extent of preoperative investigation for other causes of pain; the presence or absence of pre- or intraoperative cholangiography; and the inclusion or exclusion of patients undergoing bile duct exploration. For example, comparison of patients who had cholecystectomy alone with those who had cholecystectomy and bile duct exploration showed an increase in the number of investigations for biliary symptoms (16 versus 3%) and in reoperation rates for CBD stones (8 versus 1%) in the group which had bile duct exploration.

A further source of variability arises from the introduction of laparoscopic cholecystectomy in 1987 and its subsequent adoption as the procedure of choice for most biliary and general surgeons, with an estimated 90% of all cholecystectomies currently performed laparoscopically in the UK

Table 43.1 Symptom relief following cholecystectomy (1987) onwards

	No. of patients	Follow-up complete	Follow-up period	Pro/ Retro	Lc/ Oc	Pain free (%)	Symptom free (%)	New symptoms (%)	Satisfied (%)	Comments
Scriven et al 1993	77	97%	1 yr	Pro	Oc	73	69	33	77	
Luman et al 1996	100	97%	6 mths	Pro	Lc	87	—	—	—	
Gui et al 1998	92	—	2.5 yrs (mean)	Retro	Oc 35/ Lc 57	86	—	16	94	
Black et al 1994	583	96%	6 wks	Pro	Oc	78	43	—	90	
Ros & Zambon 1987	130	75%	2 yrs	Pro	Oc	99	53	—		
Gilliland & Traverso 1990	650	81%	4 yrs (mean)	Retro	Oc	—	88	—	—	90% OTC/ excluded CBD expl
Vander-Velpen 1993	160	76%	6 mths	Retro	Lc 80 Oc 80	82	94 improvement (Oc 98, Lc 93)		93	
Wilson & Macintyre 1993	315	85%	1 yr	Retro	Lc 115 Oc 200	Lc 94 Oc 93	94/94 improved or cured		Lc 94 Oc 95%	Preop ERCP < 5%
Bates et al 1991	292	94/73%	1–2 yrs	Pro	Oc	66 1 yr				OTC – 'most'
Jorgensen et al 1991	122	115	6–12 mths	Pro	Oc	78	—	—	—	24/122% CBD expl
Fenster et al 1995	225	—	3 mths	Pro	Lc	82	76	—	—	
Quereshi et al 1993	100	—	1 yr median	Retro	Lc	87	75	13	84	OTC/ERCP (preop) 12%
McMahon et al 1995	299	86%	1 yr	Pro	Lc 151 Oc 148		90 improved		93	Exluded CBD stones
Konsten 1993	351	93%	10 yrs median	Retro	Oc	—	82	—	—	
Mühe 1992	230	97%	5 yrs	Retro	Lc 94 Oc 136	74	74	3		Excluded CPB expl
Sand et al 1996	296	—	20–30 yrs	Retro	Oc	76	61	19	—	40% had CBD expl

Key: Pro, prospective   Retro, retrospective
Oc, open cholecystectomy   Lc, laparoscopic
CBD expl, common bile duct exploration

(Motson & Menzies 1997). Several studies have compared laparoscopic and open cholecystectomy on the incidence of PCP but none has shown a difference in the relief of preoperative symptoms nor the development of new abdominal symptoms, with the exception of an increase in wound pain following open cholecystectomy (Mühe 1992, McMahon et al 1995, Wilson & Macintyre 1993, Vander-Velpen et al 1993, Gui et al 1998).

When relief of biliary pain (i.e. right upper quadrant or epigastric pain) is used as the main outcome measure, 73 to 99% of patients are improved or cured by cholecystectomy. However, if cure is defined as the relief of all symptoms then the success rate falls to 43 to 94% of patients improved or cured. The relationship of the symptoms of fatty food intolerance, flatulent dyspepsia and bloating in the presence of gallstones and their response to cholecystectomy remains unclear. Evidence suggests that these symptoms are common in the general population and the relationship between dyspepsia and gallstones is purely fortuitous. In a population study in England and Scotland, Jones et al (1990) showed that the prevalence of dyspepsia in the general population was 33 to 40%, of whom only 17 to 29% sought medical advice. Price (1963) showed the incidence of dyspepsia (defined as various combinations of flatulence, fatty-food intolerance, nausea, abdominal discomfort) to be approximately 50% irrespective of the presence of gallstones. A large prevalence study from Denmark found that only 6% of 3608 subjects with dyspeptic symptoms had gallstones (Jorgensen 1989). Studies of 655 hospitalized patients, and a prevalence study in a South Wales town showed no difference in food intolerance between those with and without gallstones (Koch 1964, Bainton et al 1976). Ros & Zambon (1987),

Bates et al (1991), Black et al (1994) and Fenster et al (1995) showed no overall benefit in relief of dyspepsia with persistent symptoms in more than 50% of patients up to 2 years after cholecystectomy. Other studies however, have shown improvement in various symptoms including fat intolerance (Scriven et al 1993), heartburn (Vander-Velpen et al 1993, Gui et al 1998), bloating (Plaisier et al 1994) and dyspepsia (Johnson 1971, Kingston & Windsor 1975, Gilliland & Traverso 1990). The mechanism by which removal of the gallbladder might relieve flatulent dyspepsia is unclear particularly in the absence of data to support a causal relationship between the presence of gallstones and dyspeptic symptoms. Fenster et al (1995) has suggested that there may be a strong placebo effect. Improvement of dyspepsia is less likely the longer the symptoms have been present (Johnson 1971) and when dyspepsia is the only indication for surgery (Ros & Zambon 1987).

ETIOLOGY

The list of causes of postcholecystectomy symptoms may be divided into biliary or non-biliary in origin (Table 43.2). Amongst the many possible causes of postcholecystectomy pain it is arguable whether any have been shown to be due to the absence of a gallbladder (Editorial 1974).

Table 43.2 Classification of causes of postcholecystectomy symptoms

Biliary	Postoperative
	Early: hematoma
	       abscess
	       minor bile leak (gallbladder bed of cystic duct)
	       main bile duct injury
	
	Late: neuroma/wound pain
	      port site hernia/incisional hernia
	
	CBD stones
	Stricture: benign
	          malignant
	Cystic duct remnant/stones
	Papillary disorders: sphincter of Oddi stenosis
	                  sphincter of Oddi dysfunction
	                  (choledochoduodenal fistula)
	
	Others

Non-biliary	Peptic ulcer disease Gastro-oesophageal reflux Irritable bowel syndrome Diverticular disease Pancreatic disease: postsurgical concurrent disease Liver disease Renal disease Postsurgical: adhesions Others Psychosomatic disorders

Complications of cholecystectomy

Symptoms may develop in the immediate postoperative period due to direct complications of the surgery or anesthetic. These include hemorrhage, bile leakage, hematoma, abscess, and injury to the bile ducts. These are dealt with in greater detail in Chapters 49 & 50.

Biliary causes

The incidence of biliary causes of PCP varies widely from 2 to 80% (Ros & Zambon 1987, McCloy et al 1984). This is partly due to the selectivity of series, with centers performing ERCP having disproportionately larger numbers of patients with biliary causes (Hunt & Blumgart 1982, Carlson et al 1982, McCloy et al 1984) than non-specialist centers. The majority of patients with PCP of biliary origin have retained or recurrent common bile duct (CBD) stones with evidence of jaundice, deranged liver function tests or dilated bile ducts on ultrasound examination. The presence of retained or new stones (Chs 39–42), strictures or leaks caused by the operation (Chs 49, 50) and coexistent tumors of the biliary system (Ch. 54) are dealt with in more detail elsewhere. The remaining biliary causes of pain are discussed under their individual headings below.

Non-biliary causes

Diseases of the upper gastrointestinal tract share a final common pathway of referred pain by virtue of their common embryological origins. Thus pain from the esophagus, stomach, duodenum, liver, pancreas, or biliary system may all be experienced as epigastric pain or discomfort. Hunt & Blumgart (1982) observed duodenal inflammation or ulceration in 32% of PCP patients at endoscopy. Pain from colonic disease, most notably diverticular disease and irritable bowel syndrome, may also present with poorly localized pain and flatulent dyspepsia. Patients presenting with epigastric or right upper quadrant pain in whom gallstones are found may not have been further investigated, and undergo a cholecystectomy when other gastointestinal tract pathology may be the cause of their pain. In series from non-specialized centers, 70 to 80% of patients were found to have non-biliary causes accounting for their postcholecystectomy pain (Burnett & Shields 1958, Bates et al 1991) most of whom had gastro-esophageal or colonic disease as the cause of their symptoms.

Concurrent disease of the pancreas is not uncommon in some series (Ruddell et al 1980, Sugawa et al 1983) which may be undetected at the time of cholecystectomy especially with the advent of laparoscopic or mini-laparotomy cholecystectomy. The importance of findings of pancreatic disease in this group of patients is uncertain. It is known that patients with cholelithiasis have a higher incidence of pancreatogram abnormalities at ERCP than other patient groups (Axon et al 1979) suggesting that cholelithiasis produces pancreatic changes in some patients. The incidence of these changes in patients without PCP who have thus not undergone ERCP, is not known. Furthermore many patients with incidental pancreatic disease recognized at surgery do not develop postoperative abdominal pain (Schofield & MacLeod 1966).

Psychosomatic factors

Psychological disorders or psychiatric problems may be associated with PCP in some patients and should be considered if no organic cause can be identified. Luman et al (1996) found a higher incidence of usage of psychotropic drugs in patients with PCP compared with patients who were symptom-free following cholecystectomy (62 versus 15%). McMahon et al (1995) found a high incidence of anxiety and depression in PCP patients, similar to those seen in patients with irritable bowel syndrome (Tallet et al 1986, Haug et al 1995). Other studies have found psychiatric problems in 40% (Christiansen & Schmidt 1971) and psychosomatic disorders in over 50% investigated for PCP (Kakizaki et al 1976). It should be noted that in most of these series psychiatric assessment was performed after surgery and during investigation of PCP which itself may affect the anxiety and depression scores. This is demonstrated in the Kakizaki et al (1976) series where although >50% had psychosomatic disorders on analysis, some of these patients were found to have biliary tract pathology which accounted for their symptoms. Thus although psychosomatic disorders may account for post-surgical symptoms they should be considered only after exclusion of organic pathology.

INVESTIGATION AND DIAGNOSIS

Several modalities of radiological and endoscopic investigation are available to evaluate symptoms suggestive of PCP. The order in which imaging is undertaken will vary according to the timing of presentation and the extent and nature of preoperative investigations, in particular whether or not the bile ducts were imaged pre- or intraoperatively. Investigations should begin with a clinical history and examination, and review of preoperative investigations and the operation note.

With over 90% of patients undergoing LC for removal of their gallbladder most patients have been discharged home within 48 hours of surgery. Return within the first 2 weeks is most commonly due to postoperative hemorrhage, infec-

tion, bile leakage or bile duct injury. Initial investigation includes full blood count and biochemical profile including liver function tests and serum amylase. A review of operative findings and difficulties may suggest a high suspicion of iatrogenic injury. Re-examination of intraoperative cholangiograms may reveal missed stones, strictures or tumor (Blumgart et al 1977) or unsuspected operative damage to the extrahepatic biliary system, especially the right hepatic duct.

Ultrasound

Ultrasound is the most useful imaging modality in the early postoperative period as it will reveal fluid collections due to hemorrhage, abscess or bile leakage, and will demonstrate biliary dilatation. Significant fluid collections should be aspirated and cultured. A drain should be left in situ if pus or bile are aspirated. In many cases this may lead to complete resolution. Patients with large bile collections or dilated bile ducts should undergo biliary imaging by percutaneous transhepatic cholangiography (PTC) or endoscopic retrograde cholangiopancreatography (ERCP).

Ultrasound has a more limited role in the investigation of PCP beyond the postoperative period. The diameter of the CBD alone is a poor discriminator of postcholecystectomy problems as there is a large overlap in bile duct diameters between populations with and without significant biliary tract disease when 7 mm is used as the upper limit of normal (Ruddel et al 1980, Hamilton et al 1982). Furthermore ultrasound is less sensitive in identifying stones located in the distal CBD (Dewbury et al 1983).

Endoscopy

Epigastric symptoms are frequently caused by diseases of the esophagus, stomach and duodenum as well as by gallstones. Unresolved, recurrent or new symptoms may therefore be due to upper gastrointestinal pathology and are best excluded by upper gastrointestinal endoscopy.

Endoscopic retrograde cholangiopancreatography (ERCP)

Endoscopic retrograde cholangiopancreatography has become the preferred technique for imaging the biliary tree in patients with postcholecystectomy pain as it allows visualization of the papilla, pancreas and biliary system. When pathology is found it permits tissue diagnosis and therapeutic interventions. The majority of patients with an organic cause for PCP have abnormalities of the biliary or pancreatic system (Table 43.3) with retained or recurrent

Table 43.3 Incidence of pathology in symptomatic patients after cholecystectomy

Reference	Number of patients	Organic disease	Non-biliary disease (%)	Pancreatic disease (%)	Total (%)	Biliary disease Stone (%)	Stricture (%)	Periampullary problems (%)[a]
Burnett & Shields (1958)	20	90	80	—	10	5	0	0
Schofield & MacLeod (1966)	74	45	37	0	8	8	0	0
Bodvall & Övergaard (1967)	764	—	—	—	9	8	—	—
Christiansen & Schmidt (1971)	77	66	53	8	13	—	—	—
Stefanini et al (1974)	249	—	—	0	14	9	0	6
Brandstätter et al (1976)	47	66	23	—	43	—	—	—
Hess (1977)	199	58	54	—	4	—	—	—
Ruddell et al (1980)	102	51	24	21	27	23	4	0
Hamilton et al (1982)	109	—	—	—	36	33	3	—
Hunt & Blumgart (1982)	157	81	18	10	63	25	9	22
Sugawa et al (1983)	164	73	22	17	34	28	5	17
McCloy & Kirwan (1983)	21	76	5	0	71	67	0	19
McCloy et al (1984)	70	96	16	4	80	35	35	19
Ros & Zambon (1987)	93	47	48	18	2	2	—	—
Bates et al (1991)	292	82	68	—	—	—	—	–
Mühe (1992)	59	12	37	—	8	8	0	—
Singh et al (1996)	239	—	—	5	78	37	22	5

[a] Periampullary problems include papillary stenosis, choledochoduodenal fistulae and ampullary tumors.

CBD stones being the commonest cause, accounting for pain in 42% of patients in a review of 1139 cases of PCP (Tondelli & Gyr 1983). In a series of 239 patients undergoing ERCP for investigation of abdominal pain or jaundice following cholecystectomy, 75% had abnormalities of the pancreatic or biliary tract, the commonest being stones (37%) and strictures (22%) (Singh et al 1996).

Ruddell et al (1980) performed ERCP on 102 patients with 'severe' PCP, 29 of whom were jaundiced. A diagnosis was made in 51%, with CBD stones in 24%. Whilst the diameter of the CBD was significantly greater in patients with CBD stones (15.9 versus 10.5 mm) there was considerable overlap making bile duct diameter of no predictive value. A further study from the Leeds group comparing non-PCP patients with normal ERCPs, PCP patients with and without stones, and jaundiced patients with stones, confirmed these findings (Hamilton et al 1982).

In a series of 466 patients with PCP undergoing ERCP over a 13-year period a diagnosis was made in 51%, with CBD stones in 41% of the total (Carlson et al 1992). The yield was highest in patients with abnormal liver function tests and/or a common bile duct diameter > 7 mm on ultrasound. However these criteria alone were not sensitive enough to select patients as 19% of patients with CBD diameter < 7 mm and normal liver function tests had a biliary cause identified, with CBD stones present in 13%. A previous history of CBD exploration was the strongest predictor of biliary pathology with a 60 to 75% incidence of CBD stones.

Magnetic resonance cholangiopancreatography (MRCP)

Magnetic resonance cholangiopancreatography (Ch. 16) is a non-invasive technique that requires no contrast and allows detection of biliary and pancreatic pathology with a high degree of sensitivity and specificity (Bearcroft & Lomas 1997). In the preoperative evaluation of patients undergoing laparoscopic cholecystectomy with abnormal liver function tests or dilated bile ducts on ultrasound, MRCP identified patients with CBD stones (Dwerryhouse et al 1998) with a sensitivity of 88% and a specificity of 93% when compared with ERCP. There are no studies specifically assessing the role of MRCP in the investigation of PCP but it will undoubtedly become a tool for screening patients to prevent a large number of unnecessary ERCPs with its attendant complications.

Endoscopic ultrasound (EUS)

Endoscopic ultrasound (EUS) is capable of visualizing the extrahepatic bile ducts and pancreas with great accuracy. It has been shown to be as effective as ERCP in identifying CBD stones without morbidity (Norton & Alderson 1997, Prat et al 1996). It is more sensitive than ERCP for identifying chronic pancreatitis (Dancygier 1995), and provides accurate diagnosis and staging of pancreatic and ampullary carcinoma (Snady 1995, Dancygier & Natterman 1994). It has a number of advantages over ERCP because duct cannulation is not required. The failure rate is lower, there is minimal risk of inducing acute pancreatitis and there is no radiation exposure. However it is not as widely available, still requires sedation (compared with MRCP) and has no therapeutic role at present in choledocholithiasis. There are no data at the present time that assesses its efficacy in the investigation of PCP.

SPECIFIC CAUSES OF PCP

WOUND PAIN

Long-term PCP attributed to the surgical scar has been reported in 24% (Ros & Zambon 1987) and 27% (Gunn & Keddie 1972) of patients undergoing open cholecystectomy. In studies including both OC and LC patients, results confirm a higher incidence of wound related problems in the open cholecystectomy group with wound pain present in 9% of OC and 5% of LC patients at 6 months (Vander-Velpin et al 1993). Stiff et al (1994) reported significantly more patients with right upper quadrant pain in the open group (10 versus 3%), and Mühe (1992) found 12% of patients with scar problems (pain or incisional hernia) following OC, compared to only 2% following LC at 5 years.

CYSTIC DUCT OR GALLBLADDER REMNANT

Historically the cystic duct remnant has been held responsible for postcholecystectomy pain in many patients, with over 500 patients reported in the literature prior to 1970 (Bodvall 1973). Garlock & Hurwitt (1951) first described the cystic duct stump syndrome, consisting of repeated attacks of biliary colic, nausea and vomiting. A number of theories for the cause of pain have been postulated: distention of the cystic duct stump by raised choledochal pressure (Bernhard 1943); a rise in the sphincter of Oddi pressure (Caroli & Mercadier 1949); inflammation within the remnant (Gray & Sharpe 1944, Peterson 1946, Morton 1954, Glenn & Johnson 1955); and development of an amputation neuroma (Comfort & Walters 1931, Stembridge 1951).

In an extensive series of 103 patients with postcholecystectomy symptoms who underwent removal of cystic duct and gallbladder remnants at reoperation, Bodvall & Hurwitt (1973) found only one patient with a true neuroma of the cystic duct stump. There was no improvement in symptoms following excision of the stump, except in the presence of cystic duct or common duct stones (Fig. 43.1). Similarly, Hopkins et al (1979) found improvement after reoperation only in patients who had stones within the

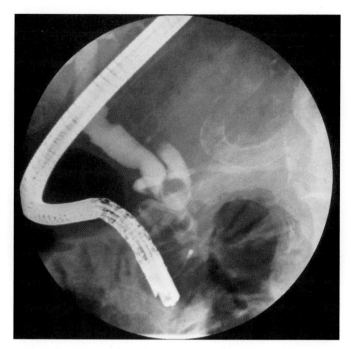

Fig. 43.1 Cystic duct stump with stone. Pain resolved following removal of stone.

cystic duct remnant. Thus it is unlikely that the cystic duct remnant per se has any clinical significance in the development of postcholecystectomy symptoms (Bodvall 1973, Hopkins et al 1979).

CHOLEDOCHODUODENAL FISTULA

Prior to the introduction of ERCP, choledochoduodenal fistulae were considered to be a relatively rare condition (Glenn & Sharpe 1957, Haff et al 1971). Their existence has been increasingly recognized with several series described (Ikeda & Okada 1975, Hunt and Blumgart 1980, Martin & Tweedle 1984). The etiology of these fistulae is due to impaction and subsequent passage of CBD stones (Tanaka & Ikeda 1982) or following CBD exploration (Hunt & Blumgart 1980, Martin & Tweedle 1984, Van Linda Rosson 1984) with the site of the fistula most commonly located in the Vaterian segment of the CBD.

The importance of these fistulae has been the subject of debate. McCloy et al (1984) described 6 patients with choledochoduodenal fistula and proposed that symptoms were due to the reflux of duodenal contents into the CBD. The proposed etiology of symptoms due to duodenobiliary reflux seems improbable now with the relative frequency of endoscopic sphincterotomy and the absence of symptoms from this. Martin & Tweedle (1984) identified 13 patients with choledochoduodenal fistula in a consecutive series of

800 ERCPs. Ten of 13 were due to iatrogenic injury following CBD exploration. However, in all cases stones were either present within the CBD (9), or had recently passed (2) or other features (e.g. chronic pancreatitis in two), were sufficient to account for the symptoms of postcholecystectomy pain. The relative frequency of choledochoduodenal fistulae diagnosed endoscopically in comparison with their rarity in surgical series, further supports the belief that the majority of such fistulae are asymptomatic and are unlikely to be a cause of postcholecystectomy pain.

SPILLED GALLSTONES

Spillage of bile and gallstones due to perforation of the gallbladder appears to have become a more common complication of cholecystectomy since the introduction of the laparoscopic technique, with an incidence of 6 to 40% (Peters et al 1991, Rice et al 1997, Schafer et al 1998, Soper & Dunnegan 1991, Strasberg et al 1992). This usually occurs during dissection of the gallbladder from the liver bed, as a result of intraoperative retraction, or during extraction of the gallbladder through the abdominal wall (Rice et al 1997). While this complication undoubtedly occurred at open surgery it rarely caused problems as stones were easily located and retrieved and few stones were left within the peritoneal cavity. A more thorough irrigation of the bile spillage could also be carried out in the open procedure.

There have been many case reports of the complications of spilled stones with the commonest problems being retro- and intraperitoneal abscesses (Rice et al 1997, Memon et al 1999) but with a wide range of presentations including discharge of stones through fistulae into the lung (Downie et al 1993) and bladder (Chia et al 1995).

Experimental studies implanting human gallstones and bile into rabbits (Welch et al 1991, Tzardis et al 1996) rats (Sax & Adams 1993, Johnston et al 1994, Cline et al 1994, Zisman et al 1995) and dogs (Cohen et al 1994) have all shown a benign course with the development of localized adhesions and some abscess formation in rats but no long-term problems. The overwhelming conclusion was that most spilled stones do not cause problems.

In a retrospective study of 10 174 LCs from Switzerland, gallbladder perforation occurred in 6% with complications arising from spilled stones in 0.08% (Schafer et al 1998). Rice et al (1997) prospectively analysed 1059 LCs performed over 3 years at the Mayo clinic and found a perforation rate of 29% with spillage of stones in 11%. Subhepatic abscesses developed in 2% of patients with perforated gallbladders (n = 6) compared with none in the intact group. Three patients required laparotomy and two thoracotomy for adequate drainages. Memon et al (1999) prospectively analysed 856 patients undergoing LC who had a gallbladder perforation rate of 16% of whom 64% were available for follow-up. Of these 106 patients, four had postoperative pyrexia attributable to local pus collections although only one required percutaneous drainage. There was only one late complication with spontaneous discharge of a stone through a cutaneous fistulae at 8 months. The overall incidence of complications attributable to retained stones was 0.6% for all patients and 3% in the patients with perforated gallbladders. Every effort should be made to retrieve stones spilled at laparoscopic cholecystectomy by use of forceps, bags and suction/irrigation. The actual rate of complications is so low that conversion to an open procedure to retrieve stones is not recommended as the additional morbidity of a laparotomy is likely to exceed any benefit for the majority of patients.

SPHINCTER OF ODDI DYSFUNCTION

Sphincter of Oddi dysfunction is a challenge from both the diagnostic and therapeutic point of view. The clinical syndrome is poorly defined, incompletely understood and difficult to diagnose. A number of terms have been used to describe the same clinical entity (e.g. papillary stenosis, sclerosing papillitis, biliary spasms, biliary dyskinesia, postcholecystectomy syndrome) and to avoid confusion it has been proposed that there are two types of sphincter of Oddi dysfunction on the basis of the pathogenic mechanism, namely stenosis and dyskinesia (Chuttani & Carr-Locke 1993, Toouli 1996).

Sphincter of Oddi stenosis is a structural abnormality with narrowing of part or all of the sphincter due to chronic inflammation and fibrosis. This may be caused by pancreatitis or injury from gallstone migration through the papilla, trauma from intraoperative manipulation of the common bile duct or non-specific inflammatory conditions e.g. adenomyosis. There is associated elevated basal sphincter pressure and alteration of phasic contractions measured by endoscopic manometry.

Sphincter of Oddi dyskinesia is an intermittent functional blockage of the high pressure zone of the sphincter. It results from spasm, hypertrophy or denervation of the sphincter muscle. This may reflect a motility disorder of the sphincter similar to motility disorders elsewhere in the gastrointestinal tract, e.g. hypertensive lower esophageal sphincter. Basal pressure is elevated but administration of smooth muscle relaxants (nitrates) causes decrease of the basal sphincter pressure in functional dyskinesia. There is significant overlap between the manometric values in these two subgroups.

Diagnosis of sphincter of Oddi dysfunction

Sphincter of Oddi dysfunction should be suspected in patients with pain of biliary or pancreatic origin, in the absence of a demonstrable organic cause revealed by conventional investigations. Hogan and Geenen (1988) have proposed a classification system for patients with suspected sphincter of Oddi dysfunction, the Milwaukee biliary group classification (Table 43.4). This system clarifies a scheme for investigation and predicts the outcome of endoscopic sphincterotomy or surgical sphincteroplasty. Sherman et al (1991) have described a similar classification for pancreatic type pain (Table 43.5).

After cholecystectomy a dilated common bile duct (CBD) detected by ultrasound scan is often a feature of sphincter of Oddi dysfunction (Venu & Geenen 1986) with high predictive value for favorable outcome after sphincterotomy (Thatcher et al 1987). However, it is a non-specific feature, and is detected in 4% of asymptomatic patients postcholecystectomy (Graham et al 1980, Mueller et al 1981). In addition, the diameter of the CBD varies with the age of the patient (Coelho & Wiederkehr 1996). Determination of the increase in duct diameter after a fatty meal or cholecystokinin octapeptide may be useful in the evaluation of sphincter of Oddi function (Fein et al 1984, Simeone et al 1982). No increase in diameter measured by ultrasound after provocation should occur in normal subjects. Changes in sphincter motility (Ch. 6) would enhance

bile flow into the duodenum and decrease the diameter of CBD (Toouli 1996). A paradoxical increase in CBD diameter reflects abnormal resistance to bile outflow and an increase of greater than 2 mm is observed in patients with sphincter dysfunction (Fein et al 1984).

Another commonly used measure of sphincter of Oddi dysfunction is delayed emptying of the common bile duct at ERCP examination which is the first line investigation of hepatobiliary and pancreatic symptoms. Reproduction of pain during injection of contrast media is not a reliable indicator of sphincter dysfunction. Dynamic hepatobiliary scintigraphy is a non-invasive method for evaluation of the sphincter of Oddi, providing indirect evidence of increased sphincter resistance by measuring a significant delay in hepatic uptake and washout (Steinberg 1988, Sostre et al 1992). It is highly sensitive when used as an early diagnostic tool to evaluate suspected sphincter dysfunction (Coelho & Wiederkehr 1996) provided a structural lesion of the common bile duct has been excluded (Steinberg 1988).

Abnormal scintigraphy is unusual when performed in a patient who is free of pain (Madacsy et al 1995). Some authors use scintigraphy techniques after stimulation with cholecystokinin and have proposed a scoring system that combines visual and quantitative criteria for the diagnosis of sphincter of Oddi dysfunction (Sostre et al 1992).

A number of pharmacological tests are available to assess sphincter function. The most widely used is the morphine-prostigmine provocation test (Nardi test) (Nardi & Acosta 1966). An intramuscular injection of 10 mg morphine and 1 mg prostigmine is given to produce simultaneously spasm of sphincter of Oddi and stimulation of exocrine pancreatic secretion. Reproduction of the pain and/or increase in pancreatic or liver-associated enzymes (amylase/lipase) are required for a positive result. This test also identifies those patients most likely to benefit from sphincteroplasty and septectomy (Nardi & Acosta 1966).

There has been interest recently in sphincter of Oddi manometry as a diagnostic tool of dysfunction (Ch. 6). Three manometric methods have been described: direct endoscopic manometry, indirect manometry and tip-transducer manometry (Coelho & Wiederkehr 1996). Several problems remain in performance and interpretation of biliary manometry. First, the procedure itself is expensive and performed in only a few specialized centers. It is difficult to perform, invasive and requires sedation, which may modify the behavior of the sphincter. A dedicated and experienced endoscopist may only achieve an adequate and complete examination in two thirds of the patients (Bar-Meir et al 1984, Neoptolemos et al 1988, Lans et al 1991). Meshkinpour & Mollot (1992) found in a series of 64 patients with postcholecystectomy syndrome that only 41%

Table 43.4 Milwaukee biliary group classification (Hogan & Geenen 1988)

	Biliary type pain	Abnormal LFTs	Dilated CBD	Delayed drainage
Group I	+	+	+	+
Group II	+	one or two of the above		
Group III	+	none of the above		

Abnormal LFTs: ALP and AST more than two times normal value, on at least two occasions
Dilated CBD: > 12 mm on ultrasound scan (or 10 mm on ERCP film)
Delayed drainage: > 45 minutes on ERCP—supine position

Table 43.5 Pancreatic type pain classification (Sherman et al 1991)

	Recurrent pancreatitis and/or typical pancreatic pain	Abnormal enzymes	Dilated PD	Delayed drainage
Group I	+	+	+	+
Group II	+	one or two of the above three		
Group III	+	none of the above three		

Abnormal enzymes: > 1.5–2 times the upper normal limit
Dilated PD: > 6 mm in the head, > 5 mm in the body, on ERCP film
Delayed drainage: > 9 min

showed a manometric abnormality. Among patients of group I-Milwaukee classification, which is the most homogenous and stringently selected group, 27% of patients had manometric values similar to those obtained from healthy volunteers.

It is difficult to know whether these manometric abnormalities correlate with pain, because the patient is sedated during the procedure. The assessment of the sphincter activity is limited to a brief period which may be misleading given the intermittent nature of the disorder (Blades & Sivak 1993). Estimates show that if endoscopic manometry is used to screen patients with postcholecystectomy pain, seven studies are required to diagnose one case of sphincter of Oddi dysfunction (Sostre et al 1992). This yield is unacceptable for an invasive procedure which is difficult to perform and has potentially dangerous complications. Although biliary manometry is an important research tool which should clarify our understanding of sphincter dysfunction it is not a viable method of routine clinical investigation.

The ideal test for sphincter of Oddi dysfunction has not yet been identified although endoscopic manometry is considered a gold standard by several authors. In a recent prospective study (Wehrmann et al 1996) the clinical outcome for 33 patients after endoscopic sphincterotomy correlated well with the Milwaukee biliary group classification. Sphincterotomy was performed on the basis of elevated basal pressure measured manometrically. The manometric findings did not correlate with either Milwaukee classification or the clinical outcome in that series of patients with suspected sphincter of Oddi dysfunction, type II (*n*: 20) and III (*n*: 13). This poor correlation between Milwaukee classification and manometric findings has been reported by others (Botoman et al 1994). In another recent prospective series with similar patients various tests were correlated with the results of sphincteromy in 23 patients with manometrically proven elevated basal pressure (Bozkurt et al 1996). A positive morphine-neostigmine test, pain induced by the injection of contrast at ERCP and delayed drainage of contrast from CBD were associated with favorable clinical outcome from endoscopic sphincterotomy in 79, 74 and 61% of patients respectively. These results were not significantly different from those of abnormal sphincter of Oddi manometry in which favorable outcome occurred in 83% of patients (Bozkurt et al 1996).

Treatment

Sphincter of Oddi dysfunction is uncommon but not life-threatening. Patients may be severely debilitated but it is difficult to select those patients who may benefit from therapy. Even if the selection is made using strict criteria the outcome may still be poor. An explanation for this conundrum is that sphincter of Oddi dysfunction, and particularly dyskinesia, may represent a generalized gastrointestinal motility disorder. Treatment directed to one part of the gastrointestinal tract would not be expected to improve or cure all symptoms (Toouli 1989, Soffer & Johlin 1994). The objective of treatment of sphincter of Oddi dysfunction is to facilitate drainage of biliary and pancreatic secretion into the duodenum. Three alternative therapies are described in the literature to achieve this goal: (a) pharmacologic treatment (b) endoscopic treatment (endoscopic sphincterotomy and/or stenting) and (c) surgical treatment (sphincteroplasty and biliary-enteric drainage). The endoscopic and surgical methods are used more frequently than medical treatment.

In a recent study, stenting was used in patients with suspected sphincter of Oddi dysfunction but no increase in basal sphincter pressure, on the assumption that these patients might have intermittent spasm (Goff 1995). There was a poor symptomatic relief associated with a high risk of stent-induced pancreatitis. Endoscopic stenting cannot be recommended as a routine method of treatment. The results

Table 43.6 Results of surgical treatment

Source	Year	n	Follow-up	Result (%)	Morbidity (%)
Moody et al	1983	83	1–10 yrs	good: 43, fair: 33, poor: 24	21
Nardi et al	1983	89*	5–20 yrs	pain free: 50	
Anderson et al	1985	28	67.5 months (mean)	good: 79, poor: 21	
Stephens & Burdrick	1986	81	6 months	pain free: 68, fair: 25, poor: 7	7
Hastbacka et al	1986	22		good: 59, moderate: 23, poor: 18	18
Williamson	1988	20	6–100 months	pain free: 60, improved: 25, poor: 15	20
Nussbaum et al	1989	29	22 months (mean)	ex/good: 62, fair: 14, poor: 24	38
Kelly & Rowlands	1996	20	9–80 months	pain free: 55, good: 10, poor: 35	10
Toouli et al	1996	26*	9–105 months	pain free: 58, mild: 30, poor: 12	8

* For recurrent acute pancreatitis exclusively

Table 43.7 Results of endoscopic treatment

Source	Year	n	Follow-up	Result (%)	Morbidity (%)
Riemann et al	1983	25	2–9 years	free: 48, improved: 32, poor: 20	
Roberts-Thomson et al	1985	46	25 months (mean)	pain free: 13, improved: 48, poor: 39	5
Thatcher et al	1987	46	15.9 months (mean)	pain free: 67	16
Neoptolemos et al	1988	30	46 months (median)	good: 63.3, poor: 36.7	25
Seifert	1988	127		pain free: 55.1, improved: 32.3, poor: 12.6	
Geenen et al*	1989	47	1 year	good: 43, fair: 35, poor: 22	
Bozkurt et al***	1996	23	19 months (mean)	pain free: 57, improved: 26, poor: 17	22
Wehrmann et al	1996	33	2.5 years (median)	improvement—II: 60	
				III: 8	

* National study, collective data from 25 German centers
** Prospective randomized trial, type II Milwaukee classification, *n*: 23 sphincterotomy, *n*: 24 sham
*** Prospective trial, type II and III Milwaukee classification, manometric criteria for sphincterotomy

of both surgical (Table 43.6) and endoscopic (Table 43.7) series in the literature of the last 15 years are presented. Poor results are still common with both endoscopic sphincterotomy (12–39%) and surgical sphincteroplasty (7–35%). This probably reflects the lack of specific objective tests for accurately diagnosing and the selection of patients for these interventions and the sphincter abnormality may be part of a more generalized smooth muscle disorder of the gastrointestinal tract.

The surgical procedure of transduodenal sphincteroplasty and transampullary septectomy has been standardized over the last two decades and is designed to provide adequate drainage of both biliary and pancreatic ducts (Fig. 43.2).

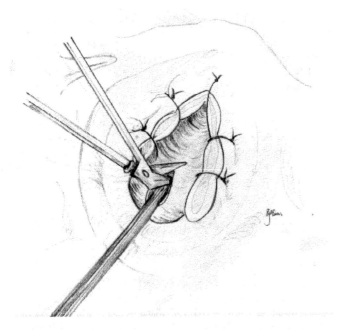

Fig. 43.2 Transduodenal sphincteroplasty. Transampullary septectomy is shown.

There are two theoretical advantages of the surgical procedure over the endoscopic sphincterotomy: namely access to the transampullary septum and accurate apposition to the duodenal and duct mucosal lining. Endoscopic sphincterotomy does not affect the transampullary septum and drainage of pancreatic duct, although there are occasional reports of endoscopic septotomy (Fuji et al 1989, Grimm et al 1989). The transampullary septum plays a primary role in the pathologic process because of the muscular interrelationships of the fibers of the sphincter. This thin veil of tissue is so strategically placed that, when thickened by inflammation or fibrosis, the outflow of bile or pancreatic juice may be compromised (Moody et al 1983). Studies have shown that separate recording from the pancreatic sphincter in patients with recurrent pancreatitis will demonstrate manometric stenosis in the absence of raised basal biliary sphincter pressure (Funch-Jenson & Kruse 1987, Rolny et al 1989). There is strong evidence that pancreatic outflow obstruction is associated with severe episodic pain in some patients and these patients benefit from TDS-TAS. In the series of Moody et al (1983), 12 out of 17 patients with adequate but unsuccessful sphincteroplasty obtained pain relief after excision of the septum (Moody et al 1990). The mucosa to mucosa apposition obtained by the surgical procedure is important since it avoids further scarring and restenosis of the ampulla (Moody et al 1990, Watanapa & Williamson 1992) contributing to a more favorable outcome.

Sphincter of Oddi dysfunction is not a common condition, but is a challenging one to diagnose and treat. Diagnosis and definition of the disorder remains often elusive or arbitrary. The high failure rate of endoscopic and surgical treatment reflects the difficulties in accurate diagnosis and the lack of specific objective criteria to select appropriate therapy. All procedures on the sphincter should be undertaken with caution after meticulous investigation, and patient selection must be based on strict objective criteria.

Patients with suspected sphincter of Oddi dysfunction are best managed by referral to centers with special expertise in the management of this condition, rather than generalists attempting to improve difficult problems without the requisite information and skill.

POSTCHOLECYSTECTOMY DIARRHEA

Although pain is the most frequently recognized postcholecystectomy problem, the existence of altered bowel habit after cholecystectomy is now accepted (Fine et al 1993, Powell 1995). The incidence of postcholecystectomy diarrhea (PCD) ranges from 5 to 18% of patients (Wilson & Macintyre 1993, Ros & Zambon 1987, Sand et al 1996, Vander-Velpen et al 1993). Fort et al (1996) found that 4 years after cholecystectomy 12% of patients suffered diarrhea (three or more watery stools per day), a further 20% had an increase in stool frequency and 5% had developed constipation.

The pathophysiology of PCD has not been fully established. Cholecystectomy removes the major storage site for the bile acid pool and therefore bile acids must be stored in the gut between meals (Hoffman 1993). When measured however, the actual effect on the bile acid pool is small and the major effect is increased dehydroxylation of the bile acids (Hoffman 1993). Bile acid malabsorption has been implicated in PCD (Hutcheon et al 1979, Krejs et al 1983). Noninvasive tests of bile acid absorption using radiolabeled ^{75}selenium homocholic acid taurine have confirmed malabsorption of bile acids following cholecystectomy (Suhr et al 1988, Sciarreta et al 1992). High levels of bile acids reaching the colon are known to induce diarrhea by acting as secretagogues within the gut and increasing the fluid load on the colon resulting in more watery stools (Hoffman 1993, Mekhjian et al 1971). Secondary bile acids, which are more common after cholecystectomy, have an even greater capacity to cause diarrhea (Berr et al 1989). Although this hypothesis is attractive, fecal bile acid levels have been reported as elevated (Breuer et al 1986, Arlow et al 1987) and normal (Fromm et al 1987). Furthermore the clinical effects of the bile acid binding agent cholestyramine on controlling PCD have been extremely varied ranging from highly effective (Arlow et al 1987), to inconsistent (Sciarreta et al 1992) and ineffective (Fromm et al 1987). Standard antidiarrheals, however, are safe and effective in the management of PCD (Phillips 1996).

An alternative hypothesis is that cholecystectomy results in increased colonic transit times. Fort et al (1996) using a modified radiopaque maker method showed an increase in colonic transit which correlated with both defecation frequency and fecal consistency. Experimental data support a dual effect of bile acids on increasing colonic transit by both secretory and motor phenomena (Mekhjian et al 1971, Flynn et al 1982, Shiff et al 1982).

SUMMARY AND CONCLUSION

The incidence of postcholecystectomy problems following laparoscopic cholecystectomy appears to be similar to that following open cholecystectomy with the exception of wound pain. Selective investigation of patients with post cholecystectomy pain by ultrasound, endoscopy and ERCP, will provide an organic cause in the majority of patients. Organic causes are most likely in patients who presented with jaundice, cholangitis or pancreatitis compared with those presenting with biliary pain and least likely in patients undergoing surgery for dyspepsia and bloating. Newer, less invasive radiological techniques, including endoscopic ultrasound and MRCP will undoubtedly become increasingly important in the diagnosis of postcholecystectomy problems.

Treatment of biliary tract pathology is usually straightforward and carries a high success rate with the exception of sphincter of Oddi dysfunction which is difficult to diagnose and treat. Patients with sphincter of Oddi stenosis with an identifiable structural abnormality and abnormalities of liver function tests have a significantly better outcome than those with sphincter of Oddi dyskinesia alone.

REFERENCES

Abu Farsakh N A, Roweily E, Steitieh M, Butchoun R, Khalil B 1995 Prevalence of *Helicobacter pylori* in patients with gallstones before and after cholecystectomy: a longitudinal study. Gut 36: 675–678

Agalar F, Sayek I, Agalar C, Cakmakci M, Hayran M, Kavuklu B 1997 Factors that may increase morbidity in a model of intra-abdominal contamination caused by gallstones lost in the peritoneal cavity. European Journal of Surgery 163(12): 909–914

Anderson T A, Pitt H A, Longmire W P 1985 Experience with sphincterotomy and sphincerotomy in pancreatobiliary surgery. Annals of Surgery 201: 399–406

Anon. 1988 Cholecystectomy: The dissatisfied customer. Lancet i: 339

Arlow F L, Dekovich A A, Priest R J, Beher W J 1987 Bile acid mediated postcholecystectomy diarrhea. Archives of Internal Medicine 147: 1327–1329

Axon A T, Ashton M G, Lintott J 1979 Pancreatogram changes in patients with calculous biliary disease. British Journal of Surgery 66: 466–470

Bainton D, Davies G T, Evans K T, Gravelle I H 1976 Gallbladder disease. Prevalence in a South Wales industrial town. New England Journal of Medicine 294: 1147–1149

Bar-Meir S, Halpern Z, Bardan E, Gilat T 1984 Frequency of papillary dysfunction among cholecystectomized patients. Hepatology 4: 328–333

Barthet M, Affriat C, Bernard J P, Berthezene P, Dagorn J C, Sahel J 1995 Is biliary lithiasis associated with pancreatographic changes? Gut 36: 761–765

Bates T, Mercer J C, Harrison M 1984 Symptomatic gallstone disease: before and after cholecystectomy. Gut 25: A579 60

Bates T, Ebbs S R, Harrison M, A'Hern R P 1991 Influence of cholecystectomy on symptoms. British Journal of Surgery 78: 964–967

Baxter J N, O'Dwyer P J 1992 Laparoscopic or minilaparotomy cholecystectomy? British Medical Journal 304: 559–560

Bearcroft P W, Lomas D J 1997 Magnetic resonance cholangiopancreatography. Gut 41: 135–137

Bergman J J, van den Brink G, Fauws E A, de Wit L, Obertop H, Huibregtse K, Tytgat G N, Gouma D J 1996 Treatment of bile duct lesions after laparoscopic cholecystectomy. Gut 38: 141–147

Bernhard F 1943 Die klinische Bedeutung der Gallenblasenneubildung nach Cholecystektomie. Chirurg 15: 510

Berr F, Stellard F, Pratschke E, Paumgartner G 1989 Effects of cholecystectomy on the kinetics of primary and secondary bile acids. Journal of Clinical Investigation 83: 1541–1550

Black N A, Thompson E, Sanderson C F 1994 Symptoms and health status before and six weeks after open cholecystectomy: a European cohort study. European Collaborative Health Services Study (ECHSS) Group. Gut 35: 1301–1305

Blades E W, Sivak M V 1993 Sphincter of Oddi manometry: how far is the leap of faith? Gastrointestinal Endoscopy 39: 593–595

Blumgart L H, Carachi R, Imrie C W, Benjamin I S, Duncan J G 1977 Diagnosis and management of postcholecystectomy symptoms: the place of endoscopy and retrograde choledochopancreatography. British Journal of Surgery 64: 809–816

Blumgart L H, Wood C B 1979 Endoscopic treatment of biliary tract disease. Lancet i: 274

Bodvall B 1973 The postcholecystectomy syndromes. Clinics in Gastroenterology 2(1): 103–126

Bodvall B, Övergaard B 1967 Computer analysis of postcholecystectomy biliary tract symptoms. Surgery, Gynecology and Obstetrics 124: 723–732

Born P, Bruhl K, Rosch T, Ungeheuer A, Neuhaus H, Classen M 1996 Long-term follow-up of endoscopic therapy in patients with postsurgical biliary leakage. Hepatogastroenterology 43(9): 477–482

Botoman V A, Kozarek R A, Novell L A, Patterson D J, Ball T J, Wechter D G et al 1994 Long-term outcome after endoscopic sphincterotomy in patients with biliary colic and suspected sphincter of Oddi dysfunction. Gastrointestinal Endoscopy 40: 165–170

Bozkurt T, Orth K H, Butsch B, Lux G 1996 Long-term clinical outcome of postcholecystectomy patients with biliary-type pain: results of manometry, non-invasive techniques and endoscopic sphincterotomy. European Journal of Gastroenterology and Hepatology 8: 245–249

Brandstätter G, Kratochvil P, Weidner F 1976 Die diagnostische Bedeutung der endoskopisch retrograden Cholangiopankreatikographie beim sogenannten postcholezystektomiesyndrom. Wiener Klinische Wochenschrift 88: 806–810

Breuer N F, Dommes S J, Goebell H 1986 Fecal bile acid excretion pattern in cholecystectomized patients. Digestive Diseases and Sciences 31: 953–960

Burnett W, Shields R 1958 Symptoms after cholecystectomy. Lancet 1: 923–925

Byrne R L, Gompertz R H, Lennard T W 1993 Symptomatic outcome after laparoscopic cholecystectomy. British Journal of Surgery 80: 1083

Carlson G L, Rhodes M, Stock S, Lendrum R, Lavelle M I, Venables C W 1992 Role of endoscopic retrograde cholangiopancreatography in the investigation of pain after cholecystectomy. British Journal of Surgery 79: 1342–1345

Caroli J, Mercadier M 1949 Les Dyskinésies Biliaires. Vigot, Paris

Catarci M, Zaraca F, Gossetti F, Scaccia M, Carboni M 1995 The fate of lost stones after laparoscopic cholecystectomy. American Journal of Surgery 169: 282

Chan S Y Y, Osborne A W, Purkiss S F 1998 Cholelithoptysus: An unusual complication following laparoscopic cholecystectomy. Digestive Surgery 15(6): 707–708

Chan Y K, Evans P R, Doswett J F, Kellow J E, Badcock C A 1997 Discordance of pressure recordings from biliary and pancreatic duct segments in patients with suspected sphincter of Oddi dysfunction. Digestive Diseases and Sciences 42: 1501–1506

Chia J K S, Ross M, Calif T 1995 Gallstones exciting the urinary bladder: a complication of laparoscopic cholecystectomy. Archives of Surgery 130: 677

Christiansen J, Schmidt A 1971 The postcholecystectomy syndrome. Acta Chirurgica Scandinavica 137: 789–793

Chuttani R, Carr-Locke D L 1993 Pathophysiology of the sphincter of Oddi. Surgical Clinics of North America 73(6): 1311–1322

Cline R W, Poulos E, Clifford E J 1994 An assessment of potential complications caused by intraperitoneal gallstones. American Surgeon 60: 303–305

Coelho J C, Wiederkehr J C 1996 Motility of Oddi's sphincter: Recent developments and clinical applications. American Journal of Surgery 48–51

Cohen R V, Pereira P R, de Barros M V, Ferreira E A, de Tolosa E M 1994 Is the retrieval of lost peritoneal gallstones worthwhile? Surgical Endoscopy 8: 1360 (letter, comment)

Comfort M W, Walters W 1931 Intermittent jaundice due to neuroma of cystic and common bile ducts. Annals of Surgery 93: 1142–1145

Dancygier H 1995 Endoscopic ultrasonography in chronic pancreatitis. Gastrointestinal Endoscopy Clinics of North America 5: 795–804

Dancygier H, Nattermen C 1994 The role of endoscopic ultrasonography in biliary tract disease: obstructive jaundice. Endoscopy 26: 800–802

Dewbury K C, Meire H B, Husband J E 1983 Ultrasound imaging and computer tomography. In: Wright R, Alberti G, Karran S R, Sadler H M (eds) Liver and Biliary Disease: a Pathophysiological Approach. London, W B Saunders Ch. 24, pp 474–495

Downie G H, Robbins M K, Souza J J, Paradowski L J 1993 Cholelithoptysis. A complication following laparoscopic cholecystectomy. Chest 103: 616–617

Dwerryhouse S J, Brown E, Vipond M N 1998 Prospective evaluation of magnetic resonance cholangiography to detect common bile duct stones before laparoscopic cholecystectomy. British Journal of Surgery 85: 1364–1366

[Editorial] 1974 Effect of Cholecystectomy. British Medical Journal 1: 72–73

Evans P R, Bak Y T, Dowsett J F, Smith R C, Kellow J E 1997 Small bowel dysmotility in patients with postcholecystectomy sphincter of Oddi dysfunction. Digestive Diseases and Sciences 42: 1507–1512

Evans P R, Dowsett J F, Bak Y, Chan Y, Kellow J E 1995 Abnormal sphincter of Oddi response to cholecystokinin in patients with irritable bowel syndrome. Digestive Diseases and Sciences 40: 1149–1156

Fein A B, Rauch R F, Bowie J D et al 1984 Intravenous cholecystokinin octapeptide: its effect on the sonographic appearance of the bile ducts in normal subjects. Radiology 153: 499–504.

Fenster L F, Lonborg R, Thirlby R C, Traverso L W 1995 What symptoms does cholecystectomy cure? Insights from an outcomes measurement project and review of the literature. American Journal of Surgery 169: 533–538

Fine K D, Krejs G J, Fordtran J S 1993 Diarrhea. In: Sleisenger MH, Fordtran JS eds. Gastrointestinal disease. 5th ed. Saunders, Philadelphia, p 1034–1071

Flynn M, Hammond V, Darby C, Taylor I 1982 Effects of bile acids on human colonic motor function 'in vitro'. Digestion 23: 211–216

Fort J M, Azpiroz F, Casellas F, Andreu J, Malagelada J R 1996 Bowel habit after cholecystectomy: physiological changes and clinical implications. Gastroenterology 111: 617–622

Friedman G D 1993 Natural history of asymptomatic and symptomatic gallstones. American Journal of Surgery 165: 399–404

Fromm J, Tunuguntla A K, Malavolti M, Sherman C, Ceryak S 1987 Absence of significant role of bile acids in diarrhea of a heterogeneous group of postcholecystectomy patients. Digestive Diseases and Sciences 32: 33–44

Fuji T, Amano H, Ohmura R, Akiyama T, Aibe T, Takemoto T 1989 Endoscopic pancreatic sphincterotomy—technique evaluation. Endoscopy 21: 27–30

Fullarton G M, Bell G 1994 Prospective audit of the introduction of laparoscopic cholecystectomy in the west of Scotland. West of Scotland Laparoscopic Cholecystectomy Group. Gut 35: 1121–1126

Funch-Jensen P, Kruse A 1987 Manometric activity of the pancreatic duct sphincter in patients with total bile duct sphincterotomy for sphincter of Oddi dyskinesia. Scandinavian Journal of Gastroenterology 22: 1067–1070

Garlock J A, Hurwitt E S 1951 Cystic duct stump syndrome. Surgery 29: 833–841

Geenen J E, Hogan W J, Dodds W J, Toouli J, Venu R P 1989 The efficacy of endoscopic sphincterotomy after cholecystectomy in patients with sphincter of Oddi dysfunction. New England Journal of Medicine 320: 82–87

Gilliland T M, Traverso L W 1990a Cholecystectomy provides long-term symptom relief in patients with acalculous gallbladders. American Journal of Surgery 159: 489–492

Gilliland T M, Traverso L W 1990b Modern standards for comparison of cholecystectomy with alternative treatments for symptomatic cholelithiasis with emphasis on long-term relief of symptoms. Surgery, Gynecology and Obstetrics 170: 39–44

Glenn F, Johnson G Jr 1955 Cystic duct remnant, a sequelae of incomplete cholecystectomy. Surgery, Gynecology and Obstetrics with International Abstracts of Surgery 113: 331–345

Glenn F, Mannix H Jr 1957 Biliary enteric fistula. Surgery, Gynaecology and Obstetrics 105: 693–705

Goff J S 1955 Common bile duct sphincter of Oddi stenting in patients with suspected sphincter dysfunction. American Journal of Gastroenterology 90(4): 586–589

Graham M F, Cooperberg P L, Cohen M M, Burhenne H J 1980 The size of the normal common hepatic duct following cholecystectomy: an ultrasonic study. Radiology 135: 137–139

Gray H K, Sharpe W S 1944 Biliary dyskinesia: the role played by a remnant of the cystic duct. Proceedings of the Staff Meetings of the Mayo Clinic 19: 164–168

Grimm H, Meyer W H, Nam V C, Soehendra N 1989 New modalities for treating chronic pancreatitis. Endoscopy 21: 70–74

Gui G P, Cheruvu C V, West N, Sivaniah K, Fiennes A G 1998 Is cholecystectomy effective treatment for symptomatic gallstones? Clinical outcome after long-term follow-up. Annals of the Royal College of Surgeons of England 80: 25–32

Gunn A, Keddie N 1972 Some clinical observations on patients with gallstones. Lancet 2: 239–241

Haff R C, Wise L, Ballinger W F 1971 Biliary enteric fistula. Surgery, Gynaecology and Obstetrics 133: 84–88

Hainsworth P J, Rhodes M, Gompertz R N, Armstrong, Lennard T W 1994 Imaging of the common bile duct in patients undergoing laparoscopic cholecystectomy. Gut 35: 991–995

Hastbacka J, Jarvinen H, Kivilaakro E, Jurunen M T 1986 Results of sphincteroplasty in patients with spastic sphincter of Oddi. Scandinavian Journal of Gastroenterology 21: 516–520

Hamilton I, Ruddell W S J, Mitchell C J, Lintott D J, Axon A T R 1982 Endoscopic retrograde cholangiograms of the normal and postcholecystectomy biliary tree. British Journal of Surgery 69: 343–345

Hammarstrom L E, Holmin T, Stridbeck H 1996 Endoscopic treatment of bile duct calculi in patients with gallbladder in situ: long-term outcome and factors. Scandinavian Journal of Gastroenterology 31: 294–301

Hammarstrom L E, Holmin T, Stridbeck H, Ihse I 1995 Long-term follow-up of a prospective randomized study of endoscopic versus surgical treatment of bile duct calculi in patients with gallbladder in situ. British Journal of Surgery 82: 1516–1521

Hammerstrom L E, Stridbeck H, Ihse I 1996 Long-term follow-up after endoscopic treatment of bile duct calculi in cholecystomized patients. World Journal of Surgery 20: 272–276

Hastier P, Buckley M J, Dumas R, Kuhdorf H, Staccini P, Demarquay J F, Caroli-Bose F X, Delmont J P 1998 A study of the effect of age on pancreatic duct morphology. Gastrointestinal Endoscopy 48: 53–57

Haug T T, Wilhelmsen I, Berstad A, Ursin H 1995 Life events and stress in patients with functional dyspepsia compared with patinets with duodenal ulcer and healthy controls. Scandinavian Journal of Gastroenterology 30: 524–530

Havard T J, Scriven M W, Lewis M H 1994 Postcholecystectomy symptoms after laparoscopic cholecystectomy. Annals of the Royal College of Surgeons of England 76: 143

Heaton K W, Parker D, Cripps H 1993 Bowel function and irritable bowel symptoms after hysterectomy and cholecystectomy—a population based study. Gut 34: 1108–1111

Hess W 1977 Nachoperationen an den Gallenwegen. In: Praktische Chirurgi, Enke, Stuttgart, Part 91

Hoffmann A F 1993 The enterohepatic circulation of bile acids in health and disease. In: Sleisenger M H, Fordtran J S eds. Gastrointestinal disease. 5th ed. Philadelphia: Saunders, 127–150

Hogan W J, Geenen J E 1988 Biliary dyskinesia. Endoscopy 20: 179–183

Hopkins S F, Bivins B A, Griffen W O 1979 The problem of the cystic duct remnant. Surgery, Gynecology and Obstetrics 148: 531–533

Horton M, Florence M G 1998 Unusual abscess patterns following dropped gallstones during laparoscopic cholecystectomy. American Journal of Surgery 175: 375–379

Hunt D R, Blumgart L H 1980 Iatrogenic choledochoduodenal fistula: an unsuspected cause of postcholecystectomy symptoms. British Journal of Surgery 67: 10–13

Hunt D R, Blumgart L H 1982 Endoscopic abnormalities in patients with postcholecystectomy symptoms. Surgical Gastroenterology 1: 155–158

Hutcheon D F, Bayless T M, Gadacz T R 1979 Postcholecystectomy diarrhea. The Journal of the American Medical Association 241: 823–824

Ikeda S, Okada Y 1975 Classification of choledochoduodenal fistula diagnosed by duodenal fiberoscopy and its etiological significance. Gastroenterology 69: 130–137

Johnson A G 1971 Gallstones and flatulent dyspepsia: cause or coincidence? Postgraduate Medical Journal 47: 767–772

Johnston S, O'Malley K, McEntee G, Grace P, Smyth E, Bouchier-Hayes D 1994 The need to retrieve the dropped stone during laparoscopic cholecystectomy. American Journal of Surgery 167: 608–610

Jones R H, Lydeard S E, Hobbs F D R et al 1990 Dyspepsia in England and Scotland. Gut 31: 401–405

Jorgensen R, Teglbjerg J S, Wille-Jorgenson P, Bille T, Thorvaldsen P 1991 Persisting pain after cholecystectomy. A prospective investigation. Scandinavian Journal of Gastroenterology 26: 124–128

Jorgensen T 1989 Abdominal symptoms and gallstone disease: an epidemiological investigation. Hepatology 9: 856–869

Kadar N, Reich H, Liu C Y, Manko G F, Gimpelson R 1993 Incisional hernias after major laparoscopic gyncecological procedures. American Journal of Obstetrics and Gynecology 168: 1493–1495

Kakizaki G, Kato E, Fujiwana K, Hasegawa N 1976 Postbiliary surgery complaints. Psychosomatic aspects. American Journal of Gastroenterology 66: 62–68

Kelly S B, Rowlands B J 1996 Transduodenal sphincteroplasty and transampullary septectomy for papillary stenosis HPB Surgery 9: 199–207

Kingston R D, Windsor C W O 1975 Flatulent dyspepsia in patients with gallstones undergoing cholecystectomy. British Journal of Surgery 62: 221–223

Koch J P 1964 A survey of food intolerances in hospitalized patients. New Engalnd Journal of Medicine 271: 657–660

Konsten J, Gouma D J, von Meyenfeldt M F, Menheere P 1993 Long-term follow up after open cholecystectomy. British Journal of Surgery 80: 100–102

Krejs G J, Fordtran J S 1983 Diarrhea. In: Sleisenger M H, Fordtran J S (eds.) Gastrointestinal Disease: Pathophysiology, Diagnosis, Management. Philadelphia, W B Saunders pp.273

Ladas S D, Tassios P S, Giorgiotis K, Rokkas T, Theodosiou P, Raptis S A 1993 Pancreatic duct width: its significance as a diagnostic criterion for pancreatic disease. Hepatogastroenterology 40(1): 52–55

Lajer H, Widecrantz S, Heisterberg L 1997 Hernias in trocar ports following abdominal laparoscopy—a review. Acta Obstetrica Gynecologica Scandinavica 76: 389–393

Lam C M, Murray F E, Cuschieri A 1996 Increased cholecystectomy rate after the introduction of laparoscopic cholecystectomy in Scotland. Gut 38: 282–284

Lans J L, Parikh N P, Geenen J E 1991 Application of sphincter of Oddi manometry in routine clinical investigations. Endoscopy 23: 139–143

Legorreta A, Silber J, Constantino G, Kobylinski R, Zata S 1993 Increased cholecystectomy rate after the introduction of laparoscopic cholecystectomy. Journal of the American Medical Association 270: 1429–1432

Luman W, Adams W H, Nixon S N, Mcintyre I M, Hamer-Hodges D, Wilson G, Palmer K R 1996 Incidence of persistent symptoms after laparoscopic cholecystectomy: a prospective study. Gut 39 863–866

Luman W, Williams A J, Pryde A, Smith G D, Nixon S J, Heading R C, Palmer K R 1997 Influence of cholecystectomy on sphincter of Oddi motility. Gut 41: 371–374

Macintyre I M, Wilson R G 1993 Laparoscopic cholecystectomy. British Journal of Surgery 80: 1220

Martin D F, Tweedle D E F 1984 The aetiology and significance of distal choledochoduodenal fistula. British Journal of Surgery 71: 632–634

McCloy R F, Jaff V, Blumgart L H 1984 Endoscopy and postcholecystectomy problems. In: Salmon PR (ed) Gastrointestinal Endoscopy, Advances in Diagnosis and Therapy. Chapman and Hall, London. Vol 1, Ch 18, 199–206

McCloy R F, Kirwan M 1983 Unpublished data

McMahon A J, Ross S, Baxter R N, Russell J N, Russell I T, Anderson J R, Morran C G, Sunderland G T, Galloway D J, O'Dwyer J R 1995 Symptomatic outcome 1 year after laparoscopic and minilaparotomy cholecystectomy: a randomised trial. British Journal of Surgery 82: 1378–1382

Madacsy L, Velosy B, Lonovics J, Csernay L 1995 Evaluation of results of the prostigmine-morphine test with quantitative hepatobiliary scintigraphy: a new method for the diagnosis of sphincter of Oddi dyskinesia. European Journal of Nuclear Medicine 22: 227–232

Memon M A, Deeik R K, Maffi T R, Fitzgibbons R J Jr 1999 The outcome of unretrieved gallstones in the peritoneal cavity during laparoscopic cholecystectomy. Surgical Endoscopy 13: 848–857

Mekhjian H S, Phillips S F, Hofmann A F 1971 Colonic secretion of water and electrolytes induced by bile acids: perfusion studies in man. Journal of Clinical Investigations 50: 1569–1577

Meshkinpour H, Mollot M 1987 Bile duct dyskinesia and unexplained abdominal pain: A clinical and manometric study. Gastroenterology 92: 1533A

Meshkinpour H, Mollot M 1992 Sphincter of Oddi dysfunction and unexplained abdominal pain: Clinical and manometric study. Digestive Diseases and Sciences 37(2): 257–261

Moody F G, Becker J M, Potts J R 1983 Transduodenal and transampullary septectomy for postcholecystectomy pain. Annals of Surgery 197: 627–636

Moody F G, Calabuing R, Vecchio R, Runkel N 1990 Stenosis of the sphincter of Oddi. Surgical Clinics of North America 70(6): 1341–1354

Morgan B, Rathod A, Crozier A, Mullick S 1996 Biliary distensibility during pre-operative cholangiography as compared to pre-operative ultrasound: a four-year follow-up study. Clinical Radiology 51: 338–340

Mort E A, Guadagnoli E, Schroeder S A et al 1994 The influence of age on clinical and patient-reported outcomes after cholecystectomy. Journal of General Internal Medicine 9: 61–65

Morton C B II 1954 Post-cholecystectomy symptoms from cystic duct remnants. Annals of Surgery 139: 679–682

Motson R W, Menzies D 1997 Gallstones. Hepatobiliary and Pancreatic Surgery 6: 175–200

Mueller P R, Ferrucci J T, Simeone J F et al 1981 Postcholecystectomy bile duct dilatation: myth or reality? American Journal of Roentgenology 136: 355–358

Mühe E 1992 Long-term follow-up after laparoscopic cholecystectomy. Endoscopy 24: 754–758

Murison M S, Gartell, P C, McGinn F P 1993 Does selective preoperative cholangiography result in missed common bile duct stones? Journal of the Royal College of Surgeons of Edinburgh 38: 220–224

Nardi G L, Acosta J M 1966 Papillitis as a cause of pancreatitis and abdominal pain: Role of evocative test, operative pancreatogram and histologic evaluation. Annals of Surgery 164: 611–621

Nardi G L, Michelassi F, Zannini P 1983 Transduodenal sphincteroplasty 5–25 year follow up of 89 patients. Annals of Surgery 198: 453–461

Neoptolemos J P, Bailey I S, Carr-Locke D L 1988 Sphincter of Oddi dysfunction: results of treatment by endoscopic sphincterotomy. British Journal of Surgery 75: 454–459

NIH Consensus Conference—Gallstones and Laparoscopic Cholecystectomy 1993 JAMA 269: 1018–1024

Norton S A, Alderson D 1997 Prospective comparison of endoscopic ultrasonography and endoscopic retrograde cholangio-pancreatography in the detection of bile duct stones. British Journal of Surgery 84: 1366–1369

Nussbaum M S, Warner B S, Sax H C, Fischer J E 1989 Transduodenal sphincteroplasty and transampullary septomy for primary sphincter of Oddi dysfunction. American Journal of Surgery 157: 38–43

O'Leary D P 1995 *Helicobacter pylori* and cholecystectomy. Gut 37: 849

Olsen D O 1993 Mini-lap cholecystectomy. American Journal of Surgery 165: 440–443

Orlando R, Russell J, Lynch J, Mattie A 1993 Laparoscopic cholecystectomy: a statewide experience. Archives of Surgery 128: 494–499

Pemberton M, Wells A D 1997 The Mirizzi syndrome. Postgraduate Medical Journal 73: 487–490

Peters J H, Gibbons G D, Innes J T et al 1991 Complications of laparoscopic cholecystectomy. Surgery 110: 769–777

Peterson F R 1946 Re-formed gallbladder; review of 42 cases. Journal of the Iowa Medical Society 36: 134–138

Phillips S F 1996 Diarrhea after cholecystectomy: if so, why? Editorial. Gastroenterology 111(3) 816–818

Plaisier P W 1997 Incidence of persistent symptoms after laparoscopic cholecystectomy. Gut 41: 579

Plaisier P W, van der Hul R L, Nijs H G T et al 1994 The course of biliary and gastrointestinal symptoms after treatment of uncomplicated symptomatic gallstones: results of a randomized study comparing extracorporeal shock wave lithotripsy with conventional cholecystectomy. American Journal of Gastroenterology 89: 739–744

Ponce J, Cutshall K E, Hodge M J, Browder W 1995 The lost laparoscopic stone. Potential for long-term complications. Archives of Surgery 130: 666–668

Powell D W 1995 Approach to the patient with diarrhea. In: Yamada T (ed.) Textbook of Gastroenterology. 2nd edn. Lippincott, Philadelphia, p 813–863

Prat F, Amouyal G, Amouyal P, Pelletier G, Fritsch J, Choury A D et al 1996 Prospective controlled study of endoscopic ultrasonography and endoscopic retrograde cholangiography in patients with suspected common bile duct lithiasis. Lancet 347: 75–79

Price W H 1963 Gallbladder dyspepsia. British Medical Journal ii: 138–141

Primbram B O C 1950 Postcholecystectomy syndromes. Journal of the American Medical Association 142: 1262

Qureshi M A, Brindley N M, Osborne D H et al 1993 Post cholecystectomy symptoms after laparoscopic cholecystectomy. Annals of the Royal College of Surgeons of England 75: 349–353

Ray C E Jr, Hibbeln J F, Wilbur A C 1993 Complications after laparoscopic cholecystectomy: imaging findings. AJR. American Journal of Roentgenology 160: 1029–1032

Reimann J F, Lux G, Forster P, Altendorf A 1983 Long-term results after endoscopic papillotomy. Endoscopy 15: 165–168

Rhodes M, Lennard T W, Farndon J R, Taylor R M 1988 Cholecystokinin (CCK) provocation test: long-term follow-up after cholecystectomy. British Journal of Surgery 75: 951–953

Rice D C, Memon Ma Jamison R L et al 1997 Long-term consequences of intraoperative spillage of bile and gallstones during laparoscopic cholecystectomy. Journal of Gastrointestinal of Surgery 1: 85–91

Roberts-Thomson I C, Toouli J 1985 Abnormal responses to morphine-neostigmine in patients with undefined biliary type pain. Gut 26: 1367–1372

Rolny P, Arleback A, Funch-Jensen P, Kruse A, Jarnerot G 1989 Clinical significance of manometric assessment of both pancreatic duct and bile duct sphincter in the same patient. Scandinavian Journal of Gastroenterology 24: 751–754

Rolny P, Geenen J E, Hogan W J 1993 Post-cholecystectomy patients with 'objective signs' of partial bile outflow obstruction: clinical characteristics, sphincter of Oddi manometry findings, and results of therapy. Gastrointestinal Endoscopy 39: 778–781

Ros E, Zambon D 1987 Postcholecystectomy symptoms. A prospective study of gallstone patients before and 2 years after surgery. Gut 28: 1500–1504

Ruddell W S J, Ashton M G, Lintott D J, Axon A T R 1980 Endoscopic retrograde cholangiography and pancreatography in investigation of postcholecystectomy patients. Lancet i: 444–447

Sand J, Pakkala S, Nordback I 1996 Twenty to thirty-year follow-up after cholecystectomy. Hepato-Gastroenterology 43: 534–537

Sax H C, Adams J T 1993 The fate of the spilled gallstone. Archives of Surgery 128: 469 (letter)

Schafer M, Suter C, Klaiber C H, Wehrli H, Frei E, Krahenbuhl L 1998 Spilled gallstones after laparoscopic cholecystectomy: a relevant problem? A retrospective analysis of 10,174 laparoscopic cholecystectomies. Surgical Endoscopy 12: 305–309

Schmalz M J, Geenen J E, Hogan W J, Dodds W J, Venu R P, Johnson G K 1990 Pain on common bile duct injection during ERCP: does it indicate sphincter of Oddi dysfunction? Gastrointestinal Endoscopy 36(5): 458–461

Sciarretta G, Furno A, Mazzoni M, Malaguti P 1992 Post-cholecystectomy diarrhea: evidence of bile acid malabsorption assessed by SeHCAT test. American Journal of Gastroenterology 87: 1852–1854

Schofield G E, MacLeod R G 1966 Sequelae of cholecystectomy. British Journal of Surgery 53: 1042–1045

Scriven M W, Burgess N A, Edwards E A, Morgan A R, Bundred N J, Lewis M H 1993 Cholecystectomy: a study of patient satisfaction. Journal of the Royal College of Surgeons of Edinburgh 38: 79–81

Seifert E 1988 Long-term follow up after endoscopic sphincterotomy (EST). Endoscopy 20: 232–235

Sherman S, Troiano F P, Hawes R H, O'Connor W O, Lehman G A 1991 Frequency of abnormal sphincter of Oddi manometry compared with the clinical suspicion of sphincter of Oddi dysfunction. American Journal of Gastroenterology 586–590

Shiff S J, Soloway R D, Snape W J Jr 1982 Mechanism of deoxycholic acid stimulation of the rabbit colon. Journal of Clinical Investigation 69: 985–992

Simeone J F, Mueller P R, Ferrucci J T et al 1982 Sonography of the bile ducts after a fatty meal: an aid in detection of obstruction. Radiology 143: 211–215

Singh V, Kumar P, Rai H S, Singh K 1996 Postcholecystectomy problems and the role of endoscopic retrograde cholangiopancreatography. British Journal of Clinical Practice 50: 183–186

Smythe A, Majeed A W, Fitzhenry M, Johnson A G 1998 A requiem for the cholecystokinin provocation test? Gut 43: 571–574

Snady H 1995 Influence of endoscopic ultrasonography on management and outcomes. Gastrointestinal Endoscopy Clinics of North America 5: 755–762

Soffer E E, Johlin F C 1994 Intestinal dysmotility in patients with sphincter of Oddi dysfunction. A reason for failed response to sphincterotomy. Digestive Diseases and Sciences 39: 1942–1946

Soper N J, Dunnegan D L 1991 Does intraoperative gallbladder perforation influence the early outcome of laparoscopic cholecystectomy? Surgical Laparoscopy and Endoscopy 1: 156–161

Soper N J, Flye M W, Brunt L M, Stockmann P T, Sicard G A, Picus D, Edmundowica S A, Aliperti G 1993 Diagnosis and management of biliary complications of laparoscopic cholecystectomy. American Journal of Surgery 165: 663–669

Sostre S, Kalloo A N, Spiegler E J, Camargo E E, Wagner H N Jr 1992 A noninvasive test of sphincter of Oddi dysfunction in postcholecystectomy patients. The scintigraphic score. Journal of Nuclear Medicine 33: 1216–1222

Stefanini P, Carboni M, Patrassi N, Loriga P, De Bernadinis G, Negro P 1974 Factors influencing the long-term results of cholecystectomy. Surgery, Gynecology and Obstetrics 139: 734–738

Steinberg W 1988 Sphincter of Oddi dysfunction: A clinical controversy. Gastroenterology 95: 1409–1415

Steiner C A, Bass E B, Talamini M A, Pitt H A, Steinberg E P 1994 Surgical rates and operative mortality for open and laparoscopic cholecystectomy in Maryland. New England Journal of Medicine 330: 403–408

Steinle E W, VanderMolen R L, Silbergleit A, Cohen M M 1997 Impact of laparoscopic cholecystectomy on indications for surgical treatment of gallstones. Surgical Endoscopy 11: 933–935

Stembridge V A 1951 Amputation neuroma following cholecystectomy. Annals of Surgery 134: 1048–1051

Stephens R V, Burdrick G E 1986 Microscopic transduodenal sphincteroplasty and transampullary septoplasty for papillary stenosis. American Journal of Surgery 152: 621–627

Stiff G, Rhodes M, Kelly A, Telford K, Armstrong C P, Rees B I 1994 Long-term pain: less common after laparoscopic than open cholecystectomy. British Journal of Surgery 81: 1368–1370

Strasberg S M, Sanabria J R, Clavien P A 1992 Complications of laparoscopic cholecystectomy. Canadian Journal of Surgery 35: 275–280

Stubbs R S, McCloy R F, Blumgart L H 1983 Cholelithiasis and cholecystitis: surgical treatment. Clinics in Gastroenterology 12(1): 179–201

Sugawa C, Clift D, Walt A J 1983 Endoscopic retrograde cholangiopancreatography after cholecystectomy. Surgery, Gynecology and Obstetrics 157: 247–251

Suhr O, Danielsson A, Nijhlin H, Truedsson H 1988 Bile acid malabsorption demonstrated by SeHCAT in chronic diarrhea, with special reference to the impact of cholecystectomy. Scandinavian Journal of Gastroenterology 23: 1187–1194

Tallet N J, Fung L H, Gilligan I J, McNeil D, Piper D W 1986 Association of anxiety, neuroticism and depression with dyspepsia of unknown cause. Gastroenterology 90: 886–892

Tanaka M, Ikeda S 1982 Multiple choledochoduodenal fistulas in the periampullary region. Endoscopy 14: 200–202

Taylor T V 1981 Postvagotomy and cholecystectomy syndrome. Annals of Surgery 194: 625–629

Thatcher B S, Sivak M V, Tedesco F J, Vennes J A, Hutton S W, Achkar E A 1987 Endoscopic sphincterotomy for suspected dysfunction of the sphincter of Oddi. Gastrointestinal Endoscopy 33: 91–95

Tondelli P, Gyr K 1983 Postsurgical syndromes. Clinics in Gastroenterology 60: 1020–1026

Tondelli P, Gyr K, Stalder G A, Allgower M 1979 The biliary tract. Clinics in Gastroenterology 8(2): 487–505

Toouli J 1989 What is sphincter of Oddi dysfunction? Gut 30: 753–761

Toouli J 1996 Sphincter of Oddi. The Gastroenterologist 4: 44–53

Traverso L W 1993 Clinical manifestations and impact of gallstone disease. American Journal of Surgery 165: 405–409

Tzardis P J, Vougiouklakis D, Lymperi M et al 1996 Septic and other complications resulting from biliary stones placed in the abdominal cavity: experimental study in rabbits. Surgical Endoscopy 10: 533–536

Van Linda B M, Rosson R S 1984 Choledochoduodenal fistula and choledocholithiasis: treatment by endoscopic enlargement of the choledochoduodenal fistula. Journal of Clinical Gastroenterology 6: 321–324

Vander-Velpen G C, Shimi S M, Cuschieri A 1993 Outcome after cholecystectomy for symptomatic gallstone disease and effect of surgical access: laparoscopic versus open approach. Gut 34: 1448–1451

Venu R P, Geenen J E 1986 Diagnosis and treatment of diseases of the papilla. Clinical Gastroenterology 15: 439–455

Wastell C 1991 Laparoscopic cholecystectomy. British Medical Journal 302: 330–304

Watanapa P, Williamson R C N 1992 Pancreatic sphincterotomy and sphincteroplasty. Gut 33: 865–867

Wehrmann T, Wiemer K, Lembecke B, Caspary W F, Jung M 1996 Do patients with sphincter of Oddi dysfunction benefit from endoscopic sphincterotomy? A 5-year prospective trial. European Journal of Gastroenterology and Hepatology 8: 251–256

Welch N, Hinder R A, Fitzgibbons R J Jr., Rouse J W 1991 Gallstones in the peritoneal cavity: a clinical and experimental study. Surgical Laparoscopy and Endoscopy 1: 246–247

Williamson R C N 1988 Pancreatic sphincteroplasty: indications and outcome. Annals of the Royal College of Surgeons of England 70: 205–211

Wilson R G, Macintyre I M 1993 Symptomatic outcome after laparoscopic cholecystectomy. Br J Surg 80: 439–441

Yoshitomi S, Martin A, Murat J, Yamamoto M, Tanaka T, Ohshio G, Manabe T, Imamura M 1996 Electrogastroenterographic examination of 22 patients before and after cholecystectomy. Digestive Diseases and Sciences 41: 1700–1705

Zeman R K, Burrell M I, Dobbins J, Jaffe M H, Choyke P L 1985 Postcholecystectomy syndrome: evaluation using biliary scintigraphy and endoscopic retrograde cholangiopancreatography. Radiology 156: 787–792

Zisman A, Loshkov G, Negri M et al 1995 The fate of long standing intraperitoneal gallstone in the rat. Surgical Endoscopy 9: 509–511

Intrahepatic stones

44

J. KAMIYA, Y. KITAGAWA, Y. NIMURA

INTRODUCTION

Intrahepatic stones are prevalent in East Asia including China, Hong Kong, Korea and Japan. Although the disease is extremely rare, it is increasingly encountered in Western countries because of increased immigration from Asia.

Intrahepatic stones include brown pigment stones (calcium bilirubinate stones), cholesterol stones and other rare stones. The majority of intrahepatic stones are brown pigment stones. Some centers, especially in Japan, have reported several cases of primary cholesterol stones originating in the liver.

DEFINITION AND SURGICAL ANATOMY

Intrahepatic stones are defined as a concretion existing in the intrahepatic bile duct. Although the confluence of the hepatic ducts is situated outside of the parenchyma of the liver an intrahepatic bile duct is, for convenience, defined as any bile duct proximal to the confluence of right and left hepatic ducts. The Japan research group for the study of hepatolithiasis has proposed a classification of intrahepatic stones focusing on the location of the stones. In this classification, patients with hepatolithiasis are separated in two groups, patients with stones only in the intrahepatic bile duct (designated 'I'), and in both intra- and extrahepatic bile duct (designated 'IE'). Additionally, a stone in the right side of the liver is designated 'R', and in the left side is designated 'L'. In 1998 a modification was made to describe stones in the caudate lobe (designated 'C').

In Japan, the proportion of type 'I' intrahepatic stones was 20.6% between the years 1975 and 1979 and increased to 45.5% between 1989 and 1992 (Tanimura et al 1994). In Hong-Kong, type 'I' occupied 51% of intrahepatic stones from 1991 to 1996 (Liu et al 1998). 18.3% was the percentage of type 'I' in Kaohsiung, Taiwan from 1980 to 1986 (Yuan et al 1990). It is interesting that many patients with intrahepatic stones are reported to have no stones in the gallbladder. Yuan reported that only 62 (30.7%) out of 202 patients with intrahepatic stones had stones in the gallbladder. As regards distribution of stones in the liver, type 'L' is reported to be dominant. In Japan the rate is 45.5% type 'L', 26.1%, 'R', and 26.3%, 'LR' between the years from 1989 to 1992. It is 52.1, 11.5 and 31.3% in Hong Kong, and 55, 18.3 and 26.7% in Taiwan, respectively, during the same period. Although stones in the caudate lobe (type 'C') have been regarded as rare, the incidence is reported to be 6.6% (Nimura et al 1998).

Hepatobiliary radiologists, endoscopists, and surgeons should have a thorough knowledge of the segmental and subsegmental branches of the intrahepatic bile ducts. A description of the subsegmental anatomy of the intrahepatic bile ducts (Fig. 44.1) was established on the basis of clinical cholangiography (Nimura 1997). This cholangiographic anatomy is related to the radiological study of the intrahepatic portal vein branches (Takayasu et al 1985). The left lateral segmental ducts (B2, lateral posterior branch; B3, lateral anterior branch) usually join just behind the umbilical portion of the left portal vein. The left medial segmental duct (B4) enters this common trunk and forms the left hepatic duct. However B3 and B4 may make a common trunk which B2 joins to form the left hepatic duct. The right anterior segmental branches are superimposed over the right posterior segmental branches, and are thus hard to distinguish from each other on clinical cholangiograms taken with the patient in a supine position. They are clearly divided by the right hepatic vein on cholangiograms taken with the patient in the right lateral position, the former in

supine position

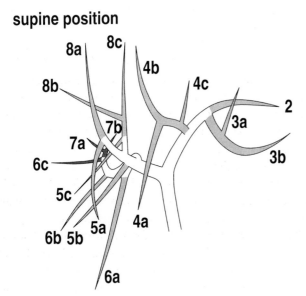

right lateral position

Fig. 44.1 Cholangiographic anatomy of the intrahepatic segmental ducts according to the patient's position. Numerals refer to Couinaud's segments. 3a superior branch; 3b inferior branch; 4a inferior branch; 4b superior branch; 4c dorsal branch; 5a ventral branch; 5b dorsal branch; 5c lateral branch; 6a ventral branch; 6b dorsal branch; 6c lateral branch; 7a ventral branch; 7b dorsal branch; 8a ventral branch; 8b lateral branch; 8c dorsal branch.

the left cranial and the latter in the right caudal area. In 20% the right posterior segmental duct joins the left hepatic duct, which may be an important factor in the distribution of intrahepatic stones.

PATHOLOGY

Intrahepatic calcium bilirubinate stones are composed mainly of bilirubin, cholesterol, fatty acid and calcium. They

are dark brown, soft and friable. On the broken surface lamellar structures can be seen (Fig. 44.2). Stones are frequently located in the large bile ducts such as the main hepatic ducts. Diffuse dilatation of the biliary tree, chiefly of the stone-containing ducts and their merging peripheral branches, as well as stenosis-like ductal lesions distal to the stones are commonly noted.

The histological changes of the bile ducts with calcium bilirubinate stones are classified into chronic proliferative, suppurative, and chronic granulomatous cholangitis (Nakanuma et al 1981). Chronic proliferative cholangitis consists of extensive proliferation of fibrous connective tissue in the ductal wall, moderate-to-severe infiltration of inflammatory cells (primarily lymphocytes) and the proliferation of mucin-producing glandular elements in the ductal wall. Suppurative cholangitis is characterized by ulceration and suppurative inflammation of the ductal wall. Chronic granulomatous cholangitis is histologically characterized by prominent granulomatous changes in the ductal wall and periductal tissues. In chronic proliferative cholangitis, histochemical observation shows that the majority of proliferative glands in the ducts have mucin-producing activity. These glands are observed to secrete large amount of acid (sialylated and sulfated) mucins into the lumen (Sasaki et al 1996, Maki et al 1971). The affected part of the liver frequently shows atrophic changes. When the whole liver is involved, patients with intrahepatic stones may develop biliary cirrhosis and portal hypertension.

Intrahepatic cholesterol stones are yellow and hard (Fig. 44.3). On the broken surface radial or crystalloid structures can be seen. Bile ducts containing cholesterol stones show milder stage of fibrosis and glandular hyperplasia than those with calcium bilirubinate stones. Foamy cell aggregates and

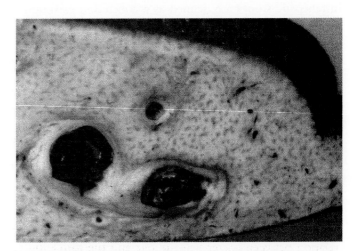

Fig. 44.2 Cut surface of a resected liver specimen shows dilated intrahepatic ducts filled with calcium bilirubinate stones. On the broken surface a lamellar-like structure is seen.

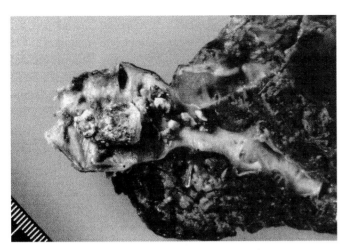

Fig. 44.3 Resected liver specimen showing dilated bile duct with cholesterol stones.

multinucleated giant cells are characteristic findings in cases with intrahepatic cholesterol stones.

Intrahepatic stones are occasionally associated with cholangiocarcinoma. Presumably, chronic irritation of the bile duct by bile stasis, infestation with parasites, or the presence of stones can lead to adenomatous hyperplasia of the epithelium and subsequently to cholangiocarcinoma. The reported incidence detected at operation varied from 1.4 to 13% (Jeng et al 1996, Liu et al 1998). Intrahepatic stones associated with intrahepatic cholangiocarcinoma are calcium bilirubinate stones in 89% of reported cases (57 of 64 cases) (Sato et al 1998). An autopsy case of intrahepatic cholesterol stones with peripheral intrahepatic cholangiocarcinoma was reported, in which the causal relationship between the stones and the carcinoma remains speculative (Terada et al 1989).

ETIOLOGY

Most intrahepatic stones appear as brown pigment stones (calcium bilirubinate stones) by visual inspection and infrared analysis. However, the chemical composition of intrahepatic calcium bilirubinate stones is not identical to that of brown pigment stones in the extrahepatic bile ducts; the former contain more cholesterol and less bilirubin and bile acid and also include lesser amounts of bile acids modified by bacterial metabolism (Yamashita et al 1988, Shoda et al 1991).

The very high incidence of bacteria in bile in cases with intrahepatic calcium bilirubinate stones suggests a close relation between bacteria in the bile and the formation of stones (Maki 1966). Among the bacteria in bile, *Escherichia coli*, *Clostridium* spp., and *Bacteroides* spp. show e-glu-

curonidase activity which is thought to be responsible for the hydrolysis of bilirubin glucuronide, the water soluble form of bilirubin in bile, to free unconjugated bilirubin. The latter is water insoluble and combines with ionized calcium in bile to form calcium bilirubinate leading to the stone formation. However, bacterial infection cannot explain solely why intrahepatic brown pigment stones contain a higher amount of cholesterol than those in the extrahepatic ducts. Up-regulated cholesterogenesis and down-regulated bile acid synthesis in the liver may be one of the etiologic factors responsible for the formation of hepatic bile substantially supersaturated with cholesterol, which leads to subsequent formation of cholesterol-rich stones (Shoda et al 1995).

The most important factors for the formation of intrahepatic calcium bilirubinate stones are considered to be biliary stasis, bacterial infection and biliary mucin, which is produced from the covering epithelium and the proliferated mucous gland epithelium of the intrahepatic bile ducts. Calcium bilirubinate and fatty acid-calcium soap occur through hydrolysis of bilirubin conjugates and lecithins by bacterial e-glucuronidase and phospholipase in bile. These salts can precipitate and form microcalculi, particularly if a nidus such as desquamated epithelium or biliary mucin is present (Forstner and Forstner 1975). These microcalculi then coalesce to form large stones. Chronic proliferative inflammation is suggested to precede bile duct deformations and the development of intrahepatic stone formation may make strictures which promote further growth of initial stones through alterations of bile flow (Nakanuma et al 1988).

A study on the biliary dynamics of ^{99m}Tc-EDTA in patients with intrahepatic stones revealed that the time activity curves of ^{99m}Tc-EDTA were prolonged significantly not only in affected *but in unaffected intrahepatic bile ducts compared with the curves in normal subjects* (Takahashi et al 1986). This result suggests bile stasis may exist in the right and left lobes of patients with only one of the two lobes affected by stones. Furthermore, the curves in the bile ducts of the left lobe were significantly longer than in those of the right lobe, even in normal subjects. The prolongation in the left intrahepatic bile ducts could explain why involvement of the left lobe are predominant. Sphincter of Oddi motility was analyzed in patients with intrahepatic stones and common bile duct stones by means of percutaneous transhepatic manometry (Yausa et al 1994). This study disclosed no significant manometric differences among three groups (intrahepatic stone group, cholecystectomy group with common bile duct stones, and noncholecystectomy group with common bile duct stones) with the exception of the higher frequencies and greater duration of the burst contractions during duodenal phase III of the migrating motor complex in the cholecystectomy group with common bile duct stones. The abnormality of the sphincter of Oddi probably plays little role in etiology of intrahepatic stones.

There is indirect evidence that metabolic factors play a more important etiologic role in intrahepatic cholesterol stones. Cholesterol supersaturation and microscopic cholesterol crystals, which are major stages recognized in the formation of cholesterol gallbladder stones (Ch. 31), have been observed in the hepatic bile of patients with intrahepatic cholesterol stones (Strichartz et al 1991, Schillio et al 1992). Activity of apolipoprotein A-1 which is one of the inhibiting factors of cholesterol nucleation in bile is reported to decrease in the hepatic segments containing cholesterol stones (Ohta et al 1993).

SIGNS AND SYMPTOMS

Abdominal pain either in the right upper quadrant or in the upper abdomen is the most frequent initial symptom and is observed in 70% of cases (Tanimura et al 1994). Jaundice and fever follow and are present in 10 to 30% of the cases. Other abdominal complaints include abdominal discomfort and vomiting. All of these symptoms are not specific to intrahepatic stones. Recently asymptomatic cases have increased in number up to 16.1% probably as a result of advances in diagnostic imaging modalities. Previous biliary surgery for calculous disease has been performed in 42.1% of patients with intrahepatic stones, and 22.2% have had two or more operations.

DIAGNOSIS

With the introduction of various new imaging modalities, intrahepatic stones are now more accurately diagnosed before surgery.

Survey by ultrasonography (US) (Ch. 13) is noninvasive and a reliable, inexpensive procedure. It may reveal features of biliary obstruction, stones in the biliary system, pneumobilia, or liver abscesses. The major findings at ultrasonography examination are hyperechoic lesions with acoustic shadows and/or ductal dilatation (Itai et al 1980). However, interpretation may be difficult owing to the presence of pnemobilia as a result of previous papillotomy or bilioenteric anastomosis. In addition, intrahepatic stones may not cast a sonic shadow and may be missed.

Computed tomography (CT) (Ch. 15) provides information on the location and components of stones and yields important information on which to base treatment. Round or oval high-density shadows in the dilated ducts are a sure sign of intrahepatic calcium bilirubinate stones (Figs 44.4A, B). The false positive rate is low (Itai et al 1980). On the other hand, cholesterol stones or pigmented stones contain

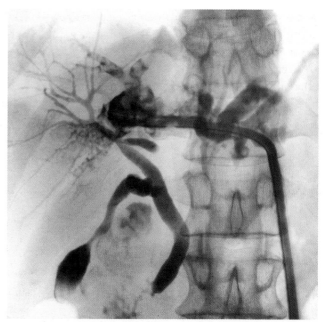

(A)

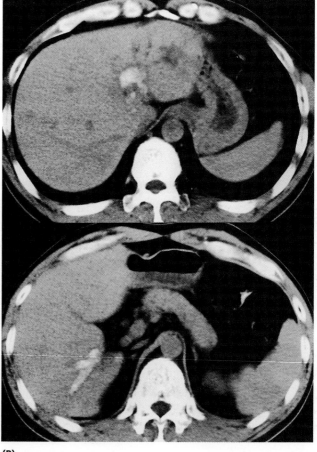

(B)

Fig. 44.4 A case of intrahepatic calcium bilirubinate stone.
(A) Cholangiography through percutaneous transhepatic biliary drainage (PTBD) catheter demonstrates multiple filling defects in the dilated intrahepatic bile ducts. **(B)** Precontrast computed tomography shows high-density shadows in the left lobe and right posterior segment.

less calcium and are hard to detect (Figs 44.5A, B). It is important to examine noncontrast films first because intrahepatic stones may be less conspicuous after parenchymal enhancement. Pneumobilia does not hinder CT evaluation of the biliary system. CT also determines the degree of atrophy of the affected part of the liver and detects segmental or subsegmental ductal involvement when cholangiography fails to visualize these ducts. In addition, CT provides accurate location of liver abscess, raises the suspicion of cholangiocarcinoma, and detects the presence of portal hypertension as a result of biliary cirrhosis. However,

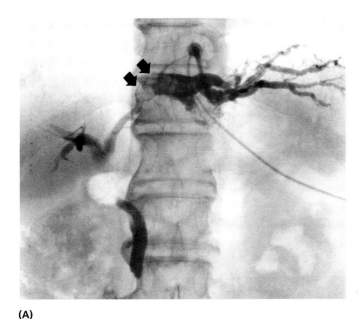

(A)

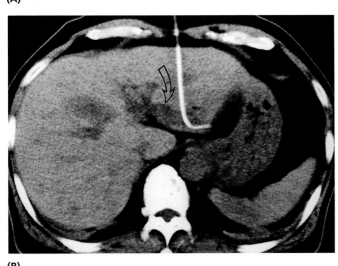

(B)

Fig. 44.5 A case of intrahepatic cholesterol stone. **(A)** Cholangiography through PTBD catheter demonstrates filling defects (arrows) in the dilated intrahepatic bile ducts of the left lateral posterior segment (S2). **(B)** Precontrast computed tomography shows low-density shadows (arrow) in S2.

accurate diagnosis of cholangiocarcinoma is difficult, as small tumors often appear as abscesses or even escape detection on CT scans. Magnetic resonance cholangiopancreatography (MRCP) (Ch. 16) is useful for diagnosis of stone location, obstructed intrahepatic segmental ducts and bile duct anatomy.

If these modalities show intrahepatic stones only in the lateral segment of the left lobe, no further imaging investigations are necessary. However, if stones are located in the right liver or bilaterally, percutaneous transhepatic biliary drainage (PTBD) followed by percutaneous transhepatic cholangioscopy (PTCS) should be carried out so as to design the most rational treatment (Nimura et al 1981). Ultrasonography, CT or MRCP provide less precise information about a segmental and subsegmental anatomy of the intrahepatic bile ducts and strictures than cholangiograms obtained by percutaneous transhepatic cholangiography (PTC), tube cholangiograms via PTBD, or selective cholangiography by PTCS. Endoscopic retrograde cholangiopancreatography (ERCP) frequently misdiagnoses intrahepatic stones because intrahepatic bile ducts peripheral to the stones or the strictures are often less well visualized. ERCP also has the disadvantage of the frequency of cholangitis after the procedure.

With the help of US, a dilated part of intrahepatic bile duct can be accurately punctured and visualized by PTC. However PTC does not always provide sufficient information due to impacted stones, mud or mucin in the intrahepatic ducts. Tube cholangiography via PTBD and selective cholangiography by PTCS are more informative than PTC because (1) they are obtained after biliary drainage which decreases mud or mucin around the stone, (2) cholangiograms from various projections such as right/left anterior oblique or right/left lateral position are available and allow an understanding of the segmental anatomy of the intrahepatic bile ducts. Percutaneous transhepatic cholangioscopy makes it possible to obtain clear selective cholangiograms before and after removal of impacted stones prior to operation. Patients with calcium bilirubinate stones frequently have biliary strictures with proximal biliary dilatation on cholangiography. However, some strictures with proximal biliary dilatation are reversible and disappear on cholangiography obtained after cholangioscopic lithotomy. A thin flow of contrast medium through the narrow space between the stones and bile duct wall yields a false image of a stricture at cholangiography. A true biliary stricture should be defined as a localized and unchanging diminution of bile duct caliber. Whether biliary strictures with proximal biliary dilatation result in stones or result from stones and repeated infections remains an open question.

The diagnosis of associated cholangiocarcinoma is difficult because intrahepatic stones and strictures hinder clear visualization of the entire intrahepatic ducts on cholangiography. As diagnostic clues the importance of filling defects and obliteration of the involved intrahepatic ducts on cholangiography, mucobilia and mucosal changes on cholangioscopy and on the gross appearance are stressed (Chen et al 1993).

TREATMENT

In acute obstructive suppurative cholangitis due to intrahepatic stone, emergency PTBD is indicated instead of urgent laparotomy or endoscopic transpapillary approach. Local rather than general anesthesia in PTBD can alleviate much of the risk to such a critically ill patient. Emergency exploration does not allow definitive treatment and usually results in incomplete biliary decompression. The endoscopic transpapillary approach is an effective and safer treatment for distal bile duct stones but more experience and further studies are required to clarify the therapeutic advantages for intrahepatic stone with acute cholangitis.

The role of cholangioscopy in the treatment of intrahepatic stones has been emphasized. With the refinement of fiberoptic cholangioscopes and the development of percutaneous transhepatic approaches to the bile ducts, PTCS has allowed nonsurgical removal of intrahepatic stones (Nimura et al 1981). However, the size of extractable stones is limited by the caliber of the PTBD sinus tract. Moreover, the presence of a biliary stricture in association with intrahepatic stones often makes stone extraction more difficult. In order to overcome these difficulties, laser cholangioscopy has been applied for intrahepatic stones with success (Hayakawa et al 1981). Furthermore, electrohydraulic lithotripsy (EHL) during cholangioscopy may solve these problems (Matsumoto et al 1987). Electrohydraulic lithotripsy is a unique method to disintegrate stones by means of shock waves generated by an electric discharge in a liquid medium. Under cholangioscopic control, the lithotriptor probe should be kept in touch with stones during application of discharge sparks so as to avoid any damage to the bile duct wall.

Hepatic resection removes not only the stones and the causative lesions but also obviates the consequences, such as recurrent stones and cholangiocarcinoma. Hepatectomy is generally indicated when segments or a lobe of the liver are grossly atrophic. In addition to the atrophic liver, indications for hepatectomy may include multiple intrahepatic strictures and/or cystic dilatation of the peripheral intrahepatic bile duct that cannot be managed by endoscopic or radiographic intervention, particularly if the left lobe or the left lateral

segment is involved. The surgical mortality is low but morbidity is substantial. When PTCS discloses that biliary stricture involves the right or left hepatic duct or the hepatic confluence and the liver parenchyma is relatively normal, an end to side hepatico-jejunostomy is performed at the confluence, or to the left hepatic or right hepatic duct according to the level of stricture. Hepatic resection with hepatico-jejunostomy may be indicated when PTCS reveals a biliary stricture at the hepatic confluence in a case with bilateral intrahepatic stone. If the function of the sphincter of Oddi deteriorates, hepatico-jejunostomy is also indicated.

With recent advances in interventional radiological management of residual or recurrent intrahepatic stone with biliary stricture, percutaneous dilatation therapy has become the treatment of choice for difficult biliary stricture. Several devices such as balloon catheters or metallic stents are available for dilatation therapy. The clinical value of percutaneous transhepatic placement of a metallic stent at the site of benign biliary strictures must be re-evaluated since clogging, recurrence of intrahepatic stones and the local effects of the material on the bile duct wall remain to be a problem.

A systemic stepwise approach is recommended in cases of difficult bilateral intrahepatic stone with bilateral biliary strictures (Nimura 1984):

1. PTBD to B3 or the left hepatic duct is performed using a direct anterior approach. This has several advantages in the management of right intrahepatic stones. Using this anterior approach there is easy access for a cholangioscope to the right intrahepatic ducts, especially to the right posterior segmental ducts. Intraoperative cholangioscopy and/or postoperative cholangioscopy through a T-tube sinus tract or jejunal loop is much more difficult.

2. The PTBD sinus tract is dilated step by step. One week after the PTBD, 6-F drainage catheter is replaced by 10 or 11-F catheter (PTCS catheters, Fig. 44.6). Then the tract is dilated by exchanging the catheter for a larger one 2 or 3 times a week and a 16-F catheter can be introduced in 2 weeks after PTBD. During this period, CT and US study of the liver is performed. A hepatectomy is indicated in the case of unilateral atrophy of the hepatic segments (vide supra).

3. Cholangioscopic lithotomy is performed in the hepatic segments or lobes which will be preserved. If intrahepatic bile duct stenoses hinder cholangioscopic lithotomy, they should be dilated by introducing a 12 or 15-F PTCS catheter. Recent advances in lithotripsy technology makes it possible to remove impacted stones without difficulty if the affected segments or lobes are not atrophic. Percutaneous transhepatic cholangioscopy

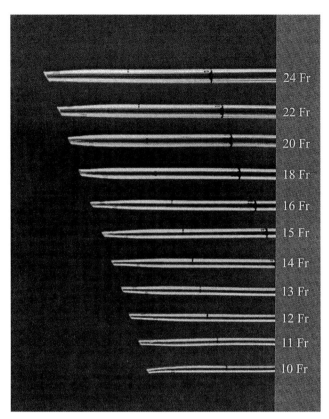

Fig. 44.6 PTCS catheters. Eleven sizes of drainage catheters (10–24 F) with a tapered tip and two side holes.

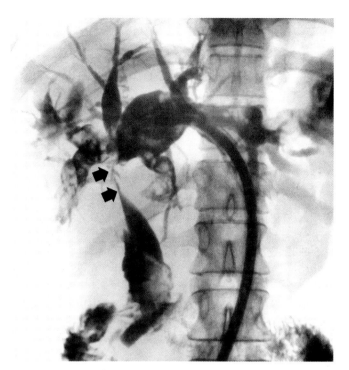

(A)

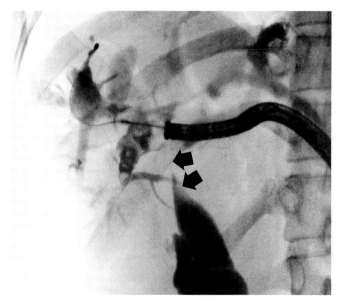

(B)

Fig. 44.7 A case of bilateral intrahepatic stones with biliary stenosis at the hepatic hilus. **(A)** Cholangiography through PTCS catheter revealed severe biliary stenosis at the hepatic hilus (arrows). The patient had undergone biliary operations twice without any clinical improvement: first, choledocho-duodenostomy; second, choledochotomy with T-tube drainage. **(B)** Cholangiography during PTCS lithotomy showed marked biliary stenosis remained after removing most stones in the liver. These findings indicate hilar bile duct resection with hepaticojejunostomy.

enables definition of biliary stenoses prior to surgical treatment. In the case of biliary stenosis at the hepatic hilus, hilar bile duct resection with hepatico-jejunostomy is indicated (Fig. 44.7).

4. If neither liver atrophy nor strictures are found after cholangioscopic lithotomy, operation is not necessary. Cholecystectomy may be indicated if the gallbladder stones are in situ. In the case of hepatic segmental or lobar atrophy without biliary stricture at the hepatic hilus, cholecystectomy, hepatectomy, choledochotomy, intraoperative cholangioscopy, and T-tube placement without bilioenteric anastomosis are recommended (Fig. 44.8). For a patient with an atrophic segment or lobe and biliary stricture at the hepatic hilus, hilar bile duct resection with hepatico-jejunostomy should be added to cholecystectomy, hepatectomy, and intraoperative cholangioscopy. If a biliary stricture is defined only at the hepatic hilus after endoscopic lithotomy by PTCS, cholecystectomy, hilar bile duct resection, intraoperative cholangioscopy, and hepaticojejunostomy are indicated.

5. In the case of surgical intervention, postoperative cholangioscopy must be performed to verify no residual stones and to observe the postoperative changes of the intra-

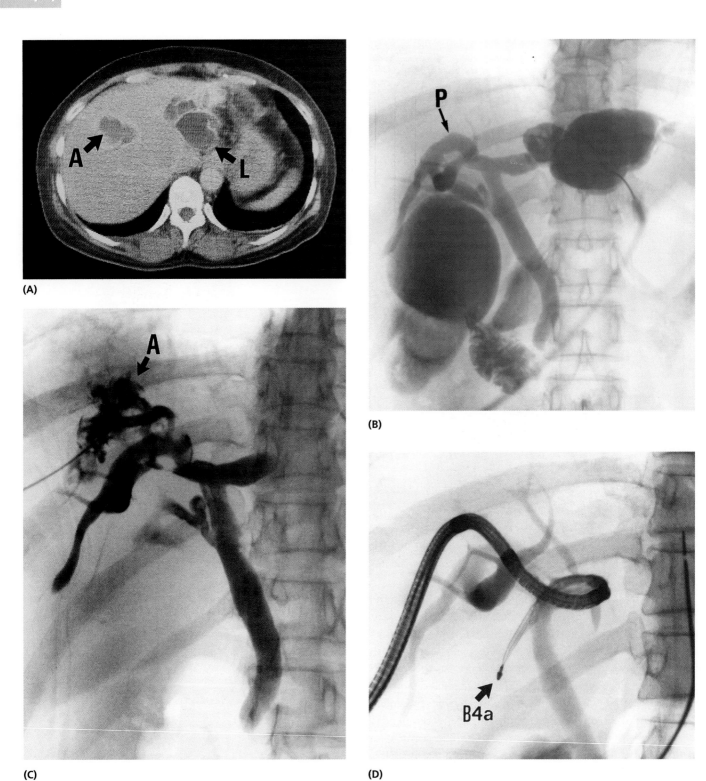

Fig. 44.8 A case of bilateral intrahepatic stone. **(A)** Computed tomography showed two low-density lesions in the left lateral segment (L) and the right anterior segment (A) where ultrasonography had revealed stones. These two segments are atrophic. **(B)** US guided percutaneous transhepatic cholangiography (PTC) revealed dilated intrahepatic segmental bile ducts of the left lateral segment. The right posterior segmental duct (P) is demonstrated, but the right anterior segmental duct is not visualized. **(C)** Selective PTC of the right anterior segmental duct (A) was carried out under US guidance. The right anterior segmental duct was occupied by many stones which made it difficult to make a definitive diagnosis of the pathology of the right anterior segmental duct. Therefore PTBD was performed into the right anterior segmental duct so as to allow a precise diagnosis. **(D)** A cholangioscope introduced into the left hepatic duct through the right anterior segmental duct, and selective cholangiograms of the left medial segment (4a, 4b) were obtained. The left medial segment was free from hepatolithiasis. After cholangioscopic lithotomy, it became possible to introduce the cholangioscope into the right and left hepatic duct. (*Continued*)

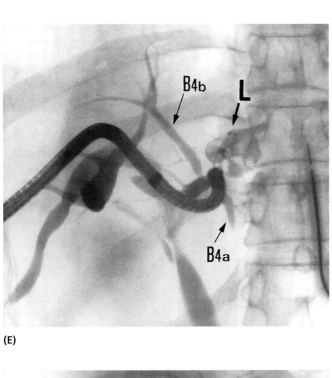

(E)

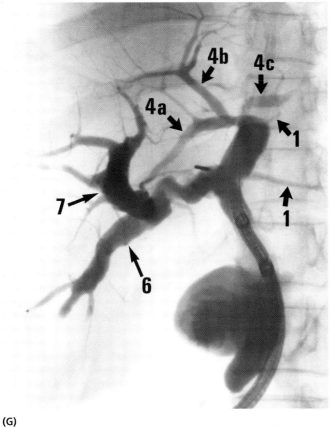

(G)

Atrophic anterior segment

P   A   M   L

Hepatic duct

1

2

3

4

(F)

Fig. 44.8 (*Continued*) A case of bilateral intrahepatic stone. **(E)** Selective cholangiography of the left lateral segmental duct (L) showed severe stricture. **(F)** Scheme of the operation. 1, A left lateral segmentectomy. The dilated left lateral segmental duct is resected proximally to the confluence of the left medial segmental (quadrate) duct. P, right posterior segment (sector); M, left medial segment (quadrate); C, caudate lobe. 2, A right anterior segmentectomy (sectorectomy). The dilated right anterior segmental duct is resected at the confluence of the right posterior segmental duct. 3, Intraoperative cholangioscopy through the opening of the right posterior segmental (sectoral) duct. 4, T-tube placement through a choledochotomy. **(G)** Postoperative cholangioscopic cholangiography showed no residual stone. The subsegmental bile ducts of the left medial segment (4a, 4b, 4c), the right posterior segment (6, 7) and the caudate lobe (1) were preserved as proposed preoperatively.

hepatic biliary strictures. If the treatment effect is not sufficient, biliary stenting with a silicon catheter should be applied.

In regard to the treatment of intrahepatic cholesterol stones, a non-surgical procedure is the treatment of choice. (Kondo et al 1995) (Fig. 44.9). Because of the inaccessibility of peripherally located stones and the absence of significant intrahepatic biliary dilatation, the success rate of cholangio-scopic lithotomy for cholesterol stones is reported to be lower than that of intrahepatic calcium bilirubinate stones. Limited partial hepatectomy with or without bilioenteric anastomosis should be applied following PTCS treatment in selected patients after defining the remaining biliary strictures and retained stones. The endoscopic retrograde approach does not seem feasible due to the inaccessible location of the intrahepatic stones. Extracorporeal shock wave lithotripsy may be effective, especially in combination with the use of dissolution therapy. Improvement in bile composition has been reported following oral dissolution

therapy in patients with intrahepatic cholesterol stones, suggesting that this therapy is probably useful as a preventive adjunctive (Strichartz et al 1991, Schillio et al 1992).

There has been controversy regarding the indications for therapy in the asymptomatic patient with intrahepatic stones. If the component of stones is diagnosed as choles-terol, there may be no indication for treatment. On the con-trary, if associated intrahepatic cholangiocarcinoma is suspected, hepatectomy should be applied. In Kami-Goto Island of Japan, a screening survey for intrahepatic stones has been performed by ultrasonography because of high incidence of this disease, and 122 asymptomatic cases of intrahepatic stones were detected and followed for 10 years (Furukawa et al 1998). Only 14 patients (11.5%) of the 122 developed symptoms, and 13 (92.9%) of the 14 had an atrophic segment or lobe of the liver. However, the inci-dence of liver atrophy was low (13.0%) in cases without symptoms. This data led us to the conclusion that treatment is not indicated for asymptomatic patients without atrophy of a hepatic segment or lobe.

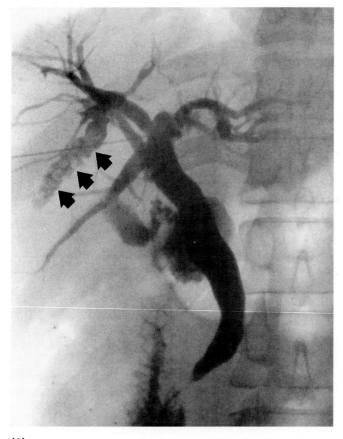

(A)

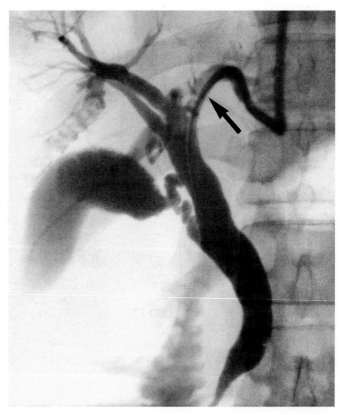

(B)

Fig. 44.9 A case of intrahepatic cholesterol stone. **(A)** Percutaneous transhepatic cholangiography disclosed stones (arrows) in the bile duct of segment V. Note the cylindrical dilatation of the stone-bearing duct. **(B)** PTBD of the left hepatic duct (arrow) was performed using a direct anterior approach. (*Continued*)

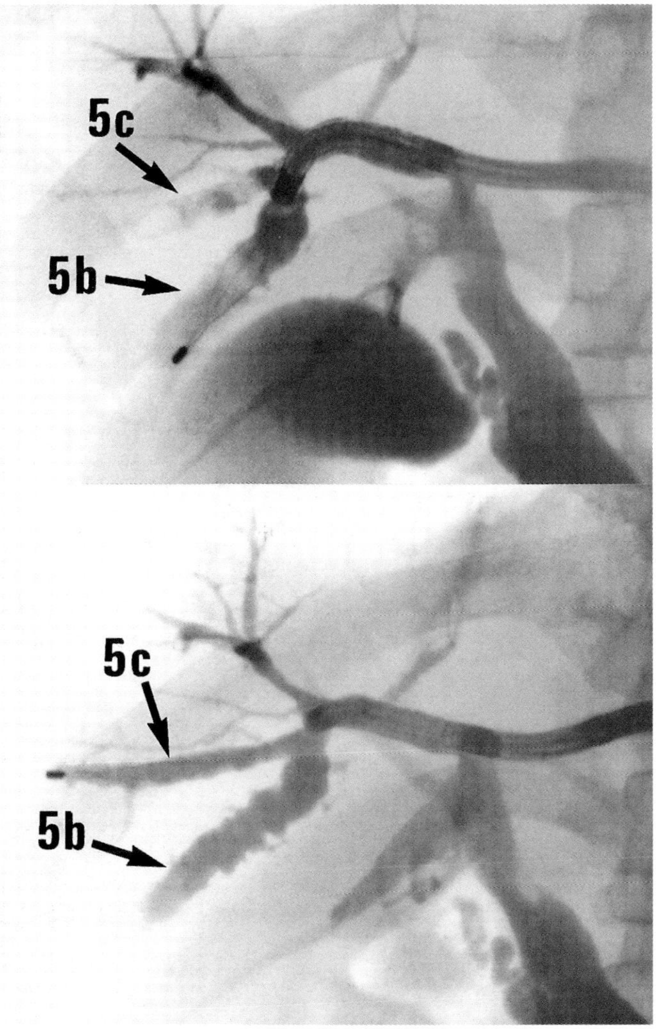

(C)

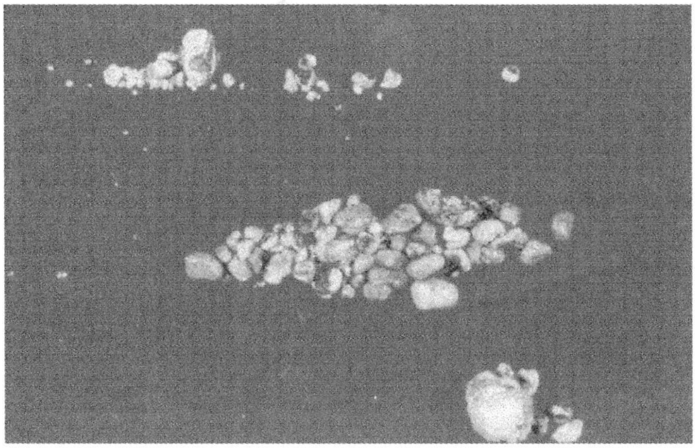

(D)

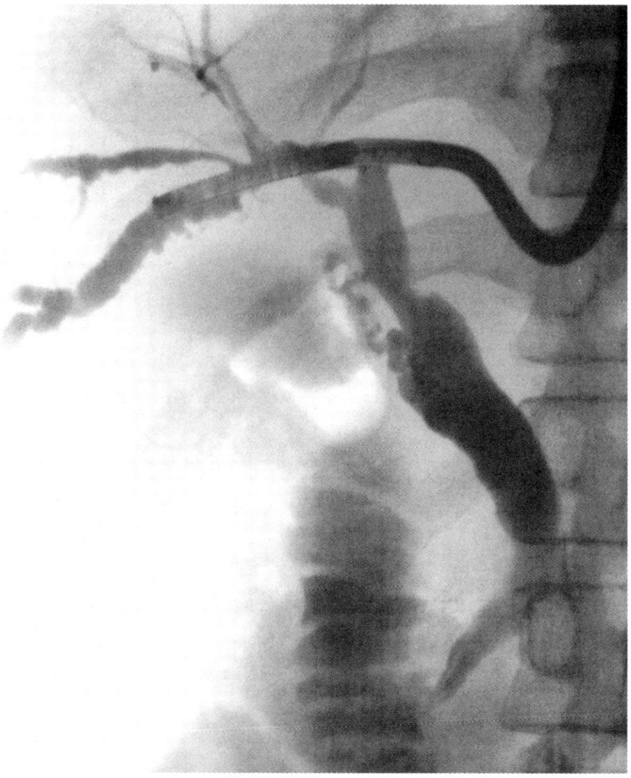

(E)

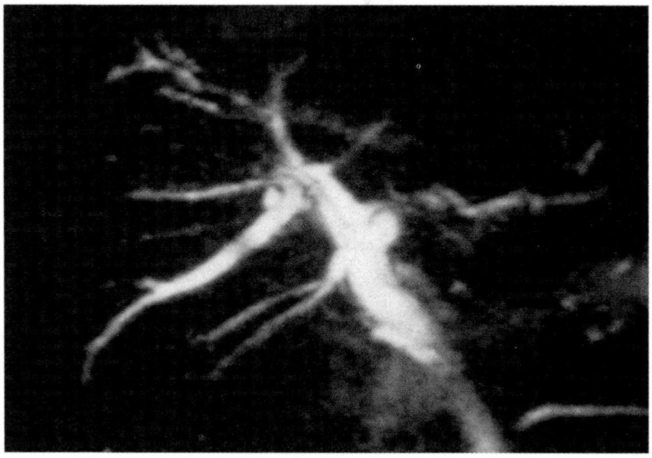

(F)

Fig. 44.9 (*Continued*) A case of intrahepatic cholesterol stone. **(C)** PTCS revealed that the stones were cholesterol stones and were located only in the subsegmental ducts of segment V (5b, 5c). Cholangioscopic lithotomy was easily carried out with a basket catheter because of absence of any biliary stenosis. **(D)** All stones were removed from 5b and 5c in three sessions of PTCS. **(E)** Selective cholangiography shows no residual stones in the subsegmental ducts of segment V. After cholangioscopic lithotomy, the patient underwent cholecystectomy which disclosed no stones in the gallbladder with mild cholesterosis. **(F)** Magnetic resonance cholangiopancreatography 17 years after the treatment showed no recurrent intrahepatic stones.

PROGNOSIS

Intrahepatic stones carry a high rate of recurrence. Of all cases treated in Japan from 1989 to 1992, the recurrence rate was 6.6% (119 of 1815 cases) (Tanimura et al 1994). It was 5.3% (38 of 719) in cases undergoing hepatectomy, 8.3% (21 of 254) after choledochojejunostomy, 6.4% (40 of 624) after choledochotomy followed by cholangioscopic lithotomy, and 9.6% (20 of 208) after PTCS, respectively. The lowest recurrence rate reported is 3.1% (3 of 96) (mean follow-up period of 26 months) in Hong Kong (Liu et al 1998). The highest is 32.6% (43 of 132) for cases undergoing lithotomy by PTCS with a mean follow-up period of 5 years (Yeh et al 1995).

The survival rate after surgery for intrahepatic cholangiocarcinoma associated with hepatolithiasis is low because most patients have advanced carcinoma at the time of surgery. Chen reported that the 1-, 2- and 4-year survival rates in 55 patients were 30, 12.7 and 3.6%, respectively (Chen et al 1993). In Japan 48% of cases of intrahepatic stones with cholangiocarcinoma died within one year of operation (Tanimura et al 1994).

REFERENCES

Chen M F, Jan Y Y, Wang C S, Hwang T L, Jang L B, Chen S C 1993 A reappraisal of cholangiocarcinoma in patients with hepatolithiasis. Cancer 71: 2461–2465

Forstner J F, Forstner G G 1975 Calcium binding to intestinal goblet cell mucin. Biochem Biophys Acta 386: 283–292

Furukawa M, Ohtsubo K, Yasaka T, Shirahama S 1998 Asymptomatic hepatolithiasis: a follow-up study. In: Japanese Government, Annual reports of the Japanese Ministry of Health and Welfare. Tokyo, Japan: 12–14 (in Japanese)

Hayakawa N, Nimura Y, Kamiya J, Hasegawa H, Maeda S, Iyomasa Y 1981 Studies on Laser cholangioscopy—application for lithotripsy of gallstones. In: Atsumi K (ed) LASER TOKYO 81, p 2316–2318

Itai Y, Araki T, Furui S, Tasaka A, Atomi Y, Kuroda A 1980 Computed tomography and ultrasound in the diagnosis of intrahepatic calculi. Radiology 136: 399–405

Jeng K S, Ohta I, Yang F S 1996 Reappraisal of the systemic management of complicated hepatolithiasis with bilateral intrahepatic biliary strictures. Archives of Surgery 131: 141–147

Kondo S, Nimura Y, Hayakawa N, Kamiya J, Nagino M, Miyachi M, Kanai M 1995 A clinicopathologic study of primary cholesterol hepatolithiasis. Hepato-Gastroenterol 42: 478–486

Liu C L, Fan S T, Wong J 1998 Primary biliary stones: diagnosis and mangement. World Journal of Surgery 22: 1162–1166

Maki T 1966 Pathogenesis of calcium bilirubinate gallstone: role of *E. coli*, β-glucuronidase and coagulation by inorganic ions, polyelectrolytes and agitation. Annals of Surgery 164: 90–100

Maki T, Matsushiro T, Suzuki N, Nakamura N 1971 Role of sulfated glycoprotein in gallstone formation. Surg Gynecol Obstet 132: 846–854

Matsumoto S, Tanaka M, Yoshimoto H, Miyazaki K, Ikeda S, Nakayama F 1987 Electrohydraulic lithotripsy of intrahepatic stones during choledochoscopy. Surgery 102: 852–856

Nakanuma Y, Ohta G, Nagakawa T, Matsubara F 1981 Histological studies on the livers with intrahepatic gallstones. Japanese Journal of Gastroenterology 78: 874–882

Nakanuma Y, Yamaguchi K, Ohta G, Terada T, Japanese Hepatolithiasis Study Group 1988 Pathologic features of hepatolithiasis in Japan. Human Pathology 19: 1181–1186

Nimura Y, Hayakawa N, Toyota S, Iyomasa Y, Nakazawa S 1981 Percutaneous transhepatic cholangioscopy (PTCS). Stomach and Intestine 16: 681–689 (in Japanese with English abstract)

Nimura Y 1984 Percutaneous transhepatic cholangioscopy (PTCS) in the treatment of intrahepatic stones. In: Sheen P C, Ker C G (eds) Gallstone and choledochoscope, Mei Yuh Co., Kaoshiung, p 71–85

Nimura Y 1997 Surgical anatomy of the biliary ducts. In: Medical radiology: biliary tract radiology, Springer-Verlag, Berlin, p 21–30

Nimura Y, Kitagawa Y, Kamiya J 1998 Intrahepatic stone in the caudate lobe. In: Japanese Government, Annual reports of the Japanese Ministry of Health and Welfare. Tokyo, Japan: 45–49 (in Japanese)

Ohta T, Nagakawa T, Takeda T, Fonseca L, Kanno M, Mori K, Kayahara M, Ueno K, Miyazaki I, Terada T 1993 Histological evaluation of the intrahepatic biliary tree in intrahepatic cholesterol stones, including immunohistochemical staining against apolipoprotein A-1. Hepatology 17: 531–537

Sasaki M, Morita T, Hoso M, Nakanuma Y, Tanimura H 1996 Carcinoembryonic antigen and blood group-related carbohydrate antigens in glycoproteins in human bile in hepatolithiasis. Hepatology 23: 258–263

Sato M, Watanabe Y, Ueda S, Ohno J, Kashu Y, Nezu K, Kawachi K 1998 Intrahepatic cholangiocarcinoma associated with hepatolithiasis. Hepato-Gastroenterology 45: 137–144

Schillio Y, Amouyal G, Gayet B, Dumont M, Degott C, Erlinger S 1992 Primary intrahepatic cholesterol stones: report of one case and treatment with ursodeoxycholic acid. Digestive Diseases and Sciences 37: 1460–1463

Shoda J, Tanaka N, Matsuzaki Y, Honda A, Osuga T, Shigematsu N, Miyazaki H 1991 Microanalysis of bile acid composition in intrahepatic calculi and its etiological significance. Gastroenterology 101: 821–830

Shoda J, He B F, Tanaka N, Matsuzaki Y, Yamamori S, Osuga T 1995 Primary dual defect of cholesterol and bile acid metabolism in liver of patients with intrahepatic calculi. Gastroenterology 108: 1534–1546

Strichartz S D, Abedin M Z, Ippoliti A F, Derezin M, Roslyn J J 1991 Intrahepatic cholesterol stones: a rationale for dissolution therapy. Gastroenterology 100: 228–232

Takahashi K, Narumi T, Fukushima N, Momota Y, Matsumoto M, Endo M, Suzuki H, Sasaki M, Ono K 1986 Biliary dynamics in patients with intrahepatic gallstones. J Bil Tract Pancr 10: 1317–1322 (in Japanese)

Takayasu K, Moriyama N, Muramatsu Y, Shima Y, Goto H, Yamada T 1985 Intrahepatic portal vein branches studied by percutaneous transhepatic portography. Radiology 154: 31–36

Tanimura H, Uchiyama K, Ishimoto K, Nagai M 1994 Epidemiology of hepatolithiasis in Japan. In: Japanese Government, Annual reports of the Japanese Ministry of Health and Welfare. Tokyo, Japan: 17–27 (in Japanese)

Terada T, Kurumaya H, Nakanuma Y 1989 Intrahepatic cholesterol stones associated with peripheral cholangiocellular carcinoma: an autopsy case. American Journal of Gastroenterology 84: 1434–1436

Yamashita N, Yanagisawa J, Nakayama F 1988 Composition of intrahepatic calculi—etiological significance. Gastroenterology 101: 821–830

Yeh Y H, Huang M H, Yang J C, Mo L R, Lin J, Yueh S K 1995 Percutaneous trans-hepatic cholangioscopy and lithotripsy in the treatment of intrahepatic stones: a study with 5 year follow-up. Gastrointestinal Endoscopy 42: 13–18

Yuan C Y, Yaun C C, Yuan T K 1990 A reevaluation of 202 patients after surgical removal of intrahepatic stones: with special emphasis on intrahepatic biliary stricture. Journal of the Formosan Medical Association 89: 373–377

Yuasa N, Nimura Y, Yasui A, Akita Y, Odani K 1994 Sphincter of Oddi motility in patients with bile duct stones: a comparative study using percutaneous transhepatic manometry. Digestive Diseases and Sciences 39: 257–267

45

Supraduodenal choledochotomy and choledochoduodenostomy—technique

L.H. BLUMGART

SUPRADUODENAL CHOLEDOCHOTOMY AND EXPLORATION OF THE COMMON BILE DUCT

Laparoscopic common bile duct exploration (Ch. 38) has become commonplace. However, open choledochotomy remains an important procedure. The operative approach to common duct stones and the results are detailed by Girard in Chapter 39.

Indications

Several studies have evaluated the importance of clinical symptoms, blood biochemistry and ultrasound findings in predicting the presence of cholelithiasis. This was important before the widespread use of intraoperative cholangiography, which is now the established intraoperative investigation for detecting bile duct calculi. The accepted absolute indications for duct exploration are obstructive jaundice, a filling defect on the operative cholangiogram and a stone, which can be palpated. However, even an experienced surgeon fails to palpate a significant percentage of stones. Dilatation of the common bile duct greater than 12 mm is, by itself, not a strong indicator for bile duct stones (Orloff 1978). However, in combination with either a raised alkaline phosphatase, minimally raised bilirubin or history of jaundice, the predictive value for common duct stones is 90 to 100% (Lacaine et al 1980). A common bile duct greater than 15 mm represents a strong indication for exploration. Multiple small stones in the gallbladder, an enlarged cystic duct and a history of jaundice are but weak indicators and may help to decide, in the presence of other positive findings, whether to explore the common bile duct or not. In biliary pancreatitis the rate of common duct stones varies between 11% and 50% depending on the time of cholecyst-ectomy (Ch. 35). The longer the period between onset of symptoms and elective cholecystectomy, the smaller the chance of finding stones on operative cholangiography. Recent biliary pancreatitis is therefore no absolute indication for common duct exploration.

These indications (Table 45.1) imply that the patients coming to exploration of the common bile duct have more serious pathology and, as a result, a higher morbidity than patients having cholecystectomy alone (McSherry and Glenn 1980). The operation of choledochotomy demands clearly defined indications and, with the increasing use of endoscopic sphincterotomy, is now required much less often, especially in older patients.

The management of retained stones after cholecyst-ectomy is most frequently in the domain of the endoscopist (Ch. 40). Nevertheless, operative ductal exploration is still of importance, particularly in patients with grossly dilated bile ducts containing multiple and large stones (Ch. 42). Choledochoduodenostomy may be indicated in such cases (vide infra). Supraduodenal choledochotomy may also be

Table 45.1 Indications for choledochotomy

Indications	Positive exploration* (%)
Absolute	
Palpable stone	98–100
Cholangitis with jaundice	94–97
Positive cholangiogram	50–85
Common bile duct > 15 mm	73–93
Relative	
Common bile duct < 12 mm	21–35
Small stones in gallbladder	10–37
History of jaundice	34–37
Pancreatitis	11–50
Abnormal liver function test	25

*Values summarized from the literature (Way 1972, Orloff 1978, Lygidakis 1984, Gunn 1988, Yip and Lam 1988).

necessary in patients in whom endoscopic approaches are difficult or compromised (e.g. the presence of duodenal diverticula, or following previous gastrectomy).

Exposure

The liver is retracted superiorly with a broad-bladed slightly curved retractor. This retractor should be deep enough to

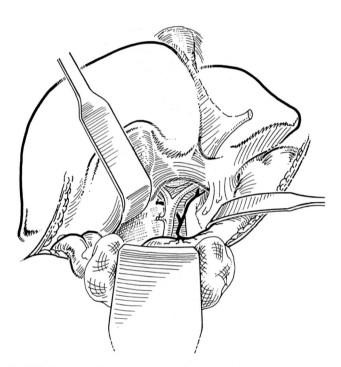

Fig. 45.1 Exposure of the common duct by packs and retractors.

displace the liver but not so curved as to traumatize it. The curved broad-based Hartmann (or 'sweetheart') retractor often serves this purpose well. A pack should be put over the hepatic flexure of the colon down to the hepatorenal pouch and the medial part of the duodenum. This pack is retracted by a similar broad bladed retractor to prevent the colon or duodenum obscuring vision (Fig. 45.1). The lesser omentum and stomach are retracted to the left after having placed another pack.

The gallbladder is usually removed prior to exploration of the common bile duct because it may obstruct vision although in some cases it can be a useful aid to retraction. Palpation of the common bile duct and handling of its lower part during exploration and subsequent choledochoscopy cannot be properly done without have performed a classic Kocher maneuver (Fig. 45.2).

Choledochotomy

The site of the choledochotomy depends on several factors. Choledochoduodenostomy (vide infra) may become necessary and therefore the opening must be in the lowest part of the supraduodenal common bile duct that is consistent with an easy subsequent anastomosis (Figs 45.3 and 45.4).

A distal choledochotomy is advocated so that as much as possible of the common duct is left proximally in case the duct is needed for some further procedure (e.g. repair of a stricture) in this part of the duct. The third reason why the choledochotomy should be placed distal and close to the duodenum is that the usual distance from this point to the papilla measures ± 7 cm. This is the exact length of the rigid choledochoscope with which common duct exploration

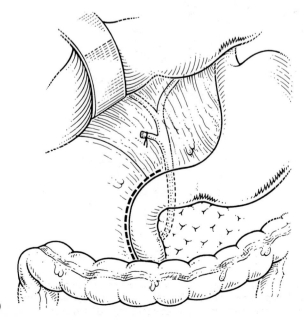

(A)

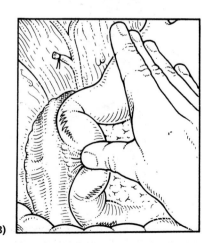

(B)

Fig. 45.2 **(A)** The gallbladder has been removed. The dotted line indicates the incision in the retroperitoneum to allow mobilization of the duodenum by the Kocher maneuver **(B)**.

may be carried out and a clear view of the papilla of Vater is obtained. The anatomy of the cystic duct is so variable that care must be exercised to open the correct duct. A cystic duct lying anterior or closely applied to the common bile duct can easily be opened in error (Fig. 45.5).

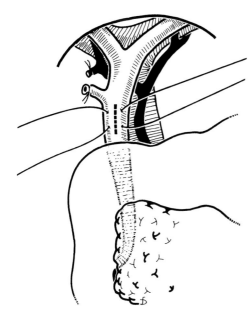

Fig. 45.3 The common bile duct is opened just above the duodenum leaving room for a choledochoduodenostomy if this is found to be necessary.

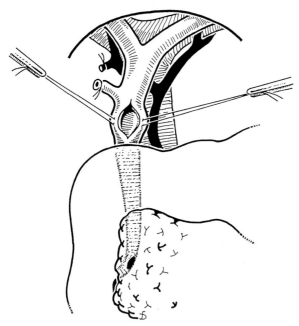

Fig. 45.4 Two fine stay sutures of 3/0 P.D.S. or 3/0 Vicryl are used to lift and render the common bile duct tense for an incision about 1–2 cm long, depending on the size of the duct and the size of the stones. If the duct is not made tense then damage can be done to the posterior wall or an irregular incision made.

Bile is aspirated by gentle suction and a specimen of the common bile duct bile should be sent for culture.

EXPLORATION OF THE DUCT

Exploration should be as atraumatic as possible. The use of rigid instruments is to be avoided (Orloff 1978, Gunn 1983). Grasping forceps of any type may catch the wall of

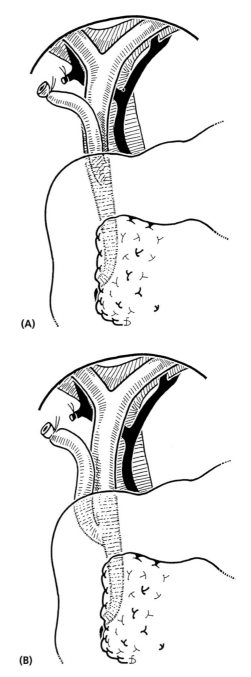

Fig. 45.5 (A) The cystic duct may lie anterior to the common duct and may be opened in error. **(B)** The cystic duct may run parallel to the common duct with a low entrance mimicking a dilated duct.

the duct with possible damage and late stricture formation. Bougies have been used traditionally but metal instruments can create a false passage into the duodenum or even into the pancreas. The Fogarty balloon catheter has been found to be suitable for common bile duct exploration (Fogarty et al 1968, Fox & Gunn 1984).

The Fogarty probe is held in long forceps and introduced into the common duct. The forceps are held in the surgeon's right hand (Fig. 45.6) and the catheter is passed into the duodenum (Fig. 45.7).

The balloon is inflated and the catheter withdrawn until it impinges against the papilla. As already mentioned, the duct is normally about 7 cm from the point of choledochotomy to the duodenum. The second part of the duodenum is palpated and the balloon identified to determine the site of the papilla in case duodenotomy is necessary. Any stone present can usually be felt against the shaft of the catheter. The balloon is deflated and gently withdrawn through the papilla. This is detected by a sudden easing of the pull on the catheter. Immediately after this happens the balloon is re-inflated. The catheter is held by the syringe in the left hand and the degree of inflation controlled by the thumb and the plunger. With gentle traction superiorly by long forceps in the surgeon's right hand the catheter is gradually pulled up to the choledochotomy site (Fig. 45.8), care being taken to prevent any stone slipping into the proximal biliary tree.

If the traction is anteriorly rather than superiorly, there is the risk of lacerating the opening into the duct (Fig. 45.9).

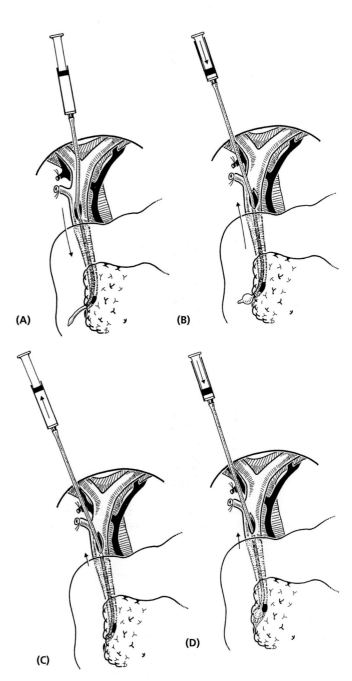

Fig. 45.7 (A) The Fogarty catheter is attached to a syringe and balloon is inflated in the duodenum. **(B)** The Fogarty catheter is retracted with the balloon against the papilla. **(C)** The balloon is deflated gently until it slips through the papilla when the balloon is reinflated. **(D)** The Fogarty is gently withdrawn with the balloon inflated.

Fig. 45.6 A Fogarty catheter is fed into the duct with forceps using the right hand. The operator's left hand grasps the mobilized duodenum and allows palpation of the passage of the catheter and of any stones within the intrapancreatic portion of the common bile duct.

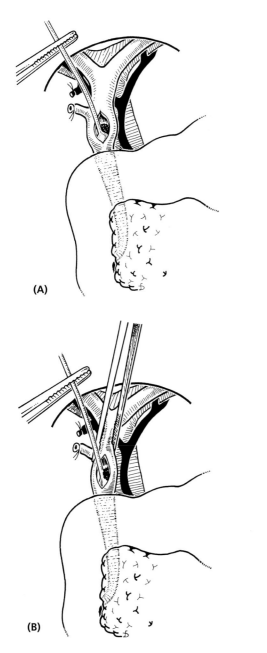

Fig. 45.8 (A) The balloon is gently withdrawn revealing the stone.
(B) Long forceps can be used to obstruct the common hepatic duct to prevent the stone from slipping upward.

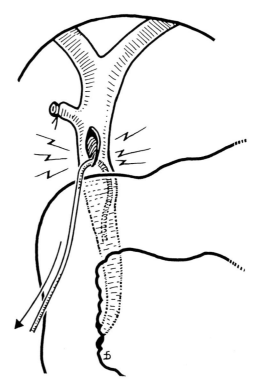

Fig. 45.9 Angled traction on the Fogarty catheter results in tearing of the lower end of the choledochotomy.

The risk is increased when the opening in the duct is longitudinal. The procedure is repeated until it is considered that the distal duct is clear.

The catheter is withdrawn and reinserted upwards into each of the main hepatic ducts and the procedure is repeated. It is important that the balloon inflation is correct; overinflation could damage the ducts and underinflation may miss any stone that is present. This can be achieved by inflating the balloon until the fingers feel the tension of the syringe plunger. This tension is maintained as the catheter is withdrawn into the gradually widening duct.

It is important to remove the stone when it appears at the choledochotomy opening and to avoid allowing it to fall into another part of the duct. The second step in common duct exploration is to irrigate the duct with saline. Small stones, sludge and debris can be flushed into the duodenum or back into the choledochotomy opening by irrigating the ductal system.

The last step in this technique is to repass the Fogarty catheter into the duodenum, inflate the balloon and retract it against the papilla. While the catheter is held in the right hand, the index and middle fingers of the left hand are placed posterior to the duodenum with the thumb anteriorly. This allows palpation of the duct against the wall of the catheter for any residual stones.

Postexploratory investigations

The surgeon must attempt to ensure that the duct system is normal even though no operative methods may be available for removing residual stones or dealing with residual strictures (Chs 40, 41, 42).

CHOLEDOCHOSCOPY (Ch. 23)

Choledochoscopy is the established method. Modern instruments are small enough to allow visualization of the major right and left hepatic ducts and intermediate hepatic ducts and to allow vision of the orifices of the smaller biliary radicals. Some surgeons experienced in choledochoscopy advocate exploration of the common duct and removal of stones under direct vision using the choledochoscope.

T-TUBE CHOLANGIOGRAPHY

After insertion of a T-tube and closure of the choledochotomy (see below), T-tube cholangiography is the remaining option of post-exploratory investigation. With proper technique and by use of fluoroscopy, it is an excellent tool for detecting residual stones after common duct exploration (Fig. 45.10).

The cystic duct stump, a possible location of residual stones, can be delineated and incorrect placement of the T-tube can be detected in order to prevent complications after the operation. In case of a residual stone, the T-tube has to

be removed and the duct re-explored. This necessitates a second suture of the common duct. In our view this is a major disadvantage of T-tube cholangiography.

T-TUBE DRAINAGE

The standard practice is to use a T-tube to allow spasm or edema of the sphincter to settle following the trauma of the exploration. Failure to drain the duct might result in a build up of pressure in the extrahepatic ductal system and leakage at or disruption of the closure of the duct with biliary peritonitis.

One other important reason for the use of T-tube is the detection and subsequent treatment of retained stones. In the event of a stone being left behind, then the T-tube can be of use later for interventional radiological techniques through the track created by the tube (Fig. 45.11).

However, the use of a T-tube creates a fistula between the skin and the lumen of the duct, both being potentially contaminated surfaces. The track of the fistula crosses the peritoneal surface. The size of the T-tube should be adapted to the diameter of the common duct, French gauge 14 being the smallest that should be used if a satisfactory track is to be left for subsequent interventional radiology. This acknowledges the fact that a significant proportion of patients who have had choledochotomy for common bile duct stones will subsequently be found to have residual stones. The use of postexploratory choledochoscopy and cholangiography will greatly reduce the number of residual stones, but the wise surgeon should accept that stones will occasionally be left.

T-TUBE PLACEMENT

The limbs of the T-tube have to be shortened (Fig. 45.12A). T-tubes can become obstructed, particularly if they are tight fitting and can be difficult to extract. This can be avoided by cutting off a strip of the wall (Fig. 45.12B). The practice of dividing the back wall of the T-tube makes subsequent interventional radiology more difficult as the guide wire lodges in the posterior defect. In the main this can be avoided by making the length of the T appropriate or by limiting the division of the T-tube. The modified T-tube is held in Desjardin's forceps, which conveniently grasps the T-junction of the tube allowing it to be slipped into the choledochotomy (Fig. 45.13). The long limb of the tube is placed at the lower end of the opening and repair commenced just above the upper apex of the incision using continuous or interrupted resorbable material. The final stitch should close the opening against the T-tube (Fig. 45.14).

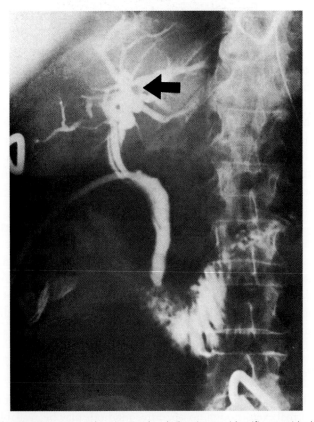

Fig. 45.10 A post-exploration T tube cholangiogram identifies a residual stone in the intrahepatic bile ducts, missed during operative exploration of the bile duct.

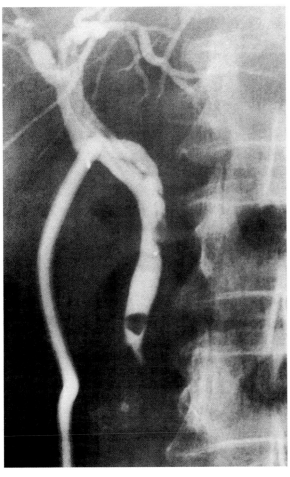

(A)

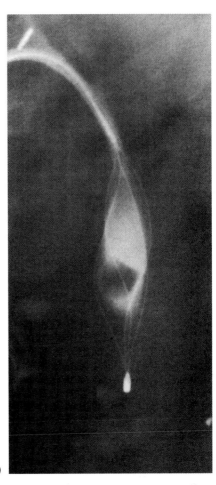

(B)

Fig. 45.11 (A) Faceted retained distal common duct stone on T-tube cholangiography 1 week after operation. Note that the T-tube is inserted in the common hepatic duct above the confluence of the cystic duct. **(B)** The retained common duct stone is ensnared in the wire basket before extraction. This stone measured 5 mm in diameter and was extracted intact through the sinus tract of a 14 Fr T-tube.

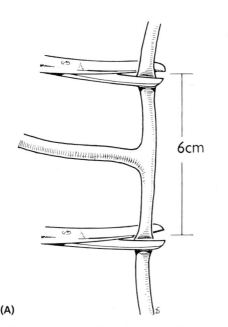

(A)

6cm

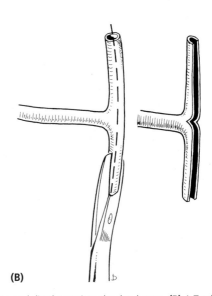

(B)

Fig. 45.12 (A) The T-tube is modified by shortening the limbs to prevent proximal obstruction and distal entry into the duodenum. **(B)** A T-tube is modified by removing half the diameter to prevent obstruction and easy removal.

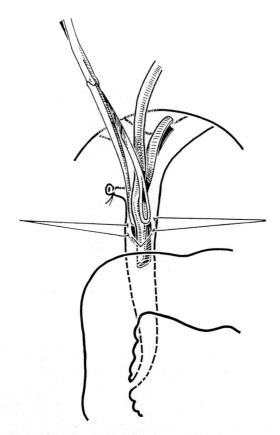

Fig. 45.13 The T-tube is introduced by Desjardins forceps.

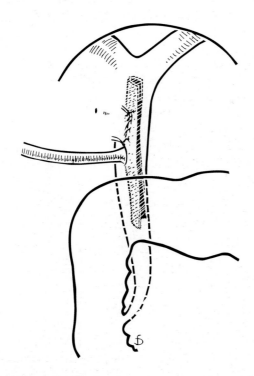

Fig. 45.14 The choledochotomy closure is commenced above with the T-tube emerging at the lower end of the repair.

AVOIDING PROBLEMS IN THE CLOSURE OF THE CHOLEDOCHOTOMY

Care must be taken that the wall of the T-tube is not caught in one of the sutures and the end of the suture should not be tied around the tube (Fig. 45.15). Either of these faults may result in the tearing of the duct when the tube is withdrawn.

The proximal limb of the T-tube should not enter one of the hepatic ducts as this can produce obstruction. The distal end must not enter the duodenum as this can act as a syphon. In addition, a tube through the papillary orifice may excite pancreatitis.

The correct position of the T-tube is with the long limb emerging under the costal margin laterally (Fig. 45.16). This facilitates radiological techniques for later postoperative removal of stones should this be necessary. A suction drain is placed on the right, within the abdomen as high as possible in the hepatorenal pouch.

Postoperative management

Initially, bile is allowed to drain freely into a bile bag to allow any spasm or edema of the sphincter to settle before testing the suture line of the choledochotomy. The volume drained varies with decreasing amounts as flow increased through the sphincter. If the volume drained remains high or increases, then the reason should be established. This may be due either to continuing distal obstruction or because the distal limb is lying within the duodenum. Similarly, there is a problem if there is no drainage of the bile or bile drains around the T-tube. This suggests that the tube has either become blocked or has become dislodged from the duct.

The answer to all these problems is revealed by T-tube cholangiography. Provided there have been no problems, the subsequent management is aimed at waiting for the bile to flow easily through the papilla into the duodenum. The bile bag should not be lifted or clamped.

A T-tube cholangiogram is taken about 5–7 days after the operation. Provided this is normal the tube is removed on day 7 or 8 by gentle traction.

If there are residual stones or unclear findings on T-tube cholangiography, it is good practice to repeat T-tube cholangiogram several days later. Should a stone still be demonstrated, this is managed initially by sending the patient home with a sealed drainage system, but with instructions to open the drain and connect it to a bag in the event of any problems. After a period of some 5 weeks, further cholangiography is carried out. If the stone is still

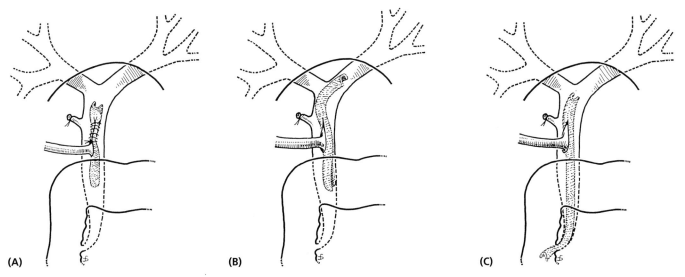

Fig. 45.15 (A) The suture must not catch the tube as shown here. **(B)** The T-tube limb should not enter the hepatic duct as shown here. **(C)** The distal end of the T-tube should not enter the duodenum.

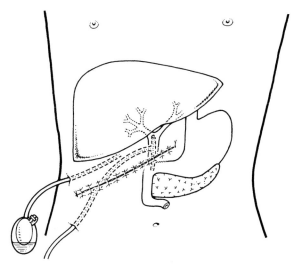

Fig. 45.16 The T-tube should be brought out lateral to the wound. A closed suction drain should be placed in the hepatorenal space beneath the liver.

present, this is extracted by means of interventional radiology. Gallstone dissolution or endoscopic papillotomy (Fig. 45.17) are reserved for such cases that fail at interventional radiological removal.

CHOLEDOCHODUODENOSTOMY

In the performance of supraduodenal choledochotomy, it may be elected to carry out choledochoduodenostomy at the conclusion of ductal exploration rather than place a T-tube. The following outline of the indications for and

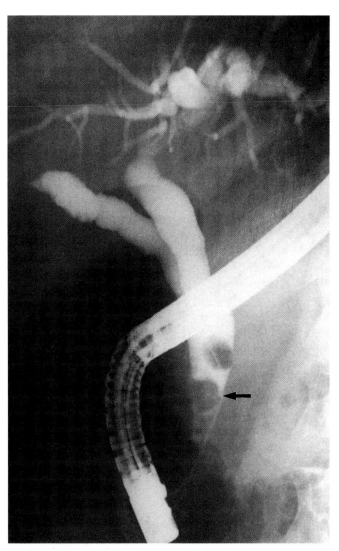

Fig. 45.17 Balloon extraction of a single stone (arrow).

techniques of the procedures owes much to the description of Gliedman in the previous edition of this book (Gliedman 1994).

Indications

A dilated duct is the sine qua non for this procedure. It should not be performed with ducts less than 1.4 cm in diameter and a duct narrower than 1.2 cm is an absolute contraindication. The circumstances in which this bypass has been effective in association with a dilated duct are:

1. Retained or recurrent calculi in the choledochus or hepatic ducts
2. Cholangitis
3. Ampullary stenosis
4. Presence of primary choledochal calculi or stasis bile
5. Tubular stricture of the transpancreatic portion of the choledochus usually due to chronic pancreatitis
6. Combinations of these
7. Low iatrogenic stricture
8. Malignant obstruction in the periampullary area.

Contraindications include duodenal ulcer and acute pancreatitis.

Technique

Two technical criteria are essential for a proper choledochoduodenostomy: a common duct of 1.4 cm in diameter at the minimum and a stoma size of 2.5 cm. A stoma size of 2.5 cm cannot be accomplished with other than a single-layer anastomosis.

The degree of satisfaction with the procedure will depend upon the development of a standard technique for the rapid

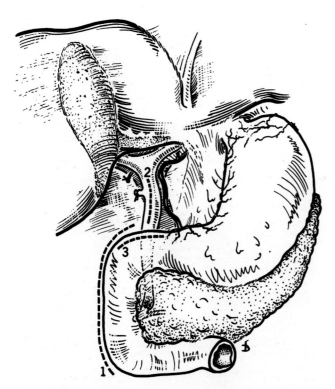

Fig. 45.18 After the gallbladder is removed, the common duct is opened through a conventional longitudinal incision following a Kocher incision (1) freeing the lateral duodenum around the common duct. Routine common duct exploration is carried out. If the indications for a choledochoduodenostomy exist, the anastomosis is performed. The incision in the common duct (2) is extended to 2.5 cm by direct measurement. In almost all instances, the incision in the duct will carry into the common hepatic duct. The incision in the post bulbar duodenum (3) is slightly smaller since the stoma in the duodenum stretches to approximate the choledochal incision.

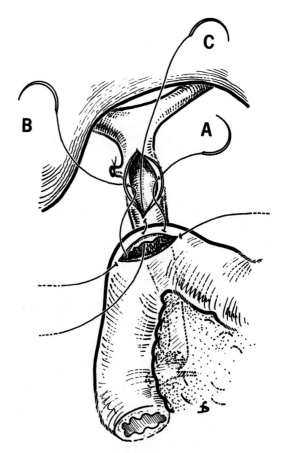

Fig. 45.19 Each side of the choledochoduodenostomy is bisected by stitch (A and B) of absorbable material (chromic catgut or polyglycolic acid) that passes from the end of the duodenal incision through the mid-point of the choledochal incision. Likewise the duodenal incision is bisected by a stitch through the posterior wall of the duodenal incision and the lower apex of the choledochal incision (C). These stitches convert part of the longitudinal choledochotomy incision into a transverse ostium. A lax approximation of the duodenal and choledochal incision occurs, with the duodenum mobilized, by placing tension on a lateral stay suture (A or B) and the middle stay suture (C).

construction of a stoma that allows free entry and egress from the common bile duct.

While attempts are made to remove stones and particulate matter from the common bile duct, impacted stones at the distal common bile duct that are not easily retrieved and stones in the hepatic duct are not too vigorously pursued prior to the anastomosis (Gliedman 1994). The detailed technical steps are shown in Figs 45.18–45.22.

An alternative technique which the author has found simple and of value is shown in Fig. 45.23. This method involves a continuous suture of 4/0 Vicryl developed with two needles—the surgeon working with each alternately.

In cases of malignancy in the periampullary region, end-to-side choledochoduodenostomy may be carried out as described in Chapter 30. However, choledochojejunostomy is the preferred approach and choledochoduodenostomy is rarely performed.

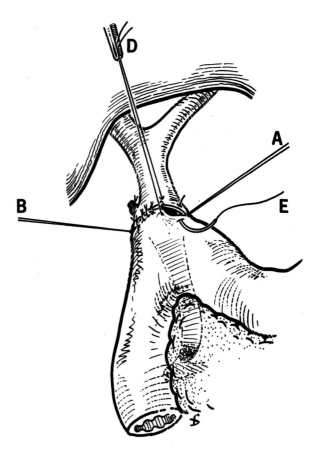

Fig. 45.21 With this bisecting suture (D) tented forwards, each of the segments, between the tied lateral stay suture and this anterior suture is similarly approximated using interrupted sutures with the knots tied on the outside. The anastomosis is completed by completing the third segment of this triangle by sutures placed between the remaining lateral stay suture and the suture 'D'. It is important in the placement of these last sutures that they do not catch the posterior suture line. The benefit of placing all the sutures in one line of the triangular closure and then tying them all following placement is that it allows an internal inspection before the lumen of the choledochoduodenostomy is obscured. A single row of sutures is all that is utilized. A second row does nothing but decrease the choledochoduodenostomy orifice size and is to be avoided. The sutures should be placed close enough so that there is a bile-tight approximation. Digital pressure on the duodenum or the common duct should give no evidence of leakage.

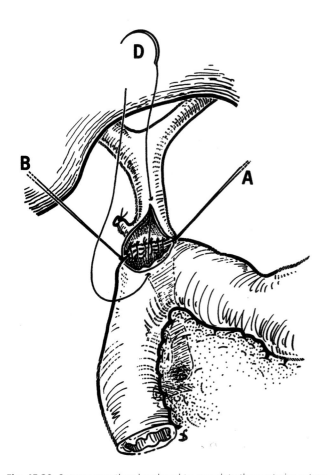

Fig. 45.20 Sutures may then be placed to complete the posterior suture line approximating the common bile duct to the posterior duodenal incision. Following placement of the sutures they are tied so that the knots are within the lumen. The anterior wall is similarly approximated utilizing a suture bisecting the anterior duodenal incision (D) and through the original apex of the bile duct incision.

Postoperative evaluation and results

Postoperative evaluation is carried out radiologically either by barium meal study or by HIDA scans (Ch. 14), which allows good anatomical visualization as well as assessment of the physiologic function of the anastomosis in emptying the biliary tree. Gliedman (1994) reports no difficulties with post-choledochoduodenostomy cholangitis or the so-called 'sump syndrome' and believes that this is a result of a commitment to a measured anastomosis of 2.5 cm or greater in the duodenum and common bile duct. The single-layer

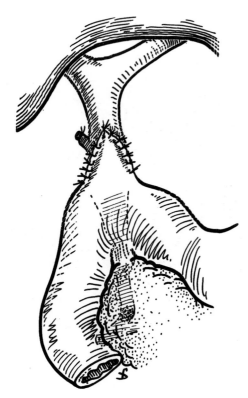

Fig. 45.22 The completed anastomosis allows a thumb-sized defect to be palpated through the duodenal tongue that has been brought on to the common bile duct and common hepatic duct. One may drain or not drain the anastomosis according to preference. There has been a 1% leak rate. The presence of a closed suction drain (Jackson-Pratt type) obviates the need for a subsequent percutaneous drainage catheter should this uncommon complication occur.

anastomosis helps to ensure that there will be no decrease of size of the opening achieved by the described technique.

The published experience supports the attitude that a properly performed choleduochoduodenostomy will serve as an effective bypass. It is simple in terms of technical performance and has a low postoperative mortality and morbidity.

Schein (1978) reports that the procedure can be safely and widely applied to all ducts that are at least 1.4 cm wide. It can be done in the presence of extensive cholangitis at either the primary or revisional operation. In 50 cases, there was only 1 death. There have been no leaks and no intraperitoneal complications. An initial wound infection rate of 12% has been reduced by the use of pre- or intraoperative antibiotics in all patients undergoing the procedure (Robson et al 1970). The technical safety of the procedure is analogous to that of gastroenterostomy for obstructed duodenal ulcer disease.

In the elderly, very sick patient, it can be performed more rapidly than the procedures required for monitoring conventional common duct exploration.

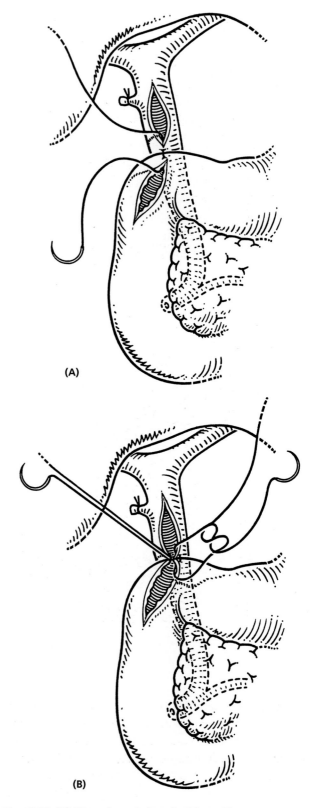

Fig. 45.23 (A) Alternative technique for side-to-side choledochoduodenostomy. The bile duct is opened longitudinally just above the duodenum and a duodenotomy is made in a slightly oblique fashion starting at almost the same point. **(B)** Two 3/0 Vicryl sutures are used to bring the lower apex together. Both needles are retained. (*Continued*)

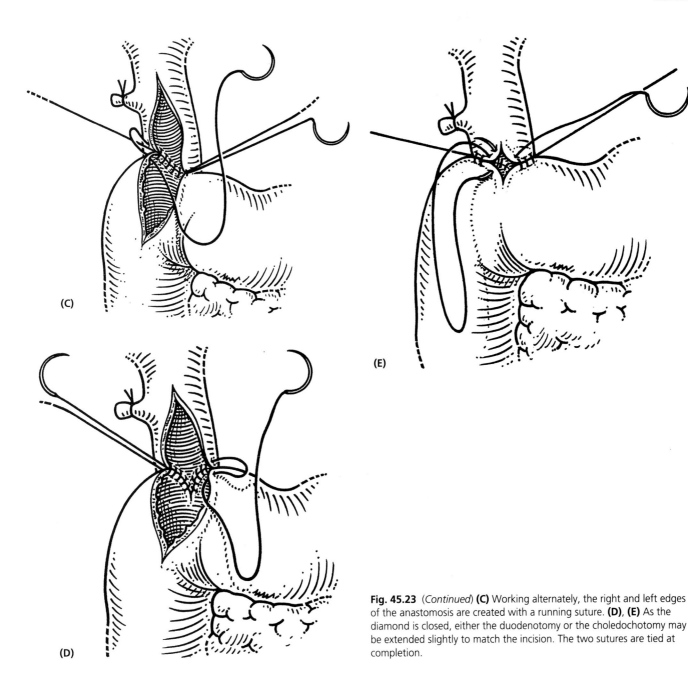

(C)

(E)

(D)

Fig. 45.23 (*Continued*) **(C)** Working alternately, the right and left edges of the anastomosis are created with a running suture. **(D)**, **(E)** As the diamond is closed, either the duodenotomy or the choledochotomy may be extended slightly to match the incision. The two sutures are tied at completion.

Madden et al's review (1970) of the collective literature reported an incidence of cholangitis of 0.4% in 1225 operations. In each of these cases, cholangitis was related to stomal stricture, which must be viewed as a technical problem. The long history and follow-up indicate there are probably few ill effects from incontinent drainage of bile into the duodenum and from possible reflux of duodenal contents into the bile duct. The possible problem of the blind segment (sump syndrome) between choledochoduodenal anastomosis and the ampulla of Vater has not been a source of difficulty in any of the major series.

REFERENCES

Braasch J W, Fender HR, Boneval M M 1980 Refractory primary common bile duct stone disease. American Journal of Surgery 139: 526–530

Degenshein G 1974 Choledochoduodenostomy, an 18-year study of 175 consecutive cases. Surgery 76: 319–324

Fogarty F J, Krippaeine W W, Dennis D L, Fletcher W S 1968 Evaluation of an improved operating technique in common duct surgery. American Journal of Surgery 116: 117–182

Fox J, Gunn A A 1984 Common bile duct exploration by balloon catheter. Journal of the Royal College of Surgeons, Edinburgh 29: 81–84

Gliedman M L 1994 Choledochoduodenostomy—technique. In Blumgart L H (ed) 2nd edn. Surgery of the liver and biliary tract, Churchill Livingstone, Edinburgh, p. 797

Gliedman M, Schein C 1980 The use and abuse of choledocho-duodenostomy. In: Najarian J, Delaney J P (eds) Hepatic, biliary and pancreatic surgery. Miami Symposia Specialists, p 91

Gliedman M, Gold M 1985 Choledochoduodenostomy. In: Schwartz S I, Ellis H (eds) 8th edn. Maingot's abdominal operations, Appleton-Century-Crofts, Norwalk, CT, p 1909–1922

Gunn A A 1983 Cholecystectomy, cholecystectomy and exploration of the common duct. In: Dudley H A, Pories W J, Carter D B (eds) 4th edn. Rob and Smith, operative surgery, Butterworth, London, p 616

Gunn A A 1988 Supraduodenal choledochotomy. In: Blumgart L H (ed) 1st edn. Surgery of the liver and biliary tract, Churchill Livingstone, Edinburgh, p 647

Jones S A 1978 The prevention and treatment of recurrent bile duct stones by transduodenal sphincterectomy. World Journal of Surgery 2: 473–485

Jones A G, Harding Rains A J 1978 Prevention and treatment of recurrent bile duct stones by choledochoduodenostomy. World Journal of Surgery 2: 487–496

Lacaine F, Corlette M, Bismuth H 1980 Preoperative evaluation of the risk of common bile duct stones. Archives of Surgery 115: 1114–1116

Lawson R, Gunn A 1970 The value of operative cholangiography. Journal of the Royal College of Surgeons of Edinburgh 15: 222–227

Lygidakis N J 1982 Surgical approaches to postcholecystectomy choledocholithiasis. Archives of Surgery 117: 481–484

Lygidakis N J 1984 The incidence and significance of common bile duct dilatation in biliary calculous disease. World Journal of Surg 8: 327–334

Madden J, Chun J, Kandalaft S, Parekh M 1970 Choledochoduodenostomy. An unjustly maligned surgical procedure? American Journal of Surgery 119: 45

McSherry C K, Glenn F 1980 The incidence and causes of death following surgery for nonmalignant biliary tract disease. Annals of Surgery 191: 271

Orloff M 1978 Importance of surgical technique in prevention of retained and recurrent bile duct stones. World Journal of Surgery 2: 403–410

Robson M, Bogart J, Heggers J 1970 An endogenous source for wound infections based on quantitative bacteriology of the biliary tract. Surgery 86: 471

Schein C, Benevato T, Jacobson H 1966 Choledochoduodenostomy—roentgen considerations. Surgery 60: 958–963

Schein C, Shapiro N, Gliedman M 1978 Choledochoduodenostomy as an adjunct to choledocholithotomy. Surgery, Gynecology and Obstetrics 146: 25–32

Schein C 1978 Postcholecystectomy syndromes. A clinical approach to etiology, diagnosis, and management, Harper and Row, Hagerstown, Maryland

Schein C, Gliedman M 1981 Choledochoduodenostomy as an adjunct to choledocholithotomy. Surgery, Gynecology and Obstetrics 152: 797–804

Way L W, Admirand W H, Dunphy J E 1972 Management of Choledocholithiasis. Annals of Surgery 176: 347–359.

Yip A, Lam K M 1988 An evaluation of routine operative cholangiography. Australian & New Zealand Journal of Surgery 58: 391–395

46

Transduodenal sphincteroplasty and exploration of the common bile duct

G. RIBOTTA, F. PROCACCIANTE

Endoscopic and laparoscopic procedures have further reduced the use of open operation to explore the common bile duct (CBD) and to operate on the papilla. Transduodenal sphincteroplasty (TSP) is still indicated for *failure of the endoscopic sphincterotomy*, in addition it is advised in *patients with Bilroth II gastrectomy*, in *papillitis* where patency of the papillotomy has to be assured long-term and in *pancreatitis* when a drainage procedure of the distal duct of Wirsung is indicated (Lehman & Sherman 1998).

Furthermore, the less frequently TSP is performed the more difficult it is for surgeons to acquire experience; it is therefore important to be well acquainted with the operative technique (Matsuoka et al 1994).

Sphincteroplasty consists of suturing the outer edge or both edges of a surgical sphincterotomy, thus avoiding possible future stenosis of the incision. The stitches achieve hemostasis of the incision margins and help to avoid possible leakage of the duodenal contents should the incision extend beyond the common portion of the sphincter thus incurring the risk of perforation of the duodenal wall.

Instrumental exploration of the CBD through the sphincteroplasty is easy and safe. Catheters and instruments may be inserted along the axis of the CBD, whereas in supraduodenal choledochotomy access they must be inserted transversely and then angled to 90°, with the resultant risk of damage to the posterior choledochal wall (Ratych et al 1991). Exploration using Randall's forceps or with Dormia or Fogarty catheters allows the surgeon to deliver stones easily. Similarly, hydatid cyst remnants and membranes are readily extracted. Exploration may extend to the left and right hepatic ducts and Randall's angled forceps are useful for this purpose.

INDICATIONS (Table 46.1)

STONES IMPACTED IN THE DISTAL AMPULLARY REGION

The stone is often readily palpable and the incision may safely be made using it as a guide. In such cases extraction through a supraduodenal choledochotomy is often impossible without undue risk of creating a false passage (Ratych et al 1991) and without significant risk of post-operative pancreatitis.

Table 46.1 Indications for sphincteroplasty

Exploration of the common bile duct
    Bile duct stones
    Hydatid cyst
Necessity or therapeutic
    Impacted ampullary stones
    Papillary stenosis
Drainage procedure
    Biliary mud and sludge
    Multiple CBD stones
    Recurrent CBD stones
    Pyogenic cholangitis
Contraindications
    CBD diameter > 2 cm
    Long sphincter stricture, more than 15 mm
    Peri-Vaterian diverticulum
    Duodenal wall and head of the pancreas severely inflamed

(Barraya et al 1974, Chigot et al 1978, Arianoff 1980)

MULTIPLE AND RECURRENT CBD STONES

In such cases sphincteroplasty should provide long-term biliary drainage. When 20 or more stones are retrieved from the CBD, it is probable that one or more stones are still present (Stain et al 1991). While choledochoduodenostomy may also be used in this situation, sphincteroplasty yields excellent results.

PAPILLARY STENOSIS

This is less frequently encountered than in the past but may be now more precisely defined. When papillary stenosis is found at operation, TSP ensures good biliary drainage and prevents stenosis (Ramirez et al 1994) since endoscopic sphincterotomy is technically successful in only 60 to 80% of cases and its mortality exceeds 1% (Seifert et al 1982). In addition, endoscopic sphincterotomy for papillary stenosis is five times more likely to develop restenosis than if the same procedure is performed for calculi (Tzovaras and Rowlands 1998).

PYOGENIC CHOLANGITIS (see Ch. 60)

This coexists with papillary stenosis and/or CBD stones and is an indication for definitive biliary drainage, and this can be obtained by TSP.

CHRONIC PANCREATITIS AND GALLSTONE ACUTE PANCREATITIS

In chronic pancreatitis some authors report good long-term results obtained with TSP alone (Hakaim et al 1994) or in addition to transampulary septectomy (Moody et al 1983) or with other drainage procedures of the duct of Wirsung (Kestens et al 1996).

The presence of a stone at the lower end of the CBD or pancreatic duct may cause biliary, pancreatic or duodenal reflux, depending where the stone is impacted. Trypsinogen activated by the reflux is a potential cause of pancreatitis (Armstrong et al 1985). TSP with clearance of the CBD represents one treatment option in this condition.

TSP is contraindicated in the presence of a large CBD (> 2 cm) or where there is a long suprasphincteric stricture. It should not be attempted in the presence of a duodenal diverticulum or when there is severe periampullary inflammation (Table 46.1).

TECHNIQUE

Sphincteroplasty consists of the incision of the common portion of the sphincter of Oddi (Fig. 46.1) with partial suture of the incision margin. By this procedure the sphinc-

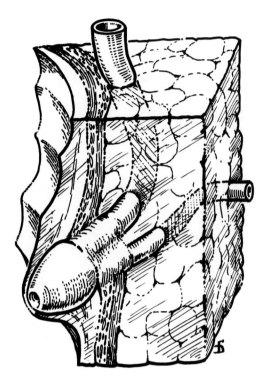

Fig. 46.1 A section of the sphincter of Oddi. Note the distinction between the papilla, the common portion of the sphincter and the sphincters of the common bile duct and duct of Wirsung.

ters of the common bile duct (CBD) and the duct of Wirsung are not involved and therefore their function is not impaired. The procedure can also be defined as 'subtotal lower sphincteroplasty' (Fig. 46.2) (Stefanini et al 1977). The approach to the sphincter of Oddi is through a minimal duodenotomy in the second part of the duodenum. The following description is of the technique recommended by the authors.

PREPARATION AND POSITIONING OF THE PATIENT

Preoperative preparation is routine. A Levin tube is introduced preoperatively and maintained until the third or fourth postoperative day. The patient is placed in a supine position on a radiotransparent operating table.

INCISION

The authors prefer a transverse incision below the right costal margin (Vogt & Hermann 1981). This allows optimal light and excellent access. This approach is particularly suitable in obese patients and the incidence of postoperative incisional hernia is probably lower than with vertical and oblique incisions.

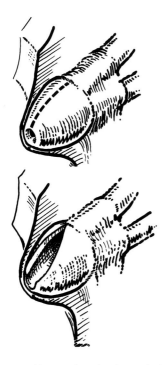

Fig. 46.2 Subtotal lower sphincteroplasty involves only the papilla while the sphincter of the common bile duct and that of the duct of Wirsung are preserved.

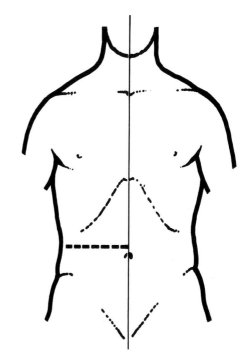

Fig. 46.3 Transverse subcostal incision. This offers excellent exposure with a low incidence of postoperative incisional hernia.

The incision of the abdominal wall follows a transverse line, from the midaxillary to the median line at the level of the 11th/12th rib (Fig. 46.3).

PREPARATION OF THE OPERATIVE FIELD

The abdomen is opened and a large retractor is positioned at the upper margin of the wound. The right flexure of the colon is displaced inferiorly and the stomach to the left by means of two surgical pads. Viscera are maintained in this position with two large curved Deaver retractors.

INTRAOPERATIVE RADIOLOGY

Intraoperative fluoroscopy and cholangiography (see Ch. 22) is always performed before TSP. It is carried out after cannulation of the cystic duct.

Image interpretation suggesting papillary stenosis is difficult and for this reason the authors, in some cases, in addition to radiological examination, perform flow measurements (Vayre & Jost 1981) and more recently, sphincter of Oddi manometry (Gilbert et al 1992, Montesani et al 1988).

In previously cholecystectomized patients, where a cystic duct remnant is present and a 5–6 mm stump can be isolated, this is employed. When this is not possible, contrast medium is injected by direct fine-needle puncture of the common bile duct.

EXPOSURE AND MOBILIZATION OF THE DUODENUM

Kocher maneuver

For the performance of sphincteroplasty, extended mobilization of the duodenum and pancreas (Kocher maneuver) is mandatory (Moody et al 1983). The assistant surgeon displaces the second portion medially and forward. The peritoneum is incised posteriorly along the curved lateral margin of the duodenum (Fig. 46.4). The mesocolon of the right colic flexure is cleared inferiorly. At this point the assistant surgeon should also displace the duodenum superiorly (Fig. 46.5). Access is thus provided to the avascular space between the posterior aspect of the head of the pancreas anteriorly and the perinephric fat and inferior vena cava posteriorly; elevation of the structures should reach the left margin of the inferior vena cava. It is very important to expose and mobilize the third portion of the duodenum so as to allow easy access to the papilla and for closure of the duodenotomy without tension (Fig. 46.6).

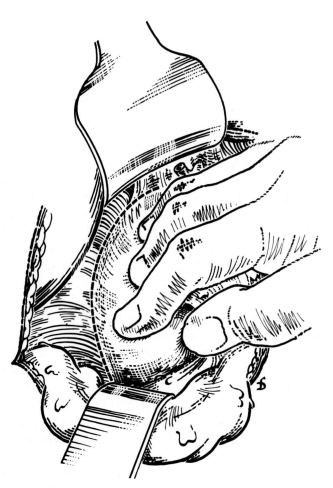

Fig. 46.4 Kocher maneuver: this commences with an incision of the peritoneum laterally at the outer margin of the second portion of the duodenum (dashed line). Mesocolon related to the right colic flexure is stripped inferiorly.

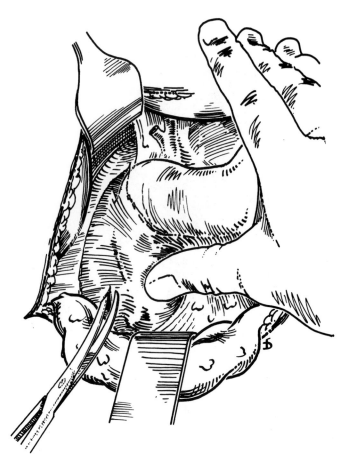

Fig. 46.5 To help mobilization of the duodenum the assistant surgeon displaces the second portion of the duodenum medially and superiorly.

Inframesocolic and extraperitoneal approaches

In some cases where the subhepatic space is obscured by adhesions as a result of previous surgery, access to the second portion of the duodenum using a different approach has been suggested. The authors are not familiar with these techniques since even in cases of extensive adhesions there has been little difficulty in access to the duodenum as described above.

In the inframesocolic approach (Villalba & Lucas 1978) the greater omentum and transverse colon are displaced superiorly and the small bowel inferiorly and to the left. Next, a transverse incision is made in the posterior peritoneum at the base of the transverse mesocolon from the superior mesenteric vessels extending laterally to expose the second and third duodenal portions.

In the extraperitoneal approach (Choi et al 1982), an incision is made in the abdominal wall below the right costal margin from the mid-axillary line to the lateral edge of the

right rectus abdominis muscle. The peritoneum is displaced superiorly and medially. The right kidney and its perinephric fat are identified and the duodenum reached extraperitoneally.

DUODENOTOMY

Duodenotomy is performed in the lateral duodenal wall by surgical diathermy. The cut is 10–15 mm long, immediately above the inferior knee of the duodenum, the surgeon taking account of the fact that the papilla is usually located at the junction of the lower third with the upper two-thirds of the second portion of the duodenum (Fig. 46.7).

The duodenal incision may be longitudinal or transverse, both types being suitable, provided that the suture of such incisions is always transverse. The authors prefer a longitudinal incision because if the retractor on the duodenum widens the duodenotomy, this occurs longitudinally; in the

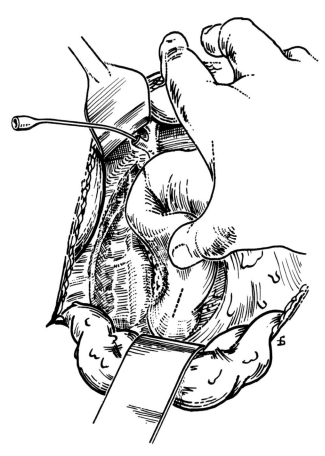

Fig. 46.6 It is important to expose and mobilize the third portion of the duodenum so as to make identification and operation on the papilla easy and to allow facile closure of the duodenotomy.

case of a transverse duodenotomy any inadvertent extension would cause a transverse enlargement of the wound.

IDENTIFICATION OF THE PAPILLA

Following the duodenal incision the papilla is readily visualized on the medial duodenal wall in some 15 to 20% of cases; it appears as a roundish elevation with a central orifice. When the papilla is not readily visible it should be detected by displacement and flattening of the mucosal folds. This should be done with great care to avoid tearing of the mucosa which would hinder good visualization. Identification of the papilla, under direct vision, is possible in 80% of cases. If this is not the case, digital palpation can be used running the forefinger, introduced through the duodenotomy, across the medial duodenal wall; the papilla is then identified as a small elevation (Fig. 46.8).

Should digital palpation fail, a small (5–6 Fr) Nelaton's catheter can be introduced via the cystic duct stump and advanced downwards to emerge at the papilla. This maneuver should never be performed with rigid catheters since they may result in the formation of false passages (Barraya et al 1974). A further recently introduced possibility consists of the passage of a 3 mm diameter fiber optic light source introduced through the cystic duct which transilluminates the common bile duct as far as the papilla, making it identifiable even prior to duodenotomy, which can then be performed exactly at the level of the trans-

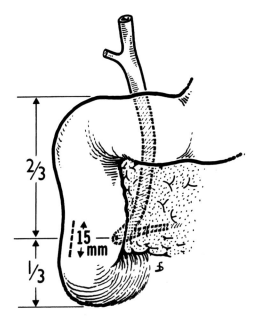

Fig. 46.7 The duodenotomy is performed above the junction of the second and third portions of the duodenum, the surgeon taking into account that the papilla is usually located at the junction of the upper two-thirds and lower third of the second part of the duodenum.

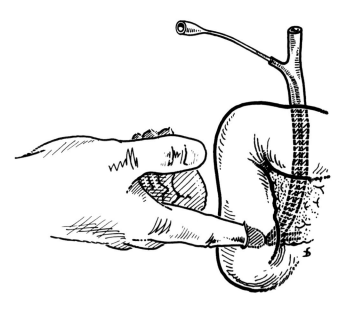

Fig. 46.8 If the papilla is not easily seen, a small Nelaton's catheter is introduced through the cystic duct stump until it is seen to protrude from the papillary orifice. The forefinger, introduced through the duodenotomy, detects the papilla as a small, thick elevation.

illumination. The authors have no personal experience of this technique.

Sometimes a very small papilla is detected and its catheterization is difficult or impossible. In such cases the orifice is probably that of the duct of Santorini, while the major papilla should be searched for in a lower position.

SPHINCTEROPLASTY

Once the papilla has been identified it is exposed by gentle extraction with an Allis's or similar clamp. This is applied laterally and never medially so as to avoid trauma to the duct of Wirsung (Partington 1977) (Fig. 46.9). A Nelaton's catheter (4–5 Fr) is introduced from the outside or via the cystic duct. Following the line of the catheter (and avoiding plastic catheters which melt when surgical diathermy is applied) make a cut using surgical diathermy. This is made superiorly (at '11 o'clock') for 4-5 mm (Fig. 46.10). The authors prefer surgical diathermy because good hemostasis

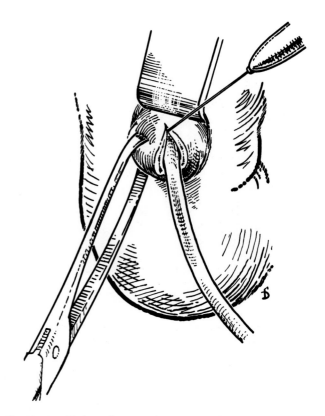

Fig. 46.10 With the Nelaton's catheter as a guide, a cut is made using surgical diathermy on the medial wall of the duodenum extending superiorly and slightly externally ('11 o'clock'). With diathermy good hemostasis is secured.

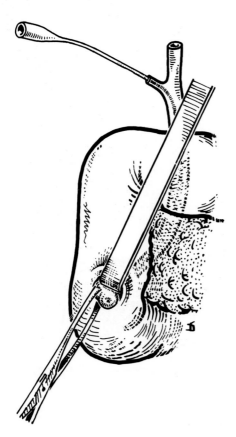

Fig. 46.9 The duodenotomy is kept open by a suitable retractor placed in the upper margin of the duodenal incision. The papilla is exposed by gentle traction with an Allis clamp placed laterally (never medially) to avoid trauma to the duct of Wirsung.

is ensured by this instrument. When a sample for biopsy is required this should be done with a scalpel and taken only from the outer margin of the incision. Possible bleeding from the cut, usually modest, can be arrested with a stitch.

After sphincterotomy two or three stitches are placed between the duodenal mucosa and the wall of the common bile duct on the outer margin using an atraumatic needle and 3–0 silk. Traction is now applied to these sutures and incision of the sphincter is extended for a further 6–7 mm with sutures placed every 2–3 mm (all laterally) until the whole common tract of the sphincter of Oddi is incised (Fig. 46.11). The incision is complete when it is 10–12 mm long and an appropriate forceps can easily be introduced (Fig. 46.12). Its entry into the CBD allows an abundant flow of bile due to distention of its sphincter.

Sutures should be placed only on the outer margin of the sphincterotomy in order to prevent the risk of damage to the duct of Wirsung. The opening of the duct of Wirsung is usually identified as a small orifice from which clear, colorless pancreatic juice flows (see Fig. 46.11).

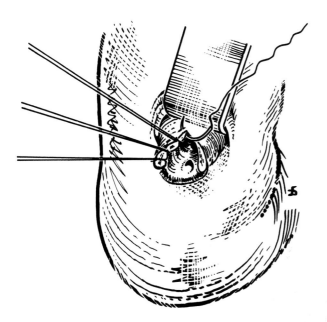

Fig. 46.11 After sphincterotomy is performed several stitches are placed between the duodenal mucosa and the wall of the common bile duct using an atraumatic needle and 3–0 silk. Sutures should be placed only on the outer margin of the sphincterotomy to avoid the risk of damaging the duct of Wirsung which in its distal portion runs inferiorly and medially along the length of the common bile duct.

INSTRUMENTAL EXPLORATION OF THE COMMON BILE DUCT

After sphincteroplasty, instrumental exploration of the CBD and extraction of stones is performed (Speranza et al 1982).

An angled Randall's forceps is introduced into the common bile duct, and the left and right hepatic ducts carefully explored. The maneuver should be repeated several times in order to extract all stones. The next step is to rinse with saline solution, introduced under slight pressure by a Nelaton's catheter (8–9 Fr) and abruptly withdrawn so that, with the siphoning, small fragments flow downstream (Fig. 46.13).

Other means of extraction of stones from the common bile duct are the Fogarty catheter and Dormia basket. The

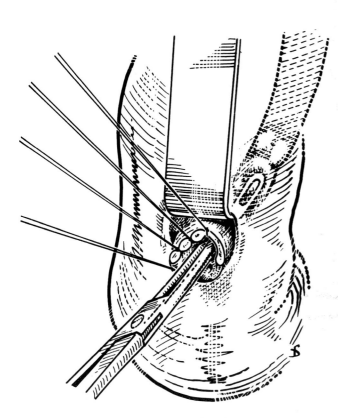

Fig. 46.12 Spincteroplasty is completed when the incision is 10–12 mm long and a Randall's forceps can be easily introduced into the common bile duct to extract stones or other foreign bodies.

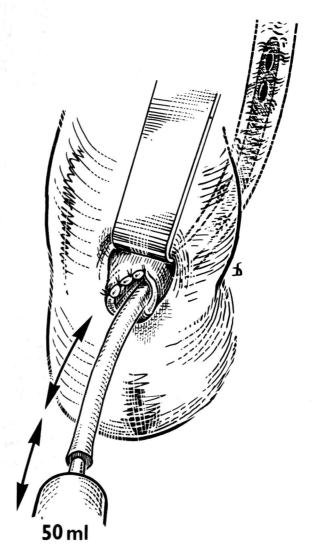

50 ml

Fig. 46.13 After the extraction of stones the common bile duct is rinsed with saline solution introduced under slight pressure with a Nelaton's catheter and with subsequent siphoning so that small fragments can run downstream.

authors have never used these instruments since Randall's forcep and rinsing and siphoning are effective.

The problem of residual stones exists and the best method of prevention is to use choledochoscopy, introducing the endoscope via the sphincteroplasty (Sheridan et al 1987).

DUODENAL CLOSURE

As already emphasized, initial longitudinal duodenotomy should always be closed transversely to avoid stenosis of the duodenum. First, the superior and inferior margins of the incision are approximated and subsequently the resulting gaps are sutured with two extra-mucosal non-adsorbable purse string sutures. Three or four non-adsorbable seromuscular sutures are then added (Fig. 46.14).

It is important that the suture should not be under tension and it is for this reason that preliminary extended mobilization of the duodenum and pancreas is mandatory. The authors have never experienced dehiscence of the duodenal suture using this procedure.

The operation is now complete and the wound is closed without abdominal drains.

COMMENT

It is emphasized that the authors do not perform TSP combined with supraduodenal choledochotomy, which has a higher associated mortality (Sheridan et al 1987). They only use the cystic duct remnant to introduce a Nelaton's catheter in order to assist recognition of the papilla. There is therefore no need to insert a T tube, which lengthens the hospital stay and may predispose the patient to stenosis and infection of the CBD (Sheridan et al 1987, Ratych et al 1991). Patients with no drain tubes and without complications may be discharged on the fifth or sixth postoperative day.

RESULTS

A total of 416 patients were operated upon between 1970 and 1992. Of these patients, 351 were treated during the 15 years between 1970 and 1984, with a mean of 23.4 TSPs each year. In the following 8 years, 65 patients were operated upon, with a mean of 8.1 TSPs per year. Of the 416 patients, 262 were females (63%) and 154 males (37%). The mean age was 54.8 (range 18–92) years. Of these patients, 27.7% were in the sixth and 13.5% in the seventh decades of life.

TSP was most frequently performed for exploration of the CBD for stones (Lechat et al 1976), although in 71 patients (17%) both stones and papillary stenosis were thought to be present. In eight cases (1.9%) primary papillary stenosis and in five cases (1.2%) gallstone pancreatitis were the indications for operation. In four cases, hydatid cyst remnants and membranes obstructing the biliary tree were found at exploration of the CBD.

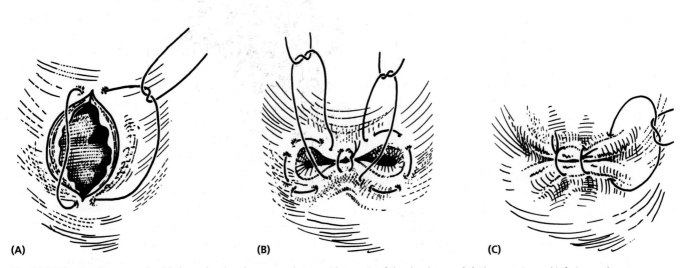

Fig. 46.14 The duodenotomy should always be closed transversely to avoid stenosis of the duodenum. **(A)** The superior and inferior angles are approximated; **(B)** the resulting lateral gaps are sutured with two extramucosal non-absorbable pursestring sutures; **(C)** 3–4 non-absorbable seromuscular stitches are added as a second layer. The sutures should not be under tension.

(A)   (B)   (C)

MORBIDITY AND MORTALITY (Table 46.2)

In 21 cases (5%), postoperative complications occurred and five of these patients (1.2%) died. The most feared complication of this operation, acute pancreatitis, was observed in six cases, two of which proved fatal. There were five cases of postoperative bleeding, resulting from the incision of the sphincter of Oddi in four, and from an acute gastric ulcer in one. Reoperation was not necessary in these cases since bleeding was arrested with conservative measures. Four bronchopulmonary complications were also observed, one of which was fatal. One fatal pulmonary embolism occurred. There was one case with an infected intra-abdominal hematoma and one case of wound infection. Residual stones in the CBD were found to be present in three cases, one of which presented with obstructive jaundice in the immediate postoperative period and required reoperation. The second one presented rapidly progressive and ultimately fatal pyogenic cholangitis, due to the presence of a retained stone. The third patient underwent endoscopic retrieval of the stone.

In those patients without complications (95%), the mean hospital stay was 8.1 (range 6–10) days.

Table 46.2 Postoperative complications and mortality in 416 patients undergoing TSP

Postoperative complications	Observed	Percentage	Deaths	Percentage
Acute pancreatitis	6	1.4	2	0.5
Bleeding				
Sphincter incision	4	1.2	–	
Acute gastric ulcer	1			
Cholangitis and				
retained stones	1	0.2	1	0.2
Retained stones	2	0.5	–	
Infection (wound/ internal abdominal				
hematoma)	2	0.5	–	
Pneumonia	4	1.0	1	0.2
Pulmonary embolism	1	0.2	1	0.2
Total	21	5.0	5	1.2

LONG-TERM RESULTS

A total of 211 patients have been followed for a period of 6 months to 16 years (median 18 years and 5 months). Follow-up clinical data were recorded and, when indicated, laboratory investigation of liver function, ultrasonography, cholangiography, barium meal, gastroduodenoscopy and liver scanning with ^{99m}Tc HIDA were carried out. In selected cases, endoscopic manometry of residual sphincter function was performed (Geenen et al 1980).

The long term results were classified (Stefanini et al 1977, Choi et al 1981) as good in 91% (192 cases) if there was a total absence of symptoms or only modest transient dyspepsia, as fair (15 cases) if dyspeptic symptoms were present, and as poor (four cases) in patients who complained of symptoms identical or worse than those preoperatively. Two of the patients in the last group exhibited duodenal reflux to the CBD at barium meal, probably causing acute pancreatitis in one case 5 years after TSP; a third patient suffered recurrent attacks of cholangitis, and a fourth presented with stenosis of the sphincteroplasty requiring hepaticojejunostomy 3 years after initial operation.

In 29 of the 61 patients followed cholangiographically, a pharmacodynamic test (Jones 1978) was performed, consisting of the intravenous injection of cholecystokinin (Toouli et al 1982) (or its synthetic analogue caerulein), following an intravenous injection of morphine hydrochloride. In 24 of these patients the administration of morphine caused interruption of the flow of contrast medium into the duodenum. This was resumed with the administration of cholecystokinin. This behaviour suggests the presence of residual biliary sphincter activity (Montesani et al 1988). In fact, when a radiological study is performed, air or barium enters the biliary tree only in a minority of patients operated on with TSP (Baker et al 1987).

REVIEW OF RESULTS

In a retrospective analysis of 25 541 TSPs carried out by 130 surgeons in different countries, the early TSP-related complications were bleeding 0.65%, acute pancreatitis 0.60%, dehiscence of duodenal closure 0.55% and cholangitis 0.50%, for an overall morbidity of 2.3% and a mortality rate of 0.8% (Negro et al 1984). In a retrospective study (Sellner et al 1988) it was found that the factors affecting mortality in 2.1% of 333 patients (but only 0.9% for sphincterotomy-related complications) were: age >70 years, bilirubin level >85 mmol/L, diabetes, renal failure and coagulopathy.

The mortality rate increases if supraduodenal choledochotomy is combined with TSP and for patients in whom a T tube is inserted (Sheridan et al 1987, Sellner et al 1988).

A 12 year retrospective study on a series of 53 patients (Baker et al 1987) shows that 90% were very well after TSP. Three patients required further intervention, one for sclerosing cholangitis (not related to transduodenal operation), and two for the development of cholangitis, one with recurrent stones. Three other patients had retained stones that were identified in the early postoperative period.

TSP alone (Hakaim et al 1994) or associated with transampullary septectomy (Kelly & Rowlands 1996), has led to good long-term results in chronic pancreatitis, in recurrent acute pancreatitis even in cases with pancreas divisum, and also in selected patients with abdominal pain of hepatobiliary origin.

REFERENCES

Arianoff A A 1980 Analysis of 607 cases of choledochal sphincterotomy. World Journal of Surgery 3: 483–487

Armstrong C P, Taylor T V, Jeacock J, Lucas S 1985 The biliary tract in patients with acute gallstone pancreatitis. British Journal of Surgery 72: 551–555

Baker A R, Neoptolemos J P, Leese T, James D C, Fossard D P 1987 Long term follow-up of patients with side to side choledochoduodenostomy and transduodenal sphincteroplasty. Annals of the Royal College of Surgeons of England 68: 253–257

Barraya L, Pujol Soler R, Yvergneaux J P, Rozes J, Chauvin P 1974 Surgery of the sphincter of Oddi—Surgical techniques. In: Modern techniques in surgery—digestive surgery. Editions Techniques, Paris, p 1–17

Chigot J P, Clot J P, Cassina I, Mercadier M 1978 La sphincterotomie oddienne, indications, complications, resultats. Annales de Chirurgie 32: 355–360

Choi T K, Wong J, Lam K H, Lim T K, Ong G B 1981 Late result of sphincteroplasty in the treatment of primary cholangitis. Archives of Surgery 116: 1173–1175

Choi T K, Lee N W, Wong J, Ong G B 1982 Extraperitoneal sphincteroplasty for residual stones. Annals of Surgery 196: 26–29

Geenen J E, Hogan W J, Dodds W J, Stewart E T, Arndorfer R C 1980 Intraluminal pressure recording from the human sphincter of Oddi. Gastroenterology 78: 317–324

Gilbert D A, DiMarino A J, Jensen D M et al 1992 Status evaluation: sphincter of Oddi manometry. Gastrointestinal Endoscopy 38: 757–759

Hakaim A G, Broughan T A, Vogt D P, Hermann R E 1994 Long-term results of surgical management of chronic pancreatitis. American Journal of Surgery 60: 306–308

Jones S A 1978 The prevention and treatment of recurrent bile duct stones by transduodenal sphincteroplasty. World Journal of Surgery 2: 473–485

Kelly S B, Rowlands B J 1996 Transduodenal sphincteroplasty and transampullary septectomy for papillary stenosis. Hepatobiliary Surgery 9: 199–207

Kestens P J, Gigot J F, Foxius A, Collard A, Gianello P 1996 Traitement chirurgical de la pancraetite chronique avec atteinte cephalique predominante par double derivation wirsungienne et repermeabilisation canalaire cephalique. Annales de Chirurgie 50: 853–864

Lechat J R, Leborgne J, LeNeel J C, Visset J, Mousseau M 1976 La place actuelle de la sphincterotomie oddienne dans la chirurgie pour lesions benignes de la voie biliaire principale chez l'adulte. Annales de Chirurgie 30: 363–369

Lehman G A, Sherman S 1998 Hypertensive pancreatic sphincter. Canadian Journal of Gastroenterology 12: 333–337

Matsuoka J, Sakagami K, Gouch A, Orita K 1994 A safe, easy technique for transduodenal sphinteroplasty. Journal of the American College of Surgeons 179: 474–476

Montesani C, De Milito R, Narilli P et al 1988 Intraoperative manometry during papillosphincterotomy. Chirurgia Epatobiliare 7: 17–19

Moody F G, Becker J M, Potts J R 1983 Transduodenal sphincteroplasty and transampullary septectomy for postcholecystectomy pain. Annals of Surgery 197: 627–636

Negro P, Tuscano D, Flati D, Flati G, Carboni M 1984 Le risque opératoire de la sphinctérotomie Oddienne. Résultats d'une enquete internationale (25 541 cas). Journal de Chirurgie 121: 133–139

Partington P F 1977 Twenty-three years of experience with sphincterotomy and sphincteroplasty for stenosis of the sphincter of Oddi. Surgery, Gynecology and Obstetrics 145: 161–168

Ramirez P, Parrilla P, Bueno F S, Abad J M, Muelas M S, Candel M F, Robles R, Aguilar J, Lujan J, Sanchez J 1994 Choledochoduodenostomy and sphincterotomy in the treatment of choledocholithiasis. British Journal of Surgery 81: 121–123

Ratych R E, Sitzmann J V, Lillemoe K D, Yeo C J, Cameron J L 1991 Transduodenal exploration of the common bile duct in patients with nondilated ducts. Surgery, Gynecology and Obstetrics 173: 49–53

Seifert E, Gali K, Weismuller J 1982 Langzeitresulate nach endoskopischer Sphinkterotomie. Deutsche Medizinische Wochenschrift 107: 610–614

Sellner F J, Wimberger M, Jelinek R 1988 Factors affecting mortality in transduodenal sphincteroplasty. Surgery, Gynecology and Obstetrics 167: 23–27

Sheridan W G, Williams H O L, Lewis M H 1987 Morbidity and mortality of common bile duct exploration. British Journal of Surgery 74: 1095–1099

Speranza V, Lezoche E, Minervini S, Carlei F, Basso N, Simi M 1982 Transduodenal papillostomy as a routine procedure in managing choledocholithiasis. Archives of Surgery 117: 875–878

Stain S C, Cohen H, Tsuishoysha M, Donovan A J 1991 Choledocholithiasis, endoscopic sphincterotomy or common bile duct exploration. Annals of Surgery 213: 627–634

Stefanini P, Carboni M, De Bernardinis G, Negro P 1977 Long-term results of papillostomy. In: Delmont J (ed) The sphincter of Oddi. Karger, Basel, p 206–212

Toouli J, Geenen J E, Hogan W J 1982 Action of cholecystokinin octapeptide on sphincter of Oddi basal pressure and phasic wave activity in human. Surgery 92: 497–503

Tzovaras G, Rowlands BJ 1998 Diagnosis and treatment of sphincter of Oddi dysfunction. British Journal of Surgery 85: 588–595

Vayre P, Jost J L 1981 La radiomanodebimetrie peroperatorie. Incidences sur la chirurgie des voies biliaires extra-epatiques pour 1600 operes depuis plus de 5 ans. Journal de Chirurgie 11: 625–635

Villalba M R, Lucas R J 1978 Inframesocolic transduodenal approach to the distal biliary-pancreatic ductal system. Archives of Surgery 113: 496–499

Vogt D P, Hermann R E 1981 Choledochoduodenostomy, choledochojejunostomy or sphincteroplasty for biliary and pancreatic disease. Annals of Surgery 193: 161–168

Biliary stricture and fistula

47

Biliary atresia

E.R. HOWARD

DEFINITION

Biliary atresia may be defined as the end result of a destructive inflammatory process of unknown etiology which may affect bile ducts of newborn infants. The condition is associated with intrahepatic changes which have been likened to sclerosing cholangitis and it is of interest that the occurrence of biliary atresia and sclerosing cholangitis has now been recorded in two siblings (Isoyama et al 1995). The incidence throughout the world is constant with a frequency of approximately one case per 12 000 live births, and in the United Kingdom there are therefore approximately 40 new cases per year. Large series of cases have shown a small preponderance of females over males in a ratio of 1.4 : 1.0 (Karrer et al 1990).

Infants with biliary atresia present with jaundice (conjugated hyperbilirubinemia) which is usually noted within the first few weeks of life and examination of the stools shows a complete absence of bile pigment. Abdominal examination may reveal hepatomegaly and splenomegaly which becomes noticeable after 8 to 10 weeks of age. Weight loss and growth retardation also occur with increasing age. Surgery before 8 weeks of age gives the best chance of good bile flow and long term survival but the apparently normal development of the infants at this stage of the disease and the absence of any of the stigmata of chronic liver disease may unfortunately lead to a delay in diagnosis. Spontaneous bleeding secondary to vitamin K malabsorption may be the presenting feature in some of the affected infants.

The delay in diagnosis of biliary atresia is illustrated in a survey of 816 cases reported from more than 100 hospitals in the USA which showed a median age at surgery of 10 weeks (Karrer et al 1990). A similar analysis of 50 consecutive cases treated at our hospital also revealed a median age at operation of 10 weeks (Mieli-Vergani et al 1989).

The best description of the inflammatory process in the bile ducts likens it to a form of sclerosing cholangitis which starts as an extrahepatic lesion of variable distribution (Hays & Kimura 1981). The inflammatory process eventually destroys the whole of the bile duct system and death from cirrhotic liver disease occurs in a majority of untreated cases before 2 years of age (Hays & Snyder 1963).

HISTORICAL

Early single case reports of infants with biliary atresia were published by Home (1813) and Cursham (1840). Thomson (1892), in the first major review of the condition, described the clinical history and gross pathology of the biliary system in 49 cases collected from published reports, and added a further personal case. His description of the typical presentation of affected infants is difficult to improve. He stated:

> 'The children themselves are either jaundiced at birth, or they become so within the first week or so of life; otherwise they are healthy and well nourished. In some cases there is a discharge of normal meconium followed by colourless motions; in others the faeces are devoid of colour from the very first.'

He went on to describe clearly the progressive nature of the inflammatory lesion and reported that most of the children died from spontaneous hemorrhage within the first few months of life.

Holmes (1916) analyzed more than 100 reported cases and stated that the condition was not as rare as was supposed at that time. His important observation was that on gross macroscopic examination at least 16% were suitable for operation with a bile duct to bowel anastomosis. He also discussed diagnosis and suggested that laparotomy was justified as soon as the diagnosis could be established with reasonable certainty—which is in complete agreement with the modern approach to treatment. From the time of Holmes' report, cases of biliary atresia were classified into 'correctable' or 'non-correctable' depending on the presence or absence of a residual segment of bile duct suitable for a conventional type of biliary-enteric anastomosis.

Ladd (1928) provided the first reports of successful surgery in six out of 11 cases submitted to laparotomy. However it now seems that the early reports often confused biliary atresia with choledochal cyst, neonatal hepatitis and inspissated bile syndrome and the overall results of surgical treatment remained extremely poor. Bill (1978), for example, found only 52 reported successes from operation on patients with biliary atresia between 1927 and 1970. A variety of techniques were attempted to try and improve these dismal results including resection and anastomosis of the left lobe of the liver (Longmire & Sandford 1948), the implantation of intrahepatic tubes (Sterling & Lowenburg 1963) and the anastomosis of hepatic lymphatics to the bowel (Fonkalsrud et al 1966). Kasai & Suzuki (1959) developed the present treatment of biliary atresia from their observation that bile drainage could be established after resection of all remnants of the obliterated extrahepatic ducts in a number of cases of 'non-correctable' atresia. Microscopic studies of residual tissue in the porta hepatis showed channels up to 300 μm in diameter which frequently communicated with intrahepatic ducts. Anastomosis of a Roux-en-Y loop of jejunum to the cut surface of the tissue in the porta hepatis is now known as the portoenterostomy procedure, and effective bile drainage has been described in large numbers of patients during the last 20 years. The oldest survivors are now in their third decade.

Liver transplantation is now widely available for patients who fail to improve after a portoenterostomy operation, or for those who progress to cirrhotic liver failure later in life and long-term survival is therefore now achievable in a majority of the patients with biliary atresia. A survey of the world results of the treatment of non-correctable biliary atresia by Carcassonne and Bensoussan in 1977 showed that of 416 patients less than 9.0% of patients survived for more than 3 years. In comparison the results after appropriate treatment with portoenterostomy or transplantation show a dramatic improvement with current long-term survival rates of over 50.0% for portoenterostomy alone. The use of transplantation for the patients who deteriorate after the portoenterostomy procedure increases the overall survival rate to over 80.0% (Davenport et al 1997, Nagral et al 1997, Van der Werf et al 1998).

ETIOLOGY

EXPERIMENTAL

Many attempts have been made to produce an experimental model of biliary atresia. Bile duct lesions have been produced but usually without the progressive hepatic disease typical of the condition.

Okamoto et al (1980) devascularized the whole length of the extrahepatic bile ducts of newborn puppies. Atretic changes with cord-like segments of bile ducts were produced with destruction of epithelium and fibrous thickening of the muscle in the duct wall, but only one animal showed intrahepatic effects. Animals operated on after 14 days of age did not develop atretic lesions, and it was suggested that they were protected by larger intramural vascular channels.

Other experiments have given conflicting results and have been reviewed in detail by Hashimoto et al (1983). Ligation and devascularization of the common bile duct in fetal rabbits, pigs and lambs may cause lesions resembling biliary atresia, but a theory of vascular catastrophe is not really borne out by the clinical observation of normal hepatic arteries and the excellent blood supply to tissue of the porta hepatis in most patients. The production of sclerosing inflammation of the biliary tract in animals is possible after the administration of toxic substances such as Sporidesmin (Ito et al 1980) and the direct injection of sodium morrhuate (Holder & Ashcraft 1967). Outbreaks of biliary atresia have been described in lambs and calves and it has been suggested that this was related to the ingestion of plant toxins by ewes and cows in the early stages of pregnancy (Harper et al 1990). Epidemiological studies in these reports revealed the presence of specific weeds (e.g. *Centipeda cunninghamii*) within the grazing areas which might have been implicated.

No link has been demonstrated with either ionizing radiation (Brent 1962) or teratogenic drugs (Gourevitch 1971), and simple ligation of the common bile duct in fetal lambs caused choledochal cysts rather than atresia (Spitz 1977).

DEVELOPMENT

Miyano et al (1979) have described an abnormally long common channel at the junction of bile and pancreatic ducts in infants with atresia similar to the abnormality found in some cases of choledochal cyst (Howard 1989). This was also demonstrated by Chiba et al (1990) in 28 cases of atresia but not in 7 infants with neonatal hepatitis. It still remains unclear whether the common channel anomaly is of etiological significance or whether it is a coincidental anatomical observation.

Biliary atresia has been reported in association with the trisomy syndromes 17–18 (Alpert et al 1969) and 21 (Danks 1965) which perhaps suggests a genetic factor in etiology. However twin studies do not indicate a simple genetic cause as biliary atresia has been reported in single siblings of both monozygotic and dizygotic pairs (Strickland et al 1985).

Associated anatomical anomalies are found in 10 to 30% of cases (Chandra 1974, Lilly and Chandra 1974, Miyamoto and Kajimoto 1983, Karrer et al 1990). These include situs inversus, polysplenia, and anomalies of the portal venous system and vena cava (Table 47.1). An association with immotile cilia in the respiratory tract has also been described (Gershoni-Baruch et al 1989).

Studies of human embryos have shown a close similarity between the appearances of the developing bile ducts during the first trimester of pregnancy and the abnormal ductules observed in the residual fibrous tissue resected from the porta hepatis during the portoenterostomy operation. It has been suggested from these observations that biliary atresia might be the end result of an interruption in the remodeling process which normally takes place in the bile ducts at the porta hepatis, and that there is a persistence of fetal-type bile ducts. The typical periductular inflammatory reaction might be secondary to bile leakage from these abnormal ducts (Tan et al 1994).

In 25 to 30% of cases the intrahepatic ducts show features which have been defined as 'ductal plate malformation' which implies a partial or complete persistence of the embryonic formation of ducts. In contrast the majority of cases possess ducts with a mature type of tubular shape but with epithelial damage and duct destruction (Desmet & Callea, 1991).

Table 47.1 Anomalies observed in 87 (11.5%) out of 758 children with biliary atresia

Anomaly	Number of patients
Gastrointestinal	
Malrotation	11
Situs inversus	5
Splenic	
Polysplenia	11
Bifid spleen	9
Asplenia	1
Vascular	
Preduodenal portal vein	5
Absent inferior vena cava	3
Cardiac	
Ventricular septal defect	11
Dextrocardia	3
Genitourinary	
Cystic kidneys	6
Hydronephrosis	2

(From Miyamoto & Kajimoto, 1983).

There are two pieces of evidence for the early onset of biliary atresia in the fetus. Redkar et al (1998) described the antenatal ultrasound detection of 3 cases as early as 16 weeks gestation, and collected five further cases from the literature. In another study MacGillivray et al (1994) reported low levels of the enzyme gamma-glutamyl-transpeptidase (GGT) in amniotic fluid samples taken from mothers whose infants were later proven to have biliary atresia. GGT, which is synthesized in the liver, is normally passed into the gut of the fetus and then into the amniotic fluid via the rectum at approximately 15 weeks of gestation. Both of these studies suggest that the biliary tract has become occluded by the end of the first trimester.

METABOLIC

Vacanti & Folkman (1979) investigated the effect of the amino acid L-proline on the development of the biliary tract of the mouse. Intraperitoneal infusion was associated with epithelial proliferation and enlargement of proximal bile ducts although there was no effect on intrahepatic structures. Investigation of four infants with biliary atresia, three with bile duct hypoplasia and one each with choledochal cyst and neonatal hepatitis revealed low levels of L-proline and high levels of the precursor L-glutamic acid. The authors postulated that reduced hepatic synthesis of the amino acid L-proline during postnatal growth of the biliary tree may result in anatomical abnormality of the bile ducts. A toxic effect of monohydroxy bile acids on the hepatobiliary system has also been proposed (Jenner & Howard 1975) and injection of lithocholic acid into pregnant rabbits was associated with obstructive lesions in the biliary tract in two of the offspring.

VIRAL STUDIES

An etiological relationship between biliary atresia, choledochal cyst and neonatal hepatitis syndrome was proposed by Landing (1974), and he suggested that all of these conditions could be included in the term 'obstructive infantile cholangiopathy'. A viral origin had previously been suggested (Strauss & Bernstein 1968) but attempts to isolate viruses from the liver and biliary tracts of patients with 'obstructive cholangiopathy' were unsuccessful. However, Morecki et al (1983) reported studies of the hepatotropic Reo 3 virus which produces antibodies detectable in 50% of adults. Phillips et al (1969) reported that 21-day-old weanling mice developed chronic liver disease and obstructive jaundice after exposure and Morecki et al (1983) studied the development of the pathological changes in the porta hepatis which have a remarkable similarity to those found in the biliary tract of infants with biliary atresia. However Reo 3 virus was not identified in a study of infants with biliary atresia, although 68% of patients possessed antibodies compared with 8% of age-matched controls. The authors suggested a causal relationship between Reo 3 virus and human biliary atresia but this has been disputed in other reports, (Brown et al 1988).

Viral particles have not been observed in biliary atresia tissue examinations with sophisticated techniques such as polymerase chain reaction (PCR), (Parashar et al 1992).

ACQUIRED BILIARY ATRESIA

Damage to the extrahepatic bile ducts in early infancy may lead to bile duct occlusion from stricturing and an erroneous diagnosis of congenital atresia. Of 3 infants presenting with obstructive jaundice, 2 were secondary to the well recognized condition of spontaneous perforation of the bile duct whilst the third case was related to previous surgery for duodenal and ileal atresias (Davenport et al 1996). In contrast to cases of congenital atresia these three infants had dilated but otherwise normal intrahepatic ducts and corrective surgery (hepatico-jejunostomy) was followed by a complete correction of liver function.

PATHOLOGY

The intrahepatic histology in infants with biliary atresia is typical of any bile duct obstruction in this age group, showing widening of all the portal tracts with edema and fibrosis and proliferation of bile ductules. Bile stasis is present within canaliculi and hepatocytes. In contrast with hepatitis the liver architecture is preserved in the first few weeks of life but unrelieved cholestasis leads eventually to hepatocellular damage associated with the formation of multinucleate giant hepatocytes. Hepatocellular necrosis, giant cell formation and inflammatory cell infiltrate in the hepatic parenchyma are classic features of hepatitis but all may be seen occasionally in biliary atresia and this reduces the accuracy of liver biopsy in the two conditions to approximately 83% (Manolaki et al 1983). Intrahepatic changes similar to those of biliary atresia are seen in alpha-1-antitrypsin deficiency which accounts for between 10 and 20% of infants presenting with the hepatitis syndrome and PAS-positive inclusions, which are characteristic of this disease in later life, may be absent. Alpha-1-antitrypsin phenotyping is therefore essential in the investigation of infants with conjugated hyperbilirubinaemia. Histological confusion may also occur with intrahepatic biliary hypoplasia which also pre-

sents as persistent jaundice in infancy and which may be associated with failure to thrive. Liver biopsy shows inflammatory changes within the parenchyma as well as the portal tracts but in contrast with biliary atresia the bile ductules are absent or sparse. A syndromic form of hypoplasia includes a characteristic facial appearance, pulmonary stenosis, vertebral anomalies, hypogonadism and other abnormalities (Alagille et al 1975).

The morphology of the extrahepatic ducts is very variable and the original description of 'correctable' or 'non-correctable' atresia which depended on the presence or absence of a residual segment of patent bile duct has now been replaced by the classification of the Japanese Society of Pediatric Surgeons (Hays & Kimura 1980) which describes 3 principal types (Fig. 47.1): atresia of the common bile duct which may be associated with a cyst in the porta hepatis (type 1); atresia of the common hepatic duct (type 2); and atresia of the right and left hepatic ducts (type 3) (Hays & Kimura 1980). The classification is extended into subtypes to indicate patency or occlusion of the distal common bile duct and gallbladder as well as the morphological features of the tissue at the porta hepatis but these subdivisions have doubtful prognostic significance on the outcome of surgery. A review of 643 cases from Japan showed a 10% incidence of type 1 and an 88% incidence of type 3 lesions. Type 2 cases were rare and represented only 2% of the series (Ohi et al 1987).

Non-communicating cystic dilatations may occur in any segment of the extrahepatic bile ducts and may suggest an erroneous diagnosis of type 1 atresia or even choledochal cyst. Unless the lumen of any cystic dilatation contains bile it must be regarded as non-communicating and must be resected during surgery.

Kasai et al (1980) have shown that during the first few weeks of life atresia patients possess patent intrahepatic bile ducts which reach the porta hepatis. Three-dimensional studies of the porta hepatis in type 3 disease have revealed that the major intrahepatic ducts divide into many small branches which terminate in the fibrous tissue which replaces the extrahepatic ducts. The number of major intrahepatic ducts progressively decreases with increasing age and this process is accompanied by a proliferation of ductules in the portal tracts which is maximal between six and 10 months of age, after which time it starts to decline. These studies suggest that attempts to establish bile drainage might be most successful if performed before six or eight weeks of age.

Microscopic examination of extrahepatic duct remnants has shown a variety of features which include duct-like structures, inflammatory cell infiltrates and fibrosis. The duct-like structures may be biliary glands, collecting

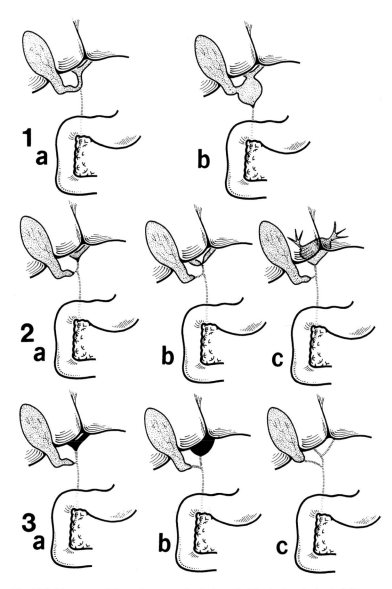

Fig 47.1 Diagrams of the main types of extrahepatic bile duct occlusion in biliary atresia. Types 1 and 2 include the 'correctable' atresias of previous classifications.

ductules, or residual lumina of true bile ducts and the latter generally show at least partial loss of the epithelial lining (Ohi et al 1984). Gautier & Eliot (1981) classified the histological appearances into three main types. Type 1 cases show a complete absence of ducts and few inflammatory cells in the surrounding connective tissue. Type 2 tissue contains small lumina, usually less than 50 µm in diameter, lined by cuboidal epithelium and thought to be biliary glands. Type 3 tissue is identified by the presence of true bile ducts, lined at least in part by epithelium of the columnar type (Fig. 47.2). Bile may be identified within macrophages in more than two-thirds of the type 3 cases.

Several authors have compared the success of biliary drainage after surgical resection of tissue from the porta

hepatis with the histological appearances of the bile duct remnants. It appears that bile flow may be anticipated when the maximum size of residual bile ducts exceeds 150 µm (Altman et al 1975, Ohi et al 1984). However postoperative bile flow has been noted in some cases with much smaller duct remnants and even in patients in whom duct structures were not identified at surgery (Lawrence et al 1981).

A larger study of bile duct remnants resected from 205 infants again analyzed the numbers of residual ductules and the severity of inflammation at the porta hepatis (Tan et al 1994). These features were related to the patient age at the time of surgery and to long-term survival. The long term follow up of the patients showed that poor results were

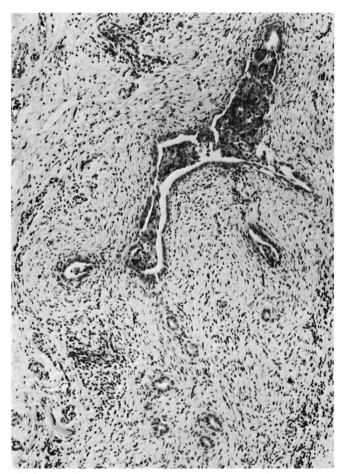

Fig 47.2 Histological appearances of tissue excised from the porta hepatis of a 10-week infant with non-correctable atresia. A large bile duct shows partial destruction of epithelium and smaller biliary ductules are surrounded by fibrous tissue. (Hematoxylin and eosin).

associated with either a small number (or a complete absence) of ductules and an absence of portal inflammation. The common hepatic and common bile ducts were variably affected by the sclerosing atretic process but the extent of the luminal obliteration did not correlate with prognosis.

The response of the hepatobiliary system to surgery must be at least partly dependent on the severity of intrahepatic inflammation and fibrosis (Tan et al 1994) as well as the morphological features of the extrahepatic bile duct tissue. Haas (1978) suggested that the rapid onset of cirrhosis is due both to the bile duct obstruction and to a 'cholangiopathic process akin to that seen in neonatal hepatitis'. The establishment of satisfactory bile drainage after surgery in patients with type 1 disease may be followed by an improvement in the histology of intrahepatic ducts. Ducts in type 3 cases, however, never become normal although there may be a reduction in the severity of hepatic fibrosis and inflammatory cell infiltrate (Ito et al 1983).

There does not seem to be any correlation between preoperative hepatic histology and the response to surgery. Dessanti et al (1985), for example, could not relate the severity of portal fibrosis to surgical results and Altman (1978) found no correlation between resolution of jaundice and the 3 histological parameters of hepatic fibrosis, inflammation and giant cell formation. Similarly there was no correlation between histological criteria and short-term surgical outcome in the author's own cases (Mieli-Vergani et al 1989).

Two studies of long-term jaundice-free survivors did show a disappointing progression of hepatic fibrosis in 73% (Altman et al 1975) and 70% (Gautier et al 1984) of the children.

A study of the innervation of the liver demonstrated a distribution of nerve fibers around the hepatic arteries, portal vein and bile ducts both in the porta hepatis and in the hepatic lobules of normal livers. In contrast an examination of biopsy specimens from 15 infants with biliary atresia showed that, in common with other liver diseases, there was a proliferation of nerve fibers around branches of the hepatic artery and portal vein but that there was a total absence of innervation in the hepatic lobules and around the proliferating bile ducts. (Iwami et al 1997). The authors suggested that this original observation of a lack of parenchymal innervation might have a role in disease progression to cirrhosis.

ASSOCIATED ANATOMICAL ABNORMALITIES (Table 47.1)

A review of ten series of operations for biliary atresia showed additional anatomical abnormalities in 21% of the patients (Silveira et al 1991). Cardiovascular, splenic (polysplenia and asplenia), gastrointestinal (malrotation and situs inversus) and genitourinary abnormalities are found most frequently and a preduodenal portal vein is not uncommon. Examples of all of these have been recorded in the author's personal series of cases but the commonest association is with the polysplenia syndrome (i.e. polysplenia, situs inversus, dextrocardia, preduodenal portal vein and anomalies of the inferior vena cava) which was present in 7.5% of 308 cases of atresia (Davenport et al 1993). In this report we suggested the term 'biliary atresia-splenic malformation', or BASM, for this constellation of abnormalities. Asplenia occurred in two cases and a double spleen in one. One of the infants with asplenia also had immotile respiratory cilia (Kartagener's syndrome), cavernous transformation of the portal vein and malrotation of the gut. The etiology of polysplenia is not known although it must result from an antenatal insult at a critical time in organ formation early in embryogenesis—probably between 30 and 40 days gestation.

Chromosomal abnormalities have been associated with biliary atresia and have included trisomy 18 (Alpert et al 1969), and trisomy 21 (Stowens 1959), and this is further evidence of an embryological origin for the condition.

INVESTIGATIONS (Table 47.2)

Accurate and rapid investigation is essential in the infant with suspected biliary atresia so that surgery can be undertaken before seven weeks of age. Obstructive jaundice in older children and adults can be readily separated from 'medical' jaundice in approximately 80% of cases by history, clinical examination and biochemical test of liver function. In early infancy, however, hepatocellular disease, intrahepatic bile duct disorders (hypoplasia) and obstructive lesions of the extrahepatic bile ducts (biliary atresia, choledochal cyst, etc) all have similar clinical and laboratory features. Jaundice, dark urine and pale stools, the signs of conjugated hyperbilirubinemia, are found in all three groups. Hepatomegaly is common and all groups are prone to bleeding (e.g. intracranial hemorrhage) from malabsorption of the fat soluble vitamin K. Liver function tests are usually unhelpful in infantile cholestasis as there is an element of hepatocellular injury in all types which is reflected in elevated serum transaminase, gamma glutamyl transpeptidase, alkaline phosphatase and alphafetoprotein levels. Further problems in diagnosis are caused by a lack of intrahepatic bile duct dilatation which limits the usefulness of ultrasonography except in the rare case of choledochal cyst. Hepatobiliary excretion scans using technetium labeled agents are now used routinely for diagnosis (Dick & Mowat 1986) and their sensitivity has been enhanced by the prior administration of a 3 day course of phenobarbitone.

A firm diagnosis of biliary atresia requires a battery of tests (Table 47.2) for the exclusion of infective, metabolic, genetic and endocrine causes of jaundice and a percutaneous liver biopsy which is often of crucial importance. Duodenal aspiration and analysis of the aspirate for bilirubin pigment is commonly used in Japan but, whilst the presence of bilirubin excludes a diagnosis of atresia, false negative results may be obtained in severe hepatitis syndromes. Laparoscopy and guided percutaneous cholangiography have also been used in infants (Sunaryo & Watkins 1983).

The difficulties in separating the causes of infantile obstructive jaundice were illustrated in an analysis of diagnostic tests in 85 jaundiced infants (Manolaki et al 1983). Serum bilirubin and liver enzyme values were unhelpful. Radioisotope excretion was reported absent in 97% of infants with biliary atresia but was also absent in 67% of the children with hepatitis syndromes. Percutaneous liver biopsy was the most reliable investigation with an accuracy greater than 82%.

Direct visualization of the biliary tract in infants is now possible with small side viewing endoscopes (PJF endoscope, Olympus Keymed, England). Takahashi et al (1987) reported an 87% diagnostic success rate with endoscopy in infants with persistent jaundice, and similar results have been obtained by Heyman et al (1988). In further studies, Guelrud et al (1991) and Ohnuma et al (1997) reported ERCP examinations in a total of 74 patients with atresia. Accurate diagnoses were obtained in 67 (90%) of the cases and the variability in the length of atretic bile duct was clearly demonstrated in both studies.

An accurate preoperative diagnosis of bile duct obstruction is extremely important in these infants as the patent extrahepatic bile ducts in hepatitis syndrome and bile duct hypoplasia are minute. Their patency may not be proven even with the most careful intraoperative cholangiography and this has led to false diagnoses of biliary atresia and unnecessary surgery on the bile ducts (Kahn & Daum 1983).

Table 47.2 Investigation of infantile cholestasis

Hematology
Liver function tests
Screening tests for infective, metabolic, endocrine and genetic causes of cholestasis
Ultrasonography
Hepatobiliary radionuclide imaging
Duodenal aspiration
Endoscopic retrograde cholangiography
Percutaneous liver biopsy
Laparoscopy
Operative cholangiography

SURGICAL TREATMENT

Before the advent of sophisticated investigations it was usual to confirm a diagnosis of biliary atresia by limited laparotomy. This was performed through a short transverse incision in the right hypochondrium when the diagnosis might be obvious from the atretic appearances of the gallbladder. Operative cholangiography through the gallbladder was performed whenever the gallbladder and cystic ducts were patent (approximately 25% of cases) and the procedure was terminated by taking a generous wedge biopsy of the liver. A more extensive laparotomy was undertaken a few days later if macroscopic appearances, cholangiography and histology suggested atresia rather than hepatitis.

Most cases of biliary atresia are now diagnosed preoperatively and the surgeon must be prepared to perform either hepaticojejunostomy for the type 1 cystic disease found in approximately 10% of cases, or the more radical portoenterostomy procedure for the remainder. Anomalies such a polysplenia, situs inversus and preduodenal portal vein, must also be expected in a significant number.

PREOPERATIVE PREPARATION

The prothrombin time can generally be corrected to normal by the intramuscular injection of vitamin K (1.0 mg/day for four days). The bowel is prepared by the oral administration of neomycin (50 mg/kg/day in six divided doses for 24 hours) and one unit of blood is crossmatched. Oral fluids are withheld for four hours before operation. The child is placed supine on a heated operating table which is thermostatically controlled and which contains facilities for intraoperative cholangiography. An adequate intravenous line is set up, a rectal temperature probe inserted and the first intravenous dose of a broad-spectrum antibiotic (e.g. a cephalosporin) is given at the induction of anesthesia.

HEPATICOJEJUNOSTOMY FOR CYSTIC TYPE 1 ATRESIA (Fig. 47.3)

The abdomen is opened through a transverse upper abdominal incision which extends across both rectus muscles and divides the falciform ligament. A record is made of the size of the spleen, the size and texture of the liver and any ascites, portal hypertension or anatomical anomalies outside of the biliary tract such as situs inversus, preduodenal portal vein or polysplenia. The gallbladder, which may be hidden within a cleft between segment V and the quadrate lobe, is examined for patency. A shrunken, fibrotic gallbladder suggests a diagnosis of atresia and precludes operative cholangiography. A patent gallbladder should be aspirated and intubated for X-ray studies. A clear mucoid fluid is generally present in the gallbladder but when bile is obtained in the aspirate the diagnosis is either a cystic type-1 lesion or a hepatitis syndrome with a patent extrahepatic biliary system and cholangiography is mandatory.

Cystic dilatation of the proximal hepatic ducts is usually visible during the examination of the gallbladder. An operative cholangiogram (Fig. 47.4) may show a communication via the cystic duct or bile may be aspirated from the cyst by direct puncture.

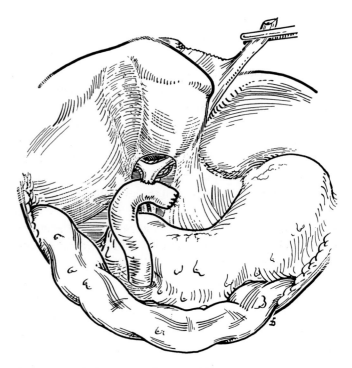

Fig 47.3 Hepaticojejunostomy for type 1 biliary atresia.

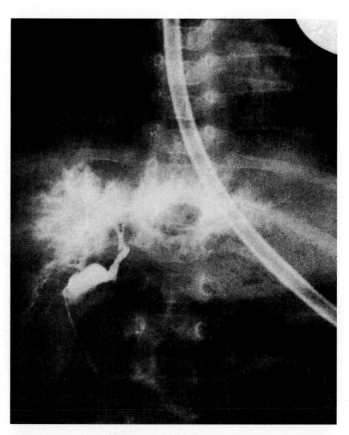

Fig 47.4 Intraoperative cholangiogram in a 3-month infant with type 1 biliary atresia. The hepatic ducts and gallbladder are patent and in communication with the intrahepatic ducts but the common bile duct is occluded.

The confirmation of a cystic type-1 lesion is followed by the operation of hepaticojejunostomy which is facilitated by mobilization of the liver. The left and right triangular ligaments are divided to allow displacement of the bulk of the liver into the abdominal wound. This maneuver gives exceptionally clear visualization of the porta hepatis in the infant (Fig 47.5). The gallbladder is dissected from its bed after division of the cystic artery between ligatures. Traction on the gallbladder allows identification of the atretic segment of distal common bile duct which is divided. The cystic segment is mobilized from the adjacent hepatic artery and portal vein and transected between stay sutures at its widest diameter. A Roux-en-Y loop of proximal jejunum, 40 cm in length, is prepared and passed in a retrocolic position to the porta hepatis. The open end of the Roux loop is closed in two layers and an end-to-side anastomosis constructed between the cyst and the bowel using interrupted sutures of 5–0 polydioxanone (PDS), in a single layer. Transanastomotic tubes are not used. A drain is placed in the subhepatic space and the abdominal wound closed in layers.

It should be emphasized that this procedure is only rarely possible in cases of biliary atresia and good communication with the intrahepatic ducts must be demonstrated on cholangiography.

PORTOENTEROSTOMY (Figs 47.7A–H)

A convenient biliary-enteric anastomosis is not possible in a majority of cases of biliary atresia, when the proximal hepatic ducts are either very narrow (type 2) or completely occluded (type 3). The demonstration of bile drainage from microscopic channels after transection of these abnormal hepatic ducts led Kasai to the development of the porto-enterostomy procedure in which a Roux-en-Y loop of jejunum is anastomosed to the edge of the area left in the porta hepatis after excision of all remnants of extrahepatic bile ducts.

The initial stages of the portoenterostomy procedure are identical to those performed for hepaticojejunostomy and include mobilization of the liver to expose the porta hepatis. In a proportion of cases the cystic and distal common bile ducts are patent and contrast medium will flow from the gallbladder into the duodenum (Fig. 47.6). However the proximal atretic ducts will not be visualized even after occlusion of the supraduodenal portion of the common bile duct with a small vascular clamp. The operation commences with complete mobilization of the gallbladder which is used as a guide to the fibrous remnant of the common hepatic duct (Fig. 47.7B and 47.7C) which may be obscured by thickened peritoneum and enlarged lymph nodes. The bile duct

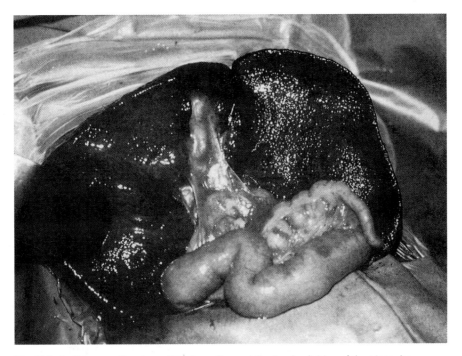

Fig 47.5 An intraoperative view of the liver after mobilization by division of the triangular ligaments. The liver has been lifted into the abdominal wound to give good access to the structures of the porta hepatis.

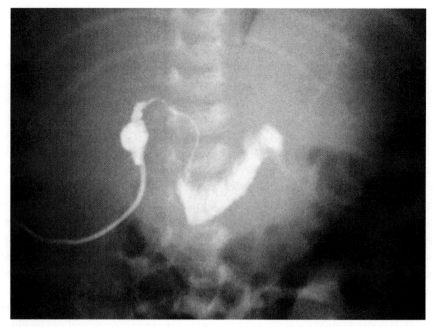

Fig 47.6 Operative cholangiogram in a 10-week infant with type 3 biliary atresia. The gallbladder and distal common bile duct are patent but the hepatic ducts are completely occluded.

remnants are dissected free of the hepatic artery and portal vein which are exposed throughout their course in the porta hepatis (Fig. 47.7D).

The distal portion of the common bile duct is divided between ligatures at the upper border of the duodenum and the gallbladder and attached ducts are dissected towards the porta hepatis. Small vessels and lymphatics are ligated meticulously to prevent postoperative ascites from a leak of lymph. The dissection continues to the bifurcation of the portal vein (Fig. 47.7E) and both left and right veins are exposed. It is necessary to divide 2 or 3 short tributaries of the portal vein which run directly from the bile duct remnants (Fig. 47.7F). The bile duct tissue is removed by a transection which is parallel to the liver capsule and which extends behind the posterior surface of the portal vein. The transection is made as wide as possible within the area bounded by the right and left portal veins (Fig. 47.7G) and the atretic gallbladder is removed in continuity with the residual bile duct tissue (Fig 47.8). Bleeding points in the porta hepatis are controlled by direct pressure.

Finally a 40 cm Roux-en-Y loop of jejunum is prepared, the distal cut end oversewn, and passed in a retrocolic position to the hilum of the liver (Fig. 47.7H). An anastomosis is constructed between the edge of the transected area at the hilum and the side of the Roux loop with interrupted sutures of 5–0 polydioxanone (PDS). All of the sutures of the posterior row are placed in position before the loop is 'rail-roaded' into position. The sutures are tied and the

anterior row completed. The operation is completed by placing a drain in the subhepatic space.

The critical part of the portoenterostomy procedure is the removal of the residual biliary tract tissue flush with the liver capsule at the porta hepatis. Microscopic biliary ductules emerging from the liver must not be damaged and dissecting scissors have been designed to facilitate the tissue excision. The points of the scissors are sharp to cut fibrous tissue and are angled at 45 degrees to allow the line of section to parallel the portal plate (Davenport & Howard 1991) (Fig. 47.9).

CUTANEOUS ENTEROSTOMY (Fig 47.10)

Episodes of ascending bacterial cholangitis occur in approximately 40% of patients after operation, although in many cases this is restricted to one attack. Surgical attempts to reduce this complication have involved the cutaneous diversion of bile to prevent high intraluminal bowel pressure and infection from reaching the portoenterostomy anastomosis. Many ingenious stomas have been described (Howard 1991) but their beneficial effect on the incidence of cholangitis has not been proven (Altman 1983, Burnweit & Coln 1986), (Table 47.3). There was no reduction in the incidence of cholangitis in a personal series of cases in which the author added a cutaneous enterostomy and he has now returned to the original Kasai operation. Furthermore, complications of dehydration, hyponatremia, intussusception and bleeding from the stoma edge were all encountered in

Table 47.3 An example of the failure of biliary diversion to modify or reduce the incidence of cholangitis after portoenterostomy

	No diversion	Diversion
Number of patients	19.0	12.0
Episodes of cholangitis	6.0 (32%)	4.0 (33%)
Two year survival	14.0 (82%)	7.0 (58%)

(From Burnweit & Coln, 1986).

the patients with cutaneous bile drainage. An analysis of 648 Japanese patients showed that 43% of the patients suffered episodes of cholangitis in spite of the almost universal use of some form of biliary diversion (Ohi et al 1987). The authors concluded that the first episode of infection usually occurred between one and three months after portoenterostomy and that there was no difference in incidence between those who were treated with the standard portoenterostomy and those who were given the Roux loop modifications.

Stomas are therefore no longer recommended. They do not prevent cholangitis and they may be complicated by episodes of dehydration and hyponatremia. The almost inevitable formation of varices at the mucocutaneous junction of the stoma may lead to frequent bleeding which can be extremely difficult to control (Smith et al 1988). The stomas also complicate hepatic transplantation surgery which may be required later in some of these patients.

PORTOCHOLECYSTOSTOMY (Fig. 47.11)

An anastomosis between the gallbladder and the transected area in the porta hepatis may be possible after patency of the gallbladder and distal common bile duct has been demonstrated with cholangiography. There does appear to be a reduced incidence of cholangitis after this operation and Karrer et al (1990), in a survey of 670 children on the North American Biliary Atresia Registry, reported a reduced incidence of 35% compared with 55% for other types of portoenterostomy. However the benefits of reduced cholangitis have to be balanced against an increase in technical complications after portocholecystostomy which include bile leaks, gallbladder obstruction and kinking of the common bile duct (Lilly 1979, Freitas et al 1987).

POSTOPERATIVE CARE

Intravenous fluids and nasogastric drainage are continued until bowel activity returns. Any unexplained pyrexia accompanied by deteriorating liver function tests suggests cholangio-hepatitis and the responsible organisms must be identified from blood and liver cultures. *E. coli*, Proteus and Klebsiella are commonly responsible for these infections.

Systemic antibiotics are continued for 5 days after operation and are then replaced by oral prophylaxis for 3 weeks.

Phenobarbitone, and cholestyramine are given to try and maximize bile flow although randomized prospective trials have not demonstrated any definite advantage (Vajro et al 1986). The fat soluble vitamins D and K are essential for metabolic and coagulation functions and are also prescribed in all cases for at least one year after surgery.

Although there have been no controlled trials on the use of post-operative steroid therapy, their use in infants who have suffered cholangitis or poor bile flow has been encouraging. Karrer and Lilly (1985), for example, compared 16 patients who received a week of treatment with 10 mg/kg/day of prednisolone with a group of 16 who received antibiotics alone. The results showed a significant early increase in bile output in the steroid-treated patients but the long-term results were not given.

When the child is discharged from hospital the parents and the referring hospitals are given full details of the operative procedure and information on the recognition, hazards and treatment of any attacks of cholangitis.

The establishment of satisfactory bile drainage and the clearance of jaundice is difficult to predict after these operations. Serum bilirubin may fall to normal at any time between three weeks and six months later and histological analysis of the tissue from the porta hepatis is of prognostic significance only if ducts greater than 150 µm in diameter are identified (Howard 1991).

Davenport and Howard (1996) studied the macroscopic appearances of the liver and bile duct remnants at the time of surgery. A scoring system was devised to take into account the consistency of the liver (soft or hard), the size of the remnant of atretic bile duct in the porta hepatis, and any associated abnormalities such as the polysplenia syndrome. Detailed analysis in 30 infants showed a correlation between the time taken for clearance of jaundice and the macroscopic appearance of the porta hepatis and the consistency of the liver.

POSTOPERATIVE COMPLICATIONS AND TREATMENT

Patients who fail to lose their jaundice after operation show a gradual deterioration in liver function, and death commonly occurs between 1 and 2 years of age. In contrast, the prognosis for children who drain bile satisfactorily can be extremely good and there are now several survivors over 20 years of age (Ohi 1991). However, the postoperative progress of patients who lose their jaundice after either

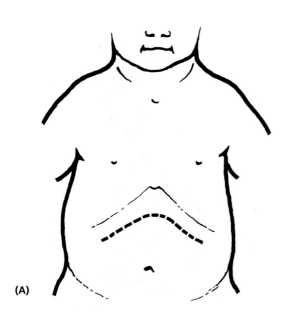

(A)

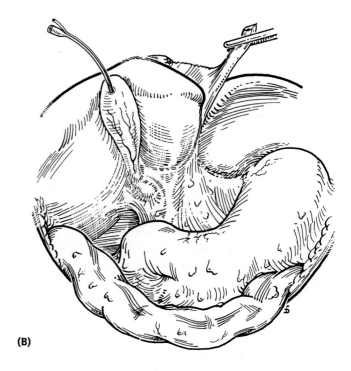

(B)

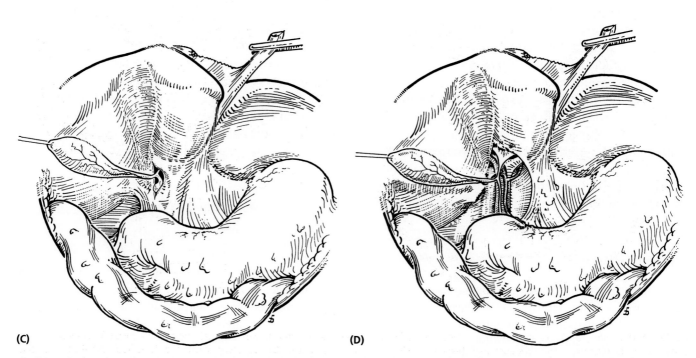

(C)

(D)

Fig 47.7 A–H **(A)** (Abdominal bilateral subcostal incision. **(B)** Mobilization of liver, exposure of gallbladder and operative cholangiogram. **(C)** Dissection of gallbladder from its bed. **(D)** Dissection of structures in the porta hepatis. (*continued*)

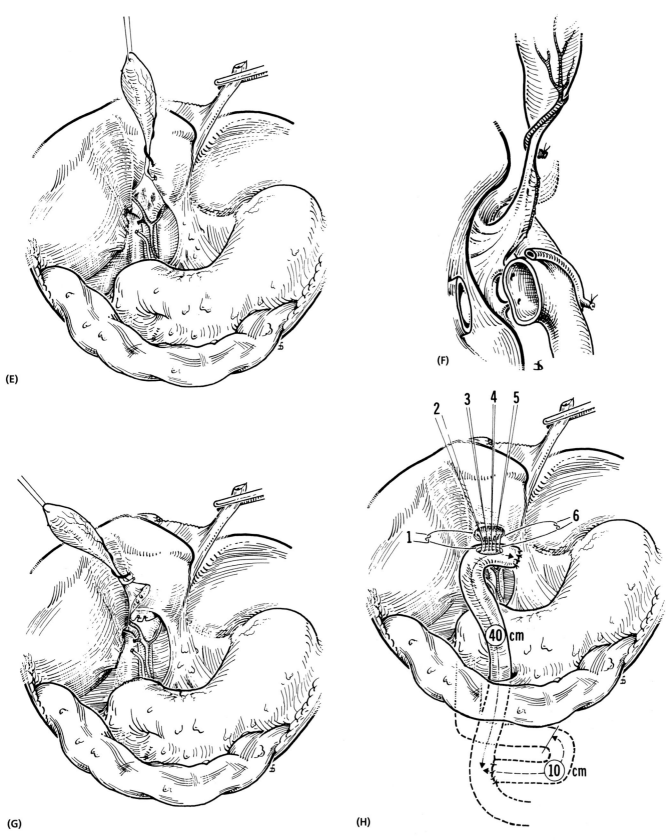

(E)

(F)

(G)

(H)

Fig 47.7 A–H (*continued*) **(E)** Elevation of the gallbladder and bile duct remnants after transection of the distal common bile duct. **(F)** Lateral view of porta hepatis showing the residual bile duct tissue behind the bifurcation of the portal vein. **(G)** Transection of bile duct tissue flush with the liver capsule in the porta hepatis. **(H)** Construction of 40 cm Roux loop of jejunum: note that all of the posterior sutures are placed in position before the Roux loop is 'railroaded' into apposition with the transected tissue of the porta hepatis.

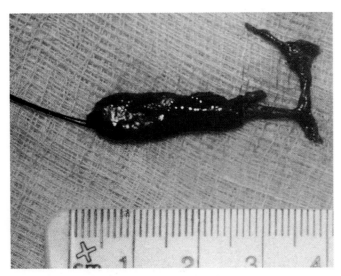

Fig 47.8 An operative specimen showing the resected gallbladder and residual, atretic bile ducts.

hepaticojejunostomy or portoenterostomy may be complicated by bacterial cholangitis, portal hypertension, or a variety of metabolic disorders, and they probably need careful follow-up for the whole of their lives.

BACTERIAL CHOLANGITIS

Infections of the biliary tract may be confidently diagnosed from the triad of pyrexia, rising serum bilirubin and recurrence of acholic stools. These infections are most likely to occur in the first 9 months after surgery but are uncommon in older age groups. The author's experience has shown that cholangitis is rare after 4 years and that the late onset of infection should arouse the suspicion of a possible mechanical cause such as Roux loop obstruction (Fig 47.12).

Ascending bacterial cholangitis is a serious complication, as a permanent deterioration in liver function may follow an attack. Houwen et al (1989) reported a 5 year survival rate of 54% in patients with documented cholangitis, compared with 91% in those who remained infection free after surgery.

It is commonly believed that cholangitis arises by a direct infection from the bowel, but other suggested portals of entry include the portal venous system (Danks et al 1974), the hilar lymphatics (Hirsig et al 1978), and the combination of an infected intestinal conduit with a partially obstructed biliary tree (Lilly 1978).

A diagnosis of intrahepatic infection may be made from blood cultures or, if these are negative, from cultures of percutaneous liver biopsy specimens, and a wide range of Gram-negative organisms may be isolated. Treatment is empirical in the early stages of the illness and usually consists of the systemic administration of a broad spectrum antibiotic such as a cephalosporin and gentamicin.

Prophylactic antibiotics have had little effect on the incidence of cholangitis (Lilly et al 1989) and cutaneous diversion of bile has proved disappointing (Hays & Kimura 1980). It must be emphasized that investigations of patients

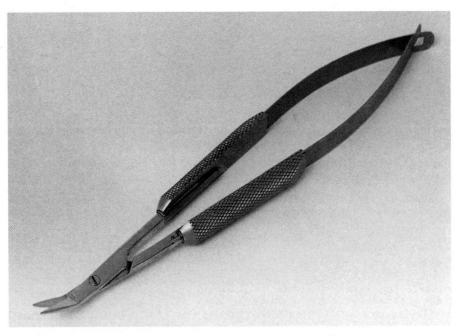

Fig 47.9 Portoenterostomy scissors showing the flat, pointed blades angled at 45°. This instrument facilitates accurate removal of the tissue in the porta hepatis.

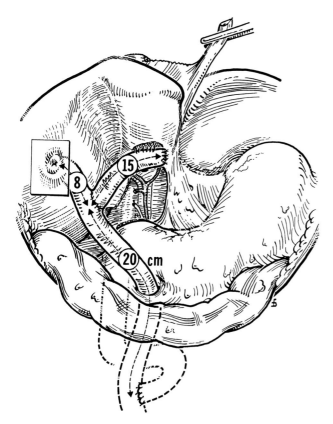

Fig 47.10 The Kasai 2 cutaneous enterostomy in which a stoma is fashioned in the Roux loop. The recommended lengths of bowel are indicated in cm.

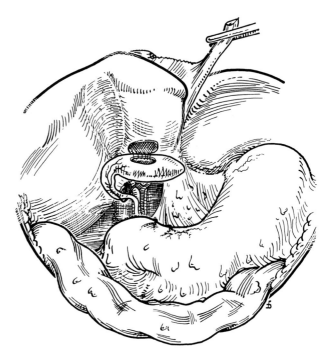

Fig 47.11 Portocholecystostomy. A patent gallbladder and distal common bile duct may be anastomosed to the transected tissue in the porta hepatis in some cases of type 3 biliary atresia.

who present with cholangitis after a long jaundice-free interval should include percutaneous cholangiography (Fig. 47.12) and radionuclide scanning to exclude a surgically correctable obstruction. Three patients in the author's series have benefited from reconstruction of the Roux loop 3 to 6 years after the original portoenterostomy.

PORTAL HYPERTENSION

Hepatic fibrosis is present at the time of diagnosis of biliary atresia and measurements of portal pressure at porto-enterostomy have confirmed the presence of portal hyper-tension in a majority of cases. The fibrotic process often progresses even after successful surgery and follow-up measurements in 16 jaundice-free survivors showed portal pressures between 44 and 135 mm of water. Higher pressures (more than 200 mm of water) were recorded in eight out of 10 in children who had suffered attacks of cholangitis (Kasai et al 1981).

Endoscopy of jaundice-free survivors has revealed oesophageal varices in a large proportion of cases and variceal haemorrhage has been a major problem in 10 to 23% (Lilly & Stellin 1984). Stringer et al (1989) found varices in 67% of children who underwent endoscopy 2.5 years or more after portoenterostomy. However only 28% had a problem with variceal bleeding and as in other reports the problems were worse in those who remained jaundiced after surgery (Ohi et al 1986).

Table 47.4 is a summary of the risk of bleeding in the larger published series of long-term survivors after porto-enterostomy. The figures confirm that the average risk of bleeding was 27%.

Surprisingly the effects of portal hypertension may dimin-ish with age (Odievre 1978), and for this reason injection

Table 47.4 The incidence of bleeding from esophageal varices more than 5 years after portoenterostomy

	Numbers of Patients	Bleeding from varices
Kobayashi et al (1984)	35	7 (20%)
Laurent et al (1990)	40	15 (37%)
Tagge et al (1991)	34	6 (18%)
Valayer et al (1996)	80	19 (24%)
Karrer et al (1996)	35	20 (55%)
Howard & Davenport (1997)	51	8 (16%)
Total	275	75 (27%)

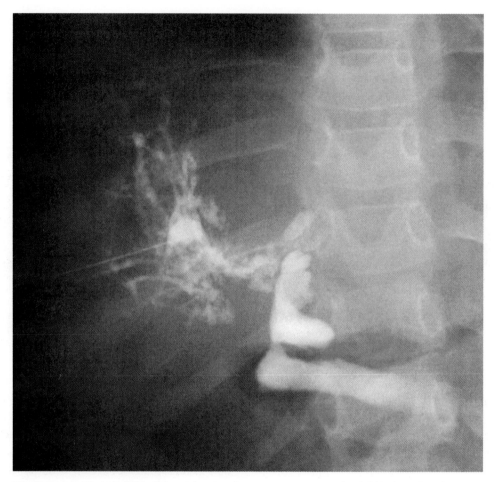

Fig 47.12 Percutaneous cholangiogram six years after portoenterostomy. The child had developed recurrent attacks of ascending cholangitis. The X-ray shows a stricture in the Roux loop of jejunum. Note the abnormal intrahepatic ducts which are typical of the long-term survivor with biliary atresia. The stricture was corrected at six years and the patient is now well at 15 years of age.

sclerotherapy is currently regarded by the author as the treatment of choice. We have demonstrated successful obliteration of bleeding varices in 12 of 16 cases presenting after portoenterostomy (Stringer et al 1989).

Portal hypertension in biliary atresia has also been treated with portosystemic shunting, and Valayer (1991) reported 14 patients treated in this way before the advent of liver transplantation. Shunting still has an occasional role in management, particularly for acute bleeding from ectopic varices distal to the esophagus such as those in the stomach or at anastomotic sites (Heaton & Howard 1993).

The use of transjugular intrahepatic portosystemic stent shunts (TIPS—see Chapter 101) has been reported in 7 cases of children with biliary atresia (Schweizer et al 1995) and as a temporary method of reducing portal pressure in an infant prior to transplantation (Cao et al 1997). Long term results of the technique in children are not yet available although a shunt occlusion rate of 50% at one year, caused

by intimal proliferation with the lumen of the stent, has been reported in adults.

Splenomegaly associated with attacks of abdominal pain, thrombocytopenia and leucopenia is seen in many of the long-term survivors after portoenterostomy and portosystemic shunts have been used for this problem. The prevalence of thrombocytopenia after 2 and 10 years after surgery has been reported as 43% and 25% by Chiba et al (1991) who used splenic embolization as an alternative method of treatment. The procedure was used in 19 children who were between 3 and 13 years of age and in whom the platelet counts varied from 26 000 to 110 000/mm^3. No serious complication was encountered after the embolization of between 45% and 90% of the splenic volume. Nine of the children were re-assessed 4 years later when 41% of the splenic tissue had regenerated in 7 although 2 of the cases showed no restoration of splenic volume. In 7 cases the platelet count showed a fourfold increase, but 2 required re-embolization for persistent thrombocytopenia.

In summary portal hypertension is a problem in many long-term survivors after portoenterostomy. Most esophageal varices can be successfully controlled with either sclerotherapy or banding but a small number of patients may require portosystemic shunting for either bleeding from ectopic varices or hypersplenism. Splenic embolization provides an alternative technique of treatment for the latter complication.

METABOLIC PROBLEMS

Abnormalities in the metabolism of fat, protein, fat and water soluble vitamins, iron, calcium, zinc and copper have all been described in children with chronic liver disease (Greene 1983). The effects are minimized by the regular administration of fat soluble vitamins, particularly D and K, and a multivitamin preparation which includes thiamine, riboflavine, pyridoxine, ascorbic acid and folic acid. Florid rickets may occur occasionally and seems to be the result of poor intestinal absorption rather than impaired metabolism of vitamin D. The condition is rapidly corrected by giving increased doses of vitamin D and ensuring that there is adequate calcium and phosphate in the diet, (Toki et al 1997).

Vitamin E deficiency is not uncommon in young children with cholestatic disease and has been associated with a progressive neurological disorder (Nelson et al 1983), which includes loss of tendon reflexes, a reduction in proprioception and sensation, abnormal eye movements and intellectual deterioration. Histological abnormalities have been described in large caliber sensory axons in the spinal cord and in peripheral nerves.

INTRAHEPATIC CYST FORMATION

Collections of bile (bile 'lakes') separate from the biliary tree are frequently found at autopsy within the central portion of the liver in patients who have never established satisfactory bile drainage. Large intrahepatic cysts, easily detected on ultrasound examination and of variable anatomy, may also occur occasionally in jaundice-free children and may be associated with attacks of jaundice and ascending cholangitis. Tsuchida et al (1994) have suggested a classification of these cysts into three types, depending on their relationship with the biliary tract, as follows: type A—single and non-communicating; type B—single and communicating through a small opening with the Roux-en-Y loop at the porta hepatis; type C—multiple cystic dilatations of irregular intrahepatic bile ducts similar to the intrahepatic dilatation of some types of choledochal cyst.

An example of a type B cyst is illustrated in Fig. 47.13. In this case percutaneous cholangiography and radionuclide

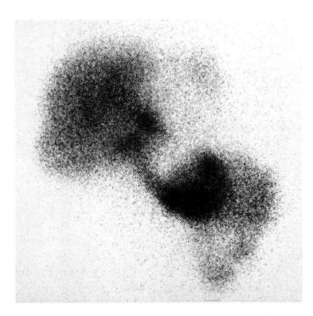

Fig 47.13 Radionuclide scan (DISIDA) four and a half years after portoenterostomy, with good excretion from the right lobe of the liver 25 minutes after injection. A 'cold' area in the left lobe represents a cystic collection of bile.

scanning showed good drainage from the right intrahepatic ducts into the Roux loop but the left lobe was almost totally occupied by a cystic collection of bile. Cystogastrostomy was followed by rapid obliteration of the cyst. Saito et al (1984) reported a similar lesion in a 13-month old child which also disappeared after surgical drainage through the abdominal wall. The origin of these cysts is not understood but they appear to be the end result of a degenerative process.

Approximately 66% of the cysts in Tsuchida's series (1994) were associated with symptoms within 4 years of the portoenterostomy operation. However symptoms did not develop in five of the type C cases until 10 to 28 years after surgery. Although symptoms may be relieved with antibiotics and either percutaneous transhepatic drainage or cyst-enterostomy, the development of this type of intrahepatic pathology is probably an indication for transplantation.

HEPATOPULMONARY SYNDROME AND PULMONARY HYPERTENSION

Hypoxia, with cyanosis which worsens on standing and exertion and which is secondary to intrapulmonary shunting and intrapulmonary vascular dilatation, may occur in patients with biliary atresia just as in patients with other forms of chronic liver disease. The complication, known as hepatopulmonary syndrome, has been observed more commonly in the group of patients with polysplenia syndrome (Valayer 1996).

Pulmonary hypertension, which is well recognized as a complication of cirrhosis in adults, may also occur in long-term survivors after portoenterostomy. The aetiology of these complications is not understood but could be related to vasoactive substances such as endothelin or prostaglandin F2 which are either not metabolized in the liver or which are secreted by endothelial cells.

MALIGNANT CHANGE

Malignant change in cirrhotic livers after portoenterostomy procedures have been reported on at least 10 occasions (Kulkarni and Beatty 1977, Starzl 1983, Valayer 1996). The lesions have included incidental hepatomas found at the time of transplantation performed for liver failure, and cholangiocarcinomas. The possibility of this complication should be borne in mind during the follow-up examinations of the increasing numbers of long-term post-portoenterostomy survivors.

REOPERATION

The results of re-operation on the porta hepatis in a patient who has undergone a correct portoenterostomy procedure are not good unless there is a mechanical problem with the Roux loop of jejunum which can be demonstrated with either radionuclide scanning or with percutaneous cholangiography. In a series of re-operations performed for persistent or recurrent jaundice after failure of portoenterostomy (Suruga et al 1982) only seven out of 33 achieved some increase in bile flow and long-term results are not available. Furthermore only three out of 30 cases responded satisfactorily to re-operation in a series reported by Saito (1983) whilst a larger review of more than 200 re-operations for persistent jaundice revealed satisfactory results in less than 30% (Ohi et al 1987).

Reoperation invariably causes increased numbers of intra-abdominal adhesions which add to the risk of morbidity in any subsequent transplant operation and in view of the poor results is no longer recommended. A failed portoenterostomy operation is now an indication for hepatic transplantation.

RESULTS OF TREATMENT

Any consideration of the current results of treatment for biliary atresia should be compared with the results achieved before the introduction of the operation of portoenterostomy in the 1960s. In a typical series of 41 cases reported by Hays and Snyder in 1963 for example, surgical correction was possible in only one infant and the average age at death was 19 months.

'Correctable' (type 1) forms of biliary atresia treatable by conventional biliary-enteric anastomosis represent only 8 to 15% of cases in most large series. Bile flow is usually seen immediately after surgery but the long-term results have often been disappointing. Kasai corrected 25 type 1 cases between 1953 and 1976 but only 49% achieved long-term jaundice-free survival (Hays & Kimura 1980) and Caccia et al (1983) reported long-term success in only two out of four type 1 cases in a series of 72 patients.

For 'uncorrectable' atresia (types 2 & 3), previously thought to be inoperable, it is now clear that portoenterostomy can result in long-term survival and the results of treatment have improved steadily over the last 25 years. Ohi et al (1990), for example, reported a gradual rise in the numbers of long-term jaundice-free children from 12% in the period 1953–61 to 85% in 1987–88. The numbers of patients surviving more than 10 years also increased from 10% of the patients who underwent operation in the period 1953–67 to 48% of those treated in 1973–77. One of the most important factors contributing to these improvements has been the age at surgery. We have observed bile flow in 86% of infants treated before eight weeks of age compared with 36% of older children (Mieli-Vergani et al 1989).

The overall 5 year survival of 184 cases of biliary atresia treated by the author between 1980 and 1989 (Howard & Davenport 1997) was approximately 39%. Although the total number of operations was much smaller it is of interest that the 10 year survival for the period 1973–1979 was very similar at 43% and collected figures from the major long-term series showed similar results for 5 and 10 year survival (Tables 47.5 & 47.6). However the collected series also showed that although survival is similar at 5 and 10 years, the numbers of children who remained free from jaundice diminished from 25% to 16%.

A further analysis of these cases showed the relationship of successful treatment to the age of infants at the time of surgery and this is illustrated in Table 47.7 which demonstrates that the success rates of operations performed before 8 weeks of age was approximately 67%. This contrasted with a success rate of 36% for those treated at an older age.

It should be emphasized that although most series have shown a greater chance of successful outcome in the younger infant, older infants should not be denied treatment providing that the synthetic ability of the liver, as measured by INR and albumen levels, is reasonable. For example, in a small series of cases Tagge et al (1991),

Table 47.5 5-year survival after portoenterostomy in 6 series

	Survivors	No jaundice
Kobayashi et al (1984)	32/132 (24%)	17 (13%)
Ohi et al (1985)	52/214 (24%)	47 (22%)
Houwen et al (1989)	17/71 (24%)	11 (15%)
Gauthier et al (1991)	31/69 (45%)	23 (33%)
Tagge et al (1991)	19/34 (56%)	7 (21%)
Howard & Davenport (1997)	71/184 (39%)	68 (37%)
Totals	222/704 (32%)	173 (25%)

Table 47.6 10-year survival after portoenterostomy in 4 series

	Survivors	No jaundice
Caccia et al (1991)	13/46 (28%)	8 (17%)
Karrer et al (1996)	23/98 (23%)	19 (19%)
Valayer (1996)	80/271 (30%)	38 (14%)
Howard & Davenport (1997)	17/39 (44%)	9 (23%)
Totals	133/454 (29%)	74 (16%)

Table 47.7 The effect of age at the time of surgery and restoration of bile flow after portoenterostomy in two series

	Under 8 weeks	Over 8 weeks
Mieli-Vergani et al (1989)	12/14 (86%)	13/36 (36%)
Gauthier et al (1991)	31/50 (62%)	52/143 (36%)
Totals	43/64 (67%)	65/179 (36%)

reported that 3 out of 12 cases who underwent operation before 8 weeks of age were alive at 5 years compared with 7 out of 9 operated after 12 weeks. Valayer (1996) also emphasized that 24 out of 38 jaundice-free patients surviving for 10 years underwent surgery later than 8 weeks of age. Therefore although successful biliary drainage is achieved more frequently in younger infants, the relationship between age at surgery and long-term survival is not consistent.

Many long-term survivors show persistently abnormal liver function tests and severe changes in liver histology despite satisfactory bile drainage. Hadchouel et al (1983) examined liver biopsies from 20 patients who had survived at least five years after satisfactory surgery. Cirrhosis was present in all specimens but the degree of fibrosis and the size of regenerative nodules varied. Severe fibrosis was present in 15 of the patients and mild to moderate fibrosis in 5. The portal tracts commonly showed inflammatory infiltrate with mononuclear cells and a surprising observation was the absence of bile ductules within the portal tracts of four patients, all of whom were anicteric.

The long-term prognosis after operation for extrahepatic biliary atresia depends on many factors. Age at operation,

histology of tissue resected from the porta hepatis, the occurrence of ascending cholangitis, the severity of portal hypertension and the progress of intrahepatic inflammatory disease are all important. The experience of the surgeon is also a factor and was highlighted in a survey of surgical results in the United Kingdom (McClement et al 1985). Centers treating one case per year achieved jaundice-free survival in 11% of their patients compared with 29% in centers managing two to five per year. The success rate rose to 43% when more than 5 cases per year were treated.

With regard to quality of life after portoenterostomy the report of Nio et al (1996) is very encouraging. Of 22 patients who have survived for more than 20 years 16 have had near normal lives. Menstruation occurred at the expected ages and normal secondary sexual characteristics were noted in males and females. Three of the women have married and one has given birth to a normal child. Successful pregnancies after portoenterostomy have been recorded by other authors (Howard 1998).

Satisfactory quality of life was reported in 16 of the patients and studies of liver function did not reveal any progressive deterioration. Importantly all of the patients were in employment.

Barkin and Lilly (1980) analyzed the stresses in the parents of children who had undergone surgery for biliary atresia. Problems included divorce, abandonment of the child, unemployment and financial pressure. However it is difficult to draw definite conclusions from this study as the results were not compared with parents looking after children with other types of chronic disease.

LIVER TRANSPLANTATION

Liver transplantation is now a recognized procedure for children in whom portoenterostomy is unsuccessful (Chs 108, 112) and biliary atresia is the single most common indication for the operation in the pediatric age group. It is now a reasonable option for infants who either do not respond to portoenterostomy or who develop intractable complications at a later age.

Biliary atresia was the major indication for pediatric transplantation in Pittsburgh between 1980 and 1986 (Iwatsuki 1987) and 67% were alive 2 to 5 years after the procedure. In the youngest age group under one year of age 12 out of 20 survived transplantation (Esquivel et al 1987).

There has been concern that a previous portoenterostomy might have a deleterious effect on the results of organ replacement but Millis et al (1988) reported no significant differences in intraoperative blood loss or postoperative biliary tract complications between a group of 28 children who had previously undergone portoenterostomy and a group of 8 in whom the transplant was not complicated by previous abdominal surgery. Interestingly the six month survival rate in the children with a previous portoenterostomy was 82% compared with 63% for those with no previous surgery.

Current results for liver transplantation in biliary atresia are summarized in Table 47.8.

Table 47.8 Results of liver transplantation in biliary atresia in three series

	Patient numbers	Survivors
Beath et al (1993)	39	28 (72%)
Valayer et al (1993)	72	62 (86%)
Goss et al (1996)	190	154 (81%)
Totals	301	244 (81%)

CONCLUSION

Advances in the treatment of biliary atresia over the last 30 years have increased the chances of long-term survival after portoenterostomy from 2% to more than 40%. Ten-year survival after portoenterostomy is no longer unusual and liver transplantation is improving the overall results still further. Portoenterostomy should continue to be regarded as the first choice of treatment, preferably before 8 weeks of age, but liver transplantation should be considered an option for children with intractable jaundice, failure to thrive or intractable portal hypertension. The best results for this rare condition will be achieved with an integrated program of management which provides for early porto-enterostomy and later liver transplantation should this be necessary.

REFERENCES

Alagille D, Odievre M, Gautier M, Dommergues J P 1975 Ductular hypoplasia associated with characteristic facies, vertebral malformation, retarded physical, mental and sexual development and cardiac murmur. Journal of Pediatrics 86: 63–71

Alpert L I, Strauss L, Hirschhorn K 1969 Neonatal hepatitis and biliary atresia associated with trisomy 17–18 syndrome. New England Journal of Medicine 280: 16–20

Altman R P 1978 The portoenterostomy procedure for biliary atresia. Annals of Surgery 188: 357–361

Altman R P 1983 Longterm results after the Kasai procedure. In: Daum F (ed) Extrahepatic biliary atresia. Marcel Dekker, New York, ch 9, p 96

Altman R P, Chandra R, Lilly J R 1975 Ongoing cirrhosis after successful porticoenterostomy in infants with biliary atresia. Journal of Pediatric Surgery 10: 685–689

Barkin R M, Lilly J R 1980 Biliary atresia and the Kasai operation: continuing care. Journal of Pediatrics 96: 1015–1019

Beath S, Pearmain G, Kelly D, McMaster P, Mayer A, Buckels J 1993 Liver transplantation in babies and children with extrahepatic biliary atresia. Journal of Pediatric Surgery 28: 1044–1047

Bill A H 1978 Biliary atresia. World Journal of Surgery 2: 557–559

Brent R L 1962 Persistent jaundice in infancy. Journal of Pediatrics 61: 111–114

Brown W R, Sokol R J, Levin M J, Silverman A, Tamaru T, Lilly J R et al 1988 Lack of correlation between infection with Reovirus type 3 and extrahepatic biliary atresia. Journal of Pediatrics 113: 670–676

Burnweit C A, Coln D 1986 Influence of diversion on the development of cholangitis after hepatoportoenterostomy for biliary atresia. Journal of Pediatric Surgery 21: 1143–1146

Caccia G, Dessanti A, Alberti D 1983 An 8 years experience on the treatment of extrahepatic biliary atresia: results in 72 cases. In: Kasai (ed) Biliary atresia and its related disorders. Excerpta Medica, Amsterdam, p 181–184

Caccia G, Dessanti A, Alberti D 1991 More than 10 years after surgery for biliary atresia. In: Ohi R (ed) Biliary atresia, ICOM Associates Inc, Tokyo, p 246–249

Cao S, Monge H, Smeba C, Cox K L, Berquist W, Concepcion W, et al 1997 Emergency transjugular intrahepatic portosystemic shunt (TIPS) in an infant: a case report. Journal of Pediatric Surgery 32: 125–127

Carcassonne M, Bensoussan A 1977 Long-term results in treatment of biliary atresia. Progress in Pediatric Surgery 10: 151–160

Chandra R S 1974 Biliary atresia and other structural anomalies in congenital polysplenia syndrome. Journal of Pediatrics 85: 649–655.

Chiba T, Ohi R, Mochizuki I 1990 Cholangiographic study of the pancreaticobiliary ductal junction in biliary atresia. Journal of Pediatric Surgery 25: 609–612

Chiba T, Ohi R, Yaoita S, Goto M, Nio Masaki, Hayashi Y et al 1991 Partial splenic embolization for hypersplenism in pediatric patients with special reference to its long-term efficacy. In Ohi R (ed). Biliary Atresia, ICOM Associates, Inc, p 154–158

Cursham G 1840 Case of atrophy of the gallbladder with obliteration of the bile ducts. London Medical Gazette 26: 388–389

Danks D M 1965 Prolonged neonatal obstructive jaundice. A survey of modern concepts. Clinical Pediatrics 4: 499–510

Danks D M, Campbell P E, Clarke A M, Jones P G, Solomon J R 1974 Extrahepatic biliary atresia. American Journal of Diseases of Children 128: 684–686

Davenport M, Howard E R 1991 Portoenterostomy scissors: a new instrument for surgery in the porta hepatis. Annals of the Royal College of Surgeons of England 74: 68–69

Davenport M, Howard E R 1996 Macroscopic appearance at portoenterostomy—a prognostic variable in biliary atresia. Journal of Pediatric Surgery 31: 1387–1390

Davenport M, Savage M, Mowat A P, Howard E R 1993 The biliary atresia-splenic malformation syndrome: an aetiological and prognostic subgroup. Surgery 113: 662–668

Davenport M, Saxena R, Howard E R 1996 Acquired biliary atresia. Journal of Pediatric Surgery 31: 1721–1723

Davenport M, Kerkar N, Mieli-Vergani G, Mowat A P, Howard E R 1997 Biliary atresia: The King's College Hospital Experience (1974–1995). Journal of Pediatric Surgery 32: 479–485

Desmet V, Callea F 1991 Ductal plate malformation (DPM) in extrahepatic bile duct atresia (EHBDA). In: Ohi R (ed) Biliary Atresia. ICOM Associates, Inc, Tokyo, p 27–31

Dessanti A, Ohi R, Hanamatsu M, Mochizuchi I, Chiba T, Kasai M 1985 Short term histological liver changes in extrahepatic biliary atresia with good postoperative bile drainage. Archives of Disease in Childhood 60: 739–742

Dick M, Mowat A P 1986 Biliary scintigraphy with DISIDA. A simpler way of showing bile duct patency in suspected biliary atresia. Archives of Disease in Childhood 61: 191–192

Esquivel C O, Koneru B, Karrer F, Todo S, Iwatsuki S, Gordon R D, et al 1987 Liver transplantation before one year of age. Journal of Pediatrics 110: 545–548

Fonkalsrud E W , Kitagawa S, Longmire W P 1966 Hepatic lymphatic drainage to the jejunum for congenital biliary atresia. American Journal of Surgery 112: 188–194

Freitas L, Gauthier F, Valayer J 1987 Second operation for repair of biliary atresia. Journal of Pediatric Surgery 22: 857–860

Gauthier F, Laurent J, Bernard O, Valayer J 1991 Improvement of results after Kasai operation: the need for early diagnosis and surgery. In Ohi R (ed), Biliary atresia, ICOM Associates Inc, Tokyo, 91–95

Gautier M, Eliot N 1981 Extrahepatic biliary atresia: morphological study of 98 biliary remnants. Archives of Pathology and Laboratory Medicine 105: 397–402

Gautier M, Valayer J, Odievre M, Alagille D 1984 Histological liver evaluation 5 years after surgery for extrahepatic biliary atresia: A study of 20 cases. Journal of Pediatric Surgery 19: 263–268

Gershoni-Baruch R, Gottfried E, Pery M, et al 1989 Immotile cilia syndrome including polysplenia, situs inversus and extrahepatic biliary atresia. American Journal of Medical Genetics 33: 390–393

Goss J A, Shackleton C R, Swenson K, Satou N L, Nuesse B J, Imagawa D K et al 1996 Orthotopic liver transplantation for congenital biliary atresia: an 11 year single-center experience. Annals of Surgery 224: 276–284

Gottrand F, Bernard O, Hadchouel M, Pariente D, Gauthier F, Alagille D 1991 Late cholangitis after successful surgical repair of biliary atresia. American Journal of Diseases of Children 145: 213–215

Gourevitch A 1971 Duodenal atresia in the newborn. Annals of the Royal College of Surgeons of England 48: 141–158

Greene H L 1983 Nutritional aspects in the management of biliary atresia. In: Daum F (ed) Extrahepatic biliary atresia. Marcel Dekker, New York, ch 14, p 133–143

Guelrud M, Jaen D, Mendoza S, Plaz J, Torres P 1991 ERCP in the diagnosis of extrahepatic biliary atresia. Gastrointestinal Endoscopy 37: 522–526

Haas J E 1978 Bile duct and liver pathology in biliary atresia. World Journal of Surgery 2: 561–569

Hadchouel M, Gautier M, Valayer J, Odievre M, Alagille D 1983 Histopathology of the liver five years after successful surgery for extrahepatic biliary atresia. In: Daum F (ed) Extrahepatic biliary atresia. Marcel Dekker, New York, ch 6, p 65–70

Harper P A W, Plant J W, Unger D B 1990 Congenital biliary atresia and jaundice in lambs and calves. Australian Veterinary Journal 67: 18–22

Hashimoto T, Yura J, Mahour G H, Warburton D, Landing B H, Stanley P et al 1983 Recent topics of experimental production of biliary atresia, and an experimental model using devascularization of extrahepatic bile duct in the fetal sheep. In: Kasai M (ed) Biliary atresia and its related disorders. Excerpta Medica, Amsterdam, p 38–45

Hays D M, Snyder W H 1963 Life-span in untreated biliary atresia. Surgery 64: 373–375

Hays D M, Kimura K 1980 Biliary atresia: the Japanese experience. Harvard University Press, Cambridge, Mass

Hays D M, Kimura K 1981 Biliary atresia: new concepts of management. Current Problems in Surgery 18: 546

Heaton N D, Howard E R 1993 Complications and limitations of injection sclerotherapy in portal hypertension. Gut 34: 7–10

Heyman M B, Shapiro H A, Thaler M M 1988 Endoscopic retrograde cholangiography in the diagnosis of biliary malformations in infants. Gastrointestinal Endoscopy 34: 449–453

Hirsig J, Kara O, Rickham P P 1978 Experimental investigations into the etiology of cholangitis following operation for biliary atresia. Journal of Pediatric Surgery 13: 55–57

Holder T M, Ashcraft K W 1967 The effects of bile duct ligation and inflammation in the fetus. Journal of Pediatric Surgery 2: 35–40

Holmes J B 1916 Congenital obliteration of the bile duct: Diagnosis and suggestions for treatment. American Journal of Diseases of Children 11: 405–431

Home E 1813 On the formation of fat in the intestine of living animals. Philosophical Transactions of the Royal Society 103: 156–157

Houwen R H J, Zwierstra R P, Severijnen R S, Bouquet J, Madern G, et al 1989 Prognosis of extrahepatic biliary atresia. Archives of Disease in Childhood 64: 214–218

Howard E R 1989 Choledochal cysts. In: Schwartz S I, Ellis H (eds) Maingot's Abdominal Operations, Appleton and Lange, Norwalk, CT, p 1365–1379

Howard E R 1991 Biliary atresia: aetiology, management and complications. In: Howard E R (ed) Surgery of liver disease in children. Butterworth-Heinemann, Oxford, p 39–59

Howard E R 1998 Biliary atresia. In: Stringer M D, Oldham K T, Mouriquand P D E, Howard E R (eds) Pediatric surgery and urology: long term outcomes. WB Saunders & Co., London, p 402–416

Howard E R, Davenport M 1997 The treatment of biliary atresia in Europe 1969–1995. Tohoku Journal of Experimental Medicine 181: 75–83

Howard E R, Davenport M, Mowat A P 1991 Portoenterostomy in the eighties: the King's College Hospital experience. In: Ohi R (ed) Biliary atresia. Professional Postgraduate Services, Tokyo, p 111–115

Isoyama K, Yamada K, Ishikawa K, Sanada Y 1995 Coincidental cases of primary sclerosing cholangitis and biliary atresia in siblings. Acta Paediatrica 84: 1444–1446

Ito T, Sugito T, Shimoji H 1980 Obstructive jaundice produced by Sporidesmin, a product of *Pithomyces chartarum*: experimental studies in the pathogenesis of biliary atresia in rabbits. In: Kasai M, Shiraki K (eds) Cholestasis in infancy. University Park Press, Baltimore, p 225–239

Ito T, Horisawa M, Ando H 1983 Intrahepatic bile ducts in biliary atresia: a possible factor determining the prognosis. Journal of Pediatric Surgery 18: 124–130

Iwami D, Ohi R, Masaki N, Shimaoka S, Sano N, Nagura H 1997 Abnormal distribution of nerve fibres in the liver of biliary atresia. Tohoku Journal of Experimental Medicine 181: 57–65

Iwatsuki S 1987 Liver transplantation for children with biliary atresia. In Biliary Atresia, edited by R. Ohi, Professional Postgraduate Services, Tokyo, p 315–319

Jenner R E, Howard E R 1975 Unsaturated monohydroxy bile acids as a cause of idiopathic obstructive cholangiopathy. Lancet 2: 1073–1074

Kahn E I, Daum F 1983 Arterio-hepatic dysplasia: evaluation of the extrahepatic biliary tract, porta hepatis and hepatic parenchyma. In: Daum F (ed) Extrahepatic Biliary Atresia, Marcel Dekker, New York, p 94

Karrer F M, Lilly J R 1985 Corticosteroid therapy in biliary atresia. Journal of Pediatric Surgery 20: 683–695

Karrer F M, Lilly J R, Stewart B A, Hall R J 1990 Biliary atresia registry, 1976 to 1989. Journal of Pediatric Surgery 25: 1076–1081

Karrer F M, Price M R, Bensard D D, Sokol R J, Markewicz M R, Smith D J et al 1996 Long-term results with the Kasai operation for biliary atresia. Archives of Surgery 131: 493–496

Kasai M, Suzuki S 1959 A new operation for 'non-correctable' biliary atresia: hepatic portoenterostomy. Shujitsu 13: 733–739

Kasai M, Ohi R, Chiba T 1980 Intrahepatic bile ducts in biliary atresia. In Kasai M, Shiraki K (eds) Cholestasis in Infancy, University Park Press, Baltimore, p 181–188

Kasai M, Okamoto A, Ohi R, Yabe K, Matsumura Y 1981 Changes of portal vein pressure and intrahepatic blood vessels after surgery for biliary atresia. Journal of Pediatric Surgery 16: 152–159

Kobayashi A, Itabashi F, Ohbe Y 1984 Long-term prognosis in biliary atresia after hepatic portoenterostomy: analysis of 35 patients who survived beyond 5 years of age. Journal of Pediatrics 105: 243–246

Kulkarni P B, Beatty E C 1977 Cholangiocarcinoma associated with biliary cirrhosis due to congenital biliary atresia. American Journal of Diseases of Children 131: 441–444

Ladd W E 1928 Congenital atresia and stenosis of the bile duct. Journal of the American Medical Association 91: 1082–1084

Landing B H 1974 Considerations of the pathogenesis of neonatal hepatitis, biliary atresia and choledochal cyst: the concept of infantile obstructive cholangiopathy. Progress in Pediatric Surgery 6: 113–139

Laurent J, Gauthier F, Bernard O, Hadchouel M, Odievre M, Valayer J et al 1990 Long-term outcome after surgery for biliary atresia: study of 40 patients surviving for more than 10 years. Gastroenterology 99: 1793–1796

Lawrence D, Howard E R, Tzanatos C, Mowat A P 1981 Hepatic portoenterostomy for biliary atresia. Archives of Disease in Childhood 56: 460–463

Lilly J R 1978 Etiology of cholangitis following operation for biliary atresia. Journal of Pediatric Surgery 13: 559–560

Lilly J R 1979 Hepatic portocholecystostomy for biliary atresia. Journal of Pediatric Surgery 14: 301–304

Lilly J R, Chandra R S 1974 Surgical hazards of co-existing anomalies in biliary atresia. Surgery, Gynecology and Obstetrics 139: 49–54

Lilly J R, Stellin G 1984 Variceal haemorrhage in biliary atresia. Journal of Pediatric Surgery 19: 476–479

Lilly J R, Karrer F M, Hall R J, Stellin G P, Vasquez-Estevez J J, Greenholz S K, et al 1989 The surgery of biliary atresia. Annals of Surgery 210: 289–296

Longmire W P, Sandford M C 1948 Intrahepatic cholangiojejunostomy for biliary obstruction. Surgery 24: 264–276

MacGillivray T E, Scott Adzick N 1994 Biliary atresia begins before birth. Pediatric Surgery International 9: 116–117

Manolaki A G, Larcher V F, Mowat A P, Barrett J J, Portmann B, Howard E R 1983 The prelaparotomy diagnosis of extrahepatic biliary atresia. Archives of Disease in Childhood 58: 591–594

McClement J W, Howard E R, Mowat A P 1985 Results of surgical treatment for extrahepatic biliary atresia in the United Kingdom, 1980–1982. British Medical Journal 290: 345–347

Mieli-Vergani G, Howard E R, Portmann B, Mowat A P 1989 Late referral for biliary atresia—missed opportunities for effective surgery. Lancet 1: 421–23

Millis J M, Brems J J, Hiatt J R, Klein A S, Ashizawa T, Ramming P K, et al 1988 Orthotopic liver transplantation for biliary atresia. Archives of Surgery 123: 1237–1239

Miyamoto M, Kajimoto T 1983 Associated anomalies in biliary atresia patients. In: Kasai M (ed) Biliary Atresia and its Related Disorders, p 13–19. Excerpta Medica, Amsterdam, p 13–19

Miyano T, Suruga K, Suda K 1979 Abnormal choledocho-pancreatico ductal junction related to the etiology of infantile obstructive jaundice diseases. Journal of Pediatric Surgery 14: 16–26

Morecki R, Glaser J H, Horwitz M S 1983 Etiology of biliary atresia: the role of reo 3 virus. In: Daum F (ed) Extrahepatic Biliary Atresia, Marcel Dekker, New York, p 1–9

Nagral S, Muisan P, Vilca-Mendez H, Mieli-Vergani G, Baker A, Karani J et al 1997 Liver transplantation for extra hepatic biliary atresia. Tohoku Journal of Experimental Medicine 181: 67–74

Nelson J S, Rosenblum J L, Keating J P, Prensky A L 1983 Neuropathological complications of childhood cholestatic liver disease. In: Daum F (ed) Extrahepatic Biliary Atresia, Marcel Dekker, New York, p 153–157

Nio M, Ohi R, Hayashi Y, Endo N, Ibrahim M, Iwami D 1996 Current status of 21 living patients surviving more than 20 years after surgery for biliary atresia. Journal of Pediatric Surgery 31: 381–384

Odievre H 1978 Long-term results of surgical treatment of biliary atresia. World Journal of Surgery 2: 589–594

Ohi R 1991 Biliary atresia: long-term results of hepatic portoenterostomy. In: Howard E R (ed), Surgery of Liver Disease in Children. Butterworth-Heinemann, Oxford, p 60–71

Ohi R, Shikes R H, Stellin G P, Lilly J R 1984 In biliary atresia duct histology correlates with bile flow. Journal of Pediatric Surgery 19: 467–470

Ohi R, Hanamatsu M, Mochizuki I, Chiba T, Kasai M 1985 Progress in the treatment of biliary atresia. World Journal of Surgery 9: 285–293

Ohi R, Mochizuki I, Komatsu K, Kasai M 1986 Portal hypertension after successful hepatic portoenterostomy in biliary atresia. Journal of Pediatric Surgery 21: 271–274

Ohi R, Chiba T, Ohkochi N, Yaoita K, Goto M, Ohtsuki S et al 1987 The present status of surgical treatment for biliary atresia: Report of the questionnaire for the main institutions in Japan. In: Ohi R (ed) Biliary Atresia, Professional Postgraduate Services, Tokyo, p 125–130

Ohi R, Nio M, Chiba T, Endo N, Goto M, Ibrahim M 1990 Long-term follow-up after surgery for patients with biliary atresia. Journal of Pediatric Surgery 25: 442–445

Ohnuma N, Takahashi H, Tanabe M, Yoshida H, Iwai J 1997 Endoscopic retrograde cholangiopancreatography (ERCP) in biliary tract disease of infants less than one year old. Tohoku Journal of Experimental Medicine 181: 67–74

Okamoto E, Okasura T, Totosaka A 1980 An experimental study on the etiology of congenital biliary atresia. In: Kasai M, Shiraki K (eds) Cholestasis in Infancy. University Park Press, Baltimore, p 217–224

Parashar K, Taplow M J, McCrae M A 1992 Experimental Reovirus type 3-induced murine biliary tract disease. Journal of Pediatric Surgery 27: 843–847

Phillips P A, Keast D, Papadimitriou J M, Walters M N I, Stanley N F 1969 Chronic obstructive jaundice induced by Reovirus type 3 in weanling mice. Pathology 1: 193–203

Redkar R, Davenport M, Howard E R 1998 Antenatal diagnosis of congenital anomalies of the biliary tract. Journal of Pediatric Surgery 33: 700–704

Saito S 1983 Reoperation for biliary atresia after hepatic portoenterostomy. In: Kasai M (ed) Biliary atresia and its related disorders. Excerpta Medica, Amsterdam, p 224–227

Saito S, Nishina T, Tsuchida Y 1984 Intrahepatic cysts in biliary atresia after successful hepatoportoenterostomy. Archives of Disease in Childhood 59: 274–275

Schweizer P, Brambs H J, Schweizer M, Astfalk W 1995 TIPS: a new therapy for esophageal variceal bleeding caused by EHBA. European Journal of Pediatric Surgery 5: 211–215

Silveira T R, Salzano F M, Howard E R, Mowat A P 1991 Congenital structural abnormalities in biliary atresia: evidence for etiopathogenic heterogeneity and therapeutic implications. Acta Paediatrica Scandinavica 80: 1192–1199

Smith S, Wiener E S, Starzl T E, Rowe M I 1988 Stoma-related variceal bleeding: an under recognized complication of biliary atresia. Journal of Pediatric Surgery 23: 243–245.

Spitz L 1977 Experimental production of cystic dilatation of the common bile duct in lambs. Journal of Pediatric Surgery 12: 39–42

Starzl T E 1983 Liver transplantation for biliary atresia. In: Daum F (ed) Extrahepatic biliary atresia. Marcel Dekker, New York, p 111–117

Sterling J A, Lowenburg K 1963 Increased longevity in congenital biliary atresia. Annals of the New York Academy of Sciences 111: 483–503

Stowens D 1959 Congenital biliary atresia. American Journal of Gastroenterology 32: 577–590

Strauss L, Bernstein J 1968 Neonatal hepatitis in congenital rubella; a histopathological study. Archives of Pathology 86: 317–327

Strickland A D, Shannon K, Coln, C D 1985 Biliary atresia in two sets of twins. Journal of Pediatrics 107: 418–419

Stringer M, Howard E R, Mowat A P 1989 Endoscopic sclerotherapy in the management of esophageal varices in 61 children with biliary atresia. Journal of Pediatric Surgery 24: 438–442

Sunaryo F P, Watkins J B 1983 Evaluation of diagnostic techniques for extrahepatic biliary atresia. In: Daum F (ed) Extrahepatic biliary atresia. Marcel Dekker, New York, ch 2, p 17

Suruga K, Miyano T, Kimura A, Arai T, Kojima Y 1982 Reoperation in the treatment of biliary atresia. Journal of Pediatric Surgery 17: 1–6

Tagge D U, Tagge E P, Drongowski R A, Oldham K T, Coran A G 1991 A long-term experience with biliary atresia: reassessment of prognostic factors. Annals of Surgery 214: 590–598

Takahashi H, Kuriyama Y, Maiae M, Ohnoma N, Eto T 1987 ERCP in jaundiced infants. In: Ohi R (ed) Biliary Atresia, Professional Postgraduate Services, Tokyo, p 110–113

Tan C E L, Davenport M, Driver M, Howard E R 1994 Does the morphology of the extrahepatic biliary remnants in biliary atresia influence survival? A review of 205 cases. Journal of Pediatric Surgery 29: 1459–1464

Tan C E L, Moscoso G J, Howard E R, Driver M 1994 Extrahepatic biliary atresia: a first trimester event? Clues from light microscopy and immunohistochemistry. Journal of Pediatric Surgery 29: 808–814

Thomson J 1892 Congenital obliteration of the bile ducts. Oliver and Boyd, Edinburgh

Toki A, Todani T, Watenabe Y, Sato Y, Ogura K, Yoshikawa M et al 1997 Bone mineral analysis in patients with biliary atresia after successful Kasai procedure. Tohoku Journal of Experimental Medicine 181: 213–216

Tsuchida Y, Honna T, Kawarasaki H 1994 Cystic dilatation of the intrahepatic biliary system in biliary atresia after hepatic portoenterostomy. Journal of Pediatric Surgery 29: 630–634

Vacanti J P, Folkman J 1979 Bile duct enlargement by infusion of L-Proline: potential significance in biliary atresia. Journal of Pediatric Surgery 14: 814–818

Vajro P, Couterier M, Lemmonier F, Odievre M 1986 Effects of post-operative cholestyramine and phenobarbital administration on bile flow restoration in infants with extrahepatic biliary atresia. Journal of Pediatric Surgery 21: 262–265

Valayer J 1991 Portosystemic shunt surgery. In: Howard E R (ed) Surgery of Liver Disease in Children. Butterworth-Heinemann, Oxford, p 171–180

Valayer J, Gauthier F, Yandza T, Lababidi A, De-Dreuzy O, Hamada H 1993 Biliary atresia results of long-term conservative treatment and of liver transplantation. Transplantation Proceedings 25: 3290–3292

Valayer J 1996 Conventional treatment of biliary atresia: long term results. Journal of Pediatric Surgery 31: 1546–1551

Van der Werf W J, D'Alessandro A M, Knechtle S J, Pilli G, Hoffmann R M, Judd R H et al 1998 Infant pediatric liver transplantation results equal those for older pediatric patients. Journal of Pediatric Surgery, 33: 20–23

Primary sclerosing cholangitis

48

R.T. PRALL, R.H. WIESNER, N.F. LaRUSSO

INTRODUCTION

'Sclerosing cholangitis' is a term used to depict a clinical syndrome characterized by recurrent fever, pain, and jaundice resulting from fibrosing and inflammatory obstruction of the bile ducts. An identifiable etiological agent is found in a portion of cases, this group of disorders collectively being termed secondary sclerosing cholangitis. This chapter will discuss the idiopathic variety of this syndrome, primary sclerosing cholangitis, a biliary disorder with its own unique features.

Primary sclerosing cholangitis (PSC) is a chronic cholestatic liver disease of unknown etiology characterized by diffuse fibrosing inflammation of the intrahepatic and extrahepatic bile ducts, leading to obliteration of the biliary tree, biliary cirrhosis, and ultimately death due to complications from liver failure if liver transplantation is not performed (Wiesner & LaRusso 1980). The syndrome was first described by Delbet in 1924 and was thought to be quite rare, with fewer than 100 cases reported prior to 1980 (Lazaridis et al 1999). The association with inflammatory bowel disease is now well known, and with the widespread use of endoscopic retrograde cholangiography and routine biochemical screening, PSC is diagnosed earlier and more frequently. Despite intense investigation, several associations but no clear etiology have been identified. With increased recognition as an important cause of cholestatic liver disease, PSC has been associated with numerous other diseases and clinicians are increasingly aware of the complications of PSC, in particular cholangiocarcinoma, a major cause of mortality in these patients. The natural history of PSC is often progressive, leading to liver failure and death. Prognostic models have been devised which allow the clinician to predict survival and determine the best time for liver transplantation. At present, there is no effective medical therapy. Surgical treatment has moved largely to orthotopic liver transplantation, which remains the only effective treatment for this disease.

DIAGNOSTIC CRITERIA

Today, PSC is readily diagnosed from its clinical presentation, biochemical profile, and characteristic radiologic appearance. This has not always been so. Previously this disease was diagnosed at celiotomy for a suspected bile duct cancer, with sclerosing cholangitis diagnosed only after biopsy excluded a neoplasm (Schwartz & Dale 1958). In the 1960s the association with inflammatory bowel disease (IBD) was recognized and PSC was diagnosed more frequently (Thorpe et al 1967). With the advent of endoscopic retrograde cholangiography (ERC) and its widespread use in the 1970s, the characteristic 'beaded' or 'pruned tree' cholangiographic appearance obviated the need for exploratory surgery to diagnose PSC and its recognition further increased (Wiesner & LaRusso 1980).

The first formal diagnostic criteria included (1) absence of previous operative trauma to the biliary system; (2) sclerosis and stenosis involving all or most of the extrahepatic bile ducts; (3) exclusion of malignant disease involving the biliary system; and (4) absence of calculi in the gallbladder and common bile duct (Holubitsky & McKenzie 1964). With ERC, it was recognized that some patients had intrahepatic disease alone and the criteria expanded to include these patients (MacCarty et al 1983). In addition, serial ERC examinations of PSC patients demonstrated the subsequent development of cholangiocarcinoma, now considered a complication or perhaps part of the natural history of PSC (Chapman et al 1980). Therefore, cholangiocarcinoma arising in the setting of sclerosing cholangitis was eliminated as an exclusionary criterion. Lastly, with modern imaging techniques, biliary tract calculi are frequently seen prospectively in patients with established PSC, causing some to suggest the removal of calculi as an exclusionary criterion as well (Kaw et al 1995).

Currently, the diagnosis of PSC relies on demonstration of the near pathognomonic cholangiographic findings in a patient with a compatible clinical history and biochemical profile after exclusion of secondary causes of sclerosing cholangitis. An archetypal presentation would be that of a jaundiced young man with a history of ulcerative colitis complaining of pruritus with an elevated alkaline phosphatase on serum biochemistries. Perhaps the most common presentation now is an asymptomatic patient with persistently elevated levels of alkaline phosphatase first noted on routine serum biochemical screening. In the proper clinical context, a characteristic cholangiogram is sufficient for diagnosis; we feel a liver biopsy is not ordinarily required. Liver biopsy can serve to (1) exclude other causes of cholestatic liver disease when the diagnosis is in doubt; (2) diagnose small duct PSC when large duct disease

Table 48.1 Differential diagnosis of primary sclerosing cholangitis

Primary biliary cirrhosis
Drug-induced cholestasis
Congenital abnormality of the biliary tract
Idiopathic adulthood ductopenia
Cholestasis associated with autoimmune hepatitis or alcoholic liver
  disease
Bile duct carcinoma or lymphoma
Extrahepatic obstruction
Secondary sclerosing cholangitis

Table 48.2 Diagnostic criteria for primary sclerosing cholangitis

Appropriate clinical history (e.g. pruritus, jaundice, inflammatory
  bowel disease)
Persistent 2- to 3-fold elevation of serum alkaline phosphatase
Characteristic cholangiographic appearance of diffusely distributed,
  multifocal strictures
Characteristic histology (fibro-obliterative cholangitis is nearly
  diagnostic but is seen in less than 5% of cases)

Exclusion of:
  Secondary causes of sclerosing cholangitis
    Bile duct carcinoma (unless found in setting of established PSC)
    Choledocholithiasis (unless found in the setting of established
      PSC)
    Ischemic strictures (more common in the post-transplantation
      setting)
    Prior biliary tract surgery or trauma
    Human immunodeficiency virus infection and concomitant
      infection with Cryptosporidium, Cytomegalovirus,
    Microsporidium, or Cyclospora
    Intra-arterial infusion of floxuridine
    Formaldehyde injection of hepatic hydatid cysts

Modified from Lazaridis KN, Wiesner RH, Porayko MK et al (1999)

is absent on cholangiography; and lastly (3) define stage to determine prognosis and assess efficacy of treatment in therapeutic trials. In the majority of patients, the history, serum biochemical profile, serology, cholangiography, and histology distinguish PSC from other causes of cholestatic liver disease. The differential diagnosis of PSC as well as diagnostic and exclusionary criteria are presented in Tables 48.1 and 48.2.

EPIDEMIOLOGY

The prevalence of PSC is not precisely known but has been estimated based on the association with chronic ulcerative colitis, with a prevalence estimated to be 40–225 cases per 100 000 in the United States (Stonnington et al 1987). PSC is thought to occur in 2.4% to 7.5% of patients with ulcerative colitis (Schrumpf et al 1988, Shepherd et al 1983). If one accepts the Olmsted County (Minnesota) data for ulcerative colitis as representative, the prevalence of PSC could be as high as 9 per 100 000 people in the United States. This is similar to the prevalence obtained from the Swedish Health Registry, which estimates the prevalence of PSC as 6.3 per 100 000 (Olsson et al 1991). Still, this may be an underestimation as approximately 30% of patients with PSC do not have inflammatory bowel disease and a smaller portion may have normal alkaline phosphatase levels or normal cholangiograms, both criteria necessary for diagnosis of PSC in most epidemiologic surveys.

Recently, an interesting correlation between non-smoking behavior and PSC has been reported. It had been noted previously that smoking may be protective against the development of ulcerative colitis. Investigators in the Netherlands interviewed patients with PSC, ulcerative colitis alone, and control subjects. They found the incidence of current smoking to be 19%, 12% and 38% respectively in these groups (van Erpecum et al 1996). In a separate American study of 184 PSC patients matched to age and sex controls, only 4.9% were current smokers compared to 26.1% of controls, with an estimated odds ratio of having PSC in current smokers compared with never-smokers of 0.13. Subanalysis showed that this difference was not attributable to the prevention of ulcerative colitis (Loftus et al 1996a). It is not known how active smoking influences disease activity, but oral nicotine trials are underway. Smoking should be strongly discouraged as a recent report suggests a very strong association between smoking and the development of cholangiocarcinoma in patients with PSC (Bergquist et al 1998).

CLINICAL MANIFESTATIONS

PSC can occur at any age. In the largest North American pediatric series of 32 patients, the median age of diagnosis was 13 years with four children diagnosed before the age of 2. Interestingly, children with PSC very frequently have characteristic features of autoimmune hepatitis and may have a variant of adult PSC (Louis et al 1995). In a large adult series, two thirds were male and the median age at diagnosis was 39.9 years (Wiesner et al 1989). PSC may develop later in women. In a Swedish study, the average age at diagnosis was 50 years for women, compared to 35 years for men (Olsson et al 1991).

Many patients, especially those with IBD, are now diagnosed at an asymptomatic stage after the detection of an elevated serum alkaline phosphatase on screening biochemistries. There are no pathognomonic signs or symptoms when the disease becomes clinically apparent. Symptoms include jaundice, pruritus, right upper quadrant pain, fatigue and intermittent fevers. Abdominal pain and fever, symptoms of bacterial cholangitis, are unusual unless there has been previous biliary surgery. Physical findings of PSC are similar to those of other cholestatic liver diseases or hepatic failure. Findings on initial physical examination vary depending on stage at time of diagnosis. In a series with a high proportion of patients symptomatic at the time of diagnosis, 50% had abnormalities at the time of initial examination; these include jaundice (44%), hepatomegaly (28%), and splenomegaly (29%) (Wiesner & LaRusso 1980). Hyperpigmentation and excoriations are frequently seen. Spider angiomata, clubbing, and xanthomas occur less often. Ascites, esophagogastric varices, and peripheral edema are found with the development of biliary cirrhosis and portal hypertension.

BIOCHEMICAL ABNORMALITIES

There are no pathognomonic or even specific biochemical tests for PSC. The great majority will have a cholestatic profile, with a serum alkaline phosphatase elevated 2–3 fold considered typical. A normal alkaline phosphatase level does not exclude the diagnosis of PSC as normal levels have been described in a report of 12 patients with cholangiographically-proven disease. In seven of these patients, levels remained normal in follow-up and fluctuated in five cases, returning to normal in four. Indeed, four patients with a normal alkaline phosphatase had histologically advanced (cirrhotic stage) disease on liver biopsy (Balasubramaniam et al 1988). Therefore, a normal alkaline phosphatase level should not dissuade further investigation if the clinical history (e.g. presence of inflammatory bowel disease) suggests liver disease.

Aminotransferase levels are usually elevated, being abnormal in more than 90% of patients. Levels are usually less than five times the upper limit of normal, increased three-fold or less on average. PSC patients with high increases in aminotransferases may show histologic features and serologic evidence of autoimmune hepatitis. Indeed, some will meet criteria for each disorder (Czaja 1998).

Bilirubin levels tend to fluctuate with the disease. They may be normal for a long period of time or a patient may present with jaundice. Bilirubin levels will eventually rise with progressive biliary cirrhosis; however an abrupt, sustained rise may herald a dominant stricture, a stone, or a cholangiocarcinoma and should prompt investigation. High bilirubin levels are a negative impact factor on survival with or without liver transplantation.

Tests evaluating hepatic copper metabolism are usually abnormal. Hepatic and urinary copper levels and serum ceruloplasmin levels are increased in 75% of patients. Hepatic copper levels can be increased to the same levels as seen in Wilson's disease and primary biliary cirrhosis and are a reflection of prolonged cholestasis (LaRusso et al 1984). A summary of biochemical test abnormalities at the time of diagnosis is shown in Table 48.3.

Table 48.3 Biochemical tests in primary sclerosing cholangitis at time of diagnosis

Test	Percent of patients with abnormal results
Serum alkaline phosphatase	98–99%
Serum transaminases	95%
Serum bilirubin	65%
Serum albumin	20%
Prothrombin time	10%
Serum copper	50%
Serum ceruloplasmin	75%
Urine copper	65%

Modified from LaRusso NF & Wiesner RH (1992)

SEROLOGIC ABNORMALITIES

Much has been learned regarding the immunology of chronic inflammatory diseases of the liver. Indeed, screening for antibodies which are highly sensitive for autoimmune liver disease has become an integral part of diagnosis.

The high prevalence of anti-nuclear, anti-smooth muscle, and anti-mitochondrial antibodies in autoimmune hepatitis and primary biliary cirrhosis (PBC), respectively, is well known. These autoantibodies can be elevated to detectable but low titers in PSC. The prevalence of anti-nuclear antibodies is not definitely known. In our experience, anti-nuclear antibodies are elevated in 6% and smooth muscle antibodies in 11% of patients. Anti-mitochondrial antibodies are seen infrequently and in low titers, in sharp distinction to primary biliary cirrhosis. These tests are used more effectively to distinguish PSC from other autoimmune liver diseases such as PBC rather than as serologic markers for PSC. Autoantibody testing may also serve to identify PSC patients with an overlap syndrome with autoimmune hepatitis who may benefit from immunosuppression. In no circumstance are antibody titers used to follow disease activity in PSC.

Other serologic markers of immunologic overactivity are known but are not useful diagnostically due to their high prevalence in autoimmune liver disease. If looked for, hypergammaglobulinemia will be noted in 30%, with a disproportionate increase in IgM in 40 to 50%. The most frequent serologic abnormality is the high prevalence of anti-neutrophil cytoplasmic antibodies with a peripheral staining distribution (pANCA), seen in 70–80% of patients with PSC (Lo et al 1992). pANCA positivity is only slightly lower in ulcerative colitis and is seen in up to 92% of patients with well-defined autoimmune hepatitis (Vidrich et al 1995). In addition, disease activity does not correlate with pANCA positivity or titer; therefore, we do not routinely obtain this test.

IMAGING

Changes of sclerosing cholangitis can be visualized using a variety of radiologic modalities. Small duct disease, which by definition is not radiologically detectable, occurs alone in only a small percentage of cases.

Ultrasonography is often able to show large duct dilatation and mural thickening of the common bile duct in patients with confirmed abnormalities on ERC (Majoie et al 1995). Ultrasound is not typically used to diagnose PSC. Its major limitation is its inability to exclude intrahepatic ductular disease. Ultrasound can be used effectively to detect gallstones or biliary tract calculi. This may be important in the evaluation of suppurative cholangitis or worsening cholestasis or jaundice when a retained large duct stone is suspected. These patients, however, will still need an ERC as part of their diagnostic evaluation or for therapy.

Nonetheless, ultrasound remains the best method to evaluate gallstones and gallbladder disease, which are much more common in patients with PSC (Brandt et al 1988).

Computed tomography (CT) is able to detect both extrahepatic and intrahepatic ductal abnormalities in sclerosing cholangitis. In addition, morphologic features of advanced cirrhosis in PSC are seen on CT, with a tendency to more marked hypertrophy of the left lateral segment and caudate lobe and more severe atrophy of the right and medial left segments than those typically seen in other types of cirrhosis (Campbell et al 1998). CT findings were compared to cholangiography in a study of 20 patients with PSC. In 16 of 19 cases of extrahepatic disease seen on cholangiography, CT demonstrated abnormalities including duct dilatation, wall thickening, and mural enhancement. In intrahepatic disease, CT findings of duct dilatation, duct stenosis, pruning, or beading were seen in all 20 cases and the investigators concluded that CT was superior to cholangiography in assessment of the intrahepatic duct system in 11 of the 20 (Teefey et al 1988). CT is also a useful complement to cholangiography in the evaluation of cholangiocarcinoma, as it has the ability to detect peripheral intrahepatic cholangiocarcinoma, and metastatic spread within the liver parenchyma. Bile duct wall thickening greater than 5 mm, delayed contrast enhancement, and peripheral hepatic soft tissue masses are characteristic features suggestive of malignancy. Perihilar lymphadenopathy is very common in PSC with or without cholangiocarcinoma and therefore cannot be taken as evidence of malignancy or metastasis (Campbell et al 1998).

Cholangiography remains the gold standard for the diagnosis of PSC. Strictures at all levels of the biliary tree are the hallmark of the disease and are seen in almost all patients. Stricture formation is diffuse but not uniform, characterized by multiple areas of alternating segmental fibrosis and ectasia resulting in the classic findings of pruning and beading of the biliary tree (see Fig. 48.1). Strictures can vary from a band-like appearance only 1–2 millimeters in length, to long, confluent, annular strictures several centimeters in length. Approximately one quarter will have outpouchings resembling diverticula, and 44% will have mural irregularities producing a shaggy appearance, varying from a 'fine brush border' to frank nodularity (MacCarty et al 1983).

In a study of cholangiographic findings in 86 patients with PSC, the intrahepatic ducts were involved in all 80 patients who had adequate visualization of the intrahepatic biliary tree. Similarly, the extrahepatic ducts were involved in 85 of 86 patients. In 20%, only the intrahepatic and proximal extrahepatic ducts were involved. A very small number of patients with PSC have only small duct involvement (i.e. normal cholangiogram, disease detectable only on histology). Gallbladder and cystic duct disease is typically less

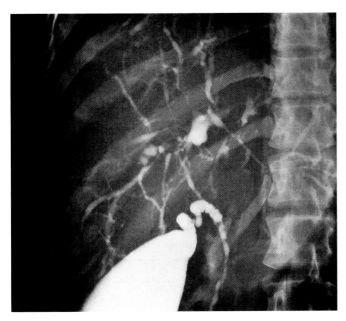

Fig. 48.1 Endoscopic retrograde cholangiogram illustrating the classical appearance of primary sclerosing cholangitis with stricturing and dilatation of the intrahepatic and extrahepatic bile ducts.

Table 48.4 Cholangiographic findings in PSC vs. PSC with carcinoma (CA)

Finding	PSC only	PSC + CA
Polypoid mass	7% (6/91)	46% (6/13)
Marked ductal dilatation*	24% (20/84)	100% (12/12)
Progressive stricture	18% (11/62)	100% (4/4)
Progressive dilatation	2% (1/53)	100% (4/4)

Expressed as percentage of cases with positive findings.

* Marked ductal dilatation defined as common duct ≥ 2.0 cm, main right hepatic duct ≥ 0.8 cm, main left hepatic duct ≥ 1.0 cm, and intrahepatic duct ≥ 0.5 cm.

Modified from MacCarty RL, LaRusso NF, May GR et al (1985)

severe and less common, with abnormalities detected in 18% and strictures in only 7 to 14%. In the same study, 40 patients had pancreatography and of these 3 (8%) had abnormalities of the pancreatic ducts (MacCarty et al 1983).

We feel endoscopic retrograde cholangiography should be performed in all patients in whom PSC is suspected. ERC accomplishes several important goals: (1) it establishes the diagnosis; (2) defines the extent and distribution of disease; (3) identifies benign dominant strictures for endoscopic dilatation or stenting; and (4) allows brushings for cytology to screen for cholangiocarcinoma. As many as 10% of cholangiocarcinomas present as a diffuse sclerosing variant with radiologic features mimicking sclerosing cholangitis. Despite this, there are cholangiographic features that suggest malignant degeneration of established PSC. These include markedly dilated ducts or ductal segments, presence of a polypoid mass 1 centimeter or greater in diameter, and progressive stricture formation or ductal dilatation. Identical features are also seen to a lesser extent in the absence of malignancy, summarized in Table 48.4 (MacCarty et al 1985).

Magnetic resonance imaging (MRI) of the liver and biliary tract has improved substantially and is reviewed in Chapter 16. The role of magnetic resonance cholangiography (MRC) in PSC is currently being determined. In a study comparing MRC findings in patients with PSC, PBC, alcoholic cirrhosis, and no liver disease, abnormalities of the

ductal system were detected in all PSC patients and in none of the control subjects without liver disease. Slightly dilated peripheral bile ducts unconnected to the central ducts in several hepatic segments were the characteristic finding. Only one of the 18 patients with other liver disease had a PSC-like pattern but it was confined to only one area (Ernst et al 1998).

Optimistically, one would hope that MRI could be used successfully and with greatest benefit for the detection of and non-invasive screening for cholangiocarcinoma in PSC patients. In a retrospective, non-blinded study of patients with known biliary tract carcinoma complicating PSC, MRI findings of a well-defined mass exhibiting abnormal signal intensity were classified as definite cholangiocarcinoma in six of the seven patients who had an MRI performed. Cholangiocarcinomas typically display low signal intensity on spin-echo T1-weighted images and high signal intensity with T2-weighting (Campbell et al 1998). When the diagnosis is not known beforehand, as it was in this study, one is less confident distinguishing the enhanced signal intensity seen with fibrosis from that of malignancy. In addition, the tumors were visualized by other modalities and also classified as definite carcinoma in all cases, causing one to question if there is any added benefit in performing this test.

MRC may someday replace diagnostic ERC, but at present it is insufficiently sensitive and does not allow for therapeutic intervention or biopsy. MRC may potentially be used to follow areas of interest non-invasively, search for calculi, guide endoscopic therapy or biopsy, or rarely as primary evaluation in patients in whom ERC is technically difficult.

HISTOPATHOLOGY

PSC affects all levels of the biliary system. In nearly all patients, disease involves some portion of the extrahepatic biliary tree. Intrahepatic disease is almost always seen at cholangiography as well. Infrequently, disease may be limited to the intrahepatic ducts, and in some cases, only the smallest ducts, detectable only on histology. Previously known as 'pericholangitis,' involvement of only microscopically identifiable (interlobular and septal) disease is now termed 'small duct PSC.' Small duct PSC is rare, but its true prevalence is unknown. In an unpublished study, 95% of patients with histologic small duct disease also had cholangiographic evidence of large duct disease. The natural history and pathogenesis of small duct PSC also remain obscure (Ludwig 1991).

Histologically, 'PSC is characterized by damage to, atrophy of, and, ultimately, loss of bile ducts' (Scheuer 1998). This histologic picture is seen in several hepatobiliary diseases, but in adults this is most commonly PSC or primary biliary cirrhosis. Involvement of the large intrahepatic and extrahepatic ducts distinguishes PSC from PBC. Complicating the histopathologic diagnosis of PSC is the need to separate changes from the disease process itself from changes seen in simple obstruction of the distal bile ducts.

Liver biopsy of an affected site will show portal tract inflammation and sclerosis. Affected bile ducts are surrounded by a cuff of lightly inflamed fibrous tissue and edema, causing the layers to separate and forming the characteristic onion skin appearance (see Figure 48.2.) These ducts will eventually atrophy, and when obliteration is complete, leave characteristic rounded scars where bile ducts were formerly found. Although uncommon, the findings of fibro-obliterative cholangitis are nearly pathognomonic for PSC. Occasionally, however, these changes have been seen in obstruction of the large bile ducts, PBC, ductopenic rejection after liver transplantation, and after intra-arterial infusion of floxuridine. Distinguishing PSC from PBC at an early stage is often very difficult, although the inflammation is typically milder than in early stage PBC (Scheuer 1998). Granulomas, thought to be classically associated with PBC, may be seen in 3 to 4% of biopsy samples from PSC patients and thus their presence alone cannot reliably distinguish PSC from PBC (Ludwig 1995).

Canalicular cholestasis is nonspecific and can occur as a result of any cause of duct obstruction. As the disease progresses, the changes of chronic cholestasis spill over into the hepatic parenchyma. Ludwig devised a histological staging system based on parenchymal changes, designating disease stages I through IV as portal, periportal, septal, and cirrhotic, respectively (Ludwig et al 1986). The Ludwig histological stage has proven to be a very useful independent predictor of prognosis and time to liver failure in PSC.

ETIOPATHOGENESIS

PSC is generally considered an immune-mediated disease and several different theories have emerged in relation to possible inciting events. As listed previously, many secondary causes have been identified but are not responsible for the clinical syndrome of primary sclerosing cholangitis. Although many different theories have been put forth, none fully explain the etiology or pathogenesis of PSC.

The possible primary role of bacteria or their metabolic products as toxins in the pathogenesis of PSC has generated considerable interest. With the strong association with IBD, it follows that a chronic, low-grade portal bacteremia may incite an immune response. Investigators have shown, however, no significant portal vein bacteremia in patients undergoing surgery for fulminant ulcerative colitis (Warren et al 1966). Similarly, histologic evidence of bacteremia manifested as portal phlebitis is mild or absent in most PSC patients (Ludwig et al 1981). Others have speculated that toxic bile salts elaborated by bacterial metabolism of primary bile acids are absorbed through the mucosa of the ulcerated colon and into the portal circulation. Studies, however, have not detected any major abnormalities in bile acid metabolism in patients with PSC or ulcerative colitis (Siegel et al 1977). Two important clinical observations cast serious doubt upon the role of colonic bacteria or toxins in the development of PSC in patients with ulcerative colitis. First, PSC occurs in the absence or prior to the diagnosis of inflammatory bowel disease in 30% of patients. Even when invasive screening of asymptomatic patients is employed, the majority will have no endoscopic or histologic evidence of inflammatory bowel disease. Second, PSC can occur in the absence of a colon, being reported years after procto-

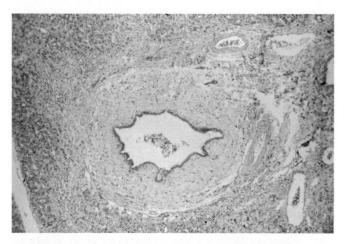

Fig. 48.2 Histologic appearance of early stage primary sclerosing cholangitis demonstrating prominent cholangiectasis and fibrosing cholangitis of an interlobular bile duct (Hematoxylin & eosin, ×100).

colectomy for ulcerative colitis. The weight of the evidence suggests that colonic bacteria or toxins they may produce are not significant causative factors in PSC.

Viral agents are inevitably sought as the inciting mechanism in immune-mediated diseases of unknown etiology. Reovirus type 3 had been shown to induce cholangitis and biliary atresia in weanling mice but this has not been established in humans as antibody titers to this virus are similar in humans with and without PSC (Phillips et al 1969, Morecki et al 1982). Cytomegalovirus has been shown to cause an obliterative cholangitis in small intrahepatic ducts (Finegold & Carpenter 1982), but extrahepatic disease occurs only in the setting of acquired human immuno-deficiency syndrome. The common hepatotrophic viruses causing hepatitis A, B, and C have been shown not to cause PSC. There is no evidence at present to implicate a viral etiology.

Genetic factors do seem to be implicated in PSC. A genetic predisposition based on HLA type has been identified in large population based studies in Europe. Moreover, there are reports of PSC occurring in siblings and twins (Quigley et al 1983). HLA associations have been well studied. There is an increased frequency of HLA B8, DR3, and DR2 in PSC compared to the expected frequency in the population (Chapman et al 1983, Donaldson et al 1991). HLA-B8 and DR3 are well recognized as being more frequent in a variety of autoimmune diseases. Associations with other alleles are continuing to appear. Several studies have claimed certain haplotypes to portend aggressive disease, however, subsequent studies failed to show this association. Most recently, a study of 124 PSC patients examined the relative risk of death or need for liver transplantation based on HLA haplotypes. The investigators found the DR3, DQ2 haplotype to be significantly associated with a poor prognosis, whereas the DR2, DQ6 haplotype was an indicator of a more favorable disease course (Boberg et al 1998).

As HLA molecules are involved in antigen processing and presentation to immune cells, it is thought that certain HLA haplotypes are more likely to present a normally innocuous antigen to the immune system in an altered, pathogenic fashion. This then may elicit an immune response against common antigenic epitopes present on the biliary tree. It has also been noted that HLA class II (HLA DR) antigens are expressed more heavily on cholangiocytes during early PSC. This is probably an epiphenomenon however, as enhanced expression of HLA class II antigens is also observed in PBC and extrahepatic biliary obstruction (Chapman et al 1988). In addition to the HLA associations, numerous other abnormalities of the immune system have been detailed. Hypergammaglobulinemia with a disproportionate increase in IgM subclass is often present. In addi-

tion, increased titers of specific autoantibodies including anti-smooth muscle, anti-nuclear, anti-colonic, anti-portal tract, anti-endothelial cell, anti-catalase, and anti-neutrophilic cytoplasmic antibodies have been described. None of these have a defined pathogenic role or are specific for PSC. A generalized activation of the complement system as well as several abnormalities of lymphocyte number, type, and activation have been observed but are too numerous to list here.

How all these possible factors relate is unclear. It seems most favor the current autoimmune hypothesis that PSC is a disease of immunologic overactivity directed against the biliary system, perhaps triggered by a pathogen, in a genetically susceptible individual. The primary factor leading to the activation of the immune response has yet to be identified.

ASSOCIATED DISEASES

The association of PSC with inflammatory bowel disease is well known. There are now also many case reports of patients with histologic, biochemical, and serologic features of both PSC and autoimmune hepatitis. Numerous other diseases with a suspected autoimmune pathogenesis have also been reported in association with PSC. It is unclear whether these associations are coincidental or represent a true increase in incidence of a rare disease. An abridged list of diseases reported to be associated with PSC is presented in Table 48.5.

Table 48.5 Diseases associated with primary sclerosing cholangitis

Chronic ulcerative colitis
Crohn's colitis
Chronic pancreatitis
Sicca syndrome
Hypereosinophilia
Reidel's thyroiditis
Celiac disease
Pulmonary infiltrates
Autoimmune hemolytic anemia
Sarcoidosis
Glomerulonephritis

INFLAMMATORY BOWEL DISEASE

The most common association with PSC by far is inflammatory bowel disease (IBD), most commonly chronic ulcerative colitis (CUC). IBD is seen in approximately 70% of patients with PSC, with CUC accounting for 90% of the

IBD in patients with PSC. Conversely, PSC is seen in approximately 2.4 to 7.5% of patients with CUC. There appear to be no major differences in PSC with or without CUC; however, colitic disease in patients with both CUC and PSC is typically milder in comparison to patients with CUC alone.

PSC is also seen in some cases of Crohn's disease, occurring in 9% of cases of Crohn's colitis in one study. This study also suggested that Crohn's-associated PSC may be milder than PSC associated with ulcerative colitis, as five of the nine patients with PSC had only small duct disease (Rasmussen et al 1997). Interestingly, PSC has not been seen in Crohn's disease involving only the small bowel.

Inflammatory bowel disease is diagnosed prior to PSC in 70% to 80% of patients, on average 8 to 10 years (Chapman et al 1980, Loftus et al 1996b). This, as well as the observation that the colon was always involved as part of the IBD suggested that perhaps the colonic disease in some way caused PSC, or that treating the colonic disease may alter the course of the biliary disease. This does not appear to be true, as PSC is sometimes diagnosed after proctocolectomy and removing the colon has no effect on the course of PSC (Cangemi et al 1989).

Conversely, intense interest has revolved around the possible effects PSC may have on ulcerative colitis since Broome and colleagues in 1992 showed an increased risk of dysplasia in ulcerative colitis patients with PSC compared to patients with ulcerative colitis alone. Multiple subsequent studies have reached different conclusions as to whether PSC is an independent risk factor for colorectal dysplasia and carcinoma in patients with PSC and CUC. Results vary greatly by study design. In one Swedish study, patients who had ulcerative colitis diagnosed prior to PSC had a cumulative risk of colon cancer ten years after the diagnosis of PSC of 25% and a risk of 33%, 20 years after the diagnosis of ulcerative colitis (Kornfeld et al 1997). Others have shown an increased risk of dysplasia but not cancer. A Mayo Clinic case control study of 171 patients with both ulcerative colitis and colorectal carcinoma and 171 patients with ulcerative colitis but no neoplasia (carcinoma or dysplasia) found a similar prevalence of PSC in both groups (Nuako et al 1998). By its design, however, this retrospective study did not answer the question of interest in a direct manner, possibly being confounded by the possibility of some patients having undiagnosed, subclinical PSC. Ideally, one would like to follow large numbers of patients with proven PSC prospectively for the development of neoplasia as compared to a control group with ulcerative colitis alone for a similar duration. A prospective study of patients undergoing colonoscopic surveillance with extensive mucosal biopsy sampling concluded that patients with both PSC and ulcer-

ative colitis were five times more likely to develop dysplasia, but that the time interval between diagnosis of colitis and dysplasia was unchanged (Brentnall et al 1996). It is uncertain whether this represents a true association or reflects the fact that PSC patients have milder, pancolonic disease of longer duration that may have remained undetected for a longer period of time. In a study of nine PSC patients without clinical signs of IBD undergoing colonoscopy, seven were found to have histologic evidence of disease (Broome et al 1995a,b). The issue of increased neoplastic potential is particularly relevant after liver transplantation with attendant prolonged immunosuppression. Several studies have found an increased risk of colorectal dysplasia and cancer in patients with ulcerative colitis after transplantation for PSC (Bleday et al 1993). In fact, at some centers it is the highest cause of post-transplant mortality (Narumi et al 1995). When examined at our institution, this increased risk did not translate into a negative impact on survival, perhaps due to frequent screening and early detection of neoplasia (Loftus et al 1998). As colorectal carcinoma threatens to be a major cause of mortality, our current practice is to perform an annual surveillance colonoscopy with biopsy sampling in patients with PSC and ulcerative colitis. If patients do not have symptoms or an established diagnosis of ulcerative colitis at the time of diagnosis of PSC, we still perform an initial screening colonoscopy searching for subclinical disease.

AUTOIMMUNE HEPATITIS

Overlap syndromes between autoimmune hepatitis and PBC have previously been described. Several groups have now reported small sets of patients with features of both PSC and autoimmune hepatitis (Gohlke et al 1996, Luketic et al 1997, McNair et al 1998). Indeed, these patients typically fulfill definite criteria for both. They may present with or without jaundice but all have elevated serum aminotransferases and alkaline phosphatase, IgG, and anti-nuclear and/or anti-smooth muscle antibody titers. On liver histology, a moderate to severe interface hepatitis is present with or without biliary features. Aminotransferase levels are elevated beyond what one would expect for simple PSC (typically five times normal or greater). Inflammatory bowel disease may be present but could be with a lower frequency than simple PSC. Patients demonstrate cholangiographic features of PSC at the time of presentation or in some cases subsequent to the diagnosis after the development of an alkaline phosphatase-predominant pattern. The key point is that the hepatitis present in these patients with an overlap syndrome may respond to immunosuppressive therapy. Conversely, in patients with autoimmune hepatitis who respond incompletely to immunosuppression and develop a cholestatic profile, a cholangiogram may reveal the presence of concomitant PSC.

NATURAL HISTORY

PSC frequently progresses to liver failure and death but in the past it was unclear how to predict this for individual patients. Several accurate natural history models have since been developed; these allow clinicians not only to give patients prognostic information but also to assess efficacy of treatment and to assist in the timing of orthotopic liver transplantation. In a prospective study of 174 patients seen at the Mayo Clinic done before liver transplantation was widely available as a therapeutic option, median survival from time of diagnosis was estimated to be 11.9 years. Of special interest is the subgroup of 45 patients who were asymptomatic at the time of diagnosis. After a mean prospective follow-up of 6.25 years, 76% had progression of their liver disease, and 31% developed liver failure requiring liver transplant or resulting in death (Porayko et al 1990). Using Cox regression multivariate analysis, the investigators determined age, serum bilirubin concentration, blood hemoglobin concentration, presence or absence of inflammatory bowel disease, and histologic stage on biopsy to be independent predictors of survival (Wiesner et al 1989). A risk score (see also Ch. 108) was determined for each patient that could then be used to estimate survival. To confirm validity of this model, a multicenter, international collaboration provided additional data to be pooled with that of the Mayo Clinic resulting in a database of 426 patients. The new model uti-

lized age, histologic stage, bilirubin, and splenomegaly to predict survival and provided accurate predictions of survival stratified by risk score (Dickson et al 1992) (see Figure 48.3.) This model still required a liver biopsy to determine histologic stage. To avoid the need for a biopsy, investigators at the Cleveland Clinic evaluated an age-adjusted Child–Pugh classification and found it had comparable accuracy to the Mayo disease-specific model at predicting survival. Seven-year Kaplan–Meir actuarial survivals for Child–Pugh class A, B, and C were 89.8%, 68%, and 24.9% respectively (Shetty et al 1997). Most recently, the Mayo investigators revised their previous model, also eliminating the need for liver biopsy, making it more clinically applicable (Kim et al 1999).

COMPLICATIONS

Complications from PSC can be broadly classified by their specificity for the disease. The most common symptoms are not specific to PSC but are a consequence of chronic cholestasis and liver failure, with other complications resulting from portal hypertension arising as the disease progresses to cirrhosis. Lastly, some complications are specific for PSC and require special awareness.

Most patients with PSC or other chronic cholestatic liver diseases will complain of fatigue and pruritus at some time. The factors responsible for the fatigue are not known. The pruritus can be extremely severe, debilitating, and itself be an indication for liver transplantation. In order of their intended use as needed, cholestyramine, rifampin, ursodeoxycholic acid, phenobarbital, and antihistamines, are usually effective in ameliorating pruritus, with plasmapheresis, and charcoal hemoperfusion being prescribed for refractory cases. Opiate receptor antagonists and serotonergic antagonists such as ondansetron may be efficacious and are under evaluation (Milano et al 1998).

Patients with cholestatic liver disease may also suffer from steatorrhea and subsequent deficiencies of fat soluble vitamins. Deficiencies of vitamins A, D, and E are present in 82%, 57% and 43% of patients with advanced PSC respectively (Jorgensen et al 1995). This can be treated with simple supplementation. Deficiencies of vitamin K result in prolongation of the prothrombin time, which may be correctable with parenteral administration of vitamin K if parenchymal damage to the liver is not too severe. Consideration should be given to the diagnosis of celiac sprue or chronic pancreatitis in patients with steatorrhea, especially in early stage disease, as they are both treatable causes of fat malabsorption and are present with increased

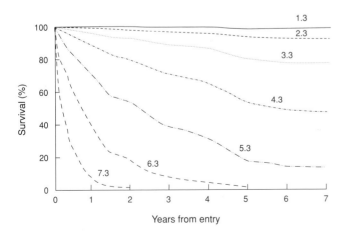

Fig. 48.3 Estimated survival for patients with primary sclerosing cholangitis (PSC), based on increasing Mayo PSC risk score. From Wiesner RH et al (1996)

frequency in PSC. As with other cholestatic liver diseases, patients with PSC frequently have hypercholesterolemia but this is not usually clinically significant. Metabolic bone disease is also extraordinarily common. Osteopenic bone disease can be severe in advanced PSC, with 50% of patients having a bone mineral density below the fracture threshold (Hay et al 1991). Biopsies reveal this to be consistent with osteoporosis, not osteomalacia. This is surprising given that two thirds of patients with PSC are male.

Patients with PSC suffer from the complications of portal hypertension just as other patients with other causes of cirrhotic liver disease. Variceal bleeding can occur anywhere along the gastrointestinal tract, complicated often by a coagulopathy. This is usually managed with sclerotic therapy or a banding procedure (Ch. 97); when ineffective a shunting procedure can be performed, but hopefully as a bridge to transplantation. Likewise, patients with cirrhotic stage PSC develop ascites, spontaneous bacterial peritonitis, and encephalopathy, but probably not with an increased frequency compared to other causes of cirrhotic liver failure. Again, liver transplantation should be considered optimal management of these symptoms.

COMPLICATIONS SPECIFIC FOR PRIMARY SCLEROSING CHOLANGITIS

Recalling that PSC is a disease primarily of young men, it is surprising that 25 to 30% will have calculi either in the gall-bladder or biliary tree. Radiologic studies have shown that intrahepatic calculi are present in 8% of patients (Dodd et al 1997). In one study of the gallbladders of 121 patients with PSC, 26% had gallstones; half on examination were pigment stones. The spectrum of pathology in the gallbladder is not limited to stones. In the same study, PSC directly involved the gallbladder in 15% (Brandt et al 1988). The gallbladder also seems to suffer an unusual form of acalculous cholecystitis characterized by a diffuse lymphoplasmacytic infiltrate in five of eleven patients with chronic cholecystitis studied (Jessurun et al 1998).

Biliary calculi can serve as a nidus for the development of bacterial cholangitis. Suppurative cholangitis is relatively uncommon in PSC in the absence of hepatobiliary stones, a dominant stricture, or prior biliary surgery and its presence should prompt an endoscopic evaluation to remove calculi and allow biliary drainage. Cholangitis as a complication of ERC occurs more commonly in patients with PSC than in those without; therefore, we routinely provide prophylactic antibiotics prior to this procedure in patients with known or suspected PSC.

Dominant strictures will occur in 15–20%, presenting with increased jaundice, pruritus, cholangitis, or right upper quadrant pain. Endoscopic retrograde cholangiography is necessary in this instance to evaluate for cholangiocarcinoma and allows therapeutic dilatation. Endoscopic therapy for dominant strictures has generally been successful in relieving symptoms of cholestasis. In a prospective study of twelve symptomatic patients with PSC and major ductal strictures treated with repeated balloon dilatation and naso-biliary catheter perfusion, eight patients showed sustained improvement. An average of three sessions was needed to obtain satisfactory reopening (Wagner et al 1996). In a retrospective study of 25 patients with symptomatic dominant strictures treated with endoscopic stent therapy from 1985 to 1994, therapeutic stenting was technically successful in 84%. After a median follow-up of 29 months, 57% remained asymptomatic with stable liver biochemistries. An additional 19% had a relapse that responded favorably to additional endoscopic therapy (van Milligen de Wit et al 1996). The same group reports that short-term stent placement (median 9 days) may be superior in reducing the rate of stent occlusion, with 81% of patients remaining symptom-free and without biochemical evidence of stent occlusion after a median follow-up of 19 months (van Milligen de Wit et al 1997).

The most dreaded complication of PSC is cholangiocarcinoma (Ch. 54), estimated to occur in 7 to 30% of patients at some time during their course (Farges et al 1995). At ten years, the cumulative risk of biliary tract malignancy was 11.2% in a Swedish study (Kornfeld et al 1997). This is consistent with pathology data showing approximately 10% of explanted livers have unsuspected cholangiocarcinoma at the time of liver transplantation. Cholangiocarcinomas associated with PSC are usually found in or near the large ducts. One quarter are intrahepatic; the remainder are distributed along the extrahepatic tree including the cystic duct and gallbladder.

The prognosis for patients with cholangiocarcinoma is grim. Rosen et al (1991) reviewed the experience of 30 patients with both PSC and cholangiocarcinoma at our institution. From the time of diagnosis of cholangiocarcinoma, median survival was 5 months; 63% of patients had metastatic disease at the time of diagnosis, and of the seventeen patients who were believed to have localized disease, eight were found to have abdominal metastasis during surgical exploration. Metastases or local extent of disease precluded curative resection in all but one patient who was disease-free more than two years later. Palliative resection, chemotherapy, and radiotherapy do not meaningfully prolong survival.

The advanced tumor stage at diagnosis reflects both the insidious nature of the tumor and the difficulty of detecting cholangiocarcinoma at an early stage. Most patients do not have recognized symptoms until the disease is too far advanced to cure. This may be because many of the symptoms are similar to those seen in PSC alone. In our experience, patients presenting with rapidly progressive jaundice, weight loss, or abdominal discomfort are more likely to have malignancy. A comparison of PSC patients who developed cholangiocarcinoma with those who did not determined that there were no clinical or biochemical features in the year prior to diagnosis which heralded the onset of malignancy. This study did show that 50% of the patients with PSC and cholangiocarcinoma seen at a single hospital were current or previous daily smokers. None of the matched PSC patients without cholangiocarcinoma had a history of smoking (Bergquist et al 1998). Prior studies have shown age, histologic stage of liver disease, and the presence of ulcerative colitis to also be risk factors for malignant degeneration, but the most recent review at our institution was unable to correlate cirrhotic stage with risk for malignancy (Rosen & Nagorney 1991). Dysplasia of the biliary epithelium may be the greatest risk factor or, indeed, a precursor of cholangiocarcinoma in PSC. A recent study examined the frequency of biliary dysplasia on liver biopsy in patients with PSC alone, PSC plus cholangiocarcinoma, and patients with PSC who later developed cholangiocarcinoma within two years of biopsy. Dysplasia was discovered in hepatic histological specimens from 5 of 5 patients with PSC and cholangiocarcinoma and none (0 of 60) of the patients who were free of malignancy after two years. After the reviewing pathologists agreed on criteria, dysplasia was seen in 9 to 26% of specimens of the 23 patients with PSC who later did develop cholangiocarcinoma within two years of the biopsy (Fleming et al 1998). Likewise, colonic dysplasia seems to be a very strong risk factor for cholangiocarcinoma in PSC, with risk increased significantly over the already increased risk seen in patients with PSC and ulcerative colitis but without dysplasia (Broome et al 1995b). Therefore, the discovery of dysplasia in either the colon or the biliary tree should encourage vigilant surveillance for cholangiocarcinoma. Indeed, under certain circumstances, biliary dysplasia may be an indication for liver transplantation. The risk factors for

the development of cholangiocarcinoma in PSC are summarized in Table 48.6.

Once suspected, most cholangiocarcinomas are visible by some form of radiographic imaging. There are some cholangiographic features suggestive of malignancy. Despite this, the distinction between benign and malignant disease is often impossible. Cytology specimens obtained at ERC are at best 50% sensitive for diagnosing malignancy. To improve detection, investigators have examined carbohydrate antigen 19-9 (CA 19-9) as a serum tumor marker for cholangiocarcinoma and found a level greater than 100 units/ml to be 89% sensitive and 86% specific for the diagnosis of bile duct carcinoma in PSC. In addition, a carcinoembryonic antigen (CEA) level greater than 5 ng/ml was 100% specific but only 38% sensitive for cholangiocarcinoma (Nichols et al 1993). Another study utilizing an index of CA 19-9 + CEA x 40 showed an 86% diagnostic accuracy. Although most of these patients had radiologically occult disease and several went on to transplantation, the great majority still died from cholangiocarcinoma (Ramage et al 1995).

Currently, there are no reliable means to detect cholangiocarcinoma at an early, curable stage. Work is being done to find molecular markers of carcinoma development. p53 mutations occur in cholangiocarcinoma arising in the setting of PSC but are probably a late event. Investigators have shown p53 mutations in 79% of tumors of patients with PSC, but not in the surrounding tissue or in the cholangiocarcinomas of patients without PSC (Rizzi et al 1996). Thus, detection of p53 mutations may be of future diagnostic use but is not able to identify patients at a preneoplastic stage. Presently, there are no effective molecular biological techniques to identify pre-cancerous lesions. This would be the ideal test because one could then offer life-saving liver transplantation prior to the development of this lethal malignancy.

Positron emission tomography (PET) (Ch. 14) may be a promising tool in the future. Based on the principle that malignant cells take up and metabolize glucose more readily than non-malignant cells, PET utilizes enhanced uptake of a radioactive glucose analogue to visualize tumors. In a small study, PET was able to detect small cholangiocarcinomas arising in the setting of PSC with 100% accuracy (Keiding et al 1998). In three of six patients with cholangiocarcinoma, the tumor was not visible by ultrasound. Whether PET is superior to other radiologic imaging modalities for the detection of cholangiocarcinoma requires further study. Conceivably, if this technology becomes more widely available, an early tumor discovered on a screening PET scan could result in earlier liver transplantation and subsequently decreased mortality from cholangiocarcinoma.

Table 48.6 Risk factors for the development of cholangiocarcinoma in primary sclerosing cholangitis

Biliary dysplasia
Colonic dysplasia
Smoking
Duration and histologic stage of liver disease
Presence and duration of ulcerative colitis
Age

PRIMARY THERAPY FOR PRIMARY SCLEROSING CHOLANGITIS

MEDICAL THERAPY

There are no effective medical therapies for primary treatment of PSC. Numerous trials involving cupruretic, anti-fibrotic, choleretic, and immunosuppressive regimens have been performed and are detailed in Table 48.7. To summarize, a number of treatment regimens have shown improvement in liver biochemical tests but none have shown a sustained histological improvement versus placebo. Similarly, none have shown increased survival or increased time to liver transplantation.

Because it is widely used in the treatment of cholestatic liver disease, ursodeoxycholic acid (UDCA) deserves discussion. UDCA is beneficial in the treatment of PBC, as manifested by improvements in liver biochemistries and transplant-free survival. Its mechanism is unknown but is speculated to be due to its replacement of other toxic bile acids in bile acid pool, a cytoprotective effect on hepatocytes and cholangiocytes, an immunomodulatory effect, or its action as a choleretic agent. Whatever the mechanism, it was hoped that UDCA would also be effective in PSC, as it was noted to improve liver biochemistries and clinical outcomes in small pilot and uncontrolled studies. A large, randomized, double-blind, placebo-controlled trial was conducted to determine the clinical benefit of UDCA in the treatment of PSC. Biochemical improvements were noted after one and two years in patients treated with UDCA but not placebo. However, there was no difference between the two groups in primary outcome, time to treatment failure

(Lindor 1997). Because it is safe and effective in PBC, we still prescribe UDCA at higher dosages and in combination with other drugs in the context of clinical trials.

SURGICAL THERAPY

The surgical approach to PSC has evolved tremendously in the past 30 years. Choledochotomy with operative cholangiography and biopsy were once required for diagnosis, the need for this being obviated by the advent of endoscopic and transhepatic cholangiography. Similarly, in the era of transplant medicine, palliative biliary reconstruction has largely been replaced by curative orthotopic liver transplantation.

Non-transplant biliary surgery

Surgical treatment of PSC is complicated by the distribution of strictures along all levels of the biliary tree. Still, there are many patients with a predominance of extrahepatic or peri-hilar disease which may be approached surgically. The early surgical approaches to treat sclerosing cholangitis advocated prolonged T-tube drainage and steroids. Schwartz (1973) reported that nine of eleven patients treated this way showed clinical, biochemical, and radiologic improvement with survival as long as twenty years. Wood & Cuschieri (1980) suggested that T-tube drainage and lavage may actually reverse the disease process. This experience was not shared in other series (Wiesner & LaRusso 1980).

Attempting to improve upon the palliation of simple T-tube drainage and alter disease course, the group at UCLA advocated a more aggressive surgical approach employing

Table 48.7 Results of trials of medical therapy for primary treatment of primary sclerosing cholangitis

Medical therapy	Investigators	Study size*	Design	Results
Corticosteroids	Burgert et al 1984	10	O	Biochemical improvement
Penicillamine	LaRusso et al 1988	70	R	No improvement and toxic
Cyclosporine	Wiesner et al 1991	34	R	No improvement
Methotrexate	Knox & Kaplan 1994	24	R	No improvement
Colchicine	Olsson et al 1995	84	R	No improvement
Tacrolimus	Van Thiel et al 1995	10	O	Biochemical improvement
Ursodeoxycholic acid (UDCA) + Methotrexate	Lindor et al 1996	19	O	No better than UDCA alone, toxicity attributed to methotrexate
Ursodeoxycholic acid	Lindor et al 1997	105	R	Biochemical improvement only, no effect on time to treatment failure

* Number of patients
O = open, R = randomized

Modified from Lindor KD (1996)

biliary–enteric anastomosis. Pitt et al (1982) reported the outcomes of 22 patients managed with surgery between 1974 and 1980; 17 of the 22 underwent choledochoenteric anastomosis. Of these, 13 had a good or excellent result after surgery.

Cameron reported the Johns Hopkins experience with extended biliary resection in combination with stenting and biliary-enteric anastomosis. The procedure involved excision of the hepatic duct bifurcation and extrahepatic biliary tree, dilatation of the intrahepatic ducts, insertion of Silastic transhepatic biliary stents, and bilateral hepaticojejunostomies. In 1988, Cameron and colleagues published the results of 31 patients who underwent this procedure for persistent jaundice or recurrent cholangitis. Twenty-nine of the 31 patients had a dominant stricture at or near the hepatic duct bifurcation; the remaining two had their major obstruction in the distal common bile duct. Five of the patients had cirrhosis. Of the 26 patients with less advanced disease, one died post-operatively and the 1-, 3-, and 5-year actuarial survival rates were 92%, 87%, and 71% respectively. The mean bilirubin in this group improved from 9.9 mg/dl to 4.3 mg/dl after five years. In contrast, two of the five patients with cirrhosis died after surgery and only one survived the first post-operative year. The authors concluded that primary biliary reconstruction should be considered in patients with severe stricturing at or near the hepatic duct bifurcation or in the distal biliary tree if cirrhosis is not present. Patients with cirrhosis, they concluded, should be referred for liver transplantation.

Over the past decade, biliary reconstructive surgery for PSC has become much less common as endoscopic techniques for dilatation and stenting and outcomes with liver transplantation have improved. In addition, hesitation arose after several centers reported increased difficulty performing liver transplantation in patients who had previous biliary surgery. Despite this, biliary–enteric anastomosis may still be indicated in non-cirrhotic patients with primarily extrahepatic disease. To compare efficacy of these different modes of therapy, Ahrendt, Pitt, and colleagues retrospectively reviewed the 146 patients with PSC seen at the Johns Hopkins Hospital from 1980 to 1994. Of these, 50 patients underwent resection of the extrahepatic bile ducts and long-term transhepatic stenting (replaced every 2.2 months on average), 54 were managed nonoperatively with endoscopic balloon dilatation with or without percutaneous stenting, 28 were treated medically, and 21 received liver transplantation (Ahrendt et al 1998). Of the 50 patients managed with resection of the extrahepatic biliary tree, ten had cirrhosis. Three of the 50 patients (6%) died prior to discharge from the hospital (two of these had cirrhosis and all three died before 1985). Four of 21 patients (19%) died after liver transplant. There were no post-procedural deaths in the endoscopically managed group. In non-cirrhotic patients managed with resection, bilirubin levels fell significantly from 8.2 mg/dL preoperatively to just over 3 mg/dL after five years. By comparison, those patients managed nonoperatively with endoscopic or percutaneous procedures had a slight lowering of their serum bilirubin levels at one and three years but then returned to pretreatment levels by five years. Most significant, however, was the improvement in five-year and transplant-free survival (85 and 78%) in patients managed with resection versus endoscopic dilatation and/or percutaneous stenting (59 and 46% five-year and transplant-free survival, respectively). Part of the difference in survival was due to the development of cholangiocarcinoma in three of the endoscopically managed patients. As the majority of cholangiocarcinomas occur in the perihilar region, this may explain why none of the patients who underwent resection died from this complication.

Myburgh (1994) reported his experience with biliary enteric bypass without the need for transanastomotic stenting in 24 patients. Utilizing the Hepp–Couinaud technique (Ch. 30), a side-to-side anastomosis 2.5 to 3.5 cm wide between a Roux-en-Y loop of jejunum and the right and left hepatic ducts at their confluence was performed. Without stents, the need for repeated stent changes and increased risk of cholangitis were eliminated. In the 16 non-cirrhotic patients who underwent bypass, actuarial survival was 100% and eleven remained free of jaundice with a median follow-up of 6.5 years. He concluded that this technique was effective in non-cirrhotic patients with dominant extrahepatic biliary strictures but patients with cirrhosis derived minimal benefit and should undergo liver transplantation.

It does appear that biliary reconstructive surgery may be an effective palliative measure for non-cirrhotic patients with primarily extrahepatic disease. However, our practice is to refer patients with dominant strictures for endoscopic dilatation given the high degree of success attained by this procedure and its relative ease compared to surgery. We would only recommend biliary reconstructive surgery for those few patients who are not candidates for liver transplantation and are not amenable to endoscopic palliation.

Orthotopic liver transplantation

Orthotopic liver transplantation (OLT) (Ch. 109) remains the most effective treatment for PSC and clearly improves survival. In patients with cirrhosis who have a high morbidity and mortality from non-transplant biliary reconstructive procedures, it is the only effective therapy. The development of natural history models clarified which patients would benefit from transplant. Indeed, patients at all risk stratifications have improvement in expected survival with transplantation. Additional models were subsequently developed that identified poor prognostic factors for post-transplant survival. This then allowed the question of optimal timing of transplant to be addressed (see also Ch. 108).

At our institution, recent one-year and five-year patient survival rates are 92% and 86% respectively. This compares favorably with results of liver transplantation for all other conditions. Wiesner and colleagues (1996) reported outcomes for patients who underwent OLT for PSC and identified risk factors that adversely affected outcome. These factors can be categorized into those which influence outcome in liver transplantation in general and those which are specific for PSC. The former include residence in the intensive care unit or being on life support prior to transplantation, age greater than 65 years, poor nutritional status, Child's class C, and renal failure requiring dialysis prior to or after transplantation. These factors are also predictive of increased blood loss, prolonged ICU stay, and major postoperative complications. Risk factors specific for PSC are disease severity, previous biliary or shunt surgery, concurrent bile duct cancer, and presence of inflammatory bowel disease. Utilizing the Mayo risk score as the measure of severity of disease, actual survival after transplantation stratified by risk is shown in Figure 48.4. This figure demonstrates that survival is improved with transplantation for all stages of disease (Abu-Elmagd et al 1993). With these data in mind, earlier transplantation has been advocated for patients with PSC as this would improve patient outcome and resource utilization. This is difficult given the current and increasing shortage of organs (Wiesner et al 1996).

Controversy surrounds the impact of prior biliary surgery on subsequent liver transplantation for PSC. There is little doubt that prior biliary surgery increases the technical difficulty of transplantation but it is unknown if this affects survival. In a series of 26 patients, Farges et al (1995) reported increased operative time, blood loss, and severe complications including death in the 12 transplant patients who had underwent previous right upper quadrant abdominal surgeries. In a combined series of 216 patients from the University of Pittsburgh and the Mayo Clinic, prior biliary tract and/or portal hypertensive surgery was associated with increased mortality the first five years after transplantation but this did not reach statistical significance (Abu-Elmagd et al 1993). At the University of California at San Francisco, increased operative time and blood loss but not mortality were found in patients with a history of prior colectomy or biliary surgery other than simple cholecystectomy (Narumi et al 1995). Ahrendt et al (1998) reported the Johns Hopkins experience with 21 patients who had undergone transplantation for PSC and found significantly increased operative time and blood loss in patients with previous biliary tract operations as well as increased operative mortality, but this did not reach statistical significance. These reports suggest that prior biliary tract surgery increases the technical difficulty of transplantation for PSC and is associated with a trend towards slightly increased mortality when performed at large transplant centers.

After transplantation, there are disease-specific complications unique to PSC patients. Increased rates of biliary strictures have been noted in patients transplanted for PSC. Probably not all of this increase represents disease recurrence as other factors may also cause biliary stricturing, such as ischemia related to chronic rejection or possible chronic low-grade bacterial cholangitis resulting from the Roux-en-Y anastomosis which is performed much more frequently in patients with PSC. However, a University of Pittsburgh study found a significantly increased incidence of strictures in allografts of patients transplanted for PSC versus other patients who also had a liver transplant and choledochojejunostomy bile duct anastomosis for other end-stage liver disease (Sheng et al 1993). Because cholangiographic and other clinical and biochemical criteria for recurrent disease have not been widely accepted, there is no consensus regarding the incidence of recurrent PSC in allografts. However, a careful analysis at our institution concluded 20% of patients transplanted for PSC have recurrent disease based on characteristic cholangiographic and histologic features (Graziadei et al 1999). In addition, several centers now report an increased incidence of rejection in patients transplanted for PSC (van Hoek et al 1992). Acute and chronic ductopenic rejection can be severe and steroid

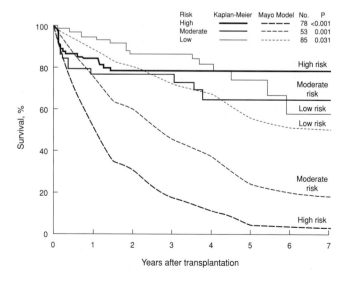

Fig. 48.4 Actual (Kaplan–Meir) survival after transplantation in three risk groups of patients with PSC. From Abu-Elmagd et al (1993)

resistant, often resulting in graft loss (Narumi et al 1995). The most recent report from Baylor University of 100 consecutive patients transplanted for PSC suggests that chronic rejection and disease recurrence occur frequently (13 and 16%, respectively) after transplantation for PSC, adversely affecting both graft and patient survival, markedly so in those patients with chronic rejection (Jeyarajah et al 1998). Five-year graft survival rates were 33 and 65% for patients with chronic rejection and disease recurrence, respectively, as compared to 76% for patients free of chronic rejection or recurrence. The authors suggested that chronic rejection and disease recurrence after transplantation for PSC are distinct entities as evidenced by the difference in outcome and should be managed accordingly.

As many patients with PSC have ulcerative colitis, concern has arisen over the possibility that OLT and attendant, prolonged immunosuppression may increase the risk of colorectal carcinoma. In a study of 108 patients with PSC and concomitant inflammatory bowel disease who underwent OLT, Loftus reported a fourfold (but not statistically significant) increase in colon carcinoma in the group that did not have a prior colectomy compared to expected in a group with comparable (pretransplantation) duration of disease. This did not affect patient survival, however (Loftus et al 1998). Goss also reported no difference in patient survival in groups with or without a prior colectomy (Goss et al 1997). Given the lack of impact on survival, we do not recommend prophylactic proctocolectomy. Nonetheless, the risk of neoplasia warrants annual surveillance colonoscopy with biopsies, and colectomy when even low-grade dysplasia is detected.

Cholangiocarcinoma in patients undergoing OLT merits additional discussion. Survival after OLT for patients with cholangiocarcinoma is dependent upon how and when the cancer is detected. In the past, in patients with PSC in whom a cholangiocarcinoma is known preoperatively, liver transplantation has been ineffective with recurrence of carcinoma occurring almost uniformly. In addition, patients with cholangiocarcinomas discovered at the time of transplantation have also fared poorly (Abu-Elmagd et al 1993). However, incidental cholangiocarcinomas, defined as tumors less than one centimeter in diameter discovered only at the time of pathological sectioning of the explanted liver portend a different prognosis. In the UCLA study, 8% of patients transplanted for PSC had an incidental cholangiocarcinoma and had five-year actuarial survivals of 83%, not significantly different from the survival of patients undergoing OLT without an incidental cholangiocarcinoma (Goss et al 1997). As our ability to detect small cholangiocarcinomas preoperatively improves, we will need to re-evaluate the surgical management of these tumors.

Lastly, our approach to selected patients with known unresectable cholangiocarcinoma may be changing. Gores and colleagues at our institution recently reported the results of a pilot study of 16 patients with unresectable cholangiocarcinoma above the cystic duct without intrahepatic or extrahepatic metastases. Patients were treated with 5-fluorouracil, external beam radiation, and brachytherapy using iridium placed within a biliary stent. Subsequently, an exploratory laparotomy was performed to exclude metastatic disease. Nine (five without and four with PSC) of the 16 patients remained eligible and underwent successful orthotopic liver transplantation, all alive and disease-free with a median follow-up of 24 months (Gores et al 1999). To our knowledge, this is the first successful treatment protocol for selected patients with unresectable cholangiocarcinoma.

Proctocolectomy

The presence of PSC in patients with chronic ulcerative colitis (CUC) affects management of this disease. Much has already been said regarding the increased risk of dysplasia and colon carcinoma. We currently recommend the removal of the colon only for colitic indications, these being severe symptoms or the presence of dysplasia. The decision to perform a Brooke ileostomy or an ileal pouch–anal anastomosis (IPAA) is greatly influenced by the presence of PSC, however. In a retrospective analysis of patients treated with either a Brooke ileostomy or an IPAA, 8 of 31 patients (26%) with the ileostomy developed peristomal varices and subsequent bleeding. None of the 40 patients who had the IPAA developed perianastomotic varices or perineal bleeding (Kartheuser et al 1996). There was a very high incidence of pouchitis in the patients who underwent IPAA, 64 versus 32% in a similar cohort of patients with CUC but not PSC (Penna et al 1996). Hence, PSC is associated with a greatly increased risk of pouchitis in patients who have this procedure. Nonetheless, in patients who need a proctocolectomy, we recommend IPAA in patients over Brooke ileostomy, as treating pouchitis is simpler than managing bleeding varices.

CONCLUSION

Primary sclerosing cholangitis is a cholestatic liver disease of unknown etiology affecting primarily young men with inflammatory bowel disease. It is characterized by a progressive, fibrous obliteration of the biliary tree leading to biliary cirrhosis, portal hypertension, and liver failure.

Patients with PSC have unique complications and are challenging to manage. There is no effective primary medical therapy but endoscopic dilatation and, occasionally, biliary reconstructive procedures, can palliate the symptoms of chronic cholestasis. Currently, orthotopic liver transplantation is the only curative procedure. Our management of PSC will improve with the elucidation of the underlying pathogenic mechanisms of this enigmatic disease.

REFERENCES

Abu-Elmagd K M, Malinchoc M, Dickson E R et al 1993 Efficacy of hepatic transplantation in patients with primary sclerosing cholangitis. Surgery, Gynecology and Obstetrics 177: 335–44

Ahrendt S A, Pitt H A, Kalloo A N et al 1998 Primary sclerosing cholangitis: resect dilate, or transplant? Annals of Surgery 227: 412–23

Balasubramaniam K, Wiesner R H, LaRusso N F 1988 Primary sclerosing cholangitis with normal alkaline phosphatase activity. Gastroenterology 95: 1395–8

Bergquist A, Glaumann H, Persson B et al 1998 Risk factors and clinical presentation of hepatobiliary carcinoma in patients with primary sclerosing cholangitis: a case control study. Hepatology 27: 311–6

Bleday R, Lee E, Jessurun J et al 1993 Increased risk of early colorectal neoplasms after hepatic transplant in patients with inflammatory bowel disease. Diseases of the Colon and Rectum 36: 908–12

Boberg K M, Rocca G, Spurkland A et al 1998 The HLA-DRB1*03, DQA1*0501, DQB1*02 (DR3, DQ2 haplotype is associated with a more rapid disease progression in primary sclerosing cholangitis: Abstract). Hepatology 28: 445A

Brandt D J, MacCarty R L, Charboneau J W et al 1988 Gallbladder disease in patients with primary sclerosing cholangitis. AJR 150: 571–4

Brentnall T A, Haggitt R C, Rabinovitch P S et al 1996 Risk and natural history of colonic neoplasia in patients with primary sclerosing cholangitis and ulcerative colitis. Gastroenterology 110: 331–8

Broome U, Lindberg G, Lofberg R 1992 Primary sclerosing cholangitis in ulcerative colitis ñ a risk factor for the development of dysplasia and DNA aneuploidy? Gastroenterology 102: 1877–80

Broome U, Lofberg R, Lundqvist K et al 1995a Subclinical time span of inflammatory bowel disease in patients with primary sclerosing cholangitis. Dis Colon Rectum 38: 1301–5

Broome U, Lofberg R, Veress B et al 1995b Primary sclerosing cholangitis and ulcerative colitis: evidence for increased neoplastic potential. Hepatology 22: 1404–8

Burgert S L, Brown B P, Kirkpatrick R B et al 1984 Positive corticosteroid response in early primary sclerosing cholangitis: Abstract. Gastroenterology 86: 1037

Cameron J L, Pitt H A, Zinner M J et al 1988 Resection of hepatic duct bifurcation and transhepatic stenting for sclerosing cholangitis. Annals of Surgery 207: 614–22

Campbell W L, Ferris J V, Holbert B L et al 1998 Biliary tract carcinoma complicating primary sclerosing cholangitis: evaluation with CT, cholangiography, US, and MR imaging. Radiology 207: 41–50

Cangemi J R, Wiesner R H, Beaver S J et al 1989 Effect of proctocolectomy for chronic ulcerative colitis on the natural history of primary sclerosing cholangitis. Gastroenterology 96: 790–4

Chapman R W G, Arborgh B A, Rhodes J M et al 1980 Primary sclerosing cholangitis: a review of its clinical features, cholangiography, and hepatic histology. Gut 21: 870–7

Chapman R W, Varghese Z, Gaul R et al 1983 Association of primary sclerosing cholangitis with HLA-B8. Gut 24: 38–41

Chapman R W, Kelly P M, Heryet A et al 1988 Expression of HLA-DR antigens on bile duct epithelium in primary sclerosing cholangitis. Gut 29: 422–7

Czaja A J 1998 Frequency and nature of the variant syndromes of autoimmune liver disease. Hepatology 28: 360–5

Delbet P 1924 Retrecissement du choledoque cholecystoduodenostomie. Bull Mem Soc Chir Paris 50: 1144–6

Dickson E R, Murtaugh P A, Wiesner R H et al 1992 Primary sclerosing cholangitis: refinement and validation of survival models. Gastroenterology 103: 1893–901

Dodd G D 3rd, Niedzwiecki G A, Campbell W L et al 1997 Bile duct calculi in patients with primary sclerosing cholangitis. Radiology 203: 443–7

Donaldson P T, Farrant J M, Wilkinson M L et al 1991 Dual association of HLA DR2 and DR3 with primary sclerosing cholangitis. Hepatology 13: 129–133

Ernst O, Asselah T, Sergent G et al 1998 MR cholangiography in primary sclerosing cholangitis. AJR 171: 1027–30

Farges O, Malassagne B, Sebagh M et al 1995 Primary sclerosing cholangitis: liver transplantation or surgery. Surgery 117: 146–50

Finegold M J, Carpenter R J 1982 Obliterative cholangitis due to cytomegalovirus: a possible precursor of paucity of intrahepatic bile ducts. Human Pathology 13: 662–5

Fleming K A, Clausen O P, Glaumann H et al 1998 Biliary dysplasia in primary sclerosing cholangitis as a marker of increased risk of cholangiocarcinoma (Abstract). Hepatology 28: 446A

Gohlke F, Lohse A W, Dienes H P et al 1996 Evidence for an overlap syndrome of autoimmune hepatitis and primary sclerosing cholangitis. Journal of Hepatology 24: 699–705

Gores G J, Steers J L, Burch P A et al 1999 Prolonged, disease free survival following orthotopic liver transplantation (OLT) for cholangiocarcinoma. Transplantation (In press)

Goss J A, Shackleton C R, Farmer D G et al 1997 Orthotopic liver transplantation for primary sclerosing cholangitis. Annals of Surgery 225: 472–83

Graziadei I W, Wiesner R H, Batts K P et al 1999 Recurrence of primary sclerosing cholangitis following liver transplantation. Hepatology (In press)

Hay J E, Lindor K D, Wiesner R H et al 1991 The metabolic bone disease of primary sclerosing cholangitis. Hepatology 14: 257–61

Holubitsky I B, McKenzie A D 1964 Primary sclerosing cholangitis of the extrahepatic bile ducts. Canadian Journal of Surgery 7: 277–83

Jessurun J, Bolio-Solis A, Manivel J C 1998 Diffuse lymphoplasmacytic acalculous cholecystitis: a distinctive form of chronic cholecystitis associated with primary sclerosing cholangitis. Human Pathology 29: 512–7

Jeyarajah D R, Netto G J, Lee S P et al 1998 Recurrent primary sclerosing cholangitis after orthotopic liver transplantation. Transplantation 66: 1300–6

Jorgensen R A, Lindor K D, Sartin J S et al 1995 Serum lipid and fat soluble vitamin levels in primary sclerosing cholangitis. Journal of Clinical Gastroenterology 20: 215–9

Kartheuser A H, Dozois R R, LaRusso N F et al 1996 Comparison of surgical treatment of ulcerative colitis associated with primary sclerosing cholangitis: ileal pouch–anal anastomosis versus Brooke ileostomy. Mayo Clinic Proceedings 71: 748–56

Kaw M, Silverman W B, Rabinovitz M et al 1995 Biliary tract calculi in primary sclerosing cholangitis. American Journal of Gastroenterology 90: 72–5

Keiding S, Hansen S B, Rasmussen H H et al 1998 Detection of cholangiocarcinoma in primary sclerosing cholangitis by positron emission tomography. Hepatology 28: 700–6

Kim W R, Lindor K D, Poterucha J J et al 1999 The Mayo risk score increases rapidly in the terminal phase of primary sclerosing cholangitis. Gastroenterology (In press.)

Knox T A, Kaplan M M 1994 A double-blind controlled trial of oral-pulse methotrexate therapy in the treatment of primary sclerosing cholangitis. Gastroenterology 106: 494–9

Kornfeld D, Ekbom A, Ihre T 1997 Survival and risk of cholangiocarcinoma in patients with primary sclerosing cholangitis. A population based study. Scandinavian Journal of Gastroenterology 32: 1042–5

LaRusso N F, Wiesner R H 1992 Sclerosing cholangitis. In: Kaplowitz N (ed) Liver and Biliary Diseases, Williams & Wilkins, pp 686–697

LaRusso N F, Wiesner R H, Ludwig J et al 1984 Primary sclerosing cholangitis. New England Journal of Medicine 310: 899–903

LaRusso N F, Wiesner R H, Ludwig J et al 1988 Prospective trial of penicillamine in primary sclerosing cholangitis. Gastroenterology 95: 1036–42

Lazaridis K N, Wiesner R H, Porayko M K et al 1999 Primary sclerosing cholangitis. In: Schiff E R, Sorrell M F & Maddrey W C (eds) Schiff's Diseases of the Liver, 8th edn, Lippincott-Raven, Philadelphia, pp 649–69

Lindor K D 1996 Management of primary biliary cirrhosis and primary sclerosing cholangitis: medical approaches. From LaRusso NF (director) AASLD Postgraduate Course: Diseases of the bile ducts: pathogenesis, pathology, and practice, pp 139–147

Lindor K D 1997 Ursodiol for primary sclerosing cholangitis. New England Journal of Medicine 336: 691–5

Lindor K D, Jorgensen R A, Anderson M L et al 1996 Ursodeoxycholic acid and methotrexate for primary sclerosing cholangitis: a pilot study. American Journal of Gastroenterology 91: 511–5

Lo S K, Fleming K A, Chapman R W 1992 Prevalence of anti-neutrophil antibody in primary sclerosing cholangitis and ulcerative colitis using an alkaline phosphatase technique. Gut 33: 1370–5

Loftus E V Jr., Sandborn W J, Tremaine W J et al 1996a Primary sclerosing cholangitis is associated with nonsmoking: a case-control study. Gastroenterology 110: 1496–502

Loftus E V Jr, Sandborn W J, Tremaine W J et al 1996b Risk of colorectal neoplasia in patients with primary sclerosing cholangitis. Gastroenterology 110: 432–40

Loftus E V Jr, Aguilar H I, Sandborn W J et al 1998 Risk of colorectal neoplasia in patients with primary sclerosing cholangitis and ulcerative colitis following orthotopic liver transplantation. Hepatology 27: 685–90

Louis P, Griffiths A M, Blendis L M et al 1995 Primary sclerosing cholangitis in 32 children: clinical, laboratory, and radiographic features, with survival analysis. Hepatology 22: 1415–22

Ludwig J 1991 Small-duct primary sclerosing cholangitis. Seminars in Liver Disease 11: 11–7

Ludwig J 1995 Granulomas in primary sclerosing cholangitis. Liver 15: 307–12

Ludwig J, Barham S S, LaRusso N F et al 1981 Morphologic features of chronic hepatitis associated with primary sclerosing cholangitis or chronic ulcerative colitis. Hepatology 1: 632–40

Ludwig J, LaRusso N F, Wiesner R H 1986 Primary sclerosing cholangitis. In: Peters R L, Craig J R (eds) Contemporary Issues in Surgical Pathology: Liver Pathology, Churchill Livingstone, New York, pp 193–213

Luketic V A C, Gomez D A, Sanyal A J et al 1997 An atypical presentation for primary sclerosing cholangitis. Digestive Diseases and Sciences 42: 2009–16

MacCarty R L, LaRusso N F, Wiesner R H et al 1983 Primary sclerosing cholangitis: findings on cholangiography and pancreatography. Radiology 149: 39–44

MacCarty R L, LaRusso N F, May G R et al 1985 Cholangiocarcinoma complicating primary sclerosing cholangitis: cholangiographic appearances. Radiology 156: 43–6

Majoie C B, Smits N J, Phoa S S et al 1995 Primary sclerosing cholangitis: sonographic findings. Abdominal Imaging 20: 109–12

McNair A N, Moloney M, Portmann B C et al 1998 Autoimmune hepatitis overlapping with primary sclerosing cholangitis in five cases. American Journal of Gastroenterology 93: 777–84

Milano C, Fassio E, Gutierrez S et al 1998 Ondansetron for treatment of pruritus in cholestasis (Abstract). Hepatology 28: 442A

Morecki R, Glaser J H, Cho S et al 1982 Biliary atresia and reovirus type 3 infection. New England Journal of Medicine 307: 481–4

Myburgh J A 1994 Surgical biliary drainage in primary sclerosing cholangitis. Archives of Surgery 129: 1057–62

Narumi S, Roberts J P, Emond J C et al 1995 Liver transplantation for sclerosing cholangitis. Hepatology 22: 451–7

Nichols J C, Gores G J, LaRusso N F et al 1993 Diagnostic role of serum CA 19-9 for cholangiocarcinoma in patients with primary sclerosing cholangitis. Mayo Clinic Proceedings 68: 874–9

Nuako K W, Ahlquist D A, Sandborn W J et al 1998 Primary sclerosing cholangitis and colorectal carcinoma in patients with chronic ulcerative colitis. Cancer 82: 822–6

Olsson R, Danielsson A, Jarnerot G et al 1991 Prevalence of primary sclerosing cholangitis in patients with ulcerative colitis. Gastroenterology 100: 1319–23

Olsson R, Broome U, Danielsson et al 1995 Colchicine treatment of primary sclerosing cholangitis. Gastroenterology 108: 1199–203

Penna C, Dozois R, Tremaine W et al 1996 Pouchitis after ileal pouch-anal anastomosis for ulcerative colitis occurs with increased frequency in patients with associated primary sclerosing cholangitis. Gut 38: 234–9

Phillips P A, Keast D, Papadimitriou J M et al 1969 Chronic obstructive jaundice induced by reovirus type 3 in weanling mice. Pathology 1: 193–203

Pitt H A, Thompson H H, Tompkins R K et al 1982 Primary sclerosing cholangitis: results of an aggressive surgical approach. Annals Surgery 196: 259–68

Porayko M K, Wiesner R H, LaRusso N F et al 1990 Patients with asymptomatic primary sclerosing cholangitis frequently have progressive disease. Gastroenterology 98: 1594–1602

Quigley E M M, LaRusso N F, Ludwig J et al 1983 Familial occurrence of primary sclerosing cholangitis and ulcerative colitis. Gastroenterology 85: 1160–5

Ramage J K, Donaghy A, Farrant J M et al 1995 Serum tumor markers for the diagnosis of cholangiocarcinoma in primary sclerosing cholangitis. Gastroenterology 108: 865–9

Rasmussen H H, Fallingborg J F, Mortensen B et al 1997 Hepatobiliary dysfunction and primary sclerosing cholangitis in patients with Crohn's disease. Scandinavian Journal of Gastroenterology 32: 604–10

Rizzi P M, Ryder S D, Portmann B et al 1996 p53 Protein overexpression in cholangiocarcinoma arising in primary sclerosing cholangitis. Gut 38: 265–8

Rosen C B, Nagorney D M 1991 Cholangiocarcinoma complicating primary sclerosing cholangitis. Seminars in Liver Disease 11: 26–30

Scheuer PJ 1998 Pathologic features and evolution of primary biliary cirrhosis and primary sclerosing cholangitis. Mayo Clinic Proceedings 73: 179–83

Schrumpf E, Fausa O, Elgjo K et al 1988 Hepatobiliary complications of inflammatory bowel disease. Seminars in Liver Disease 8: 201–9

Schwartz S I 1973 Primary sclerosing cholangitis. Surgical Clinics of North America 53: 1161–1168

Schwartz S I, Dale W A 1958 Primary sclerosing cholangitis: review and report of six cases. Arch Surg 77: 439–51

Sheng R, Zajko A B, Campbell W L et al 1993 Biliary strictures in hepatic transplants: prevalence and types in patients with primary sclerosing cholangitis vs. those with other liver diseases. AJR. American Journal of Roenterology 161: 297–300

Shepherd H A, Selby W S, Chapman R W G et al 1983 Ulcerative colitis and persistent liver dysfunction. Quarterly Journal of Medicine 52: 503–13

Shetty K, Rybicki L, Carey W D 1997 The Child–Pugh classification as a prognostic indicator for survival in primary sclerosing cholangitis. Hepatology 25: 1049–53

Siegel J H, Barnes S, Morris J S 1977 Bile acids in liver disease associated with inflammatory bowel disease. Digestion 15: 469–81

Stonnington C M, Phillips S F, Melton L J I et al 1987 Chronic ulcerative colitis: incidence and prevalence in a community. Gut 28: 402–9

Teefey S A, Baron R L, Rohrmann C A et al 1988 Sclerosing cholangitis: CT findings. Radiology 169: 635–9

Thorpe M E C, Scheuer P J, Sherlock S 1967 Primary sclerosing cholangitis, the biliary tree, and ulcerative colitis. Gut 8: 435–48

van Erpecum K J, Smits S J, van de Meeberg P C et al 1996 Risk of primary sclerosing cholangitis is associated with nonsmoking behavior. Gastroenterology 110: 1503–6

van Hoek B, Wiesner R H, Krom R A et al 1992 Severe ductopenic rejection following liver transplantation: incidence, time of onset, risk factors, treatment, and outcome. Seminars in Liver Disease 12: 41–50

van Milligen de Wit A W, van Bracht J, Rauws E A et al 1996 Endoscopic stent therapy for dominant extrahepatic bile duct strictures in primary sclerosing cholangitis. Gastrointestinal Endoscopy 44: 293–9

van Milligen de Wit A W, Rauws E A, van Bracht J et al 1997 Lack of complications following short-term stent therapy for extrahepatic bile duct strictures in primary sclerosing cholangitis. Gastrointest Endosc 46: 344–7

Van Thiel D H, Carroll P, Abu-Elmagd K et al 1995 Tacrolimus (FK 506), a treatment for primary sclerosing cholangitis: results of an open-label preliminary trial. Am J Gastroenterol 90: 455–9

Vidrich A, Lee J, James E et al 1995 Segregation of pANCA antigenic recognition by DNase treatment of neutrophils: ulcerative colitis, type 1 autoimmune hepatitis, and primary sclerosing cholangitis. Journal of Clinical Immunology 15: 293–9

Wagner S, Gebel M, Meir P et al 1996 Endoscopic management of biliary tract strictures in primary sclerosing cholangitis. Endoscopy 28: 546–551

Warren K W, Athanassiades S, Monge J I 1966 Primary sclerosing cholangitis. A study of 42 cases. American Journal of Surgery 111: 23–38

Wiesner R H, LaRusso N F 1980 Clinicopathologic features of the syndrome of primary sclerosing cholangitis. Gastroenterology 79: 200–6

Wiesner R H, Grambsch P M, Dickson E R et al 1989 Primary sclerosing cholangitis: natural history, prognostic factors and survival analysis. Hepatology 10: 430–6

Wiesner R H, Steiner B, LaRusso N F et al 1991 A controlled clinical trial evaluating cyclosporin in the treatment of primary sclerosing cholangitis. (Abstract). Hepatology 14: 63A

Wiesner R H, Porayko M K, Hay J E et al 1996 Liver transplantation for primary sclerosing cholangitis: impact of risk factors on outcome. Liver Transplant Surgery 2(5): suppl 1, pp. 99–108

Wood R A B, Cuschieri A 1980 Is sclerosing cholangitis complicating ulcerative colitis a reversible condition? Lancet 2: 716–8

Benign biliary strictures

49

W.R. JARNAGIN, L.H. BLUMGART

A COMBINED SURGICAL AND RADIOLOGICAL APPROACH TO BENIGN BILE-DUCT STRICTURES AND OTHER BILIARY PROBLEMS

A.S. LIVINGSTONE, D.G. HUTSON

INTRODUCTION

Benign biliary strictures remain difficult management problems. Unlike malignant biliary obstruction, in which short-term palliation is often the goal of therapy, benign strictures require durable repair since most patients are in otherwise good health and are expected to survive for years. Many of these strictures result from iatrogenic injuries, often in young patients in the most productive years of life. Improper management may result in disastrous complications, such as biliary cirrhosis, portal hypertension or recurrent cholangitis. Furthermore, repeated intervention greatly reduces the likelihood of a successful outcome. It is therefore imperative that any attempt at repair be carried out in a precise and expert manner in the setting of a specialist center. The best results are achieved through early diagnosis, mature clinical judgement and technical expertise at the first attempt at repair.

Benign biliary strictures may affect the intrahepatic and/or extrahepatic bile ducts and may be solitary or multiple. Several causes of benign biliary strictures have been described (Table 49.1). Iatrogenic injuries after cholecystectomy are by far the most commonly reported and best characterized, however, and this topic will be emphasized in this chapter to illustrate the principals of diagnosis and management. Strictures and other injuries may also occur after common bile duct exploration or biliary reconstruction. Other procedures in the upper abdomen may put the biliary tract in harm's way, especially those involving the liver, pancreas and stomach/duodenum. The true incidence of biliary injury after these procedures is difficult to assess but appears to be substantially lower than after cholecystectomy.

Table 49.1 Causes of benign biliary strictures

1. Congenital strictures
   a. Biliary atresia (see Ch. 47)
2. Bile duct injuries
   a. Postoperative strictures
      (i) Cholecystectomy and/or common bile duct exploration
      (ii) Biliary-enteric anastomosis
      (iii) Hepatic resection
      (iv) Portacaval shunt
      (v) Pancreatic surgery
      (vi) Gastrectomy
      (vii) Liver transplantation (see Ch. 115)
   b. Strictures following blunt or penetrating trauma (see Ch. 68)
   c. Strictures following endoscopic or percutaneous biliary intubation
3. Inflammatory strictures
   a. Cholelithiasis or choledocholithiasis
   b. Chronic pancreatitis
   c. Chronic duodenal ulceration
   d. Abscess or inflammation of liver or subhepatic space
   e. Parasitic infection (see Chs 62, 63)
   f. Recurrent pyogenic cholangitis (Oriental cholangiohepatitis) (see Ch. 64)
4. Primary sclerosing cholangitis (see Ch. 48)
5. Radiation-induced stricture
6. Papillary stenosis

BILE DUCT INJURY AT CHOLECYSTECTOMY

Incidence

Because of the great frequency with which the operation is performed, cholecystectomy remains the greatest source of postoperative biliary injuries. Open cholecystectomy has long been associated with a modest incidence of biliary injuries. In a review of over 42 000 open cholecystectomies performed in the United States in 1989, Roslyn et al documented a 0.2% incidence of biliary injuries (Roslyn et al 1993), while Strasberg et al reported a 0.3% incidence of injuries in a literature review of over 25 000 open cholecystectomies since 1980 (Strasberg et al 1995). However, the advent of laparoscopic cholecystectomy (Ch. 38) has refocused attention on this issue because of the significant increase in the number of injuries. Several studies worldwide have documented a marked increase in the frequency of bile duct injuries associated with the laparoscopic approach, ranging from 0.4 to 1.3% (Adamsen et al 1997, Deziel et al 1993, Fletcher et al 1999, MacFadyen et al 1998, Richardson et al 1996, Wherry et al 1996). Also, in a review of nearly 125 000 laparoscopic cholecystectomies reported in the literature from 1991 through 1993, Strasberg and associates reported an overall incidence of biliary injuries of 0.85% and a 0.52% incidence of major injuries (Strasberg et al 1995). Given the inherent difficulties in collecting data on postcholecystectomy biliary injuries, the true incidence at any one time may never be known precisely. However, it is clear that the figures reported for laparoscopic cholecystectomy represent a substantial increase over historical controls reported for open cholecystectomy.

There are several reasons that the bile duct is at increased risk of injury during laparoscopic cholecystectomy compared with open cholecystectomy (vide infra). It has long been argued that surgeon inexperience is a major culprit, and that with increased familiarity with the procedure, the number of injuries will decrease: the so-called 'learning curve effect' (The Southern Surgeons Club 1991). There is considerable evidence to support this view. Several authors have shown an inverse relationship between the incidence of bile duct injuries and number of cases performed (Deziel et al 1993, Gigot et al 1997, Woods et al 1994). Also, large population-based reviews have documented a decline in injuries over time (Richardson et al 1996, Russell et al 1996), and some authors have noted a decline in the number of injuries referred for repair (Woods et al 1994). These trends, while encouraging, have not been observed by all investigators, however. Several contemporary reports have suggested no change in the incidence of bile duct injuries over time (Adamsen et al 1997, Fletcher et al 1999, Wherry et al 1996), and the number and complexity of cases referred for repair has remained static at some specialist units (Walsh et al 1998). Moreover, reports of major bile duct injuries inflicted by surgeons with considerable experience continue to appear (Carroll et al 1996, Gigot et al 1997). The data would therefore suggest that postcholecystectomy bile duct injuries will remain a significant problem for the forseeable future.

Pathogenesis

There are several factors associated with an increased risk of bile duct injury at cholecystectomy, some of which are general and some unique to the laparoscopic approach. Ultimately, however, the final common pathway of most injuries is either a technical error or misinterpretation of the anatomy (Table 49.2) (Olsen 1997, Strasberg et al 1995). Many authors classify biliary injuries as major, such as transection of the common bile duct, or minor, such as biliary leak, but the line separating the two is often blurred. In general, major injuries are more serious and usually require reoperation to repair. However, minor injuries are not always trivial and may require operative intervention. The classification of biliary injuries is discussed later in the chapter.

Table 49.2 Classification of causes of laparoscopic biliary injuries

Misidentification of the bile ducts as the cystic duct
   Misidentification of the common bile duct as the cystic duct
   Misidentification of an aberrant right sectoral hepatic duct as the cystic duct

Technical causes
   Failure to occlude securely the cystic duct
   Plane of dissection away from gallbladder wall into the liver bed
   Injudicious use of electrocautery for dissection or bleeding control
   Excessive traction on cystic duct with tenting upwards of common hepatic duct
   Injudicious use of clips to control bleeding
   Improper techniques of ductal exploration

(Modified from Strasberg et al 1995, reprinted with permission)

Anatomical variations. Any surgeon operating on the biliary tree must be familiar with the wide range of anatomical variations that may be encountered (see Ch. 1). Anomalies of the cystic duct insertion into the common hepatic duct are seen most commonly (Fig. 49.1). The cystic duct may join the common hepatic duct quite high, almost at the biliary confluence, or may run parallel to the common hepatic duct for a long distance before joining it very low, occasionally at the level of the ampulla. In a large number of patients, perhaps as high as 25%, the right hepatic duct per se is absent, and the right anterior and posterior sectoral hepatic ducts join the left hepatic duct independently. In some cases, one of the right sectoral hepatic ducts (usually the anterior) may follow a prolonged extrahepatic course and enter the common hepatic duct quite low and may also receive drainage from the cystic duct (Fig. 49.1D). Such unrecognized, low-entry right sectoral hepatic ducts (Bismuth type 5) are at particular risk of injury during laparoscopic cholecystectomy (Wherry et al 1996) (Fig. 49.2).

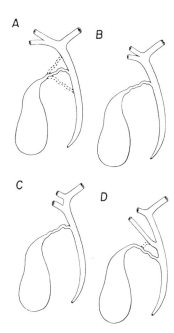

Fig. 49.1 Schematic representation of the manner of junction of the cystic duct with the main extrahepatic biliary channel. **(A)** The cystic duct may join the main bile duct either very high, almost at the confluence of the hepatic ducts, or it may run parallel to the common hepatic duct before entering almost at the level of the ampulla of Vater. Note that in this illustration, the right anterior and posterior sectoral hepatic ducts join to form a main right hepatic duct. **(B)** The right anterior and posterior sectoral hepatic ducts may join the left hepatic duct at a common confluence. **(C)** The right anterior and posterior sectoral hepatic ducts may join the left hepatic duct independently. **(D)** The right anterior or posterior sectoral hepatic duct may join the common hepatic duct at a much lower level. The cystic duct may drain into such a duct. Another variation, not shown and probably not relevant for postcholecystectomy injuries, is entry of the right anterior or posterior sectoral hepatic duct into the left hepatic duct.

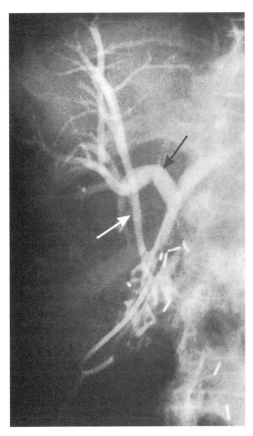

Fig. 49.2 The right anterior sectoral hepatic duct (white arrow) drains into the common hepatic duct and the right posterior sectoral hepatic duct (black arrow) joins a main left hepatic duct. The situation is as illustrated in Fig. 49.1D. In this patient, cholecystectomy was accompanied by a biliary injury at the point of confluence of the common hepatic duct and the right anterior sectoral hepatic duct (Bismuth type 5). Repair has been carried out by hepaticojejunostomy Roux-en-Y.

In some cases, the cystic duct is quite short, and misinterpretation of the anatomy can easily occur. This is especially true if, on intraoperative cholangiography, the catheter has been advanced well into the common bile duct and the proximal ducts are not visualized. The surgeon may then mistake the common duct for the cystic duct, ligate it and remove it with the attached gallbladder (Fig. 49.3). This type of injury appears to be much more common after laparoscopic rather than open cholecystectomy and is well-described (Davidoff et al 1992). A related situation can occur in cases of long-standing cholelithiasis and chronic cholecystitis, resulting in obliteration of the cystic duct (vide infra).

Vascular anomalies are also common, occurring in up to 20% of patients (see Ch. 1). In the most common of these, the right hepatic arterial supply arises in part or in whole from the superior mesenteric artery. Such an aberrant vessel usually courses to the right of the portal vein, lateral and somewhat posterior to the common bile duct. During cholecystectomy, this vessel is prone to injury at the cystic duct/common hepatic duct junction. Of course, vascular injuries are not limited to patients with anatomical anomalies. The 'classic' biliary injury during laparoscopic cholecystectomy, in which the surgeon mistakes the common bile duct for the cystic duct, is not infrequently associated with injury to the right hepatic artery (vide infra) (Davidoff et al 1992). Hepatic artery injury may not be apparent at the initial operation but rather may come to attention later as a hepatic artery pseudoaneurysm (Balsara et al 1998).

Ischemia. Late biliary stricture formation, in the absence of overt injury, may result from extensive periductal dissection and consequent interruption of the major ductal arterial supply (see Ch. 1). Most of the arterial supply to the extrahepatic bile duct is provided by two small arteries traveling along the lateral duct borders, in the 3 o'clock and 9 o'clock

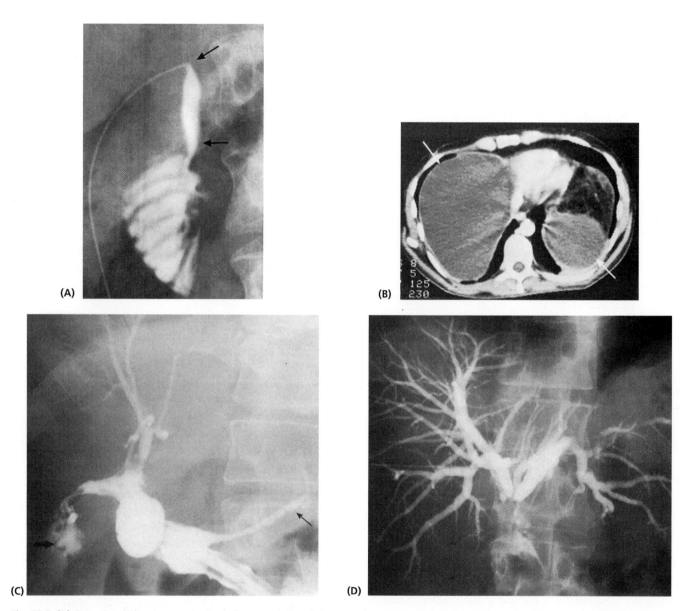

Fig. 49.3 (A) Operative cholangiogram obtained after cannulation of the cystic duct. Note that the cannula has entered the common bile duct (upper arrow) and that only the common bile duct has been outlined (lower arrow). The common hepatic duct has not been visualized. The surgeon proceeded with cholecystectomy in the belief that he had cannulated the cystic duct. **(B)** The patient became extremely ill after operation and was referred. CT scan revealed massive collections of intraperitoneal bile (arrows) which were drained. **(C)** A subsequent fistulogram revealed a fistulous tract with connections to both the right and left abdomen (arrow). The right anterior sectoral hepatic duct is also visualized. The patient, now well and free of jaundice, was followed. **(D)** Percutaneous transhepatic cholangiogram obtained after the patient returned with jaundice demonstrated that the fistula is now closed and there is a stricture just below the biliary confluence (Bismuth type 3). Repair was performed by hepaticojejunostomy Roux-en-Y using an approach to the left hepatic duct and extending the dissection to the right.

positions. Sixty percent of the blood supply runs upward from the major inferior vessels (retroduodenal, gastroduodenal) and approximately 38% runs downward from the right hepatic artery (Northover & Terblanche, 1979). Extensive circumferential dissection of the duct may thus disrupt this axial blood flow and has been proposed as a major mechanism of biliary stricture formation. Although there is no direct evidence to support this, it would seem reasonable not to pursue extensive dissection of the common duct during cholecystectomy. Also, damage to these vessels is likely as a contributing if not a central factor in the formation of strictures attributed to electrocautery use.

Pathological factors. Patients with acute cholecystitis may have severe inflammation in the porta hepatis and Calot's triangle, which greatly distorts the anatomy. In addition, the gallbladder is often friable and difficult to grasp, and persistent oozing of blood often obscures the field. Some or all of these factors may conspire to preclude safe laparoscopic cholecystectomy. That is not to say that laparoscopic cholecystectomy cannot be performed safely in patients with acute cholecystitis. On the contrary, several reports document that laparoscopic approach is not only possible but safe in selected cases of acute cholecystitis (Adamsen et al 1997, Fletcher et al 1999, Kum et al 1996, Wherry et al 1996). However, these studies have also revealed a greater potential for biliary injury when laparoscopic cholecystectomy is performed for acute cholecystitis. Fletcher et al reported that complex cases, which included patients with acute cholecystitis, cholangitis and gallstone pancreatitis, are associated with a dramatically increased incidence of bile duct injuries (1.7%), although acute cholecystitis alone was not an independent risk factor (Fletcher et al 1999). Others have shown that acute cholecystitis increases the incidence of bile duct injuries two- to three-fold above baseline (Adamsen et al 1997, Russell et al 1996). An attempt at laparoscopic cholecystectomy is certainly reasonable in patients with acute inflammation, since many will benefit. However, given the increased risk of biliary injury in this setting, the threshold for conversion to an open procedure should be low.

Occasionally, the inflammatory reaction is so severe that even conversion to an open procedure does not clarify the anatomy. Fibrosis and inflammation within Calot's triangle makes dissection of the cystic duct particularly hazardous. In severe cases, the gallbladder neck and cystic duct may be fused to the common duct within a sheath of scar tissue. This finding should lead the surgeon away from an extensive dissection to define the cystic duct, which risks a major biliary injury. Placement of a cholecystostomy tube may be a safer approach (Dawson 1981). An alternative option is partial cholecystectomy with amputation of the gallbladder well away from the cystic duct/common hepatic duct junction and placement of a drain (Grey-Turner 1944). In such heavily fibrosed cases, the cystic duct is nearly always obliterated, and postoperative biliary leak is infrequent.

A potentially more difficult problem is the small, contracted, fibrotic gallbladder with extensive surrounding inflammation, sometimes partially embedded into the liver, and obliterating Calot's triangle such that the gallbladder neck and cystic duct are adherent to the common hepatic duct (Fig. 49.4). In such cases, the cystic duct is obliterated and safe dissection in Calot's triangle is impossible. With long-standing disease, particularly associated with large impacted gallstones in the gallbladder neck, a cholecystocholedochal fistula is not uncommon. Moreover, there may very well be a common hepatic duct stricture resulting from

an impacted stone and the subsequent inflammatory response (see Fig. 54.8) (Mirizzi 1948). A cholecystocholedochal fistula should be suspected in any patient with gallstones, jaundice, cholangitis and imaging studies or operative findings to suggest such an inflamed and contracted gallbladder. In these cases, an attempt to perform a total cholecystectomy should be abandoned, as this will lead the surgeon directly into the common hepatic duct (Sharma et al 1998). Rather, partial cholecystectomy with extraction of the stones allows inspection of the depths of the gallbladder and is preferable. A rush of bile into the operative field at this point is strong evidence for a cholecystocholedochal fistula since the cystic duct is nearly always obliterated. Because there is often a biliary stricture distal to the fistula, direct closure of the defect should be avoided but rather reconstructed as a cholecystocholedochoduodenostomy (Fig. 49.4B).

Technical factors

General. Cholecystectomy is performed so commonly that it is easy to adopt a casual attitude toward the procedure. This is unwise, however, since some of these cases can be quite challenging. Also, while it is true that many bile duct injuries are committed by inexperienced or poorly trained

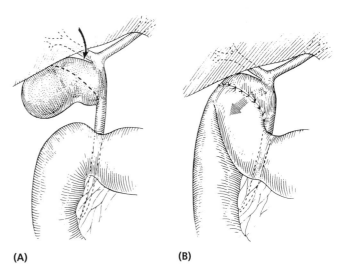

(A) **(B)**

Fig. 49.4 (A) Obliteration of Calot's triangle (curved arrow) by the inflammatory process accompanying severe chronic cholecystitis. The gallbladder is contracted around two large gallstones, one of which has eroded into the common hepatic duct producing a cholecystocholedochal fistula. Such cases often present with obstructive jaundice or cholangitis. There should be no attempt at complete cholecystectomy since this will lead inevitably to biliary injury. Partial cholecystectomy (dotted line) can be performed with extraction of the calculi.
(B) Cholecystocholedochoduodenostomy can be carried out with safety and adequate drainage of bile.

surgeons (see above), not even the best-trained and most experienced surgeons are exempt from bile duct injury. It is imperative, therefore, that the surgeon adhere strictly to the basic tenets of cholecystectomy, either laparoscopic or open, to minimize the risk of biliary injury (see Chs 37 and 38).

Safe cholecystectomy requires clear visualization of the relevant anatomy, which in turn demands proper exposure. Adequate assistance and retraction must be available, and the incision must be adequate in length or the trochars properly placed. It is absolutely imperative that no structure be ligated or divided unless its identity is known unequivocally.

Early reports of laparoscopic biliary injury cited bleeding and subsequent attempts to achieve hemostasis as major contributing factors to bile duct injury (Davidoff et al 1992, Rossi et al 1992). At laparoscopy, even a small amount of blood obscures the field and hinders dissection. However, hemorrhage must be controlled precisely, regardless of the approach, and blind placement of clips or indiscriminate use of electrocautery must be avoided. Early demonstration of the cystic artery is desirable, and it should be divided close to the gallbladder in order to avoid injury to the right hepatic or common hepatic artery.

Excessive traction on the gallbladder during cholecystectomy may tent the common duct upwards, putting it at risk of injury if unrecognized. This mechanism does not appear to be as common at laparoscopic cholecystectomy, although other problems related to retraction may predispose to biliary injury at laparoscopy (vide infra). Some authors have argued that the cystic duct/common hepatic duct junction should be precisely demonstrated before it is ligated and divided, even if this requires separating an adherent cystic duct and tracing it to its termination (Kune & Sali 1981). We firmly believe that this is unnecessary and potentially hazardous. The risk of biliary injury with such extensive dissection is high and greatly outweighs the risk of a retained cystic duct stone.

The plane of dissection should be maintained as close to the gallbladder wall as possible to avoid entering the liver parenchyma. This is especially important when there is significant inflammation or fibrosis and the ductal anatomy is unclear. Straying off the gallbladder wall may result in entry into the liver parenchyma and bleeding, further obscuring the field, or injury to a low-entry sectoral hepatic duct or a replaced right hepatic artery. In addition, it is important to realize that the major right portal pedicles may be quite superficial in the liver substance with respect to the gallbladder fossa, and damage to these structures can occur if the plane of dissection is too deep. During a difficult open cholecystectomy, one has an advantage over the laparo-scopic approach in that a finger can be inserted into the gall-bladder to help define the proper plane.

The observation of bile draining from the gallbladder fossa must always suggest the possibility of a biliary injury, perhaps to an aberrant right sectoral hepatic duct. It is tempting to ascribe such a finding to drainage from a subvesical duct of Lushka, a slender, 1–2 mm in diameter duct that passes from the right lobe in the gallbladder fossa to join the right hepatic or common hepatic duct (McMahon et al 1995).

Cholangiographic studies identify a subvesical duct in only 1 to 2% of patients (Taniguchi et al 1993), thus making it an unlikely cause of bile leak. In this situation, a major bile duct injury must be considered the leading diagnosis until disproved, and the surgeon is compelled to convert to an open procedure or to place a drain and investigate the cause postoperatively.

The utility of routine cystic duct cholangiography remains controversial (Ch. 22), particularly with respect to reducing the incidence of biliary injury at laparoscopic cholecystectomy (vide infra). Occasionally, operative cholangiography reveals a very small common bile duct with a filling defect suggesting a small stone. In this situation, simple cholecystectomy without exploration of the common duct is probably safer than operative pursuit of a tiny stone in a small duct. Postoperative endoscopic cholangiography with stone extraction is nearly always possible if subsequently indicated. In general, exploration of a small caliber, otherwise normal-appearing common duct is frequently unrewarding, potentially dangerous, and more likely to result in postoperative symptoms than if such a stone were left in situ. Moreover, biliary strictures are more than just a theoretical concern after exploration of a small bile duct (Fig. 49.5).

When indicated at cholecystectomy, exploration of the common bile duct should be performed through a supraduodenal choledochotomy with careful exposure of a sufficient length of duct but without excessive dissection (see Chs 39 and 42). Exploration must be gentle and performed only with soft bougies, Fogarty-type balloon catheters or a choledochoscope (rigid or flexible). Metal bougies such as Bake's dilators or stone forceps should be used with caution and should never be forced through the papilla of Vater into the duodenum; otherwise, secondary postinflammatory papillary stenosis may occur or a false passage into the duodenum or pancreas may be created. After bile duct exploration, the choledochotomy should be closed with care since this is also a potential cause of biliary stricture (see Chs 39 and 42).

Transduodenal sphincteroplasty is probably best reserved for patients with stones impacted in the distal bile duct (see

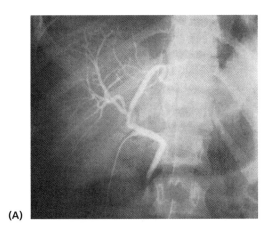

(A)

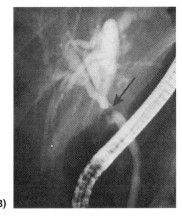

(B)

Fig. 49.5 (A) Cystic duct cholangiogram obtained at the time of cholecystectomy. A stone was suspected in a small-caliber common bile duct. Bile duct exploration was performed but no stone identified. **(B)** Postoperatively, the patient developed recurrent attacks of cholangitis. Endoscopic cholangiogram demonstrated a bile duct stricture at the previous choledochotomy site (arrow).

a long length of the common duct is excised up to the proximal common hepatic duct, which is either occluded or left to drain bile into the peritoneal cavity. This devastating injury, referred to as the 'classic' laparoscopic injury and rarely seen at open cholecystectomy, may also be associated with damage to the right hepatic artery (Davidoff et al 1992, Strasberg et al 1995). Less severe injuries may also occur, such as lacerations of the duct wall or near complete transections.

Proper exposure is essential to avoid injuries arising from such anatomical misinterpretations. Maximum cephalad traction on the gallbladder fundus is necessary to expose the cystic duct and Calot's triangle. However, concomitant lateral traction on the infundibulum is equally important to open the angle between the cystic and common hepatic ducts. If lateral traction is inadequate, Calot's triangle is not opened sufficiently and the course of the common duct is placed directly in line with that of the cystic duct (Fig. 49.6) (McMahon et al 1995, Rossi et al 1992). The common duct may then be damaged during dissection of the cystic duct, because of its proximity, or because it is misidentified. Before any structures are divided, Calot's triangle must be cleared of all fatty and areolar tissue. The peritoneal reflection along the posterolateral aspect of the gallbladder should be opened to expose fully the junction of the gallbladder neck and cystic duct. At the completion of the dissection, only the cystic artery and cystic duct should be seen

Chs 39 and 46). Stenosis or stricture of the distal common bile duct may result after surgical or endoscopic sphincteroplasty or sphincterotomy. Side-to-side choledochoduodenostomy is an option that should be considered in patients with multiple stones, primary stasis stones, or distal obstruction by stricture or papillary stenosis. The results are generally good provided that the common bile duct is dilated to at least 15 mm in diameter and a stoma of at least 2 cm can be created (Schein & Glieddman 1981). On the other hand, choledochoduodenostomy performed to a decompressed duct is more likely to result in stricture formation and cholangitis (Johnson & Stevens 1969) (see Ch. 45).

Laparoscopic specific. Several technical factors, specific to laparoscopic cholecystectomy, predispose to biliary injury. Mistaking the common duct for the cystic duct is a frequent technical error (Davidoff et al 1992, Gigot et al 1997, Olsen 1997). In the most common sequence of events that follow,

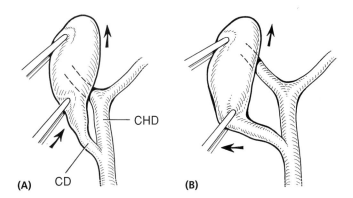

(A) CD   CHD   (B)

Fig. 49.6 Area of the triangle of Calot as it appears during laparoscopic cholecystectomy. **(A)** Upward traction on the gallbladder, with insufficient lateral traction on the infundibulum, fails to open Calot's triangle adequately. This causes the cystic (CD) and common hepatic ducts (CHD) to become aligned within the same plane. Injury to the common duct can occur during dissection of the cystic duct, because of its proximity, or as a result of mistaking the common duct for the cystic duct. **(B)** Proper lateral traction on the infundibulum opens the triangle of Calot, allowing safer dissection of the cystic duct. In some cases, obliteration of Calot's triangle by dense fibrosis prevents adequate exposure of this area, even with adequate traction (see Fig. 49.4).

entering the gallbladder, and the bottom of the gallbladder fossa should be visible. The use of a 30° laparoscope has been advocated to improve visualization of this area (Hunter 1991). The dissection should be maintained close to the gallbladder wall, and the cystic duct should be divided as close as possible to its junction with the gallbladder.

Routine intraoperative cholangiography has been advocated by many to minimize the incidence of laparoscopic biliary injuries (Asbun et al 1993, Moossa et al 1992, Way 1992) but remains a point of controversy. In a large review of cholecystectomies from Western Australia, Fletcher et al reported that intraoperative cholangiography reduced the incidence of biliary injury two-fold overall and eight-fold in complex cases (acute cholecystitis, cholangitis, pancreatitis) (Fletcher et al 1999). In addition, a strong inverse correlation between biliary injury and non-performance of cholangiography has been noted by some authors (Torkington et al 1998). On the other hand, cholangiography is clearly not preventative if the injury occurs after a normal study or if the study serves only to identify an injury that has already been inflicted (Andren-Sandberg et al 1985). Several reports have suggested, however, that routine cholangiography may not reduce the incidence of biliary injury but may minimize injury severity and allow immediate recognition and definitive repair (Carroll et al 1996, Gigot et al 1997, Russell et al 1996, Woods et al 1994). Of course, this is critically dependent on proper interpretation of the study. In a review of 177 biliary injuries, Olsen found that only two of 32 cholangiographies were correctly interpreted, despite evidence of impending bile duct transection in the vast majority (Olsen 1997). The most common error was accepting an incomplete study, without opacification of the right and left hepatic ducts, as normal. Failure to opacify the proximal bile ducts in their entirety should prompt immediate open conversion. Laparoscopic ultrasonography has been described as an alternative to cholangiography, both for delineation of the cystic duct and identification of common duct calculi (Tomonaga et al 1999) but is not widely used.

Bile leakage occurs with greater frequency after laparoscopic cholecystectomy than after open cholecystectomy, which may be related to the use of clips rather than ties or (McMahon et al 1995). Clips are less secure than sutures and may become dislodged if improperly placed or if manipulated after placement (Nelson et al 1992). Also, incomplete occlusion may occur if clips are placed across a thickened, rigid cystic duct or a cystic duct containing stones or if other tissues are included. When placing clips, it is important that the tips meet in order to ensure adequate occlusion. If both tips cannot be visualized as the clip is being applied, damage to adjacent structures may occur.

Furthermore, if the clip does not fit across the entire width of the cystic duct, the surgeon must consider the possibility that the structure about to be divided is in fact not the cystic duct but rather the common duct. On the other hand, if the anatomy is clear and the cystic duct is simply thickened, placement of a ligature may be more appropriate (Michalowski et al 1998). Also, using electrocautery in areas adjacent to clips should be avoided as this may result in conduction of thermal energy to the adjacent common duct and delayed biliary structure.

Location and classification

The ease of management, operative risk, and outcome of biliary injuries vary considerably and are dependent on the type of injury and its location (Chapman et al 1995). It has long been recognized that strictures involving the common bile duct or distal common hepatic duct are easier to repair than are more proximal injuries. The anatomical classification of Bismuth has been widely adopted in recognition of this fact (Fig. 49.7) (Bismuth 1982). In this classification scheme, five stricture types are recognized, reflecting the location with respect to the hepatic duct confluence (Types 1–4) or the involvement of an aberrant right sectoral hepatic duct with or without a concomitant hepatic duct stricture (Type 5) (Table 49.3).

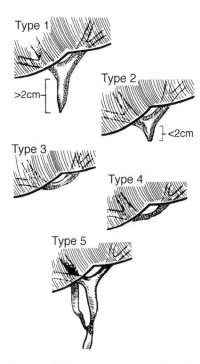

Fig. 49.7 Classification of bile duct strictures based on location with respect to the hepatic duct confluence (After Bismuth 1982). (See also Table 49.3.)

Table 49.3 Bismuth classification of biliary stricture

1. Low common hepatic duct stricture – hepatic duct stump > 2 cm
2. Proximal common hepatic duct stricture – hepatic duct stump < 2 cm
3. Hilar stricture with no residual common hepatic duct – hepatic duct confluence intact
4. Destruction of hepatic duct confluence – right and left hepatic ducts separated
5. Involvement of aberrant right sectoral hepatic duct alone or with concomitant stricture of the common hepatic duct

The Bismuth classification is useful for localization and for offering prognosis after repair but does not encompass the entire spectrum of injuries that are possible. For example, no provision is made for biliary leaks or major ductal injuries without stricture. Indeed, even within the group of patients with biliary leaks there are varying degrees of severity. In an effort to fill this gap, Strasberg et al have proposed a comprehensive classification system that incorporates Bismuth's scheme but is much broader in scope (Fig. 49.8) (Strasberg et al 1995). Injuries are classified as Type A to Type E, with the latter representing biliary strictures and further subdivided as E1 to E5 according to the Bismuth classification. Type A injuries are bile leaks from minor ducts still in continuity with the common bile duct. This encompasses the most common causes of biliary leaks seen after laparoscopic cholecystectomy, namely leakage from the cystic duct and from a subvesical duct of Luschka. Type B injuries involve occlusion of part of the biliary tree, which for practical purposes almost always is an aberrant right sectoral hepatic duct. When this duct is transected without ligation, the injury is termed Type C, reflecting the differences in presentation and management between the two. A lateral injury to an extrahepatic bile duct is termed type D, which is similar to Type A injuries in that the extrahepatic biliary tree remains in continuity but is classified separately to underscore the greater severity and potential need for major reconstruction.

The incidence of each type of biliary injury is difficult to ascertain with certainty. The majority of literature reports are derived from tertiary referral centers and are therefore biased towards the more severe injuries. Most surgical series focus on management of Type E biliary strictures while endoscopic and radiologic reports are mainly concerned with the treatment of biliary leaks. Type A injuries may be the most common, but it would appear that many are managed successfully without referral and are thus underrepresented in reports from major centers (Strasberg et al 1995).

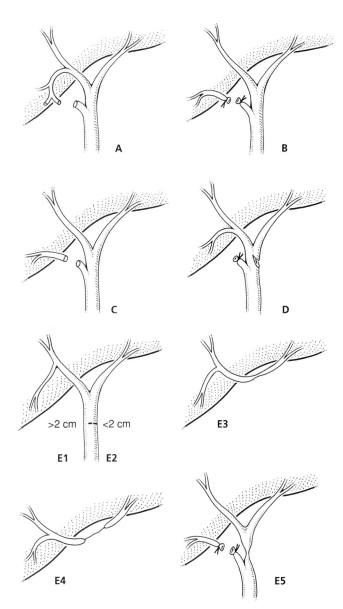

Fig. 49.8 Classification of laparoscopic biliary injuries according to Strasberg et al. Injuries are stratified from type A to type E. Type E injuries are further subdivided into E1 to E5 according to the Bismuth classification system.

Clinical presentation

Most patients with postcholecystectomy biliary injuries, if not diagnosed at operation, present early in the postoperative period. After open cholecystectomy, only about 10% of injuries are suspected after the first week but nearly 70% are diagnosed within the first 6 months after operation (Pitt et al 1982). By contrast, injuries after laparoscopic cholecystectomy appear to be recognized somewhat earlier (Davidoff et al 1992, Lillemoe et al 1997). This probably reflects differences in the pattern of injuries between the two approaches combined with a heightened awareness of the potential for injury at laparoscopy (Strasberg et al 1995).

The clinical presentation depends on the type of injury, and conversely, one may infer the type of injury based on the clinical picture at presentation. Patients with significant bile leaks (Types A, C and D) generally present within the first week after operation but some may not become apparent for several weeks and very few are diagnosed intraoperatively (Strasberg et al 1995). Most patients have abdominal pain coupled with fever or other signs of sepsis, which is most common, or bile leakage from an incision. A small number of patients have neither of these signs and symptoms but rather have non-specific complaints of weakness, fatigue or anorexia. Elevated alkaline phosphatase levels are characteristic as is mild hyperbilirubinemia but markedly elevated serum bilirubin levels (>3 mg/dL) are uncommon (Brooks et al 1993, vanSonnenberg et al 1993).

Major injuries to the common duct (type E injuries) are more likely to be discovered intraoperatively, although the majority remain unrecognized until after operation. Like bile leaks, these injuries are more often diagnosed within the first few postoperative weeks. However, patients with a slowly evolving stricture may not come to attention for several months (Strasberg et al 1995), which is distinctly uncommon for patients with bile leaks. Most patients with these injuries present with jaundice, often coupled with pain and occasionally sepsis. It is important to recognize, however, that jaundice is not always present early in the course of the illness. In some patients, the stricture may evolve slowly or cause only partial obstruction. Such patients may have non-specific complaints, pruritis, or derangements in liver function tests, any or all of which should prompt an investigation. In addition, patients with an isolated right sectoral hepatic duct injury (Type B) or an internal bilary fistula may present with a history of unexplained fevers, pain or general debilitation.

The findings on physical examination are often non-specific. Jaundice, if present, is usually obvious and there may be multiple skin excoriations from pruritis. Abdominal distention and pain may be seen in patients with bile peritonitis, whereas focal tenderness is more suggestive of a localized collection or abscess. Hepatomegaly may be seen with longstanding biliary obstruction. Splenomegaly or other signs of portal hypertension are uncommon but, if present, should alert the surgeon to the possibility of concomitant portal venous injury or severe underlying hepatocellular damage. The presence of portal hypertension in association with a biliary stricture portends a poor outcome (vide infra), and its identification is important not only for planning management but also in a medicolegal context.

Pathological consequences

Fibrosis. Biliary obstruction is associated with the formation of high local concentrations of bile salts at the canalicular membrane, and these initiate pathological changes in the liver (Schaffner et al 1971). Bile thrombi form within dilated centrilobular bile canaliculi and secondary changes develop in adjacent hepatocytes. A complex cascade of molecular and cellular events ensue, collectively termed fibrogenesis (Friedman 1997), that ultimately lead to the deposition of collagen and other extracellular matrix proteins and eventually fibrosis and scarring around bile ducts and ductules (Friedman 1997, Jarnagin et al 1994, Maher & McGuire 1990). As this process progresses, mechanical interference to the flow of bile develops in these intrahepatic biliary radicles and perpetuates cholestasis.

Fibrosis is accompanied by liver cell hyperplasia (Weinbren et al 1985). This is not necessarily true in secondary biliary cirrhosis since the lobular structure of the liver is usually well-preserved (Fig. 49.9), and the marked fibrosis that occurs in advanced cases only rarely proceeds to true cirrhosis (see Ch. 7). This knowledge is of importance in planning therapy since many of these pathological changes are potentially reversible, and there may be a slow return to near-normal liver function following relief of biliary obstruction (Blumgart 1978). Fibrosis may also develop in the extrahepatic ducts proximal to the stricture, and this is especially likely after biliary intubation. Upward retraction of the ducts is accompanied by a sequence of mucosal atrophy, squamous metaplasia, inflammatory infiltration, and further fibrosis in the subepithelial layers of the ducts.

Evidence of liver fibrosis and portal hypertension usually takes several years to become evident, although it may present as early as 2 years after the development of the stricture. Major stigmata of hepatocellular dysfunction such as spider angiomata or encephalopathy are uncommon in benign biliary obstruction and should raise the possibility of pre-existing parenchymal disease (e.g. chronic hepatitis, alcoholic liver disease). If liver biopsy reveals significant primary hepatocellular disease in association with a benign stricture, then the prognosis is especially poor.

Atrophy (see Chapter 3). The distribution of liver mass is regulated by a poorly understood balance in which bile flow, portal venous flow, and hepatic venous flow are the main factors. Segmental or lobar atrophy may result from portal venous obstruction or bile duct occlusion in the affected area. Unilobar atrophy is associated with hypertrophy of the contralateral lobe and may present diagnostic and operative difficulties. Liver lobe atrophy and compensatory

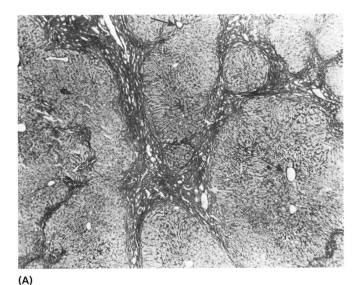

(A)

(B)

Fig. 49.9 (A) Photomicrograph showing the effect of long-standing biliary obstruction due to benign biliary stricture. There is hepatic fibrosis present but preservation of the basic hepatic architecture, with the portal tract (white arrow) and hepatic venous radicles (black arrows) maintaining their normal relationships. The fibrosis extends between the lobules but the pattern is not one of true cirrhosis in which there is destruction of the basic hepatic architecture. **(B)** Extensive fibrosis with substantially normal relation of hepatic venous radicles (black arrows) to portal tracts (white arrow) in a patient with portal hypertension (Weinbren et al 1985).

hypertrophy is frequently found in benign strictures and may be associated with asymmetrical involvement of lobar or sectoral hepatic ducts, interference with portal venous blood supply, or decreased portal perfusion due to secondary fibrosis. In benign strictures, the dilated ducts within the atrophic segments are often filled with infected bile and debris, and even though drainage of an atrophic segment will not be effective in relieving jaundice, continued cholangitis may continue unabated unless satisfactory drainage of the atrophic and the hypertrophic segments is achieved.

The presence of significant atrophy and compensatory hypertrophy will significantly influence the approach to repair. The most common situation is gross hypertrophy of the left lobe accompanied by right lobe atrophy (Czerniak et al 1986). Anastomosis in the region of the hilum is made difficult by the rotational deformity and anatomical distortion imposed by this condition (see Chs 3 and 30). A thoracoabdominal approach to such strictures provides more direct exposure and access for repair by allowing rotation of the liver to the left (Bismuth & Lazorthes 1981). Similar problems may occur in bile duct strictures following right hepatic resection.

Portal hypertension. Patients with biliary strictures may develop portal hypertension as a result of secondary hepatic fibrosis or direct damage to the portal vein. Alternatively, portal hypertension may be due to pre-existing liver disease. It is important that these patients undergo further work-up, including a liver biopsy, to exclude underlying chronic parenchymal disease. Many patients with iatrogenic biliary injuries are the subject of medicolegal proceedings. Precise documentation of all injuries is, therefore, essential in order to provide an accurate assessment of the causation of symptoms and prognosis. The outcome of patients with biliary strictures and portal hypertension is much worse than for patients without portal hypertension, with a hospital mortality of 25 to 40% (Blumgart et al 1984, Chapman et al 1995). However, it has been suggested that adequate biliary drainage may be followed by some resolution of fibrosis and perhaps a reduction in portal pressure (Blumgart 1978). Recently, the concept of mild to moderate 'latent' portal hypertension has been introduced that may affect patients with biliary stricture but no vascular injury (Ibrarullah et al 1996). Significant elevations of portal venous pressure were seen in some of these patients which did not correlate with duration of obstruction, serum bilirubin or measured pressure within the biliary tree. The elevations in portal pressure were noted to normalize after operative correction and were not otherwise associated with clinical features of portal hypertension. Mild to moderate cholestatic changes were not uncommon but hepatic architecture was generally maintained. The results of this study support the view that hepatic hemodynamic and pathologic changes may occur, without concomitant vascular injury, and are reversible if treated early (Ibrarullah et al 1996).

Management

Successful management of patients with postcholecystectomy bile duct injuries requires careful planning. The importance of thorough investigation and patient preparation cannot be overemphasized. Before any intervention, the surgeon must define completely the type and extent of injury and treat coexisting conditions that are a threat to life and reduce the likelihood of a successful outcome (i.e. sepsis, cholangitis, ongoing biliary leakage, abscess). Hasty treatment decisions based on incomplete data are more likely to exacerbate an already difficult situation. Imaging studies play a central role in assessing patients with biliary injuries and should be directed at answering the following questions: is there a subhepatic bile collection or abscess?; is there ongoing bile leakage?; what is the level and extent of injury in the biliary tree?; are there associated vascular injuries?; and, is there evidence of lobar atrophy?

Radiological investigations. Duplex ultrasonography is an excellent, non-invasive means of demonstrating intrahepatic ductal dilatation and may also reveal a subhepatic fluid collection or evidence of vascular damage. While ultrasound (US) may provide valuable information regarding the level of biliary injury, it is of little value in assessing the extent of a stricture and is of no value if the biliary tree is decompressed. Computed tomography (CT) is probably the best initial study, the results of which will help direct further investigations. A good quality CT scan will demonstrate a dilated bilary tree and help localize the level of ductal obstruction in patients with strictures. In addition, CT will identify fluid collections or ascites, may suggest the possibility of vascular damage, and will reveal lobar atrophy, if present (vide infra). In patients with biliary strictures, complete delineation of the level and extent of injury is necessary. All branches of the right and left intrahepatic biliary tree must be outlined, particularly in cases of high bile duct stricture and recurrent stricture after previous reconstruction. Displaying the hepatic duct confluence (if intact) and the left ductal system and its branches is especially important in selecting the appropriate reconstruction (vide infra). Percutaneous transhepatic cholangiography (PTC) is much more likely than endoscopic cholangiography (ERCP) to provide this information and remains the standard investigation in this setting (Fig. 49.10). The risk of cholangitis can be reduced with prophylactic antibiotics. Recently, magnetic resonance cholangiopancreatography (MRCP) has emerged as a potentially valuable tool in evaluating proximal bile duct injuries (Coakley et al 1998). This non-invasive modality provides striking images of the biliary tree, and yields anatomical information in a single study that was previously obtainable only with CT and PTC (Fig. 49.11).

Endoscopic cholangiography is seldom of value in the precise diagnosis of complete proximal bile duct strictures since there is often discontinuity of the common bile duct preventing visualization of the intrahepatic ductal system.

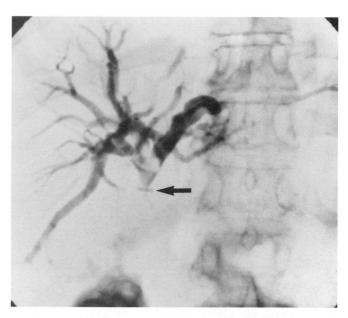

Fig. 49.10 Percutaneous transhepatic cholangiogram showing a surgical clip occluding the common hepatic duct just below the confluence (arrow). Note that all major branches of the proximal biliary tree are outlined.

Endoscopic cholangiography may be more helpful for incomplete strictures (stenoses) and is appropriate for patients with a history of sphincteric damage at previous common duct exploration or if there is a question of papillary stenosis or other periampullary pathology. Endoscopic cholangiography also has a role in the diagnosis and treatment of patients with bile leakage from the cystic duct stump or from a laceration of the common duct (Brooks et al 1993). These patients will have evidence of an intra-abdominal fluid collection on CT. After percutaneous drainage, biliary scintigraphy (e.g. HIDA scan) can be used to establish the presence of a persistent bile leak. Endoscopic cholangiography may then be applied to identify the location of the leak, and placement of a stent may reduce or eliminate bile leakage. It is important to recognize, however, that many bile leaks resolve with percutaneous drainage alone, and ERCP is probably unnecessary in the absence of radiographic or clinical evidence of ongoing bile drainage (Brooks et al 1993).

Isotopic scanning techniques may also be of value in assessing bile duct strictures, particularly the functional assessment of incomplete strictures, previous biliary reconstructions and isolated sectoral hepatic duct strictures (see Ch. 14). HIDA scanning offers a dynamic and quantitative assessment of liver function and of the clearance of bile across anastomoses and stenoses (Fig. 49.12) (McPherson et al 1983). In patients with hepatocellular disease, HIDA scanning may be of value in distinguishing the contribution of the biliary obstruction from that of the intrinsic liver disease to the overall biochemical and symptomatic picture. In such cases, the bilirubin level may be normal but the alkaline phosphatase level is raised. HIDA scanning is also valuable during follow-up of patients after surgical repair. Since it can be repeated and is non-invasive, it is of particular value in demonstrating anastomotic patency and function when

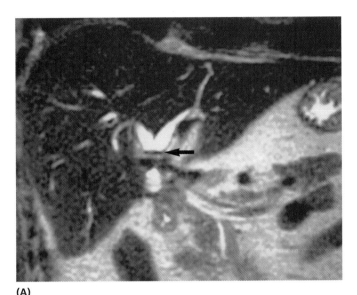

(A)

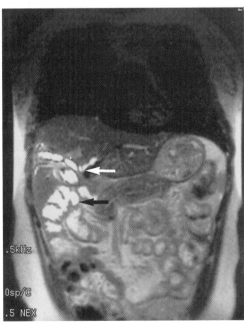

(B)

Fig. 49.11 (A) Coronal single-shot fast spin-echo magnetic resonance cholangiographic section showing a surgical clip (arrow) occluding the common hepatic duct just below the confluence (from Coakley et al 1998). **(B)** Coronal single-shot fast spin-echo magnetic resonance cholangiographic section in a young woman with recurrent cholangitis after multiple attempts to repair a postcholecystectomy bile duct injury. The hepatic duct confluence (white arrow) is shown. There is also excess fluid noted in the adjacent colon (black arrow), suggesting a fistula from the biliary tree to the hepatic flexure. Surgical findings confirmed a fistula from the right posterior sectoral hepatic duct, which had been excluded from the anastomosis (adapted from Coakley et al 1998).

no tube has been left across the anastomosis at the time of repair (Fig. 49.12). An isolated sectoral hepatic duct stricture is suggested by delayed clearance of isotope from a portion of the liver.

Arteriography and delayed-phase portography should be obtained if there is any evidence of vascular injury on the initial studies, a suspicion of portal hypertension from the history and physical exam, or a history of excessive bleeding at the time of cholecystectomy. A biliary injury in the setting of portal hypertension dramatically increases the morbidity and mortality of operative intervention, and its presence should therefore redirect the management approach (Chapman et al 1995). The combination of biliary and vascular injuries often leads to segmental or lobar atrophy but may also be seen with longstanding biliary obstruction alone. An atrophic lobe may be evident on the initial US or CT scan and appears as a small, often hypoperfused area with dilated, irregular and crowded bile ducts (Fig. 49.13). Isotopic scanning may show what appears to be a filling defect in the affected area. It is important to recognize lobar atrophy on the cross-sectional imaging studies, not only because it is an indicator of concomitant vascular injury needing further evaluation but also because it will change the operative approach during repair (see Ch. 30). In addition, patients with combined bile duct and hepatic artery injuries appear to be at increased risk for severe complications after reconstructive surgery, such as hepatic necrosis and abscess. In addition, biliary reconstruction in the setting of hepatic artery occlusion may be at greater risk of late stricture recurrence (Gupta et al 1998).

Occasionally, injection of contrast into an established biliary fistula or percutaneous drain will outline the ductal system (Fig. 49.14). Such studies may complement information provided by formal percutaneous cholangiography, particularly if the fistula or tube tract drains an excluded sectoral duct. Since bacterial colonization or biliary infection is inevitable in such cases, it is wise to administer prophylactic antibiotics before and after these studies.

Preoperative preparation. In general, operative repair of bile duct injuries need not be rushed, the exceptions being for bile duct injuries recognized at the time of initial cholecystectomy or, rarely, for emergency treatment of suppurative cholangitis or peritonitis. For the vast majority of patients, there is ample time to treat coexisting conditions and to perform a full investigation, both of which increase the likelihood of a successful outcome (Chapman et al 1995, Stewart & Way 1995).

Cholangitis is not infrequent in patients with bile duct strictures, especially after ductal intubation. Administration of intravenous antibiotics is important as a preliminary to

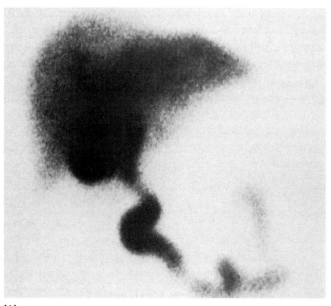

(A)

surgical treatment, and the results of bile cultures, obtained at the time of PTC, should be used to direct therapy. Patients with severe cholangitis and sepsis are unlikely to respond to antibiotics alone and should be submitted to percutaneous drainage before surgery. On the other hand, preoperative antibiotics are usually adequate in managing milder attacks and should also be used in patients with no clinical evidence of cholangitis, given the high incidence of bacterial contamination. Antibiotic regimens should take into account the frequent presence of anaerobic organisms and enterococci in patients with biliary obstruction (Hochwald et al 1998, Thompson et al 1990). It is the authors' practice to begin antibiotics immediately before operation and to continue appropriate treatment for 5 to 7 days postoperatively if cholangitis is a preoperative feature. Although no firm data exist to guide the duration of treat-

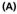

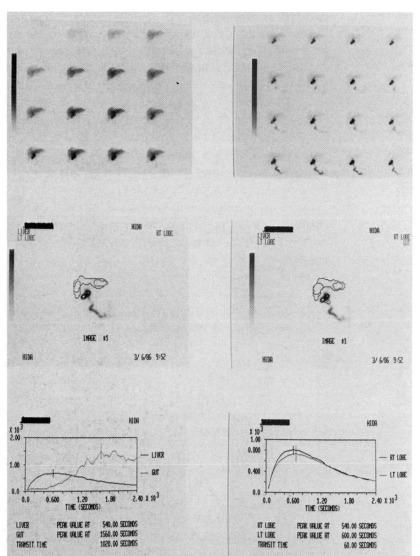

Fig. 49.12 **(A)** Anterior view of the liver at 2 minutes after the intravenous injection of 120 MBq (3mC) of 99mTc HIDA (dimethyl imino diacetic acid) in a patient after hepaticojejunostomy for a benign stricture. This shows tracer in the liver, major bile ducts and in the upper small bowel. **(B)** Upper images show 32 6.25 second sequential frames on the same patient as in part **(A)** Regions of interest have been selected over the right and left lobes of the liver, and also the gut (shown on central images). Time-activity curves (lower left and right) show prompt uptake of tracer and rapid clearance with a rising curve over the bowel. These are normal findings.

(B)

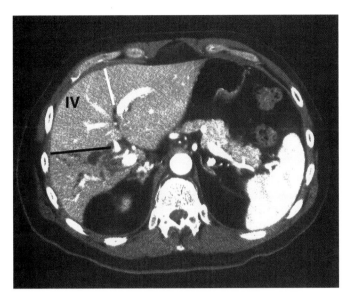

Fig. 49.13 CT scan showing severe atrophy of the right lobe. The right lobe is hypoperfused and small and is clearly demarcated from the left lobe (black line). Notice the markedly increased size of segment IV and the left lateral segment (white line) and the dilated and crowded ducts in the small right lobe.

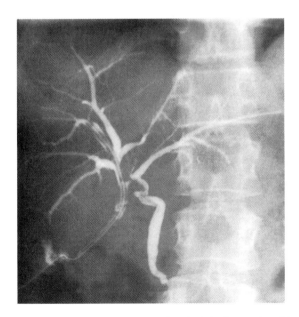

Fig. 49.14 Injection of contrast into a tube which had been placed into the ductal system following a hilar ductal injury recognized at operation. The patient was referred draining approximately 200 ml of bile per day but with normal liver function tests and no fever. Note that the tube has been passed into the right hepatic ductal system, but there is filling of the entire intrahepatic biliary tree. There appears to be a complete division of the common hepatic duct. A fistulous connection has developed between the left hepatic ductal system and the common hepatic duct. The tube was withdrawn and no repair was performed. There was subsequent atrophy of the right liver but the patient was well and symptom-free with normal liver function tests over a 4-year follow-up.

ment, the markedly increased incidence of postoperative infectious complications in patients with endoscopic or percutaneous stents suggests that a prolonged course of treatment is justified (Hochwald et al 1998). These data would further suggest that jaundice without evidence of cholangitis is not an indication for biliary intubation.

Anemia should be corrected, if necessary, by blood transfusion, and coagulation defects, typically manifest as a prolongation of the prothrombin time, should be treated with vitamin K or fresh frozen plasma. Patients with a prolonged illness may present with malnutrition (see Ch. 26). Enteral feedings through a fine-bore nasal catheter may be successful in some cases but may not be tolerated in sufficient amounts, and parenteral nutrition may be necessary. Despite these measures, however, weight gain is sometimes difficult to achieve, and to date no prospective randomized trials have demonstrated a benefit from short-term preoperative nutritional support. A significant external bile fistula predisposes to excessive fluid and electrolyte loss, and may lead to hyponatremia and acidosis (McPherson et al 1982). It is imperative to correct fluid deficits and electrolyte imbalances prior to operation (see Ch. 26).

The preoperative management of complications of biliary injury, such as biliary peritonitis, subphrenic or subhepatic abscess, hemorrhage from erosive gastritis or esophageal varices, or hepatic failure secondary to fibrosis, is important and usually must be addressed before biliary reconstruction can be considered. In general, drainage of intra-abdominal abscesses and control of gastrointestinal hemorrhage takes priority. If there is systemic sepsis arising from an obstructed biliary tree (a factor which may contribute to other complications), then immediate biliary drainage is essential. In such desperately ill patients, it is preferable to perform a rapid percutaneous drainage to allow further resuscitative measures with intravenous antibiotics and hydration to prevent renal insufficiency. The question of management of portal hypertension and external bile fistula occurring in association with stricture are addressed below.

Surgical treatment. The most appropriate management of bile duct injuries depends on the injury type and whether or not the injury is diagnosed immediately or at some time after operation.

Injury recognized at initial operation. If injury to the extrahepatic biliary tree is recognized at the time of initial cholecystectomy, then the surgeon should immediately consider his or her experience and ability to repair it immediately. The advice of a more experienced surgeon should be sought, if possible. The situation is not immediately desperate, and there is always time to wait a short while for another opinion and for additional assistance. There is substantial evidence to suggest that immediate open conversion and repair by an experienced surgeon is associated with reduced morbidity, shorter duration of illness and lower cost (Savader et al 1997, Stewart and Way 1995). It must be emphasized, however, that each failed repair is associated with some loss of bile duct length (Tocchi et al 1996) and greatly exacerbates an already difficult situation. This is particularly true of injuries involving the biliary confluence, where failure of the initial repair and loss of bile duct length may result in isolation of the right and left hepatic ducts. Repair becomes more difficult, and the likelihood of a successful outcome is reduced (Chapman et al 1995). If the surgeon cannot effect a reasonable repair and competent help is not available, then drains should be placed to control any biliary leak and the patient referred to a specialist center.

The damaged area of bile duct requires careful dissection to define the extent of injury. To accomplish this without making matters worse, the laparoscopic approach must be abandoned in favor of a generous right subcostal, an extended subcostal or a chevron incision, and additional assistance to aid in exposure should be obtained. Operative cholangiography may be helpful at this point to delineate the anatomy and the type of injury.

Regardless of the location of the lesion, initial repair of the damage recognized at the time of cholecystectomy should have two basic aims:

1. Maintenance of ductal length below the hilus without sacrifice of tissue
2. Avoidance of uncontrolled postoperative bile leakage.

It is important to point out that the initial intervention may not be the final definitive reconstruction. This is particularly true of injury to small ducts where repair may be difficult and the prime aims of maintaining length and preventing fistulation should guide the surgeon rather than elaborate attempts at reconstruction under adverse circumstances. It is probably safer to provide external drainage by means of a tube inserted proximally into the bile duct and to refer the patient for specialist treatment than to complicate the situation with a repair that is likely to fail and lead to further damage.

Unfortunately, the injury in most cases involves complete transection with or without excision of a length of common duct. Occasionally, only an aberrant right sectoral hepatic duct is involved (Bismuth type 5), although this too may be associated with concomitant injury to the common hepatic or common bile duct. Durable re-establishment of biliary-enteric continuity is indeed difficult when the ducts are small and decompressed, and referral to a specialist unit is all the more important in this situation.

There are two options for repairing a complete duct tran-section. The first is end-to-end repair over a T tube. This is feasible only if the transected ends can be apposed without tension, which usually requires full mobilization of the duodenum and head of pancreas. The anastomosis is created using a single layer of interrupted absorbable sutures with the T-tube brought out of the bile duct away from the anastomotic line. Silk sutures should be avoided for all biliary reconstructions since they can promote an inflammatory reaction and act as a nidus for stone formation. It must be recognized, however, that end-to-end anastomoses are associated with a high incidence of late stricture formation, as high as 50 to 60% in some reports (Pellegrini et al 1984, Rossi & Tsao 1994, Stewart & Way 1995, Csendes et al 1989). Roux-en-Y hepaticojejunostomy (vide infra) is therefore more likely to give better long-term results and is the recommended approach.

An injury to the lateral duct wall may be amenable to direct suture repair. Relatively small and simple lacerations may be repaired with interrupted 4-0 or 5-0 absorbable suture. The area of injury should be adequately exposed but extensive dissection risks further injury and late stricture formation. Some authors recommend T tubes for all such repairs, but they are probably unnecessary for small lacerations, and their placement into a decompressed bile duct may exacerbate the injury (Rossi & Tsao 1994). An analogous situation is primary choledochorrhaphy after common bile duct exploration, with several authors reporting excellent results without using T tubes (Sheen-Chen & Chou 1990, Sorensen et al 1994, Tu et al 1999), On the other hand, long lateral injuries, which are not circumferential, may be impossible to repair transversely without compromising the lumen, and direct repair over a T tube likely will result in future stenosis. Some authors have suggested that vein patches may be used to cover such defects (Belzer et al 1965, Ellis & Hoile 1980) while others have described using the cystic duct stump or pedicled flaps of jejunum (Okamura et al 1985). The authors have no experience with these techniques but prefer instead to use a Roux-en-Y loop of jejunum as a serosal patch (Fig. 49.15). A T tube is placed across the defect and its long limb led out through the Roux loop and exteriorized through the abdominal wall. This approach has several advantages. First, bile duct length is maintained. Second, the jejunal serosa is used to cover the defect, secured in place with fine interrupted absorbable sutures to the bile duct wall without attempting direct approaches to the ragged edge of the damaged duct. Finally, the T tube provides biliary decompression across the jejunum so that, when it is removed, any leaking bile will drain into the bowel lumen rather than the abdominal cavity. This method may be particularly useful to the inexperienced surgeon caught in a difficult situation.

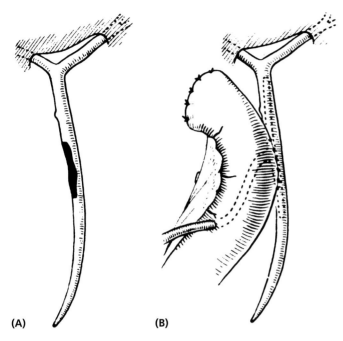

(A)   (B)

Fig. 49.15 Method of repair of a non-circumferential laceration to the bile duct wall. **(A)** There is a lateral injury with loss of ductal wall over some considerable length. **(B)** A Roux-en-Y loop of jejunum is prepared and brought up. A T tube is placed within the injured bile duct and the long limb led out across the jejunal loop, which is secured to the bile duct as a serosal patch over the defect.

Injury recognized in the immediate postoperative period. Biliary injuries not appreciated intraoperatively may present in the first few days following operation. The mode of presentation may be bile drainage through the wound, bile peritonitis or progressive jaundice, depending on the injury type.

In the setting of an external biliary fistula (Ch. 50), the essential consideration in management is to avoid early re-operation. It is wiser to take full stock of the situation, to carry out appropriate investigations (as described above), to keep the patient well-nourished and free of infection. If fistulography or other studies reveal continuity between the biliary system and the gastrointestinal tract, then a prolonged period of drainage is warranted and may result in spontaneous closure, provided there is no distal obstruction to bile flow. This is particularly true of bile leakage from the cystic duct or a subvesical duct of Lushka (Type A) or from a non-circumferential laceration (Type D). More severe lacerations or complete transections of the common duct or an aberrant right sectoral hepatic duct with ongoing bile leakage require careful consideration. Since the biliary tree is decompressed, the proximal ducts are small in caliber. Immediate surgical treatment of these injuries is far from simple. Adequate repair requires exposing healthy bile duct mucosa within a sufficiently dilated proximal duct to allow precise anastomosis. In the setting of a decompressed biliary tree and significant inflammation, this can be quite demanding or even impossible. A delayed approach remains the most appropriate course of action, since such fistulae may also close without operative intervention and this may be associated with eventual proximal ductal dilatation and easier subsequent repair (see Fig. 49.3). If fluid losses from the biliary fistula remain high over a prolonged period, a useful but rarely used technique is creation of a temporary internal fistulojejunostomy, with definitive repair deferred for a later date (Smith et al 1982). Alternatively, placement of an endoscopic or percutaneous stent across the defect may reduce output from the fistula, hasten closure and make management easier. Some authors advocate early endoscopic sphincterotomy to decrease the relative resistance of transpapillary bile drainage to promote closure (Abdel et al 1996, Fujii et al 1998, Inui et al 1998, Liguory et al 1991). While these approaches are occasionally useful, there is no evidence that they provide a significant advantage, and a waiting period of 2–3 weeks is recommended since most fistulae will close or decrease substantially.

Patients with bile peritonitis are often desperately ill, especially if the bile is infected, although some patients with sterile bile may accumulate large volumes without overt signs of sepsis (see Fig. 49.3B). Drainage of the bile collection and control of ongoing bile leak is the primary objective, and often requires percutaneous abscess drains in combination with percutaneous biliary catheters. Definitive repair is seldom possible initially, with the bile ducts collapsed, deeply bile stained and friable, and is best delayed until the biliary leak has been completely controlled and the patient has been resuscitated fully.

Injury presenting at an interval after initial operation. Many patients presenting at a long interval from the time of cholecystectomy have biliary strictures. The principles of managing late bile duct stenoses and strictures are as follows:

1. Exposure of *healthy proximal bile ducts draining all areas of the liver*
2. Preparation of a suitable segment of distal mucosa for anastomosis
3. Creation of a mucosa-to-mucosa sutured anastomosis of the bile ducts to the distal conduit (almost always a Roux-en-Y loop of jejunum).

It may be necessary to consider a staged approach to stricture repair in the presence of intra-abdominal infection, portal hypertension, or poor general condition of the patient. Repair attempts in the face of uncontrolled local infection, acute complications of portal hypertension or general debilitation are doomed to fail. The initial approach in such cases should be limited to establishing external bile drainage, controlling sepsis and treating other co-existing conditions that are a threat to life. In this manner, the clinical condition of the patient may be improved before attempts at definitive repair (Cattell & Braasch 1959). In the patient with portal hypertension, initial interventional radiological management by percutaneously placed biliary drainage catheters is probably safer than operation, given the danger of intraoperative hemorrhage (Pellegrini et al 1984).

Technical approaches to biliary repair

End-to-end duct repair. Excision of the stricture with end-to-end anastomosis was one of the earliest techniques used for reconstruction (Cattell & Braasch 1959). This repair re-establishes normal anatomical continuity and drainage via an intact sphincter of Oddi. Such an approach has been tried even for high strictures after extensive mobilization of the duodenum and common duct. It has become apparent, however, that end-to-end repair is associated with a 50 to 60% incidence of long-term failure (Csendes et al 1989, Pellegrini et al 1984, Stewart & Way 1995). It is worth emphasizing that these figures reflect the failure rates in the most favorable of cases, since patients with more extensive injuries usually were submitted to biliary-enteric anastomosis (Rossi & Tsao 1994). These data suggest that end-to-end repair has a limited role in the surgical treatment of benign biliary strictures.

Biliary-enteric repair procedures. For most cases of bile duct transection or stricture, biliary-enteric anastomosis is the procedure of choice. For strictures of the retropancreatic or immediate supraduodenal portion of the common bile duct, choledochoduodenostomy is an ideal procedure. The anastomosis may be performed either side-to-side or end-to-side (see Ch. 45). This technique is appropriate only in the setting of a dilated bile duct and will almost certainly result in recurrent stricture if created to a decompressed duct. Most postcholecystectomy strictures are not amenable to choledochoduodenostomy, since such low injuries are unusual in contrast to postgastrectomy strictures, which often involve the distal bile duct.

Strictures involving the common hepatic duct are more difficult to manage, especially those involving the biliary confluence, and almost always require Roux-en-Y hepatico-jejunostomy for reconstruction. The technical aspects of biliary-enteric anastomosis have been described (Blumgart & Kelley 1984, Voyles & Blumgart 1982) and are outlined in Chapter 30.

There are a variety of approaches to the proximal hepatic ducts. When the stricture is below the confluence (Bismuth type 1 or type 2), then a direct anastomosis to the hepatic duct stump is usually straightforward. By contrast, when the stricture encroaches upon the confluence of the right and left hepatic ducts (type 3) or extends proximally so as to isolate the ducts (type 4), the problem becomes more complex and good results are more difficult to achieve. The choice of surgical approach should be tailored to the height and extent of the lesion. The technical descriptions that follow should be read in conjunction with Chapter 30.

An important feature is early division of the falciform ligament back to the diaphragm and freeing the liver of adhesions. Dissection should begin in the right subhepatic area, and it is usually necessary to mobilize completely the hepatic flexure of the colon, starting from below and working upward and medially. The duodenum is often adherent to the undersurface of the liver and to the hilar structures, particularly in the area of the stricture. Indeed, the surgeon may encounter an internal bile fistula to the duodenum or may injure the duodenal wall during this portion of the dissection, either of which will require repair.

Attempts to identify the duct below the stricture are unnecessary, since the distal duct generally cannot be used for anastomosis. Moreover, the duct in this area is usually encased in dense scar tissue and extensive dissection to free it risks injury to the hepatic artery and portal vein. The essential point is identification of the bile ducts proximal to the stricture. A systematic, careful and patient approach is necessary. Dissection in the area lateral to the hepatic artery pulsation will allow identification of the common hepatic duct. While this approach is reasonable in patients with relatively low strictures (Bismuth type 1), it is not appropriate in most cases. It is generally much easier and safer to expose the left hepatic duct by lowering the hilar plate at the base of segment IV (quadrate lobe). Often, this area has not been disturbed by the previous surgeon and is likely to be relatively free of adhesions. This maneuver delivers the left hepatic duct and the biliary confluence from the under surface of the liver and makes identification of the strictured area much easier. Adhesions posterior to a damaged duct may be dense, and extensive dissection in this situation risks injury to the underlying portal vein. It is generally unnecessary to come around the scarred area completely, provided that the posterior wall of the duct above the stricture can be elevated sufficiently for anastomosis.

Strictures at or above the level of the biliary confluence are much more challenging. Adequate exposure of the bile ducts is usually achievable by dissecting the left hepatic duct system. This approach is based on the anatomical studies of Couinaud (Couinaud 1953, 1955, Hepp & Couinaud 1956) and is well-described (Bismuth et al 1978, Blumgart

& Kelley 1984). For Type 2 and 3 strictures, biliary-enteric anastomosis to the left hepatic duct will provide complete drainage of both the left and right ductal systems. For type 4 strictures, however, there is obliteration of the confluence and it is necessary to provide drainage of the right lobe as well, often by dissection across the stricture and creation of a second anastomosis to the right duct system. Occasionally, mobilization or even partial excision of the quadrate lobe may be necessary in some type 4 strictures.

While the vast majority of high strictures may be approached and managed as described above, it is occasionally difficult to expose the left hepatic duct due to adhesions or fibrosis. Excessive bleeding may be encountered or a large, overhanging quadrate lobe may prevent access to the left duct. Occasionally, the extrahepatic length of the left duct, normally much greater than the right, is short and access to it is therefore difficult. In such instances, repair can be effected by dissection of the left duct within the umbilical fissure (*ligamentum teres or round ligament approach*) (Fig. 49.16) (Soupault & Couinaud 1957). This approach is rarely indicated for benign strictures and should not be

used unless the biliary confluence is intact so that a left-sided anastomosis will drain the entire liver.

The mucosal graft procedure of Smith (Smith 1969, 1979) has largely fallen out of favor. This method was introduced for treating high strictures in which hilar dissection was thought to be impossible and the proximal ducts could not be delivered for mucosa-to-mucosa anastomosis. The object of the procedure is to utilize a transhepatic tube to draw the jejunal mucosa high up into the hepatic ducts and thus allow apposition. The procedure was claimed to be easier and quicker since no sutures were inserted. The transhepatic tube was left in place for 2–6 months, occasionally longer for difficult cases. Initially hailed as an important advance in technique (Kune & Sali 1981), it is now clear that the dome of the jejunal mucosa, drawn into the hepatic ducts, may actually block significant secondary intrahepatic ducts, thus occluding and isolating segments of liver tissue (Blumgart 1978, Blumgart et al 1984). Indeed, it is possible for the surgeon to erroneously 'graft' only one sectoral duct, leaving the main stricture untouched. In addition, the mucosa may slip away postoperatively and the jejunal loop become detached (Fig. 49.17). Recurrent stricture at the site of previous mucosal grafting is not uncommon, and the senior author (LHB) has observed 15 of 22 cases of re-stricture at the site of biliary-enteric apposition in patients with failed grafts. Finally, it must be emphasized that short segments of the right hepatic duct and up to 4 cm of the left duct are extrahepatic structures and may be approached by lowering the hilar plate. In a series of 78 patients with complex high biliary strictures, 67 of whom came to operation, mucosa-to-mucosa anastomosis was achieved in all but two despite the fact that 20 had been subjected to prior mucosal grafting (Blumgart et al 1984). Moreover, several series of complex biliary strictures have documented good to excellent long-term results using biliary-enteric anastomotic techniques without using the mucosal graft approach (Chapman et al 1995, Lillemoe et al 1997, McDonald et al 1995, Nealon & Urrutia 1996, Schol et al 1995, Stewart & Way 1995, Tocchi et al 1996).

Liver split and liver resection. In order to expose the bile ducts for repair, it is sometimes necessary to open the liver tissue as a hepatotomy (Blumgart 1980). The most frequent situations involve opening the umbilical fissure for access to the segment III duct or extending the subhepatic approach so as to expose the origin of the right hepatic duct. This latter approach involves opening the liver in the line of the gallbladder fossa. Upward mobilization of the entire quadrate lobe by this maneuver combined with opening the umbilical fissure facilitates access for selected type 4 strictures, especially where there is difficulty in approaching the right hepatic ducts. A similar approach has been described

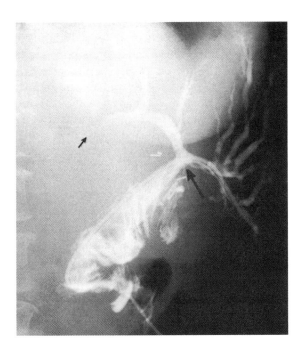

Fig. 49.16 Hepaticojejunostomy Roux-en-Y to the segment III duct following postcholecystectomy stricture initially treated by hepaticojejunostomy using the mucosal graft technique with a transhepatic tube through the right liver. At referral, the patient had a grossly atrophic right lobe and a high bile duct stricture (small arrow). At operation, the left hepatic duct was exposed using the ligamentum teres approach and anastomosis carried out (large arrow). Subsequent re-stricture occurred 1 year later and was treated by refashioning of the anastomosis and subsequent transtubal balloon dilatation with a satisfactory outcome. The patient was well and symptom-free 2 years after operation.

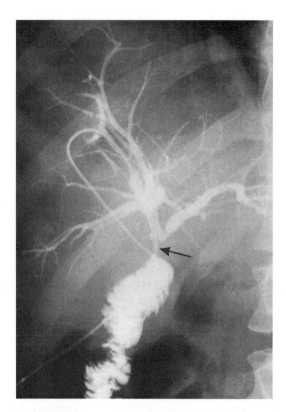

Fig. 49.17 Cholangiogram obtained by injection of a U tube used to develop a mucosal graft repair of a high bile duct stricture carried out 2 weeks before this radiograph was obtained. It was considered that there were no ducts visible at the hilus of the liver which would allow formal anastomosis. Note that the mucosal graft is already widely separated from the biliary confluence (arrow). Repair was carried out by an approach to the left hepatic duct. A wide anastomosis was easily obtained and the patient was well, symptom-free and with normal liver function tests 3.5 years after operation.

by Fiddian-Green et al (Fiddian-Green et al 1988). Division of liver tissue in this setting must be accomplished patiently as it may be accompanied by significant hemorrhage. These techniques are unnecessary if approaches to the left duct are possible.

Actual liver resection is rarely necessary for exposure of the bile ducts in benign postcholecystectomy strictures. Most often, this involves excision of the anterior portion of the quadrate lobe if exposure of the umbilical fissure and incision in the gallbladder bed is insufficient to expose the ducts in difficult type 4 strictures.

More rarely, benign strictures may be treated by means of an intrahepatic hepaticojejunostomy as described by Longmire and Sandford (Longmire Jr. & Sandford 1949), which involves resection of a portion of the left lateral-segment (segments II and III) and anastomosis to ducts exposed on the cut surface of the liver. In general, this procedure is difficult and potentially dangerous, since the liver is often fibrous and resection is met by a fair degree of hem-

orrhage. Furthermore, the bleeding vessels are generally in close proximity to the ducts needed for anastomosis. The use of this procedure is limited to cases in which there is left-sided hypertrophy (Czerniak et al 1986) and is rarely the only option available to secure access to the bile ducts.

Isolated sectoral hepatic duct injuries. Injuries to aberrant or 'low entry' right sectoral hepatic ducts can be particularly difficult to diagnose and to manage. Patients with a stricture but no bile leak (Type B) may remain asymptomatic for months or even years after the injury and only then present with pain or evidence of cholangitis. Some patients may remain essentially asymptomatic and come to attention because of abnormal liver function tests. These injuries are not associated with jaundice unless there is concomitant stricture of the common hepatic duct (Type E5). Longstanding obstruction may result in atrophy of the corresponding hepatic sector drained by the occluded duct (right anterior or right posterior). Some of these patients will have had ERCP in the course of their evaluation which is interpreted as normal, but in retrospect actually shows partial non-filling of the right biliary tree. Biliary drainage to a Roux-en-Y loop of jejunum should be done in symptomatic patients. In those with symptoms, especially recurrent cholangitis, and evidence of liver atrophy, drainage alone may not be sufficient and resection of the atrophic sector may be required. Asymptomatic patients may not require intervention, especially if the injury was remote and there is already evidence of significant atrophy; however, those with a relatively recent injury and no atrophy are probably best served with operative drainage in order to prevent future problems (Strasberg et al 1995).

Patients with sectoral hepatic duct injuries associated with biliary leak (Type C) are a particularly difficult group to manage. After appropriate initial investigation, control of biliary leak and resuscitation, reconstruction to a Roux-en-Y jejunal loop should be performed. Because the transected duct is small and decompressed, achieving good results is difficult even in experienced hands, and restenosis is not uncommon. It has been suggested that percutaneous transhepatic drainage of the affected duct before operation (Lillemoe et al 1999, Strasberg et al 1995) and prolonged postoperative anastomotic stenting are critical for successful management (Lillemoe et al 1999). The authors believe that neither of these maneuvers is necessary as a matter of routine but may be helpful in selected cases only.

Combined modality approaches. The standard surgical techniques of biliary reconstruction described above are suitable for the majority of cases. However, in the most complex and difficult strictures, and especially in the presence of intrahepatic strictures and stones, even optimal surgical management is met with a disappointingly high incidence of postoperative intrahepatic stone formation, cholangitis, and recurrent stricture. Interventional radiological and endoscopic techniques, used as primary therapy in this setting, are similarly unsuccessful because of recurrent cholangitis associated with stent occlusion or recurrent stricture after balloon dilatation. Often, non-operative techniques are technically impossible because of limited access.

Under such adverse circumstances, when the risk of recurrent stricture or stone formation is believed to be high, hepaticojejunostomy may be performed over a trans-jejunal tube brought to the exterior across the blind end of the Roux limb. The defunctionalized Roux limb is deliberately left long and the end is secured subcutaneously or subperitoneally (Fig. 49.18) (vide infra). This allows easy subsequent access for cholangiography, cholangioscopy, dilatation or stone removal. The blind end of the Roux-en-Y limb may be re-accessed by percutaneous puncture under fluoroscopic guidance or a small incision under local anesthetic for late diagnostic or therapeutic procedures long after the trans-jejunal tube has been remove. In the authors' experience, this approach provides an excellent chance of excellent outcome in very difficult cases and may spare the patient the need for repeated major surgical intervention months or years later (Schweizer et al 1991). It is generally unnecessary to add the morbidity of a formal stoma, although such an approach has been reported (Barker & Winkler 1985). Details of this approach are described below by Dr Alan Livingstone.

Liver transplantation. Only rarely does secondary biliary fibrosis due to long-standing biliary obstruction progress to true cirrhosis. In such cases, orthotopic liver transplantation should be considered as an alternative to biliary reconstruction. However, to date, there are no series reporting the results of transplantation for benign bile duct strictures, and thus it is impossible to make any definitive comments regarding guidelines for selection. Suffice it to say that, even in experienced transplantation centers, surgical reconstruction is preferred for the vast majority of patients with benign strictures.

Portal hypertension and biliary stricture. Patients with co-existing portal hypertension and biliary strictures represent an especially difficult group to manage. This combination has been reported in 10 to 20% of patients at the time of referral (Blumgart & Kelley 1984, Chapman et al 1995). Portal hypertension may result from secondary biliary fibrosis or direct injury to the portal vein or there may be coincident hepatocellular disease from alcohol abuse, chronic hepatitis or other causes. The presence of splenomegaly or a history of gastrointestinal bleeding in a patient with biliary stricture should prompt further investigation with esophagogastroduodenoscopy and angiography with delayed-phase splenoportography. Bleeding esophageal varices, particularly if accompanied by hypersplenism or ascites, renders the overall prognosis far worse (Chapman et al 1995, Way & Dunphy 1972). Furthermore, collateral venous channels in the subhepatic region and within adhesions makes dissection difficult and bloody. Patients with portal hypertension very often have a proximal stricture and multiple previous attempts at repair, further reducing the likelihood of a successful outcome.

In seriously ill patients with jaundice and portal hypertension, it is advisable to attempt non-operative stenting or balloon dilatation than to proceed to immediate definitive repair (Fig. 49.19) (Molnar & Stockum 1978, Pellegrini et al 1984, Schwarz et al 1981, Teplick et al 1980, Toufanian et al 1978). In the face of severe gastrointestinal bleeding, initial measures must be directed at stopping the hemorrhage and resuscitation (see Chs 95 and 97). If bleeding continues, then consideration should be given to immediate splenorenal or transjugular intrahepatic portosystemic shunting (TIPS) (Ch. 101) to achieve control, with bile duct reconstruction deferred until a later date. The best and most convenient form of operative shunt is the splenorenal (see Chs 100 and 102). Transjugular intrahepatic portosystemic shunts have a limited patency and are used most often as a bridge to transplantation (see Ch. 101). Moreover, the risk of biliary injury and subsequent biliary-venous fistula is high in the setting of a dilated biliary tree and appears to be a major mechanism of early shunt failure (Jalan et al 1996, Saxon et al 1996, Saxon et al 1998). TIPS is thus unlikely to

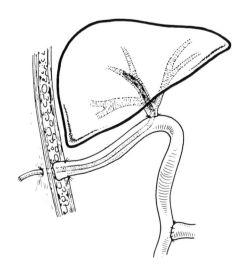

Fig. 49.18 Hepaticojejunostomy with a long defunctionalized Roux limb with the end secured subcutaneously or subperitoneally. This allows access for future diagnostic or therapeutic studies.

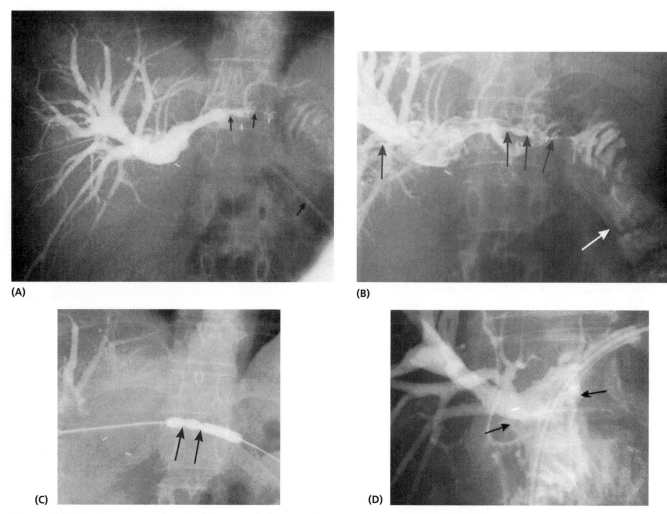

(A)

(B)

(C)

(D)

Fig. 49.19 (A) Percutaneous transhepatic cholangiogram showing a high (Type 3) postcholecystectomy biliary stricture in a patient after cholecystectomy during which there had been excision of the entire common hepatic duct. This was followed by two attempts at a mucosal graft repair and then by a left-sided hepaticojejunostomy by the Longmire-Sandford procedure. On failure of this operation, percutaneous intubation of the biliary ductal system was undertaken from the right side with attempted balloon dilatation of the hepaticojejunostomy on three consecutive occasions. The radiograph shows the area of the hilus (marked by a surgical clip), two strictures in the left hepatic ductal system, one just proximal to and the other at the hepaticojejunostomy (black arrows). A free endoprosthesis is seen (small black arrow) lying in the jejunum. **(B)** Cholangiogram obtained during attempted balloon dilatation of the stricture reveals the passage of the catheter (black arrows) and the biliary system full of clot. The guide-wire crosses the stricture. A free endoprosthesis lies within the jejunal loop (white arrow). This procedure was followed by a severe episode of hemobilia requiring blood transfusion. **(C)** Radiograph obtained during balloon dilatation clearly shows the two strictures (arrows). **(D)** Hepaticojejunostomy Roux-en-Y was performed using the left hepatic duct approach and a very wide anastomosis obtained (between the arrows). The previous hepaticojejunostomy to the left lobe was dismantled and the new anastomosis splinted by a tube passed through the left hepatic ductal system. The tube was removed 2 months later. The patient was well and symptom-free with normal liver function tests 2 years after operation.

play a major role in the management of this patient population. Percutaneous drainage or balloon dilatation may be used in association with the above measures.

If hemorrhage is encountered during the course of stricture repair, then hepaticostomy drainage may be performed as an initial measure and a splenorenal shunt undertaken at a later date. Bile duct stricture repair carried out at the time of the shunting procedure can be extremely difficult and, in any event, is unwise at a time of severely compromised liver function. Occasionally, patients present with variceal hem-

orrhage after otherwise successful previous stricture repair (Fig. 49.20). In these instances, portal-systemic shunting may be indicated, either as an emergency measure or, preferably, after initial conservative management. Injection sclerotherapy may successfully control the bleeding and obviate the need for operative intervention (see Ch. 97).

Results of biliary reconstruction. Given the wide spectrum of injuries that are possible at laparoscopic cholecystectomy, it is difficult to fully assess the results of operative

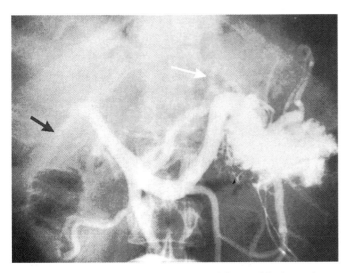

Fig. 49.20 Splenoportography in a patient with benign bile duct stricture and a history of vascular injury at the time of initial operation. The patient presented with portal hypertension and bleeding esophageal varices. Note that only a portion of the right portal venous vasculature is outlined (black arrow). Note varices in the area of the gastric fundus (white arrow). Percutaneous transhepatic cholangiography revealed a stenosis near the biliary confluence but not a complete obstruction. Liver biopsy demonstrated hepatic fibrosis. The patient was managed with a splenorenal shunt; biliary reconstruction was not undertaken. She has remained well for several years after the shunt and repair of the stricture has never been necessary.

repair. Most surgical series report results of repair of biliary strictures (Type E) and do not address operative intervention for other injury types. In addition, many patients are subjected to immediate repair at the time of initial injury; the more difficult cases and the failures are generally referred to specialist units but the long term outcome of the others is often not reported. Thus, most literature reports, generated from tertiary referral centers, include significant numbers of patients requiring difficult reconstructions or with multiple previous repair attempts and may underestimate the overall success rate. Furthermore, relatively few reports with sufficient follow-up focus on the results of repair of laparoscopic injuries alone (Table 49.4). It remains to be determined if the results of repair of bile duct strictures after open cholecystectomy or other procedures can be extrapolated to repair of laparoscopic injuries. It has been suggested that laparoscopic bile duct injuries may have a less satisfactory outcome because of the more complex nature of many of these injuries and the frequent inflammation and fibrosis secondary to bile leakage (Lillemoe 1997).

Operative morbidity and mortality. Several previous studies suggested significant morbidity associated with repair of benign (Blumgart et al 1984, Kune & Sali 1981). The most common postoperative complications seen were intra-abdominal abscess, wound infection, cholangitis, sepsis, biliary fistula, postoperative hemorrhage and pneumonia. Indeed, the perioperative mortality in many series ranged from 5 to 8% (Cattell & Braasch 1959, Warren et al

Table 49.4 Selected recent series reporting outcome after repair of benign biliary strictures. The vast majority of repairs were performed as hepatico- or choledocho-jejunostomy, Roux-en-Y. Previous repair attempt refers to the number and percentage of patients referred after at least one attempt at repair. Successful outcome refers to the percentage of patients requiring no further intervention after initial, definitive surgical management at the reporting institution; most series reported salvaging some of the initial failures with interventional radiological or further surgical intervention.

Author	N	Mechanism of injury	Previous repair attempt	Morbidity/ mortality	Successful outcome	Mean follow-up
Chapman et al 1995	122	OC (all)	80 (66%)	NR / 1.8%*	76%	86 months
McDonald et al 1995	45	OC – 26 LC – 16 Other – 3	11 (24%)	36% / 0	95%†	55 months
Stewart & Way 1995	45	LC (all)	27 (60%)	4% / 0	94%	NR
Tocchi et al 1996	84	OC – 60 CBDE – 4 Trauma – 4 Other – 16	4 (5%)	21% / 2.2%	83%**	108 months
Lillemoe 1997	59	LC (all)	15 (25%)	NR / 0	92%**	33 months

OC, open cholecystectomy; LC, laparoscopic cholecystectomy; CBDE, common bile duct exploration; NR, not reported
* Postoperative deaths in 2 patients subjected to mucosal grafts; no deaths occurred in patients submitted to direct biliary-enteric repair
** Includes patients with excellent or good outcomes
† Includes some asymptomatic patients with mild elevations of liver function tests

1982, Way & Dunphy 1972). In the past decade, however, several authors have documented a considerable decline in mortality, with many citing no perioperative deaths (Table 49.4). These figures generally do not take into account patients who die of biliary tract-related sepsis while awaiting definitive treatment. Factors frequently associated with perioperative death include advanced age, significant co-morbid medical conditions and biliary sepsis. Significant underlying liver disease is perhaps the most important predictor of adverse outcome. Chapman et al reported a perioperative mortality of 23% in patients with biliary strictures and portal hypertension subjected to any operative procedure (Chapman et al 1995).

One must bear in mind that a significant proportion of patients in many reports were referred after one or more repair attempts. Failed repairs nearly always render subsequent more difficult and negatively impact on the ultimate outcome (vide infra). The reported morbidity and mortality figures reflect this point and underscore the serious nature of these injuries. Nevertheless, in experienced hands, operative repair of biliary strictures is a relatively safe procedure, and this fact must be considered when comparing surgery to non-operative techniques.

Long-term results and follow-up. Several factors must be considered when analyzing the long-term results of biliary reconstruction. First, there is no consistently used algorithm for postoperative investigation. Likewise, the measures used to assess outcome vary considerably. Approaches to follow-up range from simple observation and measurement of liver function tests to performance of cholangiography or HIDA scans. Consistency in analyzing long term results is important and should include an assessment of symptoms and liver function tests as well as radiographic studies. Such a triad of criteria is useful for clarifying the results and is the only way to accurately compare the results from different series or different interventions (Table 49.5) (Schweizer et al 1991). In addition, length of follow-up is critically important in analyzing the final results of any series or when comparing two different treatment modalities. Pitt et al reported that two-thirds of recurrent strictures were apparent within

2 years but 20% were diagnosed 5 or more years after the initial repair (Pitt et al 1982). Similarly, Tocchi et al observed that 40% of re-strictures were identified more than 5 years after the initial operation (Tocchi et al 1996). Thus, complete and accurate assessment of the results of surgery or any other intervention requires a minimum follow-up of 5-years and probably longer (Bismuth 1982).

Several specialist centers have reported satisfactory outcomes in 80 to 90% of patients reconstructed with a biliary-enteric anastomosis, Roux-en-Y (Table 49.4). Many of these studies have also identified factors associated with an adverse outcome (Table 49.6). Chapman et al found that long-term failure and the need for reintervention were significantly greater in patients with injuries involving the biliary confluence and those subjected to three or more repair attempts prior to referral (Chapman et al 1995). Tocchi et al observed that the best results correlated directly with the degree of biliary ductal dilatation, independent of stricture location (Tocchi et al 1996). Surgeon experience and the type of repair are also important determinants of outcome. In the series reported by Stewart and Way, primary end-to-end repairs over a T tube were always unsuccessful when the duct had been completely transected (Stewart & Way 1995). Likewise, the mucosal graft procedure is associated with a recurrence rate of 15% at 2 years, and many patients without obvious stenoses have persistently elevated alkaline phosphatase levels (Smith 1969, 1979).

The use of anastomotic stents has been advocated by many authors (Crist et al 1987, Lillemoe et al 1997, Smith 1969) but their impact on long-term patency is questionable. It should be noted that many, including the authors, rarely use stents and achieve excellent results (Bismuth et al 1978, Bismuth 1982, Stewart & Way 1995, Tocchi et al 1996). Thus, transanastomotic stents appear to have little impact on outcome and probably should not be used

Table 49.5 Suggested criteria for assessing the late results of biliary stricture management

Classification	Symptoms	Biochemistry[a]	Radiology[b]
Excellent	None	Normal	Normal
Good	None	± Elevated	± Abnormal
Fair	Improved	Elevated	Abnormal
Poor	Persistent/Worse	Elevated	Abnormal

[a] Serum bilirubin and alkaline phosphatase
[b] HIDA scan and/or cholangiography

Table 49.6 Factors associated with stricture recurrence or poor outcome after operative reconstruction

- Proximal stricture (Bismuth Type 3 and 4)
- Multiple prior attempts at repair
- Portal hypertension
- Hepatic parenchymal disease (cirrhosis or hepatic fibrosis)
- End-to-end biliary anastomosis
- Surgeon inexperience
- Intrahepatic or multiple strictures
- Concurrent cholangitis or hepatic abscess
- Intrahepatic stones
- External or internal biliary fistula
- Intra-abdominal abscess or bile collection
- Hepatic lobar atrophy
- Advanced age or poor general health

routinely. While stents may be useful in selected cases, it is clear that they cannot prevent the inevitable failure of a poorly constructed anastomosis.

The results of surgical reconstruction for injuries other than strictures of the principal extrahepatic bile duct have not been reported in great numbers and is therefore not known precisely. Recently, Lillemoe et al reported the results of 9 cases of reconstruction for isolated sectoral hepatic duct strictures over an 18-year period (Lillemoe et al 1999). All patients in this series incurred injuries to aberrant right sectoral hepatic ducts at laparoscopic or open cholecystectomy, and all had associated bile leaks. After Roux-en-Y hepaticojejunostomy, six of nine patients (67%) had a successful outcome, while three patients developed late strictures requiring re-intervention.

Patients with recurrent strictures after reconstruction at a specialist unit may be salvaged with further intervention, either anastomotic revision or balloon dilatation. Several authors have reported some measure of success with these patients (Chapman et al 1995, Lillemoe et al 1997, Stewart & Way 1995, Tocchi et al 1996). However, the likelihood of a good outcome decreases. In the series reported by Chapman et al, 11 of 22 operative failures (50%) were successfully re-treated and had satisfactory outcomes but this was substantially lower than the nearly 80% success rate after their initial repair. As discussed above, the loss of bile duct length associated with a failed repair is a major factor that limits the success of subsequent interventions.

Duodenal ulceration has been reported in as high as 10% of patients after Roux-en-Y biliary-enteric reconstruction and constitutes an additional cause of late morbidity (McArthur & Longmire Jr 1971, Pappalardo et al 1982, Sato et al 1982). The majority will respond to anti-ulcer medication but some may develop significant hemorrhage.

Non-operative approaches. Advances in the field of interventional radiology have resulted in a broader application of non-operative approaches to bile duct strictures. The largest reported experience has been with percutaneous balloon dilatation. With this technique, the biliary tree is accessed percutaneously and a guidewire is passed through the stricture. The stricture is then dilated with an angioplasty-type balloon catheter, following which a transhepatic stent is left in place for follow-up cholangiography and repeat dilatation. In most cases, multiple dilatations and prolonged biliary intubation are required.

Early results have been encouraging, with several authors reporting good results in 55 to 85% of patients (Lillemoe et al 1997, Moore et al 1987, Mueller et al 1986, Pitt et al 1989, Vogel et al 1985, Williams et al 1987). These results must be viewed with considerable caution, however. First,

the mean follow-up in most of these studies was less than 3 years, which is insufficient to make a definitive comment regarding long-term efficacy. Second, balloon dilatation is limited in its application to cases in which biliary continuity is intact or has been restored by a previous attempt at repair, but has no role for strictures at or above the confluence and cannot be used if the bile duct has been transected (Lillemoe et al 1997). Third, complications related to balloon dilatation or to the percutaneous catheter are not infrequent and include hemobilia, bile leak and cholangitis in up to 20% of patients.

Comparing the results of balloon dilatation with operative reconstruction is difficult because of differences in the types of injuries selected for each type of treatment, inconsistencies in defining successful outcomes and differences in reporting complications and length of follow-up. To date, there have been no randomized studies comparing the two techniques. In two retrospective analyses, biliary reconstruction was more likely to result in a successful outcome, 89% versus 52% (Pitt et al 1989) and 92% versus 64% (Lillemoe et al 1997), respectively. Moreover, because balloon dilatation requires multiple readmissions and repeat interventions, the overall cost and morbidity appears to be similar to that of operatively treated patients (Pitt et al 1989). The data would suggest that, in most cases, biliary-enteric anastomosis is more effective and provides more durable relief of symptoms than balloon dilatation. However, balloon dilatation is preferable in patients who would otherwise not tolerate an operation and may be tried as an initial treatment in patients with biliary anastomotic strictures where the success rate appears to be greater than for primary bile duct strictures (Millis et al 1992).

BILE DUCT INJURY AFTER OTHER OPERATIONS

Biliary reconstructive operation

Procedures requiring biliary-enteric anastomoses may be complicated by postoperative stricture or fistula. Such procedures include reconstruction after pancreaticoduodenectomy, bile duct resection for mid-bile duct tumors, or after excision of choledochal cysts. Typically, these procedures involve choledocho- or hepatico-enteric anastomosis. Late strictures after such procedures are most likely to occur when enteric anastomosis is performed to a normal-caliber duct or when the duct itself is diseased, as in cases of choledochal cysts. When biliary-enteric anastomosis has been performed for long-standing biliary obstruction, the duct is dilated and thickened. In these cases, the anastomosis is usually easy to construct and late stenosis is uncommon (Tocchi et al 1996). Indeed, in most cases, stricture of a biliary-enteric anastomosis following resections for malignancy are the result of cancer recurrence.

Late stricture after side-to-side choledochoduodenostomy performed for choledocholithiasis or as a bypass procedure for chronic pancreatitis may also occur. This complication is rare if the anastomosis is performed to a sufficiently dilated duct (at least 1.5 cm) and the final diameter of the anastomosis is at least 2–2.5 cm (Escudero-Fabre et al 1991, Schein & Glieddman 1981). The so-called 'sump syndrome' after choledochoduodenostomy, in which particulate matter, stones and food debris accumulate and stagnate in the distal 'blind' end of the common duct, is an occasional cause of recurrent cholangitis which can result in anastomotic stricture (Matthews et al 1993). Endoscopic management, consisting of sphincterotomy with or without balloon dilatation of the anastomosis has been reported for this condition (Baker et al 1985). However, this approach may not be adequate to remove the thick, infected debris which is often densely adherent to the wall of the inflamed distal common bile duct, and re-stricture of the anastomosis is not infrequent. The authors prefer reoperation, with end-to-side hepaticojejunostomy, Roux-en-Y in order to prevent persistent regurgitation of intestinal contents and to permanently remove the 'sump' (Matthews et al 1993). In cases where dissection in the hilus is rendered hazardous because of dense scarring, an alternative maneuver is to perform a pyloric exclusion and gastrojejunostomy, which accomplishes the same objective of preventing reflux of intestinal contents into the biliary tree.

Recurrent cholangitis after biliary-enteric anastomosis is almost invariably attributed to anastomotic stricture; however, this assumption has been questioned (Goldman et al 1983). Some patients develop repeated episodes of cholangitis despite apparently free drainage of bile through the anastomosis in the absence of a clear stricture. In these cases, there may be an overlooked intrahepatic stricture or intrahepatic stone disease (Matthews et al 1993).

Gastric resection

Injury to the bile duct at gastrectomy is particularly likely when the pyloric region and duodenal bulb are severely distorted or inflamed (Florence et al 1981). The most common situation is biliary injury during Billroth II gastrectomy. Such cases may present in the postoperative period with jaundice or biliary fistula, and one may mistakenly attribute this to a duodenal stump leak. Less commonly, bile duct injury occurs during a Billroth II gastrectomy (Fig. 49.21).

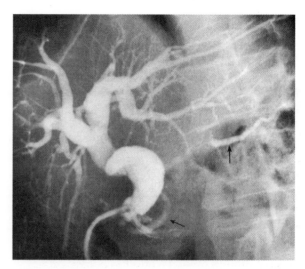

Fig. 49.21 A patient with ampullary disconnection which occurred during Billroth I gastrectomy. The duodenal loop was completely detached from the periampullary area. A fistulogram obtained through a T tube which had been left in situ demonstrates both the bilary tree and the pancreatic duct (arrows). (From Dr H. Gooszen, University of Leiden, The Netherlands.)

Repair of the damaged bile duct following Billroth II gastrectomy is usually not difficult. The stricture typically lies close to the proximal divided end of the duodenum, and it is a simple matter to identify the biliary tree and perform a direct anastomosis at or near the duodenal stump. Occasionally, the entire first and second portion of the duodenum has been disconnected from the pancreatic head. The senior author (LHB) has managed three such cases by bringing up a retrocolic Roux-en-Y segment and enveloping the pancreatic head in the open end of the jejunum.

Hepatic resection

Biliary injury during hepatic resection is uncommon in experienced hands but certainly can occur, particularly when carried out for lesions near the hilus (Fig. 49.22). If there is a suspicion of ductal injury inflicted during operation that cannot be readily identified or if the biliary anatomy is unclear, then intraoperative cholangiography should be performed; deliberate choledochotomy with passage of fine bougies into the right and left ducts may assist identification. If a choledochostomy has been performed, a T tube is usually inserted.

The management of injuries that present following partial hepatectomy can be extremely difficult (Johnson et al 1979, Matthews et al 1991, Smith et al 1982), the problems being similar to those encountered with liver atrophy (vide supra). It should be emphasized that a biliary fistula after liver resection should be treated expectantly for a long period, since

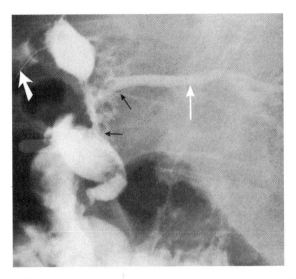

Fig. 49.22 Complex biliary stricture and fistula following right hepatic lobectomy for hydatid disease. There was a biliary fistula through the right chest wall (large white arrow). The radiograph was obtained by injection of a tube within the fistulous tract. A cavity in the right chest and one below the diaphragm were both outlined and there was an associated right empyema. There is complete disruption of the biliary ductal system (black arrows). The left hepatic duct in the regenerated liver remnant is shown (white arrow) and a fistula is filling the low common bile duct and the duodenum independently. The patient was managed by drainage of the empyema, antibiotics and parenteral nutrition. Subsequently, repair of the duodenal fistula and hepaticojejunostomy Roux-en-Y to the exposed bile duct were successfully carried out. The patient recovered and was without symptoms 3 years after operation.

to offer no significant benefit (Vougas et al 1996) and their routine use has been discontinued in many centers (Macfarlane et al 1996, Vougas et al 1996). Hepatic artery thrombosis is an uncommon but well-recognized cause of biliary stricture after liver transplantation (Colonna et al 1992, Orons et al 1995, Sanchez-Urdazpal et al 1993). Late stricture is seen in as high as 10 to 15% of cases (Macfarlane et al 1996, Vougas et al 1996), which is much lower than the reported rate of recurrent stricture after direct anastomosis for bile duct injuries. Many of these patients require operative revision but some may be managed successfully with endoscopic or interventional radiologic approaches (Colonna et al 1992, Lemmer et al 1997, Macfarlane et al 1996).

BILE DUCT INJURY DUE TO BLUNT OR PENETRATING INJURY

Hepatic and biliary injuries from trauma are discussed more fully in Chapter 68. The gallbladder or biliary tree may be damaged by blunt (Fig. 49.23) or penetrating abdominal injuries. The common bile duct is susceptible to disruption from deceleration injuries usually at the level of the pancreaticoduodenal junction, where it is relatively fixed compared

many resolve spontaneously. Operative repair should only be undertaken for persistent fistula despite continued observation or for jaundice or recurrent episodes of cholangitis.

Other procedures

Late biliary stenosis may follow any other procedure requiring dissection in or near the porta hepatis, such as portocaval shunt or lymphadenectomy (Ishizuka et al 1998). Biliary strictures have also been described after external beam radiation therapy (Schmets et al 1996) and after endoscopic injection of sclerosant into a bleeding duodenal ulcer (Luman et al 1994).

Bile duct strictures may also complicate orthotopic liver transplantation (Ch. 115), although their frequency appears to have decreased over the past several years (Calne 1976, Colonna et al 1992, Lemmer et al 1997, Macfarlane et al 1996, Vougas et al 1996). Direct end-to-end choledochostomy) has been the preferred method of reconstruction but Roux-en-Y choledochojejunostomy is also used (Lopez-Santamaria et al 1999). The use of T tubes after biliary reconstruction, once considered essential, has been shown

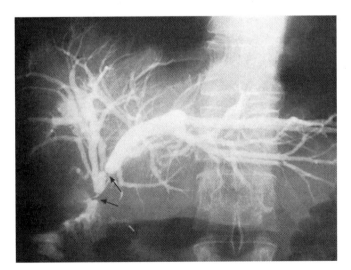

Fig. 49.23 Percutaneous transhepatic cholangiogram in a young man with recurrent attacks of cholangitis 1 year after repair of a biliary stricture at the site of damage to the common hepatic duct associated with a liver injury necessitating right hepatectomy. Note that there are two strictures present—one at the site of previous hepaticojejunostomy and the other in the main left hepatic duct. Rotation of the liver had made an approach to the left duct difficult. Hepaticojejunostomy was refashioned in the area of the confluence and the stricture within the left hepatic duct was treated by subsequent balloon dilatation with a good result.

to the more proximal duct. Delayed common duct stricture has been reported after blunt abdominal trauma (Horiguchi et al 1998; Yoon et al 1998). Late problems may also arise after hepatic trauma, where prolonged fistulization occurs from a segment of liver isolated by the injury, particularly when there is bile drainage from a large portion of the liver through the fistulous tract.

Management of ductal injuries will depend on the extent of associated injuries. Major hemorrhage and other life-threatening injuries obviously take priority, and in this setting external diversion of bile flow through a tube passed proximally into the duct will prevent bile leak and allow later definitive repair. Roux-en-Y biliary-enteric reconstruction is the preferred approach for complete ductal transections. Traumatic strictures are also probably best approached in this manner, although successful dilatation has been reported (Horiguchi et al 1998). Management of persistent bile leak after liver injury is a much more difficult problem; the fistula may persist even after a prolonged period of observation. One should exclude the possibility of an associated distal stricture, which will perpetuate bile drainage. One approach to management is by anastomosis of a well-developed fistula tract to a loop of jejunum (fistulojejunostomy) or to the gallbladder. Fistulojejunostomy may yield a permanent cure, although late stenosis or stricture may still develop for which secondary repair must be performed (Smith et al 1982). Resection of an isolated segment of liver that is the source of the drainage is difficult and seldom warranted. Direct oversewing of the fistula is rarely successful.

POSTINFLAMMATORY BILIARY STRICTURES

LONG-STANDING CHOLELITHIASIS

Repeated attacks of cholecystitis may result in progressive fibrosis and shrinking of the gallbladder that ultimately obliterates the triangle of Calot (vide supra). The inflammatory process may thereby spread to involve the common hepatic duct, causing inflammatory stenosis and resulting in jaundice and cholangitis (Mirizzi 1948). The presentation may be associated with a history of acute or chronic cholecystitis and an overt stricture may be present at the time of cholecystectomy. Intraoperative cholangiography may be difficult to obtain and inadvertent bile duct injury may ensue during attempts to remove the gallbladder. A large stone in the region of Hartmann's pouch may erode in the common hepatic duct to cause a cholecystocholedochal fistula (see Figs 54.8 and 49.4). In such cases, attempts to remove the gallbladder will result in injury to the common

hepatic duct or even removal of a portion of the duct. Therefore, patients with longstanding gallstones and jaundice should never be submitted to operation without preliminary percutaneous or endoscopic cholangiography.

Inflammatory strictures of the common hepatic duct in association with chronic cholelithiasis may present with radiological features that are indistinguishable from cholangiocarcinoma (see Fig. 54.9) (Ch. 54). This possibility must be considered in all patients suspected of harboring a tumor at the biliary confluence in whom there is coincident choledocholithiasis (Hadjis et al 1985, Standfield et al 1989, Wetter et al 1991). Biliary cytology and percutaneous biopsy are generally not helpful, since a benign result never excludes a malignancy, and the diagnosis is usually established at operation.

CHRONIC DUODENAL ULCER

Chronic duodenal ulcer can cause inflammation and fibrosis in the entire periampullary area, resulting in distal biliary stricture or choledochoduodenal fistula. The presentation is typically jaundice and cholangitis in a patient with a long history of duodenal ulcer. The advent of H_2-receptor antagonists and acid-reducing agents has greatly reduced the incidence of complications related to peptic ulcer disease and such problems are now rarely seen.

RECURRENT PYOGENIC CHOLANGITIS

Recurrent pyogenic cholangitis, also known as oriental cholangiohepatitis, is addressed in detail in Chapter 64. This condition is seen mainly in Southeast Asia and is associated with intrahepatic calcium bilirubinate stones and intrahepatic strictures (Chen et al 1984, Choi et al 1982, Maki et al 1972, Ong, 1962). Recurrent episodes of cholangitis and sepsis is a major threat to life in these patients; there is also a significantly increased risk of cholangiocarcinoma (Chijiiwa et al 1995, Chu et al 1997, Sato et al 1995, Sato et al 1998). Hepatic resection combined with Roux-en-Y biliary-enteric reconstruction is effective in relieving symptoms and clearing stones. This is particularly true if the disease is unilateral but even patients with bilateral disease may benefit from a combination of resection and postoperative balloon dilatation and stone extraction (Jeng et al 1996). Because of the high incidence of recurrent stricture and stone formation, a team approach that includes experienced surgeons and interventional radiologists is required to obtain the best results (Kim et al 1998). Some authors have reported some success using balloon dilatation in combination with transhepatic choledochoscopic lithotripsy, either as initial therapy or for recurrent stones after surgery

(Sheen-Chen et al 1998, Yoshida et al 1998). A large number of patients have advanced parenchymal disease at presentation and die of related complications, despite aggressive intervention (Chijiiwa et al 1995).

CHRONIC PANCREATITIS

Chronic pancreatitis is a well-known cause of distal bile duct stenosis and stricture. The incidence of biliary stricture in these patients is difficult to know with certainty but has been reported in up to 30% (Sarles et al 1976). The characteristic lesion is a long, narrow stricture involving the retropancreatic portion of the common bile duct (Fig. 49.24), but other variants have been described (Barthet et al 1994, Sarles and Sahel 1978). Although more common in association with chronic alcohol-related pancreatitis, it may occur in chronic pancreatitis unrelated to alcohol use. In addition to jaundice, pain is common, which may be intermittent and similar to biliary colic but cholangitis and fever are less frequent (Barthet et al 1994, Kalvania et al 1989, Stabile et al 1987).

The diagnosis of bile duct stricture is usually made at ERCP, but occasionally by PTC. The radiological appearance is typically a long stenosis of the retropancreatic por-

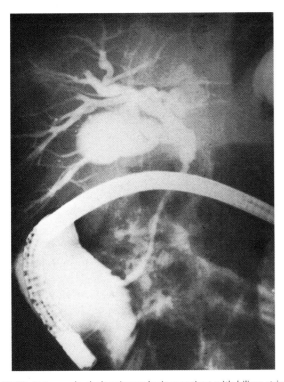

Fig. 49.24 Retrograde cholangiography in a patient with biliary stricture related to pancreatitis. Note the long stricture in the common bile duct as it passes through the head of a calcified pancreas. The stricture is a result of pancreatitis form alcohol ingestion and the patient's symptoms were of intermittent attacks of jaundice and pain. The pancreatic duct could not be delineated. Management included laparotomy and choledochojejunostomy.

tion of the common bile duct. The fibrotic process may also affect the proximal duct gradually over a prolonged period so that it is relatively non-distensible, and the proximal duct may exhibit little dilatation as one would expect from a stricture from other causes. Occasionally, however, the stenosis is shorter in length or may only involve the immediate papillary area. Contrast medium usually but not always traverses the stenosis and flows into the duodenum. Differentiating a stricture related to pancreatitis from malignant obstruction may be very difficult. While the long, tapering, narrow stricture of the bile duct is characteristic of chronic pancreatitis, especially when associated with demonstrable pancreatic ductal abnormality on ERCP, carcinoma may still be present and one must use extreme caution to avoid an erroneous diagnosis.

The presence of a bile duct stenosis or stricture in association with chronic pancreatitis is not necessarily an indication for therapy. Quite severe stenosis may be found in the presence of absolutely normal liver function tests and in whom there has never been jaundice. If, however, cholestasis or cholangitis occurs, then biliary bypass becomes necessary. Occasionally, operation is necessary in the management of chronic pancreatitis itself and, if it is known that a high grade biliary stricture is present, biliary bypass may be performed concomitantly. Thus, in the senior author's (LHB) series of 240 patients with chronic pancreatitis, 39 of whom came to operation, nine had symptomatic biliary obstruction and a total of 13 were subjected to some form of biliary-enteric anastomosis, either alone or associated with excisional surgery for pancreatic disease (Blumgart et al 1982). It is important to emphasize, however, that the majority of patients with common bile duct stenosis associated with chronic pancreatitis may be managed without biliary bypass (Kalvania et al 1989, Smits et al 1996). Temporary endoscopic biliary stenting may be useful in some cases and may be definitive therapy in 10 to 25% (Barthet et al 1994, Itani & Taylor 1995, Smits et al 1996).

For patients requiring biliary bypass, side-to-side choledochoduodenostomy may be used, but this is often not the best option since the surrounding inflammatory reaction may render the duodenum rigid and less mobile; also, the common bile duct may also be involved in periductal fibrosis and thus only minimally dilated. Roux-en-Y choledochojejunostomy is the preferred reconstructive approach. Cholecystojejunostomy should not be used, and transduodenal sphincteroplasty is generally not suitable because of the great length of the stricture. Biliary-enteric anastomosis generally affords excellent long-term relief of obstruction, but relief from chronic pain associated with the pancreatitis itself is unusual (Barthet et al 1994, Blumgart et al 1982, Stabile et al 1987).

A combined surgical and radiological approach to benign bile duct strictures and other biliary problems

A. LIVINGSTONE, D.G. HUTSON

The preceding chapter (vide supra) has masterfully summarized the options for managing benign biliary strictures. The plethora of procedures is testimony to the challenge of definitively treating these problems, for if one technique were uniformly successful, there would be no need to develop alternatives. Recent technological developments in interventional radiology have led to the development of innovative techniques for diagnosis as well as stricture dilatation, stone extraction, and bile duct perfusion (Ferrucci & Mueller 1982, Gallacher et al 1985, Molnar & Stocktum 1978, Pereiras et al 1979). As with surgery, radiological approaches often require repeated interventions to be successful. The solution was to develop and evaluate a surgical procedure that would allow safe, easy, repeated radiologic access to the biliary tree for the diagnosis and treatment of a variety of biliary tract problems, thereby avoiding reoperation.

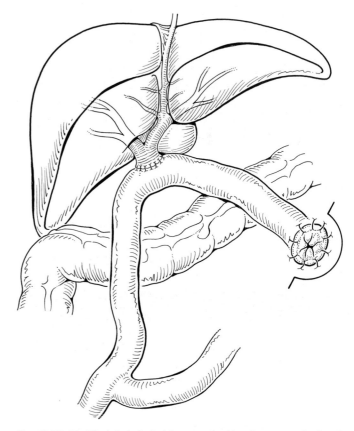

Fig. 49.25 Modified choledochojejunostomy with subcutaneously placed afferent limb.

SURGICAL TECHNIQUE

The surgical procedure is a simple modification of a standard Roux-en-Y choledocho- or hepaticojejunostomy creating a long afferent jejunal limb (LAJL) the end of which is placed either subfascially or beneath the skin of the abdominal wall (see also Ch. 30). We modified our original technique (Hutson et al 1984) by placing the subcutaneous segment of the jejunal limb beneath a skin incision (Fig. 49.25). This clearly identifies the subcutaneous segment, and because the puncture is through normal skin rather than scar tissue, post dilatation leakage of bile is minimized (Fig. 49.26). Leakage is not a problem if the jejunal segment is subfascial, but it must be marked with clips to facilitate its future localization. If a Roux-en-Y choledocho- or hepaticojejunostomy is already present at the time of reoperation, it can be converted by one of several techniques to a LAJL without revising the biliary anastomosis (Hutson et al 1984). One must remember that the surgical procedure is designed for postoperative use by the invasive radiologist; therefore, their technical needs must be considered when constructing the form of the jejunal extension.

The following overview is based on a personal experience of over 190 patients with a LAJL.

RADIOLOGICAL TECHNIQUES

Our technique for diagnosing and managing biliary pathology through the LAJL has remained constant since the original report (Russell et al 1985). The jejunal limb can be accessed in the ambulatory patient using sedation and local anesthesia at the skin puncture site. Transhepatic access is rarely required. The almost 100% success rate is true regardless of whether the limb is placed subcutaneously or sub-

Our general policy is to dilate any residual stricture intra-operatively and to restudy patients through the LAJL at 4 months, even if asymptomatic. Of course, an earlier study would be performed should the patient become symptomatic or if the liver function tests deteriorates. Subsequently, further dilatations are determined by three factors: the radiographic appearance of the stricture at the time of dilatation (severe strictures are dilated more frequently), the development of cholangitis, or an elevation of the liver function tests (LFT) (particularly the alkaline phosphatase). During lifelong follow-up, if a stricture recurs it should be dilated and the patient returned to 4 month restudy intervals. This schedule should continue until recurrence of the stricture is minimal, or it is felt that the procedure has failed and operative intervention is indicated. Once the stricture is stable, the patient may be followed with monthly LFT and a repeat study at 8 months. If after 2×8-month studies there is no recurrence, the patient may be followed symptomatically and with LFT. Most patients develop a characteristic periodicity to their recurrences, with some requiring dilatation every few months and others only once a year.

BENIGN DISEASE

IATROGENIC INJURIES

Historically, the treatment of biliary strictures following iatrogenic injuries, whether primary or recurrent, has been surgical. While most reports continue to favor a surgical approach, it is now apparent that recurrent strictures secondary to bile duct injuries can be effectively managed by balloon dilatation, and the need for repeated operation is unusual (Hutson et al 1998). While a single dilatation is effective in the short-term treatment of many of these problems, it is unlikely to be durable over the life of the patient; thus, the need for repeated, easy access to the bile ducts.

The operative technique varies depending on the level of injury, patency of the distal duct, stricture length, the presence of a biloma, or previous surgery. If continuity of the distal duct is preserved and the stricture is short, we would recommend an aggressive trial of endoscopic dilatation. If there is discontinuity of the duct or if the stricture is long, a bypass (LAJL) above the stricture is recommended. In mature, very high strictures involving the right or left hepatic ducts, where continuity of the distal duct is preserved, we would consider anastomosing the jejunum to the distal duct below the stricture, relying solely on dilatation for initial and long term control of recurrence problems (Hutson et al 1998). Transjejunal cholangiography (Fig. 49.27) demonstrates recurrence of a

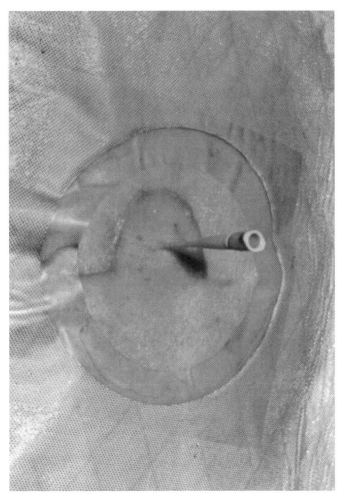

Fig. 49.26 Access of subcutaneous limb through omega-shaped skin incision.

fascially. These jejunal limbs have been accessed over 400 times without a death or major complication (Hutson et al 1998). Patients are routinely pretreated with antibiotics as transient bacteremia after dilatation is not uncommon. A distinct advantage of this approach is that retrograde cannulation uniformly allows access to the entire biliary tree. An antegrade approach, as with a percutaneous transhepatic approach, often requires multiple punctures to manage hilar or bilateral strictures.

FREQUENCY OF DILATATIONS DURING FOLLOW UP

The need for repeat studies and dilatations must be individualized and, therefore, the approach is flexible and responsive to the patient's condition. However, certain guidelines have been developed.

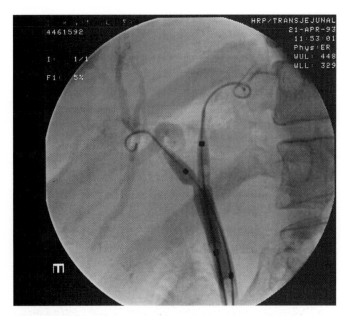

Fig. 49.27 Stricture of right hepatic duct at the bifurcation.

right hepatic stricture in such a case. This patient has been followed over 8 years, undergoing dilatations as determined by the appearance of the stricture. Occasional elevations of the alkaline phosphatase prompted radiologic evaluation through the LAJL. With several dilatations, the patient has remained asymptomatic, and her most recent study demonstrated no recurrence.

When a patient with a previous Roux-Y limb becomes symptomatic we would consider converting this to a LAJL without necessarily revising the biliary jejunal anastomosis. The decision would be made intraoperatively. If conditions in the sub-hepatic area are favorable, we might elect to revise the anastomosis and develop a LAJL. If it were unfavorable and the stricture could be traversed with guide wires, conversion to a LAJL without revision of the anastomosis would be elected. In our experience there is no difference in the long-term results of these two approaches. Further surgery is avoided, although more dilatations are necessary if the anastomosis is distal to the stricture.

Because of the significant failure rate of initial surgery, we recommend that all patients undergoing repair of a bile duct injury, or stricture related to an injury, have a LAJL constructed at the initial operation. This conclusion is based on a prospective study of 33 patients with bile duct injuries treated by repeat dilatations through an LAJL (Hutson et al 1998). The patients were followed over 13 years and there were no re-operations for recurrent strictures in this group. An additional group of patients has undergone the procedure, but, detailed follow-up is incomplete. In our total

experience, there has not been a single reoperation for recurrent stricture when a LAJL has been used. In addition there were no operative deaths, development of cirrhosis, or liver failure. These results were attained regardless of the classification of the injury (Bismuth 1982). Similar outcomes over a 10-year period were reported by McPherson et al (1998).

As an adjunct to other surgical problems

Although infrequently used today, we believe the Rodney Smith procedure (Smith 1964) (vide supra) to be a viable approach to difficult hilar strictures provided it is combined with a LAJL. The operation allows facile access to the entire biliary tree.

Similarly, constructing a LAJL as part of a Longmire procedure (Longmire & Sanford 1948) is technically straightforward (Fig. 49.28). However, the angles developed as part of this operation are not as favorable for access to the entire biliary tree as when the approach is at the hilum. Nevertheless, we have effectively dilated strictures and extracted stones in this situation. A patient who demonstrates the need for repeated easy access to the biliary tree is a 48-year-old woman who developed biliary

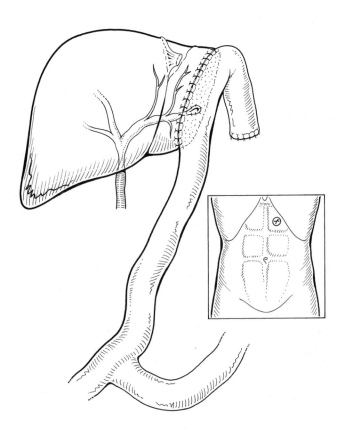

Fig. 49.28 Conversion of Longmire procedure to include LAJL.

obstruction 17 years following a standard Longmire operation. A right transhepatic cholangiogram was required to define the obstruction at the hepaticojejunostomy (Fig. 49.29). The stricture was traversed and dilated; however, the end result (Fig. 49.30, arrow) suggests that repeated dilatations will be required. Had a LAJL been constructed initially, it would have facilitated repeat dilatation at 4 months thus avoiding further surgery. In a second patient, a LAJL was constructed at the time of the original Longmire procedure. This patient required two dilatations over the next 5 years. He remained asymptomatic for 12 years when he developed cholangitis. Studies through the jejunal limb demonstrated multiple intrahepatic stones, a stricture at the biliary-jejunal anastomosis, and strictures in the right ductal system. The LAJL was accessed (Fig. 49.31), the strictures were dilated, and the majority of the stones were extracted. However, the approach for these manipulations were difficult.

SCLEROSING CHOLANGITIS

Strictures associated with sclerosing cholangitis are most often multiple involving both the intra- and extrahepatic biliary tree (Fig. 49.32). While dilatation of these strictures is technically feasible, recurrence is the rule in all patients; thus, repeated, easy access to all ducts over the life-span of the patient is essential. If this therapeutic pathway is chosen,

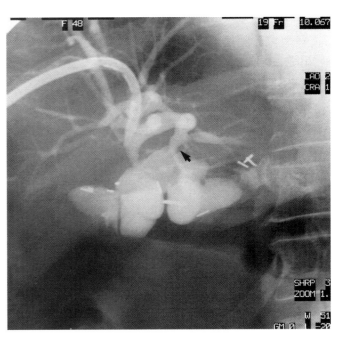

Fig. 49.30 Stricture (arrow) of hepaticojejunostomy (Longmire anastomosis) following dilatation.

we recommend construction of a LAJL. While the interval between dilatations can be individualized, in most cases it is required every 6 months regardless of the LFT or the symptoms. The alkaline phosphatase is a poor indicator of the need for repeat studies since it remains elevated in all patients, even following successful dilatation.

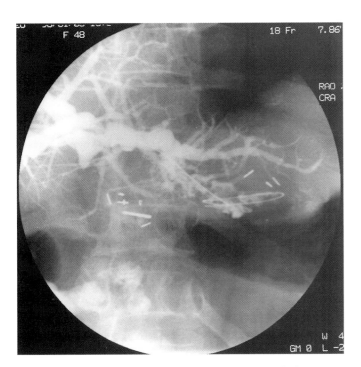

Fig. 49.29 Transhepatic cholangiogram demonstrating marked stricture of the hepaticojejunostomy (Longmire).

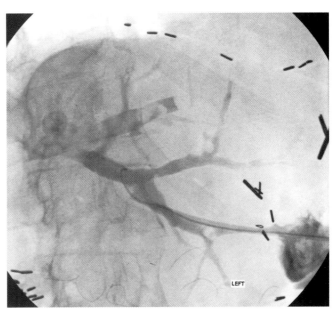

Fig. 49.31 Access of hepaticojejunostomy (Longmire) through subcutaneous jejunal limb.

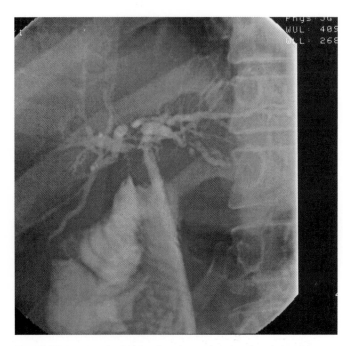

Fig. 49.32 Intra- and extrahepatic strictures in sclerosing cholangitis.

Our recommendations are based on a 15-year follow-up of 35 patients with sclerosing cholangitis who we treated with repeat dilatations through a LAJL. All patients were symptomatic prior to surgery. Several had advanced cirrhosis and/or near total obliteration of the entire intrahepatic biliary tree (Fig. 49.33). The actual 5-year survival of the entire group was 74%. If those patients with advanced cirrhosis and/or obliteration of the intrahepatic biliary tree are withdrawn, the survival increases to 84%. In addition, the

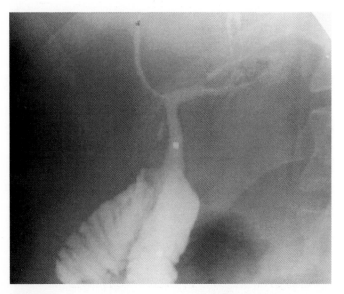

Fig. 49.33 Marked obliteration of ducts in sclerosing cholangitis

15-year analysis strongly suggests that, in selected patients, a combination of dilatation followed by transplantation is the treatment of choice. The operative mortality for liver transplantation is unaffected by previous biliary procedures, even though the operation is somewhat more difficult (McEntee et al 1991).

CAROLI'S DISEASE

The fact that we can repeatedly access the biliary tree and extract stones through the LAJL suggests that the procedure may be useful in the treatment of bilateral, diffuse Caroli's disease. We have treated two such patients, but both were lost to long-term follow-up. It was demonstrated, however, that over the short term, the biliary tree could be completely cleared of stones with control of cholangitis (Reddy et al 1988). The treatment of choice for unilateral Caroli's is liver resection (Ramond et al 1984); however, our practice is to develop a LAJL at the same time for future studies, and stone extraction should this becomes necessary.

TRANSPLANTATION

The two most widely used techniques for reconstructing the biliary tree after transplantation are a choledochocholedochostomy (CDC) and a Roux-en-Y choledochojejunostomy (CDJ). They result in a significant incidence of complications including anastomotic disruption, leaks, strictures (both early and late), and stone formation. In the early postoperative period, these complications present both a diagnostic and a therapeutic dilemma. If a Roux-en-Y reconstruction is used, we recommend fashioning a LAJL. This expedites diagnosis and treatment of both early and late complications of biliary reconstruction.

Our experience suggests that the LAJL has all of the advantages of transhepatic cholangiography as a diagnostic or therapeutic tool, eliminating many of the disadvantages. It is safe and simple to construct and adds little to the operative time or the complexity of the transplantation procedure. It provides easy access to the entire biliary tree for the purpose of diagnosis and treatment.

The major long-term complication of biliary reconstruction in transplant patients is the development of strictures, either anastomotic or intrahepatic, and the LAJL provides expeditious access for dilatation. Experience with balloon dilatation in the long-term treatment of extrahepatic strictures strongly suggests that extrahepatic post-transplant strictures can be effectively managed in this manner. Whether posttransplant intrahepatic strictures can be managed by repeated balloon dilatation is less clear.

HILAR CHOLANGIOCARCINOMA (Ch. 54)

Operation can provide excellent palliation and cure of adenocarcinoma at the bifurcation of the hepatic ducts (Ch. 54). If patency of the major ducts is maintained thus preventing cholangitis and jaundice, excellent long-term palliation may be expected. Over the last dozen years, 24 of 84 patients we treated for bile duct cancer had a LAJL as part of their management. An analysis of these patients supports our bias that a LAJL is not only simple and safe, but beneficial. In these 24 patients, microscopically negative margins were obtained in only nine. Sometimes the tumor was resected leaving positive hepatic duct margins, and in five the anastomosis was performed distal to the obstruction, leaving the unresectable tumor in situ. Overall median survival was 22 months. However, no patient with unresectable disease lived longer than 27 months, whereas 3- and 5-year survival rates with resectable tumors were 31 and 13%, respectively. Local recurrence can be anticipated in the majority of these patients, and if significant palliation is to be achieved, the treatment strategy must be able to maintain ductal patency.

We recommend that a LAJL be constructed in all patients even if resected for cure, since recurrence is common in this group. The limb facilitates dilatation if strictures develop, as well as provides a route for brachytherapy. An additional benefit of the limb is that brachytherapy through the LAJL can achieve excellent palliation and an occasional long term survivor (Hutson et al 1995).

In reviewing our experience with this approach, it is apparent that in many of these patients the indication for repeat dilatation was the development of clinical jaundice. Jaundice is often a late manifestation of recurrence and if used as the only indicator for repeat study, effective dilatation may be impossible. We now recommend that these patients be studied, and dilated if necessary, every 6 months regardless of the LFTs. Excellent palliation of patients with Klatskin tumors can be provided by repeat dilatation through a LAJL, if a rigid schedule for dilatation is followed.

REFERENCES

Abdel W M, el-Ebiedy G, Sultan A, el-Ghawalby N, Fathy O, Gad el-Hak N, Abo E A, Abo Z M, Ezzat F 1996 Postcholecystectomy bile duct injuries: experience with 49 cases managed by different therapeutic modalities. Hepato-Gastroenterology 43: 1141–1147

Adamsen S, Hansen O H, Funch-Jensen P, Schulze S, Stage J G, Wara P 1997 Bile duct injury during laparoscopic cholecystectomy: a prospective nationwide series. Journal of the American College of Surgeons 184: 571–578

Andren-Sandberg A, Alinder G, Bengmark S 1985 Accidental lesions of the common bile duct at cholecystectomy: pre- and perioperative factors of importance. Annals of Surgery 201: 328–332

Asbun, H J, Rossi R L, Lowell J A, Munson J L 1993 Bile duct injury during laparoscopic cholecystectomy: mechanism of injury, prevention, and management. World Journal of Surgery 17: 547–552

Baker A R, Neoptolemos J P, Carr-Locke D L, Fossard D P 1985 Sump syndrome following choledochoduodenostomy and its endoscopic treatment. British Journal of Surgery 72: 433–435

Balsara K P, Dubash C, Shah C R 1998 Pseudoaneurysm of the hepatic artery along with common bile duct injury following laparoscopic cholecystectomy. A report of two cases. Surgical Endoscopy 12: 276–277

Barker E M, Winkler M 1985 Permanent-access hepaticojejunostomy. British Journal of Surgery 71: 181–191

Barthet M, Bernard J P, Duval J L, Affriat C, Sahel J 1994 Biliary stenting in benign biliary stenosis complicating chronic calcifying pancreatitis. Endoscopy 26: 569–572

Belzer F O, McKay W J, Ross H B, Dunphy J E 1965 Autoreconstruction of the common bile duct after venous patch graft. Annals of Surgery 162: 346–355

Bismuth H 1982 Postoperative strictures of the bile duct. In: Blumgart L H (ed) The biliary tract. Clinical surgery international. Churchill Livingstone, Edinburgh, p 209–218

Bismuth H, Franco D, Corlette M B 1978 Long term results of Roux-en-Y hepaticojejunostomy. Surgery, Gynecology & Obstetrics 146: 161–167

Bismuth H, Lazorthes F 1981 Les traumiatismes operatoires de la voie biliarire principale. Masson, Paris

Blumgart L H 1978 Biliary tract obstruction—new approaches to old problems. American Journal of Surgery 135: 19–31

Blumgart L H 1980 Hepatic resection. In: Taylor S (ed) Recent advances in surgery. Churchill Livingstone, Edinburgh, p 1–26

Blumgart L H, Imrie C W, McKay A J 1982 Surgical management of chronic pancreatitis. Journal of Clinical Surgery 1: 229–235

Blumgart L H, Kelley C J 1984 Hepaticojejunostomy in benign and malignant high bile duct stricture: approaches to the left hepatic ducts. British Journal of Surgery 71: 257–261

Blumgart L H, Kelley C J, Benjamin I S 1984 Benign bile duct stricture following cholecystectomy: critical factors in management. British Journal of Surgery 71: 836–843

Blumgart LH, Benjamin I S 1994 Cancer of the bile ducts. In Blumgart L H (ed) Surgery of the liver and biliary tract. 2nd edn. Churchill Livingstone, New York, p 967–995

Brooks D C, Becker J M, Connors P J, Carr-Locke D L 1993 Management of bile leaks following laparoscopic cholecystectomy. Surgical Endoscopy 7: 292–295

Calne R 1976 A new technique for biliary drainage in orthotopic liver transplantation utilizing the gallbladder as a pedicle graft between the donor and recipient common bile ducts. Annals of Surgery 184: 605–609

Carroll B J, Friedman R L, Liberman M A, Phillips E H 1996 Routine cholangiography reduces sequelae of common bile duct injuries. Surgical Endoscopy 10: 1194–1197

Cattell R B, Braasch J W 1959 Two-stage repairs of benign strictures of the bile duct. Surgery, Gynecology and Obstetrics 109: 691–696

Chapman W C, Halevy A, Blumgart L H, Benjamin I S 1995 Postcholecystectomy bile duct strictures. Archives of Surgery 130: 597–604

Chen H H, Zhang W H, Wang S S 1984 Twenty-two-year experience with the diagnosis and treatment of intrahepatic calculi. Surgery, Gynecology and Obstetrics 159: 519–524

Chijiiwa K, Yamashita H, Yoshida J, Kuroki S, Tanaka M 1995 Current management and long-term prognosis of hepatolithiasis. Archives of Surgery 130: 194–197

Choi T K, Wong J, Ong G B 1982 The surgical management of primary intrahepatic stones. British Journal of Surgery 69: 86–90

Chu K M, Lo C M, Liu C L, Fan S T 1997 Malignancy associated with hepatolithiasis. Hepato-Gastroenterology 44: 352–357

Coakley F V, Schwartz L H, Blumgart L H, Fong Y, Jarnagin W R, Panicek D M 1998 Complex postcholecystectomy biliary disorders: preliminary experience with evaluation by means of breath-hold MR cholangiography. Radiology 209: 141–146

Colonna J O, Shaked A, Gomes A S, Colquhoun S D, Jurim O, McDiarmid S V, Millis J M, Goldstein L I, Busuttil R W 1992 Biliary strictures complicating liver transplantation. Incidence, pathogenesis, management, and outcome. Annals of Surgery 216: 344–350

Couinaud C 1953 Les hepato-cholangiostomies digestives. La Presse Medicale 61: 468–470

Couinaud C 1955 Recherches sur la chirurgie du confluent biliaire superieur et des canaux hepatiques. La Presse Medicale 63: 669–674

Crist D W, Kadir S, Cameron J L 1987 The value of preoperatively placed percutaneous biliary catheters in reconstruction of the proximal part of the biliary tract. Surgery, Gynecology and Obstetrics 165: 421–424

Csendes A, Diaz J C, Burdiles P, Maluenda F 1989 Late results of immediate primary end to end repair in accidental section of the common bile duct. Surgery, Gynecology and Obstetrics 168: 125–130

Czerniak A, Soreide O, Gibson R N, Hadjis N S, Kelley C J, Benjamin I S, Blumgart L H 1986 Liver atrophy complicating benign bile duct strictures. Surgical and interventional radiologic approaches. American Journal of Surgery 152: 294–300

Davidoff A M, Pappas T N, Murray E A, Hilleren D J, Johnson R D, Baker M E, Newman G E, Cotton P B, Meyers W C 1992 Mechanisms of major biliary injury during laparoscopic cholecystectomy. Annals of Surgery 215: 196–208

Dawson J L 1981 Cholecystostomy. In: Lord Smith of Marlow and Dame Sheila Sherlock (eds) Surgery of the gallbladder and bile ducts, 2nd edn. Butterworth, London, p 329

Deziel D J, Millikan K W, Economou S G, Doolas A, Ko S T, Airan M C 1993 Complications of laparoscopic cholecystectomy: a national survey of 4,292 hospitals and an analysis of 77,604 cases. American Journal of Surgery 165: 9–14

Ellis H, Hoile R W 1980 Vein patch repair of the common bile duct. Journal of the Royal Society of Medicine 73: 635–637

Escudero-Fabre A, Escallon A, Sack J, Halpern N B, Aldrete J S 1991 Choledochoduodenostomy: analysis of 71 cases followed for 5 to 15 years. Annals of Surgery 213: 635–644

Ferrucci J T, Mueller P R 1982 International radiology of the biliary tract. Gastroenterology 82: 974–985

Fiddian-Green R G, Siviski P R, Karol S V 1988 Median hepatotomy using ultrasonic dissection for complex hepatobiliary problems. Archives of Surgery 123: 901–907

Fletcher D R, Hobbs M S T, Tan P, Valinsky L J, Hockey R L, Pikora T J, Knuiman M W, Sheiner H J, Edis A 1999 Complications of cholecystectomy: risks of the laparoscopic approach and protective effects of operative cholangiography. Annals of Surgery 229: 449–457

Florence M G, Hart M J, White T T 1981 Ampullary disconnection during the course of biliary and duodenal surgery. American Journal of Surgery 142: 100–105

Friedman S L 1997 Molecular mechanisms of hepatic fibrosis and principles of therapy. (Review) (37 refs). Journal of Gastroenterology 32: 424–430

Fujii T, Maguchi H, Obara T, Tanno S, Itoh A, Shudo R, Takahashi K, Saito H, Ura H, Kohgo Y 1998 Efficacy of endoscopic diagnosis and treatment for postoperative biliary leak. Hepato-Gastroenterology 45: 656–661

Gallacher D, Kird S, Kaufman S et al 1985 Nonoperative management of benign postoperative biliary strictures. Radiology 156: 625–629

Gigot J, Etienne J, Aerts R, Wibin E, Dallemagne B, Deweer F, Fortunati D, Legrand M, Vereecken L, Doumont J, Van Reepinghen P, Beguin C 1997 The dramatic reality of biliary tract injury during laparoscopic cholecystectomy. An anonymous multicenter Belgian survey of 65 patients. Surgical Endoscopy 11: 1171–1178

Goldman L D, Steer M L, Silen W 1983 Recurrent cholangitis after biliary surgery. American Journal of Surgery 145: 450–454

Grey-Turner R G 1944 Injuries to the main biliary duct. Lancet i: 621–622

Gupta N, Solomon H, Fairchild R, Kaminski D L 1998 Management and outcome of patients with combined bile duct and hepatic artery injuries. (Review) (20 refs). Archives of Surgery 133: 176–181

Hadjis N S, Collier N A, Blumgart L H 1985 Malignant masquerade at the hilum of the liver. British Journal of Surgery 72: 659–661

Hepp J, Couinaud C 1956 L'abord et l'utilisation du canal hepatique gauche dans les reparations de la voie biliaire principale. La Presse Medicale 64: 947–948

Hochwald S N, Burke E C, Jarnagin W R, Fong Y, Blumgart L H 1999 Preoperative biliary stenting is associated with increased post-operative infectious complications in proximal cholangiocarcinoma. Archives of Surgery 134: 261–6

Horiguchi J, Ohwada S, Tanahashi Y, Sawada T, Ikeya T, Ogawa T, Aiba S, Shiozaki H, Yokoe T, Iino Y, Morishita Y 1998 Traumatic biliary stricture successfully treated by percutaneous transhepatic bile duct dilatation: a case report. Hepato-Gastroenterology 45: 2038–2041

Hunter J G 1991 Avoidance of bile duct injury during laparoscopic cholecystectomy. American Journal of Surgery 162: 71–76

Hutson D, Russell E, Yrizarry J et al 1998 Percutaneous dilatation of biliary strictures through the afferent limb of a modified Roux-en-Y choledochojejunostomy or hepaticojejunostomy. American Journal of Surgery 175:108–113

Hutson D, Russell E, Levi J, Livingstone A et al 1995 Balloon dilatation through the subcutaneously placed afferent limb of a hepaticojejunostomy in patients with resected Klatskin tumors. The American Surgeon 61: 518–520

Hutson D, Russell E, Schiff E et al 1984 Balloon dilatation of biliary strictures through a choledochojejuno-cutaneous fistula. Annals of Surgery 199: 637–647

Ibrarullah M, Sikora S S, Agarwal D K, Kapoor V K, Kaushik S P 1996 'Latent' portal hypertension in benign biliary obstruction. HPB Surgery 9: 149–152

Inui H, Kwon A H, Kamiyama Y 1998 Managing bile duct injury during and after laparoscopic cholecystectomy. Journal of Hepato-Biliary-Pancreatic Surgery 5: 445–449

Ishizuka D, Shirai Y, Hatakeyama K 1998 Ischemic biliary stricture due to lymph node dissection in the hepatoduodenal ligament. Hepato-Gastroenterology 45: 2048–2050

Itani K M, Taylor T V 1995 The challenge of therapy for pancreatitis-related common bile duct stricture. American Journal of Surgery 170: 543–546

Jalan R, Harrison D J, Redhead D N, Hayes P C 1996 Transjugular intrahepatic portosystemic stent-shunt (TIPSS) occlusion and the role of biliary venous fistulae. Journal of Hepatology 24: 169–176

Jarnagin W R, Rockey D C, Koteliansky V E, Wang S S, Bissell D M 1994 Expression of variant fibronectins in wound healing: Cellular source and biological activity of the EIIIA segment in rat hepatic fibrogenesis. Journal of Cell Biology 127: 2037–2048

Jeng K S, Ohta, I, Yang F S 1996 Reappraisal of the systematic management of complicated hepatolithiasis with bilateral intrahepatic biliary strictures. Archives of Surgery 131: 141–147

Johnson A G, Lyon I M, Blumgart L H 1979 Stricture of common hepatic duct after right hepatic lobectomy treated by Longmire's operation. Journal of the Royal Society of Medicine 72: 136–139

Johnson A G, Stevens A E 1969 The importance of the size of the stoma in choledochoduodenostomy. Gut 10: 68–70

Kalvania I, Bornman P C, Marks I N, Girdwood A H, Banks L, Kottler R E 1989 The spectrum and natural history of common bile duct stenosis in chronic alcohol-induced pancreatitis. Surgery, Gynecology and Obstetrics 165: 121–126

Kim K H, Sung C K, Park B G, Kim W G, Ryu S K, Kim K S, Paik I S, Oh C H 1998 Clinical significance of intrahepatic biliary stricture in efficacy of hepatic resection for intrahepatic stones. Journal of Hepato-Biliary-Pancreatic Surgery 5: 303–308

Kum C K, Eypasch E, Lefering R, Paul A, Neugenbauer E, Troidl H 1996 Laparoscopic cholecystectomy for acute cholecystitis: is it really safe? World Journal of Surgery 20: 43–49

Kune G A, Sali A 1981 Benign biliary strictures. In: The practice of biliary surgery, 2nd edn. Blackwell, Oxford

Lemmer E R, Spearman C W, Krige J E, Millar A J, Bornman P C, Terblanche J, Kahn D 1997 The management of biliary complications following orthotopic liver transplantation. South African Journal of Surgery 35: 77–81

Liguory C L, Bitole G C, Lefebvre J F, Bonnel D H, Corand F 1991 Endoscopic treatment of postoperative biliary fistulae. Surgery, Gynecology and Obstetrics 110: 779–783

Lillemoe K D 1997 Benign post-operative bile duct strictures. (Review) (48 refs). Baillières Clinical Gastroenterology 11: 749–779

Lillemoe K D, Martin S A, Cameron J L, Yeo C J, Talamini M A, Kaushal S, Coleman J, Venbrux A C, Savader S J, Osterman F A Jr, Pitt H A 1997 Major bile duct injuries during laparoscopic cholecystectomy: follow-up after combined surgical and radiologic management. Annals of Surgery 225: 459–471

Lillemoe K D, Petrofski J A, Choti M A, Venbrux A C, Cameron J L 1999 Isolated right segmental hepatic duct injury: a diagnostic and therapeutic challenge. Journal of Gastrointestinal Surgery in press,

Longmire WP, Sandford MC 1948 Intrahepatic cholangiojejunostomy with partial hepatectomy for biliary obstruction. Surgery 128: 330–347

Longmire W Jr, Sandford M C 1949 Intrahepatic cholangiojejunostomy for biliary obstruction—further studies: report of 4 cases. Annals of Surgery 130: 455–460

Lopez-Santamaria M, Martinez L, Hierro L, Gamez M, Murcia J, Camarena C, De la Vega A, Frauca E, Jara P, Diaz M, Berrocal T, Prieto C, Garzon G, Tovar J A 1999 Late biliary complications in pediatric liver transplantation. Journal of Pediatric Surgery 34: 316–320

Luman W, Hudson N, Choudari C P, Eastwood M A, Palmer K R 1994 Distal biliary stricture as a complication of sclerosant injection for bleeding duodenal ulcer. Gut 35: 1665–1667

MacFadyen J B, Vecchio, R, Ricardo A E, Mathis C R 1998 Bile duct injury after laparoscopic cholecystectomy. The United States experience. (Review) (74 refs). Surgical Endoscopy 12: 315–321

Macfarlane B, Davidson B, Dooley J S, Dawson K, Osborne M J, Rolles K, Burroughs A K 1996 Endoscopic retrograde cholangiography in the diagnosis and endoscopic management of biliary complications after liver transplantation. European Journal of Gastroenterology and Hepatology 8: 1003–1006

Maher J J, McGuire R F 1990 Extracellular matrix gene expression increases preferentially in rat lipocytes and sinusoidal endothelial cells during hepatic fibrosis in vivo. Journal of Clinical Investigation 86: 1641–1648

Maki T, Sato T, Matsushiro T 1972 A reappraisal of surgical treatment for intrahepatic gallstones. Annals of Surgery 175: 155–165

Matthews J B, Baer H U, Schweizer W P, Gertsch P, Carrel T, Blumgart L H 1993 Recurrent cholangitis with and without anastomotic stricture after biliary-enteric bypass. Archives of Surgery 128: 269–272

Matthews J B, Gertsch P, Baer H U, Schweizer W P, Blumgart L H 1991 Biliary stricture following hepatic resection. HPB Surgery 3: 181–90; discussion 190–1

McArthur M S, Longmire W Jr 1971 Peptic ulcer disease after choledochojejunostomy. American Journal of Surgery 122: 155–158

McDonald M L, Farnell M B, Nagorney D M, Ilstrup D M, Kutch J M 1995 Benign biliary strictures: repair and outcome with a contemporary approach. Surgery 118: 582–591

McEntee G, Wiesner RH, Rosen C et al 1991 A comparative study of patients undergoing liver transplantation for primary sclerosing cholangitis and primary biliary cirrhosis. Transplant Proceedings 23: 1563–1564

McMahon A J, Fullarton G, Baxter J N, O'Dwyer P J 1995 Bile duct injury and bile leakage in laparoscopic cholecystectomy. (Review) (95 refs). British Journal of Surgery 82: 307–313

McPherson G A, Benjamin I S, Habib N A, Bowley N B, Blumgart L H 1982 Percutaneous transhepatic drainage in obstructive jaundice: advantages and problems. British Journal of Surgery 69: 261–264

McPherson G A, Fitzpatrick M, Benjamin I S, Blumgart L H 1983 Can HIDA scanning provide a functional assessment of biliary-enteric anastomosis? British Journal of Surgery 70: 306

McPherson S, Gibson R, Collier N et al 1998 Percutanous transjejunal biliary intervention: 10-year experience with access via Roux-en-Y loops. Radiol 206: 665–672

Michalowski K, Bornman P C, Krige J E, Gallagher P J, Terblanche J 1998 Laparoscopic subtotal cholecystectomy in patients with complicated acute cholecystitis or fibrosis. British Journal of Surgery 85: 904–906

Millis J M, Tompkins R K, Zinner M J, Longmire W P J, Roslyn J J 1992 Management of bile duct strictures. An evolving strategy. Archives of Surgery 127: 1077–1082

Mirizzi P L 1948 Sidrome del conducto hepatico (sindrome hepaticiano). Journal of International Surgery 8: 731–734

Molnar W, Stockum A E 1978 Transhepatic dilatation of choledochoenterostomy strictures. Radiology 129: 59–64

Moore A V J, Illescas F F, Mills S R, Wertman D E, Heaston D K, Newman G E, Zuger J H, Salmon R B, Dunnick N R 1987 Percutaneous dilation of benign biliary strictures. Radiology 163: 625–628

Moossa A R, Easter D W, van Sonnenberg E, Casola G, D'Agostino H 1992 Laparoscopic injuries to the bile duct: a cause for concern. Annals of Surgery 215: 203–208

Mueller P R, vanSonnenberg E, Ferrucci J T J, Weyman P J, Butch R J, Malt R A, Burhenne H J 1986 Biliary stricture dilatation: multicenter review of clinical management in 73 patients. Radiology 160: 17–22

Nealon W H, Urrutia F 1996 Long-term follow-up after bilioenteric anastomosis for benign bile duct stricture. Annals of Surgery 223: 639–645

Nelson M T, Nakashima M, Mulvihill S J 1992 How secure are laparoscopically placed clips? An in vitro and in vivo study. Archives of Surgery 127: 718–720

Northover J M A, Terblanche J 1979 A new look at the arterial blood supply of the bile duct in man and its surgical implications. British Journal of Surgery 66: 379–384

Okamura T, Orii, K, Ono A, Ozaki A, Iwasaki Y 1985 Surgical technique for repair of benign strictures of the bile ducts, preserving the papilla of Vater. World Journal of Surgery 9: 619–625

Olsen D 1997 Bile duct injuries during laparoscopic cholecystectomy. Surgical Endoscopy 11: 133–138

Ong G B 1962 A study of recurrent pyogenic cholangitis. Archives of Surgery 84: 199–225

Orons P D, Sheng R, Zajko A B 1995 Hepatic artery stenosis in liver transplant recipients: prevalence and cholangiographic appearance of associated biliary complications. American Journal of Roentgenology 165: 1145–1149

Pappalardo G, Correnti S, Mobarhan S, Frattoroli F, Castrini G 1982 Long term results of hepaticojejunostomy and hepaticoduodenostomy. Annals of Surgery 196: 149–152

Pellegrini C A, Thomas M J, Way L W 1984 Recurrent biliary stricture: patterns of recurrence and outcome of surgical therapy. American Journal of Surgery 147: 175–180

Pereiras R, Schiff E, Barbin J et al 1979 Role of interventional radiology in diseases of the hepatobiliary system and pancreas. Radiological Clinics of North America 17: 555–608

Pitt H A, Kaufman S L, Coleman J, White R I, Cameron J L 1989 Benign postoperative biliary strictures. Operate or dilate? Annals of Surgery 210: 417–425

Pitt H A, Miyamoto T, Parapatis S K, Tompkins R K, Longmire W P Jr 1982 Factors influencing outcome in patients with postoperative biliary strictures. American Journal of Surgery 144: 14–21

Ramond M, Huguet C, Danan G et al 1984 Partial hepatectomy in the treatment of Caroli's disease. Report of a case and review of the literature. Dig Dis Sci 29: 367–370

Richardson M C, Bell G, Fullarton G M 1996 Incidence and nature of bile duct injuries following laparoscopic cholecystectomy: an audit of 5913 cases. West of Scotland Laparoscopic Cholecystectomy Audit Group (see comments). British Journal of Surgery 83: 1356–1360

Reddy K R, Hutson D G, Russell E, et al 1988 Case report: Combined surgical and radiologic approach to recurrent cholangitis and intrahepatic pigment stones. Gastroenterology 95: 1383–1387

Roslyn J J, Binns G S, Hughes E F, Saunders-Kirkwood K, Zinner M J, Cates J A 1993 Open cholecystectomy. A contemporary analysis of 42,474 patients. Annals of Surgery 218: 129–137

Rossi R L, Schirmer W J, Braasch J W, Sanders L, Munson L 1992 Laparoscopic bile duct injuries: risk factors, recognition, repair. Archives of Surgery 127: 596–602

Rossi R L, Tsao J I 1994 Biliary reconstruction. Surgical Clinics of North America 74: 825–841

Russell E, Hutson D, Guerra J et al 1985 Dilatation of biliary strictures through a stomatized jejunal limb. Acta Radiologica Diagnostica 26: 283–286

Russell J C, Walsh S J, Mattie A S, Lynch J T 1996 Bile duct injuries, 1989–1993: a statewide experience—Connecticut laparoscopic cholecystectomy registry. Archives of Surgery 131: 382–388

Sanchez-Urdazpal L, Gores G J, Ward E M, Maus T P, Buckel E G, Steers J L, Wiesner R H, Krom R A 1993 Diagnostic features and clinical outcome of ischemic-type biliary complications after liver transplantation. Hepatology 17: 605–609

Sarles H, Payan N, Tasso F, Sahel J 1976 Chronic pancreatitis, relapsing pancreatitis, calcifications of the pancreas. In: Bochus H L (ed) Gastroenterology. W B Saunders, Philadelphia, p 1040

Sarles H, Sahel J 1978 Cholestasis and lesions of the biliary tract in chronic pancreatitis. Gut 19: 851–857

Sato M, Watanabe Y, Horiuchi S, Nakata Y, Sato N, Kashu Y, Kimura S 1995 Long-term results of hepatic resection for hepatolithiasis. HPB Surgery 9: 37–41

Sato M, Watanabe Y, Ueda S, Ohno J, Kashu Y, Nezu K, Kawachi K 1998 Intrahepatic cholangiocarcinoma associated with hepatolithiasis. Hepato-Gastroenterology 45: 137–144

Sato R, Imamura M, Sasaki I, Kameyama J 1982 Biliary reconstruction and gastric acid secretion. American Journal of Surgery 144: 549–553

Savader S J, Lillemoe K D, Prescott C A, Winick A B, Venbrux A C, Lund G B, Mitchell S E, Cameron J L, Osterman F A Jr 1997 Laparoscopic cholecystectomy-related bile duct injuries: a health and financial disaster. Annals of Surgery 225: 268–273

Saxon R R, Mendel-Hartvig J, Corless C L, Rabkin J, Uchida B T, Nishimine K, Keller F S 1996 Bile duct injury as a major cause of stenosis and occlusion in transjugular intrahepatic portosystemic shunts: comparative histopathologic analysis in humans and swine. Journal of Vascular and Interventional Radiology 7: 487–497

Saxon R S, Ross P L, Mendel-Hartvig J, Barton R E, Benner K, Flora K, Petersen B D, Lakin P C, Keller F S 1998 Transjugular intrahepatic portosystemic shunt patency and the importance of stenosis location in the development of recurrent symptoms. Radiology 207: 683–693

Schaffner F, Bacchin P G, Hutterer F, Scharnbeck H H, Sarkozi L L, Denk, Popper H 1971 Mechanism of cholestasis. 4. Structural and biochemical changes in the liver and serum in rats after bile duct ligation. Gastroenterology 60: 888–897

Schein C J, Glieddman M L 1981 Choledochoduodenostomy as an adjunct to choledocholithotomy. Surgery, Gynecology and Obstetrics 152: 797–804

Schmets L, Delhaye M, Azar C, Deviere J, Cremer M 1996 Postradiotherapy benign biliary stricture: successful treatment by self-expandable metallic stent. Gastrointestinal Endoscopy 43: 149–152

Schol F P, Go P M, Gouma D J 1995 Outcome of 49 repairs of bile duct injuries after laparoscopic cholecystectomy. World Journal of Surgery 19: 753–756

Schwarz W, Rosen R J, Fitts W T J, Mackie J A, Oleaga J A, Freiman D B, McLean G K, Ring E J 1981 Percutaneous transhepatic drainage preoperatively for benign biliary strictures. Surgery, Gynecology and Obstetrics 152: 466–468

Schweizer W P, Matthews J B, Baer H U, Nudelmann L I, Triller J, Halter F, Gertsch P, Blumgart L H 1991 Combined surgical and interventional radiological approach for complex benign biliary tract obstruction. British Journal of Surgery 78: 559–563

Sharma A K, Rangan H K, Choubey R P, Thakur S K, Kumar A 1998 Pitfalls in the management of Mirizzi's syndrome. Tropical Gastroenterology 19: 72–74

Sheen-Chen S M, Cheng Y F, Chen F C, Chou F F, Lee T Y 1998 Ductal dilatation and stenting for residual hepatolithiasis: a promising treatment strategy. Gut 42: 708–710

Sheen-Chen S M, Chou F F 1990 Choledochotomy for biliary lithiasis: is routine T-tube drainage necessary? A prospective controlled trial. Acta Chirurgica Scandinavica 156: 387–390

Smith E E, Bowley N, Allison D J, Blumgart L H 1982 The management of post-traumatic intrahepatic cutaneous biliary fistulas. British Journal of Surgery 69: 317–318

Smith R 1964 Hepaticojejunostomy with transhepatic intubation: a technique for very high strictures of the hepatic ducts. British Journal of Surgery 51: 186–195

Smith R 1969 Strictures of the bile ducts. Proceedings of the Royal Society of Medicine 62: 131–137

Smith R 1979 Obstructions of the bile duct. British Journal of Surgery 66: 69–79

Smits M E, Rauws E A, van Gulik T M, Gouma D J, Tytgat G N, Huibregtse K 1996 Long-term results of endoscopic stenting and surgical drainage for biliary stricture due to chronic pancreatitis. British Journal of Surgery 83: 764–768

Sorensen V J, Buck J R, Chung S K, Fath J J, Horst H M, Obeid F N 1994 Primary common bile duct closure following exploration: an effective alternative to routine biliary drainage. American Surgeon 60: 451–454

Soupault R, Couinaud C 1957 Sur un procede nouveau de derivation biliaire intra-hepatique. La Presse Medicale 65: 1157–1159

Stabile B G, Calabria R, Wilson S E, Passaro E 1987 Stricture of the common bile duct from chronic pancreatitis. Surgery, Gynecology and Obstetrics 165: 121–126

Standfield N J, Salisbury J R, Howard E R 1989 Benign non-traumatic inflammatory strictures of the extrahepatic biliary system. British Journal of Surgery 76: 849–852

Stewart L, Way L W 1995 Bile duct injuries during laparoscopic cholecystectomy: factors that influence the results of treatment. Archives of Surgery 130: 1123–1129

Strasberg S M, Hertl M, Soper N J 1995 An analysis of the problem of biliary injury during laparoscopic cholecystectomy. Journal of the American College of Surgeons 180: 101–125

Taniguchi Y, Ido K, Kimura K, Yoshida Y, Ohtani M, Kawamoto C, Isoda N, Suzuki T, Kumagai M 1993 Introduction of a 'safety zone' for the safety of laparoscopic cholecystectomy. American Journal of Gastroenterology 88: 1258–1261

Teplick S K, Goldstein R C, Richardson P A, Haskin P H, Wilson A R, Corvasce J M, Ring E J, Wolferth C C Jr 1980 Percutaneous transhepatic choledochoplasty and dilatation of choledochoenterostomy strictures. JAMA 244: 1240–1242

The Southern Surgeons Club 1991 A prospective analysis of 1,518 laparoscopic cholecystectomies performed by Southern US surgeons. New England Journal of Medicine 324: 1073–1078

Thompson J E, Pitt H A, Doty J E, Coleman J, Irving C 1990 Broad spectrum penicillin as an adequate therapy for acute cholangitis. Surgery, Gynecology and Obstetrics 171: 275–282

Tocchi A, Costa G, Lepre L, Liotta G, Mazzoni G, Sita A 1996 The long-term outcome of hepaticojejunostomy in the treatment of benign bile duct strictures. Annals of Surgery 224: 162–167

Tomonaga T, Filipi C J, Lowham A, Martinez T 1999 Laparoscopic intracorporeal ultrasound cystic duct length measurement: a new technique to prevent common bile duct injuries. Surgical Endoscopy 13: 183–185

Torkington J, Pereira J, Chalmers R T, Horner J 1998 Laparoscopic cholecystectomy, bile duct injury and the British and Irish surgeon. Annals of the Royal College of Surgeons of England 80: 119–121

Toufanian A, Carey L C, Martin E T Jr 1978 Transhepatic biliary dilatation: an alternative to surgical reconstruction. Current Surgery 35: 70–73

Tu Z, Li J, Xin H, Zhu Q, Cai T 1999 Primary choledochorrhaphy after common bile duct exploration. Digestive Surgery 16: 137–139

vanSonnenberg E, D'Agostino H B, Easter D W, Sanchez R B, Christensen R A, Kerlan R K J, Moossa A R 1993 Complications of laparoscopic cholecystectomy: coordinated radiologic and surgical management in 21 patients. Radiology 188: 399–404

Vogel S B, Howard R J, Caridi J, Hawkins I F Jr 1985 Evaluation of percutaneous transhepatic balloon dilatation of benign biliary strictures in high-risk patients. American Journal of Surgery 149: 73–79

Vougas V, Rela M, Gane E, Muiesan P, Melendez H V, Williams R, Heaton N D 1996 A prospective randomised trial of bile duct reconstruction at liver transplantation: T tube or no T tube? Transplant International 9: 392–395

Voyles C R, Blumgart L H 1982 A technique for the construction of high biliary-enteric anastomoses. Surgery, Gynecology and Obstetrics 154: 885–887

Walsh R M, Henderson J M, Vogt D P, Mayes J T, Grundfest-Broniatowski S, Gagner M, Ponsky J L, Hermann R E 1998 Trends in bile duct injuries from laparoscopic cholecystectomy. Journal of Gastrointestinal Surgery 2: 458–462

Warren K W, Christophi C, Armendari Z R 1982 Surgical Gastroenterology 1: 141–154

Way L W 1992 Bile duct injury during laparoscopic cholecystectomy. Annals of Surgery 215: 195

Way L W, Dunphy J E 1972 Biliary stricture. American Journal of Surgery 124: 287–295

Weinbren K, Hadjis N S, Blumgart L H 1985 Structural aspects of the liver in patients with biliary disease and portal hypertension. Journal of Clinical Pathology 38: 1013–1020

Wetter L A, Ring E J, Pellegrini C A, Way L W 1991 Differential diagnosis of sclerosing cholangiocarcinomas of the common hepatic duct (Klatskin tumors). American Journal of Surgery 161: 57–62; discussion 62–63

Wherry D C, Marohn M R, Malanoski M P, Hetz S P, Rich N M 1996 An external audit of laparoscopic cholecystectomy in the steady state performed in medical treatment facilities of the department of defense. Annals of Surgery 224: 145–154

Williams H J J, Bender C E, May G R 1987 Benign postoperative biliary strictures: dilation with fluoroscopic guidance. Radiology 163: 629–634

Woods M S, Traverso L W, Korzareck R A, Tsao J I, Rossi R L, Gough D, Donohue J H 1994 Characteristics of biliary tract complications during laparoscopic cholecystectomy: a multi-institutional study. American Journal of Surgery 167: 27–34

Yoon K H, Ha H K, Kim M H, Seo D W, Kim C G, Bang S W, Jeong Y K, Kim P N, Lee M G, Auh Y H 1998 Biliary stricture caused by blunt abdominal trauma: clinical and radiologic features in five patients. Radiology 207: 737–741

Yoshida J, Chijiiwa K, Shimizu S, Sato H, Tanaka M 1998 Hepatolithiasis: outcome of cholangioscopic lithotomy and dilation of bile duct stricture. Surgery 123: 421–426

50

External biliary fistula

A. CZERNIAK

INTRODUCTION

A biliary fistula is an abnormal, persistent discharge of bile or bile containing fluid. An 'uncontrolled fistula' denotes fistula formation but with intraperitoneal leakage and collections of bile. 'Controlled fistula' denotes a fistula with drainage to the exterior, through the abdominal wall, but without significant intraperitoneal collection.

Biliary fistulae may be intentionally created by the surgeon, as for example in the creation of a cholecystostomy or a choledochostomy. These fistulae are of significance only when they continue to discharge bile unexpectedly.

Almost all clinically significant biliary fistulae follow some type of surgical procedure on or in the neighborhood of the biliary system. The persistent biliary discharge is the result of some unrecognized pathology in the bile ducts, of an unexpected complication of the surgical procedure or, importantly, of a surgical error. Bile duct injuries and fistulae are of importance because they are preventable, but once they occur they may be associated with considerable morbidity and mortality.

The initial management of these lesions greatly influences the course and outcome and demands a team approach consisting of an experienced interventional radiologist, an endoscopist and a surgeon.

ETIOLOGY AND PREVENTION

When grouping the causes of biliary fistulae it is useful to classify them according to the type of previous intervention performed. The following procedures are the more commonly associated surgical antecedents of fistula.

FISTULA FOLLOWING CHOLECYSTOSTOMY

Cholecystostomy is now infrequently performed. A persistent biliary fistula from the biliary system after cholecystostomy is usually due to distal biliary tract obstruction either as a result of a retained bile duct stone or an unrecognized malignancy. A retained gallstone lodged within Hartmann's pouch (Fig. 50.1) may result in a persistent mucous or biliary fistula.

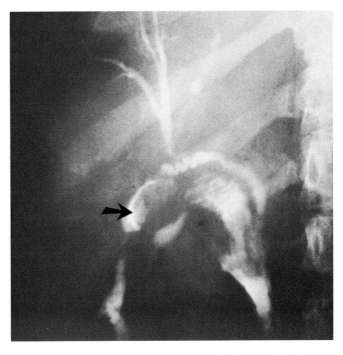

Fig. 50.1 Postcholecystostomy external mucus fistula caused by a large retained gallstone in Hartmann's pouch (arrow) as demonstrated by a fistulography.

FISTULA FOLLOWING LAPAROSCOPIC CHOLECYSTECTOMY (see also Ch. 49)

Laparoscopic cholecystectomy is currently the standard procedure for symptomatic cholelithiasis and for all forms of cholecystitis. Indeed, laparoscopic cholecystectomy is now the standard procedure for acute cholecystitis and is performed even in instances of gangrenous cholecystitis (Kiviluoto et al 1998). However, it is associated with an increased incidence of bile duct injuries including fistula which may rise to 1.3% (Adamsen et al 1997) and to as high as 5.5% (Kum et al 1996). Under these difficult circumstances, the procedure should be performed or at least supervised by an experienced surgeon and a high conversion rate, of up to 40% in instances of gangrenous cholecystitis should be expected (Eldar et al 1998).

The operative treatment of Mirizzi syndrome now includes laparoscopic option (Silecchia et al 1995). However, it is the author's belief that once the presence of Mirizzi syndrome, and particularly type II, is suspected or realized—safety demands that the laparoscopic procedure be converted to an open one (Moser et al 1993).

Small amounts of bile leakage may occur occasionally in the immediate postoperative period after inadvertent damage to a subvesical duct (Viikari 1960), which is present in normal subjects in 20 to 50% of cases (Kune & Sali 1980). Removal of an intrahepatic gallbladder may also be followed by a transient biliary leak caused by damage to tiny bile ducts in the liver around the gallbladder fossa.

Biliary fistula following laparoscopic cholecystectomy may occur either as a result of injury to the extrahepatic biliary tree, or it may originate from the cystic duct stump. A leak from the cystic duct stump may occur from burn injury, pressure necrosis of a metal clip, but in most instances, from distal bile duct obstruction caused by a retained stone resulting in a build up of pressure with a resultant blow out of the cystic stump. It is therefore important to differentiate those patients at risk of having choledocholithiasis. Patients having deranged liver function tests and/or dilated bile ducts on ultrasound should undergo endoscopic cholangiography prior to cholecystectomy. Sphincterotomy and stone extraction should be performed if choledocholithiasis is established.

The majority of ductal injuries are not recognized during the initial laparoscopic cholecystectomy (Lillemoe et al 1997), or indeed in the immediate postoperative period mainly because drains are usually not left in the abdomen and the patient leaves the hospital usually within 24–48 h. The resulting uncontrolled biliary fistula becomes evident within days or sometimes even weeks after the operation, with the clinical presentation of abdominal pain, fever and jaundice and the demonstration of an intra-abdominal fluid collection which produces bile on puncture.

Compared to open cholecystectomy, laparoscopic cholecystectomy is associated with an increased rate of bile duct injuries (Davidoff et al 1992) (Ch. 49). Such injuries are common to most reported series of laparoscopic cholecystectomy, and may reach an incidence as high as 0.9%. Reviews by Strasberg (Strasberg et al 1995) and Vecchio (Vecchio et al 1998) encompassing more than 100 000 patients from multiple hospitals found the incidence of major bile duct injuries to be around 0.5%, and this incidence has reached a 'steady state' (Wherry et al 1996, Walsh et al 1998).

The mechanisms resulting in bile duct injury are now well recognized (Ch. 38). The most common injury is caused by misidentification of the common duct for the cystic duct resulting in complete transection of the common duct, often with some portion of the biliary tree (Fig. 50.2). A traction injury results from inadvertent lateral traction of the gallbladder and 'tenting' of the cystic duct–common duct junction. In this instance the common bile duct may be occluded by the clip intended for the cystic duct, or a portion of the common bile duct may be removed between clips.

An unrecognized anomalous biliary system, in particular a cystic duct emptying directly into the right hepatic duct, or a low-inserted right hepatic sectoral duct may result in similar damage (Chs 1 and 49). (Lillemoe et al 1997, Davidoff et al 1992) (Fig. 50.3). Other less common mechanisms include thermal injury due to excessive use of the cautery or laser, and the application of excessive clips to control bleeding in the triangle of Calot.

The role of operative cholangiography in the prevention of bile duct injuries is controversial (Ch. 22). Intraoperative cholangiography may supply information regarding the presence of unsuspected choledocholithiasis and unexpected anomalous anatomy, and its routine use is recommended by several authors (Stuart et al 1998, Fletcher et al 1999). However, there is no evidence that it may prevent major bile duct injury (Wright & Wellwood 1998). Indeed, the use of operative cholangiography has not increased and in a recent review of forty series of laparoscopic cholecystectomy in the United States, intraoperative cholangiography was performed in only 40% (MacFadyen et al 1998). The author uses operative cholangiography selectively, when ductal anatomic variations or anomalies or bile duct injuries are suspected. Early conversion to laparotomy is favored if the ductal anatomy remains unclear. It should be stressed that operative cholangiography cannot replace meticulous technique and cannot be relied upon to prevent biliary injuries.

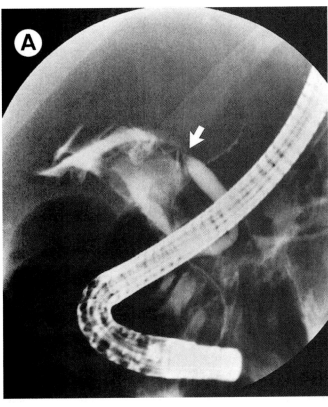

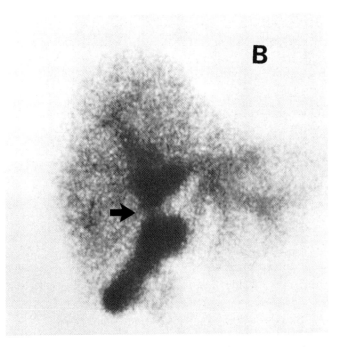

Fig. 50.2 Injury to the bile duct at laparoscopic cholecystectomy. The common bile duct was misidentified for the cystic duct, resulting in a transection of the common bile duct between the clips. **(A)** Endoscopic retrograde cholangiographic study demonstrating a transected bile duct at the level of a clip (arrow) with extravasation of contrast. **(B)** HIDA scan showing a total uncontrolled fistula originating from the proximal cut end of the choledochus.

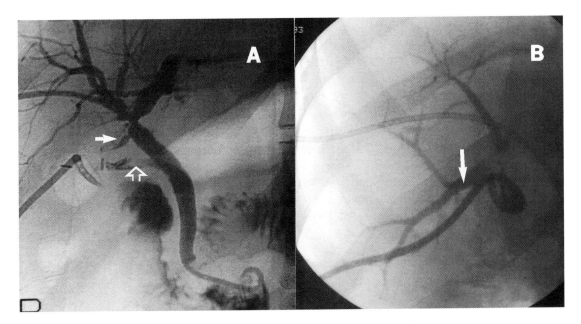

Fig. 50.3 Injury to a right sectoral hepatic duct at laparoscopic cholecystectomy. **(A)** Percutaneous transhepatic cholangiography. Note the remnant of the duct draining into the common bile duct (arrow), cystic stump (framed arrow). Note the low entry of this duct into the common bile duct. **(B)** Tube fistulography. The biliary ductal system of the cut sectoral duct is outlined.

FISTULA FOLLOWING OPEN CHOLECYSTECTOMY (see also Ch. 49)

The occurrence of unexpected biliary fistula after chole-cystectomy almost always indicates operative injury to a major bile duct. Such fistulation may arise from damage to the common bile duct (Fig. 50.4) or to an anomalous sectoral right hepatic duct (Ch. 1). A 0.21% incidence of bile duct injuries has been found in a recent study of 42 474 patients who had undergone an open cholecystec-tomy (Roslyn et al 1993). Bile duct injury is recognized at the time of cholecystectomy in only a minority of patients. In about 25 to 40% of patients with unrecog-nized bile duct injury the injury becomes apparent only when the presence of a controlled or an uncontrolled biliary fistula is recognized (Sandberg et al 1985). In the remaining patients the injury is recognized only later, when a biliary stricture develops (Blumgart et al 1984). The recognition of biliary ductal anomalies and preven-tion of biliary injury at cholecystectomy is detailed in Chapter 49. Inadequately ligated or sloughed ligatures on the cystic duct are responsible for biliary fistula in rare instances, and for this reason transfixion suturing of the cystic stump is recommended. However, the presence of an unrecognized significant distal obstruction may be followed by a blowout of the cystic duct stump, resulting in a biliary fistula or bile peritonitis.

Cholecystectomy is sometimes performed under difficult circumstances, as in the presence of a gangrenous gallblad-der associated with fibrosis and inflammation in the region of the triangle of Calot. In these instances, proper identifi-cation and transfixion of the cystic stump may not be possi-ble and the patient is left with a temporary biliary fistula (Fig. 50.5). The presence of a type II Mirrizi syndrome may pose significant technical difficulties, and specific surgical techniques have been devised to deal with this situation (Baer et al 1990) (Ch. 49). However, in instances where the anatomy is not clear, it is better not to attempt direct repair of the defect in the common bile duct which may result in further damage or stricture formation, but rather to end the procedure with adequate drainage expecting a future con-trolled fistula. *In all these difficult instances where a biliary fistula is anticipated, it is most important to insure controlled and adequate drainage of bile and to exclude the presence of a distal obstruction to biliary-enteric bile flow.* Under these cir-cumstances most fistulae will close spontaneously following conservative treatment.

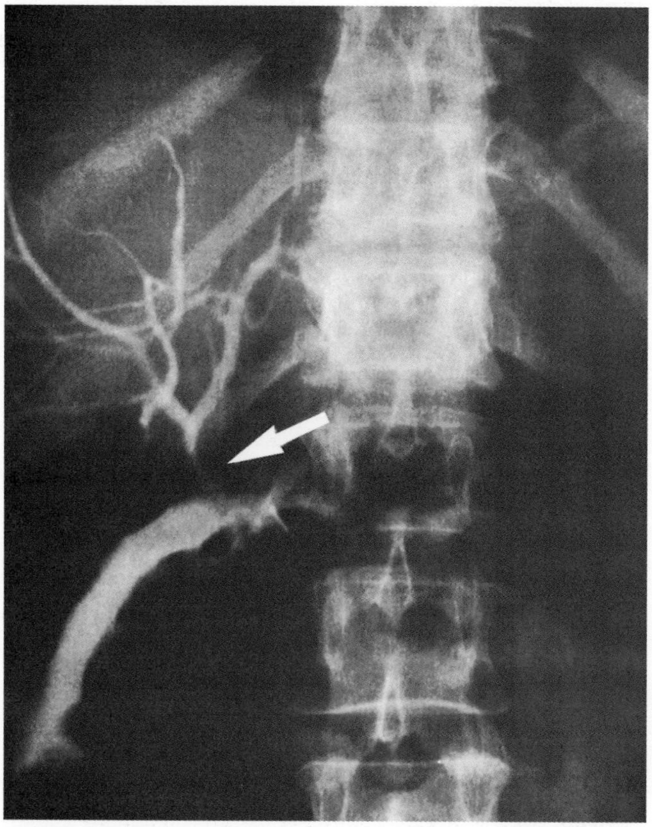

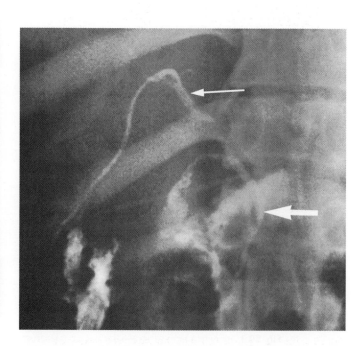

Fig. 50.4 Postcholecystectomy fistulography. Biliary fistula caused by accidental transection of the common hepatic duct (arrow), the commonest cause of a persistent external biliary fistula.

Fig. 50.5 Postcholecystectomy fistulography outlining large irregular cavity (bottom arrow) and connecting with a faintly outlined, but apparently normal, biliary ductal system (top arrow).

FISTULA FOLLOWING COMMON DUCT EXPLORATION

Replaced by laparoscopic and endoscopic techniques, the classic open common duct exploration is now less frequently performed (Csendes et al 1998). However, a biliary fistula whether after open or laparoscopic exploration of the common bile duct, or a biliary fistula persisting after removal of a T-tube is almost always due to a residual bile duct gallstone (Fig. 50.6). It is therefore essential to perform cholangiography and rule out the presence of retained stones before removal of a T-tube or a biliary stent placed at exploration.

Less commonly, an overlooked malignant distal obstruction is the causative factor (Fig. 50.7). The passage of metal bougies through the papilla during common duct explo-

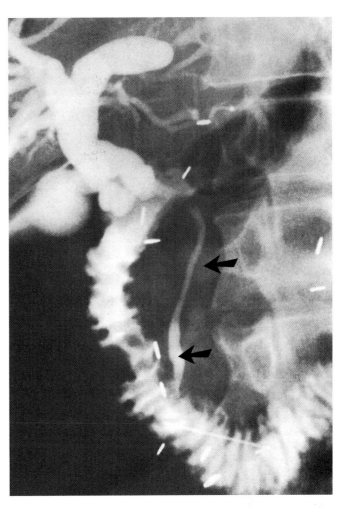

Fig. 50.7 Postcholecystectomy fistulography showing the external biliary fistula was caused by an extrinsic compression of the pancreatic portion of the bile duct (arrows). At reoperation, choledochal compression was shown to be due to cancer of the head of the pancreas.

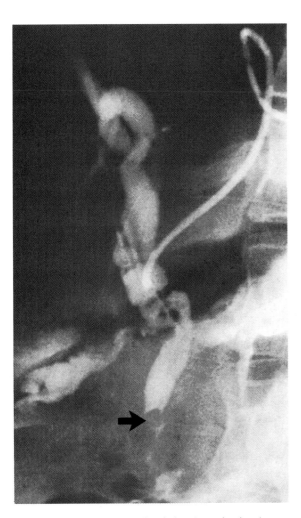

Fig. 50.6 Postcholecystectomy T-tube cholangiography showing a retained stone obstructing the distal bile duct (arrow). The stone was removed 6 weeks after surgery by the instrumental basket extraction through the T-tube track, preventing a persistent external biliary fistula.

ration may result in the creation of a false tract, particularly when there is a papillary stenosis. This may result in a choledochoduodenal fistula. This situation may cause jaundice, ascending cholangitis, and acute or chronic recurrent pancreatitis. Treatment consists essentially of a papillotomy or sphincterotomy, thereby joining the fistulous orifice with the papillary opening. This treatment may now be attempted endoscopically (Jorge et al 1991).

FISTULA FOLLOWING BILIARY-INTESTINAL ANASTOMOSIS

A major biliary fistula following biliary-intestinal anastomosis, though relatively uncommon, does occur. Anastomoses created well below the hilus, as for example choledochoduodenostomy or choledochojejunostomy, are very rarely associated with fistulae (Parilla et al 1991), while biliary fistula following hilar hepaticojejunostomy is more common. When fistulae do occur, a technical error such as suture line disruption or failure to incorporate a significant bile duct within the anastomosis, must be suspected. Failure of the surgeon to appreciate ductal anatomy is particularly likely to occur in the hilar region, where the mode of confluence of the right and left ducts and caudate lobe ducts is extremely variable (Ch. 1). In these instances the fistula becomes evident immediately after surgery. Meticulous technique with mucosa-to-mucosa anastomosis (Ch. 30) obviates most such leakage.

Alternatively, suture line disruption may also be caused by local factors such as abscess or ischemic necrosis of the bile duct or bowel wall. Such fistulae may become evident some days after surgery. It is important to ascertain whether the fistula is purely biliary or whether it also contains duodenal and/or pancreatic juice.

BILIARY FISTULA AFTER LIVER INJURY AND LIVER SURGERY

Liver injury

Liver injury may be followed by the formation of a biliary fistula. Such fistulation may occur in association with damage to the liver (Fig. 50.8) as well as the bile ducts, or it may follow sequestration and infection of areas of liver necrosis. Blunt or penetrating Grade III or IV liver trauma may be complicated by bilomas and biliary fistula in around 5% of instances (Shahrudin & Noori 1998, Glaser et al 1994). Emergency partial hepatectomy for major liver trauma may result in an injury to the bile ducts at the confluence with an early biliary leak and, later, a biliary stricture (Bismuth et al 1986). Complete transection of the common bile duct requires immediate hepaticojejunostomy, while lacerations of the main biliary channel may be sutured after placement of a T-tube.

A persistent biliary fistula may occur from a segment of the liver isolated by the injury. Management of this situation is difficult, particularly when the fistula is associated with a distal stricture. Rarely, the fistula can be identified at operation and oversewn. Alternatively, a well-developed fibrous fistulous tract may be anastomosed to a jejunal loop or to the gallbladder (Fig. 50.8) (Smith et al 1982).

Biliovenous fistula with subsequent leakage of bile into the venous system is a rare but serious complication of liver trauma. Following the formation of a necrotic cavity within the liver, an open connection between a vein and an intrahepatic bile duct may follow allowing bile to leak into the venous circulation (Haberlik et al 1992) (Ch. 70).

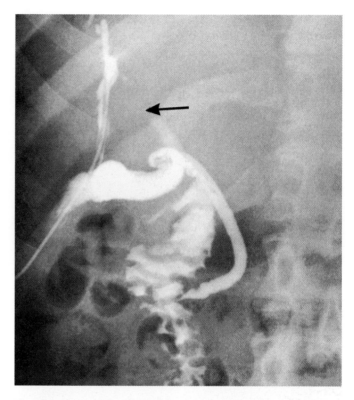

Fig. 50.8 External biliary fistula following blunt injury to the right lobe of the liver and subsequent drainage of a large right intrahepatic hematoma. The injury was associated with damage to the right hepatic duct and a subsequent intrahepatic stricture (arrow). Following external drainage a high-output biliary fistula developed. The tubogram illustrated was obtained after anastomosis of the fistulous track issuing from the liver to the adjacent mobilized gallbladder. Note that the cavity within the liver has collapsed and that the gallbladder fills and subsequently outlines the common bile duct. The tube was removed and postoperative recovery was uneventful. The patient remains symptom free and with normal liver function tests 5 years after surgery (Smith et al 1982).

Liver resection

Liver resection carried out for tumor (Ch. 83) may be followed by biliary fistula which may result from inadequate ligation of the bile ducts at the cut liver surface (Thompson et al 1983), or failure to secure the bile ducts at the hilus. This is more likely following right hepatectomy where the anatomy of the right sectoral hepatic ducts is variable in the hilar region. Extended left hepatic lobectomy has also been associated with a high incidence of biliary fistula (Starzl et al 1982) (Ch. 83).

Operative injury to the biliary tract likely to result in fistulation is more common following resection of lesions involving or close to the hilar structures (Fig. 50.9). It is also more likely to occur after resection of lesions involving the caudate lobe ducts—since the anatomy of these ducts is significantly variable in the hilar region. Resection of hilar cholangiocarcinoma, utilizing major hepatic resections, combined with biliary-enteric reconstruction may be complicated by a biliary fistula originating usually either from caudate lobe ducts or from the biliary-enteric anastomosis (Ch. 83).

Hepatic cryotherapy (Ch. 80) which may be used either at the cut liver surface following hepatectomy or for ablation of deep intrahepatic lesions may be complicated by biliary fistula (Sarantou et al 1998). It may be prudent to leave a drain in-situ following this procedure.

HYDATID DISEASE OF THE LIVER

Hydatid disease of the liver (Ch. 63) is associated with biliary involvement by the disease in around 10% of instances (Erguney et al 1991). A live expanding cyst results in compression and stretching of adjacent liver tissue, including the bile ducts. It may then erode into a stretched bile duct with the establishment of continuity between the cyst cavity and the biliary system. Hydatid material may enter into the biliary tree or, conversely, bile may leak into the cyst.

Biliary fistula develops after operation for hydatid disease in three situations. Firstly, a communication between the cyst cavity and the biliary system is missed at operation and is not directly secured (Fig. 50.10). It is therefore prudent to drain all cyst cavities, particularly multiloculated hydatid cysts, in order to ensure that if a biliary fistula develops, it will be controlled. Indeed, unless a distal obstruction is present, these fistulae usually close spontaneously. Secondly, and rarely, the presence of hydatid material within the biliary tract produces biliary ductal obstruction (Fig. 50.11), resulting in a persistent biliary fistula which is only relieved once the hydatid material passes or is removed. This is achieved either by exploration of the common bile duct with or without a bypass procedure (Ozmen et al 1992) or by endoscopic methods (Iscan & Duren 1991). Assessment of the biliary tree, preferably by

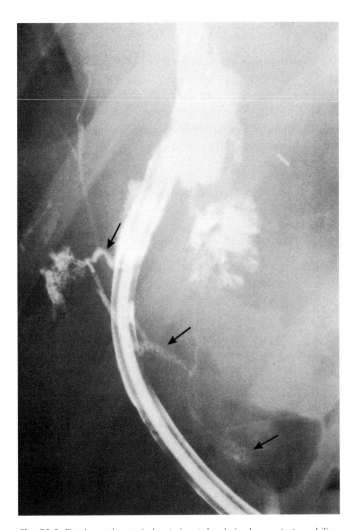

Fig. 50.9 Fistulography carried out via a tube drain demonstrates a biliary fistula following extended left hepatic lobectomy for primary hepatocellular cancer. The tumor was large and involved the hilar ducts in that tumor extension was demonstrated within the left hepatic duct. The fistula was managed conservatively and closed within 4 weeks. Arrows indicate the fistula and the course of the right hepatic duct and common bile duct.

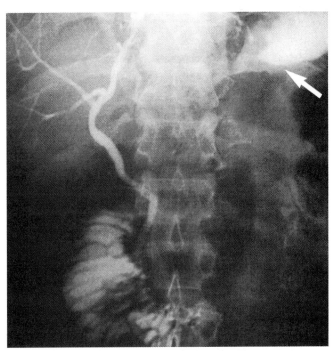

Fig. 50.10 Persistent external biliary fistula following external drainage of a hydatid cyst cavity (arrow) in the left lobe of the liver. The fistulography shows clear communication between the cyst cavity and the left hepatic duct.

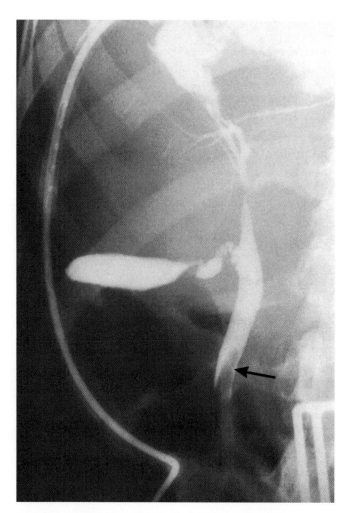

Fig. 50.11 Fistulography obtained after excision of a right hepatic hydatid cyst. Note the persistent fistula consequent upon retained hydatid material in the common bile duct (arrow). Treatment was by exploration of the common bile duct and surgical removal of the retained hydatid material. The fistula rapidly closed.

endoscopic cholangiography, should therefore be performed prior to surgery in patients with a history of jaundice or cholangitis or in the presence of a large cyst located centrally and abutting the hilar structures. Once a cystobiliary communication is demonstrated, the biliary system should be cleared of all debris and cyst remnants, and endoscopic sphincterotomy performed prior to surgical intervention (Kornaros & Aboul-Nour 1996).

Percutaneous treatment of hydatid cysts (Men et al 1999) is associated with a 10% incidence of biliary fistula. Such fistulae usually close spontaneously once biliary distal obstruction, when present, is relieved.

Finally, although liver resection is not the preferred method of treatment for liver hydatid disease, it is occasionally performed and such patients are prone to all the complications of liver resection carried out for other reasons.

FISTULA AFTER LIVER TRANSPLANTATION

Biliary leak and fistula are a continuing source of morbidity and mortality following liver transplantation. Pathogenesis is usually related to technical and vascular considerations and, in particular, to hepatic artery thrombosis (Ch. 115).

BILIARY FISTULA AFTER GASTRECTOMY

Injury to the bile duct may occur during gastrectomy, and is more common in polyagastrectomy, particularly when the pyloric region or the first part of the duodenum is grossly distorted and inflamed (Florence et al 1981). Such an injury becomes apparent either as a biliary fistula or at a later stage with the development of a stricture (Ch. 49).

BILIARY FISTULA AFTER INVASIVE RADIOLOGICAL PROCEDURES

Biliary leak and fistulae may follow most invasive radiological procedures on the hepatobiliary system.

The creation of transjugular intrahepatic portosystemic stent-shunt may be complicated by biliary-venous fistulae, when a large-caliber intrahepatic bile duct is transected. The resulting biliary leak plays an important role in the stenosis and occlusion of the portosystemic shunt (Jalan et al 1996).

CLINICAL PRESENTATION

The clinical presentation of a biliary fistula may be of an excessive, abnormal biliary drainage from the drain site or wound or, alternatively, of a localized or generalized peritonitis resulting from an intra-abdominal collection of bile. Once a diagnosis of a biliary fistula has been established, it is most important to assess clinically the adequacy of bile drainage.

In *controlled* fistulae there is adequate external biliary drainage, with no signs of localized or generalized peritonitis, and the adverse pathophysiological features associated with cholestasis are not present.

In an *uncontrolled* biliary fistula there is inadequate biliary drainage resulting in an intra-abdominal bilious collection. Since the bile is usually or soon becomes infected, the presentation is mostly of either a subphrenic or subhepatic abscess or generalized peritonitis. The situation may further be complicated by cholangitis with or without intrahepatic abscess and septicemia demanding urgent treatment. It must be stressed that in some patients with sterile bile, huge volumes may accumulate within the peritoneal cavity with minimal clinical findings apart from a distended abdomen (Fig. 50.12).

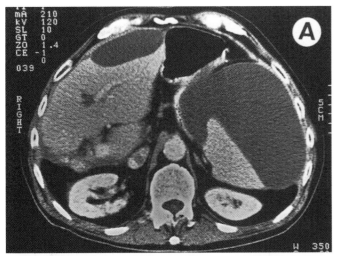

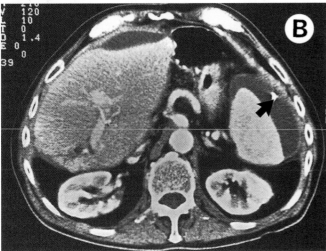

Fig. 50.12 (A) Huge asymptomatic biloma 3 weeks after partial hepatectomy for hepatocellular cancer. The patient complained of abdominal distension only. **(B)** Computerized-tomography-guided puncture and drainage (arrow) converted the uncontrolled fistula into a controlled one. The fistula closed spontaneously after 17 days.

It is therefore important to observe patients having had laparoscopic cholecystectomy at 24 h after the operation at which time the liver function tests are checked. A high index of suspicion is important since minimal abdominal symptoms and slightly deranged liver function tests may be the only indicators of biliary damage. The presence of skin excoriation and digestion implies that activated digestive enzymes are present in the fistula effluent, since bile alone contains no digestive enzymes.

PATHOLOGICAL CONSEQUENCES OF EXTERNAL BILIARY FISTULA

The important pathophysiological effects of an external biliary fistula depend on the volume of bile drained daily, the length of time the fistula has been present and the degree to which bile is diverted from the gastrointestinal tract. Consequences of biliary fistula are mainly due to depletion of electrolytes and fluid, to the absence of bile from the gut and to the possibility of ascending exogenously acquired biliary infection. The important practical considerations are that the volume of bile secreted daily by the liver is of the order of 1000 ml and that the electrolyte composition of bile is equal to that of blood.

Total biliary loss for short periods of up to 3 weeks may not result in a serious depletion of electrolytes and fluid since the body is able to compensate for this loss. Long-term total external biliary fistula results in fluid and electrolyte disturbances if replacement therapy is not instituted. Sodium loss is usually in excess of chloride loss, leading to metabolic acidosis (Cass et al 1955). The serum potassium level is initially lowered, but the accompanying fluid loss may lead to a decrease in plasma volume, low-output renal failure and hyperkalaemia (Knochel et al 1962). Absence of bile from the gastrointestinal tract causes interference in the absorption of fat-soluble vitamins A, D and K. Vitamin A and D deficiency is associated with long-term total biliary fistula and is rarely seen today, while vitamin K deficiency is evident earlier. Clinically, patients with an external biliary fistula even in the short term, feel unwell, weak and lethargic. In advanced and neglected cases, caloric and protein malnutrition results in gradual weight loss while the electrolyte changes may result in stupor and vasomotor collapse.

DIAGNOSTIC PROCEDURES AND INITIAL TREATMENT

The presence of a biliary fistula may first become apparent at reoperation. More commonly and particularly after laparoscopic cholecystectomy the biliary fistula becomes apparent at endoscopic cholangiography or, following percutaneous drainage of a perihepatic collection.

Reoperation is usually done either for peritonitis or for drainage of an intra-abdominal collection (Fig. 50.6). Such collections may be a complication from previous surgery on the hepatobiliary system, the pancreas or, rarely, the stomach or duodenum. They may rarely follow a spontaneously occurring pathological process such as hemorrhagic pancreatitis or rupture of a liver cyst. Once the presence of an uncontrolled biliary fistula has been realized, initial management demands conversion of the fistula into a controlled one, usually by means of tube drainage. No attempt at definitive repair should be made at this early stage, since the involved bile duct(s) are collapsed, friable and are usually embedded within a severe local inflammatory reaction. Moreover, it is virtually impossible to expose healthy bile ducts for any form of long-lasting definitive repair, and such an attempt, which is bound to fail, will render further operation more difficult (Czerniak et al 1988).

The early demonstration, within 24–48 h of laparoscopic cholecystectomy, of an uncontrolled biliary fistula together with a transected or completely occluded common bile duct bile is an indication for early surgical intervention. Decision regarding definitive repair is based on operative findings. Rarely, removal of a misplaced clip intended for the cystic stump and causing complete obstruction of the common bile duct is all that is necessary.

Alternatively, percutaneous computerized tomography (CT) or ultrasound-guided drainage of a subphrenic or infrahepatic fluid collection may be followed by the establishment of an external biliary fistula. It is then most important to ensure adequate drainage and that the fistula is indeed controlled. Biliary drainage is ideally carried out using a sealed drainage bag system (Blenkarn et al 1981). Drainage should, at least initially, be under a low pressure, closed suction system which is valuable in reducing the cavity of the intra-abdominal bile collection or abscess to a fistula track. Improvement of the clinical picture together with repeat ultrasound or CT studies should eventually demonstrate proper positioning of the drain and no residual collection or abscess. HIDA scintigraphy (Ch. 14) and tubography are helpful in this respect (Fig. 50.7).

Once the fistula is controlled, conservative treatment is instituted, the patient is nourished, deficits of electrolytes and vitamins (mostly vitamin K) are corrected and infection is treated. It is important to know whether the biliary fistula contains bile only or whether it also contains duodenal, pancreatic or intestinal juice. When the latter is present, appropriate measures to protect the skin should be taken. Parenteral nutrition is an essential element in the management of duodenal and pancreatic fistulae, where total prohibition of oral intake is important in allowing healing to occur. It has been shown that treatment with somatostatin can significantly reduce bile secretion (Nyberg 1990). Somatostatin has also been used successfully in the management of pancreatic and small intestinal fistulae (Rosenberg & Brown 1991) and may be of value in the management of combined biliary-pancreatic-duodenal fistulae.

Following the establishment of a controlled fistula, various radiological investigations are then performed with the aim of assessing:

- The origin of the fistula
- The presence and extent of an injury to the extrahepatic biliary system

- Adequacy of drainage
- The presence of biliary-enteric bile flow.

The anatomy of the *entire* intrahepatic and extrahepatic biliary tree should be demonstrated, and this is achieved by a variety of radiological studies. All contrast examinations should be covered with antibiotic prophylaxis to minimize the risk of a bacteremic episode.

Tube cholangiography should be performed routinely prior to removal of a cholecystostomy or choledochostomy tubes or tubal drainage across biliary-enteric anastomoses. Whenever an obstruction to free biliary-enteric bile flow is present, it should be treated. Removal of such a tube in the presence of a distal stricture or a retained bile duct stone will invariably result in a persistent biliary fistula.

Fistulography is a simple and effective means of finding out whether biliary drainage is adequate and whether a fistulous cavity, has indeed converted to a fistulous track. The site and underlying cause of the biliary fistula can also be clearly demonstrated by fistulography (Figs 50.1 to 50.3, 50.8, 50.9, 50.11 and 50.13).

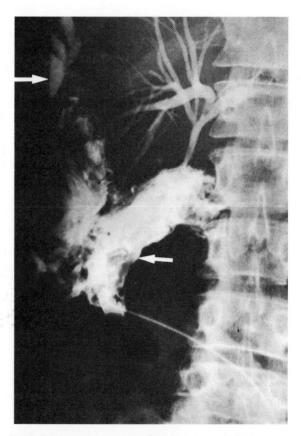

Fig. 50.13 Fistulography in a case of neglected postcholecystectomy biliary fistula due to accidental transection of the common hepatic duct with associated subphrenic (top arrow) and subhepatic (bottom arrow) collections of infected bile.

Percutaneous transhepatic cholangiography (PTC) is used when the findings of fistulography are equivocal and when the intrahepatic biliary tract, in particular the right system, is not fully demonstrated. Iatrogenic damage to a right sectoral hepatic duct is an example of this problem and PTC is the only diagnostic modality to yield accurate definition.

Endoscopic retrograde cholangiography (ERC) is a most useful diagnostic and therapeutic tool in instances where there is a continuity of the extrahepatic biliary system (Davids et al 1992), particularly following laparoscopic cholecystectomy (Kozarek et al 1994) and in liver transplanted patients (Sherman et al 1993). The value of ERC is limited in fistulation arising at the hilus and resulting from iatrogenic bile duct injury.

HIDA scintigraphy (Ch. 14) is a useful non-invasive method of evaluating liver function and bile secretion (Holbrook et al 1991) (Ch. 16). Though it may not supply accurate anatomical details, information regarding the presence of a fistula, its origin (liver or extrahepatic biliary system) (Fig. 50.14), adequacy of drainage (controlled or uncontrolled) (Fig. 50.15), and mode of biliary-enteric bile flow (McPherson et al 1984) can all be clearly obtained.

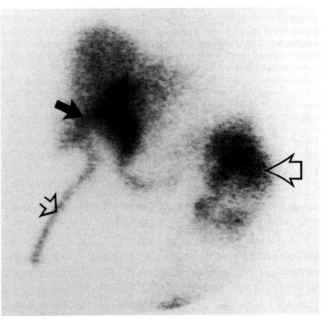

Fig. 50.15 HIDA scan (right lateral view) demonstrating a controlled biliary fistula (incomplete open arrow) resulting from an incomplete closure of a wide cystic stump (filled arrow) at laparoscopic cholecystectomy. A free biliary-enteric bile flow is demonstrated (open arrow). The fistula closed spontaneously after 2 weeks.

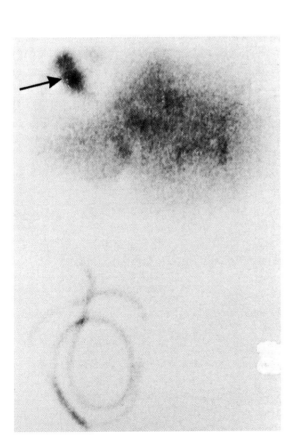

Fig. 50.14 HIDA scan demonstrating a fistula issuing from the liver surface (arrow). Same case as Fig. 50.11. Note that the drainage tube is also demonstrated (McPherson et al 1984). (Reproduced with permission of Surgical Gastroenterology).

TREATMENT

The principles of management of a postoperative biliary fistula are essentially the same regardless of the initial surgical procedure, and are outlined in Figure 50.16. These principles are modified slightly according to the initial surgical procedure and to the individual patient. Endoscopic cholangiography and endoscopic techniques now play an integral and indispensable part in the management of biliary fistula. The individual treatment plan should therefore be made and agreed upon jointly by all members of the team involved in the treatment of the patient.

As stated above, it is most important to establish a controlled fistula. This can be achieved initially by ultrasonography or CT-guided drainage of the abscess or collection. Operation is indicated when non-operative measures are not suitable such as in diffuse bile peritonitis, a septic patient with an intra-abdominal abscess too large to be drained by the percutaneous route, or the presence of necrotic material and debris within the abscess. Early surgery is also indicated when percutaneous drainage has failed. It must be stressed again that, during the operation, one should not be tempted to attempt primary repair at this stage, but rather to establish good drainage only. Occasionally, drainage of large amounts of bile with significant fluid and electrolyte

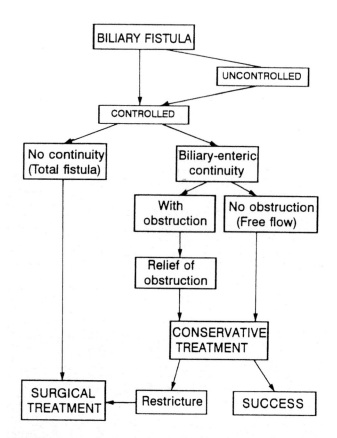

Fig. 50.16 Proposed management plan for postoperative biliary fistula. The initial treatment is most important and includes the establishment of a 'controlled' fistula. This is achieved either radiologically (percutaneous drainage of a collection) or surgically, at which time no attempt at primary repair is made. The fistula is then evaluated for biliary-enteric continuity. Once a total fistula has been diagnosed it is most important to insure that it is controlled. Definitive surgical repair is attempted following a reasonable period of conservative treatment. When biliary-enteric continuity is present, and there is free biliary-enteric bile flow, conservative treatment is instituted and will result in spontaneous closure in most cases. The presence of a biliary-enteric continuity with a distal obstruction calls for some form of treatment to relieve the obstruction and this is done either endoscopically or, preferably, percutaneously by balloon dilatation. Following the establishment of free biliary-enteric bile flow, patients are treated conservatively. In suitable cases, nasobiliary intubation is followed up carefully after fistula closure for early signs of stricture. High complex hilar fistulae are treated conservatively with prolonged periods of drainage. The fistula is expected to close and this usually occurs together with the development of stricture. Once a stricture has developed it is treated surgically.

loss may necessitate early operation when the external fistula may be converted to an internal fistulojejunostomy using a mobilized and approximated Roux-en-Y jejunal loop (Smith et al 1982) (Fig. 50.8). In this procedure the drainage tube is led from the fistula origin through the jejunal loop to the exterior allowing initial control, but an almost certain necessity of reoperation for restenosis at a later stage.

It is most important to identify the presence or absence of a biliary-enteric bile flow. This differentiates a total biliary fistula, from a partial fistula with some residual biliary-enteric continuity. This significantly influences subsequent management, since in the first case, operation is usually unavoidable, whereas in the latter case non-operative approach may be successful. Occasionally, and rarely, a total biliary fistula closes spontaneously when an internal fistula develops between the divided upper duct and the gut (Collins & Gorey 1984).

When biliary-enteric continuity is present and there is *no obstruction to bile flow* distal to the origin of the fistula, a prolonged period of conservative treatment is indicated as spontaneous closure of the fistula is usual. The mainstay of this conservative treatment is the adequate and timely application of endoscopic techniques. Fistula closure may be facilitated by *temporary* placement of a stent across the fistulous opening in the bile duct thus excluding bile flow through the fistula. This method may be attempted in instances where there is an intact common bile duct above the fistula origin and the defect in the bile duct is not too large. It may be particularly helpful in instances of cystic stump fistula and may facilitate early closure. Stenting may be achieved by endoscopic placement of an endoprosthesis or a nasobiliary tube with its tip above the origin of the fistula. When a short period of stenting is anticipated, nasobiliary intubation is preferred since it enables follow-up cholangiography, damage to the papilla is minimal and a second endoscopic procedure is avoided. Using this method, some fistulae will close within 2 weeks (Toriumi et al 1989). This method is most useful in patients with a liver transplant who have undergone duct-to-duct biliary reconstruction. However, the nasobiliary tube may be uncomfortable for the patient. It may dislodge and it may enhance metabolic acidosis resulting from bile loss if used for prolonged periods of time.

In most instances a biliary endoprosthesis is used and is left in place usually for several weeks until fistula closure. Closure is verified by HIDA scan prior to removal of the stent.

Some recommend endoscopic sphincterotomy alone with the intention of reducing the pressure gradient between the biliary system and the duodenum (Ponchon et al 1989). This is unnecessary, since the fistula will close in any event if no distal obstruction is present. Sphincterotomy may also be associated with short- and long-term septic and obstructive complications (Kracht et al 1986) and should therefore be avoided unless specifically indicated, as for example in patients with a papillary stricture. It has also been shown that stenting is more effective than sphincterotomy alone in the resolution of biliary fistulae (Marks et al 1998).

Once an *obstruction distal to the fistula* has been diagnosed it should be dealt with since the fistula will not close spontaneously. Obstruction is usually caused by a retained stone or a stricture. Retained stones are usually removed by endoscopic means. Relief of a benign stricture can be achieved using balloon dilatation applied either endoscopi-

cally or by interventional radiology following PTC. The patient is then treated conservatively and expectantly—either for fistula closure or for restricture which, once it occurs, is then treated operatively. Thus, fistula closure can be facilitated by *temporary stenting* (Fig. 50.17), if the location and the size of the defect in the bile duct are suitable.

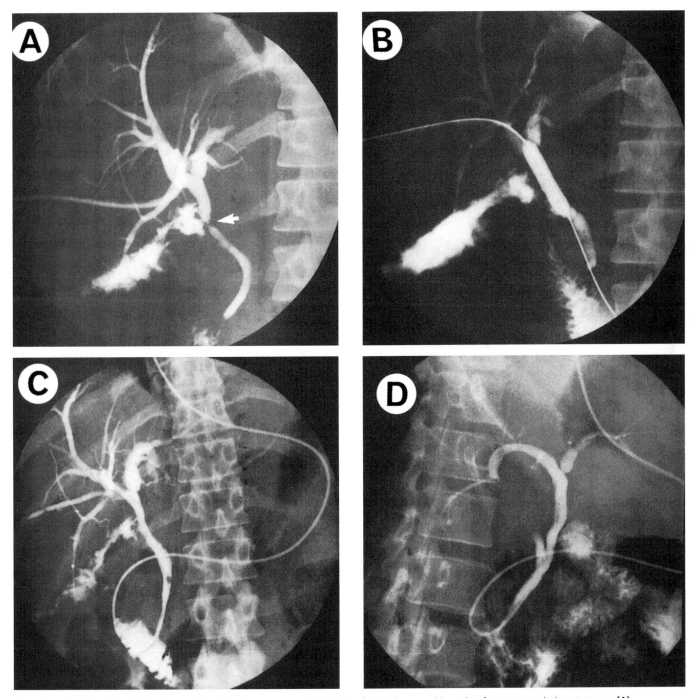

Fig. 50.17 Combined surgical/endoscopic/ radiologic management of a biliary fistula diagnosed 3 weeks after an open cholecystectomy. **(A)** Percutaneous transhepatic cholangiographic study demonstrating a biliary fistula with a significant distal stricture (arrow). **(B)** Percutaneous transhepatic balloon dilatation of the stricture. **(C)** A percutaneous transhepatic guide is exchanged for a nasobiliary tube which is placed endoscopically with its tip above the origin of the fistula. Free biliary-enteric bile flow is obtained. The fistula is still present but is smaller. **(D)** Check-up cholangiography (lateral view) after 2 weeks of nasobiliary drainage, demonstrating fistula closure. The nasobiliary drain was therefore removed.

The use of temporary stenting is limited in high complex hilar fistulae combined with stricture(s), particularly those with separation of a right and left ductal system. Some authors place an endoprosthesis across the stricture and leave it for months (Ponchon et al 1989) and even for more than a year with periodic replacements (Davids et al 1992). This is not only unnecessary but it may be harmful, resulting in obstruction and septic complications. The endoprosthesis, if placed, should be removed when the fistula has closed.

Management of biliary fistula following laparoscopic cholecystectomy follows the same principles. Since early recognition of biliary fistula or bile duct damage significantly affects treatment, a high index of suspicion is important. Initial evaluation includes abdominal ultrasound and HIDA scan to rule out the presence of an abnormal collection and establish the presence of free biliary-enteric bile flow. Abnormal findings at either study calls for an endoscopic cholangiography. Treatment of biliary fistula with or without biliary enteric continuity follows the guidelines outlined.

A biliary fistula associated with malignant distal obstruction, is treated with reoperation and surgical excision of the neoplasm or the creation of an appropriate biliary-enteric bypass (Chs 30 and 55).

Following closure of the fistula, patients are followed up carefully with regular liver function tests and HIDA scan, in order to detect early signs of the development of a biliary stricture. This may take months and sometimes years, and is likely to occur particularly in instances where a stricture has already been present or when the fistula was associated with an injury to a major bile duct (Blumgart et al 1984).

The proposed plan may involve relatively prolonged management, but improves the chances of a successful and long-lasting bile duct repair particularly in instances following injury at cholecystectomy. In this situation, early and untimely surgical attempts at definitive repair carry a high risk of biliary leak and anastomotic stricture.

REFERENCES

Adamsen S, Hansen O H, Funch-Jensen P et al 1997 Bile duct injury during laparoscopic cholecystectomy: a prospective nationwide series. Journal of the American College of Surgeons 184: 571–578

Baer H U, Matthews J B, Schweizer W P, Gertsch P, Blumgart L H 1990 Management of the Mirizzi syndrome and the surgical implications of cholecystocholedochal fistula. British Journal of Surgery 77: 743–745

Bismuth H, Smadja C, Houssine D 1986 Liver injuries: the late cases. Clinical Surgery International 12: 139–145

Blenkarn J J, McPherson G A D, Blumgart L H 1981 An improved system for external biliary drainage. Lancet ii: 781–782

Blumgart L H, Kelley C J, Benjamin I S 1984 Benign bile duct strictures following cholecystectomy: critical factors in management. British Journal of Surgery 71: 836–843

Branum G, Schmitt C, Baillie J et al 1993 Management of major biliary complications after laparoscopic cholecystectomy. Annals of Surgery 217: 532–541

Cass M H, Robson R, Rundle F F 1955 Electrolyte losses in biliary fistula: postcholecystectomy acidotic syndrome. Medical Journal of Austria 1: 165–168

Cates J A, Tompkins R K, Zinner M J, Busuttil R W, Kallman C, Roslyn J J 1993 Biliary complications of laparoscopic cholecystectomy. The American Surgeon 59: 243–247

Collins P G, Gorey T F 1984 Iatrogenic biliary stricture: presentation and management. British Journal of Surgery 71: 900–902

Csendes A, Burdiles P, Diaz J C 1998 Present role of classic open choledochostomy in the surgical treatment of patients with common bile duct stones. World Journal of Surgery 22: 1167–1170

Czerniak A, Thompson J N, Soreide O, Benjamin I S, Blumgart L H 1988 The management of fistulas of the biliary tract after injury to the bile duct during cholecystectomy. Surgery, Gynecology and Obstetrics 167: 33–37

Davidoff A M, Pappas T N, Murray E A et al 1992 Mechanisms of major biliary injury during laparoscopic cholecystectomy. Annals of Surgery 215: 196–202

Davids P H P, Rauws E A J, Tytgat G N J, Huibregtse K 1992 Postoperative bile leakage: endoscopic management. Gut 33: 1118–1122

Eldar S, Sabo E, Nash E et al 1998 Laparoscopic cholecystectomy for the various types of gallbladder inflammation: a prospective trial. Surgical Laparoscopy and Endoscopy 8: 200–207

Erguney S, Tortum O, Taspinar A H, Ertem M, Gazioglu E 1991 Complicated hydatid cysts of the liver. Annals de Chirurgie 45: 584–589 (in French)

Fletcher D R, Hobbs M S, Valinsky T P et al 1999 Complications of cholecystectomy: risks of laparoscopic approach and protective effects of operative cholangiography: a population-based study. Annals of Surgery 229: 449–457

Florence M G, Hart M J, White T T 1981 Ampullary disconnection during the course of biliary and duodenal surgery. American Journal of Surgery 142: 100–105

Glaser K, Wetscher G, Pointner R 1994 Traumatic bilhemia. Surgery 116: 24–27

Haberlik A, Cendron M, Sauer H 1992 Biliovenous fistula in children after blunt liver trauma: proposal for a simple surgical treatment. Journal of Pediatric Surgery 27: 1203–1206

Holbrook R F, Jacobson F L, Pezzuti R T, Howel D A 1991 Biliary patency imaging after endoscopic retrograde sphincterotomy with gallbladder in situ. Archives of Surgery 126: 739–741

Iscan M, Duren M 1991 Endoscopic sphincterotomy in the management of postoperative complications of hepatic hydatid disease. Endoscopy 23: 282–283

Jorge A, Diaz M, Lorenzo J, Jorge O 1991 Choledochoduodenal fistulae. Endoscopy 23: 76–78

Jalan R, Harrison D J, Redhead D N et al 1996 Transjugular intrahepatic portosystemic stent-shunt (TIPPS) occlusion and the role of biliary venous fistulae. Journal of Hepatology 24: 169–176

Kiviluoto T, Siren J, Luukkonen P et al 1998 Randomised trial of laparoscopic versus open cholecystectomy for acute and gangrenous cholecystitis. Lancet 31; 351(9099): 321–325

Knochel J P, Cooper E B, Barry K G 1962 External biliary fistula: A study of electrolyte derangements and secondary cardiovascular and renal abnormalities. Surgery 51: 746–754

Kozarek R A, Ball T J, Patterson D J, Brandabur J J, Raltz S, Traverso L W 1994 Endoscopic treatment of biliary injury in the era of laparoscopic cholecystectomy. Gastrointestinal Endoscopy 40: 10–16

Kracht M, Thompson J N, Bernhoft R A et al 1986 Cholangitis following endoscopic sphincterotomy in patients with high biliary stricture. Surgery, Gynecology and Obstetrics 163: 324–326

Kornaros S E, Aboul-Nour T A 1996 Frank intrabiliary rupture of hydatid hepatic cyst: diagnosis and treatment. Journal of the American College of Surgeons 183: 466–470

Kune G A, Sali A 1980 The practice of biliary surgery, 2nd edn. Blackwell Scientific, Oxford, ch 1, p 9

Kum C K, Eypasch E, Lefering R et al 1996 Laparoscopic cholecystectomy for acute cholecystitis: is it really safe? World Journal of Surgery 20: 43–49

Lillemoe K D, Martin S A, Cameron J L et al 1997 Major bile duct injuries during laparoscopic cholecystectomy. Annals of Surgery 225: 459–471

Marks J M, Ponsky J L, Shillingstad R B, Singh J 1998 Biliary stenting is more effective than sphincterotomy in the resolution of biliary leaks. Surgical Endoscopy 12: 327–330

MacFadyen J B V, Vecchio R, Ricardo A E, Mathis C R 1998 Bile duct injury after laparoscopic cholecystectomy. The United States experience. Surgical Endoscopy 12: 315–321

McPherson G A D, Collier N, Lavender J P et al 1984 The role of HIDA scanning in the assessment of external biliary fistula. Surgical Gastroenterology 3: 77–80

Men S, Hekimoglu B, Yucesoy C, Arda I S, Baran I 1999 Percutaneous treatment of hepatic hydatid cysts: an alternative to surgery. American Journal of Roentgenology 172: 83–89

Moser J J, Baer H U, Glattli A, Schweizer W, Blumgart L H, Czerniak A 1993 Mirizzi syndrome—a contraindication for laparoscopic surgery. Helvetica Chirurgica Acta 59: 577–580

Nyberg B 1990 Bile secretion in man. The effects of somatostatin, vasoactive intestinal peptide and secretin. Acta Chirurgica Scandinavica Supplementum 557: 1–40

Ozmen V, Igci A, Kebudi A, Kecer M, Bozfakioglu Y, Parlak M 1992 Surgical treatment of hepatic hydatid disease. Canadian Journal of Surgery 35: 423–427

Parrila P, Ramirez P, Sanchez-Bueno F et al 1991 Long-term results of choledochoduodenostomy in the treatment of choledocholithiasis: assessment of 225 cases. British Journal of Surgery 78: 470–472

Ponchon T, Gallez J P, Valette P J, Chavaillon A, Bory R 1989 Endoscopic treatment of biliary tract fistulas. Gastrointestinal Endoscopy 35: 490–498

Rosenberg L, Brown R A 1991 Somatostatin in the management of nonendocrine gastrointestinal and pancreatic disorders: a preliminary study. Canadian Journal of Surgery 34: 223–229

Roslyn J J, Binns G S, Hughes E P X et al 1993 Open cholecystectomy. A contemporary analysis of 42 474 patients. Annals of Surgery 218: 129–137

Sandberg A A, Johansson S, Bengmark S 1985 Accidental lesion of the common bile duct at cholecystectomy: II. Results of treatment. Annals of Surgery 209: 452–455

Sarantou T, Bilchik A, Ramming K P 1998 Complications of hepatic cryosurgery. Seminars of Surgical Oncology 14: 156–162

Shahrudin M D, Noori S M 1997 Biloma and biliary fistula associated with hepatorrhaphy for liver injury. Hepatogastroenterology 44: 519–521

Sherman S, Shaked A, Cryer H M, Goldstein L, Busuttil R W 1993 Endoscopic management of biliary fistulas complicating liver transplantation and other hepatobiliary operations. Annals of Surgery 218: 167–175

Silecchia G, Materia A, Bezzi M et al 1995 Minimally invasive approach in Mirizzi syndrome. Journal of Laparoendoscopic Surgery 5: 151–156

Smith E E J, Bowley N, Allison D J, Blumgart L H 1982 The management of post-traumatic intrahepatic cutaneous biliary fistulas. British Journal of Surgery 69: 317–318

Starzl T E, Iwatzuki S, Shaw B W et al 1982 Left hepatic trisegmentectomy. Surgery, Gynecology and Obstetrics 155: 21–27

Strasberg S M, Hertl M, Soper N J 1995 An analysis of the problem of biliary injury during laparoscopic cholecystectomy. Journal of the American College of Surgeons 180: 101–125

Stuart S A, Simpson T I, Alvord L A, Williams M D 1998 Routine intraoperative laparoscopic cholangiography. American Journal of Surgery 176: 632–637

Thompson H H, Tompkins T K, Longmire W P 1983 Major hepatic resections—a 25-year experience. Annals of Surgery 197: 365–337

Toriumi D, Ruchim M, Goldberg M et al 1989 Transnasal biliary drainage for treatment of common bile duct leakage and bile peritonitis. Digestive Diseases and Sciences 34: 315–319

Vecchio R, MacFadyen BV, Latteri S 1998 Laparoscopic cholecystectomy: an analysis on 114,005 cases of United States series. International Surgery 83: 215–219

Viikari S J 1960 Operative injuries to the bile ducts. Acta Chirurgica Scandinavica 119: 83–92

Walsh R M, Henderson J M, Vogt D P et al 1998 Trends in bile duct injuries from laparoscopic cholecystectomy. Journal of Gastrointestinal Surgery 2: 458–462

Wherry D C, Marohn M R, Malanosky M P et al 1996 An external audit of laparoscopic cholecystectomy in the steady state performed in medical treatment facilities of the Department of Defense. Annals of Surgery 224: 145–154

Wright K D, Wellwood J M 1998 Bile duct injury during laparoscopic cholecystectomy without operative cholangiography. British Journal of Surgery 85: 191–194

Biliary tumors

51

Tumors of the bile duct – pathologic aspects

A. ZIMMERMANN

Several cell types have been described in the epithelial lining of major intrahepatic and extrahepatic bile ducts together with subepithelial mucous glands and, hypothetically, different varieties of tumor may arise from any. The majority, however, appear to be microscopically and histogenetically similar, resembling to some extent the most common lining cells of the bile ducts.

For many years the nature of bile duct tumors was difficult to define as most of the material for study was derived either from small biopsy fragments, the orientation of which was often difficult, or from autopsy material which, because of concomitant jaundice and sepsis, was severely affected by autolysis (Willis 1960). Recently with more radical surgery, tumors of the ducts have been resected together with the ducts bearing them and it has been possible to observe the characteristics of the tumors (Takasan et al 1980, Weinbren & Mutum 1983). In general, the tumors are mainly mucin-producing adenocarcinomas, benign epithelial neoplasms being distinctly unusual although certain special varieties will be discussed; they are found more frequently in some sites of the biliary tract, show certain associations with other ductal lesions, appear to be less aggressive than hepatocellular carcinomas and in most parts of the world have a lower incidence than hepatocellular carcinomas (Cruickshank 1961). Tumors arising from other cell types than biliary epithelial cells are occasionally reported.

CHOLANGIOCARCINOMA OF THE EXTRAHEPATIC BILE DUCTS (Ch. 54)

Cholangiocarcinomas (CCCs) are rare tumors, with an autopsy incidence of 0.01 to 0.5%, mainly occurring in the 50 to 70 years age group (for recent reviews, see Vauthey &

Blumgart 1994, Carriaga & Henson 1995). Apart from apparently spontaneously evolving CCCs, several conditions are known to favor their development, including ulcerative colitis, malformations such as choledochal cyst, and anomalies of the pancreatico-choledochal junction. In this section, important aspects of the gross and microscopic presentation of extrahepatic CCCs are discussed.

MACROSCOPIC FEATURES

Tumors are found mainly in three sites in the bile ducts: (1) proximal to the junction of the cystic duct, including the hilar region (Klatskin 1965); (2) distal to the junction with the cystic duct (the lower mid-region); and (3) at the lower end of the common bile duct (van Heerden et al 1967, Weinbren & Mutum 1983). The usual appearance of proximal and hilar lesions (Klatskin tumors; for a review see Bosma 1990) is that of a sclerosing mass of tumor, up to approximately 4 cm in length with an increase in ductal wall thickness to 1 cm (Figs 51.1 and 51.2). This often extends into surrounding liver tissue, forming a spherical mass up to about 5 cm diameter. It is usually clearly demarcated from surrounding liver tissue, but there is sometimes an extension along the duct wall. Based on computed tomographic (CT) scanning and angiography, several growth patterns have been proposed, i.e. infiltrative and exophytic types, with a nodular and a periductal subtype for the latter (Yamashita et al 1992). By the time that medical advice is sought, the duct bearing the tumor is occluded, although, if the tumor is confined to the right or left branches, jaundice may not be present (Meyerowitz & Aird 1962).

Depending on the exact site of the tumor and the degree of involvement of the common hepatic duct, symptoms may occur earlier in the course of the development of the

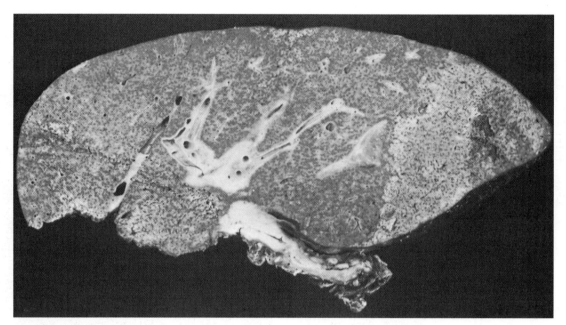

Fig. 51.1 Sclerosing cholangiocarcinoma in the common hepatic duct at the hilum. Resection.

tumor and so lesions at the hilum may become evident when they are only 2 or 3 cm in diameter. All, however, are dense and usually clearly demarcated from surrounding hepatic parenchyma (Fig. 51.3). Occasionally, Klatskin tumors are polypoid and protrude into the lumen of the bile duct. Based on the anatomical location of the tumor, Bismuth & Corlette (1975) classified carcinomas of the hepatic confluence as: type I, unobstructed primary confluence (tumor located in the main hepatic duct); type II, obstruction limited to the primary confluence (tumor located exactly at the confluence); and type III, obstruction of the primary confluence with extension to the right or left secondary confluence. Tumors in the lower middle region of the ductal system, that is, involving the common bile duct immediately proximal to the pancreas, are generally discrete tumors, causing thickening of the ductal wall, but often presenting an intraluminal, sharply demarcated spherical mass (Fig. 51.4). These may be up to 2 cm in diameter, but generally cause jaundice and therefore probably represent an earlier stage in the development of the tumor. The

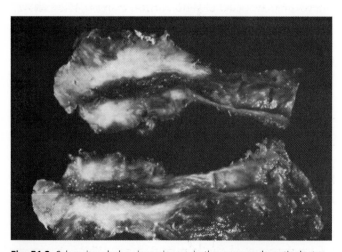

Fig. 51.2 Sclerosing cholangiocarcinoma in the common hepatic duct 1 cm distal to hilum. Resection.

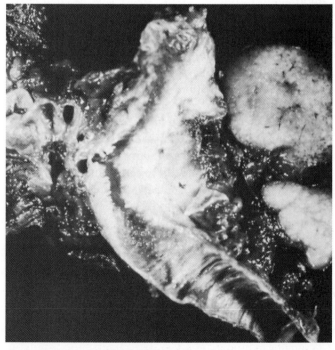

Fig. 51.3 Sclerosing cholangiocarcinoma at junction of the common hepatic and common bile ducts. Reactive lymph nodes on the right, cystic duct on the left. Resection.

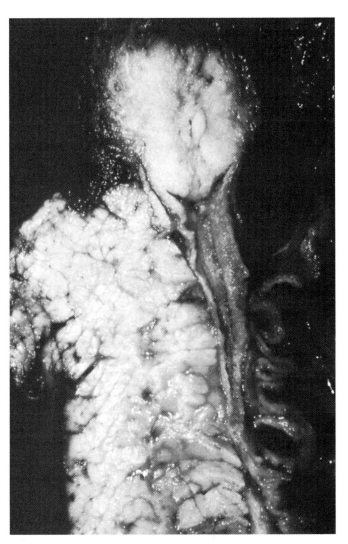

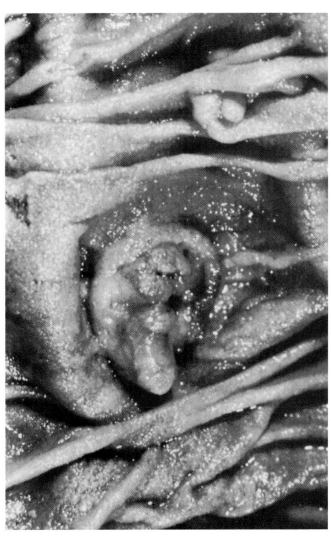

Fig. 51.4 Nodular cholangiocarcinoma in the suprapancreatic part of the common bile duct. Note tumor thickening of the duct wall. Resection.

Fig. 51.5 Papillary cholangiocarcinoma protruding at the ampullary orifice. The pancreatic duct orifice is to the upper right. Resection.

luminal surface of the duct wall is usually irregular. The tumors in the distal 2 cm of the common bile duct are papillary adenocarcinomas, usually friable, pink or greyish-white masses. They may be seen within the duodenum surrounding the orifice of the papilla of Vater (Figs 51.5 and 51.6). Most ductal tumors fall into these three categories, with annular sclerosing tumors proximally, globular or nodular sclerosing tumors at the lower mid-region, and papillary tumors in the region of the papilla. Allocation of carcinomas of the bile ducts to one of these three categories of gross presentation is important in a clinical setting, may be more significant than the histological subtype, and should be specified at pathological examination. In addition to the site, the pathologist should inform the surgeon as to the major growth pattern found at examination of specimens. Growth is generally of three types, and these patterns mostly occur at distinct sites, as exemplified above, with exceptions. Papillary lesions represent an intraluminal growth pattern, and there may be a field change with multiple tumor sites. It has been suggested that multiple tumors may be found in 7% of patients with such bile duct tumors (Tompkins et al 1976). As specified above, papillary growth patterns clearly predominate in the low bile duct and in the region of the sphincter of Oddi, but high lesions may also occur. In situations of extended papillary growth at a distal level it may be difficult to differentiate primary bile duct carcinomas from tumors involving the duodenal mucosa. Moreover, invasion of the duodenal mucosa of ductal papillary adenocarcinoma may induce gross mucosal surface changes that can give rise to uncertainty as to what lesion is present (Weinbren & Mutum 1983). A second gross growth pattern, the nodular type of tumor, can be sclerosing or nodular with projection into the bile duct lumen. Most of these occur in the upper and mid-duct, the sclerosing variant being typical of the Klatskin tumor (see above). The diffuse growth pattern shows a duct wall which is thickened over an extensive area, with narrow lumen and inflammatory change in the surrounding tissues. Lesions of this type may be very difficult to differentiate from reactive changes, in particular sclerosing cholangitis.

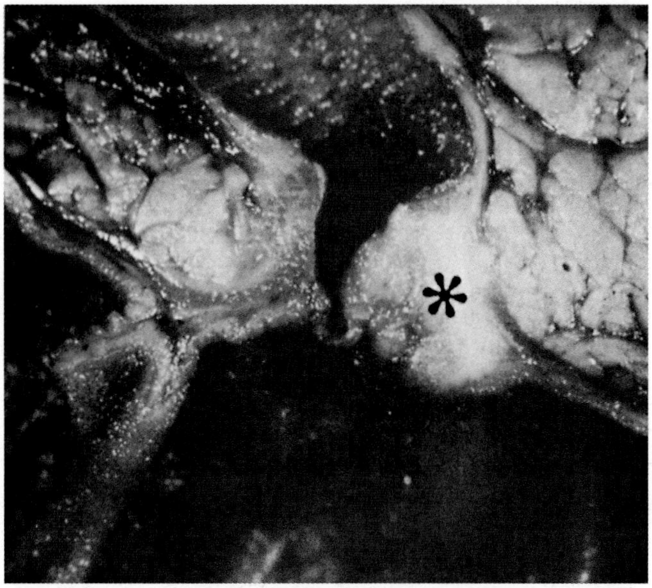

MICROSCOPIC FEATURES

The tumors are generally adenocarcinomas consisting of acinar and solid structures (Fig. 51.7). The individual cells are larger than normal duct cells, varying in height from 12 to 25 mm. Between acini and trabecula there is usually a striking fibrosis (desmoplastic or sclerosing reaction of stroma; Fig. 51.8). The acini themselves vary in size, with a preponderance of smaller structures involving narrow elongated or spherical lumina, as opposed to the large acini with intraluminal necrotic tumor frequently found in metastatic adenocarcinoma. Single tumor cells or small groups of tumor cells, sometimes with associated mucin, may be found within the stroma, and occasionally free mucin lakes are noted (Fig. 51.9). These features are not invariable and occur in approximately 50% of sclerosing or nodular cholangiocarcinomas. Striking cytological features are the very high incidence of prominent nucleoli in large tracts of cells (about 80% of tumors) and a notable heterogeneity of lining cells within single acini (about 50% of tumors) (Fig. 51.10). Apart from hepatic cystadenocarcinoma (see below; Short et al 1975, Ishak et al 1977, Nakajima et al 1992), the juxtaposition of normal and tumor cells is usually not remarked in other tumors.

Fig. 51.6 Section through a small tumor at the papilla with a proximal dilated duct. The dilated common bile duct is above, the duodenum below and the tumor is marked by an asterisk.

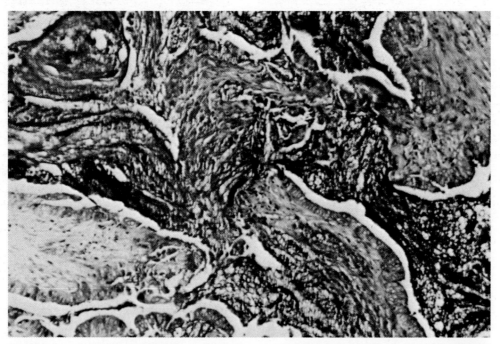

Fig. 51.7 Irregular mucin-containing tumor acini in fibrous stroma (Alcian blue [AB], periodic acid-Schiff [PAS], diastase x150).

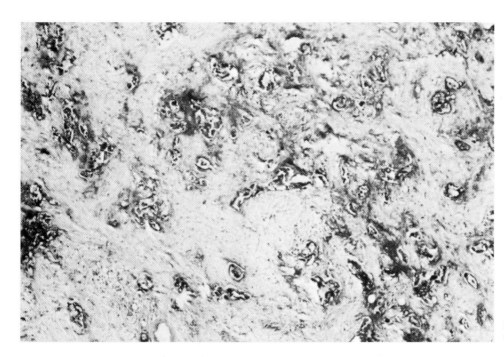

Fig. 51.8 Abundant fibrosis between tumor acini (AB, PAS, diastase x 60).

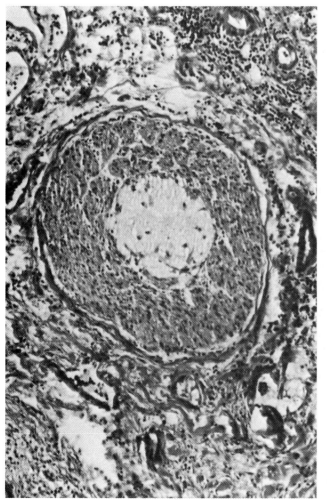

Fig. 51.9 Free mucin lake within a nerve (Hematoxylin & eosin (H and E), x150).

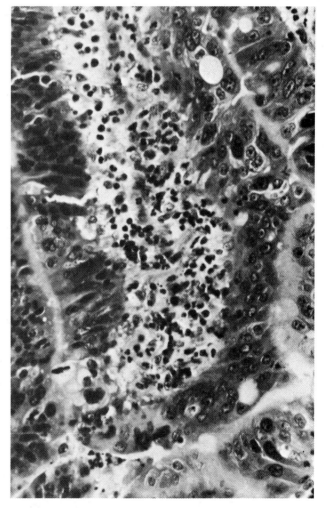

Fig. 51.10 Large cholangiocarcinoma cells with striking nucleoli (right) lining the same lumen as relatively normal-appearing bile duct epithelial cells (left). (H and E, x150).

VARIANTS OF EXTRA- AND INTRAHEPATIC CHOLANGIOCARCINOMAS

Several histological variants of CCCs have been described, and some of these exhibit a different biological behavior and may, therefore, also be of clinical significance. Most of these variants have been defined in the WHO histological typing of tumors (Gibson 1978, Albores-Saavedra et al 1991); a commentary to the second WHO edition has recently been published (Albores-Saavedra et al 1992). Variants comprise distinct forms of adenocarcinoma (papillary, intestinal, mucinous, clear cell, signet-ring cell and adenosquamous types), and squamous cell, small cell and undifferentiated carcinomas.

A distinct variant, which is easily identifiable at gross examination already is mucin-producing CCC (MPCCC), which amounted to 12.9% of CCCs in a large series (Chen et al 1998), and which resulted in better survival rates after hepatic resection. MPCCC has been reported as a complication of hepatolithiasis and recurrent pyogenic cholangitis (Chow et al 1997). Some cases present microcystic features (Sonobe et al 1995), and the mucinous component may be associated with extensive peri- and intraneural invasion (neurotropic MPCCC). Intrahepatic CCC can present as a circumscribed nodular lesion and has been described under the term, minute nodular intrahepatic CCC (Yamamoto et al 1998). CCCs composed of medium-sized cells with vesicular nuclei and poor stromal formation are termed, medullary type CCC. Interestingly, these tumors may preferentially occur in liver fluke endemic areas (Shirai et al 1992). Cholangiocarcinomas with a lymphoepithelial component have been observed in association with Epstein-Barr virus infection (Hsu et al 1996). Of relevance with respect to histopathological differential diagnosis is an unusual variant of peripheral cholangiocarcinoma, clear cell papillary carcinoma of the liver (Tihan et al 1998), because it may mimick clear cell hepatocellular carcinoma or intrahepatic metastases of renal cell carcinoma. Intestinal type CCC, which is mainly composed of goblet cells, colonic-like epithelium, or both, often contains a population of endocrine cells and, rarely, clusters of Paneth cells (Albores-Saavedra et al 1991).

INVASION AND SPREAD OF CHOLANGIOCARCINOMAS

The spread of CCCs as seen within biopsy or resection material depends to some extent on the site of the tumor,

ampullary tumors usually showing no evidence of venous invasion and more proximal sclerosing (desmoplastic) and nodular tumors exhibiting involvement of veins in approximately 20% of tumors and involvement of nerves (peri- and/or intraneural invasion) in about 80% of instances (Fig. 51.11). CCC cells can spread, sometimes superficially, along intrahepatic bile ducts (Kato et al 1997) and are well known to invade the peribiliary capillary plexus, the latter probably representing a major pathway for the intrahepatic extension of disease, whereas invasion of the peri- and intraneural tissue compartment is a crucial factor for local recurrence in the case of hilar and other extrahepatic tumors (Bhuiya et al 1993). Spread has been demonstrated to also occur via the sinusoidal spaces, and overall CCCs with a vascular involvement presented a higher tendency of

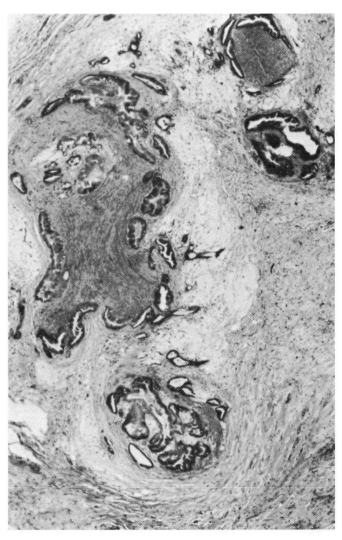

Fig. 51.11 Cholangiocarcinomatous invasion of nerve trunks. (H and E, x40).

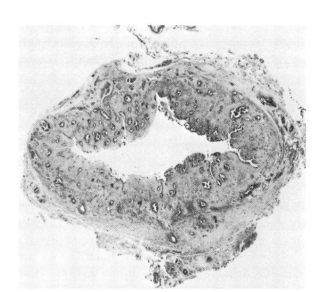

Fig. 51.12 Subepithelial spread of cholangiocarcinoma (H and E).

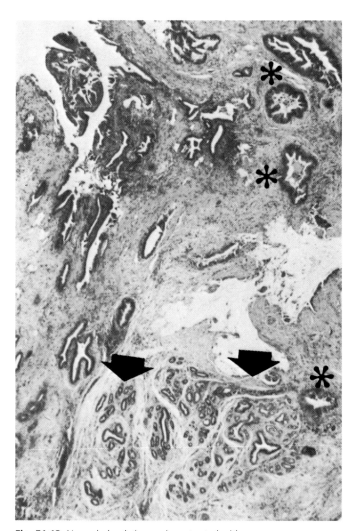

Fig. 51.13 Normal glands (arrows) contrasted with cholangiocarcinomatous acini (asterisk). (H and E, x40).

intrahepatic as well as extrahepatic metastases (Nakajima et al 1988). A systematic study on hilar tumors has shown that, with respect to extramucosal infiltration, invasion extended more frequently and further to the hepatic side than to the duodenal side, usually by the route of the extramural layer (Hayashi et al 1994), an observation which has also an impact on the sampling and interpretation of intraoperative frozen sections.

Within the liver, expansion can be identified by atrophy of adjacent hepatocytes, frequently associated with direct invasion of liver sinusoids by tumor cells, the latter phenomenon being visualized in about half of the cases. Subepithelial spread in bile ducts is noted in about 10%, which may be difficult to recognize during operations, because of the overlying intact and smooth lining epithelium (Figs. 51.12 and 51.13; Weinbren and Mutum 1983).

SPECIAL CHARACTERISTICS AND VARIATIONS AS A FUNCTION OF THE ANATOMICAL SITE

The features which generally reflect a form of mucin-secreting adenocarcinoma are observed in tumors arising in any part of the biliary tree but there are sometimes differences between tumors at different sites. Some of these differences may be observed on naked-eye examination and some are microscopic.

At the hilum of the liver, about 70% of cholangiocarcinomas are predominantly sclerosing (desmoplastic) tumors, but macroscopically papillary tumors are described (Fig. 51.14). Most of these papillary tumors appear to be associated with other lesions involving the biliary system. The lesions so far reported include cystic dilatation of ducts with papillomatosis (Newmann et al 1976, Helpap 1977), benign cysts and choledochal cysts (Caroli & Corcos 1964, Caroli 1973) although occasional papillary tumors at the hilum are found without associated abnormalities (Fig. 51.15; Madden & Smith 1974). Choledochal cysts may occur anywhere in the extrahepatic biliary system (Kagawa et al 1978). Biliary papillomatosis (see below) may also arise in non-obstructive intrahepatic (biliary) dilatations seen in other situations, such as congenital hepatic fibrosis (Nakanuma et al 1982) and adult polycystic disease of the liver and kidneys (Terada & Nakanuma 1988), or may rarely occur in intrahepatic non-obstructive bile duct dilatations not related to one of the hereditary polycystic diseases (Terada et al 1991). The papillary tumors vary in size between approximately 1 and 3 cm, sometimes occlude the ductal lumen and may be associated with non-invasive

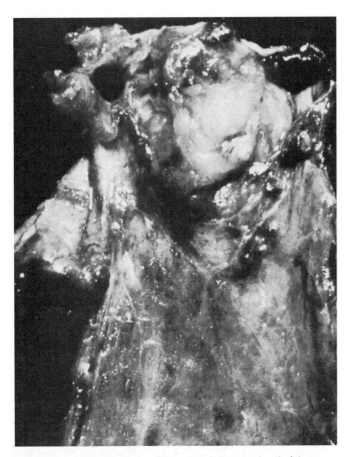

Fig. 51.14 Papillary cholangiocarcinoma at the proximal end of the common hepatic duct.

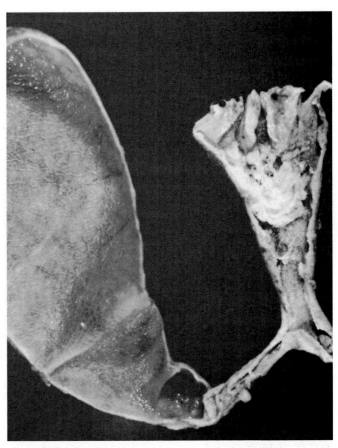

Fig. 51.15 Papillary cholangiocarcinoma at the proximal part of the common hepatic duct, 1 cm distal to the hilum.

neoplastic change or carcinoma in situ (Fig. 51.16). At the base of papillary tumors, fibrosis may be seen within the wall of the duct, but this is not necessarily the case in tumors associated with choledochal cysts or with papillomatosis (Figs 51.17, 51.18, 51.19 and 51.20).

Tumors situated at the choledochoduodenal junction are either papillary or ulcerating, or a combination of these two forms. Ulcerating lesions are usually frankly duodenal or pancreatic in origin, but all periampullary papillary tumors do not necessarily arise in the bile duct. It is sometimes difficult to distinguish the site of origin of papillary tumors, and the structural relationships are sometimes severely distorted. The folds of epithelium of the bile duct at the papilla of Vater, which appear to be redundant at different degrees of contraction of the sphincteric mechanism, ought to be distinguished from any papillary tumor tissue at the site (Ch. 52) (Baggenstoss 1938). In addition, carcinoma of the small intestine, on the whole an unusual tumor, nonetheless occurs most frequently in the duodenum, and the mucosal site of origin may be close to and sometimes inseparable from the papilla. It may therefore be difficult to define the

site of origin without multiple sections of carefully oriented tissue, fixed after resection and before blocks are taken (Figs 51.21, 51.22 and 51.23). Villous adenomas of the duodenum are encountered, and carcinoma in situ and invasive carcinoma are associated with these lesions, but it is rare to find villous adenomas of the biliary epithelium. Structures resembling parts of villous adenoma arising from the end of the bile duct are usually derived from the normal biliary epithelium and may not represent what have been called 'residuals of villous adenoma' (Okuda et al 1977). The basis for this contention is that the cytological features of these structures are entirely normal, no nuclear enlargement, cellular crowding or loss of polarity being reported. A form of intestinal metaplasia has sometimes been reported in bile ducts bearing tumors (Kozuka et al 1984) but this is not a constant feature. Tumors extending down from the bile duct are not usually ulcerated, whereas both duodenal and pancreatic tumors frequently are (Blumgart & Kennedy 1973).

Owing to their clinical and pathologic complexity, features of ampullary carcinoma are summarized here in some

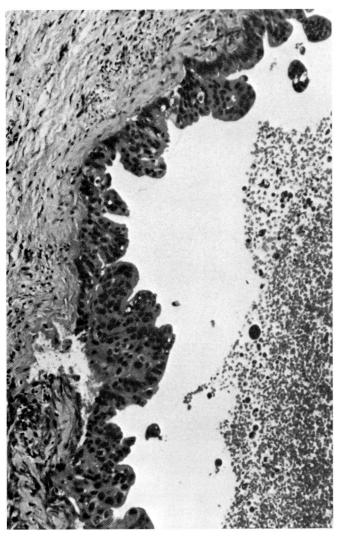

Fig. 51.16 Carcinoma in situ in a communicating cyst at the hilar region from the same patient as in Fig. 51.14.

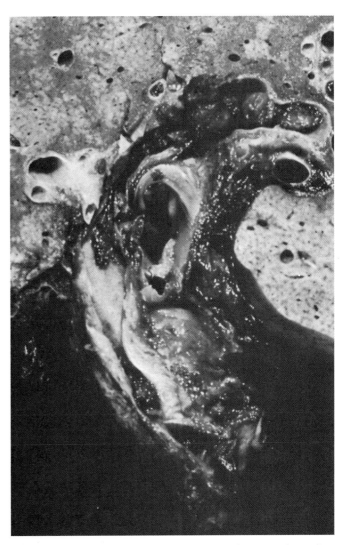

Fig. 51.17 Duct papillomatosis showing small papillary tumors extending from the left hepatic to the common hepatic duct.

more detail. Most of these tumors are adenocarcinomas, but special types or variants comprise signet-ring cell carcinoma (Gardner et al 1990), undifferentiated carcinoma (Sato et al 1995), and tumors showing variable degrees of neuroendocrine differentiation, including small-cell neuroendocrine carcinoma and tumors strongly expressing somatostatin (Stamm et al 1986, Stommer et al 1987, Sarker et al 1992). Adenocarcinoma of the ampullary region represents about 1% of all epithelial malignancies and about 5% of all carcinomas of the gastrointestinal tract, and the main morphologic pattern is either of the intestinal or papillary type (Talbot et al 1988). Several reports refer to the particular biology of these tumors (Yamaguchi & Enjoji 1987, Hayes et al 1987, Nakao et al 1994, Farrell et al 1996), and long-term survival after resection has been

demonstrated to be associated independently with tumor grade and a new staging classification that assesses local invasiveness (Neoptolemos et al 1988). As outlined above, differential diagnosis from carcinomas of the most distal part of the common bile duct may be difficult, and a special protocol for the examination of these tumors has been developed by the Cancer Committee of the College of American Pathologists (Compton 1997). Ampullary carcinomas can be spatially associated with adenomas (see below; Seifert et al 1992), the latter sometimes associated with familial adenomatous polyposis (Alexander et al 1989, Noda et al 1992, Bertoni et al 1996), remnants of adenoma, and/or dysplastic epithelium, in particular flat duct epithelial dysplasia (Baczako et al 1985, Talbot et al 1988, Kimura & Ohtsubo 1988).

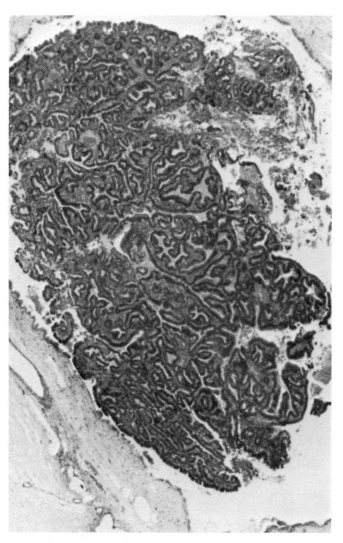

Fig. 51.18 Section of a papillomatous lesion showing papillary fronds. (H and E, x40).

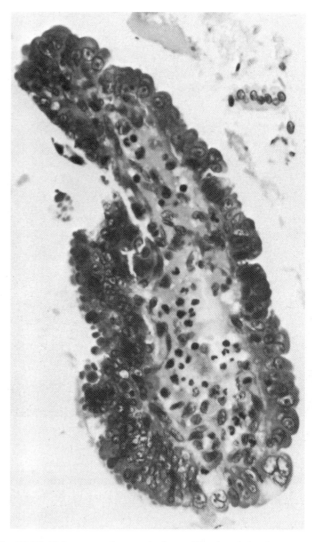

Fig. 51.19 High-power micrograph of a papillary frond showing dysplasia (H and E, x200).

LESIONS ASSOCIATED WITH CHOLANGIOCARCINOMA

Changes proximal to the tumor involve the epithelium and subepithelial mucous glands of proximal ducts and also the substance of the liver. Some changes develop as an effect of obstruction to the biliary system and some of the changes noted may antedate and possibly predispose to the development of cholangiocarcinoma.

The changes in the liver following obstruction to the common hepatic or common bile duct have been well described (Desmet 1972) and, in general, the occurrence of intracanalicular cholestasis, inflammation, edema of portal tracts and ductular proliferations is agreed upon by most workers (Gall & Dobrogorski 1964), but there is some con-

flict of opinion about more chronic changes in the liver of patients suffering from duct obstruction. Cirrhosis (so-called secondary biliary cirrhosis) is frequently reported, especially when there is evidence of portal hypertension (Ruebner & Montgomery 1982), but a recent analysis suggests that the liver in most patients with portal hypertension and chronic obstructive biliary disease is not really cirrhotic but has retained normal vascular relations and developed a diffuse thickening of hepatocyte plates, the latter probably resulting from hepatocyte hyperplasia (Weinbren et al 1985). The difference in these two interpretations of the lesions in chronic obstructive biliary disease is significant and material to the possibility of restoration of normal portal venous pressure after relief of the obstruction. It is generally acknowledged that cirrhosis is probably irreversible, so that portal hypertension may remain a problem even after

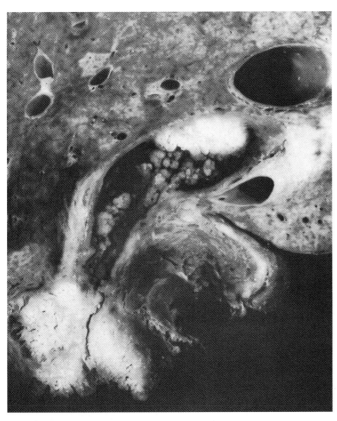

Fig. 51.20 Ductal papillomatosis with invasion by cholangiocarcinoma through the duct wall at several points.

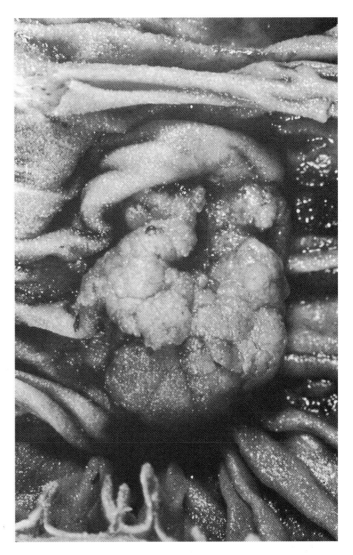

Fig. 51.21 Ampullary tumor seen from the duodenum.

the free flow of bile is restored, but that the venous pressure change observed in patients without cirrhosis may possibly be reversible and that even recovery from portal hypertension may be contemplated (Weinbren et al 1985). In the light of the distinct structural changes occurring in bile duct obstruction, 'biliary fibrosis with hyperplasia and/or atrophy' may be a term more appropriate than 'cirrhosis' in these conditions. That a hyperplastic reaction of parenchymal cells occurs is supported by the observation that bile duct ligation in the rat induces a significant hepatocellular proliferation, in part related to increased nuclear expression of epidermal growth factor receptor (Zimmermann et al 1995). It is still unclear to what extent these alterations are reversible by biliodigestive anastomosis in humans, but reversibility of secondary biliary fibrosis by biliodigestive anastomosis in the rat has recently been demonstrated (Zimmermann et al 1992). Fibrosis is also, in some instances, a morphological element of liver atrophy, the incidence of which in hilar carcinoma of the bile ducts is around 20%. Atrophy may be associated with compensatory hypertrophy of uninvolved parts of the liver (atrophy/hypertrophy complex, AHC; Lory et al 1994). Under experimental situations, however, reduced portal

vein blood flow is a more important driving force for atrophy than the biliary obstruction alone (Schweizer et al 1995).

Changes within proximal ducts include proliferations of subepithelial mucous glands. In a recent study, the prevalence of hyperplasia of extramural mucous acini was high in biliary obstruction (Terada & Nakanuma 1992), but also occurred in cirrhosis, cholangitis and systemic infection. Obstruction may be associated with papillary formations of the duct epithelium and collections of lymphocytes in the wall of the duct. These lesions are usually distinguishable from tumors and occur in non-neoplastic chronic inflammatory diseases of the bile ducts, the most notable example being Asiatic pyogenic cholangitis (Gibson 1971).

Apart from ductular proliferations, fibrosis and nodular change, bile infarction may occur in livers with obstructed

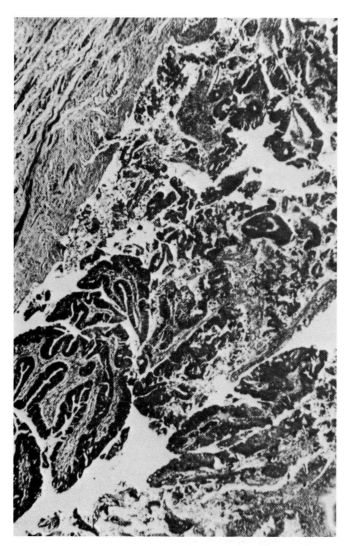

Fig. 51.22 Sections showing papillary adenocarcinoma (H and E, x40).

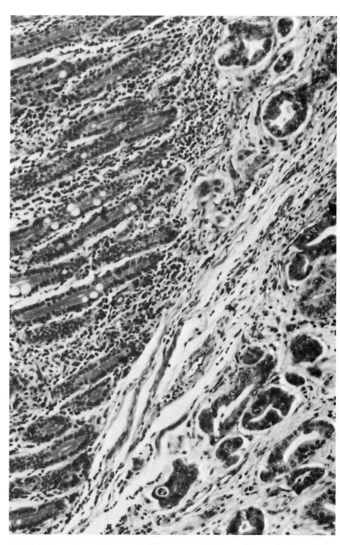

Fig. 51.23 Invasion from same tumor as in Fig. 51.22 into the tunica propria of the duodenum (H and E, x150).

bile ducts. It was generally thought that the development of bile infarction requires two pathogenic factors, i.e. a toxic chemical factor (the stagnant bile) and a mechanical factor (the raised biliary pressure), but recent studies suggest that bile infarction is caused by the toxic action of bile constituents other than bilirubin and bile acids, absorbed into the blood from the obstructed biliary system (Shibayama 1990).

At the site of the tumor in the ductal system it may be difficult to identify underlying changes which may have preceded neoplastic development, but such changes are sometimes found elsewhere in the ductal system (Inglis & Farmer 1975). This is observed in patients in whom cholangiocarcinoma is found to be accompanied by changes generally considered to represent different stages of primary sclerosing cholangitis, the latter condition a known associa-

tion of ulcerative colitis in 5% of patients (Ross & Braasch 1973). While the structural changes in primary sclerosing cholangitis are only partly defined, the replacement of part of the biliary tract, both intra- and extrahepatic segments, by fibrosis and the destruction of the epithelial lining appear to be accepted (Chapman et al 1980, Ludwig 1989, Lindor et al 1990). Periductal fibrosis, noted also in primary sclerosing cholangitis, is probably non-specific, as such changes are also observed in chronic duct obstruction (Weinbren & Mutum 1983). An association between primary sclerosing cholangitis and cholangiocarcinoma was first suggested on an epidemiological basis. It is estimated that at least 10% of patients with primary sclerosing cholangitis also develop cholangiocarcinoma (Converse et al 1971), but the actual risk of developing this tumor in patients with primary sclerosing cholangitis is difficult to ascertain (Rosen &

Nagorney 1991). In a prospective clinical trial, cholangiocarcinoma occurred in 42% of autopsy patients and in at least 7% of patients with pre-existing primary sclerosing cholangitis in the study (Rosen et al 1991). Pathological reviews of bile duct tumors arising in patients with chronic ulcerative colitis further support the association between primary sclerosing cholangitis and cholangiocarcinoma. Cholangiocarcinoma can mimic the radiographic features of primary sclerosing cholangitis through extensive periductal infiltration or multicentricity (Rosen & Nagorney 1991). Cholangiocarcinomatous invasion of periductal tissue is usually radial from its origin and limited to 5 cm. This extent of periductal infiltration was present in only four of 22 patients with sclerosing cholangiocarcinoma in the detailed pathological study performed by Weinbren & Mutum (1983), and these authors found no multicentric tumors. In contrast, another study on eight patients with chronic ulcerative colitis and cholangiocarcinoma showed multicentric origins of tumor, presence of carcinoma in situ in areas of fibrous cholangitis, and histological evidence of longstanding inflammatory hepatobiliary disease prior to the diagnosis of tumor (Wee et al 1985). It has been suggested that patients with chronic ulcerative colitis are 10–30 times more prone to developing cholangiocarcinoma, than members of the general population (Rosen & Nagorney 1991), and that primary sclerosing cholangitis appears to precede a pattern of biliary epithelial atypia probably corresponding to dysplasia (Haworth et al 1989).

Other forms of ductal disease are reported as occurring together with cholangiocarcinoma. These include certain forms of non-parasitic cystic disease; but not all varieties of liver cysts are associated with cholangiocarcinoma. In about 20% of patients with polycystic disease of the liver (Melnick 1955), small foci of microscopical cysts enmeshed in mature fibrous tissue are found abutting on portal tracts. These lesions are termed von Meyenburg complexes or biliary hamartomas/microhamartomas (see below). A report in which tumors are described in association with these microhamartomas (Homer et al 1968) has been challenged, but bile duct carcinomas associated with multiple biliary microhamartomas have since been reported (Honda et al 1986, Burns et al 1990). In contrast, no substantive and acceptable report of the association of cholangiocarcinoma and simple non-communicating cysts appears to have been published. Even the condition of cystadenoma within the liver substance is structurally different from a simple cyst (see below; Ishak et al 1977). What is agreed, however, is that, in general, extrahepatic cysts (e.g. choledochal cysts), especially if calculus-containing, are sometimes associated with some forms of cholangiocarcinoma (Fieber & Nance, 1997) and the same holds true for Caroli's disease (Gallagher et al

1972) and for congenital hepatic fibrosis (Yamato et al 1998) (Ch. 66). Cholangiocarcinoma has also been reported in the context of hereditary nonpolyposis colorectal carcinoma (Mecklin et al 1992).

CAUSES OF CHOLANGIOCARCINOMA

In autopsy material the incidence of cholangiocarcinoma is reported as lying between 0.089 and 0.42% of necropsies carried out in general hospitals (Kuwayti et al 1957). The tumor is reported more frequently after the sixth decade and it is unusual under the age of 40 years, although a cholangiocarcinoma has been described in a 33-year-old man (Weinbren & Mutum 1983). Almost twice as many men as women are affected by cholangiocarcinomas. The associated ductal lesions have been referred to, but it is not yet fully clear how the changes in primary sclerosing cholangitis or choledochal or other communicating cysts predispose to the development of this tumor, hyperplasias and atypical hyperplasias (Kurashina et al 1988) or dysplasia (Haworth et al 1989) probably representing timely distant lesions within the carcinogenic sequence already. Parasitic infestation is regarded as a serious cause of cholangiocarcinoma, especially affecting populations in Hong Kong, south-east China and Thailand (Gibson 1971). The liver flukes *Clonorchis sinensis* and *Opisthorchis viverrini* are frequently the cause of the parasitic infestation, but infestation by *Fasciola hepatica* and *Schistosoma* sp. does not appear to have similar carcinogenic effects.

A raised incidence of bile duct cancer has also been reported in patients who had received thorium dioxide (thorotrast) in the past (Visfeldt & Poulsen 1972, Altmann 1978). Experimental induction of cholangiocarcinoma has been achieved in several species, notably the hamster, using dimethylnitrosamine and *Opisthorchis viverrini* (Flavell & Lucas 1982), and the rat, using high doses of nitrosomorphyline (Bannasch 1978).

In order to obtain a deeper insight into the pathogenesis of human cholangiocarcinomas, several studies have focused on oncogenes. There has been progress in understanding the genesis and the cell biology of cancers from the study of the expression of proto-oncogenes, and the expression of proteins encoded by the *ras, myc* and *erbB-2* oncogenes has been investigated in patients with cholangiocarcinoma. The c-myc gene product is thought to play a significant role in the control of cell proliferation and cell differentiation. Its expression is, for example, elevated in hepatic regeneration (Fausto & Shank 1983), but aberrant expression of the c-myc gene has been detected in malignant cell lines and in several human tumors (Slamon et al 1984). The *ras* genes encode a protein (p21^{ras} protein) which binds nucleotides, possesses intrinsic GTPase activity, and may play an important role in cellular signal-transducing pathways (Barbacid 1987). The *ras* gene appears to be involved in liver regeneration (Fausto & Shank 1983), and increased p21^{ras} protein expression was observed in many human cancers (Tanaka et al 1986). The *c-erbB-2* gene (the *neu* oncogene located on chromosome 17) encodes a protein which is highly homologous to the sequence of the epidermal growth factor receptor (Yamamoto et al 1986) and which has tyrosine kinase activity. Amplification of this gene has been found in several human malignant tumors (Zhou et al 1987). In a recent study, 95% of human cholangiocarcinomas expressed p62^{c-myc}, 75% expressed p21^{c-ras} and 73% expressed p190$^{c-erbB-2}$ (Voravud et al 1989). The expression of c-myc and *c-ras,* but not of c-erB2, correlated directly with tumor differentiation based on morphology, and no difference was observed in oncogene expression between intrahepatic and extrahepatic cholangiocarcinomas. As expression of c-myc and *c-ras* in normal growing liver was only observed until 5 years of age, testing of oncogene expression may be used to distinguish neoplastic from non-neoplastic biliary tissues (Voravud et al 1989), in particular by testing K-ras codon 12 mutations (Hruban et al 1997). However, the relationship between oncogene expression and biology in biliary cancers is still far from clear. For example, there was no correlation between the expression of p21^{ras} in cholangiocarcinomas and the production of two export proteins, human chorionic gonadotrophin and α-fetoprotein (Nonomura et al 1989), although it is known that human chorionic gonadotrophin production by cholangiocarcinomas occurs in a minority of cases and is preferentially restricted to a poorly differentiated subset of cells (Nonomura et al 1989). Similarly, a correlation between the expression of p21^{ras} antigen and the production of carcinoembryonic antigen, which may be an important molecule for cellular interaction, has not been found in cholangiocarcinomas (Nonomura et al 1987). K-ras codon 12 mutations are common in distal bile duct carcinomas, but were of no prognostic value in a recent study (Rijken et al 1998). Similar K-ras mutation patterns were observed in perihilar carcinomas (Sturm et al 1998). Alterations of this gene may be involved in periductal extension and a spicula-like growth pattern, but not for mass-forming tumor types, suggesting that K-ras may influence the local presentation of neoplastic disease (Ohashi et al 1995), probably by exerting a regulatory action on proliferation activity (Ohashi et al 1996). Other agents operational in the regulation of proliferation include interleukin-6; the expression of IL-6 in CCCs is inversely related to proliferation and positively

related to differentiation (Sugawara et al 1998). Besides factors modulating the proliferative behaviour of CCCs, current interest also focuses at tumor suppressors and factors inducing or modulating apoptosis in these tumors. The tumor suppressor, p53, is variably expressed in CCCs (Washington & Gottfried 1996, Rizzi et al 1996), and it has been shown that p53 protein is related to both, higher grade of malignancy and shorter survival in at least a subset of these tumors (Diamantis et al 1995). In contrast, analysis of the p53 mutation pattern in Klatskin tumors has uncovered no apparent clinicopathological impact (Jonas et al 1998). The potential role of p53 with respect to carcinogenesis, biology and, in particular, regulation of apoptosis has, therefore, to be investigated in more detail. In the context of modulation of programmed cell death in CCC it is of interest to note that the apoptosis protector, bcl-2, appears to be overexpressed in a cholangiocarcinoma cell line (Harnois et al 1997).

CHOLANGIOCARCINOMA: DIFFERENTIAL DIAGNOSIS

Lesions which may resemble cholangiocarcinoma include other tumors invading the ductal wall (or lumen) (Kojiro et al 1982), tumors arising from cells other than epithelial cells and non-neoplastic changes.

Both metastatic adenocarcinoma and hepatocellular carcinoma are described as invading the ductal wall and extending along the lumen. The hilar region is particularly affected in this way and tumors presenting within the ductal lumen may require microscopical examination in order to be identified. Hepatocellular carcinoma is reported as invading the bile duct in 2–9% of instances (Kojiro et al 1982).

Cholangiocarcinoma is recognizable in most instances by the characteristic acid glycoprotein-secreting acini, cytological characteristics and associated fibrosis (desmoplasia) but there is the possibility of confusion between CCC and other tumors involving ducts, both in the hilar region and also in the extrahepatic ducts. Acinar structures are encountered in hepatocellular carcinomas, which can invade ductal structures, and bile may be trapped in cholangiocarcinoma, rendering differential diagnosis difficult in some situations. Cells of bile duct carcinomas can express carcinoembryonic antigen (CEA) (Nakajima & Kondo 1989), but CEA may also be present on the luminal (apical) border of some hepatocellular carcinoma cells. However, CEA expression is usually stronger in cholangiocarcinomas. Well-differentiated biliary adenocarcinomas express CEA along the apical surfaces of the cells. With the dedifferentiation of the cells, CEA expression extends to the whole cell surface and to the cytoplasm (Nonomura et al 1987). Testing of cytokeratin profiles (Johnson et al 1988), in particular cytokeratins 7 and 19, of carbohydrate antigen 19-9 (Nakajima & Kondo 1989) and of glyco-conjugate expression (Zhang et al 1989) may be of some utility in difficult situations.

HEPATOCELLULAR CARCINOMA

A form of sclerotic hepatocellular carcinoma is described (MacSween 1974) which resembles cholangiocarcinoma. Cytological characteristics may be confusing, particularly since hepatocellular tumor cells often contain prominent nucleoli and cytoplasm may be sparse. In addition, striking acinar formation may be found in hepatocellular carcinoma and immunohistochemical reactions for α-fetoprotein may be negative. The most important distinguishing feature is the presence of acid mucin, which has not generally been reported in hepatocellular carcinoma, although mucin is demonstrated in the fibrolamellar variant (Goodman et al 1985). This finding has led the authors to consider the fibrolamellar variant to be a mixed tumor, composed of both hepatocellular and cholangiocellular components. Arrangements of cells on a stalk of fibrous connective tissue is usual for cholangiocarcinoma and distinctly unusual for hepatocellular carcinoma.

METASTATIC ADENOCARCINOMA

The chances of a metastatic deposit of adenocarcinoma involving the extrahepatic bile ducts are remote but, because of the marked proclivity of many tumors to metastasize to the liver, cholangiocarcinoma arising within the liver may be simulated by metastatic adenocarcinoma.

It is acknowledged that it may be impossible to distinguish metastatic adenocarcinoma from cholangiocarcinoma in every instance, and particularly if the metastatic tumor arises from the pancreas, but there are general features which may be helpful. On the macroscopic level, metastatic tumors are usually centrally depressed, a result of the combination of tumor necrosis and the retention of an intact although umbilicated Glisson's capsule, and are recognized on the basis of the microscopic features already recounted. In the main, large tumor acini with intraluminal necrotic masses favor metastases and small acini consisting of tumor cells with striking nucleoli tend to favor cholangiocarcinoma. Due to lack of specificity, immunohistochemical techniques available so far may not help much in the differential diagnosis because, e.g. with regards metastases of

ductal pancreatic carcinomas, more or less the same pattern ensues.

OTHER INTRAHEPATIC HILAR MASSES

These include hepatocellular adenoma, focal nodular hyperplasia, bile duct adenoma and cystadenoma or cystadenocarcinoma, all of which may be sharply demarcated but do not cause obstruction to the biliary system unless there is a chance and most exceptional siting of the tumor. The first two lesions mentioned are composed mainly of well-differentiated hepatocytes. Bile duct, adenoma may theoretically develop at the hilar region, although it is usually subcapsular; but it does resemble cholangiocarcinoma because its dense-white, sharply demarcated gross appearance represents intertwined well-differentiated duct-like structures enmeshed in relatively mature fibrous stroma. The regular and well-differentiated epithelial cells do not give the appearance of carcinoma cells and form the basis for the distinction between the two lesions (Edmondson 1976).

OTHER BENIGN AND MALIGNANT EPITHELIAL TUMORS OF THE BILE DUCTS

BILIARY CYSTADENOMA AND CYSTADENOCARCINOMA

These tumors (synonyms: hepatobiliary cystadenoma and cystadenocarcinoma) more frequently affect the liver substance itself than the bile duct walls, but instances of direct bile duct involvement have been reported (Short et al 1975), and the tumors may even have a relationship to the gallbladder. In such circumstances and also when the tumors may be encountered in the hilar region, a distinction from cholangiocarcinoma may be required.

Biliary cystadenoma (BCA; WHO: intrahepatic bile duct cystadenoma) is, per definition, a benign cystic tumor lined by mucus-secreting epithelium which may include goblet cells and typically shows papillary infoldings. The cells may express carcinoembryonic antigen (Tomioka et al 1986). The tumor is usually multilocular and, at gross examination, well-defined by a fibrous capsule. The cavities of BCA contain a thin, opalescent or glairy fluid, or a mucinous viscous material. Two histological variants of BCA are recognized: a mucinous type (the more common variant) and the rare serous type (review: Colombari & Tsui 1995). Mucinous BCA usually occurs in middle-aged women, and about 80% of the patients are more than 30 years old (Ishak et al 1977). Fifty per cent are located in the right lobe, 40% in the left lobe, 10 to 20% occupy both lobes. A simultaneous occurrence with pancreatic mucinous cystic neoplasms has been reported (O'Shea et al 1987). Cyst diameters range from a few cm to almost 30 cm (mean: 15 cm). The immunohistochemical phenotype (cytokeratins, epithelial membrane antigen and carcinoembryonic antigen) is similar to that of bile duct epithelia, but cells with neuroendocrine features may also occur (Devaney et al 1994). Endocrine cells were found in BCA with or without mesenchymal stroma (see below), and were located beneath and among the columnar epithelial cells (Terada et al 1997). The finding of BCA with neuroendocrine differentiation may be related to the presence of neuro-endocrine cells in bile ducts and the capability of duct and ductule epithelia to undergo neuroendocrine differentiation (Kurumaya et al 1989, Roskams et al 1990, Roskams et al 1993). Furthermore, epithelial dysplasia has been noted suggesting transition to more aggressive forms of this tumor (Devaney et al 1994). Intracystic gallstones may be formed (Lei et al 1994). In female patients, BCA can show a distinct type of mesenchymal 'ovarian-like' stroma immunoreactive for vimentin, actin and desmin (hepatobiliary cystadenoma with mesenchymal stroma, CMS; Wheeler & Edmondson 1985, Weihing et al 1997). This stromal reaction may be related to the action of sex steroids, because there have been reports of such BCAs occurring in oral contraceptive users (Scully et al 1976, Suyama et al 1988), and immunostaining has demonstrated estrogen receptor (Scott et al 1995) or progesterone receptor expression (Grayson et al 1996, Weihing et al 1997) in the mesenchymal cells of the stroma.

BCA of the serous type is very rare, representing about 5% of the total number of intrahepatic cystic lesions of bile duct origin, but also showing a potential for malignant transformation. The tumor consists of numerous small cystic spaces lined by a single layer of cuboidal cells, thus being similar to serous cystadenoma of the pancreas. Rarely, BCA can ensue as a syndromatic disease, occurring together with renal and pancreatic cysts (Kennedy et al 1991).

Hepatobiliary cystadenocarcinoma (BCAC) with mesenchymal 'ovarian-like' stroma is observed in female patients; it may arise from preexisting BCA with stroma, and is believed to have a favorable prognosis. In contrast, BCAC without specific stroma is not associated with preexisting BCA, is found both in female and male patients, and is thought to be more aggressive (Devaney et al 1994). Cells of the latter variant may show considerable atypia, and transition zones between benign-looking epithelium and dysplastic areas occur. Apart from clinically manifest spread, histological invasion may be demonstrated in aggressive forms. Unusual situations include BCACs with squamous differentiation (Iemoto et al 1983), with foci of adeno-squamous carcinoma (Moore et al 1984) or with features of hepatocytes (Tomimatsu et al 1989).

BILE DUCT ADENOMA (Ch. 52)

Bile duct adenomas (synonyms: benign cholangioma, cholangioadenoma) are benign intrahepatic epithelial tumors of a few mm up to about 2 cm size (mean in a series of 152 cases: 5.8 mm; Allaire et al 1988), that are well circumscribed, nonencapsulated and usually subcapsular lesions. They are typically composed of small bile duct-like structures lined by normal-looking epithelium set in a fibrous stroma containing lymphocytes. Portal tract remnants, but not hepatocytes, may be enclosed. Cystic structures or bile are lacking. The tumor clinically presents as a nodule (mostly solitary) in an asymptomatic patient, frequently male, and not associated with polycystic disease (Allaire et al 1988, Cho et al 1978, Govindarajan & Peters 1984). Multiple bile duct adenomas containing alpha-1-antitrypsin inclusions have been reported in heterozygous (MZ) deficiency of the alpha-1-proteinase inhibitor (Scheele et al 1988). The tumors may contain an endocrine component (endocrine differentiation) as it has also been demonstrated in small bile ducts (O'Hara et al 1992). With respect to the pathogenesis of bile duct adenomas, it has been suggested that such tumors may either be neoplastic ('neoplastic type of adenoma') or hamartomas taking their origin from peribiliary glands ('hamartomatous adenoma'; Bhathal et al 1996). The question as to whether bile duct adenomas may represent precancerous lesions has not yet been settled, but there are larger lesions exhibiting cellular atypia, and few cases associated with cholangiocarcinoma have been reported (Foucar et al 1979, Hasebe et al 1995, Colombari & Tsui 1995).

Unusually large lesions with a predominance of fibrous stroma have been listed under the term, biliary adenofibroma (Tsui et al 1993). Problems arising with respect to the proper classification of biliary adenomas and hamartomas have recently been addressed (Tsui 1998).

A very rare bile duct tumor of still uncertain dignity is the hepatobiliary solid-papillary tumor (papillary cystic tumor) which has its counterpart in the pancreas (Kim et al 1990).

BILIARY MICROHAMARTOMA

Biliary microhamartoma (BMH; synonyms: biliary hamartoma, microhamartoma, von Meyenburg complex) is a benign lesion consisting of a collection of bile ducts set in a fibrous stroma which may be hyalinized. This definition is almost identical with that of biliary adenoma, but BMHs may contain bile and may be associated with polycystic disease, which is not the case in biliary adenoma. Furthermore, these lesions are usually multiple and rarely exceed 5 mm in size (Chung 1970, Thommesen 1978, Tsui 1998), but the benign lesions may nevertheless have clinical significance due to their possible interpretation as metastases, because they frequently come as bilateral nodules (Eisenberg et al 1986, Tan et al 1989). The prevalence in surgical specimens appears to be about 0.6%, in autopsy specimens about 0.7%, the prevalence apparently increasing with age. This may be due to the fact that the disorder manifests in the finest branches of the intrahepatic biliary tree, which develop in postnatal and adult life. It has been proposed that BMHs result from a faulty remodeling or arrest of the ductal plate (Desmet 1985). This hypothesis is underlined by the observation that BMHs are a frequent finding in other types of biliary disease related to a disordered development, such as polycystic disease, congenital liver fibrosis and Caroli's disease (Ramos et al 1990, Redston & Wanless 1996), leading to the suggestion that patients with numerous BMHs may have a very mild form of autosomal dominant polycystic kidney disease (ADPKD). Therefore, two types of BMH may exist, one sporadic and one associated with genetic polycystic disease.

The possible malignant potential of BMHs has not been sufficiently clarified so far, even though few reports demonstrated a transformation of the lesions or at least an association with cholangiocarcinoma (Homer et al 1968, Dekker et al 1989, Burns et al 1990).

BILIARY PAPILLOMATOSIS

Biliary papillomatosis (WHO: papillomatosis/adenomatosis; Figs 51.17, 51.18) refers to an entity that has already been addressed in a previous section, and which represents a condition characterized by either solitary or multiple recurring papillary adenomas that may involve extensive areas of bile ducts. Even though the diffuse type with multiple lesions may start with a single tumor, there are patients exhibiting solitary papillomas not showing a tendency for generalized disease and thus having a better prognosis. Overall, it is a rare disorder usually occurring in middle-aged men and women, males being about twice as frequently involved (Madden & Smith 1974, Gouma et al 1984, Brönnimann et al 1996; review: Colombari & Tsui 1995). More than 50% of the patients exhibit diffuse involvement of both, extrahepatic and intraheptic ducts, while close to 30% had exclusively intrahepatic, and close to 20% exclusively extrahepatic duct disease.

Solitary papillomas are most frequently located at the level of Vater's papilla, followed in frequency by the choledochal duct and the common hepatic duct. In case of diffuse disease, the pancreatic duct may be involved as well (Hubens et al 1991). Microscopy shows a papillary adenoma with mucus-forming cells of columnar shape. Complex glandular structures may be found, and an admixture with neuroendocrine cells may be observed. The major difficulties arising in the assessment of such lesions, and particularly in case of diffuse disease, is the judgment with respect to malignancy. Similar to the situations of dysplastic changes occurring in the papillary duct hyperplasias evolving in primary sclerosing cholangitis (Ludwig et al 1992) and in recurrent pyogenic cholangitis (Tsui & Tse 1994), variable degrees of cellular atypia or dysplasia may develop in papillomatosis (Fig. 51.19), but it is hardly possible to morphologically predict which patient will develop malignancy. Few cases were reported to show a metachronous development of cancer, whereas about 12% of the patients exhibited synchronous carcinoma (Fig. 51.20; review: Brönnimann et al 1996), resulting in the view that biliary papillomatosis might, in principle, be some sort of low-grade adenocarcinoma (Helpap 1977). More research is clearly needed to better define potential risk groups, and new methods such as the assessment of oncogene mutations may be of additional help (Ohta et al 1993).

NONTUMOROUS HYPERPLASTIC AND DYSPLASTIC LESIONS

Hyperplastic lesions associated with dysplasia and occurring in patients with ulcerative colitis have already been discussed (Haworth et al 1989). Several studies reported an increased incidence of peripheral cholangiocarcinoma in the presence of hepatolithiasis. In these situations, chronic proliferative (hyperplastic) cholangitis caused by the stones may progress through atypical epithelial hyperplasia to carcinoma (Falchuk et al 1976, Nakanuma et al 1985, Koga et al 1985). Recently, is has been suggested that mucosal dysplasia observed near stones may represent a precursor lesion of the so-called intraductal spreading type of peripheral cholangiocarcinoma in the presence of hepatolithiasis (Ohta et al 1991). Papillary hyperplasia of bile ducts may, however, also develop without any signs of atypia, and is thought to be a primary lesion of uncertain evolution (Albores-Saavedra et al 1990). Whether metaplastic bile duct changes, such as the squamous metaplasia developing in AIDS patients with cryptosporidial cholangitis (Kline et al 1993), may enter a carcinogenic pathway is not yet known.

BENIGN AMPULLARY TUMORS

This group of tumors comprises adenoma, distal variants of biliary papillomatosis, ampullary hamartoma, adenomyoma, granular cell schwannoma, neural tumors, ampullary stromal tumors, inflammatory pseudotumors, and heterotopias. Ampullary adenoma is a rare lesion, which exhibits, depending on the site, either a more tubular or more papillary growth pattern, and is a putative precancerous lesion. It affects both sexes equally and is uncommon before the age of 50. It has been reported to occur in association with familiary adenomatous polyposis and polycystic disease (Anderson & Gregor 1961, Yamaguchi & Enjoji 1991, Cattel & Pyrtek 1950, Norton et al 1995).

RARE TUMORS OF THE BILIARY TRACT

Some biliary tract carcinomas can show a neuroendocrine differentiation, and particularly in the extrahepatic biliary tract this phenomenon appears to be more frequent than generally recognized (Hsu et al 1991). Neuroendocrine patterns range from predominantly exocrine carcinoma with occasional neuroendocrine cells to neuroendocrine tumors with few epithelial cells of ductal type. The presence of predominant neuroendocrine differentiation in carcinomas of the extrahepatic biliary tract seems to be associated with shorter survival time than purely or predominantly exocrine carcinomas (Hsu et al 1991). Rarely, bile duct adenomas contain, in addition to small-caliber ducts, periductular nests and clusters of uniform round cells. These cells may elaborate several endocrine markers, and benign tumors of this type, different from conventional bile duct adenomas, have been reported under the term 'bile duct adenoma with endocrine component' (O'Hara et al 1992). One may suggest that tumors of this type and some of the neoplasms described below are derived from argyrophil and, in part, somatostatin containing cells, which are physiologically present in the biliary tree (Kurumaya et al 1989).

Primary biliary carcinoid tumors are exceedingly rare (Judge et al 1976, Barron-Rodriguez et al 1991, Rugge et al 1992). When gallbladder carcinoids are excluded, no more than about ten cases have ever been reported. Embryologically, the gallbladder and the bile ducts are derived from the endodermal lining of the foregut, so that carcinoid tumors in these structures may be classified as foregut carcinoids (Williams & Sandler 1983). This is underlined by the observation that bile duct carcinoids may show tubular and trabecular patterns as most foregut carcinoids (Soga's mixed type B/C; Soga & Tazawa 1971). A malignant counterpart of carcinoid tumors, small cell neuroendocrine (oat cell) tumors, has been observed in the common bile duct (Van der Wal et al 1990), and neuroendocrine carcinomas can occur in the ampullary region (Sanchez-Sosa et al 1991).

On rare occasions, biliary tract carcinomas may show a histology clearly different from that of classical adenocarci-noma. Differentiation of neoplastic biliocytes into squamous epithelium can occur, thus leading to the morphology of adenosquamous carcinoma, which has been encountered in intrahepatic bile ducts (Nakajima & Kondo 1990) and in a biliary cystadenocarcinoma (Moore et al 1984). Squamous differentiation associated with formation of mucus-containing cells is typical for mucoepidermoid carcinoma, well defined as a common tumor of salivary glands, but also, rarely, arising in the biliary tract (Koo et al 1982). Malignant melanoma can metastasize to the bile ducts (O'Connel et al 1984), but bile ducts can also be the site of apparently primary malignant melanoma (Carstens et al 1986, Deugnier et al 1991). Bile duct tumors with sarcomatoid features may contain considerable numbers of giant cells, and may in fact correspond to unusual variants of carcinomas with partial giant cell transformation (Haratake et al 1992). In contrast, true sarcomas occur in infants, and usually are rhabdomyosarcomas (Davis et al 1969). Another mesenchymal tumor known to arise in bile ducts is the granular cell tumor (LiVolsi et al 1973, Whisnant et al 1974). Notwithstanding the fact that the biology of these lesions is benign, attention has to be drawn to the finding that some granular cell tumors of the extrahepatic bile ducts are multicentric (Aisner et al 1982), and may extend into the periductal connective tissue and adjacent lymph nodes, closely simulating malignancy. Moreover, hyperplasia of the overlying epithelium may lead to confusion with epithelial neoplasms (Eisen et al 1991). Paraganglioma, a benign tumor also listed in the recent classification of tumors by the WHO (Albores-Saavedra et al 1991), is composed of chief cells and sustentacular cells, and is rare, but may give rise to biliary obstruction when developing in extrahepatic bile ducts.

A curious lesion at the distal extremity of the common bile duct at the papilla is adenomyoma. This entity consists of a dense mass of intertwined muscle bands, collagen and epithelial structures forming distorted lumina. This is a benign lesion, and its origin is unclear, but the possibility of duct occlusion with the development of obstructive jaundice remains.

Finally, the common bile duct can be involved by multiple eosinophilic granuloma (Jones et al 1981), and several tumor-like lesions may occur, of which 15 are included in the second edition of the WHO classification of tumors (Albores-Saavedra et al 1991) .

ACKNOWLEDGMENT

The author wishes to acknowledge the contribution made by Agnes Gorrisen, who was responsible for most of the photography and the excellent secretarial help of Erna Müller.

REFERENCES

Aisner S C, Khaneja S, Ramirez O 1982 Multiple granular cell tumors of the gallbladder and biliary tree. Archives of Pathology and Laboratory Medicine 106: 470–471

Albores-Saavedra J, Defortuna SM, Smothermon WE 1990 Primary papillary hyperplasia of the gallbladder and cystic and common bile ducts. Human Pathology 21: 228–231

Albores-Saavedra J, Henson D E, Sobin L H 1991 Histological typing of tumours of the gallbladder and extrahepatic bile ducts. 2nd edn, International Histological Classification of Tumours, WHO, Springer-Verlag, Berlin

Albores-Saavedra J, Henson D E, Sobin L H 1992 The WHO histological classification of tumors of the gallbladder and extrahepatic bile ducts. A commentary on the Second Edition. Cancer 70: 410–414

Alexander J R, Andrews J M, Buchi K N, Lee R G, Becker J M, Burt R W 1989 High prevalence of adenomatous polyps of the duodenal papilla in familial adenomatous polyposis. Digestive Diseases Sciences 34: 167–170

Allaire G S, Rabin L, Ishak K G, Sesterhenn IA 1988 Bile duct adenoma. A study of 152 cases. American Journal of Surgical Pathology 12: 708–715

Altmann H W 1978 Pathology of human liver tumors. In: Remmer H, Bolt H M, Bannasch P, Popper H (eds) Primary liver tumors. MTP Press, Lancaster, ch 4, p 53–71

Anderson MC, Gregor WH 1961 Adenoma of the ampulla of Vater. American Journal of Surgery 102: 865–871

Baczako K, Büchler MW, Beger H-G, Kirkpatrick CJ, Haferkamp O 1985 Morphogenesis and possible precursor lesions of invasive carcinoma of the papilla of Vater: Epithelial dysplasia and adenoma. Human Pathology 16: 305–310

Baggenstoss A H 1938 Major duodenal papilla. Archives of Pathology 26: 853–868

Bannasch P 1978 Cellular and subcellular pathology of liver carcinogenesis. In: Remmer H, Bolt H M, Bannasch P, Popper H (eds) Primary liver tumors. MTP Press, Lancaster ch 6, p 87–111

Barbacid M 1987 Ras genes. Annual Review of Biochemistry 56: 779–827

Barron-Rodriguez L, Manivel J C, Mendez-Sanchez N, Jessurun J 1991 Carcinoid tumor of the common bile duct: evidence for its origin in metaplastic endocrine cells. American Journal of Gastroenterology 86: 1073–1076

Bertoni G, Sassatelli R, Nigrisoli E, Pennazio M, Tansini P, Arrigoni A, Ponz de Leon M, Rossini FP, Bedogni G 1996 High prevalence of adenomas and microadenomas of the duodenal papilla and periampullary region in patients with familial adenomatous polyposis. European Journal of Gastroenterology and Hepatology 8: 1201–1206

Bhathal P S, Hughes N R, Goodman Z D 1996 The so-called bile duct adenoma is a peribiliary gland hamartoma. American Journal of Surgical Pathology 20: 858–864

Bhuiya M R, Nimura Y, Kamiya J et al 1993 Clinicopathological studies on perineural invasion of bile duct carcinoma : Multivariate statistical analysis. World Journal of Surgery 14: 653–657

Bismuth H, Corlette M B 1975 Intrahepatic cholangiocentric anastomosis in carcinoma of the hilus of the liver. Surgery, Gynecology and Obstetrics 140: 170–178

Blumgart L H, Kennedy A 1973 Carcinoma of the ampulla of Vater and duodenum: a clinical and pathological study of 31 cases. British Journal of Surgery 60: 33–40

Bosma A 1990 Surgical pathology of cholangiocarcinoma of the liver hilus (Klatskin tumor). Seminars in Liver Disease 10: 85–90

Brönnimann S, Zimmermann A, Baer H U 1996 Die diffuse Gallengangspapillomatose: Hohe Rezidivrate und grosses Entartungspotential. Chirurgie 67: 93–97

Burns C D, Kuhns J G, Wieman T J 1990 Cholangiocarcinoma in association with multiple biliary microhamartomas. Archives of Pathology and Laboratory Medicine 114: 1287–1289

Caroli J 1973 Diseases of the intrahepatic biliary tree. Clinical Gastroenterology 2: 147–161

Caroli J, Corcos V 1964 La dilatation congenitale des voies biliaires intrahepatiques. Revue Medico-Chirurgical des Maladies du Foie, de la Rate et du Pancreas 39: 1–70

Carriaga M T and Henson D E 1995 Liver, gallbladder, extrahepatic bile ducts, and pancreas. Cancer 75: 171–190

Carstens P H, Ghazl C, Carnighan R H, Brenner M S 1986 Primary malignant melanoma of the common bile duct. Human Pathology 17: 1282–1285

Cattel R B, Pyrtek L J 1950 Premalignant lesions of the ampulla of Vater. Surgery, Gynecogy and Obstetrics 90: 21–30

Chapman R W, Marborgh B A, Rhodes J M et al 1980 Primary sclerosing cholangitis: a review of its clinical features, cholangiography and hepatic histology. Gut 21: 870–877

Chen M F, Jan Y Y, Chen T C 1998 Clinical studies of mucin-producing cholangiocellular carcinoma. A study of 22 histopathology-proven cases. Annals of Surgery 227: 63–69

Cho C, Rullis I, Rogers L S 1978 Bile duct adenomas as liver nodules. Archives of Surgery 113: 272–274

Chow L T C, Ahuja A T, Kwong K H, Fung K S C, Lai C K W, Lau J W Y 1997 Mucinous cholangiocarcinoma: an unusual complication of hepatolithiasis and recurrent pyogenic cholangitis. Histopathology 30: 491–494

Christopherson W M, Mays E T, Barrows G 1978 Hepatocellular carcinoma in young women on oral contraceptives. Lancet ii: 38–39

Chung E B 1970 Multiple bile-duct hamartomas. Cancer 26: 287–296

Colombari R and Tsui W M S 1995 Biliary tumors of the liver. Seminars in Liver Disease 15: 402–413

Compton C C 1997 Protocol for the examination of specimens from patients with carcinoma of the ampulla of Vater. A basis for checklists. Archives of Pathology and Laboratory Medicine 121: 673–677

Converse C F, Reagan J W, deCosse J J 1971 Ulcerative colitis and carcinoma of the bile ducts. American Journal of Surgery 121: 39–45

Cruickshank A H 1961 The pathology of 111 cases of primary hepatic malignancy collected in the Liverpool region. Journal of Clinical Pathology 14: 120–131

Davis G L, Kissane J M, Ishak K G 1969 Embryonal rhabdomyosarcoma (sarcoma botryoides) of the biliary tree. Cancer 24: 333–342

Dekker A, Ten Kate FJW, Terpstra OT 1989 Cholangiocarcinoma associated with multiple bile-duct hamartomas of the liver. Digestive Diseases and Sciences 34: 952–958

Desmet V J 1972 Morphologic and histochemical aspects of cholestasis. In: Popper H, Schaffner F (eds) Progress in liver disease. Grune and Stratton, New York, vol 4, p 97–132

Desmet V J 1985 Intrahepatic bile ducts under the lens. Journal of Hepatology 1: 545–559

Deugnier Y, Turlin B, Lehry D et al 1991 Malignant melanoma of the hepatic and common bile ducts. A case report and review of the literature. Archives of Pathology and Laboratory Medicine 115: 915–917

Devaney K, Goodman Z D, Ishak K G 1994 Hepatobiliary cystadenoma and cystadenocarcinoma. A light microscopic and immunohistochemical study of 70 patients. American Journal of Surgical Pathology 18: 1078–1091

Diamantis I, Karamitopoulou E, Perentes E, Zimmermann A 1995 p53 protein immunoreactivity in extrahepatic bile duct and gallbladder cancer. Correlation with tumor grade and survival. Hepatology 22: 774–779

Edmondson H A 1976 Benign epithelial tumors and tumorlike lesions of the liver. In: Okuda K, Peters R L (eds) Hepatocellular carcinoma. Wiley, New York, ch 13, p 309–330

Eisen R N, Kirby W M, O'Quinn J L 1991 Granular cell tumor of the biliary tree. American Journal of Surgical Pathology 15: 460–465

Eisenberg D, Hurwitz L, Yu A C 1986 CT and sonography of multiple bile-duct hamartomas simulating malignant liver disease (case report). AJR 147: 279–280

Falchuk K R, Lesser P B, Galdabini J J, Isselbacher K J 1976 Cholangiocarcinoma is related to chronic intrahepatic cholangitis and hepatolithiasis. American Journal of Gastroenterology 66: 57–61

Fausto N, Shank P R 1983 Oncogene expression in liver regeneration and hepatocarcinogenesis. Hepatology 3: 1016–1023

Farrell R J, Noonan N, Khan I M, Goggins M, Kelleher D P, Keeling P W N 1996 Carcinoma of the ampulla of Vater: a tumour with poor prognosis? European Journal of Gastroenterology and Hepatology 8: 139–144

Fieber S S, Nance FC 1997 Choledochal cyst and neoplasm. A comprehensive review of 106 cases and presentation of two original cases. American Surgeon 63: 982–987

Flavell D J, Lucas S B 1982 Potentiation by the human liver fluke, *Opisthorchis viverrini*, of the carcinogenic action of N-nitrosodimethylamine upon the biliary epithelium of the hamster. British Journal of Cancer 46: 985–989

Foucar E, Kaplan L R, Gold J H et al 1979 Well-differentiated peripheral cholangiocarcinoma with an unusual clinical course. Gastroenterology 77: 347–353

Gall E A, Dobrogorski O 1964 Hepatic alterations in obstructive jaundice. American Journal of Clinical Pathology 41: 126–139

Gallagher P J, Millis R R, Mitchinson M J 1972 Congenital dilatation of the intrahepatic bile ducts with cholangiocarcinoma. Journal of Clinical Pathology 25: 804–808

Gardner H A R, Matthews J, Ciano P S 1990 A signet-ring cell carcinoma of the ampulla of Vater. Archives of Pathology and Laboratory Medicine 114: 1071–1072

Gibson J B 1971 Parasites, liver disease and liver cancer. In: Liver, cancer. IARC Scientific Publications, Lyon, p 42

Gibson J B 1978 Histological typing of tumours of the liver, biliary tract and pancreas. World Health Organization, Geneva

Goodman Z D, Ishak K G, Laneloss J M, Sesterhenn I A, Rabin L 1985 Combined hepatocellular cholangiocarcinoma. A histologic and immunochemical study. Cancer 55: 124–135

Gouma DJ, Mutum SS, Benjamin IS, Blumgart LH 1984 Intrahepatic biliary papillomatosis. British Journal of Surgery 71: 72–74

Govindarajan S, Peters R L 1984 The bile duct adenoma. A lesion distinct from Meyenburg complex. Archives in Pathology and Laboratory Medicine 108: 922–924

Grayson W, Teare J, Myburgh J A, Paterson A C 1996 Immunohistochemical demonstration of progesterone receptor in hepatobiliary cystadenoma with mesenchymal stroma. Histopathology 29: 461–463

Haratake J, Yamada H, Horie A, Inokuma T 1992 Giant cell tumorlike cholangiocarcinoma associated with systemic cholelithiasis. Cancer 69: 2444–2448

Harnois D M, Que F G, Celli A, LaRusso N F, Gores G J 1997 Bcl-2 is overexpressed and alters the threshold for apoptosis in a cholangiocarcinoma cell line. Hepatology 26: 884–890

Hasebe T, Sakamoto M, Mukai K, Kawano N, Konishi M, Ryu M, Fukamachi S, Hirohashi S 1995 Cholangiocarcinoma arising in bile duct adenoma with focal area of bile duct hamartoma. Virchows Archiv 426: 209–213

Haworth A C, Manley P N, Groll A, Pace R 1989 Bile duct carcinoma and biliary tract dysplasia in chronic ulcerative colitis. Archives of Pathology and Laboratory Medicine 113: 434–436

Hayashi S, Miyazaki M, Kondo Y, Nakajima N 1994 Invasive growth patterns of hepatic hilar ductal carcinoma. A histologic analysis of 18 surgical cases. Cancer 73: 2922–2929

Hayes D H, Bolton J S, Willis G W, Bowen J C 1987 Carcinoma of the ampulla of Vater. Annals of Surgery 206: 572–577

Helpap B 1977 Malignant papillomatosis of the intrahepatic bile ducts. Acta Hepatogastroenterologica 24: 419–425

Homer L W, White H J, Read R C 1968 Neoplastic transformation of v. Meyenburg complexes of the liver. Journal of Pathology and Bacteriology 96: 499–502

Honda N, Cobb C, Lechago J 1986 Bile duct carcinoma associated with multiple von Meyenburg complexes in the liver. Human Pathology 17: 1287–1290

Hruban R H, Sturm P D J, Slebos R J C, Wilentz R E, Musler A R, Yeo C J, Sohn T A, Van Velthuysen M L F, Offerhaus G J A 1997 Can K-ras codon 12 mutations be used to distinguish benign bile duct proliferations from metastases in the liver? A molecular analysis of 101 liver lesions from 93 patients. Am J Pathol 151: 943–949

Hsu H C, Chen C C, Huang G T, Lee P H 1996 Clonal Epstein–Barre virus associated cholangiocarcinoma with lymphoepithelial component. Human Pathology 27: 848–850

Hsu W, Deziel D J, Gould V E et al 1991 Neuroendocrine differentiation and prognosis of extrahepatic biliary tract carcinomas. Surgery 110: 604–611

Hubens G, Delvaux G, Willems G et al 1991 Papillomatosis of the intra- and extrahepatic bile ducts with involvement of the pancreatic duct. Hepatogastroenterology 38: 413–418

Iemoto Y, Kondo Y, Nakano T et al 1983 Biliary cystadenocarcinoma diagnosed by liver biopsy performed under ultrasonographic guidance. Gastroenterology 84: 399–403

Inglis D A, Farmer R G 1975 Adenocarcinoma of the bile ducts. Relationship of anatomic location to clinical features. Digestive Diseases 20: 253–261

Ishak K G, Willis G W, Cummins S D, Bullock A A 1977 Biliary cystadenoma and cystadenocarcinoma. Report of 14 cases and review of the literature. Cancer 39: 322–338

Johnson D E, Herndier B G, Medeiros L J et al 1988 The diagnostic utility of the keratin profiles of hepatocellular carcinoma and cholangiocarcinoma. American Journal of Surgical Pathology 12: 187–197

Jonas S, Springmeier G, Tauber R, Wiedenmann B, Lobeck H, Gessner R, Kreft B, Kling N, Moelling K, Neuhaus P 1998 p53 mutagenesis in Klatskin tumors. Human Pathology 29: 955–960

Jones M B, Voet R, Pagani J, Lotysch M, O'Connell T, Koretz R L 1981 Multiple eosinophilic granuloma involving the common duct histologic and cholangiographic findings. Gastroenterology 80: 384–389

Judge D M, Dickman P S, Trapukdi S 1976 Nonfunctioning argyrophylic tumor (APUDoma) of the hepatic duct: simplified methods of detecting biogenic amines in tissue. American Journal of Clinical Pathology 66: 40–45

Kagawa Y, Kashihara S, Kuramoto S, Maetani S 1978 Carcinoma arising in a congenitally dilated biliary tract. Gastroenterology 74: 1286–1294

Kato M, Nimura Y, Kamiya J, Kondo S, Nagino M, Miyachi M, Kanai M, Igaki H, Maeda S 1997 Carcinoma of the common bile duct with superficial spread to the intrahepatic segmental bile ducts: A case report. American Surgeon 63: 943–947

Kennedy S M, Hashida Y, Malatack J J 1991 Polycystic kidneys, pancreatic cysts, and cystadenomatous bile ducts in the oral-facial-digital syndrome type I. Archives of Pathology and Laboratory Medicine 115: 519–523

Kim Y I, Kim S T, Lee G K, Choi B I 1990 Papillary cystic tumor of the liver. Cancer 65: 2740–2746

Kimura W, Ohtsubo K 1988 Incidence, sites of origin, and immunohistochemical and histochemical characteristics of atypical epithelium and minute carcinoma of the papilla of Vater. Cancer 61: 1394–1402

Klatskin G K 1965 Adenocarcinoma of the hepatic duct at its bifurcation within the porta hepatis. American Journal of Medicine 38: 241–256

Kline T J, De Las Morenas T, O'Brien M, Smith B F, Afdhal N H 1993

Squamous metaplasia of extrahepatic biliary system in an AIDS patient with cryptosporidia and cholangitis. Digestive Diseases and Science 38: 960–962

Koga A, Ichimiya H, Yamaguchi K, Miyazaki K, Nakayama F 1985 Hepatolithiasis associated with cholangiocarcinoma. Cancer 55: 2826–2829

Kojiro M, Kawabata K, Kawano Y, Shirai F, Takemoto N, Nakashima T 1982 Hepatocellular carcinoma presenting as intrabile duct tumor growth. A clinicopathologic study of 24 cases. Cancer 49: 2144–2147

Koo J, Ho J, Wong J, Ong G B 1982 Mucoepidermoid carcinoma of the bile duct. Annals of Surgery 196: 140–148

Kozuka S, Kurashina M, Tsubone M, Hachisuka K, Yasui A 1984 Significance of intestinal metaplasia for the evolution of cancer in the biliary tract. Cancer 54: 2277–2285

Kurumaya H, Ohta G, Nakanuma Y 1989 Endocrine cells in the intrahepatic biliary tree in normal livers and hepatolithiasis. Archives of Pathology and Laboratory Medicine 113: 143–147

Kurashina M, Kozuka S, Nakasima N et al 1988 Relationship of intrahepatic bile duct hyperplasia to cholangiocellular carcinoma. Cancer 61: 2469–2474

Kuwayti K, Baggenstoss A H, Stauffer M H, Priestley J T 1957 Carcinoma of major intrahepatic and extrahepatic bile ducts exclusive of papilla of Vater. Surgery, Gynecology and Obstetrics 104: 357–375

Lei S, Domenico D R, Howard J M 1994 Intrahepatic biliary cystadenoma with intracystic gallstone formation. HPB Surgery 7: 241–247

Lindor K D, Wiesner R H, MacCary R L et al 1990 Advances in primary sclerosing cholangitis. American Journal of Medicine 89: 73–80

LiVolsi V A, Perzin K H, Badder E M, Price J B, Porter M 1973 Granular cell tumors of the biliary tract. Archives of Pathology 95: 13–17

Lory J, Schweizer W, Blumgart LH, Zimmermann A 1994 The pathology of the atrophy/hypertrophy complex (AHC) of the liver. A light microscopic and immunohistochemical study. Histology and Histopathology 9: 541–554

Ludwig J 1989 Surgical pathology of the syndrome of primary sclerosing cholangitis. American Journal of Surgical Pathology 13: 43–49

Ludwig J, Wahlstrom HE, Batts KP, Wiesner RH 1992 Papillary bile duct dysplasia in primary sclerosing cholangitis. Gastroenterology 102: 2134–2138

MacSween R N M 1974 A clinicopathological review of 100 cases of primary malignant tumours of the liver. Journal of Clinical Pathology 27: 669–682

Madden J J, Smith G W 1974 Multiple biliary papillomatosis. Cancer 34: 1316–1320

Mecklin J P, Jarvinen H J, Virolainen M 1992 The association between cholangiocarcinoma and hereditary nonpolyposis colorectal carcinoma. Cancer 69: 1112–1114

Melnick P J 1955 Polycystic liver; analysis of 70 cases. Archives of Pathology 59: 162–168

Meyerowitz B R, Aird I 1962 Carcinoma of the hepatic ducts within the liver. British Journal of Surgery 50: 178–184

Moore S, Gold R P, Lebwohl O et al 1984 Adenosquamous carcinoma of the liver arising in biliary cystadeno-carcinoma: clinical, radiologic and pathologic features with review of literature. Journal of Clinical Gastroenterology 6: 267–275

Nakajima T, Kondo Y, Miyazaki M, Okui K 1988 A histopathologic study of 102 cases of intrahepatic cholangiocarcinoma: Histologic classification and modes of spreading. Human Pathology 19: 1228–1234

Nakajima T, Kondo Y 1989 Well-differentiated cholangiocarcinoma: diagnostic significance of morphologic and immunohistochemical parameters. American Journal of Surgical Pathology 13: 569–573

Nakajima T, Kondo Y 1990 A clinicopathologic study of intrahepatic cholangiocarcinoma containing a component of squamous cell carcinoma. Cancer 65: 1401–1404

Nakajima T, Sugano I, Matsuzaki O et al 1992 Biliary cystadenocarcinoma of the liver. A clinicopathologic and histochemical evaluation of nine cases. Cancer 69: 2426–2432

Nakanuma Y, Terada T, Ohta G et al 1982 Caroli's disease in congenital hepatic fibrosis and infantile polycystic disease. Liver 2: 346–354

Nakanuma Y, Terada T, Tanaka Y, Ohta G 1985 Are hepatolithiasis and cholangiocarcinoma aetiologically related? Virchows Archiv (A) 406: 45–58

Nakao A, Harada A, Nonami T, Kishimoto W, Takeda S, Ito K, Takagi H 1994 Prognosis of cancer of the duodenal papilla of Vater in relation to clinicopathological tumor extension. Hepatogastroenterology 41: 73–78

Neoptolemos J P, Talbot I C, Shaw D C, Carr-Locke D L 1988 Long-term survival after resection of ampullary carcinoma is associated independently with tumor grade and a new staging classification that assesses local invasiveness. Cancer 61: 1403–1407

Newmann R D, LiVolsi V A, Rosenthal N S, Burreli N, Ball T J 1976 Adenocarcinoma in biliary papillomatosis. Gastroenterology 70: 779–782

Noda Y, Watanabe H, Iida M, Narisawa R, Kurosaki I, Iwafuchi M, Sato M, Ajioka Y 1992 Histologic follow-up of ampullary adenoma in patients with familial adenomatosis coli. Cancer 70: 1847–1856

Nonomura A, Ohta G, Hayasi M et al 1987 Immunohistochemical localization of ras p21 and carcinoembryonic antigens (CEA) in cholangiocarcinoma. Liver 7: 142–148

Nonomura A, Mizukami Y, Matsubara F et al 1989 Human choriogonadotropin and alpha-fetoprotein in cholangiocarcinoma in relation to the expression of ras p21: an immunohistochemical study. Liver 9: 205–215

Norton I D, Pokorny C S, Painter D M, Johnson J R, Perkins K W 1995 Fraternal sisters with adult polycystic kidney disease and adenoma of the ampulla of Vater. Gastroenterology 109: 2007–2009

O'Connel J B, Whittemore D M, Russel J et al 1984 Malignant melanoma metastatic to the cystic and common bile ducts. Cancer 53: 184–186

O'Hara B J, McCue P A, Miettinen M 1992 Bile duct adenomas with endocrine component. Immunohistochemical study and comparison with conventional bile duct adenomas. American Journal of Surgical Pathology 16: 21–25

Ohashi K, Nakajima Y, Kanehiro H, Tsutsumi M, Taki J, Aomatsu Y, Yoshimura A, Ko S, Kin T, Yagura K, Konishi Y, Nakano H 1995 Ki-ras mutations and p53 protein expressions in intrahepatic cholangiocarcinomas : relation to gross tumor morphology. Gastroenterology 109: 1612–1617

Ohashi K, Tsutsumi M, Nakajima Y, Nakano H, Konishi Y 1996 Ki-ras point mutations and proliferation activity in biliary tract carcinomas. British Journal of Cancer 74: 930–935

Ohta H, Yamaguchi Y, Yamakawa O et al 1993 Biliary papillomatosis with the point mutation of K-ras gene arising in congenital choledochal cyst. Gastroenterology 105: 1209–1212

Ohta T, Nagakawa T, Ueda N, Nakamura T, Akiyama T, Ueno K, Miyazaki I 1991 Mucosal dysplasia of the liver and the intraductal variant of peripheral cholangiocarcinoma in hepatolithiasis. Cancer 68: 2217–2223

Okuda K, Kubo Y, Okazaki N, Arishima T, Hashimoto M, Jinnouchi S et al 1977 Clinical aspects of intrahepatic bile duct carcinoma including hilar carcinoma: a study of 57 autopsy-proven cases. Cancer 39: 232–246

O'Shea J S, Shah D, Cooperman A et al 1987 Biliary cystadenocarcinoma of extrahepatic duct origin arising in previously benign cystadenoma. American Journal of Gastroenterology 82: 1306–1310

Ramos A, Torres V E, Holley K E et al 1990 The liver in autosomal dominant polycystic kidney disease. Archives of Pathology and Laboratory Medicine 114: 180–184

Redston M S, Wanless I R 1996 The hepatic von Meyenburg complex with hepatic and renal cysts. Modern Pathology 9: 233–237

Rijken A M, Van Gulik T M, Polak M M, Sturm P D J, Gouma D J,

Offerhaus G J A 1998 Diagnostic and prognostic value of incidence of K-ras codon 12 mutations in resected distal bile duct carcinoma. Journal of Surgical Oncology 68: 187–192

Rizzi P M, Ryder S D, Portmann B, Ramage J K, Naoumov N V, Williams R 1996 p53 protein overexpression in cholangiocarcinoma arising in primary sclerosing cholangitis. Gut 38: 265–268

Rosen C B, Nagorney D M 1991 Cholangiocarcinoma complicating primary sclerosing cholangitis. Seminars in Liver Disease 11: 26–30

Rosen C B, Nagorney D M, Wiesner R H et al 1991 Cholangiocarcinoma complicating primary sclerosing cholangitis. Annals of Surgery 213: 21–25

Roskams T, van den Oord J, De Vos R, Desmet VJ 1990 Neuroendocrine features of reactive bile ductules in cholestatic liver disease. American Journal of Pathology 137: 1019–1025

Roskams T, Campos R V, Drucker D J, Desmet V J 1993 Reactive human bile ductules express parathyroid hormone-related peptide. Histopathology 23: 11–19

Ross A P, Braasch J W 1973 Ulcerative colitis and carcinoma of the proximal bile ducts. Gut 14: 94–97

Ruebner B H, Montgomery C K 1982 Pathology of the liver and biliary tract. Wiley, New York, p 211

Rugge M, Sonego F, Militello C et al 1992 Primary carcinoid tumor of the cystic and common bile ducts. American Journal of Pathology 16: 802–807

Sanchez-Sosa S, Angeles A A, Orozco H, Larriva-Sahd J 1991 Neuroendocrine carcinoma of the ampulla of Vater. A case of absence of somatostatin in a vasoactive intestinal polypeptide-, bombesin-, and cholecystokinin-producing tumor. American Journal of Clinical Pathology 95: 51–54

Sarker A B, Hoshida Y, Akagi S, Hayashi K, Murakami I, Jeon H J, Takahashi K, Akagi T 1992 An immunohistochemical and ultrastructural study of case of small-cell neuroendocrine carcinoma in the ampullary region of the duodenum. Acta Pathologica Japonica 42: 529–535

Sato T, Yamamoto K, Ouchi A, Imaoka Y, Tokumura H, Matsushiro T 1995 Undifferentiated carcinoma of the duodenal ampulla. Journal of Gastroenterology 30: 517–519

Scheele P M, Bonar M J, Zumwalt R, Mukunda B, Ray B 1988 Bile duct adenomas in heterozygous (MZ) deficiency of alpha1-protease inhibitor. Archives of Pathology and Laboratory Medicine 112: 945–947

Schweizer W, Duda P, Tanner S, Balsiger D, Höflin F, Blumgart L H, Zimmermann A 1995 Experimental atrophy/hypertrophy complex (AHC) of the liver: portal vein, but not bile duct obstruction, is the main driving force for the development of AHC in the rat. Journal of Hepatology 23: 71–78

Scott F R, More L, Dhillon A P 1995 Hepatobiliary cystadenoma with mesenchymal stroma: expression of oestrogen receptors in formalin-fixed tissue. Histopathology 26: 555–558

Scully R E, Galdabini J J, McNeely B U 1976 Case records of the Massachusetts General Hospital. New England Journal of Medicine 295: 268–275

Seifert E, Schulte F, Stolte M 1992 Adenoma and carcinoma of the duodenum and papilla of Vater: a clinicopathologic study. American Journal of Gastroenterology 87: 37–42

Shibayama Y 1990 Factors producing bile infarction and bile duct proliferation in biliary obstruction. Journal of Pathology 160: 57–62

Shirai T, Pairojkul C, Ogawa K, Naito H, Thamavit W, Bhudhisawat W, Ito N 1992 Histomorphological characteristics of cholangiocellular carcinomas in northeast Thailand, where a region infection with the liver fluke, *Opisthorchis viverrini*, is endemic. Acta Pathologica Japonica 42: 734–739

Short W F, Nedwick A, Levy H A, Howard J M 1975 Biliary cystadenoma. Archives of Surgery 102: 78–80

Slamon D J, deKernion J B, Verma I M et al 1984 Expression of cellular oncogenes in malignancies. Science 224: 256–262

Soga J, Tazawa K 1971 Pathological analysis of carcinoids. Cancer 28: 990–998

Sonobe H, Enzan H, Ido E, Furihata M, Iwata J, Ohtsuki Y, Watanabe R 1995 Mucinous cholangiocarcinoma featuring a unique microcystic appearance. Pathology International 45: 292–296

Stamm B, Hedinger CE, Saremaslani P 1986 Duodenal and ampullary carcinoid tumors. A report of 12 cases with pathological characteristics, polypeptide content and relation to MEN I syndrome and von Recklinghausen's disease (neurofibromatosis). Virchows Archiv A Pathol Anat Histopathol 408: 475–489

Stommer P E, Stolte M, Seifert E 1987 Somatostatinoma of Vater's papilla and of the minor papilla. Cancer 60: 232–235

Sturm P D J, Baas I O, Clement M J, Nakeeb A, Offerhaus G J A, Hruban R H, Pitt H A 1998 Alterations of the p53 tumor-suppressor gene and K-ras oncogene in perihilar cholangiocarcinomas from a high-incidence area. Indian Journal of Cancer 78: 695–698

Sugawara H, Yasoshima M, Katayanagi K, Kono N, Watanabe Y, Harada K, Nakanuma Y 1998 Relationship between interleukin-6 and proliferation and differentiation in cholangiocarcinoma. Histopathology 33: 145–153

Suyama Y, Horie Y, Suou T et al 1988 Oral contraceptives and intrahepatic cystadenoma having an increased level of oestrogen receptor. Hepato-gastroenterol 35: 171–174

Takasan H, Kim C 1, Arii S et al 1980 Clinicopathologic study of seventy patients with carcinoma of the biliary tract. Surgery, Gynecology and Obstetrics 150: 721–726

Talbot I C, Neoptolemos J P, Shaw D E, Carr-Locke D 1988 The histopathology and staging of carcinoma of the ampulla of Vater. Histopathology 12: 155–165

Tan A, Shen J F, Hecht A H 1989 Sonogram of multiple bile duct hamartomas. Journal of Clinical Ultrasound 17: 667–669

Tanaka T, Slamon D J, Battifora H et al 1986 Expression of p21 *ras* oncoproteins in human cancers. Cancer Research 46: 1465–1470

Terada T, Kitamura Y, Ohta T, Nakanuma Y 1997 Endocrine cells in hepatobiliary cystadenomas and cystadenocarcinomas. Virchows Archiv 430: 37–40

Terada T, Nakanuma Y 1988 Congenital biliary dilatation in autosomal dominant adult polycystic disease of the liver and kidneys. Archives of Pathology and Laboratory Medicine 112: 1113–1116

Terada T, Nakanuma Y 1992 Pathologic observations of intrahepatic peribiliary glands in 1000 consecutive autopsy livers. IV. Hyperplasia of intramural and extramural glands. Human Pathology 23: 483–490

Terada T, Mitsui T, Nakanuma Y et al 1991 Intrahepatic biliary papillomatosis arising in nonobstructive intrahepatic biliary dilatations confined to the hepatic left lobe. American Journal of Gastroenterology 86: 1523–1526

Thommesen N 1978 Biliary hamartomas (von Meyenburg complexes) in liver needle biopsies. Acta Pathologica Microbiologica Scandanavica (Sect A) 86: 93–99

Tihan T, Blumgart L H, Klimstra D S 1998 Clear cell papillary carcinoma of the liver: An unusual variant of peripheral cholangiocarcinoma. Human Pathology 29: 196–200

Tomimatsu M, Okuda H, Saito A et al 1989 A case of biliary cystadenocarcinoma with morphologic and histochemical features of hepatocytes. Cancer 64: 1323–1328

Tomioka T, Tsuchiya R, Harada N et al 1986 Cystadenoma and cystadenocarcinoma of the liver: localization of carcinoembryonic antigen. Japanese Journal of Surgery 16: 62–67

Tompkins R K, Johnson J, Storm F K, Longmire W P Jr 1976 Operative endoscopy in the management of biliary tract neoplasm. American Journal of Surgery 132: 174–182

Tsui W M S 1998 How many types of biliary hamartomas and adenomas are there? Advances in Anatomy and Pathology 5: 16–20

Tsui W M S, Loo KT, Chow LTC, Tse CCH 1993 Biliary adenofibroma. A heretofore unrecognized benign biliary tumor of the liver. American Journal of Surgical Pathology 17: 186–192

Tsui W M S, Tse C C H 1994 Biliary epithelial dysplasia in recurrent pyogenic cholangitis (Abstract) International Journal of Surgical Pathology 2: 205

Van der Wal A C, Van Leeuwen D J, Walford N 1990 Small cell neuroendocrine (oat cell) tumour of the common bile duct. Histopathology 16: 398–400

Van Heerden J A, Judd E S, Dockerty M B 1967 Carcinoma of the extrahepatic bile ducts. American Journal of Surgery 13: 49–55

Vauthey J N and Blumgart L H 1994 Recent advances in the management of cholangiocarcinomas. Seminars in Liver Diseases 14: 109–114

Visfeldt J, Poulsen H 1972 On the histopathology of liver and liver tumours in thorium-dioxide patients. Acta Pathologica et Microbiologica Scandinavica, Section A: Pathology 80: 97–108

Voravud N, Foster S, Gilbertson J A et al 1989 Oncogene expression in cholangiocarcinoma and in normal hepatic development. Human Pathology 20: 1163–1168

Washington K, Gottfried M R 1996 Expression of p53 in adenocarcinoma of the gallbladder and bile ducts. Liver 16: 99–104

Wee A, Ludwig J, Coffey R J et al 1985 Hepatobiliary carcinoma associated with primary sclerosing cholangitis and chronic ulcerative colitis. Human Pathology 16: 719–726

Weihing R R, Shintaku I P, Geller S A, Petrovic L M 1997 Hepatobiliary and pancreatic mucinous cystadenocarcinomas with mesenchymal stroma: Analysis of estrogen receptors/progesterone receptors and expression of tumor-associated antigens. Modern Pathology 10: 372–379

Weinbren K 1984 Precancerous states in the liver. In: Carter R L (ed) Precancerous states. Oxford University Press, London, p 266

Weinbren K, Mutum S S 1983 Pathological aspects of cholangiocarcinoma. Journal of Pathology 139: 217–238

Weinbren K, Hadjis N, Blumgart L H 1985 Structural aspects of the liver in patients with biliary disease and portal hypertension. Journal of Clinical Pathology 38: 1013–1020

Wheeler D A, Edmondson H A 1985 Cystadenoma with mesenchymal stroma (CMS) in the liver and bile ducts. A clinicopathologic study of 17 cases, 4 with malignant change. Cancer 56: 1424–1445

Whisnant J D, Bennett S E, Huffman S R, Weiss D L, Parker J C, Griffen W O 1974 Common bile duct obstruction by granular cell tumor (Schwannoma). American Journal of Digestive Diseases 19: 471–476

Williams E D, Sandler M 1983 The classification of carcinoid tumors. Lancet ii: 238–239

Willis R A 1960 Pathology of tumours, 3rd edn. Butterworth, London, p 444

Yamaguchi K, Enjoji M 1991 Adenoma of the ampulla of Vater: putative precancerous lesion. Gut 32: 1558–1561

Yamaguchi M, Enjoji M 1987 Carcinoma of the ampulla of Vater. A clinicopathologic study and pathologic staging of 109 cases of carcinoma and 5 cases of adenoma. Cancer 59: 506–512

Yamamoto M, Takasaki K, Nakano M, Saito A 1998 Minute nodular intrahepatic cholangiocarcinoma. Cancer 82: 2145–2149

Yamamoto T, Ikawa S, Ahyama T et al 1986 Similarity of protein encoded by the human *c-erbB-2* gene to epidermal growth factor receptor. Nature 319: 230–234

Yamashita Y, Takahashi M, Kanazawa S, Charnsangavej C, Wallace S 1992 Hilar cholangiocarcinoma. An evaluation of subtypes with CT and angiography. Acta Radiologica 33: 351–355

Yamato T, Sasaki M, Hoso M, Sakai J, Ohta H, Watanabe Y, Nakanuma Y 1998 Intrahepatic cholangiocarcinoma arising in congenital hepatic fibrosis: report of an autopsy case. Journal of Hepatology 28: 717–722

Zhang S, Wu M, Chen H, Zhang X 1989 Expression of glycoconjugates in intrahepatic cholangiocellular carcinoma. Virchows Archiv. A, Pathological Anatomy 415: 395–401

Zhou D, Battifora H, Yokota J et al 1987 Association of multiple copies of the *c-erbB-2* oncogene with spread of breast cancer. Cancer Research 47: 6123–6125

Zimmermann H, Ganz P, Zimmermann A, Oguey D, Marti U, Reichen J 1995 The overexpression of proliferating cell nuclear antigen in biliary cirrhosis in the rat and its relationship with epidermal growth factor receptor. Journal of Hepatology 23: 459–464

Zimmermann H, Reichen J, Zimmermann A et al 1992 Reversibility of secondary biliary fibrosis by biliodigestive anastomosis in the rat. Gastroenterology 103: 579–589

52

Benign tumors and pseudotumors of the biliary tract

R.M. BEAZLEY, L.H. BLUMGART

Benign biliary tumors are clinical rarities which in the past have been the subject of infrequent case reports, usually combined with a review of the literature. Benign bile duct tumors have been reported in 0.1% of all biliary tract operations and constitute only 6% of all extrahepatic bile duct neoplasms (Burhans & Myers 1971). To date, less than 200 cases of benign bile duct tumor have been reported in the English literature. As a further measure of their infrequent occurrence, only two operations for benign extrahepatic tumors were performed during a total experience of 4200 biliary tract operations at the Charity Hospital in New Orleans (Farris & Faust 1979).

As a result of their rarity, benign tumors of the bile ducts are seldom considered in the differential diagnosis of obstructive jaundice. Symptoms may be present for a few days to several years, while the clinical presentation may mimic cholecystitis, biliary calculi, or ampullary, pancreatic or bile duct cancer, all of which are infinitely more frequent. In addition, true benign bile duct neoplasms must be differentiated from a number of inflammatory conditions which may mimic them not only in presentation but in their cholangiographic features and even in their appearance at laparotomy. Indeed, preoperative diagnostic and laboratory studies almost never suggest a benign lesion, so that the surgeon is likely to be surprised by the operative findings.

It is essential that a tissue diagnosis be established in all patients with biliary tract obstruction thought to be secondary to tumor since most benign lesions are entirely curable by resective surgery. It is thus inappropriate to treat such lesions, on the assumption of malignancy, by simple intubational techniques which may not only lead to infection of a previously sterile biliary tree with long-term deleterious effects but may compromise the subsequent performance of adequate surgical resection.

Biliary lesions due either to benign neoplasms or to

benign conditions presenting as localized masses and causing biliary obstruction may be classified as follows:

1. Papilloma, adenoma and multiple biliary papillomatosis
2. Granular cell myoblastoma
3. Neural tumors
4. Leiomyoma
5. Endocrine tumors

Pseudotumors, inflammatory masses and heterotopic tissue present in the biliary tract require separate consideration.

Biliary cystadenoma will not be covered in this chapter since the lesion usually presents as a liver cell mass, difficult to differentiate from cystadenocarcinoma. Indeed, there is frequent coexistence of benign and malignant epithelium, and histological diagnosis is extremely difficult (Marsh et al 1974, Ishak et al 1977, Woods 1981, Moore et al 1984). These lesions are further considered in Chapters 51, 54, 66 and 83.

EMBRYOLOGICAL AND ANATOMICAL FACTORS

Benign tumors of a variety of histological types have been observed to occur in the extrahepatic ductal system. The embryology and anatomy of the region accounts for this to a large degree. Embryologically, the extrahepatic biliary tree develops in close relationship to the liver, arising from a thickened area of endoderm on the ventral surface of the primitive gastrointestinal tract at the junction of the foregut and hindgut in the 3 mm (fifth week of intra-uterine life) human embryo. This small outpouching is the anlage of the liver, extrahepatic biliary ducts, gallbladder and the ventral bud of the pancreas.

A diverticulum evolves from this thickened area which

divides into a superior and inferior bud as it grows into the ventral mesogastrium (Fig. 52.1A). The ventral pancreatic bud develops from the superior surface of the diverticulum, proximal to the enlarging terminal sacculations. The cranial sacculation, the larger of the two, pushes ventrally and cranially into the septum transversum which separates the thoracic from the celomic cavity. Composed of a solid mass of endodermal cells, it spreads out into the substance of the septum transversum, eventually forming the right and left lobes of the liver. Cephalad growth and extension of the cranial sacculation results in stretching of the endodermal

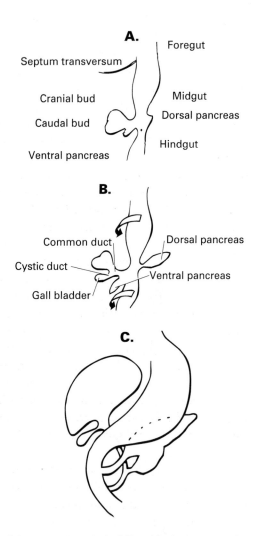

Fig. 52.1 (A) At approximately the fifth week of intrauterine life a diverticulum evolves near the junction of the mid- and hindgut and grows into the ventral mesogastrium. The ventral pancreatic bud develops from the superior surface as the cranial sacculation and pushes cephalad into the septum transversum. **(B)** The gallbladder and extrahepatic ducts develop from the caudal bud and the liver from the cranial bud. The ventral pancreas evolves in close relationship to the developing common bile duct. **(C)** At the 7 mm stage, left-to-right rotation occurs, resulting in subsequent fusion of the pancreas, gallbladders, duodenum and extrahepatic bile ducts in their normal anatomical relationship.

cell mass from the duodenum to the liver, which eventually evolves into the extrahepatic biliary tree. At approximately the seventh week of intrauterine life, vacuolization takes place within the solid mass of cells of the primitive extrahepatic biliary tree resulting in the development of a ductal lumen.

Prior to the 7 mm stage the common bile duct is attached to the ventral surface of the duodenum close to the ventral pancreatic bud. At the 7 mm stage, left-to-right rotation of the ventral pancreas and duodenum takes place so that the common bile duct eventually enters on the posteromedial surface of the duodenum (Fig. 52.1B and C). The gallbladder and cystic duct develop concurrently from the caudal portion of the primitive hepatic diverticulum during the same period (Lindner & Green 1964).

The common bile duct lies in the right border of the hepatoduodenal ligament between serosal surfaces. The ductal wall is composed of mucosa, fibrous tissue and serosa. Rare smooth muscle fibers may be found in the duct wall but muscular tissue in not a prominent component. The thickness of duct wall varies from 0.8 to 1.5 mm with an average of about 1.1 mm (Mahour et al 1967). The terminal end of the duct is invested with muscle fibers, as elegantly described by Boyden (1957). At this point the common bile duct usually joins with the major pancreatic duct, but they may fail to unite and enter the duodenum separately (Dowdy et al 1961; see Chs 2 and 9).

The mucosa lining the extrahepatic biliary tree consists of a single layer of columnar epithelium and a tunica propria containing mucous glands. Scattered chromogranin-positive cells can be formed in glands of the normal gallbladder neck, and rare cells immunoreactive for somatostatin have been found between the lining epithelium of the hepatic duct in patients with biliary disease (Dancygier et al 1984). It has been observed that chronic inflammation of the biliary tract may result in the intestinal metaplasia of the mucosa which seems to result in an increase in the number of argentaffin cells (Kulchitsky's cells). Barron-Rodriguez et al (1991) have suggested that these changes may be the basis for the development of carcinoid tumors of the biliary tree. The epithelial surface of the duct is generally flat except for tiny pits in the mucosa known as sacculi of Beale, which are luminal openings for the intramural mucous glands. As the duct penetrates the wall of the duodenum the mucosa appears to become thickened and the surface roughened by longitudinal folds of mucosa or 'valvules', particularly at the terminal end of the duct. The valvules, according to Boyden (1936), were first described in the Fabrica of Vesalius (1543) and followed by a more detailed description by Santorini (1724). A more frequent occurrence of transversally oriented flaps or valvules, which face towards the

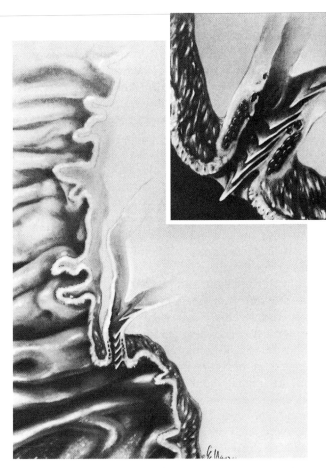

Fig. 52.2 Artist's representation of the macroscopic anatomy of the choledochoduodenal junction depicting the transverse valvules as described by Brown (1964), which probably serve to prevent reflux from the duodenum.

duodenal lumen and probably function to prevent reflux of duodenal contents into the biliary tree and pancreatic ducts were described by Brown & Echenberg (1964; Fig. 52.2). Baggenstoss (1983) has also reported that free folds of ductal epithelium in the form of papillary processes may extend from 2 to 3 mm beyond the Vaterian orifice.

Microscopically, a definite transition exists between the mucosa of the duct within the ampulla and the surrounding duodenal mucosa. The ductal mucosa exhibits numerous papillary processes which are much larger than the adjacent duodenal villi.

CLINICAL PRESENTATIONS AND DIAGNOSIS

Patients with benign biliary tract tumors and often those with inflammatory masses masquerading as neoplasms almost invariably present with clinical manifestations of jaundice. The onset of icterus may be insidious or intermittent with few other symptoms. On the other hand, the presentation may be sudden and associated with colicky epigastric pain referred to the back or shoulder, nausea and vomiting. There is seldom any significant weight loss. As these tumors are relatively slow-growing, some of the clinical symptoms may be intermittent or gradually progressive over an extended period of time only to culminate with obstructive jaundice. There are no clinical symptoms which can assist the physician in differentiating a benign biliary tract tumor from the other more common causes of biliary tract obstruction.

Physical findings are likewise non-specific: liver enlargement, a palpable gallbladder, tenderness to palpation in the right hypochondrium and, of course, jaundice. Indeed, because of the lack of characteristic symptoms and physical findings, benign biliary tumors are usually not diagnosed preoperatively or antemortem (Chu 1950).

Reports since the early 1970s have emphasized the usefulness of percutaneous transhepatic cholangiography (PTC) and, more recently, endoscopic retrograde cholangiopancreatography (ERCP) in the establishment of a preoperative diagnosis of extrahepatic obstruction (see Ch. 20) and in distinguishing between calculus and tumor as a cause (Hossack & Herron 1972, Kittredge & Baer 1975). Jain et al (1979) in their report of a patient with granular cell myoblastoma, suggested that an eccentric, short stenosis might be associated with a benign biliary tumor. However, obstructive changes identical to those seen in malignant neoplasms are not uncommon and indeed may be produced by inflammatory masses (Stamatakis et al 1979, Hadjis et al 1985). While PTC and ERCP will not distinguish between a benign tumor and a malignant one, adequate visualization of the ductal system will provide vital information concerning tumor location, extension and size, as well as the status of the intrahepatic ductal system. However, currently there is no preoperative diagnostic study capable of reliably distinguishing benign from malignant tumorous obstruction of the biliary ducts.

It is important to sound a cautionary note regarding PTC (see Ch. 17) in the diagnosis of biliary tract obstruction in that, although highly accurate in predicting tumorous involvement of the biliary tree, there are recorded instances of a tumor suggested to be at the confluence of the hepatic ducts which was not found later at surgery (Li et al 1981). Such misinterpretation at PTC is almost always due to poor radiological technique and, in particular, failure to place the patient in an upright position; late films should be repeated at an interval of up to 3 hours. This serves to allow complete mixing of contrast material with stagnant and often viscous bile. Failure to demonstrate dilated intrahepatic ducts does not preclude a diagnosis of partial obstruction of the biliary tract but should at the least lead to questioning and stimulate further studies.

PAPILLOMA AND ADENOMA

The most common variety of benign tumor of the extrahepatic biliary tree is that arising from the glandular epithelium lining the ducts. Roughly two-thirds of the benign neoplasms reported fall into the category of polyps, adenomatous papilloma or adenoma. Chu, in his classic review of benign biliary neoplasms, found that 26 out of 30 cases studied were either papillomas or adenomas (Chu 1950). Later, Dowdy et al (1962) made a related observation in that 36 of the 43 cases they reviewed were similarly classified. Since 1962, 53 additional patients have been added to the English literature (Bahuth & Winkley 1966, Short et al 1971, Sull & Brown 1972, Archie & Murray 1978, Lukes et al 1979, Bergdahl & Andersson 1980, Austin et al 1981, Gouma et al 1984, Van Steenbergen et al 1984, Thomsen et al 1984, Byrne et al 1989). Presently the authors have traced a total of 115 patients reported with either benign polyps, adenoma or cystadenoma.

There is a slight female predominance in the incidence of these lesions (1.3 : 1) and, while the average age at diagnosis is 58 years, the youngest recorded occurrence was in a 3-year-old child (Wardell 1969). Leriche (1934) reported a massive papillomatous tumor weighing 750 g arising from the common bile duct of a 4-year-old child.

The anatomical distribution of papillomas or adenomatous lesions reported to date may be found in Figure 52.3. The majority are found either in the ampulla or in close proximity to the Vaterian system (47%) while the common bile duct (27%) is the second most frequent site.

The onset of symptoms may vary from a few weeks to 35 years. Jaundice, a presenting symptom in over 90% of patients (McIntyre & Pay-Zen 1968), occurs intermittently in approximately 40% of patients. Most patients complain of right upper-quadrant pain associated with the jaundice. Wright (1958) reported a patient with relapsing pancreatitis who was cured by excision of a common bile duct polyp, which had prolapsed into the ampulla of Vater. Gallstones or biliary calculi are reported in only 20% of patients found to have benign extrahepatic ductal tumors. Cattell & Pyrtek (1950) suggest that recurrence of symptomatology following cholecystectomy should suggest the possibility of a tumor in the ampullary area rather than biliary dyskinesia. A benign adenomatous tumor should be included on the differential list in all secondary operations of the biliary tree

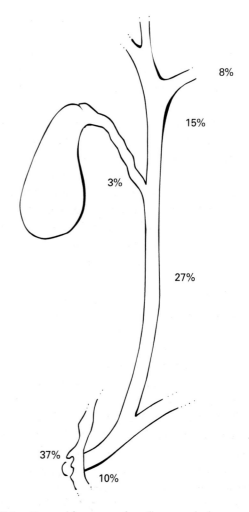

Fig. 52.3 Location and frequency of papillomas and adenomas reported between the hepatic duct confluence and the ampulla of Vater.

performed for obstruction. These lesions are generally soft, difficult to palpate and present little or no resistance to exploring ductal probes and are thus difficult to detect at the operating table. They are more frequently detected by intraoperative cholangiography, ultrasonography or choledochoscopy. Lesions developing in the lower common bile duct near the ampulla may actually protrude through the papilla and be visible endoscopically; the authors have seen such a case. In contrast, malignant lesions developing in the ampullary area tend to be infiltrative, are usually larger, firmer and more likely to be ulcerated at presentation. Presenting symptoms related to bleeding in association with benign adenomatous polyps of the bile ducts are exceedingly rare, although Teter (1954) recorded a death due to massive hemorrhage secondary to such a lesion.

Kozuka et al (1984) has suggested that most polypoid or papillary cancers of the extrahepatic duct arise from pre-existing adenomas. In a review of 43 carcinomas of the extrahepatic tree, Kozuka identified an adenomatous residue in nine (21.4%). Certainly others have suggested that suprapapillary ductal papillomatous lesions may be precancerous (see Ch. 54). Gouma et al (1984) reported a case of intrahepatic bile duct papillomata associated with changes of nuclear atypia and reviewed the literature suggesting that it is reasonable to regard these lesions as of low grade malignant potential (see below). The rarity of benign lesions of the extrahepatic bile ducts make substantiation of this theory difficult. Although the etiology of bile duct adenomas is uncertain, these lesions have been produced experimentally by performing a choledochopancreatostomy in puppies, a model for anomalous choledochopancreatic ductal junction. After several years, mucosal hyperplasia was observed in 100% of the dogs with almost one-half having bile duct adenomas (Miyano et al 1989).

Austin et al (1981) reported two patients who presented with obstructive jaundice and solitary non-parasitic liver cysts. At reoperation, the first was found to have a papillary adenoma in the common hepatic duct, which was totally excised. The second patient at reoperation had an obstructing polypoid cystadenoma of the left hepatic duct compressing the right biliary system. It was proposed that there is a possible association between non-parasitic solitary liver cysts and adenomas of the ductal system (Austin et al 1981). The clinical course of these two patients underscores the difficulty in detection of soft adenomatous tumors obstructing the extrahepatic biliary tree. There is a described association between non-parasitic cystic biliary disease and the development of cholangiocarcinoma (Schiewe et al 1968, Jones & Shreeve 1970, Gallagher et al 1972, Dayton et al 1983, Nasu et al 1971, Leroy et al 1979) and the authors have seen four such cases (see Chs 54, 65 and 66). Any association between these overt malignancies and the presence of pre-existing adenoma or papilloma within biliary cyst is difficult to prove.

TREATMENT

In 1962, Dowdy et al reviewed the literature and detailed the operative procedures for 37 patients with papillomas or adenomas. They reported that four out of the five recognized tumor recurrences were in patients who had had local tumor excision as primary therapy. Since that time, 37 additional patients have been reported in whom both the operative procedure and follow up data are available. Fifteen patients underwent local excision, presumably including the stalk and/or base of the polyp, two of whom had recurrences which necessitated re-operation. Fourteen patients with lesions in or near the ampulla had local excision by way of transduodenal papillotomy without recorded tumor

recurrence. There were 3 additional patients in whom curettage of a polypoid tumor was accomplished without recurrence. One patient had local resection of the duct and one had local resection of the duct wall without recurrence. Three patients had a Whipple resection for a low-lying tumor initially thought to be malignant.

Based upon reported experience, it appears that the choice of operative procedure is dependent upon the patient's age, medical condition and the location of the tumor but should include total resection of the lesion preferably with some duct wall. Lesions arising in the ampulla can successfully be managed by wide local excision in most instances.

MULTIPLE BILIARY PAPILLOMATOSIS

Multiple biliary papillomatosis presenting as diffuse intrahepatic and extrahepatic biliary papillomata is extremely rare. Most patients with intrahepatic papillomatosis present with obstructive jaundice, frequently intermittent and often complicated by cholangitis. This complication is a result of partial and intermittent obstruction of the bile duct by fragments which have become detached from the villous tumor. In some patients, however, the only symptom has been abdominal pain. The history may extend for more than 20 years and be associated with anemia as a result of bleeding. In only two cases has associated cholelithiasis and choledocholithiasis been reported.

Preoperative diagnosis is made radiologically and may be made more frequently now since the widespread availability of direct cholangiography. Nonetheless, filling defects seen have in the past been attributed to air bubbles or intrabiliary blood clot. Tompkins and colleagues (1976) have emphasized the value of intraoperative endoscopy in the evaluation of the biliary tree for multiple lesions. Caroli et al (1959) first reported the occurrence of diffuse papillomatosis in both the intrahepatic and extrahepatic ducts of a 42-year-old male. While the presenting symptoms were of abdominal pain and jaundice, the patient was also noted to be anemic secondary to hemobilia. A T tube was placed in the biliary tree through which 10 L of mucoid secretions were drained in the first 24 hours following surgery. The patient died 48 hours later. It was noted that the biliary secretions had a high potassium content, which the authors postulated might be analogous to the mucoid diarrhea and hypokalemia associated with villous adenoma of the colon. In the same report, a second patient, who presented with cholangitis, was reported cured following a left hepatectomy for papillomatosis confined to the left intra-hepatic ducts.

Borner (1960) reported a 62-year-old patient in whom

diffuse papillomatosis was found at operation. The extrahepatic ducts were resected and a choledochojejunostomy was performed which resulted in bile peritonitis from an anastomotic leak and the patient's death. At autopsy the intrahepatic ducts were filled with numerous small papillomas. Histologically benign polypoid lesions were also noted throughout the colon and rectum.

A total of 31 patients have been reported in the literature to have had benign papillary neoplasms of the extrahepatic biliary tree including 19 males with an average age of 62 and 12 females with an average age of 70.5 years. The most common presentation was that of obstructive jaundice secondary to occlusion of the extrahepatic bile ducts by soft polypoid tumor material. Cattell et al (1962) reported successful placement of a T tube for a similar problem, but obstructive jaundice recurred within a year. The authors suggested these lesions had a low-grade malignant potential. Indeed, there is a significant risk of malignant transformation with nuclear atypia or carcinoma in-situ being commonly observed in papillary lesions. Ohta has reported point mutations of the K-ras gene in benign papillary lesions (Ohta et al 1993). Padfield et al documented basement membrane discontinuities in three patients consistent with patterns accompanying malignant tumors and cautioned that papillary neoplasms while histologically benign should be considered premalignant (Padfield et al 1988). The authors (Gouma et al 1984) reported a similar case in which intrahepatic bile duct papillomata were (Fig. 52.4A) associated with changes of nuclear atypia. The patient was treated by left hepatic resection, including the base of the papillomatous lesions, and biliary–enteric continuity was established by hepatico-jejunostomy to the residual right liver (Fig. 52.4B). The patient was symptom-free and without recurrence 4 years after surgery. The authors concur with Cattell's view that it is reasonable to regard these lesions as of low-grade malignant potential. A further patient has been reported who lived approximately 5 years before dying of cholangitis (Madden & Smith 1974). Treatment had included partial hepatic resection, choledochoduodenostomy and weekly courses of BCNU. Some decrease in the amount of tumour was observed following therapy. Although cellular atypia was reported, no malignant changes could be documented at autopsy. Of the two recently reported patients, an 80-year-old male died after choledochoduodenostomy because of variceal bleeding, while the second reported by Gertsch was reported alive and well 15 months after curretage (Gertsch et al 1990, Hubens et al 1991).

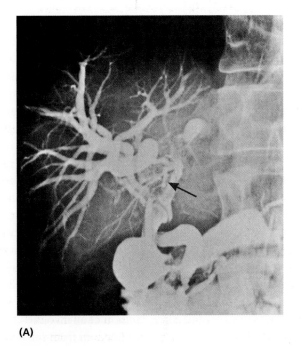

(A)

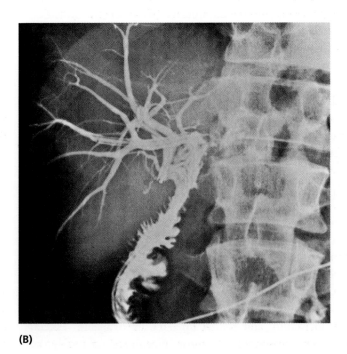

(B)

Fig. 52.4 (A) T tube cholangiogram obtained after initial choledochotomy in a patient who presented with intermittent attacks of jaundice. At operation, loose tumor particles were found in the common bile duct and proved to be fragments of papilloma. The T tube enters the main right hepatic duct and a residual filling defect is seen in the left ducts (arrow). **(B)** Tube cholangiogram following subsequent left hepatic lobectomy and reconstruction by hepaticojejunostomy Roux-en-Y. The anastomosis is widely patent. The tube was removed and the patient was alive and well 4 years later. (Reproduced, with permission, from The British Journal of Surgery 71: 72–74, 1984.)

The extent, distribution and secondary obstructive changes induced by these soft lesions present management challenges. If the lesions are limited and confined to one liver lobe, liver resection should be strongly considered although attempted radical surgery by means of hepatic lobectomy has been reported in only five cases. One of these (Gouma et al 1984) was alive and well at 4 years. One further case was reported alive 6 months after surgery with no evidence of recurrence, and one died 6 years after resection with diffuse malignant tumors in the right lobe of the liver after initial left hepatic lobectomy. The remaining two patients had multiple papillomatosis apparently localized to the left hepatic duct at operation but both had recurrence in the common and right hepatic duct 6 months and 3 years after lobectomy and died 5 and 6 years, respectively, after first operation. It seems clear, therefore, that even major resectional surgery for this lesion has a high recurrence rate and, indeed, Gouma et al (1984) were able to trace 12 patients for whom adequate follow-up figures were available (mean age 54 years), the mean survival being 28 months. It should be noted, however, that although no patient survived more than 6 years, the only 5-year survivals were in three cases submitted to radical surgery.

A recent report by Helling and Strobach documents a patient with papillomatosis with high-grade dysplasia occluding the left hepatic duct in a 67-year-old female who was successfully managed by a left hepatic lobectomy. The patient was disease free 20 months following resection. The authors reviewed the literature and commented on 3 important features of this lesion. Firstly, a high recurrence rate with approximately 50% of patients requiring re-operation. Secondly, copious mucin production which may lead to fluid electrolyte imbalances and lastly, malignant transformation which is observed in a significant percentage of patients (Helling & Strobach 1996). Since this report, four additional extrahepatic benign papillary lesions have been recorded (Loh et al 1994, Lam et al 1996, Meng et al 1996 and Khan et al 1998).

Papillomatosis affecting the entire biliary tree appears to be best managed by an intubational approach (Fig. 52.5), although the number of cases so treated are few. Employment of the approach described by Hutson et al (1984) and by Barker & Winkler (1984), whereby a Roux-en-Y hepaticodochojejunostomy is fashioned in such a manner as to allow a jejunal fistula for access to the biliary tree post-operatively and permit repeated curettage or intubation, seems reasonable. Meng et al reported on the use of the holmium-YAG laser therapy via choledochoscopy and successful ablation after curettage. Following four sessions of choledochoscopy and laser therapy, all tumor was ablated and there were no signs of tumor recurrence at 6 months

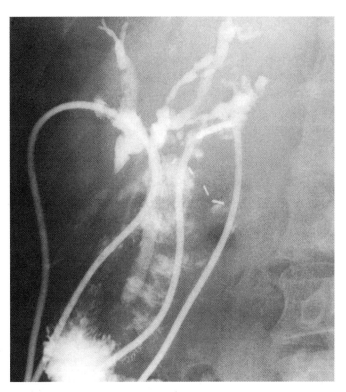

Fig. 52.5 Bilateral U tubes placed through hepaticojejunostomy to the right and left hepatic ducts in a patient with multiple intrahepatic biliary papillomatosis. The patient (a middle-aged woman) presented with chronic iron deficiency, anemia, followed by the onset of jaundice. At initial operation, papillomata at the orifice of the right and left hepatic ducts were curettaged and bilateral U tubes placed. Satisfactory palliation of jaundice was obtained for 18 months but malignancy supervened and the patient died of recurrent biliary obstruction and liver failure.

(Meng et al 1996). Lastly, consideration might be given to the employment of chemotherapy, especially with agents excreted by the liver (Madden & Smith 1974).

In summary, a reasonable approach to this rare condition includes preoperative and operative cholangiographic diagnosis, early choledochotomy and assessment of the intrahepatic biliary tree by choledochoscopy. If the tumor is bulky, curettage is performed in order to identify the sites of origin within the bile duct. Care must be taken to perform choledochoscopy of as many intrahepatic ducts as possible. When the papillomatosis appears to be confined to one lobe it is reasonable to perform a radical resection consisting of partial hepatectomy including excision of all involved ducts. Although this does not guarantee freedom from recurrence it offers good palliation and carries the best possibility of long-term cure. In cases of papillomatosis involving both right and left ductal system, radical surgery is not applicable. It seems best to avoid long-term external drainage as a preliminary palliative procedure, and curretage or internal bypass is indicated. Some form of hepaticojejunostomy which allows access percutaneously to the biliary tract may be helpful (see Ch. 30). Nevertheless, the prognosis should be regarded as poor if complete removal of the tumor is impossible.

GRANULAR CELL MYOBLASTOMA

Granular cell myoblastoma is a very rare benign tumour of uncertain etiology occasionally encountered in the extrahepatic biliary tree. Indeed, the lesion constitutes less than 10% of all benign tumors of the extrahepatic biliary tree (Dursi et al 1975). While reported in anatomical locations as varied as the pituitary and appendix, the lesions are most commonly encountered in the tongue, breast and subcutaneous tissues, with less than 1% of granular cell myoblastomas occurring in the extrahepatic biliary tree (Paskin et al 1972, Dursi et al 1975). Over 80% of documented cases have occurred in females, 66% of whom are black. Fifteen percent of the patients have multiple lesions (Vance & Hudson 1969).

Since Coggin's original autopsy report, 57 additional patients have been reported with this lesion. Thirty patients had lesions arising from the common hepatic or common bile duct, 18 from the cystic duct, five from the cystic duct and common hepatic duct and one from the hepatic duct (Kittredge & Baer 1975, Mauro & Jacques 1981, Cheslyn-Curtis et al 1986, Lewis et al 1993, MacKenzie et al 1994, Yazdanpanah et al 1993, Ferri Romero et al 1994, Foulner 1994). In addition, one patient had lesions involving the cystic duct and the hepatic duct (Sanchez & Nauta 1991), one involving the cystic duct, gallbladder and common bile duct (Aisner et al 1982), two cystic duct, common hepatic and common bile duct (Balart et al 1983, Butler & Brown 1998). The average age of patients with this tumour is 34.5 years.

The fact that extrahepatic ductal granular cell myoblastomas are found more commonly in black females is attested to in that 34 of 48 females recorded in the literature are black, nine are Caucasian, three oriental and three of unspecified racial origin. Two black males and a single male child of unspecified race have been reported. Multiple tumors within the extrahepatic biliary tree have been reported in six patients (Kittredge & Baer 1975, Mauro & Jaques 1981, Aisner et al 1982, Sanchez & Nauta 1991, Cheslyn-Curtis et al 1986, MacKenzie et al 1994). Multifocal tumors have been noted in seven patients with bile duct lesions, two patients with separate gastric tumors,

four with synchronous skin lesions, an individual with lesions in the mesentery and trachea and a single patient with simultaneous lesions in the trachea and common hepatic duct (Mulhollan et al 1992, LiVolsi et al 1973, Whisnant et al 1974, Assor 1979, Manstein et al 1981, Orenstein et al 1984, Yang & Ortiz 1993). Clinical symptoms associated with granular cell myoblastoma arising in extrahepatic biliary ducts tend to be those of painless jaundice while a presentation of upper abdominal pain and colic is more commonly associated with lesions arising in the cystic duct. Other described symptoms include anorexia, weight loss, nausea, and vomiting. Granular cell myoblastoma might be included in the differential diagnosis of obstructive jaundice presenting in a black female, especially if she has a tumor nodule in the tongue, breast or subcutaneous tissue. However, this clinical presentation would be extraordinarily rare.

The majority of tumors have been described as firm to palpation, localized, confined to the wall of the common bile duct or cystic duct, and generally less than 3 cm in diameter. Usually they do not invade surrounding structures. The mucosa overlying the tumor has generally been intact and histologically normal. On cut section, granular cell myoblastoma is yellowish-white in colour while microscopically it consists of fibrous tissue diffusely infiltrated by elongated large polygonal cells or cells containing small, dark nuclei and an abundant eosinophilic granular cytoplasm. The cytoplasmic granules are markedly positive with the periodic acid–Schiff reaction (Fig. 52.6). Frozen-section diagnosis has been shown to be adequate for delineating these lesions. While this tumor usually does not metastasize, local recurrence may occur, especially if excision is incomplete.

The histogenesis is uncertain and is marked by controversy. The tumor was initially termed granular cell myoblastoma because it was thought to be derived from 'myoid cells'. Indeed, characteristics of the cells in tissue culture suggest a myogenic origin (Murray 1951). Moreover, it is now generally regarded that granular cell tumors arise from the Schwann cell in that the tumor cells react to antibodies with S-100 protein normally found in the central nervous system and in peripheral Schwann cells. (Armin et al 1983).

Treatment

Treatment should consist of total excision of the bile duct segment containing the lesion with reconstruction by Roux-en-Y choledochojejunostomy or hepaticojejunostomy for lesions arising in the common hepatic duct (Manstein et al 1981). Chandrasoma & Fitzgibbons (1984) and Manstein et al (1981) have reported successful management of lesions

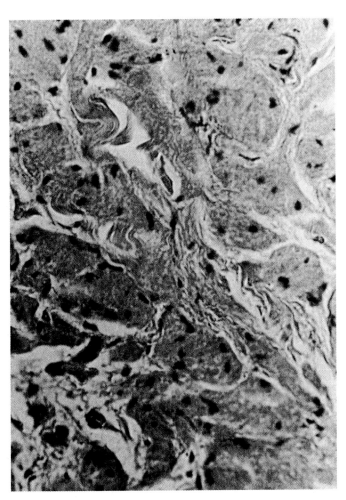

Fig. 52.6 Granular cell myoblastoma excised from the common bile duct showing large polygonal cells with indistinct cell borders. Also typically demonstrated are uniform, small, round nuclei surrounded by finely granular, eosinophilic cytoplasma. (Haematoxylin and eosin, × 120.)

demonstrated in the extrahepatic ducts are somatostatin containing D cells (Dancygier et al 1984). However, it has been postulated that metaplastic changes in the biliary epithelium, perhaps resulting from inflammation may lead to the development and appearance of argyrophile cells (Barron-Rodriguez et al 1991). Since the biliary system is derived embryologically from the foregut, it is not surprising that cells which are immunoreactive for gastrin, serotonin and somatostatin have been demonstrated in the biliary tree (Angeles-Angeles et al 1991). Only a handful of cases have been reported, most of which have been hormonally non-functional. These lesions have occurred in middle age, more commonly in females and locally metastatic in approximately a third of cases. Reported tumors fall into the category of carcinoid, gastrinoma and somatostatinoma. A clinical picture of obstructive jaundice is the usual presentation although a carcinoid was found incidentally in the unobstructive common bile duct of an explanted cirrhotic liver following orthotopic liver transplant (Hao et al 1996). To date only one patient has been recorded as having a functioning endocrine tumor, a 52-year-old female with a 2-year history of recurrent duodenal ulcer whose peptic disease was cured when her gastrinoma was excised from the common bile duct (Mandujano-Vera et al 1995).

Since Pilz's original report in 1961, a total of 17 documented cases of carcinoid tumors arising in the extrahepatic bile ducts have been reported (Hao et al 1996). The presenting symptoms were pain, jaundice, weight loss, nausea and vomiting. No case was associated with the carcinoid syndrome. Metastases were reported in five instances but in general these lesions have not been aggressive with recorded survivals of 10 and 20 years (Davies 1959; Little et al 1968).

Eleven cases have been observed in the common bile duct (Davies 1959, Pilz 1961, Little et al 1968, Bergdahl 1976, Gerlock & Muhletaler 1979, Vitaux et al 1981, Bickerstaff & Ross 1987, Angeles-Angeles et al 1991, Barron-Rodriquez et al 1991, Mandujano-Vera et al 1995, Hao et al 1996). While three have involved the common hepatic or hepatic duct (Judge et al 1976, Baum 1990, Jutte et al 1986) and three the cystic duct (Goodman & Ra 1984, Chittal 1989, Rugge et al 1992), two of the common duct tumors were found to be producing gastrin and serotonin on immunohistochemical staining (Mandujano-Vera et al 1995, Hao et al 1996).

occurring in the intrapancreatic duct by pancreaticoduodenectomy. There is one documented local recurrence and two patients required second operations because of incomplete local excision (Dursi et al 1975, Manstein et al 1981, Butler & Brown 1998). Four patients have been successfully managed by pancreaticoduodenectomy for lesions occurring in the intrapancreatic common bile duct (Chandrasoma & Fitzgibbons 1984, Manstein et al 1981, Raia et al 1978, Mackenzie et al 1994). To date malignancy has not been observed in any reported extrahepatic glandular cell tumor.

ENDOCRINE TUMORS

Endocrine tumors of the extrahepatic bile ducts are exceedingly rare. The only endocrine cells that have been normally

NEURAL TUMOURS

The incidence of neural tumors appears to be lower than expected when one considers the abundant network of neural tissue which normally surrounds the extrahepatic bile ducts. In 1955, Oden reported the occurrence of a neurinoma in a 40-year-old woman who presented with jaundice and mild epigastric discomfort. At operation a cystic tumor was found displacing the common bile duct medially. The cyst was extirpated but the wall contiguous to the common bile duct was left in situ. Several common duct stones were also removed. The patient was asymptomatic 18 months later.

Von Recklinghausen's neurofibromatosis is well recognized to produce gastrointestinal symptoms. Although bleeding, perforation and obstruction due to intussusception, volvulus or stenosis have been reported, there is only one instance of obstructive jaundice secondary to visceral neurofibromatosis recorded in the literature. Curry & Gray (1972) reported the autopsy finding of a 25 mm diameter submucosal nodular tumor protruding into the duodenum around the ampullary opening.

Sarma et al (1980) reported a hilar tumor arising in the left hepatic duct and surrounding the right hepatic duct which was deemed unresectable. The biopsy submitted at that time was interpreted as poorly differentiated carcinoma. A tube was placed through the lesion and the patient readmitted with cholangitis several times over the next 7 years. A second exploration revealed total obstruction of the left hepatic duct, partial obstruction of the right hepatic duct as well as cystic degeneration of the left lobe of the liver. A further tube was placed through the tumor into the right hepatic duct and the cystic left liver lobe drained by a Roux-en-Y jejunal loop. Review of the fresh biopsies and the original material were each interpreted as paraganglioma. While these tumors commonly arise in the adrenal gland as pheochromocytoma, extra adrenal lesions are more commonly found in the neck, the mediastinum and around the aorta. Paragangliomas have been observed in the gallbladder, gastrointestinal tract and the genitourinary tract; this appears to be the first lesion reported in the extrahepatic biliary tree.

LEIOMYOMA

Leiomyomas are the most common benign tumors of the esophagus, stomach and small intestine, while in the extrahepatic biliary tree they are among the least common. The scanty presence of muscle fibers in the normal common bile duct probably accounts for the fact that only five such lesions have been reported. Each of these patients presented with progressive jaundice, itching, nausea, vomiting and weight loss. The first patient reported had a tumor confined to the intrapancreatic segment of of the common bile duct, which was locally excised along with some of the overlying pancreatic tissue and ligation of the duct of Santorini. The proximal bile duct was anastomosed to the jejunum. This patient was reported well 3 years following surgery (Archambault & Archambault 1952). A second patient, reported by Kune & Polgar (1976), was a 49-year-old male treated by pancreaticoduodenectomy for a 4 cm tumour in the intrapancreatic segment of the common bile duct which was assumed to be a pancreatic carcinoma at surgery. Microscopically the lesion was observed to arise from the bile duct wall. The patient was well 28 months after operation. The third patient died of septicemia following ERCP demonstration of a tumor obstructing the lower part of the common bile duct seemingly as a result of external compression. Autopsy examination revealed an angioleiomyoma of the common bile duct. The mucosa overlying the tumor was observed to be intact (Ponka et al 1983). A fourth recorded leiomyoma occurred at the ampulla of Vater (Fernandez & Ganzales-Bueno 1974). Recently, Mandeville & Stawski (1991) reported a fifth patient in whom a leiomyoma of the hepatic duct bifurcation was treated.

PSEUDOTUMORS

Non-malignant lesions which may cause obstruction of the extrahepatic biliary ductal system and which may closely resemble neoplasms at investigation and even at laparotomy occur frequently enough to be seriously considered in the differential diagnosis of any lesion suspected to be a bile duct tumor (see Ch. 54). Lesions should not be assumed to be neoplastic without histological proof and certainly a presumed diagnosis of neoplasm should not be the signal for incomplete drainage procedures carried out surgically, percutaneously or endoscopically. Such maneuvers are inevitably followed by infection, necessitate tubal exchange and compromise effective surgery.

INFLAMMATORY TUMORS

Stamatakis et al (1979) reported the occurrence of a benign inflammatory mass of the common bile duct in a 13-year-old girl who presented with obstructive jaundice and abdominal pain. PTC demonstrated complete obstruction of the common hepatic duct with intraluminal shouldering, suggesting a tumor. At operation a 3 cm spherical mass was found to be closely applied to the porta hepatis, necessitating excision of the confluence, common hepatic duct and common bile duct with reconstruction by Roux-en-Y hepaticojejunostomy. Pathological examination demonstrated nearly complete obstruction of the common hepatic and common bile ducts by an encapsulated yellowish-brown mass. Microscopically, the encased bile duct exhibited loss of muscular coat, loss of ductal epithelium and replacement by collagenous fibrous tissue. Scattered throughout the fibrous tissue were foci of acute inflammatory cells. These authors concluded that the mass represented an excessive inflammatory reaction to some local chemical or infective irritant and further speculated that the lesion might represent a form of localized sclerosing cholangitis. The child was reported as fit and active 1 year post-treatment.

Haith et al (1964) published a somewhat similar clinical occurrence in a 6-year-old male, with a lesion located in the distal common bile duct, treated successfully by pancreaticoduodenectomy. A similar case has been reported by Golematis et al (1982). The patient reported was a 23-year-old man who presented with obstructive jaundice and a lesion at the confluence of the hepatic ducts. The lesion was successfully resected and histologically thought to represent a localized area of sclerosing cholangitis. One further such case has been reported by Heuser & Polk (1983).

Standfield et al (1989) reported an interesting group of 12 patients with localized strictures of the extrahepatic biliary system. No patient had a history of trauma, gallbladder stones or antecedent diseases generally associated with sclerosing cholangitis. All patients were found to have histological evidence of chronic inflammation, fibrosis and epithelial ulceration. These authors felt that this entity was distinct from sclerosing cholangitis in that the mucosa remained intact in that disease.

Hadjis et al (1985) showed eight out of 104 patients at the Hammersmith Hospital, London, submitted to surgery with a clinical diagnosis of malignant obstruction at the confluence of the bile ducts, to have benign disease. The benign nature of the lesion was not certain in six of these patients even at the time of laparotomy. Comprehensive investigation had failed to give an accurate preoperative diagnosis although biliary obstruction was accurately shown in all patients and preoperative assessment using cholangiographic and angiographic data (see Ch. 54) indicated that all were potentially resectable. For this reason and in view of the safety of local excisional surgery and excellent quality of life obtained (Beazley et al 1984, Blumgart et al 1984), palliation by intubational methods was not attempted. In all patients the obstructing lesion was removed and biliary reconstruction was by means of hepticojejunostomy Roux-en-Y. Liver biopsy was obtained in all patients.

Microscopical examination of the biopsies taken from the bile ducts of these patients showed an extensive increase of fibrous tissue in all instances. Subepithelial mucous glandular proliferation was evident in, but not in every specimen from, all patients and the glandular cells were always well-differentiated with elongated to round nuclei showing normal polarity. Most glands were surrounded but not replaced by fibrous tissue. In some instances, glands appeared to be distorted by fibrous tissue coursing between acini. Striking nerve trunks were observed in four of the patients but not in all the specimens, some of which were very small. Accumulations of lymphocytes were present in most specimens sometimes perivascular and sometimes perineural, but not diffusely infiltrating the wall of the bile duct. There was little adventitial inflammation. Sections of associated lymph nodes and of the gallbladder were unremarkable. No vascular changes were identified. In particular in no specimen was there evidence of dysplastic, neoplastic or preneoplastic cytological change. Nuclei were normal, no single epithelial cells were encountered within connective tissue and no pools of mucin were found. Similar changes are reported by Ikei et al (1989).

One patient with overt signs of peritonitis following previous laparotomy was operated upon as an emergency and found to have a loculated intra-abdominal bile collection and a subhepatic abscess which was drained; renal function was impaired at the time of laparotomy and the patient subsequently died of multiple system failure. No tumor was found at the hilum of the liver but a sclerotic lesion (see above) was confirmed together with proximal large duct obstruction.

There were no operative deaths in the eight patients submitted to elective surgery and seven were alive and asymptomatic from 16 to 46 months after operation. One patient required reoperation for a further stricture and remained reasonably well for 2 years, at which time she developed recurrent episodes of cholangitis with cholangiographic evidence of progression of intrahepatic sclerosing cholangitic lesions, and died 30 months after her second operation.

Although the cholangiographic picture of diffuse sclerosing cholangitis is usually characteristic (see Ch. 48) this is not true of the localized form of the disease. The diagnostic difficulty is compounded in that cholangiocarcinoma has been described in association with or as a complication of primary sclerosing cholangitis. It is important to emphasize that, in the presence of a localized high bile duct stricture and in the absence of angiographic involvement, it is impossible, without specific biopsy or cytology, to make a definitive diagnosis in this situation. The marked desmoplastic reaction that even small hilar cholangiocarcinoma often excites, together with the ductular and glandular hyperplastic changes consequent on long-standing obstruction and severe secondary cholangitic changes, are the main pathological factors responsible for histological difficulty in differentiating benign from malignant disease (Weinbren & Mutum 1983). Indeed, some believe that cases of sclerosing cholangitis localized at the hilum may be instances of slow-growing sclerosing carcinoma and that it is only a matter of time before such a lesion declares its malignant potential. However, extensive studies at the Royal Postgraduate Medical School have demonstrated characteristic features of malignant biliary disease (see Ch. 51; Weinbren & Mutum 1983), and these were found to be absent in all cases in the series reported by Hadjis et al (1985). Six patients remained symptom-free with normal liver function at a mean follow-up period of 28.3 months.

Malignant masquerade as termed by the authors has been observed by others since the original report. Table 52.1 records the reports in the literature since 1987 related to benign inflammatory lesions occurring in the extrahepatic biliary tree. The authors draw attention to the fact that these lesions should not be allowed to masquerade in the guise of malignant tumors but it is equally important that they are not mistaken for benign tumors.

HETEROTOPIC TISSUE

Symptomatic heterotopic tissue arising in the biliary tree is an exceedingly rare finding. In 1967, Whittaker et al first observed heterotopic gastric mucosa in a cystic duct which had obstructed the gallbladder. Welling et al (1970) have since recorded a similar mucosal mass obstructing the common bile duct at the level of the cystic duct. More recently, Kalman et al (1981) reported a 1 cm papillary tumor arising in the common hepatic duct, which on microscopic examination demonstrated gastric fundal mucosa replacing the full thickness of the bile duct wall.

Heterotopic gastric mucosa occurring at the ampulla of Vater was observed to be the basis for biliary tract obstruction by Blundell et al (1982). Although occurrence elsewhere in the gastrointestinal tract is well documented, this appears to be the first documented ampullary obstruction secondary to heterotopic gastric mucosa.

Kalman cites two hypotheses for the etiology of heterotopia (Kalman et al 1981). First, metaplasia with heterotopic differentiation is suggested. Several authors have described metaplastic gastric replacement of the gallbladder mucosa in cases of chronic cholecystitis. Usually the metaplastic glands resemble pyloric and Brunner's glands while specialized chief and parietal cells are absent. A second, and perhaps more tenable, theory is one which is based upon observation that embryologically the epithelial lining of the foregut together with parenchyma of the liver and pancreas all arise from the same primitive endoderm (see above). Kalman states that because of the 'common origin of these structures lined by multipotential cells capable of differentiation along several cell lines, it is not unreasonable to conclude that the heterotopic gastric replacement may have resulted from congenitally replaced tissue'.

Heterotopic pancreatic tissue has been observed to occur from the stomach to the ileum, as well as in the omentum, spleen, gallbladder and common bile duct. Seven cases have been reported in which heterotopic pancreatic tissue was found in the common bile duct or ampulla of Vater (Barbosa et al 1946, Weber et al 1968, Sabini et al 1970, Laughlin et al 1983).

Table 52.1 Malignant masquerade tumors of the extrahepatic biliary tree reported since 1987

Reference	Number	Location	Etiology	Treatment
Schroyens et al (1987)	1	CBD	Selerosing cholangitis	Liver transplant
	1	CBD	Selerosing cholangitis	Autopsy
Standfield et al (1989)	12		Non-traumatic inflammatory structures	Excision Roux-en-Y (7) Hepatojejunostomy (3) Intubation (2)
Wetter et al (1990)	2		Mirizzi syndrome	
	3		Granulomas	
	3		Focal stenosis	
Tsunoda et al (1991)	1	Confluence	Sclerosing cholangitis	Partial hepatectomy
Oren et al (1991)	1	CHD	Selerosing cholangitis	Stent and liver transplant

CBD, common bile duct; CHD, common hepatic duct.
For data prior to 1987 see text.

REFERENCES

Abrikossof A I 1931 Weitere untersuchungen uber myobastenmyome. Virchows Archiv für Pathologische Anatomie und für Klinische Medizin 180: 723–740

Abt A B, Feinberg E, Kunitz S 1971 Granular cell myoblastoma of the extrahepatic biliary tract. Mount Sinai Journal of Medicine 38: 457–461

Aisner S C, Khaneja S, Ramirez O 1982 Multiple granular cell tumors of the gallbladder and biliary tree: report of a case. Archives of Pathology and Laboratory Medicine 106: 470–471

Angeles-Angeles A, Quintanilla-Martinez, Larriva-Sahd J 1991 Primary Carcinoid of the common bile duct. American Journal of Clinical Pathology 96: 341–344

Archambault H, Archambault R 1952 Leiomyoma of the common bile duct. Archives of Surgery 64: 531–534

Archie J P, Murray H M 1978 Benign polypoid adenoma of the ampulla of Vater. Archives of Surgery 113: 180–181

Armin A, Connelly E M, Rowden F 1983 An immunoperoxidase investigation of S-100 protein in granular cell myoblastoma. Evidence for Schwann cell derivation. American Journal of Clinical Pathology 79: 37–44

Assor D 1979 Granular cell myoblastoma involving the common bile duct. The American Journal of Surgery 137: 180–181

Austin E H et al 1981 Solitary hepatic cyst and benign bile duct polyp: A heretofore unheralded association. Surgery 89: 359–363

Baggenstoss AH 1983 Major duodenal papilla. Archives of Pathology 26: 353–368

Bahuth J J, Winkley J H 1966 Benign tumor of the common bile duct. California Medicine 104: 307–309

Balart L A, Hines C, Mitchell W 1983 Granular cell schwannoma of the extrahepatic biliary system. American Journal of Gastroenterology 78: 297–300

Barbosa J J, Dockerty M, Waugh J 1946 Pancreatic heterotopia. Surgery, Gynecology and Obstetrics 82: 527–547

Barker E M, Winkler M 1984 Permanent-access hepaticojejunostomy. British Journal of Surgery 71: 188–191

Barron-Rodriguez L, Manivel J C, Mendez-Sanchez N, Jessurun J 1991 Carcinoid tumor of the common bile duct: evidence for its origin in metaplastic endocrine cells. American Journal of Gastroenterology 86: 1073–1076

Beazley R M, Hadjis N, Benjamin I S, Blumgart L H 1984 Clinicopathological aspects of high bile duct cancer. Annals of Surgery 199: 623–636

Bergdahl L 1976 Carcinoid tumours of the biliary tract. Australian and New Zealand Journal of Surgery 46: 136–138

Bergdahl L, Andersson A 1980 Benign tumors of the papilla of Vater. American Surgeon 46: 563–566

Bickerstaff D R, Ross W B 1987 Carcinoid of the biliary tree. Journal of the Royal College of Surgeons of Edinburgh 32: 48–51

Blumgart L H, Hadjis N S, Benjamin I S, Beazley R 1984 Surgical approaches to cholangiocarcinoma at confluence of hepatic ducts. Lancet i: 66–70

Blundell C R, Kanun C S, Earnest D L 1982 Biliary obstruction by heterotopic gastric mucosa at the ampulla of Vater. American Journal of Gastroenterology 77: 111–114

Borner P 1960 Eine papillomatose der intra and extrahepatischen gallenwege. Zeitschrift fur Krebsforschung 63: 474–480

Boyden E A 1936 The pars intestinalis of the common bile duct as viewed by the older anatomists (Vesalius, Glisson, Bianchi, Vater, Haller, Santorini, etc). The Anatomical Record 66: 217–232

Boyden E A 1957 The anatomy of the choledochoduodenal junction in man. Surgery, Gynecology and Obstetrics 104: 641–652

Brown J O, Echenberg R J 1964 Mucosal reduplications associated with the ampullary portion of the major duodenal papilla in humans. The Anatomical Record 150: 293–302

Brown W M, Henderson J M, Kennedy J C 1990 Carcinoid tumor of the bile duct. American Surgeon 56: 343–346

Bumin L, Ormenci N, Dolapci M, Gungor S 1990 Carcinoid tumors of the biliary duct. International Surgery 75: 262–264

Burhans R, Myers R T 1971 Benign neoplasms of the extrahepatic biliary ducts. The American Surgeon 37: 161–166

Butler J D, Brown K 1998 Granular cell tumor of the extrahepatic biliary tract. American Surgeon 64: 1033–1036

Butterly L F, Schapiro R H, LaMuraglia G M, Warshaw A L 1988 Biliary granular cell tumor: a little-known curable bile duct neoplasm of young people. Surgery 103: 328–334

Byrne D J, Walker M A, Pringle R, Ramesar K 1989 Extraheptic biliary cystadenoma: report of a case and review of the literature. Journal of Royal College of Surgeons, Edinburgh 34: 223–224

Caroli J 1959 Papillomes et papillomatoses de la voie bilaire principale. Reveu Medco – Chirurgicale Des Maladies Du Foie 34: 191–230

Cattell R B, Pyrtek L J 1950 Premalignant lesions of the ampulla of Vater. Surgery, Gynecology and Obstetrics 90: 21–30

Cattell R B, Braasch J W, Kahn F 1962 Polypoid epithelial tumors of the bile ducts. The New England Journal of Medicine 266: 57–61

Chandrasoma P, Fitzgibbons P 1984 Granular cell tumor of the intrapancreatic common bile duct. Cancer 53: 2178–2182

Cheslyn-Curtis S, Russell R C G, Rode J, Dhillon A P 1986 Granular cell tumor of the common bile duct. Postgraduate Medical Journal 62: 961–963

Chittal S M, Ra P M 1989 Carcinoid of the cystic duct. Histopathology 15: 643–646

Chu P T 1950 Benign neoplasms of the extrahepatic bile ducts. Archives of Pathology 50: 84–97

Coggins R P 1952 Granular-cell myoblastoma of common bile duct—report of a case with autopsy findings. Archives of Pathology 54: 398–402

Curry B, Gray N 1972 Visceral neurofibromatosis. British Journal of Surgery 59: 494–496

Dancygier H, Klein W, Leuschner W, Hubner K, Classen M 1984 Somatostatin-containing cells in the extrahepatic biliary tract of humans. Gastroenterology 86: 892–896

Davies A J 1959 Carcinoid tumor (argentaffinomata). Annals of the Royal College of Surgeons of England 25: 277–280

Dayton M T, Longmire W P Jr, Tompkins R K 1983 Caroli's disease: A premalignant condition? American Journal of Surgery 145: 41–48

Dewar J, Dooley J S, Lindsay I, George P, Sherlock S 1981 Granular cell myoblastoma of the common bile duct treated by biliary drainage and surgery. Gut 22: 70–76

Dowdy G S, Waldron G W, Brown W F 1961 Surgical anatomy of the pancreaticobiliary ductal system. Archives of Surgery 84: 93–110

Dowdy G S, Olin W G, Shelton E L, Waldron G W 1962 Benign tumors of the extrahepatic bile ducts: report of three cases and review of the literature. Archives of Surgery 85: 503–513

Duncan J T, Wilson H 1957 Benign tumor of the common bile duct. Annals of Surgery 145: 271–274

Dursi J F, Hirschl S, Gomez R, Mersheimer W L 1975 Granular cell myoblastoma of the common bile duct: report of a case and review of the literature. Review of Surgery 32: 305–310

Eisen R N, Kirby W M, O'Quinn J L 1991 Granular cell tumor of the biliary tree. A report of two cases and a review of the literature. American Journal of Surgical Pathology 15: 460–465

Eiss S, MiMaio D, Caedo J P 1960 Multiple papillomas of the entire biliary tract: case report. Annals of Surgery 152: 320–324

Farris K B, Faust B F 1979 Granular cell tumors of the biliary ducts. Archives of Pathology and Laboratory Medicine 103: 510–512

Fernandez J M C, Gonzales-Bueno C M 1974 Leiomyoma of the ampulla of Vater. Revista Espanola De Las Enfermedades Del Aparato Digestivo 47: 165–172

Ferri Romero J, Carrión Tomás A, Estrada Caballero J L, Fernández Giménez F, Ceballos Gil S, Camuñas Mohinelo F 1994 Tumor de celulas granulosas en la vía hiliar una localizacion poco fecuente. Rav Esp Enf Digest 85: 217–219

Foulner D 1994 Granular cell tumor of the biliary tree—the sonographic appearance. Clinical Radiology 49: 503–504

Gallagher P J, Millis R R, Michinson M J 1972 Congenital dilatation of intrahepatic bile ducts with cholangiocarcinoma. Journal of Clinical Pathology 25: 804–808

Gerlock A J J, Muhletaler C A 1979 Primary common bile duct carcinoid. Gastrointestinal Radiology 4: 263–264

Gertsch P, Thomas P, Baer H, Lerut J, Zimmermann A, Blumgart L H 1990 Multiple tumors of the biliary tract. American Journal of Surgery 159: 386–388

Golematis B, Giannopoulos A, Papachristou D N, Dreiling D A 1982 Sclerosing cholangitis of the bifurcation of the common hepatic duct. Mount Sinai Journal of Medicine 49: 38–40

Goodman Z D, Albores-Saavedra J, Lundblad D M 1984 Somatostatinoma of the cystic duct. Cancer 53: 498–502

Gouma D J, Mutum S S, Benjamin I S, Blumgart L H 1984 Intrahepatic biliary papillomatosis. British Journal of Surgery 71: 72–74

Hadjis N S, Collier N A, Blumgart L H 1985 Malignant masquerade at the hilum of the liver. British Journal of Surgery 72: 659–661

Haith E E, Kepes J J, Holder T M 1964 Inflammatory pseudotumor involving the common bile duct of a six-year-old boy: successful pancreatico-duodenectomy. Surgery 56: 436–441

Hao L, Friedman A L, Navarro V J, West B, Robert M E 1996 Carcinoid tumor of the common bile duct producing gastrin and serotonin. J Clinical Gastroenterology 23: 63–65

Helling T S, Strobach R S 1996 The surgical challenge of papillary neoplasia of the biliary tract. Liver Transplant Surgery 2: 290–298

Heuser L S, Polk H C Jr 1983 Proximal hepatic duct lesion. Surgical Rounds 48–52

Hossack K F, Herron J J 1972 Benign tumors of the common bile duct: report of a case and review of the literature. Australian New Zealand Journal of Surgery 42: 22–26

Hubens G, Delvaux G, Willems G, Bourgain C, Kloppel G 1991 Papillomatosis of the intra and extrahepatic bile ducts with involvement of the pancreatic duct. Hepatogastroenterology 38: 413–418

Hutson D, Russel E, Schiff E, Levi J, Jeffers L, Zeppa R 1984 Balloon dilatation of biliary strictures through a choledochojejunocutaneous fistula. Annals of Surgery 199: 637–647

Ikei S, Mori K, Yamane T, Katafuchi S, Hirota M, Akagi M 1989 Adenofibromyomatous hyperplasia of the extrahepatic bile duct—a report of two cases. Japanese Journal of Surgery 19: 576–582

Ishak K G, Willis G W, Cummins S D, Bullock AA 1977 Biliary cystadenoma and cystadenocarcinoma. Report of 14 cases and review of the literature. Cancer 39: 322–338

Jain K M, Hastings O M, Rickert R R, Swaminathan A P, Lazaro E J 1979 Granular cell tumor of the common bile duct. American Journal of Gastroenterology 71: 401–407

Jones A W, Shreeve D R 1970 Congenital dilatation of intrahepatic biliary ducts with cholangiocarcinoma. British Medical Journal 2: 277–278

Judge D M, Dickman P S, Trapukdi S 1976 Nonfunctioning argyrophilic tumor (Apudoma) of the hepatic duct. American Journal of Clinical Pathology 66: 40–50

Jutte D L, Bell R H, Penn I M, Powers J, Kolinjivadi J 1986 Carcinoid tumor of the biliary system. Digestive Diseases and Sciences 32: 763–769

Kalman P G, Stone R M, Philips M J 1981 Heterotopic gastric tissue of the bile duct. Surgery 89: 384–386

Khan A N, Wilson I, Sherlock D J, DeKrester D, Chisholm R M 1998 Sonographic features of mucinous biliary papillomatosis: Case report and review of imaging findings. Journal of Clinical Ultrasound 26: 141–154.

Kienzle H F, Bahr R, Stolte M 1986 Granularzell tumor des ductus choledochus. Deustche Medizinische Wochenschrift 111: 197

Kittredge R D, Baer J W 1975 Percutaneous transhepatic cholangiography: problems in interpretation. American Journal of Roentgenology, Radium Therapy and Nuclear Medicine 125: 35–46

Kozuka S, Tsubone M, Hachisuka K 1984 Evolution of carcinoma in the extrahepatic bile ducts. Cancer 54: 65–72

Kune G A, Polgar V 1976 Leiomyoma of the common bile duct causing obstructive jaundice. The Medical Journal of Australia 1: 698–699

Lam C M, Yuen S T, Yuen W K, Fan S T 1996 Biliary papillomatosis. British Journal of Surgery 83: 1712–1715

Laughlin E, Keown M, Jackson J 1983 Heterotopic pancreas obstructing the ampulla of Vater. Archives of Surgery 118: 979–980

Leriche R 1934 Volomineuse tumeur papillomateuse du choledoque chez un enfant. Lyons Chirurgical 31: 598–602

Leroy J P, Charles J F, Diveres B, Bellet M 1979 Carcinome biliaire developpe sur maladie de Caroli, Archives d'Anatomie, et de Cytologie Pathologique 27: 121–125

Lewis W D, Buell J F, Jenkins R L, Burke P A 1993 Biliary duct granular cell tumor: A rare but surgically curable benign tumor HPB Surgery 6: 311–317

Li A K C, Warshaw A L, Malt R A 1981 Pseudotumor at the confluence of the hepatic ducts as a pitfall of percutaneous transhepatic cholangiography. Surgery, Gynecology and Obstetrics 152: 59–62

Lindner H H, Green R B 1964 Embryology and surgical anatomy of the extrahepatic biliary tract. North American Clinics of Surgery 44: 1273–1284

Little J M, Gibson A A M, Kay A W 1968 Primary common bile duct carcinoid. British Journal of Surgery 55: 147–149

LiVolsi V A, Perzin K H, Badder E M, Price J B, Porter M 1973 Granular cell tumors of the biliary tract. Archives of Pathology 95: 13–17

Loh A, Kamar S, Dickson G H, 1994 Solitary benign papilloma (papillary adenoma) of the cystic duct: A rare cause of biliary colic. British Journal of Clinical Practice 48: 167–168

Lukes P J, Nilson A E, Rolny P, Gamklou R 1979 Premalignant lesions of the papilla of Vater and the common bile duct. Acta Chirurgica Scandinavica 145: 545–548

McIntyre J A, Pay-Zen C 1968 Adenoma of the common bile duct causing obstructive jaundice. The Canadian Journal of Surgery 11: 215–218

MacKenzie D J, Klapper E, Gordon L A, Silberman A W 1994 Granular cell tumor of the biliary system. Medical Pediatric Oncology 23: 50–56

Madden J J, Smith G W 1974 Multiple biliary papillomatosis. Cancer 34: 1316–1320

Mahour G H, Wakim K G, Ferris D E 1967 The common bile duct in man: its diameter and circumference. Annals of Surgery 165: 415–419

Mandeville G A, Stawski W S 1991 Obstructing leiomyoma of the common bile duct bifurcation simulating a Klatskin tumor. American Surgeon 57: 676–678

Mandujano-Vera G, Angeles-Angeles A, Cruz-Hernandez J, Sansores-Perez M, Larriva-Sahd J 1995 Gastrinoma of the common bile duct: Immunohistochemical and ultrastructural study of a case. Journal of Clinical Gastroenterology 20: 321–324

Manstein M E, McBrearty F X, Pellechia P E, Paskin D L 1981 Granular cell tumor of the common bile duct. Digestive Diseases and Sciences 26: 938–942

Marsh J L, Dahms B, Longmire W P Jr 1974 Cystadenoma and cystadenocarcinoma of the biliary system. Archives of Surgery 109: 41–43

Mauro M A, Jaques P F 1981 Granular cell tumors of the esophagus and common bile duct. Journal of the Canadian Association of Radiologists 32: 254–256

Meng W C S, Lau W Y, Choi C L, Li A K C 1996 Laser therapy for multiple biliary papillomatosis via choledochoscopy. Australian and New Zealand Journal of Surgery 67: 664–666

Miyano T, Tadaaki T, Suzuki F, Suda K 1989 Adenoma and stone formation of the billiary tract in puppies that had choledochopancreatic anastomosis. Journal of Pediatric Surgery 24: 539–542

Moore S, Palmer Gold R, Lebwohl O, Price J B, Lefkowitch J H 1984 Adenosquamous carcinoma of the liver arising in biliary cystadenocarcinoma: Clinical, radiologic, and pathologic features with review of the literature. Journal of Clinical Gastroenterology 6: 267–275

Mulhollan T J, Ro T Y, El-Naggar A K, Sahin A A, Ayala A G 1992 Granular cell tumor of the biliary tree. Letters to the editor. American Journal of Surgical Pathology 16: 204–209

Murray M R 1951 Cultural characteristics of three granular cell myoblastomas. Cancer 4: 857–865

Nasu S, Sakurai M, Miyagi T 1971 Cholangiocarcinoma arising in intrahepatic bile duct cyst. Nihonrinsho 29: 3075–3081

Oden B 1955 Neurinoma of the common bile duct. Acta Chirurgica Scandinavica 108: 393–397

Ohta H, Yamaguchi Y, Yamakawa O, Watanabe H, Satomura Y, Motoo Y, Okai T, Terada T, Sawabu N 1993 Biliary papillomatosis with point mutation of K-ras gene arising in congenital choledochal cyst. Gastroenterology 105: 1209–1212

Oren R, Goldin E, Harats N, Libson E, Shouval D 1991 Localized primary sclerosing cholangitis mimicking a cholecystectomy stricture relieved by an endoprosthesis. Postgraduate Medicine Journal 67: 482–484

Orenstein H H, Brenner L H, Nay H R 1984 Granular cell myoblastoma of the extrahepatic biliary system. American Journal of Surgery 147: 827–831

Padfield C J H, Ansell I D, Furness P N 1988 Mucinous biliary papillomatosis: A tumor in need of wider recognition. Histopathology 13: 687–694

Paskin D L, Hull J D, Cookson P J 1972 Granular cell myoblastoma: a comprehensive review of 15-years experience. Annals of Surgery 175: 501–504

Pilz E 1961 Uber ein karzinoid des ductus choledochus. Zentrabl Chir 86: 1588–1590

Ponka A, Laasonen L, Strengell-Usanov L 1983 Angioleiomyoma of the common bile duct. Acta Medica Scandinavica 213: 407–410

Raia A A, Saad W A, DaSilva A T, Madi R, Waitzberg D L 1978 Myoblastoma of the common bile duct: Presentation of a case. Revista Da Associaco Medica Brasileria 24: 379–380

Rugge M, Sonego F, Militello C, Guido M, Ninfo V 1992 Primary carcinoid tumor of the cystic and common bile ducts. American Journal of Surgical Pathology 16: 802–807

Sabini A, Baden J, Norman J, Martin J 1970 Heterotopic pancreatic tissue in the common bile duct or ampulla of Vater. The American Surgeon 36: 662–666

Sanchez J A, Nauta R J 1991 Resection of granular cell tumor at the hepatic confluence. A precarious location for benign tumor. American Surgeon 57: 446–450

Santorini J D 1724 Observationes anatomicae. Venetiis.

Sarma D P, Rodriguez F H, Hoffman E O 1980 Paraganglioma of the hepatic duct. Journal of the Southern Medical Association 73: 1677–1678

Savage A, Devitt P 1977 Granular cell myoblastoma of the biliary tree. Postgraduate Medical Journal 53: 574–577

Schiewe R, Baudisch E, Erhhardt G 1968 Angeborene intrahepatische gallengangzyste mit Steinbildung und maligner entartung. Bruns Beitraege zur Klinischen Chirurgie 216: 264–271

Schroyens W, Bleiberg H, Peetrons P 1987 Pseudotumoral primary sclerosing cholangitis. Report of two cases and review of the literature. Acta Gastroenterologica Belgia 1: 436–444

Short W F, Nedwich A, Levy H A, Howard J M 1971 Biliary cystadenoma. Archives of Surgery 102: 78–80

Smadja C, Bowley N B, Benjamin I S, Blumgart L H 1983 Idiopathic localised bile duct strictures: relationship to primary sclerosing cholangitis. American Journal of Surgery 146: 404–408

Stamatakis J D, Howard E R, William R 1979 Benign inflammatory tumour of the common bile duct. British Journal of Surgery 66: 257–258

Standfield N J, Salisbury J R, Howard E R 1989 Benign non-traumatic inflammatory strictures of the extrahepatic biliary system. British Journal of Surgery 76: 849–852

Sull W J, Brown H W 1972 Benign extrahepatic biliary tumor associated with acute diverticulitis. International Surgery 57: 330–333

Teter L F 1954 Massive hemorrhage from benign adenoma of the biliary duct causing death. Journal of Michigan Medical Society 53: 62–63

Thomsen P, Vasehus Madsen P, Moesgaard F, Lykkegaard Nielsens M C 1984 Biliary cystadenoma of the common bile duct with secondary biliary cirrhosis. Acta Medica Scandinavica 216: 327–330

Tompkins R K, Johnson J, Storm K F et al 1976 Operative endoscopy in the management of biliary tract neoplasms. American Journal of Surgery 132: 174–182

Tsunoda T, Eto T, Yamada M et al 1991 Segmental primary sclerosing cholangitis mimicking bile duct cancer—report of a case and review of the Japanese literature. Japanese Journal of Surgery 21: 329–334

Vance S F, Hudson R P 1969 Granular cell myoblastoma. The American Journal of Clinical Pathology 52: 208–211

Van Steenbergen W, Ponette E, Marchal G et al 1984 Cystadenoma of the common bile duct demonstrated by endoscopic retrograde cholangiography: an uncommon cancer of extrahepatic obstruction. American Journal of Gastroenterology 79: 466–471

Vesalius A 1543 De humani corporis fabrica libri septum. Basileae

Vitaux J, Salmon R J, Langville O, Buffet C, Martin E, Chaput J C 1981 Carcinoid tumor of the common bile duct. American Journal of Gastroenterology 76: 360–362

Wardell 1969 Small fatty growths obstructing cystic and common ducts. Lancet 2: 407

Weber C, Zito P, Becker S 1968 Heterotopic pancreas: an unusual cause of obstruction of the common bile duct. The American Journal of Gastroenterology 49: 153–159

Weinbren K, Mutum S S 1983 Pathological aspects of cholangiocarcinoma. Journal of Pathology 139: 217–238

Welling R E, Krause R J, Alamin K 1970 Heterotopic gastric mucosa in the common bile duct. Archives of Surgery 101: 626–627

Wetter L A, Ring E J, Pellegrini C A, Way L W 1990 Differential diagnosis of sclerosing cholangiocarcinomas of the common hepatic duct (Klatskin tumors). American Journal of Surgery 161: 57–63

Whisnant J D, Bennett S E, Huffman S R, Weiss D L, Parker J C, Griffen W O 1974 Case report: common bile duct obstruction by granular cell tumor (Schwannoma). Digestive Diseases 19: 471–476

Whitmore J T, Whitley J P, LaVerde P, Cerda J J 1969 Granular cell myoblastoma of the common bile duct. American Journal of Digestive Diseases 14: 516–520

Whittaker L D, Lynn H B, Dockerty M B, Stickler G B 1967 Heterotopic gastric mucosa in the wall of the cystic duct: Report of a case. Surgery 62: 382–385

Woods G L 1981 Biliary cystadenocarcinoma: Case report of hepatic malignancy originating in benign cystadenoma. Cancer 47: 2936–2940

Wright R B 1958 Relapsing pancreatitis: report of a case with unusual features. The British Journal of Surgery 45: 394–395

Yang K L, Ortiz L 1993 Granular cell myoblastoma involving multiple organs. Southern Medical Journal 86: 478–479

Yazdanpanah Y, Maunoury V, Saudemont A, Bouchind'Homme B, Houcke P, Lecomte-Houcke M, Paris J C 1993 Tumour a cellules granuleuses du canal cholédoque. Gastroenterologie Clinique et Biologique 17: 607

Zvargulis J E, Keating J P, Askin F B, Termberg J L 1978 Granular cell myoblastoma. American Journal of Diseases of Children 132: 68–70

53

Tumors of the gallbladder

D.L. BARTLETT, Y. FONG

INTRODUCTION

Gallbladder cancer has had a sinister reputation since its first description in 1778 (Kato et al 1994). DeStoll described the gross appearance and invasive nature of gallbladder cancer based on his study of two autopsy cases. The clinical pessimism surrounding gallbladder cancer is due to its late presentation and lack of effective therapy. In addition, gallbladder cancer spreads early by lymphatic metastasis, hematogenous metastasis, and direct invasion into the liver. It has a unique, high propensity to seed the peritoneal surfaces after tumor spillage and cause tumor implants in biopsy tracts, abdominal wounds, and the peritoneal cavity. Blalock recommended in 1924 that surgery be avoided for gallbladder cancer if the diagnosis could be made preoperatively (Blalock, 1924).

This attitude persists to the present day. The five-year survival in most large series is less than 5%, and the median survival is less than six months (Perpetuo et al 1978, Piehler and Crichlow 1978). Nevertheless, the role of radical surgery is becoming more clearly defined. It is critical for the surgeon to understand the natural history, biology, staging and surgical treatment of this tumor, so that appropriate decisions are made at the time of initial diagnosis, especially given the high chance of these lesions being found incidentally at the time of cholecystectomy. Inappropriate procedures may allow spread of tumor throughout the abdominal cavity, to laparoscopic port sites, or biopsy needle tracts, rendering the disease untreatable. On the other hand, it is important to understand the limitations of surgical resection so that operations with unreasonably high morbidity but minimal chance of success are avoided.

EPIDEMIOLOGY

The incidence of gallbladder cancer is extremely variable by geographic region and racial-ethnic groups. Comparison of incidence rates from international cancer registries show that gallbladder cancer is up to 25 times more common in some geographical regions compared to others (Diehl 1980). The highest incidences are reported in Chileans, northeastern Europeans, Israelis, American Indians, and Americans of Mexican origin. It has recently been reported that gallbladder cancer is the main cause of death from cancer among women in Chile (Roa et al 1993). Although overall, Japan has an intermediate incidence rate, it has been reported to have the highest mortality from gallbladder carcinoma in males (Yamaguchi & Enjoji 1988). The lowest rates are seen in black Zimbabweans and black Americans, and the people of Spain and India. Within the United States and the United Kingdom, urban areas show higher incidences than rural regions (Diehl 1980, Zatonski et al 1993). It has been suggested that lower socioeconomic status may lead to delayed access to cholecystectomy which may increase gallbladder cancer rates (Serra et al 1996).

Women are two to six times more commonly afflicted by gallbladder cancer than men. The incidence steadily increases with age, reaching its maximum in the seventh decade of life (Nakayama 1991). Nevertheless, reports exist of a 21-year old Chilean female (De Aretxabala et al 1994) and an 11 year-old American Indian girl (Rudolph & Cohen 1972) with the diagnosis of gallbladder cancer. Trends in gallbladder cancer mortality from 1965 to 1989 show a variable pattern. Germany and the Netherlands both have relatively high mortality rates from gallbladder cancer and have shown appreciable declines in most age groups. Sweden, France, and Bulgaria began with relatively low gallbladder cancer mortality rates and showed steady upward trends (Zatonski et al 1993). Gallbladder cancer incidence in the United States, Britain and Canada has stabilized or declined, coincident with the rise in the number of cholecystectomies.

Overall in the United States gallbladder cancer is the

most common biliary tract malignancy and the fifth most common gastrointestinal malignancy. Pancreatic cancer is about five times more common. Last SEER (Surveillance, Epidemiology, and End Results) program estimates revealed an incidence of 1.2 cases per 100 000 population per year in the United States (Carriaga & Henson 1995). Based on SEER data there are approximately 2800 deaths per year secondary to gallbladder cancer in the United States.

It is important to consider risk factors for gallbladder cancer and their influence on the variable incidence rate reported for gallbladder cancer. The most obvious risk factor is gallstone disease. Seventy-five to ninety-eight percent of all patients with carcinoma of the gallbladder have cholelithiasis (Wanebo & Vezeridis, 1994). Gallbladder cancer is usually associated with cholesterol-type stones. The epidemiology of gallbladder cancer is closely linked to the epidemiology of gallbladder stones (Zatonski et al 1997), however it is still not agreed as to whether this represents cause and effect or common risk factors.

Case control studies have only identified a history of biliary problems, older age, and female sex as risk factors for the development of gallbladder cancer (Ghadirian et al 1993, Kodama & Kodama 1994). The presence of an anomalous pancreaticobiliary duct junction has been suggested in numerous reports to be a risk factor for gallbladder cancer independent of the presence of gallstones (Chijiiwa et al 1993). This may establish a chronic inflammatory state of the gallbladder. Typhoid carriers may also suffer chronic inflammation of the gallbladder and have a six-fold higher risk of gallbladder cancer (Welton et al 1979). Other rare associations with gallbladder cancer include inflammatory bowel disease (Joffe & Antonioli 1981) and polyposis coli (Willson et al 1987). Reports of family clusters of gallbladder cancer exist in the literature (Trajber et al 1982), but any inherited predisposition has not been found in large series of gallbladder cancer (Fernandez et al 1994).

ETIOLOGY

Epidemiologic data implicate gallstones and chronic inflammation of the gallbladder in the pathogenesis of this tumor. Nevertheless, the incidence of gallbladder cancer in a population of patients with gallstones is from 0.3 to 3%, which is quite low if this is the only factor to consider. Calcification of the gallbladder (porcelain gallbladder) is associated with gallbladder cancer in 10 to 25% of cases (Berk et al 1973). The significance of this from an etiologic standpoint is not clear. Calcification is considered the end stage of a long-standing inflammatory process, and it may be that the addi-

tive effects of inflammation over a long period of time leads to carcinogenesis. It has also been suggested that the association of gallbladder cancer and calcification may be the phenomenon of scar cancer. It may be the process of scar formation as opposed to inflammation which results in transformation. The porcelain gallbladder is associated with significant scarring and fibrosis (Albores-Saavedra et al 1986).

Since infection usually accompanies chronic cholecystitis, it has been proposed that bacteria may be important in the pathogenesis of carcinoma. Both bacterial infection without stones and stones without bacterial colonization have been associated with gallbladder cancer. It is likely to be the chronic inflammation that predisposes to neoplasia, regardless of the cause of inflammation. Nevertheless, it has been difficult experimentally to induce gallbladder cancer in animals with chronic irritation alone. Fortner and Randall (1961) placed gallstones of patients with and without carcinoma of the gallbladder into the gallbladders of 126 cats. After four to five years they found carcinoma in three cats, one of which was from a patient without carcinoma.

An appealing hypothesis is that chronic inflammation acts as a promoter for some other carcinogenic exposure. Experimentally, Kowalewski and Todd (1971) showed that carcinoma of the gallbladder was induced in 68% of hamsters who had cholesterol pellets inserted into the gallbladder and were given the carcinogen dimethylnitrosamine versus only 6% of controls fed the carcinogen alone. Similar results have been reported by others (Enomoto et al 1999, Piehler & Crichlow 1978). An attempt to identify carcinogens active in human gallbladder cancer has been made. The composition of bile has been studied for the presence of carcinogens. A higher concentration of free radical oxidation products (Shukla et al 1994) and a higher concentration of secondary bile acids (biliary deoxycholate) (Shukla et al 1993) were found in patients with gallbladder cancer compared to controls with cholelithiasis alone. Strom et al (1996) found a higher concentration of biliary versus sodeoxycholate compared to controls without cancer. Chemicals implicated in carcinogenesis include methyldopa (Broden & Bengtsson 1980), oral contraceptives (Ellis et al 1978), isoniazid (Lowenfels & Norman 1999) and occupational exposure in the rubber industry (Mancuso & Brennan 1970), but none of these associations have been proven.

ANATOMIC CONSIDERATIONS

The anatomy of the gallbladder is reviewed in detail elsewhere, but certain considerations are important in the management of gallbladder cancer. The location of the primary tumor within the gallbladder and the proximity of the portal vein, hepatic artery, and bile duct are important considerations in the surgical management. The gallbladder lies on segments IVb and V of the liver and these segments are involved early in tumors of the fundus and body. A limited segmental liver resection is often possible in these patients. Tumors of the infundibulum or cystic duct readily obstruct the common bile duct and/or portal vein. This may make the tumor unresectable at an early time point. Tumors in this region often require extended liver resections because of the proximity to or invasion of the portal pedicles. In addition, tumors of the infundibulum or cystic duct usually necessitate resection of the common bile duct.

The lymphatic drainage of the gallbladder has been described in detail (Shirai et al 1992). A diagram of the principal routes of lymphatic drainage as determined by dye injection into the gallbladder lymphatics or proximal lymph nodes is shown in Figure 53.1. Importantly, the dye never ascended towards the hepatic hilum, whereas it stained node-bearing adipose tissue posterior to the head of the pancreas and portal vein as an early event. In general, the lymph descends around the bile duct and involves cystic and pericholedochal nodes first. From there connections are made to nodes posterior to the pancreas, portal vein, and common hepatic artery. Finally, the flow reaches the interaortocaval, celiac, and superior mesenteric artery lymph nodes. There is evidence that some connections are made directly from the pericholedochal nodes to interaortocaval nodes which explains the difficulty in controlling this disease with a regional lymph node dissection. It also shows the importance of full mobilization of the duodenum and pancreas with dissection of the retropancreatic and interaortocaval lymph nodes as a routine in the management of gallbladder cancer.

PATHOLOGY

Pre-neoplastic lesions

As with most tumors, gallbladder epithelium progresses from dysplasia to carcinoma in situ to invasive carcinoma (Albores-Saavedra et al 1986). If the entire gallbladder mucosa is sectioned in cases of gallbladder cancer, severe dysplasia and carcinoma in situ will be identified in over 90% of cases. In general it is easy to differentiate the cellular atypia associated with cholecystitis from dysplasia and

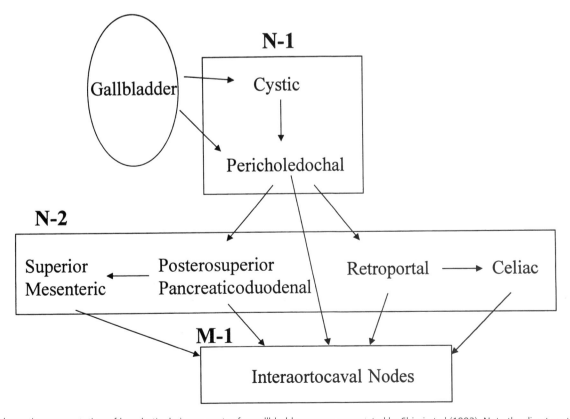

Fig. 53.1 Schematic representation of lymphatic drainage routes for gallbladder cancer as reported by Shirai et al (1992). Note the direct route from N-1 pericholedochal lymph nodes to M-1 interaortocaval lymph nodes.

carcinoma in situ (Fig. 53.2). It is likely that areas of dysplasia and carcinoma in situ are often missed in routine cholecystectomy specimens as there are no associated gross characteristics that would target an area for histologic section. It is important for the pathologist to realize that carcinoma in situ may appear within the Rokitansky-Aschoff sinuses and be mistaken for invasive carcinoma. The rate of progression of precursor lesions to invasive carcinoma has been estimated to be around 15 years (Roa et al 1996). In another series there was a five-year difference between the mean ages of patients with dysplasia and those with carcinoma in situ and a 10-year difference between the mean ages of patients with carcinoma in situ and those with invasive carcinoma (Albores-Saavedra et al 1986).

The precancerous nature of adenomas of the gallbladder are more controversial. Adenomas have been reported to be present in up to 1.1% of cholecystectomy specimens (Aldridge & Bismuth 1990). Evidence for the adenoma–adenocarcinoma sequence comes from the description of seven adenomas showing traceable histologic change into malignancy and from the finding that 19 percent of invasive carcinomas had adenomatous components (Kozuka et al 1982). Another explanation is that all well-differentiated papillary carcinomas simply show a spectrum of cytologic abnormalities that vary from minimal nuclear atypia to overt malignant changes (Albores-Saavedra et al 1986). Benign adenomas do not have the same association with cholecystitis as do invasive carcinomas therefore it is unlikely that the majority of carcinomas arise in adenomas. Nevertheless, it may be that some tumors arise in this manner, specifically papillary cancers may represent malignant degeneration of papillary adenomas.

Gross morphology

Carcinomas are difficult to differentiate grossly from chronic cholecystitis at early stages, and are often found incidentally on pathologic section. At later stages the gallbladder may be distended by the tumor, or contracted and collapsed (Fig. 53.3). Obstruction of the neck or cystic duct may lead to a hydrops. Approximately 60% of tumors originate in the fundus of the gallbladder, 30% in the body, and 10% in the neck (Albores-Saavedra et al 1986). Tumors that arise in the neck and Hartmann's pouch may infiltrate the cystic and common bile duct making it clinically and radiographically indistinguishable from hilar bile duct tumors.

In general, these tumors can be categorized into infiltrative, nodular, combined nodular-infiltrative, papillary, and combined papillary-infiltrative forms (Sumiyoshi et al 1991). The most common form is the infiltrative or combined nodular-infiltrative forms. The infiltrative tumors cause thickening and induration of the gallbladder wall, sometimes extending to involve the entire gallbladder (Fig. 53.4). They seem to spread in a subserosal plane which is the same as the surgical plane used for routine cholecystectomy. If the tumor is unrecognized at the time of surgery, it is easy to see how this leads to regional dissemination of tumor. As the infiltrative tumor becomes more advanced it invades the liver and can result in a thick wall of tumor encasing the gallbladder.

Nodular types can show early invasion through the gallbladder wall into the liver or neighboring structures. Despite this invasiveness, it may be easier to control surgically than the infiltrative form where the margins are less

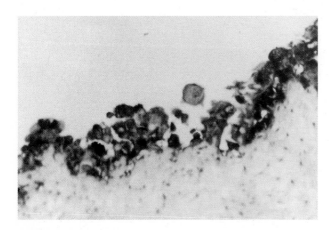

Fig. 53.2 Light micrograph of gallbladder carcinoma in situ after PAP and CEA antibody staining. Reproduced with permission from the AFIP Atlas of Tumor Pathology (Albores-Saavedra & Henson 1986).

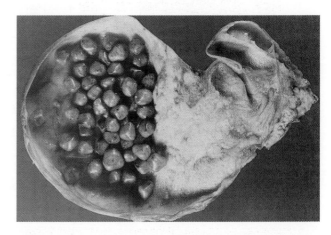

Fig. 53.3 Oat cell carcinoma of the gallbladder: This infiltrative tumor arose in the body of the gallbladder and is associated with many stones. Reproduced with permission from the AFIP Atlas of Tumor Pathology (Albores-Saavedra & Henson 1986).

defined. Papillary carcinomas exhibit a polypoid or cauliflower-like appearance (Fig. 53.5). They have a much better prognosis than the other types. The papillary tumor may be quite large and fill the lumen of the gallbladder with only minimal invasion of the gallbladder wall.

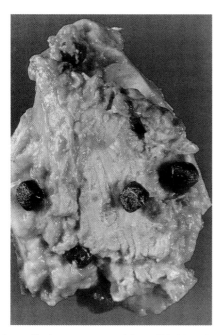

Fig. 53.4 Giant cell adenocarcinoma of the gallbladder: This tumor has an infiltrative nature, but fills most of the lumen of the gallbladder. Reproduced with permission from the AFIP Atlas of Tumor Pathology (Albores-Saavedra & Henson 1986).

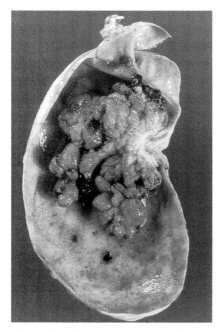

Fig. 53.5 Papillary adenocarcinoma of the gallbladder: this tumor has a cauliflower-like appearance and protrudes into the lumen with minimal invasion of the gallbladder wall. These tumors have the best prognosis. Reproduced with permission from the AFIP Atlas of Tumor Pathology (Albores-Saavedra & Henson 1986).

HISTOLOGY

The classification of malignant tumors of the gallbladder is displayed in Table 53.1. The histologic types and incidences of gallbladder cancer as recorded in the Surveillance, Epidemiology, and End Results (Carriaga and Henson, 1995) Program of the National Cancer Institute are listed in Table 53.2. While nearly all tumors can be classified into one of the histologic categories, most tumors exhibit more than one histologic pattern.

The only histologic type with clear prognostic significance is the papillary adenocarcinoma which has a markedly improved survival compared to all other histologic types (Carriaga & Henson 1995). There is some evidence to suggest that oat cell carcinomas (Henson et al 1992) and adenosquamous tumors (Yamaguchi & Enjoji 1988) have a poorer survival rate, but these conclusions are based on small numbers of patients. Recently gallbladder cancers have been separated into metaplastic and non-metaplastic types based on the presence or absence of metaplastic changes in the tumour tissues. This is similar in concept to the classification of gastric carcinoma into intestinal and

Table 53.1 Classification of malignant tumors of the gallbladder. Adapted from Table 1 in the AFIP Atlas of Tumor Pathology (Albores-Saavedra et al 1986)

Malignant epithelial tumors	Malignant mesenchymal tumors
Adenocarcinoma	Embryonal rhabdomyosarcoma
Well-differentiated	Leiomyosarcoma
Papillary	Malignant fibrous histiocytoma
Intestinal type	Angiosarcoma
Pleomorphic giant cell	Oat cell carcinoma
Poorly-differentiated, small cell	
Signet ring cell	
Clear cell	
Colloid	
With choriocarcinoma-like areas	
Squamous	
Adenosquamous	
Oat cell carcinoma	

Table 53.2 Relative incidence of gallbladder cancer by histologic type as reported by Carriaga and Henson (1995).

Histologic type	Relative incidence
Carcinoma	99%
Adenocarcinoma	89.4%
Papillary	5.7%
Mucinous and mucin-producing	5.3%
Squamous cell	1.8%
Other and unspecified	7.8%
Sarcoma	0.2%
Other and unspecified	0.9%

diffuse types. The metaplastic type showed a significantly improved survival rate (Yamamoto et al 1989).

Primary malignant mesenchymal tumors have been described including embryonal rhabdomyosarcoma, leiomyosarcoma, malignant fibrous histiocytoma, angiosarcoma, and Kaposi's sarcoma. Other primary rare tumors of the gallbladder which have been described in the literature include carcinosarcoma, carcinoid, lymphoma, and melanoma. In addition, the gallbladder can be involved with metastatic cancers from numerous sites.

Gallbladder cancers undergo histopathologic grading from G1-well differentiated to G4-undifferentiated. It is not clear that this has any prognostic significance over the observation that the papillary cancers which tend to be well differentiated have a better prognosis. For adenocarcinoma not specified as to type in the SEER data, there was a statistically significant linear association between grade and survival, such that the higher grade tumors had a worse prognosis (Henson et al 1992). The majority of patients present with grade 3, poorly differentiated tumors. It is clear that the stage of disease is the most reliable predictor of outcome over and above grade or histology. In addition, DNA ploidy has been studied for prognostic significance (Baretton et al 1994). While DNA ploidy corresponds to the grade of the tumor, it also has no prognostic significance compared to conventional staging.

Tumor biology

Multiple genetic changes are associated with the development of many tumors, and these changes usually represent activation of proto-oncogenes or inactivation of tumor suppressor genes. Recent studies have begun to describe the presence of p53 and K-ras mutations in gallbladder cancer (Itoi et al 1996). P53 is identifiable by immunohistochemistry, and if found generally represents a mutation and cellular accumulation of the P53 protein. It is found in 92% of invasive carcinomas, 86% of carcinoma in situ, and 28% of dysplastic epithelium (Wee et al 1994). K-ras mutations are identified in 39% of gallbladder carcinomas studied (Imai et al 1994). An average of 2.1 allele-specific mutations were found in invasive gallbladder carcinomas with 91% loss of heterozygosity at the p53 locus in a study of patients from Chile (Wistuba et al 1995). It is felt that allele-specific deletions of the p53 and DCC genes and of chromosome 9p play an important and early role in the pathogenesis of endemic gallbladder cancer in Chile. Other genetic abnormalities identified which may play an important role in pathogenesis include overexpression of the c-erbB-2 gene (Chow et al 1995) and decreased expression of the nm23 gene product (Fujii et al 1995).

Pattern of spread

Gallbladder cancer can spread by many routes and has a remarkable propensity to seed and grow in the peritoneal cavity, as well as along needle biopsy sites and in laparoscopic port sites. The tumor can spread early by direct extension into the liver and other adjacent organs. This predilection may be attributed to the anatomy of the gallbladder. The gallbladder has a thin wall, a narrow lamina propria, and only a single muscle layer. Tumor invades into the liver at a thickness where in other organs it would be encountering a second muscle layer. Once it penetrates the thin muscle layer it has access to major lymphatic and vascular channels. Gallbladder cancer therefore tends to have early lymphatic and hematogenous spread.

An autopsy study revealed a 94.4% incidence of lymphatic metastasis and 64.8% incidence of hematogenous dissemination (Kimura et al 1989). Hematogenous metastasis tend to be from small veins extending directly from the gallbladder into the portal venous system of the gallbladder fossa leading to segments IV and V of the liver, or via larger veins to the portal venous branch of segments V and VIII (Boerma, 1994). The incidence of regional invasion and metastasis at the time of diagnosis and treatment has been recently reviewed and is summarized in Table 53.3. There is a high propensity for intra-abdominal recurrence after resection with distant metastasis occurring late in the course. At post mortem examination, Perpetuo et al (Perpetuo et al 1978) reported that 91% of patients have liver metastasis and 82% have intra-abdominal lymph node involvement. Sixty percent had peritoneal spread, 32% had lung metastasis, and 5% had brain metastasis. The only common extra-abdominal site of metastasis is the lung. It is rare, however, to have metastasis to the lung in the absence of advanced local-regional disease.

Table 53.3 Incidence of regional invasion and metastasis at the time of diagnosis and treatment based on a literature review by Boerma (1994).

Pathologic finding	Relative incidence
Confined to gallbladder wall	10%
Liver invasion	59%
Common bile duct infiltration	35%
Lymphatic invasion and regional lymphatic metastases	45%
Gallbladder vein infiltration	39%
Portal vein or hepatic artery invasion	15%
Adjacent organ invasion (excluding liver)	40%
Perineural invasion	42%
Liver metastasis	34%
Distant metastasis (excluding liver)	20%

CLINICAL PRESENTATION

The clinical presentation of gallbladder cancer is identical to the more prevalent symptoms of biliary colic and/or chronic cholecystitis, making it difficult to suspect the diagnosis pre-operatively. Certainly for patients greater than 70 years old with a history of recent weight loss and steady right upper quadrant pain the diagnosis should be suspected. Careful history taking may reveal patients with gallbladder cancer to have a more continuous, diffuse abdominal pain compared to the crampy right upper quadrant pain associated with biliary colic. Jaundice and anorexia tend to be a sign of advanced disease (Oertli et al 1993). In a review from Thorbjarnarson and Glenn (1959), the presence of a right upper quadrant mass in association with gallbladder cancer reflected unresectability in 23 of 25 patients. Clinical jaundice represented unresectability in 18 of 18 patients. The incidence of symptoms and signs are summarized from 4 large studies in Table 53.4. The duration of symptoms does not seem to provide any clues to the presence of tumor.

Laboratory examination does not identify abnormalities specific for gallbladder cancer which may help in the diagnosis. Increased alkaline phosphatase and/or bilirubin levels are found in cases of advanced tumors. A trend towards anemia and leukocytosis has also been identified as an indicator of advanced disease (Thorbjarnarson and Glenn 1959). Serum CEA and CA19-9 levels have been studied as to their screening potential in gallbladder carcinoma. A CEA greater than 4 ng/ml is 93% specific for the diagnosis of gallbladder cancer compared to controls undergoing cholecystectomy or upper abdominal surgery for benign conditions. However, it is only 50% sensitive for detecting the diagnosis of cancer (Strom et al 1990). Ca 19-9 is a better serum marker for gallbladder cancer (Ritts et al 1999). At a serum level greater than 20 units/ml the test has 79.4% sensitivity and 79.2% specificity. Using the tests in series or parallel did not significantly improve the results. It appears that serum Ca 19-9 levels are a useful adjunct to ambiguous or indeterminate radiologic imaging.

RADIOLOGIC INVESTIGATION

Before the routine use of computed tomography (CT) and ultrasound, the preoperative diagnosis rate for gallbladder carcinoma was only 8.6%. In the 1980s, CT scanning and real-time ultrasonography increased the preoperative diagnosis rate to between 75% and 88% (Chijiiwa et al 1991). It is not clear, however, whether this increase in the preoperative diagnosis rate has had any positive impact on treatment results. In general, the tumors diagnosed pre-operatively by CT scan or ultrasound are already quite advanced and may not be amenable to curative resection. Nevertheless, accurate radiologic diagnosis combined with percutaneous fine needle aspiration cytology may avoid an unnecessary laparotomy in many patients.

A comparison of ultrasonographic features of early malignancy and benign gallbladder disease revealed some findings that were important in the differentiation. Discontinuous gallbladder mucosa, echogenic mucosa, and submucosal echolucency were significantly more common in gallbladder cancer than in benign gallbladder disease. A polypoid mass was present in 27% and a gallbladder-replacing/invasive mass was present in 50% of cases of gallbladder cancer examined (Wibbenmeyer et al 1995). These findings were specific for gallbladder cancer. Other studies confirm that the most common finding on ultrasound is an inhomogenous mass replacing all or part of the gallbladder (Franquet et al 1991, Bach et al 1998). Diffuse thickening of the gallbladder wall is also a common finding described for gallbladder cancer on both ultrasound and CT scans, but this is also found commonly in benign conditions and probably does not aid in the diagnosis.

In a recent study, computed tomography scanning revealed a mass almost filling the gallbladder lumen in 42% of cases, a polypoidal mass in 26%, and diffuse wall thickening in 6% of gallbladder cancer patients (Kumar and Aggarwal 1994) (see Fig. 53.6). Twenty-six percent of patients had a mass in the gallbladder fossa without a recognizable gallbladder. The preoperative diagnosis of

Table 53.4 Summary of symptoms and signs from 5 large reviews.

Symptoms/signs	North (1998) (North et al 1998)	Chao (1991) (Chao & Greager 1991)	Thorbjarnarson (1959) (Thorbjarnarson & Glenn 1959)	Burdette (1957) (Burdette 1957)	Perpetuo (1978) (Perpetuo et al 1978)
Abdominal pain	62%	54%	86%	82%	97%
Jaundice	13%	46%	23%	50%	44%
Weight loss	7%	28%	35%	47%	77%
Anemia	NR	8%	5%	3%	NR

NR = not reported

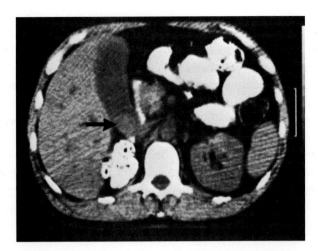

Fig. 53.6 CT scan showing a filling defect in the neck of the gallbladder (arrow) representing an early carcinoma (Collier & Blumgart 1994).

metastatic tumor in lymph nodes may alter the surgeon's decision to operate, or change the operative approach. The CT scan may be useful in this regard. A positive node on CT scan is described as a soft tissue mass with an anteroposterior dimension of at least 10 mm showing a ringlike or heterogeneous enhancement. These criteria result in an accuracy of 89% in diagnosing regional lymph nodes replaced with metastatic gallbladder cancer, with the highest false positive rate being in the cystic duct nodes (Ohtani et al 1993). Overall only 38% of pathologically positive nodes were identified preoperatively by CT scan.

The use of MRI scanning for the diagnostic work-up of gallbladder cancer has been reported (Wilbur et al 1988). Improving MR hardware and software has resulted in wide availability of magnetic resonance cholangiopancreatography (MRCP) (Ch. 16). MRCP may provide more detailed information than can be provided by ultrasound or CT scan, and at many centers have even replaced the more invasive PTC or ERCP (Schwartz et al 1998). Oral and intravenous cholangiography are not currently felt to be useful studies for diagnosing gallbladder cancer. Angiography is rarely indicated prior to attempted resection of advanced gallbladder cancer. A finding of portal vein or hepatic artery encasement may avoid an unnecessary laparotomy. Duplex ultrasonography often yields the necessary information. Endoscopic ultrasound is a good examination for peripancreatic and periportal adenopathy and may be helpful as an adjunct to other imaging modalities. Unfortunately, large inflammatory lymph nodes are difficult to differentiate from metastatic tumor without pathologic confirmation. Endoscopic ultrasound directed needle biopsy may be useful if the information would prevent a laparotomy.

Gallbladder cancer can cause obstructive jaundice by direct invasion of the common hepatic duct, or by compression and involvement of the common hepatic duct by pericholedochal lymph nodes. A high correlation between Mirizzi syndrome and gallbladder cancer exists (Redaelli et al 1997). Tumors may also cause limited obstruction of intrahepatic bile ducts leading to a high alkaline phosphatase level without a rise in bilirubin. Endoscopic or percutaneous cholangiographs (Ch. 17) may be indicated for the investigation of obstructive jaundice in cases of advanced tumors, and may be important in the planning of palliative management of gallbladder cancer. In addition these studies may be indicated in atypical cases with vague symptoms and abnormal liver function tests where other imaging modalities have not yielded a diagnosis. The pattern of changes seen on percutaneous transhepatic cholangiography (PTC) or endoscopic retrograde cholangiopancreatography (ERCP) within the intrahepatic bile ducts may differentiate gallbladder cancer from other tumors and benign disease. A malignant mid-common bile duct onstruction has to be assumed to be a gallbladder cancer until proven otherwise. Gallbladder cancer may lead to stricturing, distortion, or non-filling of bile ducts draining segments IV and V, with no effect on other segmental ducts (Collier et al 1984) (see Fig. 53.7).

In summary, the majority of patients will present with symptoms of biliary colic or chronic cholecystitis and undergo an ultrasound of the right upper quadrant. The ultrasonographer should be careful to look for any evidence

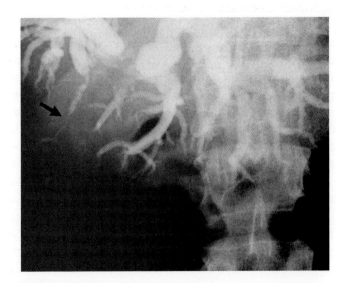

Fig. 53.7 Percutaneous transhepatic cholangiogram demonstrating malignant obstruction of the bile duct confluence and stricturing and distortion of the duct draining the segment V area of the liver (arrow). This is due to a gallbladder cancer directly invading segment V. From Collier and Blumgart (1994).

of a mass, abnormal mucosal findings, or segmental ductal dilatation. The index of suspicion should be high for elderly patients, patients with atypical symptoms, and patients with suspicious laboratory findings such as anemia, hypoalbuminemia or abnormal liver function tests. Any suspicious information should be conveyed to the surgeon and further work-up considered. Many patients in our personal series who are found incidentally at the time of cholecystectomy to have gallbladder cancer are found retrospectively to have had suspicious lesions on pre-operative ultrasound. If a suspicious finding is noted on ultrasound, a CT scan may provide complementary information. If there is laboratory or radiologic evidence of ductal obstruction an MRCP, ERCP, or PTC should be considered. Advanced masses encroaching on the porta hepatis can be further studied with duplex ultrasonography or arteriography to define major vessel involvement.

Pre-operative pathologic diagnosis

Once a mass suspicious for gallbladder cancer has been identified, it is controversial as to whether a biopsy should be performed prior to definitive exploration and resection. It is clear that cholecystectomy as a diagnostic biopsy prior to definitive resection is unacceptable, and all emphasis should be placed on being prepared for definitive resection at the time of initial exploration. The reason for controversy is that gallbladder tumors tend to seed and grow along needle biopsy tracts, along drain tracts after cholecystectomy, as drop metastasis in the peritoneal cavity, in abdominal wounds after cholecystectomy (Merz et al 1993), and in laparoscopic port sites (Fong et al 1993).

Diagnosis by examination of bile cytology is one way to avoid violating the tumor and seeding cells in the peritoneal cavity or abdominal wound. If sensitive, bile cytologic examination would be a good means for screening high risk patients for cancers of the hepatobiliary tract. The diagnostic accuracy of combined ERCP and bile cytology was reported at 50% for gallbladder cancers (Harada et al 1977). In more recent studies the sensitivity of bile cytology alone for the diagnosis of gallbladder cancer has been reported at 73% (Mohandas et al 1994) and 50% (Akosa et al 1995). The false positive rate is less than 1%. Any patient suspected of having gallbladder cancer undergoing ERCP or PTC should have bile collected for cytology. In addition, while it has not yet been shown to be effective as a general screening modality, consideration should be made for collection of bile for cytology prior to surgical exploration in high risk patients.

Percutaneous fine needle aspiration should be performed for masses which are not considered for surgical resection. It provides an easy method for obtaining tissue and an accurate pathologic diagnosis. Percutaneous core needle biopsy has a higher chance of resulting in needle tract seeding than the fine needle aspiration and should be kept in reserve for cases where fine needle aspiration is unsuccessful. The accuracy of percutaneous fine needle aspiration has been reported recently at 88% for gallbladder cancers. The false positive rate is negligible (Akosa et al 1995). In cases where a diagnosis of gallbladder cancer would result in referral to another institution for definitive surgical management, bile cytology or percutaneous fine needle aspiration cytology is preferable to any form of operative or laparoscopic biopsy.

STAGING

Multiple staging systems have been described for gallbladder cancer taking into account pathologic and clinical characteristics with prognostic significance. The different staging systems create confusion when attempting to compare the treatment results of different series in the literature. It is essential to standardize the staging system for the purpose of reporting and comparing treatment results. The main staging systems referred to in the literature over the past five years include the modified Nevin system (Donohue et al 1990, Nevin et al 1976), the Japanese Biliary Surgical Society system (Onoyama et al 1995) and the AJCC/UICC TNM staging system (Beahrs & Myers 1983) (Table 53.5). It is the latter that should be reported uniformly for standardization.

Nevin et al (1976) originally classified patients into five stages based primarily on the thickness of invasion, and combined patients with direct liver extension or distant metastasis into stage V. Donahue et al (Donohue et al 1990) modified the Nevin system to include tumors with contiguous liver invasion as stage 3 and noncontiguous liver involvement as stage 5. Stage 4 continued to include lymph node metastasis. The disadvantage of this system is that it does not differentiate tumors which invade through muscle without invading the liver from those with minimal invasion of the liver (< 2 cm) or invasion of the liver (> 2 cm). This seems to have significant prognostic significance.

The Japanese Biliary Surgical Society staging system separates tumors into four stages according to the degree of lymph node metastasis, serosal invasion, peritoneal dissemination, hepatic invasion, and bile duct infiltration. No differentiation is made between T-1 and T-2 tumors, and lymph node metastasis are considered in the same stage as microinvasion of the liver. As discussed previously, the gallbladder wall is quite thin, and a tumor of the fundus which microscopically invades the liver at an early stage would be expected to have a better prognosis than a tumor with established lymph node metastasis.

Table 53.5 Summary of most commonly used staging systems.

Stage	TNM	Modified Nevin	Japanese	Proposed new staging*
I	Mucosal or muscular invasion (T1N0M0)	In situ carcinoma	Confined to gallbladder capsule	Mucosal or muscular invasion
II	Transmural invasion (T2N0M0)	Mucosal or muscular invasion	N1 lymph nodes; minimal liver or bile duct invasion	Transmural invasion
III	Liver invasion < 2cm; lymph node metastasis (T3N1M0)	Transmural direct liver invasion	N2 lymph nodes; marked liver or bile duct invasion	(A) Liver invasion < 2 cm (T3N0M0) (B) Liver invasion > 2 cm; N1 disease (T4N0M0, TxN1M0)
IV	(A) Liver invasion > 2 cm (T4N0M0, TxN1M0) (B) Distant metastasis (TxN2M0, TxNxM1)	Lymph node metastasis	Distant metastasis	distant metastasis
V	—	Distant metastasis	—	—

*(Bartlett et al 1996)

The TNM system includes tumors invading the mucosa or muscle layer in stage I. It is important to realize that tumors can arise in Rokitanski-Aschoff sinuses and be considered stage I in a subserosal position. Tumors with invasion into the perimuscular connective tissue is considered stage II, and liver invasion less than 2 cm is stage III. In addition, nodal metastasis to the hepatoduodenal ligament are included in stage III. In contrast, stage IV includes patients with liver invasion of greater than 2 cm and no lymph node or distant metastasis. In a recent review of the gallbladder cancer experience at the Memorial Sloan-Kettering Cancer Center (MSKCC) it was clear that patients with fundal carcinomas with liver invasion > 2 cm had a better prognosis compared to those with nodal metastasis (Bartlett et al 1996). It is our impression, therefore, that stage III should be divided into IIIA and IIIB. Stage IIIA would include tumors with liver invasion less than 2 cm and no nodal metastasis (T3N0), and stage IIIB would include any N1 nodal metastasis and liver invasion greater than 2 cm (T4N0, AnyTN1). Stage IV would include only N2 nodal or distant metastasis, where there is no reasonable chance for cure.

SURGICAL MANAGEMENT

Benign polyps

Benign tumors of the gallbladder are common and can be detected on ultrasound. There remains controversy as to the malignant potential of these lesions as discussed above. They can be classified into epithelial tumors (adenoma), mesenchymal tumors (fibroma, lipoma, hemangioma) or pseudotumors (cholesterol polyps, inflammatory polyps, and adenomyoma). The majority of polyps are cholesterol polyps (Shinkai et al 1998). In addition, adenomyomatosis (extension of Rokitansky-Aschoff sinuses through the muscular wall) of the gallbladder can be picked up ultrasonographically. The question remains as to the indication for cholecystectomy if these lesions are picked up in an asymptomatic patient with or without coexistent cholelithiasis.

In a recent review of polypoid lesions of the gallbladder, ultrasound demonstrated a sensitivity of 90.1% and a specificity of 93.9% in making the diagnosis (Yang et al 1992). Out of 182 patients with polypoid lesions, malignancy was diagnosed in 13. Malignant lesions were significantly more likely to be found in patients over 50 years old, and more likely to be present as a solitary lesion > 1.0 cm in diameter. Based on these findings, the indication for cholecystectomy for asymptomatic benign polyps includes any solitary polyp greater than 1.0 cm in diameter in a patient over 50 years old. Shinkai et al (1998) reviewed 134 polypoid lesions of the gallbladder, identifying 6 cancers. Their recommendation is for cholecystectomy in patients with < 3 polyps regardless of size. For lesions that do not fit these characteristics, it is reasonable to obtain follow-up scans every six to 12 months, and any suspicious findings (focal thickening of the gallbladder wall) should be an indication for further work-up as described above. Patients with adenomyomatosis can also be followed with ultrasound screening (Aldridge & Bismuth 1990). Obviously the need for follow-up must be weighed against the morbidity of a laparoscopic cholecystectomy.

Prophylactic cholecystectomy

The incidence of gallbladder cancer is quite low compared to the incidence of gallstones in the population, and prophylactic cholecystectomy for asymptomatic cholelithiasis to prevent the development of carcinoma is not indicated. If a population at high risk is identified in the future (e.g. genetic susceptibility) then that recommendation would change. Likewise, the current recommendation for asymptomatic gallstones discovered incidentally on diagnostic imaging is that no follow-up is indicated unless symptoms develop. The risk of developing gallbladder carcinoma should not enter into this decision as it is quite low. Nevertheless, any abnormality in the gallbladder wall consistent with an early cancer needs to be taken seriously and consideration made for further work-up. Only early diagnosis and treatment of gallbladder cancer is currently able to alter its natural history.

Prophylactic cholecystectomy for gallbladder polyps is discussed in the previous section. The question of whether laparoscopic cholecystectomy is appropriate given that it is becoming clear that insufflation and laparoscopic manipulation leads to tumor cell dissemination and port site recurrences from gallbladder cancer (Wibbenmeyer et al 1995) has been addressed in a recent review by Kubota et al (1995). They recommend that polyps greater than 18 mm should be managed with open cholecystectomy and extended resection considered if carcinoma is identified.

A calcified or 'porcelain' gallbladder is an indication for cholecystectomy in the asymptomatic patient as up to 25% of cases will be associated with gallbladder cancer (Berk et al 1973). Special attention should be made to pre-operative imaging and any suspicious areas should be considered cancerous and managed accordingly. It may be in these high risk situations that serum CA19-9 evaluation and bile cytology will be helpful in making a pre-operative diagnosis of cancer. Laparoscopic cholecystectomy is not reasonable in this setting for the reasons discussed.

Extent of resection by stage

A rational approach to surgery for gallbladder carcinoma was introduced by Glenn and Hays in 1954, and included wedge resection of the gallbladder bed and regional lymphadenectomy of the hepatoduodenal ligament. Unfortunately, the overall poor prognosis, the late presentation of the tumor, and the rarity of the disease in any single institution has led to continued controversy in the surgical management. Surgeons recommend operations ranging from simple cholecystectomy alone to combined extended hepatectomy, common bile duct resection and

pancreaticoduodenectomy (Nimura et al 1991) for the same stage disease. There is currently no consensus as to the extent of surgery and the indications for radical resection. A recent survey of prominent gastrointestinal surgeons in the United States indicated that 49% recommended lymph node dissection and 64% recommended some form of liver resection for stage T2–4 disease. Twenty-one percent recommended simple cholecystectomy alone for node positive disease (Gagner & Rossi 1991). Definitive resection for gallbladder cancer depends on the stage and location of the tumor as well as whether or not it is a re-resection after a previous simple cholecystectomy.

In general, our recommendations based on results reported in the literature and our own series are as follows (see Figs 53.10 and 53.11). Stage I tumors can be treated with simple cholecystectomy. Any suspicious nodes should be removed for a frozen pathologic diagnosis. Stage II, III, and selected IVa (T4,N0) tumors should be treated with en bloc resection of the gallbladder, segments IVb and V of the liver, and regional lymph node dissection. Stage IVb tumors should be treated with appropriate palliation where indicated. Because of the high incidence of local-regional recurrence, strict operative principles should be maintained for liver resection and lymph node dissection. A diagrammatic representation of the extent of dissection in an extended cholecystectomy is shown in Fig. 53.8.

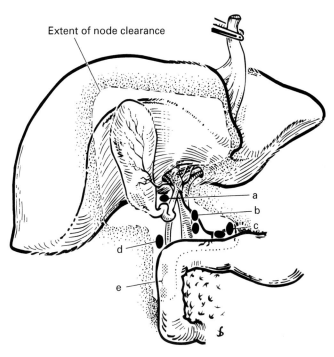

Fig. 53.8 Diagrammatic representation of the extent of dissection in an extended cholecystectomy (a–e, lymph node field) (Collier & Blumgart 1994).

Liver resection

Recommendations for liver resection for gallbladder cancer have ranged from a limited wedge excision of 2 cm of liver around the gallbladder bed to routine extended right hepatic lobectomy. It is our opinion that a limited wedge excision of the gallbladder bed is not appropriate. It is difficult to perform a wedge excision and maintain a consistent thickness around the gallbladder or gallbladder bed. In addition, such nonanatomic resection can be associated with significant bleeding and bile leaks, adding to the morbidity of the procedure. We prefer an anatomic segment IVb and V resection. The vessels to segment IVb can be controlled in the umbilical fissure in advance allowing vascular demarcation of the segment, and lessening the potential for blood loss.

Intraoperative ultrasound is helpful in defining the segmental anatomy and defining tumor margins. The resection plane is marked with the electrocautery through the liver capsule. Parenchymal dissection is then performed with intermittent inflow occlusion and the use of a Kelly clamp as described elsewhere (Ch. 83). Care must be taken to ligate the middle hepatic vein at the resection plane between segments IVa and VIII. The segmental portal triad of segment V should be encountered during the parenchymal dissection. Care must be taken to avoid injury to the anterior sectoral trunk or the segment VIII vessels, compromising blood flow to that segment.

In cases where segmental resection will result in an inadequate resection margin right hepatic lobectomy (right trisegmentectomy) should be performed. This is also true for a tumor of the gallbladder body or neck which is close to or compromises the right portal triad. In addition, sometimes after prior cholecystectomy or biliary procedures it can be difficult to differentiate scar and tumor in the portahepatis. The best management in these cases may also be a right hepatic lobectomy (Ch. 83). The complication rate for extended resection can be as high as 50% with a mortality rate of 5%. The potential gain of the procedure must justify the risk. Good patient and tumor selection are essential in these cases.

Lymph node dissection

Studies of lymphatic spread of gallbladder cancer have been published and recently reviewed (Boerma 1994). Recommendations for lymph node dissection for gallbladder cancer has ranged from excision of the cystic duct node alone to en bloc pancreaticoduodenectomy to clear the pancreaticoduodenal lymph nodes (Matsumoto et al 1992). Justification for more radical procedures comes from there being a propensity for early spread to superior anterior and posterior pancreaticoduodenal nodes, and it is assumed that nodal clearance is improved with pancreaticoduodenectomy. The benefit probably does not justify the added morbidity as the presence of N2 nodal metastasis is presumed to be an indicator of poor prognosis regardless of the extent of resection.

The real controversy lies in whether or not to routinely resect the common bile duct. It is logical to assume that resection of the common bile duct may allow more reliable complete lymphatic clearance of the hepatoduodenal ligament, but in our own experience it adds to the operative morbidity (Bartlett et al 1996). In thin patients who have not had previous biliary procedures and whose tumors arise in the fundus, it may be very easy to skeletonize the porta of all lymphatic tissue without resection of the bile duct. On the other hand, if the tumor is in the gallbladder neck and there is suspicion of spread into the common bile duct, or if inflammation and scarring compromise adequate skeletonization of the porta lymphatics, then resection of the common bile duct with subsequent Roux-en-Y hepaticojejunostomy should be performed. The technique is very similar to that employed for radical resection of hilar cholangiocarcinoma (Chs 54, 83).

In general, a full Kocher maneuver should be performed and lymphatic tissue should be dissected behind the duodenum and pancreas and swept superiorly. Any interaortocaval nodes or superior mesenteric nodes should be included in the specimen if possible. Also the soft tissue anterior to the duodenum and pancreas should be swept superiorly. The common bile duct should be transected as it courses posterior to the duodenum into the pancreas. The portal vein and hepatic artery should be skeletonized and all tissue swept superiorly along with the transected duct. At the confluence of the hepatic ducts, dissection of the porta should be continued and the relevant hepatic duct (usually the common hepatic duct or the left hepatic duct in the case of right hepatectomy) transected. A Roux-en-Y hepaticojejunostomy should be performed as described elsewhere in the text (Ch. 30). Tumors invading the porta hepatis necessitate extensive resection of the right hepatic duct, artery, and/or portal vein. In these cases a right hepatectomy lobectomy (right trisegmentectomy) should be performed with Roux-en-Y left hepaticojejunostomy for reconstruction of biliary enteric continuity (Ch. 83).

RESULTS

The natural history of gallbladder cancer has been defined through many retrospective reviews and large surveillance programs. The overall 5-year survival is consistently less than 5% with a median survival of 5 to 8 months. Piehler et al (Piehler & Crichlow 1978) reviewed 5836 cases in the world's literature from 1960 to 1978. They reported an overall 5-year survival of 4.1% and a one-year survival of 11.8%. Only about 25% were resectable for cure, and of those resected for cure, 16.5% survived 5 years. Furthermore, 5-year survival for patients found only on pathologic examination to have gallbladder cancer was 14.9%. This percentage drops to 2.9% if the surgeon identified a tumor at the time of exploration. This data illustrates the minimal impact that surgical treatment has had on this disease. The only long-term survivors were among the group where the tumor was small enough not to be recognized at the time of cholecystectomy, and even then only 14.9% survived 5 years.

Perpetuo et al (1978) reviewed the M.D. Anderson experience with gallbladder cancer over 36 years and reported a 5-year survival rate of less than 5% and median survival of 5.2 months. Cubertafond et al (1994) recently reported the results of a French Surgical Association Survey of 724 carcinomas of the gallbladder. They reported a median survival of 3 months, a 5-year survival rate of 5%, and a 1-year survival rate of 14%. They observed no differences among the different surgical procedures adopted, and concluded that no progress had been made in the treatment of gallbladder cancer. A survey of gallbladder cancer in Wessex, United Kingdom, revealed only 4 patients out of 95 surviving a duration ranging from 8 to 72 months from the time of diagnosis (Carty & Johnson 1991). A review of gallbladder cancer from Australia revealed a 12% 5-year survival rate with all survivors having stage I or II disease. The median survival for patients with stage III or IV disease was only 46 days (Wilkinson 1995).

Recent SEER data from the United States demonstrates similar unsatisfactory results with only marginal improvement over earlier studies (Carriaga & Henson 1995). Overall 5-year survival was reported at 12.3% in 2330 patients. A multi-institutional review from Japan on the other hand recently reported a 50.7% 5-year survival for 984 patients undergoing radical resection versus 6.2% for 702 patients undergoing more conservative management (Ogura et al 1991). These results suggest that it may be possible for surgery to have a role in changing the natural history of this tumor. It is again important to emphasize that there is no good prospective data on the treatment of gallbladder cancer, and no randomized trials comparing extended resection to conservative management.

Tumors confined to muscular coat (Adamsen et al 1997)

The surgical management of gallbladder carcinoma which on pathologic examination does not penetrate through the muscular layer of the gallbladder is simple cholecystectomy. In general, these lesions are noted incidentally on pathologic examination after cholecystectomy for acute or chronic cholecystectitis. No further therapy is indicated. If the lesion is recognized intra-operatively, then a cystic duct lymph node and pericholedochal lymph node may be sampled to rule out metastatic disease. Tsukada et al (1997) demonstrated 0 of 15 T-1 lesions with lymph node metastasis. Table 53.6 summarizes results of resection for stage I disease.

In a report from Japan of 31 patients with gallbladder carcinomas incidentally identified by microscopic pathologic examination, only six had stage I disease. All six were still without evidence of recurrence with a follow-up from 10 to

Table 53.6 Actuarial survival results reported in retrospective reviews after resection of stage I gallbladder cancers.

Author	Year	n	Procedure	3-year survival	5-year survival
Ouchi et al	1987	14	Not specified	78%	71.4%
Yamaguchi & Enjoji	1988	11	Not specified	100%	Not reported
Donohue et al	1990	6	83% simple cholecystectomy	100%	100%
Gall et al	1991	7	Simple cholecystectomy	86%	86%
Ogura* et al	1991	366	Not specified	87%	78%
Shirai et al	1992	39	Simple cholecystectomy	100%	100%
Yamaguchi & Tsuneyoshi	1992	6	Simple cholecystectomy	100%	100%
Shirai et al	1992	56	Simple cholecystectomy	100%	100%
		38	Extended cholecystectomy	100%	100%
Matsumoto et al	1992	4	Extended cholecystectomy	100%	100%
Oertli et al	1993	6	Simple cholecystectomy	100%	100%
Cubertafond* et al	1994	20	Simple cholecystectomy	28%	Not reported
de Aretxabala et al	1997	32	69% simple cholecystectomy	94%	94%

* – multiinstitutional survey

84 months (Yamaguchi & Tsuneyoshi 1992). In another review, of 98 inapparent carcinomas of the gallbladder, 39 patients had stage I disease (Shirai et al 1992). After cholecystectomy alone the 5-year survival rate was 100%. In an update from the same institution, patients with stage I disease were treated with simple cholecystectomy alone (56 patients) or extended cholecystectomy (33 patients) (Shirai et al 1992). With long-term follow-up only two patients recurred and went on to die of their disease. Both of these had submucosal spread of the tumor to involve the cystic duct margin. de Aretxabala et al (1997) reported 2/13 deaths in T-1 lesions that invade into muscle compared to 0/19 for the remainder of T-1 lesions. It is essential that negative margins are obtained even for stage I disease. This may necessitate a re-operation and common bile duct resection in some patients. On the other hand, radical or extended cholecystectomy is not indicated for stage I disease.

Tumor invading into subserosal layer (stage II)

The recommended management for stage II disease is an extended or radical cholecystectomy to include a liver resection and regional lymph node dissection as described above. Unfortunately, most of these lesions are also discovered incidentally at the time of pathologic examination. It is likely that a routine cholecystectomy which utilizes the subserosal plane of dissection will leave a positive margin and not be adequate treatment. In the review by Yamaguchi and Tsuneyoshi (1992), 25 patients had tumor extending into the subserosal layer and 11 of these had positive microscopic margins after simple cholecystectomy. Of those patients who had tumors with negative margins the 5-year survival rate was only 65%. This dropped to 0% for a positive margin.

It is this group of T-2 lesions who have the best chance of benefitting from definitive extended re-resection (Paquet 1998). Unfortunately, violating the subserosal tumor margin at the time of cholecystectomy may result in tumor dissemination within the peritoneal cavity and abdominal wounds. Nevertheless an attempt at curative re-resection seems justified. In the review by Shirai et al (1992), the 5-year survival rate after radical re-resection for stage II tumors was 90% which was significantly higher than that after simple cholecystectomy alone (40% 5-year survival). Tsukada et al (1997) reports 46% of T-2 tumors were associated with lymph node metastasis. In our own series, 6 of 13 patients with T-2 disease had metastatic disease to regional lymph nodes, emphasizing that regional lymph node dissection may be important for these tumors (Bartlett et al 1996). De Aretxabala (1997) compared 20 patients undergoing curative re-resection for T-2 tumors with 18 patients undergoing simple cholecystectomy alone and demonstrated a 50% improved 5-year survival rate (70% vs 20%). *If re-operation is decided upon, the patient should be advised that radical operation will be performed even should there be no evidence of residual disease at laparotomy. Indeed there may be no identifiable disease on detailed histology of the resected specimen.* (See Table 53.7.)

Ideally, if this lesion can be recognized intra-operatively, then definitive management can be undertaken and the gallbladder removed en bloc with segments IVb and V of the liver without tumor spillage. Certainly intra-operative cytologic examination of a fine needle aspirate of a suspicious thickening could make the diagnosis of cancer, but it is not possible to differentiate between T-1 and T-2 lesions without removing the gallbladder and examining it microscopically. Any suspicion of serosal invasion should be treated with definitive resection at the original operation with the gallbladder removed en bloc with the liver. The

Table 53.7 Actuarial survival results reported in retrospective reviews after resection of stage II gallbladder cancers.

Author	Year	n	Procedure	3-year survival	5-year survival
Yamaguchi & Enjoji	1988	73	Not specified	40.1%	Not reported
Donohue et al	1990	12	67% extended cholecystectomy	58%	22%
Ogura* et al	1991	499	Not specified	53%	37%
Gall et al	1991	7	86% simple cholecystectomy	86%	86%
Shirai et al	1992	35	Simple cholecystectomy	57%	40.5%
		10	Extended cholecystectomy	90%	90%
Yamaguchi & Tsuneyoshi	1992	25	Simple cholecystectomy	36%	36%
Matsumoto et al	1992	9	Extended cholecystectomy	100%	100%
Oertli et al	1993	17	Simple cholecystectomy	29%	24%
Cubertafond* et al	1994	52	88% simple cholecystectomy	20%	Not reported
Bartlett et al	1996	8	Extended cholecystectomy	100%	88%
Paquet et al	1998	5	Extended cholecystectomy	100%	80%

* – multiinstitutional survey

routine use of laparoscopic cholecystectomy will lessen the chance for intra-operative recognition of an early gallbladder cancer prior to violating the subserosal plane and potentially seeding tumor cells. While this cannot be avoided, it becomes more important to scrutinize pre-operative ultrasound for findings suspicious for cancer. In addition, the gallbladder should routinely be examined closely by the surgeon after removal and any suspicious areas marked for frozen section diagnosis. Definitive management at the time of the initial cholecystectomy is preferred.

Advanced tumors (stage III and IV)

The most significant controversy in the surgical management of gallbladder cancer lies in the treatment of advanced tumors. The debate lies in whether or not radical surgery is justified for advanced disease given the poor prognosis and low chance of long-term survival. Recently the literature abounds with reviews of radical surgery for advanced disease, and many centers report long-term survivors after aggressive surgical management. Table 53.8 provides a review of these studies.

Onoyama et al (1995) recently reported on 66 patients undergoing extended cholecystectomy in Japan. They report a 63.6% 5-year survival for Japanese Biliary Surgical Society stage II and 44.4% 5-year survival for stage III disease after extended cholecystectomy (these stages combined represent AJCC stage III). An 8.3% 5-year survival for stage IV disease was recorded. In addition, they noted a 5-year survival rate of 60% for patients having metastatic disease to N-1 nodes. These results represent a marked therapeutic alteration of the natural history of this tumor. Similarly, Nakamura et al (1989) reported 13 radical resections for tumors of Nevin's stage V with 54% alive at 1-year and two patients alive over 7 years. Five patients underwent combined pancreaticoduodenectomy and liver resection, and 3 underwent portal vein resection and reconstruction. Shirai et al (1992) reported a 45% 5-year survival for patients with node positive tumors, documenting 9 patients surviving over 5 years after radical resection.

The Japanese survival results for gallbladder cancer in general are better than those reported elsewhere. As with the results of gastric surgery this may represent stage migration from more radical operations and more careful staging, a different tumor biology, or represent improved results secondary to more standardized aggressive surgical procedures. Recently results from other countries have also demonstrated improved survival with radical surgery. Our data from the Memorial Sloan Kettering Cancer Center New York reveal a 67% actuarial 5-year survival for patients with completely resected Stage III and 33% 5-year survival for patients with completely resected stage IV tumors (Bartlett et al 1996). Gall et al (1991) in Germany also report encouraging results from radical surgery for gallbladder cancer. Four of 8 patients undergoing curative resection for AJCC stage III and IV gallbladder carcinoma at the initial operation were alive after 81, 50, 13, and 8 months. They report a median survival of 42 months for patients undergoing a curative resection at the first operation versus 12.5 months for those undergoing a curative resection at a second operation. It is clear that the best chance for success lies in appropriate initial management.

Table 53.8 Actuarial survival results reported in retrospective reviews after extended resection of stage III and IV gallbladder cancers.

Author	Year	N	Stage	3-yr surv	5-yr surv	Comments
Matsumoto et al	1992	8	III	38%	–	Majority with common bile duct (cbd) resection
Chijiiwa et al	1994	12	III	80%	–	Extended resections only
Onoyama et al	1995	12	III	44%	44%	Extended resections only
Bartlett et al	1996	8	III	63%	63%	Extended resections only
Ouchi et al	1987	12	III/IV	17%	–	Extended resections only
Nakamura et al	1989	13	III/IV	16%	16%	Includes 5 HPD, 10 extended hepatectomy
Donohue et al	1990	17	III/IV	50%	29%	Extended resections only
Gall et al	1991	8	III/IV	50%	–	Includes only curative resection at initial surgery
Shirai et al	1992	20	III/IV	–	45%	All patients have lymph node metastasis
Ogura et al	1991	453	IV	18%	8%	Multiinstitutional series with 25% simple cholecystectomy
Todoroki et al	1991	27	IV	7%	–	All patients had IORT
Nimura et al	1991	14	IV	10%	–	All patients underwent HPD
Matsumoto et al	1992	27	IV	25%	–	Includes 3 HPD, 6 extended hepatectomy, 11 cbd resection
Chijiiwa et al	1994	11	IV	11%	–	Extended resections only
Onoyama et al	1995	14	IV	8%	8%	Japanese staging
Bartlett et al	1996	7	IV	25%	25%	Long-term survivors with no lymph node metastases

HPD = hepatopancreatoduodenectomy; IORT = intraoperative radiation therapy

Suspicious findings on preoperative imaging should allow the surgeon and patient to be prepared in advance for an extended radical cholecystectomy. The diagnosis can be confirmed intraoperatively with a fine needle biopsy (to minimize the chance of tumor spillage) and an en bloc liver and lymph node dissection can be performed as the first procedure. In our series of 17 patients re-explored for gallbladder cancer after simple cholecystectomy, 8 had evidence of peritoneal or wound seeding consistent with implants from the initial procedure. None of these patients were long-term survivors even after complete resection of all disease (Bartlett et al 1996).

Laparoscopically-discovered gallbladder cancer

First described in 1985, the technique of laparoscopic cholecystectomy has become the standard procedure for treatment of patients with symptomatic gallstone disease (The Southern Surgeons Club, 1991) (Ch. 38). It is estimated that approximately 70 000 laparoscopic cholecystectomies are performed each year and that there is a decreasing perioperative morbidity traditionally associated with the surgical treatment of stone disease of the biliary tract (Grace et al 1991). With the proliferation of laparoscopic cholecystectomy, a new clinical scenario in the treatment of gallbladder cancer is now encountered, namely gallbladder cancer discovered at or after laparoscopic cholecystectomy. A number of groups (Drouard et al 1991, Pezet et al 1992, Clair et al 1993) have reported inadvertent dissemination of incidentally discovered gall bladder cancer. The utility of repeat operation for incompletely excised, laparoscopically-discovered gallbladder cancer is strongly debated.

Scant data address the utility of re-exploration and completion excision for laparoscopically discovered gallbladder cancer. A recent study examined 42 consecutive patients with laparoscopically discovered gallbladder cancer seen over a five-year period at Memorial Sloan-Kettering Cancer Center (Fong et al 1998). These were patients with advanced stage cancer, including 16 T3 and 16 T4 tumors. At re-exploration, twenty-two of the patients were found to have nodal, peritoneal, or bilateral liver disease precluding reresection. Nineteen patients had liver resection (13 right hepatic lobectomy trisegmentectomy, six bisegmentectomy), portal lymphadenectomy and hepatico-jejunostomy as the definitive operation. There was a significant survival advantage for the re-resected patients. Seventeen of the twenty-two non-resected patients have died, with a median survival of five months. With a follow-up of sixteen months, only three of the resected patients had died. These data would indicate that aggressive reresection of gallbladder cancers discovered laparoscopically is safe and effective.

A major concern about gallbladder cancer that has been discovered laparoscopically is the potential for the laparoscopic procedure to disseminate disease. Careful inspection of the abdominal cavity for dissemination of cancer should be performed during the laparotomy for re-resection of tumor. Furthermore, a number of studies in the literature have documented the potential for tumor growth in port sites after laparoscopic resection of the tumor (Fong et al 1993, Drouard et al 1991, Pezet et al 1992, Clair et al 1993, Landen 1993, Fligelstone et al 1993, Nduka et al 1994, Nally & Preshaw 1994, Kim & Roy 1994). It has therefore become our standard practice to excise laparoscopic port sites at the reexploration. Whether this will be helpful, or whether port site recurrence represents only an early indication of widely disseminated disease is unclear. Because of the potential for laparoscopic cholecystectomy to disseminate cancer, patients suspected preoperatively to have gallbladder cancer should not be subjected to a laparoscopic procedure, but rather have an open exploration with immediate potentially definitive resection. Pre-operative imaging performed in preparation for cholecystectomy should be scrutinized with vigilance for any signs of cancer. Patients with laparoscopic discovered gallbladder cancers should have conversion to an open procedure if the surgeon feels capable of performing the necessary definitive operation. If not the gallbladder should not be violated and the patient should be referred for radical resection.

Complications

An important consideration in the recommendation for radical surgery is the operative complication rate. The majority of patients undergoing treatment for gallbladder cancer are in at least their seventh decade of life, and often at increased risk for radical surgery as a consequence of concomitant medical problems. The morbidity and mortality rate of major liver resections has decreased in recent reports, even in the aged population (Fong et al 1995). The major morbidity after resection for gallbladder cancer has ranged from 5% to 54% and mortality from 0 to 21% (Table 53.9). In our series at MSKCC (Bartlett et al 1996) the complication rate was highest for those undergoing a bile duct resection.

In a multiinstitutional review of 1686 gallbladder cancer resections from Japan, a comparison of morbidity by procedure was made (Ogura et al 1991). They report 12.8% morbidity for cholecystectomy, 21.9% for extended cholecystectomy, and 48.3% for hepatic lobectomy. The mortality rates were 2.9%, 2.3%, and 17.9% respectively. They report 150 hepatopancreatoduodenectomies for galbladder cancer with a 54% morbidity and 15.3% mortality rate. The most common complications are bile collections, liver

Table 53.9 Morbidity and mortality rates after extended resection for gallbladder cancer. 'Extended procedures' refers to a variety of procedures including common bile duct resection and major liver resection in many cases.

Author	Year	n	Procedure	Morbidity	Mortality
Ouchi	1987	12	Extended procedures	–	21%
Nakamura et al	1989	13	Extended procedures	46%	0%
Donohue et al	1990	17	Extended procedures	5%	0%
Todoroki et al	1991	27	Extended chole + IORT	–	7.4%
Nimura et al	1991	14	Hepatopancreatoduodenectomy	–	21%
Gall et al	1991	8	Extended procedures	–	0%
Ogura et al	1991	659	Extended procedures	22%	2%
		302	Hepatic lobectomy	48%	18%
		150	Hepatopancreatoduodenectomy	54%	15%
de Aretxabala	1992	25	Extended procedures	–	0%
Matsumoto et al	1992	35	Extended procedures	15%	4%
Chijiiwa	1994	30	Extended procedures	–	3%
Bartlett et al	1996	23	Extended procedures	26%	0%

IORT = intraoperative radiation therapy

failure, intra-abdominal abscess, and respiratory failure. The risk of resection for each patient and for each type of resection needs to be weighed against the chance of benefit based on the stage of disease.

ADJUVANT THERAPY

Because of the rarity of this disease, as well as the rarity of completely resected gallbladder cancer, there are no prospective, randomized studies examining the utility of adjuvant therapy. The tumor has been resistant to most forms of chemotherapy, and the mode of spread does not lend itself to radiotherapy. Nevertheless, a multimodality approach with effective chemotherapy and radiotherapy would provide the best chance for long-term survival. As part of many large retrospective studies, the issue of adjuvant therapy has been addressed. In general, these include intra-operative or external beam radiation therapy and chemotherapy including 5-FU and/or mitomycin C. Other chemotherapy agents used include adriamycin and the nitrosoureas.

Chao et al (1995) reported 15 patients who received some form of chemotherapy and/or radiation therapy after resection for gallbladder cancer. There was no significant difference or trend towards improved survival compared to 7 patients who did not receive adjuvant therapy. Oswalt and Cruz (1977) reported a median survival of 20 weeks in 13 patients treated with adjuvant chemotherapy compared to 8 weeks in patients treated with surgery alone. Morrow et al (1983) from the University of Minnesota reported a median survival of 4.5 months for those receiving adjuvant chemotherapy and/or radiation therapy versus 3 months in those treated with surgery alone. It seems that it is the

patients with better performance status who receive adjuvant therapy, and it is impossible to credit minimal improvements in survival to chemotherapy without a large randomized trial.

More data has accrued on adjuvant radiation therapy, but similarly the results are inconclusive. Todoroki et al (1991) examined intraoperative radiation therapy after complete resection for stage IV gallbladder cancer. They report a 10.1% 3-year survival for patients receiving intraoperative radiation therapy versus 0% for surgery alone. Similarly Bosset et al (1989) examined post-operative external beam irradiation after complete resection in 7 patients and concluded that it was a safe treatment—5 of 7 patients were still alive at a median follow-up of 11 months. Hanna & Rider (1978) reported survival to be significantly longer in patients receiving postoperative radiotherapy compared with those who had surgery alone. In a retrospective review from Finland, the median survival of patients receiving postoperative radiation was 63 months compared with 29 months for patients receiving surgery alone (Vaittinen, 1970). While the data is encouraging, it remains inconclusive. Nevertheless, given the high incidence of local recurrence, and the minimal complications related to radiotherapy, it is not unreasonable to recommend some form of radiotherapy for selected patients, namely those with advanced T-stage or node-positive tumors.

PALLIATIVE MANAGEMENT

Given the high percentage of unresectable cases, the issue of palliative management becomes important. The median survival for patients presenting with unresectable disease is 2 to 4 months with a 1-year survival rate of less than 5%

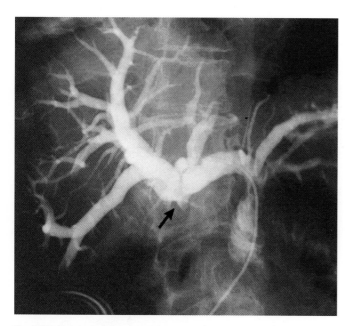

Fig. 53.9 Tubogram showing a segment III hepaticojejunostomy. The anastamosis is well away from the malignant obstructing lesion in the liver hilus (arrow). (From Collier & Blumgart 1994).

(Oertli et al 1993, Wanebo et al 1982). This aggressive course needs to be considered when deciding upon palliative management. The goal of palliation should be relief of pain, jaundice, and bowel obstruction and prolongation of life. These should be achieved as simply as possible. Resection of gross disease probably provides the best palliation and a chance for cure in some instances, but is usually not possible.

In the event of a preoperative diagnosis of advanced, unresectable gallbladder cancer in the jaundiced patient, a non-operative radiologic approach to biliary drainage is justified. Biliary enteric bypass for obstruction can be difficult because of advanced disease in the porta hepatis. For this purpose a segment III bypass is ideal (Bismuth and Corlett 1975) (Ch. 30) and can be performed at the time of initial laparotomy (Fig. 53.9). Kapoor et al (1996) report on 41 patients undergoing segment III bypass for gallbladder cancer with 87% success (12% 30-day mortality rate). The Longmire operation which includes removing a portion of the lateral segment of the left lobe to identify dilated intrahepatic ducts for anastamosis is associated with a high complication rate (Longmire et al 1973) and is not indicated since the segment III bypass provides safer and more effective decompression. In jaundiced patients with advanced disease *and without itching* it may be best to avoid biliary decompression by any means.

Chemotherapy has been used for palliation of unresectable disease. An EORTC cooperative study examined bolus mitomycin C in advanced gallbladder and biliary tree carcinoma with no significant activity identified (Taal et al 1993). Others have examined 5-FU, adriamycin, and nitrosureas alone and in combination for gallbladder cancer, with some reports of minimal responses (Perpetuo et al 1978). Regional therapy has recently been examined using intra-arterial mitomycin C for gallbladder cancer. A 48% overall response rate and a prolongation of median survival from 5 months to 14 months compared to historical controls was reported (Makela & Kairaluoma 1993).

Radiation therapy has also been examined for the palliation of gallbladder cancer. The results (Houry et al 1989) suggest that radiotherapy may increase survival. The benefit is minimal with a median survival of only 6 to 8 months. However radiotherapy does appear to be well tolerated and although of unproven benefit may improve symptoms and prolong survival in selected patients.

SUMMARY

Gallbladder cancer is an aggressive disease with a dismal prognosis. It should not, however, be approached with a nihilistic attitude. Appropriate investigation and extended resection can result in a cure. Careful pre-operative imaging for patients undergoing cholecystectomy for symptoms of cholecystitis and appropriate investigation of all suspicious lesions is mandatory. Definitive surgical treatment at the initial procedure allows the best chance for cure. Appropriate intraoperative decision making is essential, and palpable suspicious thickenings of the gallbladder wall should be diagnosed with intraoperative fine needle aspiration cytology. Positive cytology confirming tumor should lead to definitive en bloc liver resection and lymph node dissection without disruption of the cystic plate which often includes tumor.

Many lesions will be found only on pathologic examination of the gallbladder specimen. In such cases, no further therapy is indicated for T-1 tumors as long as the cystic duct margin is negative. T-2 and T-3 tumors deserve re-exploration. Evidence of N-2 disease on pre-operative investigation precludes a curative resection. These patients should be treated only as symptoms develop without re-operation. Those re-explored for resection should undergo a standard extended cholecystectomy including an extensive nodal dissection to include the superior pancreaticoduodenal nodes and a skeletonization of the vessels in the porta hepatis. If the nodal dissection is compromised by the presence of the common bile duct, then this should be resected. In addition a segment IVb and V resection or extended resection of the liver should be included as dictated by the location of the tumor and surrounding inflammation and scar tissue.

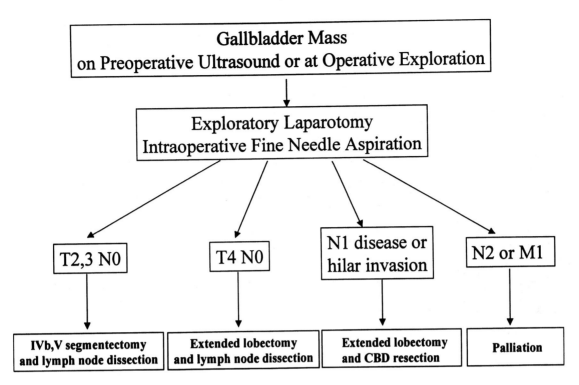

Fig. 53.10 This schematic represents an algorithm for management of gallbladder cancer found as a suspicious mass or thickening on pre-operative imaging or at the time of cholecystectomy. T-1 lesions will most likely not be recognized until after cholecystectomy. If there is a strong suspicion of a T-1 papillary lesion then a simple cholecystectomy should be performed with a pathologic frozen section for examining depth of invasion and the cystic duct margin. Otherwise recognized masses will be at least T-2 in thickness and should be treated as shown. CBD, common bile duct.

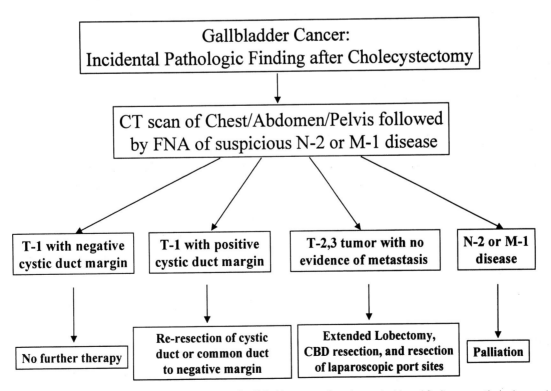

Fig. 53.11 This schema represents an algorithm for management of gallbladder cancer found as an incidental finding on pathologic examination of a cholecystectomy specimen. CBD, common bile duct.

Advanced tumors recognized on pre-operative radiologic imaging or at the time of laparotomy can be treated with aggressive surgical resection and result in long-term survival. This approach needs to be individualized and based on the patient's general health and extent of disease. Resection of hematogenous metastasis is not justified, nor is resection of N-2 nodal disease. Reports of long-term survival after resection of locally advanced T-4 lesions and N-1 metastasis justify an aggressive surgical resection in selected patients. This may include bile duct resection and extended hepatic lobectomy. An algorithm for management is shown in Figure 53.10 and Figure 53.11.

It is important to identify an effective adjuvant treatment as surgery alone does not provide satisfactory results. To date an effective regimen has not been determined. Radiation therapy is well tolerated and should be considered, although ideally in the context of a clinical trial. Likewise, it is reasonable to use adjuvant chemotherapy in the context of a clinical trial.

This aggressive disease requires new approaches and new chemotherapeutic agents for the delivery of adjuvant therapy. Given the high propensity for intraperitoneal seeding, intraperitoneal adjuvant chemotherapy delivered at the time of complete resection may have a place. Regional intra-arterial therapy may be reasonable for palliation or as a neoadjuvant to improve resectability.

REFERENCES

Adamsen S, Hansen O H, Funch-Jensen P, Schulze S, Stage J G, Wara P 1997 Bile duct injury during laparoscopic cholecystectomy: a prospective nationwide series. Journal of the American College of Surgeons 184: 571–578

Akosa A B, Barker F, Desa L, Benjamin I, Krausz T 1995 Cytologic diagnosis in the management of gallbladder carcinoma. Acta Cytologica 39: 494–498

Albores-Saavedra J, Henson D E 1986 Tumors of the gallbladder and extrahepatic bile ducts. In: Anonymous Atlas of Tumor Pathology, Second Series, Armed Forces Institute of Pathology, Bethesda

Albores-Saavedra J, Nadji M, Henson D E 1986 Intestinal-type adenocarcinoma of the gallbladder. A clinicopathologic study of seven cases. American Journal of Surgical Pathology 10: 19–25

Aldridge M C, Bismuth H 1990 Gallbladder cancer: the polyp-cancer sequence. Review, 11 refs. British Journal of Surgery 77: 363–364

Bach A M, Loring L A, Hann L E, Illescas F F, Fong Y, Blumgart L H 1998 Gallbladder cancer: can ultrasonography evaluate extent of disease? Journal of Ultrasound in Medicine 17: 303–309

Baretton G, Blasenbreu S, Vogt T, Lohrs U, Rau H, Schmidt M 1994 DNA ploidy in carcinoma of the gallbladder. Prognostic significance and comparison of flow and image cytometry on archival tumor material. Pathology, Research & Practice 190: 584–592

Bartlett D L, Fong Y, Fortner J G, Brennan M F, Blumgart L H 1996 Long-term results after resection for gallbladder cancer. Annals of Surgery 224: 639–46

Beahrs O H, Myers M H 1983 Manual for Staging of Cancer, 2nd edn. J B Lippincott & Company, Philadelphia

Berk R N, Armbuster T G, Saltzstein S L 1973 Carcinoma in the porcelain gallbladder. Radiology 106: 29–31

Bismuth H, Corlett M B 1975 Intrahepatic cholangioenteric anastomosis in carcinoma of the hilus of the liver. Surgery, Gynecology and Obstetrics 140: 170–176

Blalock A A 1924 A statistical study of 888 cases of biliary tract disease. Johns Hopkins Hosp.Bull. 35: 391–409

Boerma E J 1994 Towards an oncological resection of gall bladder cancer. Review, 61 refs. European Journal of Surgical Oncology 20: 537–544

Bosset J F, Mantion G, Gillet M, Pelissier E, Boulenger M, Maingon P, Corbion O, Schraub S 1989 Primary carcinoma of the gallbladder. Adjuvant postoperative external irradiation. Cancer 64: 1843–1847

Broden G, Bengtsson L 1980 Carcinoma of the gallbladder. Its relation to cholelithiasis and to the concept of prophylactic cholecystectomy. Acta Chirurgica Scandinavica—Supplementum 500: 15–18

Burdette W J 1957 Carcinoma of the gall bladder. Annals of Surgery 145: 832–847

Carriaga M T, Henson D E 1995 Liver, gallbladder, extrahepatic bile ducts, and pancreas. Cancer 75: 171–190

Carty N J, Johnson C D 1991 Carcinoma of the gallbladder: a survey of cases in Wessex 1982–1989. Review, 23 refs. Journal of the Royal College of Surgeons of Edinburgh 36: 238–241

Chao T C, Greager J A 1991 Primary carcinoma of the gallbladder. Journal of Surgical Oncology 46: 215–221

Chao T C, Jan Y Y, Chen M F 1995 Primary carcinoma of the gallbladder associated with anomalous pancreaticobiliary ductal junction. Journal of Clinical Gastroenterology 21: 306–308

Chijiiwa K, Sumiyoshi K, Nakayama F 1991 Impact of recent advances in hepatobiliary imaging techniques on the preoperative diagnosis of carcinoma of the gallbladder. World Journal of Surgery 15: 322–327

Chijiiwa K, Tanaka M, Nakayama F 1993 Adenocarcinoma of the gallbladder associated with anomalous pancreaticobiliary ductal junction. American Surgeon 59: 430–434

Chijiiwa K, Tanaka M 1994 Carcinoma of the gallbladder: an appraisal of surgical resection. Surgery 115: 751–756

Chow N H, Huang S M, Chan S H, Mo L R, Hwang M H, Su W C 1995 Significance of c-erbB-2 expression in normal and neoplastic epithelium of biliary tract. Anticancer Research 15: 1055–1059

Clair D G, Lautz D B, Brooks D C 1993 Rapid development of umbilical metastases after laparoscopic cholecystectomy for unsuspected gallbladder carcinoma. Surgery 113: 355–358

Collier N A, Blumgart L H 1994 Tumours of the gallbladder. In: Blumgart L H (Ed) 2nd edn. Surgery of the liver and biliary tract, p 955–966

Collier N A, Carr D, Hemingway A, Blumgart L H 1984 Preoperative diagnosis and its effect on the treatment of carcinoma of the gallbladder. Surgery, Gynecology & Obstetrics 159: 465–470

Cubertafond P, Gainant A, Cucchiaro G 1994 Surgical treatment of 724 carcinomas of the gallbladder. Results of the French Surgical Association Survey (see comments). Annals of Surgery 219: 275–280

De Aretxabala X, Roa I, Araya J C, Burgos L, Flores P, Wistuba I, Villaseca M A, Sotomayor F, Roa J C 1994 Gallbladder cancer in patients less than 40 years old. British Journal of Surgery 81: 111

De Aretxabala X, Roa I S, Burgos L A, Araya J C, Villaseca M A, Silva J A 1997 Curative resection in potentially resectable tumours of the gallbladder. European Journal of Surgery 163: 419–426

Diehl A K 1980 Epidemiology of gallbladder cancer: a synthesis of recent data. JNCI 65: 1209–1213

Donohue J H, Nagorney D M, Grant C S, Tsushima K, Ilstrup D M, Adson M A 1990 Carcinoma of the gallbladder. Does radical resection improve outcome? Archives of Surgery 125: 237–241

Drouard F, Delamarre J, Capron J 1991 Cutaneous seeding of gallbladder cancer after laparoscopic cholecystectomy. New England Journal of Medicine 325: 1316

Ellis E F, Gordon P R, Gottlieb L S 1978 Oral contraceptives and cholangiocarcinoma. Lancet i: 207–208

Enomoto M, Naoe S, Harada M 1999 Carcinogenesis in extrahepatic bile duct and gallbladder; carcinogenic effect of N-Hhydroxy-2-Acetamidofluorene in mice fed a 'gallstone-inducing' diet. Japanese Journal of Experimental Medicine 44: 37–45

Fernandez E, La Vecchia C, D'Avanzo B, Negri E, Franceschi S 1994 Family history and the risk of liver, gallbladder, and pancreatic cancer. Cancer Epidemiology, Biomarkers & Prevention 3: 209–212

Fligelstone L, Rhodes M, Flook D, Puntis M, Crosby D 1993 Tumour inoculation during laparoscopy (letter, comment). Lancet 342: 368–369

Fong Y, Blumgart L H, Fortner J G, Brennan M F 1995 Pancreatic or liver resection for malignancy is safe and effective for the elderly. Annals of Surgery 222: 426–437

Fong Y, Brennan M F, Turnbull A, Coit D G, Blumgart L H 1993 Gallbladder cancer discovered during laparoscopic surgery—potential for iatrogenic dissemination. Archives of Surgery 128: 1054–1056

Fong Y, Heffernan N, Blumgart L H 1998 Gallbladder carcinoma discovered during laparoscopic cholecystectomy: aggressive reresection is beneficial. Cancer 83: 423–427

Fortner J G, Randall H T 1961 On the carcinogenicity of human gallstones. Surgical Forum 12: 155–156

Franquet T, Montes M, Ruiz D A, Jimenez F J, Cozcolluela R 1991 Primary gallbladder carcinoma: imaging findings in 50 patients with pathologic correlation. Gastrointestinal Radiology 16: 143–148

Fujii K, Yasui W, Shimamoto F, Yokozaki H, Nakayama H, Kajiyama G, Tahara E 1995 Immunohistochemical analysis of nm23 gene product in human gallbladder carcinomas. Virchows Archives 426: 355–359

Gagner M, Rossi R L 1991 Radical operations for carcinoma of the gallbladder: present status in North America. World Journal of Surgery 15: 344–347

Gall F P, Kockerling F, Scheele J, Schneider C, Hohenberger W 1991 Radical operations for carcinoma of the gallbladder: present status in Germany. World Journal of Surgery 15: 328–336

Ghadirian P, Simard A, Baillargeon J 1993 A population-based case-control study of cancer of the bile ducts and gallbladder in Quebec, Canada. Revue d Epidemiologie et de Sante Publique 41: 107–112

Grace P A, Quereshi A, Coleman J, Keane R, McEntee G, Broe P, Osborne H, Bouchier Hayes D 1991 Reduced postoperative hospitalization after laparoscopic cholecystectomy. British Journal of Surgery 78: 160–162

Hanna S S, Rider W D 1978 Carcinoma of the gallbladder or extrahepatic bile ducts: the role of radiotherapy. Canadian Medical Association Journal 118: 59–61

Harada H, Sasaki T, Yamamoto N, Tanaka J, Tomiyama Y 1977 Assessment of endoscopic aspiration cytology and endoscopic retrograde cholangio-pancreatography in patients with cancer of the hepato-biliary tract. Part II. Gastroenterologia Japonica 12: 59–64

Henson D E, Albores-Saavedra J, Corle D 1992 Carcinoma of the gallbladder. Histologic types, stage of disease, grade, and survival rates. Cancer 70: 1493–1497

Houry S, Schlienger M, Huguier M, Lacaine F, Penne F, Laugier A 1989 Gallbladder carcinoma: role of radiation therapy. British Journal of Surgery 76: 448–450

Imai M, Hoshi T, Ogawa K 1994 K-ras codon 12 mutations in biliary tract tumors detected by polymerase chain reaction denaturing gradient gel electrophoresis. Cancer 73: 2727–2733

Itoi T, Watanabe H, Ajioka Y, Oohashi Y, Takel K, Nishikura K, Nakamura Y, Horil A, Saito T 1996 APC, K-ras codon 12 mutations and p53 gene expression in carcinoma and adenoma of the gall-bladder suggest two genetic pathways in gall-bladder carcinogenesis. Pathology International 46: 333–340

Joffe N, Antonioli D A 1981 Primary carcinoma of the gallbladder associated with chronic inflammatory bowel disease. Clinical Radiology 32: 319–324

Kapoor V K, Pradeep R, Haribhakti S P, Sikora S S, Kaushik S P 1996 Early carcinoma of the gallbladder: an elusive disease. Journal of Surgical Oncology 62: 284–287

Kato S, Nakagawa T, Kobayashi H, Arai E, Isetani K 1994 Septum formation of the common hepatic duct associated with an anomalous junction of the pancreaticobiliary ductal system and gallbladder cancer: report of a case. Surgery Today 24: 534–537

Kim H J, Roy T 1994 Unexpected gallbladder cancer with cutaneous seeding after laparoscopic cholecystectomy. Southern Medical Journal 87: 817–820

Kimura W, Nagai H, Kuroda A, Morioka Y 1989 Clinicopathologic study of asymptomatic gallbladder carcinoma found at autopsy. Cancer 64: 98–103

Kodama M, Kodama T 1994 Epidemiological peculiarities of cancers of the gall-bladder and larynx that distinguish them from other human neoplasias. Anticancer Research 14: 2205–2214

Kowalewski K, Todd E F 1971 Carcinoma of the gallbladder induced in hamsters by insertion of cholesterol pellets and feeding dimethylnitrosamine. Proceedings of the Society for Experimental Biology and Medicine 136: 482–489

Kozuka S, Tsubone N, Yasui A, Hachisuka K 1982 Relation of adenoma to carcinoma in the gallbladder. Cancer 50: 2226–2234

Kubota K, Bandai Y, Noie T, Ishizaki Y, Teruya M, Makuuchi M 1995 How should polypoid lesions of the gallbladder be treated in the era of laparoscopic cholecystectomy? (see comments). Surgery 117: 481–487

Kumar A, Aggarwal S 1994 Carcinoma of the gallbladder: CT findings in 50 cases. Abdominal Imaging 19: 304–308

Landen S M 1993 Laparoscopic surgery and tumor seeding (letter, comment). Surgery 114: 131–132

Longmire W P, McArthur M S, Bastounis E A, Hiatt J 1973 Carcinoma of the extrahepatic biliary tract. Annals of Surgery 178: 333–345

Lowenfels A B, Norman J 1999 Isoniazid and bile duct cancer. JAMA 240: 434–435

Makela J T, Kairaluoma M I 1993 Superselective intra-arterial chemotherapy with mitomycin for gallbladder cancer. British Journal of Surgery 80: 912–915

Mancuso T F, Brennan M J 1970 Epidemiological considerations of cancer of the gallbladder, bile ducts and salivary glands in the rubber industry. Journal of Occupational Medicine 12: 333–341

Matsumoto Y, Fujii H, Aoyama H, Yamamoto M, Sugahara K, Suda K 1992 Surgical treatment of primary carcinoma of the gallbladder based on the histologic analysis of 48 surgical specimens. American Journal of Surgery 163: 239–245

Merz B J, Dodge G G, Abellera R M, Kisken W A 1993 Implant metastasis of gallbladder carcinoma in situ in a cholecystectomy scar: a case report. Surgery 114: 120–124

Mohandas K M, Swaroop V S, Gullar S U, Dave U R, Jagannath P, Desouza L J 1994 Diagnosis of malignant obstructive jaundice by bile cytology: results improved by dilating the bile duct strictures [see comments]. Gastrointestinal Endoscopy 40: 150–154

Morrow C E, Sutherland D E, Florack G, Eisenberg M M, Grage T B 1983 Primary gallbladder carcinoma: significance of subserosal lesions and results of aggressive surgical treatment and adjuvant chemotherapy. Surgery 94: 709–714

Nakamura S, Sakaguchi S, Suzuki S, Muro H 1989 Aggressive surgery for carcinoma of the gallbladder. Surgery. 106: 467–473

Nakayama F 1991 Recent progress in the diagnosis and treatment of carcinoma of the gallbladder—introduction. World Journal of Surgery 15: 313–314

Nally C, Preshaw R M 1994 Tumour implantation at umbilicus after laparoscopic cholecystectomy for unsuspected gallbladder carcinoma. Canadian Journal of Surgery 37: 243–244

Nduka C C, Monson J R T, Menzies-Gow N, Darzi A 1994 Abdominal wall metastases following laparoscopy. British Journal of Surgery 81: 648–652

Nevin J E, Moran T J, Kay S, King R 1976 Carcinoma of the gallbladder: staging, treatment, and prognosis. Cancer 37: 141–148

Nimura Y, Hayakawa N, Kamiya J, Maeda S, Kondo S, Yasui A, Shionoya

(1991 Hepatopancreatoduodenectomy for advanced carcinoma of the biliary tract. Hepato-Gastroenterology 38: 170–175

North J H J, Pack M S, Hong C, Rivera D E 1998 Prognostic factors for adenocarcinoma of the gallbladder: an analysis of 162 cases. American Surgeon 64: 437–440

Oertli D, Herzog U, Tondelli P 1993 Primary carcinoma of the gallbladder: operative experience during a 16 year period. European Journal of Surgery 159: 415–420

Ogura Y, Mizumoto R, Isaji S, Kusuda T, Matsuda S, Tabata M 1991 Radical operations for carcinoma of the gallbladder: present status in Japan. World Journal of Surgery 15: 337–343

Ohtani T, Shirai Y, Tsukada K, Hatakeyama K, Muto T 1993 Carcinoma of the gallbladder: CT evaluation of lymphatic spread. Radiology 189: 875–880

Onoyama H, Yamamoto M, Tseng A, Ajiki T, Saitoh Y 1995 Extended cholecystectomy for carcinoma of the gallbladder. World Journal of Surgery 19: 758–763

Oswalt C E, Cruz A B, Jr 1977 Effectiveness of chemotherapy in addition to surgery in treating carcinoma of the gallbladder. Review of Surgery 34: 436–438

Ouchi K, Oioada Y, Matsumo S, Sato T 1987 Prognostic factors in the surgical treatment of gallbladder carcinoma. Surgery 101: 731–737

Paquet K J 1998 Appraisal of surgical resection of gallbladder carcinoma with special reference to hepatic resection. Journal of Hepato-Biliary-Pancreatic Surgery 5: 200–206

Perpetuo M D, Valdivieso M, Heilbrun L K, Nelson R S, Connor T, Bodey G P 1978a Natural history study of gallbladder cancer: a review of 36 years experience at MD Anderson Hospital and Tumor Institute. Cancer 42: 330–335

Perpetuo M D C M O, Valdivieso M, Heilbrun L K, Nelson R S, Connor T, Bodey G 1978b Natural history of gallbladder cancer. Cancer 42: 330–335

Pezet D, Fondrinier E, Rotman N, Guy L, Lemesle P, Lointier P, Chipponi J 1992 Parietal seeding of carcinoma of the gallbladder after laparoscopic cholecystectomy. British Journal of Surgery 79: 230–230

Piehler J M, Crichlow R W 1978 Primary carcinoma of the gallbladder. Review, 193 refs. Surgery, Gynecology & Obstetrics 147: 929–942

Redaelli C A, Buchler M W, Schilling M K, Krahenbuhl L, Ruchti C, Blumgart L H, Baer H U 1997 High coincidence of Mirizzi syndrome and gallbladder carcinoma. Surgery 121: 58–63

Ritts R E, Nagorney D M, Jacobson D J, Talbot R W, Zurawski V R Jr 1999 Comparison of preoperative serum CA19-9 levels with results of diagnostic imaging modalities in patients undergoing laparotomy for suspected pancreatic or gallbladder disease. Pancreas 9: 707–716

Roa I, Araya J C, Shiraishi T, Yatani R, Wistuba I, Villaseca M, de and Aretxabala X 1993 DNA content in gallbladder carcinoma: a flow cytometric study of 96 cases. Histopathology 23: 459–464

Roa I, Araya J C, Villaseca M, de A X, Riedemann P, Endoh K, Roa J 1996 Preneoplastic lesions and gallbladder cancer: an estimate of the period required for progression. Gastroenterology 111: 232–236

Rudolph R, Cohen J J 1972 Cancer of the gallbladder in an 11-yr-old Navajo girl. Journal of Pediatric Surgery 7: 66–67

Schwartz L H, Coakley F V, Sun Y, Blumgart L H, Fong Y, Panicek D M 1998 Neoplastic pancreaticobiliary duct obstruction: Evaluation with breath-hold MR cholangiopancreatography. American Journal of Roentgenology 170: 1491–5

Serra I, Calvo A, Baez S, Yamamoto M, Endoh K, Aranda W 1996 Risk factors for gallbladder cancer. An international collaborative case-control study (letter, comment). Cancer 78: 1515–1517

Shinkai H, Kimura W, Muto T 1998 Surgical indications for small polypoid lesions of the gallbladder. American Journal of Surgery 175: 114–117

Shirai Y, Yoshida K, Tsukada K, Muto T 1992a Inapparent carcinoma of the gallbladder. An appraisal of a radical second operation after simple cholecystectomy. Annals of Surgery 215: 326–331

Shirai Y, Yoshida K, Tsukada K, Muto T, Watanabe H 1992b Radical surgery for gallbladder carcinoma. Long-term results. Annals of Surgery 216: 565–568

Shirai Y, Yoshida K, Tsukada K, Ohtani T, Muto T 1992 Identification of the regional lymphatic system of the gallbladder by vital staining. British Journal of Surgery 79: 659–662

Shukla V K, Shukla P K, Pandey M, Rao B R, Roy S K 1994 Lipid peroxidation product in bile from patients with carcinoma of the gallbladder: a preliminary study. Journal of Surgical Oncology 56: 258–262

Shukla V K, Tiwari S C, Roy S K 1993 Biliary bile acids in cholelithiasis and carcinoma of the gall bladder. European Journal of Cancer Prevention 2: 155–160

Strom B L, Maislin G, West S L, Atkinson B, Herlyn M, Saul S, Rodriguez-Martinez H A, Rios-Dalenz J, Iliopoulos D, Soloway R D 1990 Serum CEA and CA 19-9: potential future diagnostic or screening tests for gallbladder cancer? International Journal of Cancer 45: 821–824

Strom B L, Soloway R D, Rios-Dalenz J, Rodriguez-Martinez H A, West S L, Kinman J L, Crowther R S, Taylor D, Polansky M, Berlin J A 1996 Biochemical epidemiology of gallbladder cancer. Hepatology 23, 1402–1411

Sumiyoshi K, Nagai E, Chijiiwa K, Nakayama F 1991 Pathology of carcinoma of the gallbladder. World Journal of Surgery 15, 315–321

Taal B G, Audisio R A, Bleiberg H, Blijham G H, Neijt J P, Veenhof C H, Duez N, Sahmoud T 1993 Phase II trial of mitomycin C (MMC) in advanced gallbladder and biliary tree carcinoma. An EORTC gastrointestinal tract cancer cooperative group study. Annals of Oncology 607–609

The Southern Surgeons Club 1991 A prospective analysis of 1518 laparoscopic cholecystectomies. New England Journal of Medicine 324: 1073–1078

Thorbjarnarson B, Glenn F 1959 Carcinoma of the gallbladder. Cancer 12, 1009–1015

Todoroki T 1997 Radiation therapy for primary gallbladder cancer. Review, 43 refs. Hepato-Gastroenterology 44, 1229–1239

Todoroki T, Iwasaki Y, Orii K, Otsuka M, Ohara K, Kawamoto T, Nakamura K 1991 Resection combined with intraoperative radiation therapy (IORT) for stage IV (TNM) gallbladder carcinoma. World Journal of Surgery 15: 357–366

Trajber H J, Szego T, de C H J, Mester M, Marujo W C, Roll S 1982 Adenocarcinoma of the gallbladder in two siblings. Cancer 50: 1200–1203

Tsukada K, Kurosaki I, Uchida K, Shirai Y, Oohashi Y, Yokoyama N, Watanabe H, Hatakeyama K 1997 Lymph node spread from carcinoma of the gallbladder. Cancer 80: 661–667

Vaittinen E 1970 Carcinoma of the gall-bladder. A study of 390 cases diagnosed in Finland 1953–1967. Annales Chirurgiae et Gynaecologiae Fenniae—(suppl) 168: 1–81

Wanebo H J, Castle W N, Fechner R E 1982 Is carcinoma of the gallbladder a curable lesion? Annals of Surgery 196: 624–631

Wanebo H J, Vezeridis M P 1994 Treatment of gallbladder cancer. (Review, 51 refs). Cancer Treatment & Research 69: 97–109

Wee A, Teh M, Raju G C 1994 Clinical importance of p53 protein in gall bladder carcinoma and its precursor lesions. Journal of Clinical Pathology 47: 453–456

Welton J C, Marr J S, Friedman S M 1979 Association between hepatobiliary cancer and typhoid carrier state. Lancet i: 791–794

Wibbenmeyer L A, Wade T P, Chen R C, Meyer R C, Turgeon R P, Andrus C H 1995 Laparoscopic cholecystectomy can disseminate in situ carcinoma of the gallbladder (see comments). Journal of the American College of Surgeons 181, 504–510

Wilbur A C, Gyi B, Renigers S A 1988 High-field MRI of primary gallbladder carcinoma. Gastrointestinal Radiology 13: 142–144

Wilkinson D S 1995 Carcinoma of the gall-bladder: an experience and review of the literature. Review, 40 refs. Australian & New Zealand Journal of Surgery 65: 724–727

Willson S A, Princenthal R A, Law B, Leopold G R 1987 Gallbladder carcinoma in association with polyposis coli. British Journal of Radiology 60: 771–773

Wistuba I I, Sugio K, Hung J, Kishimoto Y, Virmani A K, Roa I, Albores-Saavedra J, Gazdar A F 1995 Allele-specific mutations involved in the pathogenesis of endemic gallbladder carcinoma in Chile. Cancer Research 55: 2511–2515

Yamaguchi K, Enjoji M 1988 Carcinoma of the gallbladder—a clinicopathology of 103 patients and a newly proposed staging. Cancer 62: 1425–1432

Yamaguchi K, Tsuneyoshi M 1992 Subclinical gallbladder carcinoma. American Journal of Surgery 163: 382–386

Yamamoto M, Nakajo S, Tahara E 1989 Carcinoma of the gallbladder: the correlation between histogenesis and prognosis. Virchows Archives—A, Pathological Anatomy & Histopathology 414: 83–90

Yang H L, Sun Y G, Wang Z 1992 Polypoid lesions of the gallbladder: diagnosis and indications for surgery. British Journal of Surgery 79, 227–229

Zatonski W, La Vecchia C, Levi F, Negri E, Lucchini F 1993 Descriptive epidemiology of gall-bladder cancer in Europe. Journal of Cancer Research & Clinical Oncology 119: 165–171

Zatonski W A, Lowenfels A B, Boyle P, Maisonneuve P, Bueno de Mesquita H B, Ghadirian P, Jain M, Przewozniak K, Baghurst P, Moerman C J, Simard A, Howe G R, McMichael A J, Hsieh C C, Walker A M 1997 Epidemiologic aspects of gallbladder cancer: a case–control study of the SEARCH Program of the International Agency for Research on Cancer. Journal of the National Cancer Institute 89: 1132–1138

54

Cancer of the bile ducts: The hepatic ducts and common bile duct

W.R. JARNAGIN, P.F. SALDINGER, L.H. BLUMGART

HILAR AND INTRAHEPATIC CHOLANGIOCARCINOMA WITH EMPHASIS ON PRESURGICAL MANAGEMENT

M. NAGINO, Y. NIMURA

INTRODUCTION

Malignant strictures involving the bile ducts remain a major challenge in biliary surgery and result either from primary biliary tract cancers or from malignancies arising from other sites that involve the bile ducts secondarily (liver, gallbladder, pancreas, papilla of Vater, duodenum or adjacent lymph nodes). This chapter deals with primary malignancy of the intrahepatic and extrahepatic bile ducts. Cancers that secondarily involve the biliary tree are covered in detail in Chapters 53, 55, 56 and 73.

The distinctive approach of Japanese surgeons to intrahepatic and hilar cholangiocarcinoma, including detailed percutaneous biliary intubation with cholangiography, cholangioscopy, angiography and often pre-operative portal vein embolization are discussed by Professor Y. Nimura.

LOCATION AND PATHOLOGY

Although cholangiocarcinoma can arise anywhere within the biliary tree, tumors involving the biliary confluence are the most common. This observation may be biased by referral patterns, since most large series are generated from tertiary centers. Nevertheless, over the past three decades, the proportion of patients with tumors involving the hilus has remained fairly constant at 40 to 60% (Table 54.1) (Burke 1998, Nagorney et al 1993, Nakeeb et al 1996a,b, Tompkins et al 1981, Fong et al 1996, Yeo et al 1997, Haswell-Elkins et al 1991, Kuo & Wu 1990). Approximately 10% of cholangiocarcinoma cases arise within the intrahepatic biliary tree (Berdah et al 1996, Chu

et al 1997, Harrison et al 1998) (vide infra) (Shimizu et al 1991, Severini et al 1981). These tumors usually present as an intrahepatic mass, and although uncommon, jaundice may result from intrabiliary tumor extension (Fig. 54.1). Less than 10% of patients will present with multifocal or diffuse involvement of the biliary tree (Saunders et al 1991).

It has long been suggested that the majority of bile duct tumors are relatively slow-growing (Klatskin 1965, Akwari and Kelly 1979, Altenmeier et al 1966); however, disease progression can be rapid in some patients. Blood-borne metastases are uncommon but nodal metastases may occur in up to one-third of cases (Tsuzuki et al 1983, Burke 1998). Direct invasion of the liver or perihepatic structures is a common feature of hilar cholangiocarcinoma (Weinbren

Table 54.1 Incidence of hilar cholangiocarcinoma in selected series. Years refers to the time interval over which patients were accumulated. MSKCC—Memorial Sloan-Kettering Cancer Center, UCLA – University of California at Los Angeles.

Institution	Years	Number of patients with cholangiocarcinoma	Number of patients with hilar cholangiocarcinoma
UCLA (Tompkins et al 1981)	24	96	47 (49%)
Mayo Clinic (Nagorney et al 1993)	9	171	79 (46%)
Johns Hopkins (Nakeeb et al 1996)	23	294	197 (67%)
MSKCC (Burke 1998)	6	225	90 (40%)

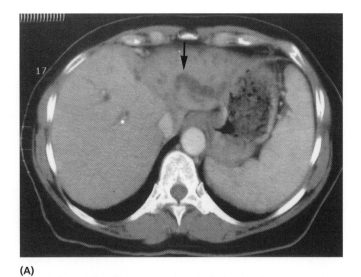

(A)

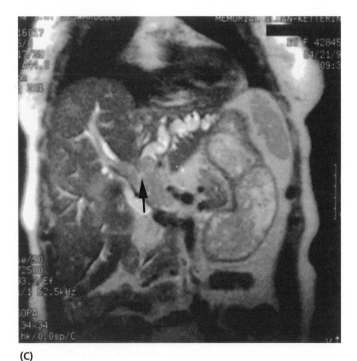

(C)

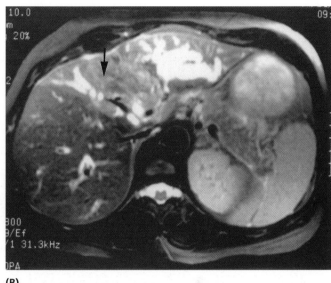

(B)

Fig. 54.1 Images from a patient with an intrahepatic cholangiocarcinoma and jaundice. **(A)** Cross-sectional CT scan image showing dilated left biliary tree (arrow) but no clearly defined mass. **(B)** Cross-sectional image from a magnetic resonance cholangiopancreatogram (MRCP) showing a heterogeneous mass in segment IV (arrow). Dilated bile ducts appear as white. **(C)** Coronal MRCP reconstruction showing the tumor growing down the left hepatic duct and extending across the right hepatic duct and into the common hepatic duct (arrow). The dilated bile ducts again appear as white.

& Mutum 1983). Special characteristics of cholangiocarcinoma include invasive spread with neural, perineural and lymphatic involvement and subepithelial extension (Weinbren & Mutum 1983).

Over 90% of extrahepatic cholangiocarcinomas are adenocarcinomas, often well-differentiated and mucin-producing (Carriaga & Henson 1995, Weinbren & Mutum 1983, Rodgers et al 1981). Many tumors express carcinoembryonic antigen (CEA) and the carbohydrate antigen CA 19-9. However, serum levels of these markers, although elevated in some patients, have little diagnostic value (Pitt et al 1995a). It has been suggested that CEA levels in hepatic

bile may help distinguish between benign and malignant strictures in patients with premalignant conditions (Nakeeb et al 1996a). The molecular changes associated with the pathogenesis of cholangiocarcinoma are not completely characterized. Multiple K-*ras* oncogene mutations at codon 12 have been identified in up to 100% of resected specimens (Levi et al 1991). However, these mutations most likely occur at some point along a stepwise progression to malignancy but probably are not the inciting genetic lesion. Moreover, there are wide epidemiological variations in the incidence of K-*ras* mutations, suggesting that other genetic changes are also involved (Lee et al 1995, Levi et al 1991, Nakamura et al 1981).

Three distinct *macroscopic* subtypes of cholangiocarcinoma are well-described: sclerosing, nodular and papillary (Weinbren & Mutum 1983). Sclerosing tumors account for the majority of all cases and are more common at the hilus than in the distal bile duct. Sclerosing tumors are very firm and cause an annular thickening of the bile duct, often with diffuse infiltration and fibrosis of the periductal tissues (Fig. 54.2). Nodular tumors are characterized by a firm, irregular nodule of tumor that projects into the lumen of the duct. Features of both types are often seen, hence the frequently used descriptor nodular-sclerosing. The papillary variant accounts for approximately 10% of all cholangiocarcinomas, and while occasionally seen at the hilus, is more common in the distal bile duct (Weinbren & Mutum 1983). These tumors are soft and friable, and may be associated with little transmural invasion. A polypoid mass that expands rather than contracts the duct (Fig. 54.3) is a characteristic feature.

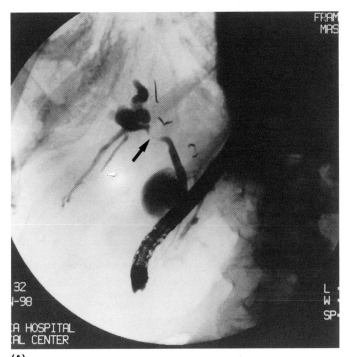

(A)

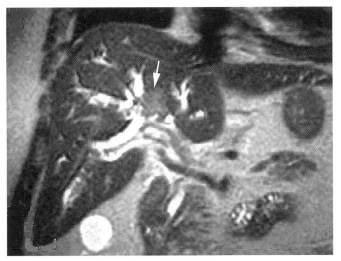

(B)

Fig. 54.2 **(A)** Endoscopic cholangiogram showing the typical, irregular biliary stricture characteristic of sclerosing adenocarcinomas (arrow). These tumors cause a circumferential thickening of the duct wall and periductal fibrosis, which ultimately obliterates the lumen. **(B)** Coronal MRCP reconstruction showing an infiltrating tumor involving the hepatic duct confluence (arrow). The right and left intrahepatic ducts, which appear white, are dilated.

Although papillary tumors may grow to significant size and appear surgically unapproachable on radiographic studies, they often arise from a well-defined stalk. Frequently, the bulk of the tumor is mobile within the bile duct. Recognition of this variant is important since they are more often resectable and have a more favorable prognosis than the other types (Pitt et al 1995).

Longitudinal spread along the duct wall and periductal tissues is an important pathologic feature of cholangiocarcinomas (Weinbren & Mutum 1983). There may be substantial extension of tumor beneath an intact epithelial lining, as much as 2 cm proximally and 1 cm distally (Shimada et al 1988). The full tumor extent may thus be underestimated by radiographic studies and may not be appreciated on palpation. This predilection for submucosal extension underscores the importance of frozen section analysis of the duct margins during resection.

While the overwhelming majority of these tumors are adenocarcinomas, in rare instances other malignant cell types may arise primarily in the biliary tree and cause biliary obstruction (e.g. carcinoid tumours [Jutte et al 1987, Rugge et al 1992, Sankary et al 1995]).

In this chapter, tumors of the extrahepatic bile ducts are discussed. The difficult group of hilar cholangiocarcinoma, lesions involving the hepatic duct confluence, are given special emphasis since they present the greatest challenge in preoperative diagnosis and management. The pathological, diagnostic and management problems related to low bile duct cancers, in particular, differentiation from benign tumors and from cancer of the pancreas, are also discussed in Chapters 51, 55 and 56. Intrahepatic cholangiocarcinoma is discussed below by Prof. Nimura.

INCIDENCE

The incidence of bile duct tumours in large autopsy series varies from 0.01 to 0.2% and may constitute about 2% of all reported cancers (Kuwayti et al 1957). It is an uncommon cancer with an incidence of one to two per 100 000 in the United States (Carriaga & Henson 1995). The advent of new diagnostic methods applicable in obstructive jaundice has led to the preoperative discovery of many more of these lesions, almost certainly misdiagnosed in the past. Thus, in a specialist referral center in the UK, 37 new cases of hilar cholangiocarcinoma were seen in one 17-month period (Voyles et al 1983). The majority of patients are greater than 65 years of age, and the peak incidence occurs in the eighth decade of life (Carriaga & Henson, 1995).

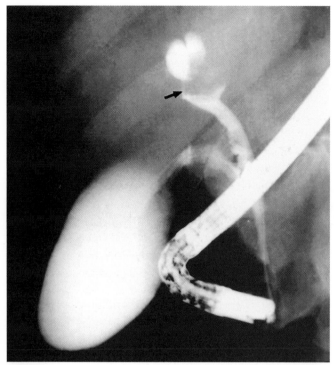

(A)

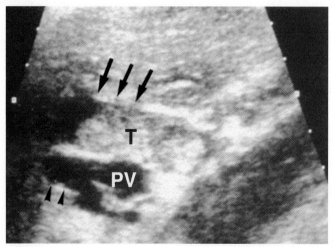

(B)

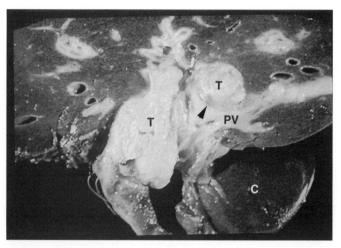

(C)

Fig. 54.3 (A) Endoscopic cholangiogram illustrating the typical features of a papillary adenocarcinoma of the bile duct. The duct is expanded rather than contracted. The contrast filling around the tumor creates the appearance of a golf ball on a golf tee. **(B)** Duplex ultrasound of a papillary tumor of the hepatic duct confluence. The tumor (T) fills the lumen of the duct (arrows) but there does not appear to be invasion of the adjacent liver parenchyma. The underlying portal vein (PV) appears uninvolved (arrowheads). **(C)** Gross appearance of a resected papillary bile duct tumor. The liver has been cut in a sagittal plane at the level of the biliary confluence. A well-circumscribed papillary tumor (T) occupies the entire lumen of the bile duct (black arrow), with little apparent invasion of the underlying portal vein. (C) caudate lobe.

NATURAL HISTORY

The vast majority of patients with unresectable bile duct cancer die within 6 months to a year of diagnosis. Death usually results from liver failure or infectious complications secondary to biliary obstruction (Kuwayti et al 1957, Sako et al 1957, Okuda et al 1977, Burke 1998). The prognosis has been considered worse for lesions affecting the confluence of the bile ducts and better for lesions close to the papilla. This probably reflects the relatively later presenta-

tion and the failure of physicians and surgeons to institute timely and effective therapy for proximal lesions rather than a difference in biologic behavior. Indeed, it has been shown that location within the biliary tree (proximal versus distal) has no impact on survival provided that complete resection is achieved (Nagorney et al 1993).

ETIOLOGY

The etiology of cholangiocarcinoma is unknown. Most cases are probably sporadic, but several conditions confer an increased risk of developing cholangiocarcinoma.

PRIMARY SCLEROSING CHOLANGITIS (see also Ch. 48)

Although most patients with cholangiocarcinoma have no obvious risk factors, several conditions are associated with an increased incidence. Perhaps the most common of these in the West is primary sclerosing cholangitis (PSC). PSC is an autoimmune disease characterized by inflammation of the periductal tissues, ultimately resulting in multifocal strictures of the intrahepatic and extrahepatic bile ducts (Broome et al 1996, Pitt et al 1995a,b, Katoh et al 1988). Seventy to eighty percent of patients with PSC have associated ulcerative colitis; by contrast only a minority of those with ulcerative colitis develop PSC (Broome et al 1996). The natural history of PSC is quite variable, and the true incidence of cholangiocarcinoma is unknown. In a Swedish series of 305 patients followed for over 5 years, 8% of patients eventually developed cancer (Broome et al 1996). On the other hand, occult cholangiocarcinoma has been reported in up to 40% of autopsy specimens and up to 36% of liver explants from patients with PSC (Broome et al 1996, Pitt et al 1995a, Katoh et al 1988). Unlike most patients with sporadic cholangiocarcinoma of the extrahepatic biliary tree, PSC patients are at risk for multifocal disease that is not amenable to resection. It is important to recognize that medical or surgical treatment of coexisting ulcerative colitis does not alter the subsequent risk of developing cholangiocarcinoma (Broome et al 1996, Pitt et al 1995a, Katoh et al 1988). Deterioration of hepatic function represents a major threat to these patients, and those without obvious or widespread malignant transformation are often considered for liver transplantation.

CONGENITAL BILIARY CYSTIC DISEASE (see also Ch. 66)

The increased risk of cholangiocarcinoma in patients with congenital biliary cystic disease (choledochal cysts, Caroli's disease) is well-described (Hewitt et al 1995, Vogt 1954). Malignant degeneration is uncommon in choledochal cysts diagnosed and excised early in life. However, the incidence of cancer increases substantially (approximately 15 to 20%) in patients who are not treated until after the age of 20 years or in those previously treated by cyst drainage (Lipsett et al 1994, Vogt 1954). The reason for the high incidence of cancer in patients with cystic diseases is not clear but appears to be related to an abnormal choledochopancreatic duct junction which predisposes to reflux of pancreatic secretions into the biliary tree, chronic inflammation and bacterial contamination (Lipsett et al 1994, Tanaka et al 1998, Vogt 1954, Jeng et al 1994). A similar mechanism may also explain the increased incidence of cholangiocarcinoma reported in patients subjected to transduodenal sphincteroplasty. In a series of 119 patients subjected to this procedure for benign conditions, Hakamada et al found a 7.4% incidence of cholangiocarcinoma over a period of 18 years (Hakamada et al 1997). There is no evidence to suggest that endoscopic sphincterotomy carries the same risk.

HEPATOLITHIASIS AND BILIARY INFESTATION (see also Chs 62 and 64)

Hepatolithiasis, also known as recurrent pyogenic cholangiohepatitis or Oriental cholangiohepatitis, is prevalent in Japan and parts of Southeast Asia. This condition is thought to result from chronic portal bacteremia and portal phlebitis, which gives rise to intrahepatic pigment stone formation. Obstruction of intrahepatic ducts leads to chronic, recurrent episodes of cholangitis and stricture formation (Chu et al 1997b, Kubo et al 1995, Winslet et al 1990, Meade et al 1994, Chu et al 1997b). Although sepsis is the major threat to life in these patients, approximately 10% will develop cholangiocarcinoma (Kubo et al 1995, Winslet et al 1990, Meade et al 1994). Biliary parasites (*Clonorchis sinensis, Opisthorchis viverrini*) are also prevalent in parts of Asia and are similarly associated with an increased risk of cholangiocarcinoma (Pitt et al 1995a,b). In Thailand, where approximately 7 million people are infested with opisthorchis, the annual incidence of cholangiocarcinoma is 87 per 100 000 (Watanapa 1996).

Finally, several radionuclides and chemical carcinogens may be associated with an increased risk of cholangiocarcinoma, including thorium, radon, nitrosamines, dioxin and asbestos.

CHOLANGIOCARCINOMA INVOLVING THE PROXIMAL BILE DUCTS (HILAR CHOLANGIOCARCINOMA)

Clinical presentation

The early symptoms of hilar cholangiocarcinoma are nonspecific. Abdominal pain or discomfort, anorexia, weight loss and pruritis are the most common but are seen only in about one-third of patients. Fever is rarely seen at initial presentation (Pitt et al 1995a, Nakeeb et al 1996b, Farley et al 1995, Katoh et al 1988, Meade et al 1994, Vatanasapt et al 1990b). Most patients have few symptoms and come to attention because of jaundice or abnormal liver function tests. Although most patients eventually become jaundiced, this finding is not present initially in cases of incomplete biliary obstruction (i.e., right or left hepatic duct) or segmental ductal obstruction. Segmental obstruction may go unrecognized for months, resulting in ipsilateral lobar atrophy without overt jaundice. These patients are often further evaluated and diagnosed because of an elevated alkaline phosphatase or gamma glutamyltransferase. In some patients, pruritis precedes jaundice by some weeks, and this symptom should prompt an evaluation, especially if associated with abnormal liver function tests. Patients with papillary tumors of the hilus may give a history of intermittent jaundice. Small fragments of tumor may detach from a friable papillary tumor of the right or left hepatic duct and pass into the common hepatic duct. Alternatively, the main tumor itself, if mobile within the lumen, may cause a ball-valve effect at the hepatic duct confluence.

In jaundiced patients, the total bilirubin level may suggest an etiology. In those with obstruction from cholangiocarcinoma, the serum bilirubin level is usually greater than 10 mg/dL and averages 18 mg/dL, whereas those with obstruction from choledocholithiasis have bilirubin levels of 2–4 mg/dL and rarely higher than 15 mg/dL (Way 1994). In patients with cholangiocarcinoma and no previous biliary intervention, cholangitis is uncommon at initial presentation, despite a 30% incidence of bacterial contamination (bacterbilia) (Hochwald et al 1999, Meade et al 1994). On the other hand, the incidence of bacterbilia is nearly 100% after biliary intubation, and cholangitis is more common (Hochwald et al 1998).

PHYSICAL EXAMINATION

The physical findings are often non-specific but may provide some useful information. Jaundice will usually be obvious. Patients with pruritis often have multiple excoriations of the skin. The liver may be enlarged and firm as a result of biliary tract obstruction. The gallbladder is usually decompressed and non-palpable with hilar obstruction. Thus, a palpable gallbladder suggests a more distal obstruction or an alternative diagnosis. Rarely, patients with long-standing biliary obstruction and/or portal vein involvement may have findings consistent with portal hypertension.

INFECTION

Bacterial contamination of the bile (bacterbilia) is relatively common in patients with hilar cholangiocarcinoma (McPherson et al 1984). However, in the absence of prior biliary intubation, frank cholangitis is uncommon at initial presentation. Endoscopic or percutaneous instrumentation as well as previous operation significantly increase the incidence of bacterial contamination and the risk of infection. Bacterial contamination of the biliary tract in partial obstruction is not always clinically apparent. The presence of overt or subclinical infection at the time of surgery is a major source of postoperative morbidity and mortality.

Escherichia coli, Kebsiella and *Enterococcal* species are the most common pathogens identified. However, this spectrum of organisms may change after endoscopic or percutaneous intubation, both of which are associated with greater morbidity and mortality following surgical resection or palliative bypass for hilar cholangiocarcinoma. We have analyzed 71 patients who underwent either a curative resection or palliative biliary bypass for proximal cholangiocarcinoma. All patients who were stented endoscopically and 62% of the patients who were stented percutaneously had bacterbilia. Postoperative infectious complications were doubly increased in those patients stented before surgery compared to non-stented patients. Non-infectious complications were equal in both groups (Hochwald et al 1998). *Enterococcus, Klebsiella, Streptococcus viridans* and *Enterobacter aerogenes* were the most common organisms isolated from intraoperative bile cultures. This spectrum of bacteria must be considered when administrating perioperative antibiotics. It is imperative to take intraoperative bile specimens for culture in order to adjust the antibiotics postoperatively.

ATROPHY (see also Ch. 3)

Portal venous inflow and bile flow are important in the maintenance of liver cell size and mass (Hadjis & Blumgart 1987). Segmental or lobar atrophy may result from a portal venous occlusion or biliary obstruction. Either or both of these findings are often present in patients with hilar cholangiocarcinoma and arise through a gradual process of involvement of the lobar hepatic ducts and portal vessels. Longstanding biliary obstruction may cause moderate atrophy while concomitant portal venous compromise results in rapid and severe atrophy of the involved segments. Appreciation of gross atrophy on preoperative imaging is important since it often influences therapy (Hadjis & Blumgart 1987). We consider atrophy to be present if cross-sectional imaging demonstrates a small, often hypoperfused lobe (Figs. 54.4 and 54.5) with crowding of the dilated intrahepatic ducts. Tumor involvement of the portal vein is usually present if there is compression/narrowing, encasement or occlusion seen on imaging studies.

Diagnosis

The diagnosis of hilar cholangiocarcinoma is usually made on evaluation of obstructive jaundice or elevated liver enzymes. Biliary cancers are usually clinically silent for long periods of time and it may be many months before a patient bearing such a tumor presents with overt clinical features. However, the first and leading symptom of biliary cancer

Fig. 54.4 (A) Cross sectional CT image of a patient with cholangiocarcinoma involving the left hepatic duct. The left lobe, clearly demarcated from the right, is shrunken and hypoperfused (arrows). The bile ducts, which appear black, are dilated and crowded. **(B)** T1-weighted, gadolinium-enhanced cross sectional MRI image of a different patient with hilar cholangiocarcinoma involving the left hepatic duct. The left lobe is small and the bile ducts (which appear black) are dilated and crowded. There is evidence of hypoperfusion of the left lobe, which appears darker. There is also evidence of hypoperfusion of the right posterior sector, which also appears darker and is clearly demarcated from the well-perfused right anterior sector (arrowheads) but does not as yet show evidence of atrophy. These radiographic features suggest that the tumor involves the left hepatic duct, the left portal vein and is beginning to involve the right portal pedicle.

is jaundice. In some patients there may be an initial attack of jaundice signifying the presence of a tumor, whereas intermittent jaundice may be seen in patients with papillary lesions. However, progressive and unremitting jaundice is usually the predominant clinical feature. Diagnostic investigations are largely related to elucidation of the cause of biliary tract obstruction.

A relative minority of patients will present with abdominal pain that may be mistakenly attributed to gallstone disease. It is important to remember that gallstones or even common bile duct stones may coexist with bile duct cancer. However, in the absence of certain predisposing conditions (e.g., primary sclerosing cholangitis, Oriental cholangiohepatitis), it is quite uncommon for choledocholithiasis to cause obstruction at the biliary confluence. It is therefore imperative to fully investigate and delineate the level and nature of any obstructing lesion causing jaundice to avoid missing the diagnosis of carcinoma.

Most patients are referred after having had some studies done elsewhere, usually a computed tomography scan (CT) and some form of direct cholangiography (PTC or ERCP) (see Ch. 17). These studies are often inadequate for full assessment of the tumor extent. Many patients will have been surgically explored prior to referral, often without reaching a definitive diagnosis (Voyles et al 1983). In our view, histologic confirmation of malignancy is not mandatory prior to exploration. In the absence of previous biliary tract surgery, the finding of a focal stenotic lesion

combined with the appropriate clinical presentation are sufficient for a presumptive diagnosis of hilar cholangiocarcinoma, which is correct in most instances (Wetter et al 1991).

RADIOGRAPHIC STUDIES

Radiographic studies are pivotal in selecting patients for resection. In the past, computed tomography (CT), percutaneous transhepatic cholangiography (PTC) and angiography were considered standard investigations. Currently, however, we rely almost exclusively on non-invasive studies, specifically magnetic resonance cholangiopancreatography (MRCP) (see Ch. 16) and duplex ultrasonography (US) (see Ch. 13), which provide the same information with less risk.

Cholangiography

Cholangiography demonstrates the location of the tumor and the biliary extent of disease, both of which are critical in surgical planning. Although endoscopic retrograde cholangiography (ERC) may provide some helpful information, percutaneous transhepatic cholangiography (PTC) displays the intrahepatic bile ducts more reliably and has been the preferred study (Pitt et al 1995a,b). More recently, however, magnetic resonance cholangiopancreatography (MRCP) has emerged as a powerful investigative tool (see below).

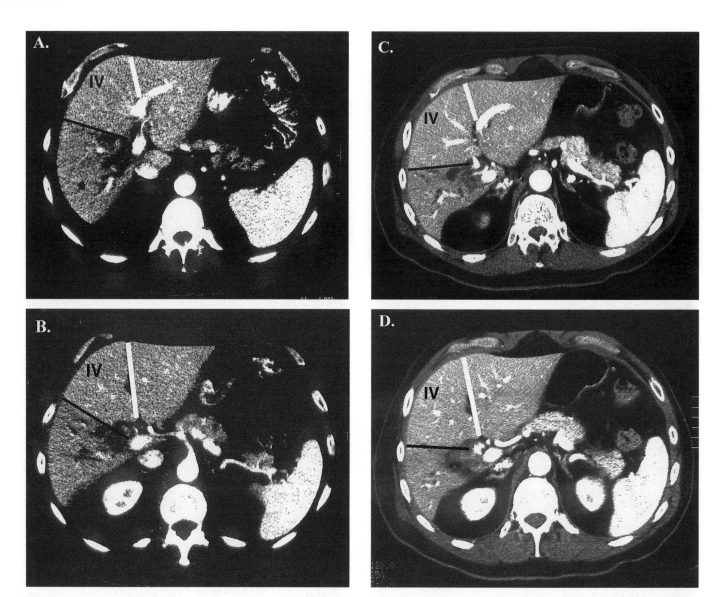

Fig. 54.5 Contiguous CT scan images of a patient with hilar cholangiocarcinoma involving the right hepatic duct and lobar atrophy. Images **A** and **B** are from a scan performed several months prior to referral; images **C** and **D** are from a later scan done prior to surgery. There is clearly atrophy of the right lobe on the early scan (**A** and **B**) which is more pronounced on a later scan (**C** and **D**). The demarcation of the right and left hemilivers is indicated by the black line while the left lateral segment lies to the left of the white line. Notice that the right lobe is significantly smaller in size and the left lateral segment (dermarcation from segment indicated by the white line) has significantly enlarged in scans **C** and **D**.

Computed tomography

Computed tomography (CT) remains an important study for evaluating patients with biliary obstruction. A high-quality CT scan can provide valuable information regarding level of obstruction, vascular involvement and liver atrophy (Figs 54.4 and 54.5). Because of its wide availability, CT scans are often done prior to referring the patient to a specialist unit.

Duplex ultrasonography

Ultrasonography is a non-invasive but operator dependent study that often precisely delineates tumor extent.

Ultrasonography may not only demonstrate the level of biliary ductal obstruction but can also provide information regarding tumor extension within the bile duct and in the periductal tissues (Figs. 54.6 and 54.7) (Gibson et al 1986, Okuda et al 1988, Hann et al 1997). Duplex ultrasonography is firmly established as a highly accurate predictor of vascular involvement and resectability. In a series of 19 consecutive patients with malignant hilar obstruction, ultrasonography with color spectral Doppler technique was equivalent to angiography and CT portography in diagnosing lobar atrophy, level of biliary obstruction, hepatic parenchymal involvement, and venous invasion (Hann et al

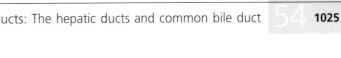

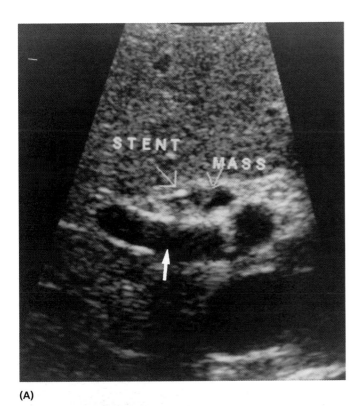

(A)

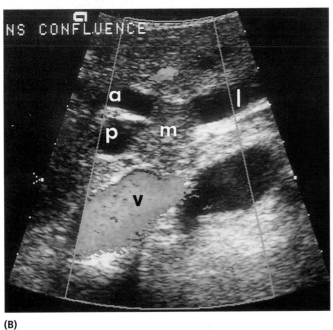

(B)

Fig. 54.6 (A) Duplex ultrasound from a patient with hilar cholangiocarcinoma. The tumor is clearly seen at the biliary confluence just above the portal vein (arrow). The mass is clearly in contact with the portal vein but there is no clear invasion or venous narrowing. A transtumoral stent is also visible. **(B)** Transverse color Doppler sonogram of the biliary confluence shows a papillary cholangiocarcinoma (m) extending into both the right anterior (a) and posterior (p) sectoral ducts and the origin of the left duct (l) The adjacent portal vein (v) is not involved and has normal flow. (Reprinted with permission from Journal of Ultrasound Medicine 15: 37–45, 1996).

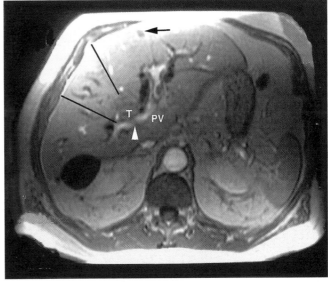

(A)

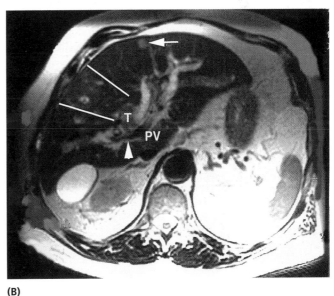

(B)

Fig. 54.7 (A) T1-weighted, gadolinium enhanced MRI image of a patient with hilar cholangiocarcinoma. In this image, the bile ducts appears black. A hilar tumor is seen (T), apparently adherent to or encasing the right portal vein branch (PV) (white arrowhead). The tumor has occluded the right anterior sectoral branch of the portal vein and the anterior sector appears atrophic (indicated by the black lines) with crowded, dilated ducts. Intrahepatic metastases are also noted (arrow). **(B)** MRCP image cut through the same area of the liver. Similar findings are indicated in this image, in which the bile ducts appears white. The vascular findings seen on MRI were confirmed on duplex ultrasonography. Biopsies of the main tumor and the intrahepatic metastases confirmed adenocarcinoma.

1997). Duplex ultrasonography is particularly useful for assessing portal venous invasion. In a series of 63 consecutive patients from Memorial Sloan-Kettering Cancer Center (MSKCC), duplex ultrasonography predicted portal vein involvement in 93% of the cases with a specificity of 99% and a 97% positive predictive value. In the same series angiography with CT angioportography had a 90% sensitivity, 99% specificity and a 95% positive predictive value (Bach et al 1996).

Magnetic resonance cholangiopancreatography (MRCP)

In our practice magnetic resonance cholangiopancreatography (MRCP) has almost replaced endoscopic and percutaneous cholangiography for the preoperative assessment of hilar cholangiocarcinoma. Several studies have demonstrated its utility in evaluating patients with biliary obstruction (Itoh et al 1992, Guthrie et al 1996, Lee et al 1997, Schwartz et al 1998). MRCP may not only identify the tumor and the level of biliary obstruction but may also reveal obstructed and isolated ducts not appreciated at endoscopic or percutaneous study (Figs 54.2, 54.4 and 54.6). MRCP also provides information regarding the patency of hilar vascular structures, the presence of nodal or distant metastases and the presence of lobar atrophy (Fig. 54.6). Furthermore, unlike other modalities, MRCP does not require biliary intubation. Biliary instrumentation and

bacterbilia, which may increase perioperative morbidity, may thus be avoided (Heslin et al 1998, Hochwald et al 1998).

Japanese surgeons extend the diagnostic process by performing detailed cholangiography with one or more percutaneous catheters placed in the intrahepatic ducts, often combined with cholangioscopy (vide infra). We have not used this approach.

Alternative diagnoses

The vast majority of patients with hilar strictures and jaundice have cholangiocarcinoma. However, alternative diagnoses are possible and can be expected in 10 to 15% of patients (Wetter et al 1991). The most common of these are gallbladder carcinoma, Mirizzi syndrome and idiopathic benign focal stenosis (malignant masquerade). Distinguishing gallbladder carcinoma from hilar cholangiocarcinoma can be difficult. A thickened, irregular gallbladder with infiltration into segment IV and V of the liver, selective involvement of the right portal pedicle, or obstruction of the common hepatic duct with occlusion of the cystic duct on endoscopic cholangiography are all suggestive of gallbladder carcinoma. Mirizzi syndrome is a benign condition resulting from a large gallstone impacted in the neck of the gallbladder (Fig. 54.8). The ensuing pericholecystic and periductal inflammation and fibrosis can obstruct the proximal bile duct, which is often difficult to distinguish from a

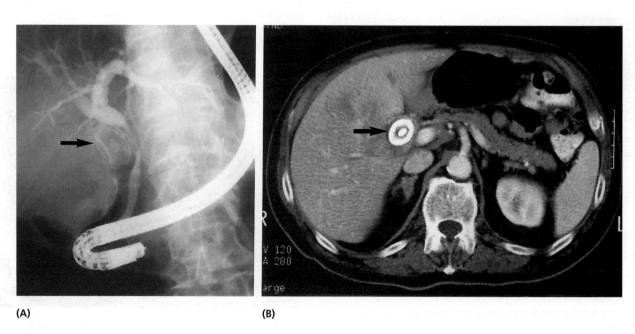

(A) **(B)**

Fig. 54.8 Endoscopic retrograde cholangiogram (ERC) and cross sectional CT scan images of a patient with Mirizzi syndrome. **(A)** The ERC shows a characteristic large gallstone impacted in the neck of the gallbladder causing obstruction of the hepatic duct just below the biliary confluence. **(B)** The CT scan confirms the presence of a large gallstone. In most cases, the diagnosis of Mirizzi syndrome is not as clear cut since the stone is not visualized.

malignant cause (Baer et al 1990, Cabooter et al 1990, Callery et al 1997). Benign focal strictures (malignant masquerade) can occur at the hepatic duct confluence but are uncommon (Wetter et al 1991, Hadjis et al 1985, Verbeek et al 1992) (Fig. 54.9) (Saldinger & Blumgart 1999, Wetter et al 1991).

The finding of a smooth, tapered stricture on cholangiography suggests a benign stricture (Fig. 54.9). However, hilar cholangiocarcinoma must remain the leading diagnosis until definitively disproved. In most cases, this cannot be done without exploration. Furthermore, the alternative conditions that one may encounter are best assessed and treated at operation. Relying on the results of percutaneous needle biopsy or biliary brush cytology is dangerous, since they are often misleading and one may miss the opportunity to resect an early cancer (Rabinovitz et al 1990, Enjoji et al 1998). We firmly believe that, in the absence of clear contraindications, exploration is indicated in all patients with suspicious hilar lesions.

Preoperative evaluation

Evaluation of patients with hilar cholangiocarcinoma is principally an assessment of resectability, since resection is the only effective therapy. First and foremost, the surgeon must assess the patient's general condition and fitness for operation, which usually includes partial hepatectomy. The presence of significant comorbid conditions, chronic liver disease and/or portal hypertension generally precludes resection. In these patients, biliary drainage is the most appropriate intervention, and the diagnosis should be confirmed histologically if chemotherapy or radiation therapy is anticipated. Patients with potentially resectable tumors occasionally present with biliary tract sepsis, frequently after intubation of the biliary tree. These patients require resuscitation and treatment of the infection before surgery can be considered.

The preoperative evaluation must address four critical determinants of resectability (Burke 1998):

1. Extent of tumor within the biliary tree
2. Vascular invasion
3. Hepatic lobar atrophy
4. Metastatic disease.

Lobar atrophy is an often-overlooked finding in patients with hilar cholangiocarcinoma. However, its importance in determining resectability cannot be overemphasized, since it often influences therapy (Hadjis & Blumgart 1987). Longstanding biliary obstruction may cause moderate atrophy, whereas concomitant portal venous compromise induces rapid and severe atrophy of the involved segments. On cross-sectional imaging, atrophy is characterized by a small, often hypoperfused lobe with crowding of the dilated intrahepatic ducts (Burke 1998) (Figs. 54.4, 54.5 and 54.10). The authors do not perform detailed cholangiography via percutaneous catheters nor do we perform angiography as described below by Professor Nimura.

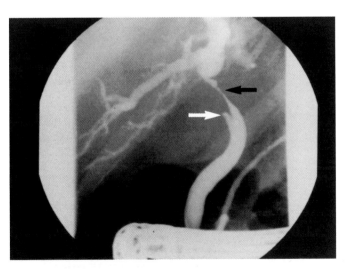

Fig. 54.9 Endoscopic cholangiogram from a patient with a benign stricture of the proximal bile duct. Note the smooth, tapered appearance (black arrow), in contrast to the irregular stricture typical of sclerosing tumors (Fig. 54.2). Non-filling of the cystic duct (white arrow) is an important finding and in the appropriate setting should raise the suspicion of gallbladder carcinoma. In this patient, the chronic inflammatory process had involved both the hepatic duct and cystic ducts. It should be pointed out that most cases of benign strictures of the proximal bile duct spare the cystic duct.

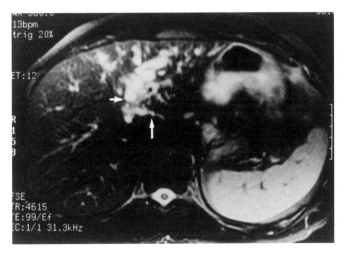

Fig. 54.10 Cross-sectional MRCP image from a patient with hilar cholangiocarcinoma extending into the left hepatic duct and left lobe atrophy. The bile ducts appear as white. The left lobe is small with dilated and crowded ducts (arrowhead). The principal caudate lobe duct, seen joining the left hepatic duct, is also dilated (arrow).

STAGING AND ASSESSMENT FOR RESECTABILTY

While it has been recognized that hilar cholangiocarcinomas are often small and apparently well-localized, few authors have remarked on the relationship between adjacent vascular involvement and the extent of spread along the bile ducts into the hepatic parenchyma. These factors may compromise complete excision of the tumor unless partial hepatectomy is performed, occasionally with reconstruction of the blood supply to the liver remnant. Adequate intraoperative assessment of vascular involvement requires extensive hilar dissection and may be technically difficult, especially if there has been prior biliary intervention. Therefore, an approach aimed at full radiological diagnosis has been made leading to a synthesis of all the available preoperative data. This allows preoperative staging and decision as to whether the patient is a potential candidate for curative resection. Previously, longitudinal ductal tumor extension has been assessed by either endoscopic retrograde cholangiopancreatography (ERCP) or percutaneous transhepatic cholangiography (PTC). Hepatic angiography with late phase portography combined with CT portography was previously used by us and others to assess radial spread of the tumor (Voyles et al 1983). At Memorial Sloan-Kettering Cancer Center (MSKCC), we favor duplex ultrasound and MRCP to stage patients before surgery (Hann et al 1997, Hann et al 1998). The radiological criteria used to define irresectability are listed in Table 54.2.

Currently, there is no clinical staging system available that stratifies patients preoperatively into subgroups based on potential for resection. The modified Bismuth-Corlette classification stratifies patients based on the extent of biliary duct involvement by tumor (Bismuth et al 1992) (Fig. 54.11). Although useful to some extent it is not indicative of resectability or survival. The current AJCC T stage system (Table 54.3) is based largely on pathological criteria and has little applicability for preoperative staging. The ideal staging system should accurately predict resectability, the need for hepatic resection and correlate with survival. Such a system would assist the surgeon in formulating a treat-

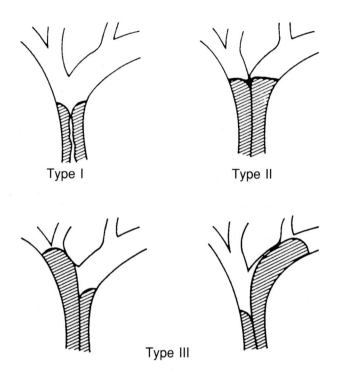

Fig. 54.11 The Bismuth-Corlette classification scheme of biliary strictures.

ment plan and help the patient understand the treatment options and outcome. We have proposed a preoperative staging system using preoperative imaging, taking into account the extent of biliary ductal involvement, vascular involvement and lobar atrophy (Burke 1998). This T staging system is based on the extent of local disease irrespective of N or M status (Table 54.4).

We have compared this new system to the AJCC classification in a series of 87 patients with cholangiocarcinoma.

Table 54.2 Criteria for irresectability

Hepatic duct involvement up to secondary biliary radicles bilaterally
Encasement or occlusion of the main portal vein proximal to its bifurcation
Atrophy of one hepatic lobe with encasement of contralateral portal vein branch
Atrophy of one hepatic lobe with contralateral involvement of secondary biliary radicles
Distant metastases (peritoneum, liver, lung)

Table 54.3 Current American Joint Commission on Cancer staging system for cancer of the extrahepatic bile ducts

Stage 0	T*is*	N0	M0
Stage 1	T1	N0	M0
Stage 2	T2	N0	M0
Stage 3	T1 or 2	N1 or 2	M0
Stage 4A	T3	Any N	M0
Stage 4B	Any T	Any N	M1

T*is*—carcinoma *in situ*; T1—tumor invades subepithelial connective tissue or fibromuscular layer; T2—tumor invades perifibromuscular connective tissue; T3—tumor invades adjacent organs (liver, pancreas, duodenum, gallbladder, colon, stomach).

N0—no regional lymph node metastases; N1—metastasis to lymph nodes within the hepatoduodenal ligament (cystic duct, pericholedochal and/or hilar lymph nodes); N2—metastasis to peripancreatic, periduodenal, periportal, celiac, superior mesenteric and/or posterior pancreaticoduodenal lymph nodes.

M0—no distant metastasis; M1—distant metastasis

Table 54.4 Proposed preoperative T-staging of hilar cholangiocarcinoma. T1 tumors are confined to the hilus with or without involvement of the right *or* left hepatic duct and are not associated with atrophy or portal vein involvement. T2 tumors are associated with ipsilateral lobar atrophy but not portal vein branch involvement. T3 tumors are characterized by ipsilateral portal venous branch involvement and may or may not be associated with lobar atrophy. T4 tumors are defined as irresectable based on tumor extension to secondary biliary radicles bilaterally or encasement/occlusion of the main portal vein (Burke 1998).

T-Stage	Biliary involvement	Ipsilateral lobar atrophy	Ipsilateral portal vein involvement	Main portal vein involvement
T1	Hilus and/or right or left hepatic duct	No	No	No
T2	Hilus and/or right or left hepatic duct	Yes	No	No
T3	Hilus and/or right or left hepatic duct	Yes/No	Yes	No
T4	Secondary biliary radicles bilaterally	Yes/No	Yes/No	Yes

Table 54.6 Proportion of patients amenable to curative resection and proportion requiring partial hepatectomy stratified by proposed T staging criteria (Burke 1998).

T-Stage	n	Resected n (%)	Hepatectomy n (%)
1	40	19 (48)	11 (58)
2	7	3 (43)	3 (100)
3	32	8 (25)	8 (100)
4	8	0	0
Total	87	30 (35)	22 (73)

Table 54.7 Percent of patients with distant or nodal metastases found on preoperative scan or at operation and survival stratified by proposed T stage (Burke 1998) (Reprinted with permission from Annals of Surgery).

T-Stage	n	Metastases n (%)	Median survival (months)	5-Year survival %
1	40	12 (30)	21±3	20
2	7	1 (14)	35±21	29
3	32	17 (52)	10±2	16
4	8	1 (13)	14±12	0
Total	87			

There was no correlation between stage and resectability or median survival using the AJCC system (Table 54.5). In the proposed staging system, resectability was highest in the T1 group (48%), and decreased progressively to 0 in the T4 group (irresectable due to extent of local disease). The percentage of patients requiring partial hepatectomy for complete resection also increased with T stage (Table 54.6). Importantly, these initial findings were confirmed prospectively in a separate group of 70 consecutive patients (unpublished data). The proposed staging system does not consider the presence of nodal or distant metastases, nevertheless the incidence of these findings on preoperative imaging and at laparotomy increased with increasing T-stage (Table 54.7). Portal vein involvement was the only independent predictor of resectability while portal vein involvement, hepatic lobar

Table 54.5 Resectability and median survival in patients with hilar cholangiocarcinoma staged according to the AJCC criteria.

Stage	n	Curative resection (%)	Median survival (months)
I	0	–	–
II	68	34	16
III	0	–	–
IV a	11	73	46
IV b	8	0	9
Total	87	36	

atrophy and hepatic ductal extension were independent predictors of the need for hepatectomy (Burke 1998). *In this context the importance of portal vein involvement and liver atrophy in relation to the extent of ductal cancer spread becomes evident. Thus ipsilateral involvement of vessels and bile ducts is usually amenable to resection while contralateral involvement is not.* These results emphasize the need for a more reliable preoperative system for selecting patients who are candidates for a potentially curative resection.

The role of laparoscopy in the staging of cholangiocarcinoma remains to be defined. A recent study, which examined the role of laparoscopy combined with laparoscopic ultrasound in a mixture of hepatobiliary and pancreatic malignancies, detected radiological occult metastases in 30% of the patients (Callery et al 1997). However, there was no mention of the number of patients with hilar cholangiocarcinoma. Hilar cholangiocarcinoma is often considered slow to metastasize. In our experience, however, many patients have radiographically occult peritoneal or nodal metastases. Preoperative imaging predicts irresectability based on local extension but is poor for assessing nodal or peritoneal metastases. In our recent series, 23 of 39 patients irresectable at laparotomy were found to have metastatic disease. Fourteen had gross metastatic disease to periportal or retroperitoneal lymph nodes (Table 54.8). CT scan only indicated lymphadenopathy in 4 of these patients. Nine patients had unsuspected metastatic disease found on explo-

Table 54.8 Summary of factors precluding a curative resection in patients at initial evaluation or at exploratory laparotomy. **Age, comorbidity, sepsis (Burke 1998) (Reprinted with permission from Annals of Surgery).

Group	n	Local extension	Nodal metastases	Distant metastases	Other**
Unresectable at presentation	21	9	0	8	4
Unresectable at laparotomy	39	8	14	9	8
Total	60	17 (28%)	14 (23%)	17 (28%)	12(20%)

ration: four had omental and/or peritoneal metastases, 3 had liver metastases, and 2 had both liver and peritoneal disease (Burke 1998). The authors have been conducting a prospective evaluation of staging laparoscopy in patients with hepatobiliary malignancies, including hilar cholangiocarcinoma. Laparoscopic detection of irresectability based on vascular involvement and biliary tumor extent remain difficult, particularly in patients with biliary stents (unpublished data).

A very detailed approach to definition of resectability based on direct cholangiography of segmental ducts and cholangioscopy is described by Professor Nimura in a comment to this chapter. This approach does not appear to have resulted in an increased resectability rate and we have no experience with it.

Treatment options

There are two objectives in the therapy of hilar cholangiocarcinoma: complete tumor excision with negative margins if possible, and restoration of biliary-enteric continuity. Patients should be fully evaluated for possible curative resection before any intervention is performed, since stent-associated infection and inflammation renders assessment and exploration difficult. If resection is clearly not feasible, then transtumoral drainage or paratumoral surgical bypass offer satisfactory palliation and can be combined with radiotherapy (vide infra).

Orthotopic liver transplantation has been attempted for irresectable hilar tumors. Klempnauer and colleagues reported 4 long-term survivors out of 32 patients submitted to transplantation for hilar cholangiocarcinoma (Klempnauer et al 1997). The same group also reported a 17.1% 5-year survival for their overall transplant group (Pichlmayr et al 1996). Comparable results were reported by Iwatsuki and colleagues (Iwatsuki et al 1998). Presently most centers do not perform liver transplantation for cholangiocarcinoma. The high incidence of lymph node metastases is of concern

and larger series taking this into account and with long-term follow-up will be required before liver transplantation can be recommended for irresectable disease (Pichlmayr et al 1995). We have not performed preoperative portal vein embolization as outlined below by Professor Nimura.

RESECTION

In patients with potentially resectable tumors based on preoperative imaging, the primary goal should be complete resection with intent to cure. Our criterion for curative resection is complete removal of all gross disease with clear histologic margins (R0 resection). However, this definition is not applied as stringently by all investigators and reported results are often not comparable.

There is now substantial evidence to support the argument that partial hepatectomy is usually required to achieve this goal. Bile duct excision and partial hepatectomy, often with en bloc caudate lobectomy (Nimura et al 1990), is frequently necessary to achieve negative margins (Ch. 83). Indeed, several recent studies show a parallel between the number of patients undergoing partial hepatectomy and negative margins (Table 54.9). We perform caudate resection in all cases with suggested tumor extension into the caudate lobe. The principal caudate lobe ducts drain into the left hepatic duct. Thus, tumors extending into the left hepatic duct almost always involve the caudate duct and usually require caudate resection (Mizumoto and Suzuki 1988). A dilated caudate duct, suggesting tumor involvement, may occasionally be visualized on preoperative imaging (Fig. 54.9). In some cases intraoperative frozen section of the caudate duct margin may help the decision to proceed to caudate resection. The importance of negative resection margins for long-term survival is confirmed by the results of our recent study (Burke 1998). Of the 90 patients

Table 54.9 Influence of partial hepatectomy on histological margins in patients who underwent a potentially curative resection for hilar cholangiocarcinoma: Summary of recent studies.

Author	Potential curative resection	Hepatectomy %	Negative margins %
Cameron (Cameron et al 1990)	39	20	15
Hadjis (Hadjis et al 1990)	27	60	56
Klempnauer (Klempnauer et al 1997)	147	79	79
Burke (Burke et al 1998)	30	73	83
Nimura (Nimura et al 1990)	55	98	83

Table 54.10 Influence of histologic margins on survival (from Burke 1998) (Reprinted with permission from Annals of Surgery)

Resection	n	Hepatic resection (%)	30-day mortality (%)	Median survival	5-year survival (%)
PCR*	30	22 (73)	2 (6)	40 ± 10	45
Neg. margins	25	20 (80)	2 (6)	not reached	56
Pos. margins	5	2 (40)	0 (0)	22 ± 10**	0

*Potentially curative resection (Burke 1998).
**$p \leq 0.01$

evaluated for resection, 69 underwent exploration and 30 had a potentially curative resection (removal of all gross disease), 22 (73%) of whom required partial hepatectomy and 2 required segmental portal vein resection. Of these 30 patients, 25 (83%) had negative histologic margins (R0) and a significantly better survival than patients with positive margins (Table 54.10, Fig. 54.12). It is of interest that in this resected group 15 patients had involvement of secondary biliary radicals by tumor, 11 had unilateral lobar liver atrophy and eight had encasement or occlusion of a major portal vein branch. In the past, these findings were considered technically insurmountable and the patients regarded as irresectable. It is now clear that this is not necessarily true, provided that the surgeon can leave behind a cancer-free and well-perfused liver remnant with adequate biliary drainage.

Patient selection

Distinguishing resectable from irresectable tumors demands careful consideration of all available data. Bilateral tumor extension to second order intrahepatic biliary radicles and encasement or occlusion of the main portal vein clearly precludes resection. By and large, however, the individual determinants of resectability must be considered within the context of all findings. Thus, ipsilateral involvement of the portal vein and bile ducts may be amenable to resection whereas contralateral involvement is usually not. Likewise, ipsilateral lobar atrophy does not preclude resection, whereas atrophy of the contralateral lobe does (Table 54.11).

Technique

Invasion of the main portal vein or its branches by tumor is a major determinant of resectability. Such vascular involvement may be documented on preoperative duplex sonography or MRCP. The preoperative analysis of vascular involvement and ductal extension of tumor is an essential part of operative planning and gives valuable information to the surgeon with respect to the extent of operation and operative strategy.

Several technical steps during the exploration and the resection of hilar cholangiocarcinoma are crucial to the success of the operation. *Local resection* for small tumors not extending beyond second order intrahepatic bile ducts and not involving the major vessels may be possible. In this

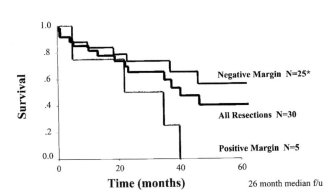

Fig. 54.12 Actuarial survival curves after resection of hilar cholangiocarcinoma, stratified by histologic margins. Median survival was 40 months in all resected patients. Projected survival exceeded 60 months in patients resected with negative histologic margins. (Burke 1998) (Reprinted with permission from Annals of Surgery).

Table 54.11 Criteria of irresectability in patients with hilar cholangiocarcinoma

Patient factors
    Medically unfit for operation
    Cirrhosis/portal hypertension
Local factors
    Hepatic duct involvement up to secondary radicles bilaterally
    Encasement or occlusion of the main portal vein *proximal to its bifurcation*
    Atrophy of one lobe with encasement of contralateral portal vein branch
    Atrophy of one lobe with contralateral involvement of secondary biliary radicles
Distant disease
    Histologically proven metastases to N2 lymph nodes.
    Liver, lung or peritoneal metastases

situation, resection must include removal of the entire supraduodenal bile duct, gallbladder, cystic duct, and extrahepatic hepatic ducts, together with clearance of the supraduodenal tissues including the related lymph nodes. In most patients, however, there is intrahepatic extension of the tumor, right or left portal vein involvement or both. In these cases, *en-bloc liver resection*, often with caudate lobectomy, is necessary to achieve tumor clearance (Ch. 83). In a small number of patients, tumor adherence to the portal vein can be managed by segmental portal vein resection and reconstruction (Blumgart et al 1984, Nimura et al 1991b, Burke 1998). This can only be done if intraoperative assessment shows that a tumor free remnant with intact biliary drainage and blood supply can be left in situ.

Some centrally located tumors may be amenable to a more limited hepatic resection. Such resections, which include segments IV and V or IV and I, are limited in their application (Grune et al 1991, Miyakawa et al 1996, Miyazaki et al 1998a,b). For example, of the 30 resected patients in our recent series, 11 had lobar atrophy and 8 had encasement or occlusion of a major portal vein branch (Burke 1998). Central hepatic resections are clearly not appropriate in the face of these findings.

Incision and exploration

The operation begins with a thorough exploration of the abdomen. Contrary to popular belief, metastatic disease is common in patients with hilar cholangiocarcinoma. In our recent series of 90 consecutive patients, 31 of 60 (52%) irresectable patients had metastases to regional lymph nodes or distant sites (Burke 1998). These findings are supported by results from other series (Lai et al 1987, Cameron et al 1990). Staging laparoscopy may help identify some irresectable patients before committing them to a laparotomy (see above). While extrahepatic disease can usually be visualized, identifying those with extensive biliary involvement is difficult on laparoscopic ultrasound.

The abdomen is entered through a bilateral subcostal incision with proximal extension to the xiphoid if necessary. Careful bimanual palpation of the liver is performed to rule out unsuspected masses in the liver. Palpation of the caudate lobe is performed after incision of the lesser omentum allowing access to the lesser sac. A Kocher maneuver is performed to allow access to the retroduodenal lymph nodes. The ligamentum teres is elevated exposing the undersurface of the liver and allowing thorough examination of the subhilar and retroduodenal area. Precise assessment of tumor extension, biopsy of any suspicious lesions or lymph nodes with frozen section analysis should be performed. Evidence of multicentricity within the liver, intrahepatic metastases,

spread to distant sites or N2 level lymph nodes (see Table 54.3) preclude resection. With any of these findings, the patient should be considered for palliative biliary drainage.

While a segmental bile duct resection and biliary reconstruction are possible in some patients, the majority require partial hepatectomy to achieve complete tumor clearance (see above). In all cases, therefore, the surgeon must be prepared to perform a liver resection. The general principals of intraoperative management are discussed in Chapter 27. Preparation for surgery includes suitable intraoperative monitoring and the possibility for rapid transfusion. The patient's central venous pressure is kept below 5 mmHg during the operation so as to keep blood loss low during retrohepatic dissection, dissection of the hepatic veins and parenchymal transection (Cunningham et al 1994, Melendez et al 1998). The patient is positioned in 15° Trendelenburg in order to avoid air embolism.

The following description summarizes the initial steps of dissection, exposure of the hilar structures, their dissection and resection, and subsequent biliary–enteric reconstruction as performed for a segmental bile duct resection. The specifics of *en bloc* liver resection, including caudate lobectomy, are discussed in Chapter 83.

Tumor assessment and resection

In order to reach the confluence of the bile ducts and assess its relation to the portal vein, the common bile duct must first be transected above the duodenum and turned upwards. The liver hilus is fully exposed anteriorly by taking down the gallbladder and lowering the hilar plate by incising Glisson's capsule along the base of segment IV (Fig. 54.13). Exposure of the left hepatic duct is improved by dividing the bridge of liver tissue that often connects the base of segment IV and the left lateral segment and which may be quite substantial in some patients (Figs 54.14 and 54.15). The entire extrahepatic biliary apparatus and adjacent lymphatic tissues are turned upwards to expose the portal vein. A plane can easily be developed between the posterior aspect of the bile duct tumor and the portal vein provided there is no tumor invasion into the vessels (Fig. 54.16). The dissection is continued upwards toward the hilus, skeletonizing the portal vein and hepatic artery.

At this point, the surgeon should assess the proximal extent of tumor by palpation and if necessary by biopsy. Segmental bile duct resection is possible only if an adequate length of the hepatic ducts can be achieved beyond the tumor and there is no vascular involvement. If the tumor extends to the second order biliary radicals unilaterally such that clearance cannot be achieved or if there is ipsilateral portal vein branch involvement, then partial hepatectomy

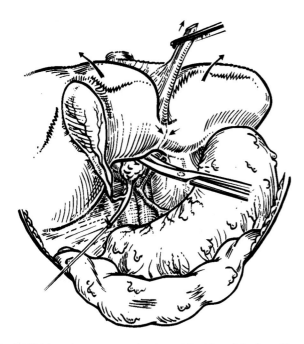

Fig. 54.13 Dissection to expose structure at the hilus of the liver. The ligamentum teres is elevated and the liver turned upwards. Dissection at the base of the quadrate lobe (scissors) lowers the hilar plate. Note that the bridge of liver tissue connecting segments III and IV is still intact (arrows). The common bile duct is divided immediately above the duodenum and its lower end has been separated from the underlying portal vein and hepatic artery and elevated together with associated connective tissue and lymph nodes.

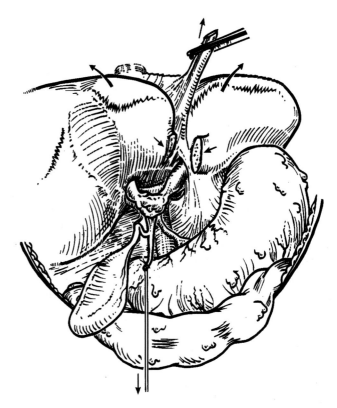

Fig. 54.14 The bridge of liver tissue at the base of the umbilical fissure has been divided (arrow). This is readily accomplished or by dividing it with diathermy (see Fig. 54.15). The gallbladder has been mobilized together with the common bile duct. The biliary confluence and left hepatic duct together with the tumor have been lowered from beneath the quadrate lobe.

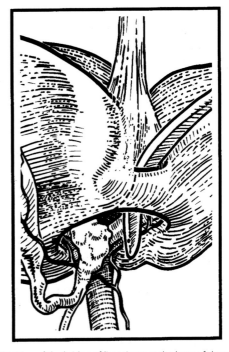

Fig. 54.15 Division of the bridge of liver tissue at the base of the umbilical fissure. A director or clamp can usually be passed beneath the liver tissue, above the pedicular structures, allowing safe division of the liver parenchyma. This opens the umbilical fissure and exposes the left hepatic duct.

must be performed (see Ch. 83). Tumors extending well into the left hepatic duct may involve the caudate ducts as well (see above) and will require en bloc caudate lobectomy (Mizumoto et al 1986, Mizumoto & Suzuki 1988). If partial hepatectomy is required, inflow control is obtained by ligation and transection of the ipsilateral branch of the portal vein and hepatic artery. Extrahepatic control and division of the ipsilateral hepatic vein is performed prior to parenchymal transection (see Ch. 83).

Once it is established that segmental bile duct excision is feasible, the left and right hepatic ducts are divided above the tumor (Fig. 54.17). Biliary–enteric continuity is restored by hepaticojejunostomy to a Roux-en-Y loop of jejunum. After removal of the tumor, the surgeon may be faced with multiple exposed duct orifices, all of which require suitable drainage. It is not infrequent that removal of the tumor results in discontinuity of the right anterior and posterior sectoral ducts and/or separation of one or more caudate ducts from the left hepatic duct. The side walls of adjacent ducts can be brought into apposition with sutures and regarded as a single duct for purposes of the anastomosis. In cases of multiple exposed ducts, it is often possible to create a situation where there are no more than two or three separate ducts to be anastomosed. A Roux-en-Y loop of jejunum

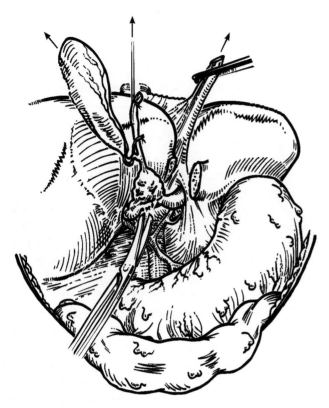

Fig. 54.16 The entire extrahepatic biliary apparatus is elevated together with associated portal connective tissue and nodes so as to allow dissection anterior to the bifurcation of the portal vein and elevation of the tumor, which is now completely mobilized. The hepatic artery and portal vein are skeletonized.

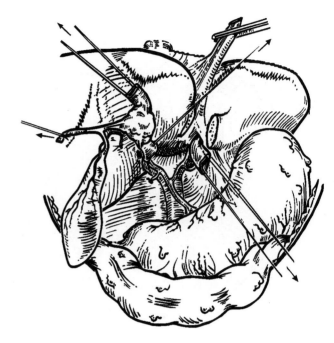

Fig. 54.17 The left hepatic duct has been divided clear of the tumor and is held on stay sutures. Its proximal end, together with the confluence of the bile ducts, common hepatic and common bile ducts and the gallbladder is turned upwards and to right and stay sutures are placed in the right hepatic duct, which is then similarly divided with subsequent removal of the tumor. The margins should be sent for frozen section histology. Note that after transection of the left hepatic duct and during the retrohilar and retrotumoral dissection towards the right, it is not infrequent to encounter obstructed and dilated ducts issuing from the caudate lobe, and for there to be two right hepatic ductal orifices representing the anterior and posterior right sectoral ducts. In this instance, each duct encountered is individually marked with stay sutures for subsequent anastomosis.

is prepared and brought up usually in a retrocolic fashion. Anastomosis is now carried out in an end-to-side fashion between the exposed ducts and the side of the jejunal loop (Fig. 54.18) using a single layer of 4–0 interrupted Vicryl sutures (Blumgart & Kelley 1985, Voyles & Blumgart 1982). Anastomotic techniques are illustrated and discussed in greater detail in Chapter 30. High biliary anastomoses to multiple ducts can be exceedingly difficult and require careful planning. Multiple disconnected ducts that cannot be approximated should similarly be viewed as a single duct for purposes of the anastomosis. It is usually impossible to perform sequential anastomoses in this location. The safest and most reliable method is to place the entire anterior row of sutures to all exposed ducts and then separately place the entire posterior row of sutures to the duct and jejunum. The jejunum is then railroaded up on the posterior sutures so that the back wall of the duct is flush with the back wall of the jejunum. The posterior layer of sutures to all exposed ducts is tied first and the previously placed anterior sutures are then passed sequentially through the anterior jejunal wall to complete the anastomosis. We routinely employ dependent drainage near the anastomosis.

RESULTS OF RESECTION

Long-term survival can be achieved with an acceptable operative mortality (Olthoff et al 1990, Lupi et al 1990, Hadjis et al 1990, Nimura et al 1990, Nagata et al 1990, Rosen et al 1991, Haswell-Elkins et al 1991, Wolber et al 1991, Nagorney et al 1993, Baer et al 1993, Nagorney et al 1993, Pichlmayr et al 1996, Nakeeb et al 1996a,b, Parc et al 1997, Klempnauer et al 1997, Burke 1998, Ahrendt et al 1998). It is clear, however, that the results of resection depend critically on the status of the resection margins. Several studies have shown that patients resected with negative histologic margins survive significantly longer than those with involved margins (Hadjis et al 1990, Lupi et al 1990, Pichlmayr et al 1996, Burke 1998, Ahrendt et al 1998) (Table 54.7). Over the past 20 years, there has been a steady increase in the use of hepatic resection in patients with hilar cholangiocarcinoma. We firmly believe that this is responsible for the increase in the percentage of R0 resections (negative histologic margins) and the observed perioperative mortality was 7.4%. The median survival after resection was 22 months (Hadjis et al 1990).

In the period from 1986 to 1990, 29 of 41 patients assessed were explored for possible curative resection. Eight of these patients were found to have unresectable disease and underwent a biliary-enteric bypass. A local tumor excision was performed in 12 patients and concomitant hepatic resection in 9. Seven patients (33%) had positive margins after resection. Operative mortality was 5%. The median survival for resected patients was 36 months (range 10–58 months) (Baer et al 1993).

More recently, at MSKCC, 90 patients with hilar cholangiocarcinoma were assessed over a 5-year period (1992 to 1997). Sixty-nine patients were explored for possible resection and 30 were resected. Thirty-nine of these patients were found to be irresectable at laparotomy. Local tumor resection was performed in eight patients and bile duct/tumor excision with concomitant hepatic resection in 22 patients, 2 of whom required portal vein resection and reconstruction. Four patients (17%) had positive margins after resection. The peri-operative mortality was 6%. The median survival for all resected patients was 40 months. Histologically positive margins significantly shortened survival (22 months). On the other hand, median survival in patients with negative margins was greater than 60 months. The 5-year survival for the latter group was 56 months (Burke 1998). The summary of this analysis is shown in Table 54.12 and reflects the current trend in the state-of-the-art treatment of hilar cholangiocarcinoma. Comparing the results from these three time periods, there is a progressive increase in the percentage of R0 resections and partial hepatectomy.

Adjuvant therapy

Several studies have investigated the benefit of postoperative adjuvant radiation therapy in patients with hilar cholangiocarcinoma. In two separate reports from Johns Hopkins, (Cameron et al 1990, Pitt et al 1995) showed no benefit of adjuvant external beam and intraluminal radiation therapy. On the other hand, Kamada et al suggested that radiation may improve survival in patients with histologically positive hepatic duct margins (Kamada et al 1996). Additionally, in a small series of patients (5 with hilar cholangiocarcinoma) from Louisville, resectability was reportedly greater in patients given neoadjuvant radiation therapy prior to exploration (McMasters et al 1997). It must be remembered, however, that none of these studies was randomized and most consist of a small, heterogeneous group of patients. At the present time, there is no data to support the routine use of adjuvant or neoadjuvant radiation therapy, except in the

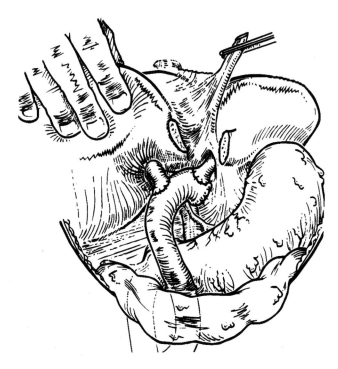

Fig. 54.18 The exposed right and left hepatic ducts are anastomosed using a single layer of 3-0 absorbable suture to a 70 cm retrocolic Roux-en-Y loop of jejunum. If there are multiple ducts exposed at the hilus, then these may be approximated one to another, if possible. In any event, all exposed ducts must be included in the anastomosis. The technique for suture is described in detail in Chapter 30.

improvement in survival after resection. These points are emphasized by the senior author's (LHB) personal series of 262 patients accumulated over a 20-year interval (Saldinger & Blumgart 1999).

From 1977 to 1985 of 131 patients who were assessed, 27 were resected with curative intent. Local bile duct excision was performed in 11 patients while 16 underwent a bile duct excision combined with hepatectomy. Twelve (44%) who underwent resection had positive margins. The

Table 54.12 Summary of the senior author's (LHB) experience with the treatment of 269 patients with hilar cholangiocarcinoma over 20 years. NA, not available

Reference	1977–1985 (Hadjis et al 1990)	1986–1990 (Baer et al 1993)	1991–1997 (Burke 1998)
Patients evaluated	131	48	90
Patients resected	27	21	30
Negative margin	15 (56%)	14 (67%)	25 (83%)
Hepatectomy	16 (60%)	9 (43%)	22 (73%)
Operative mortality	7.4%	5%	6%
Median survival	25 months	36 months	40 months
5-yr survival	22%	NA	56%

context of a controlled trial. Likewise, there is currently no role for adjuvant chemotherapy.

PALLIATION

The majority of patients with hilar cholangiocarcinoma are not suitable for resection. In this setting, the management options include some form of biliary decompression or supportive care. Jaundice alone is not necessarily an indication for biliary decompression, given the associated morbidity and mortality. Our current indications for biliary decompression in inoperable patients are intractable pruritus, cholangitis, the need for access for intraluminal radiotherapy and to allow recovery of hepatic parenchymal function in patients receiving chemotherapeutic agents. Supportive care alone is probably the best approach for elderly patients with significant comorbid conditions, provided that pruritis is not a major feature. Patients who are found to be unresectable at operation represent a different group and operative biliary decompression is usually performed successfully (Burke 1998) and can be so constructed as to provide access to the biliary tree for postoperative irradiation (Kuvshinoff et al 1995).

Assessment of palliative biliary drainage procedures is difficult since the spectrum of patients ranges from the critically ill and irresectable to those in relatively good health with potentially resectable tumors. All patients should be properly assessed by experienced personnel with a view toward possible resection. This point cannot be over emphasized. If the patient is deemed irresectable, the diagnosis should be confirmed with a biopsy. Biliary decompression can be obtained either by percutaneous transhepatic puncture or by endoscopic stent placement. It is important to realize that these patients have a short life expectancy and periprocedural complications extends hospital stay and consumes time. Hilar tumors are more difficult to transverse with the endoscopic technique. Moreover, the failure rates and incidence of subsequent cholangitis are high (Liu et al 1998). Thus, most patients with irresectable hilar tumors are not candidates for endoscopic biliary drainage.

Percutaneous biliary drainage (see also Ch. 58)

Percutaneous transhepatic biliary drainage and subsequent placement of a self-expandable metallic endoprosthesis (Wallstent) can be successfully performed in most patients with hilar obstruction. However, satisfactory results, even with experienced interventional radiologists, are more difficult to achieve in patients with hilar tumors than in those with distal biliary obstruction (Cheung & Lai 1995, Becker et al 1993, Miyazaki et al 1998a,b). Frequently, hilar tumors isolate all 3 major hilar ducts (left hepatic, right anterior sectoral hepatic and right posterior sectoral hepatic), and 2 or more stents must be placed for adequate drainage (Schima et al 1997) (Fig. 54.19). One must also consider that jaundice may result from hepatic dysfunction secondary to portal vein occlusion. Jaundice in this setting, without intrahepatic biliary dilatation, is not correctable with biliary stents. In addition, lobar atrophy is an important factor when considering palliative biliary procedures. Percutaneous drainage through an atrophic lobe usually does not relieve jaundice and should be avoided. The presence of multiple intrahepatic metastases or ascites may also add to the technical difficulty of the procedure.

The median patency of metallic endoprostheses at the hilus is approximately 6 months (Glattli et al 1993), significantly lower than that reported for similar stents placed in the distal bile duct. Becker et al reported one-year patency rates of 46% and 89% for Wallstents placed at the hilus and the distal bile duct, respectively (Becker et al 1993). Similarly, Stoker et al documented occlusion in 36% of patients with Wallstents at the hilus compared with 6% of patients with Wallstents in the distal bile duct (Stoker & Lameris 1993). In most series of Wallstents placed for hilar obstruction, documented stent occlusion requiring reintervention occurs in 25% of patients (Becker et al 1993, Schima et al 1997, Stoker & Lameris 1993, Rossi et al 1994, Glattli et al 1993, Bergquist et al 1998, Hurlimann &

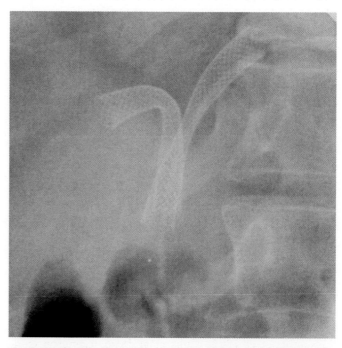

Fig. 54.19 This patient with hilar cholangiocarcinoma had isolation of all major hilar bile ducts and required two expandable metallic stents for adequate biliary drainage.

Gardiol 1991). This concurs with our findings of a mean patency of 6.1 months in 35 patients palliated for malignant high biliary obstruction by placement of expandable metallic endoprostheses. The periprocedural mortality was 14% at 30 days and seven patients (24%) had documented stent occlusion requiring repeated intervention (Glattli et al 1993).

Intrahepatic biliary-enteric bypass (see also Ch. 30)

Patients found to be irresectable at operation may be candidates for intrahepatic biliary-enteric bypass. The segment III duct is usually the most accessible and is our preferred approach, but the right anterior or posterior sectoral hepatic ducts can also be used (Jarnagin et al 1998). Typically, segment III bypass is used to restore biliary-enteric continuity after the bile duct has been divided and a locally invasive, irresectable tumor has been discovered. Segment III bypass provides excellent biliary drainage and is less prone to occlusion by tumor than are Wallstents (Stoker & Lameris 1993), since the anastomosis can be placed at some distance away from the tumor (Fig. 54.20). Relief of jaundice will be achieved if at least one-third of the functioning hepatic parenchyma is adequately drained. Communication between the right and left hepatic ducts is not necessary, provided that the undrained lobe has not been percutaneously drained or otherwise contaminated (Baer et al 1994). In this circumstance, there is a high risk of persistent biliary fistula and cholangitis. Bypass to an atrophic lobe or a lobe heavily involved with tumor is generally not effective. In our recent report of 55 consecutive bypasses in patients with malignant hilar obstruction, segment III bypass in patients with hilar cholangiocarcinoma (*n* = 20) yielded the best results. The one-year bypass patency in this group was 80% and there were no perioperative deaths (Jarnagin et al 1998).

Palliative radiation therapy

Patients with irresectable, locally advanced tumors but without evidence of widespread disease may be candidates for palliative radiation therapy. A combination of external beam radiation (5000–6000 cGy) and intraluminal iridium-192 (2000 cGy) delivered percutaneously is typically used. Several authors have demonstrated the feasibility of this approach but improved survival compared with biliary decompression alone has not been documented in a controlled study (Cameron et al 1990, Bowling et al 1996, Kuvshinoff et al 1995, Vallis et al 1996, Cameron et al 1990, Vatanasapt et al 1990a, Nagano et al 1990). In a group of 12 patients treated with this regimen over a 3-year

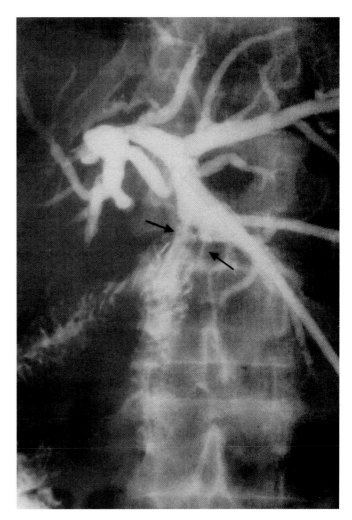

Fig. 54.20 Transhepatic cholangiogram obtained via a temporary percutaneous drainage tube showing a widely patent anastomosis from the segment III duct to a Roux-en-Y loop of jejunum (arrows).

period at MSKCC, the median survival was 14.5 months. Episodes of cholangitis and intermittent jaundice were relatively common but the incidence of serious complications was low and there were no treatment-related deaths (Kuvshinoff et al 1995). Cameron et al reported improved survival in irradiated patients compared to a group of patients not irradiated; however, the median survival in both groups was less than one year (Cameron et al 1990). Others have reported no benefit and question its routine use, given the increased incidence of complications and greater time spent in hospital (Bowling et al 1996). Radiation therapy is clearly not appropriate in patients with widespread disease. Systemic chemotherapy is the only option for these patients but response rates are low and no study has shown a survival benefit compared with biliary drainage alone (Patt et al 1996).

Photodynamic therapy

Ortner and colleagues have recently evaluated the efficacy of photodynamic therapy in unresectable hilar cholangiocarcinoma (Ortner et al 1998). This method has previously been used in the treatment of tumors of the esophagus, colon, stomach, bronchus, bladder and brain. It is a two-step procedure. First a photosensitizer is injected then direct illumination via cholangioscopy activates the compound causing tumor cell death. The authors treated nine patients in this fashion who had failed endoscopic stenting. They report a 0% mortality for the procedure, however there was a 25% mortality related to the initial endoscopic stenting, which must be considered. The authors do not mention their indication for biliary drainage. This information is important in order to assess the extent of disease prior to therapy. Detailed reasons for irresectability are not discussed, and the reported median survival of 439 days is therefore difficult to interpret. The data presented in this report, including decrease in bilirubin and some improved quality of life does not suffice to advocate routine use of this method. Comparison in a randomized controlled fashion to other palliative modalities will be needed to define its real value.

Chemotherapy

Chemotherapy has been investigated in uncontrolled studies. No benefit has been demonstrated in the uncontrolled series published to date. Two phase II studies analyzing the effect of 5-FU combined with interferon alpha-2b and the effect of paclitaxel failed to show any benefit (Patt et al 1996, Jones Jr et al 1996).

SUMMARY

The treatment of hilar cholangiocarcinoma continues to evolve. Judicious use of preoperative investigations using duplex ultrasound, CT scan and especially MRCP and improvements in surgical techniques have allowed better patient selection and the performance of appropriately radical operations with an acceptable mortality.

Long-term survival and possible cure, rather than palliation, is now the primary aim. Recent results presented in this chapter justify an aggressive approach in attempting resection with negative margins. It should be recognized that partial hepatectomy is usually necessary to achieve this goal. The detailed diagnostic approach with preoperative biliary drainage, cholangiography via multiple drainage tubes and cholangioscopy practiced by Japanese surgeons (vide infra) may offer an advantage but to date has not been proven to increase resectability, reduce perioperative mortality or improve long term survival.

All methods of biliary–enteric decompression, whether surgical or intubational, have considerable morbidity but allow reasonable palliation in some patients. Radiotherapy and photodynamic therapy may have a role in increasing stent patency and possibly survival. However, further study is required to establish their position within the current armamentarium.

Hilar cholangiocarcinoma should not be approached with therapeutic nihilism. Diagnostic and therapeutic approaches to these lesions require special expertise and patients should be referred to centers where adequately trained teams are available.

CHOLANGIOCARCINOMA INVOLVING THE DISTAL BILE DUCT (see also Chs 51, 55 and 56)

Tumors of the lower bile duct are classified according to their anatomical location, although there may be considerable overlap. Mid-bile duct tumors arise below the confluence in the common bile duct between the upper border of the duodenum and the cystic duct; distal bile duct tumors are those arising anywhere from the duodenum to the papilla of Vater (Tompkins et al 1981). Tumors of the distal bile duct represent approximately 20 to 30% of all cholangiocarcinomas and 5 to 10% of all periampullary tumors (Fong et al 1996, Nakeeb et al 1996a,b, Wade et al 1997, Yeo et al 1997). True mid-duct tumors are distinctly uncommon. Nakeeb et al proposed an alternative classification scheme that divides cholangiocarcinomas into intrahepatic, perihilar and distal subgroups, thus eliminating the mid-duct group which are often difficult to accurately classify (Nakeeb et al 1996b). There are approximately 2000 new cases of distal bile duct cancer in the United States each year (Fong et al 1996). As is true for hilar cholangiocarcinoma, adenocarcinoma is the principal histologic type in the lower bile duct; however, papillary tumors are more common in the distal bile duct than at the hilus (Tompkins et al 1981).

Clinical presentation and diagnosis

The clinical presentation of distal bile duct cancer is generally indistinguishable from that of proximal cholangiocarcinoma or other periampullary malignancies. Progressive jaundice is seen in 75 to 90% of patients. Abdominal pain, weight loss, fever or pruritis occur in one-third or fewer

(Fong et al 1996, Nakeeb et al 1996a,b). The occasional patient will present with intermittent jaundice, and this is particularly true if the lesion is papillary in nature. Lesions in the periampullary region may mimic choledocholithiasis; the level of the serum bilirubin may provide a clue as to the etiology of the obstruction (Way 1994) (see above).

Distal bile duct tumors are frequently mistaken for adenocarcinoma of the pancreatic head, the most common periampullary malignancy. In a series of 119 periampullary tumors, the site of origin was incorrectly diagnosed in 28% of patients preoperatively and in 20% of patients intraoperatively (Jones et al 1985). Nevertheless, endoscopic retrograde cholangiopancreatography (ERCP) can provide valuable information regarding the level of obstruction and may show clearly that the obstruction is arising from the bile duct and does not involve the pancreatic duct. ERCP may also be useful in cases where choledocholithiasis is suspected and may be therapeutic in these patients. Percutaneous transhepatic cholangiography is generally less useful for tumors of the distal bile duct. A good quality cross-sectional imaging study is also required, usually a CT scan, to assess for vascular involvement and/or metastatic disease. It is not uncommon that CT scan does not reveal a mass, however, since these tumors are frequently small at the time of presentation. Increasingly, magnetic resonance cholangiopancreatography (MRCP) is being used to evaluate periampullary tumors. As is true for hilar lesions, MRCP can provide images of the distal bile duct previously obtainable only with ERCP and CT scan and without the need for invasive procedures (Georgopoulos et al 1999) (Figure 54.21).

In patients with a stricture of the distal bile duct and a clinical presentation consistent with cholangiocarcinoma, histologic confirmation of malignancy is generally unnecessary, unless non-operative therapy is planned. Benign strictures do occur in the lower bile duct but these are difficult to differentiate definitively from malignant strictures without resection. Percutaneous needle biopsy is difficult and often impossible because of the small size of these tumors. In addition, endoscopic brushings of the bile duct have an unacceptably low sensitivity, making a negative result virtually useless (Ryan 1991). Excessive reliance on the results of percutaneous or brush biopsies will serve only to delay therapy. Additional discussion regarding the evaluation of patients with distal bile duct cancers can be found in Chapter 55.

Treatment options

Complete resection is the only effective therapy for cancers of the lower bile duct (Fong et al 1996, Nagorney et al

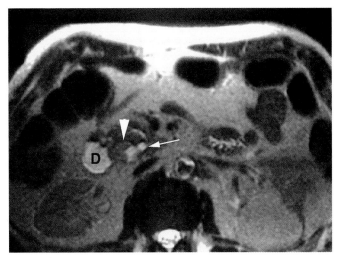

(A)

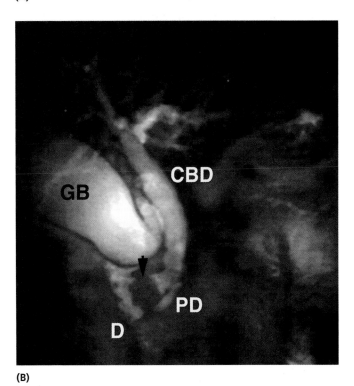

(B)

Fig. 54.21 (A) Cross sectional MRI image showing a filling defect within the distal bile duct (arrowhead) just at the point where it meets the pancreatic duct (arrow). D, duodenum. **(B)** Coronal MRCP reconstruction showing clearly a papillary mass in the distal bile duct (arrowhead). GB, gallbladder; CBD, common bile duct; PD, pancreatic duct; D, duodenum.

1993, Nakeeb et al 1996b, Tompkins et al 1981, Wade et al 1997, Yeo et al 1997). Meaningful experience with these relatively uncommon tumors has been limited to a few centers. However, in reports containing significant numbers of patients, 5-year survival rates of up to 40% have been reported after complete resection (Table 54.13). In most studies, survival beyond one year was uncommon in patients

Table 54.13 Recently published series of patients with adenocarcinoma of the distal bile duct

Author	Year	Length of study (years)	Number of patients	Number of patients resected	Median survival (months)	5-year survival
Nagorney et al	1993	10	39	22	24	40%
Fong et al	1996	10	104	45	33	27%
Wade et al*	1997	4	156	34	22**	14%
Yeo et al†	1997	6	–	65	20	16%‡

* Combined data from 159 U.S. Department of Veterans Affairs Hospitals.
** Indicates mean survival.
† Data derived from a study of patients undergoing pancreaticoduodenectomy for   benign and malignant periampullary diseases.
‡ Indicates survival at 3 years.

subjected to palliative bypass or biliary intubation (Fong et al 1996, Nakeeb et al 1996b, Tompkins et al 1981, Wade et al 1997).

Resection of most distal bile duct cancers requires pancreaticoduodenectomy (see Ch. 56). In the series from Memorial Sloan-Kettering Cancer Center (MSKCC), only 13% of patients (6 of 45) were amenable to bile duct excision alone (Fong et al 1996), while in the Veterans Hospital study this figure was 8% (3 of 34) (Wade et al 1997). In comparison to patients with pancreatic cancer, patients with distal bile duct cancer are more often amenable to resection, less often have microscopic disease at the resection margin and less frequently have spread of tumor to adjacent lymph nodes (Fong et al 1996, Nakeeb et al 1996a,b, Yeo et al 1997). However, in addition to completeness of resection, lymph node status is a critical determinant of outcome. Fong et al found that lymph node status was the only independent predictor of long-term survival in resected patients, with positive nodes conferring a 6.7 times greater likelihood of recurrence and death (Fong et al 1996). Similarly, Wade et al identified no survivors beyond 3 years with involved regional lymph nodes (Wade et al 1997), and Nakeeb et al found that lymph node status and tumor differentiation were independent predictors of outcome (Nakeeb et al 1996a,b).

The combined data from the literature would suggest that survival after resection of adenocarcinoma of the distal bile duct is at least as good and probably better than that for pancreatic cancer (Fong et al 1996, Wade et al 1997). Moreover, it has long been assumed that survival after resection of distal bile duct tumors is greater than after resection of hilar cholangiocarcinomas (Tompkins et al 1981). This assumption is almost certainly erroneous and likely evolved from older reports that did not take into account the status of resection margins in patients with hilar tumors. If adjusted for stage and completeness of resection, the survival rates appear to be comparable (Nagorney et al 1993). Adjuvant therapy after resection (chemotherapy and radiation therapy) has not been proven to improve survival, although this issue has not been evaluated in a prospective fashion (Nakeeb et al 1996a,b).

Palliating biliary obstruction in unresectable patients can be achieved with a surgical bypass (hepatico-jejunostomy or choledochojejunostomy) or biliary endoprostheses. Endoprostheses for distal biliary obstruction (Ch. 59) are easier to place and have a greater long term patency than those placed for hilar obstruction (Becker et al 1993). Surgically created bypasses provide excellent relief of jaundice and can be done with an acceptably low morbidity and mortality. It has been suggested that surgical bypass is more appropriate for patients expected to survive greater than 6 months (van den Bosch et al 1994). The authors generally use biliary endoprostheses in patients with clear cut metastatic disease, discovered preoperatively or at staging laparoscopy, and in those unfit for operation.

Hilar and intrahepatic cholangiocarcinoma with emphasis on presurgical management

M. NAGINO, Y. NIMURA

INTRODUCTION

Hepatobiliary resection has become common in treating patients with cholangiocarcinoma (Tsuzuki et al 1983, Blumgart et al 1984, Bengmark et al 1988, Nimura et al 1990, Miyagawa et al 1995, Pichlmayr et al 1996, Miyazaki et al 1998a,b, Iwatsuki et al 1998, Burke 1998)) and combined portal vein and liver resection (Blumgart et al 1984, Sakaguchi & Nakamura 1986, Nimura et al 1991a, Miyazaki et al 1998a,b, Burke 1998) or hepatopancreatoduodenectomy (Nimura et al 1991b, Mimura et al 1991, Nakamura et al 1994, Tsukada et al 1994, Miyagawa et al 1996) has been used in Japan, Korea, Europe and the USA. The safe performance of such high-risk procedures remains a major challenge for hepatobiliary surgeons (Nagino et al 1993a,b, Hamahata et al 1998). Thus, it is of particular importance that the preoperative management of patients who are to undergo liver resection is optimized. In this section, we outline our methods of and recommendations for preoperative management of intrahepatic cholangiocarcinoma and especially focus on carcinoma involving the hepatic hilus. Further details are described in Chapter 83.

Macroscopic typing of intrahepatic cholangiocarcinoma

In 1997 the *Liver Cancer Study Group of Japan* developed a new classification of primary liver cancer.

According to this classification, intrahepatic cholangiocarcinoma are classified into the following three macroscopic types: *Mass-forming, Periductal-infiltrating, Intraductal growth*, and others (Fig. 54.22). The mass-forming type is characterized by the presence of a round-shaped mass in the liver parenchyma with a distinct border. The periductal-infiltrating type is distinguished by tumor infiltration along the intrahepatic bile duct: this variant occasionally involves the surrounding blood vessels or hepatic parenchyma. The intraductal growth type is characterized by papillary and/or granular growth within the bile duct lumen, occasionally associated with superficially spreading carcinoma. When more than one type is found, all of the types involved are recorded, in order of the degree of involvement; the first-recorded type is the predominant type, for example, 'Mass-forming type + Periductal infiltrating type' or 'Periductal infiltrating type + Intraductal growth type'.

PREOPERATIVE MANAGEMENT

In contradiction to the approach described by the editors of this book (see above), we outline here an approach which relies heavily on percutaneous intubation, cholangioscopy and preoperative angiography with portal venous embolization.

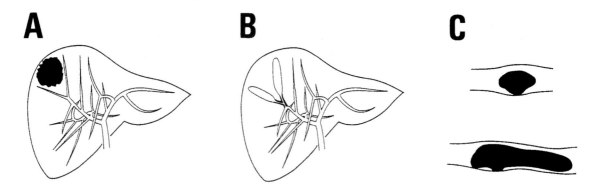

Fig. 54.22 Schematic illustration of macroscopic types of intrahepatic cholangiocarcinoma according to the Classification of Primary Liver Cancer, developed by the Liver Cancer Study Group of Japan. **(A)** Mass-forming type. **(B)** Periductal infiltrating type. **(C)** Intraductal growth type with papillary growth (*top*) or intraductal growth type forming a tumor thrombus (*bottom*).

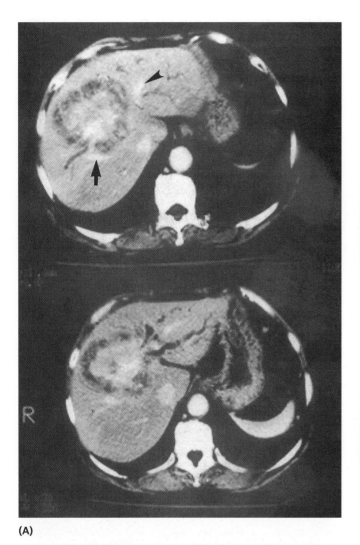

(A)

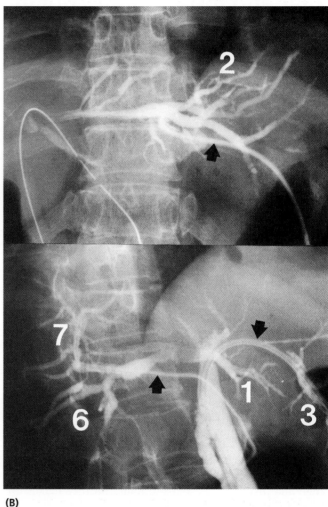

(B)

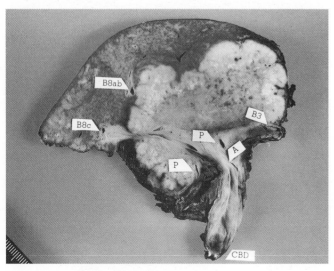

(C)

Fig. 54.23 A patient with mass forming type intrahepatic cholangiocarcinoma involving the hepatic hilus. The tumor was curatively resected by central hepatic bisegmentectomy with en bloc resection of the caudate lobe and extrahepatic bile duct. **(A)** Computed tomography showing a large tumor occupying the right anterior sector and the left medial segment. The middle hepatic vein was not visualized and the right (arrow) and the left (arrow head) hepatic veins are adjacent to the tumor. Note that intrahepatic bile ducts are dilated. **(B)** Cholangiograms through percutaneous transhepatic biliary drainage catheters show strictures at the hepatic hilus. Three catheters (arrows) are placed in the left lateral posterior (2), the left lateral anterior (3), and the right posterior sectoral (6+7) bile ducts, respectively. **(C)** Cut surface of the resected specimen shows a nodular whitish tumor involving the hepatic hilus. A, right anterior bile duct; P, right posterior bile duct; CBD, common bile duct; B3, resected stump of the left lateral anterior bile duct; B8ab, ventral and lateral branches of the right antero-superior bile duct; B8c, a dorsal branch of the right antero-superior bile duct.

Percutaneous transhepatic biliary drainage (PTBD)

Cholangiocarcinoma, including both extrahepatic and intrahepatic cholangiocarcinoma, frequently separates the intrahepatic biliary tree into several units, which necessitates multiple biliary drainage, i.e. drainage of each isolated intrahepatic bile duct (Nagino et al 1992, Nimura et al 1995a). Many authors (Speer et al 1987, Gholson & Burton 1991, Polydorou et al, 1992) have stressed the advantages of endoscopic retrograde biliary drainage (ERBD) because it is associated with technical success, a low procedure-related morbidity and mortality, and a shorter hospital stay. However, ERBD is also associated with a high incidence of cholangitis, due to catheter blockage and/or inability to perform multiductal biliary drainage (Cotton 1984, Andersen et al 1989). In addition, the endoscopic approach does not allow the diagnosis of proximal extent of carcinoma in separate intrahepatic segmental ducts.

Our preferred method of PTBD is Takada's direct anterior approach under fluoroscopic guidance (Takada et al 1976). Usually, the left hepatic duct is punctured perpendicularly in the ventrodorsal direction. When the intrahepatic bile ducts are separated into several units in advanced disease additional PTBD is simultaneously performed into the right anterior, the right posterior or other subsegmental branches (Nagino et al 1992, Nimura et al 1995a,b) (Fig. 54.23). One week after PTBD, the inner 6F tube and the outer Teflon tube are replaced with a 9F polyvinyl catheter (PTCS catheter; Sumitomo Bakelite Co., Tokyo) to prevent catheter dislodgment and to provide a sinus tract as rapidly as possible. If 'segmental' cholangitis (Kanai et al 1996) develops in patients with PTBD catheters, urgent additional puncture into the affected segmental duct should be performed (Iyomasa et al 1994, Sakamoto et al 1995) (Fig. 54.24).

Clinical studies of biliary decompression have demonstrated that external drainage has limited benefits and that the internal drainage is useful with respect to bile flow (Clements et al 1993). Therefore, when internal drainage is difficult, oral intake of the externally drained bile is recommended.

Although the clinical utility of preoperative biliary drainage has been debated over the last decades, this issue still remains controversial. Many retrospective reports (Nakayama et al 1978, Denning et al 1981, Norlander et al 1982, Gundy et al 1994) support preoperative PTBD, while several prospective randomized studies (Hatfield et al 1982, McPherson et al 1984, Pitt et al 1985) concluded that PTBD did not reduce operative morbidity and mortality. These reports discouraged the transhepatic approach in treating malignant obstructive jaundice. Our series of over

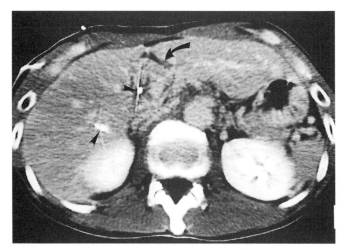

(A)

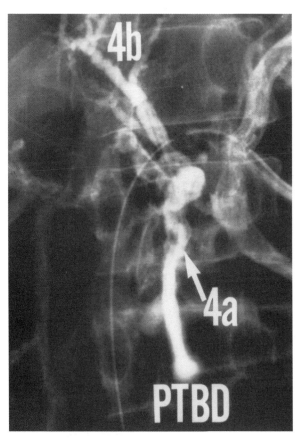

(B)

Fig. 54.24 A cholangiocarcinoma patient with segmental cholangitis after percutaneous transhepatic biliary drainage (PTBD). High fever, leukocytosis, and the presence of undrained segmental bile duct represent the 'triad' of segmental cholangitis. **(A)** Computed tomography taken two weeks after the initial PTBD in which two catheters (arrowhead) were placed. The left medial segmental bile duct (curved arrow) is dilated. **(B)** The left medial segmental bile duct was successfully drained by additional selective PTBD. 4a, an inferior branch of the left medial segmental bile duct; 4b, a superior branch of the left medial segmental bile duct.

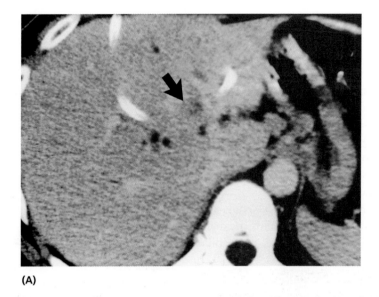

(A)

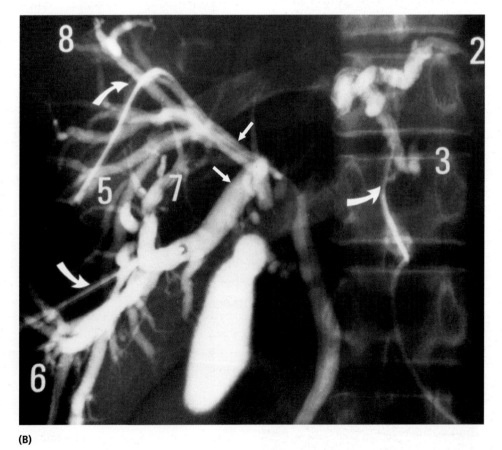

(B)

Fig. 54.25 A patient with periductal infiltrating intrahepatic cholangiocarcinoma involving the hepatic hilus. The tumor was curatively resected by left hepatic lobectomy with en bloc resection of the caudate lobe and extrahepatic bile duct. **(A)** Computed tomography showing a small low-density area (arrow) with obscure margin. **(B)** Selective cholangiography through multiple percutaneous transhepatic biliary drainage (PTBD) catheters demonstrates obstruction of the left hepatic duct and the confluence. The right anterior and posterior segmental bile ducts are separated, however, cancer invasion of these ducts is limited. A cholangiogram allows us to define the resection line of these bile ducts (arrow). Note that three PTBD catheters (curved arrows) were placed. Numerals indicate the number of Couinaud's hepatic segments. (*Continued*)

100 patients with multiple PTBD (Nimura et al 1995a,b) have demonstrated satisfactory results with a success rate of 100% and no fatal complications. It is our opinion that PTBD is safe and indeed indispensable in patients with proximal cholangiocarcinoma who are scheduled to undergo liver resection.

High quality cholangiography is essential for accurately diagnosing the extent of cancer (Nimura 1997) (Fig. 54.25). This, in turn, permits a rational surgical approach. Although bile duct cancer can usually be diagnosed by conventional cholangiography, either via endoscopic retrograde cholangiography (ERC) or PTC, these procedures do not precisely delineate the segmental anatomy of the intrahepatic bile ducts or the proximal extent of cancer spread into each segmental bile duct. By contrast, PTBD allows repeated cholangiography in several projections. Furthermore, multiple PTBD can provide selective cholangiograms of the separated hepatic segments which leads to accurate preoperative diagnosis extent of the cancer along the biliary branches (Kamiya et al 1994, Nimura et al 1995a,b, Nimura 1997). Therefore, PTBD should be considered not only an effective method of relieving jaundice but also as an important diagnostic modality.

Percutaneous transhepatic cholangioscopy (PTCS)

Despite the advent of new diagnostic modalities, cholangioscopic examination with biopsy plays an important role in diagnosing biliary malignancies (Nimura & Kamiya 1996). Peroral cholangioscopy is less invasive and allows rapid inspection of the biliary tree but has a limited value in preoperative staging of bile duct cancer. Percutaneous transhepatic cholangioscopy (PTCS) is more applicable and reliable: differentiation between malignant and benign lesions, definition of proximal and distal cancer extent, and early detection of small lesions and multiple foci, can be accomplished by cholangioscopic observation followed by biopsy and histological confirmation (Nimura et al 1988). PTCS is unrivaled in identification of superficially spreading bile duct carcinoma (Bhuiya et al 1993, Sano et al 1997, Kato et al 1997, Iwahashi et al 1998). At PTCS irregularly dilated and tortuous tumor vessels within the bile duct are a characteristic finding of malignancy; and a fine granular and papillary mucosa extending continuously from a main lesion, eroding the normal ductal epithelium, is indicative of the superficial spread of carcinoma (Nimura 1993).

PTCS is carried out through the sinus tract of a prior PTBD. One week after PTBD, the 6 F drainage catheter is replaced by 9 or 10 F catheter (PTCS catheter); then, the sinus tract is gradually dilated by replacing the existing catheter with a larger one 2 or 3 times a week. A small caliber cholangioscope (3.9 mm in outside diameter) can be introduced into the sinus tract of 12 F catheter, while standard type cholangioscope (4.9 mm in outside diameter) requires placement of 15 F catheter. An important preparation for PTCS is dilatation of the sinus tract within the shortest time period possible. The PTCS catheters we use are of varying caliber and are radiopaque and tapered at the tip; these catheters allow easier and safer changing. In addition the material is polyvinyl chloride which has a stronger tissue reaction than polyethylene or silicon, therefore a firm sinus tract is formed in a short time period.

Most intrahepatic cholangiocarcinomas are mass-forming

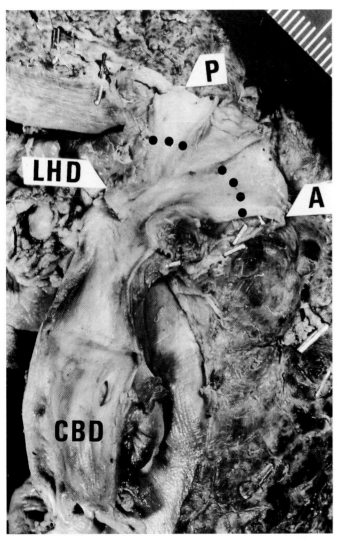

(C)

Fig. 54.25 (*Continued*) **(C)** A resected specimen reveals that the right anterior (A) and posterior (P) segmental bile ducts were resected with enough surgical margins, respectively. Closed circles express the proximal extension of carcinoma. CBD, common bile duct; LHD, orifice of the left hepatic duct.

(Fig. 54.23) or of diffusely periductal infiltrating type (Fig. 54.25). In these tumors, cancer is apt to extend more predominantly in the submucosal layer than in the mucosal layer (Sakamoto et al 1998). In addition, both direct and lymphatic invasion are proven to be common routes of submucosal extension, and are usually accompanied by marked fibrosis and infiltration (Weinbren & Mutum 1983). These histologic changes cause the findings of rigidity, narrowing, tapering, and obstruction of the bile duct seen on cholangiograms. Thus, a careful search for these findings on high-quality selective cholangiograms leads to an accurate diagnosis of cancer extent. By contrast, mucosal extension is a characteristic of the leading edge of intraductal growth type tumors, which present as protruding lesions in the intrahepatic bile duct (Fig. 54.26) or sometimes in cystic lesions communicating with the intrahepatic bile duct (Fig. 54.27).

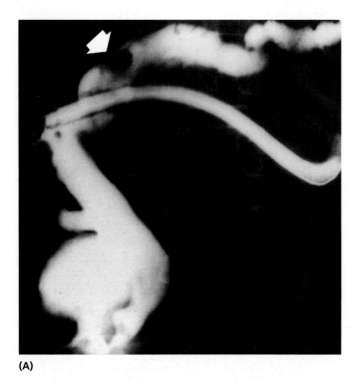

(A)

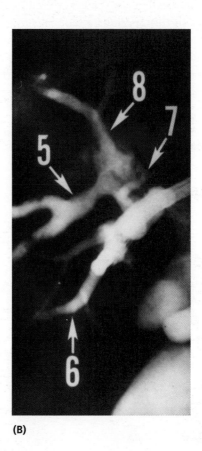

(B)

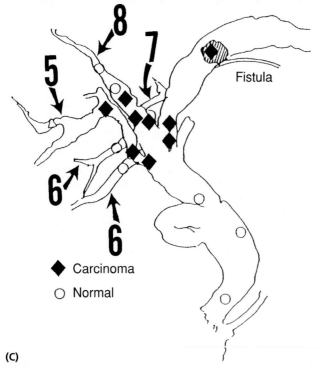

◆ Carcinoma

○ Normal

(C)

Fig. 54.26 A patient with intraductal growth type intrahepatic cholangiocarcinoma. **(A)** A cholangiogram through percutaneous transhepatic biliary drainage catheter showing a protruding tumor (arrow) in the left lateral posterior bile duct. Note that the other bile ducts are not opacified due to a lot of mucin secreted by the tumor. **(B)** Percutaneous transhepatic cholangioscopy (PTCS) depicted granular mucosa continuously extending from the protruding tumor. Numerals indicate the number of Couinaud's hepatic segments. **(C)** Mapping of biopsy examination under PTCS reveals that superficial spread of cancer markedly extends in the right anterior sectoral bile duct. Based on this biopsy information, a left hepatic trisegmentectomy with caudate lobectomy was selected as a curative resection procedure. Numerals indicate the number of Couinaud's hepatic segments.

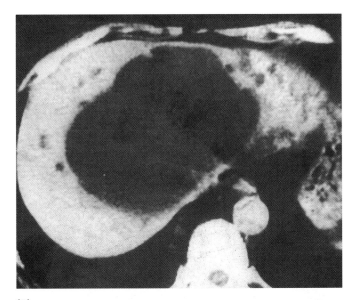

(A)

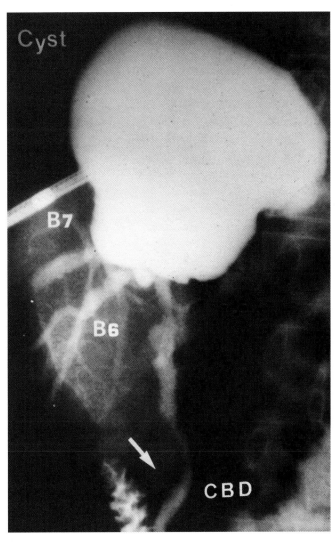

(B)

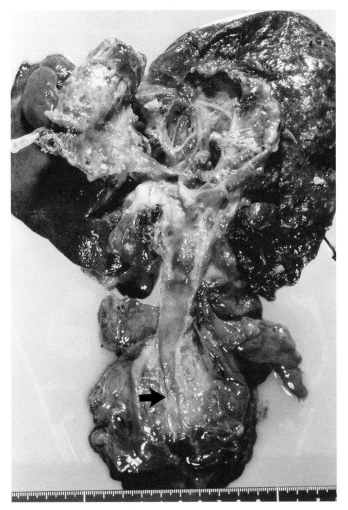

(C)

Fig. 54.27 A patient with intraductal growth type (cystic type) intrahepatic cholangiocarcinoma. **(A)** Computed tomography demonstrates a giant cystic lesion occupying the left lobe and the right anterior sector. **(B)** Drainage of the cystic lesion was performed for percutaneous transhepatic cholangioscopy (PTCS). PTCS with biopsy revealed that (1) this cystic lesion was communicated with the left hepatic duct, (2) the cyst wall was granular and was studded with small nodules, (3) all of biopsies taken from the cyst wall were positive for cancer, and (4) granular mucosa extended down to the common bile duct (arrow). **(C)** Left hepatic trisegmentectomy with caudate lobectomy and pancreatoduodenectomy was performed. A diagnosis of so-called cystadenocarcinoma was made. A resected specimen shows superficial spread of cancer extending from the cystic lesion to near the distal end of the common bile duct (arrow).

Intraductal growth type tumors are often associated with the superficial spread of carcinoma. Mucosal extension is easily detectable through PTCS (Nimura 1993). However, because fibrosis in the submucosal layer is rarely seen with mucosal extension, cholangiograms are of less diagnostic value. Taking these facts into consideration, it is practical that PTCS, aimed at preoperative diagnosis of cancer extent, is indicated in patients with the intraductal growth type of cholangiocarcinoma. Attention should be paid not only to the intrahepatic extension but also to the distal (downstream) extension of the tumor. We have experienced several cases of proximal or intrahepatic cholangiocarcinoma with superficially spreading carcinoma which extended down to near the distal end of the common bile duct (Fig. 54.27).

Neuhaus and Hoffmann (1993) have reported that PTCS improves the preoperative selection of completely resectable carcinomas of the hepatic hilum and that the mapping of the tumor extension into individual hepatic segments allows curative operations to be carried out with the smallest necessary hepatic resection. However, they have emphasized that the value of PTCS for hilar cholangiocarcinoma must be evaluated in future controlled trials.

ARTERIOGRAPHY

Selective celiac and superior mesenteric arteriography are essential preoperative diagnostic methods. The distribution of the hepatic arteries is clearly shown and information on resectability and precise planning of resectional procedure is provided. We recommend arteriography in two projections, that is, anteroposterior and right anterior oblique projections.

Three-dimensional understanding of the main hepatic artery distribution expedites skeletonization resection of the hepatoduodenal ligament, and that of the intrahepatic artery branching is helpful during resection of segmental or subsegmental bile ducts as the final step of hepatobiliary resection (see Ch. 83). Hepatobiliary surgeons must appreciate two variations of the hepatic artery distribution (Fig. 54.28): one is a left hepatic artery running *right* to the umbilical portion of the left portal vein; and the other is a posterior branch of the right hepatic artery running *cranially* to the right portal trunk. Careful attention should be paid to the former variant in extended right hepatic resection with caudate lobectomy and the same applies to the latter variant in extended left hepatectomy with caudate lobectomy. These variations can be seen on arteriograms prior to surgery.

Unilateral involvement of the hepatic artery is compatible with resection (Williamson et al 1980). Bilateral involvement of the hepatic artery is always associated with irre-

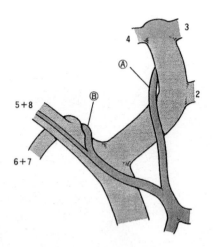

Fig. 54.28 Schematic illustration of two different types of rare variation of the hepatic artery distribution: the left hepatic artery running to the right of the umbilical portion of the left portal vein **(A)**; and the right posterior hepatic artery running cranially to the right portal trunk **(B)**.

sectability, when the tumor is located mainly on the right. We have never carried out right side hepatectomy with resection and reconstruction of the left hepatic artery. When the tumor is located mainly on the left, however, left side hepatectomy with resection and reconstruction of the right hepatic artery is indicated in some selected patients (Fig. 54.29). To date, we have performed this type of resection in 4 patients all of whom underwent left hepatic lobectomy and caudate lobectomy. The resected right hepatic artery was reconstructed with direct end-to-end anastomosis in two patients and with a great saphenous vein graft in the remaining two. Two patients died of cancer recurrence 8 and 10 months after surgery, respectively, and the remaining two are alive at 12 and 14 months. The technique of hepatic artery reconstruction is now well established, but it remains to be proven whether or not combined hepatic artery and liver resection offers a better chance of long-term survival.

Percutaneous transhepatic portography (PTP)

There has been a persistent belief that involvement of the main trunk portal vein denotes irresectability of cholangiocarcinoma (Williamson et al 1980, Blumgart et al 1984). Hoevels & Ihse (1979) have emphasized that portography showing portal vein invasion suggests irresectability. Launois et al (1979) have also reported that the main reason for unresectability of hilar cholangiocarcinoma is invasion of the portal bifurcation. However, as described by the editor (LHB) (vide supra) (Ch. 83), portal vein resection for tumor involvement at the bifurcation has been reported as early as 1984 (Blumgart et al 1984) and several surgeons

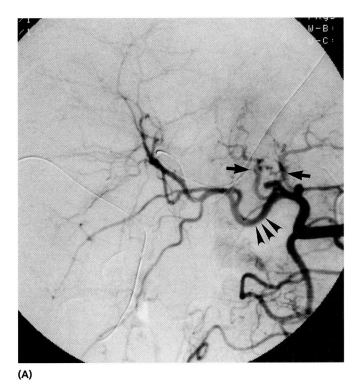

(A)

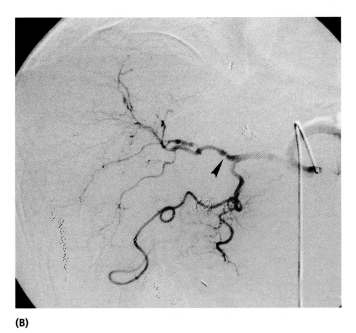

(B)

Fig. 54.29 A patient with cholangiocarcinoma invading bilateral hepatic arteries. The tumor was curatively resected by a left lobectomy and caudate lobectomy with resection and reconstruction of the right hepatic artery. **(A)** An arteriogram delineating narrowed right hepatic artery (arrowheads) and encasement of branches of the middle and left hepatic arteries (arrow). **(B)** Postoperative arteriogram demonstrating good patency of the right hepatic artery which was resected and reconstructed with direct end-to-end anastomosis (arrowhead).

have reported portal vein resection for advanced biliary tract carcinoma (Sakaguchi & Nakamura 1986, Nimura et al 1991b, Miyazaki et al 1998a,b). We have carried out combined portal vein and hepatobiliary resection in 45 patients with advanced cholangiocarcinoma, and have demonstrated significantly better survival in patients who underwent portal vein resection than in those with an unresectable carcinoma (Nimura et al 1991b). The presence of portal vein invasion is now not a contraindication for resection.

For such an aggressive surgical strategy, we consider portography essential to clearly demonstrate the portal distribution and tumor extension along the portal vein. High-quality portograms make it possible to estimate the part and the length of the portal vein to be resected, and in turn, to design the resection and reconstruction procedure. In this context, percutaneous transhepatic portography (PTP) is superior to standard arterial late-phase portography which may not provide sufficient opacification of the portal vein (Williamson et al 1980). The recent advent of digital subtraction angiography (DSA) has reduced the volume of contrast medium required. Using DSA, only 10 ml of contrast medium is enough per portogram, allowing for two or more projections. PTP is safe, easy to perform, and can produce high-quality portograms in several projections. We consider that these advantages outweigh the disadvantage of the invasive nature of the procedure.

For PTP, a 5 F catheter is advanced into the superior mesenteric vein, over the guidewire introduced by ultrasound-guided puncture of the right anterior portal vein. Portograms are taken in antero-posterior and right anterior oblique projections. Right anterior cranial oblique, right anterior caudal oblique, or lateral projections are also obtained as needed (Fig. 54.30). The image intensifier is tilted 30° to the patient's right for the right anterior oblique projection, 30° to the patient's right and 20° cranial for the right anterior cranial oblique projection, and 30° to the patient's right and 20° caudal for the right anterior caudal oblique projection. Portograms taken in several projections are helpful in the three-dimensional display of portal distribution.

Whether or not hilar cholangiocarcinoma invades the portal bifurcation is a matter of surgical importance because involvement of the portal bifurcation is a determinant of the operative indication and of the surgical procedure. Therefore, it is important to focus on the portal bifurcation on portograms. We emphasize, as do others (see Ch. 83) that portographic findings of involved bifurcation do not preclude resection but define the need for combined portal vein and liver resection. In cases of a markedly involved right portal vein, if contralateral involvement does not reach the umbilical portion of the left portal vein, curative resec-

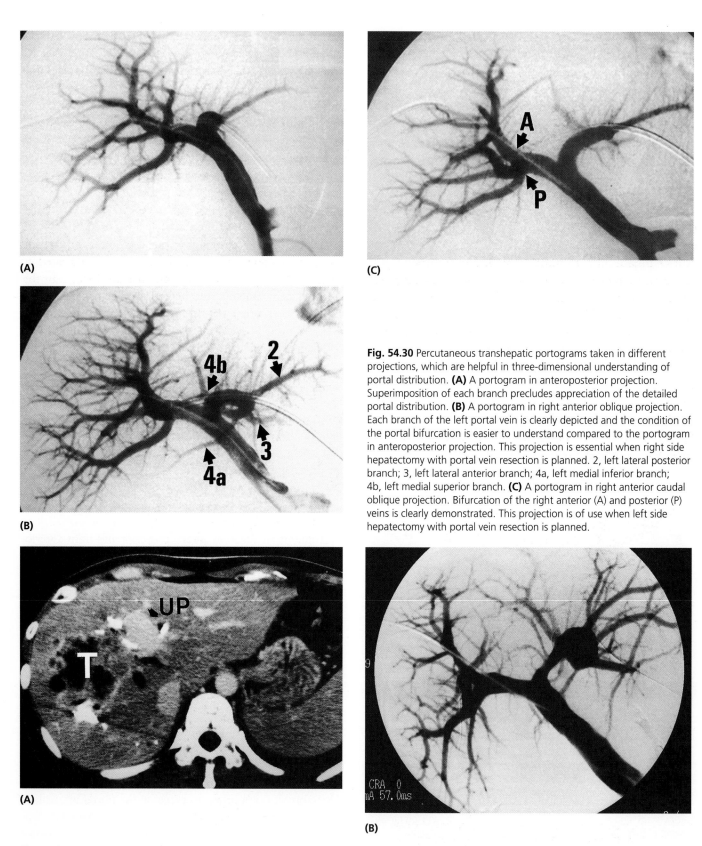

Fig. 54.30 Percutaneous transhepatic portograms taken in different projections, which are helpful in three-dimensional understanding of portal distribution. **(A)** A portogram in anteroposterior projection. Superimposition of each branch precludes appreciation of the detailed portal distribution. **(B)** A portogram in right anterior oblique projection. Each branch of the left portal vein is clearly depicted and the condition of the portal bifurcation is easier to understand compared to the portogram in anteroposterior projection. This projection is essential when right side hepatectomy with portal vein resection is planned. 2, left lateral posterior branch; 3, left lateral anterior branch; 4a, left medial inferior branch; 4b, left medial superior branch. **(C)** A portogram in right anterior caudal oblique projection. Bifurcation of the right anterior (A) and posterior (P) veins is clearly demonstrated. This projection is of use when left side hepatectomy with portal vein resection is planned.

Fig. 54.31 A patient with mass forming type intrahepatic cholangiocarcinoma involving the hepatic hilus. The tumor was curatively resected by right hepatic trisegmentectomy and caudate lobectomy with portal vein resection and reconstruction. **(A)** Computed tomography demonstrating a large mass (T) in the right anterior and the left medial segments. UP—umbilical portion of the left portal vein. **(B)** A percutaneous transhepatic portogram taken in right anterior oblique projection shows that both the left and right portal veins including the bifurcation are involved. The proximal side of the portal vein was cut at the main trunk and the distal side was cut at the transverse portion near the left portal elbow, followed by direct end-to-end anastomosis.

tion is still possible using a right hepatectomy with portal vein resection and reconstruction (Fig. 54.31). On the contrary, when the left portal vein is considerably involved, if *contralateral involvement is limited* within the right portal trunk, a left side hepatectomy with portal vein resection and reconstruction is indicated (Fig. 54.32).

PORTAL VEIN EMBOLIZATION

Portal vein embolization, devised by Makuuchi et al (1990) (Ch. 87) and Kinoshita et al (1986), has become important in the presurgical management of patients who are to undergo extensive liver resection. The purpose of portal vein embolization is to initiate compensatory hypertrophy in the future remnant of the liver and thus minimize postoperative liver dysfunction and to prevent liver failure (Nagino et al 1995b). There are two different types of approach for portal vein embolization: one is the percutaneous approach (percutaneous transhepatic portal vein embolization, PTPE) (Kinoshita et al 1986, Baere et al 1993); and the other is transileocolic approach (transileocolic portal vein embolization, TIPE) (Makuuchi et al 1990). Evidently the former is superior to the latter because TIPE requires laparotomy under general anesthesia, consequently increasing the burden to the patient.

Performance of PTPE via the portal vein branch in the nonembolized lobe has been reported (Kinoshita et al 1986, Baere et al 1993). Usually, the umbilical portion of the left portal vein is punctured and the right lobe is embolized. This *contralateral* approach for PTPE is somewhat dangerous, as the puncture is made in the lobe that is not to be embolized. Such puncture may cause complications such as hemobilia, arterioportal shunt formation, or portal thrombosis and may even lead to irreparable damage, which would make liver resection impossible.

We developed a different approach for PTPE that we have termed the *ipsilateral* approach (Nagino et al 1993a,b, 1996) (Fig. 54.33). In this approach the portal branch designated for embolization is punctured. PTPE is indicated in patients who are to undergo right hepatic lobectomy or extended right or left hepatic resections. *In such procedures,*

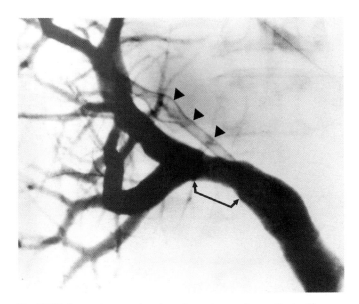

Fig. 54.32 A percutaneous transhepatic portogram in a patient with intrahepatic cholangiocarcinoma involving the hepatic hilus. The left portal vein is occluded and the right portal trunk is markedly involved (arrow). Left hepatic trisegmentectomy with caudate lobectomy was done. The proximal side of the portal vein was cut at the main trunk and the distal side was cut at the right posterior portal branch, followed by direct end-to-end anastomosis. Arrowheads indicate an endoprosthesis in the right anterior segmental bile duct which was placed at a local hospital.

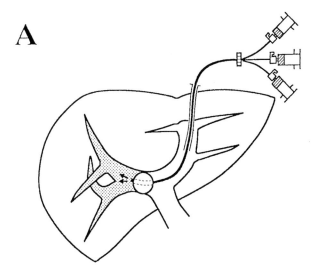

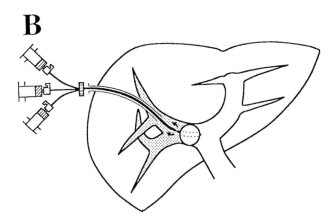

Fig. 54.33 Schematic illustration of two different types of approach for percutaneous transhepatic portal vein embolization. **(A)** *Contralateral* approach in which the portal vein in the nonembolized segment is punctured. **(B)** *Ipsilateral* approach in which the portal vein designated for embolization is punctured.

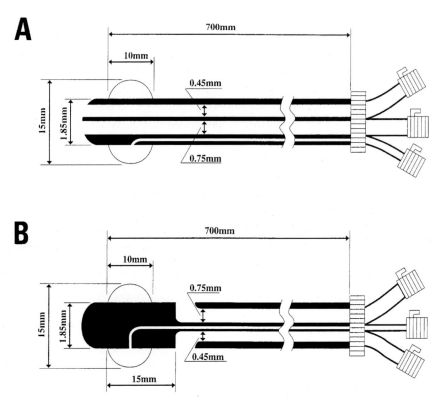

Fig. 54.34 Schematic illustration of two 5.5 F triple lumen balloon catheters. **(A)** Type I (distal end hole) catheter. **(B)** Type II (proximal side hole) catheter.

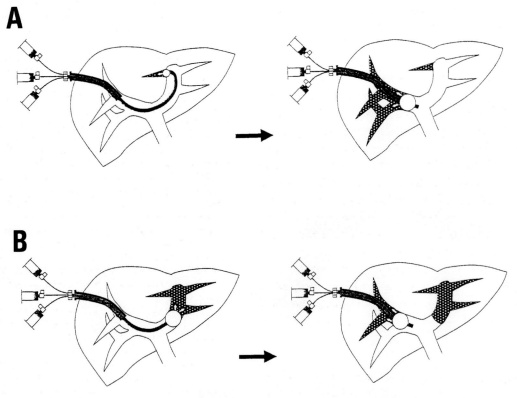

Fig. 54.35 Schematic illustration of trisegment portal vein embolization. **(A)** Right trisegment portal vein embolization. The left medial portal branch is first embolized by using the Type I catheter. Then after the catheter is exchanged, the right portal vein is embolized by using the Type II catheter. **(B)** Left trisegment portal vein embolization. The left portal vein is first embolized by using the Type I catheter. Then the right anterior portal branch is embolized by using the Type II catheter.

the right anterior sector of the liver is always the sector resected. Consequently, the right anterior portal branch is the preferred access site for embolization with the ipsilateral approach. Use of the ipsilateral approach does not result in complications serious enough to deter liver resection, as treatment involves the hepatic lobe to be resected. Further, when the ipsilateral approach is used, the catheter sheath can be removed soon after embolization without any fear of posttreatment bleeding. In addition, the ipsilateral approach with two types of balloon catheters (Fig. 54.34) allows selective embolization of each intrahepatic portal vein branch and makes it possible to conduct right or left trisegmental portal vein embolization through a single portal puncture (Nagino et al 1995a) (Fig. 54.35). It is extremely difficult or impossible to perform trisegmental portal vein embolization with use of a contralateral approach. Thus, the ipsilateral approach is safer and clinically more useful than the conventional contralateral approach.

PTPE can produce a sizable compensatory hypertrophy of the nonembolized segments of the liver (Baere et al 1993, Kawasaki et al 1994, Nagino et al 1995a,b). In right portal vein embolization, the volume of the left lobe increases by 130 cm³ on average within 2 weeks after embolization, and the estimated resection volume decreases by an average of approximately 10% (Nagino et al 1995b). It has been reported that portal vein embolization accelerates hepatic mitochondrial function and induces hepatocyte proliferation in the nonembolized segments, probably in a way similar to partial hepatectomy (Lee et al 1993, Shimizu et al 1995, Takeuchi et al 1996). On the other hand, the atrophy of the embolized segments is proven to be induced by apoptosis of hepatocyte (Harada et al 1997, Tsugane et al 1999). The hypertrophy rate of nonembolized segments after PTPE is predictable from the extent of increase in the portal blood flow velocity. This extent can be estimated easily and noninvasively by Doppler ultrasound, indicating that Doppler study has clinical utility for monitoring patients after PTPE (Goto et al 1998). As to postembolization hepatic function, we have demonstrated that the functional gain in the nonembolized segments is greater than the volume gain in the corresponding segments, at least within 2 weeks after PTPE (Uesaka et al 1996). However, further study is required to elucidate changes in hepatic function after embolization.

CONCLUSION

The diagnosis and treatment of intrahepatic cholangiocarcinoma with or without hilar invasion requires a full under-standing of the three-dimensional anatomy of the liver and the intrahepatic bile duct, in-depth knowledge of liver function, and advanced skill in interventional radiology and hepatobiliary surgery. We recommend that the preoperative management, including PTBD, PTCS, arteriography, PTP and PTPE, is essential to making a precise and accurate preoperative diagnosis and to design a definitive resection procedure.

REFERENCES

Ahrendt S A, Pitt H A, Kalloo A N, Venbrux A C, Klein A S, Herlong H F, Coleman, J, Lillemoe K D, Cameron J L 1998 Primary sclerosing cholangitis: resect, dilate, or transplant? Annals of Surgery 227: 412–423

Akwari O E, Kelly K A 1979 Surgical treatment of adenocarcinoma. Location: junction of the right, left, and common hepatic biliary ducts. Archives of Surgery 114: 22–25

Altemeier W A, Gall E A, Culbertson W R, Inge W W 1966 Sclerosing carcinoma of the intrahepatic (hilar) bile ducts. Surgery 60: 191–200

Andersen J R, Sorensen S M, Kruse A, Rikkjaer M, Matzen P 1989 Randomized trial of endoscopic endoprosthesis versus operative bypass in malignant obstructive jaundice. Gut 30: 1132–1135

Bach A M, Hann L E, Brown K T, Getrajdman G I, Herman S K, Fong Y, Blumgart L H 1996 Portal vein evaluation with US: comparison to angiography combined with CT arterial portography. Radiology 201: 149–154

Baer H U, Matthews J B, Schweizer W P, Gertsch P, Blumgart L H 1990 Management of the Mirizzi syndrome and the surgical implications of cholecystcholedochal fistula (see comments). British Journal of Surgery 77: 743–745

Baer H U, Rhyner M, Stain S C, Glauser P W, Dennison A R, Maddern G J, Blumgart L H 1994 The effect of communication between the right and left liver on the outcome of surgical drainage for jaundice due to malignant obstruction at the hilus of the liver. Hepato-Biliary Surgery 8: 27–31

Baer H U, Stain S C, Dennison A R, Eggers B, Blumgart L H 1993 Improvements in survival by aggressive resections of hilar cholangiocarcinoma. Annals of Surgery 217: 20–27

Baere T, Roche A, Vavasseur D, Therasse E, Indushekar S, Elias D, et al 1993 Portal vein embolization: Utility for inducing left hepatic lobe hypertrophy before surgery. Radiology 188: 73–77

Becker C D, Glattli, A, Maibach R, Baer H U 1993 Percutaneous palliation of malignant obstructive jaundice with the Wallstent endoprosthesis: follow-up and reintervention in patients with hilar and non-hilar obstruction. Journal of Vascular and Interventional Radiology 4: 597–604

Bengmark S, Ekberg H, Evander A, Klofver-Stahl B, Tranberg K G 1988 Major liver resection for hilar cholangiocarcinoma. Annals of Surgery 207: 120–125

Berdah S V, Delpero J R, Garcia S, Hardwigsen J, Le Treut Y P 1996 A western surgical experience of peripheral cholangiocarcinoma. British Journal of Surgery 83: 1517–1521

Bergquist A, Glaumann H, Persson B, Broome U 1998 Risk factors and clinical presentation of hepatobiliary carcinoma in patients with primary sclerosing cholangitis: a case–control study. Hepatology 27: 311–316

Bhuiya M M R, Nimura Y, Kamiya J, Kondo S, Nagino M, Hayakawa N 1993 Carcinoma of the hepatic hilus with superficial spreading to the intrahepatic segmental bile duct. Journal Hepato-Biliary-Pancreatic Surgery 1: 22–26

Bismuth H, Corlette MB 1975 Intrahepatic cholangioenteric anastomosis in carcinoma of the hilus of the liver. Surgery, Gynecology Obstetrics 140: 170–178

Bismuth H, Nakache R, Diamond T 1992 Management strategies in resection for hilar cholangiocarcinoma. Annals of Surgery 215: 31–38

Blumgart L H, Hadjis N S, Benjamin I S, Beazley R 1984 Surgical approaches to cholangiocarcinoma at confluence of hepatic ducts. Lancet i: 66–70

Blumgart L H, Kelley C J 1985 Hepaticojejunostomy in benign and malignant high bile duct stricture. Approaches to the left hepatic ducts. Schweizerische Rundschau fur Medizin Praxis 74: 1238–1244

Bowling T E, Galbraith S M, Hatfield A R, Solano J, Spittle M F 1996 A retrospective comparison of endoscopic stenting alone with stenting and radiotherapy in non-resectable cholangiocarcinoma. Gut 39: 852–855

Broome U, Olsson R, Loof L, Bodemar G, Hultcrantz R, Danielsson A, Prytz H, Sandberg-Gertzen H, Wallerstedt S, Lindberg G 1996 Natural history and prognostic factors in 305 Swedish patients with primary sclerosing cholangitis. Gut 38: 610–615

Burke E C 1998 Hilar cholangiocarcinoma: patterns of spread, the importance of hepatic resection for curative operation, and a presurgical clinical staging system. Annals of Surgery 228: 385–394

Cabooter M, Sas S and Laukens P 1990 Mirizzi syndrome. Nederlands Tijdschrift voor Geneeskunde 134: 708–711

Callery M P, Strasberg S M, Doherty G M, Soper N J, Norton J A 1997 Staging laparoscopy with laparoscopic ultrasonography: optimizing resectability in hepatobiliary and pancreatic malignancy. Journal of the American College of Surgeons 185: 33–39

Cameron J L, Pitt H A, Zinner M J, Kaufman S L, Coleman J 1990 Management of proximal cholangiocarcinomas by surgical resection and radiotherapy. American Journal of Surgery 159: 91–98

Carriaga M T, Henson D E 1995 Liver, gallbladder, extrahepatic bile ducts, and pancreas. Cancer 75: 171–190

Cheung K L, Lai E C 1995 Endoscopic stenting for malignant biliary obstruction. Archives of Surgery 130: 204–207

Chu K M, Lai E C, Al-Hadeedi S, Arcilla C E, Jr, Lo C M, Liu C L, Fan S T, Wong J 1997a Intrahepatic cholangiocarcinoma. World Journal of Surgery 21: 301–306

Chu K M, Lo C M, Liu C L, Fan S T 1997b Malignancy associated with hepatolithiasis. Hepato-Gastroenterology 44: 352–357

Clements W B D, Diamond T, McCrory D C, Rowlands B J 1993 Biliary drainage in obstructive jaundice: Experimental and clinical aspects. British Journal of Surgery 80: 834–842

Cotton P B 1984 Endoscopic methods for relief of malignant obstructive jaundice. World Journal of Surgery 8: 854–861

Cunningham J D, Fong Y, Shriver C, Melendez J, Marx W L, Blumgart L H 1994 One hundred consecutive hepatic resections. Blood loss, transfusion, and operative technique. Archives of Surgery 129: 1050–1056

Denning D A, Ellison E C, Carey L C 1981 Preoperative percutaneous transhepatic biliary decompression lowers operative mortality in patients with obstructive jaundice. American Journal of Surgery 141: 61–65

Enjoji M, Sakai, H, Nakashima M, Nawata H 1998 Integrins: utility as cell type- and stage-specific markers for hepatocellular carcinoma and cholangiocarcinoma (letter). In Vitro Cellular & Developmental Biology Animal 34: 25–27

Farley D R, Weaver A L, Nagorney D M 1995 'Natural history' of unresected cholangiocarcinoma: patient outcome after noncurative intervention. Mayo Clinic Proceedings 70: 425–429

Fong Y, Blumgart L H, Lin E, Fortner J G, Brennan M F 1996 Outcome of treatment for distal bile duct cancer. British Journal of Surgery 83: 1712–1715

Georgopoulos S K, Schwartz L H, Jarnagin W R, Gerdes H, Breite I, Fong Y, Blumgart L H, Kurtz R C 1999 A comparison of magnetic resonance cholangiopancreatography (MRCP) and endoscopic retrograde cholangiopancreatography (ERCP) in malignant pancreaticobiliary obstruction. Archives of Surgery 134: 1002–1007

Gibson R N, Yeung, E, Thompson J N, Carr D H, Hemingway A P, Bradpiece H A, Benjamin I S, Blumgart L H, Allison D J 1986 Bile duct obstruction: radiologic evaluation of level, cause, and tumor resectability. Radiology 160: 43–47

Gholson C F, Burton F R 1991 Obstructive jaundice: Nonsurgical options for surgical jaundice. Postgraduate Medicine 90: 107–110

Glattli, A, Stain S C, Baer H U, Schweizer, W, Triller J and Blumgart L H 1993 Unresectable malignant biliary obstruction: treatment by self-expandable biliary endoprostheses. (Review 16 refs). Hepato-Biliary Surgery 6: 175–184

Goto Y, Nagino M, Nimura Y 1998 Doppler estimation of portal blood flow after percutaneous transhepatic portal vein embolization. Annals of Surgery 228: 209–213

Grune S, Mullhaupt B, Moradpour D, Munch R, Siegenthaler-Zuber G, Siegenthaler W 1991 Primary sclerosing cholangitis. Deutsche Medizinische Wochenschrift 116: 1095–1100

Gundy S R, Strodel W E, Knol J A, Eckhause F E, Thompson N W 1994 Efficacy of preoperative biliary tract decompression in patients with obstructive jaundice. Archives of Surgery 119: 703–708

Guthrie J A, Ward J, Robinson P J 1996 Hilar cholangiocarcinomas: T2-weighted spin-echo and gadolinium-enhanced FLASH MR imaging. Radiology 201: 347–351

Hadjis N S, Blenkharn J I, Alexander, N, Benjamin I S, Blumgart L H 1990 Outcome of radical surgery in hilar cholangiocarcinoma. Surgery 107: 597–604

Hadjis N S, Blumgart L H 1987 Role of liver atrophy, hepatic resection and hepatocyte hyperplasia in the development of portal hypertension in biliary disease. Gut 28: 1022–1028

Hadjis N S, Collier N A, Blumgart L H 1985 Malignant masquerade at the hilum of the liver. British Journal of Surgery 72: 659–661

Hakamada K, Sasaki M, Endoh M, Itoh T, Morita T, Konn M 1997 Late development of bile duct cancer after sphincteroplasty: a ten- to twenty-two-year follow-up study. Surgery 121: 488–492

Hamahata N, Nagino M, Nimura Y 1998 APACHE III, unlike APACHE II, predicts posthepatectomy mortality in patients with biliary tract carcinoma. Critical Care Medicine 26: 1671–1676

Hann L E, Greatrex K V, Bach A M, Fong Y, Blumgart L H 1997 Cholangiocarcinoma at the hepatic hilus: sonographic findings. AJR American Journal of Roentgenology 985–989

Hann L E, Schwartz L H, Panicek D M, Bach A M, Fong Y, Blumgart L H 1998 Tumor involvement in hepatic veins: comparison of MR imaging and US for preoperative assessment. Radiology 206: 651–656

Harada H, Imamura H, Miyagawa S, Kawasaki S 1997 Fate of the human liver after hemihepatic portal vein embolization: Cell kinetics and morphometric study. Hepatology 26: 1162–1179

Harrison L E, Fong, Y, Klimstra D S, Zee S Y, Blumgart L H 1998 Surgical treatment of 32 patients with peripheral intrahepatic cholangiocarcinoma. British Journal of Surgery 85: 1068–1070

Haswell-Elkins M R, Sithithaworn P, Mairiang E, Elkins D B, Wongratanacheewin S, Kaewkes S, Mairiang P 1991 Immune responsiveness and parasite-specific antibody levels in human hepatobiliary disease associated with *Opisthorchis viverrini* infection. Clinical & Experimental Immunology 84: 213–218

Hatfield A R W, Terblanche J, Fataar S, Kernoff L, Tobias R, Girdwood A H, et al 1982 Preoperative external biliary drainage in obstructive jaundice: A prospective controlled trial. Lancet ii: 896–899

Heslin M J, Brooks A D, Hochwald S N, Harrison L E, Blumgart L H, Brennan MF 1998 A preoperative biliary stent is associated with increased complications after pancreatoduodenectomy. Archives of Surgery 133: 149–154

Hewitt P M, Krige J E, Bornman P C, Terblanche J 1995 Choledochal cyst in pregnancy: a therapeutic dilemma. Journal of the American College of Surgeons 181: 237–240

Hochwald S N, Burke E C, Jarnagin W R, Fong Y, Blumgart L H 1999 Preoperative biliary stenting is associated with increased post-operative infectious complications in proximal cholangiocarcinoma. Archives of Surgery 134: 261–266

Hoevels J, Ihse I 1979 Percutaneous transhepatic portography in bile duct carcinoma: Correlation with percutaneous transhepatic cholangiography and angiography. Fortesch Roentgenstr 131: 140–150

Hurlimann J, Gardiol D 1991 Immunohistochemistry in the differential diagnosis of liver carcinomas (see comments). American Journal of Surgical Pathology 15: 280–288

Itoh K, Fujita N, Kubo K, Ogawa H, Satoh Y, Tomita M, Hasegawa T, Irie G 1992 MR imaging of hilar cholangiocarcinoma—comparative study with CT. Nippon Igaku Hoshasen Gakkai Zasshi—Nippon Acta Radiologica 52: 443–451

Iwatsuki S, Todo S, Marsh J W, Madariaga J R, Lee R G, Dvorchik I, Fung J J, Starzl T E 1998 Treatment of hilar cholangiocarcinoma (Klatskin tumors) with hepatic resection or transplantation. Journal of American College of Surgeons 187: 358–364

Iyomasa S, Kato T, Nimura Y, Kamiya J, Kondo S, Nagino M 1994 Successful management of preoperative cholangitis by percutaneous transhepatic biliary drainage: Case report of advanced gallbladder carcinoma with severe cholangitis. Journal of Hepato-Biliary-Pancreatic Surgery 1: 424–428

Iwahashi J, Hayakawa N, Yamamoto H, Maki A, Kawabata Y, Murayama A, et al 1998 Mucosal bile duct carcinoma with superficial spread. Journal of Hepato-Biliary-Pancreatic Surgery 5: 221–225

Jarnagin W R, Burke E C, Powers C, Fong Y, Blumgart L H 1998 Intrahepatice biliary enteric bypass provides effective palliation in selected patients with malignant obstruction at the hepatic duct confluence. American Journal of Surgery 175: 453–460

Jeng K S, Ohta I, Yang F S, Liu T P, Shih S C, Chang W S, Wan H Y, Huang SH 1994 Coexisting sharp ductal angulation with intrahepatic biliary strictures in right hepatolithiasis. Archives of Surgery 129: 1097–1102

Jones B A, Langer B, Taylor B R, Girotti M 1985 Periampullary tumours: which ones should be resected? American Journal of Surgery 149, 46–51

Jones D V, Jr, Lozano R, Hoque A, Markowitz A, Patt Y Z 1996 Phase II study of paclitaxel therapy for unresectable biliary tree carcinomas. Journal of Clinical Oncology 14: 2306–2310

Jutte D L, Bell R H Jr, Penn I, Powers J, Kolinjivadi J 1987 Carcinoid tumor of the biliary system. Case report and literature review. Digestive Diseases & Sciences 32: 763–769

Kamada T, Saitou H, Takamura A, Nojima T, Okushiba S I 1996 The role of radiotherapy in the management of extrahepatic bile duct cancer: an analysis of 145 consecutive patients treated with intraluminal and/or external beam radiotherapy (see comments). International Journal of Radiation Oncology, Biology, Physics 34: 767–774

Kamiya J, Nimura Y, Hayakawa N, Kondo S, Nagino M, Kanai M 1994 Preoperative cholangiography of the caudate lobe: Surgical anatomy and staging for biliary carcinoma. Journal of Hepato-Biliary-Pancreatic Surgery 1: 385–389

Kanai M, Nimura Y, Kamiya J, Kondo S, Nagino M, Miyachi M et al 1996 Preoperative intrahepatic segmental cholangitis in patients with advanced carcinoma involving the hepatic hilus. Surgery 119: 498–504

Kato M, Nimura Y, Kamiya J, Kondo S, Nagino M, Miyachi M, et al 1997 Carcinoma of the common bile duct with superficial spread to the intrahepatic segmental bile ducts: A case report. American Surgeon 63: 943–947

Katoh H, Shinbo T, Otagiri H, Saitoh M, Saitoh T, Ishizawa S, Shimizu T, Satoh A, Tazawa K, Fujimaki M 1988 Character of a human cholangiocarcinoma CHGS, serially transplanted to nude mice. Human Cell 1: 101–105

Kawasaki S, Makuuchi M, Miyagawa S, Kakazu T 1994 Radical operation

after portal embolization for tumor of hilar bile duct. Journal of American College of Surgeons 178: 480–486

Kinoshita H, Sakai K, Hirohashi K, Igawa S, Yamasaki O, Kubo S 1986 Preoperative portal vein embolization for hepatocellular carcinoma. World Journal of Surgery 10: 803–808

Klatskin G 1965 Adenocarcinoma of the hepatic duct at its bifurcation within the porta hepatis. American Journal of Surgery 38: 241–256

Klempnauer J, Ridder G J, von Wasielewski R, Werner M, Weimann A, Pichlmayr R 1997 Resectional surgery of hilar cholangiocarcinoma: a multivariate analysis of prognostic factors. Journal of Clinical Oncology 15: 947–954

Klempnauer J, Ridder G J, Werner M, Weimann A, Pichlmayr R 1997 What constitutes long-term survival after surgery for hilar cholangiocarcinoma. Review, 50 refs. Cancer 79: 26–34

Kubo S, Kinoshita H, Hirohashi K, Hamba H 1995 Hepatolithiasis associated with cholangiocarcinoma. World Journal of Surgery 19: 637–641

Kuo Y C, Wu C S 1990 Spontaneous cutaneous biliary fistula: a rare complication of cholangiocarcinoma. Journal of Clinical Gastroenterology 12: 451–453

Kuvshinoff B W, Armstrong J G, Fong Y, Schupak K, Getradjman G, Heffernan N, Blumgart L H 1995 Palliation of irresectable hilar cholangiocarcinoma with biliary drainage and radiotherapy. British Journal of Surgery 82: 1522–1525

Kuwayti K, Baggenstoss A H, Stauffer M H, Priestly J I 1957 Carcinoma of the major intrahepatic and the extrahepatic bile ducts exclusive of the papilla of Vater. Surgery, Gynecology & Obstetrics 104, 357–366

Lai E C, Tompkins R K, Mann L L, Roslyn J J 1987 Proximal bile duct cancer. Quality of survival. Annals of Surgery 205: 111–118

Launois B, Campion J P, Brissot P, Gosselin M 1979 Carcinoma of the hepatic hilus: Surgical management and the case for resection. Annals of Surgery 190: 151–157

Lee K C, Kinoshita H, Hirohashi K, Kubo S, Iwasa R 1993 Extension of surgical indications for hepatocellular carcinoma by portal vein embolization. World Journal of Surgery 17: 109–115

Lee J C, Lin P W, Lin Y J, Lai, J, Yang H B, Lai M D 1995 Analysis of K-ras gene mutations in periampullary cancers, gallbladder cancers and cholangiocarcinomas from paraffin-embedded tissue sections. Journal of the Formosan Medical Association 94: 719–723

Lee M G, Lee H J, Kim M H, Kang E M, Kim Y H, Lee S G, Kim P N, Ha H K, Auh Y H 1997 Extrahepatic biliary diseases: 3D MR cholangiopancreatography compared with endoscopic retrograde cholangiopancreatography. Radiology 202: 663–669

Levi S, Urbano-Ispizua A, Gill R, Thomas D M, Gilbertson J, Foster C, Marshall C J 1991 Multiple K-ras codon 12 mutations in cholangiocarcinomas demonstrated with a sensitive polymerase chain reaction technique. Cancer Research 51: 3497–3502

Lipsett P A, Pitt H A, Colombani P M, Boitnott J K, Cameron J L 1994 Choledochal cyst disease. A changing pattern of presentation. Annals of Surgery 220: 644–652

Liu C L, Lo C M, Lai E C, Fan S T 1998 Endoscopic retrograde cholangiopancreatography and endoscopic endoprosthesis insertion in patients with Klatskin tumors. Archives of Surgery 133: 293–296

Liver Cancer Study Group of Japan 1997 Classification of primary liver cancer. Tokyo: Kanehara & Co, Ltd

Lupi L, Bighi S, Cervi P M, Marzola A 1990 The CT and US aspects in hepatic cholangiocarcinoma due to thorium dioxide (thorotrast). A case report and review of the literature. Review, 10 refs. Radiologia Medica 79: 399–401

Makuuchi M, Thai B L, Takayasu K, Takayama T, Kosuge T, Gunven P, et al 1990 Preoperative portal embolization to increase safety of major hepatectomy for hilar bile duct carcinoma: A preliminary report. Surgery 107: 521–527

McMasters K M, Tuttle T M, Leach S D, Rich, T, Cleary K R, Evans D B, Curley S A 1997 Neoadjuvant chemoradiation for extrahepatic cholangiocarcinoma. American Journal of Surgery 174: 605–609

McPherson G A, Benjamin I S, Hodgson H J, Bowley N B, Allison D J, Blumgart L H 1984 Pre-operative percutaneous transhepatic biliary drainage: the results of a controlled trial. British Journal of Surgery 71: 371–375

Meade C J, Birke F, Metcalfe S, Watson C, Jamieson N, Neild G 1994 Serum PAF-acetylhydrolase in severe renal or hepatic disease in man: relationship to circulating levels of PAF and effects of nephrectomy or transplantation. Journal of Lipid Mediators & Cell Signalling 9: 205–215

Melendez J A, Arslan V, Fischer M E, Wuest D, Jarnagin W R, Fong Y, Blumgart L H 1998 Perioperative outcomes of major hepatic resections under low central venous pressure anesthesia: blood loss, blood transfusion, and the risk of postoperative renal dysfunction. Journal of the American College of Surgeons 187: 620–625

Mimura H, Takakura N, Kim H, Hamazaki K, Tsuge H, Ochiai Y 1991 Block resection of the hepatoduodenal ligament for carcinoma of the bile duct and gallbladder: Surgical technique and a report of 11 cases. Hepato-Gastroenterology 38: 561–567

Miyagawa S, Makuuchi M, Kawasaki S 1995 Outcome of extended right hepatectomy after biliary drainage in hilar bile duct cancer. Archives of Surgery 130: 759–763

Miyagawa S, Makuuchi M, Kawasaki S, Hayashi K, Harada H, Kitamura H, et al 1996 Outcome of major hepatectomy with pancreatoduodenectomy for advanced biliary malignancies. World Journal of Surgery 20: 77–80

Miyakawa S, Horiguchi A, Hayakawa M, Mizuno K, Ishihara S, Miura K 1996 Arterial reconstruction of the posterior segment after central bisegmentectomy and caudate lobectomy. Hepato-Gastroenterology 43: 225–228

Miyazaki M, Ito H, Nakagawa K, Ambiru S, Shimizu H, Shimizu Y, Kato A, Nakamura S, Omoto H, Nakajima N, Kimura F, Suwa T 1998a Aggressive surgical approaches to hilar cholangiocarcinoma: hepatic or local resection? Surgery 123: 131–136

Miyazaki M, Ito H, Nakagawa K, Ambiru S, Shimizu H, Shimizu Y, Okuno A, Nozawa S, Nukui Y, Yoshitomi H, Nakajima N 1998b Segments I and IV resection as a new approach for hepatic hilar cholangiocarcinoma. American Journal of Surgery 175: 229–231

Mizumoto R, Kawarada Y, Suzuki H 1986 Surgical treatment of hilar carcinoma of the bile duct. Surgery, Gynecology & Obstetrics 162: 153–158

Mizumoto R, Suzuki H 1988 Surgical anatomy of the hepatic hilum with special reference to the caudate lobe. World Journal of Surgery 12: 2–10

Nagano H, Sasaki Y, Imaoka S, Masutani S, Ohashi I, Ishikawa O, Oohigashi H, Yasuda T, Furukawa H, Fukuda I, et al 1990 Intraarterial and intraportal chemotherapy combined with decollateralization for cholangiocellular carcinoma and metastatic liver cancer. Gan to Kagaku Ryoho (Japanese Journal of Cancer & Chemotherapy) 17: 1758–1762

Nagata Y, Hiraoka M, Akuta K, Abe M, Takahashi M, Jo S, Nishimura Y, Masunaga S, Fukuda M, Imura H 1990 Radiofrequency thermotherapy for malignant liver tumors. Cancer 65: 1730–1736

Nagino M, Hayakawa N, Nimura Y, Dohke M, Kitagawa S 1992 Percutaneous transhepatic biliary drainage in patients with malignant biliary obstruction of the hepatic confluence. Hepato-Gastroenterology 39: 296–300

Nagino M, Nimura Y, Hayakawa N, Kamiya J, Kondo S, Sasaki R, et al 1993a Logistic regression and discriminant analyses of hepatic failure after liver resection for carcinoma of the biliary tract. World Journal of Surgery 17: 250–255

Nagino M, Nimura Y, Hayakawa N 1993b Percutaneous transhepatic portal embolization using newly devised catheters: Preliminary report. World Journal of Surgery 17: 520–524

Nagino M, Nimura Y, Kamiya J, Kondo S, Uesaka K, Kin Y, et al 1995a Right or left trisegmental portal vein embolization before hepatic trisegmentectomy for hilar bile duct carcinoma. Surgery 117: 677–681

Nagino M, Nimura Y, Kamiya J, Kondo S, Uesaka K, Kin Y, et al 1995b Changes in hepatic lobe volume in biliary tract cancer patients after right portal vein embolization. Hepatology 21: 434–439

Nagino M, Nimura Y, Kamiya J, Kondo S, Kanai M 1996 Selective percutaneous transhepatic embolization of the portal vein in preparation for extensive liver resection: The ipsilateral approach. Radiology 200: 559–563

Nagorney D M, Donohue J H, Farnell M B, Schleck C D, Ilstrup D M 1993 Outcomes after curative resections of cholangiocarcinoma. Archives of Surgery 128: 871–879

Nakamura S, Nishiyama R, Yokoi Y, Serizawa A, Nishiwaki Y, Konno H, et al 1994 Hepatopancreatoduodenectomy for advanced gallbladder carcinoma. Archives of Surgery 129: 625–629

Nakayama T, Ikeda A, Okuda K 1978 Percutaneous transhepatic bile drainage. Gastroenterology 74: 554–559

Neahaus H, Hoffmann W 1993 Hilares Gallengangkarzinom: Diagnostische und therapeutische strategien. Bildgebung 60 (Suppl 1): 51–56

Nakamura K, Andoh H, Komuro K, Nagayama A, Hirasawa M, Kobayashi T, Gotoh M, Kido Y, Eguchi F, Hara Y, Hashiguchi F, Sakamoto R, Shimada A, Yamanouchi T, Gomi M 1981 Combined use of surgical treatment and postoperative radiotherapy for carcinoma of the extrahepatic bile ducts (author's transl). Nippon Gan Chiryo Gakkai Shi (Journal of Japan Society for Cancer Therapy) 16: 194–203

Nakeeb A, Lipsett P A, Lillemoe K D, Fox-Talbot M K, Coleman J, Cameron JL, Pitt H A 1996a Biliary carcinoembryonic antigen levels are a marker for cholangiocarcinoma. American Journal of Surgery 171: 147–153

Nakeeb A, Pitt H A, Sohn T A, Coleman J, Abrams R A, Piantadosi S, Hruban R H, Lillemoe K D, Yeo C J, Cameron J L 1996b Cholangiocarcinoma. A spectrum of intrahepatic, perihilar, and distal tumors. Annals of Surgery 224: 463–475

Nimura Y, Shionoya S, Hayakawa N, Kamiya J, Kondo S, Yasui A 1988 Value of percutaneous transhepatic cholangioscopy. Surgical Endoscopy 2: 213–217

Nimura Y, Hayakawa N, Kamiya J, Kondo S, Shionoya S 1990 Hepatic segmentectomy with caudate lobe resection for bile duct carcinoma of the hepatic hilus. World Journal of Surgery 14: 535–544

Nimura Y, Hayakawa N, Kamiya J, Maeda S, Kondo S, Yasui A, Shionoya S 1991a Combined portal vein and liver resection for carcinoma of the biliary tract. British Journal of Surgery 78: 727–731

Nimura Y, Hayakawa N, Kamiya J, Maeda S, Kondo S, Yasui A, et al 1991b Hepatopancreatoduodenectomy for advanced carcinoma of the biliary tract. Hepato-Gastroenterology 38: 170–175

Nimura Y 1993 Staging of biliary carcinoma: cholangiography and cholangioscopy. Endoscopy 25: 76–80

Nimura Y, Kamiya J, Kondo S, Nagino M, Kanai M 1995a Technique of inserting multiple biliary drainage and management. Hepato-Gastroenterology 42: 323–331

Nimura Y, Hayakawa N, Kamiya J, Kondo S, Nagino M, Kanai M 1995b Hilar cholangiocarcinoma—Surgical anatomy and curative resection. Journal of Hepato-Biliary-Pancreatic Surgery 2: 239–248

Nimura Y, Kamiya J 1996 Cholangioscopy. Endoscopy 28: 138–146

Nimura Y 1997 Surgical anatomy of the biliary ducts. In: Rossi P, ed. Biliary tract radiology. Springer-Verlag, Berlin, Heidelberg 21–30

Norlander A, Kalin B, Sundblad R 1982 Effect of percutaneous transhepatic drainage upon liver function and postoperative mortality. Surgery, Gynecology and Obstetrics 155: 161–166

Okuda K, Kubo Y, Okazaki N, Arishima T, Hashimoto M 1977 Clinical aspects of intrahepatic bile duct carcinoma including hilar carcinoma: a study of 57 autopsy-proven cases. (Review) Cancer 39: 232–246

Okuda K, Ohto M, Tsuchiya Y 1988 The role of ultrasound, percutaneous transhepatic cholangiography, computed tomographic scanning, and magnetic resonance imaging in the preoperative assessment of bile duct cancer. World Journal of Surgery 12: 18–26

Olthoff K M, Millis J M, Rosove M H, Goldstein L I, Ramming K P, Busuttil R W 1990 Is liver transplantation justified for the treatment of hepatic malignancies? (Review) Archives of Surgery 125: 1261–1268

Ortner M A, Liebetruth J, Schreiber S, Hanft M, Wruck U, Fusco V, Muller J M, Hortnagl H, Lochs H 1998 Photodynamic therapy of nonresectable cholangiocarcinoma (see comments). Gastroenterology 114: 536–542

Parc Y, Frileux P, Balladur P, Delva E, Hannoun L, Parc R 1997 Surgical strategy for the management of hilar bile duct cancer. British Journal of Surgery 84: 1675–1679

Patt Y Z, Jones D V Jr, Hoque A, Lozano R, Markowitz A, Raijman I, Lynch P, Charnsangavej C 1996 Phase II trial of intravenous flourouracil and subcutaneous interferon alfa–2b for biliary tract cancer. Journal of Clinical Oncology 14: 2311–2315

Pichlmayr R, Weimann A, Klempnauer J, Oldhafer K J, Maschek H, Tusch G, Ringe B 1996 Surgical treatment in proximal bile duct cancer. A single-center experience. (Review) Annals of Surgery 224: 628–638

Pichlmayr R, Weimann A, Oldhafer K J, Schlitt H J, Klempnauer J, Bornscheuer A, Chavan A, Schmoll E, Lang H, Tusch G, et al 1995 Role of liver transplantation in the treatment of unresectable liver cancer. World Journal of Surgery 19: 807–813

Pitt H A, Gomes A S, Lois J F, Mann L L, Deutsch L S, Longmire W P Jr 1985 Does preoperative percutaneous biliary drainage reduce operative risk or increase hospital cost? Annals of Surgery 201: 545–552

Pitt H A, Dooley W C, Yeo C J, Cameron J L 1995a Malignancies of the biliary tree. (Review) Current Problems in Surgery 32: 1–90

Pitt H A, Nakeeb A, Abrams R A, Coleman J, Piantadosi S, Yeo C J, Lillemore K D, Cameron J L 1995b Perihilar cholangiocarcinoma. Postoperative radiotherapy does not improve survival. Annals of Surgery 221: 788–798

Polydorou A A, Cairns S R, Dowsett J F, Hatfield A R W, Salmon P R, Cotton P B, et al 1992 Palliation of proximal malignant biliary obstruction by endoscopic endoprosthesis insertion. Gut 32: 685–689

Rabinovitz M, Zajko A B, Hassanein T, Shetty B, Bron K M, Schade R R, Gavaler J S, Block G, Van Thiel D H, Dekker A 1990 Diagnostic value of brush cytology in the diagnosis of bile duct carcinoma: a study in 65 patients with bile duct strictures. Hepatology 12: 747–752

Rodgers C M, Adams J T, Schwartz S I 1981 Carcinoma of the extrahepatic bile ducts. Surgery 90: 596–601

Rosen C B, Nagorney D M, Wiesner R H, Coffey R J Jr, LaRusso N F 1991 Cholangiocarcinoma complicating primary sclerosing cholangitis. Annals of Surgery 213: 21–25

Rossi P, Bezzi M, Rossi M, Adam A, Chetty N, Roddie M E, Iacari V, Cwikiel W, Zollikofer C L, Antonucci F 1994 Metallic stents in malignant biliary obstruction: results of a multicenter European study of 240 patients. J Vasc Interv Radiol 5: 279–285

Rugge M, Sonego F, Militello C, Guido M, Ninfo V 1992 Primary carcinoid tumor of the cystic and common bile ducts. (Review) American Journal of Surgical Pathology 16: 802–807

Ryan M E 1991 Cytologic brushings of ductal lesions during ERCP. Gastrointestinal Endoscopy 37: 139–142

Sakaguchi S, Nakamura S 1986 Surgery of the portal vein in resection of cancer of the hepatic hilus. Surgery 99: 344–349

Sakamoto E, Nimura Y, Hayakawa N, Kamiya J, Kondo S, Nagino M, et al 1995 Case of bile duct carcinoma of the hepatic hilus with segmental obstructive cholangitis. Hepato-Gastroenterology 42: 501–505

Sakamoto E, Nimura Y, Hayakawa N, Kamiya J, Kondo S, Nagino M, et al 1998 The pattern of infiltration at the proximal border of hilar bile duct carcinoma. Annals of Surgery 227: 405–411

Sako K, Seitzinger G L, Garside E 1957 Carcinoma of the extra-hepatic bile ducts: review of the literature and report of six cases. Surgery 41: 416–437

Saldinger P F, Blumgart L H 1999 Resection of hilar cholangiocarcinoma— a European and United States experience. Journal of Hep Bil Pancr Surg (in press)

Sankary H N, Foster P, Frye E, Williams J W 1995 Carcinoid tumors of the extrahepatic bile duct: an unusual cause of bile duct obstruction. Liver Transplantation & Surgery 1: 122–123

Sano T, Nimura Y, Hayakawa N, Kamiya J, Nagino M, Kanai M, et al 1997 Clinical utility of percutaneous transhepatic cholangioscopy in defining tumor extent: A case of mucin-producing bile duct carcinoma originating in the left caudate lobe. Gastrointestinal Endoscopy 46: 455–458

Saunders K, Longmire W Jr, Tompkins R, Chavez M, Cates J, Roslyn J 1991 Diffuse bile duct tumors: guidelines for management. American Surgeon 57: 816–820

Schima W, Prokesch R, Osterreicher C, Thurnher S, Fugger R, Schofl R, Havelec L, Lammer J 1997 Biliary Wallstent endoprosthesis in malignant hilar obstruction: long-term results with regard to the type of obstruction. Clinical Radiology 52: 213–219

Schwartz L H, Coakley F V, Sun Y, Blumgart L H, Fong Y, Panicek D M 1998 Neoplastic pancreaticobiliary duct obstruction: evaluation with breath-hold MR cholangiopancreatography. American Journal of Roentgenology 170: 1491–1495

Severini A, Bellomi M, Cozzi G, Pizzetti P, Spinelli P 1981 Lymphomatous involvement of intrahepatic and extrahepatic biliary ducts. PTC and ERCP findings. Acta Radiologica: Diagnosis 22: 159–163

Shimada H, Niimoto S, Matsuba A, Nakagawara G, Kobayashi M, Tsuchiya S 1988 The infiltration of bile duct carcinoma along the bile duct wall. International Surgery 73: 87–90

Shimizu, Y, Iwatsuki S, Herberman R B, Whiteside T L 1991 Effects of cytokines on in vitro growth of tumor-infiltrating lymphocytes obtained from human primary and metastatic liver tumors. Cancer Immunology, Immunotherapy 32: 280–288

Shimizu Y, Suzuki H, Nimura Y, Onoue S, Nagino M, Tanaka M, et al 1995 Elevated mitochondrial gene expression during rat liver regeneration after portal vein ligation. Hepatology 22: 1222–1229

Speer A G, Russel R C, Hatfield A R W, MacRae K D, Cotton P B, Mason R R, et al 1987 Randomized trial of endoscopic versus percutaneous stent insertion in malignant obstructive jaundice. Lancet ii: 57–62

Stoker J, Lameris J S 1993 Complications of percutaneously inserted biliary Wallstents. Journal of Vascular and Interventional Radiology 4: 767–772

Takada T, Hanyu F, Kobayashi S, Uchida Y 1976 Percutaneous transhepatic cholangial drainage. Journal of Surgical Oncology 8: 83–97

Takeuchi E, Nimura Y, Mizuno S, Nagino M, Kawaguchi M, Izuta S, et al 1996 Ligation of portal vein branch induces DNA polymerases, , and alpha, delta, epsilon in nonligated lobes. Journal of Surgical Research 65: 15–24

Tanaka K, Ikoma A, Hamada N, Nishida S, Kadono J, Taira A 1998 Biliary tract cancer accompanied by anomalous junction of pancreaticobiliary ductal system in adults. American Journal of Surgery 175: 218–220

Tompkins R K, Thomas, D, Wile A, Longmire W P Jr 1981 Prognostic factors in bile duct carcinoma: analysis of 96 cases. Annals of Surgery 194: 447–457

Tsugane K, Koizumi K, Nagino M, Nimura Y, Yoshida S 1999 A possible role of nuclear ceramide and sphingosine in hepatocyte apoptosis in rat liver. Journal of Hepatology 31: 8–17

Tsukada K, Yoshida K, Aono T, Koyama S, Shirai Y, Uchida K, et al 1994 Major hepatectomy and pancreatoduodenectomy for advanced carcinoma of the biliary tract. British Journal of Surgery 81: 108–110

Tsuzuki, T, Ogata Y, Iida S, Nakanishi I, Takenaka Y, Yoshii H 1983

Carcinoma of the bifurcation of the hepatic ducts. Archives of Surgery 118: 1147–1151.

Uesaka K, Nimura Y, Nagino M 1996 Changes in hepatic lobar function after right portal vein embolization: An appraisal by biliary indocyanine green excretion. Annals of Surgery 223: 77–83

Vallis K A, Benjamin I S, Munro A J, Adam A, Foster C S, Williamson R C, Kerr G R, Price P 1996 External beam and intraluminal radiotherapy for locally advanced bile duct cancer: role and tolerability. Radiotherapy & Oncology 41: 61–66

van den Bosch R P, van der Schelling G P, Klinkenbijl J H.G, Mulder P G H, van Blankenstein M, Jeekel J 1994 Guidelines for the application of surgery and endoprostheses in the palliation of obstructive jaundice in advanced cancer of the pancreas. Annals of Surgery 219: 18–24

Vatanasapt V, Tangvoraphonkchai V, Titapant V, Pipitgool V, Viriyapap D, Sriamporn S 1990b A high incidence of liver cancer in Khon Kaen Province, Thailand. Southeast Asian Journal of Tropical Medicine & Public Health 21: 489–494

Vatanasapt V, Uttaravichien T, Mairiang E O, Pairojkul C, Chartbanchachai W, Haswell-Elkins M 1990a Cholangiocarcinoma in north-east Thailand (letter). Lancet 335: 116–117

Verbeek P C, van Leeuwen D J, de Wit L T, Reeders J W, Smits N J, Bosma A, Huibregtse K, van der Heyde M N 1992 Benign fibrosing disease at the hepatic confluence mimicking Klatskin tumors. Surgery 112: 866–871

Vogt D P 1954 Current management of cholangiocarcinoma. (Review) Oncology 2: 37–44

Voyles C R, Blumgart L H 1982 A technique for the construction of high biliary-enteric anastomoses. Surgery, Gynecology & Obstetrics 154: 885–887

Voyles C R, Bowley N J, Allison D J, Benjamin I S, Blumgart L H 1983 Carcinoma of the proximal extrahepatic biliary tree radiologic assessment and therapeutic alternatives. Annals of Surgery 197: 188–194

Wade T P, Prasad C N, Virgo K S, Johnson F E 1997 Experience with distal bile duct cancers in U.S. Veterans Affairs hospitals: 1987–1991. Journal of Surgical Oncology 64: 242–245

Watanapa P 1996 Cholangiocarcinoma in patients with opisthorchiasis. British Journal of Surgery 83: 1062–1064

Way L W 1994 Biliary Tract. In: Way L W (Ed.) Current Surgical Diagnosis and Treatment, 10 edn. Appleton and Lange, Norwalk p 537–566

Weinbren K, Mutum S S 1983 Pathological aspects of cholangiocarcinoma. Journal of Pathology 139: 217–238

Wetter L A, Ring E J, Pellegrini C A, Way L W 1991 Differential diagnosis of sclerosing cholangiocarcinomas of the common hepatic duct (Klatskin tumors). American Journal of Surgery 161: 57–63

Williamson B W, Blumgart L H, McKellar N J 1980 Management of tumors of the liver: Combined use of arteriography and venography in the assessment of resectability especially in hilar tumours. American Journal of Surgery 139: 210–215

Winslet M C, Bramhall S, Neoptolemos J P, Harding L K, Hesslewood S R 1990 Diffuse increase in renal uptake of technetium 99m methylene diphosphonate in association with disseminated cholangiocarcinoma. European Journal of Nuclear Medicine 17: 372–373

Wolber R A, Greene C A, Dupuis B A 1991 Polyclonal carcinoembryonic antigen staining in the cytologic differential diagnosis of primary and metastatic hepatic malignancies. Acta Cytologica 35: 215–220

Yeo C J, Cameron J L, Sohn T A, Lillemoe K D, Pitt H A, Talamini M A, Hruban R H, Ord S E, Sauter P K, Coleman J, Zahurak M L, Grochow L B, Abrams R A 1997 Six hundred fifty consecutive pancreaticoduodenectomies in the 1990s: pathology, complications, and outcomes. Annals of Surgery 226: 248–257

Periampullary and pancreatic cancer

M.F. BRENNAN

55

INTRODUCTION

Peripancreatic carcinoma is a common entity in the United States. Approximately 28 000 cases will be seen in 2000. It should be remembered that islet cell tumors, distal bile duct tumors, ampullary tumors and duodenal tumors, as well as other less common tumors, make up about 30% of all the malignant lesions that involve the head of the pancreas. It is important to be aware that surgical resection is the only therapeutic option that offers a potential cure for all patients with peripancreatic neoplasms, but the life expectancy is variable depending on the underlying histopathology. For pancreatic adenocarcinoma the deaths/cases ratio is approximately 99%. Even for patients resected, long term survival is of the order of 10%.

EPIDEMIOLOGY, RISK FACTORS AND GENETICS

In the United States, the mortality rate is overall approximately 10/100 000 for men and 7/100 000 for women. Although, increased mortality rates are found in Black males which may rise to 15/100 000.

Mortality rates in other parts of the world vary, with mortality rates 5/100 000 in Spain to 10/100 000 in Hungary and Czechoslovakia. This disease is clearly a disease of increasing age with cases under the age of 50 uncommon and the majority developing malignancy after their 65th year (Fig. 55.1). Our own age based incidence at Memorial Sloan Kettering Cancer Center (MSKCC) reflects that of the National Database (Fig. 55.2).

ASSOCIATED FACTORS

There are only limited known risk factors for the development of pancreatic and peripancreatic cancer. It is a disease

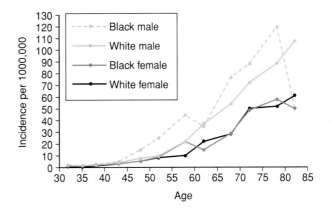

Levin DL. Cancer 31:1231, 1973

Fig. 55.1 Pancreatic adenocarcinoma is clearly a disease of increasing age with cases under the age of 50 uncommon and the majority developing malignancy after their 65th year.

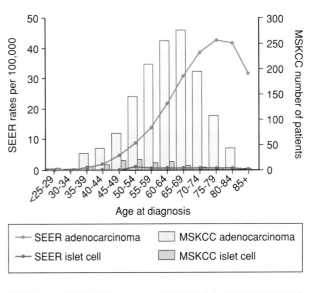

SEER data 1983-1987   MSKCC data 10/15/83-1/15/95

Fig. 55.2 Age of patients referred to MSKCC for consideration of operation, compared to age of patient in the SEER data.

of the older population with an increase in the United States in black males and some limited association with hereditary non-polyposis colon cancer (HNPCC), familial breast cancer, the familial atypical multiple mole melanoma syndrome and hereditary pancreatitis. Peutz-Jeghers syndrome and ataxia-telangiectasia have also been associated. There is evidence demonstrating increased risk of developing pancreatic cancer in patients with diabetes, but the association is of insufficient power to be of much help in screening. Environmental factors are poorly elucidated, although it is clear that there is a linear increase in the risk of pancreatic cancer with increasing pack years of cigarette smoking.

The association with heavy cigarette smoking is sufficiently well established that studies have now been completed that suggest that long-term smoking cessation (greater than 10 years) can reduce the risk by approximately 30% relative to the risk of patients who continue to smoke. Dietary associations have been widely promulgated and are confusing at best. As with other malignancies, high caloric intake, high fat intake and high cholesterol intake have all been implicated. These are supported by laboratory-based studies as showing additive effects in carcinogenesis models. Multitudinous studies have looked at the association of coffee consumption with widely varying results. The association between pancreatitis and the development of pancreatic cancer has been investigated and documented in a number of studies and appears to be a real association. Overall, however, the number of patients with pancreatic cancer in which chronic pancreatitis is an etiological agent remains small, perhaps reaching as high as 5% of all patients with pancreatic cancer. All of the positive and real associations are infrequent, preventing the identification of high risk populations.

GENETICS

Pancreatic genetics have been reviewed and there is clearly a high prevalence of expression of tumor-suppressor genes, including p53 and p16 (Hruban et al 1998).

Chromosomal loss has been reported on chromosomes 18, 13, 12, 17 and 6 with chromosomal gain on chromosomes 12 and 7. The p53 tumor-suppressor gene on 17p and the tumor suppressor gene p16 on 9p are frequently lost in pancreatic cancer. The continuing expansion and identification of tumor oncogenes in pancreatic cancer gives some prospect for therapeutic options in the future. The examination of these genetic abnormalities in familial pancreatic cancer and genetic syndromes associated with cancer continues to be a major area of investigation.

DEFINITIONS

Pancreatic cancer is often considered one disease, when in fact it is a multitude of pathological entities each with differing presentations, behavior and outcome.

The most common malignant pancreatic tumor is a pancreatic ductal adenocarcinoma. However, it is often hard to diagnose whether or not a lesion situated in the pancreas, particularly in the head of the pancreas, is a distal bile duct lesion, an ampullary lesion, a duodenal lesion, or, indeed, an islet cell lesion. On rare occasions metastatic lesions can involve the pancreas.

Based on our recent experience of approximately 3 000 admissions for expected or proven peripancreatic malignancy, it is clear that approximately 65% of patients will have pancreatic adenocarcinoma once the definitive diagnosis has been established (Fig. 55.3). It is important that this be appreciated, as any therapeutically nihilistic approach to pancreatic adenocarcinoma will mean that 30% of patients will be denied the chance of operative resection and cure for more favorable lesions of the duodenum and ampulla or islet cell neoplasms.

Cystic neoplasms, both serous and mucinous cystadenoma and cystadenocarcinoma are more common than previously suspected, and should be aggressively diagnosed so as to be resected where appropriate, for cure. The philosophy when confronted with a lesion involving and apparently arising from the pancreas proper, is to try to determine the pathologic type and anatomical origin of such lesions, with definition and accuracy.

EARLY DETECTION

Early detection of pancreatic adenocarcinoma remains elusive. Unfortunately, all tests require a suspicion for the diagnosis and aggressive invasive investigation: ERCP, biliary cytology, and CA 19-9 antigen analysis used as screening tools are not cost-effective at present (Riker et al 1997). With the identification of small familial aggregates of pancreatic adenocarcinoma, these aggressive efforts at early diagnosis or malignant transformation of benign precursors are being further investigated to establish a high risk population.

PATHOLOGY

Numerous possibilities exist for pathological classification of pancreatic tumors. A standard classification taken from the AFIP Atlas of Pathology based on the WHO classification is shown in Table 55.1 (Solcia et al 1997). It should be noted that some benign lesions such as the intraductal papillary, and

Peripancreatic Cancer
Site

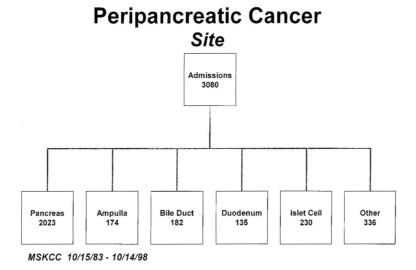

Fig. 55.3 Diagnosis of patients admitted to our Institution from 1983 to 1998 with suspected or proven peripancreatic malignancy.

Table 55.1 Classification of tumors of the pancreas and peripancreatic area

Primary tumors
Benign	Cystadenoma
	Serous
	Mucinous
	Intraductal papillary—mucinous
	Cystic teratoma
	Adenoma
	Ampulla
	Duodenum
Malignant	
	Adenocarcinoma
	Mucinous
	Signet ring cell
	Adenosquamous
	Anaplastic (undifferentiated)
	Mixed ductal—endocrine
	Duodenal adenocarcinoma
	Ampullary carcinoma
	Distal bile duct carcinoma
	Cystadenocarcinoma
	Serous
	Mucinous
	Intraductal papillary
	Giant cell
	Acinar cell
	Pancreatoblastoma

Endocrine tumors
Benign
Malignant

It should be noted that some benign lesions such as the intraductal-papillary, mucinous types can have variable malignant potential and may be difficult to describe as purely benign or frankly malignant.
Modified from: Solcia et al, Tumors of the Pancreas (1997)

mucinous types can have malignant potential that is difficult to quantify by histopathology and may be described as such.

Histopathological confirmation is absolute when reporting outcome data based on treatment strategies, as survival is highly site and histopathology dependent.

TUMOR MARKERS

The role of markers in the diagnosis of pancreatic adenocarcinoma has received increasing emphasis. Tumor markers tend to be remarkably non-specific.

The most commonly valued marker is CA 19-9. In a situation where a reference value exceeds 200 u/ml in the non-jaundiced patient with a consistent CT, then CA 19-9 has strong predictive value, but exceptions exist, i.e. patients with cystadenoma, with very high CA 19-9 and patients with advanced malignancy with low CA 19-9. In our own studies, while CA 19-9 was a discriminant for resectability based on median values, individual values showed wide confidence limits. Although a rising level was a relatively consistent marker of relapse following resection, it does appear that a normalization of CA 19-9 after resection is a predictor of improved outcome (Ritts & Pitt 1998).

Unfortunately, the finding of elevated CA 19-9 levels in jaundiced patients is less specific, presumably because metabolism of the antigen is altered by liver dysfunction.

In a comprehensive study (Safi et al 1996) 2119 patients were examined and a high sensitivity for pancreatic cancer (*n* = 347) was found for CA 19-9. Ca 19-9 levels were significantly lower in those patients who proved to have resectable tumors. In the same study, patients whose CA 19-9 levels returned to normal after resection had improved survival over those that did not. This finding was quite marked with, in Stage I, a difference in survival between 33 and 11.3 months and in Stage II, a difference between 41 and 8.6 months.

A recent comparative study of CA 195 and CEA suggested that CA 195 was more sensitive for detection of pancreatic carcinoma than CEA. However as a diagnostic tool, CA 195 is relatively poor with specificity of 73% (Andicoechea et al 1999).

K-*ras* and p53 mutations occur in approximately 90% and 50% of pancreatic cancers, respectively (Friess et al 1997). Because there is such a high prevalence of K-*ras* mutations, it is at least theoretically possible that these could be identified in blood, stool or bile samples.

Interestingly, widespread genetic analysis is being utilized to search for potentially new tumor markers. A recent manuscript examined 45 000 genes identified in pancreatic adenocarcinoma, of which 183 were found to be expressed at significantly higher levels (Zhou et al 1998). One of these genes was tissue inhibitor of metalloproteinase Type 1 (TIMP-1) and these authors found significant increases of TIMP-1 in pancreatic cancer patients' serum. However, as with other single markers such as CA 19-9 and CEA, TIMP-1 was an inadequate specific marker. A combination of markers was able to detect carcinoma of the pancreas in 60% of patients.

Clinical suspicion

Patients with pancreatic adenocarcinoma commonly present at a time at which the tumor is already far advanced. The majority of patients present with tumors that are inoperable for any chance of complete resection. This is a consequence of the close proximity of the pancreas to important intra-abdominal vascular structures and the ease with which progress can occur in the retroperitoneum prior to any symptoms, and the frequency of early metastasis to peripancreatic nodes and liver.

The symptoms are nonspecific and often associated with vague discomfort, dyspepsia, bloating and disturbance in bowel habit with diarrhea. Jaundice is often a late manifestation. Weight loss, a common accompaniment to the presence of pancreatic adenocarcinoma unfortunately often predicates a far advanced tumor. The presence of pain, particularly back pain, is usually an indication of unresectability because of the site of the tumor, around the body of the pancreas with celiac plexus and vascular invasion. Back pain,

however, is not an absolute contraindication to consideration of operation. For pancreatic adenocarcinoma we found that significant back pain resulted in a 9% resection rate as opposed to minimal back pain with a 31% resectability rate (Kelsen 1994). A very common accompaniment is anorexia, loss of appetite, weakness and lethargy. Vomiting, as opposed to nausea, is relatively uncommon and further indicative of advanced disease. The association of pancreatitis with the development of malignancy should always be suspected. Pancreatitis not associated with the presence of any known causative factor such as alcohol or gallstones should raise the suspicion of an underlying obstructive malignancy. In addition, patients with longstanding chronic pancreatitis have an increased incidence of pancreatic adenocarcinoma. The onset of adult diabetes of mild form always raises the suspicion of underlying pancreatic carcinoma in patients over the age of 60.

The only common physical finding is jaundice. In the presence of a malignancy this is accompanied by a distended gallbladder (Courvoisier's sign). Should a tumor be palpated, then it is almost certainly a cystadenoma or islet cell tumor as adenocarcinoma is rarely palpable prior to demise.

The laboratory findings are limited. Liver function tests indicate the degree of bile obstruction and duration, and other tests confirm the degree of electrolyte imbalance and nutritional impairment. Adult onset diabetes is common, with at best glucose intolerance and usually mild elevation of fasting blood sugar, often responsive to oral hypoglycemics. The need for insulin to control the mild diabetes associated with pancreatic cancer is uncommon.

DIAGNOSIS

The important aspect following clinical suspicion is a high quality helical computed tomographic (CT) scan (Fig. 55.4). This scan, carefully done and interpreted, can give a great deal of information about the underlying diagnosis, the prospects for curative resection, the presence or absence of metastatic disease and the potential for resectability.

Cystic lesions are often benign or of low malignancy (Fig. 55.5). Large lesions are not necessarily lesions of poor prognosis. Often islet cell tumors can gain quite significant size without metastatic disease. Similarly, cystic degeneration in an islet cell tumor does not preclude resection. Cystic change, in fact, is often a favorable observation suggesting a cystic neoplasm or an islet cell carcinoma. In reviewing the CT scan, very careful attention to detail is important. First, are there any metastases? These are often best appreciated first in the liver and then in peripancreatic nodal tissue. Obvious nodal disease from advanced disease can sometimes be discerned as an omental mass. Similarly, the presence of even small quantities of ascites is highly suspicious for peritoneal disease. More subtle presence of nodal metastasis is seen between the aortal-caval window and to the left of the aorta, involving the base of the superior mesenteric artery and extending into the small bowel mesentery. On a normal CT scan, nodal enlargement is not commonly seen in this area and the presence of enlarged lymph nodes here or between aorta and vena cava is a

worrisome factor for the presence of an advanced malignant lesion. The presence of varices clearly presupposes venous obstruction of either portal, splenic or superior mesenteric vein.

The site of the lesion in the pancreas is often a potential predictor both of histopathology and the likelihood of resection. Lesions in the head, which are small and difficult to appreciate, are often ampullary or distal bile duct lesions (Fig. 55.6). Larger lesions with any significant involvement with the head of the pancreas are usually pancreatic adenocarcinomas. Often the site of pancreatic duct obstruction can be clearly identified by tracing the dilated pancreatic duct, or bile duct, or both, to the site of occlusion. If pancreatic duct dilatation is present without bile duct occlusion, then the site of the obstruction is usually in the neck of the gland. In similar fashion, if there is no pancreatic duct obstruction but bile duct obstruction, then a distal bile duct lesion can be suspected. If no mass is seen, then the possibility of a benign stricture or stone disease must be considered.

Duodenal carcinomas commonly present with gastrointestinal bleeding and may be detected because of the extent of duodenal encroachment and the minimal change seen in the head of the pancreas. Lesions with any significant degree of involvement of either the head of the pancreas or the body and tail are usually adenocarcinomas of the pancreas or, less commonly, islet cell tumors. As mentioned previously, islet cell tumors can be quite large and often cystic degeneration is present.

Lesions that involve the entire pancreas are usually cystic neoplasms. On many occasions, with careful attention to

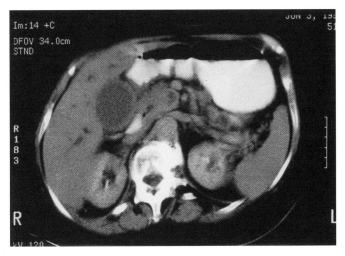

Fig. 55.4 CT scan showing early T2N0M0 pancreatic adenocarcinoma with distended gallbladder.

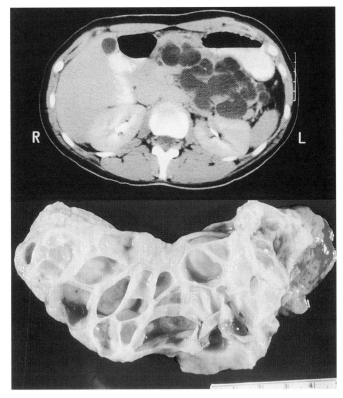

Fig. 55.5 Large cystadenoma of the distal pancreas.

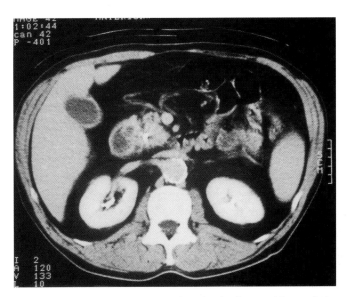

Fig. 55.6 Small ampullary tumor invading the duodenum with stent in place.

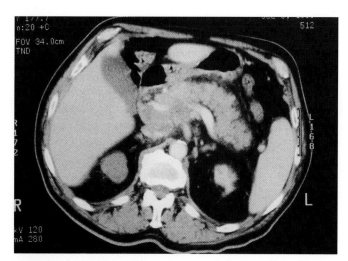

Fig. 55.7 Obvious vascular encasement on CT precludes any consideration of resection.

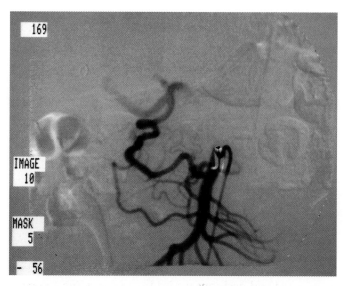

Fig. 55.8 Median accurate ligament syndrome demonstrated by arteriography.

histopathological examination, mucous cystic adenomas will be found to have areas of mucous cystic adenocarcinoma. In patients with apparently localized lesions to the head or body of the pancreas, if the patient has intermittent obstruction, then a periampullary lesion is more likely the cause. Obvious vascular encasement on CT precludes any consideration of resection (Fig. 55.7).

Angiography

It is clear from the information obtained from angiography that it is, in our opinion, rarely indicated for pancreatic neoplasia. On occasions when an islet cell tumor or a large vascular microcystic adenoma is suspected, angiography may be considered. For islet cell tumors, however, the important issue is often that an adequate examination arteriographically of the liver becomes at least as important as the vascular supply to the primary tumor. Islet cell tumors can have multiple diffuse small highly vascular lesions within the liver, not seen even on good contrast enhanced CT. This precludes resection for cure and should be identified prior to consideration of exploration.

It has been argued that arteriography is needed because of the importance of the venous phase in identifying superior mesenteric or portal vein venous encroachment. In our opinion, this is almost always identified by a high quality helical CT scan and so cannot be the justification for arteriography. The need for arteriography to determine aberrant arteries is redundant in the hands of the experienced surgeon. The low risk of median arcuate syndromes (< 1%) (Fig. 55.8) combined with careful examination of the proximal hepatic artery before division of the gastroduodenal

artery is insufficient to justify routine use of angiography (see also Ch. 56).

Magnetic resonance cholangiography (MRCP)

MRCP (Ch. 16) is a relatively new and non-invasive imaging technique utilized to evaluate pancreas and bile ducts. It is proving to be a valuable tool in the evaluation of common bile duct obstruction. Its reported accuracy is 85 to 100% for assessing the site and level of obstruction (Pavone et al 1998).

It is particularly applicable to the patient with pancreatitis with a suspected underlying neoplasm with some ability to differentiate small mass lesions not seen on more conventional studies. There are certainly situations where it can replace ERCP. Some reports have included a false positive diagnosis of ductal narrowing due in part to the way in which the images are processed or in the presence of gas or metal hemoclips. More recently a new instrument, magnetic resonance endoscopy, has been introduced, but it is too soon to be certain of its relative value (Inui et al 1998).

Some information can be gained as to histopathology. For example, endocrine tumors tend to be low-signal intensity on T1 images and high-signal intensity on T2 images and additionally enhance on post-gadolinium images. Conversely, pancreatic ductal carcinomas are generally low-signal intensity on T1 and T2 images and enhance poorly on post-gadolinium images (Kelekis & Semelka 1997).

Endoscopic retrograde cholangiography (ERCP)

ERCP with or without the use of endoscopic stenting, is an area of some significant controversy. When a small ampullary distal bile duct or duodenal lesion is suspected, ERCP can often provide the histopathological diagnosis. Conversely, an ERCP may provide a clear 'cut off' of both distal bile duct and proximal pancreatic duct, highly suggestive of pancreatic adenocarcinoma (Fig. 55.9), the classic 'double duct' sign. If the patient has intermittent jaundice, then ERCP may be clearly diagnostic, as it is often caused by a periampullary polypoid lesion (Ch. 17).

While it can provide the diagnosis when small lesions are suspected, it is not by any means mandatory in large lesions identified on the CT scan in the head of the pancreas. While we may employ ERCP, the important issue is that ERCP be considered and decisions made about proceeding to operation or to endoscopic stenting *before* the procedure is embarked on. We are frustrated when ERCP and a stent are automatically placed in patients who have minimal jaundice and minimal dilatation of the bile duct. If the patients are going to go on to resection, this is rarely of value and can only introduce infection to the biliary tree and complicate the procedure. *ERCP should be employed but with great care and consideration, preferably with prior consultation with the surgeon who will care for the patient.*

In particular, the decision as to whether a stent should be placed should be made prior to ERCP and based particularly on a decision to proceed to relatively urgent operation. In patients with minimal degrees of obstruction and minimal elevation of bilirubin, random application of stents can only complicate management. Based on prospective randomized studies, it would appear clear that preoperative biliary drainage does not improve the operative morbidity or mortality of pancreatic resection. (Povoski et al 1999a,b, McPherson et al 1984). The injudicious use of biliary stents is accompanied by increased postoperative infectious complications (Povoski et al 1999a,b) (see also Ch. 56).

Percutaneous transhepatic cholangiography (PTC)

PTHC for lesions of the head of the pancreas and the distal bile duct is rarely, if ever, indicated. Such studies introduce infection into the biliary tree, and provide little information about anatomical constraints. They should be reserved for delineation of proximal bile duct obstruction or for the establishment of permanent internal biliary drainage for more distal lesions, when no operative intervention is contemplated, and retrograde endoscopy has failed (Chs 17 & 58).

Preoperative biopsy

Preoperative biopsy is only rarely indicated, non-operative biopsy should be reserved for those patients where the potential diagnosis is unclear (e.g. lymphoma) or for patients clearly unresectable, who are to receive radiation, chemotherapy or investigational agents.

STAGING

Clinical and pathological staging of pancreatic cancer

Staging of pancreatic cancer is variable among groups and mainly relies on the American Joint Committee on Cancer (AJCC) and the TNM Committee of the International Union for the Control of Cancer (IUCC) with a combined stage group as described in Table 55.2. While reasonable, this approach to staging is unwieldy, and it is difficult to utilize based solely on preoperative evaluation. As prognosis is heavily influenced by resectability, the staging system is of

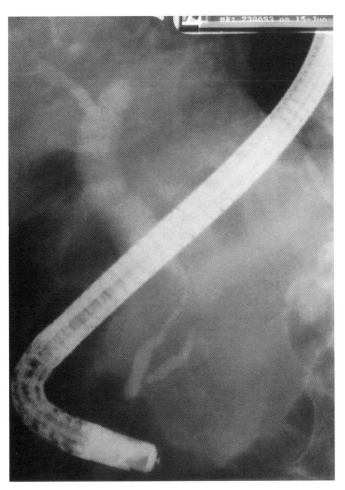

Fig. 55.9 The classical ERCP 'double duct' sign of pancreatic adenocarcinoma.

Table 55.2 AJCC staging of cancer of the pancreas

DEFINITIONS

Primary tumor (T)

TX	Primary tumor cannot be assessed
T0	No evidence of primary tumor
Tis	Carcinoma in situ
T1	Tumor limited to the pancreas 2 cm or less in greatest dimension
T2	Tumor limited to the pancreas more than 2 cm in greatest dimension
T3	Tumor extends directly into any of the following: duodenum, bile duct, peripancreatic tissues
T4	Tumor extends directly into any one of the following: stomach, spleen, colon, adjacent large vessels

Regional lymph nodes (N)

NX	Regional lymph nodes cannot be assessed
N0	No regional lymph node metastasis
N1	Regional lymph node metastasis
pN1a	Metastasis in a single regional lymph node
pN1b	Metastasis in multiple regional lymph nodes

Distant metastasis (M)

MX	Distant metastasis cannot be assessed
M0	No distant metastasis
M1	Distant metastasis

Stage grouping

0	Tis	N0	M0
I	T1	N0	M0
	T2	N0	M0
II	T3	N0	M0
III	T1	N1	M0
	T2	N1	M0
	T3	N1	M0
IVA	T4	Any N	M0
IVB	Any T	Any N	M1

From: Fleming ID et al AJCC Cancer Staging Manual, 5th Edition 1997

limited value. The correlation between clinical and pathological systems is clearly difficult, as the incidence of nodal positivity may not be determined unless a complete resection with node dissection is undertaken, and so patients are classified in a variable manner dependent on whether the staging is clinical or pathological.

Laparoscopy/laparoscopic ultrasound (Ch. 20)

As the majority of patients continue to present with advanced disease, i.e. at most 20% of all patients with pancreatic cancer are resectable, techniques of identifying the unresectable have become increasingly important. As described, CT and MRI can help discriminate these patients, but in many centers they still undergo surgical exploration despite findings suggestive of unresectability. Laparoscopy has the attraction that it can visualize small volume metastatic disease (< 5 mm), diagnose extent of nodal metastasis and identify small, superficial peritoneal disease, most of which cannot be identified by any other study.

Early studies by Cuschieri et al (1978) and Warshaw et al (1986) suggested that unsuspected liver or peritoneal metastases were seen in 40 to 70% of patients and that resectability was improved to 40 to 44% if the laparoscopy was negative. We have felt strongly that this technique can be further developed and a recent analysis (Conlon et al 1996) has suggested that resectability after a negative laparoscopy and laparoscopic ultrasound can be as high as 90%. Even in the absence of laparoscopic ultrasound, resectability rates following a negative laparoscopy should exceed 75%. Clearly, excellent CT scanning has decreased the number of patients needing to come to operation, but in our opinion laparoscopy still improves the resectability rate by the order of 20% with laparoscopic ultrasound adding a further 10%. In a recent analysis at our institution of 221 patients with radiologically resectable peripancreatic tumors, laparoscopic staging found 79 who were unresectable (36%). The predominant reason for this was unsuspected hepatic metastases. Of the 141 patients who were considered to have resectable disease by laparoscopy, resection was performed in 129 or 90% (Conlon et al 1996). We believe this has important implications for patient safety and comfort and is cost effective, as patients who undergo laparotomy will have prolonged hospital stay compared to a laparoscopic procedure which may be performed as an outpatient or with a single day of hospitalization.

OPTIONS FOR TREATMENT

Surgical resection remains the only effective treatment for pancreatic adenocarcinoma and certainly should be considered as a potentially curative procedure in patients with duodenal, islet cell and ampullary tumors.

Unfortunately, the majority of patients are not resectable for potential cure. In a recent experience (Fig. 55.3) with 3000 patients admitted with peripancreatic malignancy, the majority had pancreatic adenocarcinoma. However, whereas two-thirds of all of the patients presenting had pancreatic adenocarcinoma, these patients made up only 48% of those patients undergoing resection (Fig. 55.10). Primary operation for pancreatic adenocarcinoma is pancreatic resection, either pancreaticoduodenectomy, distal pancreatectomy or rarely total pancreatectomy (see Ch. 56).

As the majority of patients with peripancreatic cancer will not be resectable, palliative procedures are important. The majority of patients can be palliated without a major open operation, and laparoscopic palliative biliary and gastric bypass can now be performed.

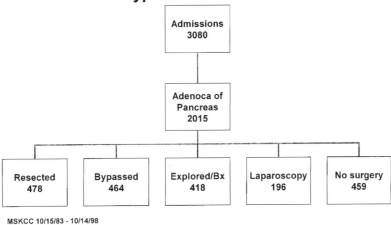

Fig. 55.10 Two-thirds of all of the patients presenting had pancreatic adenocarcinoma, but these patients made up only 40% of those patients undergoing resection.

Palliative procedures

Endoscopic or percutaneous transhepatic stenting can be performed in the patients that are clearly unresectable with internalization of the stent and good palliation from jaundice for limited life expectancy. The issue of prophylactic gastrojejunostomy remains a matter of some debate with some authors suggesting that as many as 10% of patients who do not undergo prophylactic bypass eventually require such a bypass. This has certainly not been our experience: in 150 patients following laparoscopically confirmed metastatic disease, only three (2%) have required bypass prior to demise (Espat et al 1999).

When open surgical biliary decompression is required, the author prefers cholecystojejunostomy unless the cystic duct is potentially involved by tumor. We have not been able to show that choledochojejunal anastomosis improves survival or improves the rate at which the bilirubin declines (de Rooij et al 1991).

Operations

The techniques for pancreaticoduodenectomy and total pancreatectomy are described in Chapter 56.

Frozen section biopsy of pancreas

In the absence of a preoperative diagnosis, some surgeons advocate intraoperative biopsy. We think this should not be a routine event, as the decision for resection should be based predominantly on the clinical findings, both preoperatively and intraoperatively. If there is high suspicion for malignancy, then resection can proceed without histological confirmation. Open biopsy of the pancreas either by Trucut needle through the duodenum or by direct biopsy is often difficult, often imprecise and we do not believe routinely justified. It is important to emphasize that preoperative discussion of this issue can often prevent postoperative confusion, among the patient, the family and some of the medical consultants.

THE RESULTS OF PANCREATICODUODENECTOMY FOR PANCREATIC CANCER

Our recent experience with operations for peripancreatic cancer is outlined in Table 55.3. For patients with adenocarcinoma of the pancreas who undergo resection, serious problems still remain. At least 60% of patients are node positive and approximately 22% of patients will prove to have a positive margin, usually the posterior pancreatic margin but still occasionally the transected pancreas. Operative mortality is markedly diminished and, in fact, in some centers 100 consecutive operations have been performed without a mortality (Trede et al 1990) (Cameron et al 1991) (see Chapter 56).

RESULTS

Overall survival for the management of pancreatic adenocarcinoma remains poor. Patients who undergo operation

Table 55.3 Perioperative mortality and morbidity for peripancreatic cancer at Memorial Sloan-Kettering Cancer Center 10/15/83–10/14/98

Site	n	Resections n (%)	30 Day mortality n (%)	Length of stay Median
Ampulla	174	139 (80)	7 (5)	17
Bile duct	182	85 (47)	3 (4)	16
Duodenum	135	75 (56)	3 (4)	14
Adenoca pancreas	2023	478 (24)	17 (4)	16
Islet cell	230	108 (47)	3 (3)	11
Other	336	191 (57)	7 (4)	16
All	3080	999 (34)		

have at least some realistic benefit for long-term survival. The recent results of 1000 pancreatic resections at our institution are outlined in Fig. 55.11 based on histopathology.

The consequence of nodal positivity in adenocarcinoma certainly results in a worse survival, but as the survival is relatively poor for pancreatic adenocarcinoma, the issue of peripancreatic node positivity should not limit attempts at palliation (Fig. 55.12). Margins, as mentioned above, are a poor prognostic factor (Fig. 55.13) but again, relative to the overall survival make only a small difference.

It has long been debated that patients with pancreatic adenocarcinoma of the body and tail fare worse than patients with lesions of the head. While it is clear that patients with body and tail lesions are less likely to be resected, when resected the long term survival is similar (Fig. 55.14).

Actual survival, as opposed to actuarial survival, provides greater insight into the disease. It is clear that even survival for patients at four years may approximate 15%. This number continues to decline subsequently and the majority of patients alive at five years go on to die of the disease at some period in the next five years (Table 55.4).

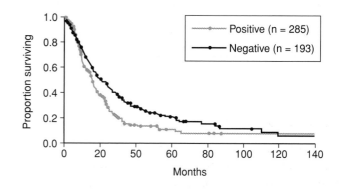

MSKCC 10/15/83 – 10/14/98   n = 478   p = 0.002

Fig. 55.12 Nodal positivity results in a worse survival.

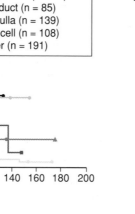

MSKCC 10/15/83 – 10/14/98   n = 1078   p < 0.01

Fig. 55.11 The recent results of 1000 pancreatic resections are outlined based on histopathology.

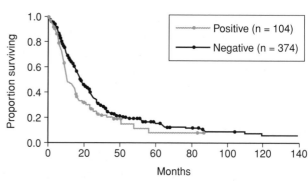

MSKCC 10/15/83 – 10/14/98   n = 478   p = 0.02

Fig. 55.13 Margins are a poor prognostic factor.

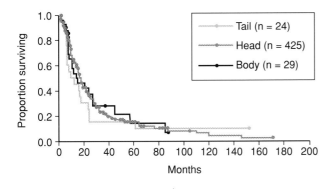

MSKCC 10/15/83 – 10/14/98 n = 478   *p* = ns

Fig. 55.14 Patients with body and tail lesions are less likely to be resected, but when resected the long term survival is the same.

Table 55.4 Actual survival after resection for peripancreatic adenocarcinoma at Memorial Sloan-Kettering Cancer Center 10/15/83–10/14/93

Site	n	Alive ≥ 4 years	Alive ≥ 5 years	DOD > 5 years
Pancreas	235	34 (14%)	25 (11%)	11
Bile duct	43	12 (28%)	7 (16%)	1
Duodenum	31	18 (58%)	15 (48%)	2
Ampulla	79	38 (48%)	25 (32%)	6
Islet cell	52	28 (54%)	20 (38%)	4

SPECIAL SITES AND HISTOPATHOLOGY

As mentioned above, the common peripancreatic malignancy is ductal adenocarcinoma. It makes up approximately two-thirds of all peripancreatic malignancies. However, within the classical pancreatic carcinoma there are a number of pathological variants with different behavior.

Adenosquamous

This rare variant of ductal adenocarcinoma shows both squamous and glandular differentiation. However, the behavior is similar to conventional adenocarcinoma of the pancreas. Some authors suggest a poorer prognosis than classical ductal adenocarcinoma.

Acinar carcinoma

This is a rare tumor with a different histological appearance. The tumor is most common in white males, usually large (mean 10 cm). The tumor has been associated with the development of subcutaneous fat necrosis and an erythematous rash, eosinophilia and polyarthralgia (Klimstra et al 1992) in 16% of patients. It has been hypothesized that this is a consequence of lipase release by the tumor, as immunohistochemical stains for lipase (77%) trypsin (100%) and amylase and chymotrypsin are commonly positive. Acinar carcinomas may present as large lesions with central necrosis on the CT scan. This diagnosis should be made and it appears that their long-term survival is somewhat better than that seen with ductal adenocarcinoma, although many present with metastasis, three year survival is 30%. In some patients there may be an endocrine component identified.

Giant cell carcinoma

Giant cell carcinomas are another rare variant seen in the pancreas. They have a characteristic appearance with, on occasion, osteoclast-like giant cells. Those with osteoclast-like cells are often well circumscribed and have a more favorable prognosis than ductal adenocarcinoma making the diagnosis imperative.

Pancreatoblastoma

This uncommon neoplasm occurs predominately in children. It is a rare variant, even in children. They are often large and can range widely from locally well encapsulated to invasive. They have a variable prognosis but are thought to be more favorable than conventional ductal adenocarcinoma.

Cystic neoplasms

Cystic change can occur in pancreatic neoplasia because of the large size of the tumor (e.g. an endocrine tumor or an acinar cell tumor) or can occur as a primary cystic neoplasm.

Primary cystic neoplasms may be difficult to differentiate from pseudocysts. However, this is an important distinction as the management is different and the prognosis for cystic neoplasms is in the main much more favorable than ductal adenocarcinoma. Several types exist:

Mucinous cystic neoplasms

These are usually large tumors often with variable malignant potential from a purely benign lesion through to invasive adenocarcinoma (mucinous cyst adenocarcinoma). The difficult lesions are those with malignant potential but not clearly invasive malignancy. Again, for all varieties of mucinous cystic neoplasms including mucinous cyst adenocarcinoma, the prognosis is much better than that seen in ductal adenocarcinoma.

Serous cystic neoplasms

These are sometimes termed 'micro cystic adenomas or glycogen-rich cyst adenomas' and are more common in women than men. Again, they can be quite large at the time of presentation, showing large amounts of contained serous fluid, the majority being entirely benign. Only rarely has serous cyst adenocarcinoma been reported and, clearly following resection, their results are far superior to that of infiltrating ductal adenocarcinoma.

Intraductal papillary mucinous neoplasms (IPMN)

This tumor with multiple names including mucinous duct ectasia, mucinous cyst adenoma, intraductal papillary neoplasm, are commonly identified by the observation of extensive mucin coming from the ampulla at the time of ERCP. An important distinction is that invasive adenocarcinoma and severe dysplasia are often identified if diligent and extensive sectioning is performed. Metastatic disease can occur but the overall prognosis is clearly superior to that of ductal adenocarcinoma.

Solid and cystic papillary neoplasms

Solid and cystic papillary neoplasms predominately occur in women in the third to fourth decade and are often large. They have associated necrosis with both solid, cystic and papillary components. They can form metastases but the prognosis again is far superior to that of infiltrating ductal adenocarcinomas.

Other rare tumors do occur in the pancreas including metastatic disease, neuro-endocrine tumors, sarcomas, and lymphoid neoplasms.

Endocrine tumors of the pancreas

This large category of tumors is not covered in detail in this volume. However, the prognosis following resection is better than adenocarcinoma (Table 55.4). Large tumors particularly if cystic at CT study and often in the absence of jaundice should lead to suspicion of an endocrine tumor.

Duodenal adenocarcinoma

Duodenal adenocarcinoma obstructing the ampulla is commonly mistaken for a pancreatic neoplasm. These, however, should be viewed as gastrointestinal tumors with behavior very similar to that of gastric carcinoma. A more extensive node dissection for staging may, therefore, be justified (Brennan et al 1997) (Rose et al 1996). Survival is shown in Fig. 55.11.

Ampullary adenocarcinoma

Ampullary carcinoma was first resected by Halsted in 1898 (Halsted 1899). Carcinoma of the ampulla is an uncommon neoplasm, accounting for approximately 6% of all peri-ampullary tumors with an incidence of approximately 5.7 cases per million population per year. Survival for resected periampullary tumor is more favorable than that for pancreatic adenocarcinoma or distal bile duct tumors, with median survival in varying series from 30–50 months (Fig. 55.11). Five year survival is approximately 40%. Recent analysis of our own experience with 123 patients presenting with carcinoma of the ampulla of Vater has been published (Howe et al 1998). The mean size of the resected ampullary carcinoma was 2.7 cm and the rate of positive nodes in patients with resected ampullary tumors was 45%. Median survival for resected patients was 58.8 months versus 9.7 months for patients who were not able to undergo resection. The major prognostic factor for outcome was the presence of positive metastatic lymph nodes. Multiple previous series have shown similar degrees of positive nodal disease and survival (Howe et al 1998).

Other unusual peripancreatic neoplasms

Pancreaticoduodenectomy for isolated metastatic or locally advanced non-periampullary tumors is, on occasion, performed. A recent analysis (Harrison et al 1997) examined 18 patients with unusual primary tumor pathology, including seven metastatic colon lesions, four gastric lesions, three renal cell, two lung cancers, a bladder cancer and metastatic melanoma. The perioperative death rate for these patients was 5.5%, seven patients having positive lymph nodes. However, median survival was 40 months, suggesting that in highly selected metastatic lesions with absence of disease elsewhere, pancreaticoduodenectomy can provide significant prolongation of survival.

CHEMOTHERAPY AND RADIATION THERAPY

Combination adjuvant therapy has been used for pancreatic cancer. The primary premise on which this was based was that the GITS Study Trial showed a benefit to the use of radiation plus 5-FU (Gastrointestinal Tumor Study Group, 1987). Unfortunately, this trial has been criticized because of the small numbers, the rather minimal prolongation of survival and comparable results in other centers with surgery alone. Attempts to reproduce this study have been performed in a number of centers.

The European study group for pancreatic cancer has developed a prospective randomized trial (Neoptolemos et al 1997) which examines whether or not postoperative treatment with 40 Gy with 5-FU or 5-FU plus folinic acid or a combination of these treatments versus a control arm of no treatment is of value. The trial commenced in 1994 and as of 1997 348 patients have been accrued into this 3-treatment arm study and we await the results with great interest.

A recent non-randomized study (Spitz et al 1997) examined the effects of preoperative versus postoperative 5-FU-based chemotherapy and radiation in the management of such patients. 142 patients with localized adenocarcinoma of the pancreatic head, who were thought to be resectable, were treated with curative intent involving either preoperative or postoperative chemoradiation. This was not a randomized trial. The preoperative approaches involved either a standard external-beam radiation to a dose of 50.4 Gy (1.8 Gy/d, 5 d/wk) or 30 Gy (3 Gy/d, 5 d/wk) combined with continuous infusion 5-FU (300 mg/m²/d, 5 d/wk). Postoperative chemoradiation combined 50.4 Gy of external-beam with continuous infusion 5-FU. 25% of patients, (6 of 25) did not receive postoperative chemoradiation because of delayed recovery after pancreaticoduodenectomy. No significant difference in survival was found and the authors have argued for preoperative therapy on the basis that it allows completion of the treatment, which is often not able to be completed after the pancreaticoduodenectomy. Unfortunately the patients who undergo preoperative treatment do not necessarily all come to operation so the fact there is no survival benefit limits the value of the approach.

RADIOTHERAPY FOR PALLIATION

Radiation therapy has been used for palliation for pancreatic adenocarcinoma that is not resectable and can result in prolongation of survival. This unfortunately is measured in months but in some studies median survivals as high as 12 months have been obtained (Prott et al 1997).

Our experience with intraoperative brachytherapy for the disease is outlined in Fig. 55.15 with a 4-month prolongation of survival by this technique. Unfortunately, this technique is not a major improvement over external-beam therapy and so has limited application.

CHEMOTHERAPY FOR ADVANCED PANCREATIC ADENOCARCINOMA

Pancreatic adenocarcinomas remain one of the most resistant and refractory malignancies to common chemotherapy. As a consequence, multiple studies have looked at new agents for example, farnesyl transference inhibitors, matrix

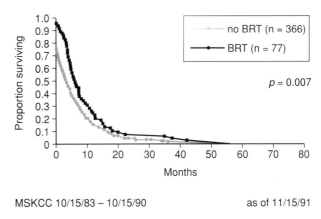

MSKCC 10/15/83 – 10/15/90   as of 11/15/91

Fig. 55.15 Our experience with intraoperative brachytherapy.

metalloproteins inhibitors (MMPI) and antibodies to various oncogenes such as Her-2 (Butera et al 1998).

The chemotherapy for advanced pancreatic cancer has recently been reviewed (Kollmannsberger et al 1998). A randomized trial of 5FU plus gemcitabine has been shown to provide clinical benefit for patients with decreased pain and some have improved performance status but limited improvement in survival. It is important to realize that because of the difficulty in evaluating outcome for advanced pancreatic cancer, the concept of clinical benefit to the patient has been utilized to assess any changes in the patient's symptoms, performance and status, rather than strictly focusing on survival. This has resulted in rather significant claims for gemcitabine in comparison to 5FU. Nevertheless, the duration of these changes is extremely short. The survival benefit in patients receiving gemcitabine is modest at best (6 weeks). The attractiveness of gemcitabine is relative lack of serious side effects in patients already suffering a devastating and debilitating disease.

MMPIs have completed phase I and II clinical trials and a national trial looking at these agents as adjuvants following resection is currently underway. Other agents such as tamoxifen have been utilized in the adjuvant settings. Agents such as octreotide and interferon have been applied in limited studies suggesting some minimal benefit in patient palliation but no major impact on survival for advanced disease. There are other potential agents such as capecitabine and the Onyx-015 adenovirus which replicate in and kill p-53 abnormal cells (Von Hoff et al 1998). There is a serious lack of well designed chemotherapy trials evaluated against best supportive care, such that all patients with advanced pancreatic cancer should be considered potential trial candidates.

REFERENCES

Andicoechea A, Vizoso F, Alexandre E et al 1999 Comparative study of carbohydrate antigen 195 and carcinoembryonic antigen for the diagnosis of pancreatic carcinoma. World Journal of Surgery 23: 227–232

Brennan M F:1991 Duodenal cancer. Asian Journal of Surgery 13: 204–209

Butera J, Malachovsky M, Rathore R, Safran H 1998 Novel approaches in development for the treatment of pancreatic cancer. Frontiers in Bioscience 3: E226–229

Cameron J L, Crist D W, Sitzman J V, Hruban R H, Boitnott J K, Seidler A J 1991 Factors influencing survival after pancreaticoduodenectomy for pancreatic resection. American Journal of Surgery 161: 120–125

Conlon K C, Dougherty E, Klimstra D S, Coit D G, Turnbull A D M, Brennan M F 1996 The value of minimal access surgery in the staging of patients with potentially resectable peripancreatic malignancy. Annals of Surgery 223: 134–140

Cuschieri A, Hall A W, Clark J 1978 Value of laparoscopy in the diagnosis and management of pancreatic carcinoma. Gut 19: 672–677

de Rooij P D, Rogatko A, Brennan M F 1991 Evaluation of palliative surgical procedures in unresectable pancreatic cancer. British Journal of Surgery 78: 1053–1058

Espat N J, Brennan M F, Conlon K C 1999 Patients with laparoscopically staged unresectable pancreatic adenocarcinoma do not require subsequent surgical biliary or gastric bypass. Journal of the American College of Surgeons 188: 649–657

Friess H, Kleeff J, Gumbs A, Buchler M W 1997 Molecular versus conventional markers in pancreatic cancer. Digestion 58: 557–563

Gastrointestinal Tumor Study Group 1987 Further evidence of effective adjuvant combined radiation and chemotherapy following curative resection of pancreatic cancer. Cancer 59: 2006–2010

Halsted W S 1899 Contributions to the surgery of the bile duct passages, especially of the common bile duct. Boston Medical and Surgical Journal 141: 645–654

Harrison L E, Merchant N, Cohen A M, Brennan M F 1997 Pancreaticoduodenectomy for non-periampullary primary tumors. American Journal of Surgery 174: 393–395

Howe J R, Klimstra D S, Moccia R D, Conlon K C, Brennan M F 1998 Factors predictive of survival in ampullary carcinoma. Annals of Surgery 228: 87–94

Hruban R H, Petersen G M, Ha P K, Kern S E 1998 Genetics of pancreatic cancer. From genes to families. Surgical Oncology Clinics of North America 7: 1–23

Inui K, Nakazawa S, Yoshino J, Ukai H 1998 Endoscopic MRI. Pancreas 16: 413–417

Kelekis N L, Semelka R C 1997 MRI of pancreatic tumors. European Radiology 7, 875–886

Kelsen D 1994 The use of chemotherapy in the treatment of advanced gastric and pancreas cancer. Seminars in Oncology 21: 58–66

Klimstra D S, Heffess C S, Oertel J E, Rosai J 1992 Acinar cell carcinoma of the pancreas. A clinicopathologic study of 28 cases. American Journal of Surgical Pathology 16: 815–837

Kollmannsberger C, Peters H D, Fink U 1998 Chemotherapy in advanced pancreatic adenocarcinoma. Cancer Treatment Review 24: 133–156

McPherson G A D, Benjamin I S, Hodgson H J F, Bowley N B, Allison D J, Blumgart L H 1984 Pre-operative percutaneous transhepatic drainage: the results of a controlled trial. British Journal of Surgery 71: 371–375

Neoptolemos J P, Kerr D J, Beger H et al 1997 ESPAC-1 trial progress report: the European randomized adjuvant study comparing radiochemotherapy, 6 months chemotherapy and combination therapy versus observation in pancreatic cancer. Digestion 58: 570–577

Pavone P, Laghi A, Panebianco V, Catalano C, Lobina L, Passariello R 1998 MR cholangiography: techniques and clinical applications. European Radiology 8: 901–910

Povoski S P, Karpeh M S Jr, Conlon K C, Blumgart L H, Brennan M F 1999 Effect of preoperative biliary drainage on postoperative outcome following pancreaticoduodenectomy. Annals of Surgery 230: 131–142

Povoski S P, Karpeh M S Jr, Conlon K C, Blumgart L H, Brennan M F 1999 Preoperative biliary drainage: Impact on intraoperative bile cultures and infectious morbidity and mortality after pancreaticoduodenectomy. Journal of Gastrointestinal Surgery 3: 496–505.

Prott F J, Schonekaes K, Preusser P et al 1997 Combined modality treatment with accelerated radiotherapy and chemotherapy in patients with locally advanced inoperable carcinoma of the pancreas: results of a feasibility study. British Journal of Cancer 75: 597–601

Riker A, Libutti S K, Bartlett D L 1997 Advances in the early detection, diagnosis, and staging of pancreatic cancer. Surgical Oncology 6: 157–169

Ritts R E, Pitt H A 1998 Ca 19–9 in pancreatic cancer. Surgical Oncology Clinics of North America 7: 93–101

Rose D M, Hochwald S N, Klimstra D S, Brennan M F 1996 Primary duodenal adenocarcinoma: A ten-year experience with 79 patients. Journal of the American College of Surgeons 183: 89–96

Safi F, Schlosser W, Falkenreck S, Beger H G 1996 CA 19-9 serum course and prognosis of pancreatic cancer. International Journal of Pancreatology 20: 155–161

Solcia E, Capella C, Kloppel G 1997 Tumors of the pancreas. In Rosai J, Sobin LH (eds) Atlas of Tumor Pathology. Armed Forces Institute of Pathology, Washington DC, p 25–28

Spitz F R, Abbruzzese J L, Lee J E et al 1997 Preoperative and postoperative chemoradiation strategies in patients treated with pancreaticoduodenectomy for adenocarcinoma of the pancreas. Journal of Clinical Oncology 15: 928–937

Trede M, Schwall G, Saeger H D 1990 Survival after pancreatoduodenectomy: 118 consecutive resections without an operative mortality. Annals of Surgery 211: 447–458

Von Hoff D D, Goodwin A L, Garcia L 1998 Advances in the treatment of patients with pancreatic cancer: improvement in symptoms and survival time. The San Antonio Drug Development Team. British Journal of Cancer 78, suppl 3: 9–13

Warshaw A L, Topper J E, Shipley W U 1986 Laparoscopy in the staging and planning of therapy of pancreatic cancer. American Journal of Surgery 151: 76–80

Zhou W, Sokoll L J, Bruzek D J et al 1998 Identifying markers for pancreatic cancer by gene expression analysis. Cancer Epidemiology, Biomarkers, & Prevention 7: 109–112

Pancreaticoduodenectomy

56

M.F. BRENNAN

INTRODUCTION

Pancreaticoduodenectomy remains the primary surgical treatment for lesions involving the head of the pancreas. In malignant disease (Ch. 55), these may be lesions arising from duodenum, ampulla or the pancreas. Prof. Michael Trede has pointed out that Allen Old Father Whipple, who was the Clinical Director of Memorial Sloan-Kettering, is commonly credited as having developed the operation of pancreaticoduodenectomy (Whipple et al 1935) prior to his association with our Institution. However, as Whipple acknowledged, Professor W. Kausch, in July 1909, performed a pancreatic and duodenal resection for a small carcinoma of the ampulla of Vater. Apparently, the patient died from acute cholangitis from a benign stricture 9 months later, and at autopsy the pathologist found no evidence of any recurrence (Kausch 1912). Prof. Trede attributes the first pancreaticoduodenectomy to Prof. Codivlla of Bologna for a distal gastric carcinoma involving the duodenum and head of the pancreas in 1898 (Trede 1985). In 1899 William Halsted removed an ampullary tumor by local excision only, and that patient died of local recurrence approximately 6 months later (Halsted 1899). Early operations were performed in two stages involving biliary and gastric diversion first, followed by subsequent resection, and have now been replaced by a one stage procedure that, in experienced hands, can be performed expeditiously and safely with a limited hospital stay and limited complications.

ANATOMICAL CONSIDERATIONS

The anatomy of the pancreas has been described in Chapter 1. The important issue for resection includes the lymphatic drainage from pancreatic head lesions, which results in a high incidence of lymph node positivity in the posterior pancreaticoduodenal region. This major drainage area should be resected taking all the tissue in front of the vena cava, the renal veins and the nodes between aorta and vena cava with the specimen.

It is essential that the surgeon be familiar with the arterial variations normally encountered to avoid injury and particularly avoid hepatic ischemia in the jaundiced patient. The important variations are those of the right hepatic artery. The right hepatic artery crosses in front of the portal vein in greater than 90% of cases. However, in a small percentage of cases the right hepatic artery passes behind the portal vein and can be felt high in the porta, which raises a suspicion, when this is palpated, of an accessory or replaced right hepatic artery which is the most common variant. This arises from the superior mesenteric artery in up to 25% of patients and passes on the right side and somewhat posterior to the common bile duct. The difference between a true right accessory or replaced hepatic artery and a right hepatic artery passing behind the portal vein can be easily validated by palpation of the porta just above the duodenum where the true ectopic artery will be felt. The relationships of the hepatic artery to the bile duct are variable. In the majority of cases, the right hepatic artery passes behind the bile duct, but a right hepatic artery passes in front of the common bile duct so commonly that one must identify it clearly particularly during mobilization of the gallbladder and cystic duct to avoid damage by inadvertent placement of a clamp on the divided bile duct, which encroaches on the right hepatic artery. The presence of an accessory or replaced right hepatic artery from the superior mesenteric artery does not preclude resection of the pancreatic head. Often the vessel will pass posteriorly and can be carefully dissected free. Unresectability is not defined by variant anatomy but rather by the local invasion of major vascular structures independent of their position.

PREOPERATIVE ASSESSMENT OF RESECTABILITY

Once metastatic disease has been excluded, the most important consideration as to resectability will be the degree of vascular involvement. Gross and obvious encroachment can often be distinguished on helical computerized tomographic (CT) scan (Fig. 56.1). More subtle degrees of involvement can be suspected and almost invariably proven when the clear fat plane surrounding the celiac axis or the superior mesenteric artery is lost and a blurring or 'fuzziness' is identified (Fig. 56.2). In questionable cases laparoscopic or endoscopic ultrasound should resolve the issue (Ch. 55). Arterial encroachment or encasement by adenocarcinoma of the pancreas, in our opinion, precludes resec-

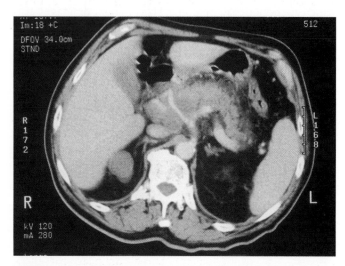

Fig. 56.1 Gross and obvious encroachment of the celiac and splenic arteries as seen on a helical CT.

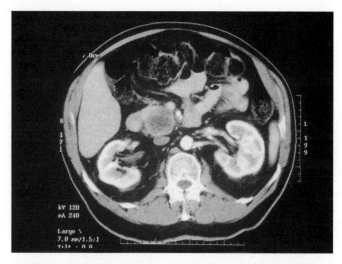

Fig. 56.2 The loss of the clear fat plane around the superior mesenteric artery indicates tumor encroachment and predicts irresectability.

tion for cure. Early experience with resection of major arteries for adenocarcinoma of the pancreas, while technically feasible, has not resulted in any significant long-term palliation (Fortner 1973).

Venous involvement is much more controversial. The presence of obvious enlarged varices on the CT scan almost always precludes any resection for cure. More subtle involvement of the superior mesenteric vein or the portal vein, however, can often be appreciated on the CT scan and is more difficult to interpret. As resection of the portal vein is not particularly technically difficult (see below), venous involvement of the superior mesenteric or portal vein does not necessarily preclude resection. Nevertheless, any significant degree of venous involvement will almost always mean that there is some degree of extension of the tumor to the arteries, usually the superior mesenteric artery, by posterior encroachment behind the superior mesenteric and portal veins. Complete obstruction of the splenic vein does not preclude resection, but proximal splenic involvement raises the issue of involvement of the base of the celiac axis, which would clearly prevent meaningful resection.

ANGIOGRAPHY

Angiography, in our opinion, is rarely indicated for malignant pancreatic neoplasia (see also Ch. 55). There remains a limited role for benign insulinoma. On occasions when a malignant islet cell tumor or a large vascular microcystic adenoma is suspected, angiography may be considered. For islet cell tumor, however, the important issue is often that an adequate examination arteriographically of the liver becomes at least as important as the vascular supply to the primary tumor. Islet cell tumors can have multiple diffuse small highly vascular lesions within the liver, not seen even on good contrast enhanced CT. This precludes resection for cure and should be identified prior to consideration of exploration.

It has been argued that arteriography is needed because of the importance of the venous phase in identifying superior mesenteric or portal vein venous encroachment. In our opinion, this is almost always identified by a high quality helical CT scan and so cannot be the justification for arteriography. The need for arteriography to determine aberrant arteries is redundant in the hands of the experienced surgeon, and the low risk of median arcuate syndromes (<1%) combined with careful examination of the proximal hepatic artery before division of the gastroduodenal artery, is sufficient to justify abandoning routine use of angiography. Should the occlusion at the gastroduodenal artery result in cessation of the pulse in the porta, then a median arcuate ligament should be searched for.

PREOPERATIVE PREPARATION

A patient with a malignancy at the head of the pancreas will often present with a certain degree of inanition. Unfortunately, the application of nutritional support prior to pancreaticoduodenectomy is of limited value and not shown to have impact on outcome. It is important, however, to restore the patient's fluids and electrolyte balance before embarking on the procedure. Anemia is uncommon and rarely will the patient need preoperative transfusion. Significant anemia associated with a duodenal pancreatic mass suggests a duodenal adenocarcinoma. We prefer a limited bowel preparation and a single dose of preoperative systemic antibiotics. We know that the primary organism in postoperative infection is the same organism identified intraoperatively in the contaminated bile. A recent paper from our group (Povoski et al 1999a) suggests that the common organisms are *Enterococcus* species, *Streptococcus viridans*, *Klebsiella* species, *Enterobacter* species, *Escherichia coli*, yeast, *Citrobacter* species and *Bacteroides* species (Table 56.1). Polymicrobial intraoperative bile cultures are found in 70% of positive cultures.

Table 56.1 Microorganisms isolated from the bile of 94 patients with a positive intraoperative bile culture

Microorganisms	Number of positive cultures (%)
Enterococcus species	50 (53)
Streptococcus viridans	26 (28)
Klebsiella species	22 (23)
Enterobacter species	19 (20)
Escherichia coli	12 (13)
Yeast	10 (11)
Citrobacter species	9 (10)
Bacteroides species	8 (9)
Clostridium perfringens	7 (7)
Pseudomonas species	6 (6)
Coagulase negative staphylococcus	6 (6)
Lactobacillus species	5 (5)

Condensed from: Povoski et al 1999a

Recent experience has suggested that the standard preoperative antibiotic designed to address wound infection such as cephalosporin is ineffective in wound infection prophylaxis. A more broad-spectrum antibiotic such as a cefotetan (cefoxitin) should be used. Newer synthetic antibiotics such as combinations of piperacillin and Tazobactam (Zosyn) can now be argued as the most appropriate prophylactic particularly in patients who have undergone antecedent biliary instrumentation with bile contamination as they cover, in addition to the coverage of cefoxitin, *Enterococcus faecalis*.

PREOPERATIVE BILIARY DRAINAGE

Prospective randomized studies (McPherson et al 1984) have not shown a benefit to preoperative biliary drainage by the transhepatic route or, in other studies, by the endoscopic route. Not only are these procedures not advantageous, but there is some evidence to suggest that, indeed, they may be harmful (Blenkharn et al 1984). While instrumentation for diagnostic purposes does not seem to be an issue, our analysis would suggest that the placement of indwelling stents inevitably contaminates the bile, prolongs peripancreatic inflammatory response, is on occasions accompanied by severe pancreatitis (Fig. 56.3) and often cannot be justified. In a recent analysis the primary indicator of postoperative morbidity, particularly infectious complications, was the placements of permanent biliary drainage (Povoski et al 1999b) (Table 56.2). A highly selective use of permanent biliary drainage for those patients who are either not going to be resected or in whom the delay between diagnosis and resection may be quite prolonged is justified. Clearly, biliary drainage has a major contribution to make in the unresected patient and in the relief of pruritus, where resection must be delayed, or is not contemplated.

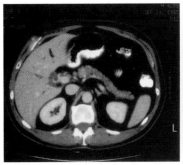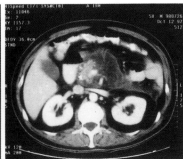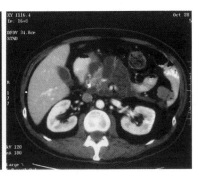

Fig. 56.3 Severe pancreatitis following unnecessary endoscopic stenting for a small periampullary lesion.

Table 56.2 Effect of preoperative biliary drainage on postoperative outcome after pancreaticoduodenectomy

	Morbidity	Infection	Abscess	Death
Biliary drainage	0.025	0.01	0.02	0.04
Biliary instrumentation	0.3	0.2	0.5	0.5
Age	0.4	0.9	0.3	0.8
Sex	0.4	0.1	0.7	0.6
Jaundice	0.9	0.9	0.6	0.8
Bilirubin > 1.8 mg%	0.4	0.2	0.1	0.8

Multivariate analysis $n = 240$
Condensed from: Povoski et al 1999b

OPERATIVE CONSENT

It is important that the primary surgeon have a discussion with the patient and, where appropriate, also a member of his/her family as to the planned procedure. In addition to the description of the procedure and the potential complications, in those patients in whom a histopathological diagnosis has not been obtained (the majority of patients), it is important to emphasize that a resection may be undertaken and the subsequent histopathology will prove to be benign. It is often difficult for the patient to accept the difficulty in making intraoperative or preoperative histopathological diagnosis and the difficulties encountered by too aggressive attempts to confirm the diagnosis are underappreciated by the patient. As long as these issues are discussed beforehand, then the procedure should be able to be performed without misunderstanding, and an unsuspected benign diagnosis, a source of great relief, rather than a cause for criticism.

PANCREATICODUODENECTOMY

The procedure usually begins with a laparoscopy (Ch. 55) in an effort to determine remote metastasis and, with the use of laparoscopic ultrasound, the presence or absence of unsuspected hepatic metastases or vascular encasement.

OPERATIVE APPROACH

If the laparoscopy is negative and the laparoscopic ports have been placed appropriately in the planned bilateral subcostal incision, the incision is then made (Fig. 56.4). Alternatively, some prefer a vertical midline incision or a right subcostal oblique incision extended to the left costal margin. The rectus is divided with the cautery, elevating the rectus muscle with packing forceps (Fig. 56.5). All muscles of the abdominal wall are divided with the cautery after the skin has been divided with the knife. The abdomen is opened and careful exploratory laparotomy performed. The liver is evaluated for metastases, which are rarely missed by laparoscopy. Invasion of the transverse mesocolon is examined and the routine examination of other organs and sites performed.

The lesion is then evaluated for resectability. An acceptable approach is the following. The colon is mobilized from the right upper quadrant (Fig. 56.6), the retroperitoneal tissues incised, and the right renal vein identified at its confluence with the inferior vena cava. The inferior vena cava is then dissected free of all tissue, preserving the gonadal vessels. The third and fourth part of the

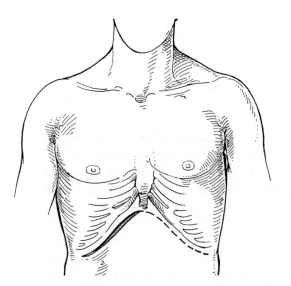

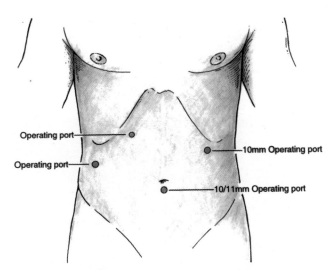

Operating port
Operating port
10mm Operating port
10/11mm Operating port

Fig. 56.4 If the laparoscopy is negative and the laparoscopic ports have been placed appropriately in the planned bilateral subcostal incision, the incision is then made to encompass the superior port sites.

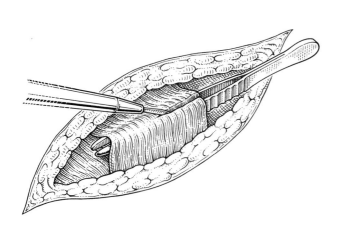

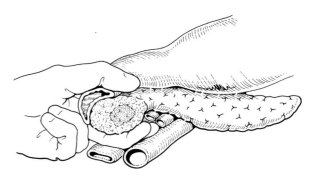

Fig. 56.7 The third and fourth part of the duodenum is reflected and the pancreas elevated so that the hand can be passed behind the pancreas to palpate the tumor mass and the superior mesenteric vessels.

Fig. 56.5 The rectus is divided with the cautery, elevating the rectus muscle with packing forceps.

duodenum is reflected and the pancreas elevated so that the hand can be passed behind the pancreas to palpate the tumor mass (Fig. 56.7). This can usually determine quite accurately whether or not the likelihood of posterior extension to the superior mesenteric artery is present. If extension of tumor from the head of the pancreas to the superior mesenteric artery is encountered, one can presuppose that mesenteric or portal venous involvement is present. Certainly gross invasion by palpation of the superior mesenteric artery presupposes venous encasement and unless the artery is completely free, we would terminate the procedure at this stage. Assuming that the artery

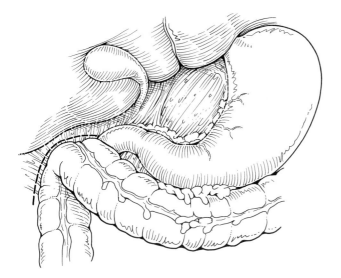

Fig. 56.6 The colon is mobilized from the right upper quadrant (dotted line).

is free by gross palpation, we then prefer to elevate the omentum and enter into the lesser sac (see also Variation 1 below). The omentum is detached from the colon, the lesser sac entered, and the inferior border of the pancreas identifed. The anterior surface of the superior mesenteric vein is identified, and the right gastric epiploic vein divided and the anterior branch of the inferior pancreatico-duodenal vein ligated just below the pancreas. We believe it is important to ligate this latter vessel directly, as tension on this vessel can cause bothersome bleeding. The middle colic vessels that drain into the superior mesenteric should be preserved. Only in rare circumstances where they are tethered to a low-lying tumor should they be divided. Conversely, traction on the mesocolon at this time can cause bothersome bleeding if this is not appreciated. The pressure of any significant varices in the omentum or colonic mesentery should raise concern as to portal vein or superior mesenteric vein obstruction. The pancreas is then elevated from the anterior surface of the superior mesenteric vein to determine whether or not there is tumor adherence. This is, in essence, an avascular plane (Fig. 56.8) so that venous bleeding from this site presupposes firm tethering by the tumor to the posterior or right side of the superior mesenteric–splenic vein confluence. If this dissection plane is free, then the dissection can continue to the superior border of the pancreas. Usually, however, before completion of the dissection from below, we turn our attention to the superior border of the pancreas, where the common hepatic artery is identified (Fig. 56.9).

At this site there are commonly enlarged, often inflammatory nodes, which if not removed with the specimen, need to be carefully dissected free, and, with the use of hemostatic clips, bothersome hemorrhage prevented. The magnitude of the common hepatic artery pulsation is

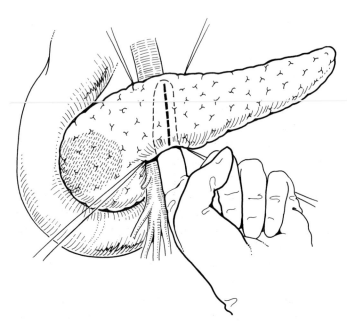

Fig. 56.8 The pancreas is then elevated from the anterior surface of the superior mesenteric vein to determine whether or not there is tumor adherence. This is, in essence, an avascular plane. Venous bleeding from this site presupposes firm tethering by the tumor to the posterior or right side of the superior mesenteric–splenic vein confluence.

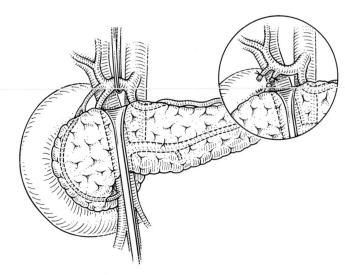

Fig. 56.9 Usually before completion of the dissection from below, we turn our attention to the superior border of the pancreas, where the common hepatic artery is identified. Inset: The gastroduodenal artery is identified and, if at this stage there is no adherence or encasement of the vessels, this vessel is doubly ligated and divided, as is the right gastric artery.

consciously examined to avoid a median arcuate ligament syndrome or for an unsuspected accessory hepatic arterial supply if the artery is found to be small. Each of the abnormalities can be then searched for and corrected or preserved. The gastroduodenal artery is identified. If at this stage there is no adherence or encasement of the common hepatic artery, the gastroduodenal artery is doubly ligated and divided, as is the right gastric artery (Fig. 56.9, inset). Prior to formal division and ligation of this vessel, temporary occlusion and palpation of the distal common hepatic ensures no retrograde flow. This provides excellent access to the superior part of the portal vein above the superior border of the pancreas (see Variation II below). The portal vein can then be dissected superiorly, retracting the common hepatic artery up to its bifurcation, to the patient's left, and isolating the common hepatic duct. At this point we usually turn our attention to the ligament of Treitz, but it is perfectly acceptable at this time to mobilize the gallbladder from the gallbladder fossa in standard fashion, reflecting the gallbladder down with the specimen, such that it is attached only by the cystic duct. This can be done later in the procedure if preferred, because ligation of the cystic artery has the theoretical prospect of devascularizing the gallbladder and allowing the potential for infected bile to leak through the ischemic gallbladder wall. If the gallbladder is in any way difficult,

or if there is a very high insertion of the cystic duct, for example into the right hepatic duct, the cystic artery can be divided and the gallbladder removed. We would normally not divide the common bile duct at this stage (see Variation II below).

At some point following this dissection, a decision as to biopsy of the pancreas should be made (see Variation IIIa below). We do not routinely biopsy the pancreas.

Attention is then turned to the ligament of Treitz, which is mobilized. This is done carefully, as far behind the mesenteric vessels as possible and identifying the inferior mesenteric vein. Small branches of the jejunal vascular arcade of the most proximal part of the jejunum are then ligated and divided, usually using hemoclips. The GI stapler is used to transect the bowel (Fig. 56.10). The small portion of the divided proximal jejunum beyond the ligament of Treitz can usually be quite safely passed behind the mesenteric vessels.

With that completed we turn our attention to the greater omentum and in a standard procedure the omentum is completely divided to the border of the stomach. The stomach is then isolated and divided. We prefer to place straight and curved Kocher clamps on the stomach wall and then divide the remaining portion of the stomach with the GI stapler. This can be oversewn with a running suture, but is not mandatory (Fig. 56.11). The divided stomach is then reflected to the patient's right and attention turned to the

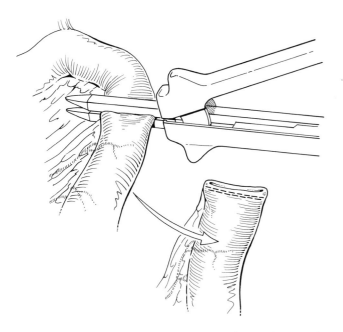

Fig. 56.10 Following dissection of the ligament of Treitz, the GI stapler is used to transect the bowel.

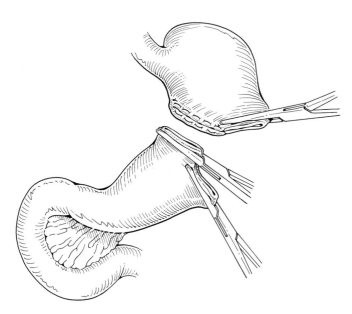

Fig. 56.11 Straight and curved Kocher clamps are placed on the stomach wall and then the remaining portion of the stomach is divided with the GI stapler. The divided stapler may be oversewn (as shown) but it is not mandatory.

common hepatic duct. This is divided just above the entrance of the cystic duct and, in patients suspected of having a distal bile duct carcinoma, a frozen section obtained at the transection site. Careful attention is paid to the commonest variation of abnormal arterial anatomy,

which is the passing of the right hepatic artery behind the common hepatic duct, to lie just to the right of the proximal hepatic duct. The dissection can continue down the side of the remaining portion of the common duct, taking all the tissue, which usually contains several nodes, from the retroperitoneum at this site. A bile culture is obtained at the time of transection.

We then prefer to place stay sutures in the inferior and superior border of the pancreas to prevent any hemorrhage and then divide the pancreas sharply with the knife so as to have a cleanly divided pancreatic mucosal division for subsequent suture (Fig. 56.12A and B). (See also Variation IV below.) On the specimen, hemorrhage from the small divided inferior and superior pancreatic vessels can be controlled with large clips or sutures. On the theoretical possibility of contamination of the intra-peritoneal wound with malignant cells from the pancreatic duct, a suture is placed in the dividend pancreatic duct on the specimen side.

There remains then only to dissect out the uncinate process which is reflected from behind the superior mesenteric vein, if this has not been performed earlier in the procedure (see also Variation I below). Careful attention is taken to dissect along the right side of the portal vein. It is often easier to commence this dissection from above, identifying the origin of the superior mesenteric artery and then dissecting along the right side wall of the artery to gain a clean dissection of all tissue running behind the portal vein. There is often adherence in the three dimensional 'corner' between the posterior lying mesenteric artery and the anteriorly placed superior mesenteric-portal vein. On occasions, the portal vein will need to be resected (see also Variation VI below). However, if there is no attachment to the vein and the arterial attachments are free, a clean dissection along the superior mesenteric artery can be obtained. Often, if the surgeon is on the patient's left side, it is possible to gain a clear dissection along the right side of the portal vein protecting the superior mesenteric artery with the fingers of the left hand for the assistant to dissect. An alternative approach from the right side is to retract the portal vein so that the operating surgeon can dissect along the right side of the superior mesenteric artery with direct vision. With this completed, the specimen is removed. A decision must now be made as to frozen section of the divided pancreas (see also Variation IIIb below).

RECONSTRUCTION

In the standard pancreaticoduodenectomy (Whipple's procedure) a standard reconstruction follows (multiple alternatives are discussed below). We have been comfortable with an end-to-side choledochojejunal anastomosis, performed first, using a running everting suture of 4/0 absorbable monofilament suture (Fig. 56.13). The duct is clearly identified and held by a small pediatric Satinsky or 'bulldog' clamp. A fixation stitch is placed at the left corner of the duct, an incision made in the serosa of the bowel and a lesser incision made in the mucosa. A running everting posterior layer is designed to prolapse mucosa of the bowel into the bile duct. This involves a greater 'bite' on the serosa of the bowel and the bile duct wall than the mucosa of the bowel. A second anterior layer, performed in similar or direct over and over fashion, ensures a patent but not cicatricial anastomosis. A direct mucosa-to-mucosa anastomosis of the pancreatic duct to the sidewall of the jejunum is similarly made. First a posterior layer of running, or interrupted 4-0 PDS sutures are placed to invaginate part of the posterior aspect of the pancreas into the sidewall of the jejunum. The serosa is then scored on the jejunum and a single posterior duct to mucosa stitch of 5-0 monofilament suture placed at the site of the anastomosis. The mucosa is incised with a small opening and an interrupted 5-0 duct to mucosa anastomosis completed. It is rare that even the smallest duct

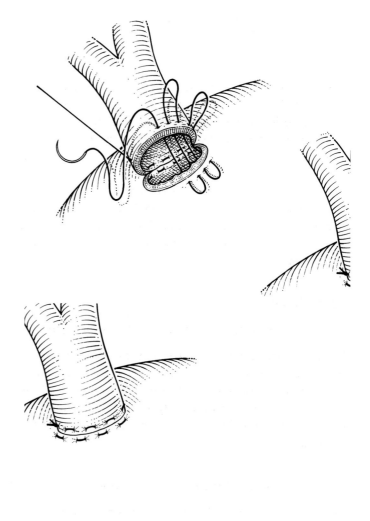

Fig. 56.12 (A) We prefer to place stay sutures in the inferior and superior border of the pancreas to prevent any hemorrhage and then divide the pancreas sharply. **(B)** We prefer to use the knife to divide the pancreas so as to have a clearly divided pancreatic mucosal division for subsequent anastomosis.

Fig. 56.13 End-to-side choledochojejunal anastomosis, performed first, using running everting sutures of 4-0 monofilament absorbable suture.

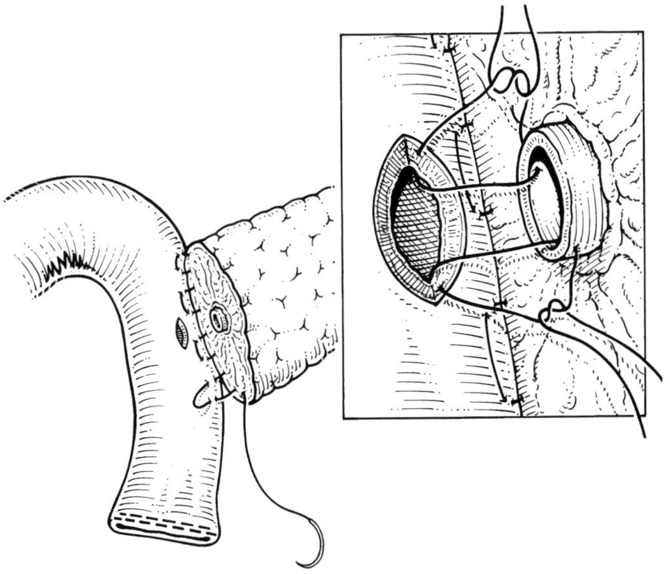

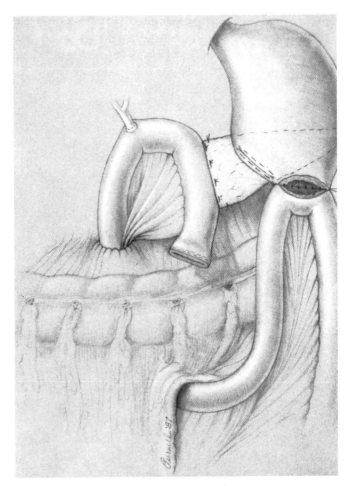

Fig. 56.14 Even the smallest duct can usually accommodate three interrupted sutures at 2, 6, and 10 o'clock.

cannot accommodate three interrupted sutures at 2, 6, and 10 o'clock (Fig. 56.14). Similarly, anterior running sutures are used to invaginate the anterior pancreatic capsule into the sidewall of the jejunum. Stents are rarely employed.

A standard antecolic gastrojejunostomy is then created, using a running 3-0 PD suture. The completed reconstruction is as shown (Fig. 56.15). A nasogastric tube may be placed into the afferent loop, but this is usually removed within 24 hours. Abdominal wall closure is by a single layer of number 1 running PDS with staples applied to the skin.

Fig. 56.15 The completed reconstruction is as shown.

VARIATIONS

I. Dissection of the mesenteric vein from the right

Often in mobilizing the third part of the duodenum, it may be easier to continue that dissection along the inferior border of the duodenum to the sidewall of the vein of the superior mesenteric vein, identifying the right sidewall at that point and mobilizing the uncinate process early in the procedure.

II. Early division of the common bile duct

Many surgeons, having determined that a biliary bypass will be required regardless of whether or not the lesion will be able to be resected, will divide the common bile duct early in the procedure (Fig. 56.16). This gives excellent access to the supra pancreatic portion of the portal vein, and should

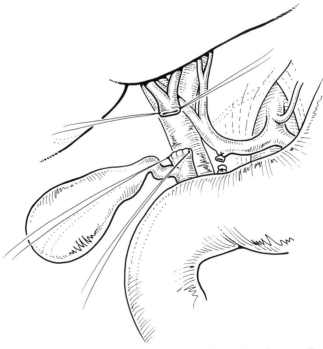

Fig. 56.16 Many surgeons, having determined that a biliary bypass will be required regardless of whether or not the lesion will be able to be resected, will divide the common bile duct early in the procedure.

always be considered an option if there is difficulty in isolating the portal vein or if the area of greatest concern is tumor attachment to the portal vein above the splenic vein confluence. If this approach is preferred, it is important to be aware of the possibility of an accessory or replaced right hepatic artery (vide supra).

III. Frozen section biopsy of the pancreas

a. In the absence of a preoperative diagnosis, some surgeons advocate intraoperative biopsy. We think this should not be routine, since the decision for resection should be based predominantly on the clinical findings, both preoperatively and intraoperatively. If there is high suspicion for malignancy, then resection can proceed without histological confirmation. Open biopsy of the pancreas either by Tru-cut needle through the duodenum or by direct biopsy is often difficult and imprecise and we do not believe routinely justified. It is important to emphasize that preoperative discussion of this issue can often prevent postoperative confusion.

b. The transected section of the pancreas should only be sent for frozen section biopsy if the surgeon plans to act on the information. If there is concern that there is a small amount of potentially malignant tissue such that a positive biopsy would result in a further 1–3 cm of resection of the pancreas with a similar safe reconstruction, then it should be considered. If, however, there is concern above extensive disease and the procedure is purely palliative, or total pancreatectomy would not be considered for multifocal disease, then frozen section becomes redundant. With increasing passage of time, we have become less and less aggressive about performing frozen section biopsies of the transected pancreas, provided that we are comfortable that we are clinically beyond the tumor and the transected duct is not involved. A positive soft tissue margin is at least as common in the posterior peripancreatic soft tissue as it is in the transected pancreas, if the duct is not involved at this site. This can often be easily decided by the caliber of the large duct and the associated appearance of the transected pancreas.

IV. Division of the pancreas

Some prefer to transect the pancreas with the GIA stapler. We prefer not to do that given the fact that while it is effective in the patient with a small atrophic pancreas, in any enlarged pancreas it tends to crush the pancreas and not achieve the goal of ensuring hemostasis. In addition, one then has to remove part of the staple line to identify the pancreatic duct. Only in the hands of the very experienced will an awareness of where the duct is, allow this to be done simply and without hemorrhage. The proposed benefit that

suturing to the staple suture line gives stability to the pancreatic jejunal anastomosis is an argument with which we have no experience.

V. Variations in reconstruction

a. The choledochojejunal anastomosis

Much debate about this revolves around suture material and technique: running continuous or interrupted sutures, the use of stents, and the need for split Roux-en-Y diversion. These are purely decisions for the operating surgeon. We are comfortable with a running suture, while others prefer interrupted sutures. A minor variation from the above technique is shown in Fig. 56.17. The author is comfortable not to use a stent through the choledochojejunal anastomosis. Most prefer monofilament absorbable suture material.

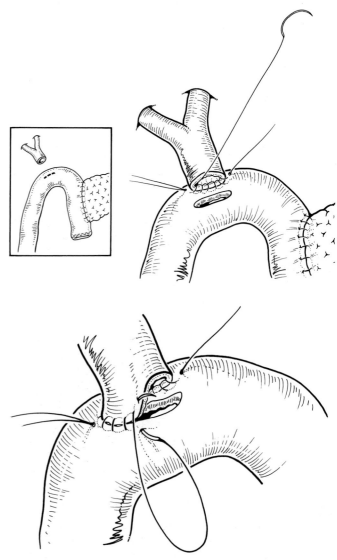

Fig. 56.17 An alternative modification of the choledochal anastomosis technique.

b. Pancreaticojejunostomy

Multiple alternatives have been proposed for the management of the pancreatic remnant. They include the description above and the following.

Alternative suture approach

A minor variation on the above technique is the use of interrupted sutures placed 'through and through' the pancreas and tied after the duct sutures are placed (Fig. 56.18).

Direct invagination of the pancreas into the jejunum

End-to-end pancreaticojejunal invagination. This is usually performed by tailoring the pancreatic remnant to the sides of the small intestine. A layer of interrupted, absorbable or non-absorbable sutures is placed between the posterior layer

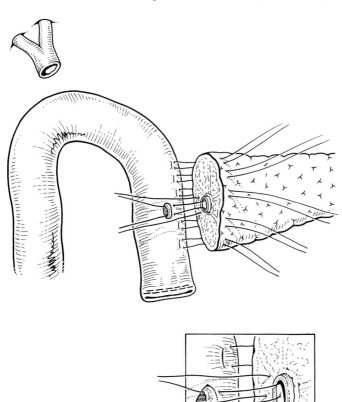

Fig. 56.18 An alternative approach to the pancreaticojejunal anastomosis using interrupted 'through and through' sutures placed first. Interrupted ductal sutures are placed before the 'through and through' pancreatic sutures are pulled up and tied. The 'through and through' sutures are tied and the anterior ductal sutures are placed. The anterior pancreaticojejunal interrupted sutures are finally placed and subsequently tied.

and the seromuscular layer of the jejunum. These are placed such that the edge of the transected pancreas and the free end of the jejunum are sewn to each other circumferentially with the sutures, including the duct, where appropriate. An anterior outer layer is then placed to further insert the pancreas into the jejunum.

Ductal ligation

Primary oversewing of the pancreatic duct. This contiguous pancreatic duct ligation technique has been accompanied by an unacceptable rate of prolonged pancreatic drainage as high as 80% and should, we believe, be abandoned.

Pancreaticogastrostomy

A recent analysis of a randomized trial examining the value of pancreaticogastrostomy as opposed to pancreaticojejunostomy has not shown any difference in outcome in terms of mortality and morbidity.

The choice of method, therefore, remains that of the surgeon and should be based on his or her personal preference.

c. Reconstruction of gastrointestinal continuity

Multiple approaches have been applied. The basic approach (above) has served us well and we think is appropriate. An important alternative is a Roux-en-Y reconstruction separating the stomach from the pancreatic and biliary anastomoses.

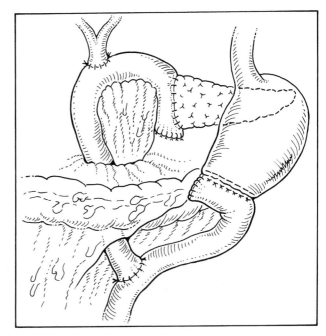

Fig. 56.19 Some prefer a Roux-en-Y reconstruction to further divert the biliary pancreatic anastomosis from the gastroenteric flow.

While we prefer the standard reconstruction, some prefer a Roux-en-Y (Fig. 56.19) reconstruction and believe that, should a pancreatic leak develop, the fistula will be more easily managed.

VI. Resection of the portal vein

Deliberate planned resection of the portal vein is only rarely considered ahead of time. If there is a major portal vein involvement, the tumor is often not resectable for cure because of arterial encroachment. Nevertheless, all surgeons should be familiar with the techniques of resecting the portal vein, if only for those situations in which unanticipated adherence either by tumor or inflammatory tissue makes sharp dissection of the right side of the vein difficult and unsafe. At least 2 cm and occasionally 3 cm of portal vein/supramesenteric vein can be resected and an end-to-end anastomosis be performed (Fig. 56.20). It will depend on where the site of the attachment exists. If below the splenic vein, then a sleeve resection allowing continuity of the portal vein is possible, and a simple end-to-end superior mesenteric vein reconstruction performed. However, this is usually only possible by ligation of the splenic vein (Fig. 56.20) and direct superior mesenteric to portal vein anastomosis. This is usually done by elevating the small bowel such that a tension free anastomosis can be performed. The vessels are clamped with pediatric vascular clamps and

anastomosis is performed with a 4-0 prolene suture. The final knot is tied so as to leave room for expansion once the clamps are released (Fig. 56.21).

There is often great temptation when there is minimal adherence to the vein, to perform some form of sleeve resection. In the majority of situations, this results in an inferior result with narrowing of the vein and incomplete tumor clearance.

Some authors have preferred the direct division and interposition of a portion of autogenous vein graft, usually from a jugular vein. We have only rarely found this necessary.

PYLORUS PRESERVING PANCREATICODUODENECTOMY

The pylorus preserving pancreaticoduodenectomy has been most recently defined (Grace et al 1986, Longmire & Traverso 1981). The argument for this operation suggests that for pancreatic adenocarcinoma the procedure is equivalent in outcome and nutritional and gastrointestinal physiology are improved.

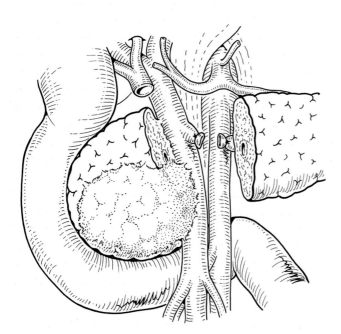

Fig. 56.20 Tumor involves 2–3 cm of the superior mesenteric vein. The portal vein, superior mesenteric vein and splenoportal junction are dissected. The splenic vein is ligated and divided at the splenoportal junction.

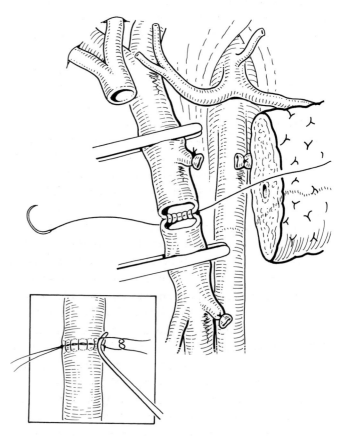

Fig. 56.21 Primary anastomosis of the veins. A running 4/0 Prolene suture is used. The final knot is tied over a nerve hook to allow for 'growth' of the anastomosis (inset).

Technically, the resection is as described above for pancreaticoduodenectomy, with the only issue being that the duodenum is divided approximately 2 cm distal to the pylorus. For this to be successful, an intact vascular blood and neural innervation of the pylorus is required. This means that the right gastric artery should be preserved as should the nerve of Laterjet.

Reconstruction, as described above, is very similar with the exception that duodenojejunostomy is necessary.

The argument made above for the pancreaticojejunostomy and the choledochojejunostomy being placed proximal to the duodenojejunostomy is to limit the consequences of gastric acid entry into the jejunum, but other alternatives such as end-to-end duodenojejunostomy, including the use of a Roux-en-Y have also been utilized.

The operation has gained greater acceptance for chronic pancreatitis and ampullary tumors than for adenocarcinoma of the pancreas.

REGIONAL SUBTOTAL AND REGIONAL TOTAL PANCREATECTOMY

Regional operations are based on the premise of a more extensive node dissection and deliberate resection of major arteries and veins with replacement. Arguments that such operations can improve outcome have undergone serious re-evaluation. At the present time the author believes that while more extended nodal dissection is clinically justified for lesions thought to be duodenal or ampullary, no good evidence can be provided that resection of major arterial structures provides any realistic improvement in cure rates for adenocarcinoma of the head of the pancreas (Fortner et al 1996). Resection of the portal vein (vide supra) is a technical procedure that, as discussed above, one must be familiar with. As best as we can tell, vein resection does not influence long-term outcome (Harrison et al 1996). In essence, therefore, the regional operations are now confined to more extended nodal dissection. Extended resection has been described for the standard pancreaticoduodenectomy (vide supra). In this approach, the nodal dissection posteriorly involves dissecting all tissue from in front of the inferior vena cava and the right and left renal veins. This is an easy plane to dissect and it is standard procedure for us. This dissection of all nodal tissue is easily extended by dissection of all the tissue between the vena cava and the aorta, skeletonizing the right side of the aorta and the origin of the superior mesenteric artery. A randomized trial examining this issue has not shown proven benefit (Michaelassi et al 1989).

In similar fashion the nodal tissue along the hepatic arteries is skeletonized as is done in a D2 dissection for gastric adenocarcinoma. The gonadal vein on the right is usually ligated in the extended resection at the base of the mesocolon and proximally as it enters the vena cava. An alternative, however, is to make the line of the genital vein the posterior lateral aspect of the inferior dissection.

The extent of the aortic dissection reported has varied widely. The original proposal was that the dissection continue to the inferior mesenteric artery. But even in the hands of those advocating the procedure, this length of dissection has become limited. The first part of the dissection allows an adequate palpation of the head of the pancreas with the contained tumor without a forced dissection in the plane of lymphatic drainage between the pancreas and the retropancreatic nodal tissue. More extended dissection superiorly involves the lymphatic vessels in association with the hepatic artery and portal vein, much as is done for a nodal dissection in gallbladder or bile duct carcinoma (Chs. 53, 54).

In the classical regional operations first advocated, arterial involvement, provided it was segmental, was not a barrier to resection. This continues to be performed by some surgeons in Japan, but has been largely abandoned by surgeons in the United States. Nevertheless, the development of such a procedure has led to the adoption of a more extensive nodal dissection by the majority of surgeons managing these neoplasms.

TOTAL PANCREATECTOMY

Despite early enthusiasm (Brooks & Culebras 1976, Moosa 1982), total pancreatectomy for adenocarcinoma of the pancreas is only rarely employed. We reserve the procedure for those patients with extensive low-grade lesions, such as cystadenocarcinoma or extensive intraductal papillary lesions involving the majority of the gland. On rare occasions, when the patient is an insulin-dependent diabetic, the procedure may be considered. Given that the majority of resections for pancreatic adenocarcinoma are palliative procedures, total pancreatectomy cannot currently be supported in an effort to improve the long-term results of surgical resection for pancreatic adenocarcinoma.

As with all operations for carcinoma of the pancreas, but even more so for total pancreatectomy, it is particularly important that the patient understands the consequences of a total pancreatectomy and the fragile diabetes that may result. For this reason, care should be taken to avoid total pancreatectomy in the elderly or medically unstable patient.

TECHNICAL CONSIDERATIONS FOR TOTAL PANCREATECTOMY

We prefer the bilateral subcostal incision, although others have used a right subcostal extended over the left costal margin. Rarely, a long midline incision may be used. The initial approach to the operative procedure is the same as for any other pancreatic resection, with careful examination of the peritoneal cavity, the placement of self-retaining retractors and assessment of the tumor for resectability.

The mobilization of the duodenum and head of the pancreas is as for pancreaticoduodenectomy. The lesser sac exploration is similar, with elevation of the pancreas from the superior mesenteric splenic vein confluence. The gastroduodenal artery division, transection of the common bile duct, and removal of the gallbladder are all as for pancreaticoduodenectomy. Mobilization of the spleen and distal pancreas is similar to that performed in distal pancreatectomy.

We prefer to first retract the pancreas and incise the peritoneum at the superior and inferior borders of the pancreatic capsule. The splenorenal and gastrosplenic attachments are then divided, and the spleen and tail of the pancreas can be elevated upwards and forwards. Some authors prefer a more extensive gastric resection than is done in pancreaticoduodenectomy to decrease the amount of acid production, given the complete removal of the alkali-producing pancreas. We, however, tend to remove a similar amount of stomach, i.e. approximately the distal third, as is done in pancreaticoduodenectomy and in the same fashion.

The inferior border of the pancreas is then dissected free, the inferior mesenteric vein being ligated as it enters the splenic vein or the splenic vein mesenteric confluence. If the inferior mesenteric vein enters directly into the superior mesenteric vein, it can be left uninterrupted. In total pancreatectomy, the splenic vein is removed with the specimen in contradistinction to operations on the distal pancreas, where, on occasion, particularly with neuroendocrine tumors, the splenic vein and artery can be preserved. The splenic vein is double-ligated at its confluence with the portal vein. The small bowel mobilization at the ligament of Treitz is as for pancreaticoduodenectomy. The superior border of the pancreas is mobilized as the tail is reflected upwards and forwards and the splenic artery is double-ligated at its origin from the celiac vessels.

On occasion, the portal vein will require resection and that is done in standard fashion as described above, if anything, with greater ease, as there is considerable mobilization of the superior mesenteric vein ad the portal vein which, with division of the splenic vein, allows easy mobilization and juxtaposition for anastomosis.

Reconstruction is as for pancreaticoduodenectomy, but there is no pancreaticointestinal anastomosis. Postoperative care is similar, with the risk of pancreatic leak obviated, but replaced with an insulin sensitive diabetes. Diabetic management becomes the central issue. With no counter regulatory hormonal responses (no glucagon, no insulin suppression with catecholamines) the patient is insulin sensitive. Long-term liver fatty infiltration is a serious problem.

DUODENAL PRESERVING RESECTION OF THE HEAD OF THE PANCREAS

It is rarely possible to resect the head of the pancreas, preserving the duodenum. This is an uncommon procedure and requires the preservation of the vascular arcade that runs in the medial aspect of the duodenum from the anterior and posterior pancreaticoduodenal vessels, both superior and inferior. More commonly, this approach is seen in a near total pancreaticoduodenectomy, where the ductal structures of the pancreas are preserved with a small rim of pancreas lying in the curvature of the medial border of the duodenum. This procedure is usually required when a patient has had a previous distal pancreatectomy for an islet cell tumor. In the circumstances where the islet cell tumor has not been found and is then found in the head of the gland. Such a procedure is designed to retain a small quantity of functional exocrine and endocrine tissue. This procedure is not appropriate for adenocarcinoma of the pancreas.

USE OF INTRAOPERATIVE BILIARY STENTING

It has been suggested that the choledochojejunal anastomosis should be stented, as should the pancreaticojejunal anastomosis. While we would have no debate with those who have found these procedures helpful, they are, in our opinion, rarely necessary. In similar fashion, routine postoperative invasive studies to look for leakage are, we think, unjustified, and these decisions can be made based on clinical progress of the patient.

POSTOPERATIVE MANAGEMENT

A nasogastric tube is placed at the time of procedure but is removed in the recovery room the morning following the procedure. Rarely, in situations of delayed gastric emptying where the patient is more comfortable with a naso-gastric tube, the tube may be reinserted, although this is rarely necessary.

The use of prokinetic agents, such as metoclopramide and erythromycin, have been advocated and in selected studies have shown a benefit in terms of measured gastric emptying. However, none have been shown to have impact on hospital stay. We, therefore, do not use them routinely.

The issue of postoperative drainage following pancreatic resection has been a matter of some debate.

The majority of surgeons advise peripancreatic and chole-dochojejunal drainage. This is usually achieved by a simple, low pressure, closed-suction system. Whether or not this drainage is useful or indeed helpful, remains an area of some debate. In a recent analysis of 89 consecutive patients who underwent pancreaticoduodenectomy, 38 had no drainage and 51 had drains placed at the conclusion of the operation (Heslin et al 1998a). Analysis of nutritional, laboratory and operating room factors in relation to complications and length of hospital stay, did not show that drainage altered significantly the risk of fistula, abscess or reoperation or the necessity for CT-guided interventional radiologic drainage after pancreaticoduodenectomy. This raises the interesting conjecture that drains may not be of value: a prospective randomized trial is underway.

USE OF SOMATOSTATIN

A number of series have examined the use of somatostatin (Jenkins & Berein 1995) and octreotide; somatostatin has gained favor in patients with acute pancreatitis. Some authors continue to use octreotide as a post-resection adjuvant following pancreaticoduodenectomy or adeno-carcinoma but we have found the benefits are insufficient to justify the routine use of such an agent.

LENGTH OF STAY

Length of stay for patients undergoing pancreaticoduo-denectomy has progressively declined in recent years (Fig. 56.22) and does not appear to depend on the underlying histopathology (Table 56.3).

Some of this decrease in length of stay has been accompanied by same-day admission for pancreaticoduodenectomy,

Table 56.3 Length of stay for peripancreatic cancers resected at Memorial Sloan–Kettering Cancer Center 10/15/83–10/14/9

		Length of stay (days)	
	n	Median	Range
Adenocarcinoma of pancreas	478	16	1–131
Ampulla	139	17	4–91
Bile duct	85	16	5–82
Duodenum	75	14	6–146
Islet cell	108	11	5–52

MSKCC 10/15/83–10/14/98

but more recently continued expertise with the operation has decreased lengths of stay to the order of 7 to 10 days. The overall median length of stay continues to fall.

POSTOPERATIVE COMPLICATIONS

The operative mortality for pancreaticoduodenectomy should be < 5%. It is clear in the majority of studies that operative mortality is related to the experience of the surgeon and institution and in some institutions mortality rates of < 1% are achieved (Heslin et al 1998b, Lieberman et al 1995, Begg et al 1998, Yeo et al 1995). It is important to emphasize that patients undergoing resection for adenocarcinoma of the pancreas, are in an older age group (in our recent experience with 500 cases, 66% were over the age of 60) (Fig. 56.23). Operative mortality does not appear to differ depending on the underlying malignant histopathology for which the oper-ation has been performed. Postoperative complications con-

Adenocarcinoma of the Pancreas - Resections

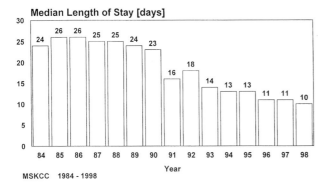

Fig. 56.22 Length of stay for patients undergoing pancreaticoduodenectomy has progressively declined in recent years.

Adenocarcinoma of the Pancreas
Resections by Age

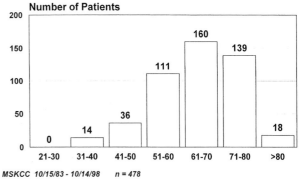

Fig. 56.23 It is important to emphasize that patients undergoing resection for adenocarcinoma of the pancreas are in an older age group, i.e. in our recent experience with 500 cases, 66% were over the age of 60.

tinue to occur in 20 to 50% of patients. The most common complications are infections, occurring in approximately 30%. Wound infection, although often minor, occurs in 15% of our patients and some form of intra-abdominal infection in 12%. The latter often requires drainage, most frequently, but percutaneous CT guided methods. A high degree of suspicion for intra-abdominal collections should be maintained. The patient with an unexplained tachycardia or delayed gastric emptying is certainly a candidate for consideration of computed tomography in an effort to identify an undrained collection. The majority of intra-abdominal collections are related to either an unappreciated anastomotic leak or to contamination at the time of operation from a previously instrumented biliary duct. In such patients, wound infection is not uncommon and should be treated at the bedside. Pancreatic anastomotic leakage continues to occur in 5 to 10% of patients, while bile duct anastomotic leakage occurs in 1 to 2%. Both of these complications can now be managed without reoperation in the majority of cases. Conversely, it is essential to consider reoperation if percutaneous drainage does not rapidly resolve the systemic effects of intra-abdominal collection or abscess.

POSTOPERATIVE NUTRITIONAL SUPPORT

As mentioned previously, many patients undergoing pancreaticoduodenectomy enter the procedure in a state of inanition. As a consequence, we performed a prospective randomized trial examining the benefits of total parenteral nutrition in such patients (Brennan & Pisters 1994). The results of this suggested that infectious complications were greater in the group undergoing total parenteral nutrition and so the routine application of total parenteral nutrition cannot be recommended. (Table 56.4). Given the concerns about the parenteral route of nutritional support in patients who are at risk of infection, we then proceeded to a prospective randomized trial of enteral feeding in patients with upper abdominal malignancy including pancreaticoduodenectomy (Heslin et al 1997). In this study we were likewise unable to show a benefit from routine application of enteral nutritional support in these patients (Table 56.5).

Parenteral and enteral nutritional support, therefore, is reserved for the patient in whom a complication develops with failure to take oral nutrients. The majority of patients will be able to take fluids within 3 or 4 days of operation and be advanced to a full diet consisting of small frequent meals by the time of discharge on the 7th to the 14th day. The results of the operation are discussed in Chapter 55.

Table 56.4 Infectious complications in a prospective randomized trial of total parenteral nutrition

	TPN (n = 60)	Morbidity Control (n = 57)	p Value
Major complications	27	13	0.02
Minor complications	32	24	0.30
Minor complications (excluding atelectasis)	23	13	0.11
Reoperation	6	3	0.18
Median length of stay (days)	16 (7–72)	14 (6–88)	

Brennan et al 1994

Table 56.5 Prospective randomized trial of enteral feeding in patients undergoing resection for upper GI malignancy

	Complications ENT	Control	p Value
Total patients	97	98	
Any major	27	25	0.71
Any complication	44	33	0.10
Any infection	20	23	0.63
LOS			
Median	11	10	0.4
Range	4–41	6–75	

Condensed from: Heslin et al 1997

REFERENCES

Begg C B, Cramer L, Hoskins W J, Brennan M F 1998 Impact of hospital volume on operative mortality for major cancer surgery. JAMA 280: 1747–1751

Blenkharn J I, McPherson G A, Blumgart L H 1984 Septic complications of percutaneous transhepatic biliary drainage. Evaluation of a new closed drainage system. American Journal of Surgery 147: 318–321

Blumgart L H (ed) 1994 Surgery of the liver and biliary tract, 2nd edn. Churchill Livingstone, London

Brennan M F, Pisters P W, Posner M, Quesada O, Shike M 1994 A prospective randomized trial of total parenteral nutrition after major pancreatic resection for malignancy. Annals of Surgery 220: 436–441

Brooks J R, Culebras J M 1976 Cancer of the pancreas. Palliative operation. Whipple procedure, or total pancreatectomy? American Journal of Surgery 131: 516–520

Fortner J G 1973 Regional resection of cancer of the pancreas: A new surgical approach. Surgery 73: 307–320

Fortner J G, Klimstra D S, Senie R T et al 1996 Tumor size is the primary prognostic factor for pancreatic cancer after regional pancreatectomy. Annals of Surgery 223: 147–153

Grace P A, Pitt H A, Tompkins R K et al 1986 Decreased morbidity and mortality after pancreatoduodenectomy. American Journal of Surgery 151: 141–149

Halsted W S 1899 Contributions to the surgery of the bile passages, especially of the common bile duct. Boston Med Surg J 141: 645–654

Harrison L E, Klimstra D, Brennan M F 1996 Isolated portal vein involvement in pancreatic adenocarcinoma: A contradiction for resection? Annals of Surgery 224: 342–349

Heslin M J, Latkany L, Leung D et al 1997 A prospective randomized trial of early enteral feeding after resection of upper GI malignancy. Annals of Surgery 226: 567–580

Heslin M J, Harrison L E, Brooks A D, Hochwald S N, Coit D G, Brennan M F 1998a Is intra-abdominal drainage necessary after pancreaticoduodenectomy. Journal of Gastrointestinal Surgery 2: 373–378

Heslin M J, Brooks A D, Hochwald S N, Harrison L E, Blumgart L H, Brennan M F 1998b Preoperative biliary stenting is associated with increased complications after pancreaticoduodenectomy. Archives of Surgery 133: 149–154

Jenkins S A, Berein A 1995 Review article: the relative effectiveness of somatostatin and octreotide therapy in pancreatic disease. Alimentary Pharmacology and Therapeutics 9(4): 349–361

Kausch W 1912 Das Carcinom de Papilla Duodeni und seine radikale Entfernung. Beltrage zur Klinischen Cirurgie 78: 439–486

Lieberman M D, Kilburn H, Lindsey M, Brennan M F 1995 The relationship of perioperative mortality to hospital volume in patients undergoing pancreatic resection for malignancy. Annals of Surgery 222: 638–645. Archives of Surgery 133: 149–154

Longmire W, Traverso L 1981 The Whipple procedure and other standard operative approaches to pancreatic cancer. Cancer 47: 1706–1711

McPherson G A D, Benjamin I S, Hodgson H J F, Bowley N B, Allison D J 1984 Preoperative percutaneous transhepatic drainage: the results of a controlled trial. British Journal of Surgery 71: 371–375

Michelassi F, Erroi F, Dawson P J et al 1989 Experience with 647 consecutive tumors of the duodenum, ampulla, head of the pancreas, and distal common bile duct. Annals of Surgery 210: 544–556

Moosa A R 1982 Pancreatic cancer—selection for surgery and choice of operation. Cancer 50: 2689

Povoski S P, Karpeh M S Jr, Conlon K C, Blumgart L H, Brennan M F 1999a Preoperative biliary drainage: Impact on intraoperative bile cultures and infectious morbidity and mortality after pancreaticoduodenectomy. Journal of Gastrointestinal Surgery 3: 496–505.

Povoski S P, Karpeh M S Jr, Conlon K C, Blumgart L H, Brennan M F 1999b Effect of preoperative biliary drainage on postoperative outcome following pancreaticoduodenectomy. Annals of Surgery (submitted)

Trede M 1985 The surgical treatment of pancreatic carcinoma. Surgery 97: 28–35

Trede M, Schwall G, Saeger H 1990 Survival after pancreatico-duodenectomy. 118 consecutive resections without an operative mortality. Annals of Surgery 211: 447–458

Whipple A O, Parsons W B, Mullins C R 1935 Treatment of carcinoma of the ampulla of Vater. Annals of Surgery 102: 763–779

Yeo C J, Cameron J L, Lillemoe K D 1995 Pancreaticoduodenectomy for cancer of the pancreas: 201 patients. Annals of Surgery 221: 721–723

Transduodenal resection of the papilla of Vater

57

Ph GERTSCH, L.H. BLUMGART

INTRODUCTION

The periampullary region represents the confluence of epithelia originating from the pancreatic and bile ducts and from the duodenal mucosa. Tumors arising in the region of the papilla of Vater may therefore have their origin from the distal bile duct, the duodenum, the ampulla of Vater itself or the pancreas. Because the epithelium of origin is often impossible to determine and because their clinical characteristics are similar, they are often described as periampullary tumors.

BENIGN TUMORS

Benign tumors of the papilla of Vater are rare (see Ch. 52). They may include lipoma, neurogenic tumors, lymphangioma, leiomyofibroma and some neuroendocrine tumors other than carcinoids (Ricci 1993). Adenomatous polyps, although being the most common tumors of this region are rare with a reported incidence of 0.04 and 0.12% (Galandiuk et al 1988, Rosenberg et al 1986); Motton et al (1996) collected 250 cases in the world literature from 1975 to 1996. The malignant potential of adenomatous polyps has been well documented, foci of malignant cells being detected in 47 to 56% of cases (Delpy et al 1983, Ryan et al 1986). Similarly, complete histological examination of malignant periampullary tumors has revealed residual adenomatous tissue in up to 80 and 91% of cases (Kozuka et al 1981, Baczako et al 1984). The author has, in a series of 16 malignant periampullary tumors, observed residual adenomatous tissue in 44% of cases (Gertsch et al 1987). Thus, the sequence of change of adenoma to carcinoma is frequent for adenomatous polyps of the periampullary region (Perzin & Bridge 1981, Sellner & Machacek 1986, Kimura & Ohtsubo 1988, Seifert et al

1992). Furthermore, the incidence of malignant degeneration of 35–85% (Schulten et al 1976, Perzin & Bridge 1981) tend to show that the risk is higher than for adenomas in other parts of the digestive tract.

Benign tumors may remain asymptomatic for long periods of time. In a systematic study of 23 patients with familial adenomatosis coli, Noda et al (1992) discovered 17 tubular adenomas of the papilla of Vater that were asymptomatic.

One can postulate that symptoms occur in a significant proportion of cases only when adenomas increase in size or when malignant changes have taken place. Symptoms, most commonly jaundice, pain or pancreatitis, are present in the majority of patients with adenomas submitted to surgery (Asbun et al 1993, Branum et al 1996, Cahen et al 1997).

MALIGNANT TUMORS

Malignant tumors of the periampullary region are, in most cases, adenocarcinomas. Carcinoids are extremely rare and should be considered as malignant tumours (Ricci, 1993). The origin of adenocarcinomas can sometimes be detected on careful macroscopic examination of the specimen. Histological characteristics rarely help in identifying their origin (Warren et al 1968, Alexander et al 1984), although it is suggested that the pattern of sulfated mucin production by the pancreatic ductal epithelium is distinct from that of the sialomucin secretion by ampullary or biliary epithelia (Dawson & Connolly 1989).

Periampullary malignant tumors become symptomatic at an early stage because of their particular location. For this reason, radical resection is possible in the majority of cases (Michelassi et al 1989, Klempnauer et al 1995, Talamini et al 1997). Early manifestations include abdominal pain, incomplete biliary obstruction causing pruritus alone, or icterus, which may fluctuate (Blumgart & Kennedy 1973,

Knox & Kingston 1986, Koch et al 1991). Chronic or acute bleeding can cause anemia or melaena and has been reported in one-third of cases (Monson et al 1991). Pancreatitis, resulting from obstruction of the duct is a less frequent manifestation of the disease (Ohmori et al 1976, Iida et al 1989, Koch et al 1991, Talamini et al 1997) but patients presenting with acute pancreatitis seem more likely to have unresectable tumors (Talamini et al 1997).

INVESTIGATIONS

Preoperative investigations are important, and have two objectives: to establish the diagnosis and to stage the extension of the tumor. Ultrasonography and computed tomography (CT) are usually the first investigations to be performed in the presence of altered liver function tests or obstructive jaundice. Dilatation of the common bile duct down to the ampullary region and also, on occasions, a dilatation of the pancreatic duct are identified. When a periampullary tumour is suspected, duodenoscopy, using a side-viewing endoscope, should be the next investigation. Endoscopy allows direct inspection of the medial wall of the duodenum and clear visualization of the papilla. Biopsy is readily performed. However, a normal-looking papilla does not rule out an occult periampullary tumor since inapparent endoluminal growth has been reported in 37% of cases; this should be suspected when an irregularity or filling defect in the distal bile duct is revealed by retrograde cholangiography (Ponchon et al 1989).

Tumour cells might be collected through catheter aspiration or transpapillary endoscopic biopsy (Nakao et al 1982), but in most cases an endoscopic sphincterotomy should be performed for direct access to the tumour and to allow biopsy (Ponchon et al 1989). However, endoscopic biopsy has been reported to miss the diagnosis in 56 to 60% of cases (Ryan et al 1986, Komorovski et al 1991). Global accuracy rate of biopsies increased from 69 to 77% when performed after endoscopic sphincterotomy (Sauvanet et al 1997).

Endoscopic sphincterotomy should be performed after endoscopic ultrasonography because it reduces its reliability. Endoscopic has been compared to transabdominal ultrasonography, CT and angiography. It has been demonstrated to be the most effective single imaging procedure for local tumor staging (Rösch et al 1992). However systematic studies have given controversial results. Some observed an accuracy of 83% and even of 100% in staging malignant tumors in absence of endoscopic stents (Quirk et al 1997); others consider that endoscopic ultrasonography is unreliable for detecting malignancy in ampullary tumors, even when combined with endoscopic biopsies (Cahen et al

1997, Sauvanet et al 1997). Furthermore, the value of endoscopic ultrasonography for preoperative evaluation of the T stage (TNM classification) has also been questioned, in particular for early stages (T1 and T2) (Rattner et al 1996, Cahen et al 1997). Endoscopic ultrasonography has proven to be significantly superior to US and CT scan in the recognition of enlarged lymph nodes (Rösch et al 1992), but the reliability of such staging is not established yet (Cahen et al 1997).

PROGNOSTIC FACTORS

It has been established that resectable periampullary carcinoma has a better prognosis than carcinoma of the head of the pancreas (Warren et al 1968, Akwari et al 1977, Nix et al 1983, Tarazi et al 1986, Shutze et al 1990, Klempnauer et al 1995).

Several characteristics of periampullary carcinomas have been shown to be of prognostic importance: origin of the tumor and histologic features, lymphatic invasion or metastasis (Jones et al 1985, Monson et al 1991). Carcinomas of ampullary origin have the best prognosis while those of pancreatic ductal origin obviously fare worse than all others (Blumgart & Kennedy 1973, Dawson & Connolly 1989, Michelassi et al 1989, Monson et al 1991). Origin from the biliary epithelium has been regarded as a good pronostic factor by some (Jones et al 1985). Others have expressed the opposite opinion (Tarazi et al 1986, Monson et al 1991). Well differentiated carcinomas or tumors with papillary characteristics have a better prognosis (Blumgart & Kennedy 1973, Akwari et al 1977, Monson et al 1991, Klempnauer et al 1995, Talamini et al 1997). Tumor size has been suspected to influence the prognosis (Nix et al 1983, Klempnauer et al 1995, Nakai et al 1997) and it seems that ulcerating tumors fare worse than those protruding (Nakai et al 1997).

Lymph node metastases, or the presence of lymphatic invasion was correlated with a significantly worse prognosis for some authors (Monson et al 1991, Talamini et al 1997), but not for others (Allema et al 1995, Matory et al 1993). Microperineural invasion seems to be another significant prognositic factor (Nakai 1997).

The adenoma–carcinoma sequence for periampullary adenomatous polyps is well established, and foci of malignant cells might be present in a benign-appearing tumor even if endoscopic biopsies are negative. The risk of malignancy seems higher in villous than in tubular adenomas and the size might also be predictive of malignant transformation. The larger the lesion, the greater the chance that carcinoma will be found on histologic examination (Perzin & Bridge 1981, Koch et al 1991). However, further studies are needed to confirm these findings which might prove to be important for selecting the treatment adapted to each particular case.

THERAPY

Periampullary tumors can be removed either by local resection, as pioneered by Halsted in 1899 or by radical cephalic pancreaticoduodenectomy, as performed by Whipple et al in 1935. Both operations have been used, and their respective places in the treatment of benign or malignant periampullary tumors has been the subject of constant debate. In the absence of a controlled study and standardized technique for local excision of the papilla of Vater, no definitive answer can be given as to which operation should be adopted in each particular situation.

Advocates of local excision for ampullary carcinomas consider that similar long-term results have been obtained after local resection and Whipple's procedure, and state that mortality is lower with local excision (Isaksson et al 1982, Chiappetta et al 1986, Robertson & Imrie 1986, Goldberg et al 1987, Farouk et al 1991) (Table 57.1). Although the last argument seems persuasive, recent results for large series of pancreaticoduodenectomy (see Chs 55 & 56) have a low mortality and offer radical clearance of tumor with a 5 year survival of up to 62%. Thus, Talamini et al (1997) report a mortality rate of 3.8% in 105 patients operated over a period of 27 years and others quote similar results (Tarazi et al 1986, Michelassi et al 1989, Monson et al 1991, Matory et al 1993, Sperti et al 1994). However, morbidity of the Whipple's procedure remains in general above 30% in particular when it is performed for tumors of the papilla of Vater (Chareton et al 1996, Böttger et al 1997, Talamini et al 1997).

Assessment of long-term results is difficult since selection of patients might well have influenced results. More reports involving large number of patients have been published after radical than after local resections of periampullary carcinomas (Table 57.1).

Because of the low mortality observed after Whipple's procedure, there is general agreement that radical resection should be preferred to local resection since it offers wide resection margins and lymphatic clearance. Indeed, microscopic lymphatic invasion has been observed in up to 51% and lymph node metastases in 39% of cases (Monson et al 1991, Talamini et al 1997, Shirai et al 1997). In the presence of lymphatic invasion or positive lymph nodes, the 5 year survival rate is less than 10% while it is superior to 60% when no lymphatic invasion is present (Monson et al 1991, Böttger et al 1997) reaching 80% in early stages (Sperti et al 1994, Chareton et al 1996, Böttger et al 1997). The bad results observed in spite of radical resection for advanced

Table 57.1 Results of radical and local resections of periampullary adenocarcinoma

Reference	Year of report	No. of patients	Hospital mortality	5-year survival
Radical resection				
Warren	1975	93	11%	32%
Nakase	1977	351	16%	6%
Akwari et al	1977	87	13%	34%
Lerut	1984	24	4%	50%
Tarazi et al	1986	46	8%	37%
Shutze et al	1990	520 (collected series)	—	40%
Monson et al	1991	104	6%	34%
Roder et al	1995	66	4.5%	35%
Klempnauer et al	1995	85	9%	38%
Talamini et al	1997	105	3.8%	38%
Böttger et al	1997	31	3%	63%
Local resection				
Wise et al	1976	8	12%	38%
Nakase et al	1977	17	0%	11%
Akwari et al	1977	4	0%	50%
Schlippert	1978	7	14%	50%
Newmann & Pittam	1982	9	11%	43%
Isakson et al	1982	13	7%	17%
Knox & Kingston	1986	25	0%	51%
Robertson & Imrie	1986	8	25%	44%
Koch et al	1991	4	0%	100%

stages or in the presence of lymphatic involvement could perhaps explain that long term survival has been similar or better after local excision in small series (Table 57.1).

A major source of confusion in analyzing the results obtained after local excision is the fact that the term ampullectomy has been applied to different operations such as simple excision of the duodenal mucosa about the ampulla of Vater or wide resection of the papilla encompassing the posterior duodenal wall, the distal end of the biliary duct and the pancreatic duct (Gertsch et al 1990, Branum et al 1996). The wide excision, which should be referred as papilloduodenectomy, provides a specimen with clear anatomical landmarks where the resection's margins can be investigated histologically. One can therefore suspect that the differences between the two types of excisions might have influenced the long-term results.

The treatment of adenomatous polyps of the papilla of Vater represents a dilemma. It is difficult to regard these tumors as benign when one knows that foci of carcinomatous cells have been observed in 30–50% of cases of 'benign' polyps (Delpy et al 1983, Ryan et al 1986). On one hand, one would hesitate to undertake a major operation such as a Whipple's procedure for a small benign-looking tumour which might be benign or harbor a carcinoma in situ, and on the other hand one would be worried leaving behind malignant cells after an incomplete local excision for a potentially curable condition. Failure to recognize malignancy may result in performing an inadequate operation. As preoperative assessment has been considered by some as unreliable both for detecting malignancy and for staging early carcinoma (Rattner et al 1996, Cahen et al 1997, Sauvanet et al 1997), intraoperative assessment of the specimen by frozen section seems of paramount importance. Branum et al (1996) reported 100% accuracy for the diagnosis of adenoma or adenocarcinoma with the combination of preoperative and frozen section biopsies. Unfortunately, other authors were unable to detect malignancy with reliability using similar diagnostic approach (Ryan et al 1986, Asbun et al 1993, Cahen et al 1997, Böttger et al 1997). This raises the question as how to proceed if the pathologist does not confirm the intraoperative diagnosis of benign tumor after local excision. Reoperative pancreaticoduodenectomy has been performed in some instances, with no operative mortality being reported in a series of 29 patients (Robinson et al 1996). It remains that the addition of the risks of two operations should not be part of a therapeutic plan.

What is the place of local resection for neoplasms of the papilla of Vater? Rattner et al (1996) consider that local resection is acceptable for benign tumors smaller than 3 cm and small neuroendocrine tumors. Carcinoids of the papilla of Vater metastatize in lymph nodes and should be resected radically (Ricci 1993).

Well-differentiated carcinomas limited to the mucosa can be treated by local excision (Rattner et al 1996, Böttger et 1997). These criteria put into focus the current difficulty for assessing the tumor characteristics before and during surgery in most institutions. Unless substantial improvements are made in obtaining precise diagnosis and staging, the place of local excision will remain limited mainly to patients unable to support a Whipple's procedure and its complications. In these circumstances papilloduodenectomy offers a reasonable chance of cure for a significant number of patients.

TECHNIQUE OF PAPILLODUODENECTOMY

This operation involves the complete resection of the papilla of Vater (with the sphincter apparatus), the distal bile duct and the pancreatic duct with the surrounding pancreatic tissue (Hunt & Budd 1935, Chatelin 1969, Gertsch et al 1990, Farouk et al 1991, Branum et al 1996) (Fig. 57.1).

Cholecystectomy is performed first, with intra-operative cholangiography so as to delineate intraductal tumor extension and define the anatomy. Leaving the gallbladder in place after resection of the papilla is contraindicated because of the risk of cholecystitis as a result of chronic duodeno-biliary reflux.

The duodenum is mobilized by the Kocher maneuver, and a longitudinal duodenotomy is performed opposite to the region of the ampulla of Vater (Fig. 57.2). Dilatation of both the bile and pancreatic ducts represents an ideal situation since reimplantation of these two structures into the

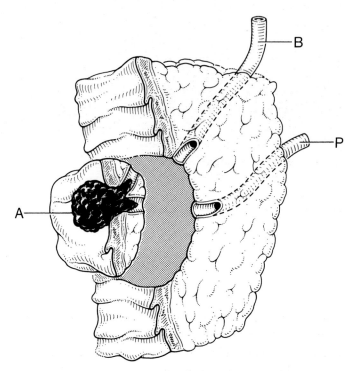

Fig. 57.1 Schematic representation of wide resection of the papilla of Vater, with complete excision of the papilla and sphincter apparatus, of the posterior duodenal wall and terminal segments of the common bile duct (B) and pancreatic duct (P). A, ampulla of Vater, and tumour.

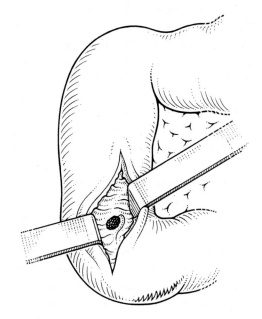

Fig. 57.2 The duodenum is mobilized by the Kocher maneuver and opened longitudinally opposite to the papilla of Vater.

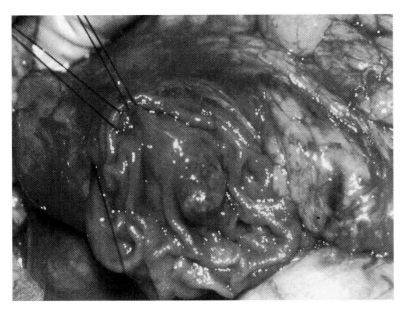

Fig. 57.3 (A) Two stay sutures are placed into the posterior duodenal wall over the distal common bile duct above the papilla.

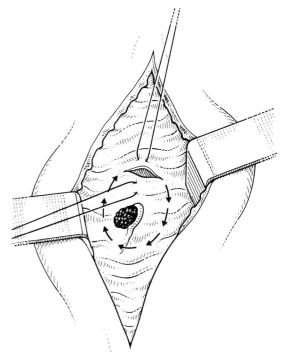

Fig. 57.3 (B) A transverse incision of the posterior duodenal wall at the point of protrusion of the distal choledochus is made between the two stay sutures.

duodenum after resection is facilitated by pre-existent dilatation. When the distal end of the common bile duct is dilated, a bulging protrusion in the suprapapillary duodenal wall can be identified. If necessary, a probe can be introduced through the cystic into the distal bile duct, which allows exact palpation of this structure in all instances.

Two stay sutures are placed into the posterior duodenal wall over the distal common bile duct, above the papilla (Fig. 57.3A). While applying gentle traction on these stay sutures, the posterior duodenal wall and underlying dilated lower bile duct are opened by a 5 mm long transverse incision using diathermy (Fig. 57.3B). The papilla and the tumor are transfixed by a strong stay suture for retraction. An absorbable suture is then passed into the transected duodenal wall and the underlying dilated lower bile duct. The duodenal wall around the papilla is incised further, progressively mobilizing the papilla and opening the bile duct until the pancreatic duct is reached. This maneuver is performed stepwise in 4 mm segments with careful hemostasis using diathermy. This is followed by placing serial interrupted stitches between the duodenal wall and the bile duct (Fig. 57.4). These sutures are not tied until after complete excision of the papilla. Once the pancreatic duct is reached, the inferior part of the common bile duct and the superior part of the pancreatic duct are progressively transected and sutured together using 4-0 polyglycolic acid sutures in order to reconstruct a common opening (Fig. 57.5).

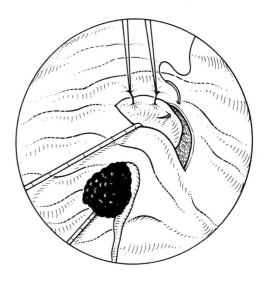

Fig. 57.4 The tumour mass and papilla are pulled downwards by a heavy stay suture. The posterior duodenal wall and underlying distal common bile duct are incised stepwise and sutured together.

During this phase of the operation, the papilla of Vater is progressively separated from its posterior attachments. The excision of the papilla and suturing of the posterior duodenal wall and inferior part of the pancreatic duct are then continued in a similar manner around the papilla to meet the initial point of dissection.

The specimen is carefully examined and frozen section of the specimen and its margin is then obtained. If the margin is not clear, further resection should be performed before the sutures are tied and cut (decision that local resection is insufficient and that radical excision of the tumor requires a duodenopancreatectomy may be taken at this stage of the procedure). Endoscopy of the dilated ducts may also be performed at this time (Fig. 57.6). Once the sutures are cut, the reimplanted ducts retract and visualization is obscured by bulging duodenal mucosa. The duodenum is then closed using continuous single-layer suture or interrupted stitches, and a soft drain is left in situ (Fig. 57.7). The cystic duct is tied; drainage of the common bile duct is

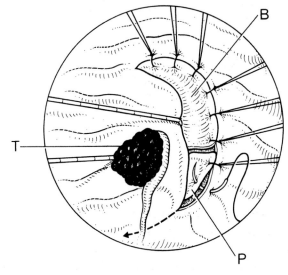

Fig. 57.5 The stepwise incision of the posterior duodenal wall and underlying biliary and pancreatic ducts continue around the papilla until the initial point of dissection is reached. t, T, tumour; p, P, pancreatic duct; b, B, bile duct.

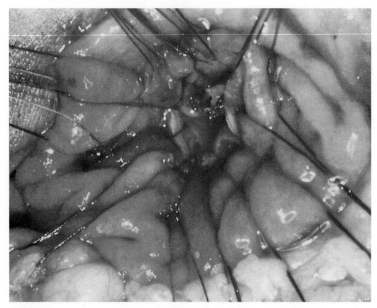

Fig. 57.6 The papilla has been completely excised. Biliary and pancreatic ducts are sutured together and fixed to the duodenal wall; the sutures are tied at the end when a frozen section of the resections margin has proven absence of residual tumour.

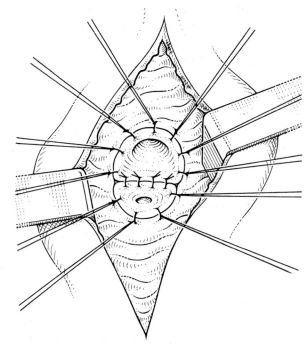

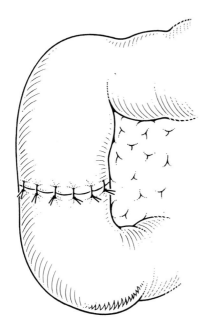

Fig. 57.7 The duodenum is closed with single layer suture.

not necessary. Approximation of the duodenal mucosa with the pancreatic and biliary ducts may be difficult in the absence of ductal dilatation. In this instance loupe magnification is useful for precise reconstruction; a small catheter may be introduced during the resection in one or both ducts, cut short and left within the duodenum (Chatelin 1969).

When papilloduodenectomy is performed for resection of a malignant periampullary tumor, choledochoduodenostomy may prevent biliary obstruction in case of local recurrence (Chatelin 1969).

Postoperative care

Nasogastric aspiration is continued for the first 2–3 days. Feeding can usually be started between the fourth and seventh postoperative days.

CONCLUSION

The technique of papilloduodenectomy presented allows a wide resection of the papilla with 0.5 to 1 cm of the distal bile and pancreatic duct, thus facilitating histologic examination for tumor clearance. Evaluation of local resection of periampullary tumors as a curative operation is thus possible and randomized studies might in future allow for refinement of the indications for this technique.

Papilloduodenectomy, when performed with a precise technique, is a safe operation, which is well suited to selected cases in elderly and frail patients. The hospital stay and costs are significantly lower than after duodenopancreatectomy (Rattner et al 1996, Quirk et al 1997). Conversion to duodenopancreatectomy during the procedure is possible and should be discussed preoperatively.

REFERENCES

Allema J H, Reinders M E, van Gulik T M, van Leeuwen D J, Verbeek P C M, de Wit L T, Gouma D J 1995 Results of pancreaticoduodenectomy for ampullary carcinoma and analysis of prognostic factors for survival. Surgery 117: 247–253

Asbun H J, Rossi R I, Munson J L 1993 Local resection for ampullary tumors. Is there a place for it? Archives of Surgery 128: 515–520

Akwari O K, Van Heerden J P, Adson M A, Baggentoss A H 1977 Radical pancreaticoduodenectomy for cancer of the papilla of Vater. Archives of Surgery 112: 451–456

Alexander F, Rossi R L, O'Brian M, Khettry U, Braash J W, Watkins E 1984 Biliary carcinoma. American Journal of Surgery 147: 503–509

Baczako K, Buchler M, Rampf W 1984 Klinik und Feinstuktur des Papillenkarziomas. Deutsche Mediznische Wochenschrift 109: 1629–1634

Böttger T C, Boddin J, Heintz A, Junginger T 1997 Clinicopathologic study for the assessment of resection for ampullary carcinoma. World Journal of Surgery 21: 379–383

Branum G D, Pappas T N, Meyers W C 1996 The management of tumors of the ampulla of Vater by local resection. Annals of Surgery 224: 621–627

Blumgart L H, Kennedy A 1973 Carcinoma of the ampulla of Vater and duodenum. British Journal of Surgery 60: 33–40

Cahen D L, Fockens P, De Wit L T, Offenhaus G J A, Obertop H, Gouma D J 1997 Local resection or pancreaticoduodenectomy for villous adenoma of the ampulla of Vater diagnosed before operation. British Journal of Surgery 84: 948–951

Chatelin C 1969 Technique de l'ampullectomie. Journal de Chirurgie 141: 645–654

Chareton B, Coiffic J, Landen S, Bardaxoglou E, Campion J P, Launois B 1996 Diagnosis and therapy for ampullary tumors: 63 cases. World Journal of Surgery 20: 707–712

Chiappetta A, Sperti C, Bonadimani B, Pasquali C, Militello C, Petrin P, Pedrazzoli S 1986 Surgical experience with adenocarcinoma of the ampulla of Vater. American Surgeon 52: 603–606.

Dawson P J, Connolly M M 1989 Influence of site of origin and mucin production on survival in ampullary cancer. Annals of Surgery 210: 173–179

Delpy J C, Bruneton J N, Aubanel D, Lecomte P 1983 Vaterian duodenal adenomas. Fortschr Röntgenstr Nuklearmed 138: 623–625

Farouk M, Niotis M, Branum G D, Cotton P B, Meyers W C 1991 Indications for and the technique of local resection of tumors of the papilla of Vater. Archives of Surgery 126: 650–652

Galandiuk S, Hermann R E, Jagelman D G, Fazio V W, Sivak M V 1988 Villous tumors of the duodenum. Annals of Surgery 207: 234–239

Gertsch Ph, Preitner J, Fontolliet C 1987 Carcinome de l'ampoule de Vater et états précurseurs. Schweizerische Medizinische Wochenschrift 117: 1098–1100

Gertsch Ph, Matthews J B, Lerut J, Baer H U 1990 The technique of papilloduodenectomy. Surgery, Gynecology and Obstetrics 170: 254–256

Goldberg M, Zamir O, Hadary A 1987 Wide local excision as an alternative treatment for periampullary carcinoma. American Journal of Gastroenterology 82: 1169–1171

Halsted W S 1899 Contributions to the surgery of the bile passages, especially of the common bile duct. Boston Medical & Surgical Journal 141: 645–654

Hunt V C, Budd J 1935 Transduodenal resection of the ampulla of Vater for carcinoma of the distal end of the common duct. Surgery, Gynecology & Obstetrics 61: 651–661

Iida M, Yao T, Itoh H, Watanabe H, Matsui T, Iwashita A, Fujishima M 1989 Natural history of duodenal lesions in Japanese patients with familial adenomatosis coli (Gardner's syndrome). Gastroenterology 96: 1301–1306

Isaksson G, Ihse I, Andrean-Sandberg A 1982 Local excision for ampullary carcinoma. Acta Chirurgica Scandinavica 148: 163–165

Jones B A, Langer B, Raylor B R, Girotti M 1985 Periampullary tumors: which ones should be resected? The American Journal of Surgery 149: 46–52

Kimura W, Ohtsubo K 1988 Incidence, sites of origin, and immunohistochemical and histochemical characteristics of atypical epithelium and minute carcinoma of the papilla of Vater. Cancer 1988; 1394–1402

Klempnauer J, Ridder G J, Pichlmayer R 1995 Prognostic factors after resection of ampullary carcinoma: multivariate survival analysis in comparison with ductal cancer of the pancreatic head. British Journal of Surgery 82: 1686–1691

Knox R A, Kingston R D 1986 Carcinoma of the ampulla of Vater. British Journal of Surgery 73: 72–73

Koch B, Hildebrandt U, Schüder G, Seitz G, Feifel G 1991 Eingeschränkte chirurgische Radikalität beim okkulten Karzinom der Papilla Vaateri. Langenbecks Archiv für Chirurgie 376: 195–198

Komorowski R A, Beggs B K, Geenan J E, Venu RP 1991 Assessment of ampulla of Vater pathology. An endoscopic approach. The American Journal of Surgery 15: 1188–1196

Kozuka S, Tsubone M, Yamagushi A, Hachisuka K 1981 Adenomatous residue in cancerous papilla of Vater. Gut 22: 1031–1034

Lerut J P, Gianello P R, Otte J B, Kestens P J 1984 Pancreaticoduodenal resection. Surgical experience and evaluation of risk factors in 103 patients. Annals of Surgery 199: 432–437

Matory Y L, Gaynor J, Brennan M 1993 Carcinoma of the ampulla of Vater. Surgery, Gynecology & Obstetrics 177: 366–370

Michelassi F, Erroi F, Dawson P J, Pietrabissa A, Noda S, Handcock M, Block G E 1989 Experience with 647 consecutive tumors of the duodenum, ampulla, head of the pancreas, and distal common bile duct. Annals of Surgery 210: 544–554

Monson J R T, Donohue J H, McEntee G P, McIlrath D C, van Heerden J A, Shorter R G, Nagorney D M, Ilstrup D M 1991 Radical resection for carcinoma of the ampulla of Vater. Archives of Surgery 126: 353–357

Motton G, Veraldi G F, Fracastoro G, Ricci F, Lateraza E, Dorucci V, Cordiano C 1996 Vater's papilla and periampullary area villous adenoma: personal experience about nine cases and review of the literature. Hepato-Gastroenterology 43: 448–455

Nakai T, Koh K, Kawabe E, Son H, Yoshikawa H, Yasutomi M 1997 Importance of microperineural invasion as a prognostic factor in ampullary carcinoma. British Journal of Surgery 84: 1399–1401

Nakao N K, Siegel J H, Stenger R J, Gelb A M 1982 Tumors of the ampulla of Vater: early diagnosis by intrampullary biopsy during endoscopic cannulation. Gastroenterology 83: 459–464

Nakase A, Matsumoto Y, Uchida K, Honjo I 1977 Surgical treatment of cancer of the pancreas and the periampullary region: cumulative results in 57 institutions in Japan. Annals of Surgery 185: 52–57

Newmann R J, Pittam M R 1982 Local excision in the treatment of carcinoma of the ampulla of Vater. Journal of the Royal College of Surgeons 27: 154–157

Nix J A J J, Wilson J H P, Schmitz P I M, Dees J, Hofwijik R 1983 Carcinoma of the papilla of Vater. Fortschr Röntgenstr 138: 531–535

Noda Y, Watanabe H, Iida M 1992 Histologic follow-up of ampullary adenomas in patients with familial adenomatosis coli. Cancer 70: 1847–1856

Ohmori K, Kinoshita H, Shiraha Y, Satake K, 1976 Pancreatic duct obstruction by a benign polypoid adenoma of the ampulla of Vater. American Journal of Surgery 132: 662–663

Perzin K H, Bridge M F 1981 Adenomas of the small intestine. A clinicopathological review of 51 cases and a study of their relationship to carcinoma. Cancer 48: 799–819

Ponchon T, Berger F, Chavaillon A, Bory R, Lambert R 1989 Contribution of endoscopy to diagnosis and treatment of tumors of the ampulla of Vater. Cancer 64: 161–167

Quirk D M, Rattner D W, Fernandez-del Castillo C, Warshaw A L, Brugge W R 1997 The use of endoscopic ultrasonography to reduce the cost for treating ampullary tumors. Gastrointestinal Endoscopy 46: 334–337

Rattner D W, Fernandez-del Castillo C, Brugge W R, Warshaw A L 1996 Defining the criteria for local resection of ampullary neoplasms. Archives of Surgery 113: 366–371

Ricci J L 1993 Carcinoid of the ampulla of Vater. Cancer 71: 686–690

Robertson J F, Imrie C W 1986 Local excision of ampullary carcinoma. Acta Chirurgica Scandinavica 152: 537–539

Robinson E K, Lee J E, Lowy A M, Fenoglio C J, Pisters P W T, Evans D B 1996 Reoperative pancreaticoduodenectomy for periampullary carcinoma. The American Journal of Surgery 172: 432–438

Roder J D, Schneider P M, Stein J H, Sievert J R 1995 Number of lymph node metastases is significantly associated with survival in patients with radically resected carcinoma of the ampulla of Vater. British Journal of Surgery 82: 1693–1696

Rösch T, Braig C, Gain T, Feuerbach S, Sievert J J, Schusdziarra V, Classen M 1992 Staging of pancreatic and ampullary carcinoma by endoscopic ultrasonography. Gastroenterology 102: 188–199

Rosenberg J, Welch J P, Pyrtek L J, Walker M, Trowbridge P 1986 Benign villous adenomas of the ampulla of Vater. Cancer 58: 1563–1568

Ryan D P, Shapiro R H, Warshaw A L 1986 Villous tumors of the duodenum. Annals of Surgery 203: 301–306

Sauvanet A, Chapuis O, Hammel P, Fléjou J-F, Ponsot P, Bernades P, Belghiti J 1997 Are endoscopic procedures able to predict the benignity of ampullary tumors? The American Journal of Surgery 174: 355–358

Schlippert W, Lucke D, Anuras S, Christensen J 1978 Carcinoma of the papilla of Vater. A review of fifty-seven cases. American Journal of Surgery 135: 763–770

Schulten M F, Oyasu R, Beal J M 1976 Villous adenoma of the duodenum. A case report and review of the literature. American Journal of Surgery 132: 90–96

Seifert E, Schulte F, Stolte M 1992 Adenoma and carcinoma of the duodenum and papilla of Vater: A clinicopathological study. The American Journal of Gastroenterology 87: 37–42

Sellner F, Machacek E 1986 Zur Entstehung der Karzinome de Papilla Vateri über eine Adenom-Karzinom-Sequenz. Viener Klinische Wochenschrift 98: 182–187

Shirai Y, Ohtani T, Tsukada K, Hatakeyama K 1997 Patterns of lymphatic spread of carcinoma of the ampulla of Vater. British Journal of Surgery 84: 1012–1016

Shutze W P, Sack J, Aldrete J S 1990 Long-term follow-up of 24 patients undergoing radical resection for ampullary carcinoma. Cancer 66: 1717–1720

Sperti C, Pasquali C, Piccoli A, Sernagiotto C, Pedrazzoli S 1994 Radical resection for ampullary carcinoma: long-term results. British Journal of Surgery 81: 668–671

Talamini M A, Moesinger R C, Pitt H A, Sohn T A, Hruban R H, Lillemoe K D, Yeo C J, Cameron J L 1997 Adenocarcinoma of the ampulla of Vater. A 28-year experience. Annals of Surgery 225: 590–600

Tarazi R Y, Hermann R E, Vogt D P, Hoerr S O, Esselstyn C B, Coopermann A M, Steiger E, Grundfest S 1986 Results of surgical treatment of periampullary tumors: a thirty-five year experience. Surgery 100: 716–723

Warren K W, Braasch J W, Thum C W 1968 Carcinoma of the pancreas. Surgical Clinics of North America 48: 601–618

Warren K W, Choe D S, Plaza J, Relihan M 1975 Results of radical resection for periampullary cancer. Annals of Surgery 181: 534–540

Whipple A O, Parsons W B, Mullins C R 1935 Treatment of carcinoma of the ampulla of Vater. Annals of Surgery 102: 763–779

Wise L, Pizzimbono C, Dehner L P 1976 Periampullary cancer. A clinicopathologic study of sixty-two patients. The American Journal of Surgery 131: 141–148

58

Percutaneous intubational techniques in biliary and periampullary cancer

R. Ó LAOIDE, E. VANSONNENBERG

Percutaneous transhepatic cholangiography (PTC) (Ch. 17) is the parent procedure from which other palliative procedures in the management of malignant biliary tract obstruction have evolved. The first PTC was performed by Huard & Do-Xuan-Hop in 1937. Subsequently, several investigators noted that the plastic cannula of the sheathed PTC needle could be left within the bile ducts for temporary decompression of an obstructed biliary tree prior to surgery, thereby avoiding intraperitoneal bile leakage. The advantages of this approach for long-term external biliary drainage were described by Carter & Saypol in 1952. Molnar & Stockum published their results with internalization of external biliary drainage in 1974. Since then, refinements in instrumentation, techniques and clinical management have increased the safety and efficacy of percutaneous biliary drainage (PBD).

TECHNIQUE OF PBD (see also Ch. 29)

PATIENT PREPARATION

The normalization of abnormal clotting studies and the use of preprocedural antibiotics are two of the factors that have led to the increased safety of PBD. The prothrombin time should not be greater than 3 seconds above control, the activated partial thromboplastin time not greater than 42 seconds, and platelets should be over $50\,000/\text{cm}^3$. Coagulation abnormalities secondary to biliary obstruction can frequently be reversed by using parenteral vitamin K. If this is not successful, or if emergency biliary drainage is required, fresh frozen plasma should be given both before and during the procedure.

Up to one-third of patients with malignant biliary stricture have infected bile. Thus, broad-spectrum parenteral antibiotics should be administered preprocedure, ideally for 24 hours. PBD may be performed under sedoanalgesia, epidural anesthesia, or general anesthesia; the preferred choice frequently reflects the local anesthetic arrangements. The presence of an anesthesiologist during epidural or general anesthesia ensures optimal monitoring of the patient, and optimal treatment of hemodynamic or respiratory complications, should they arise.

PBD PROCEDURE

Traditionally, biliary drainage is performed using fluoroscopic guidance. The biliary tract is punctured blindly using a fine 22 gauge needle and subsequently is opacified with dilute contrast medium. Multiple passes are commonly required before a duct is punctured when fluoroscopic guidance alone is used. Overdistention of the biliary tree is avoided by injecting an amount of contrast medium just sufficient to make a diagnosis. The subsequent cholangiogram is then used to select an appropriate duct for biliary drainage. In most patients, a right hepatic duct is punctured using a right intercostal approach. Occasionally, segmental or lobar biliary obstruction, ascites or a previous history of surgery on the right ductal system dictates that a left duct be punctured using a left subxiphoid approach. The target duct is punctured using an 18 gauge sheath needle, allowing a one-step introduction of a 0.038 inch (0.965 mm) guidewire.

More recently, ultrasound has been used as a guidance modality for biliary drainage (Fig. 58.1). In contrast to fluoroscopically guided PBD, ultrasound-guided PBD is usually performed via the left hepatic duct rather than a right duct. Although ultrasound-guided PBD through the right hepatic system has been described, it is more difficult to perform. The advantage of ultrasound is that a horizontally oriented dilated duct can be selected and punctured

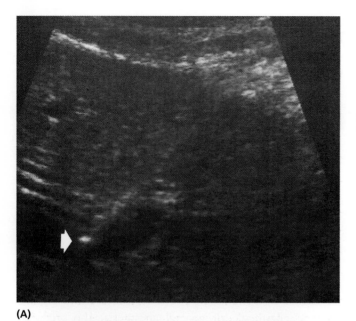

(A)

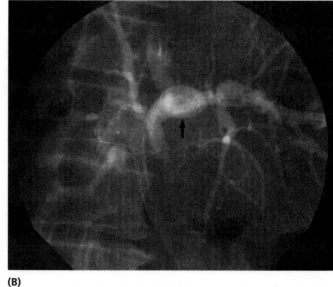

(B)

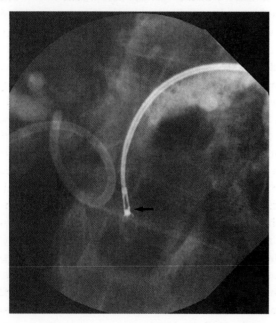

(C)

Fig. 58.1 Right and left-sided PBD for high malignant obstruction. **(A)** A dilated left-sided bile duct is punctured under ultrasound guidance using a 22 gauge needle (arrow). **(B)** A cholangiogram confirms obstruction of the left hepatic ductal system and external drainage from the left side was performed. The locking pigtail catheter (arrow) is identified with a dilated duct. **(C)** Right-sided PBD is then performed. A biopsy forceps were placed (arrow) through the left tract. Final diagnosis was hilar cholangiocarcinoma.

peripherally, using a fine 22 gauge needle. A cholangiogram can then be performed. Using a coaxial access system, the same puncture site can be used for biliary drainage. The coaxial access system is used so that a working 0.038 inch guide-wire can be advanced into the bile duct. Initially, a 0.018 inch (0.457 mm) guide-wire is inserted through the 22 gauge needle; using a variety of tapered dilators and sheaths over the 0.018 inch guide-wire, the system can be converted to one that utilizes a 0.038 inch guide-wire. This method avoids blind PTC in most patients, obviating the need for multiple punctures. The use of a coaxial access system rather than direct puncture with a large 18 gauge

sheathed needle probably helps to reduce the incidence of bleeding and sepsis.

The advantages of a left subxiphoid approach include the ability to use ultrasound guidance, and utilization of the more frequently horizontal orientation of the left ductal system compared to the right. The latter facilitates catheterization, permits better purchase into the duct, and allows for a 'downhill' cholangiogram as contrast medium flows from left to right in the supine position. In addition, the left-sided approach is preferable in patients with ascites as technical difficulties during the procedure, such as buckling of guide-wires or catheters in the ascitic fluid, and the risk of postprocedure pericatheter leakage are reduced. Finally, use of the left-sided approach markedly reduces the chances of traversing the pleura. A relative disadvantage of the left-sided approach is the increased risk of radiation exposure to the hands of the operator. By placing the patient in an oblique position, or by using a C arm, this risk can be minimized. Ultrasound-guided PBD using a left-sided approach is currently the preferred method of PBD in our institution.

After a 0.038 inch guide-wire has been advanced into the biliary system, a decision must be made as to whether the obstruction should be crossed or not. In patients with suspected cholangitis, no attempt should be made to cross the stricture; in these patients, the goal is generally to provide external drainage with a minimal amount of manipulation within the biliary tract. This allows drainage of the biliary tree proximal to the site of obstruction. If cholangitis is not a concern, an attempt should be made to cross the stricture to provide internal/external drainage. Internal/external catheters have side-holes positioned above and below the stricture; this allows bile to flow in an antegrade fashion into the duodenum. In difficult cases, a hydrophilic-coated guide-wire (Terumo) is particularly useful to negotiate an obstruction. Occasionally the stricture cannot be passed at the first session; however, after a 3–4 day period of external drainage, most strictures can be traversed.

POSTPROCEDURE CARE

After an external or internal/external biliary catheter has been placed, it is connected to a drainage bag. The patient is observed closely on the ward for evidence of hemorrhage, bile leak, or sepsis. Patients are generally maintained on antibiotics for at least 48–72 hours after the procedure. The catheter is placed to external drainage until hemobilia has cleared and cholangitis has resolved. Most patients can be discharged from the hospital within 48 hours. After discharge, catheter irrigation should be performed daily with sterile saline. Patients are usually seen for follow-up at 2–4 monthly intervals as out-patients.

INDICATIONS FOR PBD

PBD may be performed either as a temporary or long-term procedure in patients with malignant biliary tract obstruction. Temporary drainage is performed in selected patients in whom further therapeutic maneuvers are being considered such as operation, chemotherapy or radiotherapy. Long-term biliary drainage is performed as a palliative procedure in those patients with advanced malignancy.

INDICATIONS FOR TEMPORARY BILIARY DRAINAGE

The notion that preoperative PBD reduces the morbidity and mortality of subsequent palliative or curative surgical operation for biliary obstruction has been seriously questioned. The risk factors in patients undergoing surgical decompression of the biliary tract include sepsis and renal failure (Cheng-His Su et al 1992). Although PBD lowers the serum bilirubin level, and improves both renal and hepatic function (Denning et al 1981, Smith et al 1985), it is controversial whether these changes translate into a better prognosis for patients undergoing palliative or curative surgery. In addition, the risks of PBD must be taken into account when assessing the potential benefits as a preoperative procedure.

Early retrospective studies strongly suggested that patients should be decompressed prior to surgery (Nakayama et al 1978, Denning et al 1981). Since then, however, there have been four prospective randomized trials, three of which demonstrated no reduction in morbidity and mortality in patients undergoing PBD prior to surgery (Hatfield et al 1982, McPherson et al 1984, Pitt et al 1985). In the majority of these patients, only external biliary drainage was used. Since absence of bile salts in the bowel promotes the growth of anaerobic bacteria and therefore the incidence of endotoxemia in jaundiced patients, it is possible that internal drainage may be more advantageous (Gouma et al 1987). Internal drainage was used in the fourth randomized prospective study by Smith et al (1985). There were fewer complications in patients undergoing surgery after PBD; however, this advantage was partially offset by the complications of PBD.

More recently, Foschi et al (1986) in a randomized prospective trial demonstrated a reduction in the post-operative morbidity and mortality in patients undergoing combined PBD and hyperalimentation compared with patients undergoing PBD alone prior to surgery. Although biliary drainage generally is not performed as a routine preoperative procedure, it does appear to have a role in patients with evidence of cholangitis, marked hyperbilirubinemia (20 mg/dL), and possibly in patients with impaired renal function (Pitt et al 1985, Smith et al 1985).

Placement of a PBD catheter also may be useful during operation in patients undergoing complex bilioenteric anastomosis. The surgeon can palpate the catheter at surgery, thereby helping identification of the structures. However, some surgeons including the editors consider that preoperative PBD increases the difficulty of operation by reducing the size of the bile ducts and makes bilœnteric anastomosis more difficult, and is, in any event, unnecessary to locate ducts (Ch. 54).

Patients with malignant biliary obstruction secondary to tumours that are responsive to chemotherapy or radiotherapy, such as lymphoma or oat cell metastases, are potential candidates for temporary PBD. The procedure may be indicated because of pruritus and/or cholangitis prior to definitive therapy. In addition, patients who require chemotherapeutic agents that are excreted into the bile also may benefit from temporary PBD.

INDICATIONS FOR LONG-TERM PBD

The indications and utilization of PBD for long-term palliative treatment of malignant biliary obstruction must be considered with respect to available surgical and endoscopic alternatives. The type of malignancy and the site of obstruction are factors influencing the appropriate palliative procedure.

Pancreatic carcinoma

Pancreatic carcinoma (Chs 55, 56) is the most frequent cause of malignancy biliary tract obstruction. Fewer than 20% of patients with pancreatic carcinoma have resectable tumours at the time of presentation. The mean duration of survival is 5–6 months (Watanapa & Williamson 1992). Advances in both pancreatic imaging and in percutaneous biopsy and in pre-exploratory laparoscopy have reduced the necessity for explorative laparotomy for the diagnosis and assessment of resectability of pancreatic carcinoma (Fig. 58.2). During PBD, percutaneous brush or forceps biopsy may be performed to confirm the clinical and radiological diagnosis of a malignant stricture. Sensitivity rates from 60 to 100% have been reported using these techniques (Mendez et al 1980, Terasaki et al 1991). Bile samples may be collected for cytological examination. This is a simple, inexpensive method to confirm a malignant stricture; however, the detection rate is only 34% (Muro et al 1983).

Patients who are unfit for laparotomy, because of extensive disease, age or general debilitation, are typically referred for PBD; surgical bypass is usually performed in fit patients. Thus, patient selection makes comparison of the efficacy of surgical versus percutaneous procedures difficult.

In a review of the literature published between 1981 and 1990, Watanapa & Williamson (1992) found that the mean

operative mortality associated with surgical bypasss for pancreatic carcinoma was 14% (range 0–26%). In general, procedure-related mortality is lower with PBD (0–6%) (Wittich et al 1985). Similarly, periprocedural morbidity is generally lower with PBD (5–20%), compared with surgical bypass (6–65%) (Wittich et al 1985, Watanapa & Williamson 1992).

The choice of PBD versus endoscopic drainage is largely dependent on the availability of local expertise. While some studies have shown fewer complications with endoscopic drainage, these data must be balanced by the realization that percutaneous drainage is frequently performed after a failed endoscopic attempt, and that PBD is more likely to be successful than endoscopic drainage. Cholangitis after failed endoscopic drainage increases the risks of percutaneous drainage.

PBD often has a role in postoperative patients for pancreatic malignancy. If laparotomy alone has been performed for assessment of resectability and biliary obstruction subsequently develops, PBD may be utilized for palliation. In addition, when surgical bypasss is not technically feasible at the time of operation, or if a recurrent obstruction develops after an initially successful surgical bypass, PBD may obviate further surgery.

Periampullary tumors and cholangiocarcinoma (Ch. 55)

Periampullary tumors (other than pancreatic head carcinoma) arise in the ampulla, distal common bile duct, or

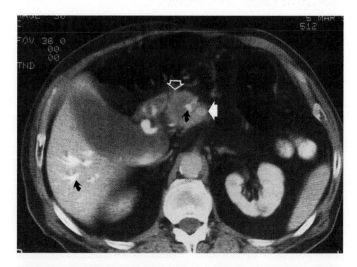

Fig. 58.2 Inoperable pancreatic carcinoma. A low-attenuated mass (open arrow) is identified in the region of the pancreatic head. A clear fat plane is not identified between the mass and the superior mesenteric artery (white arrow), indicating inoperability. Residual contrast medium is identified within the pancreatic and biliary ducts after endoscopic retrograde cholangiopancreatography (curved black arrows).

duodenum. Patients with such lesions have a better prognosis than patients who have pancreatic carcinoma; 5 year survival rates of 20–40% have been reported (Jones et al 1985). Because these tumors are often resectable, an aggressive surgical approach is advocated (Jones et al 1985, Michelassi et al 1989).

The prognosis for cholangiocarcinoma in the proximal biliary tract (Ch. 54) is not as favorable as for periampullary adenocarcinoma (Braasch 1973). Tumor extension or a high surgical risk precludes resection in about 80% of patients (Ottow et al 1985). Extension of tumor proximally, leading to bilateral involvement of the hepatic ducts beyond the second-order branches, contraindicates resection (Bismuth et al 1988). In such patients, PBD is advantageous because drainage of both the right and left lobes can be achieved. Complete drainage of both the left and the right lobe using endoscopy is accomplished in only 25% of patients (Huibregtse & Tytgat 1989). An undrained or partially undrained segment leaves the patient at risk of developing cholangitis. When multisite intrahepatic obstruction exists, the quality of life may be so compromised by the presence of multiple catheters that the risk of cholangitis is outweighed (Fig. 58.3). When segmental obstruction is associated with an atrophic liver segment or with extensive tumor involvement of a segment, percutaneous drainage of that segment is not usually performed. Percutaneously placed catheters may also be used as a conduit for the application of local radiotherapy, such as iridium-192 wires (Lameris et al 1991).

Metastatic biliary obstruction

Metastatic biliary obstruction may be secondary to lung, breast or ovarian carcinomas. Such patients usually have widespread malignancy and are therefore inoperable and have a dismal prognosis. Biliary drainage is therefore a strictly palliative procedure, and is only indicated in the context of severe pruritus or cholangitis.

CONTRAINDICATIONS

BLEEDING DIATHESIS

As bleeding is one of the possible major complications of PBD, the procedure should not be performed in the presence of a bleeding diathesis. As previously mentioned, parenteral vitamin K or fresh frozen plasma should be given prior to the procedure to correct coagulation abnormalities.

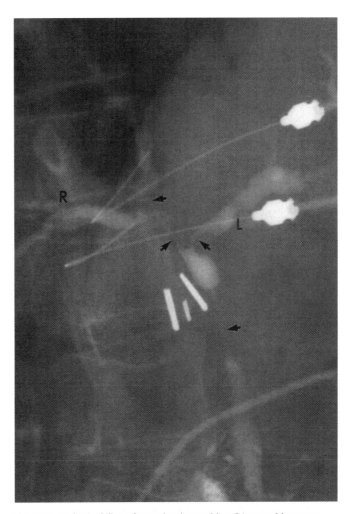

Fig. 58.3 Multi-site biliary obstruction (arrows) in a 31-year-old woman with metastatic breast carcinoma. L, left hepatic duct; R, right hepatic duct.

ASCITES

Ascites is a relative contraindication to PBD. When performing right-sided PBD, the procedure is technically more difficult due to buckling of guide-wires and catheters in the ascitic fluid. This leads to an increased risk of hemorrhage and intraperitoneal bile leakage. After the procedure, pericatheter leakage of ascites may occur, especially if relief of obstruction does not lead to some resolution of the ascites. This may be a chronic and bothersome problem. As previously mentioned, left-sided drainage may help to avoid these difficulties.

RESULTS

As a rule, effective biliary drainage is achieved in over 90% of patients (Ferrucci et al 1980, Clark et al 1981, Mueller et al

1982, Ogelvie et al 1992). The bilirubin level usually falls to 50% of the initial value within 10 days of the procedure. Diffuse metastatic disease of the liver or underlying hepatic dysfunction may, however, preclude a good response. Pruritus usually disappears within 24–48 hours following drainage. In patients with cholangitis, clinical improvement with deeffervescence is generally seen within 24–48 hours (Ferrucci et al 1980).

COMPLICATIONS

Complications after PBD may be classified as acute or delayed. Acute complications occur in 5–20% of patients, and include bleeding (1–4%), septicemia (3–10%), bile peritonitis (1–2%) and procedure-related death (0–5%) (Ferrucci et al 1980, Mueller et al 1985, Wittich et al 1985). Preventive measures to avoid hemorrhage include correction of coagulation abnormalities, the use of small caliber coaxial access systems, and puncturing a peripheral duct to prevent damage to a central large vessel.

Hemorrhage into the bile duct (Ch. 70) is frequently due to undesired retrograde catheter movement that results in side-holes communicating with portal or hepatic veins. Repositioning of the catheter so that the side-holes are within the duct will alleviate this problem. Rarely, hepatic angiography is required for bleeding; embolization may be indicated if a defined bleeding source is demonstrated.

Sepsis is avoided by the use of periprocedural antibiotics, avoidance of overdistension of the biliary tree during PTC and PBD, and minimal manipulation in a known infected system. Antibiotics and external drainage are usually effective treatments in these cases. The incidence of bile peritonitis is reduced by avoiding an extrahepatic puncture and by performing a PBD if a PTC shows a high-grade obstruction. The risk of bile peritonitis is also reduced by performing a PBD when biliary pressures are elevated above 35–40 cm of saline. In addition, correct positioning of the catheter side-holes, so that none are extrahepatic, prevents bile peritonitis.

Delayed complications of PBD include cholangitis secondary to catheter occlusion (4–45%), catheter dislodgement (10–20%), and pericatheter leakage (10–30%) (Ferrucci et al 1980, Mueller et al 1985, Wittich et al 1985). These problems are relatively easy to remedy with an internal/external catheter. Regular irrigation with 3–5 ml of sterile saline, the use of large-caliber catheters (10–14F), elective catheter exchanges every 2–4 months, and preprocedural antibiotics during catheter exchange help to reduce the incidence of delayed complications. In addition, locking catheters effectively prevent dislodgement. Local skin infections, granulomas and tumor tracking at the catheter entry site may occur occasionally.

Infrequent complications after PBD include pseudo-aneurysms, pneumothorax, intra or perihepatic abscess, or pancreatitis. Electrolyte imbalance may occasionally be a problem in the acute situation after PBD when there is external drainage only; however, this is relieved after the catheter is clamped and antegrade drainage into the duodenum is achieved with internal drainage. Tumor implantation into the skin and peritoneum have been reported, but is exceedingly rare (Oleaga et al 1980, Miller et al 1983).

BILIARY ENDOPROSTHESES

By definition, external/internal catheter drainage requires a protruding catheter; this system has potential associated problems that include local pain, irritation, infection, peritubal leakage, and catheter dislodgement. To overcome these problems, an indwelling stent (endoprosthesis) was proposed as an alternative to internal/external catheter drainage (Pereiras et al 1978, Burcharth et al 1978, Fig. 58.4). The ideal stent should bypass the obstruction, remain in place, and maintain patency. After initial enthusiasm for stent placement, it soon became clear that these devices were far from ideal (Mendez et al 1984). The advantage of an internalized bypass is counterbalanced by the disadvantages of migration, poor long-term patency, and the necessity for repeat biliary drainage or endoscopy to remedy these problems periodically. More recently, expandable metal stents have been introduced as an alternative to conventional plastic endoprostheses to reduce the aforementioned problems.

INDICATIONS FOR BILIARY ENDOPROSTHESES

The decision to place an indwelling biliary endoprosthesis rather than an external/internal biliary drainage requires an individual approach for each patient. The mean duration of stent patency using conventional plastic endoprotheses is 5–6 months (Mueller et al 1985, Lammer & Neumayer 1986); therefore, a patient with a short life expectancy is more suitable for this technique. Other indications for endoprosthesis placement include ascites, inability to perform catheter care, and patient choice. Some patients see a protruding catheter as a constant reminder of their disease, while other patients see it as a potential lifeline and elect for internal/external catheter drainage.

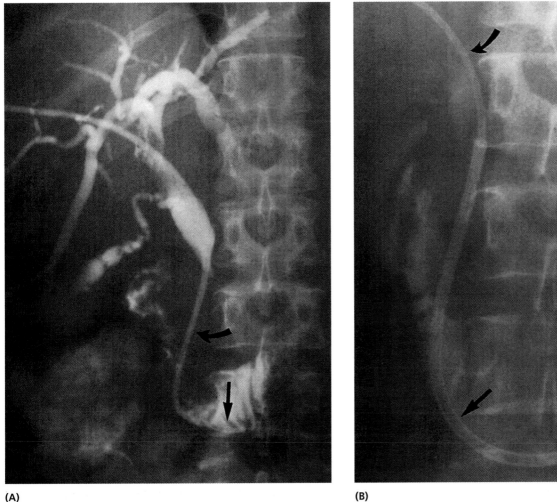

(A)

(B)

Fig. 58.4 Internal/external drainage and placement of a plastic endoprosthesis in a patient with biliary obstruction secondary to pancreatic carcinoma. **(A)** An internal/external catheter, with its distal end in the duodenum (straight arrow) traverses a distal common bile duct structure secondary to pancreatic carcinoma (curved arrow). **(B)** Subsequently, the internal/external catheter was exchanged for a plastic endoprosthesis (straight arrow). There is a proximal protective catheter (curved arrow) that was removed 3 days after the procedure.

CONVENTIONAL PLASTIC ENDOPROSTHESES

After a catheter cholangiogram has been performed, a stiff guide-wire is advanced through the external/internal catheter into the duodenum and the catheter is removed. Subsequently, the tract is widened either with serial or coaxial dilators or by balloon dilatation. The final size of the tract needs to be as large as the outer diameter of the proposed plastic endoprosthesis; this is usually 13–16 Fr. The endoprosthesis is positioned across the obstruction through a transhepatically placed peel-away sheath with a pusher catheter system. Following insertion of the endoprosthesis, percutaneous access is maintained via a 'protective catheter' until hemobilia has cleared and clamping of the protective catheter has been well tolerated.

Major complications of biliary endoprostheses are really those of PBD. In addition, there are two further complications of endoprostheses – occlusion and migration. The incidence of occlusion is 6–23%, with a mean duration of patency of 5–6 months (Mueller et al 1985, Lammer & Neumayer 1986). Occlusion is primarily caused by bile encrustation and/or biliary sludge. Factors that influence occlusion include stent material and inner diameter. Experiments by Lammer et al (1986) suggested that polyurethane and perculflex are the least likely materials to occlude, and teflon and polyethylene the most likely to occlude. Endoprostheses with a smaller inner diameter are associated with a higher rate of obstruction. Other factors related to occlusion include the presence of infection, the local biochemical environment, and whether the distal end of the endoprosthesis is within the duodenum. Attempts to manipulate these variables have included the use of antibiotic-impregnated endoprostheses and alteration of bile pH.

Migration of plastic endoprostheses occurs in 3–6% of patients (Mueller et al 1985, Lammer & Neumayer 1986). Several retention devices have been used to prevent migration; these include V-shaped notches, Malecot tips, and subcutaneous anchoring devices.

EXPANDABLE METALLIC ENDOPROSTHESES

Metal stents are currently being used increasingly in the treatment of malignant biliary tract obstruction (Fig. 58.5). The rationale for their use is the capability to introduce a large-diameter stent over a small introducer system.

The stents are compressed prior to insertion and expand to their full diameter only after deployment. Metallic endoprostheses have several theoretical advantages. The expanded luminal diameter of metallic stents is 10–12 mm. This compares favorably with the diameter of conventional plastic stents (4–7 mm). In view of the recognized correlation between luminal diameter and patency rates in plastic endoprostheses, the larger diameter of metallic stents might be expected to improve the patency rates.

Early results however did not match this expectation, with stent occlusion reported in 42–50% of patients (Irving et al 1989, Gilliams et al 1990). Subsequent studies cited lower occlusion rates of 7–15% and a mean duration of patency of 4–8 months (Adam et al 1991, Lameris et al 1991, Rossi et al 1994). These figures are similar to previous results reported with the use of conventional plastic endoprostheses. More recent studies have reported a mean duration of patency of 10–12 months (Mathieson et al 1994, Lee et al 1997) possibly reflecting an increased understanding of the technical requirements for optimal stent insertion.

Metal stents are introduced via a 7–10 Fr tract, depending on the type of metal stent that is deployed and whether or not a protective outer sheath is used. In contrast, tract dilatation up to 16 Fr may be required to insert a 14 Fr plastic endoprostheses. The smaller delivery system for metallic stents offers several potential advantages including a reduction in pain and discomfort during tract dilatation, a decrease in the number of early complications, and an ability to perform biliary drainage and stent insertion at one sitting. The incidence of early complications associated with plastic endoprostheses has been reported to be 9–17%, while the incidence of early complications associated with metallic stents is 6–16% (Mueller et al 1985, Lammer et al 1990, Lameris et al 1991, Rossi et al 1994, Lee et al 1997).

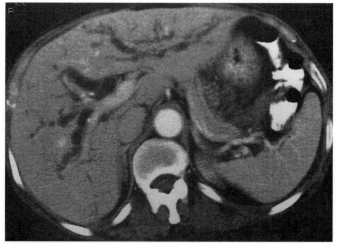

(A)

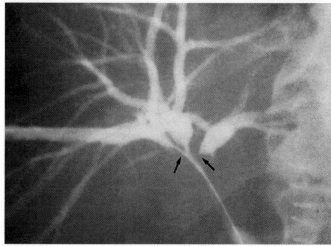

(B)

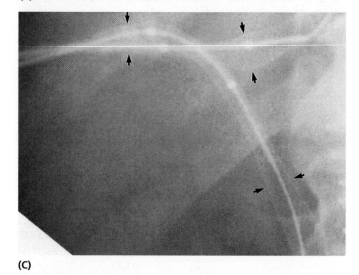

(C)

Fig. 58.5 Percutaneous metal stents for palliation of inoperable cholangiocarcinoma in an elderly man. **(A)** A computed tomography (CT) scan demonstrates dilatation of both left and right intrahepatic bile ducts. **(B)** A cholangiogram shows evidence of obstruction of the left and right hepatic ducts (arrows). **(C)** Two Wallstents (arrows) have been placed via the right hepatic duct.

Some, but not all, authors have placed metallic stents during the initial procedure in up to 88% of patients (Gordon et al 1992).

Metal stents are composed of a mesh of stainless steel wires. The surface area of their wall is compared to plastic endoprostheses. In addition, metal stents may be incorporated into the bile duct wall, further reducing the exposed surface area. This has the potential advantage of reducing the rate of infection, as bacteria deposition on the stent wall is thought to be an initiating factor in cholangitis. Some studies have demonstrated a reduction in the incidence of late cholangitis in patients with metallic stents when compared to the incidence in patients with plastic stents (Knyrim et al 1993, Wagner et al 1993, Rossi et al 1994). In contrast to plastic endoprostheses, migration has not been a problem with metal stents.

The cause of occlusion in metallic stents primarily is tumor overgrowth, rather than bile encrustation as occurs in plastic endoprostheses. The longest possible stent should be used, as this reduces the likelihood of tumor overgrowth at either end of the stent. Stents are available in various lengths and may be used coaxially to elongate the distance they bridge.

Metal stents are much more expensive than plastic endoprostheses. The advocates of metal stents suggest that the shorter hospital stay associated with insertion of a metal stent at one sitting, and the reduced incidence of delayed complications necessitating further hospital readmissions, may make their use cost effective (Lee et al 1992, Knyrim et al 1993, Wagner et al 1993, Rossi et al 1994). The final role of metal stents in the treatment of malignant biliary obstruction has yet to be ascertained, and larger series with more extended follow-up periods are necessary to evaluate their overall role.

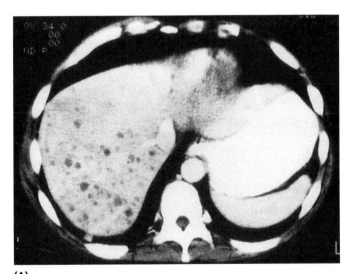

(A)

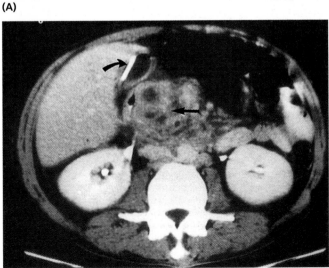

(C)

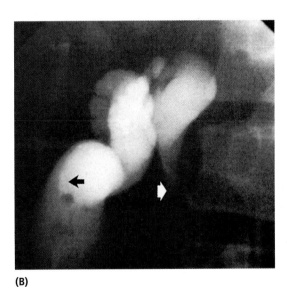

(B)

Fig. 58.6 Percutaneous cholecystostomy for biliary decompression in a 40-year-old man with pancreatic carcinoma, who has obstructive jaundice and extrahepatic bile duct dilatation. **(A)** A CT scan shows multiple areas of low attenuation within the liver, representing cholangitic abscesses. Dilated intrahepatic bile ducts are difficult to identify and therefore decompression was performed via the gallbladder. **(B)** A catheter (black arrow) is identified within the gallbladder. A subsequent catheter cholecystocholangiogram shows a stricture of the distal end of the dilated common bile duct (white arrow). **(C)** A follow-up CT scan shows the catheter within the gallbladder (curved arrow). A complex mass is seen in the pancreatic head consistent with a pancreatic carcinoma (straight arrow).

PERCUTANEOUS CHOLECYSTOSTOMY FOR BILIARY DISEASE (see also Ch. 41)

Decompression of the biliary tract via the gallbladder is useful in selected patients (vanSonnenberg et al 1990). When there is distal biliary obstruction with negligible or minimally dilated bile ducts and a dilated gallbladder, this method is superior to transhepatic biliary drainage for rapid decompression (Fig. 58.6). Percutaneous cholecystostomy (PC) is preferable because difficulty in accessing and cannulating a non-dilated system by the transphepatic route may result in a prolonged, painful and poorly tolerated procedure. Most radiologists prefer to defer standard PBD until the ducts are dilated. However, in the presence of cholangitis or severe pruritus, urgent drainage may be required. Although endoscopic drainage may be used in these situations, it fails in 10–20% of attempted patients. In such patients, or where endoscopic drainage is not available, PC is extremely useful. Drainage by PC can be achieved in 5–15 minutes. Because internalization via the cystic duct is difficult, the procedure is best reserved for preoperative patients or if patients are acutely ill.

REFERENCES

Adam A, Chetty N, Roddie M, Yeung E, Benjamin I S 1991 Self expandable stainless steel endoprostheses for treatment of malignant bile duct obstruction. American Journal of Roentgenology 156: 321–325

Bismuth H, Castaing D, Traynor O 1988 Resection or palliation: priority of surgery in treatment of hilar cancer. World Journal of Surgery 12: 39–47

Braasch J W 1973 Carcinoma of the bile duct. Surgical Clinics of North America 53: 1217–1227

Burcharth F 1978 A new endoprosthesis for nonoperative intubation of the biliary tree in the malignant obstructive jaundice. Surgery, Gynecology and Obstetrics 146: 76–78

Carter R F, Saypol M G 1952 Transabdominal cholangiography. Journal of the American Medical Association 148: 253–255

Cheng-His S U, Fang-Ku P, Wing-Yiu L 1992 Factors affecting morbidity and mortality in biliary tract surgery. World Journal of Surgery 16: 536–540

Clark R A, Mitchell S E, Colley D P, Alexander E 1981 Percutaneous catheter biliary decompression. American Journal of Roentgenology 137: 503–509

Denning D A, Ellison E C, Carey L C 1981 Preoperative percutaneous transhepatic biliary decompression lowers operative morbidity in patients with obstructive jaundice. American Journal of Surgery 141: 61–65

Ferrucci J T, Mueller P R, Harbin W P 1980 Percutaneous transphepatic biliary drainage. Radiology 135: 1–13

Foschi D, Cavagna G, Callioni F, Morandi E, Rovati V 1986 Hyperalimentation of jaundiced patients on percutaneous transhepatic biliary drainage. British Journal of Surgery 73: 716–719

Gilliams A, Dick R, Dooley J S, Wallsten H, El-Din A 1990 Self-expandable stainless steel braided endoprosthesis for biliary strictures. Radiology 174: 137–140

Gordon R L, Ring E J, LaBerge J M, Doherty M M 1992 Malignant biliary obstruction: treatment with expandable metallic stent – follow-up of 50 consecutive patients. Radiology 182: 697–701

Gouma D J, Coelho J C U, Schlegel J F, Li Y F, Moody F G 1987 The effect of preoperative internal and external biliary drainage on mortality of jaundiced rats. Archives of Surgery 122: 731–734

Hatfield A R W, Terblanche J, Fataar S et al 1982 Preoperative external biliary drainage in obstructive jaundice. Lancet ii: 896–899

Huard P, Do-Xuan-Hop 1937 La ponction transhepatique des canaux biliares. Bulletin de la Societe Medico-chirugicale de l'Indochine 15: 785–803

Huibregtse K, Tytgat G U 1989 Endoscopic biliary drainage (Amsterdam). In: Lygidakis N J, Tytgat J U (eds) Hepatobiliary and pancreatic malignancies: diagnosis, medical and surgical management. Thieme Verlag, Stuttgart, p 429–438

Irving J D, Adam A, Dick R, Dondelinger R F, Lunderquist A, Roche A 1989 Gianturco expandable metallic biliary stents: results of a European clinical trial. Radiology 172: 321–326

Jones B A, Langer B, Taylor B R, Girotti M 1985 Periampullary tumors: which ones should be resected? American Journal of Surgery 149: 46–52

Knyrim K, Wagner H J, Pausch J, Vakil N 1993 A prospective, randomized, controlled trial of metal stents for malignant obstruction of the common bile duct. Endoscopy 25: 207–212

Lameris J S, Stoker J, Nijs H G T et al 1991 Malignant biliary obstruction: percutaneous use of self expandable stents. Radiology 179: 703–707

Lammer J, Neumayer K 1986 A biliary drainage endoprostheses: experience with 201 placements. Radiology 159: 625–629

Lammer J, Stoffler G, Petek W W, Hofler H 1986 In vitro long term perfusion of different materials for biliary endoprostheses. Investigative Radiology 21: 329–331

Lammer J, Klein G E, Kleinert R, Hausegger K, Einspieler R 1990 Obstructive jaundice: use of expandable metal endoprosthesis for biliary drainage. Work in progress. Radiology 177: 789–792

Lee M J, Dawson S L, Mueller P R, Thornsten L K, Saini S, Hahn P F 1992 Palliation of malignant bile duct obstruction with metallic biliary endoprostheses: technique, results and complications. Journal of Vascular and Interventional Radiology 3: 665–671

Lee B H, Choe D H, Lee J H, Kim K H, Chin S Y 1997 Metallic stents in malignant biliary obstruction: prospective long-term clinical results. AJR. American Journal of Roentgenology 168: 741–745

Mathieson J R, McLoughlin R F, Cooperberg P L et al 1994 Malignant obstruction of the common bile duct: long term results of Gianturco-Rosch metal stents used as initial treatment. Radiology 192: 663–667

McPherson G A D, Benjamin I S, Hodgson H J F, Bowley N B, Allison D J, Blumgart L H 1984 Preoperative percutaneous transhepatic biliary drainage; the results of a controlled trial. British Journal of Surgery 71: 371–375

Mendez G, Russell E, Levi J U, Koolpe H, Cohen M 1980 Percutaneous brush biopsy and internal drainage of biliary tree through endoprosthesis. American Journal of Roentgenology 134: 653–659

Mendez G, Russell E, LePage J R, Guerra J J, Posniak R A, Trefler M 1984 Abandonment of endoprosthetic drainage technique in malignant biliary obstruction. American Journal of Roentgenology 143: 617–622

Michelassi F, Erroi F, Dawson P J et al 1989 Experience with 647 consecutive tumors of the duodenum, ampulla, head of the pancreas, and distal common bile duct. Annals of Surgery 210: 544–556

Miller G A Jr, Heaston D K, Moore A V Jr, Mills S R, Dunnick N R 1983 Peritoneal seeding of cholangiocarcinoma in patients with percutaneous biliary drainage. American Journal of Roentgenology 141: 561–562

Molnar W, Stockum A E 1974 Relief of obstructive jaundice through percutaneous transhepatic catheter – a new therapeutic method. American Journal of Roentgenology 122: 356–367

Mueller P R, vanSonnenberg E, Ferrucci J T 1982 Percutaneous biliary drainage: technical and catheter related problems in 200 procedures. American Journal of Roentgenology 138: 17–23

Mueller P R, Ferrucci J T Jr, Teplick S K et al 1985 Biliary stent endoprosthesis: analysis of complications in 113 patients. Radiology 156: 637–639

Muro A, Mueller P R, Ferrucci Jr J T, Taft P D 1983 Bile cytology – a routine addition to percutaneous biliary drainage. Radiology 149: 846–847

Nakayama T, Ikeda A, Okuda K 1978 Percutaneous transhepatic drainage of the biliary tract: technique and results in 104 cases. Gastroenterology 74: 554–559

Ogelvie S B, vanSonnenberg E, D'Agostino H B, Sanchez R, O'Laoide R, Fundell L 1992 Recent experience with percutaneous biliary drainage. Radiology 185(P): 112

Oleaga J A, Ring E J, Freiman D B, McLean G K, Rosen R J 1980 Extension of neoplasm along the tract of a transhepatic tube. American Journal of Roentgenology 135: 841–842

Ottow R T, August D A, Sugarbaker P H 1985 Treatment of proximal biliary tract carcinoma: an overview of techniques and results. Surgery 97: 251–262

Pereiras R V Jr, Rheingold O J, Hutson D et al 1978 Relief of malignant obstructive jaundice by percutaneous insertion of a permanent prosthesis in the biliary tree. Annals of Internal Medicine 89: 589–593

Pitt H A, Gomes A S, Lois JF, Mann L L, Deutsch L S, Longmire W P 1985 Does preoperative percutaneous biliary drainage reduce operative risks or increase hospital costs? Annals of Surgery 201: 545–553

Rossi P, Bezzi M, Rossi M et al 1994 Metallic stents in malignant biliary obstruction: results of a multicenter European study of 240 patients. Journal of Vascular and Interventional Radiology 281: 279–285

Smith R C, Pooley M, George C R P, Faithful G R 1985 Preoperative percutaneous transhepatic internal drainage in obstructive jaundice: a randomized controlled trial examining renal function. Surgery 97: 641–647

Terasaki K, Wittich G R, Lycke G et al 1991 Percutaneous transluminal biopsy of biliary strictures with a bioptome. American Journal of Reontgenology 156: 77–78

VanSonnenberg E, D'Agostino H B, Casola G, Varney R R, Taggart S C, May S R 1990 The benefits of percutaneous cholecystostomy for decompression of selected cases of obstructive jaundice. Radiology 176: 15–18

Wagner H J, Knyrim K, Vakil N, Klose K J 1993 Plastic endoprostheses versus metal stents in the palliative treatment of malignant hilar biliary obstuction. A prospective and randomized trial. Endoscopy 25: 213–218

Watanapa P, Williamson R C N 1992 Surgical palliation for pancreatic cancer: developments during the past two decades. British Journal of Surgery 79: 8–20

Wittich G R, vanSonnenberg E, Simeone J F 1985 Results and complications of percutaneous biliary drainage. Seminars in Interventional Radiology 2: 39–49

59

The endoscopic management of biliary and periampullary cancer

R.C. KURTZ

INTRODUCTION

Endoscopic retrograde cholangiopancreatography (ERCP) was first used in the late 1960s and has remained an important diagnostic modality frequently used by gastroenterologists and surgeons in the management of patients with hepatobiliary and pancreatic diseases (Ch. 17). The 1980s saw the introduction of endoscopic therapeutic approaches to disease of the biliary tract and pancreas. With the advent of endoscopic stenting, during which a polyethylene endoprosthesis is inserted into the bile duct, across the stricture, in order to restore the natural flow of bile in patients suffering from malignant biliary obstruction (Soehendra & Reynders-Frederix 1980, Huibregtse & Tytgat 1982, Classen & Hagenmuller 1984, Siegel 1984). More recently, refinements in technique, new video duodenoscopes, advances in biliary stent design, and new digital fluoroscopic equipment have made therapeutic endoscopy routinely available in gastrointestinal endoscopy units throughout the world. The therapeutic use of endoscopy continues its rapid growth and in many endoscopy units, therapeutic approaches to biliary and pancreatic disease now supersedes diagnostic ERCP. In the Gastrointestinal Endoscopy Unit at Memorial Sloan-Kettering Cancer Center (MSKCC), the ratio of therapeutic to diagnostic procedures is about five to one. The procedures performed include endoscopic sphincterotomy, bile duct stone extraction, and insertion of endobiliary stents for the palliative, nonsurgical management of malignant biliary obstruction due to periampullary and distal bile duct cancers. Nonsurgical biliary drainage is an important treatment option to palliate the pruritus associated with malignant biliary obstruction, and to lower serum bilirubin levels so that aggressive chemotherapeutic programs can be instituted.

TECHNIQUE

All endoscopic therapeutic procedures involving the biliary system start with diagnostic retrograde cholangiopancreatography (Ch. 17). This is an endoscopic procedure first, with careful evaluation of the stomach and duodenum. These structures are inspected for compression or invasion by tumor. Biopsies may be taken from any mucosal abnormality or ulceration and can give histological confirmation of the underlying malignancy rapidly and accurately. Then the ampulla is approached, inspected, and cannulated. Both cholangiography and pancreatography are performed to document tumor involvement of the biliary and pancreatic ductal systems. Not uncommonly, cannulation may be difficult or even impossible due to duodenal narrowing or displacement of the distal bile duct by the tumor. A periampullary cancer may obstruct the ampulla or may cause narrowing and atrophy due to disuse. In difficult cannulations, our practice at MSKCC is to use a double-channel sphincterotome through which contrast can be injected, to gain initial access to the bile duct. This allows for increased maneuverability of the cannula tip, which can be a great help. In a small number of patients, a precut sphincterotomy may be needed to gain access to the biliary tree. Once cannulation has been successfully performed, a guidewire is then inserted through the catheter to maintain access to the biliary system. We will often use a hydrophilic guidewire, which makes passage across a tight malignant biliary stricture easier. We do not use routine endoscopic sphincterotomy in our endoscopy unit, prior to endoscopic biliary stent placement. Sphincterotomy is done in less than 15% of patients, and only when it is felt that it will aide in passage of large-bore polyethylene endoprosthesis. The newer, self-expandable metal stents are packaged in an 8-French delivery system and endoscopic sphincterotomy is usually not necessary for insertion of this device through the ampulla. The theory that endoscopic sphincterotomy prevents occlusion of the pancreatic duct by the biliary endoprosthesis, and thus minimizes the risk of post-procedure pancreatitis, is probably not correct. Many endoscopists successfully manage patients with bile duct malignancies with endobiliary prostheses, without the use of a sphincterotomy and have not experienced a higher frequency of pancreatic complications. Biopsy of ampullary tumors may, however, be facilitated by an initial endoscopic sphincterotomy. It may be difficult to obtain an accurate biopsy of an ampullary mass without a small sphincterotomy, as the actual malignancy may be deep in the mass or within the bile duct, and superficial biopsies will show only adenomatous tissue. In addition, the associated obstructive jaundice may also be temporarily relieved by this procedure. Bourgeois and colleagues obtained the correct histologic diagnosis in all 55 patients with periampullary cancer after endoscopic sphincterotomy, but in only half of the patients before sphincterotomy (Bourgeois et al 1984).

When the decision is made to use a polyethylene stent, a 6 French teflon catheter is inserted over the guidewire to give the guidewire additional support. Under fluoroscopic guidance, the wire is maneuvered through the stricture, closely followed by the catheter, the end result being the advancement of the catheter well beyond the level of the stricture up into either the right or left biliary system. The rigid assembly of catheter and guidewire now serves as a firm guide for final insertion of the polyethylene endoprosthesis. The endoprosthesis is pushed over the catheter with the help of a pushing tube (Fig. 59.1). Fluoroscopy is criti-

cal to the proper positioning of the stent, that is, to insure that the proximal stent flap and opening lies proximal to the malignant stricture and that the distal flap is seen distal to the ampullary orifice. Once the endoprosthesis has been properly inserted, it is kept in position with the pushing catheter while the catheter assembly containing the guidewire is withdrawn out of the side-viewing endoscope. The distal end of the endoprosthesis is seen protruding from the ampulla into the duodenum, often with bile flowing from it (Fig. 59.2). The endoscope is then removed, leaving the endoprosthesis in place. We employ a 10 French, 5 or 7 cm straight polyethylene endoprostheses for distal biliary strictures, and 10 French, 9 cm straight polyethylene endoprostheses for strictures that are in the mid-common hepatic duct. At MSKCC, we rarely use endoscopy and endobiliary stents for bile duct bifurcation tumors, but rather palliate these patients either by surgical biliary bypass at the time of laparotomy or percutaneous transhepatic biliary drainage (PTD) when the patients are clearly not resectable (Ch. 54).

Self-expanding metal stents are being used more frequently. The self-expanding metal stent is composed of surgical-grade stainless steel filaments woven together to form a wire mesh (Fig. 59.3). It is pliable and flexible in the longitudinal axis. A stent with a length of 10 cm and a diameter of 8-French gauge in the constrained form shortens to 6.8 cm and expands to 30-French gauge when deployed. The delivery system consists of an 8-French gauge coaxial catheter with an invaginated membrane to constrain the stent. When self-expanding metal stents are used, the technique of deployment is similar to that described for polyethylene endoprostheses. However, the insertion of a teflon overtube is not needed. The stent delivery system is inserted directly over the 0.035 inch guide wire, positioned appropriately with fluoroscopic guidance, and deployed. Deployment of the endoprostheses involves

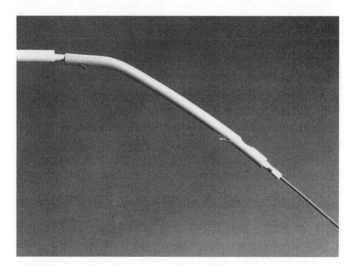

Fig. 59.1 Three layer system for introduction of biliary duct stent consisting of guidewire, guiding catheter, pusher tube and straight endoprosthesis with side flaps (Wilson-Cook Med. Inc., Winston-Salem, NC, USA).

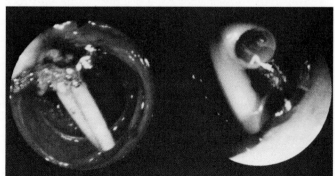

Fig. 59.2 A double prosthesis. An endoscopic view of two endoprostheses with obvious flow of bile.

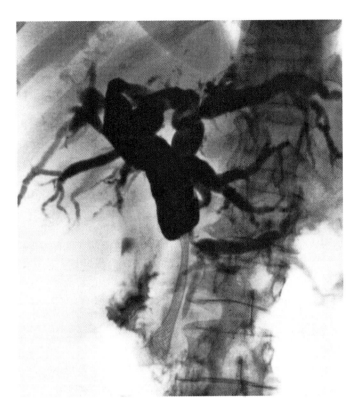

Fig. 59.3 A metal self-expanding Wallstent (Schneider Inc., Switzerland) is inserted in a distal bile duct stricture caused by pancreatic cancer.

peeling off the outer membrane after the system has been introduced into the appropriate portion of the bile duct.

If biliary endoprosthesis placement is unsuccessful, the endoscopist may consider the combined or rendezvous approach (Dowsett et al 1989a,b,c). This technique entails the percutaneous placement of a guidewire, under fluoroscopic guidance, into a biliary radicle, from whence it is manipulated into the common bile duct and through the ampulla of Vater. The wire is then retrieved by the endoscopist and the endobiliary stent is placed over the wire from below. In Dowsett's series of 72 patients published in 1989, the authors were successful with this combined approach in 60 cases. The total morbidity and 30-day mortality were 33% and 0% respectively. The theoretical advantage of this combined procedure over conventional percutaneous stent placement is that a much smaller puncture tract through the liver can be employed. Even so, the inherent risks of the percutaneous route (subcapsular hemorrhage, bile leakage) remain. We stopped using this approach several years ago at MSKCC, and now refer patients in whom endobiliary stent placement is not possible for percutaneous cholangiography and drainage (Ch. 29).

PATIENT SELECTION FOR ENDOSCOPIC BILIARY DRAINAGE

The location or level of the malignant biliary stricture is important in determining success and complication rates associated with the placement of endobiliary stents. Endoscopic biliary drainage (EBD) and percutaneous biliary drainage (PTD) are complementary procedures, and we select them based on the level of the biliary obstruction. We routinely use endoscopic biliary drainage for palliation of inoperable ampullary (Fig. 59.4), periampullary cancer, gallbladder cancer, and bile duct cancer up to the level of the mid-common hepatic duct (Fig. 59.5). For the palliative management of bile duct cancers or metastatic disease that

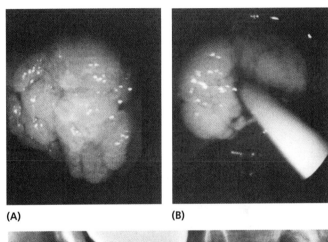

(A)   **(B)**

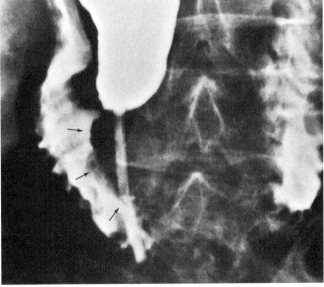

(C)

Fig. 59.4 Papillary tumor. **(A)** Endoscopic photograph of a large papillary neoplasm. **(B)** Endoprosthesis visible in the duodenum after placement. **(C)** Mass effect in duodenum (small arrows) and the endoprosthesis in place with good drainage.

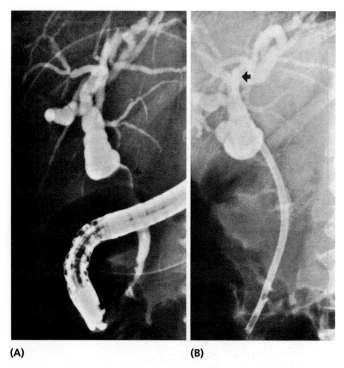

(A)   **(B)**

Fig. 59.5 Mid-common-duct tumor. **(A)** Obstruction in mid-common duct with dilated proximal biliary tract. **(B)** Placement of a single 15-cm long endoprosthesis (arrow denotes tumor).

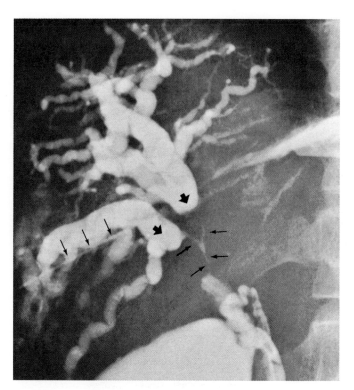

Fig. 59.6 Transhepatic cholangiogram in a bifurcation tumor. A fine needle (thin arrows) has entered the dilated right hepatic duct system (large arrows). A marked stricture is noted at the bifurcation. The left intrahepatic biliary tract is not filled.

cause proximal biliary obstruction at the hilus of the liver, percutaneous drainage is our procedure of choice (Fig. 59.6). There have been several studies that demonstrate that endoscopic drainage of hilar biliary obstruction is less likely to be successful and has a higher rate of cholangitis and sepsis. In one such study, 70 patients with malignant hilar strictures were stratified by Deviere and associates into three groups. Twenty patients had common hepatic duct lesions (type I), and 50 patients had bifurcation or intrahepatic strictures (type II and III). The type I patients required only one stent, and were likely to be completely drained. Approximately 50% of the type II and III patients could have only one stent placed. These patients had a higher 30-day mortality, a higher rate of early cholangitis, a higher death rate from sepsis, and a shorter post-procedure survival than those patients in whom adequate drainage was established. Success in adequately draining common bile duct and common hepatic duct strictures is about 90% following endoscopy, ERCP and the placement of a large-bore endoprosthesis. The success rate for establishing drainage by EBD in bifurcation or intrahepatic strictures is much lower. Even when one stent is successfully inserted, in only 30% of patients will a second stent be successfully placed. Using an aggressive approach, with multiple attempts and combining EBD with PTD only increased the success rate of insertion

of two or more stents to about 50% of patients with hilar strictures (Fig. 59.7).

In an MSKCC series (Kurtz et al 1988) that studied PTD after failed EBD, the rate of sepsis for patients with intrahepatic and bifurcation strictures was significantly greater than for those with common hepatic or common bile duct lesions (75% versus 17%; $p = 0.04$).

SURGICAL VERSUS ENDOSCOPIC BILIARY DRAINAGE

Stent placement should be successful in approximately 90% of cases (Table 59.1) (Huibregtse et al 1986, Huibregtse 1988, Speer at al 1988, Dowsest et al 1989c). Figure 59.8 demonstrates the typical 'double-duct' sign (Freeny et al 1976) of obstructing pancreatic carcinoma, and subsequent endoprosthesis insertion. Until the advent of radiological and, later, endoscopic stenting techniques, palliative treatment took the form of bilioenteric bypass. Biliary bypass is associated in some series with up to a 20% 30-day mortality, high morbidity and a hospital stay that may in some cases

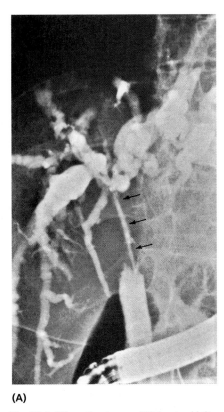

(A)

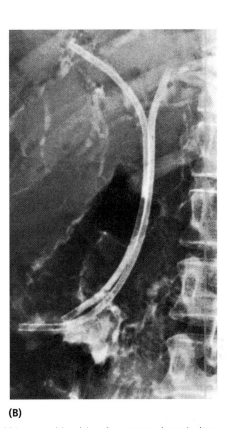

(B)

Fig. 59.7 Bifurcation tumor. **(A)** Proximal biliary tract stricture (thin arrows) involving the common hepatic duct and the bifurcation. **(B)** Endoprostheses are placed in both the left and the right hepatic ducts.

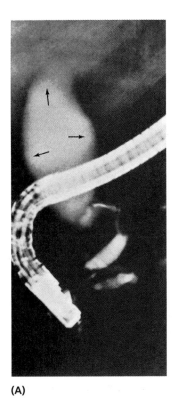

(A)

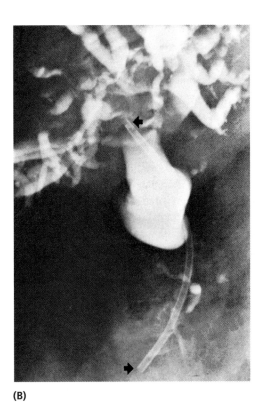

(B)

Fig. 59.8 Pancreatic tumor. **(A)** Obstruction of both the pancreatic duct and the common bile duct ('double duct sign') with dilated biliary tract proximally (small arrows). **(B)** A 12-cm long endoprosthesis in place (large arrows denote the proximal and distal ends).

Table 59.1 Results of endoscopic stents in patients with carcinoma of the pancreas in two large series

	University of Amsterdam*	Middlesex Hospital†
No. of patients	632	403
Mean age (years)	71	NA
Successful drainage (%)	87	85
30-day mortality (%)	10.8	17
Median survival (months)	5	4.5
Duodenal stenosis (%)	9	5
Stent blockage (%)	29	16

NA, not available.
*Coene (1990).
†Dowsett et al (1989a,b,c).

patients required rehospitalization (average charge of $4029), and about one-quarter of the surgical patients were readmitted (average charge of $6776). An average of 1.7 stent changes (average charge $1190) were required. Mean survival was longer for the stented group (9.7 versus 7.3 months, $p = 0.13$). The authors concluded that endoscopic stenting for unresectable pancreatic cancer provides equivalent duration of survival at reduced cost and shorter hospital stay. When curative resection is not possible, endoscopic biliary drainage should be considered the first choice for palliative management. In light of these findings, endoscopic endobiliary prosthesis placement should replace surgical biliary enteric anastomosis for nonresectable cancers of the pancreas or for those patients of advanced age or with severe comorbid medical conditions. Only in instances of impending duodenal obstruction should an operative approach be recommended. The surgical procedure should then consist of a double bypass procedure, where both biliary and enteric bypasses are performed.

last more than 4–6 weeks (Sarr & Cameron 1984, LaFerla & Murray 1987, Warshaw & Swanson 1988, Carter 1990). Three prospective, randomized studies have compared the results of endoscopic stenting and surgical bypass (Table 59.2) (Shepherd et al 1988, Andersen et al 1989, Dowsett et al 1989b). All show a lower immediate mortality rate and lower frequency of complications in the endoscopically treated patients. The early advantages of stent placement are counterbalanced somewhat by the need for re-admission for endoprosthesis changes and operative surgical bypass for late duodenal obstruction. Mean survival remains approximately 6 months for those who have undergone either method of therapy. In a Mayo Clinic study (Raikar et al 1996) of patients with adenocarcinoma of the pancreas, endoscopic biliary drainage was shown to be more cost effective than surgery. The initial hospital stay was significantly longer for surgical patients (mean 14 versus 7 days, $p < 0.001$), with higher average charges ($18 325 versus $9663). About one-third of the endobiliary stented

OUTPATIENT THERAPEUTIC EBD

Since 1996, at MSKCC, medically stable patients requiring therapeutic endoscopic procedures, have been managed as outpatients whenever possible. We reviewed our institution's experience and compared outpatient vs. inpatient treatment for endobiliary stent placement in patients with malignant common bile duct (CBD) obstruction (Cvetkovski et al 1999). We found no significant difference between the outpatients and inpatients with regard to: age, gender, procedure success rate, complication rate, the need for endoscopic sphincterotomy, and initial stent vs. stent

Table 59.2 Results of three prospective randomized trials comparing endoscopic stenting with surgical bypass for obstructive jaundice

	Shepherd et al (1988)		Andersen et al (1989)		Dowsett et al (1989c)	
	Stent	Surgery	Stent	Surgery	Stent	Surgery
No. of patients	23	25	25	19	101	103
Successful drainage (%)	91	92	96	84	94	91
Complications	22	40	NA	NA	10	28*
30-day mortality (%)	9	20	NA	NA	7	17
Duodenal bypass (%)	0	0	0	0	6	1*
Recurrent jaundice (%)	17	2	28	16	18	3*
Median survival	152 days	125 days	84 days	100 days	5 months†	5 months†
Range	39–411	52–354	3–498	10–642		

NA, not available.
*Statistically significant.
†Mean survival.

replacement. Inpatients had no procedure related complications; outpatients had two. Only one outpatient out of 31 required hospital admission. There was no procedure related mortality in either the inpatient or outpatient groups. Therapeutic endoscopy for palliation of malignant CBD obstruction can be safely and successfully performed on an outpatient basis in selected patients. This should result in better quality of life in these patients with advanced cancer by keeping them out of the hospital, as well as a cost savings.

RESULTS (Table 59.3)

The success rate of introducing an endoprosthesis endoscopically varies from 75% to 90%. In general, success is highest with ampullary tumors (95–100%), followed by pancreatic and distal common bile duct lesions (90%) and mid-common-duct and bifurcation tumors (70–75%) (Coene 1990). Failure to place an endoprosthesis in patients with distal biliary obstruction, may be due to duodenal compression by tumor, inability to deeply cannulate the bile duct, or lack of success in passing a guidewire beyond the stricture. Nearly all patients with ampullary, pancreatic and distal common duct tumors experience a decline in serum bilirubin following proper placement of an endoprosthesis, while patients with bifurcation tumors show a drop in bilirubin only 70% of the time. Hospital mortality in patients with ampullary cancer is under 5%, while with distal strictures it is 7–12%. Patients with mid-common-duct and bifurcation tumors have a 30-day hospital mortality rate of 20–25%.

COMPLICATIONS

Complications of endoscopic management of periampullary and biliary cancers can be divided into those which occur early, within the first 48 to 72 hours after stent insertion, and those which occur late, usually after 30 days or more.

EARLY COMPLICATIONS OF ENDOPROSTHESIS PLACEMENT (Table 59.4)

Early complications may be related to the method required to obtain deep cannulation (straightforward catheter

Table 59.3 Clinical results of endoscopic endoprosthesis placement in patients with cancer

Type of tumour	Success rate (%)	Disappearance of jaundice (%)	Hospital mortality (%)	Median survival (months)
Ampullary	95–100	100	5	13
Pancreatic, distal CBD	90	95	7–12	6
Mid-CBD, bifurcation	70–75	70	20–25	5–6

CBD, common bile duct.

Table 59.4 Early complications of endoprosthesis placement (within 1 week)

Complication	Rate (%)
Papillotomy related	
Bleeding	1–2
Pancreatitis	0–1
Perforation (duodenal, biliary)	0–1
Endoprosthesis related	
Cholecystitis	0–1
Early clogging (blood clots)	1–2
Acute cholangitis	0–27
Papillary tumour	0
Pancreatic tumour	8
Mid-CBD tumour	14
Bifurcation tumour	27
Mortality	2

insertion, standard sphincterotomy, or precut papillotomy) or to the endoprosthesis itself. Normally deep cannulation of the bile duct and pancreatography seldom cause complications. The smaller sphincterotomies performed in conjunction with stent placement yield a complication rate much lower than the 6–8% generally quoted for endoscopic sphincterotomy in the setting of bile duct gallstone disease. Bleeding may be seen in 1–2% of patients, and pancreatitis in 0–1%; perforation of the duodenum or bile duct is a rarity. Precut sphincterotomy using the needle knife is more traumatic and carries a complication rate of 3–5%. Endoprosthesis-related complications are primarily infectious and center largely around acute cholangitis. Acute cholangitis is unusual in the case of ampullary cancers and malignant distal common bile duct obstruction, but occurs with an increasing frequency of 8–27% for other obstructing malignant bile duct cancers, the more proximal lesions showing a higher rate of infection. Cholangitis is a serious complication and, although it usually responds to antibiotic administration, it may lead to overwhelming sepsis and death. ERCP is not a sterile procedure, and it is impossible to avoid the introduction of bacteria into the biliary tree during catheter insertion and contrast injection. Attempts to completely fill the intrahepatic biliary system with contrast in order to obtain detailed cholangiography should be avoided in this setting. Ideally, any obstructed biliary segment that has been filled with contrast should be drained.

In one study of 200 patients with pancreatic carcinoma, the overall incidence of cholangitis was 8% following endoprosthesis placement. However, it was only 2.7% if successful drainage was achieved at the first attempt, but over 22% if drainage could be achieved only after a second or third attempt (Huibregtse et al 1986). It is likely that bacterial contamination was introduced into the biliary tract during the first attempt, leading to the development of cholangitis. Antibiotics should be administered to all patients following an unsuccessful attempt at endoprosthesis placement or if complete drainage cannot be obtained. Polydorou et al (1991), following a policy of prophylactic antibiotics and limited contrast injection, were able to report a postprocedure cholangitis rate of only 7% in 190 patients with hilar tumours treated by insertion of an endoprosthesis. Deviere et al (1988) emphasized the need for complete drainage of all segments opacified at cholangiography and more recently (Motte et al 1991) have come to recommend giving prophylactic antibiotics to all jaundiced patients prior to ERCP.

Levine et al (1990) reviewed the microbiological data on septic episodes after EBD and compared the results with septic episodes after PTD. Both groups had enteric gram-negative organisms as the predominate cause for sepsis.

However, there were significantly more gram positive organisms noted in the PTD group ($p < 0.0005$). Other endoprosthesis-related complications are more unusual and consist of acute cholecystitis due to blockage of the cystic duct by the stent and clogging of the endoprosthesis by clots or tumor. Mortality directly related to the sphincterotomy and endoprosthesis procedure is an acceptable 2%, but 30-day mortality in these patients with, often advanced, cancer ranges from 10 to 20%.

LATE COMPLICATIONS OF ENDOPROSTHESIS PLACEMENT (Table 59.5)

Ever since endoscopic biliary stenting has become a standard palliative treatment for obstructive jaundice due to malignant disease of the pancreas and the hepatobiliary system, the procedure has been limited by clogging of biliary stents. This usually occurs four to five months after placement, due to formation of adherent bacterial biofilm (Coene 1990).

This leads to microcolony formation and the development of a biofilm which promotes bile salt crystallization and eventual occlusion by biliary sludge (Groen et al 1987, Speer et al 1988). When endobiliary stents occlude, patients present with malaise, low-grade fever and elevated serum bilirubin and alkaline phosphatase. Prompt recognition of these symptoms and laboratory findings should lead to removal and replacement of the clogged stent. It is of little or no value to attempt irrigation of the clogged polyethylene stent. Indeed, replacement is usually technically simple, and should take no longer than 15–20 minutes. It is nearly always followed by subsidence of the symptoms of cholangitis and jaundice. Occasionally, recurrent jaundice may be due to progression of the cancer in the liver. Non-invasive imaging studies should clearly demonstrate this and no clinical benefit would be gained by endobiliary stent replacement.

A number of methods have been investigated for the prolongation of stent patency, including prophylactic antimicrobial agents and bile salts, new stent materials, and new

Table 59.5 Late complication of endoprosthesis placement (over 1 week)

Complication	Rate (%)
Clogging (cholangitis, jaundice)	20–25 (mean 5 months)
Acute cholecystitis	0–1
Migration	1–2
Duodenal or biliary perforation	1–2
Duodenal stenosis (tumor related)	7–10 (mean 10 months)
Mortality	Unusual

stent designs. Stent size may play a role in the occlusion rate. As early as 1985 (Siegel et al 1985) it was shown that larger caliber stents remain patent for longer periods of time. Although the development of a 4.2-mm instrumentation channel duodenoscope now allows the routine placement of 10–12 French gauge endoprostheses, late clogging remains a problem, occurring in 21–31% of cases. Pereira-Lima and co-workers in a retrospective, nonrandomized fashion, compared different stent lengths and diameters in the palliation of jaundice caused by pancreatic cancer. They compared a 10-French versus 11.5-French stents and of 'short' (< or = 8 cm) versus 'long' (> or = 9 cm) stents. Median stent patency was 3 and 4 months for 10-French and 11.5-French stents, respectively ($p > 0.05$). Jaundice was reduced or eliminated (bilirubinemia < 3 mg %) in 85% of their patients. Hospital mortality was 2.7%. The commonest long-term complication was stent occlusion, which occurred 66 times in 33 patients. When analyzing the patients who were alive 6 months after therapy, the stent occlusion rate was 46% and 55% for 10-French and 11.5-French stents. Stent length did not influence stent patency. The only risk factor, which independently predicted survival, was the presence of distant metastases. Median survival for patients with metastatic disease was 2.5 months and 9 months for those without metastases ($p = 0.0015$).

The major factor limiting stent diameter has been the fixed size of the working channel of the duodenoscope. This problem has been addressed by development of self-expandable metal stents which have an 8-French diameter prior to their being deployed. Most experience has been obtained using the Wallstent (Fig. 59.3). The use of the Wallstent has significantly improved the duration of stent patency but the initial cost of the stent is considerably higher. Thus the optimal stent choice for palliation of inoperable malignant biliary strictures has remained controversial. In a recent study addressing this issue, Prat and colleagues studied (Prat et al 1998) 101 patients with malignant strictures of the common bile duct. The patients included those with pancreatic cancer (65), cholangiocarcinomas (21), ampullary tumors (3), and metastatic lymph nodes in the porta hepatis (12). Patients were randomized to receive either an 11.5-French polyethylene stent to be exchanged only when it failed, (group 1, $n = 33$), an 11.5-French stent exchanged regularly every 3 months (group 2, $n = 34$), or a self-expanding metallic Wallstent (group 3, $n = 34$). The procedures were successful in 97.1% of cases. Procedure-related morbidity was 11.9%, and mortality was 2.9%. The level of serum bilirubin after 48 hours did not differ between the three groups. Overall survivals were not different between groups, but complication-free survival for groups 2 and 3 was longer than that of group 1 ($p < 0.05$). Cumulated hospital days

were 7.4 ± 1.5, 10.6 ± 1.7, and 5.5 ± 1.4, respectively ($p < 0.05$). Cost analysis showed that metallic stents were cost effective in patients who survived for more than six months. Polyethylene stents were cost effective in patients surviving for six months or less. Metallic stents should be used in patients with the longest life expectancy. When patients receive polyethylene stents, they should be changed routinely, approximately every three months, to prevent cholangitis, sepsis, and hospitalizations.

A problem unique to Wallstents is that the open weave of the stent has rendered it susceptible to tumor ingrowth, a complication that occurs in at least 7% of patients (Huibregtse et al 1992). Tumor ingrowth can be successfully treated by the placement of a 10-French gauge plastic endoprosthesis through the Wallstent (Fockens et al 1992, O'Brien et al 1995) by diathermic cleaning or balloon trawling (Cremer et al 1990). The most cost effective method appears to be insertion of a plastic stent inside the Wallstent (Tham et al 1998) by either endoscopy or percutaneous means. Once fully expanded, the Wallstent can no longer be removed.

A much rarer complication is erosion of the proximal duodenal wall by the stent, leading to gastrointestinal hemorrhage (Ee & Laurence 1992). It has also been suggested that Wallstents may cause life-threatening hemobilia when there are bile duct varices due to portal vein obstruction by pancreatic malignancies (Cvetkovski et al 1999). This is probably an unusual occurrence.

Duodenal stenosis, although a direct complication of the tumor, is listed as a late complication. It is a relatively common problem in patients with ampullary carcinoma and pancreatic carcinoma. The incidence of late duodenal stenosis in pancreatic carcinoma is 7.5% and it occurs at a mean of about 300 days following endobiliary stent insertion. Duodenal stenosis may occur in 7–10% of patients treated by an endoprosthesis. It is much less common with mid common duct and bifurcation tumors. If a patient has significant duodenal compression at the time of endoscopy for endobiliary stent placement we recommend operative gastroenterostomy plus biliary bypass. Mortality related to late complications (Table 59.5) is rare, but prompt recognition and appropriate treatment are essential.

CONCLUSION

The advent of endoscopic biliary endoprosthesis placement has revolutionized the palliative management of biliary and periampullary cancer. The success rate of stent placement ranges from approximately 70% for hilar strictures to over

90% for distal obstructions. Endoscopic therapy, in properly selected patients, offers a lower degree of morbidity and mortality than comparable surgical treatment. The principal drawback of stent use, namely, occlusion of the endoprosthesis by biliary sludge or tumor, has recently been addressed by the development of the expandable metal stent. The search for the perfect endoprosthesis continues and we look forward to many new developments in endoprosthesis material and design.

REFERENCES

Andersen J R, Sorensen S M, Kruse A, Rokkjaer M, Matsen P 1989 Randomized trial of endoscopic versus operative bypass in malignant obstructive jaundice. Gut 30: 1132–1135

Bourgeois N, Dunham F, Verhest A, et al 1984 Endoscopic biopsies of the ampulla of Vater at the time of endoscopic sphincterotomy: difficulties in interpretation. Gastrointestinal Endoscopy 30: 163–166

Carter D C 1990 Cancer of the pancreas. Gut 31: 494–496

Classen M, Hagenmuller F 1984 Endoscopic biliary drainage. Scandinavian Journal of Gastroenterology 19 (Suppl 102): 76–83

Coene P P L O 1990 Endoscopic biliary stenting – mechanisms and possible solutions of the clogging phenomenon. Kripps Repro, Meppel

Cremer M, Deviere J, Sugai B, Baize M 1990 Expandable biliary stents for malignancies: endoscopic insertion and diathermic cleaning for tumor ingrowth. Gastrointestinal Endoscopy 36: 451–457

Cvetkovski B, Gerdes H, Kurtz R C 1999 Outpatient therapeutic ERCP with endobiliary stent placement for malignant common bile duct obstruction. Gastrointestinal Endoscopy (in press)

Deviere J, Baize M, de Toeuf J, Cremer M 1988 Long-term follow-up of patients with hilar malignant stricture treated by endoscopic internal drainage. Gastrointestinal Endoscopy 34: 95–101

Dowsett J F, Vaira D, Hatfield A R W et al 1989a Endoscopic biliary therapy using the combined percutaneous and endoscopic technique. Gastroenterology 96: 1180–1186

Dowsett J F, Williams S J, Hatfield A R W et al 1989b Endoscopic management of low biliary obstruction due to unresectable primary pancreato-biliary malignancy: a review of 463 consecutive cases. Gastroenterology 96: A129

Dowsett J F, Russell R C G, Hatfield A R W et al 1989c Malignant obstructive jaundice; a prospective randomised trial of surgery versus endoscopic stenting. Gastroenterology 96: A128

Ee H, Laurence B H 1992 Hemorrhage due to erosion of a metal biliary stent through the duodenal wall. Endoscopy 24: 431–432

Fockens P, Waxman I, Davids P H P, Huibregtse K, Tytgat G N J 1992 Early recurrence of obstructive jaundice after placement of a self-expanding metal endoprosthesis. Endoscopy 24: 428–430

Freeny P C, Bilbao M K, Katon R M et al 1976 Blind evaluation of endoscopic retrograde cholangiopancreatography (ERCP) in diagnosis of pancreatic carcinoma: the 'double duct' and other signs. Radiology 119: 271–274

Groen A K, Out T, Huibregtse K, Delzenne B, Hoek F J, Tytgat G N J 1987 Characterization of the content of occluded biliary endoprostheses. Endoscopy 19: 57–59

Huibregtse K 1988 Endoscopic biliary and pancreatic drainage. Georg Thieme Verlag, 78–85

Huibregtse K, Tytgat G N J 1982 Palliative treatment of obstructive

jaundice by transpapillary introduction of a large bore bile duct endoprosthesis. Gut 23: 371–375

Huibregtse K, Katon R M, Coene P P, Tytgat G N J 1986 Endoscopic palliative treatment in pancreatic cancer. Gastrointestinal Endoscopy 32: 334–338

Huibregtse K, Carr-Locke D L, Cremer M et al 1992 Biliary stent occlusion – a problem solved with self-expanding metal stents? European Wallstent Study Group. Endoscopy 24: 391–394

Kurtz R C, Botet J B, Gerdes H, et al 1988 Percutaneous biliary drainage following failed endoscopic drainage in malignant biliary obstruction. Gastroenterology 34: 189

LaFerla G, Murray W R 1987 Carcinoma of the pancreas: bypass surgery in unresectable disease. British Journal of Surgery 74: 212–213

Levine J G, Botet J, and Kurtz R C 1990 Microbiological analysis of sepsis complicating non-surgical biliary drainage in malignant obstruction. Gastrointestinal Endoscopy 36: 364–368

Motte S, Deviere J, Dumonceau, Serruys E, Thys J P, Cremer M 1991 Risk factors for septicemia following endoscopic biliary stenting. Gastroenterology 101: 1374–1381

O'Brien S, Hatfield A R, Craig P I, Williams S P 1995 A three year follow up of self expanding metal stents in the endoscopic palliation of longterm survivors with malignant biliary obstruction. Gut 36: 618–621.

Polydorou A A, Chisholm E M, Romanos A A et al 1989 A comparison of right versus left hepatic duct endoprosthesis insertion in malignant hilar biliary obstruction. Endoscopy 21: 266–271

Polydorou A A, Cairns S R, Dowsett J F et al 1991 Palliation of proximal malignant biliary obstruction by endoscopic endoprosthesis insertion. Gut 32: 685–689

Prat F, Chapat O, Ducot B, Ponchon T, Fritsch J, Choury A D, Pelletier G, Buffet C 1998 Predictive factors for survival of patients with inoperable malignant distal biliary strictures: a practical management guideline. Gut 42: 76–80.

Raikar G V, Melin M M, Ress A, Lettieri S Z et al 1996 Cost-effective analysis of surgical palliation vs. endoscopic stenting in the management of unresectable pancreatic cancer. Annals of Surgical Oncology 3(5): 470–475

Sarr M G, Cameron J L 1984 Surgical palliation of unresectable carcinoma of the pancreas. World Journal of Surgery 4: 906–918

Shepherd H A, Royle G, Ross A P R, Diba A, Arthur M, Colin-Jones D 1988 Endoscopic biliary endoprosthesis in the palliation of malignant obstruction of the distal common bile duct: a randomized trial. British Journal of Surgery 75: 1166–1168

Siegel J H 1984 Interventional endoscopy in disease of the biliary tree and pancreas. Mount Sinai Medical Journal 51: 535–542

Siegel J H, Pullano W E, Wright G 1985 The ultimate large caliber endoprosthesis – 12 F: Poisseuille was right – bigger is better. Gastrointestinal Endoscopy 31: 158

Soehendra N, Reynders-Frederix V 1980 Palliative bile duct drainage. A new endoscopic method of introducing a transpapillary drain. Endoscopy 12: 8–11

Speer A G, Cotton P B 1988 Endoscopic treatment of pancreatic cancer. International Journal of Pancreatology 3: 147–158

Speer A G, Cotton P B, Rode J et al 1988 Biliary stent blockage with bacterial biofilm. Annals of Internal Medicine 108: 546–553

Tham T C K, Carr-Locke D L, Vandervoort J, Wong R C K et al 1998 Management of occluded biliary wallstents. Gut 42: 703–707.

Venu R P, Rolny P, Geenen J E, Hogan W J, Johnson G K, Schmalz M 1990 Is there a need for multiple stents in hilar strictures? Gastrointestinal Endoscopy 36: 197

Warshaw A L, Swanson R S 1988 Pancreatic cancer in 1988: possibilities and probabilities. Annals of Surgery 208: 541–553

Index